SECOND EDITION

Metabolic Bone Disease

and Clinically Related Disorders

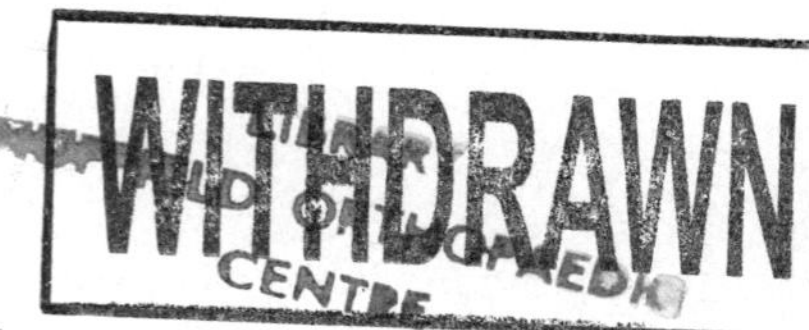

Louis V. Avioli, M.D.

Sydney M. and Stella H. Schoenberg Professor of Medicine
Professor of Cell Biology and Physiology
Washington University School of Medicine
Jewish Hospital of St. Louis
St. Louis, Missouri

Stephen M. Krane, M.D.

Persis, Cyrus and Marlow B. Harrison Professor of Medicine
Harvard Medical School
Physician and Chief, Arthritis Unit
Massachusetts General Hospital
Boston, Massachusetts

W.B. Saunders Company ▪ 1990
HARCOURT BRACE JOVANOVICH, INC.
Philadelphia ▪ London ▪ Toronto ▪ Montreal ▪ Sydney ▪ Tokyo

W. B. SAUNDERS COMPANY
Harcourt Brace Jovanovich, Inc.
The Curtis Center
Independence Square West
Philadelphia, PA 19106–3399

Library of Congress Cataloging-in-Publication Data

Metabolic bone disease and clinically related disorders / [editors]
Louis V. Avioli, Stephen M. Krane. — 2nd ed.
p. cm.
Rev. ed. of: Metabolic bone disease. 1977–1978.
Includes bibliographical references.
ISBN 0-7216-2766-8
1. Bones—Metabolism—Disorders. 2. Bones—Diseases. I. Avioli, Louis V.
II. Krane, Stephen M. III. Metabolic bone disease.
[DNLM: 1. Bone and Bones—Metabolism. 2. Bone Diseases.
3. Metabolic Diseases. WE 225 M587]
RC931.M45M468 1990
616.7′16—dc20
DNLM/DLC 89–70120

Editor: W. B. Saunders Staff
Designer: Terri Siegel
Production Manager: Linda R. Turner
Manuscript Editor: RoseMarie Klimowicz
Illustration Coordinator: Lisa Lambert
Indexer: Alexandra Nickerson

METABOLIC BONE DISEASE AND
CLINICALLY RELATED DISORDERS, Second Edition ISBN 0-7216-2766-8

Printed in the United States of America

Last digit is the print number: 9 8 7 6 5 4 3 2 1

Contributors

JOHN S. ADAMS, M.D.

Associate Professor of Medicine, UCLA School of Medicine, Los Angeles, California; Director, Mineral Metabolism Laboratory, Cedars-Sinai Medical Center, Los Angeles, California

Vitamin D Metabolism and Biological Function

CONSTANTINE S. ANAST, M.D.*

Late Professor of Pediatrics, Harvard Medical School, Boston, Massachusetts; Late Senior Associate in Medicine (Endocrinology), Children's Hospital, Boston, Massachusetts
*Deceased

Metabolic Bone Disorders in Children

LOUIS V. AVIOLI, M.D.

Sydney M. and Stella H. Schoenberg Professor of Medicine and Professor of Cell Biology and Physiology, Washington University School of Medicine, St. Louis, Missouri; Jewish Hospital of St. Louis, St. Louis, Missouri

Pathophysiology of Calcium and Phosphate Absorptive Disorders; The Female Osteoporotic Syndrome(s)

JOHN A. BARRANGER, M.D., Ph.D.

Professor of Biochemistry and Pediatrics, University of Southern California, Los Angeles, California; Head, Division of Medical Genetics, Children's Hospital of Los Angeles, Los Angeles, California

Metabolic Bone Disease in Patients with Gaucher's Disease

NORMAN H. BELL, M.D.

Professor of Medicine and Pharmacology, and Director, Division of Bone and Mineral Metabolism, Medical University of South Carolina, Charleston, South Carolina; Staff Physician, Veterans Administration Medical Center, Charleston, South Carolina

Sarcoidosis and Related Disorders

STANLEY J. BIRGE, M.D.

Associate Professor of Medicine, Washington University School of Medicine, St. Louis, Missouri; Clinical Director, Program on Aging, Jewish Hospital of St. Louis, St. Louis, Missouri

Pathophysiology of Calcium and Phosphate Absorptive Disorders

THOMAS O. CARPENTER, M.D.

Assistant Professor of Pediatrics, Yale University School of Medicine, New Haven Connecticut; Attending Physician, Yale–New Haven Hospital, New Haven, Connecticut

Metabolic Bone Disorders in Children

JACK W. COBURN, M.D.

Adjunct Professor of Medicine, UCLA School of Medicine, Los Angeles, California; Staff Physician, Veterans Administration, Wadsworth Medical Center, Los Angeles, California

Renal Osteodystrophy

S. H. COHN, Ph.D.

Retired Director, Medical Physics Medical Research Center, Brookhaven National Laboratory, Upton, New York; Former Professor of Medicine, Medical Center, State University of New York, Stony Brook, New York; Consulting Professor of Medicine, Medical Center, Stanford University, Stanford, California

Noninvasive Measurements of Bone Mass

LEONARD J. DEFTOS, M.D.

Professor of Medicine, University of California, San Diego, California; Chief, Section on Bone and Mineral Research, San Diego VA Medical Center, San Diego, California

The Thyroid Gland in Calcium and Skeletal Metabolism

SAMUEL H. DOPPELT, M.D.

Assistant Professor of Orthopaedic Surgery and Medicine, Harvard Medical School, Boston, Massachusetts; Chief of Orthopaedic Surgery, Cambridge Hospital, Cambridge, Massachusetts; Assistant Orthopaedic Surgeon and Clinical Assistant in Medicine, Massachusetts General Hospital, Boston, Massachusetts

Metabolic Bone Disease in Patients with Gaucher's Disease

MARIE-CLAUDE FAUGERE, M.D.

Pathologist, Division of Nephrology, Bone and Mineral Metabolism, Department of Medicine, University of Kentucky Medical Center, Lexington, Kentucky

Bone Biopsies—Histology and Histomorphometry of Bone

MARK C. GEBHARDT, M.D.

Assistant Professor of Orthopaedic Surgery, Harvard Medical School, Boston, Massachusetts; Associate Orthopaedic Surgeon, Massachusetts General Hospital and The Children's Hospital, Boston, Massachusetts

The Diagnosis and Management of Bone Tumors

MELVIN J. GLIMCHER, M.D.

Harriet M. Peabody Professor of Orthopaedic Surgery, Harvard Medical School, Boston, Massachusetts; Director, Laboratory for the Study of Skeletal Disorders and Rehabilitation, Children's Hospital, Boston, Massachusetts

The Nature of the Mineral Component of Bone and the Mechanism of Calcification

JOEL F. HABENER, M.D.

Professor of Medicine, Harvard Medical School, Boston, Massachusetts; Chief, Laboratory of Molecular Endocrinology, Massachusetts General Hospital, Boston, Massachusetts

Fundamental Considerations in the Physiology, Biology, and Biochemistry of Parathyroid Hormone; Primary Hyperparathyroidism

MICHAEL F. HOLICK, M.D.

Professor of Medicine, Boston University School of Medicine, Boston, Massachusetts; Attending Staff, Massachusetts General Hospital, University Hospital, and Boston City Hospital, Boston, Massachusetts

Vitamin D Metabolism and Biological Function

KEITH A. HRUSKA, M.D.

Ira M. Lang Professor of Medicine and Associate Professor of Cell Biology and Physiology, Washington University School of Medicine, St. Louis, Missouri; Chief, Renal Division, Jewish Hospital of St. Louis, St. Louis, Missouri

Regulation of Renal Phosphate Transport

L. LYNDON KEY, JR., M.D.

Associate Professor of Pediatrics, Bowman-Gray School of Medicine, Winston-Salem, North Carolina; Staff Physician, North Carolina Baptist Hospital, Winston-Salem, North Carolina

Metabolic Bone Disorders in Children

STEPHEN M. KRANE, M.D.

Persis, Cyrus and Marlow B. Harrison Professor of Medicine, Harvard Medical School, Boston, Massachusetts; Massachusetts General Hospital, Boston, Massachusetts

Paget's Disease of Bone

BRENDA R. C. KURNIK, M.D.

Assistant Professor of Medicine, University of Medicine and Dentistry of New Jersey, Robert Wood Johnson Medical School, Newark, New Jersey; Attending Physician for Department of Medicine, University of Medicine and Dentistry of New Jersey University Hospital, Newark, New Jersey

Regulation of Renal Phosphate Transport

ROBERT LINDSAY, M.B., Ch.B., Ph.D., F.R.C.P.

Professor of Clinical Medicine, College of Physicians and Surgeons, Columbia University, New York, New York; Chief, Internal Medicine, Helen Hayes Hospital, West Haverstraw, New York

The Female Osteoporotic Syndrome(s)

HARTMUT H. MALLUCHE, M.D.

Director, Division of Nephrology, Bone and Mineral Metabolism, College of Medicine, University of Kentucky Medical Center, Lexington, Kentucky; Professor of Medicine, University of Kentucky Medical Center, Lexington, Kentucky

Bone Biopsies—Histology and Histomorphometry of Bone

HENRY J. MANKIN, M.D.

Edith M. Ashley Professor of Orthopaedic Surgery, Harvard Medical School, Boston, Massachusetts; Chief of the Orthopaedic Surgery Service, Massachusetts General Hospital, Boston, Massachusetts

Metabolic Bone Disease in Patients with Gaucher's Disease; The Diagnosis and Management of Bone Tumors

T. J. MARTIN, M.D., D.Sc., F.R.A.C.P.

Professor of Medicine, University of Melbourne, Department of Medicine, St. Vincent's Hospital, Melbourne, Australia; Director, St. Vincent's Institute of Medical Research, Melbourne, Australia

Calcitonin

J. M. MOSELEY, Ph.D.

Senior Research Fellow, National Health and Medical Research Council, University of Melbourne, Department of Medicine, St. Vincent's Hospital, Melbourne, Australia

Calcitonin

GREGORY R. MUNDY, M.D.

Professor of Medicine, University of Texas Health Science Center, San Antonio, Texas; Chief, Frederic C. Barrter Clinical Research Unit, Audie Murphy Memorial Veterans Hospital, San Antonio, Texas

Hypercalcemia of Malignancy

WILLIAM A. MURPHY, M.D.

Professor of Radiology, Washington University School of Medicine, St. Louis, Missouri; Radiologist, Barnes Hospital and Children's Hospital, St. Louis, Missouri; Co-Director, Musculoskeletal Radiology, Mallinckrodt Institute of Radiology, St. Louis, Missouri

Osteopetrosis and Other Sclerosing Bone Disorders

CHARLES Y. C. PAK, M.D.

University Distinguished Chair in Mineral Metabolism, Southwestern Medical School, University of Texas Southwestern Medical Center at Dallas, Dallas, Texas; Attending Staff, Parkland Memorial Hospital, University Medical Center, Dallas, Texas

Kidney Stones: Pathogenesis, Diagnosis, and Therapy

A. M. PARFITT, M.D., B.Chir.

Director, Bone and Mineral Research Laboratory, Henry Ford Hospital, Ann Arbor, Michigan; Clinical Professor of Medicine, University of Michigan Medical School, Ann Arbor, Michigan

Osteomalacia and Related Disorders

JOHN T. POTTS, JR., M.D.

Jackson Professor of Clinical Medicine, Harvard Medical School, Boston, Massachusetts; Chief, General Medical Services, Massachusetts General Hospital, Boston, Massachusetts

Fundamental Considerations in the Physiology, Biology, and Biochemistry of Parathyroid Hormone; Primary Hyperparathyroidism

LAWRENCE G. RAISZ, M.D.

Professor of Medicine, University of Connecticut School of Medicine, Farmington, Connecticut; Head, Division of Endocrinology, University of Connecticut Health Center, Farmington, Connecticut

Cellular Basis for Bone Turnover

PAMELA GEHRON ROBEY, Ph.D.

Research Biologist, Bone Research Branch, National Institute of Dental Research, National Institutes of Health, Bethesda, Maryland

Biochemical Markers of Metabolic Bone Disease

GIDEON A. RODAN, M.D., Ph.D.

Adjunct Professor, Department of Pathology, University of Pennsylvania Medical School, Philadelphia, Pennsylvania; Executive Director, Department of Bone Biology/Osteoporosis, Merck Sharp & Dohme Research Laboratories, West Point, Pennsylvania

Cellular Basis for Bone Turnover

ANDREW E. ROSENBERG, M.D.

Instructor, Harvard Medical School, Boston, Massachusetts; Assistant Pathologist, Massachusetts General Hospital, Boston, Massachusetts

Metabolic Bone Disease in Patients with Gaucher's Disease

DAVID W. ROWE, M.D.

Professor of Pediatrics, University of Connecticut Health Center, Farmington, Connecticut; Attending Staff, John Dempsey Hospital, Farmington, Connecticut

Osteogenesis Imperfecta

JAY R. SHAPIRO, M.D., F.A.C.P.

Professor of Medicine, University of Massachusetts Medical School, Worcester, Massachusetts; Chief of Endocrinology, St. Vincent Hospital, Worcester, Massachusetts

Osteogenesis Imperfecta

FREDERICK R. SINGER, M.D.

Visiting Professor of Medicine, UCLA School of Medicine, Los Angeles, California; Director, Bone Center, Cedars-Sinai Medical Center, Los Angeles, California

Paget's Disease of Bone

EDUARDO SLATOPOLSKY, M.D.

Professor of Medicine, Washington University School of Medicine, St. Louis, Missouri; Attending Physician, Barnes Hospital, St. Louis, Missouri; Director, Chromalloy American Kidney Center, St. Louis, Missouri

Renal Osteodystrophy

JOHN D. TERMINE, Ph.D.

Chief, Bone Research Branch, National Institute of Dental Research, National Institutes of Health, Bethesda, Maryland

Biochemical Markers of Metabolic Bone Disease

MICHAEL P. WHYTE, M.D.

Associate Professor of Medicine and Pediatrics, Departments of Medicine and Pediatrics, Washington University School of Medicine, St. Louis, Missouri; Director, Metabolic Research Unit, Shriners Hospital for Crippled Children, St. Louis, Missouri

Osteopetrosis and Other Sclerosing Bone Disorders

Preface

When we first conceived of assembling a series of invited papers for the purpose of presenting a treatise on metabolic bone diseases, our primary goal was to present an up-to-date review on the diagnosis and treatment of well-established clinical disorders, and to integrate the clinical facts with current knowledge of the pathophysiology of calcium-phosphate metabolism, calciotropic hormones, and skeletal disease. Volume I of *Metabolic Bone Disease*, published in 1977, contained reviews of "Bone Metabolism and Calcium Regulation," "Kidney Function in Calcium and Phosphate Metabolism," "Alkaline Phosphatase and Metabolic Bone Disorders," "The Diagnostic Value of Bone Biopsies," "Vitamin D Rickets and Osteomalacia," "Osteoporosis," and "Nephrolithiasis." Volume II, which appeared in 1979, offered reviews of "Parathyroid Physiology and Primary Hyperparathyroidism," "Renal Osteodystrophy," "Hypoparathyroidism," "The Thyroid Gland in Skeletal and Calcium Metabolism," "Paget's Disease of Bone," "Disorders of Mineral Metabolism in Malignancy," and "Metabolic Bone Disease in Children." At that time, we apologized for not including every skeletal disorder that some of our potential readers might have deemed appropriate and expressed our intention to extend our horizons in future editions.

Thirteen years have elapsed since the publication of the first volume of *Metabolic Bone Disease*. During this interval, publications of many important discoveries relevant to the biochemistry, physiology, and molecular biology of the formation and function and hormonal control of skeletal tissues have appeared, examples of which are as follows: one form of osteoporosis has been linked to a deficiency of carbonic anhydrase II; molecular defects have been identified in collagen genes in patients with osteogenesis imperfecta (type I collagen), spondyloepiphyseal dysplasia (type II collagen), and the Ehlers-Danlos syndrome (type III collagen). It has now been established that structural mutations occasionally coding for single amino acid substitutions in the triple-helical region and the carboxypropeptide of type I collagen can result in abnormalities in skeletal metabolism resulting in short stature, osteopenia, and increased fracture potential. These observations reflect the extent of the remarkable growth in our knowledge of skeletal tissue, since in the classic textbook published in 1948, *The Parathyroid Glands and Metabolic Bone Disease: Selected Studies*, by Fuller Albright and Edward C. Reifenstein, "collagen," which composes 90 to 95 per cent of the organic bone matrix, was never mentioned!

In this new edition, we have attempted to present a correlated view of metabolic bone disease and related topics stressing the relationship between genetics, molecular biology, biochemistry, pathology, and clinical syndromes, in a single volume. We reasoned that this approach not only would afford a more integrated and cohesive presentation of the accumulated experience of our authors, but also would minimize redundancy and facilitate editing and cross-referencing among chapters. The overall format of this new edition is similar to that of the original Volumes I and II, although all chapters retained from our original volumes have been completely rewritten and new topics added.

The first 10 chapters provide an updated version of the current state of our knowledge regarding the cellular basis of bone turnover, biological mineralization, and the role of the intestine and kidney in modulating the day-to-day control of calcium and phosphate metabolism. Reviews of the metabolism of vitamin D, parathyroid hormone, and calcitonin are current, and the use of histological methodology in the diagnoses of bone disorders is presented in a refreshingly new style. Current interest in noninvasive methods of diagnosing the severity of a skeletal disorder and/or the response to therapeutic intervention should be amply satisfied by the "new" chapters "Noninvasive Measurements of Bone Mass" and "Biochemical Markers of Metabolic Bone Disease." The subsequent 14 chapters are presented primarily to summarize those clinical disorders that either present to the practicing physician as a "primary skeletal disorder" or, as in the case of medullary carcinoma, malignant hypercalcemia, and hypercalciuric stone syndromes, result from either alterations in the production and action of calciotropic hormones or the intestinal-renal handling of calcium and phosphate.

Bone tumors are rare, and physicians who care for adults with metabolic bone disease usually do not have the chance to develop any experience in the diagnosis or management of these neoplasms. Even in patients with Paget's disease, osteosarcomas develop as a complication of the skeletal lesions with a frequency of less than 1 per cent. Nevertheless, these are still important cancers in pediatric orthopedic practice, and as noted in the chapter "The Diagnosis and Management of Bone Tumors," there has been considerable improvement in prognosis as a result of better procedures to evaluate the lesions and proper appreciation of the usefulness of surgery and chemotherapy. Moreover, understanding the biology of osteosarcomas will provide us with additional information about the formation, function, and activity of osteoblasts as detailed in the first chapter, "Cellular Basis for Bone Turnover."

As detailed in each of the Prefaces to the two volumes of the first edition, there is a difference in the approach, emphasis, and style of the contributors to this new edition. We recognize that constraints imposed by editors and publishers can mitigate the stylistic effects that each author hopes to achieve. We are grateful to our publisher who has been unusually patient and tolerant in this regard.

Finally, in an effort to minimize the delay between submission and publication, authors were given the opportunity to add additional comments during the review of the final galley proofs. The new information and appropriate references, when inserted, appear in the Bibliography by letter designations, e.g., 10a, 10b. We apologize for the lack of bibliographical continuity that resulted from these insertions, but feel that the addition of the material was essential to our primary objective of offering the most current knowledge in the field to our readers.

We congratulate our 38 authors for their dedication and understanding and for their continued and timely responses to our editorial provocations and "threats." We regard their efforts as outstanding, essential, and classic contributions! We acknowledge Ms. Linda Repa-Eschen for her untiring efforts in preparing this volume, and Ms. Agnes (Babe) Kelly for her constant editorial assistance. While we mourn the death of one of our authors, Dr. Constantine Anast, a dear friend, we applaude the diligence and scholarship that produced his chapter, "Metabolic Bone Disorders in Children," and gratefully acknowledge the efforts of those who completed the chapter's final revisions.

LOUIS V. AVIOLI
STEPHEN M. KRANE

Contents

LAWRENCE G. RAISZ
GIDEON A. RODAN

1

Cellular Basis for Bone Turnover

In the introductory chapter to the first edition of *Metabolic Bone Disease*, the important advances in the field of bone and mineral metabolism that had occurred during the previous 25 years were summarized. Logarithmic growth has continued, particularly in our knowledge of the cell biology of bone and the identification of new chemical entities, both as bone constituents and as regulators. An understanding of bone metabolism at the molecular level has just begun, and this field is also rapidly expanding. The change in both concepts and emphasis has been so great that the present chapter has been largely rewritten. Moreover, the present edition contains chapters on matrix synthesis, mineralization, and bone morphology so that these areas are covered only briefly here. As in the first edition, the synthesis, secretion, and action of the calcium-regulating hormones are reviewed in detail elsewhere. In this chapter, we review the cellular physiology of skeletal tissue, summarize the effects of calcium-regulating hormones on bone cells, and compare these with the effects of other systemic and local regulators.

Brief Review of Embryology and Anatomy of Bone

The cellular sequence of steps that result in bone formation not only is seen in embryogenesis,[1] but can be recapitulated in adult animals when new ectopic bone formation is induced by the implantation of appropriate inducers.[2] In either case, the initial steps are proliferation and condensation of fibroblastic or mesenchymal cells that differentiate into a cartilage phenotype. This cartilage then forms a template for bone, and osteoblasts differentiate on its surface. The differentiation may be associated with calcification of the cartilage as in endochondral bone formation or with extension of the bone tissue around the cartilage template such as occurs in membranous bone formation in the skull. The earliest bone that appears both in the fetus and in induction models is woven; that is, the collagen is not laid down in well-defined lamellae. However, a more orderly form of lamellar deposition of collagen occurs later in fetal life, and woven bone formation reappears only in fracture repair and certain pathologic states. Surface modeling and remodeling of bone continues throughout life in all mammals, both on periosteal and endosteal surfaces and on the surface of trabeculae. In larger mammals, haversian remodeling becomes a dominant process, and a large proportion of the cortical bone consists of osteons that have been formed in haversian canals. This system of osteons may increase bone strength and also provides a mechanism for vascular penetration and nutrition of the interior of relatively thick skeletal structures. It is not clear whether the remodeling that occurs on the surface of bone trabeculae increases strength. It may be that this process is determined more by metabolic functions of the skeleton. Both cortical and trabecular remodeling may help to repair the damage produced by stress-induced microfractures.[3,4]

Dual Function and Regulation of the Skeleton

The mammalian skeleton must serve two different sets of needs that are not necessarily compatible. For its role as a structural framework for the body, the skeleton must be strong, light, mobile, able to protect vital organs, and capable of orderly growth and remodeling. At the same time, the skeleton is the reservoir for almost all of the body's calcium and most of its phosphorus and magnesium. Moreover, it is an additional source of sodium, carbonate, and hydroxyl ions, which may be useful in dealing with excesses or deficits of these elements in extracellular and intracellular fluid. In fulfilling its metabolic roles, the skeleton is responsive to the calcium-regulating hormones, particularly parathyroid hormone (PTH) and 1,25-dihydroxyvitamin D_3 [$1,25(OH)_2D_3$]. It is important to distinguish between the functions of these hormones at relatively low physiologic concentrations, under conditions when exogenous calcium and phosphate supplies are abundant, and at the increased concentrations that occur when supplies are decreased. PTH increases when there is a calcium deficit and maintains serum and tissue calcium levels by its actions on bone to increase resorption and decrease formation. This increases the amount of both calcium and phosphate available, but the net effect is on calcium concentration because the phosphate is largely excreted owing to the phosphaturic effect of PTH on the kidney. In contrast, $1,25(OH)_2D3$ increases in response to either calcium or phosphate deficits and acts to maintain the supply of both ions. This might be achieved by increasing intestinal absorption, but when there is no calcium or phosphate intake, the supply of these ions needed can be obtained only by stimulation of bone resorption, by inhibition of bone formation, and possibly also by slowing of mineralization. The increase in mineralization and growth of bone seen with physiologic concentrations of 1,25-dihydroxyvitamin D_3 is probably not the result of a direct action on bone, but due to the increase in calcium and phosphate supply, since this hormone is essential for normal absorption of these elements in the intestine. Both PTH and $1,25(OH)_2D_3$ can be considered as hormones that maintain bone turnover or remodeling. However, under physiologic conditions, it seems likely that PTH is more important. When there is a decreased production of $1,25(OH)_2D_3$ in renal disease, the increase in PTH maintains a high rate of resorption and remodeling, and when $1,25(OH)_2D_3$ is supplied exogenously, bone resorption and turnover actually decrease.

It has been more difficult to assign a physiologic role for calcitonin. Calcitonin can exert an intermittent inhibitory effect on bone resorption. This may be most important in rapidly growing animals during suckling, when large calcium loads are ingested and rapidly absorbed. Under these conditions, because of either the resultant hypercalcemia or an induced reflex, calcitonin secretion will increase and produce transient inhibition of bone resorption. This would prevent excessive increases in serum concentration and urinary excretion of calcium and prevent loss of this valuable element.

The structural adaptations of the skeleton are under both systemic and local control. Overall rates of skeletal growth are controlled by systemic hormones.[5,6] Insulin and growth hormone, acting through somatomedins, stimulate bone formation, whereas glucocorticoids inhibit skeletal growth. Before puberty, the effects of growth factors may be exerted largely on cartilage growth. After the epiphyses have closed, effects on the skeleton must be exerted directly on bone cells. There are a number of other hormones that may have effects on skeletal growth *in vitro*, but have no established physiologic role, including epidermal, fibroblast, and platelet-derived and beta-transforming growth factors (EGF, FGF, PDGF, and TGF-beta). The sex hormones clearly have important effects on skeletal growth and development, but little is known about their mechanisms.

Whereas systemic hormones can affect overall growth, there must also be local control. The shape, size, and trabecular pattern of bone are in part genetically predetermined, but are modified by changes in the mechanical forces applied to the skeleton. These may be exerted not only by changes in gravitational or muscular stress, but also by changes in local blood vessels or parenchymal organs, particularly the marrow. Thus, hyperplastic hematopoietic tissue can produce an increase in marrow space and even an expansion of the periosteal diameter of long bones.[7] If local strain is responsible for cellular responses, this could be mediated by local hormones that serve as autocrine or paracrine regulators. The paracrine or intercellular mediators could modulate adjacent cells of the same phenotype, or alter the behavior of entirely different cell types with different functions. The hypotheses that the function of osteoclasts is determined by osteoblasts and lining cells, either through changes in their shape or through local secretion,[8] and that hematopoietic cells, including both lymphocytes and macrophages, regulate bone cell function are particularly attractive.

A number of potential local mediators have been identified. Chemically, the oxygenated fatty acids are the best defined. Bone is an abundant source of cyclo-oxygenase products of arachidonic acid, particularly prostaglandin E_2 (PGE_2) and prostacyclin (PGI_2). PGE_2 is a potent stimulator of bone resorption although it can also be an inhibitor of osteoclast function. It has a biphasic effect on bone formation, stimulating at low and inhibiting at high concentrations. Systemic hormones may act in part through prostaglandins. Glucocorticoids have been shown to inhibit PGE_2 production, and PTH, EGF, PDGF, and FGF all can stimulate prostaglandin synthesis *in vitro*. Biological assays of conditioned medium from cultured bone and extracts of bone matrix have yielded other factors that act on bone tissue. These include a local somatomedin that appears to be under growth hormone control, mitogens for bone cells, a stimulator of bone resorption, and a factor that appears to act as a competitive inhibitor of PTH. The source of these factors has not been elucidated, and some may be products of hematopoietic rather than bone cells. For example, macrophages can produce prostaglandins, interleukin-1 and a bone cell growth factor.[9] Lymphocytes are probably the source of another osteoclast-activating factor, which is a potent stimulator of bone resorption, tumor necrosis factor beta, or lymphotoxin.[10] Some product of mast cells may be involved in the regulation of bone resorption. Despite the substantial evidence for the existence of local factors, their specific roles in the regulation of bone metabolism have not yet been established.

I. METHODS FOR STUDYING BONE CELL FUNCTION

Before presenting a more detailed description of factors influencing bone metabolism, it is useful to review the major methods used to develop our knowledge and consider their limitations. Much information has been obtained *in vitro* using cell and organ culture. These methods have the advantage that the perturbations can be more carefully controlled and the results are not confounded by secondary responses of extraskeletal regulatory systems.

A. Cell Culture

The study of cells isolated from osseous tissue has used primarily the following models: (1) cells isolated by enzymatic digestion from embryonic calvaria; (2) outgrowth of cells from tissue explants; (3) cells obtained by mechanical dispersion (primarily osteoclasts); and (4) cell lines obtained from osteosarcoma. All cell culture methods have the advantage of isolating the experimental variables and provide controlled conditions for (1) characterizing factors that act on bone cells, (2) identifying the target cells of such factors, (3) studying mechanism of action, and (4) recognizing features and products of specific cell types.

It should be borne in mind that all cell culture experiments deal with a situation in which the balance between cell types, the tissue geometry, and the structure and composition of the extracellular environment have been altered for experimental purposes. Following are some of the advantages and disadvantages of these models.

1. Cells obtained by enzymatic digestion from embryonic calvaria have been extensively used for studying osteoblastic cells, which are very abundant in that tissue. Sequential digestion protocols yield fairly reproducible cell populations highly enriched in osteoblasts. Osteoblastic cells obtained by this method were shown to produce bone in Millipore filter chambers implanted in animals[11] and to produce matrix that mineralizes *in vitro* in the presence of beta-glycerophosphate.[12-15] Most of the biochemical information on hormone interaction with osteoblastic cells was derived from studies in this system. Nonosteoblastic cells have been obtained from calvaria by collecting cells released during the first 10 to 20 minutes of the enzymatic digestion, or by stripping the periosteum and digesting it separately.[16-19] Disadvantages of cells digested from calvaria include the heterogeneity of the cell population, the change in cell phenotype during culture and with subsequent passages, and the inconvenience of starting experiments each time with whole animals.

2. Cell outgrowth from tissue explants had been used 50 years ago to grow bone cells in culture and has recently been successfully used to establish cultures from human biop-

sies.[20-22] One advantage of this method is the small amount of starting material required, which makes it particularly suited for studying cells derived from biopsies. This method could thus prove useful in the study of cellular and molecular defects associated with human diseases, such as osteogenesis imperfecta or hypophosphatasia. However, due to the limited amount of material and the probable change of phenotype with subculture, it may not provide sufficient material for studying basic mechanisms and for purifying cell products.

3. Mechanical dispersion has recently been successfully used for obtaining viable osteoclasts, which can be maintained in culture for up to 2 weeks.[23-25] Isolated osteoclasts can be used to study the resorption process and its control.[26,27] Studies of this system promise to fill a significant gap in our knowledge of osteoclastic function and its regulation by external factors.

4. Osteosarcoma cell lines[28] obtained by cloning have the advantage of providing large amounts of genotypically homogeneous cells that retain their phenotype over multiple passages in culture. They are therefore suited for mechanistic studies and isolation of cell products. They are, however, transformed and differ in their growth control features, cytoskeletal organization, oncogene expression, and growth factor production. They are easier to grow in serum-free medium and hence can be used to examine effects of single factors in defined media.

B. Organ Culture

Organ cultures are particularly useful for studying bone resorption.[29] They contain both fully differentiated osteoclasts and their precursors and resorption rates can be quantitated by measuring the release of stable or labeled calcium or matrix products. Organ cultures are also useful for the study of matrix synthesis. They contain fully differentiated osteoblasts that can produce large amounts of collagen in an organized fashion as well as precursor cells. However, good organ culture systems have not yet been developed for the study of mineralization. This may be one of the reasons that so little is known about the regulation of this process.

In organ culture, with multiple cell types present, the measured response to a particular agent may not indicate a direct effect since local mediators are often involved, for example, agents that stimulate bone resorption by increasing local prostaglandin production. Moreover, since multiple cell types are present in organ culture, it may not be possible to identify the target and effector cells. However, isolation techniques have been applied to organ cultures such as mechanical stripping, which yields populations enriched in particular cell types.

C. In Vivo Studies

Whatever is found in cell or organ culture must be tested *in vivo* to determine its applicability to the intact organism. Unfortunately, accurate quantitative methods for the measurement of bone formation and resorption *in vivo* are limited. Much of our knowledge is based on morphologic methods, which are discussed in detail in Chapter 10. Bone formation rates can be assessed for mineralized bone using sequential labels of tetracycline or other agents that bind to mineral[30] and for matrix using labeled matrix precursors such as [^{3}H]-proline.[31] In animals, large samples of cortical and trabecular bone can be analyzed by these methods, but in humans it is usually possible to obtain biopsies of limited areas, such as the iliac crest, and only mineral apposition rates can be measured using tetracycline labels, since administration of labeled proline would result in excessive radiation exposure.

Overall measurements of the rates of bone formation and resorption can be obtained using radioactive calcium or other bone-seeking isotopes.[32] These kinetic measurements do give useful information on the overall rates of mineral accretion and resorption if appropriate corrections are made for exchange. However, their use is limited by the amount of isotope that is needed. Use of stable isotopes of calcium has been explored, but this method is not yet fully developed.

There has been great interest in the development of better noninvasive methods for the assessment of bone formation and resorption based on measurements of bone cell products released into the blood or excreted in the urine. Values for fasting urinary calcium and hydroxyproline excretion show a rough correlation with the rate of bone resorption.[33] Although no better simple method for the measurement of bone resorption has yet been developed, it is possible that a specific product of bone matrix degradation released during the resorptive process could be identified and measured. Among measures of bone formation, serum alkaline phosphatase levels may be useful when extreme changes in bone formation occur, but the correlation between osteoblastic activity determined morphologically and alkaline phosphatase levels is relatively weak. A better correlation has been observed recently with measurements of serum concentration of the bone gamma-carboxyglutamic acid–containing protein (BGP or osteocalcin).[34,35] This protein is probably synthesized and released by osteoblasts, and its blood level appears to reflect the rate of bone formation. In addition, bone formation may be reflected by the release of procollagen peptides in the circulation. Comparison of the serum concentrations of the procollagen peptides for type I collagen, which predominates in bone, and for type III collagen, which also reflects collagen synthesis in nonskeletal tissues, may give useful index of bone formation rate.

II. BONE CELLS

The tissues of the mammalian organism can be divided into three groups regarding their capability to regenerate: (1) nonregenerating tissues such as brain; (2) conditionally regenerating tissues, such as liver; and (3) tissues that regenerate continuously and have the ability to accelerate regeneration following trauma. The last include blood, skin, intestinal mucosa, and bone. Bone is subject to continuous deposition of new tissue and removal (resorption) of existing tissue, resulting in shape changes during growth, and in the increase of the diameter of long bones throughout life. There is also continuous replacement of packets of bone across the tissue. This process is subject to local and systemic influences and provides the basis for the functional adaptation of bone to mechanical stimuli and the response of bone tissue to homeostatic demands for calcium, phosphate, bicarbonate, and so on. Most of the pathologic change of bone is related to the processes of bone formation and resorption: an imbalance between the two results in thinning of the bone leading to fractures (osteoporosis) or thickening of the bone and crowding out of the marrow (osteopetrosis). This imbalance can also be localized, as in Paget's disease. Other defects include failure to mineralize the matrix during formation (osteomalacia, rickets). Bone formation and resorption are carried out by two groups of specialized cells, the osteoblasts and the osteoclasts, respectively.

A. Osteoblastic Lineage (Fig. 1–1)

1. Osteoprogenitor Cells

Regenerating tissues possess progenitor cells that can undergo asymmetric division, resulting in another progenitor cell and a differentiated or predifferentiated cell. In the case of bone, these cells are called osteoprogenitor cells. Osteoprogenitor cells have a spindle-shaped, fibroblastic appearance and have been operationally divided into two groups: the determined osteoprogenitor cells (DOPCs) and the inducible osteoprogenitor cells (IOPCs).[36] DOPCs can form bone (judged by histologic appearance) in Millipore filter chambers implanted into animals. These chambers allow free diffusion of molecules, including macromolecules, but no penetration of cells.[37-39] IOPCs can form bone in such chambers only in the presence of "inducing" influences, provided, for example, by bladder epithelium.[40,41] DOPCs are found in the periosteum and in the bone marrow where they are thought to be the reticular cells abundant next to endosteal surfaces.[42,43] Among bone marrow cells, the reticular cells are the only ones to survive and proliferate in

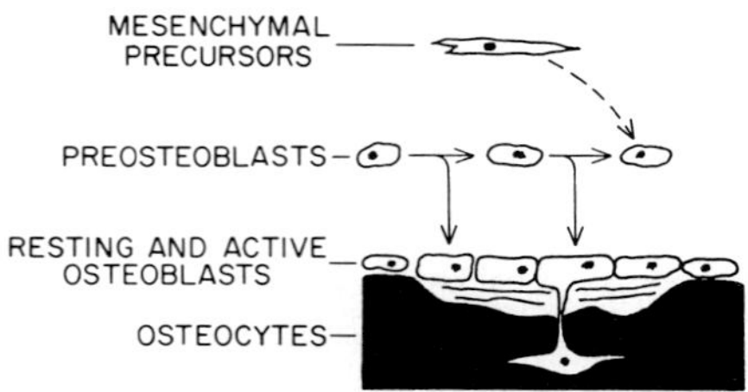

Figure 1–1. Origin of osteoblasts. The fully differentiated osteoblasts are probably derived largely from adjacent, partially differentiated preosteoblasts. However, under certain circumstances, undifferentiated mesenchymal precursors can be induced to form bone. Presumably this occurs when new bone formation is induced at ectopic sites by implantation of demineralized matrix.

culture and they do not lose their osteogenic potential in the process.[37,44] It is not clear whether reticular cells of the osteoprogenitor type are continuously generated from hematopoietic stem cells in the adult, or whether they belong to a pool of cells that separated during development. The limited evidence currently available favors the latter view. The bone marrow osteogenic reticular cells have not been extensively studied and their responses to chemotactic factors, hormones, and growth and differentiation factors have not been characterized. Nor are any of the genetic features that may distinguish them from other fibroblast-type cells known at this time. The osteogenic nature of periosteal precursor cells has been demonstrated by histologic and autoradiographic evidence following [^{3}H]-thymidine incorporation into DNA.[45]

Inducible osteogenic precursor cells have been found in thymus, spleen, and lymph nodes.[37] Cells with osteogenic potential have been also present in muscle and dermis, where endochondral bone formation can be initiated by the implantation of decalcified bone matrix.[46-48] Recent evidence suggests that the inductive principle is a peptide or a couple of peptides of molecular weight of around 20,000 daltons.[49-53] These precursor cells are probably induced during pathologic ossification in muscle or skin. It is not known whether there are one or several groups of IOPCs, in what way they differ genetically from the DOPCs, and what are the mechanisms of induction. Most progenitor cells are usually quiescent, a small fraction being activated during normal bone modeling (shape change during growth) and remodeling and a larger fraction in response to injury or other stimuli.

2. Preosteoblasts

The preosteoblasts are in a transitional state of 2 to 3 days' duration between the osteoprogenitor cell and the differentiated osteoblast. They express proliferative activity and an increase in the features associated with the osteoblastic phenotype.

The first detectable changes toward the differentiated state are (1) rounding-up, (2) organization into a contiguous layer, and (3) a rise in alkaline phosphatase levels. At this stage the cells are still proliferating,[45] and most of the progeny will become matrix-producing osteoblasts. One or two rounds of DNA synthesis are frequently associated with the differentiation of progenitor cells; however, it is not known whether this is an absolute requirement for osteoblastic cells. It is also not known what regulatory influences act on the preosteoblasts. By analogy to other differentiating systems, the genetic events set into motion in the progenitor cells probably follow a "programmed" course. In the differentiation of 3T3 fibroblasts into fat cells, it was shown that several phenotype-specific macromolecules were expressed sequentially rather than concurrently and were influenced by the state of the actomyosin cytoskeleton.[54] Locally produced growth and differentiation factors, such as insulin-like growth factor–1 and transforming growth factor beta (TGF-beta), could act in an autocrine or paracrine fashion to promote osteoblast maturation.[55,56]

3. Osteoblasts (Fig. 1–2)

Osteoblasts are actively synthesizing and secreting the matrix that mineralizes about 24 hours later to become the major constituent (by mass or volume) of bone tissue. Morphologically, osteoblasts are cuboidal cells organized as a contiguous layer above the matrix that they secrete. They have eccentric nuclei separated from the secretory surface by abundant rough endoplasmic reticulum and Golgi, characteristic features of protein-synthesizing secretory cells.[57] Osteoblasts are connected by gap junctions,[58] which may also link them to lining cells and to osteocytes (see later), creating an extensive cellular network capable of electrical[59] or cross-junction chemical communication. In addition, three features characterize differentiated cells: (1) their secretory products, (2) their enzymatic profile, and (3) their response to hormones and other signals.

4. Collagen

The osteoblasts synthesize and secrete the vast majority of the organic constituents of the bone matrix. Some constituents, such as alpha-2HS-sialoprotein, are synthesized elsewhere and are taken up from the plasma. Type I collagen amounts to 95% of the organic material in bone matrix and can account for 65% of the total protein synthesis in bone-

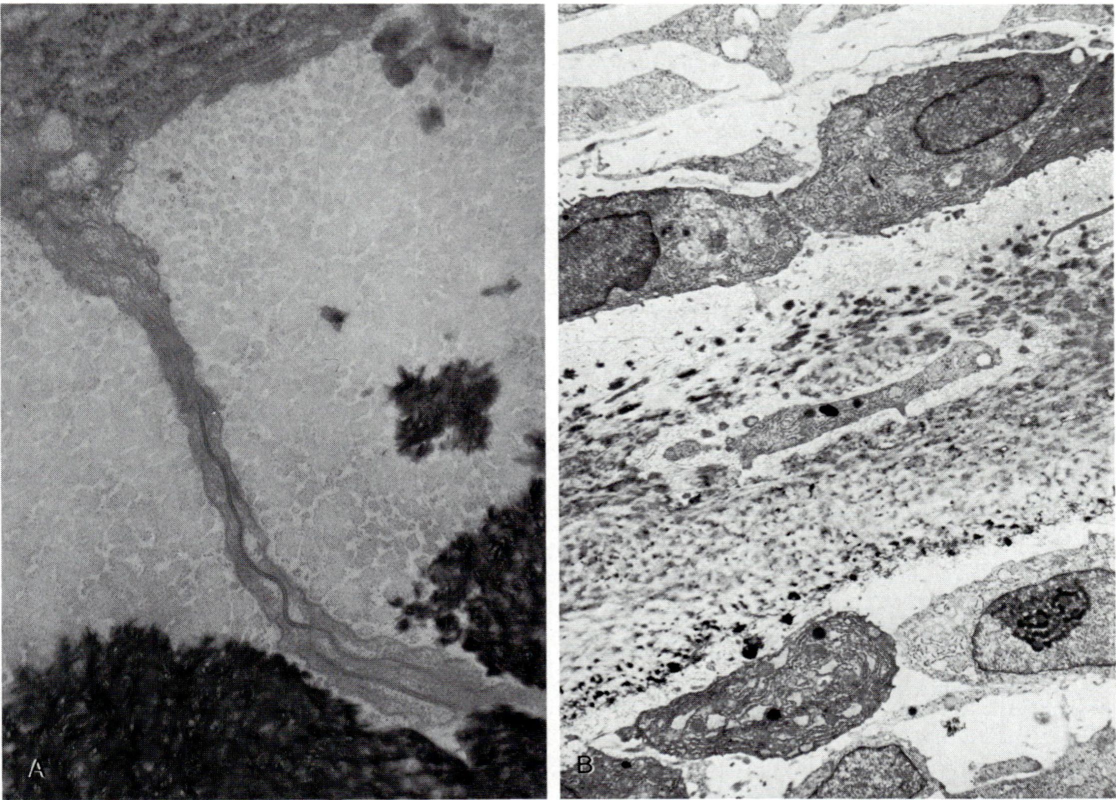

Figure 1–2. Morphology of osteoblasts. *A*, In the low-power electron micrograph, a layer of osteoblasts that are tightly connected to each other forming a syncytium is seen on the upper (forming) side of the bone; on the lower side, cells that may represent either inactive osteoblasts or precursor cells are less tightly connected to each other so that there is no true syncytium on the bone surface. A relatively inactive osteocyte is seen within the bone. *B*, A higher power view shows one of the processes extending from an osteoblast toward the mineralized bone and connecting through gap junctions with a process from an internal osteocyte. The unmineralized osteoid contains collagen bundles of increasing size. Mineralization is at first spotty, but ultimately there is a dense and continuous mineralization front. (Kindly provided by Dr. M. Holtrop.)

forming cells.[60] There is significant information available today on the complex sequence of events leading from transcription of the collagen genes to the spatial organization of collagen fibers in the extracellular matrix and the subsequent deposition of mineral. These events include the transcription of genes for type I collagen located on chromosomes 7 and 17, coding for the pro-alpha$_1$ and pro-alpha$_2$ chains, respectively; processing of the mRNA and its translation; posttranslational modifications, which include glycosylation and hydroxylation of proline and lysine; assembly of two alpha$_1$ chains and one alpha$_2$ chain into a triple helix; translocation from the site of synthesis via the Golgi to the cell membrane and secretion; deployment in the extracellular space in a specific spatial arrangement and cleavage of the NH_2-terminal and COOH-terminal extension peptides; cross-linking and specific interaction with other extracellular macromolecules, such as fibronectin, osteonectin, and proteoglycans; mineralization; and eventually degradation and removal during bone resorption (for a review, see reference 61). These steps involve multiple enzymes and co-factors and the participation of the cytoskeleton, and are subject to hormonal control (see section V). Defects at various points in the sequence of events can produce pathologic manifestations in the skeleton. For example, genetic defects affecting the amino acid sequence of the extension peptides were found to be associated with osteogenesis imperfecta. These defects are believed to retard helix formation and increase glycosylation (see Chapter 17).

5. Noncollagenous Bone Proteins

Several noncollagenous macromolecules have been isolated and purified from bone and were recently shown to be synthesized by osteoblasts. Osteocalcin (or bone gamma-carboxyglutamic acid–containing protein [BGP]) amounts to 1% to 2% of the bone protein in all vertebrates.[62,63] It has been highly conserved in evolution, has a molecular weight of 5800, and has three gamma-carboxyglutamic acid (GLA) residues that endow it with a strong affinity for hydroxyapatite.[64] The gamma-carboxylation is a vitamin K–dependent posttranslational modification of the protein. Like all secreted proteins, it is synthesized as a precursor with a leader sequence of molecular weight of about 3000.[65] The function of this protein is not known. Treatment of rats with warfarin, the vitamin K antagonist, can deplete the skeletal BGP content by over 95% without apparent ill effects on skeletal growth, remodeling, or calcium homeostasis. A significant fraction of synthesized BGP is not retained by bone and finds its way into the circulation. The level of circulating BGP is used as an index of osteoblastic activity. The usefulness of this parameter in various metabolic bone diseases is being investigated. BGP synthesis is enhanced several-fold by $1,25(OH)_2D_3$.[66] There is a separate matrix GLA protein, which is less soluble and is also regulated by vitamin D.[67,68]

Another very abundant noncollagenous protein synthesized by osteoblasts and found in bone is osteonectin. Osteonectin is a phosphoprotein, with an apparent molecular weight of around 32,000 (by electrophoresis).[69] It binds strongly to hydroxyapatite as well as collagen. *In vivo* its abundance is increased upon vitamin D repletion in vitamin D–deficient animals,[70] but its function is not known. Its use as an index of osteoblastic activity is being explored.[71,72] In bovine osteogenesis imperfecta, the amount of osteonectin in bone was found to be significantly reduced.[73] It is not an exclusive bone protein, and is present in platelets as well.[74]

Osteopontin or sialoprotein I is another noncollagenous protein purified from bone matrix, whose structure was recently elucidated.[75-77] In the rat osteopontin mRNA is found primarily in bone and kidney.[78]

Other noncollagenous proteins found in bone, which are probably synthesized by osteoblasts, include phosphoproteins with molecular weights of 12,000 (from chicken)[79,80] and 24,000 and 62,000 (from calf).[81] Bone also contains a small molecular weight proteoglycan that has a core protein with a molecular weight of about 35,000 and two chondroitin sulfate chains each with a molecular weight of about 40,000.[75] This small proteoglycan, also found in other tissues, is different from the large proteoglycan found in cartilage. Other macromolecules produced and secreted by osteoblasts include bone morphogenetic protein[49] and bone-derived growth factors.[82]

6. Alkaline Phosphatase

Among the enzymes associated with osteoblastic differentiation, alkaline phosphatase is the most prominent. Alkaline phosphatase has long been recognized as an osteoblastic marker,[83] and its level is also elevated in calcifying cartilage and dentin. This enzyme cleaves organophosphate bonds, has limited specificity, and presumably participates in the mineralization process. The enzyme is located in the plasma membrane of the osteoblast and its active site is accessible from the extracellular fluid.[84] Highest level of activity is seen in mature, matrix-synthesizing osteoblasts.[28] In humans there are several structurally different isoenzymes of alkaline phosphatase encoded by separate genes, distinguishable on the basis of heat lability and susceptibility to inhibitors: the placenta (a group of at least three),[85] the intestine (probably two),[86] and the liver-kidney-bone type.[87-89] The alkaline phosphatase is a glycoprotein dimer of molecular weight about 140,000.[90] The liver, kidney, and bone enzymes exhibit electrophoretic differences, presumably due to differences in glycosylation. The enzyme is released into the bloodstream, and elevated levels correlate with increased osteoblastic (bone-forming) activity.

7. *Hormones Acting on Osteoblasts*

Another characteristic feature of differentiated cells is the response to tissue-specific hormones. Several hormones that influence bone metabolism and calcium homeostasis were shown to act on osteoblasts, albeit not exclusively. Osteoblasts respond to parathyroid hormone (PTH) by an elevation in cyclic AMP.[16,17,19,91,92] Receptors for PTH have been demonstrated in osteoblastic cells by radioligand-binding studies.[93,94] In proliferating embryonic calvaria and osteosarcoma osteoblastic cells, PTH inhibits alkaline phosphatase[18,91,95] and collagen synthesis.[96] *In vivo* and in organ culture,[97] PTH causes bone resorption, and it was proposed that cells from the osteoblastic lineage participate in this response.[8,98]

Receptors for $1,25(OH)_2D_3$, the active metabolite of vitamin D, are also present in osteoblasts[99] and osteoblast-like osteosarcoma cells.[100,101] It was recently shown that the local action of this hormone is not necessary for mineralization,[102,103] and its role in osteoblasts is still uncertain. *In vitro*, in calvaria or osteosarcoma osteoblastic cells, $1,25(OH)_2D_3$ inhibits collagen synthesis[18,91,104] and was reported both to stimulate and to inhibit alkaline phosphatase, probably depending on the state of differentiation of the cells.[105,106] $1,25(OH)_2D_3$ was recently shown to modulate differentiation in tumor cells from many tissues,[107,108] and it may have similar effects on the growth and differentiation of cells of the osteoblastic lineage. Like all steroid hormones, $1,25(OH)_2D_3$ probably acts on transcription.[109] The recently elucidated structure of the $1,25(OH)_2D_3$ receptor contains the typical zinc-binding "finger-shaped" domain, presumed to interact with DNA.[110]

Another steroid hormone that may have similar effects is hydrocortisone (or its analogues). This hormone acts on a large number of tissues, has multiple effects on the same cell (pleiotropic action), and different effects at different stages of development or differentiation. Recent studies have demonstrated the interaction of glucocorticoid receptor with promotor sequences in the genome.[111,114] *In vivo,* glucocorticoid treatment is one of the most common causes of iatrogenic osteopenia. In rat osteoblastic cells in culture (plated at low density),[115] glucocorticoids inhibit proliferation. They also increase abundance of $1,25(OH)_2D_3$ receptors[115] and the response to PTH,[117-119] the bone-resorbing hormones. It is not known whether this would lead to enhanced bone resorption at the physiologic concentrations of these hormones. Histomorphometric studies have shown a significant increase in osteoclastic resorption surfaces in corticosteroid-treated patients and patients with Cushing's syndrome, which could also be due to secondary hyperparathyroidism caused by decreased absorption of calcium from the gut.[120] Glucocorticoids also promote the expression of osteoblastic cell-differentiated functions including collagen synthesis[121] and alkaline phosphatase activity.[122,123] These effects observed *in vitro* are also consistent with histomorphometricfindingsshowingincreasedtrabecular osteoid surface. However, the dominant effect of glucocorticoids on osteoblastic cells is inhibition of cell proliferation, leading to a reduction in the overall rate of bone formation.[124] The additional effects of the hormone observed *in vitro* illustrate the complexity governing the regulation of cellular function. Thus glucocorticoids can stimulate collagen synthesis and alkaline phosphatase while at the same time increasing the susceptibility for inhibition of these functions by $1,25(OH)_2D_3$ and PTH. The balance of these influences that interact with each other will determine the response of the cell.

Osteoblasts are also target cells for insulin, epidermal growth factor, and prostaglandins, which also act on many other mesenchymal cells.

8. *Prostaglandin Synthesis*

Osteoblasts and osteoblast-like cell lines also produce prostaglandins, primarily PGE and PGI_2.[125,126] The regulation of osteoblastic prostaglandin production and its role *in vivo* have not been fully elucidated; however, available evidence suggests that they may play a significant role in local control of bone metabolism. In organ culture, PGE_1 and PGE_2 are potent stimulators of bone resorption as well as DNA synthesis and collagen synthesis. *In vivo,* bone resorption associated with certain experimental tumors[127] and a small fraction of human tumors is dependent on prostaglandin synthesis.[128] On the other hand, experimental and therapeutic administration of prostaglandin has been shown to produce enhanced bone formation. Osteoblastic cell cultures from embryonic calvaria or osteosarcoma produce up to 2.5 ng PGE_2 per milligram protein per 24 hours, sufficiently high quantities to produce biological effects. Among rat osteosarcoma cell lines, only those with osteoblastic properties have the ability to synthesize prostaglandins,[119] the others lacking cyclo-oxygenase.

Several factors have been shown to stimulate prostaglandin synthesis in osteoblastic cells, including mechanical perturbation produced by stretching the substrate for cell growth, plastic dishes,[129] or collagen fibers.[130] Recent findings show that a quasiphysiologic strain of 5–7 *mstrain* (unpublished observation) and the disruption of microtubules increase prostaglandin synthesis in rat calvaria cells more than 2-fold.[131] PTH also stimulates PGE synthesis in calvaria-derived osteoblasts[132] and in calvaria explants and in long bones. EGF and complement-containing serum have similar effects.[133,134]

Prostaglandins stimulate cyclic AMP in osteoblastic cells, an action similar to that of PTH. The cAMP stimulatory effect of various prostanoids parallels their bone-resorbing activity.[135] This correlation and the similarity of PGE and PTH effects on osteoblasts suggested the participation of these cells in hormonal control of bone resorption.[8] Differences in prostaglandin production and in the response to prostaglandins were observed among clonal cell lines obtained from rat calvaria and osteosarcoma.[119,126,136] If this diversity is present *in vivo,* it may represent subspecialization among differentiated osteoblastic cells. Similar diversity has been observed in other cell types, including fibroblasts,[137] and is probably essential for the effective function of complex tissues. It is possible that certain cells are specifically endowed to perceive external stimuli, which are then amplified and transmitted to neighboring cells, via prostaglandin E, for example, to produce the biological response.

9. Lining Cells and Osteocytes (Fig. 1–2)

The calcified bone matrix is covered by a contiguous layer of polygonal bone lining cells.[138] These cells are flat, contain small amounts of endoplasmic reticulum, and do not proliferate. Histologic evidence suggests that they represent quiescent osteoblast-derived cells, which have completed matrix production. Their alkaline phosphatase content is significantly lower than that of osteoblasts. The bone lining cells are connected by gap junctions,[139,140] and although no tight junctions are present, it has been postulated that these cells form an effective barrier between the bone mineral and the extracellular fluid.[141] Morphologically they are not as tightly connected as are active osteoblasts. PTH produces rapid effects on the shape of these cells.[142,143] On the endosteal surfaces of long bones, PTH causes cell rounding, resulting in less tight packing as well as distention of endoplasmic reticulum and swelling of the Golgi, suggesting secretion. It has been proposed that the bone lining cells participate in the control of calcium homeostasis.[142] Some of the osteoblasts become embedded in the matrix that they produce and are surrounded by it. These cells are called osteocytes and are probably similar, functionally, to the bone lining cells. They have multiple cell processes, which connect them to other osteocytes, forming a communicating network throughout the tissue. These processes may also connect osteocytes to blood vessels, which are never farther than 100 μm away. The periosteocytic lacunae, the spaces surrounding the osteocytes are increased in hyperparathyroidism.[120]

B. Osteoclastic Lineage (Fig. 1–3)

1. Osteoclasts (Fig. 1–4)

Osteoclasts are undoubtedly the cells responsible for the resorption of bone during modeling (shape changes during growth) and remodeling (continuous replacement of bone packets) of the skeleton. It is not known to what extent other cells, such as osteocytes and lining cells, participate in the removal of calcium, phosphate, and other electrolytes from bone and whether other cells such as macrophages actively resorb bone *in vivo.*[144]

Osteoclasts are very large multinucleated cells measuring several hundred microns in diameter. They are formed by the fusion of mononuclear cells rather than cell division,

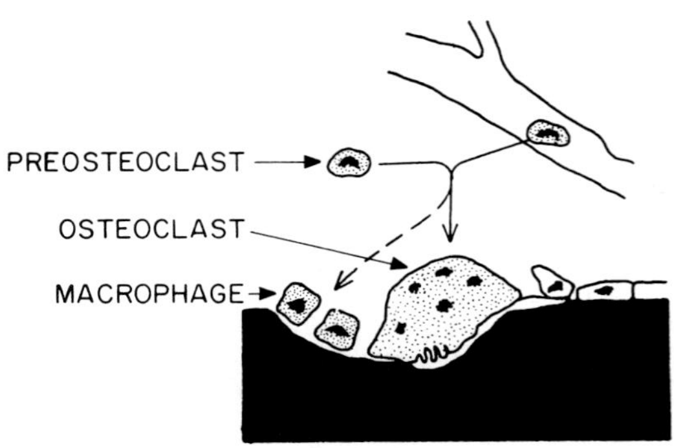

Figure 1–3. Origin and activation of osteoclasts. There is considerable evidence that osteoclasts are derived from mononuclear cells, which can be present either in the circulation or in the marrow. Their coalescence and activation may depend on a prior change in a surface resting osteoblast as indicated on the right. Monocytes that differentiate into macrophages probably also play a role in bone resorption. Whereas there is evidence that they represent a separate cell line, macrophages appear to migrate to bone-resorbing sites after osteoclastic bone resorption has removed the bulk of mineral and matrix. They may be involved in removal of residual matrix, in deposition of the noncollagenous materials that produce the "cement line," and in the release of factors that initiate osteoblastic replacement at the resorption site.

since no mitotic figures or [^{3}H]-thymidine can be seen in newly formed osteoclasts following bone-resorbing stimuli.

Nuclear kinetic studies on osteoclasts in dogs have shown that the rate of osteoclast turnover is about 8% per day, assuming steady state. The osteoclasts appear to be 20 to 40 times more efficient (per nucleus) in removing bone than osteoblasts are in forming bone during the remodeling process.[145] Morphologically, osteoclasts have indented nuclei with prominent nucleoli, abundant mitochondria with large cristae, very little rough endoplasmic reticulum, many lysosomes, and most typically, a large amount of folded plasma membrane called ruffled border, surrounded by a clear zone. The clear zone attaches to the resorption surface like a suction cup generating an enclosed space that contains the ruffled border and may function as a very large, confined, extracellular lysosomal space. A characteristic enzymatic activity found in osteoclasts is tartrate-resistant acid phosphatase.

Carbonic anhydrase, the enzyme that catalyzes the reversible hydration of CO_2 into carbonic acid, was shown to be present in osteoclasts and to change its cellular distribution following treatment with calcitonin, an inhibitor of osteoclastic activity.[146,147] Several additional recent findings support the assumption that acidification is associated with osteoclast function. A vacuolar proton pump has been identified in the osteoclast;[148,148a] and a local decrease in pH can be detected by acridine orange fluorescence[149] and direct sampling.[150]

The biochemical mechanism for osteoclastic bone resorption has not been fully elucidated. There is no evidence that osteoclasts produce collagenase. This enzyme is made by osteoblasts,[151-153] but its role in bone resorption has not been conclusively established. The bone mineral can be solubilized by acidification of its environment, and it was proposed that the matrix could be digested by lysosomal proteases such as cathepsin B or other serine proteases.[154] The release of lysosomal enzymes in response to resorptive stimuli in organ culture[155] supports this possibility.

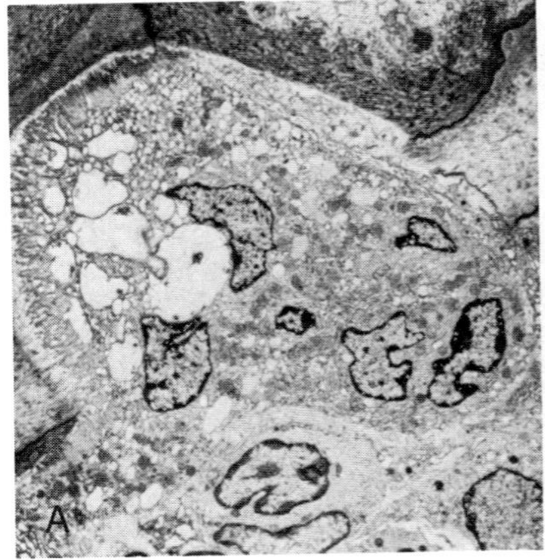

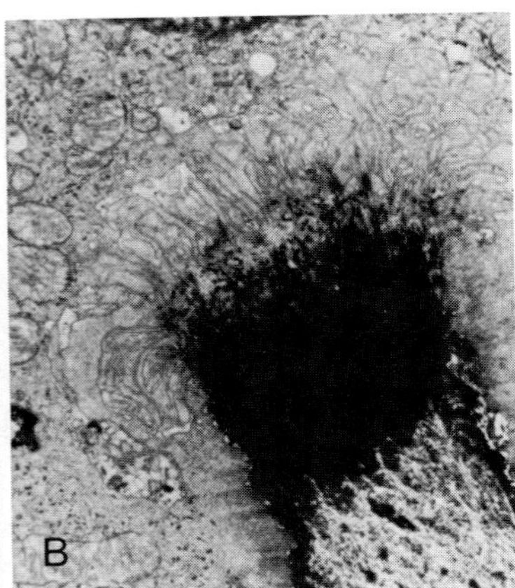

Figure 1–4. Morphology of osteoclasts. *A*, An osteoclast from PTH-stimulated bone *in vivo*. Notice the many nuclei, the large vacuoles at the site of resorption on the left, and the abundant mitochondria. *B*, A high-power view of the ruffled border in the act of degrading a spicule of bone. It is surrounded by a clear zone that attaches the osteoclast to the bone and separates the ruffled border area from the surrounding extracellular fluid. (Kindly provided by Dr. M. Holtrop.)

Osteoclasts have been isolated from the tissue and studied *in vitro*. It was shown that they are able to resorb bone when exposed to mineralized bone surfaces, but were ineffective in removing demineralized bone.[156] Some investigators proposed that the matrix might be degraded by collagenase released from osteoblast-derived cells in response to PTH,[98,156,157] thus exerting their facilitating effect on osteoclast action. These studies also showed that the isolated mature osteoclasts did not respond to parathyroid hormone or $1,25(OH)_2D_3$, but were inhibited by physiologic concentrations of calcitonin, dibutyryl cAMP, and paradoxically, prostaglandins.[158] However, addition of osteoblastic cells and a stimulator of resorption can increase osteoclastic activity in such systems.[26] This observation supports the assumption that these hormones may stimulate bone resorption indirectly by acting on other cells, such as the osteoblast-derived lining cells.[8,98] It was also shown that the isolated osteoclasts fuse with circulating monocytes, suggesting a possible monocytic origin.[159]

2. Osteoclast Origin

There is a large amount of evidence indicating that osteoclasts and osteoblasts do not originate from the same precursor cells. Whereas osteoblasts are derived from resident mesenchymal osteoprogenitor cells (see earlier), osteoclasts are most likely derived from migrating monocytes of the macrophage type. This idea was first proposed by Hancox on the basis of similarities between osteoclasts and macrophages[160] and has since received considerable support from direct and indirect experimental evidence. Fishmann and Hay showed that during limb regeneration in the newt, $[^3H]$-thymidine appeared first in mononuclear leukocytes and subsequently in osteoclasts, while mesenchymal cells remained unlabeled.[161] Jee and Nolan used charcoal particles to mark mononuclear phagocytes and showed that they gave rise to osteoclasts.[162] Similarly, macrophages from a donor rat labeled with thorium dioxide were shown to form osteoclasts in bone fractures of a recipient rat.[163] Gothlin and Ericsson also showed that in parabiotic rats in which one animal was irradiated with a dose that was lethal for mononuclear cells, osteoclasts were formed by cells from the second animal that had been labeled with $[^3H]$-thymidine.[164] However, in mice that had 40% $[^3H]$-thymidine-labeled monocytes and were treated with 1-α-hydroxycholecalciferol, only 8% of nuclei in osteoclasts were labeled, suggesting an additional source of precursor cells.[165] Similar findings were obtained by Buring, who showed that in bone grafted to the abdominal wall of rats, osteoclasts were of host origin.[166] Analogous evidence was obtained from studies of chick/quail chimera, in which the origin of nuclei can be distinguished by the nucleolar pattern, and in which it was shown that bone rudiments from one species grafted on the chorioallantoic membranes of the second one were populated by osteoclasts originating from the circulation of the host.[167,168]

Another line of evidence supporting the hematopoietic origin of osteoclasts is provided by observations on osteopetrosis. This is a group of genetic disorders in humans and animals characterized by osteoclast dysfunction and impaired bone resorption. Walker has shown that this defect can be corrected in mice by parabiosis with normal littermates or by injection of hematopoietic cells from neonatal liver or spleen following irradiation of the recipient animal.[169] Spleen cells were also shown to cure osteopetrosis in a rat.[170] Conversely, the injection of hematopoietic cells from mutant animals into normal irradiated littermates produced the osteopetrotic phenotype.[171] Monocytic rather than lymphocytic cells were shown to have the curative function. In humans it was shown that in an osteopetrotic female child cured by a bone marrow graft from a male donor, osteoclasts contained male chromosomes.[172] In osteopetrotic microphthalmic mice, it was also shown that bone-resorbing osteoclasts were of donor origin. After grafting bone marrow from beige mice, which have giant lysosomes in their monocytes, the giant lysosomes were found in the osteoclasts of the cured recipient animals.[173] In certain cases of human and murine osteopetrosis, monocytic functions were defective.

Recent studies of osteoclast formation *in vitro* also support their hematopoietic origin. Ko and Bernard showed that bone marrow mononuclear cells, co-cultured with osteoclast-free bone from fetal mouse calvaria, gave rise to osteoclasts.[174] Burger et al showed that osteoclasts could form from bone marrow mononuclear phagocytes co-cultured with periosteum-free bone rudiments, but not from peritoneal exudate cells.[175] Live bone-forming cells were required for osteoclast formation in these experiments. Several recent studies suggest that the osteoclast precursor cells may be the GM-CFC.

These findings strongly indicate that osteoclasts are derived from hematopoietic precursor cells. Osteoblast-lineage lining cells may participate in osteoclastic bone resorption by: (1) shape changes that uncover the matrix and expose it to osteoclastic activity; (2) the secretion of factors that attract preosteoclasts and stimulate their differentiation and/or activity; or (3) removal of factors that inhibit osteoclastic activity. There is good evidence for changes in lining cell shape following PTH and $1,25(OH)_2D_3$ stimulation,[142,176-178] and histologic changes consistent with secretion. Other evidence supporting osteoblast-osteoclast interaction in resorption is circumstantial. For example, live mesenchymal cells were needed for the differentiation of bone marrow monocytes into osteoclasts,[175] and osteoblastic cells restored mobility to calcitonin-treated osteoclasts.[179] $1,25(OH)_2D_3$ stimulates in osteoblastic cells the synthesis and secretion of osteocalcin,[180] which was shown to be chemotactic for monocytes.[181] However, warfarin treatment, which reduces osteocalcin content in bone by 95%, did not prevent calcium mobilization from bone.[182] On the other hand, the presence of osteocalcin in subcutaneous implants promoted their degradation by osteoclast-like cells.[183] The molecular details for osteoblast-osteoclast interaction in bone resorption, as well as bone formation, in which osteoblastic differentiation and matrix production follow the osteoclastic cutting cone, await further elucidation.

Recently, increasing consideration has been given to the immune system as a potential factor in the control of bone resorption, based on the following evidence. Bone resorption is associated with inflammation in rheumatoid arthritis and in periodontitis. Cells related to monocytes are likely precursors of osteoclasts (see earlier) and mature macrophages have been shown to resorb bone. Questions that remain to be answered include: (1) Are osteoclasts the progeny of a common stem cell, which in the adult also gives rise to macrophages, or the progeny of a subpopulation of precursor cells committed during development to the osteoclastic phenotype? (2) What is the sequence of events, molecular and cellular, leading from precursor cells to osteoclasts? and (3) What are the conditions and factors, humoral and physical, that control this process? Currently, there are just a few clues toward answering these questions. For example, osteoclasts lack surface Fc receptors, which are present in macrophages;[184] bone marrow–derived monocytes are much more effective osteoclast progenitors than are peritoneal exudate cells;[175] $1,25(OH)_2D_3$, which is a bone-resorbing hormone, has been shown to stimulate the differentiation of HL–60 cells into macrophages,[108] to promote the fusion of lung macrophages into polykarion giant cells[185] and the generation of osteoclastic cells from bone marrow.[186,187] Other studies along these lines should provide answers to these questions in the near future.

C. The Role of Other Cell Types in Bone Resorption

A potential role for cells of the osteoblastic lineage in bone resorption was mentioned previously. Osteocytes were implicated in mineral extraction from bone, since osteocytic lacunae are enlarged during increased bone resorption, such as hyperparathyroidism and glucocorticoid treatment.[188] The periosteocytic space is also rapidly labeled following radioactive calcium injection, indicating active mineral exchange. There is no evidence, however, that osteocytes can degrade matrix in ways that would contribute to bone remodeling.

Bone lining cells have been implicated in a number of ways in bone resorption. As mentioned, it was proposed that they participate in the control of calcium fluxes to and from bone in response to homeostatic needs, similar to osteocytes.[142] Other mononuclear cells have also been implicated as mediators of hormonal stimulation of osteoclastic resorption. Macrophages were shown to degrade devitalized bone *in vitro*.[189,190] Monocytic cells are chemotactically attracted by the products of bone resorption.[191] Lymphocytes activated by lectins produce factors that stimulate osteoclastic bone resorption.[192] Recently, interleukin-1, the monokine that stimulates T cell proliferation, was also shown to enhance bone resorption in organ culture.[193] IL-1 appears to be the major bone-resorbing factor in osteoclast-activating factor (OAF) from normal leukocytes.[194,195] IL-1 and lymphotoxin (TNFβ) are probably responsible for the activation of bone resorption in multiple myeloma.[196,197] In mice this activity was shown to be produced by the interaction of T lymphocytes and macrophages.[198] Stimulation of bone resorption by OAF is not dependent on prostaglandin synthesis. Serum complement was also shown to stimulate bone resorption in organ culture.[134,199] Osteopetrosis is sometimes associated with defects in monocyte or lymphocyte function,[172] and T lymphocyte–deficient mice (nude) showed reduced bone remodeling activity whereas B lymphocyte–deficient mice (moth eaten) showed accelerated bone remodeling.

Receptors for hormones that stimulate bone resorption are found in lymphocytes,[200,201] and these hormones may control growth and differentiation in those cells. For example, PTH was shown to promote T cell proliferation, and $1,25(OH)_2D_3$ was shown to inhibit the proliferation of HL–60 cells and promote their differentiation into macrophages.[107,108]

Although this evidence is often circumstantial and the molecular detail is still lacking, it strongly indicates the possible involvement of the immune system in bone resorption. It is not known at present if the immune system is only developmentally related to bone resorption, if it participates in normal bone remodeling, if it is associated with pathologic conditions that cause systemic bone loss (osteoporosis), or if it is primarily responsible for local bone loss caused by inflammation (in rheumatoid arthritis and periodontal disease).

III. BONE RESORPTION

A. Biochemical Mechanisms

Biochemical analysis of the process of bone resorption has been limited because only recently has it been possible to isolate sufficient numbers of active osteoclasts to measure chemical changes. However, as described previously, detailed morphologic studies on osteoclasts, biochemical analyses of resorbing bone in organ culture, and inferences derived from the effects of inhibitors do permit us to provide a general description of the resorptive process. The initial steps of formation of osteoclasts, migration and adherence to the bone surface, and development of the ruffled border, which is the active bone-resorbing apparatus, are less well understood. Hyaluronic acid may be involved in the initial migration of osteoclasts and their precursors, since increased hyaluronic acid synthesis precedes the increase in bone resorption seen in hormone-stimulated organ cultures. Early stimulation of cell replication by some stimulators of bone resorption and chemotactic effects of bone cell products have also been described.[202]

Once the active osteoclast has adhered to the bone surface via its clear zone and formed a ruffled border within that zone, it is possible to carry out resorption in a region that is isolated from the circulating extracellular fluid. In this region, the concentration of hydrogen ions and hydrolytic enzymes can be increased locally to dissolve bone mineral and degrade the organic matrix.[149,150] This process may depend on the formation of a large amount of folded cell membrane and a fusion of lysosomes to this membrane with subsequent release of hydrogen ions and enzymes into the extracellular space. Thus, we have likened the area between bone and ruffled border to a giant exteriorized phagolysosome. The evidence for hydrogen ion secretion is cited previously. A physicochemical hypothesis to explain the dissolution of bone mineral by hydrogen ion has been presented involving the formation of hydrogen phosphate on the crystal surface, which results in increased solubility.[203]

There is a close correlation between lysosomal enzyme release and bone resorption, whether stimulated or inhibited.[155] One of the few circumstances in which lysosomal enzyme release and changes in bone resorption are dissociated is when the phosphate concentration of the growth medium is increased in organ culture.[204] Here, inhibition of bone resorption could be explained by a physicochemical effect of phosphate to buffer hydrogen ion and prevent dissolution of hydroxyapatite crystals.

Under conditions of low pH, the hydrolytic enzymes present in lysosomes could degrade all the components of bone matrix. Phosphatases and glycosidases may be responsible for degradation of phosphoproteins and proteoglycans, while the cathepsins can break inter- and intramolecular collagen bonds. Moreover, cathepsins can degrade the collagen chains themselves at low pH, although perhaps not as effectively as mammalian collagenase. The role of a typical mammalian collagenase in bone resorption is much debated.[154,205] It has not been possible to identify collagenase in osteoclasts by immunochemical methods; yet this enzyme is abundant in osteoblasts and in macrophages and is present in resorbing bone organ cultures. Plasminogen activator is also released by osteoblast-like cells under hormonal control.[206] Studies of the surface of trabecular bone indicate that macrophages are present at the deepest sites of resorption.[207] These collagenase-producing cells may be involved in the final removal of collagen after the resorption has been initiated by osteoclasts. Macrophages may also play a role in the "reversal phase" by releasing factors that stimulate osteoblastic activity and by preparing the bone surface for the initiation of osteoblastic new bone formation. Thus, macrophages might produce the so-called cement line, which presumably is due to the deposition of noncollagen proteins or proteoglycans on the bone surface at the completion of the resorption process.

IV. FACTORS REGULATING BONE RESORPTION

A. Stimulators of Bone Resorption

A remarkably large number of factors have been found to stimulate bone resorption.[208] The most important stimulators are probably PTH, 1,25(OH)$_2$D$_3$, prostaglandins, and interleukins. Tumor-derived resorbing factors have been identified in humoral hypercalcemia of malignancy, and a PTH-related peptide has now been characterized. The leukocyte products that can stimulate bone resorption include a factor from monocytes that is probably interleukin-1 and one from lymphocytes that is probably TNF. EGF and PDGF have been shown to stimulate bone resorption *in vitro,* dependent in part on stimulation of endogenous prostaglandin synthesis. Other stimulators of prostaglandin synthesis such as bradykinin and thrombin may also stimulate bone resorption. Heparin has been described as a co-factor that enhances the response to PTH. Stimulation of bone resorption by vitamin A and thyroid hormone has been demonstrated *in vitro* and may be important for their pathologic effects. Endotoxins and other bacterial products can stimulate bone resorption, and this may be important in the pathogenesis of alveolar bone loss in periodontal disease.

1. Parathyroid Hormone

Direct stimulation of bone resorption by parathyroid hormone was first demonstrated *in vivo* by Barnicot, who showed that transplanted parathyroid glands produced local bone resorption,[209] and confirmed by Gaillard in organ culture.[210,211] PTH produces a rapid increase in both the number and activity of osteoclasts, both *in vivo* and in organ culture. Stimulation of osteoclastic bone resorption can be observed as early as 15 minutes after the administration of PTH.[212,213] The proportion of osteoclasts that show a ruffled border and the size of this resorbing apparatus as well as the total number of osteoclasts and the number of nuclei per osteoclasts can all increase with PTH. In organ culture, PTH stimulation of resorption probably depends not on the replication of osteoclast precursors but on cells derived from existing precursors, since it is not abrogated by hydroxyurea at concentrations that block DNA synthesis.[214] Nevertheless, in the absence of inhibitor, recently divided cells appear to be preferentially incorporated into active osteoclasts in PTH-treated bones. The effects on bone resorption have been demonstrated using high concentrations of the hormone (1–100 nM) in the pharmacologic or pathophysiologic range. The dose-response curve is steep, going from no effect to maximal with a 10-fold increase in concentration, and rapid, with a measurable effect at 3 hours and a maximal increase in resorption rate at 24 to 48 hours. It has been possible to obtain resorptive responses with PTH at concentrations below 0.1 nM, especially in the presence of cationic peptides, which appear to protect the hormone,[215] but this is still two orders of magnitude above the concentration of active hormone that is normally present in the circulation. Hence it is not clear how important stimulation of bone resorption is for the physiologic response to PTH.

Almost all of the biochemical responses observed when bone resorption is stimulated were first found using PTH, but such responses may also occur with other stimulators. There is a good correlation between calcium mobilization, matrix degradation, lysosomal enzyme release, and morphologic changes in osteoclasts during the resorptive response. Hyaluronic acid synthesis is also stimulated by PTH, and this effect precedes calcium release.[216] Effects on collagen synthesis, citrate decarboxylation, and cell replication do not appear to be as closely linked to resorption.[217]

PTH-stimulated resorption is presumably mediated by interaction with a cell surface receptor. Brief exposure to PTH can produce a long-lasting resorptive effect.[218] The time of exposure required for this response is only 1 to 2 hours when PTH is removed by simple washing, but 6 hours of exposure is needed for a full resorptive response when the tissue is washed with an antibody to the hormone that presumably can compete with the cell surface receptor for binding. However, it is not known which cells in bone have the receptors that mediate stimulation of resorption and what the second messengers are for this response. The hypothesis that PTH does not act directly on osteoclasts is based on negative results. There is conflicting evidence concerning the presence of PTH receptors on osteoclasts,[219,220] and it has not been possible to show stimulation by PTH when osteoclasts are isolated from other bone cells.[221] Mixtures of osteoclasts or osteoclast-like cells and other bone cells do show a response to PTH not only in organ culture, but in reconstituted cell cultures.[179,221,222] PTH could act by stimulating the production of a local bone resorber. PTH does stimulate PGE_2 production in bone (Fig. 1–5),[223,224] but the hormone still acts in the presence of cortisol and indomethacin, which are potent inhibitors of PGE_2 production.[214,225] It has been suggested that the PTH response requires vitamin D, but PTH stimulates resorption in the bones of fetuses of vitamin D–deficient mothers.[226] Other local bone-resorbing factors may be involved (see later), but these have not yet been demonstrated to be PTH responsive. One possibility is that PTH acts directly on osteoclast precursor cells to stimulate their differentiation and fusion into active osteoclasts. The increase in ruffled borders might then occur when these cells were incorporated into existing osteoclasts that had previously been relatively inactive.

PTH stimulates cAMP production in bone cells; however, this effect may be decreased in populations that have been depleted of osteoblast-like cells and enriched in either osteoclasts or their precursors.[91,227] Other stimulators of adenylate cyclase as well as cAMP analogues, phosphodiesterase inhibitors, and activators of cAMP-dependent protein kinase have all been shown to increase bone resorption under some experimental conditions,[228-231] but the response is seldom as large or as rapid as that to PTH. This could be explained in part by the fact that cAMP can also mediate inhibition of bone resorption by calcitonin. Thus, when agents that raise cAMP concentration are added to actively resorbing systems, their effects are often inhibitory.[232]

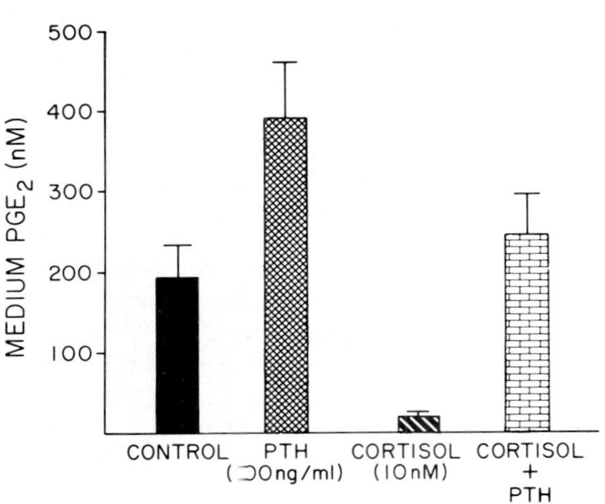

Figure 1–5. Effect of PTH on PGE_2 production. PGE_2 concentration was measured in 24-hour cultures of neonatal rat calvaria. PTH stimulated PGE_2 production about 2-fold in control cultures. PGE_2 production was markedly reduced in cultures treated with a physiologic concentration of cortisol, but the PTH response was as great as that observed in the absence of cortisol. (From Raisz LG, Simmons HA: Endocr Res 11:59–74, 1985.)

Intracellular calcium could also be the mediator of PTH-stimulated bone resorption. The observation that a calcium ionophore, A23187, can stimulate bone resorption supports this possibility.[233-236] However, inhibition of bone resorption by A23187 has also been reported.[237] Moreover, a PTH analogue, bovine 3–34 PTH, which does not stimulate cAMP production in bone, can still stimulate bone resorption and increase cell calcium concentration.[238,239] Such an effect could be related to the increase in phosphatidyl inositol turnover in bones stimulated to resorb by PTH.[240] This could activate a protein kinase C–mediated pathway independent of cAMP and provide an alternative second messenger for intracellular effects of PTH on bone-resorbing cells.

2. *Vitamin D*

Although the primary physiologic role of vitamin D appears to be to promote skeletal growth and mineralization, the active hormonal form, $1,25(OH)_2D_3$, is a potent direct stimulator of bone resorption in organ culture (Fig. 1–6)[241,242] and *in vivo*.[243] This effect occurs at concentrations as low as 10 pM, which are within the physiologic range under conditions of calcium or phosphate deprivation. The teleologic role for stimulation of bone resorption by vitamin D could be to provide calcium and phosphate from the storehouse in bone when an insufficient amount was available from the diet. In contrast, when there is a deficiency of $1,25(OH)_2D_3$, for example, in renal disease, calcium absorption is impaired and serum calcium is maintained by an increase in bone resorption due to secondary hyperparathyroidism. Repletion with vitamin D results in an increase in calcium absorption, a reversal of secondary hyperparathyroidism, and a reduction in bone resorption.

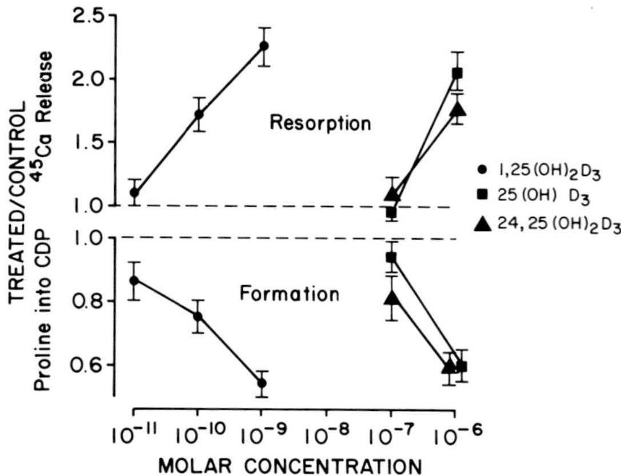

Figure 1–6. Effect of vitamin D metabolites on bone resorption and formation. 1,25-Dihydroxyvitamin D is a potent stimulator of bone resorption as indicated by its ability to stimulate release of previously incorporated ^{45}Ca from fetal rat long bones. It also inhibits collagen synthesis as measured by the incorporation of proline into collagenase digestible protein. 1,25 $(OH)_2D_3$ (●), $25(OH)D_3$ (■), and $24,25(OH)_2D_3$ (▲) were all much less potent but had the same qualitative effects. Smaller doses of these metabolites (not shown) had no significant effect on bone resorption or collagen synthesis. (From Raisz LG, et al: Calcif Tissue Int 32:135–138, 1980.)

The resorptive response to $1,25(OH)_2D_3$ is similar to the response to PTH, although the time course appears to be slower and the dose-response curve less steep than that for the peptide hormone. Induction of a prolonged resorptive response can occur after an even briefer exposure to vitamin D metabolites than is required for PTH, presumably because they enter the cell and are bound to cytoplasmic or nuclear receptors. As with PTH, no osteoclast receptor has yet been identified, but many other bone cells do have receptors for $1,25(OH)_2D_3$. In addition, monocytes and activated lymphocytes bear receptors for this hormone, supporting the possibility that these cells are involved either in the production of mediators or in the differentiation of cells of the monocyte-macrophage series into osteoclasts.[107,108,185] $1,25(OH)_2D_3$ can increase the production of interleukin-1, which may be a mediator of bone resorption.[244] $1,25(OH)_2D_3$ does not appear to stimulate prostaglandin production in bone cells.

Whereas $1,25(OH)_2D_3$ is clearly the most potent stimulator of bone resorption among the natural vitamin D metabolites thus far tested, many other analogues can stimulate bone resorption and their potency parallels their affinity for the $1,25(OH)_2D_3$ receptor. However, it is also possible that some compounds, such as 25-hydroxyvitamin D_3 and 24,25-dihydroxyvitamin D_3, could be converted by 1-hydroxylation in bone to the more active forms. These compounds are bound much more tightly to the circulating vitamin D–binding protein (DBP) than $1,25(OH)_2D_3$, and evidence from bone organ culture indicates that DBP binding can reduce the biological activity of the tightly bound metabolites but not that of $1,25(OH)_2D_3$.[245]

3. *Thyroid Hormones*

Both thyroxin and triiodothyronine can produce direct stimulation of bone resorption in organ culture.[246,247] The effect is relatively small, but fits well with *in vivo* observations. In hyperthyroidism, bone turnover is increased but PTH activity appears to be decreased as evidenced by decreased serum concentrations, low rates of nephrogenous cAMP excretion, and increased rather than decreased tubular reabsorption of phosphate.[248,249]

4. Vitamin A

The first organ culture study demonstrating direct stimulation of bone resorption was with vitamin A.[250] Retinoids have been shown to stimulate cartilage degradation, and this has been attributed to stimulation of the release of lysosomal enzymes.[251] While vitamin A also enhances lysosomal enzyme release from bone, its precise mechanism for stimulating osteoclastic resorption is not clear. The responses are quite variable in different culture systems. Vitamin A can increase the number of receptors for 1,25$(OH)_2D_3$ in cultured osteosarcoma cells.[252] The interaction between these two agents has not yet been carefully studied. *In vivo,* vitamin A can produce substantial skeletal lesions. Whereas degradation of cartilage matrix is a striking early response, hypercalcemia and decreased bone mass, presumably related to stimulation of bone resorption, can be observed with chronic vitamin A intoxication.

5. Prostaglandins

In the initial studies demonstrating that PTH increases bone cAMP content, Chase and Aurbach showed that prostaglandin E_2 (PGE_2) was also effective.[253] Subsequent studies demonstrated that PGE_2 was a potent stimulator of bone resorption in organ culture.[228] The structure/activity relations and pattern of response to prostanoids have been examined in considerable detail.[254-257] The response differs from that to PTH in being slower and more dependent on cell replication. Hydroxyurea can decrease the PGE_2 response, particularly at low concentrations.[258] Among the prostaglandins tested, PGE_2 and PGE_1 have generally been found to be the most potent, whereas PGFs are usually less active. PGE_2 and the 15-keto metabolic products of prostaglandins are relatively inactive. Other metabolic products are more active, such as 13,14-dihydro PGE_2 and 6-keto PGE_1,[259] but these are not very abundant *in vivo.* It has been difficult to assess the role of prostacyclin (PGI_2), largely because of its short half-life in physiologic solutions. Stimulation of bone resorption has been observed with this compound and with its stable analogues, but they appear to be less potent than PGEs. Other products of fatty acid oxidation have been examined less extensively, but so far there is no evidence that thromboxane, leukotrienes, or other hydroxylated unsaturated fatty acids have a potent effect on bone resorption.

Despite the abundant evidence that prostanoids stimulate bone resorption, there is evidence that they may have the opposite effect when added directly to isolated osteoclasts. In osteoclasts isolated on glass or bone surfaces, PGI_2 and its stable analogues, as well as PGEs, have a transient inhibitory effect on motility that resembles the response to calcitonin, although its duration is considerably shorter.[158,260] Attempts to demonstrate this inhibitory effect in organ culture show only a small effect.[261]

In vivo studies tend to confirm the resorptive effect of prostanoids.[257] This is true for animal tumor models in which prostaglandin production is associated with hypercalcemia and for studies of the effects of inhibitors of prostaglandin cyclo-oxygenase on bone turnover and repair in experimental fractures and on bone loss in periodontal disease. However, studies of prostaglandin administration have been difficult to interpret because of the rapid inactivation of PGE_2 *in vivo,* and with prolonged administration serum concentrations may be normal or low.

Endogenous production of prostaglandins in bone was first demonstrated in a pathologic model in which resorption was stimulated by antibodies to cell surface antigens in the presence of complement.[134,199,262] Subsequently, a large number of compounds and factors have been shown to stimulate prostaglandin synthesis in bone.[133,263-265] PGE_2 production can also be stimulated by mechanical stress on bone cells,[129] and this has led to the hypothesis that the effects of mechanical forces might be mediated by changes in local prostaglandin production. Other prostanoids are also produced, particularly PGI_2,[125,256,266] but their effects on bone appear to be smaller than those of PGE_2. It is not certain which if any of these agents and processes is important in physiologic regulation, largely because it is so difficult to measure local prostaglandin concentrations *in vivo.* Changes in prostaglandin concentration may occur after the tissue has been excised. For example, prostaglandins have been thought to mediate bone resorption in periodontal disease and are produced by inflamed gingiva, but the concentrations are much lower when the tissues are quickly frozen and dried and subsequently extracted than when less rapid methods of sampling are used.[267]

Assessment of the role of prostaglandins in regulating bone resorption and turnover *in vivo* is complicated not only by the difficulty in measurement, but also by the complex nature of the response to these agents. As indicated, there may be a transient inhibitory effect on bone resorption. Moreover, the dose-response curve for stimulation of resorption by PGE_2 is biphasic with inhibition at extremely high concentrations (10^{-4} M). A similar biphasic response has been observed for bone formation in organ culture, with stimulation at 10^{-8} and 10^{-7} M and inhibition at 10^{-6} and 10^{-5} M (Fig. 1–7).

Clearly, much more work needs to be done on the role of arachidonic acid metabolites in bone. The emphasis to date has been on PGE_2, and other compounds may be of considerable importance. Moreover, the nature of the effect may depend not only on the pattern of hydroxy fatty acid production, but on its location. For example, PGE_2 production in the marrow could have its greatest effect on osteoclast precursors and result in increased bone resorption, whereas periosteal PGE_2 production might have its greatest effect on preosteoblasts and stimulate bone formation.

6. *Osteoclast Activating Factors: Interleukins*

Although there is substantial evidence that products of lymphocytes and monocytes can influence bone resorption, the precise pathways and relations of these activities have not yet been established. Human peripheral blood mononuclear cell cultures containing both monocytes and lymphocytes, stimulated by plant lectins or by antigens to which the donor had cell-mediated immunity, were found to produce a bone-resorbing factor that was designated osteoclast-activating factor (OAF).[192] Subsequent studies have shown that this material is a low molecular weight peptide,[216,268] a potent stimulator of bone resorption, and probably an inhibitor of bone collagen synthesis, thus resembling PTH in its action.[269] Although OAF was believed to be a lymphocyte product, probably from T cells,[198] it has now been shown to be IL-1 beta, more likely derived from contaminating cells of the monocyte-macrophage line.[194,195] TNF is also a potent bone-resorbing factor and may be important in lipopolysaccharide-mediated bone resorption.[270] Normally B cells may not produce OAF, but malignant B cells in myeloma, as well as T cell leukemias, produce bone-resorbing factors that resemble OAF in biological and chemical properties.[196,197] Complete chemical characterization of OAF has not yet been accomplished; hence it is not certain whether this material is different from one of the characterized interleukins. OAF does not appear to be interleukin-2, since the latter material does not stimulate bone resorption.

Interleukin-1 has been shown to stimulate bone resorption in organ cultures of neonatal mouse calvaria. It is not clear whether interleukin-1 acts through stimulation of endogenous prostaglandin synthesis or more directly. There may be dual effects, such as have been described for EGF.

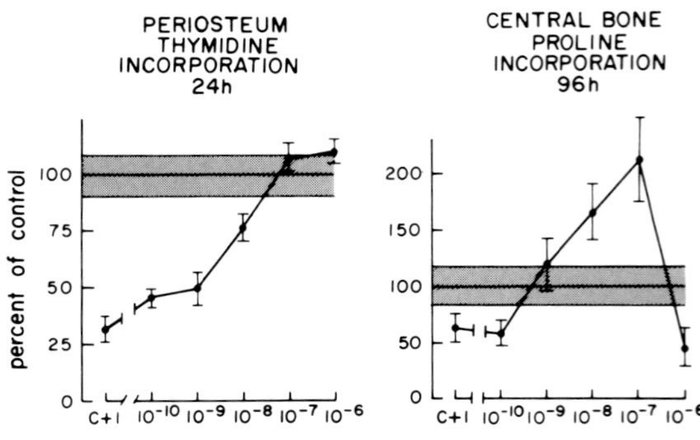

Figure 1–7. Effects of prostaglandin E_2 on DNA and collagen synthesis. In the left panel cortisol (10^{-7} M) and indomethacin (10^{-5} M) (C + I) produced a substantial reduction in thymidine incorporation into DNA at 24 hours (control ± SE is shown as the cross-hatched band). Increasing concentrations of PGE_2 increased thymidine incorporation. In the right panel this is reflected at 96 hours in a marked increase in proline incorporation (10^{-9} to 10^{-7} M), but the effect is biphasic, and proline incorporation into collagen is inhibited at 10^{-6} M and higher. (Chyun and Raisz, unpublished observations.)

7. *Epidermal Growth Factor (EGF) and Other Stimulators of Prostaglandin Synthesis*

Although it has not yet been assigned a physiologic role, EGF has powerful effects on bone resorption that appear to involve at least two different pathways. In neonatal mouse calvaria, EGF stimulates bone resorption by a prostaglandin-dependent mechanism.[133] In fetal rat long bones, EGF produces a marked increase in cell replication and a prostaglandin-independent stimulation of bone resorption.[271] However, when cell replication is blocked with hydroxyurea, EGF is still a potent resorber in fetal long bones, but now its action appears to depend on endogenous prostaglandin synthesis.[272] Both human and mouse EGF have been shown to have these effects at concentrations that approximate those found in serum. EGF-like compounds may be important in the humoral hypercalcemia of malignancy. Tumor-derived transforming growth factors of the alpha type have EGF-like activity, bind to EGF receptors, and stimulate bone resorption.[273,274] Platelet-derived growth factor (PDGF) has also been shown to stimulate resorption of neonatal mouse calvaria by a prostaglandin-dependent mechanism.[265] It is possible that some of these preparations are contaminated with a transforming growth factor. Other substances can stimulate prostaglandin synthesis in neonatal mouse calvaria, including bradykinin and thrombin.[263,264] Thus, there are a number of possible ways that injury could produce local prostaglandin synthesis in bone. Another factor that stimulates bone resorption and has been implicated in hypercalcemia of malignancy is vasoactive intestinal polypeptide.[231]

8. Humoral Hypercalcemia of Malignancy Factors

In addition to the agents that stimulate prostaglandin synthesis, bone-resorbing activity that acts like PTH has been isolated from the culture medium and tissue extracts of tumors from animals and patients with humoral hypercalcemia of malignancy.[273,275-277] This factor has recently been purified,[278] has been cloned from breast[279] and renal[280,281] cancer cells, and was found to have 60% structural homology with PTH in its first 13 amino acids. The rest of the molecule, which has a Mr of 16 kDa, was largely different from PTH. An NH_2-terminal fragment of 34 to 40 amino acids produced in rats or rat cells biological effects similar to those of PTH 1–34,[282-285] suggesting that this factor is responsible for the symptoms of hypercalcemia of malignancy. It is likely that the factors found in malignancy are the consequence of ectopic, unregulated production of a physiologic regulator of bone resorption. It is also possible that these factors have a physiologic role as the local mediators of the response to systemic stimulators of bone resorption.

9. Heparin

The resorptive response to parathyroid hormone in neonatal mouse calvaria is increased when heparin is added to the culture medium.[286] Heparin also enhances resorption of implanted bone particles.[287] The development of osteoporosis in patients given long-term heparin therapy[288] may be related to this effect. Increased numbers of mast cells have been found in the marrow of patients with postmenopausal osteoporosis.[289] In systemic mastocytosis, both osteoporosis and osteosclerosis have been reported.[290] However, it is not clear whether heparin is the factor responsible for the association between changes in the bone metabolism and mast cell proliferation since mast cells produce many other mediators.[291]

10. Bacterial Products

Bone resorption can be stimulated by several bacterial products including lipopolysaccharides and muramyl dipeptide.[292,293] These effects do not appear to depend on endogenous prostaglandin synthesis. A synergistic enhancement of the effects of PTH and PGE_2 by endotoxin has been reported,[294] which could explain the correlation between the low levels of PGE_2 and the resorptive activity found in dog gingiva.[267] These effects could be important in the pathogenesis of bone loss in periodontal disease and osteomyelitis.

B. Inhibitors of Bone Resorption

There are relatively few physiologic inhibitors of bone resorption. Calcitonin is the only known systemic hormonal inhibitor, but there is evidence for a local inhibitor of PTH-stimulated bone resorption.[295] Gamma-interferon can also inhibit bone resorption *in vitro*.[296] Phosphate is a potent inhibitor of bone resorption and may act as a regulator *in vivo*. Many pharmacologic agents have been shown to inhibit bone resorption,[208] and some of these, such as the diphosphonates, have been used clinically. Nerve growth factor has been shown to inhibit PTH-stimulated bone resorption *in vitro*, possibly by a mechanism depending on the proteolytic component of the NGF complex.[297]

1. Calcitonin

Calcitonin appears to be a direct inhibitor of osteoclast activity. It produces a rapid decrease in bone resorption, both *in vivo* and *in vitro*, associated with a loss of the active ruffled border in osteoclasts.[298] There is evidence that calcitonin binds to osteoclasts and increases cAMP production in cell populations enriched in osteoclast-like cells or their precursors.[91,299] The possibility that cAMP mediates the inhibitory effect is supported by studies showing that stimulators of adenyl cyclase, cyclic nucleotide analogues, and inhibitors of cAMP phosphodiesterase can all produce inhibition of bone resorption and mimic the effects of calcitonin, particularly in systems in which resorption has been stimulated by PTH.[232,300]

There is some controversy concerning the fate of osteoclasts that have been inhibited by calcitonin. Osteoclasts with inactive ruffled borders are still attached to bone surfaces with ample clear zones in organ cultures of fetal rat long bones after calcitonin treatment.[298] However, *in vivo* the osteoclast population may move away from the bone surface and the number of osteoclasts can decrease rapidly.

Whatever the initial fate of the osteoclasts, the inhibitory action of calcitonin may not persist.[301] In organ cultures and in patients with hypercalcemia of malignancy, continuous administration of calcitonin at high concentrations produces only a transient inhibition of resorption that is followed by escape. The mechanism of escape is not established. Desensitization to calcitonin through loss of receptors has been postulated,[302] but the number of receptors still present in desensitized bone would seem to be enough to sustain a response.[303] Prior irradiation of bone can prevent escape.[304] This led to the hypothesis that replication of a new population of calcitonin-resistant cells might be responsible. However, escape is not abrogated by treatment with hydroxyurea at concentrations that markedly inhibit DNA synthesis and cell replication (Conaway and Lorenzo, unpublished observations). The most effective way of delaying escape appears to be treatment with glucocorticoids. In organ culture, its addition to bones that have already been treated with PTH produces little inhibition of resorption, but when added simultaneously with calcitonin, can prevent escape.[301] A similar observation has been made in patients with hypercalcemia of malignancy. Treatment with calcitonin alone produces only a transient decrease in serum calcium concentration, whereas the combination of glucocorticoids and calcitonin results in a more prolonged effect.[305]

2. Other Endogenous Inhibitors

A potential physiologic inhibitor of resorption has been identified in conditioned medium from fetal and neonatal rat bone organ culture.[295] This material appears to be a macromolecule that competitively inhibits the action of PTH on bone resorption. Such a factor could provide a local mechanism for protecting portions of the skeleton from being affected by circulating PTH. This protection could then be overcome when the PTH level is extremely high and the metabolic need for calcium preempts local structural needs. An inhibitor of IL-1 activity has recently been identified in human urine.[306,307] The inhibitor blocks the bone resorption response and IL-1.[308] Gamma-interferon can also inhibit IL-1–stimulated bone resorption.[296]

3. Pharmacologic Inhibitors of Bone Resorption

There are a number of pharmacologic agents that can inhibit bone resorption. Among the most effective inhibitors are the diphosphonates, which are stable analogues of pyrophosphate.[309] Certain diphosphonates appear to inhibit osteoclasts selectively. The simplest explanation is that they coat the bone surface by binding to hydroxyapatite and that their selective effect is based on the fact that osteoclasts take up and concentrate these compounds as they dissolve mineral and that they then inhibit lysosomal enzymes and other functions.[310,311] Pyrophosphate absorbed to bone crystals may have a similar effect; however, it is easily hydrolyzed to phosphate and its effects may be due to the changing concentration of phosphate that results.

The other pharmacologic inhibitors include a wide variety of compounds. Mithramycin is a potent inhibitor that is used in hypercalcemia of malignancy and probably acts by inhibiting DNA-dependent RNA synthesis.[312] The fact that one of its earliest effects in humans is to inhibit osteoclastic bone resorption and produce hypocalcemia gives some indication of the intense metabolic activity of bone-resorbing cells. Thiophene 2-carboxylic acid, originally identified as a hypoglycemic agent, is also hypocalcemic.[313] An analogue, thionapthene 2-carboxylic acid, appears to be even more potent as an inhibitor of bone resorption.[314] Protamine, a cationic protein, has been found to inhibit bone resorption *in vivo*.[315,316] However, other cationic proteins, including poly-L-lysine and cationized albumin, have been found to enhance the response to PTH in organ culture.[215]

Some agents that inhibit bone resorption *in vitro* have provided insight into the mechanisms of the resorptive process, but have not been effective antihypercalcemic agents *in vivo*. Colchicine decreases bone resorption and causes loss of ruffled borders, suggesting that microtubules are involved in maintaining this structure.[298] Colchicine also decreases lysosomal enzyme release but increases the amount of collagenase in bone organ culture medium. Other lysosomal enzyme inhibitors, including ammonium chloride and chloroquine, can inhibit PTH-stimulated bone resorption.[317-319] A number of membrane-stabilizing agents, including phenytoin, verapamil, and procainamide, can inhibit bone resorption at high concentration.[320-322] It is not clear whether specific blockade of calcium channels is involved in these effects. Ouabain can also inhibit bone resorption and this may indicate a role for Na-Ca exchange in the resorptive process.[323,324] Amrinone also inhibits the PTH response but the mechanism may be different from that of ouabain.[325] Carbonic anhydrase inhibitors can block bone resorption,[326] presumably by interfering with the ability of osteoclasts to generate acid.

C. The Effects of Ions on Bone Resorption

Since one of the most important functions of the regulators of bone resorption is to maintain the serum calcium concentration, it is not unexpected that cell-mediated bone resorption is relatively independent of the ambient Ca^{2+} concentration *in vitro*. However, intracellular calcium may mediate the cellular response to some stimulators. PTH can increase calcium uptake in bone cells,[327] and the ability of PTH to induce a prolonged resorptive response after brief exposure is calcium dependent.[[illegible]8] Calcium ionophores can stimulate bone resorption, and inhibitors of calcium transport can block resorption. However, the concentration of inhibitors required is high and the effect could be due to nonspecific stabilization of cell membranes.

Changes in the phosphate concentration have a marked effect on bone resorption over the physiologic range of 0.5 to 4 mM.[97] Inhibition of bone resorption by phosphate can be seen both *in vivo* and *in vitro* and may be more of a physicochemical than metabolic effect. The decrease in calcium release is not associated with loss of ruffled borders or a decrease in lysosomal enzyme release, such as occurs with calcitonin and with pharmacologic inhibitors.[204]

Magnesium can affect bone resorption. In magnesium-deficient bones, the resorptive response to PTH and $1,25(OH)_2D_3$ may be impaired.[328] Hydrogen ion probably has its greatest effect on mineral dissolution. In organ culture, cell-mediated bone resorption and responses to PTH can occur over a wide range of hydrogen ion concentrations, but there are limits of alkalosis and acidosis beyond which bone resorptive responses are blunted.[329] However, *in vivo* the calcium loss that occurs with acidosis appears to be cell mediated as indicated by the inhibitory effects of colchicine and calcitonin.[330-332] High concentrations of potassium can stimulate bone resorption in organ culture.[333] This effect may be related to stimulation of prostaglandin synthesis. Copper has been shown to inhibit bone resorption. This may also involve changes in prostaglandin synthesis.[334] Finally, manganese has been shown to enhance the sensitivity of cultured bone to PTH stimulation of resorption at low concentrations and to inhibit at high concentrations.[335]

VI. FACTORS REGULATING BONE GROWTH

A. Calcium-Regulating Hormones

The calcium-regulating hormones influence the supply and concentration of calcium and phosphate largely through their effects on bone resorption, intestinal absorption, and renal tubular reabsorption of these ions. In addition, these agents have complex effects on bone formation and mineralization. Experimental data may be difficult to interpret because the effects vary with dose and duration of treatment as well as with the type of cells being studied. Moreover, there are indirect mechanisms that may be both local and systemic.

1. Parathyroid Hormone

PTH can produce both inhibitory and stimulatory effects on bone formation. There is good evidence for the presence of PTH receptors on osteoblast-like cells.[93,219] The primary direct effect on osteoblasts in organ and cell culture, and an early effect *in vivo,* is inhibition of collagen synthesis.[336,337] This inhibition is associated with a decrease in the levels of procollagen mRNA in osteoblasts and osteoblast-like cells and hence is presumed to involve transcriptional control.[96] The dose-response relations for inhibition of collagen synthesis in central osteoblast-rich bone in organ culture and in rat osteosarcoma cells are similar, although the osteosarcoma cells show a substantially lower relative rate of collagen synthesis as a percentage of total protein than that noted for the fully differentiated osteoblasts.[104]

The relation of this effect on collagen synthesis, which occurs after several hours, to immediate effects of PTH on cAMP production, osteoblast cell shape, and protein kinase activation is unknown. A role for cAMP is supported by the observation that inhibitors of phosphodiesterase can mimic the action of PTH on bone collagen synthesis.[336,338] Calcium entry may also play a role, but calcium ionophores produce an inhibition of both DNA and protein synthesis in bone and hence show a different pattern of response from that to PTH.[339] PTH can also decrease alkaline phosphatase activity,[95] and oppose the effect of $1,25(OH)_2D_3$ to stimulate BGP synthesis in cultured human osteoblast-like cells[20,21] and in fetal rat calvaria.[340] PTH may also stimulate collagenase production and release from osteoblast-like cells.[151-153]

Despite the inhibitory effect, there are many experimental models in which the administration of PTH is associated with increased bone formation as evidenced by an increase in collagen synthesis, alkaline phosphatase activity, and mineral apposition rate (Fig. 1–8).[30,341] This anabolic effect has been easiest to demonstrate when PTH is administered intermittently and at relatively small doses, which may not produce hypercalcemia.[342]

There are a number of possible mechanisms for the anabolic effect. PTH may stimulate precursor cell proliferation. Data on DNA synthesis in bone cell and organ cultures treated with PTH are not consistent, but this may be because we cannot examine the response in a homogeneous population of osteoblast precursor cells. Several indirect mechanisms have been proposed. PTH stimulation of bone resorption could result in an increased number of sites for the initiation of remodeling. This would increase total bone formation rate but could not account for the increase in trabecular bone mass that is seen in young animals treated with PTH. This increase may be due to an increase in the production or release of a bone mitogen, either a matrix-derived factor or a cell product.[343] In addition, PGE_2, the production of which is stimulated by PTH *in vitro,* could mediate an increase in osteoblast precursor cell replication and a later stimulation of bone formation;[344] however, indomethacin does not block the anabolic response to PTH in rats.[345]

2. $1,25(OH)_2D_3$ (see Fig. 1–6)

The initial effect of active vitamin D metabolites, particularly $1,25(OH)_2D_3$, on bone collagen synthesis is also inhibitory.[271,346] The structure/activity relations for the inhibitory effect on collagen synthesis appear to cor-

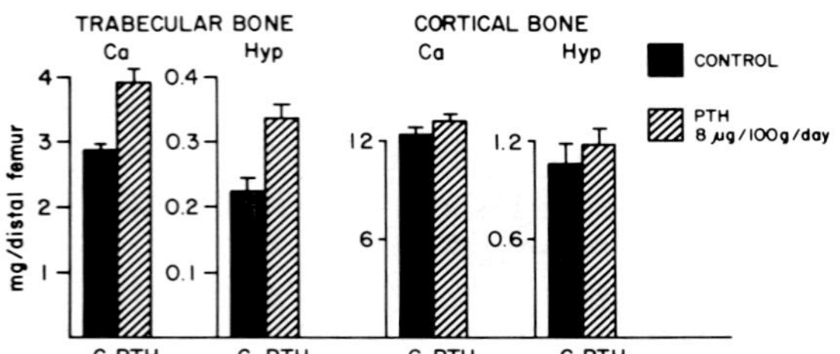

Figure 1–8. Anabolic effect of parathyroid hormone. Young rats were treated with human 1–34 PTH for 12 days. Trabecular and cortical bone of the distal half of femur were analyzed separately. Note that both calcium and hydroxyproline increase roughly in parallel in both cortical and trabecular bone; thus, there is a generalized anabolic effect. This occurred despite the fact that the dose of PTH given did not produce hypercalcemia in these animals at any time. (From Gunness-Hey M, Hock JM: Metab Bone Dis Rel Res 5:177–191, 1984.)

respond reasonably well with the affinity of different vitamin D metabolites for the intracellular 3.6S receptor that has been identified in bone as well as in many other tissues.[347] The time course in organ culture shows no lag and there is significant inhibition at 3 hours.[109] There is a close correspondence between the change in collagen synthesis and procollagen mRNA levels. Dose-response curves show gradual effects of $1,25(OH)_2D_3$ from 10^{-11} to 10^{-8} M and are similar for organ cultures and cell cultures. The inhibitory effects of $1,25(OH)_2D_3$ and PTH are not additive in organ culture but are additive in rat osteosarcoma cells.[348]

The anabolic effects of $1,25(OH)_2D_3$ on bone formation are not as clearly established as those of PTH. Vitamin D does not appear to be necessary for bone growth and mineralization in rats.[102,103] Whereas these processes are severely impaired in vitamin D deficiency, simultaneous infusion of calcium and phosphate can restore growth and mineralization to rates close to those obtained in replete animals. Trabecular bone mass may even be somewhat increased in vitamin D-depleted calcium- and phosphate-infused animals, perhaps because resorption of metaphyseal bone is decreased in the absence of $1,25(OH)_2D_3$. Administration of small doses of vitamin D or its metabolites may lead to an increase in bone mass under some experimental conditions, but this has not been a consistent finding. Administration of toxic doses of $1,25(OH)_2D_3$ or vitamin D to experimental animals results in a stimulation of bone matrix production with impaired mineralization.[349] Thus, vitamin D–intoxicated rats show a paradoxical histologic picture of osteomalacia associated with hypercalcemia. Impaired renal function in these animals may play a role in the mineralization defect. Serum BGP concentrations are increased, and this might also play a role.[350]

Studies of the effects of vitamin D metabolites on bone cell replication and differentiation have given variable results. For example, $1,25(OH)_2D_3$ may increase or decrease levels of alkaline phosphatase, depending on dose and duration of treatment and probably also on the growth rate of the target cells.[106] In mixed cell populations, $1,25(OH)_2D_3$ could have complex indirect effects, possibly mediated by changes in the production of interleukins.

There is suggestive evidence, but no conclusive proof, that other metabolites of $1,25(OH)_2D_3$ can regulate bone growth. It has been postulated that either $25(OH)D_3$ or $24,25(OH)_2D_3$ may play that role.[351] Some of the differences in the effects of these metabolites *in vivo* may be due to pharmacokinetic differences or to further metabolism by bone cells.[352]

3. Calcitonin

Calcitonin has relatively little effect on osteoblasts in organ and cell culture.[336] *In vivo,* both inhibition and stimulation of bone formation and mineralization have been reported, and in many studies no clear-cut effects were observed. Calcitonin can stimulate cAMP production in certain bone-derived cells, but not in others. It appears to be less effective in bone cell populations that are selectively enriched in osteoblasts and their precursors.[91] *In vivo,* the end result of calcitonin treatment might depend on indirect effects mediated through changes in bone resorption and serum calcium concentration. A role in mineralization has been suggested by the fact that calcium content of demineralized bone powder implants is increased after calcitonin treatment.[316] The increase in bone mass seen in patients with osteoporosis treated with calcitonin is probably due to its inhibitory effect on bone resorption, rather than stimulation of bone formation.

B. Systemic Growth Factors

1. Growth Hormone

Clinically and in experimental animals, the hormone that can be shown most clearly to regulate skeletal growth is growth hormone. Skeletal growth is stimulated in gigantism and acromegaly, with the chief difference between the two clinical pictures being the stimulation of cartilage growth before epiphyseal closure in gigantism and of bone growth together with growth of soft tissues in acromegaly. Growth hormone deficiency is associated with impaired skeletal growth in children, but its role in the maintenance of skeletal mass in adults is not established. There is some evidence for diminished growth hormone secretion in osteoporosis, but somatomedin levels are apparently not decreased.[353] The effects of growth hormone on the skeleton appear to be mediated largely through the production of somatomedins, particularly somatomedin-C or IGF-1.

2. Somatomedins (Insulin-like Growth Factors)

In older animals, IGF-1 production is probably produced largely in the liver and possibly also in the kidney, but in young animals, other tissues may be an important source.[354] Thus, growth hormone may act indirectly on the skeleton in the sense that IGF-1 production is a necessary intermediate, but a local indirect action is probable since growth hormone can stimulate skeletal growth when infused locally[355] and can increase IGF-1 production in organ cultures of fetal rat bone.[356]

Direct stimulation of bone formation by IGF-1 and related factors has been demonstrated in organ culture.[357-359] The effects occur at relatively low concentrations (10^{-8} M) and are pleiotypic in that both the periosteum and the central bone are affected and cell replication, total protein synthesis, and collagen synthesis all increase.[360,361] In rats, multiplication-stimulating activity (MSA), which appears to be the counterpart of IGF-2, a non–growth hormone–dependent circulating growth factor in humans, has an effect similar to that of IGF-1. However, it is not known whether its action is mediated by an IGF-1 or IGF-2 receptor. The possibility that it is an IGF-1 receptor is supported by the observation that high concentrations of insulin, which bind relatively poorly to IGF-2 receptors, have a similar effect. Glucocorticoids enhance the ability of IGF-1 and MSA to stimulate collagen synthesis and increase the amount of IGF-1 receptor in cultured bone cells.[362] The effects of IGF-1 and MSA appear to be independent of prostaglandin synthesis, since they are not blocked by indomethacin. There is a decrease in the response when cell replication is blocked with hydroxyurea.[363] However, stimulation of protein synthesis is not completely blocked, and this could be due to a direct action of these compounds mediated by IGF-1 receptors on osteoblasts or to an interaction with the insulin receptors in these cells.[364] Although early attempts were unsuccessful, recent studies *in vivo* have confirmed that IGF-1 can stimulate bone formation.[365] Thus, both growth hormone and IGF-1 are potential therapeutic agents in the treatment of osteopenia.

3. Insulin

Insulin has a selective effect on osteoblastic collagen synthesis at physiologic concentrations (10^{-9} M) in organ culture (Fig. 1–9).[338,363] This effect develops relatively slowly, appearing at about 12 hours with a peak at 24 hours. The stimulation of collagen synthesis is about 2-fold and is selective for the osteoblast-rich central portion of fetal calvarial cultures and for type I collagen synthesis. At low concentrations there is little effect on the periosteum and on the synthesis of type III collagen presumably derived from periosteal fibroblasts. The insulin effect is sustained as long as the hormone is present in the culture medium, but removal of insulin results in a rapid decrease in collagen synthesis. Both the slow and the rapid decrease are associated with parallel changes in type I procollagen mRNA levels.[366] This may involve changes in both transcription and degradation of collagen mRNA. High concentrations of insulin (10^{-6} M) produce a pleiotropic response that cannot be differentiated from that seen with IGF-1. The

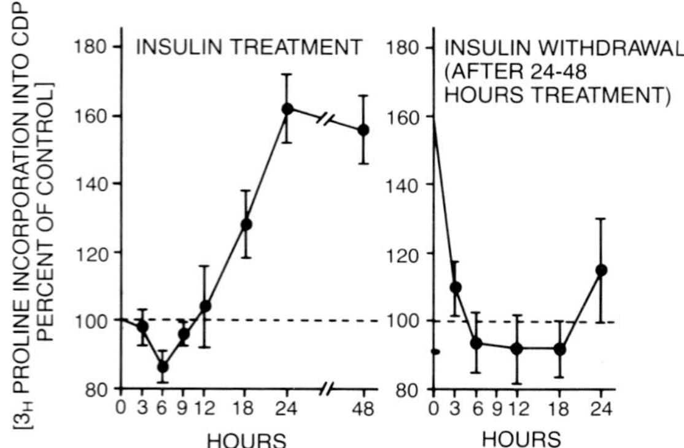

Figure 1–9. Time course of the effect of insulin on bone formation. Fetal rat calvaria were treated with insulin for the indicated periods of time. Increased collagen synthesis was seen only after 12 hours; however, when insulin was removed from the medium after 24 or 48 hours of prior treatment, there was a rapid decrease in collagen synthesis. (From Canalis EM, et al: Endocrinology 100:668–674, 1977.) An increase in collagen messenger RNA level preceded the stimulation of collagen synthesis and paralleled the decrease after insulin withdrawal.[366]

simplest explanation for this is that insulin binds to IGF-1 receptors at these concentrations.

It has been difficult to assess the importance of the direct effect of insulin on osteoblasts *in vivo*. Many other factors may affect skeletal growth in diabetic animals including changes in nutrition,[367] IGF-1 production,[368] and calcium-regulating hormones.[369,370] Whatever the mechanism, diabetes is often associated with decreased skeletal mass.[371,372]

4. Glucocorticoids

The effects of glucocorticoids on tissue growth and differentiation are complex, and the response in skeletal tissue is no exception. Glucocorticoids have a dual effect on bone formation (Fig. 1–10). In organ culture, physiologic concentrations of glucocorticoids can increase collagen synthesis.[121,373] This is not a dose-related effect—it occurs at cortisol concentrations of as low as 10^{-8} M — and may indicate a permissive role for the differentiated function of osteoblasts. There are other effects of glucocorticoids on bone cells that

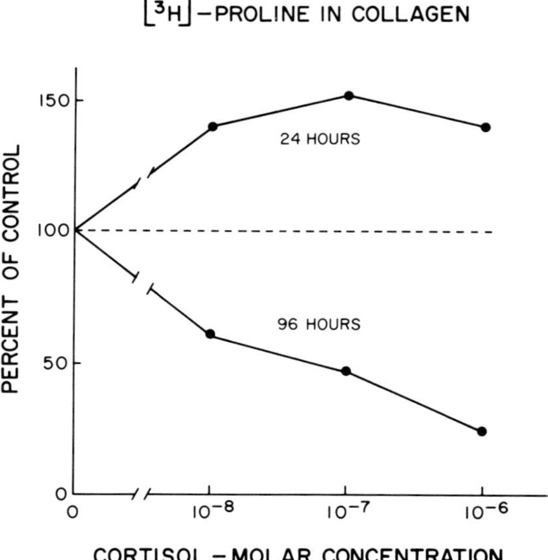

Figure 1–10. Dual effect of cortisol on bone formation. In organ cultures of fetal rat calvaria, addition of cortisol produces an increase in the incorporation of proline into collagen at 24 hours. This effect occurs at physiologic concentrations (10^{-8} M) and probably represents a permissive effect for osteoblast differentiation. With continued cortisol administration for 96 hours, there is a decrease in collagen synthesis that is dose-dependent and may be dependent on decreased cell replication.

support this possibility. Increases in receptors for IGF-1, PTH, and $1,25(OH)_2D_3$ have been described as well as in alkaline phosphatase activity.[116,117,122,123]

In vitro, the major effect of glucocorticoids is inhibition of bone formation that occurs with prolonged administration.[121,124] This effect is dose related and may begin in the periosteum as an inhibition of cell replication. Such an effect on preosteoblasts would impair osteoblast renewal, and bone growth would progressively decrease. Glucocorticoids decrease prostaglandin production in bone, and it is possible that some of their effect on cell renewal is mediated through a change in endogenous prostaglandin synthesis.[224] However, it has not been possible to reproduce the glucocorticoid response with inhibitors of prostaglandin synthase.[344]

5. Sex Hormones

The importance of sex hormones in regulating skeletal growth is well established on the basis of clinical observations, but poorly understood. An increase in androgen at puberty is associated with increased skeletal growth, and androgen-deficient males have a decreased bone mass. In women, high concentrations of estrogen probably accelerate epiphyseal closure at puberty but may stimulate skeletal growth earlier when the concentration is lower. Small doses of estrogen can increase somatomedin production, although large doses cause a decrease.[374] An important function of estrogen appears to be the maintenance of skeletal mass in women. While bone mass begins to decrease in women before the menopause, there is an accelerated loss with estrogen withdrawal. This is observed most clearly when estrogen is withdrawn rapidly by surgical oophorectomy. Estrogen withdrawal is associated with an increase in bone resorption and a smaller increase in bone formation so that bone mass decreases.[375] In rats this response could be related to endogenous PGE_2 production, which can be inhibited by estradiol administered *in vivo* and increased by oophorectomy.[376]

It is possible that these effects are indirect. *In vitro*, neither androgens nor estrogens have potent effects on bone collagen synthesis in organ culture.[377] Progesterone at high concentrations can inhibit bone collagen synthesis, but this may represent an effect on the glucocorticoid receptor. However, bone cell receptors and responses to estrogen have been reported recently.[378] There are some suggestions from clinical and animal studies for effects of prolactin or gonadotropins on bone metabolism,[379] independent of any effects on sex steroids, but these have not been clearly identified in organ or cell culture systems.

6. Other Circulating Factors

Epidermal and fibroblast growth factors stimulate cell replication in organ cultures of fetal rat calvaria and isolated osteoblastic cells, but this effect is associated with a decrease in alkaline phosphatase levels and in collagen synthesis.[380-383] In contrast, preparations of platelet-derived growth factor stimulate cell replication and produce a modest increase in collagen and noncollagen protein synthesis.[384] Interleukin-1 appears to have an effect similar to that of PDGF, and it is possible that the PDGF preparations originally studied were contaminated with interleukin-1.[385] None of these factors has yet been shown to have any important physiologic or pathologic role in the regulation of bone formation, but they certainly deserve further study.

C. Local Bone Growth Regulators

The existence of local regulators of bone formation can be assumed on the basis of the ability of the skeleton to respond to mechanical stress and other influences with changes in modeling and remodeling that result in appropriate local alterations in skeletal mass and structure. Perhaps the most striking response is the increase in skeletal mass that occurs in response to increased mechanical stress, for example, in the medial cortex of a bowed femur or in the bones of the playing arm of world-class tennis players. Another example of local regulation is the increase in bone formation behind and the increase in bone resorption in front of a tooth that is made to move by the application of orthodontic devices.

The formation of bone at ectopic sites, particularly after implantation of demineralized matrices, may represent a different form of local regulation. Here, the response seems to recapitulate ontogeny with migration of mesenchymal cells, followed by condensation into cartilage, calcification of the cartilage, formation of bone, and ultimately the development of a marrow cavity at this ectopic site. A number of factors produced by bone cells or extracted from bone matrices have been implicated in these responses, but none of them has at this time proved unequivocally to be a local regulator *in vivo.* It is possible that local bone formation responses depend on the concerted action of several factors rather than any one individual regulator.

1. Prostaglandins

Among the prostaglandins, PGE_2 is the only compound that has been studied in detail. It has both stimulatory and inhibitory effects on bone formation, depending on dose and experimental model employed (see Fig. 1–7).[124,386] In organ cultures of fetal rat calvaria, high concentrations of PGE_2 (10^{-6} to 10^{-5} M) inhibit collagen synthesis. However, PGE_2 at a lower concentration (10^{-7} to 10^{-8} M), particularly in the presence of cortisol, can stimulate periosteal cell replication acutely, and this is followed by a late increase in collagen synthesis. PGE_2 may selectively stimulate the replication of preosteoblasts that subsequently differentiate into osteoblasts and initiate new collagen synthesis. This would be reflected in increased collagen synthesis only after existing osteoblasts had completed their activity and either have become resting osteoblasts on the bone surface or have become buried in their own matrix as osteocytes. The lower concentrations of PGE_2 that stimulate formation are well within the range that can occur *in vivo.* Medium PGE_2 concentration can reach values of 10^{-7} M and higher in half calvaria from neonatal rats incubated for 24 hours in 1 ml of chemically defined medium.[224] The effects of other products of fatty acid oxidation on bone formation have not been carefully studied. It is quite possible that compounds other than PGE_2 are important local regulators.

In vivo, there is striking evidence for a stimulation of periosteal bone formation after infusions of PGE_1 both in infants who have received infusions of this compound to maintain patency of the ductus arteriosus and in experimental animals. In dogs given PGE_1 the new bone formed was a peculiar woven periosteal tissue.[387] In the infants, in whom only radiologic examination is available, the periosteal hyperostosis could be incorporated into a widened bone shaft when the PGE_1 infusion was discontinued.[388] There is some evidence that endogenous prostaglandin synthesis may be important in normal bone remodeling and in fracture repair, based on studies using inhibitors of prostaglandin synthase, but many more data are needed to resolve these possibilities.[257]

2. Bone-Derived Growth Factors

Conditioned medium for bone cell and organ cultures and extracts of bone matrix contain macromolecular factors that can stimulate bone cell replication, increase collagen and noncollagen protein synthesis in bone, and stimulate induction of new bone formation at ectopic sites.[2,47,50,82,389-393] The term "bone-derived growth factors" (BDGFs) seems to be appropriate, since it involves no assumptions. These materials have also been designated "bone morphogenetic proteins," "skeletal growth factors," and "coupling factors." They are probably not specific for bone cells; for example, a matrix factor was found to stimulate cartilage growth[394] that was either identical[395] or homologous with TGF-beta.[396] The concept that such factors are involved in coupling because they are released during the resorptive process and stimulate subsequent osteoblast proliferation or differentiation is attractive, but has not yet been proved. Among the factors thus far identified, there appears to be a large amount of higher molecular weight material that is TGF-beta and a mixture of low molecular weight factors in the culture medium of fetal rat calvaria that closely resemble IGF-1 and IGF-2 (Fig. 1–11) but also includes β_2 microglobulin.[397,398] TGF-

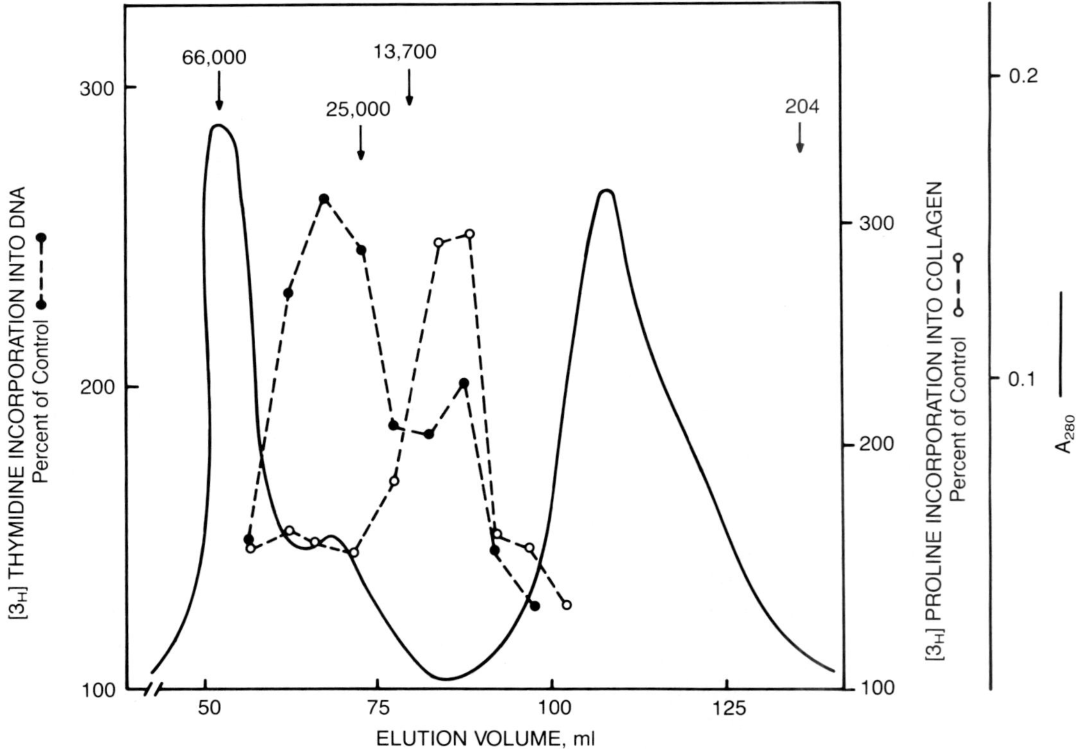

Figure 1–11. Bone-derived growth factors. Medium from fetal rat calvaria was dialyzed, lyophilized, and chromatographed on Sephadex G–100 and two peaks of biological activity were observed. The peak that eluted first had a greater effect on thymidine incorporation into DNA than on proline incorporation into collagen and probably represents TGF-beta, whereas the late eluting peak showed the reverse pattern and probably represents IGF. The late eluting peak also reacted with receptors and antibodies to insulin-like growth factor–1. (From Canalis E, et al: Science 210:1021–1023, 1980.)

beta has mitogenic activity not only in bone, but also for cartilage and normal rat kidney fibroblasts. It has complex effects on bone formation and resorption and its production can be affected by bone-resorbing hormones.[399,400] A bovine protein complex that induces ectopic bone formation contains one component of approximately 17,000 daltons, which may be the active fraction.[50] This has been isolated on the basis of its ability to induce new bone formation when reconstituted and implanted subcutaneously in rats. Using a similar assay, Wang et al. have purified three proteins from demineralized bone, and cDNAs were also isolated.[52] All three recombinant proteins induced cartilage formation *in vivo,* suggesting that "bone morphogenetic protein" may be the result of combined activities of these proteins. Recently a fraction obtained from extracts of bovine bone that stimulates the proliferation of chick osteoblasts in culture was shown to be IGF-2.[401] Human osteosarcoma cells have been found to produce a factor resembling PDGF.[402] The cell of origin of the other factors has not been identified. It is possible that some of these factors are derived from leukocytes rather than bone cells.

3. Leukocyte-Derived Factors

A stimulator of bone cell replication has been identified in the culture medium of macrophages that is felt to be different from interleukin-1.[9] However, interleukin-1 itself may have the ability to stimulate bone cells as well as fibroblasts.[21] Partially purified osteoclast-activating factor was shown to inhibit collagen synthesis in a manner similar to other potent resorbing factors such as PTH,[269] and most pure cytokines have a similar inhibiting effect.[403] The inhibition of bone formation by OAFs is consistent with the clinical observation that some patients with myeloma show lytic lesions in which there is no coupled increase in bone formation, as indicated by their failure to take up technetium diphosphonate in bone scans. Leukocytes may also be a source of prostaglandins in bone. The possibility that mast cells produce a stimulator of bone formation has been suggested clinically because some patients with mastocytosis show osteosclerosis rather than osteoporosis, but the responsible factor has not been further identified.

D. Effect of Ions on Bone Formation

There is an interesting correlation between serum phosphate concentrations and the net rate of skeletal growth, both within species at different phases of their growth curve and between species. For example, young rats that show a very high proportional increment in skeletal mass have high phosphate levels, newborn humans have higher phosphate levels than those in children, and there is a secondary increase in phosphate concentration at puberty with the lowest concentrations in adults when the overall rate of skeletal growth decreases. The possibility that these changes in phosphate concentration have a regulatory function is supported by *in vitro* observations that increasing phosphate concentration from 1 to 3 mM can enhance not only mineralization but also matrix formation in organ cultures of whole fetal long bones.[404] This effect of phosphate appears to be selective for bone to the extent that there is no stimulation of cartilage growth in the same explants. Phosphate can also stimulate bone growth *in vivo.*[405] In contrast, calcium appears to have a generalized, nonspecific role in tissue growth that involves bone and cartilage in organ culture, as well as many other replicating tissues. Different cell types have different calcium requirements for growth. In the case of bone, growth effects appear to occur over the pathophysiologic range of calcium ion concentration (0.5–2.0 mM). *In vivo,* the impairment of skeletal growth that occurs in vitamin D deficiency appears to be dependent at least in part on the reduction in serum calcium or phosphate concentrations, and administration of these ions can restore skeletal growth in vitamin D–deficient animals.[102,406]

The role of magnesium in regulating skeletal growth is less well defined. In magnesium deficiency, there may be an increased rate of mineralization, but a decreased rate of protein synthesis. Fluoride is a potent stimulator of skeletal growth *in vivo* and recently has been shown to stimulate replication of bone cells *in vitro.*[407] The effect of fluoride does not appear to be on coupling or turnover, since new bone may be formed at sites where resorption had not occurred previously. Aluminum may impair bone growth and mineralization.[408] Aluminum deposition has been associated with development of osteomalacia in patients with renal failure. This ion accumulates in bone because of treatment with aluminum-containing antacids or dialysis with aluminum-containing water. Similar changes have been observed in patients who were given total parenteral nutrition solutions contaminated with aluminum.

CONCLUSION

This chapter has emphasized recent developments in our understanding of the cell biology of bone and tried to provide a review of the many factors that have now been identified as influencing bone formation and resorption. Chapters in this volume will detail information on mineralization, regulation of collagen synthesis, and the complex control of bone formation and resorption at the tissue level in the adult when metabolism is dominated by processes involving sequential remodeling. Aspects of the regulation of bone metabolism remain unresolved. In particular, the relative importance of the various local factors, which have now been identified, has not been elucidated *in vivo;* in fact, none of them has yet been proved to be important in physiologic regulation. Clearly bone formation and resorption will occur as the integrative sum of a number of simultaneous influences. These two processes are in turn integrated in a complex system of bone turnover in which modeling may result in net gains or losses in bone mass at particular sites while remodeling may alter bone strength and improve cellular function and nutrition without actually changing bone mass or shape. There are many open questions that we need to resolve. Our understanding of the pathogenesis of metabolic bone disease is limited by the fact that we do not know what determines age-related bone loss and its menopausal acceleration. It will be particularly important to determine how estrogen acts on bone. The anabolic effects of PTH need to be understood if we are to use this phenomenon to develop new approaches to therapy. The factors that influence bone metabolism in malignancy and inflammation are being elucidated quite rapidly, but the final proof that these factors are involved in a particular clinical disorder has not yet been achieved. Nevertheless, new methods of cell and molecular biology are now being applied to these problems, and a more precise assignment of physiologic and pathologic roles for both systemic hormones and local factors that regulate bone turnover appears to be in sight.

Acknowledgment: We thank Dr. Sevgi B. Rodan for her advice and editorial help and Ms. Dianne McDonald and Ms. Jeannie Arizin for their skillful secretarial assistance.

References

1. Osdoby P, Caplan AI: First bone formation in the developing chick limb. Dev Biol 85:147–156, 1981.
2. Reddi AH, Gay R, Gay S, et al: Transitions in collagen types during matrix-induced cartilage, bone and bone marrow formation. Proc Natl Acad Sci USA 74:5589–5592, 1977.
3. Marcus R: Normal and abnormal bone remodeling in man. Annu Rev Med 38:129–141, 1987.
4. Parfitt AM: Trabecular bone architecture in the pathogenesis and prevention of fracture. Am J Med 82:68–72, 1987.
5. Raisz LG, Kream BE: Regulation of bone formation (first of two parts). N Engl J Med 309:29–35, 1983.
6. Raisz LG, Kream BE: Regulation of bone formation (second of two parts). N Engl J Med 309:83–89, 1983.
7. Raisz LG: What marrow does to bone. N Engl J Med 304:1485–1486, 1981.
8. Rodan GA, Martin TJ: Role of osteoblasts in hormonal control of bone resorption—a hypothesis. Calcif Tissue Int 33:349–351, 1981.
9. Rifas L, Shen V, Mitchell K, et al: Macrophage-derived growth factor for osteoblast-like cells and chondrocytes. Proc Natl Acad Sci USA 81:4558–4562, 1984.
10. Garrett RI, Durie BGM, Nedwin GE, et al: Production of lymphotoxin, a bone-resorbing cytokine, by cultured human myeloma cells. N Engl J Med 317:526–532, 1987.
11. Simmons DJ, Kent GN, Jilka RL: Formation of bone by isolated cultured osteoblasts in Millipore diffusion chambers. Calcif Tissue Int 34:291–294, 1982.
12. Ecarot-Charrier B, Glorieux FA, Van Der Rest M, Pereira G: Osteoblasts isolated from mouse calvaria initiate matrix mineralization in culture. J Cell Biol 96:639–643, 1983.
13. Bellows CG, Aubin JE, Heersche JNM, Antosz ME: Mineralized bone nodules formed in vitro from enzymatically related rat calvaria cell populations. Calcif Tissue Int 38:143–154, 1986.
14. Tenenbaum HC, Heersche JNM: Differentiation of osteoblasts and formation of mineralized bone in vitro. Calcif Tissue Int 34:76–79, 1982.
15. Gerstenfeld LC, Chipman SD, Glowacki J, Lian JB: Expression of differentiated function by mineralizing cultures of chicken osteoblasts. Dev Biol 122:49–60, 1987.
16. Wong G, Cohn DV: Separation of parathyroid hormone and calcitonin–sensitive cells from nonresponsive bone cells. Nature 252:713–715, 1974.
17. Wong GL, Cohn DV: Target cells in bone for parathormone and calcitonin are different: Enrich-

ment for each cell type by sequential digestion of mouse calvaria and selective adhesion to polymeric surfaces. Proc Natl Acad Sci USA 72:3167–3171, 1975.

18. Wong GL, Luben RA, Cohn DV: 1,25-Dihydroxycholecalciferol and parathormone: Effects on isolated osteoclast-like and osteoblast-like cells. Science 197:663–665, 1977.
19. Peck WA, Burks JK, Wilkins J, et al: Evidence for preferential effects of parathyroid hormone, calcitonin and adenosine on bone and periosteum. Endocrinology 94:148–154, 1977.
20. Beresford JN, Gallagher JA, Poser JW, Russell RGG: Production of osteocalcin by human bone cells in vitro. Effects of $1,25(OH)_2D_3$, $24,25(OH)_2D_3$ parathyroid hormone, and glucocorticoids. Metab Bone Dis Rel Res 5:229–234, 1984.
21. Beresford JN, Gallagher JH, Gowen M, et al: The effects of monocyte-conditioned medium and interleukin 1 on the synthesis of collagenous and noncollagenous proteins by mouse bone and human bone cells in vitro. Biochim Biophys Acta 801:58–65, 1984.
22. Robey PG, Termine JD: Human bone cells in vitro. Calcif Tissue Int 37:453–460, 1985.
23. Osdoby P, Martini MC, Caplan AI: Isolated osteoclasts and their presumed progenitor cells, the monocyte, in culture. J Exp Zool 224:331–344, 1982.
24. Zambonin-Zallone A, Teti A, Primavera MV: Isolated osteoclasts in primary culture: First observations on structure and survival in culture media. Anat Embryol 165:405–413, 1982.
25. Chambers TJ, Revell PA, Fuller K, Athanasou NA: Resorption of bone by isolated rabbit osteoclasts. J Cell Sci 66:383–399, 1984.
26. McSheehy PMJ, Chambers TJ: 1,25-Dihydroxyvitamin-D stimulates rat osteoblastic cells to release a soluble factor that increases osteoblastic bone resorption. J Clin Invest 80:425–429, 1987.
27. Blair HC, Kahn AJ, Crouch EC, et al: Isolated osteoclasts resorb the organic and inorganic components of bone. J Cell Biol 102:1164–1172, 1986.
28. Rodan GA, Rodan SB: Expression of the osteoblastic phenotype. *In* Peck WA (ed): Bone and Mineral Research Annual II. Amsterdam, Excerpta Medica, 1984, pp 244–285.
29. Stern PH, Raisz LG: Organ culture of bone. *In* Simmons DJ, Kunin AS (eds): Skeletal Research: An Experimental Approach. New York, Academic Press, 1979, pp 21–59.
30. Tam CS, Bayley A, Cross EG, et al: Increased bone apposition in primary hyperparathyroidism: Measurements based on short interval tetracycline labeling of bone. Metabolism 31:759–765, 1982.
31. Hock JM, Kream BE, Raisz LG: Autoradiographic study of the effect of 1,25-dihydroxyvitamin D_3 on bone matrix synthesis on vitamin D replete rats. Calcif Tissue Int 34:347–351, 1982.
32. Reeve J, Arlot M, Bernat M, et al: Calcium-47 kinetic measurements of bone turnover compared to bone histomorphometry in osteoporosis: The influence of human parathyroid fragment (hPTH 1–34) therapy. Metab Bone Dis Rel Res 3:23–30, 1981.
33. Lauffenburger T, Olah AJ, Dambacher MA, et al: Bone remodeling and calcium metabolism: A correlated histomorphometric, calcium, kinetic, and biochemical study in patients with osteoporosis and Paget's disease. Metab Clin Exp 26:589–605, 1977.
34. Delmas PD, Wahner HW, Mann KG, et al: Assessment of bone turnover in postmenopausal osteoporosis by measurement of serum bone Gla-protein. J Lab Clin Med 102:470–476, 1983.
35. Delmas PD, Demiaux B, Malaval L, et al: Serum bone gamma carboxyglutamic acid–containing protein in primary hyperparathyroidism and in malignant hypercalcemia. J Clin Invest 77:985–991,1986.
36. Friedenstein AJ: Determined and inducible osteogenic precursor cells. *In* Hard Tissue Growth, Repair and Remineralization. Ciba Foundation Symposium II. New York, Elsevier, 1973, pp 169–181.
37. Friedenstein AJ: Precursor cells of mechanocytes. Int Rev Cytol 47:327–355, 1976.
38. Ashton BA, Allen TD, Howlett CR, et al: Formation of bone and cartilage by marrow stromal cells in diffusion chambers in vivo. Clin Orthop Rel Res 151:294–307, 1980.
39. Bab I, Ashton BA, Gazit D, et al: Kinetics and differentiation of marrow stromal cells in diffusion chambers *in vivo*. J Cell Sci 84:139–151, 1986.
40. Friedenstein AJ: Induction of bone tissue by transitional epithelium. Clin Orthop Rel Res 59:21–35, 1968.
41. Owen M: The origin of bone cells in the postnatal organism. Arthritis Rheum 23:1073–1080, 1980.
42. Owen M: Bone growth at the cellular level: A perspective. *In* Dixon AD, Sarnat BG (eds): Factors and Mechanisms Influencing Bone Growth. Progress in Clinical and Biological Research Series, Vol 101. New York, Alan R. Liss, 1982, pp 19–28.
43. Menton DN, Simmons DJ, Orr BY, et al: A cellular investment of bone marrow. Anat Rec 203:157–164, 1982.
44. Friedenstein AJ, Chailakhjan RK, Lalykina KS, et al: The development of fibroblast colonies in monolayer cultures of guinea-pig bone marrow and spleen cells. Cell Tissue Kinet 3:393–402, 1970.
45. Young RW: Cell proliferation and specialization during endochondral osteogenesis in young rats. J Cell Biol 14:357–370, 1962.
46. Urist MR, Nakagawa M, Nakada N, et al: Experimental myositis ossificans: Cartilage and bone formation in muscle in response to a diffusible bone matrix–derived morphogen. Arch Pathol Lab Med 102:312–316, 1978.
47. Reddi AH: Collagenous bone matrix and gene expression in fibroblasts. *In* Slavkin HC, Grenlich RC (eds): Extracellular Matrix Influences on Gene Expression. New York, Academic Press, 1975, pp 619–625.
48. Reddi AH: Regulation of bone differentiation by local and systemic factors. *In* Peck WA (ed): Bone and Mineral Research Annual III. Amsterdam, Excerpta Medica, 1985, pp 27–47.
49. Sampath TK, Reddi AH: Dissociative extraction and reconstitution of extracellular matrix components involved in local bone differentiation. Proc Natl Acad Sci USA 78:7599–7603, 1981.
50. Urist MR, Huo YK, Brownell AG, et al: Purification of bovine bone morphogenetic protein by hydroxyapatite chromatography. Proc Natl Acad Sci USA 81:371–375, 1984.
51. Takaoka K, Yoshikawa H, Shimizu N, et al: Purification of a bone-inducing substance (osteogenic factor) from a murine osteosarcoma. Biomed Res 2:466–471, 1981.

52. Wang EA, Kriz M, Luxenberg D, et al: Purification and characterization of cartilage and bone inducing factors. Calcif Tissue Int 42(S):A37,1988.
53. Sampath TK, Muthukumaren N, Reddi AH: Isolation of osteogenin, an extracellular matrix-associated, bone-inductive protein, by heparin affinity chromatography. Proc Natl Acad Sci USA 84:7109–7113, 1987.
54. Spiegelman BM, Ginty CA: Fibronectin modulation of cell shape and lipogenic gene expression in 3T3 adipocytes. Cell 35:657–660, 1983.
55. Heine UI, Munoz EF, Flanders KC, et al: Role of transforming growth factor-beta in the development of the mouse embryo. J Cell Biol 105:2861–2876, 1987.
56. Noda M, Rodan GA: Type beta transforming growth factor (TGFbeta) regulation of alkaline phosphatase expression and other phenotype-related mRNAs in osteoblastic rat osteosarcoma cells. J Cell Physiol 133:426–437, 1987.
57. Holtrop ME: The ultrastructure of bone. Ann Clin Lab Sci 5:264–271, 1975.
58. Doty SB: Morphological evidence of gap junctions between bone cells. Calcif Tissue Int 33:509–512, 1981.
59. Jeansonne BG, Feagin FF, McMinn RW, et al: Cell-to-cell communication of osteoblasts. J Dent Res 58:1415–1423, 1979.
60. Moen RC, Rowe DW, Palmiter RD: Regulation of procollagen synthesis during the development of chick embryo calvaria. J Biol Chem 254:3526–3530, 1979.
61. Nimni ME: Collagen. Semin Arthritis Rheum 13:1–186, 1983.
62. Hauschka PV, Lian JB, Gallop PM: Direct identification of the calcium binding amino acid γ-carboxyglutamate, in mineralized tissue. Proc Natl Acad Sci USA 72:3925–3929, 1975.
63. Price PA, Otsuka AS, Poser JW, et al: Characterization of carboxyglutamic acid–containing protein from bone. Proc Natl Acad Sci USA 73:1447–1451, 1976.
64. Price PA, Poser JW, Roman N: Primary structure of the carboxyglutamic acid containing protein from bovine bone. Proc Natl Acad Sci USA 73:3374–3375, 1976.
65. Nishimoto SK, Price PA: Secretion of the vitamin K–dependent protein of bone by rat osteosarcoma cells. Evidence for an intracellular precursor. J Biol Chem 255:6579–6583, 1980.
66. Price P: Osteocalcin. *In* Peck WA (ed): Bone and Mineral Research Annual I. Amsterdam, Excerpta Medica, 1983, pp 157–190.
67. Price PA, Urist MR, Otawara Y: Matrix Gla protein, a new γ-carboxyglutamic acid containing protein which is associated with the organic matrix of bone. Biochem Biophys Res Commun 117:765–771, 1983.
68. Fraser JD, Otawara Y, Price PA: 1,25-dihydroxyvitamin D_3 stimulates the synthesis of matrix γ-carboxyglutamic acid protein by osteosarcoma cells. Mutually exclusive expression of vitamin K–dependent bone protein by clonal osteoblastic cell lines. J Biol Chem 263:911–916, 1988.
69. Termine JD: Osteonectin and other newly described proteins of developing bone. *In* Peck WA (ed): Bone and Mineral Research Annual I. Amsterdam, Excerpta Medica, 1983, pp 144–156.
70. Wientraub S, Fisher LW, Reddi AH, Termine JD: Non collagenous bone proteins in experimental rickets in the rat. Mol Cell Biochem 74:157–162, 1986.
71. Whitson SW, Harrison W, Dunlap MK, et al: Fetal bovine bone cells synthesize bone specific matrix proteins. J Cell Biol 99:607–614, 1984.
72. Otsuka K, Yao K-L, Wasi S, et al: Biosynthesis of osteonectin by fetal porcine calvarial cells in vitro. J Biol Chem 259:9805–9812, 1984.
73. Termine JD, Robey PG, Fisher LW, et al: Osteonectin, bone proteoglycan and phosphoryn defects in a form of bovine osteogenesis imperfecta. Proc Natl Acad Sci USA 81:2213–2217, 1984.
74. Stenner DD, Tracy RP, Riggs BL, Mann KG: Human platelets contain and secrete osteonectin, a major protein of mineralized bone. Proc Natl Acad Sci USA 83:6892–6896, 1986.
75. Fisher LW, Termine JD, Dejter SW, et al: Proteoglycans of developing bone. J Biol Chem 258:6588–6594, 1983.
76. Oldberg A, Franzen A, Heinegard D: Cloning and sequence analysis of rat bone sialoprotein (osteopontin) cDNA reveals an Arg-Gly-Asp cell binding sequence. J Biol Chem 83:8819–8823, 1986.
77. Prince CW, Oosawa T, Butler WT, et al: Isolation, characterization and biosynthesis of a phosphorylated glycoprotein from rat bone. J Biol Chem 262:2900–2907, 1987.
78. Yoon K, Buenega R, Rodan GA: Tissue specificity and developmental expression of rat osteopontin. Biochem Biophys Res Commun 148:1129–1136, 1987.
79. Lee SL, Glimcher MJ: Purification, composition and ^{31}PNMR spectroscopic properties of a non collagenous phosphoprotein isolated from chicken bone matrix. Calcif Tissue Int 33:385–394, 1981.
80. Landis WJ, Sanzone CF, Brickley-Parsons D, et al: Radioautographic visualization and biochemical identification of O-phosphoserine- and O-phosphothreonine-containing phosphoproteins in mineralizing embryonic chick bone. J Cell Biol 98:986–990, 1984.
81. Termine JD, Belcourt AB, Conn AM, et al: Mineral and collagen-binding proteins of fetal calf bone. J Biol Chem 256:10403–10408, 1981.
82. Canalis E, McCarthy T, Centrella M: Growth factors and the regulation of bone remodeling. J Clin Invest 81:277–281, 1988.
83. Robison R: The possible significance of hexosephosplionic esters in ossification. Biochem J 17:286–293, 1923.
84. Doty SB, Schofield BH: Enzyme histochemistry of bone and cartilage cells. Prog Histochem Cytochem 8:1–38, 1976.
85. Henthorn PS, Knoll BJ, Raducha M, et al:Products of two common alleles at the locus for human placental alkaline phosphatase differ by seven amino acids. Proc Natl Acad Sci USA 83:5597–5601, 1986.
86. Henthorn PS, Raducha M, Edwards YH, et al: Nucleotide and amino acid sequences of human intestinal alkaline phosphatase: Close homology to placental alkaline phosphatase. Proc Natl Acad Sci USA 84:1234–1238, 1987.
87. Goldstein DJ, Rogers CE, Harris H: Expression of alkaline phosphatase loci in mammalian tissues. Proc Natl Acad Sci USA 77:2857–2860, 1980.
88. Stigbrand T, Fishman WH: Human Alkaline Phosphatases. New York, Alan R. Liss, 1984.

89. Weiss M, Henthorn PS, Lafferty MA, et al: Isolation and characterization of a cDNA encoding a human liver/bone/kidney-type alkaline phosphatase. Proc Natl Acad Sci USA 83:7182–7186, 1986.
90. Nair BC, Majeska RJ, Rodan GA: Rat alkaline phosphatase. I. Purification and characterization of the enzyme from osteosarcoma: Generation of monoclonal and polyclonal antibodies. Arch Biochem Biophys 254:18–27, 1987.
91. Luben RA, Wong GL, Cohn DV: Biochemical characterization with parathormone and calcitonin of isolated bone cells: Provisional identification of osteoclasts and osteoblasts. Endocrinology 99:526–534, 1976.
92. Rodan SB, Rodan GA: The effect of parathyroid hormone and calcitonin on the accumulation of cyclic adenosine 3′,5′-monophosphate in freshly isolated bone cells. J Biol Chem 249:3068–3074, 1974.
93. Silve CM, Hradek GT, Jones AL, et al: Parathyroid hormone receptor in intact embryonic chicken bone: Characterization and cellular localization. J Cell Biol 94:379–386, 1982.
94. Rizzoli RE, Somerman M, Murray TM, et al: Binding of radioiodinated parathyroid hormone to cloned bone cells. Endocrinology 113:1832–1838, 1983.
95. Majeska RJ, Rodan GA: Alkaline phosphatase inhibition by parathyroid hormone and isoproterenol in a clonal rat osteosarcoma cell line. Possible mediation by cyclic AMP. Calcif Tissue Int 34:59–66, 1982.
96. Kream BE, Rowe DW, Gworek SC, et al: Parathyroid hormone alters collagen synthesis and procollagen mRNA levels in fetal rat calvaria. Proc Natl Acad Sci USA 77:5654–5658, 1980.
97. Raisz LG, Niemann I: Effect of phosphate, calcium, and magnesium on bone resorption and hormonal responses in tissue culture. Endocrinology 85:446–462, 1969.
98. Chambers TJ: The cellular basis of bone resorption. Clin Orthop Rel Res 151:283–293, 1980.
99. Chen TL, Hirst MA, Feldman D: A receptor-like binding macromolecule for 1,25-dihydroxycholecalciferol in cultured mouse bone cells. J Biol Chem 254:7491–7494, 1979.
100. Manolagas SC, Haussler M, Deftos LJ: 1,25-Dihydroxyvitamin D_3 receptor-like macromolecule in rat osteogenic sarcoma cell lines. J Biol Chem 255:4414–4417, 1980.
101. Partridge NC, Frampton RJ, Eisman JA, et al: Receptors for 1,25$(OH)_2$-vitamin D_3 enriched in cloned osteoblast-like rat osteogenic sarcoma cells. FEBS Lett 115:139–142,1980.
102. Underwood JL, DeLuca HF: Vitamin D is not directly necessary for bone growth and mineralization. Am J Physiol 246:E492–E494, 1984.
103. Weinstein RS, Underwood JL, Hutson MS, et al: Bone histomorphometry in vitamin D deficient rats infused with calcium and phosphorus. Am J Physiol 246:E499–E505, 1984.
104. Kream BE, Rowe D, Smith MD, et al: Hormonal regulation of collagen synthesis in a clonal rat osteosarcoma cell line. Endocrinology 119:1922–1928, 1986.
105. Manolagas SC, Burton DW, Deftos LJ: 1,25-Dihydroxyvitamin D_3 stimulates the alkaline phosphatase activity of osteoblast-like cells. J Biol Chem 256:7115–7117, 1981.
106. Majeska RJ, Rodan GA: The effect of 1,25$(OH)_2D_3$ on alkaline phosphatase in osteoblastic osteosarcoma cells. J Biol Chem 257:3362–3365, 1982.
107. Abe E, Miyaura C, Sakagami H, et al: Differentiation of mouse myeloid leukemia cells induced by 1,25-dihydroxyvitamin D_3. Proc Natl Acad Sci USA 78:4990–4994, 1981.
108. Bar-Shavit Z, Teitelbaum SL, Reitsma P, et al: Induction of monocytic differentiation and bone resorption by 1,25-dihydroxyvitamin D_3. Proc Natl Acad Sci USA 80:5907–5911, 1983.
109. Rowe DW, Kream BE: Regulation of collagen synthesis in fetal rat calvaria by 1,25-dihydroxyvitamin D_3. J Biol Chem 257:8009–8115, 1982.
110. McDonnell DP, Mangelsdorf DJ, Pike JW, et al: Molecular cloning of complementary DNA encoding the avian receptor for vitamin D. Science 235:1214–1217, 1987.
111. Payvan F, Wrange O, Carlstedt-Duke J, et al: Purified glucocorticoid receptors bind selectively in vitro to a cloned DNA fragment whose transcription is regulated by glucocorticoids in vivo. Proc Natl Acad Sci USA 78:6628–6632, 1981.
112. Payvan F, DeFranco D, Firestone GL, et al: Sequence-specific binding of glucocorticoid receptor to MTV DNA at sites within and upstream of the transcribed region. Cell 35:381–392, 1983.
113. Renkawitz R, Schutz G, von der Ahe D, et al: Sequences in the promoter region of the chicken lysozyme gene required for steroid regulation and receptor binding. Cell 37:503–510, 1984.
114. Gustafson JA, Carlstedt-Duke J, Poellinger L, et al: Biochemistry, molecular biology and physiology of the glucocorticoid receptor. Endocr Rev 8:185,234, 1987.
115. Chen TL, Cone CM, Feldman D: Glucocorticoid modulation of cell proliferation in cultured osteoblast-like bone cells: Differences between rat and mouse. Endocrinology 112:1739–1745, 1983.
116. Chen TL, Cone CM, Morey-Holton E, et al: 1,25-Dihydroxyvitamin D_3 receptors in cultured rat osteoblast-like cells. J Biol Chem 258:4350–4355, 1983.
117. Chen TL, Feldman D: Glucocorticoid potentiation of the adenosine 3′,5′-monophosphate response to parathyroid hormone in cultured rat bone cells. Endocrinology 102:589–596, 1978.
118. Rodan SB, Fischer ML, Egan JJ, et al: The effect of dexamethasone on parathyroid hormone stimulation of adenylate cyclase in ROS 17/2.8 cells. Endocrinology 115:951–958, 1984.
119. Rodan SB, Wesolowski G, Rodan GA: Clonal differences in prostaglandin synthesis among osteosarcoma cell lines. J Bone Mineral Res 1:213–220,1986.
120. Meunier P, Bressot C: Endocrine influences on bone cells and bone remodeling evaluated by clinical histomorphometry. *In* Parsons JA (ed): Endocrinology of Calcium Metabolism. New York, Raven Press, 1982, pp 445–465.
121. Dietrich JW, Canalis EM, Maina DM, et al: Effects of glucocorticoids on fetal rat bone collagen synthesis in vitro. Endocrinology 104:715–721, 1979
122. Canalis E: Effect of glucocorticoids on Type I collagen synthesis, alkaline phosphatase activity and deoxyribonucleic acid content in cultured rat calvariae. Endocrinology 112:931–939, 1983.
123. Majeska RJ, Nair BC, Rodan GA: Glucocorticoid regulation of alkaline phosphatase in the osteoblastic osteosarcoma cell line ROS 17/2.8. Endocrinology 116:170–179, 1985.

124. Chyun YS, Kream BE, Raisz LG: Cortisol decreases bone formation by inhibiting periosteal cell proliferation. Endocrinology 114:447–480, 1984.
125. Nolan RD, Partridge NC, Godfrey HM, et al: Cyclo-oxygenase products of arachidonic acid metabolism in rat osteoblasts. Calcif Tissue Int 35:294–297, 1983.
126. Rodan SB, Rodan GA, Simmons HA, et al: Bone resorptive factor produced by osteosarcoma cells with osteoblastic features in PGE_2. Biochem Biophys Res Commun 102:1358–1365, 1981.
127. Tashjian AH Jr, Voelkel EF, Levine L, et al: Evidence that the bone resorption stimulating factor produced by mouse fibrosarcoma cells is prostaglandin E_2. A new model for the hypercalcemia of cancer. J Exp Med 136:1329–1343, 1972.
128. Seyberth HW, Segre GV, Moyan JL, et al: Prostaglandins as mediators of hypercalcemia associated with certain types of cancer. N Engl J Med 293:1278–1283, 1975.
129. Somjen D, Binderman I, Berger E, et al: Bone modeling induced by physical stress is prostaglandin mediated. Biochim Biophys Acta 629:91–100, 1980.
130. Yeh CK, Rodan GA: Tensile forces enhance prostaglandin E synthesis in osteoblastic cells grown on collagen ribbons. Calcif Tissue Int 36:567–571, 1984.
131. Yeh C-K, Rodan GA: Microtubule disruption enhances prostaglandin E_2 production in osteoblastic cells. Biochim Biophys Acta 927:315–323, 1987.
132. Feyen JHM, Vanderwilt G, Moonen P, et al: Stimulation of arachidonic acid metabolism in primary cultures of osteoblast-like cells by hormones and drugs. Prostaglandins 28:769–783, 1984.
133. Tashjian AH Jr, Levine L: Epidermal growth factor stimulates prostaglandin production and bone resorption in cultured mouse calvaria. Biochem Biophys Res Commun 85:966–975, 1978.
134. Raisz LG, Sandberg AL, Goodson JM, et al: Complement-dependent stimulation of prostaglandin synthesis and bone resorption. Science 185:789–791, 1974.
135. Atkins D, Martin TJ: Rat osteogenic sarcoma cells: Effects of some prostaglandins, their metabolites and analogues on cyclic AMP production. Prostaglandins 13:861–871, 1977.
136. Aubin JE, Heersche JNM, Merrilees MJ, Sodek J: Isolation of bone cell clones with differences in growth hormone responses and extracellular matrix production. J Cell Biol 92:452–461, 1982.
137. Korn H: Substrain heterogeneity in prostaglandin E_2 synthesis of human dermal fibroblasts. Arthritis Rheum 28:315–322, 1985.
138. Vander Wiel CJ, Grubb SA, Talmage RV: The presence of lining cells on surfaces of human trabecular bone. Clin Orthop Rel Res 134:350–355, 1978.
139. Cooper RR, Malgniom JW, Robinson RA: Morphology of the osteon. An electron microscopic study. J Bone Joint Surg 48A:1239–1271, 1966.
140. Doty SB, Morey-Holton E: Changes in osteoblast activity due to simulated weightless conditions. Physiologist 25:5141–5142,1982.
141. Talmage R: Calcium homeostasis—calcium transport—parathyroid action: The effects of parathyroid hormone on the movement of calcium between bone and fluid. Clin Orthop 67:210–224, 1969.
142. Norimatsu H, Vander Wiel CJ, Talmage RV: Morphologic support of a role for cell lining bone surfaces in maintenance of plasma calcium concentration. Clin Orthop Rel Res 138:254–262, 1979.
143. Jones SL, Boyde A: Scanning electron microscopy of bone cells in culture. *In* Copp DH, Talmage RV (eds): Endocrinology of Calcium Metabolism. Amsterdam, Excerpta Medica, 1978, pp 97–104.
144. Mundy G: Monocyte-macrophage system and bone resorption. Lab Invest 49:119–121, 1983.
145. Jaworski ZGF, Duck B, Sekaly G: Kinetics of osteoclasts and their nuclei in evolving secondary Haversian system. J Anat 133:397–405, 1981.
146. Anderson RE, Schraer H, Gay CV: Ultrastructural immunocytochemical localization of carbonic anhydrase in normal and calcitonin-treated chick osteoclasts. Anat Rec 204:9–20, 1982.
147. Gay CV, Mueller WJ: Carbonic anhydrase and osteoclasts: Localization by labeled inhibitor autoradiography. Science 183:432–434, 1974.
148. Baron R, Neff L, Roy C, et al: Evidence for a high and specific concentration of (Na^+, K^+) ATPase in the plasma membrane of the osteoclast. Cell 46:311–320, 1986.
149a. Blair H, Teitelbaum S, Ghiselli R, et al: Osteoclastic bone resorption by a polarized vacuolar proton pump. Science 245:855–857, 1989.
149. Baron R, Neff L, Louvard D, Courtoy PJ: Cell-mediated extracellular acidification and bone resorption: Evidence for a low pH in resorbing lacunae and localization of a 100-kD lysosomal membrane protein at the osteoclast ruffled border. J Cell Biol 101:2210–2222, 1985.
150. Fallon MD: Bone resorbing fluid from osteoclasts in acidic in vitro micropuncture study. *In* Cohn DV, Fujita T, Potts JT Jr, Talmage RV (eds): Endocrine Control of Bone and Calcium, vol 8A. Metabolism. Amsterdam, Elsevier Science Publishers, 1984, pp 144–146.
151. Puzas JE, Brand JS: Parathyroid hormone stimulation of collagenase secretion by isolated bone cells. Endocrinology 104:559–562, 1979.
152. Otsuka K, Sodek J, Limeback H: Synthesis of collagenase and collagenase inhibitors by osteoblast-like cells in culture. Eur J Biochem 145:123–129, 1984.
153. Heath JK, Atkinson SJ, Meikle MC, et al: Mouse osteoblasts synthesize collagenase in response to bone resorbing agents. Biochim Biophys Acta 802:151–154, 1984.
154. Vaes G: Collagenase, lysosomes and osteoclastic bone resorption. *In* Wooley DE, Evanson JM (eds): Collagenase in Normal and Pathological Connective Tissues. New York, John Wiley and Sons, 1980, pp 185–207.
155. Eilon G, Raisz LG: Comparison of the effects of stimulators and inhibitors of resorption on the release of lysosomal enzymes and radioactive calcium from fetal bone in organ culture. Endocrinology 103:1969–1975, 1978.
156. Chambers TJ, Thomson BM, Fuller K: Effect of substrate composition on bone resorption by rabbit osteoclasts. J Cell Sci 66:383–399, 1984.
157. Sakamoto S, Sakamoto M: Bone collagenase, osteoblasts and cell-mediated bone resorption. *In* Peck WA (ed): Bone and Mineral Research Annual 4. Amsterdam, Elsevier, 1986, pp 49–102.
158. Chambers TJ, Dunn CJ: Pharmacological control of osteoclastic motility. Calcif Tissue Int 35:566–570, 1983.
159. Zambonin Zallone A, Teti A, Primavera MV:

Monocytes from circulating blood fuse in vitro with purified osteoclasts in primary culture. J Cell Sci 66:335–342, 1984.
160. Hancox NM: The osteoclast. Biol Rev 24:448–467, 1949.
161. Fishmann DA, Hay ED: Origin of osteoclasts from mononuclear leukocytes in regenerating newt limbs. Anat Rec 143:329–334, 1962.
162. Jee WSS, Nolan PD: Origin of osteoclasts from the fusion of phagocytes. Nature 200:225–226, 1963.
163. Gothlin G, Ericsson JLE: Electron microscopic studies on the uptake and storage of thorium dioxide molecules in different cell types of fracture callus. Acta Pathol Microbiol Scand A81:523–542, 1973.
164. Gothlin G, Ericsson JLE: The osteoclast, review of ultrastructure, origin and structure-function relationship. Clin Orthop 120:201–231, 1976.
165. Tinkler SMB, Williams DM, Johnson NW: Kinetics of osteoclast formation: The significance of blood monocytes as osteoclast precursors during 1-hydroxycholecalciferol-stimulated bone resorption in mice. J Anat 137:335–340, 1983.
166. Buring K: On the origin of cells in heterotopic bone formation. Clin Orthop 110:293–302, 1975.
167. Kahn AJ, Simmons DJ: Investigation of cell lineage in bone using a chimera of chick and quail embryonic tissue. Nature 258:325–327, 1975.
168. Jotereau FV, LeDouarin NM: The developmental relationship between osteocytes and osteoclasts. A study using quail-chick nuclear marker in endochondral ossification. Dev Biol 63:253–265, 1978.
169. Walker DG: Control of bone resorption by hematopoietic tissue; the induction and reversal of congenital osteopetrosis in mice through use of bone marrow and splenic transplants. J Exp Med 142:651–663, 1975.
170. Marks SC, Schneider GB: Evidence for a relationship between lymphoid cells and osteoclasts: Bone resorption restored in ia (osteopetrotic) rats by lymphocytes, monocytes, and macrophages from a normal littermate. Am J Anat 152:331–342, 1978.
171. Walker DG: Spleen cells transmit osteoporosis in mice. Science 190:785–787, 1975.
172. Coccia PF, Krivit W, Cervenka J, et al: Successful bone marrow transplantation for infantile malignant osteopetrosis. N Engl J Med 302:701–708, 1980.
173. Ash P, Loutit JF, Townsend KMS: Osteoclasts derive from hematopoietic stem cells according to marker, giant lysosomes of beige mice. Clin Orthop 155:249–258, 1981.
174. Ko JS, Bernard GW: Osteoclast formation in vitro from bone marrow mononuclear cells in osteoclast-free bone. Am J Anat 161:415–425, 1981.
175. Burger EH, Van Der Meer JWN, Nijweide PJ: Osteoclast formation from mononuclear phagocytes: Role of bone-forming cells. J Cell Biol 99:1901–1906, 1984.
176. Miller SS, Wolf AM, Arnaud CD: Bone cells in culture. Morphological transformation by hormones. Science 192:1340–1343, 1976.
177. Egan JJ, Gronowicz G, Rodan GA: The effect of parathyroid hormone (PTH) on the cytoskeleton of osteoblastic cells. Calcif Tissue Int 36:457, 1984.
178. Gronowicz G, Egan JJ, Rodan GA: The effect of 1,25-Dihydroxyvitamin D_3 on the cytoskeleton of rat calvaria and rat osteosarcoma (ROS17/2.8) osteoblastic cells. J Bone Mineral Res 1:441–455, 1986.
179. Chambers TJ: Osteoblasts release osteoclasts from calcitonin-induced quiescence. J Cell Sci 57:247–260, 1982.
180. Price PA, Baukol SA: 1,25-Dihydroxyvitamin D_3 increases synthesis of the vitamin K–dependent bone protein by osteosarcoma cells. J Biol Chem 255:11660–11663, 1980.
181. Malone JD, Teitelbaum SL, Griffin GL, et al: Recruitment of osteoclast precursors by purified bone matrix constituents. J Cell Biol 92:227–230, 1982.
182. Price PA, Williamson MK: Effects of warfarin on bone. Studies on the vitamin K–dependent protein of rat bone. J Biol Chem 256:12754–12759, 1981.
183. Lian JB, Tassinari M, Glowacki J: Resorption of implanted bone prepared from normal and warfarin-treated rats. J Clin Invest 73:1223–1228,1984.
184. Jones SL, Hogg NM, Shapiro IM, et al: Cells with Fe receptors in the cell layer next to osteoblasts and osteoclasts on bone. Metab Bone Dis Rel Res 2:357–362, 1981.
185. Abe E, Miyaura C, Tanaka H, et al: 1,25-Dihydroxyvitamin D_3 promotes fusion of mouse alveolar macrophages both by a direct mechanism and by a spleen cell-mediated indirect mechanism. Proc Natl Acad Sci USA 80:5583–5587, 1983.
186. Ibbotson KJ, Roodman GD, McManus LM, et al: Identification and characterization of osteoclast-like cells and their progenitors in cultures of feline marrow mononuclear cells. J Cell Biol 99:471–480, 1984.
187. Roodman GD, Ibbotson KJ, MacDonald BR, et al: 1,25-Dihydroxyvitamin D_3 causes formation of multinucleated cells with several osteoclast characteristics in cultures of primate marrow. Proc Natl Acad Sci USA 82:8213–8217, 1985.
188. Bressot C, Meunier PJ, Chapuy MC, et al: Histomorphometric profile, pathophysiology and reversibility of corticosteroid-induced osteoporosis. Metab Bone Dis Rel Res 1:303–311, 1979.
189. Mundy GR, Altman AJ, Gondek MD, et al: Direct resorption of bone by human monocytes. Science 196:1109–1111, 1977.
190. Kahn AJ, Stewart CC, Teitelbaum SL: Contact mediated bone resorption by human monocytes in vitro. Science 199:988–990, 1978.
191. Mundy GR, DeMartino S, Rowe DW: Collagen and collagen fragments are chemotactic for tumor cells. J Clin Invest 68:19–22, 1981.
192. Horton JE, Raisz LG, Simmons HA, et al: Bone resorbing activity in supernatant fluid from cultured human peripheral blood leukocytes. Science 177:793–795, 1972.
193. Gowen M, Wood DD, Ihrie EJ, et al: An interleukin 1 like factor stimulates bone resorption in vitro. Nature 306:378–380, 1983.
194. Dewhirst FE, Stashenko PP, Mole JE, Tsurumachi T: Purification and partial sequence of human osteoclast-activating factor: Identity with interleukin 1beta. J Immunol 135:2562–2568, 1985.
195. Lorenzo JA, Sousa SL, Alander C, et al: Comparison of the bone-resorbing activity in the supernatants from phytohemagglutinin-stimulated human peripheral blood mononuclear cells with that of cytokines through the use of an antiserum to interleukin 1. Endocrinology 121:1164–1170, 1987.
196. Mundy GR, Luben RA, Raisz LG, et al: Bone-resorbing activity in supernatants from lymphoid cell lines. N Engl J Med 290:867–871, 1974.
197. Mundy GR, Raisz LG, Cooper RA, et al: Evidence

for the secretion of an osteoclast stimulating factor in myeloma. N Engl J Med 291:1041–1046, 1974.
198. Horowitz MS, Vignery A, Gershon RK, et al: Requirement for T-lymphocytes and their interaction with macrophages in the production of the lymphokine osteoclast activating factor (OAF) in the mouse. Proc Natl Acad Sci USA 81:2181–2185, 1984.
199. Sandberg AL, Raisz LG, Goodson JM, et al: Initiation of bone resorption by the classical and alternative C pathways and its mediation by prostaglandins. J Immunol 119:1378–1381, 1977.
200. Perry HM, Chappel JC, Bellorin-Font E, et al: Parathyroid hormone receptors in circulating human mononuclear leukocytes. J Biol Chem 259:5531–5535, 1984.
201. Provvedini DM, Tsoukas CD, Deftos LJ: 1,25-Dihydroxyvitamin D_3 receptors in human leukocytes. Science 221:1181–1183, 1983.
202. Bingham PJ, Brazell IA, Owen M: The effect of parathyroid extract on cellular activity and plasma calcium levels in vivo. Endocrinology 45:387–400, 1969.
203. Christoffersen J: Dissolution of calcium hydroxyapatite. Calcif Tissue Int 33:557–560, 1981.
204. Lorenzo JA, Holtrop ME, Raisz LG: Effects of phosphate on calcium release, lysosomal enzyme activity in the medium, and osteoclast morphometry in cultured fetal rat bone. Metab Bone Dis Rel Res 5:187–190, 1984.
205. Francois-Gillet C, Delaisse JM, Eeckhout Y, et al: Immunoreactive collagenase and bone resorption. Biochim Biophys Acta 667:1–9, 1981.
206. Hamilton JA, Lingelback SR, Partridge NC, et al: Stimulation of plasminogen activator in osteoblast-like cells by bone-resorbing hormones. Biochim Biophys Res Commun 122:230–236, 1984.
207. Tran Van P, Vignery A, Baron R: An electron-microscopic study of the bone remodeling sequence in the rat. Cell Tissue Res 225:283–292, 1982.
208. Martin TJ: Drug and hormone effects on calcium release from bone. Pharmacol Ther 21:209–228, 1983.
209. Barnicot NA: The local action of the parathyroid and other tissues on bone in intracerebral grafts. J Anat 82:233, 1948.
210. Gaillard P: Parathyroid gland tissue and bone in vitro (1). Cell Res 3[Suppl]:154, 1955.
211. Gaillard PJ, Herrmann-Erlee MPM, Hellelman JW, et al: Skeletal tissue in culture. Hormonal regulation of metabolism and development. Clin Orthop Rel Res 142:196–214, 1979.
212. Holtrop ME, King GJ: The ultrastructure of osteoclast and its functional implications. Clin Orthop Rel Res 123:177–196, 1977.
213. Holtrop ME, King GJ, Cox KA, et al: Time-related changes in the ultrastructure of osteoclasts after injection of parathyroid hormone in young rats. Calcif Tissue Int 27:129–135, 1979.
214. Lorenzo JA, Raisz LG, Hock J: DNA synthesis is not necessary for osteoclastic responses to parathyroid hormone in cultured fetal rat long bones. J Clin Invest 72:1924–1929, 1983.
215. Bergmann PS, Simmons HA, Viget A, et al: Cationized serum albumin enhances response of cultured fetal rat long bones to parathyroid hormone. Endocrinology 116:1729–1734, 1985.
216. Luben RA, Goggins JF, Raisz LG: Stimulation by parathyroid hormone of bone hyaluronate synthesis in organ culture. Endocrinology 94:737–745, 1974.
217. Luben RA, Cohn DV: Effects of parathormone and calcitonin on citrate and myoluronate metabolism in cultured bone. Endocrinology 98:413–419, 1976.
218. Raisz LG, Trummel CL, Simmons H: Induction of bone resorption in tissue culture: Prolonged response after brief exposure to parathyroid hormone or 25-hydroxycholecalciferol. Endocrinology 90:744–751, 1972.
219. Pliam NB, Nyiredy KO, Arnaud CD: Parathyroid hormone receptors in avian bone cells. Proc Natl Acad Sci USA 79:2061–2063, 1982.
220. Rao LG, Murray TM, Heersche JNM: Immunohistochemical demonstration of parathyroid hormone binding to specific cell types in fixed rat bone tissue. Endocrinology 113:805–810, 1983.
221. Chambers TJ, Athanasou NA, Fuller K: Effect of parathyroid hormone and calcitonin on the cytoplasmic spreading of isolated osteoclasts. J Endocrinol 102:281–284, 1984.
222. Wong GL: Studies on osteoblast and bone-derived factor(s) that confer competence to respond to PTH on osteoclasts. Calcif Tissue Int 36:475, 1984.
223. MacDonald BR, Gallagher JA, Ahnfelt-Ronne I, et al: Effects of bovine parathyroid hormone and 1,25-dihydroxyvitamin D_3 on the production of prostaglandins by cells derived from human bone. FEBS Lett 169:49–52, 1984.
224. Raisz LG, Simmons HA: Effects of parathyroid hormone and cortisol on prostaglandin production by neonatal rat calvaria in vitro. Endocr Res 11:59–74, 1985.
225. Raisz LG, Trummel CL, Wener JA, et al: Effect of glucocorticoids on bone resorption in tissue culture. Endocrinology 90:961–967, 1972.
226. Stern PH, Halloran BP, DeLuca HF, et al: Responsiveness of vitamin D–deficient fetal rat limb bones to parathyroid hormone in culture. Am J Physiol 244:E421–E424, 1983.
227. Peck WA: Cyclic AMP as a second messenger in the skeletal actions of parathyroid hormone: A decade-old hypothesis. Calcif Tissue Int 29:1–4, 1979.
228. Klein DC, Raisz LG: Prostaglandins: stimulation of bone resorption in tissue cultures. Endocrinology 86:1436–1440, 1970.
229. Lerner U, Gustafson GT: Delayed stimulatory effect of cyclic AMP on bone resorption in vitro. Acta Endocrinol 99:281–288, 1981.
230. Tashjian AH Jr, Ivey JL: Stimulation of bone resorption in organ culture by cholera toxin. Biochem Biophys Res Commun 102:1055–1064, 1981.
231. Hohmann EL, Levine L, Tashjian AJ Jr: Vasoactive intestinal peptide stimulates bone resorption via a cyclic adenosine 3′,5′-monophosphate-dependent mechanism. Endocrinology 112:1233–1239, 1983.
232. McLeod JF, Raisz LG: Comparison of inhibition of bone resorption and escape with calcitonin and dibutyryl 3′,5′ cyclic adenosine monophosphate. Endocrinol Res Commun 8:49–59, 1981.
233. Dziak R, Stern PH: Responses of fetal rat bone cells and bone organ cultures to the ionophore A23187. Calcif Tissue Res 22:137–147, 1976.
234. Stern PH, Orr MF, Brull E: Ionophore A23187 promotes osteoclast formation in bone organ culture. Calcif Tissue Int 34:31–36, 1982.
235. Lorenzo JA, Raisz LG: Divalent cation ionophores stimulate resorption and inhibit DNA synthesis in cultured fetal rat bone. Science 212:1157–1159, 1981.
236. DeBartolo TF, Pegg LE, Shasserre C, et al: Com-

parison of parathyroid hormone and calcium ionophore A23187 effects on bone resorption and nucleic acid synthesis in cultured fetal rat bone. Calcif Tissue Int 34:495–500, 1982.

237. Ivey JL, Wright DR, Tashjian AH Jr: Bone resorption in organ culture and inhibition by the divalent cation ionophores A23187 and X-537A. J Clin Invest 58:1327–1338, 1976.
238. Herrmann-Erlee MPM, Nijweide PJ, van der Meer JM, et al: Action of bPTH and bPTH fragments on embryonic bone in vitro: Dissociation of the cyclic AMP and bone resorbing response. Calcif Tissue Int 35:70–77, 1983.
239. Lowik CWGM, van Leeuwen JPTM, Feyen JHM, et al: Cytosolic free Ca^{2+} in UMR 106 osteogenic sarcoma cells measured by quin 2: Effects of PTH and different drugs. Calcif Tissue Int 2:S26, 1984.
240. Rappaport MS, Stern PH: Parathyroid hormone enhances inositol incorporation into phospholipids in bone organ culture. Calcif Tissue Int 36:507, 1984.
241. Stern PH: The D vitamins and bone. Pharmacol Rev 32:47–80, 1981.
242. Raisz LG, Kream BE, Smith MD, et al: Comparison of the effects of vitamin D metabolites on collagen synthesis and resorption of fetal rat bone in organ culture. Calcif Tissue Int 32:135–138, 1980.
243. Maierhofer WJ, Gray RW, Cheung HS, et al: Bone resorption by elevated serum 1,25$(OH)_2$ vitamin D concentrations in healthy men. Kidney Int 24:555–560, 1983.
244. Amento EP, Bhalla AK, Kurnick JT, et al: 1,25-Dihydroxyvitamin D_3 induces maturation of the human monocyte cell line U937, and, in association with a factor from human T lymphocytes, augments production of the monokine, mononuclear cell factor. J Clin Invest 73:731–739, 1984.
245. Diez L, Van Baelen H, Bouillon R, et al: Effect of vitaminDbindingproteinonboneresorptionby1,25-dihydroxyvitamin D. Calcif Tissue Int 36:513, 1984.
246. Mundy GR, Shapiro JL, Bandelin JG, et al: Direct stimulation of bone resorption by thyroid hormones. J Clin Invest 58:529–534, 1976.
247. Hoffmann O, Klaushofer K, Koller K, et al: Indomethacin inhibits thrombin-, but not thyroxin-stimulated resorption of fetal rat limb bones. Prostaglandins 31:601–608, 1986.
248. Melsen F, Mosekilde L: Morphometric and dynamic studies of bone changes in hyperthyroidism. Acta Pathol Microbiol Scand 85:141–150, 1977.
249. Mosekilde L, Christensen MS: Decreased parathyroid function in hyperthyroidism: Interrelationships between serum parathyroid hormone, calcium-phosphorus metabolism and thyroid function. Acta Endocrinol 84:566–575, 1977.
250. Fell HB, Mellanby E: The effect of vitamin A ions on embryonic limb bones cultivated in vitro. J Physiol 116:320–340, 1952.
251. Kistler A: Structure activity relationship of retinoids in fetal rat bone cultures. Calcif Tissue Int 33:249–254, 1981.
252. Petkovich PM, Heersche JNM, Tinker DO, et al: Retinoic acid stimulates 1,25 dihydroxyvitamin D_3 binding in rat osteosarcoma cells. J Biol Chem 259:8274–8280, 1984.
253. Chase LR, Aurbach GD: The effect of parathyroid hormone on the concentration of adenosine 3′,5′-monophosphate in skeletal tissue in vitro. J Biol Chem 245:1520–1526, 1970.
254. Dietrich JW, Goodson JM, Raisz LG: Stimulation of bone resorption by various prostaglandins in organ culture. Prostaglandins 10:231–240, 1975.
255. Raisz LG, Dietrich JW, Simmons HA, et al: Effect of prostaglandin endoperoxides and metabolites on bone resorption in vivo. Nature 267:532–534, 1977.
256. Raisz LG, Vanderhoek JY, Simmons HA, et al: Prostaglandin synthesis by fetal rat bone in vitro: Evidence for a role of prostacyclin. Prostaglandins 17:905–994, 1979.
257. Raisz LG, Martin TJ: Prostaglandins in bone and mineral metabolism. *In* Peck WA (ed): Bone and Mineral Research, Annual 2. Amsterdam, Excerpta Medica, 1984, pp 286–310.
258. Lorenzo JA, Quinton J: The effects of prostaglandin E_2 on bone resorption and DNA synthesis. Calcif Tissue Int 35:646, 1983.
259. Tashjian AH Jr, Tric JE, Sides K: Biological activities of prostaglandin analogs and metabolites on bone in organ culture. Nature 266:645–647, 1977.
260. Chambers TJ, Fuller K, Athanasou NA: The effect of prostaglandins I_2, E_1, E_2 and dibutyryl cyclic AMP on the cytoplasmic spreading of rat osteoclasts. Br J Exp Pathol 65:557–566, 1984.
261. Conaway HH, Diez LF, Raisz LG: Effects of prostacyclin and prostaglandin E_1 (PGE_1) on bone resorption in the presence and absence of parathyroid hormone. Calcif Tissue Int 38:130–134, 1986.
262. Sandberg AL, Raisz LG, Wahl LM, et al: Enhancement of complement-mediated prostaglandin synthesis and bone resorption by arachidonic acid and inhibition by cortisol. Prostaglandins Leukotrienes Medicine 8:419–427, 1982.
263. Gustafson GT, Lerner U: Thrombin, a stimulator of bone resorption. Biosci Rep 3:255–261, 1983.
264. Gustafson GT, Lerner U: Bradykinin stimulates bone resorption and lysosomal enzyme release in cultured mouse calvaria. Biochem J 219:329–332, 1984.
265. Tashjian AH Jr, Hohmann EL, Antoniades HN, et al: Platelet-derived growth factor stimulates bone resorption via a prostaglandin-mediated mechanism. Endocrinology 111:118–124, 1982.
266. Voelkel EF, Tashjian AH Jr, Levine L: Cyclooxygenase products of arachidonic acid metabolism by mouse bone in organ culture. Biochim Biophys Acta 620:418–428, 1980.
267. Hopps RM, Nuki K, Raisz LG: Demonstration and preliminary characterization of bone resorbing activity in freeze-dried gingiva of dogs. Calcif Tissue Int 31:239–245, 1980.
268. Luben RA, Mundy GR, Trummel L, et al: Partial purification of osteoclast-activating factor from phytohemagglutinin-stimulated human leukocytes. J Clin Invest 53:1473–1480, 1974.
269. Raisz LG, Luben RA, Mundy GR: Effect of osteoclast activating factor from human leukocytes on bone metabolism. J Clin Invest 56:408–413, 1975.
270. Bertolini DR, Nedwin GE, Bringman TS, et al: Stimulation of bone resorption and inhibition of bone formation in vitro by human tumor necrosis factors. Nature 319:516–518, 1986.
271. Raisz LG, Simmons HA, Sandberg AL, et al: Direct stimulation of bone resorption by epidermal growth factor. Endocrinology 107:270–273, 1980.
272. Lorenzo JA, Quinton J, Sousa S, Raisz LG: Effects of DNA and prostaglandin synthesis inhibitors on the

stimulation of bone resorption by epidermal growth factor in fetal rat long-bone cultures. J Clin Invest 77:1897–1902, 1986.
273. Mundy GR, Ibbotson KJ, D'Souza SM, et al: The hypercalcemia of cancer: Clinical implications and pathogenic mechanism. N Engl J Med 310:1718–1727, 1984.
274. Ibbotson KJ, Harrod J, Gowen M, et al: Human recombinant transforming growth factor stimulates bone resorption and inhibits formation in vitro. Proc Natl Acad Sci USA 83:2228–2232, 1986.
275. D'Souza SM, Ibbotson KJ, Smith DD, et al: Production of a macromolecular bone-resorbing factor by the hypercalcemic variant of the walker rat carcinosarcoma. Endocrinology 115:1746–1752, 1984.
276. Stewart SF, Insogna KL, Goltzman D, et al: Identification of adenylate cyclase–stimulating activity and cytochemical glucose-6-phosphate dehydrogenase-stimulating activity in extracts of tumors from patients with humoral hypercalcemia of malignancy. Proc Natl Acad Sci USA 80:1454–1458, 1983.
277. Rodan SB, Insogna KL, Vignery AMC, et al: Factors associated with humoral hypercalcemia of malignancy stimulate adenylate cyclase in osteoblastic cells. J Clin Invest 72:1511–1515, 1983.
278. Moseley JM, Kubota M, Diefenback-Jagger H, et al: Parathyroid hormone–related protein purified from a human lung cancer cell line. Proc Natl Acad Sci USA 84:5048–5052, 1987.
279. Suva LJ, Winslow GA, Wettenhall REH, et al: A parathyroid hormone–related protein implicated in malignant hypercalcemia: Cloning and expression. Science 237:893–896, 1987.
280. Magnin M, Webb, AC, Dreyer BE, et al: Identification of a cDNA encoding a parathyroid hormone–like peptide from a human tumor associated with humoral hypercalcemia of malignancy. Proc Natl Acad Sci USA 85:597–601, 1988.
281. Thiede MA, Strewler GJ, Nissenson RA, et al: Human renal carcinoma expresses two messages encoding a parathyroid hormone–like peptide: Evidence for the alternate splicing of a single-copy gene. Proc Natl Acad Sci USA 85:4605–4609, 1988.
282. Horiuchi N, Caulfield MP, Fisher JE, et al: Similarity of synthetic peptide from human tumor to parathyroid hormone *in vivo* and *in vitro*. Science 238:1566–1568, 1987.
283. Rodan SB, Noda M, Wesolowski G, et al: Comparison of postreceptor effects of 1-34 human hypercalcemia factor and 1–34 human parathyroid hormone in rat osteosarcoma cells. J Clin Invest 81:924–927, 1988.
284. Kemp BE, Moseley JE, Rodda C, et al: Parathyroid hormone–related protein of malignancy: Active synthetic fragments. Science 238:1568–1570, 1987.
285. Yates AJ, Gutierrez GE, Smolens P, et al: Effects of a synthetic peptide of a parathyroid hormone-related protein in calcium homeostasis, renal tubular calcium reabsorption, and bone metabolism *in vivo* and *in vitro* in rodents. J Clin Invest 81:932–938, 1988.
286. Goldhaber P: Heparin enhancement of factors stimulating bone resorption in tissue culture. Science 147:407–408, 1965.
287. Glowacki J: The effects of heparin and protamine on resorption of bone particles. Life Sci 33:1019–1024, 1983.
288. Griffith GC, Nichols G, Asher JD, et al: Heparin osteoporosis. JAMA 193:91–94, 1965.
289. Frame B, Nixon RK: Bone marrow mast cells in osteoporosis of aging. N Engl J Med 279:626–630, 1968.
290. Fallon MD, Whyte MP, Teitelbaum SL: Systemic mastocytosis associated with generalized osteopenia. Histopathological characterization of the skeletal lesion using undecalcified bone from 2 patients. Hum Pathol 12:813–820, 1981.
291. Yoffe JR, Taylor DJ, Woolley DE: Mast cell products stimulate collagenase and prostaglandin production by cultures of adherent rheumatoid synovial cells. Biochem Biophys Res Commun 122:270–276, 1984.
292. Hausmann E, Nair BC, Knox KW, et al: Partial purification and characterization of the bone resorption factor from Actinomyces viscosus. Calcif Tissue Int 34:49–53, 1982.
293. Raisz LG, Alander C, Eilon G, et al: Effects of two bacterial products, muramyl dipeptide and endotoxin, on bone resorption in organ culture. Calcif Tissue Int 34:365–369, 1982.
294. Raisz LG, Nuki K, Alander C, et al: Interactions between bacterial endotoxin and other stimulators of bone resorption in organ culture. J Periodont Res 16:1–7, 1981.
295. Raisz LG, Woodiel FN, Alander CB: Rat bone cultured in the presence of cortisol produces a macromolecular inhibitor of parathyroid hormone stimulated bone resorption. Calcif Tissue Int 36:469, 1984.
296. Hoffmann O, Klaishofer K, Gleispach H, et al: Gamma interferon inhibits basal and interleukin 1–induced prostaglandin production and bone resorption in neonatal mouse calvaria. Biochem Biophys Res Commun 143:38–43, 1987.
297. Teitelbaum SJ, Andras RY, Cooke NE, et al: Inhibition of parathyroid hormone–induced fetal rat bone resorption in vitro by nerve growth factor. Calcif Tissue Res 26:203–208, 1978.
298. Holtrop ME, Raisz LG, Simmons HA: The effects of parathyroid hormone, colchicine, and calcitonin on the ultrastructure and the activity of osteoclasts in organ culture. J Cell Biol 60:346–355, 1974.
299. Warshawsky H, Goltzman D, Rouleau MF, et al: Direct in vivo demonstration by radioautography of specific binding sites for calcitonin in skeletal and renal tissues of the rat. J Cell Biol 85:682–694, 1980.
300. Ransjo M, Lerner UH: Effects of cholera toxin on cyclic AMP accumulation and bone resorption in cultured mouse calvaria. Biochim Biophys Acta 930:378–391, 1987.
301. Wener JA, Gorton SJ, Raisz LG: Escape from inhibition of resorption in cultures of fetal bone treated with calcitonin and parathyroid hormone. Endocrinology 90:752–759, 1972.
302. Findlay DM, DeLuise MA, Michelangeli VP, et al: Independent down regulation of insulin and calcitonin receptors in a human tumor cell line. J Endocrinol 88:271–281, 1981.
303. Tashjian AH Jr, Wright DR, Ivey JL, et al: Calcitonin binding sites in bone: Relationships to biological response and "escape." Recent Prog Horm Res 34:285–334, 1978.
304. Krieger NS, Feldman RA, Tashjian Jr AH: Parathyroid hormone and calcitonin interactions in bone: irradiation-induced inhibition of escape in vitro. Calcif Tissue Int 34:197–203, 1982.
305. Binstock ML, Mundy GR: Effect of calcitonin and

glucocorticoids in combination on the hypercalcemia of malignancy. Ann Intern Med 93:269–272, 1980.
306. Belavoine JF, deRochemonteix B, Williamson K, et al: Prostaglandin E_2 and collagenase production by fibroblasts and synovial cells is regulated by urine-derived human interleukin and inhibitor(s). J Clin Invest 78:1120–1124, 1986.
307. Seckinger P, Lowenthal JW, Williamson K, et al: A urine inhibitor of interleukin 1 activity that blocks ligand binding. J Immunol 139:1546–1549, 1987.
308. Seckinger P, Alander C, Dayer JM, Raisz LG: Effects of a urine-derived inhibitor of interleukin-1 on resorption of fetal rat long bones in organ culture. Calcif Tissue Int 425:A25, 1988.
309. Douglas DL, Duckworth T, Russell RGG, et al: Effect of dichloromethylene diphosphonate in Paget's disease of bone in hypercalcemia due to primary hyperparathyroidism or malignant disease. Cancer 39:1559–1562, 1980.
310. Felix R, Russell RGG, Felisch H: The effect of several diphosphonates on acid phosphohydrolases and other lysosomal enzymes. Biochim Biophys Acta 429:429–438, 1976.
311. Fast DK, Felix R, Dowse C, et al: The effects of diphosphonates on the growth and glycolysis of connective-tissue cells in culture. Biochem J 172:92–97, 1978.
312. Kiang DT, Loken MK, Kennedy BJ: Mechanism of the hypocalcemic effect of mithramycin. J Clin Endocrinol Metab 48:341–344, 1979.
313. Lloyd W, Fang VS, Wells H, et al: 2-Thiopenecarboxylic acid: A hypoglycemic, antilipolytic agent with hypocalcemic and hypophosphatemic effects in rats. Endocrinology 85:763–768, 1969.
314. Johannesson AJ, Onkelinx C, Rodan GA, Raisz LG: Thionapthene-2-carboxylic acid: A new antihypercalcemic agent. Endocrinology 117:1508–1511, 1985.
315. Potts M, Poppelt S, Taylor S, et al: Protamine; a powerful in vivo inhibitor of bone resorption. Calcif Tissue Int 36:189–193, 1984.
316. Glowacki J, Deftos LJ: The effects of calcitonin on bone formation. *In* Gennari C, Segree G (eds): The Effects of Calcitonin in Man. Milan, Italia Editori, 1983, pp 133–137.
317. Delaisse J-M, Eeckhout Y, Vaes G: Inhibition of bone resorption in culture by inhibitors of thiol proteinases. Biochem J 192:365–368, 1980.
318. Johannesson AJ, Raisz LG: Effects of ammonium chloride on resorption of fetal rat bones in organ culture. Am J Physiol 246:E516–E518, 1984.
319. Eilon G, Raisz LG: Chloroquine, hydroxystilbamidine, and dapsone inhibit resorption of fetal rat bone in organ culture. Calcif Tissue Int 34:506–509, 1982.
320. Dietrich JW, Mundy GR, Raisz LG: Inhibition of bone resorption in tissue culture by membrane-stabilizing drugs. Endocrinology 104:1644–1648, 1979.
321. Hermann-Erlee MPM, Guillard PJ, Hekkelman JW, et al: The effect of verapamil on the action of parathyroid hormone on embryonic bone in vitro. Eur J Pharmacol 46:51–58, 1977.
322. Goldhaber P, Rabadjija L: Inhibition of bone resorption in tissue culture by H_1-receptor antagonists. Am J Physiol 244:E141–E144, 1983.
323. Krieger NS, Tashjian AH Jr: Inhibition by ouabain of parathyroid hormone stimulated bone resorption. J Pharmacol Exp Ther 21:586–591, 1981.
324. Hahn TJ, DeBartolo TF, Halstead LR: Ouabain effects on hormonally-stimulated bone resorption and cyclic AMP content in cultured fetal rat bones. Endocr Res Commun 7:189–200, 1980.
325. Krieger NS, Stern PH: Interaction between amrinone and parathyroid hormone on bone in culture. Am J Physiol 243:E499–E504, 1982.
326. Hall GE, Kenny AD: Role of carbonic anhydrase in bone resorption: Effect of acetazolamide on basal and parathyroid hormone–induced bone metabolism. Calcif Tissue Int 40:212–218, 1987.
327. Dziak R, Stern P: Calcium transport in isolated bone cells. III. Effects of parathyroid hormone on cyclic 3′,5′-AMP. Endocrinology 97:1265–1274, 1975.
328. Johannesson AJ, Raisz LG: Effects of low medium magnesium concentration on bone resorption in response to parathyroid hormone and 1,25-dihydroxyvitamin D in organ culture. Endocrinology 113:2294–2298, 1983.
329. Dominguez JH, Raisz LG: Effects of changing hydrogen ion, carbonic acid and bicarbonate concentrations on bone resorption in vitro. Calcif Tissue Int 29:7–13, 1979.
330. Arruda JAL, Alla V, Rubinstein H, et al: Parathyroid hormone and extrarenal acid buffering. Am J Physiol 239:F333–F338, 1980.
331. Arruda JAL, Alla V, Rubinstein H, et al: Metabolic and hormonal factors influencing extrarenal buffering of an acute acid load. Mineral Electrolyte Metab 8:36–43, 1982.
332. Kraut JA, Mishler DR, Kurokawa K: Effect of colchicine and calcitonin on calcemic response to metabolic acidosis. Kidney Int 25:608–612, 1984.
333. Krieger NS, Stern PH: Potassium effects on bone: Comparison to two model systems. Am J Physiol 245:E303–E307, 1983.
334. Wilson T, Katz JM, Gray DH: Inhibition of active bone resorption by copper. Calcif Tissue Int 33:35–39, 1981.
335. Stern PH: Biphasic effects of manganese on hormone-stimulated bone resorption. Endocrinology 117:2044–2049, 1985.
336. Dietrich JW, Canalis EM, Maina DM, et al: Hormonal control of bone collagen synthesis in vitro: Effects of parathyroid hormone and calcitonin. Endocrinology 98:943–949, 1976.
337. Bringhurst FR, Potts JT Jr: Bone collagen synthesis in vitro: Structure/activity relations among parathyroid fragments and analogs. Endocrinology 108:103–108, 1981.
338. Canalis EM, Dietrich JW, Maina DM, et al: Hormonal control of bone collagen synthesis in vitro—effects of insulin and glucagon. Endocrinology 100:668–674, 1977.
339. Dietrich JW, Paddock DN: In vitro effects of ionophore A23187 on skeletal collagen and noncollagen protein synthesis. Endocrinology 104:493–499, 1979.
340. Lian JB, Coutts M, Canalis E: Studies of hormonal regulation of osteocalcin synthesis in cultured fetal rat calvaria. J Biol Chem 260:8706–8710, 1985.
341. Gunness-Hey M, Hock JM: Increased trabecular bone mass in rats treated with human synthetic parathyroid hormone. Metab Bone Dis Rel Res 5:177–191, 1984.
342. Podbesek R, Edouard C, Meunier PJ: Effects of two treatment regimens with synthetic human parathyroid hormone fragment on bone formation

and the tissue balance of trabecular bone in greyhounds. Endocrinology 112:1000–1006, 1983.
343. Howard GA, Bottemiller BL, Turner RT, et al: Parathyroid hormone stimulates bone formation and resorption in organ culture—evidence for a coupling mechanism. Proc Natl Acad Sci USA 78:3204–3208, 1981.
344. Chyun YS, Raisz LG: Stimulation of bone formation by prostaglandin E_2. Prostaglandins 27:97–103, 1984.
345. Gera I, Hock JM, Gunness-Hey M, et al: Indomethacin does not inhibit the anabolic effect of parathyroid hormone on the long bones of rats. Calcif Tissue Int 40:206–211, 1987.
346. Bringhurst FR, Potts JT Jr: Effects of vitamin D metabolites and analogs of bone collagen synthesis in vitro. Calcif Tissue Int 34:103–110, 1982.
347. Kream BE, Jose M, Yamada S, et al: A specific high-affinity binding macromolecule for 1,25-dihydroxyvitamin D_3 in fetal bone. Science 197:1086–1088, 1977.
348. Rosen V, Smith M, Kream B: Comparison of the effects of parathyroid hormone and 1,25-dihydroxyvitamin D_3 on collagen synthesis in calvaria and osteosarcoma cells. Calcif Tissue Int 36:470, 1984.
349. Boyce RW, Weisbrode SE: Effect of dietary calcium on the response of bone to $1,25(OH)_2D_3$. Lab Invest 48:683–689, 1983.
350. Hock J, Gunness-Hey M, Poser J, et al: Stimulation of undermineralized matrix formation by pharmacologic doses of 1,25-dihydroxyvitamin D_3 in long bones of rats. Calcif Tissue Int 38:79–86, 1986.
351. Corvol M, Ulmann A, Garabedian M: Specific nuclear uptake of 24,25-dihydroxycholecalciferol, a vitamin D_3 metabolite biologically active in cartilage. FEBS Lett 116:273–276, 1980.
352. Turner RT, Puzas JE, Forte MD, et al: In vitro synthesis of 1,25-dihydroxycholecalciferol and 24,25-dihydroxycholecalciferol by isolated calvarial cells. Proc Natl Acad Sci USA 77:5720–5724, 1980.
353. Bennett AE, Wahner HW, Riggs BL, et al: Insulin-like growth factors I and II: Aging and bone density in women. J Clin Endocrinol Metab 59:701–704, 1984.
354. D'Ercole AJ, Applewhite GR, Underwood LE: Evidence that somatomedin is synthesized by multiple tissue in the fetus. Dev Biol 75:315–328, 1980.
355. Schlechter NL, Russell SM, Greenberg S, et al: A direct growth effect of growth hormone in rat hindlimb shown by arterial infusion. Am J Physiol 250:E231–235, 1986.
356. Stracke H, Schulz A, Moeller D, et al: Effect of growth hormone on osteoblasts and demonstration of somatomedin-C/IGF I in bone organ culture. Acta Endocrinol 107:16–24, 1984.
357. Canalis EM, Hintz RL, Dietrich JW, et al: Effect of somatomedin and growth hormone on bone collagen synthesis in vitro. Metabolism 26:1079–1087, 1977.
358. Canalis E, Raisz LG: Effect of multiplication-stimulating activity on DNA and protein synthesis in cultured fetal rat calvaria. Calcif Tissue Int 29:33–39, 1979.
359. Canalis E: Effect of insulin-like growth factor I on DNA and protein synthesis in cultured rat calvaria. J Clin Invest 66:709–719, 1980.
360. Schmid CH, Steiner TH, Froesch ER: Insulin-like growth factor stimulates synthesis of nucleic acids and glycogen in cultured calvaria cells. Calcif Tissue Int 35:578–585, 1983.
361. Schmid C, Steiner T, Froesch ER: Insulin-like growth factor I supports differentiation on cultured osteoblast-like cells. FEBS Lett 173:48–52, 1984.
362. Bennett A, Chen T, Feldman D, et al: Characterization of insulin-like growth factor I receptors on cultured rat bone cells: Regulation of receptor concentration by glucocorticoids. Endocrinology 115:1577–1583, 1984.
363. Kream B, Smith MD, Canalis E, et al: Characterization of the effect of insulin on collagen synthesis in fetal rat bone. Endocrinology 116:296–302, 1985.
364. Hock JM, Centrella M, Canalis E: Insulin-like growth I factor has independent effects on bone matrix formation and cell replication. Endocrinology 122:254–260, 1988.
365. Schoenle E, Zapf J, Humbel RE, Froesch ER: Insulin-like growth factor I stimulates growth in hypophysectomized rats. Nature 296:252–253, 1982.
366. Craig RG, Rowe DW, Patersen DN, Kream BE: Insulin increases the steady state level of alpha 1 (I) procollagen mRNA in osteoblast-rich segment of fetal rat calvaria. Endocrinology 25:1430–1437, 1989.
367. Shires R, Avioli LV, Bergfeld MA, et al: Effects of semistarvation on skeletal homeostasis. Endocrinology 107:1530–1535, 1980.
368. Phillips LS, Belosky DC, Reichard LA: Nutrition and somatomedin action and measurement of somatomedin inhibitors in serum from diabetic rats. Endocrinology 104:1513–1518, 1979.
369. Hough S, Avioli LV, Bergfeld MA, et al: Correction of abnormal bone and mineral metabolism in chronic streptozotocin-induced diabetes mellitus in the rat by insulin therapy. Endocrinology 108:2228–2234, 1981.
370. Hough S, Russell JE, Teitelbaum SL, et al: Calcium homeostasis in chronic streptozotocin-induced diabetes mellitus in the rat. Am J Physiol 242:E451–E456, 1982.
371. Wiske PS, Wentworth SM, Norton JA Jr, et al: Evaluation of bone mass and growth in young diabetics. Metabolism 31:848–854, 1982.
372. Hui SL, Epstein S, Johnston CC Jr: Prospective study of bone mass in patients with Type I diabetes. J Clin Endocrinol Metab 60:74–80, 1985.
373. Hahn TJ, Westbrook SL, Halstead LR: Cortisol modulation of osteoblast metabolic activity in cultured neonatal rat bone. Endocrinology 114:1864–1870, 1984.
374. Copeland KC, Johnson DM, Kuehl TJ, et al: Estrogen stimulates growth hormone and somatomedin-C in castrate and intact female baboons. J Clin Endocrinol Metab 58:698–703, 1984.
375. Heaney RP, Recker RR, Saville PD: Menopausal changes in bone remodeling. J Lab Clin Med 92:964–970, 1978.
376. Feyen JHM, Raisz LG: Prostaglandin production by calvariae from Sham operated and oophorectomized rats: Effects of 17beta-estradiol in vivo. Endocrinology 121:819–821, 1987.
377. Canalis EM, Raisz LG: Effect of sex steroids on bone collagen synthesis in vitro. Calcif Tissue Res 25:105–110, 1978.
378. Gray TK, Flynn TC, Gray KM, Nabell LM: 17Beta-estradiol acts directly on the clonal osteoblastic cell line UMR106. Proc Natl Acad Sci USA 84:6267–6271, 1987.

379. Pahuja DN, DeLuca HF: Stimulation of intestinal calcium transport and bone calcium mobilization by prolactin in vitamin D deficient rats. Science 214:1038–1039, 1981.
380. Canalis E, Raisz LG: Effect of epidermal growth factor on bone formation in vitro. Endocrinology 104:862–869, 1979.
381. Canalis EM, Raisz LG: Effect of fibroblast growth factor of cultured fetal rat calvaria. Metabolism 29:108–114, 1980.
382. Canalis E, Centrella M, McCarthy T: Effects of basic fibroblast growth factor in bone formation *in vitro*. J Clin Invest 81:1572–1577, 1988.
383. Rodan SB, Wesolowski G, Thomas K, Rodan GA: Growth stimulation of rat calvaria osteoblastic cells by acidic fibroblast growth factor. Endocrinology 121:1917–1923, 1987.
384. Canalis E: Effect of platelet-derived growth factor on DNA and protein synthesis in cultured rat calvaria. Metabolism 30:970–975, 1981.
385. Canalis E: Interleukin-1 has independent effects on DNA and collagen synthesis in cultures of rat calvaria. Endocrinology 118:74–81, 1986.
386. Raisz LG, Koolemans-Beynen AR: Inhibition of bone collagen synthesis by prostaglandin E_2 in organ culture. Prostaglandins 8:377–385, 1974.
387. Lund JE, Brown WP, Tregerman L: The toxicity of PGE and PGI_2. *In* Wu KK, Rossi EC (eds): Prostaglandins in Clinical Medicine: Cardiovascular and Thrombotic Disorders. Chicago, Year Book Medical Publishers, 1982, pp 93–109.
388. Ueda K, Saito A, Nakano H: Cortical hyperostosis following long-term administration of prostaglandin E_1 in infants with cyanotic congenital heart disease. J Pediatr 97:834–836, 1980.
389. Urist MR, DeLange RJ, Finerman GAM: Bone cell differentiation and growth factors. Science 220:680–686, 1983.
390. Farley JR, Baylink DJ: Purification of a skeletal growth factor from human bone. Biochemistry 21:3502–3507, 1982.
391. Canalis E, Peck WA, Raisz LG: Stimulation of DNA and collagen synthesis by autologous growth factor in cultured fetal rat calvaria. Science 210:1021–1023, 1980.
392. Drivdahl RH, Puzas JE, Howard GA, et al: Regulation of DNA synthesis in chick calvaria cells by factors from bone organ culture. Proc Soc Exp Biol Med 168:143–150, 1981.
393. Hauschka PV, Mavrakos AE, Iafrati MD, et al: Growth factors in bone matrix. Isolation of multiple types by affinity chromatography on heparin-sepharose. J Biol Chem 261:12665–12674, 1986.
394. Seyedin SM, Thompson AY, Rosen DM, et al: In vitro induction of cartilage-specific macromolecules by a bone extract. J Cell Biol 97:1950–1953, 1983.
395. Seyedin SM, Thompson AT, Bentz H, et al: Cartilage inducing factor. Apparent identity to transforming growth factor-beta. J Biol Chem 261:5693–5695, 1986.
396. Seyedin SM, Segarini PR, Rosen DM, et al: Cartilage-inducing factor-beta is a unique protein structurally and functionally related to transforming growth factor-beta. J Biol Chem 262:1946–1949, 1987.
397. Canalis E, McCarthy T, Centrella M: A bone-derived growth factor isolated from rat calvaria is $beta_2$ microglobulin. Endocrinology, 121:1198–1200, 1987.
398. Canalis E, McCarthy T, Centrella M: Isolation and characterization of insulin-like growth factor I (somatomedin C) from cultures of fetal rat calvaria. Endocrinology 122:22–27, 1988.
399. Centrella M, McCarthy TL, Canalis, E: Transforming growth factor beta is a bifunctional regulator of replication and collagen synthesis in osteoblast-enriched cell cultures from fetal rat bone. J Biol Chem 262:2869–2874, 1987.
400. Pfeilschifter J, Mundy GR: Modulation of type beta transforming growth factor activity in bone cultures by osteotropic hormones. Proc Natl Acad Sci USA 84:2024–2028, 1987.
401. Mohan S, Jennings JC, Linkhart TA, et al: Primary structure of human skeletal growth factor (SGF): Homology with TGF-II. J Bone Mineral Res 3:S218, 1988.
402. Heldin C-H, Westermark B, Wasteson A: Chemical and biological properties of a growth factor from human-cultured osteosarcoma cells: Resemblance with platelet-derived growth factor. J Cell Physiol 105:235–246, 1980.
403. Smith DD, Gowen M, Mundy GR: Effects of interferon- and other cytokines on collagen synthesis in fetal rat bone cultures. Endocrinology 120:2494–2499, 1987.
404. Bingham PJ, Raisz LG: Bone growth in organ culture: Effects of phosphate and other nutrients on bone and cartilage. Calcif Tissue Res 14:31–48, 1974.
405. Harris WH, Heaney RP, Davis LA, et al: Stimulation of bone formation in vivo by phosphate supplementation. Calcif Tissue Res 22:85–98, 1976.
406. Liu CC, Ivey JL, Baylink DJ: The effect of vitamin D deficiency on bone repletion. Proc Soc Exp Biol Med 167:554–562, 1981.
407. Farley AR, Wergedal JE, Baylink DJ: Fluoride directly stimulates proliferation and alkaline phosphatase activity in bone-forming cells. Science 222:330–332, 1983.
408. Maloney NA, Ott SM, Alfrey C, et al: Histological quantitation of aluminum in iliac bone from patients with renal failure. J Lab Clin Med 99:206–216, 1982.

2

MELVIN J. GLIMCHER

The Nature of the Mineral Component of Bone and the Mechanism of Calcification

The questions that will be pursued in this chapter are:

1. *What* is the nature of the mineral phase in bone, that is, the chemical composition and crystal *structure* of the solid Ca-P mineral phase in bone, and what are the changes that occur *in the mineral phase per se* with time and maturation?
2. *Where* is the mineral phase located ultrastructurally?
3. *What,* if any, are the structural and chemical *relationships* between the Ca-P mineral phase and the individual components of the matrix?
4. *Why and how* is a solid mineral phase deposited? That is, what are the factors involved in the mechanism of calcification and its regulation?

I. BIOLOGICAL FUNCTIONS OF THE MINERAL PHASE

The Ca-P mineral phase in bone performs two major functions, both of which are to a significant extent dependent on the exact size, shape, chemical composition, and crystal structure of the mineral crystallites; it acts on the one hand as an *ion reservoir* and on the other hand as an excellently designed *structural material* that determines in large part the mechanical properties of bone substance, of bone tissue, and of bone as an organ. The importance of the role of bone mineral as an ion reservoir can be appreciated from the fact that ~99% of the body calcium, ~85% of the body phosphorus, and from 40% to 60% of the total body Na and Mg are associated with the bone crystals that consequently serve as the major source for the transport of these ions to and from the extracellular fluids. As a result, the bone crystals play a critical role in maintaining the extracellular fluid concentrations (ECFs) of these ions, which are critical for a variety of physiologic functions (nerve conduction and muscle contraction, for example) and a number of important biochemical reactions, and, for some of them like Ca^{2+}, maintaining their serum concentrations within a physiologically necessary narrow range.

From a structural standpoint, the impregnation of the otherwise soft, pliable organic matrix of bone tissues by the rocklike Ca-P crystals of apatite converts the soft organic matrix to a relatively hard, rigid material that now possesses the necessary mechanical properties that permit it to withstand the forces, stresses, and strains imposed on it by the mechanical forces generated by gait, prehension, respiration, and so on. Moreover this relatively inflexible and rigid material is now able to preserve the shape of the organism as a whole and to protect vital organs such as the brain, spinal cord, lungs, and heart. The mechanical properties of bone as a structural material are clearly highly dependent on both the physical and chemical properties of the mineral phase, on its three-dimensional disposition within the bone substance and bone tissue, and on its ultra-structural and molecular relationships to specific structural components of the organic matrix.

This work was supported in part by the New England Peabody Home for Crippled Children, Inc., National Institutes of Health grants AM 34078 and AM 34081, and National Science Foundation grant PCM-8216959.

Although not a direct function of bone mineral or of bone *tissue*, bone as an *organ* does provide for another important general physiologic function: it acts as host to the precursors of the blood cells (marrow).

It is precisely because both of the two major biological functions of the bone mineral ultimately depend to a great extent on the precise chemical composition, physicochemical properties, and crystal structure of the mineral phase that so much attention has been directed at elucidating these characteristics. It is important to keep in mind that significant changes in both the chemical composition and structure occur in the mineral phase with time, that is, the mineral phase changes with time after its initial deposition in the tissue. Not only must this fact be kept in mind when attempting to understand the changes in mineral metabolism as a function of the age of the organism, but, equally important, one must take this into account when trying to explain the serum and other changes (^{47}Ca uptake and disappearance, for example) observed in normal subjects and patients with metabolic bone diseases. This is especially true in instances in which the rates of bone formation and resorption have been significantly altered and consequently the amount and proportion of new bone and old bone (and therefore of young bone and old bone crystals) have also markedly changed. This in turn significantly alters the population distribution of bone mineral as a function of *bone mineral age* (as opposed to animal age). Unfortunately, such considerations are rarely taken into account in clinical studies and may in part account for some of the discrepancies noted in metabolic studies between predicted serum values and bone turnover values and those actually observed.

II. THE NATURE OF THE MINERAL PHASE IN BONE AND THE CHANGES THAT OCCUR WITH TIME

The bone mineral has been known by chemical analyses to contain calcium and phosphorus as its principal constituents for over 150 years and since 1894 to be a calcium-phosphate-carbonate.[1] The first reports of its crystal structure were published by DeJong[2] and Roseberry et al.[3] Both groups of investigators identified the bone mineral as a hydroxyapatite (HA) based on the reflections generated by x-ray diffraction. Unfortunately, progress in identifying in detail the exact chemical composition and specific spatial arrangement of its constituents at any stage of its development, that is, from its initial deposition to the final mature mineral, has been very slow. Indeed, these parameters are still not known in detail 60 years after the bone mineral was first identified as hydroxyapatite by DeJong.[2] The obstacles that have prevented a definite resolution of the problem are many—biological, crystallographic, and technical. (For some recent reviews, see references 4 to 11.) In the first place, the apatite phase in bone is very poorly crystalline, generating only a few broad peaks that by themselves do not permit one to assign to it a unique crystal structure or composition, that is, one cannot differentiate by x-ray diffraction and chemical composition between a number of similar apatitic or apatite-like structures. Indeed, a number of what appear to be closely related but distinct chemical and structural Ca-P compounds give the same apatitic x-ray diffraction pattern. The poor x-ray diffraction pattern generated by the bone mineral has also precluded the detection of small amounts of Ca-P compounds other than hydroxyapatite that might be present in addition to HA, that is, the x-ray diffraction data fail to distinguish whether such nonapatitic mineral phases are present. Bone mineral is also known by chemical and physical analyses to contain small but significant amounts of extraneous ions such as HPO_4^{2-}, Na^+, Mg^{2+}, citrate, carbonate, K^+, and others whose positions and configurations are not completely known. The ideal stoichiometry (Ca/P molar ratio of 1.67) is also rarely found in bone, especially in young bone mineral, which usually has a Ca/P ratio of less than 1.67. The bone mineral has also been shown to contain strongly bound or possibly even crystalline water. The latter cannot be a true constituent of HA, since it has the structural formula $[Ca_{10}(PO_4)_6(OH)_2]$. Both the composition of bone mineral and its x-ray diffraction characteristics change with maturation: the mineral phase becomes more crystalline with age and maturation[12] but never approaches the highly crystalline state of naturally occurring, geologic HA or synthetic HA made by precipitation and refluxing of Ca-P *in vitro*.

Electron micrographs of bone, which have revealed the very small size of the bone crystals (about (15–35 Å) × (50–100 Å) × (400–500 Å),[13,14] help to explain the poor x-ray diffraction pattern generated by the bone mineral. However, other characteristics of bone mineral such as crystal strain, vacancies, additions to (for example, carbonate) and adsorption into the lattice of other ions (Na^+, Mg^{2+}) also represent significant differences between bone mineral and crystalline HA and may also contribute to its specific x-ray diffraction characteristics. Most important, progressive changes occur in the x-ray diffraction patterns of bone mineral as a function of the age of the tissue, of the age of the animal, and principally of the age of the mineral itself. These x-ray diffraction changes are also accompanied by significant changes in the chemical composition of the mineral phase, namely, an increase in the Ca/P ratio, an increase in the content of carbonate, and a decrease in the concentration of HPO_4^{2-} and H_2O.[15,16] Recognition that the mineral phase undergoes extensive structural and chemical changes after its initial formation has led investigators to explore the nature of the first solid phase of Ca-P deposited and the detailed changes that it undergoes during aging and maturation, and to search for the reasons these x-ray and compositional changes occur. It is important to note that there is also no general agreement as to the exact structure and location of all of the carbonate ions even in synthetically prepared carbonato apatites, an indication of the technical and conceptual difficulties of determining the exact crystal structure of this class of Ca-P compounds.

Biologically, one of the major difficulties to be overcome in obtaining bone samples for structural and compositional studies, especially in studying the initial Ca-P solid phase deposited and the changes that occur in the mineral with time, is the preparation of macroscopic samples that are homogeneous with respect to the age of the bone mineral. This is due to the fact that at any age there is continuous bone formation and resorption. Depending on both the absolute and relative rates of these two processes, a sample of bone will contain different proportions of bone mineral of different ages. Since the chemistry and structure of the bone mineral changes with the age of the bone mineral, sampling techniques need to overcome this difficulty if the nature of the initial mineral phase formed is to be studied as well as the changes that occur in the mineral with time and maturation. Failure to accomplish this and the use of whole bone samples in general results in the data's reflecting only the average properties of a *heterogeneous* sample of bone mineral ranging in age from the very youngest to the very oldest crystals.

III. RECENT THEORIES OF THE NATURE OF THE BONE MINERAL

A. Amorphous Calcium-Phosphate (ACP) Theory

The first major new concept concerning the nature of the mineral phase in bone was provided in 1966 and in subsequent years by a group of scientists led by Dr. Aaron Posner of Cornell Medical School.[17-20] In essence, they reasoned that it should be possible to follow both the chemical composition and the x-ray diffraction characteristics of synthetic Ca-P solid phases as a function of time after their precipitation *in vitro*. When this was done, they found that the initial solid phase of Ca-P formed after *in vitro* precipitation of Ca and P at alkaline pH was not crystalline but rather an *amorphous* calcium phosphate (ACP); the solid phase of Ca-P did not generate a coherent x-ray diffraction pattern, indicating that there was no long-range order of the Ca-P and other ions in the Ca-P solid phase.

To explore the possibility that the same sort of kinetic processes and phase changes were occurring in the bone mineral, calculations were carried out comparing the predicted x-ray diffraction intensities of bone mineral, based on the Ca-P contents of the bone specimen used for x-ray diffraction with the intensities of the x-ray diffraction reflections found experimentally. According to these calculations, it was found that a very significant amount of the Ca-P solid phase of bone was not contributing to the x-ray diffraction reflections. This was consistent with the conclusion that a significant fraction of the Ca-P solid phase in bone was in a noncrystalline, nondiffracting, amorphous state (amorphous calcium phosphate, ACP). Further work using bone of various ages and using other techniques such as infrared spectroscopy (later found to be of doubtful or no value) supported their hypothesis that, like the precipitation of Ca-P *in vitro*, the initial Ca-P solid phase deposited in bone is an ACP that gradually transforms with time to poorly crystalline hydroxyapatite (PCHA). Thus, they concluded from their experiments that the initial Ca-P mineral phase in young, developing bone was ACP, and that with age the amount of ACP decreased and the amount of PCHA increased. The rate of ACP formation was postulated to be greater than the rate at which ACP was converted to PCHA, so that in young bone containing a large proportion of newly formed bone and therefore of newly deposited bone mineral, the *major* Ca-P solid phase was ACP. The ACP theory was a very attractive hypothesis: it accounted for the progressive change in chemical composition with age and maturation as the proportions of ACP and PCHA changed. It explained the increasing intensity of the x-ray diffraction intensities with time as more and more of the ACP (which does not generate or contribute to the intensities of the x-ray diffraction reflections at all) was converted to PCHA. The ACP formed *in vitro* also had a low Ca/P ratio, contained tightly bound or crystalline H_2O, and had other characteristics of newly deposited bone mineral. It is not surprising, therefore, that the ACP theory of the nature of the initial deposits of Ca-P in bone and the changes that occur in the mineral during maturation received very wide international acceptance for almost 20 years. However, as more and more experimental data were compiled and other structural and compositional factors were taken into account, which, like the presence of an ACP phase, would also be expected and were found experimentally to reduce the x-ray diffraction intensity of a poorly crystalline substance like bone mineral, the calculated proportion of the bone mineral in the form of ACP decreased. Indeed, the ACP content of some samples of very young bone previously calculated to contain 60% to 70% or more of ACP was now recalculated to be one half or less of this value. Similarly, the ACP of adult mature bone, earlier calculated to account for at least 35% of the bone mineral, was no longer even detectable within the limits of the methods used. Note that the critical point of the ACP theory is that the initial solid phase of Ca-P formed in bone is ACP. Consequently, as expected, and as experimentally found by these methods and calculations, the major Ca-P solid phase in young bone is ACP; indeed, in the very earliest bone mineral deposited in very rapidly turning over young bone, one would predict that the bone mineral would consist entirely or almost entirely of ACP. The finding that no ACP was detected in mature bone is not as significant as it might seem since it is consistent with the ACP theory; namely, by the time this stage of maturity of the bone mineral is reached, the ACP theory might predict that all of the ACP could have reasonably been expected to convert to PCHA.

B. Problems with the ACP Theory—Alternative Theories

The increasing reservations toward the ACP theory expressed by a number of research workers prompted a complete conceptual and experimental reevaluation of the ACP theory. Since the critical point in the ACP theory is the prediction that ACP is by far the major and in the beginning the only Ca-P solid phase in very young bone mineral, it was necessary to prepare homogeneous bone samples containing only the very youngest and most homogeneous (with respect to age) bone crystals, as well as a series of bone samples containing homogeneous (age) mineral phases of increasing age and maturation.

Another point to emphasize here is that the age of the mineral and the age of the animal are not synonymous, since in bone of any age both new bone formation and bone resorption are occurring simultaneously. Whole bone samples will therefore contain bone mineral of very widely different ages, and data from such samples will represent values based on the average age of the bone mineral in the particular samples. In many instances, bone from widely different aged animals will provide widely varying proportions of the very youngest and very oldest bone crystals, in which case the *average* age of the mineral phase varies considerably. Data from such widely different aged animals before and after long bone growth has ceased and bone turnover has decreased will provide qualitative differences in the age of the bone mineral *per se*. However, except for the very youngest embryonic bone, such samples cannot provide samples of bone mineral that are relatively homogeneous with respect to the age of the bone mineral, and clearly cannot provide the narrow homogeneous (with respect to age) samples of the very early and youngest Ca-P solid phase deposited.

Bone containing relatively homogeneous samples of very young bone mineral was obtained, first by using very young embryonic chick bone that was turning over very rapidly so that the age of the bone tissue and consequently of the bone mineral spanned at most 48 hours, and second, by fractionating bone powder from such young embryonic bones by density centrifugation. Density centrifugation produced samples of bone of different densities and therefore of different mineral content, and consequently of different bone mineral age (Fig. 2–1).[21] Not only were the ages of the bone mineral in such samples produced by this technique even more homogeneous with respect to age of the bone mineral than whole bone samples, but since the samples were derived from very young chick embryos (16–17 days),[22] and more recently 11-day-old embryonic chicks, and because of the very young age and rapid turnover of the embryos and consequently of the *whole* bone mineral in the bone tissue, the low-density samples from such preparations represent the youngest macroscopic bone mineral samples ever obtained and studied by gross physicochemical means.

As has been alluded to earlier, the amounts of ACP in various *in vitro* Ca-P preparations and in bone mineral were originally determined by the Cornell group using an *indirect*[17-20] method. The exact amount and proportion of ACP was later found to depend on how one precisely assigned values to various chemical and structural functions. To avoid this potential pitfall, in the more recent work on embryonic chick bone, the samples were analyzed for the presence of ACP by a *direct* method using a procedure referred to as x-ray radial distribution function analysis (RDF).[22,23] The important and critical findings were that *no* ACP was found in even the very earliest bone mineral, at an age at which one would predict on the basis of the previous studies of ACP calculated by the indirect method that essentially *all* of the solid Ca-P mineral phase should be in the form of ACP. Since *no* ACP was found in bone mineral of any age, the two major postulates of the ACP theory could not be substantiated experimentally: (1) that the initial Ca-P solid phase deposited and remaining in bone as the major, solid Ca-P mineral phase was an ACP, and (2) that this ACP phase gradually transformed to PCHA with time.

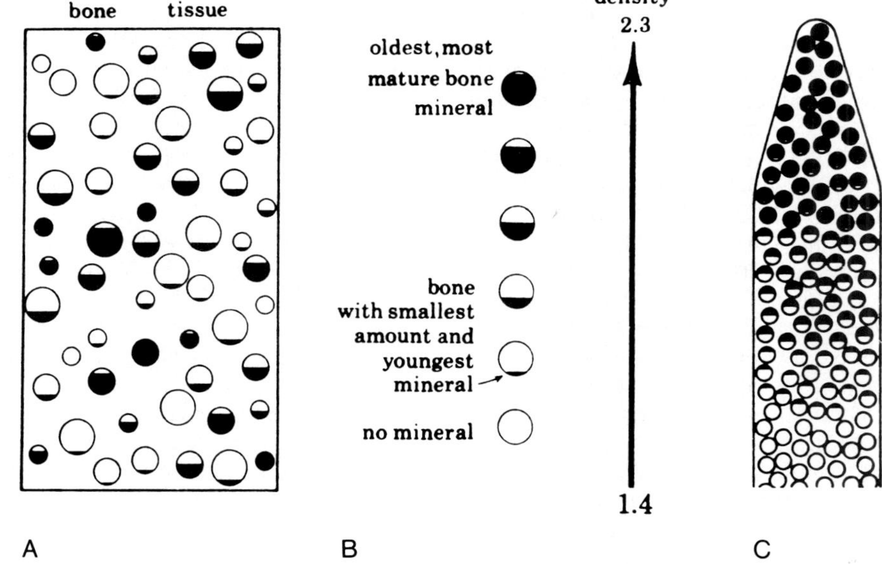

Figure 2–1. Schema for separating bone powder on the basis of mineral content. The younger mineral phase is in the low-density particles and the oldest mineral phase is in the highest-density particles. A, Bone tissue is never homogeneous with respect to the age of its mineral particles. B, Bone tissue is never homogeneous with respect to the age of its mineral particles. C, To obtain specimens of bone containing mineral particles of relatively the same ages, bone is first ground to fine powder and then separated according to its density by centrifugation. (From Glimcher MJ: Philos Trans R Soc Lond [Biol] 304:479, 1984.)

Although the failure to detect ACP in the very youngest bone mineral effectively rules out the premises of the original ACP theory, it does not mean that ACP does not occur as the (or one of the) initial solid Ca-P phases(s) formed. It is conceivable that the rate of the ACP to PCHA transformation is so rapid with respect to the formation of ACP that very little or no ACP ever appears in the tissue. Under these circumstances, ACP would not be a detectable solid phase constituent of the Ca-P mineral phase of bone. Such a concept, however, is completely different from the original ACP theory and from the calculations made from the experimental findings using this concept, namely, that ACP is the *major* solid phase constituent of the bone mineral in young developing bone. Indeed, if the ACP theory is projected to the bone mineral in very young chick embryos, it predicts that ACP constitutes ~100% of the bone mineral when indeed *none* can be demonstrated.

Recent studies using ^{31}P nuclear magnetic resonance (NMR) have also failed to detect the presence of ACP.[24,25] In addition, the ^{31}P NMR studies both of synthetic Ca-P solid phases and of bone mineral have revealed the presence of noncrystalline HPO_4^{2-} groups in a brushite ($CaHPO_4 \bullet 2H_2O$)–like configuration in addition to apatite. The amount of the noncrystalline brushite decreases with age of the bone mineral. The ^{31}P NMR spectrum of bone could be almost completely duplicated by computer modification of synthetic samples of apatite containing ~5% CO_3^- and ~5% to 10% of noncrystalline HPO_4^{2-} in a brushite-like configuration.

Complementary findings were obtained from several other studies. In one comparison study, the crystallinity or crystal index of the bone mineral was studied as a function of age and maturation.[12] These data showed that from the beginning, the Ca-P solid phase is a PCHA, whose crystallinity increases with time. However, even in the oldest bone samples studied, the PCHA, although more crystalline than younger bone mineral, remains poorly crystalline.

^1H NMR and Fourier transform-infrared spectroscopy studies have not been able to detect any hydroxyl groups in the bone mineral of very young to very old animals. What substitutes for the hydroxyl groups in these vacancies has not been determined.[26]

In summary, at the present moment, the bone mineral can be briefly described as follows: The bone mineral appears to be deposited from the beginning as a (very) poorly crystalline type B (carbonato) apatite (not hydroxyapatite), containing ~5% CO_3^- and ~5% to 10% HPO_4^{2-}, the latter in a noncrystalline brushite configuration. With time, the Ca/P increases to values approximating pure apatite (Ca/P=1.67); the content of CO_3^- increases while that of HPO_4^{2-} decreases slightly. The crystallinity of the apatite crystals increases but never beyond a poorly crystalline state.

IV. LOCATION OF THE MINERAL PHASE IN BONE

The ultrastructural location of the mineral phase in bone is a very important parameter in determining its biological functions: how it functions as an ion reservoir, its effectiveness in changing the mechanical properties of the tissue, and, as it turns out, the mechanism of calcification, that is, how and why the Ca-P crystals form at all.

Electron micrographs of osteoid and of calcified bone tissue that has been decalcified show that the volume of space between collagen fibrils accounts for at best ~10% to 15% (or less) of the volume of the extracellular space in most bone, and up to 15% to 20% in certain bone, the remaining volume of the extracellular space being occupied by the collagen fibrils. It is clear from such information alone that the vast majority of the bone mineral must reside within the collagen fibrils; there is nowhere nearly enough room to house the amount of bone mineral present in the tissue except within the collagen fibrils. This has been confirmed by electron microscopy of undecalcified tissue sections that on cross section show collagen fibrils impregnated with the mineral crystallites (Figs. 2–2 to 2–5). In these electron micrographs of the early and late stages of mineralization of fish bone, in which tissue the collagen fibrils are widely separated, thus permitting one to clearly observe the collagen fibrils and the extracellular space between them, the mineral phase is observed to be located almost entirely within the collagen fibrils, with the extracellular spaces between the collagen fibrils free of the mineral crystals. In some instances, at the very last stages of calcification, some mineral may be observed outside the collagen fibrils. A similar situation exists in chick bone and the bones of other species.

Text continued on page 52

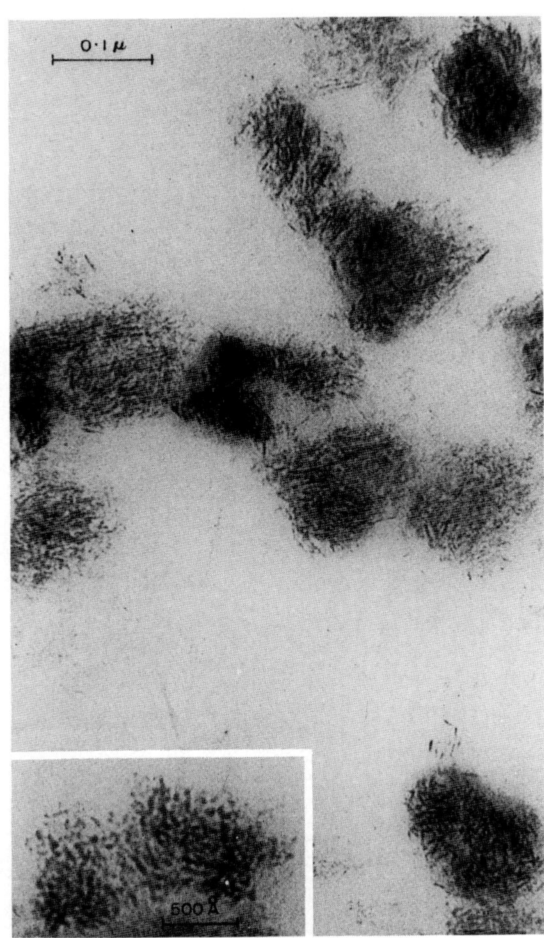

Figure 2–2. Electron micrograph of unstained fish bone, which was not decalcified. The dense particles, identified by electron diffraction as Ca-P apatite crystals, are located essentially within the collagen fibrils, as observed in this electron micrograph in which collagen fibrils are seen primarily in cross-sectional profile. Inset shows two adjacent collagen fibrils in cross-sectional profile at higher magnification. Mineral particles are located within the collagen fibrils. (From Glimcher MJ: Rev Mod Phys 31:359, 1959.)

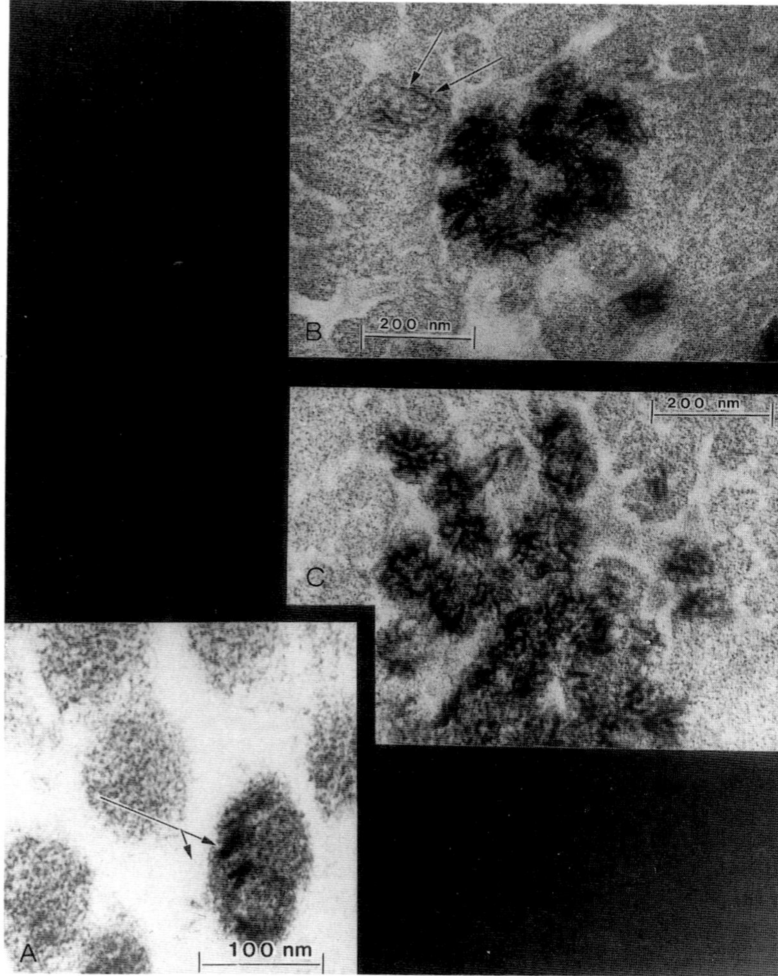

Figure 2–3. A series of high-voltage electron micrographs illustrating the successive stages of mineral deposition in herring bone tissue. Thick (1 μ) cross sections of collagen fibrils were treated completely anhydrously for specimen preparation. A, The very first electron-dense deposits (arrows) are seen to occur within the boundary of the collagen fibril. B and C, As the mineralization progresses further, it is apparent that no mineral particles have been deposited in the extracellular spaces between the fibrils. The deposition of mineral particles in the adjacent collagen fibrils demonstrates that the nucleation of Ca-P crystals in each of the fibrils is an independent physicochemical event. (D.D. Lee et al., unpublished.)

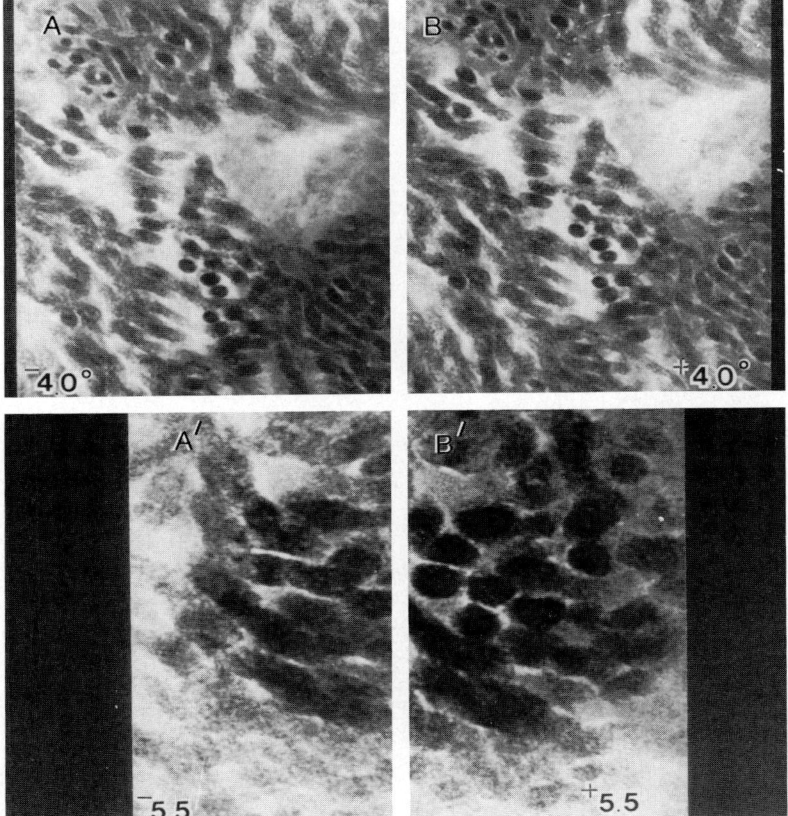

Figure 2–4. A and B, High-voltage electron stereomicrographs of a pickerel fish bone prepared anhydrously seen in cross-sectional profile. A′ and B′, Higher magnification of the same regions illustrating the electron-dense Ca-P particles located within collagen fibrils. Three-dimensional localization of these mineral crystallites can be fully appreciated by stereoscopic examination, eliminating the possibility that these minerals are located on the surface of the section. (D.D. Lee et al., unpublished.)

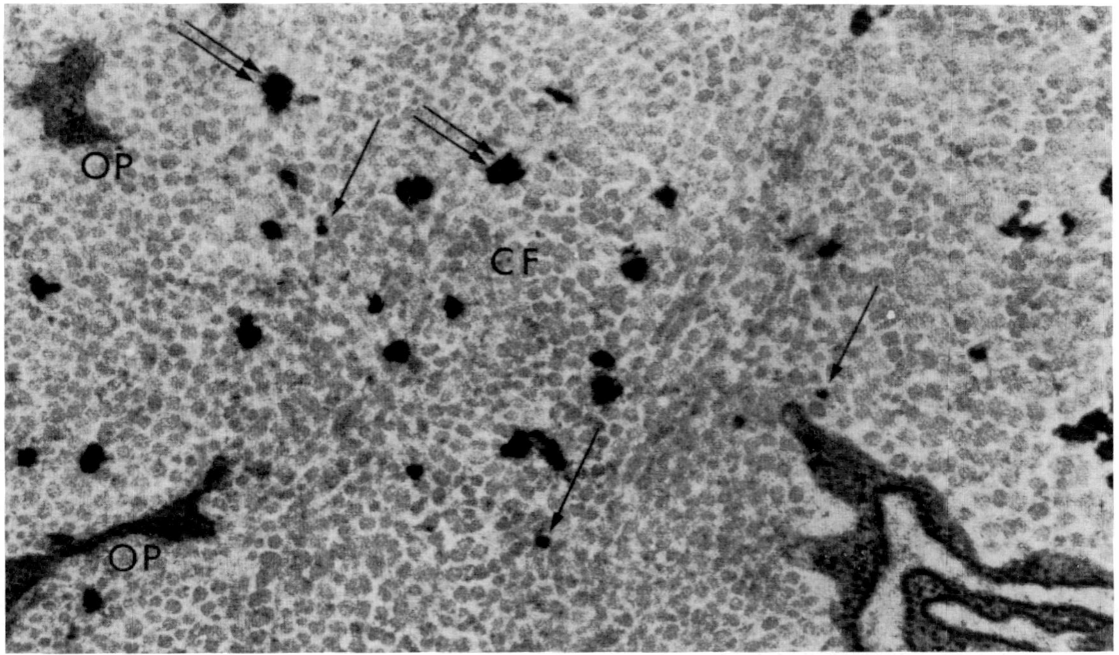

Figure 2–5. Electron micrographs of early stages of calcification of embryonic chick bone. Collagen fibrils are seen in cross section. Note mineral-free collagen fibrils (CF) and fibrils in varying stages of mineralization, that is, impregnated with a solid phase of calcium phosphate. The spaces between the fibrils are essentially free of mineral particles. The calcification of each of the fibrils and of the separate sites along the axial length of a single fibril is a physicochemical independent event. Two osteoblast processes (OP) are indicated. (From Landis WJ, Paine MC, Glimcher MJ: J Ultrastruct Res 59:1, 1977.)

The Ca-P crystals are not randomly distributed within the collagen fibrils. Electron micrographs, especially of the early stages of mineralization, have shown that the Ca-P crystals are first deposited within the hole zone region of the fibrils, essentially "staining" the fibrils and imparting an ~700 Å axial period to the fibrils (Figs. 2–6 and 2–7). Later, as more and more mineral is deposited within the collagen fibril, the ~700 Å axial periodicity of the mineral phase is gradually lost, presumably owing to the fact that with increasing calcification the crystals are also being deposited in the pores of the fibril.

Electron microscopy and electron diffraction of the mineral phase *from the beginning of collagen calcification* show that the long axes (crystalline c-axes) of the crystals within a single fibril are relatively parallel to one another and to the long axes of the fibril *in which they are located*. The localization of the earliest deposited crystals to the hole zone regions of the collagen fibrils by electron microscopy (Figs. 2–6 and 2–7)[27,28] has been confirmed by the elegant low-angle neutron and x-ray diffraction study of intact calcified turkey tendon tissue[29,30] and by reconstruction of the location of the mineral phase in collagen fibrils by optical transforms of low-angle x-ray diffraction data.[31]

Another electron microscopic observation of the early stages of calcification that is very important in eventually formulating a hypothesis of the mechanism of calcification is that the Ca-P crystals are initiated at sites distinct from one another *with unmineralized regions* separating the mineralization sites, not only in adjacent fibrils but even within a single collagen fibril. This makes it clear that the eventual deposition of the crystals within the whole length of a single collagen fibril or of groups of fibrils does not occur by a propagation from one site, but rather that there are *independent nucleation sites* along the length of individual fibrils where mineralization is initiated, namely, in the hole zone regions of the fibrils. This is not to say that secondary crystal formation does not occur locally and extend locally in the hole spaces and to the pores from the initial sites where the Ca-P crystals are first initiated, but only that each of the spaces corresponding to the hole zone regions has the potential of being an independent site where the heterogeneous nucleation of crystals can begin.

V. CURRENT THOUGHTS ABOUT THE MECHANISM OF CALCIFICATION

Regardless of the tissue involved (bone, dentin, enamel, cartilage), and indeed of the organism involved and the nature of the mineral phase (Ca-P, $CaCO_3$, $SrSO_4$), physicochemical principles dictate that the formation of a solid phase from a solution phase represents a *phase transformation* (in this case

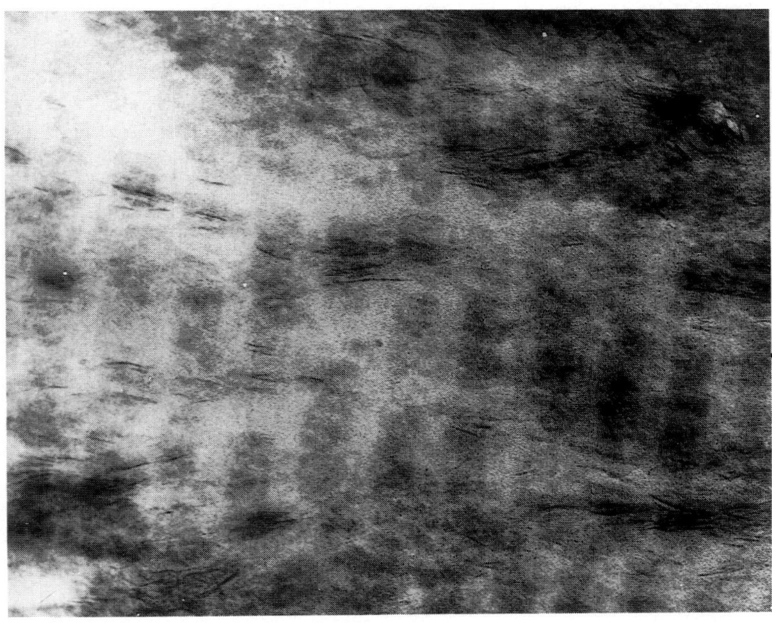

Figure 2–6. Electron micrograph of an unstained, longitudinal section of young undecalcified embryonic chick bone. The dense mineral phase appears to "stain" the collagen fibril at regular intervals along its axial length. In some areas, the inorganic crystals can be seen on edge as dark lines. Most of the mineral phase is not resolvable into individual crystals. (From Glimcher MJ: A basic architectural principle in the organization of mineralized tissues. *In* Milhaud G, Owen M, Blackwood HJJ (eds): Proceedings of the 5th European Symposium on Calcified Tissues, 1967. Paris, Societe d'Edition d'Enseignement Superieur, 1968.)

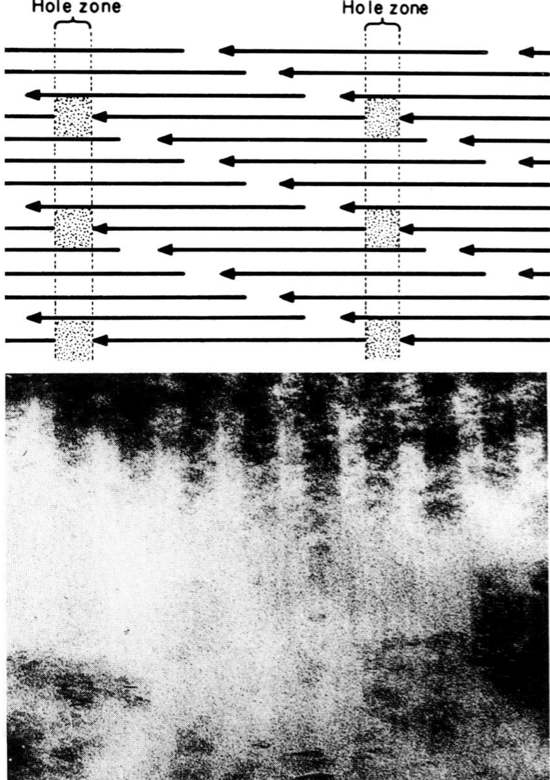

Figure 2–7. The identification of the location of the mineral phase in bone collagen between the a^3 and c^3 bands places the crystals in the hole zone. (From Glimcher MJ, Krane SM: The organization and structure of bone, and the mechanism of calcifications. *In* Ramachandran GN, Gould BS (eds): Treatise on Collagen, vol 7B. New York, Academic Press, 1968.)

solution → solid) and is not, as it was once thought to be, a chemical reaction. Biological mineralization, the formation of an inorganic solid phase in biological tissues, regardless of the nature of the mineral phase, must therefore be governed by the laws of thermodynamics concerned with the stability of phases, and with the kinetics of such phase changes. The simplest example illustrating what a phase change is and how it is distinguished from a chemical reaction is the freezing of H_2O: $H_2O_{(liq)} \rightarrow H_2O_{(solid)}$.[5,10,13]

No chemical reaction is occurring; there are no chemical reaction products. The H_2O molecules simply change their *state of aggregation* from water in a liquid state [$H_2O_{(liq)}$] to H_2O molecules in a solid (ice) state [$H_2O_{(solid)}$]. To accomplish this phase transformation, the water molecules must interact to form aggregates ("embryos") until they reach a critical size, after which an increase in size is accompanied by a decrease in free energy and continued growth of the aggregates until a solid state is reached.[13,32] If this is accomplished by gradually lowering the temperature in the absence of any external particles, there occurs the formation of a sufficient number of critically sized aggregates of H_2O liquid molecules called *embryos*, which grow by the addition of more $H_2O_{(liq)}$ molecules to form critically sized embryos called nuclei, which then grow with a decrease in free energy to form the first particles of the new phase (ice). This process is called *homogeneous nucleation*. If one carries out the experiment with AgI (or CuI) added to the water before cooling, the process differs in several very important respects from homogeneous nucleation. In the first place, the extent to which the temperature needs to be dropped before the crystals are formed is substantially less when AgI (or CuI) is present: to ~39° C without AgI and to only ~4° to 5° C with AgI or CuI present from the start. Second, without AgI the ice crystals form in one mass throughout the whole vessel. With AgI present, the ice crystals begin to form on the surface of the AgI (or CuI) crystals. The lattice parameters, especially of the basal planes of AgI (and CuI), closely match those of ice. This complementarity of crystal lattice structure between ice and AgI allows the AgI to initiate the phase change from water to ice at a higher temperature (more easily) than occurs in the absence of any particles. This process of initiating a phase change *by and on an outside agent or substance* is called *heterogeneous nucleation*, and the substance (AgI) that initiates the heterogeneous nucleation is termed a (heterogeneous) nucleator, nucleation agent, or nucleation substrate. In order for a *nucleator* to initiate *heterogeneous* nucleation, for example, of a solid phase from a solution phase, the solution phase must be in *metastable equilibrium* with respect to the components in solution that will ultimately make up the solid phase. In conceptual thermodynamic terms, a fluid or any other phase may be stable with regard to adjacent states that differ infinitesimally in their intensive properties from the given state but unstable in regard to states that differ finitesimally in their intensive properties from the given state. Such a fluid is stable with respect to *continuous* changes in state but *unstable* with respect to *discontinuous* changes in state. This is called a *metastable* state (as opposed to stable state or unstable state), and a fluid in such a state would be in *metastable equilibrium*. A *metastable solution* therefore refers to a state in which the solution phase is stable for an infinitely long time but still has the potential to form a solid phase under the right conditions, for example, by the intervention of a nucleation agent. *In vitro* nucleation experiments with a variety of solid salts and inorganic crystals have demonstrated that even under the most careful conditions and despite every effort to remove all solid particles that might act as heterogeneous nucleators, it is virtually impossible to obtain true homogeneous nucleation. That is, even under the most stringent and careful conditions, nucleation of the solid phase almost always takes place by the heterogeneous route and not by the homogeneous mechanism. The nucleation agents (dust and other particles, surface defects in the vessels) need not be and in almost all cases are not highly specific or effective catalysts; nevertheless, they are sufficiently effective to induce heterogeneous nucleation before homogeneous nucleation can occur. These data are important in formulating any mechanism for the calcification of bone or any of the other biologically mineralized tissues. Thus, considering the complexity of any biological tissue that contains a multitude of highly ordered intra- and extracellular structures and components, any or all of which can act as heterogeneous nucleators, it would hardly be possible for homogeneous nucleation of a mineral phase to occur in a biological tissue. Instead, any one or a combination of structures or macromolecular components could and would undoubtedly serve as heterogeneous nucleators long before homogeneous nucleation could occur. Indeed, if the phenomenon of calcification follows all other important biological processes, one would expect in most instances that the heterogeneous nucleation agent or substrate would be quite specific, chemically, structurally, and spatially.

Based on the observations that in some tissues and in some organisms the inorganic crystals are not highly organized but appear to be randomly dispersed with regard to their spatial disposition, and further that in some instances the crystal size and habit are very closely like those observed in *in vitro* precipitation, a general hypothesis of biological mineralization has been recently proposed.[33] Biological mineralization is divided into two general categories: (1) matrix-mediated mineralization, by which is meant that certain organic matrix components (principally extracellular) induce and control the deposition of the mineral crystals, their orientation and organization, and their growth and habit; and (2) *biologically induced* mineralization, by which the hypothesis appears to imply that unlike matrix-mediated mineralization, the intracellular or extracellular organic (matrix) constituents do not play this role. At first glance, this subdivision of biological mineralization on the descriptive level does have certain attractive features. However, on close inspection, both the semantics and, most important, the biological and physicochemical concepts underlying the thesis and used as an explanation for the differences observed morphologically can be seriously questioned. In the first instance, the separation of the two putative classes of biological mineralization into matrix-mediated and biologically induced on the basis of crystal orientation or the lack of it and the shape and size of the crystals is misleading. Clearly, if one examines many different mineralized biological tissues, one is struck with the marked difference in how the crystals are organized: in highly organized tissue the crystals are almost completely parallel with one another in an almost perfect two-dimensional array, while in others the crystals appear to be essentially randomly oriented over macroscopic areas. We believe that *all* biological mineralization is *biologically induced*, that is, crystal nucleation by organic constituents in the tissue. Only the organic constituents that act as mediators or heterogeneous nucleators vary from tissue to tissue both intra- and extracellularly. As noted in the preceding paragraph, it would hardly be possible for homogeneous nucleation of a mineral phase to occur in a biological tissue. Thus, the critical and basic underlying physicochemical mechanism of mineralization in both the classes (biologically induced and matrix-mediated) is the same. There is no physicochemical basis for separating the mineralized tissues on the basis of whether the crystals are oriented or not with the implication that this reflects some underlying difference in how and why the crystals are nucleated. The same is true for size and shape (habit) of the crystals. The separation of the biologically mineralized tissues and the cellular and extracellular components of these tissues into two broad classes based on the organization, orientation, and habit of the crystals is potentially an important one, and investigations into the underlying bases for such phenomena are likely to shed light on the mechanism of crystal deposition and crystalline growth and development. However, the author does not believe that there is any physicochemical, biological, or biochemical basis that allows one to use these morphologic observations to formulate the basis for the initiation of mineralization. Indeed, the failure to distinguish between the phenomena of crystal growth and crystal habit and both from crystal nucleation may seriously confuse a number of issues related to the initial and basic underlying mechanism of how and why crystals form at all. The important and critical fact to stress is that in both cases, biologically induced and matrix-mediated calcification, the underlying mechanism of crystallization, namely, how and why the crystals form at all, is the same: heterogeneous nucleation by a biological substrate or nucleator. To label one group biologically induced and the other matrix-mediated based on crystal orientation or habit (size and shape) is to obscure this most important point and to confuse factors that may control the subsequent growth and orientation of the crystals, which are themselves completely independent from each other, and with why the crystals are formed at all.

In the first place, whereas it is true that the crystals of many mineralized tissues are not oriented or organized parallel to one another over any significant distance, it does not follow that this lack of crystal alignment precludes their having been initiated by heterogeneous nucleation. In general, formation of crystals by a nucleation agent or substrate in no way implies or demands theoretically or experimentally that the forming crystals and eventually the formed crystals be oriented or aligned with respect to each other or to the nucleation substrate. Although the two phenomena (nucleation and oriented overgrowth or epitaxy) overlap in some instances, they are independent processes, and heterogeneous nucleation can occur with or without oriented overgrowth (epitaxy) of the crystals. Indeed in some cases, relatively poor nucleation substrates readily produce epitaxial growth (orientation) of the nucleated crystals, that is, the nucleated crystals grow with an absolutely perfect alignment along selected planes of the heterogeneous substrate with perfect co-orientation of certain planes of the forming crystals and the nucleation substrate (epitaxy). Moreover, in the tissues in question, since the exact three-dimensional architecture of the intra- or extracellular matrix and each of its components and therefore of the potential nucleation sites of the components is not known, it is possible that the nucleation sites are themselves relatively randomly organized with respect to the three-dimensional morphology of the tissue or tissue component. In such cases, even if oriented overgrowth (epitaxy) did occur after heterogeneous nucleation, one would still observe a relatively random organization of the inorganic crystals. Knowledge of the orientation of the exact molecular or macromolecular component of the organic matrix involved and of the presumptive nucleation sites is critical in trying to assess the role of organic matrices on the basis of crystal disposition and orientation. At a somewhat higher morphologic level, for example, the collagen fibrils of newly deposited, very young bone in young embryonic animals, which is being rapidly deposited and resorbed, are almost randomly oriented, the extent depending in part on the age and rate of bone synthesis. X-ray diffraction and large-field electron diffraction studies show no preferred orientation of the crystals, and routine electron microscopy likewise reveals no distinctive ordering of the crystals over long distances (in relatively large regions) of the tissue. However, careful high-resolution electron microscopy reveals that in local regions where one can visualize only a few collagen fibrils in good longitudinal profile, the crystals are indeed aligned with their long axes (c-axis) roughly parallel to the individual fibrils within which they are located.[13]

Another of the many other possibilities to explain lack of long-range order of the crystals is that there may be only a few nucleation sites within the matrix or intracellular component where crystal formation is initiated by heterogeneous nucleation, the rest and vast majority of the crystals being formed by secondary nucleation from the initial inorganic crystals formed by heterogeneous nucleation. Unless there were physical constraints within the organic matrix or its components that tended to physically direct crystal growth in a specific direction, the majority of the crystals formed by secondary nucleation would be randomly oriented.

Although there are undoubtedly many factors that together control the orientation of the crystals in tissues, one of the most important appears to be the organization of the organic substrate in which the crystals are nucleated and grow. In the case of collagen or the enamel matrix and in certain invertebrate shells, the structural organic matrix molecules are themselves assembled into highly ordered macromolecular aggregates (fibrils, enamel tubules, compartments) that structurally, architecturally, and possibly stereochemically direct the *alignment and orientation* of the crystals during their growth.[27,34] If such tertiary or quaternary structure is absent, then it is clearly possible, and in fact probable, that once nucleated by such organic molecules or structures, the crystals would be randomly oriented. Thus, the orientation of the crystals in a tissue appears to be more a function of the secondary, tertiary, and possibly quaternary structure of the organic molecules composing the nucleation substrate than any basic difference in the underlying physical chemistry or biology of the basic process of mineralization.

The hypothesis also suggests that the size and shape of the crystals are also an indication of whether mineralization is biologically induced or matrix-induced. For example, it is pointed out that in instances of biologically induced calcification, the size and shape of the crystals closely resemble those prepared *in vitro,* while in matrix-mediated calcification, the size and shape of the crystals are quite different from crystals prepared *in vitro.* Whereas this may be true in some instances, it does not hold true of the major vertebrate calcified tissues. For example, the apatite crystals in bone, dentin, and cementum, which are considered to be initiated by components in their organic matrices (matrix-mediated), are for the most part indistinguishable from those precipitated in the test tube, whereas enamel, which also falls in the class of matrix-mediated mineralization, contains highly oriented crystals several orders of magnitude greater than those precipitated at 37° C *in vitro.* In short, there is no general rule that the habit of inorganic crystals formed by clear-cut heterogeneous nucleation via an organic matrix *in vivo* must differ from the habit of crystals formed by homogeneous nucleation *in vitro* or *in vivo.* Moreover, even *in vitro,* minor changes in the solution phase can markedly alter the habit of crystals formed by either homogeneous or heterogeneous nucleation.

VI. POSTULATED ROLE OF COLLAGEN IN BONE CALCIFICATION

Based on the physicochemical principle that calcification of bone is a phase transformation, namely, that calcium, carbonate, and inorganic phosphate P_i *in solution* in the ECF aggregate form a *solid mineral phase* of Ca, P_i, and carbonate and other ions, and that it is almost certainly initiated by heterogeneous nucleation, and based on the ultrastructural data that have revealed a most striking and intimate relationship between the mineral crystals and the highly ordered, essentially two-dimensional liquid crystals of collagen fibrils, it is easy to take the next step and hypothesize that the heterogeneous nucleation sites reside in some unique location of the collagen fibril having specific physical, chemical, electrical, steric, and spatial properties.[13,28]

Experiments to test this hypothesis have been done both *in vitro* and *in vivo. In vitro,* solutions of Ca-P experimentally demonstrated to be in metastable equilibrium, that is, stable for at least one month (no crystals formed spontaneously), were exposed to purified reconstituted soft tissue collagens and to decalcified bone collagen. Both preparations nucleated apatite crystals within 24 to 48 hours.[13,32,34] A variety of other proteins failed to nucleate Ca-P crystals from the identical solutions. Electron microscopy showed that the initial crystals were formed within the collagen fibrils in a very orderly pattern with an axial period of ~700 Å, that is, once per collagen period. Later analyses revealed that this location within the collagen fibrils corresponded with the hole zone region similar to what is found in native *in vivo* calcified bone.[27,28] When the collagen molecules were polymerized into fibrils in which the molecules were aggregated differently than they are in the native fibrils of bone, skin, and tendon, these fibrils were not capable of nucleating Ca-P crystals from the metastable solutions of Ca-P *in vitro.* This demonstrated that the ability of collagen fibrils to nucleate Ca-P crystals *in vitro* was ultimately dependent on the tertiary structure of collagen; there was something about the specific three-dimensional packing of the collagen molecules in native type fibrils (~700 Å axial period) that resulted in the formation of highly specific chemical, steric, electrochemical, and spatial properties within a particular portion of the fibril (the hole zone region), which together constituted a *heterogeneous nucleation site* for apatite crystals. Further experimental evidence that particular regions within the collagen fibrils act as specific heterogeneous nucleation sites for apatite crystals comes from *in vivo* experiments in which reconstituted soft tissue collagen fibrils prepared from the skin of animals, placed back in the peritoneal cavity and subcutaneous regions of the same animals or littermates, were found to calcify *in vivo*, and in the same manner that they do *in vitro* and in native bone: the crystals are first deposited within the hole zone regions of the collagen fibrils.[35,36]

Several points need to be made, however. The first is that the initiation of calcification of reconstituted soft tissue collagens both *in vitro* and especially *in vivo* is much slower than the recalcification of decalcified bone collagen fibrils *in vitro*. But even *in vitro*, the length of time between the exposure of decalcified bone collagen fibrils to a metastable solution of Ca-P and the nucleation of a Ca-P solid phase of apatite is longer than one would expect for a very potent nucleation substrate. This raises the possibility that while the collagen fibrils of bone and other mineralized tissues are heterogeneous nucleation substrates and are *necessary* for the initiation of apatite formation, they may not be *biologically* sufficient.[10]

It will prove useful at this point to distinguish between the chemical nature of the components and other factors (structural, electrochemical, steric) that define a *nucleation site*, which is the basic *mechanism* of heterogeneous nucleation and the underlying basis for the *initiation* of calcification, and those ancillary factors that can *control* or *regulate* the nucleation process, the subsequent crystal growth, and so on. These would include factors that might facilitate or inhibit nucleation but not be part of the structural nucleation site *per se* (decreasing or increasing the lag time, for example), either directly by affecting the nucleation site or indirectly by altering the metastability of the extracellular fluids in the immediate vicinity of the nucleation substrate. Failure to make the distinction between the two categories, namely, components that are part of the nucleation site *per se* which are directly related to the mechanism of nucleation, and those components that regulate and control the rate of nucleation, for example, has caused a certain amount of confusion in the literature. This has been especially true in the assessment of the possible roles of certain tissue components in the nucleation of apatite crystals in certain tissue compartments and in the tissue as a whole, as opposed to their potential function as regulators.

In discussing and exploring some of the factors that may influence the local nucleation of apatite crystals within selected areas of the collagen fibrils, we distinguish between calcification of the tissue and calcification of specific intracellular or extracellular compartments and components within the tissue. Tissue calcification includes all of the compartments and components that are calcified (Fig. 2–8). In addition to collagen fibrils, in which the vast majority of the crystals in bone are located, Ca-P particles have been observed intracellularly in the mitochondria of osteoblasts (and in the chondroblasts of cartilage) and extracellularly in so-called matrix vesicles, compartments formed by the budding off of portions of the plasma membrane of osteoblasts and chondroblasts.

Lehninger,[37] Shapiro,[38-41] and Brighton and Hunt[42] have demonstrated that the mitochondria of differentiating cartilage cells in the epiphyseal plate (chondroblasts) as well as the osteoblasts of developing bone[14] contain a significant number of dense granules composed principally of Ca and P_i. Using specific staining for calcium in the mitochondrial granules of epiphyseal cartilage cells, it was shown that the number of such granules decreased with increasing maturation of the cartilage cells and with the onset and progression of extracellular calcification. Because the concentration and eventual virtual disappearance of these Ca-P granules in the mitochondria coincide with the appearance and progressive increase of extracellular calcification in the tissue, investigators[37,42] have suggested that the mitochondrial granules in some way help to initiate calcification of the extracellular matrix. For example, Lehninger[37] has suggested that the solid phase particles of Ca-P in the mitochondria of bone and cartilage cells are extruded into and traverse the extracellular space, eventually becoming lodged in the hole zone regions of the collagen fibrils.[37]

In a similar vein, Anderson[43-45] and Bonucci[46] have described plasma membrane–de-

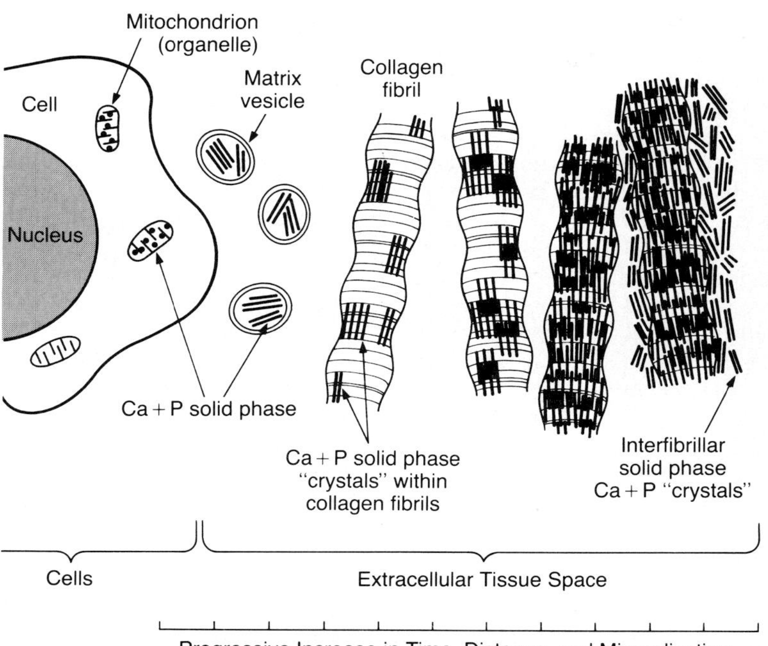

Figure 2–8. Diagrammatic representation of bone tissue calcification and of the putative calcification of several of its intra- and extracellular compartments and components. The exact and specific physical chemical roles of mitochondria and matrix vesicles in tissue calcification of bone have not yet been defined. (From Glimcher MJ: Philos Trans R Soc Lond [Biol] 304:479, 1984.)

rived vesicles in the extracellular matrices of both bone and cartilage, many of which appear to contain crystals of HA when observed electromicroscopically (matrix vesicles).

Because calcification of these vesicles appears to occur prior to the calcification of the collagen fibrils, several hypotheses have been presented that postulate that the solid phase particles or crystals of Ca-P themselves, which are deposited in the matrix vesicles, *directly* cause the mineralization of the collagen fibrils.[43-49] Several different theories have been advanced as to how crystals in one compartment (matrix vesicles) can induce nucleation of new, *de novo* crystals in *specific locations* of another compartment (collagen fibrils) spatially separated from the first compartment. In one proposal,[44,49,50] it is suggested that Ca-P particles in the matrix vesicles pierce the membrane of the matrix vesicles and are extruded in the extracellular space. The extruded crystals then act as nucleation catalysts for the formation of additional crystals of Ca-P by secondary nucleation and multiplication. The continuous formation of new crystals progressively fills the extracellular tissue spaces between the collagen fibrils with inorganic crystals. When the newly forming crystals reach the collagen fibrils, the crystals enter (and/or form) only within the hole zone regions of the collagen fibrils. Later, continued secondary nucleation and multiplication within the collagen fibrils cause new additional crystals to form within the pore spaces of the collagen as well. In this schema, collagen fibrils are simply a passive repository for the deposition of Ca-P crystals and subsequent secondary multiplication of Ca-P crystals, which eventually results in the almost complete impregnation of the fibrils with a solid mineral phase of Ca-P. Neither the collagen fibrils nor any of the noncollagenous macromolecules associated with them are considered to play any role in the formation of the crystals of Ca-P within the fibrils.

Such an explanation seems completely improbable from the standpoints of both physical chemistry and electron microscopic observations.

As pointed out, calcification of the collagen fibrils consists of a large number of independent nucleation events, at *independent* nucleation sites, which are independent from each other even within the same fibril, and which therefore must clearly be completely independent of the direct influence of crystals deposited in compartments spatially separated from the collagen nucleation sites such as matrix vesicles[51] or mitochondria.[39-42]

In the matrix vesicle theory, one would expect to find masses of crystals occupying the space in ECF between the fibrils before calcification of the collagen fibrils started. The theory suffers from the fact that the suggested sequence of events does not in any way correspond to what is actually observed during the calcification of bone (or dentin or cementum) by electron microscopy. Indeed, just the opposite is seen. In our extensive studies of embryonic chick bone by nonaqueous as well as aqueous techniques for the preparation of the tissue samples[14,27,52,53] and in countless published and unpublished electron micrographs of others, as well as recent studies of fish bone by high voltage stereoscopic electron microscopy, we have never observed a stage of calcification in which the extracellular spaces were filled with bone mineral at a time when the collagen fibrils were unmineralized. Indeed, even in the earliest stages of embryonic bone or dentin calcification, at a time when the collagen fibrils are just beginning to mineralize, the most common picture observed is of partially and completely mineralized collagen fibrils separated from one another by *unmineralized* space (see Figs. 2–2 to 2–5). At a stage when there are numerous well-mineralized collagen fibrils, there is still little or no mineral phase present between the fibrils.

Moreover, the proposal that crystals of Ca-P, formed randomly by secondary nucleation and multiplication in the extracellular spaces, are somehow able to find their way in the extracellular spaces selectively to *only* the hole zone regions of the collagen fibrils is thoroughly improbable from both the physicochemical and biological standpoints. Instead, if the sequence of events did occur as envisaged by the matrix vesicle theory, it would follow that at the early stages the collagen fibrils would become encrusted in a random fashion by the self-propagating and multiplying mineral phase particles, which would fill the extracellular tissue spaces. Collagen fibril calcification would then proceed *without* the localization of the crystals to the hole zone regions of the fibrils. This does not correspond to what is actually observed by electron microscopy[27,54] and x-ray and neutron diffraction.[29-31]

Electron microscopic studies have shown that matrix vesicles are observed in only the very early stages of embryonic chick bone development. In later stages of embryonic development, matrix vesicles either are not observed at all or are only few in number. These data are consistent with our own observations. Thus, the collagen fibrils of all the new bone laid down after this early embyonic bone has been resorbed[51] are calcified in the absence of matrix vesicles.[50,55] Matrix vesicles are therefore *not obligatory* for the calcification of bone tissue. Indeed, if they do play any role in the calcification of bone, their action must be limited to a brief period during the early stages of embryonic development, since bone that is synthesized after this very early stage calcifies in the absence of matrix vesicles.

There are, of course, indirect ways that calcification in one compartment like the mitochondria and matrix vesicle can influence the formation of solid phase mineral particles in another spatially distinct compartment: dissolution of the crystals in one compartment (matrix vesicles or mitochondria, for example) and the pumping out and *specifically* directed transport of the Ca^{2+} and P_i ions to and within the second compartment. If sufficient amounts of Ca^{2+} and P_i are transported, the metastability of the fluid within the second compartment may be increased to the point that a nucleation substrate within the second compartment is capable of initiating the formation of apatite crystals by heterogeneous nucleation more easily. Whereas this scenario is theoretically possible, it may not be a likely one, since there does not appear to be a sufficient amount of mineral in either the mitochondria or matrix vesicles so that when dissolved, the tissue ECF concentration of Ca^{2+} and P_i will have been raised significantly. Further work and measurements need to be pursued. Another suggestion has been offered by Thyberg and Friberg,[56] that the matrix vesicles may function by releasing enzymes that degrade the proteoglycans surrounding the collagen fibrils. The degradation and removal of the proteoglycans, thought by many to be inhibitors of calcification, would then permit the collagen fibrils to initiate calcification.[57]

The normal calcification of turkey tendon provides further confirmation that calcification occurs in distinct nucleation sites within the collagen fibrils, each an *independent* event—the calcification of collagen fibrils does not "spread like a wave" throughout a single fibril from a single nucleation site, but rather occurs by nucleation of crystals at multiple *independent*, spatially separated and distinct sites (hole zone region) within a single fibril and then secondary nucleation within the pores.

In bone (as with tendon), the initial deposition of the crystals within the holes of the collagen leads to an axial periodicity of the crystals along the long axes of the fibrils identical to that of the collagen itself.[13,58] With time and with increasing mineralization, more and more crystals are deposited within the pore space, eventually obliterating the initial axial periodicity of the mineral phase.

The calcifying tendon system also provided additional information. Matrix-bound mineral, presumably in matrix vesicles, was clearly observed. The mineral phase was clearly spatially separated from the sites in the collagen where mineral was initiated. It is clear that in this tissue, the mineral crystals in the putative matrix vesicles do not play any direct role in the initiation of calcification of the collagen fibrils, the crystals in the collagen being formed at a distance from the crystals in the matrix vesicles as events totally independent from the matrix vesicle crystals.

Indeed, there is no evidence that there is even an indirect effect of the mineral crystals of the matrix vesicles on collagen calcification, that is, that there is dissolution of the matrix vesicle crystals with Ca^{2+} and P_i ions pumped out to increase the metastability of the extracellular fluid in the close vicinity of the collagen fibrils. The crystals in the putative vesicles remain in the vesicles during the initiation of collagen calcification. Like the observations in bone, the calcification of the collagen fibrils in loci separated from one another implies that the initiation of calcification in each of the hole zone regions represents an independent event.

The fact that there is neither a physicochemical basis nor experimental evidence by electron microscopy or other techniques that solid phase particles of Ca-P in either mitochondria or matrix vesicles *directly* induce calcification of collagen fibrils in no way diminishes the importance of their discovery. The identification of these Ca-P particles and of the membrane-bound matrix vesicles has opened up a whole new field of investigation in the mineralized tissues that promises to shed significant information on important biological phenomena in mineralized tissues.

VII. OTHER FACTORS AND COMPONENTS THAT MAY REGULATE CALCIFICATION OF COLLAGEN FIBRILS

As already mentioned, although the specific stereochemistry and spatial organization of the collagen fibrils of bone, dentin, and cementum result in the formation of nucleation sites within the hole zone regions, these factors, although necessary, may not be sufficient *in vivo*.[10] Even if the conditions in the extracellular fluids are adequate (extent of metastability) for nucleation by the collagen fibrils, there may be other structural and chemical factors intimately related to the collagen fibrils, that, together with the collagen fibrils, constitute the necessary and biologically sufficient conditions for heterogeneous nucleation of Ca-P crystals. For example, although purified collagen fibrils in dialysis bags[35] or Millipore chambers[59] do calcify *in vivo* when placed in the peritoneum or subcutaneously, calcification does not occur for several weeks compared with the rapid calcification (hours) of collagen fibrils in the osteoid of bone.

There are a number of organic components that have been conceptually postulated to be an integral part of the nucleation site and therefore to be involved directly in the mechanism of nucleation or to regulate collagen calcification, and in support of which experimental data have been obtained.

The role of the phosphoproteins in the initiation of calcification has been projected. Reasons why organically bound phosphorus (rather than Ca^{2+}) better meets the requirements as the critical ion, which is either an integral part of the nucleation or interacts with the nucleation site in the organic matrix, have been presented in some detail.[5,27,34] In brief, (1) unlike ionic Ca^{2+} bound electrostatically to the organic matrix, the organic phosphate residues would not be randomly oriented but rather rigidly disposed and sterically organized according to the stereochemistry of the protein(s) it was associated with. Such organic phosphate groups might therefore be in sterically oriented positions according to the stereochemistry of the protein, and therefore in a three-dimensional array resembling certain planes of the apatite lattice. They would therefore be an integral part of the heterogeneous nucleation site. (2) Although covalently bound to the protein, the organic phosphate groups would still be able to react strongly with free Ca^{2+} in a way that would permit the bound Ca^{2+} to also react further with additional inorganic phosphate ions, thus building up a cluster of Ca^{2+} and phosphate ions that could function as nuclei of apatite crystals. (3) The phosphorylation of certain amino acid residues in particular locations in the protein would also be possible enzymatically by protein kinases and ATP, thus assuring exquisite biological control and localization of the process. This precise cellular control and molecular localization of the calcification process make the potential role of organically bound phosphorus very attractive from both physicochemical and biological standpoints.

Experimentally, the first step was to determine whether phosphoproteins were present in bone and other mineralized tissues. To date, all calcified tissues, both normal and pathologic, have been shown to contain phosphoproteins.[60-66] All of the phosphoproteins contain O-phosphoserine [Ser(P)]. Bone, cartilage, and cementum in addition contain significant amounts of O-phosphothreonine [Thr(P)].[64,67-70] Protein kinases have been isolated from several connective tissues that specifically phosphorylate the Ser(P) residues *in vitro* using ATP as a source for the phosphoryl groups.[27]

Functionally, the phosphoproteins have met a number of the criteria necessary if they are to function to facilitate the nucleation of apatite crystals within the collagen fibrils. For example, the phosphoproteins of dentin strongly bind large amounts of Ca^{2+},[71] and ^{31}PNMR studies have in addition shown that the Ser(P) residues are able to form ternary complexes with Ca^{2+} and inorganic phosphate ions:[72]

$$\text{protein—O—P} \begin{matrix} \text{O} \\ \text{O} \end{matrix}\text{—}Ca^{2+}\text{—}P_i$$

ternary complex

Similarly, careful calcium ion–binding studies of dentinal collagen by Li and Katz[73] have clearly shown a significant increase in the number of bound Ca^{2+} ions as a function of the number of phosphoprotein molecules complexed with collagen, and consequently the concentration of Ser(P) in the collagen-phosphoprotein complexes.

Although the physicochemical data demonstrate that the physicochemical properties of the phosphoproteins will permit them to participate in the mineralization of the collagen fibrils, there were at least three important and critical biological questions that had to be answered before any hypothesis could be formulated: (1) Are the phosphoproteins of bone synthesized by bone cells, that is, are they truly bone proteins, or like albumin and others, are they synthesized elsewhere and bound and concentrated in bone? (2) If synthesized by bone cells, by which cells? (3) Where were they located in the tissue? Were they in the region where initiation of mineralization *in vivo* occurred? Appropriate answers to all three questions were necessary as minimum requirements if phosphoproteins were even to have the potential for participating in calcification.

Tissue and then cell culture experiments established that the phosphoproteins were synthesized by bone, and in particular by the osteoblasts.[74,75] Further, when animals were given ^{33}P,[76,77] light and electron microscopy autoradiography showed that the ^{33}P [identified chemically as Ser(P) and Thr(P)] was first located within the osteoblast (and odontoblast in dentin) and then excreted and concentrated at the sites where mineralization was initiated. These findings demonstrating that the phosphoproteins were synthesized in bone and by the appropriate cells and were located in the appropriate place in the tissue, namely, where mineralization was first occurring, at least met the minimum number of biological requirements necessary for them to even be considered to function as facilitators of the heterogeneous nucleation of apatite crystals by collagen fibrils, or to be an integral part of the nucleation site itself.

Analyses of uncalcified and calcifying turkey tendon (before ossification occurs) have shown that there are no detectable phosphoproteins in regions of turkey tendon or in specific "never-to-be-calcified" turkey tendon that was placed in potentially calcifiable turkey tendons prior to calcification. However, once mineralization begins, phosphoproteins are detected and increase in concentration as increasing amounts of mineral are deposited.[68]

Recent experiments in which the lag time, (time to induce nucleation of a Ca-P solid phase) was measured during *in vitro* calcification of bone collagen were consistent with a positive role for the phosphoproteins in facilitating nucleation of apatite crystals by bone collagen fibrils.[78] In these experiments, decalcified bone collagen fibrils are placed in metastable Ca-P solutions, and the time it takes to initiate Ca-P deposition is measured. Collagen preparations complexed with varying amounts of phosphoprotein containing Ser(P) were used. The results clearly demonstrated that there was a very striking correlation of the lag time (time to initiate nucleation) and the amount of phosphoprotein complexed to the collagen as measured by the Ser(P) concentration (Fig. 2–9).

In summary, whereas the potential role of the phosphoproteins in facilitating calcification remains a hypothesis and not a proven fact, their theoretical and experimental physicochemical properties and their biological characteristics—the fact that they are synthesized by the osteoblasts in cell culture and *in vivo*, and excreted *in vivo* at sites in the native tissue where calcification is initiated—and their marked influence in facilitating nucleation by collagen fibrils *in vitro*, all are strong supporting data for their projected role in the initiation of calcification.

There are several other components and factors that have also been implicated in the initiation or facilitation of mineralization or in its inhibition.

Proteolipids and complexed acidic phospholipids[79] have been prepared from a variety of sources, and their ability to initiate calcification from metastable solutions of Ca-P *in vitro* was examined. These lipid components have been found to be very effective heterogeneous nucleators of apatite *in vitro*.[80-82] Although there has been no ultrastructural localization of these lipid components, the most likely source of these components would appear to be cell (plasma) membranes. Therefore one might expect that they are present in the membranes of the matrix vesicles, which themselves are derived from the plasma membrane. Thus, it is possible that they are involved in the calcification of matrix vesicles. Their ability to nucleate apatite crystals *in vitro*

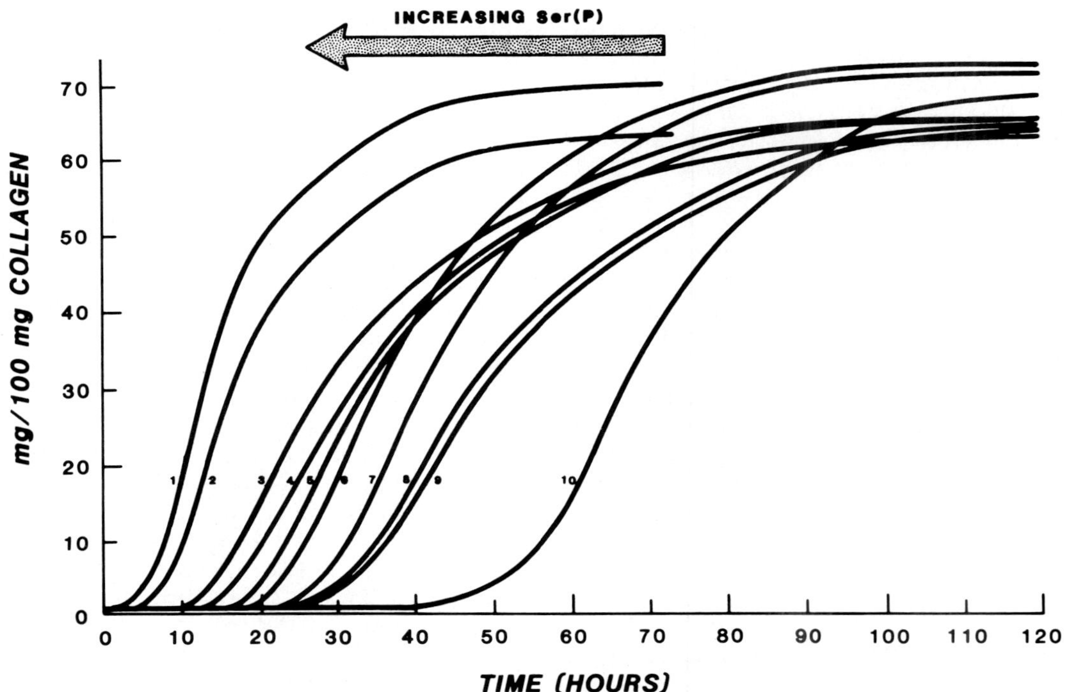

Figure 2–9. Lag time in hours of *in vitro* nucleation of a Ca-P solid phase from a metastic solution of Ca-P as a function of the amount of phosphoprotein complexed to collagen as measured by Ser(P) concentrations. Lag time, that is, time for a collagen phosphoprotein complex to initiate mineralization *in vitro*, decreases with increasing amounts of phosphoprotein complexed to the collagen. (A. Endo et al., unpublished.)

without any additional components suggests that they may be nucleation substrates *per se* rather than facilitators.

It seems clear that there must also be a number of factors that control calcification of the individual components and of the tissue as a whole in a negative sense, that is, they delay or tend to inhibit the deposition of Ca-P, either by influencing the rate of nucleation (lag time), number of nucleation sites, or both, diminishing or abolishing secondary nucleation and multiplication, decreasing the metastability of the extracellular fluids bathing the collagen fibrils of bone or, in the case of other tissues, other structural nucleators,[51] or all or some combination of these factors. The components that have received most of the attention conceptually, and which have been most intensely studied experimentally, are the proteoglycans.

The *proteoglycans*, constitutents of all of the vertebrate mineralized tissues, especially cartilage, are a good example of how important it is, when attempting to postulate whether an organic constituent acts as a nucleation agent, not to rely solely on the point of whether or not the component in question binds Ca^{2+}.[5,13,27,34] Among the factors that are equally as important as Ca^{2+}-binding ability *per se* are its configuration, whether the component exists in solution or in the solid state, the stereochemistry of the reactive groups, and most, important, *whether the Ca^{2+} in the reactive groups that form complexes with Ca^{2+} can still react with inorganic phosphate ions.* If not, the bound Ca^{2+} will essentially be chelated or clathrated and, being unable to react with inorganic phosphate ions, be unable to take part in the formation of embryos or nuclei of Ca^{2+} and P_i and thus in nucleation or calcification. Indeed, such components would *prevent* or *inhibit* nucleation and other steps in calcification, rather than facilitate it. The state of aggregation is particularly important. Aggregates of a macromolecule packed in a very particular way in the solid state might easily form a highly specific three-dimensional steric and electrical array of side chain groups derived from adjacent macromolecules that would constitute a nucleation site.[5,13] The bound Ca^{2+} ions might even be reactive enough to bind P_i ions. However, no futher reaction to build up embryos and eventually nuclei occurs because of the lack of the necessary specific three-dimensional steric array of side chains from a significant number of adjacent closely and specifically packed macromolecules. Thus, it is perfectly possible that some components may act to *block* nucleation when they are in solution, yet *facilitate* nucleation when in the solid state and vice versa. Failure to take such factors into account has led to a great deal of confusion in the literature.

The phosphoproteins are examples of such components: when dissolved in a metastable solution of Ca-P, a phosphoprotein essentially delays the onset of spontaneous precipitation,[83] whereas bound to collagen fibrils in the solid state, the phosphoprotein (in the solid state) facilitates the nucleation of Ca-P from solutions of Ca-P in metastable equilibrium.[78]

In the early literature of calcification, the ability of the proteoglycans to bind Ca^{2+} via their carbonyl and sulfate side chain groups led most investigators to postulate that these components somehow directly initiated the formation of the crystals or at least facilitated calcification (see, for example, references 84 to 86). Later, it was pointed out that this same physicochemical characteristic (Ca^{2+} binding) could serve just as well in making the proteoglycans an inhibitor, namely, by preventing the Ca^{2+} concentration in the extracellular fluid from reaching a level sufficient for heterogeneous nucleation to occur in the collagen fibrils.[13,34] The phenomenon was likened to that of tanning skin collagen,[34] in which case the process was markedly facilitated when the proteoglycans and other noncollagenous substances were first removed from the skin before tanning was begun.[87] The physicochemical similarities between the tanning and calcification of collagen (availability of collagen side chains for chemical and physical interactions with other chemical components) was demonstrated when it was shown that the collagen in native skin failed to calcify *in vitro* when exposed to metastable solutions of Ca-P, whereas skin first treated with hyaluronidase and other enzymes and/or extracted with salt solutions of high ionic strength did mineralize.[13,34]

The proteoglycans have a number of other physicochemical characteristics that theoretically would also tend to inhibit calcification. In addition to binding Ca^{2+} ions, proteoglycan gels inhibit the diffusion of Ca^{2+} and exclude inorganic phosphate ions.[5,27]

Biological evidence also exists that supports an inhibitory role for the proteoglycans in calcification. During the calcification of cartilage in endochondral ossification, the amount of proteoglycans in the tissue progressively decreases starting from the completely uncalcified regions to the regions undergoing calcification.[88] Moreover, during this time, the proteoglycan macromolecules are degraded and reduced in size.[89] Not only the decrease in size but the decrease in molecular weight and chain length[34] will decrease the number of Ca^{2+} ions that can be bound by the proteoglycans, thus "exposing" the collagen fibrils and permitting them to function as heterogeneous nucleators for the formation of apatite crystals. On the basis of analyses from direct puncture of the epiphyseal cartilage fluid, similar conclusions have been reached by Howell and Pita and their colleagues[90-96] and by Posner and colleagues,[97-99] who have conducted extensive experiments on the function of proteoglycans in *in vitro* calcification. Similarly, electron probe microanalysis of bone has shown more sulfate in the relatively sparsely mineralized osteoid of bone than in the more mineralized mature regions.[100,101] The "protective" function of the proteoglycans in inhibiting the reaction between extracellular fluid components and collagen fibrils by binding and decreasing diffusion is also illustrated in the case of cartilage by the marked enhancement of the intensity of reactions between antibodies to type II collagen after reaction of the tissue with hyaluronidase.

On the other hand, there still persists some strong feeling that the proteoglycans are directly involved in the nucleation and initiation of calcification based principally on extensive electron micrographic studies.[46,102,103] These include studies that showed that a particular protein component, the alpha(II) C-terminal propeptide ("chondrocalcin"),[104] was intimately associated with the mineral crystals in growth plate cartilage, and in the initial deposits of the mineral phase with proteoglycan as well.[104]

As for other structural factors, Katz and Li[73,105] have demonstrated that the collagen molecules in rat tail tendon are so closely packed that the diffusion of ions such as phosphate must be seriously limited. In contrast, the pathways in bone collagen are much larger, allowing diffusion of the hydrated phosphate ions to and within the collagen fibrils of bone without restriction. These structural factors would therefore have a tendency to inhibit calcification in some normally uncalcified tissues like tendon, while facilitating it in bone.

There are a large number of other substances that allegedly are also able to decrease or inhibit mineralization *in vitro* and *in vivo.* These include pyrophosphate, fluoride, polypeptides containing phosphorus, Mg^{2+}, and others.[5,27] Presumably many of these substances decrease or inhibit calcification by interacting with and effectively decreasing the number of or "inactivating" the Ca-P nuclei of the metastable solution phase,[5] rather than by binding Ca^{2+} alone (Fig. 2–10).[27]

VIII. CALCIFICATION IN SUMMARY

From the physicochemical standpoint, the formation of a solid phase of Ca-P in bone represents a *phase transformation,* a process exemplified by the formation of ice from liquid water. Considering the structural complexity and abundance of highly organized macromolecules in the cells and extracellular tissue spaces of mineralized tissues generally and in bone particularly, it is inconceivable that this phase transformation occurs by homogeneous nucleation, that is, without the active participation, initiation, and induction by an

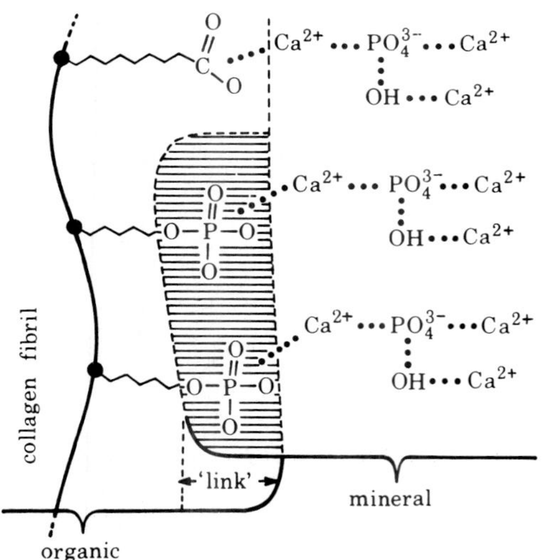

Figure 2–10. Schematic diagram illustrating how protein-bound phosphomonoester groups may be constituents of both the organic and the mineral phases and thus serve as a bridge, chemically and physically linking the organic structural molecules of the organic matrix to the inorganic mineral crystals. (From Glimcher MJ: Philos Trans R Soc Lond [Biol] 304:479, 1984.)

organic component acting as a nucleation agent. This is almost surely true in biological mineralization in general. Electron micrographs and low-angle neutron and x-ray diffraction studies clearly show that calcification of collagen fibrils occurs in an extremely intimate and highly organized fashion: initiation of crystal formation within the collagen fibrils in the hole zone region, with the long axis (c-axis) of the crystals aligned roughly parallel to the long axis of the fibril within which they are located. Crystals are initially formed in hole zone regions within individual fibrils at distances from one another with unmineralized regions separating them, that is, *spatially* distinct nucleation sites where calcification is initiated. This indicates that such regions within a single, unidirectional fibril represent *independent* sites for heterogeneous nucleation. Clearly, sites at which mineralization is initiated in adjacent collagen fibrils are even further spatially separated, emphasizing even more clearly that the process of progressive calcification of the collagen fibrils and therefore of the *tissue* is characterized principally by the presence of increasing numbers of independent nucleation sites within additional hole zone regions of the collagen fibrils. The additional increase in the mass of Ca-P apatite accrues principally by multiplication of more crystals, mostly by secondary nucleation from the crystals initially deposited in the hole zone region. Very little additional growth of the crystals occurs with time, the additional increase in mineral mass being principally the result of *multiplication* (increase in the number of crystals, not the size of the crystals [crystal growth]). The progressive increase in the number of crystals within the collagen fibrils and possibly the slow growth of the crystals extend to include the overlap zone of the collagen fibrils ("pores") so that all of the available space within the fibrils (possibly expanded in volume from its uncalcified level) is eventually occupied by the mineral crystals.

It is absolutely critical for one to recognize that the calcification of each of the tissue components and compartments *which are spatially separated* (collagen, mitochondria, matrix vesicles) *must* be an *independent physicochemical event*. That is, there is *no way* in which the solid phase Ca-P *crystals* of one component can *directly* cause or influence the initiation of calcification (nucleation) in another component *from which it is physically separated*.

References

1. Levy M: Chemische Untersuchungen über osteomalacische Knochen. Hoppe-Seylers Z Physiol Chem 19:239–270, 1894.
2. DeJong WF: La substance minerale dans les os. Recl Trav Chim Pays-Bas Belg 45:445–448, 1926.
3. Roseberry HH, Hastings AB, Morse JK: X-ray analysis of bone and teeth. J Biol Chem 90:395–407, 1931.
4. Glimcher MJ, Bonar LC, Grynpas MD, et al: Recent studies of bone mineral: Is the ACP theory valid? J Crystal Growth 53:100–119, 1981.
5. Glimcher MJ: Composition, structure, and organization of bone and other mineralized tissues and the mechanism of calcification. *In* Greep RO, Astwood EB (eds): Handbook of Physiology: Endocrinology, vol. 7. Washington, DC, American Physiological Society, 1976, pp 25–116.
6. Brown WE, Chow LC: Chemical properties of bone mineral. Annu Rev Mater Sci 6:213–236, 1976.
7. Wadkins CL, Luben R, Thomas M, Humphreys R: Physical biochemistry of calcification. Clin Orthop 99:246–266, 1974.
8. Termine JD: Mineral chemistry and skeletal biology. Clin Orthop 85:207–241, 1972.
9. Posner AS: Crystallite chemistry of bone mineral. Physiol Rev 49:760, 1969.
10. Glimcher MJ: Recent studies of the mineral phase in bone and its possible linkage to the organic matrix by protein-bound phosphate bonds. Philos Trans R Soc Lond [Biol] 304:479–508, 1984.
11. Elliot JC: The problems of the composition and structure of the mineral components of the hard tissues. Clin Orthop 93:313–345, 1973.
12. Bonar LC, Roufosse AH, Sabine WK, et al: X-ray diffraction studies of the crystallinity of bone mineral in newly synthesized and density fractionated bone. Calcif Tissue Int 35:202–209, 1983.
13. Glimcher MJ: Molecular biology of mineralized tissues with particular reference to bone. Rev Mod Phys 31:359–393, 1959.
14. Landis WJ, Glimcher MJ: Electron diffraction and electron probe microanalysis of the mineral phase of bone tissue prepared by anhydrous techniques. J Ultrastruct Res 63:188–223, 1978.
15. Woodward HQ: The composition of human cortical bone. Clin Orthop 37:187–193, 1964.
16. Pellegrino ED, Biltz RM: Mineralization in the chick embryo. I. Monohydrogen phosphate and carbonate relationships during maturation of the bone crystal complex. Calcif Tissue Res 10:128–135, 1972.
17. Eanes ED, Harper RA, Gillessen IH, Posner AS: An amorphous component in bone mineral. *In* Gaillard PJ, van der Hoff A, Steendyk R (eds): 4th European Symposium on Calcified Tissues. Amsterdam, Excerpta Medica, 1966, pp 24–26.
18. Termine JD: Amorphous calcium phosphate: The second mineral of bone. PhD Thesis, Cornell University, 1966.
19. Termine JD, Posner AS: Infrared analysis of rat bone: Age dependency of amorphous and crystalline mineral fractions. Science 153:1523–1525, 1966.
20. Termine JD, Posner AS: Amorphous/crystalline inter-relationships in bone mineral. Calcif Tissue Res 1:8–23, 1967.
21. Roufosse AH, Landis WJ, Sabine WK, Glimcher MJ: Identification of brushite in newly deposited bone

mineral from embryonic chicks. Ultrastruct Res 68:235–255, 1979.
22. Grynpas MD, Bonar LC, Glimcher MJ: Failure to detect an amorphous calcium phosphate solid phase in bone mineral. Calcif Tissue Int 36:291–301, 1984.
23. Fawcett RW: A radial distribution function analysis of an amorphous calcium phosphate with calcium to phosphate molar ratio of 1.42. Calcif Tissue Res 13:319–325, 1973.
24. Aue WP, Roufosse AH, Roberts JE, et al: Solid state ^{31}P NMR studies of synthetic solid phases of calcium phosphate: Potential models of bone mineral. Biochemistry 23:6110–6114, 1984.
25. Roufosse AH, Aue WP, Glimcher MJ, Griffin RG: An investigation of the mineral phases of bone by solid state ^{31}P magic angle sample spinning NMR. Biochemistry 23:6115–6120, 1984.
26. Roberts JE, Bonar LC, Grynpas MD, et al: Characterization of the youngest mineral phases of bone by solid state phosphorus-31 magic angle sample spinning nuclear magnetic resonance and x-ray diffraction (in preparation).
27. Glimcher MJ, Krane SM: The organization and structure of bone, and the mechanism of calcification. *In* Ramachandran GN, Gould BS (eds): Treatise on Collagen, vol 7B. New York, Academic Press, 1968, pp 68–251
28. Glimcher MJ: A basic architectural principle in the organization of mineralized tissues. *In* Milhaud G, Owen M, Blackwood HJJ (eds): Proceedings of the 5th European Symposium on Calcified Tissues, 1967. Paris, Societe d'Edition d'Enseignement Superieur, 1968, pp 3–26.
29. White SW, Hulmes DJS, Miller A, Timmins PA: Collagen-mineral axial relationship in calcified turkey leg tendon by X-ray and neutron diffraction. Nature (London) 266:421–425, 1977.
30. Berthet-Colominas C, Miller A, White SW: Structural study of the calcifying collagen in turkey leg tendons. J Mol Biol 134:431–445, 1979.
31. Engstrom A: Apatite-collagen organization in calcified tendon. Exp Cell Res 43:241–245, 1966.
32. Glimcher MJ, Hodge AJ, Schmitt FO: Macromolecular aggregation states in relation to mineralization: The collagen-hydroxyapatite system as studied *in vitro*. PNAS USA 43:860–867, 1957.
33. Lowenstam HA: Minerals formed by organisms. Science, 211:1126–1131, 1981.
34. Glimcher MJ: Specificity of the molecular structure of organic matrices in mineralization. In Sognnaes RF (ed): Calcification in Biological Systems. Washington, DC, American Association for the Advancement of Science, 1960, pp 421–487.
35. Mergenhagen SE, Martin GR, Rizzo AA, et al: Calcification *in vivo* of implanted collagen. Biochim Biophys Acta 43:563–565, 1960.
36. Glimcher MJ, Barr J, Goldhaber P: Unpublished data.
37. Lehninger AL: Mitochondria and calcium ion transport. Biochem J 119:129–138, 1970.
38. Shapiro IM, Greenspan JS: Are mitochondria directly involved in biological mineralization? Calcif Tissue Res 3:100–102, 1969.
39. Shapiro IM, Lee NH: Calcium accumulation by chondrocyte mitochondria. Clin Orthop 106:323–329, 1975.
40. Shapiro IM, Wuthier RE: A study of the phospholipids of bovine dental tissue. II. Arch Oral Biol 11:513–519, 1966.
41. Shapiro IM, Wuthier RE, Irving JT: A study of the phospholipids of bovine dental tissues. I. Arch Oral Biol 11:501–512, 1966.
42. Brighton CT, Hunt RM: Mitochondrial calcium and its role in calcification. Clin Orthop 100:406–416, 1974.
43. Anderson HC: Vesicles associated with calcification in the matrix of epiphyseal cartilage. J Cell Biol 41:59–72, 1969.
44. Anderson HC: Calcium-accumulating vesicles in the intercellular matrix of bone. *In* Elliott K, Fitzsimons DW (eds): Ciba Foundation Symposium, Hard Tissue Growth, Repair and Remineralization. Amsterdam, Elsevier, 1973, pp 213–246.
45. Morris DC, Vaananen HK, Anderson HC: Matrix vesicle calcification in rat epiphyseal growth plate cartilage prepared anhydrously for electron microscopy. Metab Bone Dis Relat Res 5:131–137, 1984.
46. Bonucci F: The locus of initial calcification in cartilage and bone. Clin Orthop 78:108–139, 1971.
47. Ali SY: Analysis of matrix vesicles and their role in the calcification of epiphyseal cartilage. Fed Proc Fed Am Soc Exp Biol 35:135–142, 1976.
48. Ali SY, Craig-Gray J, Wisby A, Phillips M: Preparation of thin cryosections for electron probe analysis of calcifying cartilage. J Microsc 111:65–76, 1977.
49. Wuthier RE: A review of the primary mechanism of endochondral calcification with special emphasis on the role of cells, mitochondria and matrix vesicles. Clin Orthop 169:219–242, 1982.
50. Anderson HC: Evolution of cartilage. *In* Slavkin HC (ed): The Comparative Molecular Biology of Extracellular Matrices. New York, Academic Press, 1972, pp 200–205.
51. Glimcher MJ: On the form and function of bone: From molecules to organs. Wolff's law revisited, 1981. *In* Veis A (ed): The Chemistry and Biology of Mineralized Connective Tissues. Amsterdam, Elsevier/North-Holland, 1981, pp 618–673.
52. Landis WJ, Hauschka, BT, Rogerson CA, Glimcher MJ: Electron microscopic observations of bone tissue prepared by ultracryomicrotomy. J Ultrastruct Res 59:185–206, 1977.
53. Landis WJ, Paine MC, Glimcher MJ: Electron microscopic observations of bone tissue prepared anhydrously in organic solvents. J Ultrastruct Res 59:1–30, 1977.
54. Glimcher MJ, Katz EP, Travis DF: The organization of collagen in bone: The role of noncovalent forces in the physical properties and solubility characteristics of bone collagen. *In* Comte P (ed): Symp Int Biochim Physiol Tissu Conjonctif, 1966. Lyon, France, Societe Ormeco et Imprimerie du Sud-Est, 1966, pp 491–503.
55. Landis WJ, Glimcher MJ: Unpublished data.
56. Thyberg J, Friberg U: Ultrastructure and acid phosphatase of matrix vesicles and cytoplasmic dense bodies in the epiphyseal plate. J Ultrastruct Res 33:554–573, 1970.
57. Landis WJ: Temporal sequence of mineralization in calcifying turkey leg tendon. *In* WT Butler (ed): The Chemistry and Biology of Mineralized Tissues. Birmingham, AL, EBSCO Media, 1985, pp 360–363.
58. Robinson RA, Watson ML: Collagen-crystal relationships in bone as seen in the electron microscope. Anat Rec 114:383–409, 1952.
59. Glimcher MJ: Unpublished data.

60. Glimcher MJ: Phosphopeptides of enamel matrix. J Dent Res 58B:790–806, 1979.
61. Veis A, Spector AR, Zamoscianyk H: The isolation of an EDTA-soluble phosphoprotein from mineralizing bovine dentin. Biochim Biophys Acta 257:404–413, 1972.
62. Linde A, Bhown M, Butler WT: Non-collagenous proteins of rat dentin: Evidence that phosphoprotein is not covalently bound to collagen. Biochim Biophys Acta 667:341–350, 1981.
63. Seyer JM, Glimcher MJ: Isolation, characterization and partial amino acid sequence of a phosphorylated polypeptide (E_4) from bovine embryonic dental enamel. Biochim Biophys Acta 493:441–451, 1977.
64. Glimcher MJ, Kossiva D, Roufosse A: Identification of phosphopeptides and gamma-carboxyglutamic acid–containing peptides in epiphyseal growth plate cartilage, proteins of bone cementum; comparison with dentin, enamel and bone. Calcif Tissue Int 27:187–191, 1979.
65. Anderson RS, Schwartz ER: Phosphorylation of proteoglycans from human articular cartilage by a cAMP-dependent protein kinase. Arthritis Rheum 27:1023–1027, 1984.
66. Oegema TR Jr, Brown N, Dziewiakowski D: The link protein in proteoglycan aggregates from the Swarm rat chondrosarcoma. J Biol Chem 252:6470–6477, 1977.
67. Cohen-Solal L, Lian JB, Kossiva D, et al: The identification of O-phosphothreonine in the soluble non-collagenous phosphoproteins of bone matrix. FEBS Lett 89:107–110, 1978.
68. Glimcher MJ, Brickley-Parsons D, Kossiva D: Phosphopeptides and carboxyglutamic acid–containing peptides in calcified turkey tendons: Their absence in uncalcified tendon. Calcif Tissue Int 27:281–284, 1979.
69. Glimcher MJ, Lefteriou B, Kossiva D: Identification of O-phosphoserine, O-phosphothreonine and carboxyglutamic acid in the noncollagenous proteins of bovine cementum; comparison with dentin, enamel and bone. Calcif Tissue Int 28:83–86, 1979.
70. Linde A, Brown M, Butler WT: Non-collagenous proteins of dentin: A re-examination of proteins from rat incisor dentin utilizing techniques to avoid artifacts. J Biol Chem 255:5931–5942, 1980.
71. Lee SL, Veis A: Studies on the structure and chemistry of dentin collagen-phosphoryn covalent complexes. Calcif Tissue Int 31:123–134, 1980.
72. Lee SL, Glonek T, Glimcher MJ: ^{31}P nuclear magnetic resonance spectroscopic evidence for ternary complex formation of fetal phosphoprotein with calcium and inorganic orthophosphate ions. Calcif Tissue Int 35:815–818, 1983.
73. Li SH, Katz E: On the state of anionic groups of demineralized matrices of bone and dentin. Calcif Tiss Res 22:275–284, 1977.
74. Glimcher MJ, Kossiva D, Brickley-Parsons D: Phosphoproteins of chicken bone matrix: Proof of synthesis in bone tissue. J Biol Chem 259:290–293, 1984.
75. Gotoh Y, Sakamoto M, Sakamoto S, et al: Biosynthesis of O-phosphoserine–containing phosphoproteins by isolated bone cells of mouse calvaria. FEBS Lett 154:116–120, 1983.
76. Weinstock M, Leblond CP: Radioautographic visualization of the deposition of a phosphoprotein at the mineralization front in the dentin of the rat incisor. J Cell Biol 56:838–845, 1973.
77. Landis WJ, Sanzone CF, Brickley-Parsons D, Glimcher MJ: Radioautographic visualization and biochemical identification of O-phosphoserine– and O-phosphothreonine–containing phosphoproteins in mineralizing embryonic chick bone. J Cell Biol 98:986–990, 1984.
78. Endo A, Glimcher MJ: The potential role of phosphoproteins in the *in vitro* calcification of bone collagen. *In* VM Goldberg (ed): Trans 32nd Mt Orthop Res Soc: Chicago, Adept Printing, 1986, p 221.
79. Raggio CL, Boyan BD, Boskey AL: In vivo induction of hydroxyapatite formation by lipid macromolecules. J Bone Joint Surg (in press).
80. Odutuga AA, Prout RES, Hoare J: Hydroxyapatite precipitator *in vitro* by lipids extracted from mammalian hard and soft tissues. Arch Oral Biol 20:311–316, 1975.
81. Boskey AL, Posner AS: The role of synthetic and bone-extracted Ca-phospholipid-PO_4 complexes in hydroxyapatite formation. Calcif Tissue Res 23:251, 1977.
82. Boyan BD: Proteolipid-dependent calcification. *In* WT Butler (ed): The Chemistry and Biology of Mineralized Tissues: Birmingham, AL, EBSCO Media, 1985, pp 125–131.
83. Nawrot CF, Campbell DJ, Shroaeder JK, van Valkenburg M: Dental phosphoproteins—Induced formation of hydroxyapatite during in vitro synthesis of amorphous calcium phosphate. Biochemistry 15:3445–3449, 1976.
84. Sobel AE: Local factors in the mechanism of calcification. Ann NY Acad Sci 60:713–732, 1955.
85. Sobel AE, Burger M: Calcification, XIV. Investigation of the role of chondroitin sulfate in the calcifying mechanism. Proc Soc Exp Biol Med 87:7–13, 1954.
86. Sylven B: Cartilage and chondroitin sulfate. II. Chondroitin sulfate and the physiological ossification of cartilage. J Bone Joint Surg 29:973–976, 1947.
87. Burton D, Reed R: Mucoid material in hides and skins and its significance in tanning and dyeing. Discussions Faraday Soc 16:195–201, 1954.
88. Lohmander S, Hjerpe A: Proteoglycans of mineralizing rib and epiphyseal cartilage. Biochim Biophys Acta 404:93–109, 1975.
89. Buckwalter JA: Proteoglycan structure and calcifying cartilage. Clin Orth 172:207–232, 1983.
90. Howell DS: Bone formation: Biochemistry of calcification. Isr J Med Sci 12:91–97, 1976.
91. Howell DS, Carlson L: The effect of papain on mineral deposition in the healing of rachitic epiphyses. Exp Cell Res 37:582–596, 1965.
92. Howell DS, Carlson L: Alterations in the composition of growth cartilage septa during calcification studied by microscopic x-ray elemental analysis. Exp Cell Res 51:185–195, 1968.
93. Howell DS, Marquez JF, Pita JC: The nature of phospholipids in normal and rachitic costochondral plates. Arthritis Rheum 8:1039–1046, 1965.
94. Howell DS, Pita J, Marquez J: Phosphate concentration and sodium activity of fluids obtained by micropuncture in epiphyseal cartilage. Fed Proc 24:566, 1965.
95. Pita JC, Cuervo LA, Madruga JE, et al: Evidence for a role of proteinpolysaccharides in regulation of mineral phase separation in calcifying cartilage. J Clin Invest 49:2188–2197, 1970.
96. Pita JC, Muller F, Howell DS. Disaggregation of proteoglycan aggregates during endochondrial cal-

cification: Physiological role of cartilage lysozyme. *In* Burleigh M, Poole R (eds): Dynamics of Connective Tissue Macromolecules. Amsterdam, Elsevier/North-Holland, 1975, pp 247–258.

97. Posner AS, Blumenthal NC, Boskey AL, Betts F: Formation and transformation of amorphous calcium phosphate to hydroxyapatite: A bone analogue in calcified tissue. *In* Czitober H, Eschberger J (eds): Calcified Tissue. Vienna, Facta Publications, 1973, pp 1–4.
98. Chen CC, Boskey AL: The effect of proteoglycans on in vitro hydroxyapatite growth. Calcif Tissue Int 36:285–290, 1984.
99. Chen CC, Boskey AL: Mechanisms of proteoglycan inhibition of hydroxyapatite growth. Calcif Tissue Int 37:395–400, 1985.
100. Baylink D, Wergedal J, Stauffer M, Rich C: Effects of fluoride on bone formation, mineralization, and resorption in the rat. *In* Vischer TL (ed): Fluoride in Medicine. Bern, Hans Huber, 1970, pp 37–60.
101. Baylink D, Wergedal J, Thompson E: Loss of proteinpolysaccharides at sites where bone mineralization is initiated. J Histochem Cytochem 20:279–292, 1972.
102. Bonucci E, Dearden LC, Mosier HD Jr: Effects of glucocorticoid treatment on the ultrastructure of cartilage and bone. Adv Exp Med Biol 171:269–278, 1984.
103. Poole AR, Pidoux I, Reiner A, Rosenberg L: An immunoelectron microscopic study of the organization of proteoglycan monomer, link protein, and collagen in the matrix of articular cartilage. J Cell Biol 93:921–937, 1982.
104. Poole AR: Personal communication.
105. Katz EP, Li S-T: Structure and function of bone collagen fibrils. J Mol Biol 80:1–15, 1973.

JOEL F. HABENER
JOHN T. POTTS, Jr.

3

Fundamental Considerations in the Physiology, Biology, and Biochemistry of Parathyroid Hormone

Parathyroid hormone (PTH) and the active forms of vitamin D constitute the principal regulators of calcium homeostasis for humans and all terrestrial vertebrates. Parathyroid hormone is the principal immediate regulator and determinant of calcium levels in extracellular fluid; the hormone raises the concentrations of extracellular fluid calcium through combined actions in several organs (Fig. 3–1). Vitamin D maintains the day-to-day and week-to-week balance of calcium in the body (see Chapter 5). The actions of vitamin D and PTH are coordinated, and each hormone influences the production of the other.[1,2]

The daily maintenance of extracellular fluid calcium at a constant level is a major homeostatic challenge in terrestrial vertebrates because calcium losses in urine and intestinal juices may exceed intake for many hours each day. By contrast, regulation of calcium in blood and tissue fluids of marine animals presents a different environmental challenge inasmuch as the concentration of calcium in the environment exceeds that in extracellular fluid so that calcium disposal is the principal challenge and not the prevention of hypocalcemia.[3]

Parathyroid glands first appear in evolution in amphibians with the migration of vertebrates from an aqueous to a terrestrial existence.[4-6] Parathyroid glands and a chemical or biological substance equivalent to PTH have not been identified in fish, although a variety of lines of evidence indicate a role for pituitary factors (possible PTH homologues) and specialized organs in calcium homeostasis in fish.[6]

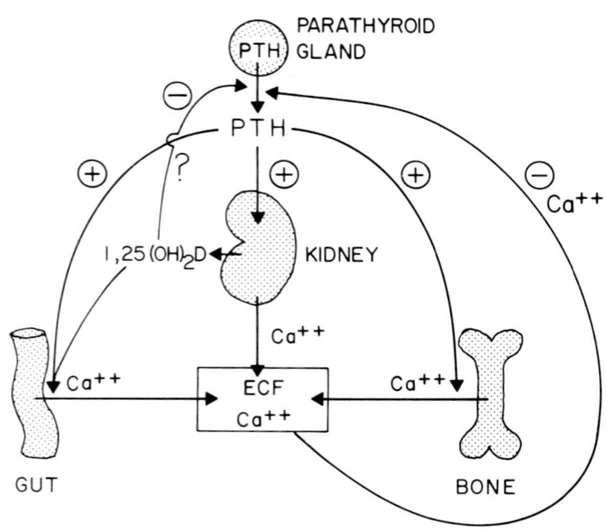

Figure 3–1. Negative feedback regulation of parathyroid hormone (PTH) secretion. Principal action of hormone is to raise calcium levels in extracellular fluid (ECF) by increasing renal tubular resorption of calcium, mobilizing calcium from bone, and increasing intestinal (gut) calcium absorption. Actions of bone and kidney are mediated directly through interactions with specific receptors. Action on gut is indirectly mediated by 1,25-dihydroxyvitamin D [1,25-$(OH)_2D$], whose synthesis in the kidney is stimulated by PTH. Extracellular calcium feeds back on parathyroid gland to inhibit further secretion of hormone. Short feedback loop involving 1,25$(OH)_2D$ has been suggested but not substantiated.

The coordinated actions of PTH on bone, kidney, and intestine increase the flow of calcium into the extracellular fluid and increase the concentration of calcium in blood.[7-10] The production of PTH is stimulated by a decrease in blood calcium, and conversely, the secretion of the hormone is inhibited by an increase in serum calcium[11] (Fig. 3–1). The biological actions of PTH and the negative feedback regulation of its production are the most important homeostatic mechanisms for the control of the concentration of calcium in extracellular fluid (Fig. 3–1).

Two rapid actions of PTH that regulate extracellular fluid calcium are increased release of calcium from bone and reduced renal clearance of calcium; these actions are central to calcium homeostasis. The third action of PTH on calcium homeostasis is the enhancement of intestinal calcium absorption indirectly through the activation of vitamin D.[1] Although physiologically important, this action affects day-by-day calcium balance rather than minute-to-minute or hour-to-hour calcium homeostasis.

It is difficult to analyze quantitatively or to contrast proportionately the relative physiologic importance of the actions of PTH on its three principal target tissues, kidney, bone, and intestine. The actions of the hormone are mediated through surface receptors and secondary messengers in specific and highly specialized cells. The complexity of bone as a tissue and the many pathways available for the exchange of calcium between the skeleton and the extracellular fluid have made the action of PTH on the skeleton particularly difficult to analyze.[7,10,12] The physical state of calcium as it exists in blood is complex; much of the calcium is present as chelates and/or bound to plasma proteins.[13] It is difficult to calculate renal clearances of calcium accurately because actual filtered loads of calcium depend on the ratio of free and bound forms of calcium.

The nature of a well-regulated homeostatic system is evident in calcium homeostasis.[1,2] Continual adjustments occur through constant, rapid changes in the rate of PTH secretion and action so that calcium, the controlled variable, remains relatively constant. Experimentally it is difficult to detect the small changes in calcium levels that are continually corrected.[12]

Parathyroid hormone also has important effects on the metabolism of inorganic phosphate.[8] From a teleologic viewpoint, the action of the hormone on phosphate metabolism is best understood as a secondary rather than homeostatic action. Phosphate is abundant in the food chain in terrestrial existence.[1,3] Unlike calcium deficiency, in the absence of renal dysfunction phosphate deficiency is unlikely to be an environmental challenge. Whenever calcium is released by dissolution of bone, phosphate is liberated simultaneously. A high blood phosphate *per se* tends to lower calcium concentration by multiple actions. Therefore, it is beneficial to eliminate in the urine the phosphate mobilized from bone while conserving the released calcium. A rise in both blood calcium (desirable homeostatically) and phosphate (undesirable) that would otherwise occur after bone dissolution is modified by the divergent actions of the hormone on the handling of the two mineral ions in the renal tubule.

The role of PTH on phosphate metabolism is not homeostatic. Phosphate ion itself, unlike calcium ion, has no effect on PTH secretion *per se*. The subsequent section reviews the direct actions of PTH on the kidney and the bone and indirect actions on the intestine, mediated through vitamin D action.

Over the past two decades, considerable advances have occurred in the techniques of polypeptide chemistry and molecular biology. These advances have led to determination of the structures of the hormonal polypeptide and the PTH gene. The work has involved the hormones from bovine, porcine, and rat origin as well as human PTH.[14-19] Multiple fragments and analogues of PTH have been chemically synthesized and used to define the region of the polypeptide required for biological activity, a sequence of some 25 residues at the amino terminus of the molecule.[20,21] Systematic structure/activity studies of the hormone have led to the design of competitive inhibitors of PTH action. The inhibitors are analogues based on the amino-terminal third of the hormone derived by progressive shortening of the sequence at the amino terminus of the molecule through removal of the first two to six amino-terminal amino acids.[22,23] The antagonists, although not yet of sufficient biological potency to be clinically useful, do inhibit the renal and certain skeletal actions of PTH and thus are useful tools for investigation of initial steps in hormone action.[23,24]

New reagents and new techniques derived from the study of the chemistry of PTH have been useful in advancing knowledge of the overall biology of the hormone's actions. The confusing heterogeneity of circulating forms of PTH, attributable to intraglandular and peripheral degradation of the native polypeptide into several fragments, has been thoroughly analyzed by several techniques including the use of antisera that recognize specific parts of the PTH sequence. The region-specific antibodies used to define the nature of circulating fragments were derived through use of peptide fragments representing discrete regions of the amino-terminal, middle, or carboxyl-terminal region of the hormone.[25-27] Recent studies have led to the conclusion that these intraglandular and peripheral degradations of PTH are not associated with the generation of biologically active, circulating fragments but rather represent catabolic hormone metabolism, exclusively a process of removal of hormone from the circulation and tissue fluids.[28] The knowledge that there is only one active molecular species of hormone in the circulation, the secreted intact polypeptide, is useful in design of radioimmunoassays that measure the physiologically and clinically relevant circulating forms of the hormone; assays that measure amino-terminal fragments separately now seem unnecessary.

Much has been learned in recent years about the nature of the hormone-receptor interaction characteristic of polypeptide hormones and the methods of signal transduction, whereby hormone-receptor interactions generate second messengers that accomplish cell-specific hormonal responses.[29,30] Parathyroid hormone has been shown to affect target cells through a receptor–guanyl nucleotide-binding protein–adenylate cyclase–cyclic AMP-dependent–kinase system.[29,31] In addition to this well-studied system of PTH signal transduction, recent studies have implicated the polyphosphoinositol second messenger system as a potential alternative pathway of hormone action.[32] The interesting question of different intracellular pathways or even different receptors in the overall mode of action of PTH is now being studied in a variety of *in vitro* systems[29,31] including the use of photo-affinity-labeled radioactive ligands[33] prepared from synthetic PTH fragments to aid efforts at purification and eventual cloning of the PTH receptors(s). Detailed analysis of the metabolism and mechanism of action of PTH and the implications of these findings for further fundamental and clinical investigations of PTH physiology and pathophysiology are reviewed in subsequent sections (VI and III).

Cloning of the DNA complementary in sequence to the messenger RNA of bovine PTH led to the determination of the nucleotide sequence of the coding portion of the parathyroid gene; this represented the initial impact of molecular biology on research on PTH.[34] There has subsequently been a great acceleration in knowledge of intracellular events in the parathyroid cell of humans and other species. Cloning of the bovine PTH cDNA was rapidly followed by cloning and structural analysis of the cDNA for human PTH and then identification and structural analysis of the complete gene for bovine, rat, and human PTH.[34-37] The techniques of molecular biology have then been applicable to analysis of the regulation of transcription and translation of the parathyroid gene that complemented earlier studies using classic techniques during incubations of parathyroid tissue *in vitro* to analyze the processes of biosynthesis of the hormone.[38] The control of PTH gene expression, the intracellular events in hormone processing and transport, and the regulation of secretion of the final glandular product, PTH, have all been studied extensively with the powerful techniques of molecular and cell biology leading to great advances in understanding the processes of biosynthesis and cellular transport of the hormone and the overall regulation of hormone biosyntheses and secretion as reviewed in detail in sections IV and V.

I. PHYSIOLOGY

A. Renal Actions

The actions of PTH on renal clearance of calcium and phosphate are the principal and homeostatically important metabolic actions of the hormone. As reviewed in Chapter 7, the hormone, however, has multiple effects on the kidney, affecting transtubular transport of sodium, potassium, bicarbonate, hydrogen ion, amino acids, glucose, cyclic AMP, calcium, and phosphate. Effects on magnesium transport in the kidney have also been demonstrated, but the direction of the effects varies.[8]

The actions of PTH on renal calcium clearance are homeostatic, but the actions on phosphate clearance are not homeostatic, although the effects of PTH on phosphate are of considerable physiologic significance in phosphate metabolism. The bulk of renal phosphate reabsorption occurs in the proximal tubule. Parathyroid hormone exerts its strongest phosphaturic actions at proximal tubular sites by direct inhibition of phosphate reabsorption through a resetting of the tubular maximum for phosphate reabsorption.[8,39] There is an additional distal tubular site(s) that is important also in overall PTH-mediated phosphate clearance.[40] In studies in dogs, Agus et al.[41] advanced the thesis that phosphate as well as calcium reabsorption in the proximal tubule is closely related to sodium transport. Studies on the kidney were interpreted to show proportionate inhibition of sodium (and calcium) reabsorption with an even greater inhibition of reabsorption of phosphate induced by PTH. Sodium rejected at the proximal tubule is reabsorbed distally but phosphate is not, leading to brisk phosphaturia. The role of the hormone in blocking distal reabsorption of phosphate was not emphasized by Agus et al.,[41] but distal action has been stressed by Knox and Lechene.[42]

The studies of Goldberg and associates,[41] as well as those of Knox and Lechene[42] and Knox et al.,[43] have clarified several aspects of interaction between volume expansion, sodium diuresis, and PTH action at both the proximal and distal tubules with regard to phosphate reabsorption. Evidence has been accumulated that the action of PTH on the proximal tubule in which inhibition of phosphate reabsorption occurs can be simulated by volume expansion or saline infusion; the magnitude of the phosphaturia caused by PTH, however, is much greater than that seen with saline infusion alone. The action of PTH on phosphate reabsorption in the proximal tubule involves inhibition of carbonic anhydrase. Other findings suggest that the greatest effect on blockade of phosphate reabsorption occurs in the distal tubule and is uninfluenced by saline infusion, volume expansion, or inhibition of carbonic anhydrase; in this view, the distal tubular locus of action is the most important overall in bringing about' phosphaturia.

It is known that most calcium reabsorption occurs in proximal tubular sites closely linked to sodium reabsorption. The overall handling of calcium by different portions of the nephron and, in particular, the anatomic site in which net calcium reabsorption actually occurs have been studied extensively.[44,45] Renal reabsorption of calcium parallels that of sodium.[46,47] The actions of PTH on distal tubular sites for calcium reabsorption are, however, the homeostatically important actions. If 7 to 10 g of calcium are filtered daily, an increase in the tubular reabsorption from 95% to 98%, as can be shown to occur under the influence of PTH action on distal tubular sites, can return an additional 200 or 300 mg of calcium to the extracellular fluid. This quantity of calcium is as large as one third of the total extracellular fluid calcium concentration and is of considerable homeostatic significance.[6-9]

These actions of PTH on renal calcium and phosphate reabsorption are mediated through a relatively small number of cells in anatomically discrete regions of the proximal and distal tubules.[48,49] The actions involve stimulation of intracellular cAMP and perhaps other second messengers as well, after interaction of the hormone with surface receptors. The details of the biochemical mechanisms of PTH action are discussed in section IV.

The effects of PTH that can be demonstrated acutely on electrolyte transport, bicarbonate reabsorption, and the transtubular transport of glucose and amino acids do not, in health, affect total body balances of sodium, potassium, nitrogen, or glucose, nor do they affect acid-base balance. The effects are either minor at physiologic concentrations of hormone or are readily overcome by homeostatic mechanisms such as those concerned with sodium and potassium balance or glucose homeostasis. Protracted excess of PTH, however, as occurs in primary hyperparathyroidism, can result in systemic acidosis through excessive bicarbonate wasting. In hyperparathyroidism, an acquired form of renal tubular acidosis of the proximal type often occurs. There is considerable retention of hydrogen ions secondary to bicarbonate diuresis, and chloride reabsorption exceeds sodium reabsorption.[39]

The other important renal physiologic action of PTH does not result in any direct action of the hormone on mineral ion metabolism in the kidney, but rather acts secondarily through later effects in the intestine. 1,25-Dihydroxyvitamin D ($1{,}25(OH)_2D$) produced in the kidney in response to PTH is the principal regulator of intestinal calcium absorption. Although many details of the control of production of $1,25(OH)_2D$, the active metabolite of vitamin D, remain unresolved, the pathways of the physiologic regulation of vitamin D metabolism are now well understood. The action of PTH is prominent among the known physiologic influences on the production of $1,25(OH)_2D$. The hormone stimulates the activity of the renal enzyme $25(OH)_2D$ 1α-hydroxylase in specific cells in the proximal tubule.[50] The 1α-hydroxylase converts the inactive substrate 25(OH)D to the active dihydroxylated metabolite. An increase in intrarenal and circulating levels of $1,25(OH)_2D$ after administration of PTH requires a few hours to become manifest. The precise relationship between the stimulation of phosphate transport and the stimulation of $1,25(OH)_2D$ production regarding cell types, receptors, and second messengers remains unclarified. Parathyroid hormone is by no means the sole regulator of the production of $1,25(OH)_2D$. Many other factors exert an influence on $1,25(OH)_2D$ formation including phosphate itself, independently of PTH. Hypophosphatemia, total body phosphorus depletion from whatever cause, or both stimulate, and hyperphosphatemia and increased tissue stores of phosphate suppress, $1,25(OH)_2D$ production. Nonetheless, in normal health with adequate nutritional intake and renal function, PTH exerts the principal physiologic regulation of $1,25(OH)_2D$ production.

B. Skeletal Actions

Several physiologically significant actions of PTH on bone have been elucidated employing multiple approaches *in vivo* and *in vitro*. Many models have been proposed and analyzed in an attempt to provide an integrative formulation of the actions of the hormone on bone.[7,10,51-54] The physiologic significance of the actions of PTH on bone comes from the important role of the hormone in preserving extracellular fluid calcium homeostasis and not the homeostasis of bone *per se*. The hormone transfers calcium and phosphate from bone to the blood by at least two distinguishable, separate mechanisms using bone as a buffer for extracellular fluid calcium maintenance. The actions of the hormone on bone, however, are inherently difficult to analyze in a temporally coherent manner whereby initial steps in hormone action can be causally related to subsequent biochemical and then physiologic events. This difficulty is largely due to the complex organization of bone as a tissue; several different cell types and a variety of patterns of tissue organization are characteristic of bone. Highly specialized cells cover bone surfaces and constitute an equivalent of a membrane lining.[10] In the interior of most bones, highly porous bone is found, consisting of interlocking spicules surrounded by marrow cells (trabecular bone), and, nearer the bone surface, a layer of dense, crystalline bone with fewer cells (cortical bone). Stimulation of bone as a tissue is a cellular response that involves complex interactions among functionally different yet interconnected cell types. The growth, development, and homeostasis of bone as a tissue involve multiple extrinsic and intrinsic coordinating factors.

Parathyroid hormone acts on certain of these cells to increase the flow of mineral ions from bone into blood. The actions of the hormone are geared to the physiologic regulation of calcium homeostasis and may perturb skeletal homeostasis. The multiple factors and cellular responses that preserve skeletal homeostasis may then counteract the original effects caused by PTH.[51] These considerations explain the difficulties in understanding the skeletal physiologic actions of PTH in precise terms.

Many *in vitro* approaches have used embryonic bone preparations in tissue culture.[7] Hormone actions can be analyzed readily, but the results are difficult to relate to the physiologic milieu *in vivo*. Responses to PTH have also been analyzed *in vivo* in humans and in several animal species.[10,54] Radioactive calcium, such as ^{45}Ca, is administered at varying times prior to administration of PTH to analyze changes in concentration of ^{45}Ca, as well as changes in total calcium during PTH-driven bone resorption. Exchanges of calcium between extracellular fluid and bone can only be described by a number of kinetic constants; the multiplicity of exchange rates of calcium reflects the complex organization of bone mineral in various sites (surface versus interior) and physical states (loosely adsorbed versus highly crystalline).[10,54]

Traditionally, osteoclasts are the cell type believed to mediate the bone-resorptive effect of the hormone.[54] Greater attention, however, is now paid to cell types in bone other than osteoclasts that respond more rapidly (less than an hour).[54] Osteoblasts, but not osteoclasts, possess receptors for PTH.[7,51,55-58] Thus, although an increase in the numbers of osteoclasts and their individual cellular activity explains much of the bone-resorbing activity of PTH, the effects on osteoclasts must be indirect and mediated through osteoblasts. Changes in osteoclast morphologic features, however, can be detected within an hour, and increased numbers of osteoclasts in response to PTH action become evident within hours.[52]

An important cellular effect of PTH on bone, not often emphasized, with respect to the maintenance of serum calcium homeostasis, is the rapid effect on a different population of hormonally responsive cells that line bone surfaces, particularly the endosteal surfaces of long bones. This action may be particularly important for calcium homeostasis.[10] Within 5 minutes after injection of PTH, bone lining cells undergo structural changes indicative of increased cellular activity.[10] These changes are also seen in osteocytes within deeper regions of bone connected with the surface by canaliculi.[10]

PTH raises calcium and phosphate levels in blood first through stimulatory effects of the hormone on cells lining endosteal surfaces and secondarily through indirect stimulation of the activity of osteoclasts.[54] The release of radiocalcium from surface pools of bone mineral can be detected (in experiments involving prior labeling of bone mineral) within less than an hour of administration of PTH. The later effect of administered hormone, detectable within several hours, is increased activity of osteoclasts, which causes resorption to occur from fully mineralized bone in the interior. (This effect is also detected by administering radiocalcium at times chosen to label primarily sites deep within bone.[10,54]) The amount of calcium mobilized increases as the numbers of osteoclasts also increase if high PTH levels are maintained for longer periods of time.[7,51,54] Both the early and later effects of PTH on bone (rapid changes in lining cells versus increased activity and number of osteoclasts) have been studied in various experimental systems, but the approaches used have not provided a comprehensive picture of the continuous spectrum of cellular changes responsible for calcium release from bone. Certain studies emphasize that the action of PTH on bone may differ as a function of variations in dose or form of hormone administration, continuous or intermittent.[7,51] Injection of large doses of PTH in dogs has been shown to lead to an initial hypocalcemia, and has been interpreted as a rapid inflow of calcium into bone cells in a manifestation of increased cellular permeability to calcium.[53] At present, it is difficult to deduce whether a single initial hormonal action on a single type of receptor present on lining cells and osteoblasts triggers a continuous chain of biochemical events that ultimately accounts for all the known physiologic actions of the hormone or whether several independent pathways are involved, using distinctive cell types and different secondary messengers within responsive cells.

Whatever the responsible cellular mechanisms, the skeletal actions of PTH provide a most effective homeostatic protection of serum calcium by continual modulation of bone calcium release to meet such physiologic challenges as overnight fasting or more serious and prolonged challenges, such as an extended period of severe nutritional deficiency, when renal and intestinal adaptive mechanisms are ineffective.

II. CHEMISTRY

The first biologically active extracts of parathyroid hormone from bovine glands were made by using hot 5% hydrochloric acid.[59] Further purification of the hormone was not achieved until much later, however, when Aurbach[60] and Rasmussen et al.[61] developed improved extraction procedures that eventually provided large quantities of relatively pure PTH. Subsequent efforts have led to the isolation and structural analysis of bovine, porcine, and human PTH. The bovine and porcine hormones were extracted and purified from parathyroid glands collected as a by-product of meat-packing centers.[59-65] The limited supplies of human tissue, however, required the development of special procedures for the extraction and purification of peptides to increase yields of the human hormone.[66] Isohormonal forms of bovine PTH were suspected to exist on the basis of fractions isolated during the final chromatography of extracts of parathyroid glands in urea.[65] However, only one hormonal form has been identified and characterized structurally in the bovine. The amino acid sequence of this major form of the bovine hormone and that of the porcine and human hormones was determined by the automated, sequential technique of Edman utilizing progressive, stepwise removal and identification of amino acids both from the amino termini of the intact polypeptides and from peptide fragments prepared by proteolytic digestions of PTH.[14-19] With the advent of recombinant DNA techniques that permit analysis of the nucleotide sequence of the coding portion of the genes for hormones and other proteins, protein sequences can be deduced from nucleotide sequence without requiring isolation of the protein *per se*. This approach has been used to provide the sequence of rat PTH.[19] The structures of the human and other mammalian molecules are shown in Figure 3–2*A*.

Nucleotide sequence analyses of the bovine and human PTH genes have confirmed the protein sequence of the hormones as our group had deduced them earlier from protein structural analysis.[34-36] Not shown in Figure 3–2 are the points of difference between our structural findings and those reported by Brewer and associates—glutamine rather than glutamic acid at position 22 in the bovine, porcine, and human hormones, and lysine and leucine rather than leucine and aspartic acid at positions 28 and 30, respectively, of the human hormone.[17,67] Despite extensive reinvestigation of the sequences by protein structural techniques,[67,68] no explanation for the discrepancy in results has been found. One theoretical explanation is the presence of isohormones in the bovine, porcine, and human species that contain the sequence differences proposed for each molecule by Brewer,[17,67] but as yet no isohormones with these structural features have been reported. Inasmuch as synthetic peptides used in parathyroid research today are based largely, if not exclusively, on the hormone sequences we reported, only these sequences are illustrated in Figure 3–2.

There is extensive sequence homology among the human, bovine, porcine, and rat hormones. The PTHs are single chain polypeptides of 84 amino acids, molecular weight approximately 9300, devoid of cysteine or substituted amino acid residues. There is a preponderance of basic residues conferring an overall positive charge to the molecule. The hormone has not been crystallized to permit analysis of secondary and tertiary structure by x-ray crystallography, but studies by circular dichroism[68] and models based on combined approaches[69] suggest the presence of some alpha-helix but extensive regions of random-coil with beta-turn structures. The middle portion of the molecule is quite hydrophobic and exhibits the greatest structural differences among species; this region is also the site of proteolytic attack in peripheral tissues as discussed in section VI. The amino acid sequence differences that are present account for the reduced reactivity of hormone from one species with antisera raised against hormone from a second species although all four forms of hormone can be detected in most radioimmunoassays. The sequence differences also account for differences in receptor affinity that partly explain the differing biological potency seen in assays *in vitro* using rat renal membrane receptors or *in vivo* with chicks (Table 3–1).

Recently, two groups have independently cloned the DNA for chicken PTH and deduced the structure of the protein based on the nucleotide sequence.[69a,b] Chicken PTH, perhaps not surprisingly in view of evolutionary distance, is the first PTH molecule to depart significantly from the basic pattern seen with the four mammalian hormones. Chicken PTH (Fig. 3–2*B*) has one deletion in the hydrophobic middle portions of the sequence and a large addition of sequence near the carbonyl-terminus. Nonetheless, there is intense homology in the amino-terminal region, associated with most known biological actions (Fig. 3–2*B*).

Also, a long sought hypercalcemic factor from squamous cell tumors has been cloned by three independent groups and the nucleotide sequence analyzed.[70a,b,c] The molecule, the product of a gene distinct from that for parathyroid hormone (located on a different chromosome), is both homologous to PTH and quite distinctive. The tumor factor is considerably larger than that of PTH, and most of the molecule bears little resemblance to PTH (Fig. 3–2*C*). Nine of the first 13 residues are identical, however, in the two polypeptides (Fig. 3–2*D*). There appears to be overall conformational homology within the first 34 residues (Fig. 3–2*C*). Both molecules bind to the same receptor, and even the sequence region 14–34 of either molecule can substiture for the other, as deduced from studies with synthetic fragments.[70d,e] The

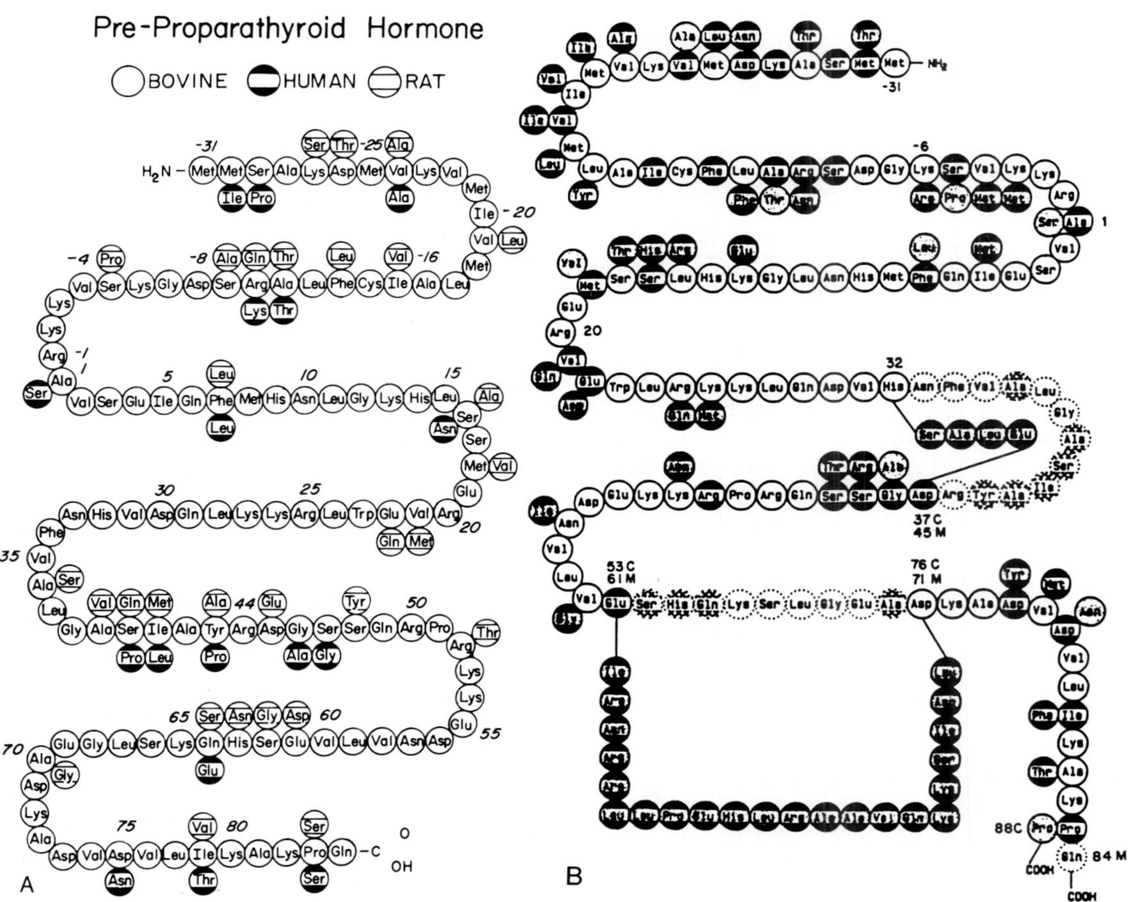

Figure 3–2. *A,* Preproparathyroid hormone. Amino acid sequences of bovine, rat, and human proteins. Differences among sequences are noted by the use of a different circle symbol opposite the residue in the bovine backbone, where sequence change is noted. (From Rosenblatt M, Kronenberg HM, Potts JT Jr: Parathyroid hormone: Physiology, chemistry, biosynthesis, secretion, metabolism and mode of action. *In* DeGroot LJ (ed): Endocrinology. Philadelphia, WB Saunders, 1989, pp 848–891.) *B,* Comparison of predicted chicken preproPTH amino acid sequence with those of the mammalian preproPTH hormones. The sequence of bovine preproPTH is shown in circles. A barred or hatched circle indicates a position at which the amino acid varies among the mammalian hormones (human, bovine, porcine, and rat); open circles indicate invariant mammalian residues. Stippled circles indicate sites where the sequence of chicken preproPTH is different from the bovine sequence but identical to that of one of the other mammalian hormones. Barred stippled circles indicate an amino acid unique to chicken preproPTH. Dotted circles represent amino acids that have apparently been deleted in the chicken sequence and replaced by unique peptides, which are joined to the rest of the sequence by lines. The first residue of mature PTH: M and C after numbers refer to the mammalian and chicken sequences, respectively. (From Khosla S, Demay M, Pines M, et al: J Bone Mineral Res 3:689–698, 1988.)

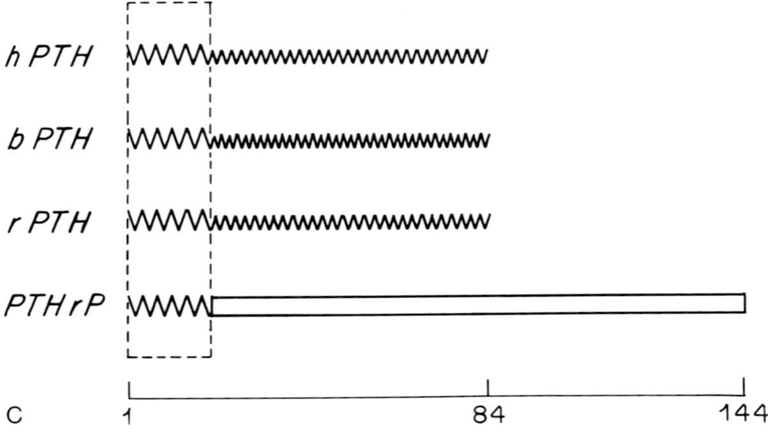

Comparison of PTH/PTHγP Sequence

1				5					10					15
H-ALA	VAL	SER	GLU	ILEU	GLN	LEU	MET	HIS	ASN	LEU	GLY	LYS	HIS	LEU
-	-	-	-	HIS	-	-	LEU	-	ASP	LYS	-	-	SER	ILEU
				20					25					30
ASN	SER	MET	GLU	ARG	VAL	GLU	TRP	LEU	ARG	LYS	LYS	LEU	GLN	ASP
GLN	ASP	LEU	ARG	-	ARG	PHE	PHE	-	HIS	HIS	LEU	ILE	ALA	GLU

D

Figure 3–2 *Continued C,* Schematic illustrating the comparative structures of the parathyroid hormone–related peptide and the mammalian parathyroid hormones. The regions of sequence homology are limited to the amino terminus of the molecule. The PTHrP peptide is much longer than the parathyroid hormone and does not have (hatched box) sequence homology beyond the limited region at the amino terminus (hatched box). *D,* Comparison of sequence of amino-terminal residues in bovine PTH (upper line) and PTHγP (lower line) over the region of sequence, position 1–30. Dash indicates identity; where PTHγP differs, the PTHγP residue is indicated (underlined sequence changes are those involving a difference in net charge).

Table 3–1. Comparison of Biological Activity of Parathyroid Peptides from Different Species

Peptide	Potency, MRC U/mg* In Vitro *Rat Renal Adenyl Cyclase Assay*	In Vivo *Chick Hypercalcemia Assay*
Native hormones		
Bovine 1–84	3000 (2500–4000)	2500 (2100–4000)
Porcine 1–84	1000 (850–1250)	4800 (3300–7000)
Human 1–84	350 (275–425)	10,000 (9060–13,400)
Synthetic fragments		
Bovine 1–34	5400 (3900–8000)	7700 (5200–11,100)
Human 1–34	1700 (1400–2150)	7400 (5200–9700)
[Ala^1]–Human 1–34	4300 (3400–5400)	—

*Values expressed as mean potency with 95% confidence limits, based on Medical Research Council research standard A for parathyroid hormone.[89] Data from Tregear et al.,[21] Keutmann et al.,[19] and Parsons et al.[116] Reprinted, by permission, from Rosenblatt M, Kronenberg HM, Potts JT Jr: *In* DeGroot L (ed): Endocrinology. Philadelphia, WB Saunders, 1989, pp 848–891.

physiologic role of the tumor peptide, produced normally by skin cells and other epithelial cells, is unknown, as is the question of use of receptors other than the PTH receptor by regions of the molecule that are nonhomologous with PTH. Evidence has been presented that the new factor, which may have endocrine or paracrine functions in normal physiology, influences placental calcium transport in sheep and milk production in the mammary gland.[70f,g]

In the following sections we summarize the extensive data on the biologically active regions of PTH and the related tumor product often referred to as PTHγP (PTH-related peptide) derived from synthesis of numerous fragments and analogues of the hormonal structures shown in Figure 3–2, particularly from the amino-terminal portion of the hormone that contains a minimum sequence sufficient for expression of biological activity.[70]

III. MECHANISM OF ACTION

The expression of peptide hormone action occurs through biochemical events initially involving binding to receptors on the surface of target cells. Parathyroid hormone interacts with hormone-specific receptors on the plasma membrane of renal tubular and bone cells. This specific interaction with receptors initiates a cascade of intracellular events including the generation of cAMP, phosphorylation of specific intracellular proteins by activated kinases, intracellular entry of calcium, stimulation of the polyphosphoinositol pathway, and activation of intracellular enzymes, transport systems, and secretion of lysosomal enzymes, and so on, that contribute to, or cause directly, a full spectrum of intracellular and extracellular metabolic consequences.[29,71-76]

Certain biologically active polypeptides have been shown to enter cells.[77,79] It is not clear whether any biological actions of peptide hormones are dependent upon intracellular entry or whether cellular uptake of hormone is simply related to hormone degradation and receptor recycling. Entry of PTH into cells has not yet been reported. Current views of the mode of action of PTH are based on the concept that the single initiating event in the expression of bioactivity is interaction of the hormone with cell surface receptors.

Multiple, complex biological actions result from the binding of peptides to receptors, and the understanding of the multiple actions of hormones presents a most difficult challenge. Many important issues related to PTH action remain to be answered. It is not known whether the specific receptors on different target tissues, such as bone and kidney, are identical or distinctive in structure or requirements for binding, or both. Differences in potency between a hormone analogue and the native peptide in responses on two different target tissues could reflect differences in binding affinity of the two peptides to receptors that are different although related structurally and functionally in the two tissues (as is known with adrenergic[80] or opiate receptors).[81]

A. Sequential Steps in Hormone Action

Models of peptide hormone action that have been developed in several endocrine systems appear to be relevant to mechanisms of PTH actions.[29,82]

1. The Receptor–Adenylate Cyclase Complex

Details of the hormone-receptor–nucleotide regulatory protein–adenylate cyclase model have been reviewed extensively.[29,82-87] (Fig. 3–3). Hormone-sensitive adenylate cyclase is composed of at least three proteins: a membrane surface receptor (R); a guanyl nucleotide–binding protein (N); and a catalytic protein (C) that is the enzyme adenylate cyclase located on the cytoplasmic side of the membrane. Some of these proteins, in turn, are themselves composed of subunits.

Binding of hormone leads to clustering of receptors in clathrin-lined coated pits.[88] The key to linkage between the receptor and the stimulation of adenylate cyclase is a multisubunit protein termed guanyl nucleotide regulatory protein. Adenylate cyclase by itself is relatively inactive. When hormone binds to receptor, a ternary complex involving hormone, receptor, and guanyl nucleotide regulatory protein forms (Fig. 3–3). The key to activation of adenylate cyclase by the receptor rests with the nucleotide regulatory component (stimulatory form) (N_s). Although PTH was originally thought to act exclusively

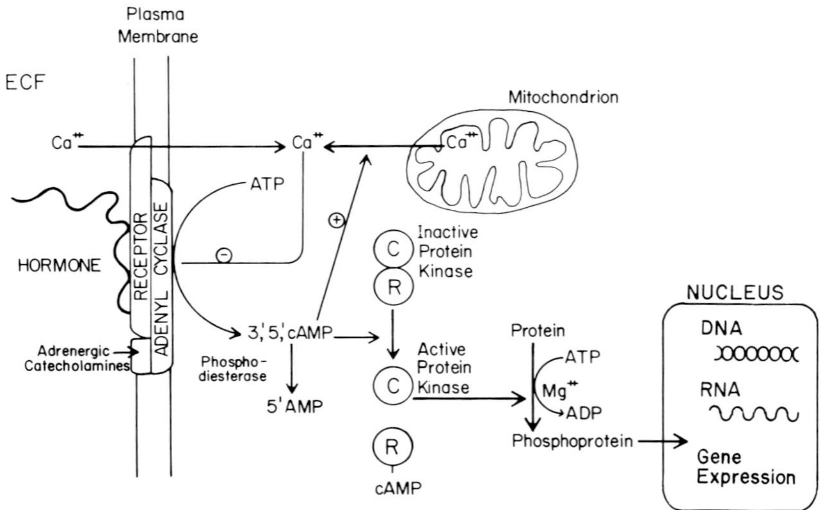

Figure 3–3. Hormone receptor and transducer system present in target cell plasma membranes illustrating the adenyl cyclase and protein kinase A pathway, a principal but probably not sole pathway of PTH action. Hormone interacts with cell surface membrane receptor. (See text for discussion of subsequent events involving adenylate cyclase and its nucleotide regulatory subunit.)

through the N_s system, there is an analogous but distinctive set of guanyl nucleotide–binding proteins to N_s present in many cells including inhibitory guanyl nucleotide regulatory protein, termed N_i.[76] N_i inhibits rather than stimulates adenylate cyclase activity after hormonal interaction with receptor. Therefore, in some cells, certain hormones (acting through their receptors) can increase cAMP levels, whereas other hormones can decrease cAMP levels via the same set of adenylate cyclase molecules, thus providing counterregulation or fine-tuning of intracellular metabolic events (Fig. 3–3).

With PTH, growing evidence for participation by the polyphosphoinositol pathway as an alternate or coordinate second messenger with cyclic AMP implies the participation of a distinctive G protein or N unit that couples the PTH-bound receptor to the phospholipase c/polyphosphoinositol/diacyglycerol and inositol triphosphate pathway of hormone mediation.[127-133]

Although many details of the system described have not yet been confirmed for PTH-sensitive adenylate cyclase in hormonally responsive target cells, research compiled from several laboratories provides evidence consistent with the overall model of cyclase-dependent hormone action for some PTH actions. Guanyl nucleotides such as the nonhydrolyzable GTP analogue Gpp(NH)p increase stimulation of adenylate cyclase in renal membranes by given doses of PTH.[29,71-76] In addition, Gpp(NH)p added to PTH-responsive renal membranes produces a stable, irreversible (holocatalytic) state of adenylate cyclase activation that cannot be inhibited by the addition of a synthetic PTH antagonist once enzyme activation occurs.[72,73]

Guanyl nucleotides also affect the efficiency of the hormone-receptor interaction that is transduced into adenylate cyclase activation. Analogues of PTH that are weak or partial agonists can be converted into highly active compounds in the presence of Gpp(NH)p. Analogues of PTH such as [desamino-Ala-1]bPTH–(1–34), which is nearly inactive in the renal membrane adenylate cyclase assay yet inhibits stimulation of adenylate cyclase by native PTH *in vitro*, can be converted into a hormone agonist *in vitro* by adding Gpp(NH)p to the assay system, thus paralleling the biological properties displayed by this analogue *in vivo*.[89] The dissociation of PTH agonist from binding to receptor sites in canine renal membranes is also facilitated by the presence of Gpp(NH)p.

Certain disease states occur as a consequence of defective receptors and provide an understanding of basic physiology. Pseudohypoparathyroidism, a disease in which the clinical manifestations are those of hypoparathyroidism, is caused by receptors that are unresponsive to biologically active PTH.[29] Hormone production is actually increased in pseudohypoparathyroidism. After administration of bioactive PTH to most patients with pseudohypoparathyroidism, no increases in urinary cAMP or mineral ion transport occur.[90] The genetic defect in these patients could lie in the receptor, in any of the subunits of the guanyl nucleotide regulatory protein, or in adenylate cyclase. Assays have been developed to measure the content and functionality of the guanyl nucleotide regulatory subunit N_s in erythrocyte membranes of normal subjects and those with pseudohypoparathyroidism. These studies reveal an average 50% reduction in N_s units in patients with the principal form of pseudohypoparathyroidism;[90] the findings point to one locus of the defective response to hormone in this disease, although several types of defects may coexist.

2. Hormone Receptors

The membrane receptor for PTH present in target tissues has been characterized indirectly by the traditional methods of competitive hormone binding and saturation analysis using hormone analogues that are agonists and antagonists. Photoaffinity labeling techniques have also been applied to analyses of the physiochemical properties of the receptor. Several different types of biologically active, highly characterized PTH analogues have been used to photoaffinity-label the PTH receptor.[91,91a-d] A single membrane component with a molecular weight of approximately 80,000 was identified.[91] The receptor present in intact cells derived from human giant cell tumors and the receptor present in human skin fibroblasts appear to be identical in molecular size to the canine renal receptor identified in fragmented membranes.[33] Parathyroid hormone receptors have also been identified on cells not conventionally regarded as derived from target tissues, such as mononuclear leukocytes[92,93] and human dermal fibroblasts.[33]

It remains unknown whether more than one form of PTH receptor is required to mediate the several specific actions of the hormone. There are as yet few firm data pointing to the existence of biochemically different receptors, but rather the evidence suggests that receptors in different target tissues are indistinguishable. Analogues of PTH have been evaluated in multiple *in vitro* and *in vivo* bioassays.[94] Both renal and skeletal-based assays reveal closely similar requirements for binding to and activation of PTH receptors. Convincing evidence for a single PTH receptor type comes from the findings that a PTH antagonist analogue effective *in vivo*, which works by competitively occupying PTH receptors, antagonizes each of the major *in vivo* parameters of PTH action: the calcemic,[23] nephrogenous cyclase,[24] and phosphaturic responses.[24]

However, one line of evidence contrary to the single receptor type hypothesis has been obtained.[94-97] This work, using native and oxidized forms of the hormone, indicates that the calcium-"preserving" actions of the hormone may be mediated by different receptors or reside within structural determinants of the PTH molecule different from those required for activation of adenylate cyclase and for phosphaturic responses. Bovine PTH, oxidized under mild conditions to generate the methionine sulfoxide form of the two methionines present in the native sequence, loses considerable activity in stimulating the excretion of urinary phosphate in the rat and activating adenylate cyclase in Japanese quail kidney membranes.[95,96] This oxidized hormone, however, still produces a hypercalcemic response in the quail, produces a hypocalciuric response in the rat, and, in quail, activates the renal 25-hydroxyvitamin D_3 1-hydroxylase and suppresses the 25-hydroxyvitamin D_3 24-hydroxylase enzymes. These studies imply the existence of more than one functional type of PTH receptor (although in some cases effects attributable to differences in animal species cannot be excluded).[98,99] The establishment of functionally distinguishable PTH receptors for different hormonal responses will require additional studies.

3. Postreceptor Cellular Responses to PTH Action

Responsive tissues may become less responsive to hormone as a result of prolonged or repeated exposure to hormone, or even a single short exposure to a large dose of hormone (tachyphylaxis). It has been shown that a decline in the number of available receptors in target tissues is responsible for the reduced sensitivity; the process is termed down-regulation. This reduction in receptor number has been shown after PTH stimulation of cells derived from human giant cell tumors of bone and canine kidney.[100-102]

Enhanced responsiveness to PTH due to increased numbers of PTH receptors can also occur. Several studies have demonstrated increased response to PTH in rat osteosarcoma cells after prior exposure to glucocorticoids.[55,103,104] An increase in number of PTH receptors on cell surfaces may occur; alternatively, the result may stem from a glucocorticoid-mediated change in the effector (guanyl nucleotide regulatory protein plus adenylate cyclase) system or an increased coupling of receptors to the effector system.

It seems likely, but has yet to be shown definitely for PTH, that the modulation of numbers of receptors may be physiologically important in hormone action and not merely a phenomenon seen only in response to pharmacologic doses of hormone.

The renal and skeletal actions of PTH have long been linked with cAMP as a second messenger.[31,105-110] Infusion of PTH increases intracellular cAMP in renal cells *in vitro*,[111,112] and excess cellular cAMP appears in the urine *in vivo*.[31,113] Cyclic AMP levels increase before hormonal metabolic effects such as phosphaturia.[31,114] An additional indication for a role of cAMP as a mediator of PTH action in the kidney is the close correlation between the potency of PTH analogues *in vivo* and their potency in an *in vitro* cell-free adenylate cyclase assay containing renal cortical plasma membranes.[115-117] Furthermore, the stable cAMP analogue dibutyryl cAMP causes PTH-like effects on the kidney.[118,119]

Parathyroid hormone stimulates adenylate cyclase at several distinct locations along the nephron as shown by micropuncture and cytochemical studies.[48,49,120,121] These PTH-responsive sites are observed predominantly in portions of the nephron that lie within the renal cortex and hence differ in location from the adenylate cyclases that are stimulated by calcitonin, vasopressin, or catecholamines.[121,123] The PTH-stimulated adenylate cyclase activity is located at the basolateral portion (anteluminal surface) of renal tubular cells, whereas the intracellular receptor proteins for cAMP are in the luminal brush border of these cells. Presumably the cAMP generated by PTH stimulation at the basolateral border of the cell migrates through the cytoplasm to activate membrane components in the brush border responsible for altered mineral ion transport.[124] For example, PTH increases the activity of the sodium-calcium exchanger in renal cortical sites.[125]

Evidence for second messengers other than cAMP have been reported to be involved in PTH action. Parathyroid hormone stimulates intracellular levels of calcium in renal cells *in vitro* without clearly involving cAMP.[126] The increased levels of intracellular calcium stimulate specific cellular responses by several mechanisms. Parathyroid hormone stimulates polyphosphoinositol metabolism by a second messenger system that utilizes diacylglycerol and the polyphosphoinositide 1,4,5-triphosphate (IP_3).[127-133] These mediators have a distinctive set of intracellular responses that might be involved in PTH action, although less is known about this pathway than about the cAMP-mediated responses.

The cytochemical assay detects the response of renal tissue to PTH as measured by several biochemical changes including enhancement of glucose-6-phosphate dehydrogenase activity and production of citrate.[305-307] The changes occur before cAMP levels are detectably increased, but adenylate cyclase activity can be demonstrated in the same tissue slices by using larger doses of PTH.[49,120,121] Hence, it is possible that cAMP is the mediator, but a rise in the nucleotide cannot be detected against a relatively high background of basal production.

Studies *in vitro* have demonstrated that exposure of bone-derived (osteosarcoma) cells to PTH at concentrations comparable to that found normally in the circulation causes increased levels of intracellular cAMP.[106] Exposure of skeletal tissue *in vitro* to dibutyryl cAMP results in biological effects that parallel stimulation of PTH.[107,108] Administration of dibutyryl cAMP *in vivo* elevates serum calcium levels as a result of the skeletal release of calcium.[109,110] Stimulation of synthesis and release of lysosomal enzymes thought to be essential for bone resorption by PTH also occurs after exposure of bone to dibutyryl cAMP.[134] These observations clearly implicate cAMP as the mediator of many of the skeletal actions of PTH.

Subsequent to the increased production of cAMP, elevation of intracellular calcium levels, or increased polyphosphoinositol mediators, the next step in the action of peptide hormones is believed to be the activation of any of several protein kinases, including cAMP-dependent kinase and protein kinase C.[126,135,136] Parathyroid hormone increases the activity of cAMP-dependent kinase in giant cell tumors of human bone.[137] Both the kinase and adenylate cyclase responses are completely abolished when PTH is added in the presence of a synthetic PTH antagonist, [N1e-8, N1e-18, Tyr-34]bPTH–(3–34)amide. Three endogenous substrates were found for the cAMP-dependent phosphokinase: phosphoproteins of molecular weights (daltons) 55,000, 43,000, and 38,000 increase their level of phosphorylation by 30%. Dephosphorylation of two proteins of molecular weights (daltons) 200,000 and 120,000 also occurs. These studies indicate that PTH action in bone may be mediated by the phosphorylation of specific substrates. Stimulation by PTH of endogenous protein phosphorylation in cAMP-dependent fashion has also been demonstrated in renal tissue. The chemical nature and biological role of these protein substrates of PTH-stimulated cAMP-dependent phosphorylation in the cellular expression of PTH action remain to be elucidated. Studies of the effects of PTH on protein kinase C have not been reported.

The early phase of stimulation of skeletal tissue by PTH produces a decrease in serum calcium levels detected *in vivo* and a concomitant increase in intracellular levels of calcium, indicating a transient, but marked, influx of calcium into bone.[53] Analogous studies *in vitro* with bone cells point to a PTH action that may be mediated by a non-cAMP mechanism.[138,139] Levels of intracellular calcium rise rapidly after stimulation by PTH. This rise in calcium levels appears to occur independently of increases in cAMP because dibutyryl cAMP does not increase cellular permeability to calcium and elevated levels of calcium intracellularly inhibit adenylate cyclase activity.[114,123] Calcium appears to serve as an independent intracellular messenger for the osteolytic response to PTH.

Increasing the intracellular level of calcium results in increased RNA synthesis and the release of lysosomal and other enzymes associated with bone resorption.[140,142] Cellular secretion of these enzymes may be mediated by binding of intracellular calcium to contractile proteins such as troponin C. Calmodulin may also be activated through the increased intracellular calcium concentration caused by PTH[143,144] and thereby mediate certain hormonal effects. Calmodulin is known to interact with and regulate the activity of a number of intracellular enzymes including protein kinases and the catalytic subunit of adenylate cyclase, stimulating its enzymic activity independently of the guanyl nucleotide regulatory subunit and phosphodiesterase (which degrades cAMP). The intracellular increase in calcium levels may also reflect PTH-induced stimulation of the polyphosphoinositide pathway and generation of inositol triphosphate, which can stimulate a wide-ranging series of metabolic events. Thus, PTH-stimulated increases in intracellular calcium may act synergistically with or independently of, or even conversely to, the effects of cAMP. A complete picture of the individual role and interplay of the several second messengers of PTH action on bone is not yet available.

Other intracellular factors besides cAMP, polyphosphoinositols, and calcium modulate PTH action. Two groups have reported substances called cytosol factors or cytosol activators that stimulate adenylate cyclase. One group partially characterized from osteosarcoma cells a substance, termed cytosol factor, that stimulates adenylate cyclase activity in plasma membrane preparations beyond the maximal activity produced by the GTP analogue Gpp(NH)p and independently of calcium concentration.[145]

Another group has also reported the presence of a cytosol activator protein (from rat reticulocytes) that enhances the adenylate cyclase response to PTH and other hormones.[146] This latter substance has a dual effect on the adenylate cyclase system; it facilitates the coupling between the stimulatory guanyl nucleotide regulatory subunit (N_s) and the catalytic subunit of adenylate cyclase, and inactivates the inhibitory subunit (N_i) by a pertussis toxin–like ADP-ribosylation mechanism.[146]

B. Actions on Target Tissue

1. Hormone Actions in Kidney

As discussed earlier, PTH exerts multiple actions on the kidney, including renal tubular transport of calcium, phosphate, sodium, potassium, and bicarbonate as well as other ions, and stimulates the production of $1,25(OH)_2D$.[161-164]

The activated subunit of the cAMP-dependent protein kinase phosphorylates specific membrane-bound proteins, resulting in altered tubular ion transport.[165] This has been most fully investigated for the PTH-mediated inhibition of phosphate reabsorption,[166] but the biochemical details of PTH mechanism of action have not been elucidated for any ion transport system. The principal PTH-modulatable calcium reabsorption occurs within the distal tubule and portions of the convoluted tubule of the nephron.[41,147-149,167] Transport in the distal segment occurs against both a calcium and an electrical gradient, indicating the presence of an active transport process, but the biochemical mechanism of PTH regulation of calcium transport is not known. As discussed earlier, two tubular sites of physiologic significance for phosphate reabsorption are known, one proximal and one distal, although the physiologic role of the proximal site in the region of the pars recta is better established.[150] The proximal tubule contains an active transport system that co-transports sodium and phosphate, and this transport system is inhibited by PTH. The hormone action appears linked to the cAMP-dependent protein kinase system described previously and PTH action can be mimicked by dibutyryl cAMP.[151]

There is heterogeneity of nephrons with regard to phosphate handling; the effect of PTH may be greater in the proximal tubules of the deep nephrons than in those of superficial nephrons.[152] Parathyroid hormone blocks phosphate accumulation by affecting the uptake of phosphate at the apical membrane, and not by promoting phosphate efflux.[153] The phosphaturic effects of PTH are also dependent on the metabolic state of the cell. Factors such as gluconeogenesis, acidosis, glucocorticoids, and starvation can all alter the phosphaturic response to PTH.[154,155]

The 1α-hydroxylase enzyme stimulated by PTH is present only in the proximal tubule at sites probably identical or closely related to the renal sites of mineral ion reabsorption.[156] The regulation of 1α-hydroxylase activity may be mediated by intracellular phosphate levels or by cAMP.[157-159] The activity of another enzyme involved in vitamin D metabolism, the 25(OH) vitamin D_3 24-hydroxylase, which biosynthesizes 24,25$(OH)_2$ vitamin D_3, is also modulated by PTH. Studies using cloned monkey kidney cell lines suggest that the effects of PTH on the 24-hydroxylase activity are also mediated by cAMP.[160]

2. *Hormone Actions in Bone*

Given the complex anatomy and the multiple cellular and metabolic processes involved in bone resorption, it is not surprising that many aspects of hormone action on bone cells are still unclear. The most striking cellular response to chronic stimulation of bone by PTH is observed among the osteoclasts.[56] However, osteoclasts lack PTH receptors and are unresponsive to PTH.[56,57] Supplementation of osteoclasts with osteoblasts *in vitro* restores PTH-responsive resorptive functions.[57] Intravenous administration of a biologically active radioligand analogue of PTH localizes by autoradiography to osteoblasts and osteoblast-like cells, and the analogue does not bind to osteoclasts.[58] The osteoblast is the direct cellular target for PTH action in bone; these cells contain PTH receptors and a PTH-stimulated adenylate cyclase response.[55] The finding that the stimulation of osteoclasts and bone resorption by PTH can be mediated only through stimulation of osteoblasts raises important questions regarding the mechanism of communication between these cells. The existence of bone-coupling factors has been postulated. Nonetheless, bone formation and bone resorption appear tightly coupled within bone as an organ. When one or the other process is stimulated, the activities of both processes increase, although one process is augmented more than the other.[168] Current theories assume the local secretion by osteoblasts of a substance active on osteoclasts. Such a factor could either stimulate osteoclast activity, negate the action of a tonic suppressor of osteoclast activity, or block the synthesis of an osteoclast inhibitor.

Osteolysis, or catabolism of bone, is accompanied by release of lysosomal hydroxylases[134] and collagenase,[169] activation of acid phosphatase and carbonic anhydrase,[170-172] activation of hydrogen-potassium-ATPase (the "proton pump"),[173] accumulation of citrate and lactate,[134,139] and increased synthesis of hyaluronate and sulfated mucopolysaccharides.[174,175] In addition, PTH may stimulate calcium release from bone by means of a sodium-calcium exchange mechanism, as demonstrated by *in vitro* experiments utilizing neonatal mouse calvaria.[176] All of these metabolic events associated with bone resorption are stimulated by PTH. The osteoclast is the exclusive bone-resorbing cell, and these findings suggest that PTH can stimulate, albeit indirectly, osteoclastic enzymes and plasma membrane ion exchangers to facilitate resorption of each of the components of bone, namely, the collagenous and protein matrices, and the mineral phase composed largely of calcium salts. In response to PTH (when osteoblasts are present), osteoclasts will release cysteine proteinases, such as cathepsin B.[177] In addition, other lysosomal enzymes appear to be involved in the resorption of organic substances.[134]

An acid environment is required for the dissolution of the mineral component of bone with release of calcium salts into the extracellular fluid.[178] The osteoclast attaches to a mineralized surface, sealing off a space between the cell and the mineralized surface in a convoluted (ruffled) border, and then filling this space with acidified fluid.[178]

The two enzymes H^+-K^+-ATPase (the proton pump) and carbonic anhydrase (type II) appear to be involved in generating a sequestered extracellular acidic microenvironment. Osteoclasts contain a membrane protein of molecular weight 100,000, similar although not identical to the proton pump in gastric parietal cells that establishes acidity of the gastric contents.[179,179a] Inhibition of this pump blocks PTH-stimulated bone resorption.[173] Other evidence indicates the importance of carbonic anhydrase (type II) in bone resorption. Patients with osteopetrosis have diminished or no carbonic anhydrase II in their tissues and fail to resorb bone.[180,181] Parathyroid hormone stimulates carbonic anhydrase activity in bone, and inhibition of carbonic anhydrase activity will block PTH-mediated bone resorption.[172,182-184] It seems probable that carbonic anhydrase may generate the necessary H^+ (from H_2O + $CO_2 \rightarrow HCO_3^- + H^+$) to supply the H^+-K^+-ATPase proton pump.

At smaller doses, particularly when administered intermittently, PTH has an anabolic effect on bone; osteoblasts increase in number, alkaline phosphatase activity (an osteoblast marker) increases, accretion of bone mineral increases, and radioactive sulfate is incorporated into cartilage.[185-187] Therapeutic applications of small doses of PTH are under evaluation as a means of reversing osteoporosis.[188]

Cellular differentiation of bone and cartilage also results from chronic exposure to PTH.[186,187] PTH may also act on cartilage cells and thus play an important role in growth and development. Labeled PTH localizes to epiphyseal growth plates, with considerable radioactivity present in regions containing hypertrophic chondrocytes undergoing the transition from cartilage to newly formed endochondrial bone.[56,188-190]

C. Structure/Activity Relations of Parathyroid Hormone

The physiologic actions of PTH represent the end stage of a multiple-step process; hence, interpretation of structure/activity relations for PTH is complicated. Changes in calcium and phosphate ion flux in blood, urine, and other tissue fluids often occur with a considerable time lag between the initial interaction between PTH and the membrane receptor and the final result. The critical steps beyond receptor binding, in analogy with a rate-limiting step in an enzyme-mediated metabolic pathway, are not known. Changes in rates of destruction of peptide during transit in the circulation may greatly modify the apparent potency of analogues in a manner not directly related to altered hormone-receptor interactions.

Extensive structure/activity studies of PTH have been performed using over 100 chemically synthesized fragments and analogues of the hormone and both *in vitro*[49,191-201] and *in vivo* assays.[115,116,202-206]

The amino-terminal third of the PTH molecule (positions 1–34) contains all the structural requirements necessary for full biological activity in multiple assay systems. This region of PTH has been synthesized and found to be nearly equipotent, on a molar basis, to native PTH in several assays, both *in vitro* and *in vivo* in several species.[21,70,116,207,208] Also, direct tests of receptor-binding affinity have shown binding of bPTH–(1–34) to renal membrane receptors is equal, on a molar basis, to binding of bPTH–(1–84).[198,199] More recently, the entire human form of the hormone hPTH–(1–84) has been successfully synthesized chemically.[209]

The presence of the carboxyl-terminal region may prolong the half-life of the hormone in tissue fluids and increase potency in certain *in vivo* bioassays, such as the rat assay based on the subcutaneous injection of hormone.[203] No discrete biological role in calcium homeostasis has yet been established for the remaining carboxyl-terminal portion of the PTH molecule (positions 35–84). Substantiation that other regions of PTH are devoid of conventional PTH-like agonist activity on mineral ion flux and stimulation of adenylate cyclase has been achieved through synthesis of middle and carboxyl-terminal segments of the hormone molecule.[210-214] There may be some small contribution to receptor binding by the mid- and carboxyl-terminal portions of the native molecule.[215-218] However, such binding does not appear to augment adenylate cyclase activity. Furthermore, the midregion and carboxyl portions of the native hormone may bind to lower affinity sites than those of the biologically active amino-terminal third of the molecule.[219]

Some evidence is accumulating indicating that other biological activities, not related to classic actions of PTH in mineral ion homeostasis, may reside in the midregion and carboxyl-terminal portions of the PTH molecule.[220] Although intriguing, none of these proposed PTH actions dependent on regions other than the amino-terminal portion of the hormone have been definitively proved. Most evidence derives from apparent differences in potency between amino-terminal fragments and the intact hormone in certain new types of test systems. Fragments of the molecule representing approximately the carboxyl-terminal two thirds of the structure accumulate in the circulation in renal failure. It has been shown in *in vitro* and *in vivo* studies[220-224] that PTH or its fragments may inhibit erythropoiesis, cardiac function, nerve conduction, and red blood cell survival times. Carboxyl-terminal peptides also may contribute to glucose intolerance in renal failure, and may exacerbate or actually be causal for many of the other toxic manifestations of the uremic state. It remains to be determined whether these actions of portions of the parathyroid molecule are mediated via PTH receptors and whether they play any role in normal physiologic functions. The precise contribution of PTH fragments to pathophysiologic changes in chronic renal failure is being studied further.

There is marked homology between the sequences of bovine[14,16,18,225] and human PTH.[14,16,19] In addition, the hormone homologue of each species is biologically active in all assay systems in which the homologues have been tested. The relative biopotency of these native forms of the hormone does differ, however, depending on the assay system utilized. In general, *in vitro* adenylate cyclase assays have shown bPTH–(1–84) to be approximately 10-fold more potent than hPTH–(1–84).[207,226,227] In general, these relations also have been supported by the evaluation of chemically synthesized human PTH–(1–84),[209] although a higher potency has been observed for the human compared with the bovine homologue *in vivo* in the chick hypercalcemia assay.[228]

The biologically active fragments of the hormone have been synthesized and evaluated. Assay of the regions bPTH–(1–34) and hPTH–(1–34) has shown that the bovine fragment is more potent than the human fragment *in vitro* in assays based on cAMP production.[115,116,202,229] In these assay systems, the rat homologue is the most potent form of the hormone.[219,225] However, in the *in vivo* chick hypercalcemia assay,[204] the human and bovine synthetic fragments were found to be nearly equal in potency.[116,229] These findings focused interest on position 1 in the native sequences, which is alanine in the bovine and rat forms, and serine in the human and porcine forms of the hormone. Most of the differences in observed biopotency in the *in vitro* activity of hPTH–(1–34) are attributable to the serine at position 1. The activity of hPTH–(1–34) could be brought nearly to the level of bPTH–(1–34) by substituting alanine at position 1. Conversely, the *in vitro* activity of bPTH–(1–34) could be diminished to the level of hPTH–(1–34) by placing serine at position 1. In general, the chick hypercalcemia assay seems less discriminating among position 1 substitutions;[116] this need not, as discussed previously, indicate a difference between kidney and bone receptors.

Studies using fragments of native PTH indicated that the fragment bPTH–(1–29) was active, but bioactivity was not present in the shorter fragment bPTH–(1–20).[230] To establish the minimum continuous sequence necessary for biological activity, multiple fragments of the fully active region, bPTH–(1–34), were synthesized,[21,116] and biopotency was tested *in vitro* in the rat renal adenylate cyclase assay, *in vivo* in the chick hypercalcemia assay, and in other bioassays.[191,194,208] Stepwise shortening of the carboxyl terminus from position 34 toward the amino terminus results in a progressive decline in biological activity *in vitro* and *in vivo* until position 25 is reached, after which point no further activity is found. The decline in potency observed with progressive truncation of the carboxyl terminus correlates with a reduction in binding affinity.[199]

Stepwise deletions at the amino terminus also caused decline in biological activity, but at a much more rapid rate.[21,115,116,231] Subsequently, studies using chemically synthesized peptides[115,232] showed that the simple deletion of position 1 caused a substantial loss of biological activity. Removal of one more residue, yielding the fragment bPTH–(3–34), caused a complete loss of bioactivity *in vitro* and *in vivo*.[21,116,232] The fragment bPTH–(3–34) is nearly inactive in all *in vitro* and *in vivo* systems.[191,194,208]

These findings delineate the minimum sequence required for biological activity as the region 2 to 25 of the hormone molecule present as a continuous sequence.[21,115,116] These studies also revealed the critical importance of position 1 for bioactivity; almost all modification of the native structure at this position causes a dramatic decline in bioactivity.[115,186,232]

Substitution with a D-amino acid–enantiomer, D-alanine, at position 1, however, causes diminished *in vitro* activity, but enhanced *in vivo* activity,[116,208,232] suggesting that resistance to degradation *in vivo* (conferred by the presence of a nonnatural amino acid) might be responsible for enhanced activity (and not an increase in avidity for the PTH receptor).

At the carboxyl terminus, simple conversion of the carboxyl-terminal carboxylic acid (COOH) to a carboxyamide ($CONH_2$), as occurs naturally in smaller hormones such as gastrin, luteinizing hormone-releasing hormone, thyrotropin-releasing hormone, and antidiuretic hormone, increases activity to approximately 250% that of PTH both *in vitro* and *in vivo*.[115,116] Although resistance to enzymic degradation may be responsible for the observed increase in activity, the data suggest greater receptor-binding avidity[199] for analogues containing the amide modification. Other single alterations or combinations of modifications can yield analogues that are four to ten times more potent than unsubstituted PTH.[197,199,233,234]

The active region of PTH can be separated into a region primarily responsible for binding to PTH receptors and a small but distinct region responsible for hormone action once receptor binding has occurred. This separation of function within the active core has permitted the design and synthesis of potent inhibitors of PTH.[23,24,101,235] It was found that removal of two amino acids from the amino terminus of the active fragment of PTH yielded a fragment, the sequence 3 to 34, which still bound (although weakly) to parathyroid hormone receptors,[199,236] but was devoid of agonist-like activity *in vitro*.

Further refinements in analogue design led to a highly effective PTH antagonist, [N1e-8, N1e-18, Tyr-34]bPTH–(3–34)amide, that was more potent than any other peptide hormone antagonist extant at the time.[237] This analogue competed for receptor occupancy with fully active PTH on an equimolar basis. In renal[137,237] and bone-derived *in vitro* assays, the analogue completely inhibited adenylate cyclase activity stimulated by PTH, and its inhibitory potency was approximately 200-fold greater than that of the unsubstituted parent peptide bPTH–(3–34).

Although this antagonist has proved potent and highly useful *in vitro*, it was found to possess weak but definite agonist properties *in vivo*.[240] The agonist-like potency of this analogue has been calculated to be 0.3% to 1% of that of PTH.[205,238,239] In other systems, the analogue had neither antagonist nor agonist properties.[240,241] Trials *in vivo* of [N1e-8, N1e-18, Tyr-34]bPTH–(3–34)amide as an antagonist were unsuccessful; the presumed reason was intrinsic agonism at the large dose used in the *in vivo* assay.

The amino-terminal region was further truncated.[242] Although stepwise deletions from the amino terminus to the carboxyl terminus led to a progressive decline in receptor affinity, fragment analogues such as 7 to 34, 10 to 34, and 15 to 34 still bound to the PTH receptor when added in high concentrations. In particular, one segment of only 10 amino acids (the segment 25 to 34)—derived from a parent peptide hormone of 84 amino acids—could occupy PTH receptors and completely block the binding of fully active radioligand. This finding, together with results from other studies, demonstrated that the principal binding domain of the hormone was located at the carboxyl terminus of the fully active fragment, removed from the activation domain at the opposite (amino) end of the molecule.

Based on these principles, a PTH antagonist effective *in vivo* and devoid of PTH-like agonist activity was generated. The antagonist, [Tyr-34]bPTH–(7–34)amide, was shown to antagonize the PTH-stimulated excretion of phosphate and cAMP by the kidney *in vivo*.[23] When the 7 to 34 analogue was administered with PTH at a molar dose ratio of 200 to 1, parathyroid hormone responses were completely inhibited. Subsequent studies demonstrated that the calcemic response to PTH *in vivo* could also be inhibited by administration of [Tyr-34]bPTH–(7–34)amide,[24] as could the *in vivo* PTH-mediated activation of the 1α-hydroxylase enzyme responsible for generating 1,25$(OH)_2$ vitamin D_3. These *in vivo* studies[23,24,243] demonstrate that each of the major indicators of PTH action *in vivo*—serum calcium, urinary phosphate, urinary cAMP response, and activation of vitamin D—can be inhibited completely with the 7 to 34 antagonist. Competitive blockade of hormone action can be useful in studies of initial events in hormone action, and might eventually find application in disease states associated with hormone excess for which surgical parathyroidectomy is not feasible.

IV. PROCESSES OF BIOSYNTHESIS AND CELLULAR TRANSPORT

During the past decade, considerable progress has been made in our knowledge of the pathways involved in the biosynthesis of parathyroid hormone (PTH). The establishment of suitable *in vitro* systems, which control for certain influences on cellular degradation of precursors and hormone secretion that may becloud results from studies done in *in vivo* systems, has made it possible to investigate in detail the pathways and specific factors involved in the regulation of the intracellular processes in the parathyroid gland. The application of a wide variety of techniques such as analysis of protein synthesis in intact tissues and cell-free systems, determination of primary protein sequence by radiomicrosequencing technology, and cloning and analysis of the nucleotide sequence of the parathyroid messenger RNA and gene has provided a comprehensive and informative view of the cellular process involved in the biosynthesis of PTH (Fig. 3–4). In the following section, evidence is reviewed that has led to an understanding of the structures, processing, and transport of biosynthetic precursors to PTH.

A. Structures of Biosynthetic Precursors

Accounts of the early studies that led to the elucidation of the biosynthetic pathways involved in the formation, cellular transport, and metabolism of PTH are provided in several reviews.[244-247] Studies of hormone biosynthesis *in vitro*, in which pulse-chase incubations of slices of parathyroid tissue with radioactive amino acids were used, led to the identification of the precursor proPTH.[38,248-252] Subsequently, the direct translation of the parathyroid mRNA in cell-free systems revealed a larger biosynthetic precursor to PTH, preproPTH.[253,256] The utilization of high sensitivity protein-sequencing techniques of the PTH precursors labeled with radioactive amino acids both in the parathyroid gland slices and in cell-free translations of mRNA prepared from parathyroid glands provided the complete primary structure of both preproPTH (115 amino acids) and proPTH (90 amino acids) (Fig. 3–5). Both preproPTH and proPTH consist of PTH with the addition of amino-terminal extension peptides of 31 and six amino acids, respectively. Specific labeling of preproPTH and not proPTH in cell-free systems containing radioactive methionine bound to the initiator methionyl transfer RNA established that the amino-terminal methionine at position 31 of preproPTH is the first amino acid incorporated into the nascent peptide during ribosomal synthesis and suggested that preproPTH is not a cleavage product of an even larger precursor with additional amino-terminal extensions.[257] The elucidation of primary structure of the messenger RNA and gene encoding preproPTH (see following) confirms that preproPTH is the initial hormonal product synthesized in the parathyroid cell and that it consists of all the protein structural information encoded in the gene for PTH (Fig. 3–5).

B. Structures of mRNAs and Genes Encoding for Preproparathyroid Hormone

The application of recombinant DNA technology has provided the complete nucleotide sequences of the preproPTH messenger RNAs from human and bovine parathyroid glands as well as the chromosomal genes for the bovine, human, and rat preproPTHs from the sequencing of recombinant lambda phage obtained from genomic DNA libraries. Decoding of the nucleotide sequences of the cDNA copies of the mRNAs reveals the presence of a termination codon immediately following the codon for glutamine at position 84 of PTH. This observation plus evidence that there is only a single gene copy per haploid genome essentially rules out the existence of additional precursors of PTH with peptide extensions at the carboxyl terminus.

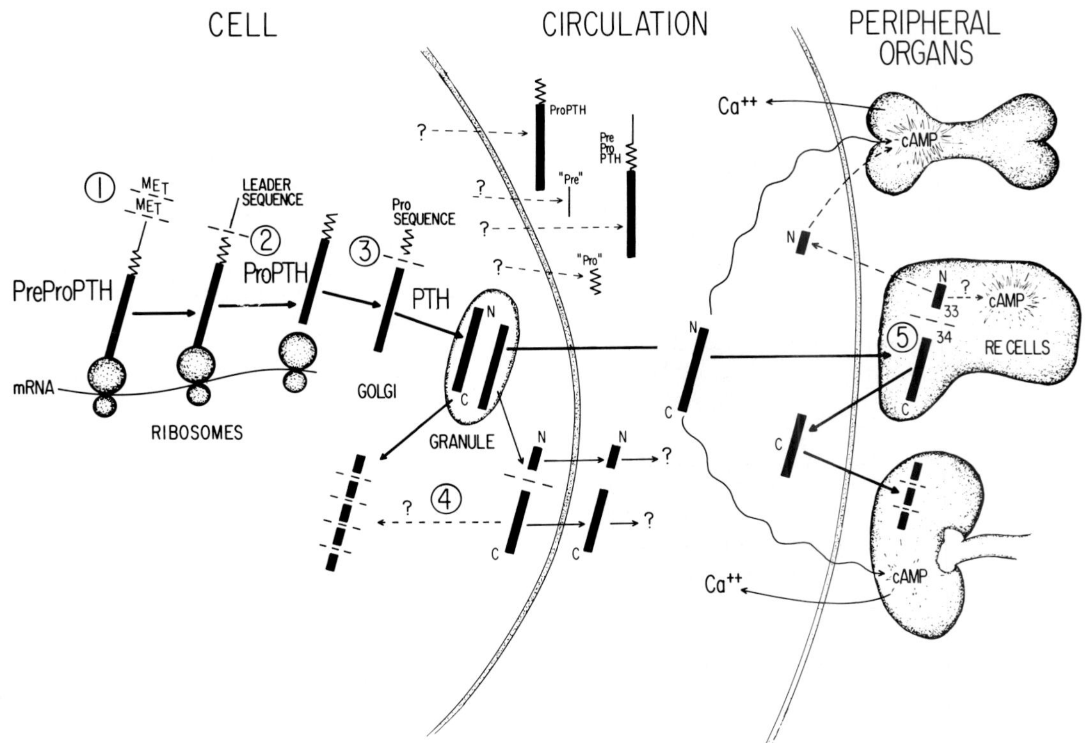

Figure 3–4. Cleavages that take place in parathyroid hormone (PTH) and its precursors during biosynthesis (cell), secretion (circulation), and metabolism (peripheral organs). Initial cellular cleavages of nascent precursor (preproparathyroid hormone [PreproPTH]) are (1) removal of two NH_2-terminal methionines (MET) and (2) removal of the remaining NH_2-terminal leader sequence of 23 amino acids. Intermediate precursor (proparathyroid hormone [ProPTH]) so formed is further cleaved in Golgi complex by removal of NH_2-terminal prosequence of six amino acids (3). Mature PTH of 84 amino acids is packaged into granules, most of which are secreted into circulation. Small fraction of PTH appears to be further cleaved (4) in parathyroid cells either by specific cathepsin B in NH_2-terminal region between amino acids 33 and 40 or by extensive proteolytic degradation. In the circulation, PTH is taken up by Kupffer cells of liver, where it is cleaved at several places between amino acids 33 and 43 into NH_2 (N) and COOH (C) fragments, carboxyl fragments that are released back into circulation. Because of these cleavages, the major form of the circulating hormone consists of COOH fragments. The intact, biologically active hormone interacts with receptors in kidney and bone. Although there have been speculations that a circulating amino-terminal fragment might be an alternate active species, no convincing evidence for this has been found. Similarly, the speculation that the precursors preproPTH and/or proPTH or precursor-specific fragments might be released into the circulation has not been confirmed.

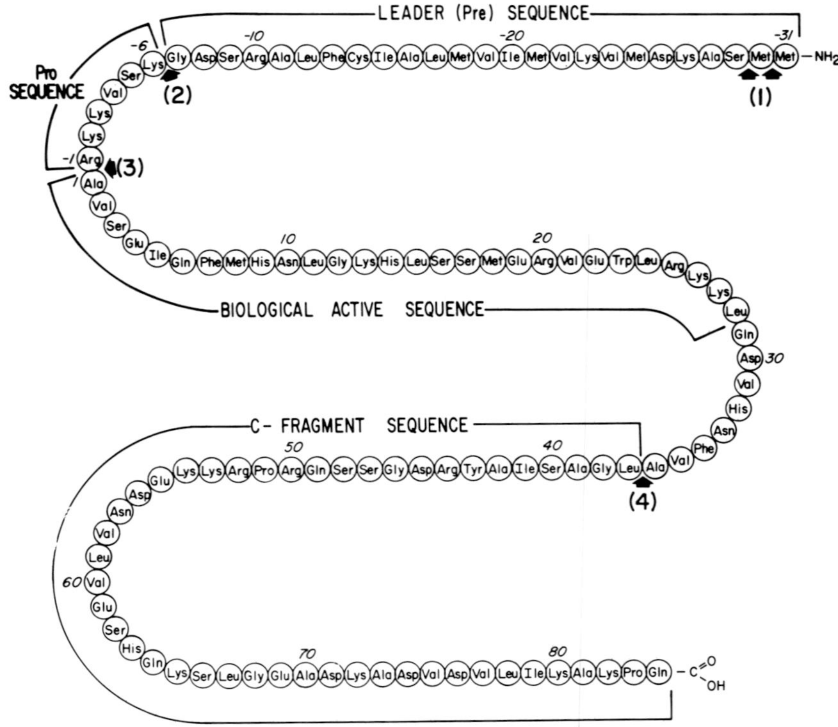

Figure 3–5. Primary structure of preproparathyroid hormone of 115 amino acids. Precursor consists of the 84–amino acid sequence of parathyroid hormone (residues 1 through 84) preceded at NH_2 terminus by precursor extension of 31 amino acids (–31 through –1). Arrows indicate peptide bonds cleaved during metabolic processing of precursor and hormone: (1) removal of NH_2-terminal methionines; (2) cleavage of leader (pre-, signal) sequence during growth of nascent polypeptide chain; (3) removal of prosequence during transport of the proparathyroid hormone through Golgi complex of parathyroid cell; and (4) cleavage of hormone into an NH_2-terminal biologically active fragment and an inactive carboxyl (C) fragment. Last-mentioned cleavage occurs in liver after uptake of hormone from circulation (see Fig. 3–4).

The nucleotide sequences of the cDNAs also established the assignment of glutamic acid to position 22 of PTH but in the human PTH necessitated a new assignment for asparagine at residue 76 and not aspartic acid, the latter being missed because of deamidation prior to protein sequence.

The topographic features of the three mammalian PTH genes that have been sequenced are similar. Each of the genes contains two introns that interrupt the transcriptional unit (mRNA) at precisely the same nucleotides. The larger first intron resides five nucleotides upstream from the methionine codon that starts the translation of preproPTH. The second smaller intron is located within the region of the gene coding for the prohormone hexapeptide sequence that separates the amino-terminal signal sequence from the sequence of parathyroid hormone. It is curious that in the majority of genes encoding polypeptide hormones, introns are located both in the 5′ untranslated tract of messenger RNAs and at or around the junction of the signal peptide with the remainder of the protein-coding sequence. The former circumstance suggests the possible existence of transcriptional regulatory elements within the more upstream intron and the latter circumstance supports the notion originally proposed by Gilbert[258] that exons encode functional domains of proteins. Inasmuch as signal sequences are essential for the intracellular transport functions of prehormones (see later), signal sequences may be considered to be functionally distinct from the extracellular functions (biological) of the hormones *per se*.

Restriction endonuclease mapping of genomic DNA obtained from the human, bovine, and rat indicate the existence of a single copy of the preproPTH gene per haploid genome.[36,37,259] The human PTH gene is located on the short arm of chromosome 11 as determined by analyses of mouse/human hybrid cell lines[260] and by *in situ* chromosomal hybridization and autoradiographic analyses.[261] Other genes that are located along with PTH genes on the short arm of chromosome 11 include calcitonin, catalase, Harvey-ras protooncogene, insulin, and beta globin. A PstI restriction fragment–length polymorphism has been found in this cluster of genes. Seventy per cent of humans carry a 2.8 kb PstI restriction fragment and 30% a 2.2 kb fragment. Approximately 40% of individuals are heterozygous for these two patterns of PstI cleavage.[262] An additional Taq I polymorphism resulting from a point mutation within the second intron of the PTH gene is also detected.[263] Inasmuch as differing alleles are inherited in mendelian fashion, they can provide useful polymorphic markers for defining familial inheritance of these alleles. This approach has potential importance for investigation of linkages in families with disorders of calcium metabolism.

C. Cellular Processing and Transport of Preproparathyroid Hormone and Proparathyroid Hormone

Studies of protein synthesis in parathyroid glands have provided an understanding of the cellular sites at which cleavages of the hormonal precursors occur and of the possible function of the precursors and the biosynthetic pathway for the hormone. Kinetic analyses of the appearances and disappearances of preproPTH, proPTH, and PTH have been based on electrophoretic characterization of the polypeptides labeled during short pulse (1–30 min) and pulse-chase incubations of parathyroid gland slices with radioactive amino acids.[38,254,264,265] Additional information has been obtained by studies of the distributions of the hormonal polypeptides and subcellular fractions[266,267] and of autoradiographic analyses of protein migration in parathyroid cells.[38]

1. Cellular Pathway for Transport

Cells that have as one of their principal functions the synthesis of proteins for export contain specialized organelles that are required for the processes of protein transport. As reviewed by Palade,[268] it is believed that the synthesis of exportable proteins, as opposed to that of proteins that remain in the cell, takes place on ribosomes bound to the membranes of the rough endoplasmic reticulum (RER) (Fig. 3–6). Newly synthesized polypeptide chains are vectorally discharged into the cistern of the RER. By this means, the proteins that are to be secreted are segregated from the proteins that are to be retained within the cell. The secreted proteins are then transported within the RER channels and the membrane-limited organelles to the Golgi region of the cell, where they are incorporated into either the secretory vesicles or granules. The protein within the granules is then either stored within the cell or transported peripherally to the plasma membrane and released by exocytosis into the extracellular fluid in response to the appropriate stimulus. A considerable body of investigative evidence has led to the development of a model whereby the initiation of preproPTH synthesis occurs on polyribosomes located within the cell matrix. When the growing polypeptide chain is approximately 20 to 30 amino acids long, the NH_2-terminus of the chain first emerges from the large subunit of the ribosome, and at this time the two NH_2-terminal methionines of preproPTH are removed by a putative methionyl aminopeptidase. As the nascent chain continues to grow, the hydrophobic NH_2-terminal sequence (the "signal," "leader," or "pre-" sequence) of preproPTH emerges and associates with the membrane of the endoplasmic reticulum in accord with the "signal" hypothesis, and the sequence of 23 amino acids of preproPTH is removed by cleavage of the glycyl-lysyl bond by enzymatic activity in or near the reticular membrane[265,269] (Figs. 3–4, 3–6, and 3–7). After a delay of approximately 10 to 15 minutes from the time of its initial formation from preproPTH in the RER, proPTH arrives at the Golgi apparatus and it there is converted to PTH by the proteolytic removal of the NH_2-terminal sequence of six amino acids specific for proPTH. Evidence that the conversion of proPTH to PTH occurs in the Golgi elements of the cell is provided by autoradiographic analyses of the migration of newly synthesized protein and by the use of pharmacologic agents that specifically disrupt the Golgi complex. Electron microscopy shows that autoradiographic grains first appear in the Golgi region of parathyroid cells 15 minutes after introduction of a pulse-label of ^{3}H[leucine] corresponding to the time at which conversion

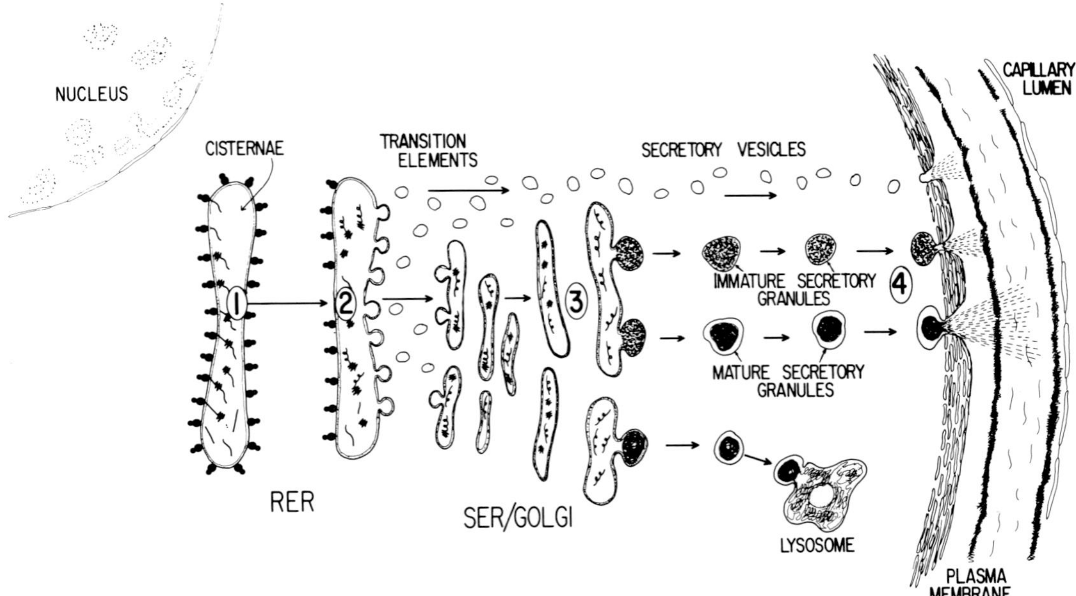

Figure 3–6. Schematic representation of subcellular organelles involved in transport and secretion of polypeptide hormones or other secreted proteins within a protein-secreting cell. RER, rough endoplasmic reticulum; SER, smooth endoplasmic reticulum; Golgi, Golgi complex. (1) Synthesis of proteins on polyribosomes attached to endoplasmic reticulum (RER), and vectoral discharge of proteins through membrane into cisterna. (2) Formation of shuttling vesicles (transition elements) from endoplasmic reticulum followed by their transport to and incorporation by Golgi complex. (3) Formation of secretory granules in Golgi complex. (4) Transport of secretory granules to plasma membrane, fusion with plasma membrane, and exocytosis resulting in release of granule contents into extracellular space. Note that secretion may occur via transport of secretory vesicles and immature granules, as well as via mature granules. Some granules are taken up and hydrolyzed by lysosomes (crinophagy). (From Habener JF: Hormone biosynthesis and secretion. *In* Felig P, et al (eds): Endocrinology and Metabolism. New York, McGraw-Hill, 1981, pp 29-59.)

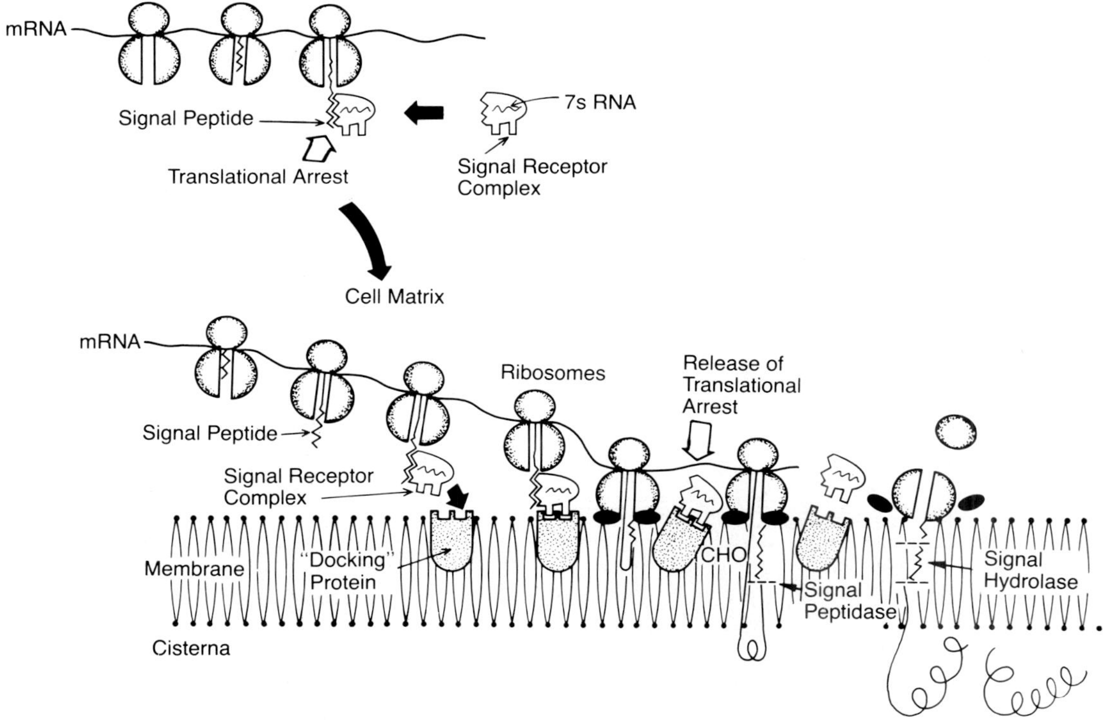

Figure 3–7. Diagram depicting cellular events in initial stages of synthesis of a polypeptide hormone according to signal hypothesis. In this schema, a signal-receptor particle, consisting of a complex of six proteins and an RNA (7S RNA), interacts with amino-terminal signal peptide of nascent polypeptide chain after approximately 70 amino acids are polymerized, resulting in arrest of further growth of polypeptide chain. Signal-receptor polyribosome–nascent chain complex remains in a state of translational arrest until it "recognizes" and binds to a "docking protein," a receptor protein located on the cytoplasmic face of endoplasmic reticular membrane. This interaction of signal-receptor complex with docking protein releases translational block, and protein synthesis resumes. Nascent polypeptide chain is discharged across membrane bilayer into cisterna of endoplasmic reticulum and is released from signal peptide by cleavage with a signal peptidase located in cisternal face of membrane. In this model, signal peptide is cleaved from polypeptide chain by signal peptidase before chain is completed (co-translational cleavage). Configuration of polypeptide during transport across membrane, and forces and mechanisms responsible for its translocation, are unknown. Loop, or hairpin, configuration of chain is shown in this arbitrary model; other models are equally possible.

of proPTH to PTH is first observed by electrophoretic analyses of the newly synthesized protein in cell extracts.[264] Amine compounds (*tris*-amino methane and related compounds) of ionophore X537A are selective inhibitors of the conversion of proPTH and produce corresponding disruptive alterations of the Golgi complex. The process of translocation of proPTH from the RER to the Golgi apparatus requires energy[270] and is probably mediated by the action of microtubules;[270,271] inhibitors of oxidative phosphorylation (dinitrophenol, antimycin A) and inhibitors of microtubular function (vinblastine, colchicine) impair the conversion of proPTH to PTH.

The efficiency of the conversion of proPTH to PTH is high, as assessed by studies of normal parathyroid tissues. Radioactive proPTH reaches a constant specific activity in the tissue within 20 minutes after a pulse-label of 3H[leucine] has been introduced into the medium bathing the parathyroid gland slices.[254,264,272] Moreover, analysis by region-specific radioimmunoassays of the amounts of proPTH and PTH in normal parathyroid glands indicates that PTH is the predominant form of the hormone stored in the gland; proPTH constitutes only 7% of the total immunoreactive hormone.[273] This quantity of prohormone approximates the amount of precursor in transit within the system of the endoplasmic reticulum to the site of cleavage in the Golgi complex. Attempts to detect proPTH in the medium bathing parathyroid gland slices incubated *in vitro* or in parathyroid effluent blood collected from calves or patients undergoing surgical removal of the parathyroid adenomas have been unsuccessful.[273] Therefore, it seems probable that little, if any, proPTH is stored within secreted granules of the parathyroid gland and that the parathyroid gland does not normally secrete proPTH. No specific functions can be attributable to proPTH, and its existence as an intermediate precursor in the formation of PTH is unknown. Perhaps its function resides in the intracellular transport of the precursor to the Golgi complex.

In this regard, studies of the expression of recombinant fusion genes with the coding sequence for the prohormone-specific hexapeptide deleted suggest that the hexapeptide sequence may be required for the accurate proteolytic cleavage of the signal sequence during the synthesis of nascent preproPTH. Proparathyroid hormone is inactive biologically on PTH receptors in target organs; removal of the NH_2-terminal hexapeptide sequence of proPTH from the sequence of PTH is necessary to generate biologically active PTH.[274] Studies *in vitro* have shown that proPTH is inactive in the renal adenylate cyclase assay and that the hexapeptide must be removed before biological activity is observed.[275]

Transport of PTH to the site of release at the plasma membrane presumably occurs via the secretory granules. Electron microscopy of parathyroid cells has shown, however, that mature membrane-limited secretory granules are few in number compared, for example, with those in pancreatic islet cells or pituitary somatotroph cells. At the same time the "immature" vesicles derived from the Golgi elements are abundant, suggesting that some fraction of PTH may be transported directly to the periphery of the cell without prior incorporation into mature secretory granules. Evidence was reported in support of the existence of two separate pathways for the secretion of PTH, one involving stored (or "mature") hormone and the other preferentially used by newly synthesized hormone.[272,276]

2. *Processing of Preproparathyroid Hormone: Functions of the Signal Sequence*

Several lines of evidence indicate that the enzymatic activity responsible for the conversion of preproPTH resides in the membranes of the endoplasmic reticulum. Particularly compelling information was obtained by comparing the products of translation of parathyroid mRNA in cell-free systems with those from systems containing pancreatic microsomal membranes derived from endoplasmic reticulum in the form of vesicles that have been stripped of ribosomes by treatment with ethylenediaminetetraacetic acid (EDTA).[277-282] PreproPTH is the only hormonal product synthesized in a microsome-free, cell-free translation system derived from extracts of wheat germ or reticulocytes,[253,256,278] whereas both preproPTH and proPTH appear as products of synthesis (proPTH dominates) under conditions in which the translation system is supplemented with or already contains microsomal vesicles.[278,279] Furthermore, the proPTH synthesized in cell-free systems supplemented with microsomal membranes is resistant to digestion when proteolytic enzymes are added, demonstrating that proPTH is sequestered inside microsomal vesicles and protected from attack by the proteolytic enzymes. The fact that only polypeptide chains undergoing synthesis and vectoral transport through the membrane bilayer into the interior of the vesicle are cleaved from proPTH[278,279] further indicates that the enzyme responsible for the cleavage of preproPTH to proPTH is associated with the inner face of the membrane. When preproPTH is synthesized, isolated, and later added to membrane-containing but cell-free extracts of either ascites tumor cells[279] or parathyroid glands,[283] it remains intact and does not convert to proPTH or PTH under conditions in which proPTH is readily converted to PTH. An assessment of the relationship of protein synthesis to protein processing in the intact parathyroid cell was accomplished by labeling cells for short periods (1–3 min) and analyzing the PTH-related protein by gel electrophoresis. After the short pulse-labeling times, virtually all the radioactivity was detected in proPTH and not preproPTH. Only a small fraction of radioactivity was detected in preproPTH. Digestion of radioactive proteins with trypsin revealed that proPTH was resistant to digestion but that preproPTH was completely degraded, indicating that proPTH was sequestered inside the reticular cisternae, whereas the preproPTH was free in the cytoplasm and accessible to digestion by proteolytic enzymes.

The preproPTH that was labeled during the short pulse incubations disappeared rapidly upon subjecting parathyroid cells to a chase incubation with nonradioactive methionine. Inasmuch as the amount of labeled prepro-PTH in the parathyroid cells was always small, it was not possible to quantitatively account for the disappearance of labeled preproPTH in the corresponding appearance of the radiolabeled proPTH during the chase incubation. The data obtained from studies in intact cells, however, are consistent with the existence of a predominant co-translational cleavage of preproPTH, and therefore support the relevance of the studies in cell-free extracts from those in the intact cell and hence support the conclusion that preproPTH is converted to proPTH co-translationally. Moreover, these findings further indicate that vectoral transport across the membrane is obligatorily coupled to synthesis and to cleavage of the signal sequence.

At present the cellular processes involved in membrane-mediated recognition of the transport of the polypeptide or in the enzymic processes that convert preproPTH to proPTH are incompletely understood. However, in a series of elegant and informative studies over the past several years, several microsomal components involved in these processes have been isolated and characterized.[284-289] At least two protein complexes are required to accomplish the translocation of the nascent polypeptide gene into the cisterna of the endoplasmic reticulum (Fig. 3–7). During the initial stages of the synthesis of the secretory proteins, the signal sequence emerges from the ribosome and is bound to an 11S ribonucleoprotein complex called the signal recognition particle.[288] This particle is composed of six proteins and a 7S RNA and its interaction with the signal sequence arrests further elongation of the nascent polypeptide chain. The complex consisting of polyribosome and the signal recognition particle then binds to a receptor protein, called the docking protein, located in the endoplasmic reticulum.[289] This binding interaction releases the inhibition of protein synthesis, amino acid polymerization resumes, and in the process the nascent precursor protein is vectorally transferred across the reticular membrane. As discussed earlier, before synthesis of the protein is complete, the signal sequence is cleaved by a "signal" peptidase.

The peptide consisting of the leader sequence of preproPTH plus the prohormone-specific region has been prepared by chemical synthesis and used as a probe to search for receptors in the endoplasmic reticulum and to investigate the processes and membrane-associated apparatus involved in the transport of nascent preproPTH to the RER.[290,291] Addition of the synthetic signal peptide to cell-free translation systems containing microsomal vesicles effectively inhibits the conversion of nascent preproPTH to proPTH as well as the sequestration of proPTH in the vesicle.[290] Similar effects of the signal peptide of preproPTH are seen with the processing of nascent pituitary and placental proteins—pre-growth hormone and pre-prolactin, and pre-placental lactogen—during the translations of the respective mRNAs encoding these hormones in cell-free systems supplemented with microsomal vesicles. Additional evidence that the inhibition of processing of preprohormones by addition of the synthetic signal sequence in the cell-free system comes about by the competitive binding and inactivation of a component of the signal receptor particle has been obtained by photochemical cross-linking of radioiodinated signal peptide to the 54 kd subunit of the signal receptor particle. These observations further indicate that this subunit may be the component of the particle that contains the signal peptide binding site.[292] Overall, these observations point to the existence in the microsomal membranes of specific saturable recognition elements (receptors) that recognize and bind nascent signal sequences of proteins destined for export from the cell. Such receptors appear to be universally found in cells that secrete proteins and appear to recognize conformational rather than primary sequence similarities common to the class of signal sequences.

An alternative hypothesis to a receptor-mediated transfer process has been suggested. Hydrophobic interactions between the hydrophobic regions of the signal sequences and the intensely hydrophobic interior of the membrane bilayer were proposed as the principal force involved in translocation of nascent polypeptides across the endoplasmic reticulum.[287,293,294] Energy derived from the hydrophobic bonding and from the processes of amino acid polymerization could theoretically provide sufficient kinetic energy to translocate the polypeptide chains across the membrane bilayer. In this regard, studies of the physical properties of the synthetic signal peptide corresponding to the NH_2-terminal sequence of preproPTH described previously have revealed that the peptide is highly structured and undergoes a marked conformational transition in changing from an aqueous to a hydrophobic environment.[295] This transitional conformation could reflect its function in the transfer of the nascent polypeptide from the aqueous cytoplasmic environment to the hydrophobic domain of the membrane. Most recent data, however, indicate that the transfer process is receptor-mediated.[284-286,288,289]

The specificity of the endopeptidase that cleaves the signal sequence from preproPTH is unusual inasmuch as it is directed toward a glycyl-lysyl bond, a bond not known to be susceptible to cleavage by the commonly recognized cellular enzymes. There is no apparent chemical homology at the site of cleavage at any of the many preproteins now studied; accurate cleavage of a preprotein produced in one tissue can be accomplished by enzymes active in microsomes obtained from another tissue (preproPTH cleaved by the pancreatic microsomes). Therefore, the responsible enzyme(s) may recognize a common three-dimensional structure shared by the signal sequences of all prehormones and preproteins. There are, however, certain topographic motifs that are shared by the signal sequences of a number of prehormones.[287] Signal sequences are usually approximately 15 to 30 amino acids in length; they begin with one to three charged residues within the first five amino acids and contain a central core sequence of eight to 12 hydrophobic amino acids. A small amino acid such as glycine, alanine, or serine usually resides at the site of cleavage of the signal peptide.[287]

More detailed information on the functions of the precursor specific sequences has come from the introduction and expression in mammalian cells of recombinant fusion genes encoding preproPTH containing mutational deletions in the regions of the signal sequence and the prohormonal hexapeptide. The intact preproPTH fusion gene was readily expressed when introduced into rat pituitary GH4 cells that secrete prolactin. Both PTH and prolactin were secreted, and analyses of the intracellular products indicate a highly efficient conversion of preproPTH to proPTH and PTH. No preproPTH was observed, presumably because the signal sequence was removed efficiently and rapidly from the precursor by co-translational processing. Several deletionally mutated fusion genes were expressed in the GH4 cells. These fusion genes lack the coding sequences for either the first six, first 10, or first 13 amino acids of the signal sequence; an additional fusion gene was constructed without the proPTH-specific hexapeptide sequence. Removal of the first six amino acids of the signal sequence had no effect on the processing of proPTH and the secretion of PTH. However, deletions of 10 and 13 amino acids led to a defect in processing and transport inasmuch as the precursor proteins were rapidly degraded without entering the secretory pathway. Expression of the mutated preproPTH fusion gene with the proPTH hexapeptide deleted resulted in a protein that functioned abnormally. The precursor crossed the endoplasmic reticulum with close-to-normal efficiency, but subsequently cleavage of the signal sequence was inefficient. The cell secreted both PTH and a molecule slightly larger than PTH. Sequence analysis revealed that the larger molecule was PTH preceded by the last two residues of the signal sequence. Several conclusions can be drawn from the results of these mutational deletion analyses. The first six amino acids of the amino-terminal region are dispensable. In contrast, the hydrophobic core of the signal sequence is vital for membrane transport. The prohormonal hexapeptide sequence for proPTH functions to optimize the accuracy of the cleavage of the signal sequence. This last observation suggests that the prohormone portion of the sequence of preproPTH can be viewed as important for the functions of the signal sequence in transmembrane transport.

Studies of hormone synthesis in intact parathyroid cells in which the fate of the signal sequence was analyzed after its cleavage from preproPTH indicate that the peptide is rapidly hydrolyzed.[269] Hence, the leader peptide appears to be destroyed within minutes after its removal from the nascent polypeptide chain, a process in keeping with the expression of the functional activity of the peptide at the earliest stages of hormone biosynthesis.

Much still remains to be learned about the biomolecular processes involved in the unidirectional transport of polypeptide precursors across the membrane bilayer. However, it appears certain that the NH_2-terminal signal sequence of preproPTH, and the comparable signal sequences of the many other precursors of secreted proteins, serve an essential function in providing the means of specifically segregating secreted proteins from nonsecreted proteins. Such a function represents an example of the role of posttranslational processes, specifically that of proteolytic cleavage, in the complex cellular events leading to the eventual expression of the biological actions of a protein.

3. Processing of Proparathyroid Hormone

The enzymatic activities that convert proPTH to PTH resemble those of trypsin followed by carboxypeptidase B. Incubation of proPTH with dilute pancreatic trypsin[249,275] or with subcellular fractions prepared from homogenates of parathyroid glands[283,296] readily and selectively results in the formation of PTH without other cleavages occurring in the hormonal molecule. The arginyl-alanyl bond (Fig. 3–5) is preferentially susceptible to cleavage by a trypsin-like enzyme. A trypsin-like activity in the parathyroid cell that accomplishes the conversion of proPTH to PTH, however, does not appear to be identical to pancreatic trypsin, inasmuch as it is not inhibited by tosyllysylchloroketone or soybean trypsin inhibitor (but it is inhibited by addition of EDTA).[283,296] The hexapeptide removed from the NH_2-terminal sequence of proPTH by trypsin-like cleavage is further modified in the cell by carboxypeptidase B–like activity.[283] Although a trypsin-like endopeptidase is sufficient by itself to convert proPTH to PTH plus the hexapeptide, combined endopeptidase and exopeptidase activity seems closely associated in the proteolytic processing of proPTH, just as it is in the processing of other prohormones or proproteins to their native form.[297] Much work has gone into attempts to isolate and characterize the specific peptidase(s) involved in the cleavages of prohormones. What remains to be determined is whether there are multiple proteases that are specific in each tissue for the cleavages of various prohormones or whether a single enzyme accomplishes the cleavage at all sites. Subsequent specificity in, for example, distinctly different cleavage products of pro-opiomelanocortin in anterior versus intermediate lobes of the pituitary could be explained by translocation of prohormones within specialized different subcellular compartments of the secretory cell. At least two enzymes have been isolated from the pituitary gland that cleave the precursor of ACTH, pro-opiomelanocortin, into specific peptides *in vitro*, in very much the same pattern as those in which they are processed during synthesis and transport in the pituitary.[298] Recent work indicates that these pituitary enzymes also accurately cleave proinsulin to insulin and provasopressin to vasopressin, findings that suggest that the enzymes have a broad substrate recognition. A carboxypeptidase, carboxypeptidase E, has been isolated from the anterior pituitary, and the sequence of the mRNA encoding the enzyme has been determined.[299] Carboxypeptidase E appears to be the enzyme that is specific for the carboxyl-terminal cleavage of proenkephalin (enkephalin convertase). Recently the gene encoding the protease that cleaves yeast alpha factor, a peptide that contains 13 amino acids and is necessary for sexual maturation in yeast, from its precursor protein has been cloned (Kex-2 gene). Of great interest has been the discovery that the co-introduction and expression of the Kex-2 and pro-opiomelanocortin genes into cells that do not normally process pro-opiomelanocortin lead to the accurate cleavages and production of authentic peptides from the precursor pro-opiomelanocortin.[298] These observations suggest that the proteases involved in the cleavages of prohormones present in cells as distant in evolutionary time as yeast and mammalian cells contain enzymes with similar structural properties. Therefore, it can be anticipated that eventually the structures of and functions for these enzymes will become understood utilizing the recombinant DNA techniques.

4. Processing of Parathyroid Hormone

In addition to the specific enzymatic cleavages responsible for the conversion of hormonal precursors to PTH, the parathyroid gland also contains cathepsins that are responsible for further cleavages of PTH into smaller fragments.[299-305] One form of the cleavage process appears to be a calcium-regulated degradation pathway within the gland involved in the turnover of newly synthesized hormone.[300] It is believed that a substantial fraction of PTH found in the gland is completely degraded, presumably by lysosomally located enzymes. Another cathepsin-mediated enzymic process, which is separate from the complete hydrolysis of hormone described previously, results in the formation of a COOH-terminal fragment (or fragments) of the hormone that is released from the gland along with the intact hormone.[304,306] One such cathepsin has been isolated from the parathyroid gland and analyzed under cell-free conditions; the enzyme cleaves PTH at a site (between residues 36 and 37) identical to one of the sites cleaved during peripheral metabolism of the hormone in the liver. Both the cleavage processes related to turnover and the process of release of PTH appear to be regulated by changes in the concentration of extracellular calcium.

V. REGULATION OF BIOSYNTHESIS AND SECRETION

A large number of studies have been conducted on analyses of the factors involved in parathyroid hormone secretion and biosynthesis. The results and interpretations of some of these studies are detailed in this section. Some general introductory comments about parathyroid gland physiology are appropriate.

Ionized calcium appears to be the major, if not the sole, physiologic regulator of PTH secretion and formation. Although a multitude of factors have been considered to be regulators of the parathyroid gland, none of them, with the exception of calcium, have been clearly implicated in the normal physiologic functioning of the gland or in the pathogenesis of pathophysiologic alterations of the gland. Unlike many endocrine glands, which undergo many-fold changes in rates of hormone secretion and biosynthesis in response to pertubations invoked by homeostatic stimuli, the parathyroid gland appears to have a limited capacity to change its rates of hormone synthesis and secretion in response to alterations in serum calcium. A possible teleologic explanation is that under normal physiologic circumstances, fluctuations in concentrations of the controlled variable, serum ionized calcium, are small. In fact, under pathophysiologic conditions of sustained hypocalcemia that occurs in chronic renal failure, the predominant response of the parathyroid gland is to enlarge. Sustained hypocalcemia appears to have a potent mitogenic effect leading to marked hyperplasia of the glands; it is not uncommon to observe growth of parathyroid glands to 100 times or greater their normal size. The processes of hormone secretion and biosynthesis appear to be coupled in parathyroid glands. Under conditions of normal fluctuations in serum ionized calcium, PTH secretion takes place in a narrow range at the lower end of the dose-response curve (Fig. 3–8). Although acute hypocalcemia can increase parathyroid hormone secretion rates as much as 5- to 10-fold, glandular stores of hormone are depleted within 1.5 to 2 hours, at which time further secretion is limited by rates of hormone biosynthesis. Chronic hypocalcemia contributes to net production at a rate twice as high as occurs in the nonstimulated condition. Hypocalcemia leads to inhibition of an intraglandular degradative pathway, which under normal circumstances prevents approximately 50% of newly synthesized hor-

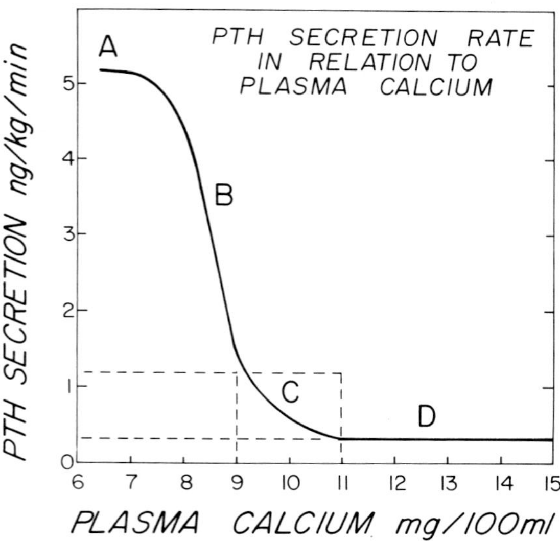

Figure 3–8. Parathyroid hormone secretion-response curve as a function of plasma calcium concentrations. Data were obtained by direct measurement of PTH levels in parathyroid gland effluent in calves during calcium or EDTA infusions. The area of the curve marked C is the normal physiologic range of regulation. A lowering of the plasma calcium levels below 9 mg/100 ml into the hypocalcemic range elicits a marked increase in secretion rate. Elevation of plasma calcium above 11 mg/100 ml into the hypercalcemic range has little effect on secretion rate. Secretion of PTH persists despite hypercalcemia, but most of what is secreted in conditions of hypercalcemia are inactive carboxyl-terminal fragments of PTH. (Adapted from Mayer GP, Hurst JG: Comparison of the effects of calcium and magnesium on parathyroid hormone secretion rate in calves. Endocrinology 102:1803–1807, 1978.)

mone from reaching a stable pool available for secretion. In any event, perhaps related to the unusual regulatable intraglandular hormone degradation, gene transcription and mRNA translation appear to be constitutively fixed at or near a maximum level. Perhaps the situation of constitutive hormone production by the parathyroid gland is not so unusual when one considers that under normal physiologic circumstances, the gland is never called upon to provide large swings in hormone production and secretion. Sustained hypercalcemia, when it develops, is usually a gradual process that takes place over weeks to months (chronic renal failure, vitamin D deficiency), and the glandular response to the pathologic overstimulation through sustained hypocalcemia is one of rapid hyperplasia.

A. Biosynthesis

Studies of the control of the biosynthesis of PTH now make it possible to draw conclusions about the cellular mechanisms of control, although much specific information yet remains to be gathered regarding several events involved in the biosynthesis of the hormone. Thus far, the most information gathered concerning the regulation of PTH biosynthesis has been obtained from studies carried out almost exclusively *in vitro*; it is not certain that regulatory responses observed under *in vitro* conditions are necessarily those expressed *in vivo*. As discussed earlier, ionized calcium is the principal factor controlling the secretion of PTH. Ultimately, however, the hormone secreted from the gland must be replenished by synthesis of the hormone, a process that requires many sequential biochemical steps, any of which could potentially be regulated (Fig. 3–9). Studies *in vitro* of the effects of varying calcium concentrations in the incubation media on the rates of labeling of preproPTH, proPTH, and PTH during pulse-chase incubations with radioactive amino acids have shown no effects on the relative rates of conversion of preproPTH to proPTH or of proPTH to PTH.[307,308] Moreover, the absolute rates of synthesis of preproPTH or proPTH change little over several hours; low calcium stimulates and high calcium suppresses synthesis of the prehormone and prohormone by 15% to 20% over a period of 4 to 5 hours.[307,308] Similar pulse-labeling analyses of the parathyroid glands removed from rats who are maintained under a mildly hypocalcemic

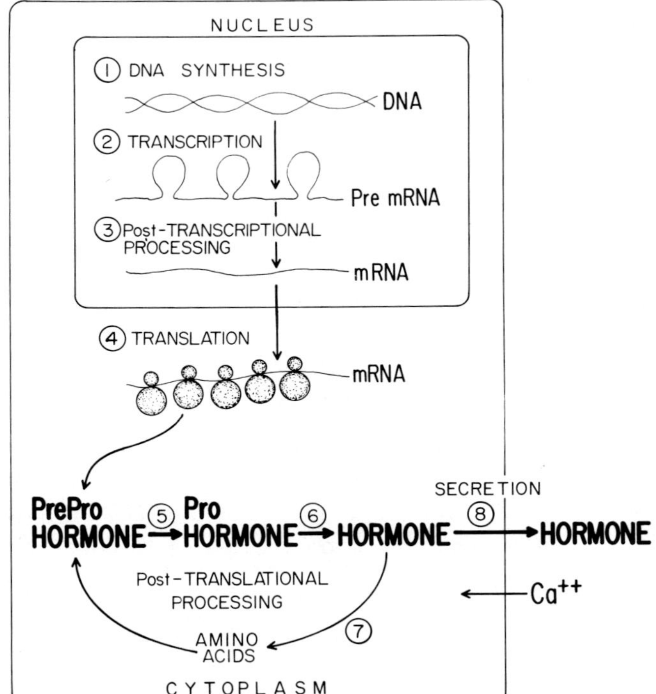

Figure 3–9. Eight potential levels in parathyroid hormone (PTH) biosynthesis that may be regulated in response to changes in levels of extracellular calcium. (See text for details.)

state for two weeks revealed no detectable differences in rates of proPTH synthesis compared with glands similarly obtained from normal calcemic rats. These observations suggest that no major regulatory effects occur at the level of translation; when protein synthesis is regulated through changes in translational activity, the effects take place much more rapidly.

Studies of the effects of extracellular calcium on parathyroid hormone gene expression have been extended back to the transcriptional and posttranscriptional levels. The stability of cytoplasmic mRNA coding for preproPTH was analyzed directly by measurements of cytoplasmic mRNA in which both (1) a cDNA hybridization-densitometric assay and endogenous translation (pulse-labeling) assays in intact cells and (2) heterologous translations of mRNA in a cell-free system derived from wheat germ were used.[309] Studies of the stability of mRNA were done in the presence and absence of actinomycin D, a potent inhibitor of RNA synthesis. Incubation of parathyroid tissues for 5 hours in the presence of actinomycin D failed to show any changes in PTH-specific mRNA levels compared with controls, whereas the synthesis of most other parathyroid gland proteins was markedly inhibited by actinomycin D. These results suggest both that the mRNA coding for preproPTH is remarkably stable and that changes in extracellular calcium do not detectably change rates of transcription of the preproPTH gene. However, in studies of dispersed bovine parathyroid cells cultured for several days in the presence of elevated calcium levels, a detectable fall in levels of hybridizable preproPTH mRNA was observed.[310] No differences in levels of preproPTH mRNA were detected in the dispersed parathyroid cells exposed to normal and low concentrations of calcium. Recently, the studies of the effects of calcium on dispersed parathyroid cell have been extended to analyses of the rates of transcription of the preproPTH gene. In nuclear run-on experiments, a decrease in gene transcription has been detected within 6 hours in response to elevated calcium concentrations.[311] In a similar model of dispersed parathyroid cells in primary culture, it has been reported that 1,25$(OH)_2D_3$ results in a fall in preproPTH mRNA levels and gene transcription as early as 2 hours after exposure to the vitamin D metabolite.[312-314] Analyses of the expression of recombinant fusion genes transferred into cultured rat pituitary cells indicate that the DNA sequences responsible for inhibiting prepro-PTH gene transcription reside within 690 base pairs of the DNA flanking the start side of transcription.[315] Further evidence that 1,25$(OH)_2D_3$ may inhibit preproPTH gene transcription is provided by showing that 1,25$(OH)_2D_3$ administration to rats leads to a substantial fall in both preproPTH gene transcription and mRNA levels in the intact animal. Although these studies demonstrated calcium and 1,25$(OH)_2D_3$ can down-regulate PTH gene expression, they do not provide a comprehensive view of the physiologic importance of the regulation of PTH gene transcription. Largely constitutive transcription of the PTH gene coupled with the existence of a remarkably stable mRNA suggests that the major control of preproPTH gene expression resides at levels other than gene transcription and mRNA stability, namely, cellular proliferation, intracellular turnover of hormone, and hormone secretion. These observations further lead one to consider that a predominant level of functional regulation of the parathyroid gland may be that of DNA synthesis, that is, cell division. Several lines of evidence lend support to this consideration, foremost of which is the fact that chronic stimulation (hypocalcemia) of the parathyroid glands invariably leads to hyperplasia of the glands, a situation almost universally encountered in patients with chronic renal failure.[40] Furthermore, studies of DNA synthesis in parathyroid glands maintained as explant cultures have shown marked increases in rates of DNA synthesis within a few hours after the introduction of hypocalcemic stimulation.[316,317] In states of chronic hypocalcemia, the numbers of cells in parathyroid glands increase. Little is known about the mechanism of these processes of cellular proliferation. For example, it is not known whether the increase in cell numbers results from increased cell division or longer survival of preexisting cells or both circumstances, whether all parathyroid cells can divide or instead only a subset of specially equipped cells can divide, or whether signals other than hypocalcemia regulate cell proliferation. Some studies have begun to define the determinants of parathyroid cell number. High concentrations of serum stimulate primary bovine parathyroid cells to divide when cultured *in vitro*, but they do not divide when cultured in the absence of serum.[318,319] The dividing parathyroid cells behave like adenoma cells in their unresponsiveness to calcium. A factor has been found in serum from patients with multiple endocrine neoplasia (MEN type I) that stimulates the proliferation of parathyroid cells maintained in long-term culture[320] (see Chapter 18). Although the relevance of this serum factor to normal parathyroid homeostasis remains to be established, parathyroid adenomas may be considered as tumors that have escaped the constraints normally placed on cell number by calcium and other regulators. It appears that sporadic parathyroid adenomas (not associated with MEN syndromes) arise by the clonal expansion of one abnormal cell.[321] Presumably, the initial abnormal cell has lost the ability to respond to the signals that maintain numbers of parathyroid cells within appropriate limits. These recent observations of the regulation of parathyroid cell division, combined with the substantial newer information concerning growth factors and their cellular targets, should provide clues to the mechanisms by which the growth of parathyroid cells is regulated.

In addition to control by calcium of the rate of secretion of preformed hormone, there is an additional cellular mechanism that supports rapid changes in secretion rates, that of a controlled degradative pathway that involves the destruction of hormone already synthesized. Thus, changes in the concentration of calcium in the extracellular fluid regulate intracellular stores of hormones through a pathway involving hormone turnover. High concentrations of extracellular calcium stimulate, and low concentrations inhibit, intracellular degradation of hormone. Perhaps the inhibition of this degradative pathway, mediated by a lowering of extracellular calcium concentrations, provides a means for a rapid increase in the amounts of hormone available for secretion.[248,307] Conversely, stimulation of the degradative pathway by elevations of extracellular calcium may be a useful mechanism for the cell to dispose of excess hormone.

At present, a reasonable but by no means proven formulation for the regulation of PTH synthesis and secretion may be summarized as follows. Hypocalcemia leads immediately (within seconds) to increased secretion of hormone owing to a release of preformed stored hormone. This rapid release of hormone may not be sustained because the limited stores of hormone that are available for secretion are readily exhausted. However, the stimulation of hypocalcemia rapidly (within minutes) inhibits the intracellular degradation of hormone, resulting in an increase in the amount of hormone available to meet secretory demands. When hypocalcemia is severe and prolonged, the chronic stimulation after several hours leads to DNA replication and eventually cell division, thereby providing more cells for the production of hormone. In this formulation, mRNA synthesis and hormone synthesis are constitutive rather than regulatory, that is, transcriptional and translational processes involving the production of hormone may not change greatly, if at all. Hence, the major levels of regulation of hormone biosynthesis in the parathyroid gland appear to be those of intracellular hormone degradation and cell division rather than changes in rates of DNA transcription and mRNA translation characteristic of many other endocrine and secretory tissues.

B. Secretion

1. Secretagogues

Calcium. Calcium is the principal regulator of parathyroid glandular activity. It has been recognized for many years that the rate of secretion of PTH is inversely dependent on the concentration of extracellular calcium ion.[322,324] Because the action of PTH is to increase the concentration of calcium in the extracellular fluid (ECF) through its effects on bone, kidney, and intestines, negative feedback inhibition of the parathyroid gland contributes to the regulation of concentrations of ECF calcium within very narrow limits. Although calcium is the potent physiologically important regulator of parathyroid hormone secretion, other secretagogues have been identified, although their physiologic role, if any, is not understood.

Cyclic AMP. Adenylate cyclase and its product, cyclic 3′,5′-AMP, appear to be intermediates in the control by calcium of PTH secretion.[325-327] Intracellular levels of cAMP change in parallel with changes in PTH secretion effected by the secretagogues epinephrine, isoproterenol, dopamine, secretin, and prostaglandin E_2 as well as by hypocalcemia.[325,334] In addition, agents that suppress secretion of PTH, such as alpha-adrenergic agonists[335] or prostaglandin F_2,[336] decrease intracellular levels of cAMP. The rise in intracellular cAMP involved by catecholamines is followed by the binding of cAMP to the regulatory unit of cAMP-dependent protein kinase, and the subsequent activation of the catalytic subunit of this kinase.[337] Further, whereas catecholamines cause a proportional stimulation of cAMP-dependent protein kinase and PTH secretion, calcium inhibits PTH secretion without affecting cAMP-dependent protein kinase.[337] Dibutyryl cAMP, forskolin, and inhibitors of phosphodiesterase (aminophylline, theophyllines) mimic the effects of hypocalcemia in eliciting a parathyroid hormone secretory response *in vitro*.[338] Several studies of the requirements for activity of adenylate cyclase prepared from parathyroid glands indicate that the enzyme is particularly sensitive to calcium. Under cell-free conditions, calcium (0.5 mM) inhibits the enzyme.[339] The adenylate cyclase from the dog and horse parathyroid glands is 200 times more sensitive to the inhibitory effect of calcium than are corresponding preparations from other tissues.[340,341] Calcium also stimulates phosphodiesterase in parathyroid tissue.[342]

As has been shown for a number of other cAMP-mediated cellular responses, maximum rates of PTH secretion appear to occur at submaximal levels of intracellular cAMP. Hormone secretion induced by norepinephrine *in vitro* reaches maximum levels at doses of norepinephrine that are not yet maximal for stimulating increased cellular levels of cAMP.

At present, the exact role of adenylate cyclase and the formation of cAMP in the secretory events involved in the release of PTH remain unknown. The observations made in studies *in vitro* that cAMP is released concomitantly with the release of PTH in response to hypocalcemia[325] suggest that the formation of cAMP is closely linked to the process of exocytosis. The biochemical nature of the reactions elicited by cAMP is unknown. It might be speculated that cAMP is in some manner involved in the phosphorylation of a substrate protein in the parathyroid gland, perhaps a membrane protein involved in the fusion of the secretory granule with the plasma membrane, resulting in discharge of hormone from the granule into the extracellular space. It has been shown that two specific proteins are phosphorylated in response to the activation of cAMP-dependent protein kinase.[343] Studies directed toward the subcellular localization of the adenylate cyclase–cAMP and a continued search for specific phosphoproteins in the parathyroid gland are indicated to gain more complex information regarding their linkage to hormone secretory responses.

Secretory Responses. The earlier suggestion that rates of PTH secretion were inversely proportional to blood calcium concentration over a wide range must be revised. In those earlier studies, measurements, by radioimmunoassay, of PTH levels in the general (peripheral) circulation of the bovine species[324,344] did not provide an accurate assessment of the control of secretion because of the presence of multiple immunoreactive forms of the hormone that gave erroneous values in plasma of hormone concentrations by radioimmunoassay. These difficulties introduced by peripheral metabolism of hormone have now been avoided by the direct measurement of hormone concentration in parathyroid effluent blood,[303,333,345-348] by studies of hormone secretion *in vitro*,[270,271,296,307,349-355] and by the use of amino-terminal radioimmunoassays that do not detect hormone fragments.

Numerous studies now support the concept of proportional control of secretion of hormone, but only over a narrow range of calcium concentrations (7.5–11 mg/100 ml). Direct measurements of PTH secretion show that a slowly induced decline of calcium concentration from 10.5 to 9.0 mg/100 ml in calves elicited small and gradual increases in secretory rate[346] (Fig. 3–8). However, a further decrease in calcium concentration from 9 to 8 mg/100 ml induced a marked rise in PTH secretion to a maximal rate. Below 8 mg/100 ml, little or no further rise in secretion occurred. The virtual constancy of secretion in normocalcemia together with the steep response in mild hypocalcemia seems to constitute a secretion-control mechanism that is appropriate for calcium homeostasis.[344] A persistent basal secretion rate was observed, even when the calcium concentration of the blood was maintained at 16 to 18 mg/100 ml for up to 24 hours.[346] A similar pattern of sustained hormone secretion at a low rate in the face of elevated concentration of extracellular calcium has been observed in studies of hormone release *in vitro*.[346,349-351,353-355] The molecular composition of the hormone secreted under these conditions of unusually high calcium concentration *in vitro* shows a predominance of biologically inactive carboxyl-terminal fragments[303] but a persistence of a smaller amount of intact, biologically active hormone.[346] This continued secretion of biologically active hormone during maximal suppression of the gland by high calcium concentrations may explain, at least in part, the abnormalities of calcium control characteristically seen in patients with hyperfunctioning tumors of the parathyroids[350,351,356,357] (in whom circulating levels of PTH remain excessively high despite sustained hypercalcemia) (see Chapter 14). The persistence of secretion of biologically active hormone, independent of blood calcium levels, is supported by experimental studies in which persistent hypercalcemia, equivalent to the state of hyperparathyroidism, was created in normal rats given multiple isologous parathyroid gland transplants.[358] The intramuscular transplantation of 20 normally functioning glands into a single rat resulted in persistent hypercalcemia and continued secretion of PTH uninhibited by hypercalcemia. Figure 3–10 illustrates the pattern of secretion of PTH in a group of normal subjects tested *in vivo* by infusions of calcium and the calcium-chelating agent EDTA to respectively raise and lower blood calcium, during which period multiple measurements of PTH were made by immunoassay. In these studies, using peripheral blood samples, the persistent PTH secretions at supranormal blood calcium levels cannot be detected. However, the persistent PTH secretion at high calcium levels was shown in normal cows by direct parathyroid gland venous sampling (the implications of persistent, calcium-independent hormone secretion for the pathophysiology of hyperparathyroidism are discussed in Chapter 14).

Changes in the rate of PTH secretion induced by reciprocal changes in the concentrations of extracellular calcium occur within one minute after application of the stimulus.[328,359] A biphasic secretion response is often observed upon induction of hypocalcemia by brief infusion of the calcium chelator EDTA. Hormone is initially released in a large spurt lasting only a few minutes, followed by a lesser response sustained for many hours.

Direct immunoassays of the hormone levels in parathyroid gland effluent blood *in vivo*[347] and measurements of the hormone content in bovine parathyroid glands[273] provided estimates of the glandular reserves of hormone potentially available for secretion. Normal bovine glands, whose total mass is of the

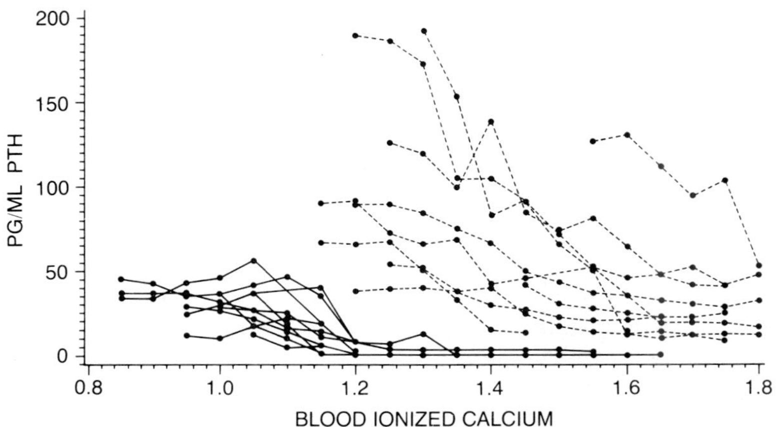

Figure 3–10. Demonstration of a "set point" defect in the PTH secretory response to blood ionized calcium in adenomatous parathyroid glands. Blood calcium levels were acutely lowered by the administration of infusions of EDTA and raised by calcium infusions in normal subjects (solid line) and patients with primary hyperparathyroidism (dotted line). Parathyroid hormone levels were measured by a radioimmunoassay that detects determinants in the amino-terminal region of PTH; calcium is plotted as ionized calcium levels (multiply by eight to convert, approximately, to total calcium concentration). (See also Figure 14–11, Chapter 14.)

order of 2 mg/kg body weight, contain approximately 200 μg of hormone per gram wet weight of tissue (0.02%). At normal secretory rates and at physiologic calcium concentrations (1.2 ng/kg/min), hormone stores could meet demands for approximately 7 hours without the need for synthesis of new hormone. Similarly, during hypocalcemic challenge, under which secretory rates rise to 5 to 6 ng/kg/min, hormone stores would become depleted in approximately 1.5 hours.

In fact, Mayer and Hurst[347] showed that during a 4-hour period of hypocalcemia, induced in a calf by continued infusion of EDTA, a maximum initial secretory rate of approximately 16 ng/kg/min fell to approximately 10 ng/kg/min after about 1.5 hours. These results are consistent with the exhaustion of hormone stores after a few hours followed by continued secretion provided by newly synthesized hormone. It appears, therefore, that the two processes of secretion and biosynthesis are closely coupled. The apparently limited stores of PTH are consistent with the observation that the numbers of secretory granules in parathyroid cells are small compared with other endocrine cells, for instance, pituitary gland or pancreatic islet cells. These observations are in keeping with the functional role of the parathyroid glands. Under normal physiologic conditions, nearly continuous release of small amounts of hormone is required (see later) rather than the episodic release of large amounts of hormone, such as can occur in the case of insulin release by the pancreatic islet beta cells.

Magnesium. Although calcium is the principal cation that influences PTH secretion, magnesium can cause similar changes, although only at concentrations several-fold higher than those found in ECF under normal physiologic conditions.[348,353] For example, it was shown in studies both *in vivo* and *in vitro* that, on a molar basis, magnesium is two to three times less effective than calcium in suppressing PTH secretion.[348,353] An earlier study[355] in which it was concluded that calcium and magnesium were equally potent in the regulation of PTH secretion *in vitro* was not borne out by subsequent analysis of the effect of these two cations.[348,353] Because the normal concentration of magnesium in the blood is lower than that of calcium, 1.0 mM compared with 1.5 mM (ionized) for calcium, and magnesium is two to three times less potent than calcium on a molar basis in effecting hormonal secretion, any contribution of magnesium to the regulation of PTH secretion is probably small under normal physiologic circumstances.

However, an adequate body store of magnesium is essential for normal function of the parathyroid gland. When blood values fall below 0.8 mEq/liter, indicative of severe magnesium depletion, an inhibition of hormone secretion results. This requirement for magnesium in hormone secretion was demonstrated first in studies in alcoholic patients,[360-362] who presented with profound hypomagnesemia, hypocalcemia, and tetany that was nearly impossible to correct by therapy with calcium alone. Blood levels of PTH were found to be inappropriately low, often below the limits of detection. Soon after the parenteral administration of magnesium salts, serum PTH levels rose dramatically with ensuing gradual increases in serum calcium.[360-362] It is unlikely that such rapid and dramatic rises in serum PTH induced by magnesium repletion could reflect anything other than a sudden release of stored hormone, and it is unlikely that the changes in PTH levels resulted from changes in peripheral metabolism of the hormone. The explanation, on a cellular basis, for such marked effects of hypomagnesemia on PTH secretion is not known but may relate in some way to the formation of intraglandular cAMP and to the process of exocytosis by which hormone is transported via the secretory granules to the ECF. Adenylate cyclase prepared from hyperplastic human parathyroid tissue is reported to require magnesium ion, all enzymic activity being lost below a concentration of 1 mM Mg.[339] Chronic, severe hypomagnesemia, found in malnourished alcoholics[360,361] and in the magnesium wasting associated with cisplatinum therapy, also causes a paradoxical decrease in PTH secretion rather than the expected increase. Current evidence indicates that the intracellular magnesium deficiency seen in these patients interferes with intracellular secretory mechanisms and blocks PTH secretion. Replenishment of magnesium immediately results in PTH secretion in these patients.[360-362]

It should be emphasized that inhibition of PTH secretion is probably not the exclusive reason for the hypocalcemia seen in association with hypomagnesemia, at least in some patients. In addition to the phenomenon of functional hypoparathyroidism, there are reports that magnesium depletion also impairs the action of PTH on the kidney and possibly the skeleton[363] and hence hypomagnesemia involves blunted response to PTH in some patients.

Catecholamines. Present evidence from studies *in vitro* and *in vivo* indicates that catecholamines modulate the secretion of PTH. Beta-adrenergic agonists (epinephrine, isoproterenol) augment the secretion of hormone induced by hypocalcemia, and this augmentation of secretion can be inhibited by antagonists of beta-adrenergic action such as propranolol.[326,364] The effects of catecholamines on the secretion of PTH are associated with changes in intracellular levels of cAMP.[326] In studies in calves *in vivo*,[328,333,365] the levels of epinephrine required to elicit secretory responses were found to be close to those occurring under normal physiologic circumstances. The effects of catecholamines on PTH secretion are additive to those of hypocalcemia, suggesting that two separate receptor-response systems may exist in the parathyroid gland—one sensitive to calcium and the other to catecholamines. Additional evidence in support of the existence of catecholamine receptors in the parathyroid gland comes from the demonstration of sympathetic nerve endings in the gland[366-368] and from the findings that propranolol inhibits the stimulation of PTH secretion due to epinephrine, but not the stimulation due to hypocalcemia. Repeated injection of epinephrine to calves *in vivo* leads to a diminishing PTH secretory response,[328] consistent with tachyphylaxis of receptors for epinephrine. The development of refractoriness of the secretory response was also observed during repeated or prolonged exposure of dispersed parathyroid cells *in vitro* to epinephrine. In these studies, however, levels of cAMP in the cells remained high at a time when the PTH secretory response of the cells was obliterated, suggesting that the resistance to beta-adrenergic stimulation is not linked directly to the formation of cAMP but rather is linked to an effect beyond cAMP formation such as protein phosphorylation.

Intradermal injections of epinephrine or propranolol to normal subjects led to prompt increases or decreases, respectively, in the secretion of PTH, providing further evidence for an effect of beta-adrenergic stimuli in the regulation of PTH secretion during hypoglycemic stress induced by the intravenous injection of insulin.[369] The increase in blood levels of PTH observed occurred 5 minutes after maximum hypoglycemia and thus before the rise in serum cortisol (30 minutes after maximum hypoglycemia), indicating that the stimulus to PTH secretion was not due to cortisol. In these experiments it was suggested that the stimulus to PTH secretion resulted from increased blood levels of epinephrine brought on by the hypoglycemic stress. Injections of either of the alpha-adrenergic agents phenylephrine[332] or methoxamine[334] elicited no parathyroid secretory response in normal subjects, supporting the conclusion that no alpha-adrenergic receptors are present in the parathyroid gland.

It should be emphasized that the catecholamines are not primary regulators of hormone secretion but rather appear to serve as modulators of PTH secretion only when secretory rates are greatly increased. When hormone secretion is basal, as it is under normal physiologic conditions, epinephrine has little, if any, effect to alter rates of hormone secretion. The role of the catecholamines in physiologic regulation and pathophysiologic processes of the parathyroid glands is uncertain. It has been suggested that excessive secretion of catecholamines in patients with pheochromocytoma of the adrenal medulla may be responsible for the hyperplasia of the parathyroid glands that frequently accompanies this disorder[370] (multiple endocrine neoplasia syndrome, type II). On the other hand, evidence presented by Pearse[371] indicates that the adrenal medulla and parathyroid gland (and the calcitonin-producing cells, C cells) arise from a common embryonic origin (neuroectoderm); clinical evidence suggests that the neoplasia-hyperplasia characteristic of the syndrome of multiple endocrine neoplasia reflects a co-independent proliferative process common to these cells rather than a primary defect in one hormonal cell type leading to adaptive changes in other cell types.

The physiologic relevance of these pharmacologic experiments with catecholamines is unclear. Definitive *in vivo* studies have been difficult to perform because the effects of catecholamines are not quantitatively impressive. In that setting it is difficult to distinguish whether changing blood levels of immunoreactive PTH reflect altered secretion or altered metabolism of the hormone. One might speculate that catecholamines could modulate PTH secretion during stress, in patients with pheochromocytomas, or perhaps in some patients with apparent primary hyperparathyroidism. Experimental studies of stress have not been definitive, largely because the models necessarily have multiple variables. Hyperventilation and metabolic acidosis, for example, cause changes in levels of ionized calcium, thus potentially obscuring effects of endogenous circulating catecholamines or effects of norepinephrine released from sympathetic terminals in parathyroid tissue. Most patients with pheochromocytoma are not hypercalcemic,[372] although hypercalcemic patients with pheochromocytoma often have concomitant primary hyperparathyroidism (multiple endocrine neoplasia, type II).[373]

Whereas definitive experiments demonstrating the importance of catecholamines in PTH physiology are lacking, the responsiveness of normal parathyroid tissue to beta-adrenergic agonists is well established. The role that catecholamines play in parathyroid pathophysiology is undefined.

Vitamin D Metabolites. Much interest has arisen as a result of the acquisition of evidence suggesting that the dihydroxylated metabolites of vitamin D, 1,25-dihydroxyvitamin D_3 [1,25$(OH)_2D_3$] and 24,25-dihydroxyvitamin D_3, may regulate the activity of the parathyroid gland (see Chapter 5). Nuclear and cytoplasmic binding components for 1,25$(OH)_2$D are found in cell-free extracts of parathyroid glands. A dose of tritium-labeled 1,25$(OH)_2$D administered to chicks has been shown to localize to the parathyroid gland (as well as to intestine and bone).[374] These findings raise the possibility of the existence of a short-loop feedback system involving the metabolites of vitamin D and the secretion of PTH.[375-377] Such a feedback loop could serve as a complement to the negative feedback loop on the parathyroid gland involving calcium and PTH. One of the physiologically important actions of parathyroid hormone is to increase the activity of the renal enzyme 25$(OH)_2$D 1α-hydroxylase, leading to increased formation of 1,25$(OH)_2$D from its precursor 25(OH)D. The actions of 1,25$(OH)_2$D in turn lead to increased intestinal absorption of calcium and a tendency to elevate blood levels of calcium. Increased blood calcium in turn feeds back on the parathyroid gland to suppress hormone secretion. Such a feedback control system, however, takes hours to complete owing to the considerable time required for 1,25$(OH)_2$D to induce the formation of intestinal calcium-binding protein and thereby increase intestinal absorption of calcium. Suppression of PTH secretion directly by 1,25$(OH)_2$D or the stimulation by 24,25$(OH)_2$D, synthesized in inverse proportion to the synthesis of 1,25$(OH)_2$D independent of changes in blood calcium levels, could theoretically shorten the time required for a feedback response on the parathyroid glands and thereby could provide a more tightly controlled feedback regulation of parathyroid hormone secretion and calcium metabolism than a system that was regulated by calcium and PTH only.

Evidence that such regulatory influences of vitamin D metabolites on PTH synthesis or secretion occur physiologically is still inconclusive. A number of studies of the effects of the vitamin D metabolites on PTH secretion have been carried out both *in vivo* and *in vitro*, and the results of the studies have been conflicting. 1,25$(OH)_2$D is reported to suppress,[375-377] stimulate,[378] or have no effect[379] on the secretion of PTH in studies done *in vivo* and *in vitro*.[380] 24,25$(OH)_2$D has also been reported to affect hormone secretion in certain test systems[378,380,381] and to have no effect on parathyroid gland function in two other studies. In one study carried out *in vivo* in the dog, suppression of PTH secretion into parathyroid effluent blood was observed within seconds after the injection of 24,25$(OH)_2$D into the thyroid artery.[378] It seems reasonable to suppose that any effects of the metabolites of vitamin D on the parathyroid gland would involve the cellular uptake of the metabolites by cytosolic receptors followed by their transport to the nucleus, where regulatory effects would be expressed at the level of RNA synthesis, an event analogous with the known mechanisms of action of the steroid hormones. These effects would likely involve regulation of PTH production at the level of synthesis of new hormone rather than at the level of secretion of preformed hormone. Such an intracellular mechanism of action of the vitamin D metabolites would not account for the reported rapid effects of the metabolites on the secretion of PTH, effects that must occur through actions at the periphery of the parathyroid cells, for example, plasma membrane and secretory granules.

Thus, the physiologic and/or pathophysiologic relevance of the effects of 1,25(OH)$_2$D on PTH secretion remains unclear. The contradictory effects observed *in vitro* may result from the difficulty of controlling and measuring the true levels of unbound vitamin D metabolites in tissue culture dishes,[382] vagaries of PTH assays, species differences, and other aspects of experimental design. *In vivo* studies may be compromised by similar problems, and also must contend with the difficulties associated with (1) using blood levels of PTH as measures of PTH secretion and (2) separating direct effects of vitamin D metabolites on the parathyroid gland from indirect effects of changing blood calcium levels, and (3) the possible consequences of further metabolism of administered vitamin D metabolites. Further experimentation will be required; the existence of a direct effect of any vitamin D metabolite on PTH secretion remains to be established.

Other Potential Regulatory Factors. A number of factors other than those indicated have been reported to influence the secretion of parathyroid hormone. For the most part, these studies have been carried out *in vitro* and the effects of the factors have been small. Whether they exert physiologically relevant regulatory effects on the parathyroid gland remains to be proved.

Calcitonin has been reported to directly stimulate the secretion of parathyroid hormone in studies using parathyroid explants *in vitro*[383] (see Chapter 4). The doses of calcitonin required to elicit a secretory response, however, were much higher than what is believed to circulate in the bloodstream *in vivo*. Some evidence, albeit indirect, suggests that markedly elevated blood levels of calcitonin may stimulate PTH secretion *in vivo* in man. Calcium infusions given to patients with medullary carcinoma of the thyroid resulted not only in the expected rise in serum calcium and calcitonin but also in a paradoxical rise in blood levels of iPTH rather than the expected suppression of PTH secretion.[384] Although not shown directly in this study, the results are consistent with the occurrence of a stimulation of PTH secretion by the large amounts of calcitonin released as a result of the calcium infusion.

Cortisol has been observed to produce elevated levels of serum PTH when administered in humans[385] and in rats[386] or when added to rat parathyroid glands maintained in organ culture.[387] Although the serum calcium levels measured in these studies remained within the normal range, the elevated levels of PTH resulting from the administration of cortisol were attributed to a transient lowering of serum calcium levels by way of the actions of cortisol to reduce intestinal absorption and renal tubular resorption of calcium. Au,[387] however, has reported finding a direct stimulatory effect of cortisol on the secretion of PTH from rat parathyroid glands maintained as explants in culture, suggesting that cortisol may influence PTH secretion by mechanisms that are independent of changes in blood levels of calcium. It was speculated that the effects of cortisol may be expressed through actions on the inhibition of the intracellular degradation of hormone, possibly by the stabilization of lysosomal membranes, and, as a consequence, may decrease release of cellular proteases.[387]

Rats given daily injections of bovine growth hormone developed enlargements of the parathyroid glands concomitant with increase in serum calcium and PTH levels.[388] These observations may help to explain the tendency for many patients with acromegaly and excessive secretion of growth hormone to develop hypercalcemia. Blood levels of PTH, however, have not been systematically evaluated in patients with acromegaly, and it remains possible that the hypercalcemia not infrequently seen in this disorder is a direct result of the growth hormone on bone resorption (or hyperparathyroidism linked to a pituitary adenoma as common components of the multiple endocrine neoplasia syndrome, type I).

Somatostatin, a polypeptide hormone located in the hypothalamus, pancreatic islets, brain, C cells of the thyroid, and gastrointestinal tract, has been shown to be a potent inhibitor of the secretion of a number of different polypeptide hormones including insulin, glucagon, growth hormone, and a number of other pituitary and gastrointestinal hormones.[389] Although a suppression of PTH levels in blood as a result of somatostatin administration has been reported in studies *in vivo* in rats and monkeys,[390] other studies done in normal human subjects and patients with parathyroid adenomas failed to show any discernible effects of somatostatin on the secretion of PTH;[334,391] the rises in blood levels of PTH observed during an infusion of EDTA with and without the concurrent administration of somatostatin were the same.

Thus, it is uncertain at the present time whether somatostatin alters secretion rates of PTH under physiologic conditions.

A number of other substances have been reported to affect PTH secretion and cellular formation of cyclic AMP in isolated bovine parathyroid cells studied *in vitro*. These substances include dopamine, nitroprusside,[392] prostaglandins,[331,336] cholera toxin,[329] and various anions.[393] The contribution of some of these substances to the physiologic regulation of PTH secretion is unknown.

Aluminum can inhibit PTH secretion *in vitro*; [394] this inhibition may actually occur in patients with end-stage renal failure who harbor large aluminum loads. Histamine stimulates release of PTH *in vitro* from bovine parathyroid slices[395] and from cells isolated from dispersed human parathyroid adenomas.[396] The effects of histamine can be blocked by cimetidine. *In vivo* studies show that acute cimetidine administration results in a modest fall in PTH levels.[395] Use of cimetidine in primary and secondary hyperparathyroidism has variably led to a fall in PTH levels, but does not affect blood calcium levels, suggesting that the changes in blood PTH levels do not necessarily reflect changes in biologically active PTH.[364]

Phosphate might be expected to influence the secretion of PTH inasmuch as one of the important actions of PTH is to inhibit the renal tubular resorption of phosphate, resulting in phosphaturia and the development of hypophosphatemia. Phosphate, however, has no apparent direct effect on the parathyroid gland.[344] Hyperphosphatemia (acute) has a stimulatory effect on PTH secretion in cows but only indirectly by virtue of lowering the ionized calcium level in blood, presumably through the formation of complexes of calcium and phosphate. Simultaneous infusions of calcium and phosphate into cows in amounts sufficient to maintain normocalcemia, despite severe hyperphosphatemia, prevents the release of PTH seen during infusions of phosphate alone.[344]

2. Mechanisms

It is believed that exocytosis is involved in the cellular processes by which parathyroid hormone gains access to the ECF. The limiting membranes of granules or vesicles that contain hormone fuse with the plasma membrane, membrane lysis occurs, and the contents of the storage vesicle are released into the bloodstream. As mentioned earlier, the studies of MacGregor et al.[276] and Morrissey and Cohn[272] suggest that more than one secretory pathway may operate in the parathyroid gland.

With the apparent exception of the parathyroid gland, the process of secretion via exocytosis in most secretory or endocrine glands is closely coupled to calcium influx into the cell.[397] Calcium serves as a "second messenger" and is required for secretion to occur. In the absence of an adequate concentration of calcium in the ECF, all secretory activity ceases. The parathyroid gland, on the other hand, appears to behave paradoxically in this regard inasmuch as increases in the concentration of ECF calcium result in an inhibition of secretion. The reason for this apparent difference in secretion control between the parathyroid gland and other glands is not understood. For that matter, very little is known about the cellular and molecular basis responsible for the coupling of extracellular stimuli and secretory events.

Calcium ionophores have been used as probes in attempts to gain an understanding of the controlling and coupling factors involved in PTH secretion.[352,398] The ionophores (X537A and A21387) bind and transport calcium (and other divalent cations) across biological membranes. The ionophores restore secretion in tissues under conditions in which ECF calcium levels are below the critical levels required for spontaneous secretion. The addition of ionophores to medium bathing parathyroid glands during *in vitro* incubations caused a suppression rather than a stimulation of the secretion of PTH (and of parathyroid secretory protein).[352]

The conclusion from these observations that cellular influx of calcium results in an inhibition of PTH secretion in a manner quite the opposite of most other secretory cells must be made with caution. In addition to effects on ion transport across the plasma membrane, the ionophores alter ion fluxes among subcellular organelles within the cell.[352] Such changes in ion flow, particularly that of potassium, are apparently responsible for the morphologic changes observed in mitochondria and in Golgi complexes in cells treated with ionophores, albeit in doses larger than those required to specifically inhibit the secretion of PTH.[169]

Moreover, studies of the uptake and release of ^{45}Ca by parathyroid gland slices *in vitro* have revealed further interesting paradoxes.[398] The parathyroid gland, in contrast to many other tissues, appears to maintain a relatively high intracellular concentration of calcium, most of which is sequestered within organelles. Although the ionophores have been found to inhibit the secretion of PTH, their effects on calcium transport result in a net efflux. Thus, there appears to be either an inhibition of cellular uptake of calcium or a release of calcium from intracellular compartments, both circumstances leading to a net outflow of the cation.

Calcium may be an important intracellular mediator of PTH secretion. Although the role of intracellular calcium in PTH secretion has not yet been clarified, a number of studies suggest that changes in intracellular calcium are involved in signaling the parathyroid cell to secrete PTH. Calcium has an important role in the metabolic processes of many cells. In most cells the level of ionized calcium free in the cytoplasm varies little in response to changes in extracellular calcium.[399] Plasma membranes are relatively impermeable to calcium. ATP-driven calcium pumps and an Na^+-Ca^{2+} exchange mechanism serve to extrude calcium from the cell; other intracellular mechanisms transport cytoplasmic calcium into mitochondria and the cisternae of endoplasmic reticulum. The interaction of these mechanisms serves to keep the intracellular calcium concentration in the 100 nM range, four orders of magnitude lower than the concentration of ionized extracellular calcium. In response to secretagogues, the concentration of intracellular calcium rises transiently in many types of cells, and this rise in calcium levels appears to be instrumental in the secretory process. The increase in intracellular calcium occurs either by influx of calcium from the extracellular fluid or by release from stores in the endoplasmic reticulum. Release of calcium from the endoplasmic reticulum is stimulated by inositol-1,4,5-triphosphate. Inositol-1,4,5-triphosphate and diacylglycerol are the products of hydrolysis of the membrane phospholipid phosphatidylinositol-4,5-diphosphate by phospholipase C. Diacylglycerol, the second product of hydrolysis of phosphatidylinositol-4,5-diphosphate, activates protein kinase C, an activation that leads to hormone secretion. Thus, in many cells, secretion is linked to the hydrolysis of phospholipids, which in turn transiently activates protein kinase C and raises the levels of ionized calcium in the cytosol.

Because calcium is required for hormone secretion from most cells, the inhibition of PTH secretion by high extracellular calcium seems to be paradoxical. Studies of intracellular calcium levels in parathyroid cells[400] appear to deepen the paradox. Parathyroid cells buffer extracellular calcium relatively poorly. Unlike many other cells, intracellular calcium levels in parathyroid cells increase several-fold in response to increases in extracellular calcium. This rise of intracellular calcium is associated not with a secretory response but rather with a decrease in PTH secretion. How precisely the rise in intracellular calcium is associated with a fall instead of a rise in PTH secretion remains an unanswered question, but current studies suggest that the relationship between intracellular calcium levels in parathyroid cells and PTH secretion is complicated. When electroshock[401] or ionophores[402] are used to raise intracellular calcium levels to the level attained in intact cells exposed to an elevation of extracellular calcium, no suppression of PTH secretion occurs. These studies suggest that the rise in total free intracellular calcium is associated with but not directly responsible for the inhibition of PTH secretion. Calcium channels seem to be involved in the regulatory process because some calcium channel agonists inhibit and others stimulate PTH secretion.[403] Calcium may act through interaction with a G protein because pertussis toxin, which ADP-ribosylates certain G proteins, antagonizes the effect of high extracellular calcium.[404] The involvement of a G protein in the secretion of PTH is further supported by studies of permeabilized cells[405] in which guanyl nucleotide analogues stimulate PTH secretion. Calcium may be linked to the activity of the phosphatidylinositol pathway. Lithium, an inhibitor of inositol-1-phosphatase, decreases the effectiveness of extracellular calcium to suppress PTH secretion. High levels of extracellular calcium lead to a rise in levels of inositol-1-phosphate in parathyroid cells, and this rise is potentiated by the presence of lithium.[406] Although these studies suggest that calcium affects the phosphatidylinositol pathway, they do not precisely define the role of this pathway in PTH secretion. Similarly, studies showing that phorbol esters, which, like diacylglycerol, can activate protein kinase C, stimulate PTH secretion[407] suggest that protein kinase C may participate in the actions of calcium. This hypothesis has been strengthened by the observation that a fall in extracellular calcium leads to a substantial increase in the level of membrane-bound protein kinase C in primary dispersed parathyroid cells.[408]

At this time, then, no coherent picture emerges to precisely explain how calcium regulates PTH secretion. The striking changes in intracellular calcium in response to changes in extracellular calcium suggest that calcium channels are involved in this regulation. Much further study will be required to shed light on these apparent differences between the secretory behavior of the parathyroid cell and that of most other secretory cells.

VI. METABOLISM

A. Heterogeneity of Circulating Forms of Parathyroid Hormone

As early as 1968 it was recognized that the hormone in plasma differed from the hormone extracted from the glands when tested in multiple immunologic assays, indicating that the secreted hormone must differ chemically from hormone stored in the gland[409] (Fig. 3–11). This important early observation has been substantiated by two decades of investigation into the heterogeneity of circulating endogenous PTH.

The heterogeneity of circulating PTH arises by proteolysis of the polypeptide of 84 amino acids into two or more fragments. This proteolysis of the hormone appears to occur at two sites: within the gland and in certain peripheral organs, for example, liver or kidney. Studies of the metabolism of PTH have produced many reports that present a confused picture, owing to the variety of methods employed and the divergence in apparent results. Studies on this problem continue, however, because delineation of the metabolism of PTH is important to understanding the relation of the chemistry of PTH to its physiologic function and the mode of action of the hormone on its target tissues.

The existence of different chemical forms of PTH in blood has complicated efforts to derive clinically useful information from measurements of circulating immunoreactive PTH; not all immunoreactive forms are biologically active or predictably related to glandular secretion. Additionally, the findings have drawn attention to the possibility that

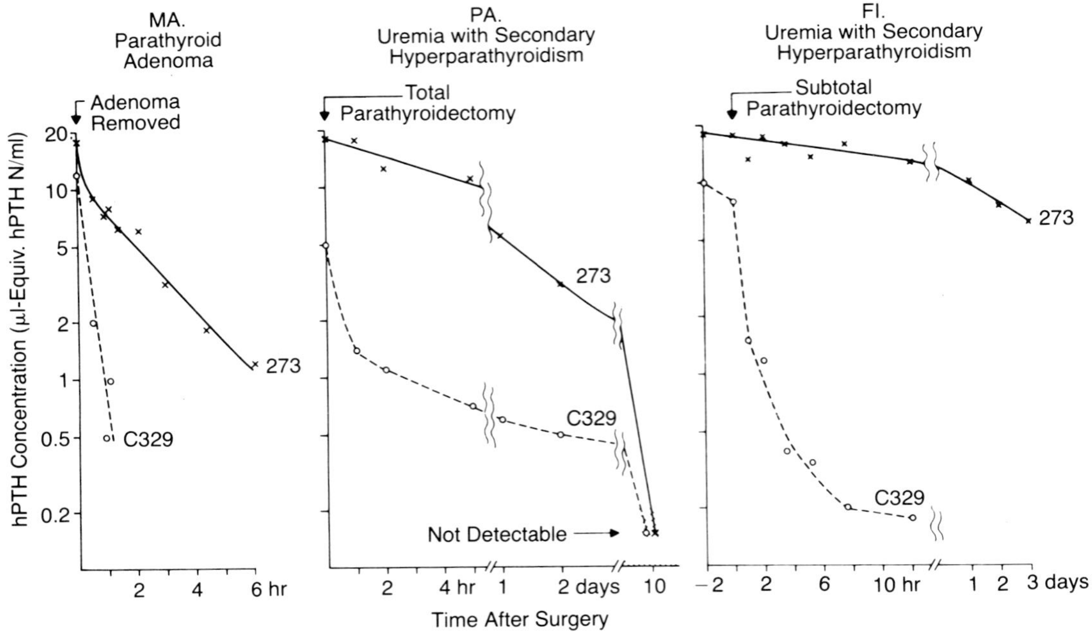

Figure 3–11. Disappearance of immunoreactive parathyroid hormone from plasma after parathyroidectomy in patients with primary or secondary hyperparathyroidism. Plasma samples were assayed with antiserum C329 and antiserum 273 using an extract of a normal human parathyroid gland as standard (hPTH N) and ^{125}I-bPTH as tracer. Plasma concentrations of hormone are given as microliter equivalents of the plasma standard of hPTH (see text). (From Berson SA, Yalow RS: J Clin Endocrinol Metab 28:1037–1047, 1968.)

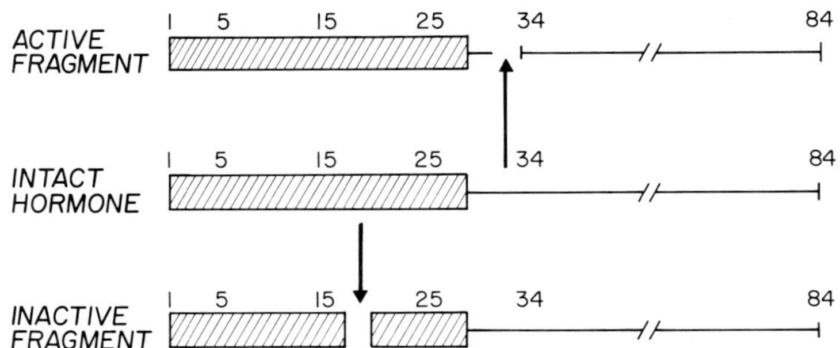

Figure 3–12. Model of the two theoretical alternate sites of metabolic cleavage of parathyroid hormone (sequence 1–84). The hatched area indicates that minimal sequence required for biological activity. (From Segre GV, Niall HD, Habener JF, et al: Am J Med 56:774, 1974.)

the metabolism of PTH might be important in the expression or overall regulation of hormone action. Structure/activity studies with parathyroid hormone indicate that amino-terminal fragments consisting of an intact sequence of 25 residues or more from the amino-terminal portion of the molecule could exert biological activity on hormonal target tissues (Fig. 3–12). It is conceivable that such biologically active fragments could constitute a unique, active molecular species, whether released from the gland or formed in peripheral sites after secretion. Physiologic alterations in the rate of intraglandular or peripheral proteolysis of PTH might complement changes in PTH secretion rate to control levels of active hormone more precisely.

Several problems have arisen in the control of experimental methods, particularly persistent concerns that some proteolysis of the hormone may be artifactual, occurring after collection of plasma samples from patients or from animals in whom PTH metabolism is studied. Much of the experimental work in animals has involved injection of hormone labeled with radioiodine, raising concerns that the metabolic fate of labeled hormone may not be the same as that of the endogenous hormone *in vivo*. In addition, supraphysiologic amounts of hormone are usually administered to generate sufficient concentrations of fragments to permit their characterization, and it is uncertain whether differences in results occur as a function of the doses of hormone used. There is the additional problem of species differences. Rats and dogs are the experimental animals most often studied, but the hormone generally available for use has been the bovine hormone or synthetic forms of human PTH. Experimental study of hormone metabolism in rats and dogs as a means of understanding hormone metabolism in humans requires the assumption that the features of proteolysis of hormone are similar among mammalian species. To date, no convincing evidence has been reported for species-specific differences in the metabolism of PTH.

Despite the overall difficulties in the interpretation of PTH metabolism, there is a general agreement that in addition to intact hormone there are at least four closely related fragment forms of immunoreactive hormone derived from the middle and carboxyl regions of the molecule[410-419] (Figs. 3–13 and 3–14). For simplicity, these biologically inactive fragments are hereafter referred to as carboxyl fragments to distinguish them from potentially biologically active, amino-terminal fragments. Differing portions of the middle and carboxyl regions of the molecule might be present in "carboxyl" fragments.

Of those groups studying the heterogeneity of circulating parathyroid hormone, some have reported evidence[410-414,417] for the existence of smaller immunoreactive forms, constituting fragments from the amino terminus, present at much lower concentrations than the fragments corresponding to the middle and carboxyl regions of the molecule.[410-414,417] Perfusion of liver or kidney *in vitro* with intact hormone leads to amino-terminal fragments that can be detected in the perfusate,[420] and in one instance the fragment was shown to be biologically active.[421] The conditions under which amino-terminal fragment(s) are detected *in vivo*, however, usually involved studies in patients with hyperparathyroidism, renal failure, or both, or administration of large doses of hormone to experimental animals in the absence or presence of renal failure. Circulating amino-terminal fragments are generally not detected by most assays in blood samples analyzed from individuals with normal parathyroid or renal function.[422,423] Biologically active fragments have

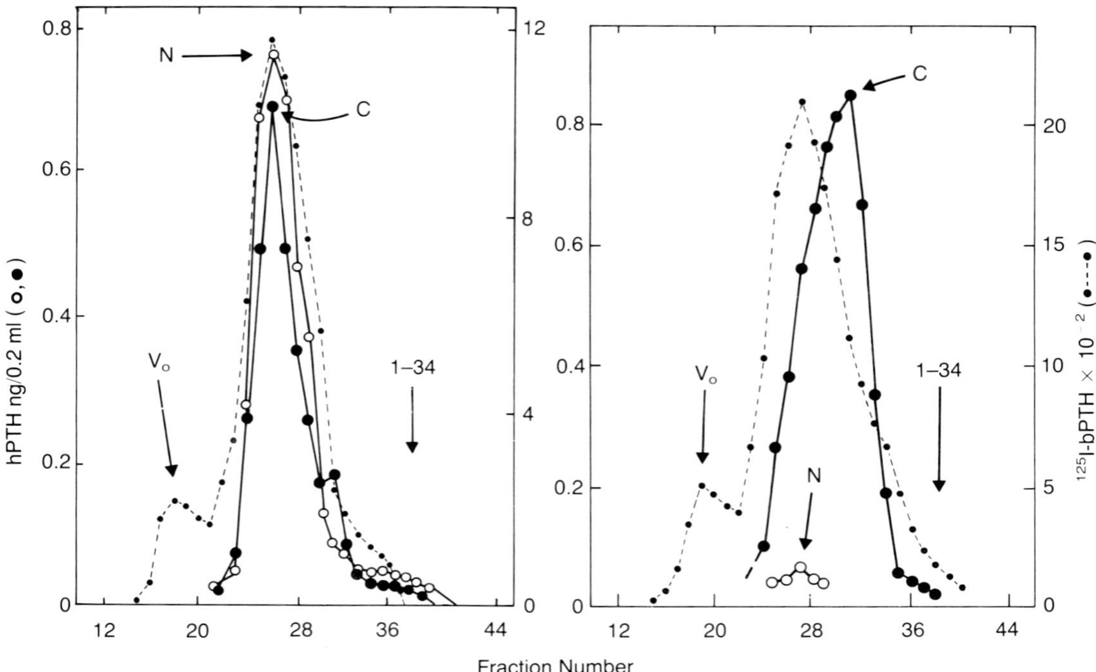

Figure 3–13. Gel filtration pattern (BioGel P–10) of immunoreactive parathyroid hormone obtained from the thyroid vein by venous catheterization (*left*) and from the general circulation by venipuncture (*right*). Plasma (0.5–0.8 ml) and 50 pg (20,000 cpm) of ^{125}I-labeled bovine parathyroid hormone (^{125}I-bPTH) consisting of native hormone purified from gland extracts were co-chromatographed. Immunoreactive parathyroid hormone was measured in aliquots of each gel fraction against a human parathyroid hormone standard using radioimmunoassays that specifically measure an amino-terminal sequence between residues 14 and 30 (amino (N) assay ○) and a carboxyl-terminal sequence between residues 53 and 84 (carboxyl (C) assay ●). Arrows indicate void volume of column (V_0) and elution position of synthetic bovine peptides 1 to 34 (1–34). (From Habener JF, Segre GV, Powell D, et al: Nature (London) New Biol 238:152, 1972.)

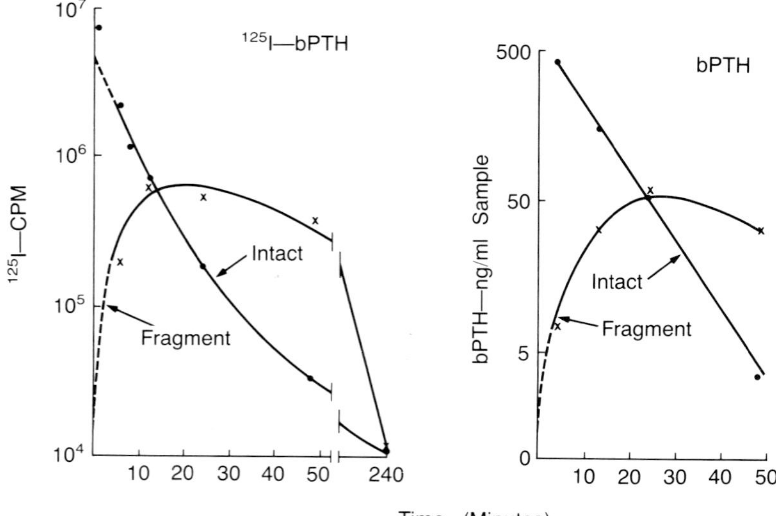

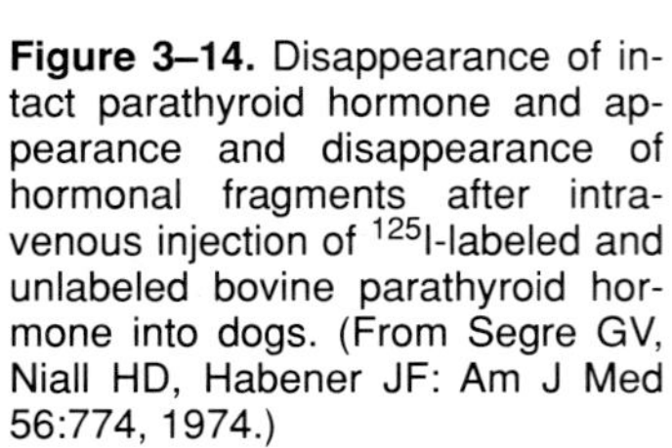
Figure 3–14. Disappearance of intact parathyroid hormone and appearance and disappearance of hormonal fragments after intravenous injection of ^{125}I-labeled and unlabeled bovine parathyroid hormone into dogs. (From Segre GV, Niall HD, Habener JF: Am J Med 56:774, 1974.)

been detected by the cytochemical bioassay in hyperparathyroid patients with renal failure.[424,425]

Because of the considerable difficulties inherent in work on PTH metabolism and the limitation of experimental approaches directly applicable to humans, different groups have addressed the heterogeneity of circulating hormone with methods that were most applicable to their laboratories, skills, and materials. Based on the evidence available, it seems most reasonable that both intraglandular cleavage and peripheral metabolism of PTH occur. One continuing line of investigation favors intraglandular cleavage as the site of origin of circulating fragments.[303,414,426-430] The direction of studies of other groups supports the existence of peripheral metabolism of hormone, which can then be invoked as the source of circulating fragments.[417,419,431-434] It is unclear, however, to what extent proteolysis within the glands and in peripheral tissues contributes quantitatively to the production of circulating fragments. It is equally unclear whether the responsible proteolytic enzymes are the same in the two sites and whether the products of cleavages are identical. Present results do at least suggest a close similarity between the fragments analyzed in extracts of glands or in venous effluent versus those generated after infusion of hormone into animals. Studies of the proteolytic processing of the hormone and, most important, the biological and physiologic significance of hormone metabolism continue in several laboratories despite the inherent difficulties in obtaining unequivocal results.

B. Intraglandular Cleavage of Hormone

Considerable evidence points toward the existence of intraglandular cleavage of hormone in humans and other mammals. If secreted along with intact hormone, the products of such intraglandular cleavage could contribute significantly to the heterogeneity of circulating PTH.[414] Three general approaches have been used to understand the nature and consequences of intraglandular cleavage of hormone. (1) Extracts of human and bovine glands have been analyzed for their content of intact hormone and hormonal fragments. (2) The nature of hormone produced by glandular tissues during incubation *in vitro* has been assessed in studies employing gland slices, gland perfusion, or primary cell cultures. (3) Parathyroid effluent blood has been assayed *in vivo* for content of hormone and fragments to detect secretion of fragments.

There have been difficulties inherent in interpretation of the data provided by each approach, but the evidence from each general technique has been complementary and reinforces the concept that fragments are indeed secreted from the gland. Two groups have reported a considerable content of carboxyl- and amino-terminal fragments when human glands saved from surgical operations are extracted to provide hormone for physiologic and biological studies.[414,435] It is not clear, however, to what extent the fragments found in the gland may have resulted from proteolysis during storage. Nonetheless, the detection of fragments in the gland in considerable abundance provides an independent line of evidence in support of intraglandular cleavage of hormone.

Direct measurement of arterial/venous differences in parathyroid effluent blood is probably the most unambiguous method of ascertaining that the parathyroid gland *in vivo* does release both intact hormone and hormonal fragments into the general circulation. Studies performed in bovines indicate secretion of carboxyl fragments in addition to intact hormone; the concentration of carboxyl fragments is higher in the venous effluent from the parathyroid glands than in the systemic circulation (particularly under conditions of systemic hypercalcemia when overall rates of hormone secretion are lower).[303] When the nature of secreted immunoreactive PTH in humans was reexamined, one group reported that the concentration of carboxyl fragments in the parathyroid effluent exceeded that present in the systemic circulation.[426,427]

Artifacts due to postcollection *ex vivo* proteolysis of hormone in plasma samples have been recognized and must be considered in any definitive interpretation of what appears to be secretion of a small concentration of fragments from the gland. Nonetheless, the overall results do indicate release of fragments of the hormone as well as intact hormone from the gland. The possible role of artifactual postcollection hormonal proteolysis seems minimal in the studies in bovines in which the concentration of fragments relative to that of intact hormone increases as the content of intact hormone falls during partial gland suppression with systemic hypercalcemia.[110] The principal interpretative advantage of studies based on analysis of the parathyroid effluent blood is that the approach largely eliminates the potential difficulty with *in vitro* studies in which incubations of glandular tissue may be associated with activation of peptidases by tissue autolysis that do not reflect true enzymic activity *in vivo*.

In fact, extended incubation of parathyroid glandular slices for periods as long as 24 hours was shown to be associated with extensive proteolysis of hormone that was subsequently shown to be largely artifactual.[354] When gland slices were used over short periods of incubation (less than 6 hours), the principal product released was intact hormone, although release of carboxyl fragments was also detected,[301,302,304,436]

Radioactive amino acids are often used in pulse-chase experiments during incubations of parathyroid tissue slices or fragments of parathyroid gland *in vitro*. One or more carboxyl-terminal fragments are released from the gland along with intact hormone.[301,302,304,436] Extensive analyses have been made of the nature and regulation of the proteases responsible for fragmentation of hormone in these experiments. Evidence has been provided in one test system that protease activity is regulated by calcium concentration in the medium.[300] A considerable body of work suggests the enzymes are cathepsins.[300,304,305,435,437] Direct analysis of the nature of the PTH cleavage by the cathepsin partially purified from parathyroid tissue indicates that the sites of cleavage are between residues 36 and 37, a site identical to one of the sites cleaved during peripheral metabolism of parathyroid hormone in the liver. Under certain conditions *in vitro*, particularly with high calcium concentration in the medium, extensive degradation of intraglandular hormone beyond the stage of carboxyl fragments to simple peptides or free amino acids has been reported; such extensive degradation may be a mechanism for the regulation of hormone stores under conditions of suppressed secretion.[307]

One group has carried out extensive studies with perfused parathyroid tissue slices, a technique felt to particularly minimize tissue anoxia and autolysis; this group also reported immunoreactive fragments, both amino- and carboxyl-terminal, as well as intact hormone, in the effluent medium.[429,430]

The overall results are clearly consistent with the secretion of fragments from the gland. Although amino-terminal fragments are detected during analyses of glandular processing *in vitro* or in glandular extracts,[414,429,435] only carboxyl-terminal fragments are detected in parathyroid effluent *in vivo*.[303,415,426,427] It is presently unknown to what extent the circulating carboxyl-terminal fragments are derived from glandular secretion versus production from metabolism in peripheral sites. This issue is not easily settled. Much of the clearance of carboxyl fragments occurs via the kidney; reduction in renal function results in a significant prolongation of the half-time of carboxyl fragments in the circulation. A quantitative estimation of the contribution of the glandular secretion of carboxyl fragments to the concentration of fragments found in the general circulation would require separate calculations of both production and clearance rates of gland-derived carboxyl fragment(s) from the circulation; such measurements have not been made and would be technically difficult to accomplish. Fragments would have to be purified or synthesized, and clearance rates would have to be estimated under varying conditions of renal function.

C. Peripheral Metabolism of Hormone: Clearance and Organ-Specific Proteolysis

The peripheral metabolism of PTH has been analyzed by injecting intact hormone into the circulation of test animals; tests have not been performed in human subjects. In the animal studies, intact hormone and hormonal fragments are detected by antisera that recognize particular epitopes in PTH representing the amino terminus or the carboxyl terminus of the molecule. As samples are analyzed following injection of a bolus of hormone into the circulation, the concentration of intact hormone falls rapidly, accompanied by a rapid increase in hormonal fragments measured exclusively by carboxyl-terminal antibodies. The overall results indicate that entry of PTH into the circulation (equivalent to secretion of intact hormone from the gland) is followed by rapid clearance of the hormone from the plasma through uptake into peripheral tissues, principally liver and kidney, where cleavage of the hormone then generates multiple peptide fragments of which the carboxyl fragments reappear in the circulation.[416-418,431,433,438-443]

The limitations in our knowledge concerning clearance rates of intact hormone and hormonal fragments impair the ability to analyze the kinetics of peripheral metabolism. It is not known whether gland-derived versus peripherally derived carboxyl fragments are similar or different; presently there is no method to detect them separately. The individual rates of clearance of the major carboxyl fragments identified in the circulation should be known in order to calculate the relative contribution of peripherally derived versus gland-derived fragments to the steady state concentration of circulating carboxyl fragments. Carboxyl fragments have not been available in sufficient quantity or purity to be infused into test animals. Some rough approximations, however, have been made of the rate of clearance of carboxyl fragments under various conditions such as after parathyroidectomy in patients with uremia; clearance was 100 times slower than that of intact hormone.[414]

Studies in animals have used approaches that permit measurements of arteriovenous differences across the circulatory beds of liver and kidney. The kidney extracted hormonal fragments as well as intact hormone and the liver extracted only intact hormone.[27,444] These studies confirmed that clearance of carboxyl fragments occurs principally by glomerular filtration, hence the critical role of renal function in concentration of carboxyl fragments.[27,444,445] Estimations of rates of clearance of carboxyl fragments after their generation in peripheral tissues following injection of intact hormone are only approximate because production and clearance of fragments occur simultaneously. Clearance T½ was at least 20 to 40 minutes in conditions of intact renal function; renal failure prolonged the clearance half-time.[446,447]

It is unknown whether hormonal clearance rates are regulated by physiologic needs, such as variations in the calcium level of the blood. There are limited, contradictory data on this point in animals. One report suggests that changes in calcium concentration do not alter the clearance rate of intact hormone in the dog,[448] but in rats it was reported that hypocalcemia enhanced skeletal and reduced renal uptake of hormone over that seen at normocalcemic levels.[449]

The formal data that exist on clearance of intact PTH are limited principally to analyses of the fate of the intact hormone in studies involving infusion or bolus injection of PTH 1–84 into either of several animal species. The overall clearance of intact hormone from plasma has been found to be very rapid (T½ of 2–3 min); the major sites of clearance are the liver and kidney.[431,433,441,450] Clearance by the liver predominates over clearance by the kidney and the two organs together account for virtually all of the clearance of intact hormone. A variety of estimations have been made of the fractional clearance of intact hormone by each organ. The studies are difficult to compare because of differences in species of test animals used and the methods employed, although hepatic clearance has been estimated to be 40% to 75% and renal clearance 20% to 30%.[431,450-452]

Organs other than liver and kidney have been implicated in clearance of the intact hormone or the biologically active synthetic peptide when the latter is injected or infused. Uptake or localization into organs other than liver and kidney has been determined by autoradiographic studies employing radioactive hormone or by organ perfusion studies. It is important in the interpretation of these studies to distinguish between two processes concerned with hormone uptake. The sites in liver and kidney responsible for the bulk of hormone clearance are high-capacity sites that are not readily saturable despite a wide range of hormone dosage administered intravenously. A low level of uptake that is readily saturable can be detected in hepatocytes but not Kupffer cells of the liver, in a small fraction of renal tubular cells, and in osteoblasts. Uptake in the last sites is characterized by selectivity for biologically active forms of the intact hormone or the synthetic fragments, as well as saturability; these sites are probably the classic PTH receptors, differing from the sites associated with bulk clearance of the peptide and proteolytic degradation. Autoradiographic studies have demonstrated specific binding of radioactive, biologically active hormone by osteoblasts in rats.[56,453] Some uptake of PTH in the kidney seems to depend on the biological activity of the hormone used as tracer in autoradiographic studies.[453] The percentage of administered dose of hormone associated with this apparent receptor-mediated uptake in bone and renal cells is less than 1%, consistent with the ready saturability of specific binding sites. A similar, probably receptor-mediated uptake is demonstrated for biologically active forms of hormone on hepatocytes.[453] In perfusion studies involving the isolated tibia in dogs, specific uptake of PTH 1–34 but not PTH 1–84 has been reported.[454] It is difficult to understand the relationship between findings in the latter studies with those in autoradiographic studies that revealed uptake of intact, biologically active hormone (PTH 1–84) by osteoblasts *in vivo*.[56,453] Despite this discrepancy, the overall results indicate that the uptake of hormone by receptors can be detected and analyzed by sensitive methods. Receptor uptake, although the most significant physiologically, is quantitatively much less than uptake by high-capacity sites on non-target cells that trap and clear hormone.

Uptake by high-capacity sites in liver and kidney has been demonstrated to be associated with significant proteolysis of PTH. As with intraglandular cleavage of hormone, organ-specific cleavage of hormone has been studied by a variety of techniques. Hormone is injected or infused into animals *in vivo*, and the tissue distribution and metabolic fate of hormone are analyzed.[416-418,431,438-443] A second approach involves perfusion of isolated organ preparations of liver or kidney; clearance across the organs and the character of modified hormone in the effluent are analyzed.[56,420,421] There is general agreement that uptake of the hormone either *in vitro* or *in vivo* is associated with extensive proteolysis. Studies *in vitro* have indicated the release of both carboxyl- and amino-terminal fragments.[420,421] In general, however, when the peripheral metabolism of PTH is analyzed by injection or infusion of hormone *in vivo*, carboxyl fragments but not amino-terminal fragments appear in the circulation following clearance and cleavage of intact hormone.

The failure to detect circulating amino-terminal fragments during analyses of peripheral metabolism in animals has remained confusing, particularly in light of evidence for the presence of circulating amino-terminal fragments in some hyperparathyroid patients with renal failure when assayed by the cytochemical bioassay[424,425] and radioimmunoassays.[410-414,417] Because renal failure is often present when amino-terminal fragments are detected, it has been proposed that very low levels of amino-terminal fragments are indeed released *in vivo* from either or both the parathyroid gland or organs involved in the peripheral metabolism of hormone. The speculation is that the presence of amino-terminal fragments in the circulation escapes detection in normal individuals but in renal failure the clearance of amino-terminal fragments is diminished, thereby raising their levels into a range of detection. The interest in this question relates to the possibility that circulating amino-terminal fragments might be an alternative active molecular species, perhaps expressing unique biological actions on one or another of the target sites of PTH. Recently, to answer this question regarding peripheral metabolism, definitive studies have been performed in animals. The release of amino-terminal fragments from liver and kidney was studied in detail during metabolism of the radioactive hormone used as tracer. These studies, discussed further in the following section, suggest that amino-terminal fragments, even at low levels, do not reenter the circulation from the liver and kidney (Bringhurst and Stern, unpublished). It is possible that amino-terminal fragments are released at low levels from the parathyroid gland and not from peripheral organs and that the fragments cannot be detected by present methods except in states of renal failure, when clearance is prolonged. It is also possible, however, that alterations associated with the uremic state interfere nonspecifically with the assays and artifactually produce evidence for the presence of circulating amino-terminal fragments *in vivo*.

Because of the obvious importance of the metabolism and clearance of PTH as a principal factor, along with rates of secretion, that determines the availability of active hormone in the circulation to interact with target organs, efforts to analyze the process have been extensive. Specific chemical techniques were developed that permitted analyses of cleavage patterns of hormone based on serial sampling of hormone and fragments in blood after hormone injection. Amino acid sequencing of hormonal fragments produced after administration of radioiodinated intact hormone to rats or dogs indicated that two major circulating carboxyl fragments result from cleavage of the hormone between residues 33 and 34 and residues 36 and 37, respectively.[446,447] This radiomicrosequencing approach was applied to analysis of labeled carboxyl fragments extracted from organs. Those found within the liver are similar to the circulating carboxyl fragments.[454] In subsequent experiments, hepatectomy but not nephrectomy was associated with disappearance of the predominant circulating carboxyl-terminal fragments with amino-terminal residues at position 34 or 37.[419] The liver is clearly responsible for the production of most of the circulating carboxyl-terminal fragments that arise from peripheral metabolism of hormone.

Several groups have examined the proteolytic specificity of various peptidases within liver and kidney to establish which enzymes cleave PTH *in vivo*. Studies with isolated hepatic cells *in vitro* have demonstrated that Kupffer cells but not hepatocytes are responsible for proteolytic modification of PTH. The products detected are identical with those found in the circulation.[434] This linkage of *in vivo* and *in vitro* studies by use of radiomicrosequencing provided assurance that valid conclusions could be drawn. In other studies, a cathepsin has been identified in liver that will cleave PTH at sites identical to at least one of the sites detected *in vivo*.[301,302] A similar but slightly different cathepsin seems responsible for intrarenal cleavage of PTH.[455] Incubations with both Kupffer cells and purified cathepsins indicate that the cleavage of PTH results in the generation of both amino- and carboxyl-terminal fragments.[301,302,434,455]

The discrepancy between these results, namely, clear evidence of cleavage of hormone into amino and carboxyl fragments *in vitro* but the detection only of carboxyl, but not amino-terminal, fragments of hormone in blood during many carefully performed analyses *in vivo*,[303,426,427] has led to a recent intensive investigation of the fate of the amino-terminal portion of the molecule during studies with radiolabeled hormone in animals *in vivo*. Analyses have been carried out of the metabolism in rats of biologically active intact hormone selectively labeled with tritium or sulfur at known sites within the hormone sequence that selectively mark the amino-terminal versus the carboxyl-terminal portions of the molecule through incorporation of radioactive amino acids during biosynthesis of the tracer hormone in gland slices. Injection of this hormone into animals led to the predictable uptake of intact hormone, approximately 50% by liver and 20% by kidney; the rapid disappearance of intact hormone was followed by the appearance of carboxyl-terminal fragments in the circulation. No convincing evidence for reentry of amino-terminal fragments into the circulation was found, despite studies in several animals using continuous infusion of hormone labeled to high specific activity in the amino-terminal portion of the molecule for periods of 10 to 30 minutes (S and B). Deliberate induction of renal failure did not change the results. The high sensitivity and specificity of these approaches argues strongly that circulating amino-terminal fragments do not originate from peripheral metabolism even in renal failure in animals. As noted, these findings suggest, since there is little evidence of major species differences in hormone metabolism, that amino-terminal fragments detected in hyperparathyroid patients with uremia, if present and not artifact, must arise from the parathyroid gland.

VII. SUMMARY

In summary, it is clear that, surprisingly, the principal fate of secreted PTH is metabolic clearance and proteolytic degradation by liver and kidney rather than specific uptake by receptors in target cells in kidney and bone. The peripheral metabolism of hormone may be subject to physiologic regulation, that is, there may be an increase or decrease in rate and efficiency of hormone uptake and cleavage as a function of various physiologic states, but there is no convincing evidence for this. Clearly, the high rates of peripheral metabolism do affect the steady state concentration of hormone and serve as an alternative route to receptor uptake of secreted hormone. Peripheral metabolism, however, does not seem to result in the generation of biologically active fragments, at least any that reenter the general circulation. The nature of the responsible enzymes is still unclarified, as is the nature of the specific cellular uptake and mechanisms of intraorgan disposal of fragments that are generated by tissue endopeptidases that seem related to cathepsins. The hormone may be metabolized by tissue degradative pathways that serve general catabolic functions and may not be of physiologic significance to PTH action *per se*. Carboxyl fragments as well as intact hormone are secreted from the parathyroid gland in humans and cows, but it remains to be proved that amino-terminal fragments are secreted, leaving unconfirmed the significance of earlier reports that there are circulating amino-terminal fragments.

References

1. Silver J, Russell J, Sherwood LM: Regulation of preproparathyroid hormone messenger RNA in bovine parathyroid cells in culture by vitamin D metabolites. *In* Norman AW, Schaefer K, Grigoleit H-G, von Herrath D (eds): Vitamin D: Chemical, Biochemical and Clinical Update. Proceedings of the Sixth Workshop Vitamin D: Merano, Italy, 1985. Berlin, de Gruyter, 1985, pp 33–34.
2. Horiuchi N, Suda T, Takahashi H, et al: In vivo evidence for the intermediary role of 3′,5′-cyclic AMP in parathyroid hormone–induced stimulation of 1α,25-dihydroxyvitamin D_3 synthesis in rats. Endocrinology 101:969–974, 1977.
3. Copp DH: Calcitonin: Comparative endocrinology. *In* DeGroot LJ (ed): Endocrinology. New York, Grune & Stratton, 1979, pp 637–640.
4. Greep RO: Parathyroid glands. *In* Von Euler US, Heller H (eds): Comparative Endocrinology, vol 1. New York, Academic Press, 1963.
5. Lange R, Van Brehm H: On the fine structure of the parathyroid gland in the toad and frog. *In* Gaillard PJ, Talmage RV, Budy AM (eds): The Parathyroid Glands. Chicago, University of Chicago Press, 1965, pp 19–26.
6. Pang PKT, Yee JA: Evolution of the endocrine control of vertebrate hypercalcemic regulation. *In* Ishii, et al (eds): Tokyo, Japanese Scientific Society Press. Berlin, Springer-Verlag, 1980, pp 103–110.
7. Reeve J, Zanelli JM: Parathyroid hormone and bone. Clin Sci 71:231–238, 1986.
8. Bijvoiet OLM: Kidney function in calcium and phosphate metabolism. *In* Avioli LV, Krane SM (eds): Metabolic Bone Disease, vol 1. New York, Academic Press, 1977, pp 49–128.
9. Nordin BEC, Peacock M, Wilkinson R: The relative importance of gut, bone and kidney in the regulation of serum calcium. *In* Talmage RV, Munson PS (eds): Calcium, Parathyroid Hormone and the Calcitonins. Amsterdam, Excerpta Medica, 1972, pp 263–272.
10. Norimatsu H, VanderWiel CJ, Talmage RV: Morphological support of a role of cells lining bone surfaces in maintenance of plasma calcium concentrations. Clin Orthop Rel Res 138:254–262, 1979.
11. Mayer GP, Habener JF, Potts JT Jr: Parathyroid hormone secretion in vivo: Demonstration of a calcium-independent, nonsuppressible component of secretion. J Clin Invest 56:678–683, 1976.
12. Neer RM: Calcium and inorganic phosphate homeostasis. *In* DeGroot LJ (ed): Endocrinology. New York, Grune & Stratton, 1979, pp 669–693.
13. Bringhurst FR, Potts JT Jr: Calcium and phosphate distribution, turnover and metabolic actions. *In* DeGroot LJ (ed): Endocrinology. New York, Grune & Stratton, 1979, pp 551–587.
14. Brewer HB Jr, Ronan R: Bovine parathyroid hormone: Amino acid sequence. Proc Natl Acad Sci 67:1862, 1970.
15. Niall HD, Keutmann HT, Sauer R, et al: The amino acid sequence of bovine parathyroid hormone I. Hoppe Seyler Z Physiol Chem 351:1586, 1970.
16. Sauer RT, Niall HD, Hogan ML, et al: The amino acid sequence of porcine parathyroid hormone. Biochemistry 13:1994, 1974.
17. Brewer HB Jr, Fairwell T, Ronan R, et al: Human parathyroid hormone: Amino acid sequence of the amino-terminal residues 1-34. Proc Natl Acad Sci 69:3585, 1972.
18. Niall HD, Sauer RT, Jacobs JW, et al: The amino acid sequence of the amino-terminal 37 residues of human parathyroid hormone. Proc Natl Acad Sci 71:384, 1974.
19. Keutmann HT, Sauer MM, Hendy GN, et al: The complete amino acid sequence of human parathyroid hormone. Biochemistry 17:552, 1978.
20. Potts JT Jr, Kronenberg HM, Rosenblatt M: Parathyroid hormone: Chemistry, biosynthesis, and mode of action. Adv Protein Chem 35:323–396, 1982.
21. Tregear GW, van Rietschoten J, Greene E, et al: Bovine parathyroid hormone: Minimum chain length of synthetic peptide required for biological activity. Endocrinology 93:1349–1353, 1973.
22. Rosenblatt M, Callahan EN, Mahaffey JE, et al: Parathyroid hormone inhibitors: Design, synthesis, and biologic evaluation of hormone analogues. J Biol Chem 252:5847–5851, 1977.
23. Horiuchi N, Holick MF, Potts JT Jr, Rosenblatt M: A parathyroid hormone inhibitor *in vivo*: Design and biological evaluation of a hormone analog. Science 220:1053–1055, 1983.
24. Doppelt SH, Neer RM, Federico P, et al: Inhibition of the *in vivo* parathyroid hormone–mediated calcemic response in rats by a synthetic hormone antagonist. Proc Natl Acad Sci USA 83:7557–7560, 1986.
25. Silverman R, Yalow RS: Heterogeneity of parathyroid hormone: Clinical and physiologic implications. J Clin Invest 52:1958–1971, 1973.
26. Habener JF, Powell D, Murray TM, et al: Parathyroid hormone secretion and metabolism *in vivo*. Proc Natl Acad Sci USA 68:2986–2991, 1971.
27. Martin KJ, Hruska KA, Freitag JJ, et al: The peripheral metabolism of parathyroid hormone. N Engl J Med 301:1092–1098, 1979.
28. Bringhurst R, Stern A, Yotts M, et al: Am J Physiol 255:E886–E893, 1989.
29. Speigel AM, Gierschik P, Levine MA, Downs RW Jr: Clinical implications of guanine nucleotide–binding proteins as receptor-effector couplers. N Engl J Med 312:26–33, 1985.
30. Ross EM, Gilman AG: Biochemical properties of hormone-sensitive adenylate cyclase. Annu Rev Biochem 49:533–564, 1980.
31. Chase LR, Aurbach GD: Parathyroid function and the renal excretion of 3′,5′-adenylic acid. Proc Natl Acad Sci USA 58:518–525, 1967.
32. Rappaport MS, Stern PH: Parathyroid hormone and calcitonin modify inositol phospholipid metabolism in fetal rat limb bones. J Bone Mineral Res 1:173–179, 1986.
33. Goldring ST, Tyler GA, Krane SM, et al: Photoaffinity labeling of parathyroid hormone receptors: Comparison of receptors across species and target

tissues and after desensitization to hormone. Biochemistry 23:498–502, 1984.

34. Kronenberg HM, McDevitt BE, Majzoub JA, et al: Cloning and nucleotide sequence of DNA coding for bovine preproparathyroid hormone. Proc Natl Acad Sci 76:4981, 1979.
35. Hendy GN, Kronenberg HM, Potts JT Jr, Rich A: Nucleotide sequence of cloned cDNAs encoding human preproparathyroid hormone. Proc Natl Acad Sci USA 78:7365, 1981.
36. Vasicek T, McDevitt BE, Freeman MW, et al: Nucleotide sequence of the human parathyroid hormone gene. Proc Natl Acad Sci USA 80:2127, 1983.
37. Heinrich G, Kronenberg HM, Potts JT Jr, Habener JF: Gene encoding parathyroid hormone: Nucleotide sequence of the rat gene and deduced amino acid sequence of rat preproparathyroid hormone. J Biol Chem 259:3320, 1984.
38. Kemper B, Habener JF, Mulligan RC, et al: Preproparathyroid hormone: A direct translation product of parathyroid messenger RNA. Proc Natl Acad Sci USA 71:3731–3735, 1974.
39. Habener JF, Potts JT Jr: Parathyroid physiology and primary hyperparathyroidism. *In* Avioli LV, Krane SM (eds): Metabolic Bone Disease, vol II. New York, Academic Press, 1977, pp 1–147.
40. Knox FG, Lechene C: Am J Physiol 229:1556, 1975.
41. Agus ZS, Gardner LB, Beck LH, Goldberg M: Am J Physiol 224:1143, 1973.
42. Knox FG, Lechene C: Am J Physiol 229:1556, 1975.
43. Knox FG, Haas JA, Lechene C: Program/Abstr Int Workshop Phosphate, 1975.
44. Nordin BEC, Marshall DH, Peacock M, Robertson WG: *In* Talmage RV, Owen M, Parsons JA (eds): Calcium-Regulating Hormones. Amsterdam, Excerpta Medica, 1975, p 239.
45. Biddulph DM, Gallimore LB Jr: Endocrinology 94:1241, 1974.
46. Lassiter WE, Gottschalk CW, Mylie M: Am J Physiol 204:771, 1963.
47. Duarte CG, Bland JH: Metab Clin Exp 14:899, 1965.
48. Chabardes D, Imbert M, Clique A, et al: PTH sensitive adenyl cyclase activity in different segments of the rabbit nephron. Pflügers Arch 354:229–239, 1975.
49. Chambers DJ, Shafer H, Laugharn JA Jr, et al: Dose-related activation by PTH of specific enzymes in various regions of the kidney. *In* Copp DH, Talmage RV (eds): Endocrinology of Calcium Metabolism. Proceedings of the Sixth Parathyroid Conference, 1977. Amsterdam, Excerpta Medica, 1978, pp 216–220.
50. Suda T, Kurukowa K: Characteristic localization of 25-hydroxyvitamin D_3 1-hydroxylase along the fetal nephron. *In* Holick MF, Gray TK, Anast CS (eds): Prenatal Calcium and Phosphorus Metabolism. Amsterdam, Elsevier, 1983, pp 57–69.
51. Raisz LG, Kream BE: Regulation of bone formation (part I). N Engl J Med 309:29–35, 1983.
52. Chambers TJ: The cellular basis of bone resorption. Clin Orthop Rel Res 151:283–293, 1980.
53. Parsons JA, Robinson CJ: Calcium shift into bone causing transient hypocalcemia after injection of parathyroid hormone. Nature 230:581–582, 1971.
54. Talmage RV, et al: The demand for bone calcium in maintenance of plasma calcium concentrations. *In* Horton, Tarpley, Davis (eds): Mechanisms of Localized Bone Resporption. Washington, DC, 1978, pp 73–92.
55. Rodan GA, Rodan SB: Expression of the osteoblastic phenotype. *In* Peck WA (ed): Bone and Mineral Research, Annual 2. Amsterdam, Elsevier Science Publishers BV, 1983, pp 244–285.
56. Barling PM, Bibby NJ: Study of the localization of [^{3}H]bovine parathyroid hormone in bone by light microscope autoradiography. Calcif Tissue Int 37:442–446, 1985.
57. McSheehy PMJ, Chambers TJ: Osteoblastic cells mediate osteoclastic responsiveness to parathyroid hormone. Endocrinology 118:824–828, 1986.
58. Rouleau MF, Warshawsky H, Goltzman D: Parathyroid hormone binding *in vivo* to renal, hepatic, and skeletal tissues of the rat using a radioautographic approach. Endocrinology 118:919–931, 1986.
59. Collip JB: Extraction of a parathyroid hormone which will prevent or control parathyroid tetany and which regulates the level of blood calcium. J Biol Chem 63:395, 1925.
60. Aurbach GD: Isolation of parathyroid hormone after extraction with phenol. J Biol Chem 234:3179, 1959.
61. Rasmussen H, Sze YL, Young R: Further studies on the isolation and characterization of parathyroid polypeptides. J Biol Chem 239:2852, 1964.
62. Rasmusssen H, Craig LC: Purification of parathyroid hormone by use of counter-current distribution. J Am Chem Soc 81:5003, 1959.
63. Rasmussen H, Craig C: The parathyroid polypeptides. Rec Prog Horm Res 18:269, 1962.
64. Aurbach GD, Potts JT Jr: Partition of parathyroid hormone on sephadex G–100. Endocrinology 75:290, 1964.
65. Keutmann HT, Aurbach DG, Dawson BF, et al: Isolation and characterization of the bovine parathyroid isohormones. Biochemistry 10:2779, 1971.
66. Keutmann HT, Barline PM, Hendy GN, et al: Isolation of human parathyroid hormone. Biochemistry 13:1646, 1974.
67. Brewer HB Jr, Fairwell T, Rittel W, et al: Recent studies on the chemistry of human, bovine and porcine parathyroid hormone. Am J Med 56:17, 1974.
68. Keutmann HT, Niall HD, O'Riordan JLH, et al: A reinvestigation of the amino-terminal sequence of human parathyroid hormone. Biochemistry 14:1842, 1975.
69. Cohn DV, Hamilton JM, MacGregor RR, et al: Parathyroid hormone: Biosynthesis and metabolism. *In* James VHT (ed): Endocrinology. Proceedings of the Fifth International Congress of Endocrinology. Amsterdam, Excerpta Medica, 1977, pp 248–255.

69a. Khosla S, Demay M, Pines M, et al: Nucleotide sequence of cloned cDNAs encoding chicken preproparathyroid hormone. J Bone Mineral Res 3:689–698, 1988.

69b. Russell J, Sherwood LM: Nucleotide sequence of the DNA complementary to avian (chicken) preproparathyroid hormone mRNA and the deduced sequence of the precursor. Mol Endocrinol 3:325–331, 1989.

70. Potts JT Jr, Tregear GW, Keutmann HT, et al: Synthesis of a biologically active N-terminal tetratriacontapeptide of parathyroid hormone. Proc Natl Acad Sci USA 68:63, 1971.

70a. Suva LJ, Winslow GA, Wettenhall REH, et al: A parathyroid hormone–related protein implicated in malignancy hypercalcemia: Cloning and expression. Science 237:893, 1987.
70b. Mangin M, Webb AC, Dreyer BE, et al: Identification of a cDNA encoding a parathyroid hormone-like peptide from a human tumor associated with humoral hypercalcemia of malignancy. Proc Natl Acad Sci USA 85:597, 1988.
70c. Nissensen RA, Strewler GJ, Stern PH, et al: Parathyroid hormone-like protein from human renal carcinoma cells: Structural and functional homology with parathyroid hormone. J Clin Invest 80:1803, 1987.
70d. Jüppner H, Abou-Samra AB, Uneno S, et al: The parathyroid hormone-like peptide associated with humoral hypercalcemia of malignancy and parathyroid hormone bind to the same receptor on the plasma membrane of ROS 17/2.8 cells. J Biochem 263:8557–8560, 1988.
70e. Abou-Samra AB, Susumu U, Jüppner H, et al: Nonhomologous sequences of parathyroid hormone and the parathyroid hormone related peptide bind to a common receptor on ROS 17/2.8 cells. Endocrinology (in press).
70f. Thiede MA, Rodan GA: Expression of a calcium mobilizing parathyroid hormone-like peptide in lactating mammary tissue. Science 242:278–280, 1988.
70g. Rodda CP, Heath JA, Ebeling PR, et al: Regulation of fetal calcium metabolism: Evidence for a novel parathyroid hormone related protein promoting placental calcium transport. J Bone Mineral Res Suppl 3:S213, 1988.
71. Hunt NH, Martin TJ, Michelangeli VP, Eisman JA: Effect of guanyl nucleotides on parathyroid hormone–responsive adenylate cyclase in chick kidney. J Endocrinol 69:401–412, 1976.
72. Goltzman D, Callahan EN, Tregear GW, Potts JT Jr: Role of 5′-guanylylimidodiphosphate in the activation of adenylyl cyclase by parathyroid hormone. Endocr Res Commun 3:407–419, 1976.
73. Michelangeli VP, Hunt NH, Martin TJ: States of activation of chick kidney adenylate-cyclase induced by parathyroid-hormone and guanyl nucleotides. J Endocrinol 72:69–79, 1977.
74. Drezner MK, Burch WM: Altered activity of nucleotide regulatory site in parathyroid hormone–sensitive adenylate-cyclase from renal cortex of a patient with pseudohypoparathyroidism. J Clin Invest 62:1222–1227, 1978.
75. Nissenson RA, Nyiredy K, Arnaud CD: Guanyl nucleotides amplify the effect of parathyroid-hormone receptor occupancy on adenylate-cyclase activation. Calcif Tissue Int 28:170 (abstract), 1979.
76. Houslay MD: A family of guanine nucleotide regulatory proteins. TIBS 9:39–40, 1984.
77. Goldfine ID, Jones AL, Hradek GT, et al: Entry of insulin into human cultured lymphocytes: Electron microscope autoradiographic analysis. Science 202:760–763, 1978.
78. Bergeron JJM, Levine G, Sikstrom R, et al: Polypeptide hormone binding sites *in vivo*: Initial localization of ^{125}I-labeled insulin to hepatocyte plasmalemma as visualized by electron microscope radioautography. Proc Natl Acad Sci USA 74:5051–5055, 1977.
79. Schlessinger J, Shechter Y, Willingham MC, Pastan I: Direct visualization of binding, aggregation, and internalization of insulin and epidermal growth-factor on living fibroblastic cells. Proc Natl Acad Sci USA 75:2659–2663, 1978.
80. Goodman AS, Gilman AG: The Pharmacological Basis of Therapeutics. 7th ed. New York, Macmillan, 1985.
81. Martin WR: Pharmacology of opioids. Pharmacol Rev 35:283–382, 1984.
82. Ross EM, Gilman AG: Biochemical properties of hormone-sensitive adenylate cyclase. Annu Rev Biochem 49:533–564, 1980.
83. Rodbell M: Role of hormone receptors and GTP-regulatory proteins in membrane transduction. Nature (London) 284:117–22, 1980.
84. Cerione RA, Sibley DR, Codina J, et al: Reconstitution of a hormone-sensitive adenylate cyclase system. J Biol Chem 259:9979–9982, 1984.
85. Robishaw JD, Russell LDW, Harris BA, et al: Deduced primary structure of the alpha subunit of the GTP-binding stimulatory protein of adenylate cyclase. Biochemistry 83:1251–1255, 1986.
86. Verkman AS, Skorecki KL, Ausiello DA: Radiation inactivation of multimeric enzymes: Application to subunit interactions of adenylate cyclase. Am J Physiol 250:C103–114, 1986.
87. Skorecki KL, Verkman AS, Jung CY, Ausiello DA: Evidence for vasopressin activation of adenylate cyclase by subunit dissociation. Am J Physiol 250:C115–123, 1986.
88. Dunn WA, Hubbard AL: Receptor-mediated endocytosis of epidermal growth factor by hepatocytes in the perfused rat liver: Ligand and receptordynamics. J Cell Biol 98:2148–2159, 1984.
89. Parsons JA, Rafferty B, Gray D, et al: Pharmacology of parathyroid hormone and some of its fragments and analogues. *In* Talmage RV, Owen M, Parsons JA (eds): Calcium-Regulating Hormones: Proceedings of the Fifth Parathyroid Conference. Amsterdam, Excerpta Medica, 1975, pp 33–39.
90. Farfel Z, Brickman AS, Kaslow HR, et al: Defect of receptor-cyclase coupling protein in pseudohypoparathyroidism. N Engl J Med 303:2317–3242, 1980.
91. Coltrera M, Rosenblatt M, Potts JT Jr: Analogs of parathyroid hormone containing D-amino acids—Evaluation of biological activity and stability. Biochemistry 19:4380–4385, 1980.
91a. Wright DS, Tyler GA, O'Brien R, et al: Immunoprecipitation of the parathyroid hormone receptor. Proc Natl Sci USA 84:26–30, 1987.
91b. Draper MW, Nissenson RA, Winner J, et al: Photoaffinity labeling of the canine renal receptor for parathyroid hormone. J Biochem 257:3714–3718, 1982.
91c. Nissenson RA, Karpf D, Bambino T, et al: Covalent labeling of a high-affinity, guanyl nucleotide sensitive parathyroid hormone receptor in canine renal cortex. Biochemistry 26:1874–1878, 1987.
91d. Shigeno C, Hiraki Y, Keutmann HT, et al: Preparation of a photoreactive analog of parathyroid hormone [NLE8, LYS (N-E-4-azido-2-nitrophenyl)13, Nle18, Tyr34 bovine parathyroid hormone-(1-34)NH_2], a selective, high-affinity ligand for characterization of parathyroid hormone receptors. Anal Biochem 179:268–273, 1989.
92. Yamamoto I, Potts JT Jr, Segre GV: Circulating bovine lymphocytes contain receptors for parathyroid hormone. J Clin Invest 71:404–407, 1983.
93. Perry HM III, Chappel JC, Bellorin-Font E, et al: Parathyroid hormone receptors in circulating

human mononuclear leukocytes. J Biol Chem 259:5531–5535, 1984.
94. Habener JF, Rosenblatt M, Potts JT Jr: Parathyroid hormone: Biochemical aspects of biosynthesis, secretion, and metabolism. Physiol Rev 64:985–1053, 1984.
95. Kenny AD, Pang PKT: Response of the renal vitamin D endocrine system to oxidized parathyroid hormone (1–34) (41497). Proc Soc Exp Biol Med 171:191–195, 1982.
96. Kenny AD, Pang PKT: Phosphaturic response to parathyroid hormone (letter). N Engl J Med 308:1362, 1983.
97. Shew RL, Kenny AD, Pang PKT: Uterine relaxing action of parathyroid hormone: Effect of oxidation and methionine substitution. Proc Soc Exp Biol Med 175:444–448, 1984.
98. Laverty G, Wideman RF Jr: Avian renal responses to oxidized and nonoxidized bPTH(1–34). Gen Compar Endocrinol 59:391–398, 1985.
99. Galceran T, Lewis-Finch J, Martin KJ, Slatopolsky E: Absence of biological effects of oxidized parathyroid hormone(1–34) in dogs and rats. Endocrinology 115:2375–2378, 1984.
100. Goldring SR, Dayer JM, Russell RGG, et al: Response to hormones of cells cultured from human giant cell tumors of bone. J Clin Endocrinol Metab 46:425–433, 1978.
101. Goldring SR, Mahaffey DE, Rosenblatt M, et al: Parathyroid hormone inhibitors: Comparison of biological activity in bone and skin-derived tissue. J Clin Endocrinol Metab 48:655–659, 1979.
102. Mahoney CA, Nissenson RA: Canine renal receptors for parathyroid hormone—down regulation *in vivo* by exogenous parathyroid hormone. J Clin Invest 72:411–421, 1983.
103. Rodan SB, Fischer MK, Egan JJ, et al: The effect of dexamethasone on parathyroid hormone simulation of adenylate cyclase in ROS 17/2.8 cells. Endocrinology 115:951–958, 1984.
104. Yamamoto I, Potts JT Jr, Segre GV: Regulation of parathyroid hormone receptor on clonal rat osteosarcoma cells. *In* Cohn DV, Fujita T, Potts JT Jr, Talmage RV (eds): Endocrine Control of Bone and Calcium Metabolism. Proceedings of the 8th International Conference on Calcium Regulating Hormones, vol 8A. Amsterdam, Excerpta Medica, 1984, pp 250–253.
105. Chase LR, Aurbach GD: Renal adenyl cyclase: Anatomically separate sites for parathyroid hormone and vasopressin. Science 159:545–547, 1968.
106. Rodan SB, Rodan GA: The effect of parathyroid hormone and thyrocalcitonin on the accumulation of cyclic adenosine 3′,5′-monophosphate in freshly isolated bone cells. J Biol Chem 249:3068–3074, 1974.
107. Raisz LG, Brand JS, Klein DC, Au WYW: Hormone regulation of bone resportion. *In* Gaul C, Ebling SG (eds): Progress in Endocrinology. Amsterdam, Excerpta Medica 1969, pp 696–703.
108. Raisz LG: *In* Handbook of Physiology, section 7. Endocrinology, vol 7. Parathyroid gland. Mechanisms of bone resorption. Washington, DC, American Physiological Society, 1976, pp 117–136.
109. Wells H, Lloyd W: Hypercalcemic and hypophosphatemic effects of dibutyryl cyclic AMP in rats after parathyroidectomy. Endocrinology 84:861–867, 1969.
110. Vaes G: Parathyroid hormone–like action of N6-2′-O-dibutyryladenosine-3′,5′-(cyclic)-monophosphate on bone explants in tissue culture. Nature 219:939–940, 1968.
111. Michelakis AM: Hormonal effects on cyclic AMP in a renal-cell suspension system. Proc Soc Exp Biol Med 135:13–16, 1970.
112. Steiner AL, Pagliara AS, Chase LR, Kipnis DM: Radioimmunoassay for cyclic nucleotides. II. Adenosine 3′,5′-monophosphate and guanosine 3′,5′-monophosphate in mammalian tissues and body fluids. J Biol Chem 347:1114–1120, 1972.
113. Kaminsky NH, Broadus AE, Hardman JG, et al: Effects of parathyroid hormone on plasma and urinary adenosine 3′,5′-monophosphate in man. J Clin Invest 49:2387–2395, 1970.
114. Aurbach GD, Chase LR: Handbook of Physiology, section 7. Endocrinology, vol VII. Parathyroid gland. Cyclic nucleotides and biochemical actions of parathyroid hormone and calcitonin. Washington, DC, American Physiological Society, 1976, pp 117–136.
115. Tregear GW, van Rietschoten J, Greene E, et al: Principles and recent applications in the solid-phase synthesis of peptide hormones. Proceedings of the Fourth International Congress of Endocrinology, 1972. Amsterdam, Excerpta Medica, 1974, pp 1–15.
116. Parsons JA, Rafferty B, Gray D, et al: Pharmacology of parathyroid hormone and some of its fragments and analogs. Calcium-Regulating Hormones. Proceedings of the Fifth Parathyroid Conference, 1974. Amsterdam, Excerpta Medica, 1975, pp 33–39.
117. Potts JT Jr, Kronenberg HM, Rosenblatt M: Parathyroid hormone: Chemistry, biosynthesis, and mode of action. Adv Protein Chem 35:323–396, 1982.
118. Rasmussen H, Pechet N, Fast D: Effect of dibutyryl cyclic adenosine 3′,5′-monophosphate, theophylline, and other nucleotides upon calcium and phosphate metabolism. J Clin Invest 47:1843–1850, 1968.
119. Russell RGG, Casey PA, Fleisch H: Simulation of phosphate excretion by the renal arterial infusion of 3′,5′-AMP (cyclic AMP)—A possible mechanism of action of parathyroid hormone. Calcif Tissue Res 2[Suppl]:54–54A, 1968.
120. Goltzman D, Henderson B, Loveridge N: Cytochemical bioassay of parathyroid hormone. J Clin Invest 65:1309–1317, 1980.
121. Sakaguchi K, Fukase M, Kobayashi I, Fujita T: Characteristics of parathyroid hormone–specific cyclic changes of glucose-6-phosphate dehydrogenase activity in the distal convoluted tubule of the guinea pig. J Bone Mineral Res 1:259–265, 1986.
122. Marx SJ, Woodward CJ, Aurbach GD: Calcitonin receptors of kidney and bone. Science 178:999–1001, 1972.
123. Marcus R, Aurbach GD: Adenyl cyclase from renal cortex. Biochim Biophys Acta 242:410–421, 1971.
124. Aurbach GD, Keutmann, Niall HD, et al: Structure, synthesis, and mechanism of action of parathyroid hormone. Recent Prog Horm Res 28:353–398, 1972.
125. Hanai H, Ishida M, Liang CT, Sacktor B: Parathyroid hormone increases sodium/calcium exchange activity in renal cells and the blunting of the response in aging. J Biol Chem 261:5419–5425, 1986.
126. Rasmussen H: The calcium messenger system. Parts 1 and 2. N Engl J Med 314:1094–1101; 1164–1170, 1986.
127. Nishizuka Y: Turnover of inositol phospholipids and signal transduction. Science 225:1365–1370, 1984.
128. Berridge MJ, Irvine RF: Inositol trisphosphate, a novel second messenger in cellular signal transduction. Nature 312:315–321, 1984.
129. Majerus PW, Wilson DB, Connolly TM, et al: Phos-

phoinositide turnover provides a link in stimulus-response coupling. TIBS 168–171, 1985.
130. Bidot-Lopez P, Farese RV, Sabir MA: Parathyroid hormone and adenosine-3′,5′-monophosphate acutely increase phospholipids of the phosphatidate-polyphosphoinositide pathway in rabbit kidney cortex tubules *in vitro* by a cycloheximide-sensitive process. Endocrinology 108:2078–2081, 1981.
131. Meltzer V, Weinreb S, Bellorin-Font E, Hruska KA: Parathyroid hormone stimulation of renal phosphoinositide metabolism is a cyclic nucleotide-independent effect. Biochim Biophys Acta 712:258–267, 1982.
132. Farese RV, Bidot-Lopez P, Sabir MA, Larson RE: The phosphatidate- polyphosphoinositide cycle: Activation by parathyroid hormone and dibutyryl-cAMP in rabbit kidney cortex. Ann NY Acad Sci 372:539–541, 1981.
133. Rappaport MS, Stern PH: Parathyroid hormone and calcitonin modify inositol phospholipid metabolism in fetal rat limb bones. J Bone Mineral Res 1:173–179, 1986.
134. Vaes G: The role of lysosomes and of their enzymes in the development of bone resorption induced by parathyroid hormone. Parathyroid Hormone Thyrocalcitonin (Calcitonin). Proceedings of the Third Parathyroid Conference, 1967. Amsterdam, Excerpta Medica 1968, pp 318–328.
135. Krebs EG: Protein kinases. Curr Top Cell Reg 5:99–133, 1972.
136. Kuo JD, Greengard P: Cyclic nucleotide-dependent protein kinases. IV. Widespread occurrence of adenosine 3′,5′-monophosphate-dependent protein kinase in various tissues and phyla of the animal kingdom. Proc Natl Acad Sci USA 64:1349–1355, 1969.
137. Ausiello DA, Rosenblatt M, Dayer JR: Parathyroid hormone modulates protein kinase in giant cell tumors of human bone. Am J Physiol 239:E144–E149, 1980.
138. Parsons JA, Neer RM, Potts JT: Initial fall of plasma calcium after intravenous injection of parathyroid hormone. Endocrinology 89:735–740, 1971.
139. Hekkelman JW, Hermann-Erlee MPM, Heersche JNM, Gaillard PJ: Studies on the mechanism of parathyroid hormone action on embryonic bone *in vitro*. Calcium-Regulating Hormones. Proceedings of the Fifth Parathyroid Conference, 1974. Amsterdam, Excerpta Medica, 1975, pp 185–194.
140. Talmage RV: Calcium homeostasis—calcium transport—parathyroid action. The effects of parathyroid hormone on the movement of calcium between bone and fluid. Clin Orthop Rel Res 67:211–234, 1969.
141. Talmage RV, Cooper CM, Park HZ: Regulation of calcium transport in bone by parathyroid hormone. Vitam Horm 28:103–140, 1970.
142. Rasmussen H, Tenenhouse A: Parathyroid hormone and calcitonin. *In* Litwack G (ed): Biochemical Action of Hormones, vol 1. New York, Academic Press, 1970, pp 365–413.
143. Klee CB, Crouch TH, Richman PG: Calmodulin. Annu Rev Biochem 49:489–515, 1980.
144. Cheung WY: Calmodulin plays a pivotal role in cellular regulation. Science 207:19–27, 1980.
145. Egan JJ, Majeska RJ, Rodan GA: Adenylate cyclase enhancing factor from rat osteosarcoma cytosol. Biochem Biophys Res Commun 80:176–182, 1978.
146. Shane E, Avioli RC, Greene VS, et al: Enhancement of parathyroid hormone–responsive renal cortical adenylate cyclase activity by a cytosol protein activator from rat reticulocytes. J Bone Mineral Res 1:41–50, 1986.
147. Nordin BEC, Peacock M: Role of kidney in regulation of plasma-calcium. Lancet 2:1280–1283, 1969.
148. Pullman TN, Lavender AR, Aho I, Rasmussen H: Direct renal action of a purified parathyroid extract. Endocrinology 67:570–582, 1960.
149. Widrow SH, Levinsky NG: Effect of parathyroid extract on renal tubular calcium reabsorption in the dog. J Clin Invest 41:2151–3259, 1962.
150. Avioli LV, Krane SM (eds): Metabolic Bone Disease, vol 2. New York, Academic Press, 1978.
151. Evers C, Murer H, Kinne R: Effect of parathyroid hormone on the transport properties of isolated renal brush-border vesicles. Biochem J 172:49–56, 1978.
152. Heramati A, Haas JA, Know FG: Nephron heterogeneity of phosphate reabsorption: Effect of parathyroid hormone. Am J Physiol 246:F155–F158, 1984.
153. Kinoshita Y, Fukaae M, Miyauchi A, et al: Establishment of a parathyroid hormone–responsive phosphate transport system *in vitro* using cultured renal cells. Endocrinology 119:1954–1963, 1986.
154. Dousa TP, Kempson SA: Regulation of renal brush border membrane transport of phosphate. Mineral Electrolyte Metab 7:113–121, 1982.
155. Kempson SA, Colon-Otero G, Ou SYL, et al: Possible role of nicotinamide adenine dinucleotide as an intracellular regulator of renal transport of phosphate in the rat. J Clin Invest 67:1347–1360, 1981.
156. Kurokawa K, Kawashima H, Torikai S: Parathyroid hormone (PTH)-sensitive and calcitonin (CT)-sensitive 25-(OH)-D_3-1-alpha-hydroxylase along the nephron—Distinct distribution and mechanisms of action. Clin Res 29:541a, 1981.
157. Horiuchi N, Suda T, Takahashi, et al: In vivo evidence for the intermediary role of 3′,5′-cyclic AMP in parathyroid hormone–induced stimulation of 1α,25-dihydroxyvitamin D_3 synthesis in rats. Endocrinology 101:969–974, 1977.
158. Kawashima H, Torikai S, Kurokawa K: Localization of 25-hydroxyvitamin D_3-1α- and -24-hydroxylase along the rat nephron. Proc Natl Acad Sci USA 78:1199–1203, 1981.
159. Kawashima H, Kurokawa K: Unique hormonal regulation of vitamin D metabolism in the mammalian kidney. Mineral Electrolyte Metab 9:227–235, 1983.
160. Matsumoto T, Kawanobe Y, Ogata E: Regulation of 24,25-dihydroxyvitamin D-3 production by 1,25-dihydroxyvitamin D-3 and synthetic human parathyroid hormone 1–34 in a cloned monkey kidney cell line (JTC–12). Biochim Biophys Acta 845:358–365, 1985.
161. Agus ZS, Puschett JB, Senesky D, Goldberg M: Mode of action of parathyroid hormone and cyclic adenosine 3′,5′-monophosphate on renal tubular phosphate reabsorption in the dog. J Clin Invest 50:617–626, 1971.
162. Froeling PGAM, Bijvoet OLM: Kidney-mediated effects of parathyroid hormone in extracellular homeostasis of calcium, phosphate and acid-base balance in man. Neth J Med 17:174–183, 1974.

163. Hellman D, Au WYW, Bartter FC, Smith G: Evidence for a direct effect of parathyroid hormone on urinary acidification. Am J Physiol 209:643–650, 1965.
164. Chabardes D, Imbert M, Clique A, et al: PTH-sensitive adenyl cyclase activity in different segments of the rabbit nephron. Pflügers Arch 354:229–239, 1975.
165. Khalifa S, Mills S, Hruska KA: Stimulation of calcium uptake by parathyroid hormone in renal brush-border membrane vesicles. J Biol Chem 258:14400–14406, 1983.
166. Aurbach GD, Keutmann HJT, Niall HD, et al: Structure, synthesis, and mechanism of action of parathyroid hormone. Recent Prog Horm Res 28:353–398, 1972.
167. Scoble JE, Mills S, Hruska KA: Calcium transport in canine renal basolateral membrane vesicles. Effects of parathyroid hormone. J Clin Invest 75:1096–1105, 1985.
168. Rodan GA, Martin TJ: Role of osteoblasts in hormonal control of bone resorption—A hypothesis. Calcif Tissue Int 33:349–351, 1982.
169. Walker DG, Lapier CM, Gross J: A collagenolytic factor in rat bone promoted by parathyroid extract. Biochem Biophys Res Commun 15:397–401, 1964.
170. Chambers TJ: The cellular basis of bone resorption. Clin Orthop 151:232–293, 1980.
171. Waite LC: Carbonic anhydrase inhibitors, parathyroid hormone and calcium metabolism. Endocrinology 91:1160–1165, 1972.
172. Mahgoub A, Stern PH: Carbon dioxide and the effect of parathyroid hormone on bone *in vitro*. Am J Physiol 226:1272–1275, 1974.
173. Tuukkanen J, Vaananen HK: Omeprazole, a specific inhibitor of H^+-K^+-ATPase, inhibits bone resorption *in vitro*. Calcif Tissue Int 38:123–125, 1986.
174. Luben RA, Goggins JF, Raisz LG: Stimulation by parathyroid hormone of bone hyaluronate synthesis in organ culture. Endocrinology 94:737–745, 1974.
175. Bernstein DS, Handler P: Effects of parathyroid extract on sulfate metabolism of cartilage and bone matrix of rachitic rats. Proc Soc Exp Biol Med 99:339–340, 1958.
176. Krieger NS, Tashjian AH Jr: Parathyroid hormone stimulates bone resorption via a Na-Ca exchange mechanism. Nature 287:843–845, 1980.
177. Delaisse J-M, Eeckhout Y, Vaes G: *In vivo* and *in vitro* evidence for the involvement of cysteine proteinases in bone resorption. Biochem Biophys Res Commun 125:441–447, 1984.
178. Blair HC, Ghandur-Mnaymneh L: Macrophase-mediated bone resorption occurs in an acidic environment. Calcif Tissue Int 37:547–550, 1985.
179. Baron R, Neff L, Louvard D, Courtoy PJ: Cell-mediated extracellular acidification and bone resorption evidence for a low pH in resorbing lacunae and localization of a 100-kilodalton lysosomal membrane protein at the osteoclast ruffled border. J Cell Biol 101:2210–2222, 1985.
179a. Blair H, Teitelbaum S, Ghiselli R, et al: Osteoclastic bone resorption by a polarized vacuolar proton pump. Science 245:855–857, 1989.
180. Sly WS, Whyte MP, Sundaram V, et al: Carbonic anhydrase II deficiency identified in 12 families with the autosomal recessive syndrome of osteopetrosis with renal tubular acidosis and cerebral calcification. N Engl J Med 131:139–145, 1985.
181. Sly WS, Hewett-Emmett D, Whyte MP, et al: Carbonic anhydrase II deficiency identified as the primary defect in the autosomal recessive syndrome of osteopetrosis with renal tubular acidosis and cerebral calcification. Proc Natl Acad Sci USA 80:2752–2756, 1983.
182. Hall GE, Kenny AD: Parathyroid hormone increases carbonic anhydrase activity in cultured mouse calvaria. Calcif Tissue Int 35:682, 1983.
183. Minkin C, Jennings JM: Carbonic anhydrase and bone remodeling: Sulfonamide inhibition of bone resorption in organ culture. Science 176:1031–1033, 1972.
184. Pierce WM, Waite LC: Acetazolamide inhibition of bone resorption: Lack of effect of phosphate release from bone *in vitro*. Horm Metab Res 13:591–592, 1981.
185. Milhaud G, Bourichon J: Calcium metabolism in man studied by means of calcium-45-hyper- and hypoparathyroidism. Compt Rend Hebd Seances Acad Sci 258:3398–3401, 1964.
186. Parsons JA: Parathyroid physiology skeleton. *In* Bourne GH (ed): The Biochemistry and Physiology of Bone. 2nd ed. New York, Academic Press, 1976, pp 159–225.
187. Parsons JA, Zanelli JM: Physiological role of the parathyroid glands. *In* von Kuhlencordt F, Bartelheimer H (eds): Handbuch der Inneren Medizin, vol 6, part 1A. Berlin, Springer-Verlag, 1980, pp 135–172.
188. Suzuki F, Yoneda T, Shimomura Y: Calcitonin and parathyroid-hormone stimulation of acid mucopolysaccharide synthesis in cultured chondrocytes isolated from growth cartilage. FEBS Lett 70:155–158, 1976.
189. Takigawa M, Takano T, Suzuki F: Effects of parathyroid hormone and cyclic AMP analogues on the activity of ornithine decarboxylase and expression of the differentiated phenotype of chondrocytes in culture. J Cell Physiol 106:259–268, 1981.
189a. Slovik DM, Rosenthal DI, Doppelt SH, et al: Restoration of spinal bone in osteoporotic men by treatment with human parathyroid hormone -(1–34) and 1,25-$(OH)_2D$. J Bone Mineral Res 4:377–381, 1986.
190. Burch WM, Lebovitz HE: Hormonal activation of ornithine decarboxylase in embryonic chick pelvic cartilage. Am J Physiol 241:E454–E459, 1981.
191. Gaillard PJ, Herrmann-Erlee MPM, Hekkelman JW: Calcif Tissue Res 21[Suppl]:70–74, 1976.
192. Goltzman D, Loveridge N, Henderson B: Biological activity of circulating forms of parathyroid hormone using a sensitive cytochemical bioassay. Program Abstracts, The 61st Endocrine Society Annual Meeting, Abstract No 171, 1979.
193. Heath DA, Aurbach GD: Studies on the binding of iodine-125 parathyroid hormone to renal cortical membranes. Calcium-Regulating Hormones. Proceedings of the Fifth Parathyroid Conference, 1974. Amsterdam, Excerpta Medica, 1975, pp 159–162.
194. Herrmann-Erlee MPM, Gaillard PJ, Hekkelman JW: Regulation of the response of embryonic bone to PTH and PTH fragments. A morphological and biochemical study. *In* Cott DH, Talmage RV (eds): Endocrinology of Calcium Metabolism. Proceedings of the Sixth Parathyroid Conference, 1977. Amsterdam, Excerpta Medica, 1978, pp 253–261.
195. McIntosh CHS, Hesch RD: Labeled antibody

membrane assay for parathyroid hormone. A new approach to the measurement of receptor bound hormone. Biochem Biophys Res Commun 64:376–383, 1975.
196. Malbon CC, Zull JE: Studies of binding of parathyroid hormone to a detergent-dispersed preparation from bovine kidney cortex plasma membranes. J Biol Chem 252:1079–1083, 1977.
197. Raisz LG, Lorenzo J, Gworek S, et al: Comparison of the effects of a potent synthetic analog of bovine parathyroid hormone with native bPTH–(1–84) and synthetic bPTH–(1–34) on bone resorption and collagen synthesis. Calcif Tissue Int 29:215–218, 1979.
198. Nissenson RA, Teitelbaum AP, Arnaud CD: Assay for parathyroid hormone receptors. Methods Enzymol 109:48–56, 1985.
199. Segre GV, Rosenblatt M, Reiner BL, et al: Characterization of parathyroid hormone receptors in canine renal cortical plasma membranes using a radioiodinated sulfur-free hormone analogue: Correlation of binding with adenylate cyclase activity. J Biol Chem 254:6980–6986, 1979.
200. Sutcliffe HS, Maetin TJ, Eisman JA, Pilczyk R: Binding of parathyroid hormone to bovine kidney cortex plasma membranes. Biochem J 134:913–921, 1973.
201. Zull JE, Malbon CC, Chuang J: Binding of tritiated bovine parathyroid hormone to plasma membranes from bovine kidney cortex. J Biol Chem 252:1071–1078, 1977.
202. Goltzman D, Callahan EN, Tregear GW, Potts JT Jr: Studies of bioactive analogs of parathyroid hormone. Proc 4th Am Pept Symp, 1975. Pept Chem Struct Biol 571–577, 1975.
203. Munson PL: Studies on the role of the parathyroids in calcium and phosphorus metabolism. Ann NY Acad Sci 60:776–796, 1955.
204. Parsons JA, Reit B, Robinson CJ: A chick bioassay for parathyroid hormone. Endocrinology 921:454–462, 1973.
205. Horiuchi N, Rosenblatt M, Keutmann HT, et al: A multiresponse parathyroid hormone assay: An inhibitor has agonist properties *in vivo*. Am J Physiol 244:E589–E595, 1983.
206. Mahaffey JE, Rosenblatt M, Shepard GL, Potts JT Jr: Parathyroid hormone inhibitors. Determination of minimum sequence requirements. J Biol Chem 254:6469–6498, 1979.
207. Di Bella FP, Arnaud CD, Brewer HB Jr: Relative biologic activities of human and bovine parathyroid hormones and their synthetic NH_2-terminal (1–34) peptides, as evaluated *in vitro* with renal cortical adenylate cyclase obtained from three different species. Endocrinology 99:429–436, 1976.
208. Herrmann-Erlee MPM, Heersche JNM, Hekkelman JW, et al: Effects of bone *in vitro* of bovine parathyroid hormone and synthetic fragments representing residues 1–34, 2–34, and 3–34. Endocr Res Commun 3:21–35, 1976.
209. Kimura T, Takai M, Masui Y, et al: Strategy for the synthesis of large peptides: An application to the total synthesis of human parathyroid hormone [hPTH(1–84)]. Biopolymers 20:1823–1832, 1981.
210. Rosenblatt M, D'Amour P, Segre GV, Potts JT Jr: Synthesis of a fragment of bovine parathyroid hormone, bPTH–(28–48): An inhibitor of hormone cleavage *in vivo*. Proc 5th Am Pept Symp, 1977, pp 232–235.
211. Rosenblatt M, Segre GV, Potts JT Jr: Synthesis of a fragment of parathyroid hormone, bPTH–(28–48): An inhibitor of hormone cleavage *in vivo*. Biochemistry 16:2811–2816, 1977.
212. Rosenblatt M, Keutmann HT, Tregear GW, Potts JT Jr: Synthesis of a fragment of human parathyroid hormone, hPTH–(44–68). J Med Chem 20:1452–1456, 1977.
213. Rosenblatt M, Segre GV, Tregear GW, et al: Human parathyroid hormone: Synthesis and chemical, biological, and immunological evaluation of the carboxyl terminal region. Endocrinology 103:978–984, 1978.
214. Rosenblatt M, Tregear GW, Shepard GL, et al: Comparison of two solid-phase peptide syntheses of a 32-amino acid carboxyl terminal fragment of human parathyroid hormone, hPTH–(53–84). Arch Biochem Biophys 199:286–296, 1980.
215. Kremer R, Bennett HPJ, Mitchell J, Goltzman D: Characterization of the rabbit renal receptor for native parathyroid hormone employing a radioligand purified by reversed-phase liquid chromatography. J Biol Chem 257:14048–14054, 1982.
216. Rizzoli RE, Murray TM, Marx SJ, Aurbach GD: Binding of radioiodinated bovine parathyroid hormone. Endocrinology 112:1303–1312, 1983.
217. Rizzoli RE, Somerman M, Murray TM, Aurbach GD: Binding of radioiodinated parathyroid hormone to cloned bone cells. Endocrinology 113:1832–1838, 1983.
218. Zull JE, Chuang J: Kidney membrane binding of native PTH compared to binding of its synthetic 1–34 fragment. Receptor Res 1:69–76, 1980.
219. Demay M, Mitchell J, Goltzman D: Comparison of renal and osseous binding of parathyroid hormone and hormonal fragments. Am J Phys 249:E437–E446, 1985.
220. Massry SG: Parathyroid hormone and uremic myocardiopathy. *In* Jahn H, Massry SG, Ritz E, Weidmann P (eds): Contributions to Nephrology. International Workshop on Cardiocirculatory Function in Renal Disease. Basel, S. Karger, 1983, pp 231–239.
221. Akmal M, Massry SG, Goldstein DA, et al: Role of parathyroid hormone in the glucose intolerance of chronic renal failure. J Clin Invest 75:1037–1044, 1985.
222. Massry SG: The toxic effects of parathyroid hormone in uremia. Semin Nephrol 3:306–328, 1983.
223. Baczynski R, Massry SG, Kohan R, et al: Effect of parathyroid hormone on myocardial energy metabolism in the rat. Kidney Int 27:718–725, 1985.
224. Akmal M, Telfer N, Ansari AN, Massry SG: Erythrocyte survival in chronic renal failure: Role of secondary hyperparathyroidism. J Clin Invest 76:1695–1698, 1985.
225. Keutmann HT, Griscom AW, Nussbaum SR, et al: Rat parathyroid hormone–(1–34) fragment: Renal adenylate cyclase activity and receptor binding properties *in vitro*. Endocrinology 117:1230–1234, 1985.
226. Martin TJ, Vakakis N, Eisman JA, et al: Chick kidney adenylate cyclase: Sensitivity to parathyroid hormone and synthetic human and bovine peptides. J Endocrinol 63:369–375, 1974.
227. O'Riordan JLH, Woodhead JS, Hendy GN, et al: Effect of oxidation on biological and immunological activity of porcine parathyroid hormone. J Endocrinol 63:117–124, 1974.
228. Zanelli JM, Lane E, Kimura T, Sakakibara S:

Biological activities of synthetic human parathyroid hormone (PTH) 1–84 relative to natural bovine 1–84 PTH in two different *in vivo* bioassay systems. Endocrinology 117:1962–1967, 1985.

229. Tregear GW, van Rietschoten J, Greene E, et al: Solid phase synthesis of the biologically active N-terminal 1–34 peptide of human parathyroid hormone. Hoppe Seyler Z Physiol Chem 355:415–421, 1974.
230. Keutmann HT, Dawson BF, Aurbach GD, Potts JT Jr: A biologically active amino terminal fragment of bovine parathyroid hormone prepared by dilute acid hydrolysis. Biochemistry 11:1973–1979, 1972.
231. Potts JT Jr, Keutmann JT, Niall HD, et al: Covalent structure of bovine parathyroid hormone in relation to biological and immunological activity. Parathyroid Hormone and Thyrocalcitonin (Calcitonin). Proceedings of the Third Parathyroid Conference, 1967. Amsterdam, Excerpta Medica, 1968, pp 44–53.
232. Tregear GW, Potts JT Jr: Synthetic analogues of residues 1–34 of human parathyroid hormone: Influence of residue number 1 on biological potency *in vitro*. Endocr Res Commun 2:561–570, 1975.
233. Rosenblatt M, Goltzman D, Keutmann HT, et al: Chemical and biological properties of synthetic, sulfur-free analogues of parathyroid hormone. J Biol Chem 251:159–164, 1976.
234. Rosenblatt M, Coltrera MD, Shepart GL, et al: Sulfur-free parathyroid hormone analogues containing D-amino acids: Biological properties *in vitro* and *in vivo*. Biochemistry 20:7246–7250, 1981.
235. Goldring SR, Dayer J-M, Rosenblatt M: Factors regulating the response of cells cultured from human giant cell tumors of bone to parathyroid hormone. J Clin Encocrinol Metab 53:295–300, 1981.
236. Goltzman D, Peytremann A, Callahan E, et al: Analysis of the requirements for parathyroid hormone action in renal membranes with the use of inhibiting analogues. J Biol Chem 250:3199–3203, 1975.
237. Rosenblatt M, Callahan EN, Mahaffey JE, et al: Parathyroid hormone inhibitors: Design, synthesis, and biologic evaluation of hormone analogues. J Biol Chem 252:5847–5851, 1977.
238. Segre GV, Rosenblatt M, Tully GL III, et al: Evaluation of an *in vitro* parathyroid hormone antagonist *in vivo* in dogs. Endocrinology 116:1024–1029, 1985.
239. Martin KJ, Bellorin-Font E, Freitag J, et al: The arterio-venous difference for immunoreactive parathyroid hormone and the production of adenosine 3′,5′ monophosphate by isolated perfused bone: Studies with analogs of parathyroid hormone. Endocrinology 109:956–959, 1981.
240. Gray DA, Parsons JA, Potts JT Jr, et al: *In vitro* studies on an antagonist of parathyroid hormone [N1e-8,N1e-18,Tyr-34]bPTH–(3–34)amide. Br J Pharmacol 76:259–263, 1982.
241. McGowan JA, Chen TC, Gragola J, et al: Parathyroid hormone: Effects of the 3–34 fragment *in vivo* and *in vitro*. Science 219:67–69, 1983.
242. Nussbaum SR, Rosenblatt M, Potts JT Jr: Parathyroid hormone renal receptor interactions: Demonstration of two receptor-binding domains. J Biol Chem 255:10183–10387, 1980.
243. Rosenblatt M, Tyler GA, Doppelt SH, et al: The design and biological evaluation of a parathyroid hormone antagonist effective *in vivo*. *In* Labrie F, Proulx L (eds): Endocrinology. Proceedings of the 7th International Congress of Endocrinology, Quebec City, Canada (July 1–7, 1984). Amsterdam, Excerpta Medica ICS, 1984, pp 579–582.
244. Cohn DV, Hamilton JW: Newer aspects of parathyroid chemistry and physiology. Cornell Vet 66:271–300, 1976.
245. Habener JF, Kemper B, Rich A, Potts JT Jr: Biosynthesis of parathyroid hormone. Recent Prog Horm Res 33:249–308, 1977.
246. Habener JF, Kronenberg HM: Parathyroid hormone biosynthesis—structure and function of biosynthetic precursors. Fed Proc 37:2561–2566, 1978.
247. Habener JF, Potts JT Jr: Biosynthesis of parathyroid hormone. N Engl J Med 299:580–585; 635–644, 1978.
248. Chu LLH, MacGregor RR, Anast JW, et al: Studies on the biosynthesis of rat parathyroid hormone and proparathyroid hormone: Adaptation of the parathyroid gland to dietary restriction of calcium. Endocrinology 93:915–924, 1973.
249. Cohn DV, MacGregor RR, Chu LLH, et al: Calcemic fraction-A: Biosynthetic peptide precursor of parathyroid hormone. Proc Natl Acad Sci USA 69:1521–1525, 1972.
250. Habener JF, Kemper B, Potts JT Jr, Rich A: Proparathyroid hormone: Biosynthesis by human parathyroid adenomas. Science 178:630–633, 1972.
251. Kemper B, Habener JF, Potts JT Jr, Rich A: Preproparathyroid hormone: Fidelity of the translation of parathyroid messenger RNA by extracts of wheat germ. Biochemistry 15:20–25, 1976.
252. MacGregor RR, Chu LLH, Hamilton JW, Cohn DV: Partial purification of parathyroid hormone from chicken parathyroid glands. Endocrinology 92:1313–1317, 1973.
253. Habener JF, Kemper B, Potts JT Jr, Rich A: Preproparathyroid hormone identified by cell-free translation of messenger RNA from hyperplastic human parathyroid tissue. J Clin Invest 56:1328–1333, 1975.
254. Habener JF, Potts JT Jr, Rich A: Pre-proparathyroid hormone: Evidence for an early biosynthetic precursor of proparathyroid hormone. J Biol Chem 251:3893–3899, 1976.
255. Habener JF, Rosenblatt M, Kemper B, et al: Preproparathyroid hormone: Amino acid sequence, chemical synthesis, and some biological studies of the precursor region. Proc Natl Acad Sci USA 75:2616–2620, 1978.
256. Kemper B, Habener JF, Mulligan RC, et al: Preproparathyroid hormone: A direct translation product of parathyroid messenger RNA. Proc Natl Acad Sci USA 71:3731–3735, 1974.
257. Kemper B, Habener JF, Ernst MD, et al: Preproparathyroid hormone: Analysis of radioactive tryptic peptides and amino acid sequence. Biochemistry 15:15–19, 1976.
258. Gilbert W: Genes in pieces. Nature 271:501, 1978.
259. Weaver CA, Gordon DF, Kissil MS, et al: Isolation and complete nucleotide sequence of the gene for bovine parathyroid hormone. Gene 28:319–329, 1984.
260. Naylor SL, Sakaguchi AU, Szoka P, et al: Human parathyroid hormone gene (PTH) is on short arm of chromosome 11. Somat Cell Gene 9:609–616, 1983.
261. Zabel BU, Kronenberg HM, Bell GI, Shows TB: Chromosome mapping of genes on the short arm of human chromosome 11: Parathyroid hormone gene is at 11p15 together with the genes for insulin, c-

Harvey-ras 1, and β-hemoglobin. Cytogenet Cell Genet 39:200–205, 1985.

262. Antonarakis SE, Phillips JA III, Mallonee RL, et al: β-Globin locus is linked to the parathyroid hormone (PTH) locus and lies between the insulin and PTH loci in man. Proc Natl Acad Sci USA 80:6615–6619, 1983.
263. Ahn TG, Antonarakis SE, Kronenberg HM, et al: Familial isolated hypoparathyroidism: A molecular genetic analysis of 8 families with 23 affected persons. Medicine 65:73–81, 1986.
264. Habener JF, Amherdt M, Ravazzola M, Orci L: Parathyroid hormone biosynthesis: Correlation of conversion of biosynthetic precursors with intracellular protein migration as determined by electron microscope autoradiography. J Cell Biol 80:715–731, 1979.
265. Habener JF, Maunus R, Dee PC, Potts JT Jr: Early events in the cellular formation of proparathyroid hormone. J Cell Biol 85:292–298, 1980.
266. Habener JF, Potts JT Jr: Subcellular distributions of parathyroid hormone, hormonal precursors, and parathyroid secretory protein. Endocrinology 104:265–275, 1979.
267. MacGregor RR, Chu LLH, Hamilton JW, Cohn DV: Studies on the subcellular localization of proparathyroid hormone in the bovine parathyroid gland: Separation of newly synthesized from mature forms. Endocrinology 93:1387–1397, 1973.
268. Palade G: Intracellular aspects of the process of protein synthesis. Science 189:347–358, 1975.
269. Habener JF, Rosenblatt M, Dee PC, Potts JT Jr: Cellular processing of pre-proparathyroid hormone involves rapid hydrolysis of the leader sequence. J Biol Chem 254:10596–10599, 1979.
270. Chu LLH, MacGregor RR, Cohn DV: Energy-dependent intracellular translocation of proparathormone. J Cell Biol 72:1–10, 1977.
271. Kemper B, Habener JF, Rich A, Potts JT Jr: Microtubules and the intracellular conversion of proparathyroid hormone to parathyroid hormone. Endocrinology 96:903–912, 1975.
272. Morrissey JJ, Cohn DV: Regulation of secretion of parathormone and secretory protein-I from separate intracellular pools by calcium, dibutyryl cyclic AMP, and (1)-isoproterenol. J Cell Biol 82:93–102, 1979.
273. Habener JF, Stevens TD, Tregear GW, Potts JT Jr: Radioimmunoassay of human proparathyroid hormone: Analysis of hormone content in tissue extracts and in plasma. J Clin Endocrinol Metab 42:520–530, 1976.
274. Goltzman D, Peytremann A, Callahan EN, et al: Interaction of parathyroid hormone with membranes of renal target cells: Analysis of intrinsic prohormone activity and actions of peptide analogues with inhibitory effects. *In* Talmage RV, Owen M, Parsons JA (eds): Calcium-Regulating Hormones: Proceedings of the Fifth Parathyroid Conference. Amsterdam, Excerpta Medica, 1975, pp 172–176.
275. Goltzman D, Callahan EN, Tregear GW, Potts JT Jr: Conversion of proparathyroid hormone to parathyroid hormone: Studies in vitro with trypsin. Biochemistry 15:5076–5082, 1976.
276. MacGregor RR, Hamilton JW, Cohn DV: The bypass of tissue hormone stores during the secretion of newly synthesized parathyroid hormone. Endocrinology 917:178–188, 1975.
277. Boime I, Szczesna E, Smith D: Membrane-dependent cleavage of the human placental lactogen precursor to its native form in ascites cell-free extracts. Eur J Biochem 73:515–520, 1977.
278. Dorner AJ, Kemper B: Conversion of pre-proparathyroid hormone to proparathyroid hormone by dog pancreatic microsomes. Biochemistry 17:5550–5555, 1978.
279. Habener JF, Kemper B, Potts JT Jr, Rich A: Parathyroid mRNA directs the synthesis of pre-proparathyroid hormone and proparathyroid hormone in the Krebs ascites cell-free system. Biochem Biophys Res Commun 67:1114–1121, 1975.
280. Jackson RC, Blobel G: Post-translational cleavage of presecretory proteins with an extract of rough microsomes from dog pancreas containing signal peptidase activity. Proc Natl Acad Sci USA 74:5598–5602, 1977.
281. Lively MO, Walsh KA: Hen oviduct signal peptidase is an integral membrane protein. J Biol Chem 258:9488–9495, 1983.
282. Perara E, Rothman RE, Lingappa VR: Uncoupling translocation from translation: Implications for transport of proteins across membranes. Science 232:348–352, 1986.
283. Habener JF, Chang HT, Potts JT Jr: Enzymic processing of proparathyroid hormone by cell-free extracts of parathyroid glands. Biochemistry 16:3910–3917, 1977.
284. Walter P, Blobel G: Purification of a membrane-associated protein complex required for protein translocation across the endoplasmic reticulum. Proc Natl Acad Sci USA 77:7112–7116, 1980.
285. Walter P, Jackson RC, Marcus MM, et al: Tryptic dissection and reconstitution of translocation activity for nascent presecretory proteins across microsomal membranes. Proc Natl Acad Sci USA 76:1795–1799, 1979.
286. Warren G, Dobberstein B: Protein transfer across microsomal membranes reassembled from separate membrane components. Nature 273:569–571, 1978.
287. Wickner WT, Lodish HF: Multiple mechanisms of protein insertion into and across membranes. Science 230:400–407, 1985.
288. Walter P, Blobel F: Translocation of proteins across the endoplasmic reticulum III. Signal recognition protein (SRP) causes signal sequence-dependent and site-specific arrest of chain elongation that is released by microsomal membranes. J Cell Biol 91:557–561, 1981.
289. Meyer DI, Krause E, Dobberstein B: Secretory protein translocation across membranes—The role of the "docking protein." Nature 297:647–650, 1982.
290. Majzoub JA, Rosenblatt M, Fennick B, et al: Synthetic pre-proparathyroid hormone leader sequence inhibits cell-free processing of placental, parathyroid, and pituitary pre-hormones. J Biol Chem 255:11478–11483, 1980.
291. Rosenblatt M, Habener JF, Tyler GA, et al: Chemical synthesis of the precursor-specific region of pre-proparathyroid hormone. J Biol Chem 254:1414–1421, 1979.
292. Caufield MP, Duong LT, O'Brien R, et al: A chemically synthesized functional radiolabeled signal peptide: Design, preparation, and biological evaluation of an iodinated analog of pre-proparathyroid hormone (in press).
293. Von Heijne G, Blomberg C: Transmembrane trans-

location of proteins: The direct transfer model. Eur J Biochem 97:175–181, 1979.
294. Wickner W: Assembly of proteins into membranes. Science 210:861–869, 1980.
295. Rosenblatt M, Callahan EN, Mahaffey JE, et al: Parathyroid hormone inhibitors: Design, synthesis, and biologic evaluation of hormone analogues. J Biol Chem 252:5847–5851, 1977.
296. MacGregor RR, Chu LLH, Cohn DV: Conversion of proparathyroid hormone to parathyroid hormone by a particulate enzyme of the parathyroid gland. J Biol Chem 251:6711–6716, 1976.
297. Steiner DF: Peptide hormone precursors: Biosynthesis, processing and significance. *In* Parsons JA (ed): Peptide Hormones. London, Macmillan, 1976, pp 49–65.
298. Marx JL: A new wave of enzymes for cleaving prohormones. Nature 235:285–286, 1987.
299. Steiner DF, Bell GI, Tager S: Chemistry and biosynthesis of pancreatic protein hormones. *In* DeGroot L (ed): Endocrinology. Philadelphia, W.B. Saunders, 1989, pp 1263–1289.
300. Fischer JA, Oldham SB, Sizemore GW, Arnaud CD: Calcium-regulated parathyroid hormone peptidase. Proc Natl Acad Sci USA 69:2341–2345, 1972.
301. MacGregor RR, Hamilton JW, Kent GN, et al: The degradation of proparathormone and parathormone by parathyroid and liver cathepsin B. J Biol Chem 254:4428–4433, 1979.
302. MacGregor RR, Hamilton JW, Shofstall RE, Cohn DV: Isolation and characterization of porcine parathyroid cathepsin B. J Biol Chem 254:4423–4427, 1979.
303. Mayer GP, Keaton JA, Hurst JG, Habener JF: Effects of plasma calcium concentration on the relative proportion of hormone and carboxyl fragments in parathyroid venous blood. Endocrinology 104:1778–1784, 1979.
304. Morrissey JJ, Hamilton JW, MacGregor RR, Cohn DV: The secretion of parathormone fragments 34–84 and 37–84 by dispersed porcine parathyroid cells. Endocrinology 107:164–171, 1980.
305. Peterson JD, Shofstall RE, MacGregor RR, Hamilton JW: The specificity of the parathormone converting protease: Studies with a synthetic double labeled substrate. Program Abstract of the 61st Annual Meeting of the Endocrine Society, Anaheim, California, 1979, 40:82.
306. Martin KJ, Hruska KA, Lewis J, et al: The renal handling of parathyroid hormone: Role of peritubular uptake and glomerular filtration. J Clin Invest 60:808–814, 1977.
307. Habener JF, Kemper B, Potts JT Jr: Calcium-dependent intracellular degradation of parathyroid hormone: A possible mechanism for the regulation of hormone stores. Endocrinology 97:431–441, 1975.
308. Habener JF, Kemper B, Potts PT Jr, Rich A: Calcium-independent intracellular conversion of proparathyroid hormone to parathyroid hormone. Endocr Res Commun 1:239–246, 1974.
309. Heinrich G, Kronenberg HM, Potts JT Jr, Habener JF: Parathyroid hormone messenger ribonucleic acid: Effects of calcium on cellular regulation in vitro. Endocrinology 112:449–458, 1983.
310. Russell J, Lettieri D, Sherwood LM: Direct regulation by calcium of cytoplasmic messenger ribonucleic acid coding for pre-proparathyroid hormone in isolated bovine parathyroid cells. J Clin Invest 72:1851–1855, 1983.
311. Russell J, Lettieri D, Sherwood LM: Direct suppression by calcium of transcription of the parathyroid hormone gene. Abstract of the 68th Annual Meeting of the Endocrine Society, June 25–27, 1986, abstract α234.
312. Silver J, Russell J, Sherwood LM: Regulation by vitamin D metabolites of messenger ribonucleic acid for preproparathyroid hormone in isolated bovine parathyroid cells. Proc Natl Acad Sci USA 82:4270–4273, 1985.
313. Russell J, Lettieri D, Sherwood LM: Direct suppression by $1,25(OH)_2D_3$ of transcription of the parathyroid hormone gene. Clin Res 34:726A, 1986.
314. Igarashi T, Muramatsu M, Ogata E, Kronenberg HM: Cis-acting regulatory elements for human parathyroid hormone gene expression. J Bone Mineral Res 1[Supp 1]:444 (abstract), 1986.
315. Okazaki T, Igarashi T, Kronenberg HM: $1,25(OH)_2$ vitamin D specifically regulates human PTH gene expression in transfected rat pituitary cells. Abstracts of the 68th Annual Meeting of the Endocrine Society, June 25–27, 1986, abstract α231.
316. Roth SI, Raisz LG: Effect of calcium concentration on the ultrastructure of rat parathyroid glands in organ culture. Lab Invest 13:331–345, 1964.
317. Roth SI, Raisz LG: The course and reversibility of the calcium effect on the ultrastructure of the rat parathyroid gland in organ culture. Lab Invest 15:1187–1211, 1966.
318. LeBoff MS, Rennke HG, Brown EM: Abnormal regulation of parathyroid cell secretion and proliferation in primary cultures of bovine parathyroid cells. Endocrinology 113:277–284, 1983.
319. LeBoff MS, Henry M, Brown EM: The association between changes in proliferation and secretory function in cultured parathyroid cells. Program and Abstracts, Sixth Annual Meeting, American Society of Bone Mineral Research, 1984, abstract αA56.
320. Brandi ML, Aurback GD, Fitzpatrick LA, et al: Parathyroid mitogenic activity in plasma from patients with familial multiple endocrine neoplasia, type I. N Engl J Med 314:1287–1293, 1986.
321. Arnold A, Staunton CE, Gaz RD, Kronenberg HM: Monoclonality of parathyroid adenomas. Clin Res 34:879A, 1986.
322. Copp DH, Davidson AGF: Direct hormonal control of parathyroid function in the dog. Proc Soc Expl Biol Med 107:342–344, 1961.
323. Patt HM, Luckhardt AB: Relationship of a low blood calcium to parathyroid secretion. Endocrinology 31:384–392, 1942.
324. Sherwood LM, Potts JT Jr, Care AD, et al: Evaluation by radioimmunoassay of factors controlling the secretion of parathyroid hormone. Nature 209:52–55, 1966.
325. Abe M, Sherwood LM: Regulation of parathyroid hormone secretion by adenyl cyclase. Biochem Biophys Res Commun 48:396–401, 1972.
326. Brown EM, Gardner DG, Windeck RA, Aurbach GD:Relationshipofintracellular3′5′-adenosinemonophosphate accumulation to parathyroid hormone release from dispersed bovine parathyroid cells. Endocrinology 103:2323–2333, 1978.
327. Williams GA, Hargis GK, Bowser EN, et al: Evidence for a role of adenosine 3′5′-monophosphate in parathyroid hormone release. Endocrinology 92:687–691, 1973.
328. Blum JW, Fischer JA, Hunziker WH, et al:

Parathyroid hormone responses to catecholamines and to changes of extracellular calcium in cows. J Clin Invest 61:1113–1122, 1978.
329. Brown EM, Gardner DG, Windeck RA, Aurbach GD: Cholera toxin stimulates 3′5′-adenosine monophosphate accumulation and parathyroid hormone release from dispersed bovine parathyroid cells. Endocrinology 104:218–225, 1979.
330. Brown EM, Hurwitz SH, Woodard CJ, Aurbach GD: Direct identification of beta-adrenergic receptors on isolated bovine parathyroid cells. Endocrinology 100:1703–1709, 1977.
331. Gardner DG, Brown EM, Windeck R, Aurbach GD: Prostaglandin E_2 stimulation of adenosine 3′5′-monophosphate accumulation and parathyroid hormone release in dispersed bovine parathyroid cells. Endocrinology 103:577–582, 1978.
332. Kukreja SC, Hargis GK, Bowser EN, et al: Role of adrenergic stimuli in parathyroid hormone secretion in man. J Clin Endocrinol Metab 40:478–481, 1975.
333. Mayer GP, Hurst JG, Barto JA, et al: Effect of epinephrine on parathyroid hormone secretion in calves. Endocrinology 104:1181–1187, 1979.
334. Metz SA, Deftos LJ, Baylink DJ, Robertson RP: Neuroendocrine modulation of calcitonin and parathyroid hormone in man. J Clin Endocrinol Metab 47:151–159, 1978.
335. Brown EM, Hurwitz SH, Aurbach GD: β-Adrenergic inhibition of adenosine 3′5′-monophosphate accumulation and parathyroid hormone release from dispersed bovine parathyroid cells. Endocrinology 103:893–899, 1978.
336. Gardner DG, Brown EM, Windeck R, Aurbach GD: Prostaglandin E_2 inhibits 3′5′-adenosine monophosphate accumulation and parathyroid hormone release from dispersed bovine parathyroid cells. Endocrinology 104:1–7, 1979.
337. Brown EM, Thatcher JG: Adenosine 3′5′-monophosphate (cAMP)-dependent protein kinase and the regulation of parathyroid hormone release by divalent cations and agents elevating cellular cAMP in dispersed bovine parathyroid cells. Endocrinology 110:1374–1380, 1982.
338. Shoback DM, Brown EM: Forskolin increases cellular cyclic adenosine monophosphate content and parathyroid hormone release in dispersed bovine parathyroid cells. Metabolism 33:509–514, 1984.
339. Rodriguez HJ, Morrison A, Slatopolsky E, Klahr S: Adenylate cyclase of human parathyroid gland. J Clin Endocrinol Metab 47:319–325, 1978.
340. Dufresne LR, Gitelman HJ: A possible role of adenyl cyclase in the regulation of parathyroid activity by calcium. *In* Talmage RV, Munson PL (eds): Calcium, Parathyroid Hormone and the Calcitonins. Proceedings of the Fourth Parathyroid Conference. Amsterdam, Excerpta Medica, 1972, pp 202–206.
341. Matsuzaki S, Dumont JE: Effect of calcium ion on horse parathyroid gland adenyl cyclase. Biochem Biophys Acta 284:227–234, 1972.
342. Willgoss D, Jacobi JM, DeJersey J, Bartley PC, Lloyd HM: Effect of calcium on cyclic nucleotide phosphodiesterase in parathyroid tissue. Biochim Biophys Res Commun 94:763–768, 1980.
343. Lasker RD, Spiegel AM: Endogenous substrates for cAMP-dependent phosphorylation in dispersed bovine parathyroid cells. Endocrinology 111:1412–1414, 1982.
344. Sherwood LM, Mayer GP, Ramberg CF, et al: Regulation of parathyroid hormone secretion: Proportional control by calcium, lack of effect of phosphate. Endocrinology 83:1043–1051, 1968.
345. Keaton JA, Barto JA, Moore MP, et al: Altered parathyroid response to calcium in hypercalcemic neonatal calves. Endocrinology 103:2161–2167, 1978.
346. Mayer GP, Habener JF, Potts JT Jr: Parathyroid hormone secretion *in vivo*: Demonstration of a calcium-dependent, non-suppressible component of secretion. J Clin Invest 57:679–683, 1976.
347. Mayer GP, Hurst JG: Sigmoidal relationship between parathyroid hormone secretion rate and plasma concentration in calves. Endocrinology 102:1036–1042, 1978.
348. Mayer GP, Hurst JG: Comparison of the effects of calcium and magnesium on parathyroid hormone secretion rate in calves. Endocrinology 102:1803–1807, 1978.
349. Arnaud CD, Sizemore GW, Oldham SB, et al: Human parathyroid hormone: Glandular and secreted molecular species. Am J Med 50:630–638, 1971.
350. Birnbaumer ME, Schneider AB, Palmer D, et al: Secretion of parathyroid hormone by abnormal human parathyroid glands *in vitro*. J Clin Endocrinol Metab 45:105–113, 1977.
351. Habener JF: Responsiveness of neoplastic and hyperplastic parathyroid tissues to calcitonin in vitro. J Clin Invest 62:436–450, 1978.
352. Habener JF, Stevens TD, Ravazzola M, et al: Effects of calcium ionophores on the synthesis and release of parathyroid hormone. Endocrinology 101:1524–1537, 1977.
353. Habener JF, Potts JT Jr: Relative effectiveness of magnesium and calcium on the secretion and biosynthesis of parathyroid hormone *in vitro*. Endocrinology 98:197–202, 1976.
354. Sherwood LM, Rodman JS, Lundberg WB: Evidence for a precursor to circulating parathyroid hormone. Proc Natl Acad Sci USA 67:1631–1638, 1970.
355. Targovnik RV, Cooper CM, Park HZ: Regulation of calcium transport in bone by parathyroid hormone. Vitam Horm 28d:103–140, 1970.
356. Habener JF, Potts JT Jr: Parathyroid physiology and primary hyperparathyroidism. *In* Avioli LV, Krane SM (eds): Metabolic Bone Disease, vol 2. New York, Academic Press, 1978, pp 1–147.
357. Murray TM, Peacock M, Powell D, et al: Nonautonomy of hormone secretion in primary hyperparathyroidism. Clin Endocrinol 1:235–246, 1972.
358. Gittes RF, Radde IC: Experimental hyperparathyroidism from multiple isologous parathyroid transplants: Homeostatic effect of simultaneous thyroid transplants. Endocrinology 78:1015–1022, 1966.
359. Blum JW, Mayer GP, Potts JT Jr: Parathyroid hormone responses during spontaneous hypocalcemia and induced hypercalcemia in cows. Endocrinology 95:84–92, 1974.
360. Anast CS, Mohs JM, Kaplan SL, Burns TW: Evidence for parathyroid failure in magnesium deficiency. Science 177:606–608, 1972.
361. Anast CS, Winnacker JL, Forte LR, Burns TW: Impaired release of parathyroid hormone in magnesium deficiency. J Clin Endocrinol Metab 42:707–717, 1976.

362. Chase LR, Slatopolsky E: Secretion and metabolic efficacy of parathyroid hormone in patients with severe hypomagnesemia. J Clin Endocrinol Metab 38:363–371, 1974.
363. Rude RK, Oldham SB, Singer FR: Functional hypoparathyroidism and parathyroid hormone end-organ resistance in human magnesium deficiency. Clin Endocrinol 5:209–224, 1976.
364. Heath H III: Biogenic amines and the secretion of parathyroid hormone and calcitonin. Endocrinol Rev 1:319–338, 1980.
365. Fischer JA, Blum JW, Binswanger U: Acute parathyroid hormone response to epinephrine *in vivo*. J Clin Invest 52:2434–2440, 1973.
366. Altenahr E: Electron microscopical evidence for involution of chief cells in human parathyroid gland. Experientia 27:1077, 1971.
367. Norberg KA, Persson B, Granberg PO: Adrenergic innervation of the human parathyroid glands. Acta Chir Scand 141:319–322, 1975.
368. Yeghiayan E, Rojo-Ortega JM, Genest J: Parathyroid vessel innervation: An ultrastructural study. J Anat 112:137–142, 1972.
369. Shah JH, Motto GS, Kukreja SC, et al: Stimulation of the secretion of parathyroid hormone during hypoglycemic stress. J Clin Endocrinol Metab 41:692–696, 1975.
370. Kukreja SC, Hargis GK, Rosenthal IM, Williams GA: Pheochromocytoma causing excessive parathyroid hormone production and hypercalcemia. Ann Intern Med 79:838–840, 1973.
371. Pearse AGE: Evolutionary and developmental relationships among the cells producing peptide hormones. *In* Parsons JA (ed): Peptide Hormones. London, Macmillan, 1976, pp 33–46.
372. Miller SS, Sizemore GW, Sheps SG, Tyce GM: Parathyroid function in patients with pheochromocytoma. Ann Intern Med 82:372–375, 1975.
373. Keiser HR, Beaven MA, Doppman J, et al: Sipple's syndrome: Medullary thyroid carcinoma, pheochromocytoma, and parathyroid disease: Studies in a large family. Ann Intern Med 78:561–579, 1973.
374. Henry HL, Norman AW: Studies on the mechanism of action of calciferol VII. Localization of 1,25-dihydroxy-vitamin D_3 in chick parathyroid glands. Biochem Biophys Res Commun 62:781–788, 1975.
375. Chertow BS, Baylink DJ, Wergedal JE, et al: Decrease in serum immunoreactive parathyroid hormone in rats and in parathyroid hormone secretion *in vitro* by 1,25 dihydroxycholecalciferol. J Clin Invest 56:668–678, 1975.
376. Oldham SB, Smith R, Hartenbower DL, et al: The acute effects of 1,25-dihydroxycholecalciferol on serum immunoreactive parathyroid. Endocrinology 104:248–254, 1979.
377. Cantley LK, Russell J, Lettieri D, Sherwood LM: 1,25-Dihydroxyvitamin D_3 suppresses parathyroid hormone secretion from bovine parathyroid cells in tissue culture. Endocrinology 117:2114–2119, 1985.
378. Canterbury JM, Lerman S, Claflin AJ, et al: Inhibition of parathyroid hormone secretion by 25-hydroxycholecalciferol and 24,25-dihydroxycholecalciferol in the dog. J Clin Invest 61:1375–1383, 1978.
379. Hurst JG, Wilson PR, Mayer GP: PTH secretory response during the administration of 1,25-dihydroxycholecalciferol (1,25-DHCC). Program Abstracts of the 61st Annual Meeting of the Endocrine Society, 1979, p 48.
380. Dietel M, Dorn G, Montz R, Altenahr E: Influence of vitamin D_3, 1,25-dihydroxyvitamin D_3, and 24,25-dihydroxyvitamin D_3 on parathyroid hormone secretion, adenosine 3′5′-monophosphate release, and ultrastructure of parathyroid glands in organ culture. Endocrinology 105:237–245, 1979.
381. Care AD, Bates RFL, Pickard DW, et al: The effects of vitamin D metabolites or their analogues on the secretion of parathyroid hormone. Calcif Tissue Res 21:142–146, 1976.
382. Spielman LL, Bancroft FC: Pregrowth hormone: Evidence for conversion to growth hormone during synthesis on membrane-bound polysomes. Endocrinology 101:651–658, 1977.
382a. Puzas JE, Brand JS: *In vitro* use of vitamin D_3 metabolites: Culture conditions determine cell uptake. Calcif Tissue Int 37:474–477, 1985.
383. Fischer JA, Oldham SB, Sizemore GW, Arnaud CD: Calcitonin stimulation of parathyroid hormone secretion *in vitro*. Horm Metab Res 3:223–224, 1971.
384. Deftos LJ, Parthemore JG: Secretion of parathyroid hormone in patients with medullary thyroid carcinoma. J Clin Invest 54:416–420, 1974.
385. Fucik RF, Kukreja SC, Hargis GK, et al: Effect of glucocorticoids on function of the parathyroid glands in man. J Clin Endocrinol Metab 40:152–155, 1975.
386. Williams GA, Peterson WC, Bowser EN, et al: Interrelationship of parathyroid and adrenocortical function in calcium homeostasis in the rat. Endocrinology 95:707–712, 1974.
387. Au WYW: Cortisol stimulation of parathyroid hormone secretion by rat parathyroid glands in organ culture. Science 193:1015–1017, 1976.
388. Lancer SR, Bowser EN, Hargis GK, Williams GA: The effect of growth hormone on parathyroid function in rats. Endocrinology 98:1289–1293, 1976.
389. Vale W, Brazeau P, Rivier C, et al: Somatostatin. Recent Prog Horm Res 31:365–388, 1975.
390. Hargis GK, Williams GA, Reynolds WA, et al: Effect of somatostatin on parathyroid hormone and calcitonin secretion. Endocrinology 102:745–750, 1978.
391. Deftos LJ, Lorenzi M, Bohanon N, et al: Somatostatin does not suppress plasma parathyroid hormone. J Clin Endocrinol Metab 43:205–207, 1976.
392. Gardner DG, Brown EM, Aurbach GD: Inhibition of adenosine 3′5′-monophosphate accumulation and parathyroid hormone release by sodium nitroprusside. Endocrinology 105:360–366, 1979.
393. Brown EM, Pazoles CJ, Creutz CE, et al: Role of anions in parathyroid hormone release from dispersed bovine parathyroid cells. Proc Natl Acad Sci USA 75:876–880, 1978.
394. Morrissey J, Slatopolsky E: Effect of aluminum on parathyroid hormone secretion. Kidney Int 29 [Suppl]:S41–44, 1986.
395. William GA, Longley RS, Bowser EN, et al: Parathyroid hormone secretion in normal man and in primary hyperparathyroidism: Role of histamine H_2 receptors. J Clin Endocrinol Metab 52:122–127, 1981.
396. Brown EM, Gardner DG, Windeck RA, et al: β-Adrenergically stimulated adenosine 3′5′-monophosphate accumulation in and parathyroid hormone release from dispersed human parathyroid cells. J Clin Endocrinol Metab 48:618–626, 1979.
397. Rubin RP: The role of calcium in the release of neurotransmitter substances and hormones. Pharmacol Rev 22:389–428, 1970.

398. Brown EM, Gardner DG, Aurbach GD: Effects of the calcium ionophore A23187 on dispersed bovine parathyroid cells. Endocrinology 106:133–138, 1980.
399. Rasmussen H, Barret PQ: Calcium messenger system: An integrated view. Physiol Rev 64:938–984, 1984.
400. Shoback DM, Thatcher J, Leobruno R, Brown EM: Relationship between parathyroid hormone secretion and cytosolic calcium concentration in dispersed bovine parathyroid cells. Proc Natl Acad Sci USA 81:3113–3117, 1984.
401. Oetting MH, LeBoff MS, Brown EM: Ca++ stimulates PTH release in permeabilized parathyroid cells. Clin Res 34:551A, 1986.
402. Morrissey J: Cytosolic calcium and parathyroid cell function. Clin Res 34:550A, 1986.
403. Fitzpatrick L, Brandi M, Aurbach G: Calcium channel agonists inhibit parathyroid hormone secretion. J Bone Mineral Res 1[Suppl]:442(abstract), 1986.
404. Fitzpatrick LA, Aurbach GD: Calcium inhibition of parathyroid hormone secretion is mediated via a guanine nucleotide regulatory protein. Program Seventh Annual Meeting of the American Society of Bone Mineral Research, 1985; abstract α320.
405. Oetting MH, LeBoff MS, Brown EM, Burrowes MTR: GppNHp elicits a dramatic stimulation of secretion in permeabilized parathyroid cells. J Bone Mineral Res 1[Suppl]:445(abstract), 1986.
406. Shoback DM, McGhee JG: Lithium and high extracellular calcium stimulate the accumulation of inositol phosphate in bovine parathyroid cells. J Bone Min Res 1[Suppl]:314(abstract), 1986.
407. Brown EM, Redgrave J, Thatcher J: Effect of the phorbol ester TPA on PTH secretion: Evidence for a role for protein kinase C in the control of PTH release. FEBS Letters 175:72–75, 1984.
408. Kobayashi N, Russell J, Lettieri D, Sherwood LM: Effects of phorbol ester on subcellular distribution of protein kinase C in bovine parathyroid cells. J Bone Mineral Res 1[Suppl]:315(abstract), 1986.
409. Berson SA, Yalow RS: Immunochemical heterogeneity of parathyroid hormone in plasma. J Clin Endocrinol Metab 28:1037–1047, 1968.
410. Arnaud CD, Goldsmith RS, Bordier PS, Sizemore GW: Influence of immunoheterogeneity of circulating parathyroid hormone on results of radioimmunoassays of serum in man. Am J Med 56:785–793, 1974.
411. Canterbury JM, Reiss E: Multiple immunoreactive molecular forms of parathyroid hormone in human serum. Proc Soc Exp Biol Med 140:1393–1398, 1972.
412. Fischer JA, Binswanger U, Dietrich FM: Human parathyroid hormone: Immunological characterization of antibodies against a glandular extract and the synthetic amino-terminal fragments 1–12 and their use in the determination of immunoreactive hormone in human sera. J Clin Invest 54:1382–1394, 1974.
413. Goldsmith RS, Furszyfer J, Johnson WJ, et al: Etiology of hyperparathyroidism and bone disease during chronic hemodialysis. III. Evaluation of parathyroid suppressibility. J Clin Invest 52:173–180, 1973.
414. Silverman R, Yalow RS: Heterogeneity of parathyroid hormone: Clinical and physiologic implications. J Clin Invest 52:1958–1971, 1973.
415. Habener JF, Powell D, Murray TM, et al: Parathyroid hormone secretion and metabolism in vivo. Proc Natl Acad Sci USA 68:2986–2991, 1971.
416. Habener JF, Segre GV, Powell D, et al: Immunoreactive parathyroid hormone in circulation of man. Nature (London) New Biol 238:152–154, 1972.
417. Hruska KA, Kopelman R, Rutherford WE, et al: Metabolism of immunoreactive parathyroid hormone in the dog: The role of the kidney and the effects of chronic renal disease. J Clin Invest 56:39–48, 1975.
418. Segre GV, Habener JF, Powell D, et al: Parathyroid hormone in human plasma: Immunochemical characterization and biological implications. JClin Invest 51:3163–3172, 1972.
419. Segre GV, D'Amour P, Hultman A, Potts JT Jr: Effects of hepatectomy, nephrectomy and nephrectomy/uremia on the metabolism of parathyroid hormone in the rat. J Clin Invest 67:439–448, 1981.
420. Hruska KA, Martin K, Mennes P, et al: Degradation of parathyroid hormone and fragment production by the isolated perfused dog kidney: The effect of glomerular filtration rate and perfusate Ca++ concentrations. J Clin Invest 60:501–510, 1977.
421. Canterbury JM, Bricker LA, Levey GS, et al: Metabolism of bovine parathyroid hormone: Immunological and biological characteristics of fragments generated by liver perfusion. J Clin Invest 55:1245–1253, 1975.
422. Canterbury JM, Reiss E: Multiple immunoreactive molecular forms of parathyroid hormone in human serum. Proc Soc Exp Biol Med 140:1393–1401, 1972.
423. Fisher JA, Binswanger U, Dietrich FM: Immunological characterization of antibodies against a glandular extract and the synthetic amino-terminal fragments 1–12 and 1–34 and their use in the determination of immunoreactive hormone in human sera. J Clin Invest 54:1382–1394, 1974.
424. Goltzman D, Henderson B, Loveridge N: Cytochemical bioassay of parathyroid hormone: Characteristics of the assay and analysis of circulating hormonal forms. J Clin Invest 65:1309–1317, 1980.
425. Grunbaum D, Wexler M, Antos M, et al: Bioactive parathyroid hormone in canine progressive renal insufficiency. Am J Physiol 247:E442–448, 1984.
426. Flueck JA, DiBella FP, Edis AJ, et al: Immunoheterogeneity of parathyroid hormone in venous effluent serum from hyperfunctioning parathyroid glands. J Clin Invest 60:1367–1375, 1977.
427. Flueck JA, Edis A, McMahon J, Arnaud C: Direct secretion of COOH-terminal fragments of human parathyroid hormone by parathyroid tumors in vivo: Contribution to immunoheterogeneity of serum PTH in hyperparathyroid man. Program Abstract, 58th Annual Meeting of the Endocrine Society, San Francisco, 1976, 15:64.
428. DiBella FP, Gilkinson JB, Flueck J, Arnaud CD: Carboxyl-terminal fragments of human parathyroid tumors: Unique new source of immunogens for the production of antisera potentially useful in the radioimmunoassay of parathyroid hormone in human serum. J Clin Endocrinol Metab 46:604–612, 1978.
429. Hanley DA, Takatsuki K, Sherwood LM: Evidence for release of fragments of parathyroid hormone during "perifusion" of bovine parathyroid glands in vitro. Program Abstract, 59th Annual Meeting of the Endocrine Society, Chicago, 1977, 255:184.

430. Hanley DA, Takatsuki K, Sultan JM, et al: Direct release of parathyroid hormone fragments from functioning bovine parathyroid glands in vitro. J Clin Invest 62:1247–1254, 1978.
431. Martin KJ, Hruska KA, Greenwalt A, et al: Selective uptake of intact parathyroid hormone by the liver: Differences between hepatic and renal uptake. J Clin Invest 58:781–788, 1976.
432. Neuman WF, Neuman MW, Sammon PJ, et al: The metabolism of labeled parathyroid hormone III studies in rats. Calcif Tissue Res 18:251–261, 1975.
433. Segre GV, D'Amour P, Potts JT Jr: Metabolism of radioiodinated bovine parathyroid hormone in the rat. Endocrinology 99:1645–1652, 1976.
434. Segre GV, Perkins AS, Witters LA, Potts JT Jr: Metabolism of parathyroid hormone by isolated rat Kupffer cells and hepatocytes. J Clin Invest 67:449–457, 1981.
435. DiBella FP, Gilkinson JB, Flueck J, Arnaud CD: Carboxyl-terminal fragments of human parathyroid tumors: Unique new source of immunogens for the production of antisera potentially useful in the radioimmunoassay of parathyroid hormone in human serum. J Clin Endocrinol Metab 46:604–612, 1978.
436. Morrissey JJ, Hamilton JW, MacGregor RR, Cohn DV: The secretion of parathormone and glycosylated proteins by parathyroid cells in culture. Biochem Biophys Res Commun 82:1279–1286, 1978.
437. Martin TJ, Greenberg PB, Melick RA: Nature of human parathyroid hormone secreted by monolayer cell cultures. J Clin Endocrinol Metab 34:437–440, 1972.
438. Davis R, Talmage RV: Evidence for liver inactivation of parathyroid hormone. Endocrinology 66:312, 1960.
439. Zull JE, Repke DW: Studies with tritiated polypeptide hormones I. The preparation and properties of an active highly tritiated derivative of parathyroid hormone: acetamidino-parathyroid hormone. J Biol Chem 247:2195, 1972.
440. Singer FR, Segre GV, Habener JF, Potts JT Jr: Peripheral metabolism of bovine parathyroid hormone in the dog. Am J Med 56:774, 1975.
441. Neuman WF, Neuman MW, Sammon PJ, et al: The metabolism of labeled parathyroid hormone III studies in rats. Calcif Tis Res 18:251, 1975.
442. Habener JF, Mayer GP, Dee PC, Potts JT Jr: Metabolism of amino- and carboxyl-sequence immunoreactive parathyroid hormone in the bovine; evidence for peripheral cleavage of hormone. Metabolism 25:385, 1976.
443. Catherwood BD, Friedler RM, Singer FR: Endocrinology 98:228, 1976.
444. Martin KJ, Hruska KA, Greenwalt A, et al: Selective uptake of intact parathyroid hormone by the liver: Differences between hepatic and renal uptake. J Clin Invest 60:808, 1977.
445. Hruska KA, Kopelman R, Rutherford WE, et al: Metabolism of immunoreactive parathyroid hormone in the dog: The role of the kidney and the effects of chronic renal disease. J Clin Invest 56:39–48, 1975.
446. Segre GV, Niall HD, Habener JF, et al: Metabolism of parathyroid hormone: Physiological and clinical significance. Am J Med 56:774, 1974.
447. Segre GV, Niall HD, Sauer RT, et al: Edman degradation of radioiodinated parathyroid hormone: Application of sequence analysis and hormone metabolism *in vivo*. Biochemistry 16:2417, 1977.
448. Fox J, Scott M, Nissenson RA, Heath H III: J Lab Clin Med 102:70, 1983.
449. Neuman WF, Schneider N, Doolittle R: *In* Cohn DV, Talmage RV, Matthews JL (eds): Hormonal Control of Calcium Metabolism: Proceedings of the Seventh Parathyroid Conference. Amsterdam, Excerpta Medica, 1981, pp 55–63.
450. Neuman WF, Neuman MW, Lane K, et al: The metabolism of labeled parathyroid hormone V. Collected biological studies. Calcif Tiss Res 18:271, 1975.
451. Hruska KA, Korkor A, Martin K, Slatopolsky E: J Clin Invest 67:885, 1981.
452. D'Amour P, Huet P, Segre GV, Rosenblatt M: Am J Physiol 241:E208, 1981.
453. Rouleau MF, Warshawsky H, Goltzman D: Endocrinology 118:919, 1986.
454. D'Amour P, Segre GV, Roth SI, Potts JT Jr: Analysis of parathyroid hormone and its fragments in rat tissues: Chemical identification and microscopical localization. J Clin Invest 63:89, 1979.
455. Zull JE, Chuang J: J Biol Chem 260:1608, 1985.

T. J. MARTIN
J. M. MOSELEY

4

Calcitonin

When it became established that parathyroid hormone (PTH) acted directly on bone to promote its resorption, the idea developed that PTH was the major hormonal factor governing calcium homeostasis in the body. This was the basis of the McLean and Urist[1] hypothesis developed in the mid 1950s, that the serum calcium was regulated by appropriate changes in secretion rate of PTH, by a negative feedback control system. In 1961 Rasmussen[2] questioned this in suggesting that if the bone were the only means of regulating serum calcium level in conjunction with the parathyroids, the resulting feedback system would lead to wide fluctuations in serum calcium. It had been known for some time that PTH lowered the urine calcium, and Rasmussen made use of this in extending the McLean-Urist theory to involve the kidney. He considered that the kidney regulator was rapid to respond, sensitive to small fluctuations in hormone concentration, and of limited capacity; the bone regulator was slow to respond, relatively insensitive, but of nearly unlimited capacity. The renal action conserved serum calcium by rapidly inhibiting urinary secretion of calcium, the skeletal action by causing a less rapid dissolution of calcium from the bone matrix to the extracellular fluid. Although this seemed a more satisfactory explanation of calcium control, Copp and his associates looked persistently for a better one. In experiments in which they perfused the thyroparathyroid apparatus of dogs and sheep, they obtained evidence for the secretion in response to a high calcium stimulus of a factor that rapidly lowered systemic plasma calcium.[3] They called this calcitonin, and suggested that it was produced by the parathyroid glands.[4]

Upon this discovery, Munson, Hirsch and their colleagues looked afresh at some observations made in their laboratory. It had been noted that in rats parathyroidectomized by cautery, a more rapid and profound fall in serum calcium occurred than in rats parathyroidectomized by surgical excision.[5] They then found that acid extracts of rat thyroid glands caused hypocalcemia when injected into rats.[6] They suggested that cautery of the thyroid gland during parathyroidectomy caused the release of a factor from the thyroid gland that provoked a greater fall in serum calcium than that which occurred following simple removal of the parathyroid glands (Fig. 4–1). They called this activity "thyrocalcitonin" and showed that it could be extracted from the thyroid glands of several species, but not from other tissues. At the same time MacIntyre's group provided support for Copp's work in demonstrating in thyroparathyroid perfusion studies in the dog that a powerful, rapidly acting calcium-lowering hormone existed.[7] Subsequent perfusion

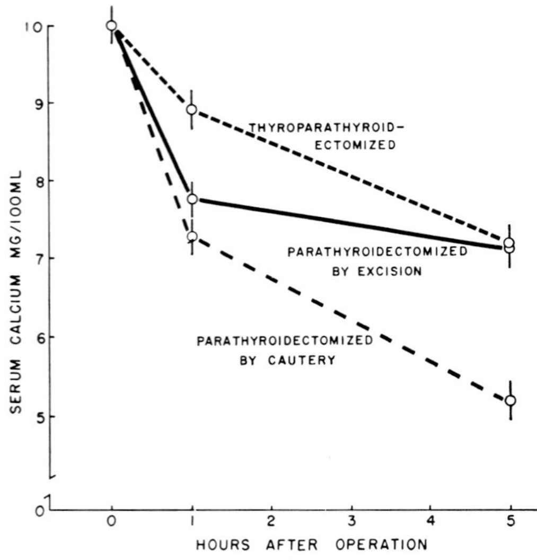

Figure 4–1. Comparison of the effects of thyroparathyroidectomy with parathyroidectomy by cautery and surgery in the rat. (From Hirsch PF, Gauthier GF, Munson PL: Endocrinology 73:244, 1963.)

studies in the goat showed that this activity was released from the thyroid gland.[8] In this species it was possible to perfuse either the external parathyroid alone or the thyroid plus parathyroid glands together (Fig. 4–2). Furthermore, autogenous thyroid extract injected into the goats rapidly lowered the systemic serum calcium.

It soon became clear that calcitonin and thyrocalcitonin were identical, were products of the thyroid gland in mammals, and probably represented an important new hormone involved in the regulation of calcium metabolism in the body.

I. NATURE OF CALCITONIN

Experiments in several species rapidly confirmed that calcitonin was a peptide released from the thyroid gland in response to a hypercalcemic stimulus and capable of rapidly lowering the calcium and phosphorus levels of plasma. It was shown to produce this effect independently of the kidney or intestine, and it acted as an inhibitor of bone resorption. Evidence for this is summarized in section V-A. The calcium-lowering effect of calcitonin was the basis for its biological assay, and indeed the convenience and sensitivity of the biological assay contributed to the fact that calcitonins of several species were isolated and sequenced within a few years of its discovery.

The recognition of calcitonin as a hypocalcemic hormone was hailed for several years as an answer to the tight control of plasma calcium. As information emerged about its action, however, it became apparent that this was not so, at least in the mature animal. The ability of calcitonin to inhibit osteoclastic bone resorption is beyond doubt, but the physiologic significance of this seems likely to vary with different stages of growth and development. Finally, the recognition of calcitonin's origin in the "C" or parafollicular cells of the mammalian thyroid drew attention to a second endocrine system in the thyroid gland, deriving its origin from the cells of the ultimobranchial bodies, which in birds and fish remain as discrete organs.

A. Embryologic Origin of Calcitonin-Producing Cells

Much of the early work on the localization of calcitonin-producing cells comes from

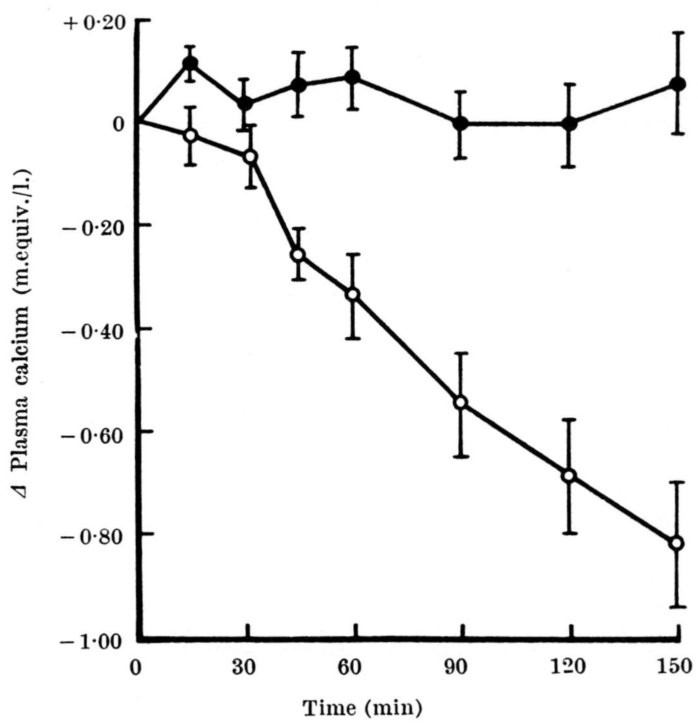

Figure 4–2. Effect on systemic plasma calcium in the goat of high calcium perfusion of parathyroid (•) and of thyroid and parathyroid glands (o). (From Foster GV, Baghdiantz A, Kumar MA, et al: Nature 202:1303, 1964. Copyright 1964, Macmillan Journals Limited.)

Pearse and his colleagues, who suggested that the "mitochondrion-rich" cells of the thyroid were responsible for calcitonin secretion.[9] When they observed electron microscopic changes in the parafollicular cells of the dog thyroid following high calcium perfusion of the gland, they ascribed to these cells the function either of synthesizing or of storing calcitonin, and gave them the name "C" cells. These cells are identical with the argyrophil parafollicular cells described in the dog by Nonidez;[10] and in other species, for example, the pig, they occupy epifollicular and follicular positions.[11] Pearse[11] produced further evidence that the "C" cells may produce a polypeptide hormone by demonstrating their property of uptake of 5-hydroxytryptophan, a faculty common to other polypeptide hormone–producing cells, for example, the pancreatic islet cells, and pituitary corticotrophs and melanotrophs (APUD cells). At the same time he pointed out that there were two possibilities for the embryologic origin of the C cells—the ultimobranchial bodies and the neural crest—and he favored the former site of origin. Subsequent cytochemical studies confirmed the ultimobranchial origin of the parafollicular C cells in the rodent thyroid,[12] and it is considered that the ultimobranchial and C cells are derived originally from the neural crest. The ultimobranchial body arises in the embryo of all vertebrates, with the exception of the cyclostomes, caudal to the last branchial arch, one on either side. Its fate in the adult is varied. In lower vertebrates it remains as a distinct structure that may persist on both sides or unilaterally. In mammals it becomes fused with the thyroid during embryonic life and here gives rise to calcitonin-secreting C cells.[12] No function had previously been ascribed to the ultimobranchial body, but seasonal changes in its structure had been observed in lizards, bats, and frogs.[13] The presence of secretory material in the follicles of the ultimobranchial bodies of reptiles, amphibians, and fish suggested an endocrine function, but there was no indication as to its nature. It was thought that the ultimobranchial body might form reserves of parathyroid or thymic tissue in conditions of stress, or possibly that it had undergone regression during evolution and lost its original function. Observations on the teleost *Astyanax mexicanus* revealed that the ultimobranchial body hypertrophied after the fish had been kept in the dark for periods of between 4 months and 2 years.[14] These changes were associated with skeletal deformities, but the authors attributed them to a parathyroid function of the ultimobranchial body. Hypertrophy of the ultimobranchial body had also been observed in frogs[15] under conditions of calcium stress and during metamorphic climax when calcium is being transferred from stores in the paravertebral lime sacs for incorporation into bone. Thus there was some evidence for involvement of the ultimobranchial body in changes in calcium metabolism, but no specific mechanisms were known. The role of ultimobranchial calcitonin in nonmammals will not be considered further in this chapter, but elucidation of that role in an endocrine control system might also have implications for our understanding of mammalian physiology.

Throughout their work, Pearse's group emphasized the variable ultimate fate of the ultimobranchial bodies in different species. After originating from the neural crest, they migrate forward during embryonic development. Although the ultimobranchial bodies remain as separate endocrine glands in birds, fish, and reptiles, in some submammalian species the cells can be found in other tissues of the neck and in the lung. In the lizard, for example, the main source of calcitonin is the lung,[16] although calcitonin-producing cells are present in other parts of the neck. Although in the rat the C cells are virtually all within the thyroid, this is not the case with several other mammals. In humans, for example, there is evidence for calcitonin-producing cells in the thymus and the lung, and it is therefore difficult to determine the result of calcitonin deficiency in mammals by experimentation, or in humans by clinical observation.

The association of calcitonin with granules in the parafollicular cells of the rat was suggested by experiments showing that administration of calcium to rats resulted in discharge from these cells of granules visible on electron microscopy.[17] In addition to the demonstration of the peptide hormone–secreting properties of C cells by histochemistry, calcitonin was identified in the C cells of the dog and the pig by immunofluorescence.[11] This was later amply confirmed, and recently the techniques of molecular biology have been used to localize calcitonin mRNA to the C cells of the thyroid.[18] In this technique of hybridization histochemistry, radiolabeled calcitonin cDNA is used to localize the tissue sections in those cells that are synthesizing calcitonin mRNA. This method has been used to demonstrate that the calcitonin cDNA probe hybridizes with C cells contained within the central portion of the thyroid gland in the rat (Fig. 4–3).

In the last few years there has been considerable interest in the discovery that immunoreactive calcitonin-like material can be identified in the nervous systems of a cyclostome and several chordate species,[19] in the pigeon,[20] in some human brain regions,[21] and in cerebrospinal fluid.[22] Immunohistochemical methods have localized calcitonin in rat pituitaries,[22-25] but efforts to identify calcitonin mRNA in pituitary using a radiolabeled calcitonin cDNA probe have been unsuccessful.[26] There has, however, been further recent confirmation of the presence of immunoreactive calcitonin in pituitary, including its demonstration in rats whose thyroid and parathyroid glands were removed some weeks previously.[27] Thus it is possible that small amounts of calcitonin are being produced in the pituitary, but that the mRNA for calcitonin is insufficient to be detected in that tissue, using current methods. Difficulty in evaluating this is further compounded by the fact that there may be wide variations between species in the amounts of pituitary calcitonin.[28] There is certainly increasing evidence for the presence of specific receptors for calcitonin in the brain, which is discussed in section VI. Together with the identification of "endogenous" brain calcitonin, this has sparked interest in the possibility of a neuromodulatory role for calcitonin.

II. CHEMISTRY

The period of time between the discovery of this peptide hormone and the determination of its amino acid sequence in several species was very short indeed. Most initial effort was made on the pig hormone, since pig thyroids provided an abundant source of calcitonin. Several groups almost simul-

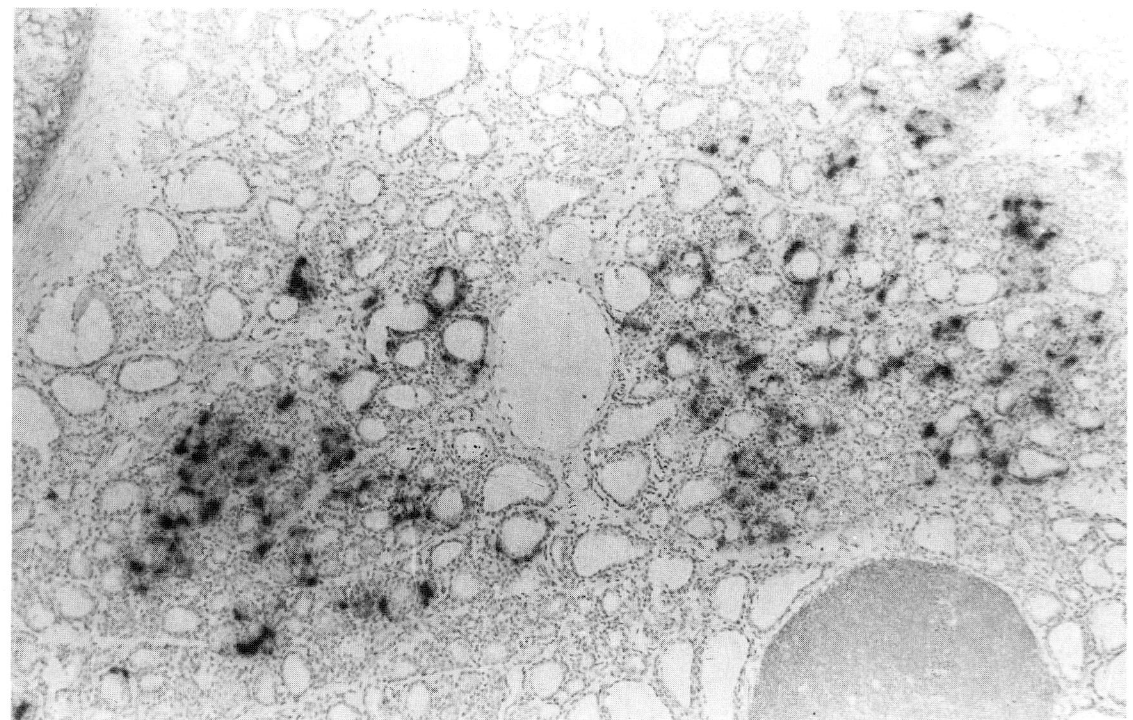

Figure 4–3. Localization by hybridization histochemistry of calcitonin mRNA in C cells of normal rat thyroid (×100). Autoradiograph kindly provided by Drs. J.P. Coghlan and J. Penschow (Howard Florey Institute, Melbourne), after preparation as described,[18] and photography by transmitted light, bright field.

taneously published the sequence of pig calcitonin[29,30] and within months pig calcitonin had been chemically synthesized.[31] It is a 32–amino acid peptide with a carboxyl-terminal proline amide, and a disulfide bridge between half cysteine residues at positions 1 and 7. The biological activity of the pure or chemically synthesized hormone is 100 to 200 units/mg.

The sequence and synthesis of salmon ultimobranchial calcitonin was to follow shortly.[32] Copp had noted in making extracts of salmon ultimobranchial glands that the hormone was extremely potent. Indeed the pure or synthetic salmon hormone, at 3000 to 5000 units/mg, is 20 to 40 times more potent than calcitonins of mammalian origin. At the same time it was pointed out that medullary carcinoma of the thyroid was most likely a tumor of cells of ultimobranchial origin. This led to the extraction and purification of human calcitonin from medullary thyroid carcinoma tissue,[33] and subsequent synthesis of the human peptide.[34]

The sequences of several mammalian and fish calcitonins are shown in Figure 4–4. They are all peptides and have in common 32 amino acids, the disulfide bridge, and the proline amide at position 32. There are very considerable differences in sequence in the distal two thirds of the molecules, and a moderate degree of homology about the amino terminus. The similarity in sequence among pig, bovine, and ovine sequences should be noted, as should that between human and rat, and between salmon and eel calcitonin.[35] On the basis of these structures, the known calcitonins fall into three main groups: (1) artiodactyl (porcine, bovine, and ovine); (2) human; and (3) teleost (salmon, eel, and probably many other nonmammalian calcitonins).[36] The teleost calcitonins have been found to be 20 to 50 times more potent than those of other species, and the most striking obvious chemical difference is their greater hydrophilicity.

A. Structure/Activity Relationships

Several chemical modifications of calcitonin and substituted analogues have been used in

–S–S– (disulfide bridge between positions 1 and 7)

			1	2	3	4	5	6	7	8	9	10	11	12	13	14	15	16
HUMAN	H_2N	-	C	G	N	L	S	T	C	M	L	G	T	Y	T	Q	D	F
PORCINE	H_2N	-	C	G	N	L	S	T	C	M	L	S	A	Y	W	R	N	L
OVINE	H_2N	-	C	G	N	L	S	T	C	M	L	S	A	Y	W	K	D	L
BOVINE	H_2N	-	C	S	N	L	S	T	C	V	L	S	A	Y	W	K	D	L
RAT	H_2N	-	C	S	N	L	S	T	C	M	L	G	T	Y	T	N	D	L
SALMON	H_2N	-	S	G	N	L	S	T	C	V	L	G	K	L	S	Q	E	L
EEL	H_2N	-	S	G	N	L	S	T	C	V	L	G	K	L	S	Q	E	L

	17	18	19	20	21	22	23	24	25	26	27	28	29	30	31	32
HUMAN	N	K	F	H	T	F	P	Q	T	A	I	G	V	G	A	P-CONH₂
PORCINE	N	N	Y	H	R	F	S	G	M	G	F	G	P	E	T	P-CONH₂
OVINE	N	N	Y	H	R	Y	S	G	M	G	F	G	P	E	T	P-CONH₂
BOVINE	N	N	Y	H	R	F	S	G	M	G	F	G	P	E	T	P-CONH₂
RAT	N	K	F	H	T	F	P	N	T	S	I	G	V	G	A	P-CONH₂
SALMON	H	K	L	Q	T	Y	P	R	T	N	T	G	S	G	T	P-CONH₂
EEL	H	K	L	Q	T	Y	P	R	T	D	V	G	A	G	T	P-CONH₂

Figure 4–4. Amino acid sequences of calcitonins of several species. The single letter code for amino acids has been used.

studies of the structural requirements for biological activity within the calcitonin molecule. Integrity of the disulfide bridge is essential for preservation of biological activity, as also is retention of the carboxyl-terminal proline amide, removal of which virtually obliterates activity.[37] It is of interest to note that preparation of an eel calcitonin analogue with aminosuberic linkage between positions 1 and 7 confers enhanced stability on the molecule.[35]

Studies of structure/activity relationships involved first the use of the biological assay in the rat,[38] but in recent years use has been made of specific calcitonin receptors linked to adenylate cyclase in certain human cancer cell lines.[39-41] Properties of the calcitonin receptor in these cells are described in section V-E, but they preserve the ability to distinguish among the calcitonins of the various species, and the relative potencies of calcitonins and analogues correlate closely with their relative potencies in the standard biological assay of calcium-lowering in the rat.[38]

Several substituted analogues of human calcitonin have been assessed in these assay systems and in the rat hypocalcemic assay,[42] and it is clear that specific changes in amino acids can be made that result in increased biological potency of the human calcitonin molecule. Some examples of such changes, with the alterations in potency, are illustrated in Table 4–1. Although in early work it had been thought that the full chain length of calcitonin was necessary for full activity, it is now known that minor deletions can be tolerated, and studies with such modified peptides have been useful in deducing chemical requirements for hormone-receptor activation. The full biological activity of des-Ser-2 and of des-Asn-3 analogues of salmon calcitonin indicated that the function of the N-terminal ring structure does not depend critically on its encompassed chain length.[43] Furthermore, deletion of Tyr-22 of salmon calcitonin had no effect on biological activity.[44] However, deletion of residue 16 from either salmon or human calcitonin resulted in 80% loss of biological activity,[45] indicating the importance of a hydrophobic residue at position 16 in the calcitonin molecule—this residue is leucine in most calcitonins and phenylalanine in human calcitonin. In all instances the 15th and 17th residues are hydrophilic in nature. Predictions[46] and observations[47] of conformation of the calcitonin molecule provide for an amphipathic helix, in which the hydrophobic and hydrophilic amino acid side chains of a peptide are on opposite faces of the helix.[46] The differences in biological activities among the calcitonins of different species or among calcitonin analogues have been correlated with their ability to form such structures of high helical content in the presence of acidic phospholipids.[48] Losses of biological potency resulting from deletion of a hydrophobic residue at position 16 might be a consequence of disruption of a normal sequence, in which hydrophobic residues are found regularly

Table 4–1. Potencies of Calcitonins and Analogues Determined in Cancer Cell Lines

Hormone or Analogue	BEN Cells		MCF 7 Cells	
	Binding	*Adenylate Cyclase*	*Binding*	*Adenylate Cyclase*
SCT	100	100	100	100
HCT	7	5	5	3
[ASU$^{1\text{-}7}$]-ECT	156	250	100	168
Des-Tyr^{22}-SCT	100	100	NT	NT
Key^{12}-HCT	12	14	12	12
Leu$^{12.16.19}$-HCT	23	26	10	30
Val^{8}-HCT	6	10	8	6
Gly^{8}-HCT	<0.2	<0.5	<0.5	<0
Arg^{24}-HCT	18	4	10	27.5
Asn^{26}-HCT	22	16	12	10
Thre^{27}-HCT	41	28	33	36
Asn^{26}-Thr^{27}-HCT	41	36	34	45
Lys^{11}-HCT	47	48	11	NT

SCT, salmon calcitonin; HCT, human calcitonin; ASU, aminosuberic acid; ECT, eel calcitonin. For adenylate cyclase and binding assays, activities of the various peptides are related to that of SCT (expressed as 100%). Data compiled from references 39–41, 44, and 45.

spaced at every third or fourth residue along the 8 to 22 residue portion of the chain. This concept implies that the distribution of hydrophobic and hydrophilic residues determines the alpha-helical structure of calcitonin. Substitutions or deletions that would destabilize the alpha-helix would be expected to result in loss of biological activity.

These and other observations[38] indicate that the site of deletions or alterations must be critical in determining the biological effectiveness of calcitonin analogues. The general conclusion is that conservation of tertiary structure is more important for biological potency than is chain length *per se*. The following major principles can be formulated to define the chemical characteristics of calcitonin that relate to biological activity:

1. Integrity of the amino-terminal ring structure is essential.
2. Increased stability of the ring (as in aminosuberic 1-7 eel calcitonin) can confer greater potency and stability.
3. Full biological activity can be preserved despite changes to the detailed sequence within the ring, and even with at least one deletion.
4. The sequence Asn-Leu-Ser at positions 3, 4, and 5 in the ring structure is invariate among the calcitonins.
5. Deletions in other parts of the molecule may or may not impair biological activity, depending on spatial arrangements of hydrophobic-hydrophilic residues.
6. Single or multiple substitutions in the human calcitonin molecule can enhance biological activity.
7. Carboxyl-terminal proline amide is essential for activity.

III. BIOSYNTHESIS

A. Calcitonin and Its Precursors

Just as the medullary carcinoma of the thyroid provided the source for studies of the amino acid sequence of human calcitonin, so this tumor has also allowed detailed analysis of the calcitonin gene in rat and humans. Without this source, the dispersed location of the normal C cells would have made study of the calcitonin gene very difficult. Messenger RNA isolated from rat medullary carcinoma of the thyroid was used to demonstrate the cell-free translation of a calcitonin precursor,[49-51] the hydrophobic leader sequence of which could be cleaved by carrying out the incubations in the presence of pancreatic microsomes. The preparation of biologically active calcitonin mRNA led to the cloning of DNA for both rat and human calcitonins, and sequence analysis of the cloned DNA revealed the amino acid sequence of the calcitonin precursor.[52,53] Thus calcitonin is synthesized as a large molecular weight precursor (136 amino acids) with a leader sequence at the amino terminus, which is cleaved during transport of the molecule into the endoplasmic reticulum. The location of dibasic amino acid residues at either end of the (1–32) calcitonin sequence in the precursor molecule ensures cleavage of the prohormone to yield mature calcitonin. In addition to cleavage, however, it is essential, as discussed earlier, that the proline residue at position 32 is amidated. The residue immediately following the proline in the precursor is glycine, which has been suggested[54] to provide the amide group for the preceding amino acids. A potentially important posttranslational modification of calcitonin is that of glycosylation.[55] It had been noted that a tripeptide sequence, Ans-Leu-Ser, found within the amino-terminal ring structure of calcitonin (Fig. 4–4) is invariate among the calcitonins of different species. This sequence is an acceptor site for the N-linked type of glycosylation, which occurs in glycoproteins. This, together with evidence for glycosylation of tumor calcitonin, led to detailed studies showing that the calcitonin precursor is indeed a glycoprotein,[56] and that the only N-linked glycosylation site in the entire precursor was within the calcitonin portion itself. The biological significance of calcitonin glycosylation has yet to be determined.

The complete sequences of the cDNA for human[57] and rat[52,58] calcitonins, and recently the DNA sequence of the full human calcitonin gene,[59] have been determined. These show that the hormone is flanked in the precursor by N- and C-terminal peptides (Fig. 4–5). The biological functions of these peptides are unknown. A molecular probe containing a 584–base pair sequence corresponding to part of the human calcitonin mRNA has been used to assign the calcitonin gene, which has been located in the p14 qter region of chromosome 11.[60]

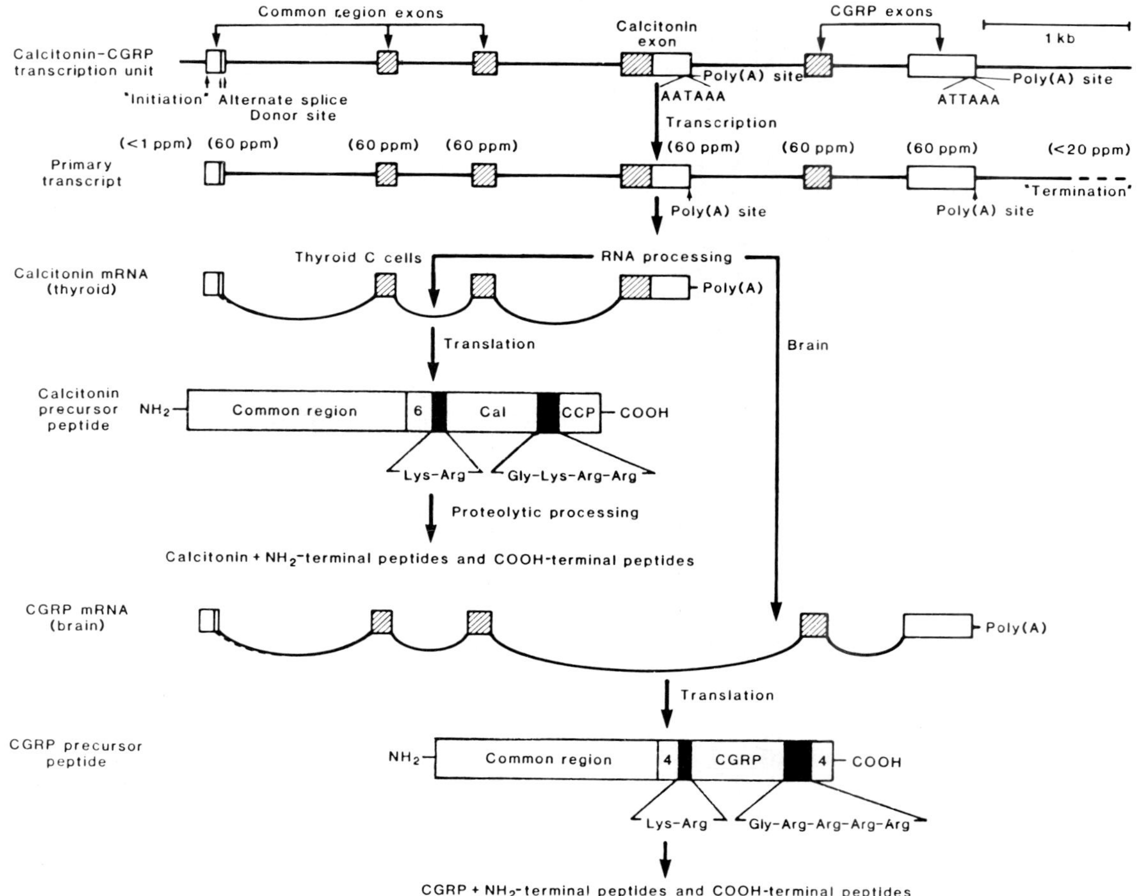

Figure 4–5. Rat calcitonin-CGRP gene, illustrating alternative patterns of RNA processing of the primary transcript. (From Rosenfeld MG, Amara SG, Evans, RM: Science 225:1315, 1984. Copyright 1984 by the AAAS.)

B. Calcitonin Gene-Related Peptide and the Gene Switching Mechanism

One of the most interesting developments out of the molecular biological approach to calcitonin biosynthesis has been the discovery of an alternative product of the calcitonin gene, and that the calcitonin gene is regulated in a tissue-specific manner. The original observation was that serially transplanted rat medullary thyroid cancers changed from states of high to low or absent calcitonin production.[61] The low producers were found to be producing different transcripts of new and structurally different mRNAs, which became known as "calcitonin gene-related peptide" (CGRP) mRNAs. The CGRP and calcitonin mRNAs share sequence identity in the amino terminal regions (Fig. 4–5), but in the carboxyl-terminal regions the nucleotide sequences are entirely different. Proteolytic cleavage sites similar to those flanking the calcitonin sequence are found flanking a 37–amino acid region within the carboxyl-terminal portion of the CGRP sequence, predicting the production of the 37–amino acid polypeptide.[62] CGRP has been located by immunochemistry in a number of cell groups in the central nervous system,[62] and occurs in thyroid tissue in animals and in humans.[63] It should be noted that alternative species of CGRP mRNA have been identified in rats and humans. The rat mRNA, which has been termed beta CGRP or CGRP-related peptide mRNA,[63] would predict a peptide sequence differing by one amino acid from rat CGRP (lysine instead of glutamate at residue 35).

The alternative human sequence identified from a medullary thyroid carcinoma differs from authentic human CGRP by three of the 37 amino acids.[64] It is not known whether this species of CGRP is expressed. Recently CGRP has been extracted from human medullary thyroid cancer tissue and its sequence determined[65] and found to be identical with that contained within the human calcitonin gene.[59]

The gene switching that has been demonstrated in the case of calcitonin and CGRP has not been recognized previously for peptide hormones, but such alternative splicing is recognized for other products, including the immunoglobulins (reviewed in reference 27). The switching between calcitonin and CGRP may occur physiologically during differentiation, resulting in CGRP expression in the nervous system and calcitonin in C cells of mammalian thyroid. The biological actions of CGRP are described in section VI.

IV. SECRETION AND METABOLISM

Calcitonin secretion from the C cells is clearly dependent on the prevailing serum calcium level. Any tendency toward lowering of the calcium level results in storage of calcitonin within the granules of the C cells; these stores are readily discharged as the serum calcium is elevated. Although there is little doubt that calcium is an important secretagogue for calcitonin in normal or tumor C cells, the exact mechanisms by which calcium provokes exocytosis of calcitonin are unknown. Reduction in numbers of granules and vesicles occurred during induced calcitonin secretion *in vivo*[17] and from thyroid slices,[66] but alteration of calcium levels did not influence the release of calcitonin from isolated pig thyroid granules,[67] consistent with the view that calcitonin release may be mediated at the cell membrane, and intracellular stores repleted from the storage granules as the intracellular concentration falls.

Agents that elevate C cell cyclic AMP may stimulate calcitonin secretion, since cAMP analogues have been shown to have this effect *in vivo*[68] and *in vitro*.[69] Probably the most important calcitonin secretagogues apart from calcium, however, are the gastrointestinal hormones. In the pig, gastrin appears to be an effective physiologic secretagogue,[70] providing part of the evidence that has led to a view of calcitonin's physiologic role as a hormone important postprandially, capable of counteracting the effect of a calcium meal and of PTH action by preventing the efflux of calcium from bone into blood.[71] Although there is some evidence in favor of this role in the pig and rat,[71] it is difficult to envisage it as being important in adult humans. However, this awaits further studies. Other gastrointestinal hormones, including glucagon, cholecystokinin, and secretin, are also capable of promoting calcitonin secretion (reviewed in reference 71). The gastrin analogue pentagastrin has been used clinically as a provocative test for calcitonin secretion in patients with medullary carcinoma of the thyroid.

Other hormones that influence calcium homeostasis may also directly or indirectly influence calcitonin secretion. $1,25(OH)_2$ vitamin D_3 administration has been reported to increase plasma calcitonin level; this was suggested to occur via specific thyroid C cell receptors for $1,25(OH)_2$ vitamin D_3, which modify secretion of calcitonin.[72] Both calcitonin and $1,25(OH)_2D_3$ levels are raised in pregnancy and lactation,[73] and it has been suggested that calcitonin may act to protect the skeleton in the face of increased calcium demand by the fetus. Estrogens may also influence plasma calcitonin levels by a direct effect on bone during pregnancy. The specific interaction of these hormones remains unclear but is reflected in the common incidence of postmenopausal osteoporosis—treatment of which will depend on a much clearer understanding of hormonal interactions in their effects on bone cells.

Most of this information on the regulation of calcitonin secretion comes from observations made during acute experiments with assays of calcitonin released into plasma or culture medium. The development of cDNA and oligonucleotide probes has allowed studies of the factors influencing calcitonin mRNA production. The serum and thyroid concentrations of calcitonin increase markedly with age in the rat, and this is associated with substantial increases in thyroid content of calcitonin mRNA.[18] The mechanisms of this are undetermined. In the same study,[18] increasing calcium concentrations did not alter hybridizable calcitonin mRNA in response to calcium, however.[74,75] Thus, in normal rats subjected to acute calcium stimulation *in vivo*, thyroid calcitonin mRNA was increased as measured in hybridization experiments and by translatable preprocalcitonin.[75] Furthermore, in a medullary thyroid carcinoma cell line, phorbol esters selectively increased calcitonin transcription while inhibiting cellular proliferation.[74] On current evidence it seems that calcium can stimulate both synthesis and secretion of calcitonin by thyroid C cells. The molecular mechanisms by which translatable calcitonin is increased by calcium will be of considerable interest.

Calcitonin is degraded by liver and kidney to inactive fragments, the half-life of the peptide in blood being only a few minutes. Teleost calcitonins are considerably more resistant to breakdown by tissue and serum enzymes than are the mammalian calcitonins. Injected salmon calcitonin, for example, has a much longer half life than either pig or human calcitonin.[76] Although this might contribute to the greater biological potency *in vivo* of salmon calcitonin, the more important factor is the greater affinity of salmon calcitonin for receptors.

Using the most specific and sensitive radioimmunoassays, the level of calcitonin in human blood appears to be less than 10 pg/ml in normal subjects. This is discussed by L. J. Deftos in Chapter 8, along with other radioimmunoassay data.

V. MECHANISM OF ACTION

Study of the mechanism of action of calcitonin has led to greater understanding of calcium and bone metabolism and to a better appreciation of the contribution made by bone to extracellular fluid calcium homeostasis. Calcitonin was found to lower calcium and phosphorus in parallel when injected into assay rats. The findings that the hypocalcemic effect of calcitonin persisted after removal of the kidneys or the gastrointestinal tract, and that the hormone had no effect on soft tissue calcium, made it seem likely that calcitonin acted on bone to alter the blood-bone calcium equilibrium in such a way as to favor the deposition of calcium and phosphate in bone. Both *in vitro* and *in vivo* evidence was obtained to show that this was so.

A. Bone Resorption

Addition of calcitonin to resorbing bone *in vitro* inhibited bone resorption,[77-79] an effect that appeared to be explained by a direct action on osteoclasts, inhibiting their production and activity. Calcitonin treatment of resorbing bone *in vitro* resulted in rapid loss of osteoclast ruffled borders and decrease of release of lysosomal enzymes. *In vivo* evidence was also consistent with an inhibitory action upon bone resorption. Thus calcitonin infused into rats resulted in an immediate reduction in the rate of excretion of hydroxyproline, consistent with the action of the hormone inhibiting the breakdown of bone collagen.[80] Furthermore, kinetic studies in rats led to similar conclusions, with no evidence to suggest any increase in the active uptake of calcium by bone.[81-83] For example, when calcitonin was infused into rats that had been injected 12 hours previously with ^{45}Ca, hormone treatment lowered plasma calcium without affecting plasma ^{45}Ca levels (Fig. 4–6). Under these experimental conditions,

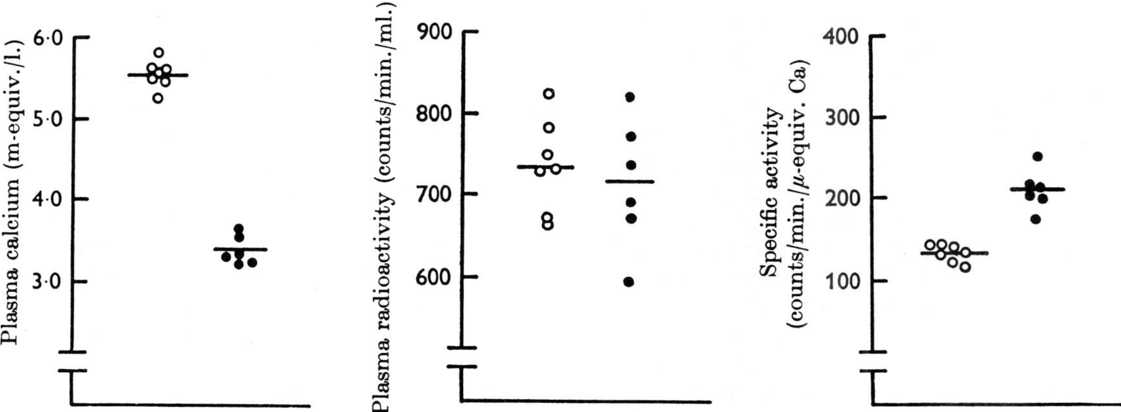

Figure 4–6. Effect of calcitonin infusion on plasma calcium, radioactivity, and specific activity in control (o) and in calcitonin-treated rats (•). ^{45}Ca was injected 12 hours before beginning the 4-hour infusion of calcitonin or control solution. (From Robinson CJ, Martin TJ, Mathews EW, et al: J Endocrinol 39:71, 1967.)

disappearance of radioactivity from the plasma reflected uptake of ^{45}Ca by the skeleton. The failure of calcitonin to influence this reflects an action of the hormone to prevent calcium efflux from bone, and is not consistent with active stimulation of calcium uptake by bone.

B. Bone Cell Targets

Calcitonin has been considered to act directly on the osteoclast, and studies in recent years of the actions of hormones on isolated bone cell populations confirm this. Autoradiographic experiments using biologically active iodinated salmon calcitonin have pointed to osteoclasts as the only discernible bone cell targets.[84] Consistent with this are the observations of its actions in organ culture, including especially the demonstration that osteoclasts in cultured mouse calvaria rapidly lost their ruffled borders.[85] A similar *in vivo* observation of loss of ruffled border in osteoclasts has been made in patients with Paget's disease, in whom bone biopsies were taken before and 30 minutes after an injection of calcitonin.[86] In the same clinical study, calcitonin was noted to decrease the number of osteoclasts in addition to altering their ultrastructure.

Both calcitonin and PTH were found to increase adenylate cyclase in bone cell membranes and cAMP production in mixed bone cell populations.[87] This seemed surprising in view of their opposing effects on bone, but could be explained if they acted upon different cell types, PTH upon osteoblasts and calcitonin upon osteoclasts. The use of sequential enzymatic digestion methods to prepare different populations of bone cells[88] has achieved a separation of calcitonin- and PTH-responsive cells. The best characterized populations of isolated bone cells are those that are osteoblast-rich, responding to PTH with an increase in cAMP, but not to calcitonin. The "osteoclast-rich" populations isolated from mouse calvaria[88] show a cAMP response to calcitonin. However, these populations are much less well characterized than the "osteoblast-rich" group. Calcitonin increases cyclic AMP production in several other target cells in which calcitonin receptors have been identified,[39-41,89,90] and it seems likely on present evidence that the cAMP target for PTH in bone is the osteoblast line of cells, whereas that for calcitonin is likely to be the osteoclast line. If this were the case it could explain some of the experimental observations that have been made relating cAMP to bone metabolism, especially that pharmacologic agents that raise intracellular cAMP concentrations can mimic the action of calcitonin on bone to inhibit resorption.[91] On the other hand, the general conclusion is that cAMP does mediate the bone-resorbing actions of both PTH and PGE_2.[92] The fact that cholera toxin, which elevates cAMP production, has been shown either to promote[93] or to inhibit[94] bone resorption *in vitro* could be explained by a calcitonin-like effect upon osteoclast cAMP, which would over-ride any PTH-like effect mediated through the osteoblast. Thus, a calcitonin effect upon cAMP in osteoclasts, not shared with PTH, can provide a convenient explanation for these observations. Recently, direct evidence has been obtained for such a direct effect on osteoclast cAMP production.

The recent studies of Chambers using isolated osteoclast preparations[95,96] point to a direct effect of calcitonin upon the osteoclast, in which the hormone rapidly inhibits the activity of osteoclasts. In further experiments[97] it was also noted that, while isolated osteoclasts remained quiescent in calcitonin as long as the hormone was present, they regained activity when osteoblasts were added to the culture. This escape of osteoclasts from inhibition by calcitonin took place at a rate proportional to the number of osteoblasts with which they were in contact. In recent studies, Chambers showed that calcitonin reduced the cytoplasmic spreading of isolated osteoclasts in a dose-dependent manner[97] (Fig. 4–7). PTH had no effect unless osteoblasts were co-cultivated with the osteoclasts, in which case addition of PTH resulted in marked increase in cytoplasmic spreading of osteoclasts. It cannot be assumed that these phenomena reflect the responses of cells in bone, but they do provide for the first time some useful direct observations of actions of hormones on isolated bone cell preparations containing osteoclasts. These observations are consistent with the view that the osteoblasts (or "lining" cells) might mediate the actions of bone-resorbing hormones by producing factors that stimulate the osteoclast[98] and also with the view that calcitonin acts directly upon the osteoclast (see Chapter 1).

The molecular mechanisms by which calcitonin decreases osteoclast function have yet

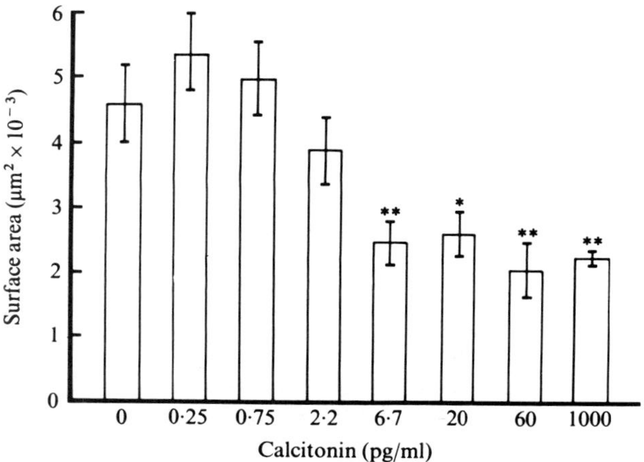

Figure 4–7. Effect of calcitonin on the surface area of isolated rat osteoclasts. (From Chambers TJ, Athanasou NA, Fuller K: J Endocrinol 102: 281, 1984.)

to be defined. The rapid effects of the hormone may be brought about through actions on a cytoskeletal function of osteoclasts, after initial events involving generation of cAMP. Early events in calcitonin action upon cyclic nucleotide metabolism have been studied in non-bone cells and are described later. With the development of improved methods of studying isolated osteoclasts, it has been possible to establish clearly that mammalian osteoclasts possess abundant specific, high-affinity receptors for calcitonin and that calcitonin stimulates cAMP formation in a sensitive and dose-dependent manner.[99] Studies in isolated cells, using immunocytochemical identification of cells in which cAMP responses occur, have confirmed that calcitonin does indeed increase cAMP production in multinucleate rat osteoclasts.[100]

On the other hand, although there has been no demonstration of calcitonin receptors in osteoblast-like cells, or of a direct biochemical effect of the hormone upon such cells, the administration of calcitonin has been observed to produce rapid changes in osteocytes, in which osteocyte shrinkage took place and was followed by the formation of hydroxyapatite crystals in the perilacunae and pericanaliculae.[101] The rapid changes in the bone lining cells produced by calcitonin are enhanced by phosphate,[102] and could be related to the possible involvement of phosphate ions in the action of calcitonin, which has been argued by Talmage (reviewed in reference 71). Most important, however, the proposal that calcitonin acts directly upon lining cells to reduce calcium efflux from bone (in direct opposition to the action of PTH) implies that these cells should possess receptors for calcitonin, but there is no direct evidence for this. PTH and the other major bone-resorbing hormones have been shown to increase plasminogen activator production by osteoblast-like cells, both normal and malignant,[103] raising the possibility of a neutral protease derived from osteoblasts contributing to the process of matrix degradation, either directly or indirectly. This increase is not influenced by calcitonin. At present there is no convincing evidence for the existence of calcitonin receptors in cells of the osteoblast lineage, but the possibility cannot be excluded that a calcitonin-responsive subpopulation exists. It is of interest to note that calcitonin receptors and cAMP response have been found to occur in late passage cultures of a PTH-responsive osteogenic sarcoma cell line that is phenotypically osteoblast. Subclones have been developed that respond both to PTH and to calcitonin.[104] It is possible that such cells reflect the existence within the osteoblast of series of cells capable of a calcitonin response.

C. "Escape"

Although calcitonin inhibits bone resorption, it has been found in organ cultures that calcitonin inhibition is followed by "escape,"[105,106] which is defined as an increase in resorption in bones stimulated by a resorptive agent, despite the continued presence of concentrations of calcitonin that initially were maximally inhibitory. Furthermore, rats treated chronically with calcitonin become refractory to the hypocalcemic action of the peptide.[107] Data from the *in vitro* experiments suggested that "escape" was due to a change in responsiveness of the bones rather than a loss of activity of the hormone. The biochemical mechanisms by which calcitonin induces refractoriness to its own action have not yet been defined. "Escape" may be due to calcitonin-induced loss of calcitonin receptors, a feature of the hormone's action in bone[107] and in other target cells, as will be discussed later. It has also been suggested that during calcitonin treatment there emerges a population of cells that are resistant to the hormone.[108] An interesting feature of the phenomenon is that the development of escape *in vitro* can be prevented by concomitant treatment of the bones with glucocorticoid.[105] Whatever the explanation, the phenomenon of "escape" is such an integral part of calcitonin action that it has to be borne in mind whenever the hormone is being used therapeutically. It would explain why calcitonin is less effective than might have been expected in the treatment of such states of excessive bone resorption as hyperparathyroidism and malignant hypercalcemia. It may also be that we should consider new experimental treatment schedules in Paget's disease that take account of the possibility of development of "escape."

D. Bone Formation

It has been stressed in earlier discussion that there is no good evidence for a stimulatory effect of calcitonin upon bone formation. Some early evidence was obtained for a stimulatory effect on osteoblasts. In rats treated chronically with calcitonin an increase in the number of osteoblasts was observed in the bones.[109] Furthermore, calcitonin treatment *in vitro* of cultures of mouse radius rudiments led to an increased net amount of bone tissue that was associated with an increased number of osteoblasts,[110] leading to the suggestion that calcitonin might have a stimulatory effect on bone formation in addition to its inhibition of resorption. It is difficult to explain such observations in the light of current views of the coupling of bone resorption to formation. It is considered that any change in bone resorption is rapidly followed by a change in formation rate in the same direction. Thus, inhibition of bone resorption by calcitonin would be expected to be accompanied by inhibition of bone formation. Indeed this is the experience, for example, in the use of calcitonin in the treatment of Paget's disease. In *in vivo* experiments, no effect of calcitonin was detected on the incorporation of labeled proline into bone hydroxyproline in rats chronically treated with calcitonin.[111] To the present time, therefore, it cannot be concluded that calcitonin has an anabolic effect on bone, and indeed it seems more likely that it would be "anti-anabolic." In normal humans, calcitonin was shown to inhibit the excretion of hydroxyproline-containing peptides, consistent with its effect of inhibiting bone resorption, but treatment also inhibited the excretion of nondialyzable hydroxyproline, which reflects bone collagen synthesis.[112] This can be interpreted as an inhibitory effect of calcitonin upon bone collagen synthesis, accompanying the decrease in breakdown in bone. It is interesting to note that in those acute experiments in humans,[112] calcitonin decreased urinary hydroxyproline excretion acutely after injection, but several hours later the rates of excretion returned to pretreatment levels. With continued treatment, however, there was a gradual fall in hydroxyproline excretion, such as is seen in Paget's disease patients treated chronically with calcitonin. This is interpreted as a dual action of calcitonin, on the one hand acutely inhibiting the function of osteoclasts, and on the other a chronic effect of inhibiting the generation of new osteoclasts.

In a bone matrix–induced bone-forming system in rats, calcitonin treatment of the animals led to increased matrix-induced bone formation.[113] This appeared to be associated with a stimulated proliferation of cartilage and bone precursor cells. The effect was seen provided the calcitonin treatment was begun before cartilage formation. After that time no effect was observed. It is not clear that this can be regarded as evidence for an anabolic effect of calcitonin upon bone formation. The conclusion at present must be that there is no direct effect of calcitonin upon bone cells resulting in increased anabolic function. Rather it seems likely that the reverse is the case, as an indirect consequence of inhibition of bone resorption by calcitonin.

E. The Calcitonin Receptor and Initial Events in Hormone Action

Although the difficulty of isolating osteoclasts in large numbers has slowed the understanding of calcitonin interaction with its bone cell target, much information on calcitonin-receptor interactions and initial events in hormone action has been obtained from studies in other target cells. These will be briefly outlined. In mammals, calcitonin receptors have been identified by direct binding studies in rat kidney,[111] pig lung,[115] human brain,[116] human lymphoid cells,[89] cultured pig kidney cells,[117] human cancer cell lines derived from lung[39,90] and breast,[40,41] and a subclone from rat osteogenic sarcoma cells.[105] In other species, calcitonin receptors have been demonstrated in trout gill.[118]

In all the calcitonin-responsive cells, specific receptors of high affinity have been demonstrated, with K_d in the range of 1 to 3 nM. In the human cancer cell lines, receptor numbers of 5000 to 30,000 were calculated. In these tissues and cell lines, calcitonin receptors are linked to activation of adenylate cyclase, although in membrane preparations from rat hypothalamus, specific calcitonin receptors have been associated with inhibition of adenylate cyclase.[119] Apart from these observations, no other initial biochemical event has been directly associated with calcitonin action. For this reason, and because a rise in cAMP in response to calcitonin has been found in some isolated bone cell populations,[88] it has been assumed that cAMP mediates the action of calcitonin on osteoclasts. This is likely to be the case but it has yet to be shown directly, and furthermore, other initial actions operate additionally. Specific calcitonin binding to osteoclasts has been shown autoradiographically.[84]

In the membrane and cell preparations in which calcitonin binding has been studied, it has been noted consistently that binding of calcitonin to its receptor has been tight, and poorly reversible. It is of interest to note that in studies of calcitonin and CGRP binding to membranes prepared from different regions of human brain, CGRP was found to bind in a readily reversible manner,[116] giving rise to the idea that calcitonin and CGRP, rather than acting upon a common receptor, might have their own specific, separate receptors. In human cancer cells[120,121] and in a pig kidney cell line[117] brief treatment with calcitonin results in activation of adenylate cyclase, which persists for several hours after washing of cells and removal of hormone. This persistent activation does not occur with alternative agonists of adenylate cyclase in the same cells, appearing to be peculiar to calcitonin. It is not known whether it is relevant to the action of calcitonin *in vivo.* It is due at least in part to persistent occupation of a small proportion of available calcitonin receptors.[121]

A particular feature of calcitonin action evident in studies of the cancer cells, and also in bone, is its ability to induce loss of its own receptors, and rapidly to desensitize the cells to its own action.[39,122,123] Desensitization and receptor loss are entirely agonist-specific, and take place in a time- and dose-dependent manner, so reminiscent of the stereospecific down-regulation and desensitization produced by beta-adrenergic catecholamines in their target cells that it seems probable that this is an integral part of calcitonin action. Thus, for example, the concentrations of calcitonin required to produce desensitization and receptor loss are the same as those required to activate the cells. The mechanisms of receptor loss have been investigated,[122] with the conclusion that initial hormone-induced loss of calcitonin receptors is primarily due to occupancy of cell-surface receptors, and later to a reduction in the concentration of cell-surface receptors mediated by an energy-requiring internalization process, analogous with the internalization of epidermal growth factor but slower than the rate required for that peptide.[124] Reappearance of receptors requires new protein synthesis.

The calcitonin receptor in cancer cell lines preserves the recognition function to be expected of a "physiologic" calcitonin receptor in that the abilities of different calcitonins and analogues to compete for binding to these receptors or to activate adenylate cyclase correlate closely with their efficacies as calcium-lowering agents in the rat.[40,41] In view of this, and because of the difficulty in obtaining osteoclasts for study, the cancer cells have provided the most abundant source of calcitonin receptor yet available for investigation of receptor chemistry. A biologically active, iodinated, photoactive derivative of salmon calcitonin has been used to identify a single molecular component (MW 85,000) of human breast cancer cells that is probably part of the calcitonin receptor.[125] No evidence was obtained for intrachain disulfide links in the receptor component. Further studies[126] indicated that the calcitonin receptor is associated with glycosyl moieties, the major contributors of which are N-acetyl-D-glucosamine residues, but N-acetyl-D-galactosamine and mannose residues are also associated.

In addition to activating adenylate cyclase in these various cell lines, calcitonin activates cAMP-dependent protein kinase.[127-130] In human breast cancer cell lines, calcitonin exclusively activated isoenzyme II of cAMP-dependent protein kinase,[127,128] whereas prostaglandin E_2, the only alternative agonist of adenylate cyclase in those cells, stimulated isoenzymes I and II approximately equally. Calcitonin also inhibited growth of the breast cancer cells, and it is worth noting that activation of isoenzyme II of cAMP-dependent protein kinase is associated with cellular processes favoring cell differentiation and growth regression. This pattern of selective activation of isoenzyme II of cAMP-dependent protein kinase is not seen with all calcitonin targets, however, since in a calcitonin-responsive human lung cancer cell line, the hormone activates both isoenzymes I and II.[129]

Such observations will provide some background to the study of calcitonin action in the osteoclast. If the hormone does indeed influence osteoclast function through initial effects on cAMP, it should be possible with techniques such as cytochemistry and immunocytochemistry to outline some steps in its action, even with osteoclasts in mixed cell populations. The possible involvement of other pathways in the early actions of calcitonin (for example, calcium fluxes phospholipid pathways) also needs to be considered.

F. Calcitonin, Bone, and Calcium Homeostasis

It is worth reflecting how the discovery of calcitonin and its mechanism of action has influenced modern views of the regulation of the extracellular fluid calcium, and the contribution to this of bone. Older concepts of calcium homeostasis that considered only PTH and bone were questioned with the suggestion that if bone were the only means of regulating the serum calcium level in conjunction with PTH, control would be inadequate. Hence the suggestion that the PTH action on the kidney might contribute. The arrival of a new calcium-lowering hormone seemed to solve the problem. However, events proved otherwise. Concepts of the role of bone in maintaining extracellular fluid calcium had relied upon observations made in the young, growing rat. Hence it was calculated that for the tibia in a young rat there was an accretion rate of 6.2% of the bone calcium per day, a resorption rate of 4.7% of the bone calcium per day, and an exchangeable fraction equivalent to 3.0% of the total calcium in the bone.[131] Thus it was clear that if accretion continued at the same rate and resorption was inhibited, the result would be a lowering of plasma calcium. The younger the animal, the more rapid is the bone resorption rate. It would therefore be expected that the calcium-lowering effect of calcitonin should be greater in younger than in older animals. This was indeed the case in the rat[132] (Fig. 4–8), in which it was noted that in the biological assay of calcitonin, which depends on the calcium-lowering effect of the hormone, the response became less marked with increasing age of the animals. It should be noted, however, that the ability of calcitonin to counteract the effect of a calcium load was not impaired in older animals, at least in the rat,[133] an observation that has not been explained and that has not been extended to other species. Dependence of the hypocalcemic action of calcitonin upon the prevailing rate of bone resorption was also noted in other species, and it soon became clear that in normal adult humans, even quite large doses

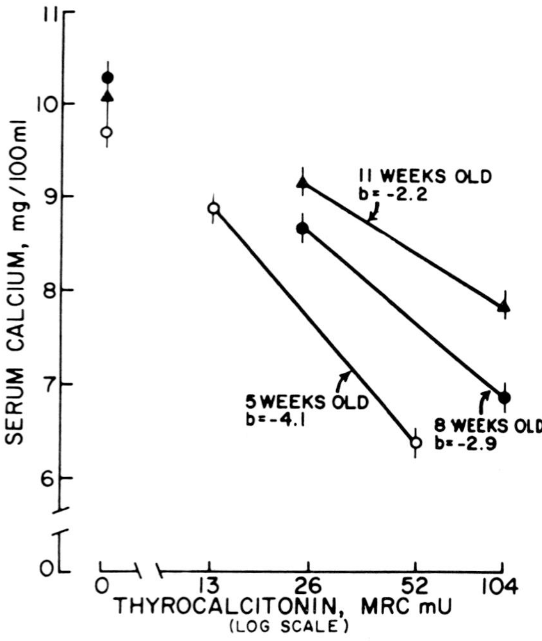

Figure 4–8. Decreasing hypocalcemic response to calcitonin with increasing age of the rat. (From Cooper CW, Hirsch PF, Toverud SV, et al: Endocrinology 81:610, 1967.)

of calcitonin had little effect on plasma calcium levels. In those subjects in whom bone turnover was increased (for example, in thyrotoxicosis, Paget's disease), calcitonin treatment acutely inhibited bone resorption and resulted in a lowering of the plasma calcium.[134]

It has been proposed that the hypocalcemic action of calcitonin is related to the availability of circulating inorganic phosphate.[71] In rats[135] and in patients with chronic renal failure,[136] the degree of calcium lowering in response to calcitonin was found to be proportional to the initial blood phosphorus concentration. It has been claimed that no hypocalcemia followed calcitonin injection in rats maintained for several weeks on a phosphorus-deficient diet.[71] In contrast, Robinson et al.[83] showed that in parathyroidectomized rats fed a low-phosphorus, high-calcium diet for 17 days, calcitonin lowered plasma calcium by a mechanism consistent with inhibition of bone resorption.

It seems that the acute effect of calcitonin on serum calcium is related to the prevailing rate of bone resorption. If that is accepted, lack of a calcium-lowering effect of the hormone in mature animal or human is not surprising, since the process of bone resorption is a slow one in maturity. It may be that the role of calcitonin in its effect on bone throughout life is that of a regulator of the bone resorptive process, whatever the overall rate of the latter. In the young, or in pathologic states of increased bone resorption in maturity (for example, Paget's disease, thyrotoxicosis), calcitonin inhibition of bone resorption can lower the serum calcium level, and there may even be a calcium homeostatic role of endogenous calcitonin in those circumstances. In a normal adult animal, however, when bone turnover is slow, no effect on serum calcium is obtained with calcitonin. The physiologic function of calcitonin in maturity may nevertheless be to regulate the bone resorptive process, in either a continuous or intermittent manner. It follows that calcitonin should not necessarily be regarded as a "calcium-regulating hormone" in maturity, but may yet be shown to be such in stages of rapid growth, for example, in the young or in states of increased bone turnover. It is nevertheless important that bone resorption be regulated, and calcitonin is the only hormone known to be capable of carrying out this function by a direct action on bone. Such a role might become more important in circumstances in which skeletal loss particularly needs to be prevented, for example, in pregnancy and lactation.[137]

G. Renal Effects of Calcitonin

Although calcitonin lowered plasma calcium in the absence of the kidneys, it was noted that in parathyroidectomized rats with very low levels of plasma calcium, calcitonin had no effect on calcium but lowered phosphorus.[136] When this phosphate-lowering effect was found to be prevented by nephrectomy[81] it was considered that in some circumstances the kidneys might be involved in the phosphate-lowering effect of calcitonin. Indeed a phosphaturic effect of thyroid extract had been shown in intact rats,[140] and infusion of calcitonin in parathyroidectomized rats led to a dose-dependent phosphaturia.[139] The effect on phosphate excretion was only a minor one in comparison with the phosphaturic effect of PTH, and although it was demonstrated in human subjects also,[134] in several species calcitonin failed to have any effect on phosphate excretion. Thus, it has seemed unlikely that the phosphaturic effect is of any major physiologic significance. The hormone was also noted to promote excretion of inorganic sulfate in rats[141] and humans,[134] probably reflecting a shared renal tubular transport system between sulfate and phosphate.

A number of other renal effects of calcitonin have been noted, including a transient increase in calcium excretion,[134,142-144] due probably to inhibition of renal tubular calcium reabsorption. Although this has not usually been regarded as an important effect of calcitonin, recent observations link it to the calcium-lowering effect of calcitonin in patients with metastatic bone disease. The use of calcitonin in the treatment of hypercalcemia due to cancer has been based exclusively on the inhibition of osteolysis by calcitonin. Some evidence has been produced that failure of the kidneys to excrete the calcium load derived from bone breakdown is a major contributor to the hypercalcemia.[145] This prompted careful studies of the relative contributions to the hypocalcemic effect of calcitonin of its renal and skeletal components.[146] It was concluded that inhibition of renal tubular reabsorption by calcitonin can induce a rapid fall in serum calcium, and that the magnitude of this effect depends upon the correction of volume depletion, which inevitably accompanies hypercalcemia. Thus, the calciuretic action of calcitonin may assume greater importance than hitherto suspected.

Calcitonin was found to produce a natriuretic effect in human subjects,[134,147] and study of the renal effects of calcitonin in rats pointed to striking increases in sodium excretion.[148] The effects were more marked with salmon calcitonin than with calcitonins of mammalian origin,[148] raising the possibility that the natriuretic property of calcitonin from lower vertebrates might be of functional significance in those species.

Calcitonin receptors have been demonstrated clearly in rat kidney,[112] and a further action on the kidney is to enhance 1-hydroxylation of 25-hydroxyvitamin D in the proximal straight tubule of the kidney.[149] The action of calcitonin upon adenylate cyclase activity has been localized in the human nephron predominantly to the medullary and cortical portions of the thick ascending limb and to the early portion of the distal convoluted tubule[151] (Fig. 4–9).

A further renal effect of calcitonin was noted as a result of studies of calcitonin effects upon a pig kidney cell line.[117] The hormone was found to stimulate greatly the production of the neutral protease, plasminogen activator.[151] This effect appeared to be related to calcitonin's actions on cAMP formation in the cells, and hormone treatment also was associated with marked inhibition of cell replication. In the same cells, calcitonin treatment was shown to enhance the transcription of plasminogen activator mRNA sequences, the data indicating that calcitonin was able to activate the plasminogen activator gene in those cells.[152] Subsequent studies in humans showed that calcitonin treatment resulted in increased urinary plasminogen activator activity.[153] The plasminogen activator/plasmin system is an important local regulator of many functions, the nature of which depends on the local tissue environment. Its involvement in the local actions of calcitonin is an intriguing possibility that merits further study. The tissue effects of plasminogen activator depend on its location—thus, they are likely to be very different in kidney from those in bone. It is worth noting that the bone-resorbing hormones have been shown to increase plasminogen activator production in osteoblast-like cells,[103] and that this effect is not influenced by calcitonin.

H. Calcitonin and the Gastrointestinal Tract

It has been suggested that the function of calcitonin is to prevent rises in plasma calcium taking place after ingestion of calcium-containing meals.[71,154] This is based on the observation made in pigs that calcium meals

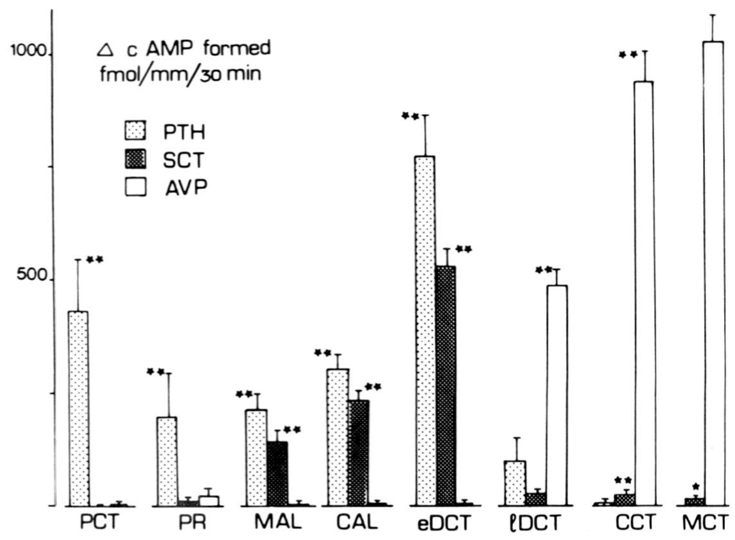

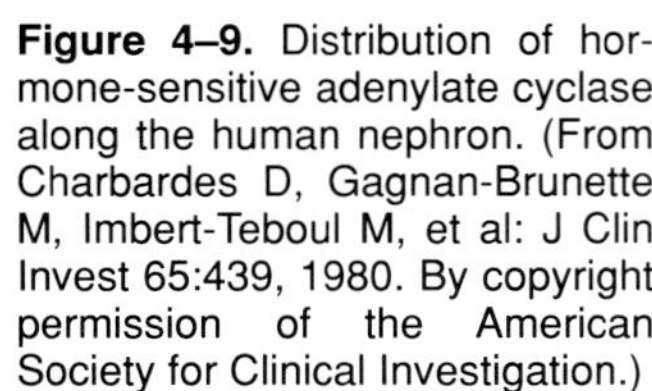
Figure 4–9. Distribution of hormone-sensitive adenylate cyclase along the human nephron. (From Charbardes D, Gagnan-Brunette M, Imbert-Teboul M, et al: J Clin Invest 65:439, 1980. By copyright permission of the American Society for Clinical Investigation.)

do not alter the plasma calcium, but that during the feeding period there is a rise in plasma calcitonin levels. This is a possible role for the hormone in humans, particularly in stages of growth, in which intermittent secretion in response to oral calcium loads could inhibit bone resorption and decrease the movement of calcium from bone to blood at a time when calcium was being absorbed from the intestine. However, much more study is needed in humans to define the relationship of calcitonin secretion to feeding and to gastrointestinal hormones. Other gastrointestinal effects of calcitonin are probably not physiologic. These include inhibition of gastric acid secretion, inhibition of pancreatic enzyme secretion, and impairment of glucose tolerance.

VI. CALCITONIN AND CGRP DISTRIBUTION AND ACTION IN THE NERVOUS SYSTEM

The origin of calcitonin-producing cells in the neural crest raised the possibility of calcitonin involvement in neural function. Both immunoreactive calcitonin and calcitonin receptors have been demonstrated in the brain and nervous system of rats, humans, and other species.[18-21,155] Immunoreactive calcitonin related antigenically to human calcitonin has been demonstrated in the nervous systems of protochordates, lizards, and pigeons.[19] Recent data, again obtained with radioimmunoassay, point to the presence of low levels of salmon calcitonin–like peptide material in the human thyroid and in the paraventricular mesencephalic region of the brain.[156] It has been suggested that this might be a vestige of a highly conserved gene for calcitonin.[156]

Specific binding sites for calcitonin have been mapped in rat[157,158] and human[20] brain, with the median eminence region of the hypothalamus showing the highest receptor concentration. This is believed to be the site of pain perception and regulation of appetite. Calcitonin administered intracerebroventricularly has been claimed to have an analgesic effect[159] and also to reduce food and water intake, gastric acid secretion, and intestinal motility. The relationship of these effects, if any, to the calcitonin binding sites in the brain remains to be elucidated. CGRP, on the other hand, may be a very important neuropeptide.

CGRP has been identified by immunocytochemistry in the central and peripheral nervous systems[63,64] and its receptors mapped in the brain.[116,160] It is especially abundant in the spinal cord,[161] where it colocalizes with substance P in the posterior horn and primary sensory neurons.[162] CGRP in the brain is found in the olfactory and gustatory systems and in the hypothalamic and limbic regions.[62,163] It is also found in the trigeminal ganglion,[62] and its calcium-dependent release has been demonstrated from cultured rat trigeminal ganglion cells.[164] CGRP has been shown by immunohistochemistry to be present in nerve fibers throughout the cardiovascular system, often associated with vascular smooth muscle.[165] The widespread distribution of CGRP in the nervous system raises the possibility that it has a neurotransmitter role, and its potent effects on the vascular system suggest that local vascular release of CGRP may be involved in the physiologic control of blood pressure.

CGRP has been shown to be remarkably potent in dilating arteries and arterioles, with its vasodilator effects on rat aortic smooth muscle requiring the presence of intact endothelium.[166,167] When it is injected intradermally in humans, it causes marked microvascular dilation.[166] Although studies of membrane adenylate cyclase in brain and other tissues indicated that CGRP had no effect,[168] the peptide does stimulate cyclic AMP formation in a sensitive and dose-dependent manner in cultured aortic smooth muscle cells,[167] indicating that in some targets at least, cyclic AMP may mediate CGRP action.

It is uncertain whether CGRP has any significant effect on calcium metabolism, but it is a widely distributed neuropeptide with potent biological effects that could indicate an important local function in several organ systems.

VII. CALCITONIN IN CLINICAL MEDICINE

The secretion of calcitonin by human thyroid and nonthyroid cancers is discussed in Chapter 15, the place of calcitonin in the treatment of Paget's disease of bone in

Chapter 17, and of malignant hypercalcemia in Chapter 12.

The discussions in this chapter of the mechanism of action of calcitonin provide background to the use of calcitonin in therapy. Its specific uses are considered in detail elsewhere in this volume, but one of the most important unanswered questions concerning the role of calcitonin in physiology, pathology, and therapeutics is whether its role as an inhibitor of bone resorption is such that calcitonin deficiency can lead to the development of osteoporosis. The corollary would be that calcitonin could be used in the treatment of osteoporosis. Initial reports that basal calcitonin levels are lower in women than in men,[169,170] fall with age in both,[171] and are reduced in osteoporotic women[172] gave rise to considerable interest in the possible use of calcitonin in the treatment of postmenopausal osteoporosis. However enthusiasm has been tempered by subsequent data showing no difference in basal calcitonin levels between postmenopausal osteoporotic and age-matched normal women.[173,174] Recent results with "calcium clamp" methods, which confirm the initial studies, are reviewed in Chapter 12. Basal calcitonin levels might be less important than stimulated levels, however, and a decreased immunoreactive calcitonin response to calcium infusion in postmenopausal osteoporotic women has been shown.[175] In an early 2-year controlled study of daily salmon calcitonin (100 units), it has been shown that calcitonin treatment resulted in a significant decrease in the loss of total body calcium as measured by neutron activation analysis. The effect was not maintained at a significant level beyond 18 months of treatment.[176] In view of the fact that calcitonin inhibition of osteoclastic bone resorption is likely to lead also to inhibited bone formation because the two processes are coupled, it may be that any role for calcitonin in the treatment of osteoporosis should be in conjunction with a treatment that will increase bone turnover.

VIII. SUMMARY

Calcitonin is a polypeptide hormone whose major effect in mammals, including humans, is to inhibit bone resorption. This it does by two means, first by acutely inhibiting osteoclast activity, and second by inhibiting the generation of osteoclasts. Because bone resorption is rapid enough to contribute to the maintenance of extracellular fluid calcium only in stages of growth or in certain disease states in maturity in which bone resorption is increased, it follows that only in those circumstances does calcitonin injection result in a significant fall in plasma calcium. Thus, although calcitonin was discovered as a calcium-lowering hormone in experiments that were carried out in young animals, it may be that its function throughout life is that of a regulator of the bone resorption process. This might not necessarily contribute to acute maintenance of plasma calcium in maturity. Consideration of the "physiologic" role of calcitonin often fails to take into account the need to regulate the bone resorptive process, however slowly that may be proceeding, and whether it contributes to maintenance of the plasma calcium level. Thus, the general role of calcitonin in skeletal metabolism may indeed be that of the most important inhibitor of the bone resorptive process, acting to prevent excessive skeletal loss throughout life, and especially at times at which skeletal loss becomes a risk, for example, in rapid growth, pregnancy and lactation, immobilization, and certain pathologic states (Paget's disease of bone, thyrotoxicosis, hyperparathyroidism). This working model of calcitonin action and function can be applied to any discussion of the hormone's role in therapy or in pathogenesis of bone disease.

The last few years have opened fascinating new aspects of calcitonin physiology. This includes particularly the discovery of calcitonin and of calcitonin receptor sites in the brain, leading to the possible role of calcitonin as a neuropeptide, perhaps concerned with pain perception. Clarification of any such role awaits further study, as does the physiologic significance of CGRP, the peptide alternate product of the calcitonin gene. This peptide is located widely throughout the body and may have important physiologic functions. Its participation with calcitonin in a "gene switching" control mechanism highlights the close relationship between the two peptides. Elucidation of their functional relationship is one of the important immediate questions in this area of biology.

Work by the authors was supported by a Program Grant from the National Health and Medical Research Council of Australia.

References

1. McLean FC, Urist MR: An Introduction to the Physiology of Skeletal Tissue. Chicago, University of Chicago Press, 1955.
2. Rasmussen H: Parathyroid hormone. Am J Med 30:112–129, 1961.
3. Copp DH, Cameron EC, Cheney BA, et al: Evidence for calcitonin—a new hormone from the parathyroid that lowers blood calcium. Endocrinology 70:638–649, 1962.
4. Copp DH, Henze KG: Parathyroid origin of calcitonin. Evidence from perfusion of sheep glands. Endocrinology 75:49–58, 1964.
5. Hirsch PF, Gauthier GF, Munson PL: Thyroid hypocalcemic principle and recurrent laryngeal nerve injury as factors affecting response to parathyroidectomy in rats. Endocrinology 73:244–251, 1963.
6. Hirsch PF, Voelkel EF, Munson PL: Thyrocalcitonin. Hypocalcemic hypophosphatemic principle of the thyroid gland. Science 146:412–414, 1964.
7. Kumar MA, Foster GV, MacIntyre I: Further evidence for calcitonin. A rapid-acting hormone which lowers calcium. Lancet 2:480–482, 1963.
8. Foster GV, Baghdiantz A, Kumar MA, et al: Thyroid origin of calcitonin. Nature 202:1303–1305, 1964.
9. Foster GV, MacIntyre I, Pearse AGE: Calcitonin production and the mitochondrion-rich cells of the dog thyroid. Nature 203:1029–1031, 1965.
10. Nonidez JF: The origin of the "parafollicular" cell, a second epithelial component of the thyroid gland of the dog. Am J Anat 49:479–493, 1932.
11. Pearse AGE: 5-Hydroxytryptophane uptake by dog thyroid "C" cells, and its possible significance in polypeptide hormone production. Nature 211:598–600, 1966.
12. Pearse AGE, Carvalheira AF: Cytochemical evidence for an ultimobranchial origin of rodent thyroid C cells. Nature 214:929–931, 1967.
13. Kingsbury B: The fate of the ultimobranchial gland in man. Proc Soc Exp Biol Med 65:333–339, 1939.
14. Rasquin P, Rosenbloom L: Endocrine imbalance and tissue hyperplasia in teleosts maintained in darkness. Bull Am Mus Nat Hist 104:362–425, 1954.
15. Robertson DR, Schwartz GE: Observations on the ultimobranchial body in Rana pipiens. Anat Rec 148:219–230, 1964.
16. Galan Galan F, Rogers RM, Girgis SI, et al: Immunochemical characterization and distribution of calcitonin in the lizard. Acta Endocrinol 97:427–432, 1981.
17. Matsuzawa T: Experimental morphological studies on the parafollicular cells of the rat thyroid gland, with special reference to the source of thyrocalcitonin. Arch Histol Jpn 27:521–534, 1966.
18. Jacobs JW, Simpson E, Penschow J, et al: Characterization and localization of calcitonin mRNA in rat thyroid. Endocrinology 113:1616–1622, 1983.
19. Girgis SI, Galan Galan F, Arnett TR, et al: Immunoreactive human calcitonin-like molecule in the nervous systems of protochordates and a cyclostome, Myxine. J Endocrinol 87:375–382, 1980.
20. Galan Galan F, Rogers RM, Girgis SI, et al: Immunoreactive calcitonin in the central nervous system of the pigeon. Brain Res 212:59–66, 1981.
21. Fischer JA, Tobler PH, Kaufmann M, et al: Calcitonin: Regional distribution of the hormone and its binding sites in the human brain and pituitary. Proc Natl Acad Sci USA 78:7801–7805, 1981.
22. Pavlinac DM, Lenhard LW, Parthemore JG, et al: Immunoreactive calcitonin in human cerebrospinal fluid. J Clin Endocrinol 50:717–720, 1980.
23. Deftos LJ, Burton BD, Catherwood BD, et al: Demonstration by immunoperoxidase histochemistry of calcitonin in the anterior lobe of the rat pituitary. J Clin Endocrinol 47:457–460, 1978.
24. Cooper CW, Peng TC, Obie JF, et al: Calcitonin-like immunoreactivity in rat and human pituitary glands. Endocrinology 107:98–105, 1980.
25. Margules DL, Flynn JJ, Walker J, et al: Elevation of calcitonin immunoreactivity in the pituitary and thyroid glands of genetically obese rats (fa/fa). Brain Res Bull 4:589–593, 1979.
26. Jacobs JW, Goltzman D, Habener JF: Absence of detectable calcitonin synthesis in the pituitary using cloned complementary DNA probes. Endocrinology 111:2014–2019, 1982.
27. Gagel RF, O'Brian DS, Voelkel EF, et al: Pituitary immunoreactive calcitonin-like material: Lack of evidence for cross-reactivity with proopiomelanocortin. Metabolism 32:686–696, 1983.
28. Rosenfeld MG, Amara SG, Evans RM: Alternative RNA processing: Determining neuronal phenotype. Science 225:1315–1320, 1984.
29. Kahnt FW, Riniker B, MacIntyre I, et al: Thyrocalcitonin. I. Isolierung und Charakterisierung wirksamer Peptide aris Schweineschilddriesen. Helv Chir Acta 51:214–217, 1968.
30. Potts JT Jr, Niall HD, Keutmann HT, et al: The amino acid sequence of porcine thyrocalcitonin. Proc Natl Acad Sci USA 59:1321–1328, 1968.
31. Rittel W, Brugger M, Kamber B, et al: Thyrocalcitonin. 3. Die Synthese des alpha-Thyrocalcitonins. Helv Chir Acta 51:924–928, 1968.
32. Niall HD, Keutmann HT, Copp DH, et al: Amino acid sequence of salmon ultimobranchial calcitonin. Proc Natl Acad Sci USA 64:771–778, 1969.
33. Neher R, Riniker B, Rittel W, et al: Thyrocalcitonin. II. Struktur von alpha-Thyrocalcitonin. Helv Chir Acta 51:1900–1917, 1968.
34. Sieber P, Brugger M, Kamber B, et al: Menschliches Calcitonin. VI. Die Synthese von Calcitonin M. Helv Chir Acta 53:2135–2150, 1970.
35. Morikawa T, Munekata E, Sakakibara S, et al: Synthesis of eel-calcitonin and [$ASU^{1,7}$]-eel-calcitonin: Contribution of the disulfide bond to the hormonal activity. Experientia 32:1104–1106, 1976.
36. Copp DH: Modern view of the physiological role of calcitonin in vertebrates. In Gennari C, Segre G (eds): The Effects of Calcitonins in Man. Milano, Masson Italia Editori, 1983, pp 3–14.
37. Rittel W, Maier R, Brugger M: Structure-activity relationship of human calcitonin. III. Biological activity of synthetic analogues with shortened or terminally modified peptide chains. Experientia 32:246–248, 1976.
38. Maier R, Riniker B, Rittel W: Analogues of human calcitonin. I. Influence of modification in amino acid positions 29 and 31 on hypocalcemic activity in the rat. FEBS Lett 48:68–71, 1974.
39. Findlay DM, DeLuise M, Michelangeli VP, et al: Properties of calcitonin receptor and adenylate cyclase in BEN cells, a human cancer cell line. Cancer Res 40:1311–1317, 1980.

40. Martin TJ, Findlay DM, MacIntyre I, et al: Calcitonin receptors in a cloned human breast cancer cell line (MCF7). Biochem Biophys Res Comm 96:150–156, 1980.
41. Findlay DM, Michelangeli VP, Eisman JA, et al: Calcitonin and 1,25-dihydroxyvitamin D receptors in several human breast cancer cell lines. Cancer Res 40:4764–4767, 1980.
42. Maier R, Kamber B, Riniker B, et al: Analogues of human calcitonin. IV. Influence of leucine substitution in positions 12, 16 and 19 on hypocalcaemic activity in the rat. Clin Endocrinol 5:327S–332S, 1976.
43. Schwartz KE, Orlowski RC, Marcus R: des-Ser[2] salmon calcitonin: A biologically potent synthetic analog. Endocrinology 108:831–836, 1981.
44. Findlay DM, Michelangeli VP, Martin TJ, et al: Conformational requirements for activity of salmon calcitonin. Endocrinology 117:801, 1985.
45. Findlay DM, Michelangeli VP, Orlowski RC, et al: Biological activities and receptor interactions of des-Leu[16] salmon and des-Phe[16] human calcitonin. Endocrinology 112:1288–1291, 1983.
46. Epand RM, Epand RF, Orlowski RC, et al: Amphipathic helix and its relationship to the interaction of calcitonin with phospholipids. Biochem Biophys Res Comm 87:455–460, 1979.
47. Merle M, Lefevre G, Milhaud G: Predicted secondary structure of calcitonin in relation to the biological activity. Biochemistry 22:5074–5080, 1983.
48. Epand RM, Epand RF, Orlowski RC: The presence of an amphipathic helical segment and its relationship to the biological potency of calcitonin analogs. Int J Pept Prot Res 25:109, 1985.
49. Jacobs JW, Potts JT Jr, Bell NH, et al: Calcitonin precursor identified by cell-free translation of mRNA. J Biol Chem 254:10600–10603, 1979.
50. Amara SG, Rosenfeld MG, Birnbaum RS, et al: Identification of the putative cell-free translation product of rat calcitonin mRNA. J Biol Chem 255:2645–2648, 1980.
51. Goodman RH, Jacobs JW, Habener JF: Cell-free translation of messenger RNA coding for a precursor of human calcitonin. Biochem Biophys Res Comm 91:932–938, 1979.
52. Jacobs JW, Chin WW, Dee PC, et al: Calcitonin messenger RNA encodes multiple polypeptides in a single precursor. Science 213:457–459, 1981.
53. Amara SG, Jonas V, O'Neill JA, et al: Calcitonin COOH-terminal cleavage peptide as a model for identification of novel neuropeptides predicted by recombinant DNA analysis. J Biol Chem 257:2129–2132, 1982.
54. Kreil G, Suchanek G, Kindas-Mugge I: Biosynthesis of a secretory peptide in honey-bee venom glands: Intermediates detected in vivo and in vitro. Fed Proc 36:2081–2086, 1977.
55. O'Neil JA, Birnbaum RS, Jacobson A, et al: A carbohydrate-containing form of immunoreactive calcitonin in transplantable rat medullary thyroid carcinomas. Endocrinology 108:1098–1100, 1981.
56. Jacobs JW, Lund PK, Potts JT Jr, et al: Procalcitonin is a glycoprotein. J Biol Chem 256:2803–2807, 1981.
57. LeMoullec JM, Jullienne A, Chenais J, et al: The complete sequence of human prepro-calcitonin. FEBS Lett 167:93–97, 1984.
58. Amara SG, Jonas V, Rosenfeld MG, et al: Alternative RNA processing in calcitonin gene expression generates mRNAs encoding different polypeptide products. Nature 298:240–244, 1982.
59. Steenbergh PH, Hoppener JWM, Zandberg J, et al: Calcitonin gene related peptide coding sequence is conserved in the human gene and is expressed in medullary thyroid carcinoma. J Clin Endocrinol Metab 59:358–360, 1984.
60. Hoppener JWM, Steenbergh PH, Zandberg J, et al: Localization of the polymorphic human calcitonin gene on chromosome II. Hum Genet 66:309–312, 1984.
61. Roos BA, Yoon MJ, Frelinger AL, et al: Tumour growth and calcitonin during serial transplantation of rat medullary thyroid carcinoma. Endocrinology 105:27–32, 11979.
62. Rosenfeld MG, Mermod JJ, Amara SG, et al: Production of a novel neuropeptide encoded by the calcitonin gene via tissue-specific RNA processing. Nature 304:129–135, 1983.
63. Tschopp FA, Tobler PH, Fischer JA: Calcitonin gene-related peptide and calcitonin in the human thyroid, pituitary and brain. Mol Cell Endocrinol 36:53–57, 1984.
64. Steenbergh PH, Hoppener JWM, Zanberg J: A second human calcitonin/CGRP gene. FEBS Lett 183:403–407, 1985.
65. Morris HR, Panico M, Etienne T, et al: Isolation and characterization of human calcitonin gene-related peptide. Nature 308:746–748, 1984.
66. Bussolati G, Monga G, Navore R, et al: Histochemical and electronmicroscopical study of C cells in organ culture. In Taylor S (ed): Calcitonin 1969. London, Heinemann, 1970, pp 240–251.
67. Greenberg PB, Martin TJ, Melick RA: Release of calcitonin from thyroid granules. Nature 233:201–202, 1971.
68. Care AD, Cooper CW, Duncan T, et al: A study of thyrocalcitonin secretion by direct measurement of in vivo secretion rates in pigs. Endocrinology 83:161–169, 1968.
69. Bell NH: Effects of glucagon, dibutyryl cyclic 3′,5′-adenosine monophosphate and theophylline on calcitonin secretion in vitro. J Clin Invest 49:1368–1373, 1970.
70. Care AD, Bates RFL, Swaminathan R, et al: The role of gastrin as a calcitonin secretagogue. J Endocrinol 51:735–744, 1971.
71. Talmage RV, Cooper CW, Toverud SV: The physiological significance of calcitonin. In Peck WA (ed): Bone and Mineral Research Annual 1. Amsterdam, Excerpta Medica, 1983, pp 74–143.
72. Freake HC, MacIntyre I: Specific binding of 1,25-dihydroxycholecalciferol in human medullary thyroid carcinoma. Biochem J 206:181–184, 1982.
73. Whitehead MI, Law G, Yaung O, et al: Interrelations of calcium-regulating hormones during normal pregnancy. Br Med J 283:10–12, 1981.
74. de Bustros A, Bayling SB, Berger CL, et al: Phorbol esters increase calcitonin gene transcription and decrease c-myc mRNA levels in cultured human medullary thyroid carcinoma. J Biol Chem 260:98–204, 1985.
75. Segond N, Jullienne A, Lesmoles F, et al: Rapid increase of calcitonin-specific mRNA after acute hypercalcemia. Eur J Biochem 139:209–215, 1984.
76. Habener JF, Singer FR, Deftos LJ, et al: Explanation for unusual potency of salmon calcitonin. Nature 232:91–93, 1971.

77. Friedman J, Raisz LG: Thyrocalcitonin: Inhibitor of bone resorption in tissue culture. Science 150:1465–1467, 1967.
78. Gaillard PU: Bone culture studies. J Bone Joint Surg 48B:386–388, 1966.
79. Aliapoulios MA, Goldhaber P, Munson PL: Thyrocalcitonin inhibition of bone resorption induced by parathyroid hormone in tissue culture. Science 51:330–332, 1966.
80. Martin TJ, Robinson CJ, MacIntyre, I: The mode of action of thyrocalcitonin. Lancet 1:900–902, 1966.
81. Johnston CC Jr, Deiss WP Jr: An inhibitory effect of thyrocalcitonin on calcium release in vivo and on bone metabolism in vitro. Endocrinology 78:1139–1146, 1966.
82. Milhaud G, Perault A-M, Moukhtar CR: Etude du mecanisme de l'action hypocalcemiante de la thyrocalcitonine. Acad Sci (Paris) 261:813–818, 1965.
83. Robinson CJ, Martin TJ, Matthews EW, et al: Mode of action of thyrocalcitonin. J Endocrinol 39:71–77, 1967.
84. Warshawsky H, Goltzman D, Rouleau MF, et al: Direct in vivo demonstration by radioautography of specific binding sites for calcitonin in skeletal and renal tissues of the rat. J Cell Biol 85:682–794, 1980.
85. Kallio DM, Garant PR, Minkin C: Evidence for an ultrastructural effect of calcitonin on osteoclasts in tissue culture. In Talmage RV, Munson PL (eds): Calcium, Parathyroid Hormone and the Calcitonins. Amsterdam, Excerpta Medica, 1972, pp 383–387.
86. Singer FR, Melvin KEW, Mills BG: Acute effect of calcitonin on osteoclasts in man. Clin Endocrinol 5:333S–340S, 1976.
87. Heersche JNM, Marcus R, Aurbach GD: Calcitonin and the formation of 3',5'-AMP in bone and kidney. Endocrinology 91:241–247, 1974.
88. Luben RA, Wong GL, Cohn DV: Biochemical characterization with parathormone and calcitonin of isolated bone cells: Provisional identification of osteoclasts and osteoblasts. Endocrinology 99:526–534, 1976.
89. Marx SJ, Woodard C, Aurbach GD, et al: Renal receptors for calcitonin. Binding and degradation of hormone. J Biol Chem 248:4797–4802, 1973.
90. Hunt NH, Ellison M, Underwood JCE, et al: Calcitonin-responsive adenylate cyclase in a calcitonin-producing human lung cancer cell line. Br J Cancer 35:777–784, 1977.
91. McLeod JF, Raisz LG: Comparison of inhibition of bone resorption and escape with calcitonin and dibutyryl 3',5' cyclic adenosine monophosphate. Endocrinol Res Comm 8:49–59, 1981.
92. Martin TJ: Drug and hormone effects on calcium release from bone. Pharmacol Ther 21:209–228, 1983.
93. Nagata N, Ono Y, Kimura N: Inhibition by cholera toxin of parathyroid hormone–induced calcium release from bone in culture. Biochem Biophys Res Comm 78:819–826, 1977.
94. Tashjian AH Jr, Ivey JL: Stimulation of bone resorption in organ culture by cholera toxin. Biochem Biophys Res Comm 102:1055–1064, 1981.
95. Chambers TJ, Magnus CJ: Calcitonin alters behaviour of isolated osteoclasts. J Pathol 136:27–39, 1982.
96. Chambers TJ: Osteoblasts release osteoclasts from calcitonin-induced quiescence. J Cell Sci 57:147–160, 1982.
97. Chambers TJ, Athanasou NA, Fuller K: Effect of parathyroid hormone and calcitonin on the cytoplasmic spreading of isolated osteoclasts. J Endocrinol 102:281–286, 1984.
98. Rodan GA, Martin TJ: The role of osteoblasts in the hormonal control of bone resorption: A hypothesis. Calcif Tissue Int 33:349–351, 1981.
99. Nicholson GC, Moseley JM, Sexton PM, et al: Abundant calcitonin receptors in isolated rat osteoclasts: Biochemical and autoradiographic characterization. J Clin Invest 78:355–361, 1986.
100. Nicholson GC, Livesey SA, Moseley JM, Martin TJ: Actions of calcitonin, parathyroid hormone and prostaglandin E_2 on cyclic AMP formation in chicken and rat osteoclasts. J Cell Biochem 31:229–238, 1986.
101. Matthews JL, Martin JH, Collins, et al: Immediate changes in the ultrastructure of bone cells following thyrocalcitonin administration. In Talmage RV, Munson PL (eds.): Calcium, Parathyroid Hormone and the Calcitonins. Amsterdam, Excerpta Medica, 1972, pp 375–382.
102. Talmage RV, Matthews JL, Martin JH, et al: Calcitonin, phosphate and the osteocyte-osteoblast bone cell unit. In Talmage RV, Owen M, Parsons JA (eds): Calcium Regulating Hormones. Amsterdam, Excerpta Medica, 1975, pp 284–296.
103. Hamilton JA, Lingelbach S, Partridge NC, et al: Stimulation of plasminogen activator in osteoblast-like cells by bone-resorbing hormones. Biochem Biophys Res Comm 122:230–236, 1984.
104. Forrest SM, Ng KW, Findlay DM, et al: Characterization of an osteoblast-like clonal line which responds to both parathyroid hormone and calcitonin. Calcif Tissue Int 37:51, 1985.
105. Raisz LG, Wener JA, Trummel CL, et al: Induction, inhibition and escape as phenomena in bone resorption. Excerpta Medica Int Congr Series No. 243:446, 1972.
106. Tashjian AH Jr, Wright DR, Ivey JL, et al: Calcitonin binding sites in bone: Relationships to biological response and "escape." Recent Prog Horm Res 34:285, 1978.
107. Messer HH, Copp DH: Changes in response to calcitonin following prolonged administration to intact rats. Proc Soc Exp Biol Med 146:643–647, 1974.
108. Krieger NS, Tashjian AH Jr: Inhibition by ouabain of parathyroid hormone–stimulated bone resorption. J Pharmacol Exp Ther 217:586–591, 1981.
109. Matrajt H, Bordier P, Tun-Chot S, et al: Histological bone changes produced by calcitonin. In Taylor SH (ed.): Calcitonin. Proc Symp Thyrocalcitonin and C cells. London, Heinemann, 1968, pp 338–346.
110. Gaillard PJ, Thesingh CW: Bone culture studies with thyrocalcitonin. In Taylor SH (ed.): Calcitonin. Proc Symp Thyrocalcitonin and C cells. London, Heinemann, 1968, pp 238–245.
111. Kalu DN, Foster GV: Effect of calcitonin on (3H) proline incorporation into bone hydroxyproline in the rat. J Endocrinol 49:233–241, 1971.
112. Krane SM, Harris ED Jr, Singer FR, et al: Acute effects of calcitonin on bone formation in man. Metabolism 22:51–58, 1973.
113. Weiss RE, Singer FR, Gorn AH, et al: Calcitonin stimulates bone formation when administered

prior to initiation of osteogenesis. J Clin Invest 68:815–818, 1981.
114. Marx SJ, Woodard CJ, Aurbach GD: Calcitonin receptors of kidney and bone. Science 178:999–1001, 1972.
115. Foucherau-Peron M, Moukhtar MS, Benson AA, et al: Characterization of specific receptors for calcitonin in porcine lung. Proc Natl Acad Sci USA 78:3973–3975, 1981.
116. Tschopp FA, Henke H, Petermann JB, et al: Calcitonin gene-related peptide and its binding sites in the human central nervous system and pituitary. Proc Natl Acad Sci USA 82:248–252, 1985.
117. Goldring SR, Dayer JM, Ausiello DA, et al: A cell strain cultured from porcine kidney increases cyclic AMP content upon exposure to calcitonin and vasopressin. Biochem Biophys Res Comm 83:434–440, 1978.
118. Fouchereau-Peron M, Moukhtar MS, Benson AA, et al: Demonstration of specific receptors for calcitonin in isolated trout gill cells. Comp Biochem Physiol 68A:417–421, 1981.
119. Rizzo AJ, Goltzman D: Calcitonin receptors in the central nervous system of the rat. Endocrinology 108:1672–1677, 1981.
120. Lamp SJ, Findlay DM, Moseley JM, et al: Calcitonin induction of a persistent activated state of adenylate cyclase in human breast cancer cells (T47D). J Biol Chem 256:12269, 1981.
121. Michelangeli VP, Findlay DM, Moseley JM, et al: Mechanisms of calcitonin induction of prolonged activation of adenylate cyclase in human cancer cells. J Cyclic Nucleotide Protein Phosphor Res 9:129–142, 1983.
122. Findlay DM, Martin TJ: Relationship between internalization and calcitonin-induced receptor loss in T47d cells. Endocrinology 115:78–83, 1984.
123. Findlay DM, DeLuise M, Michelangeli VP, et al: Independent down regulation of insulin and calcitonin receptors in human tumour cell line. J Endocrinol 88:271–281, 1981.
124. Findlay DM, Ng KW, Niall M, et al: Processing of calcitonin and epidermal growth factor after binding to receptors in human breast cancer cells (T47D). Biochem J 206:343–350, 1982.
125. Moseley JM, Findlay DM, Martin TJ, et al: Covalent cross-linking of a photoactive derivative of calcitonin to human breast cancer cell receptors. J Biol Chem 257:5846–5851, 1982.
126. Moseley JM, Findlay DM, Gorman JJ, et al: The calcitonin receptor on T47D breast cancer cells. Evidence for glycosylation. Biochem J 212:609–616, 1983.
127. Ng KW, Livesey SA, Larkins RG, et al: Calcitonin effects on growth and on selective activation of Type II isoenzyme of cyclic AMP-dependent protein kinase in human breast cancer cells. Cancer Res 43:794–800, 1983.
128. Livesey SA, Collier G, Zajac JD, et al: Characteristics of selective activation of cyclic AMP-dependent protein kinase isoenzymes by calcitonin and prostaglandin E_2 in human breast cancer cells. Biochem J 224:361–370, 1984.
129. Zajac JD, Livesey SA, Martin TJ: Selective activation of cyclic AMP-dependent protein kinase by calcitonin in a calcitonin secreting human lung cancer cell line. Biochem Biophys Res Comm 122:1040–1046, 1984.
130. Ausiello DA, Hall DH, Dayer J-M: Modulation of cAMP-dependent protein kinase by vasopressin and calcitonin in cultured renal LLC-PK_1 cells. Biochem J 186:773–780, 1980.
131. Bauer GCH, Carlsson A, Lindquist B: Evaluation of accretion, resorption and exchange reactions in the skeleton. Kungl Fysiog Gallsk Und Forhandl Bank 25:3–22, 1955.
132. Cooper CW, Hirsch PF, Toverud SV, et al: An improved method for the biological assay of thyrocalcitonin. Endocrinology 81:610–617, 1967.
133. Harper C, Toverud SV: Ability of thyrocalcitonin to protect against hypercalcaemia in adult rats. Endocrinology 93:1354–1359, 1973.
134. Martin TJ, Melick RA: The acute effects of porcine calcitonin in man. Aust Med 18:258–263, 1969.
135. Kennedy JW, Talmage RV: Effects of thyrocalcitonin on bone phosphate without concurrent effects on calcium. In Talmage RV, Munson RL (eds): Calcium, Parathyroid Hormone and the Calcitonins. Amsterdam, Excerpta Medica, 1972, pp 416–421.
136. Cochran M, Hillyard CJ, Dew GJ, et al: Acute responsiveness to calcitonin in chronic renal failure. Br Med J 2:396–398, 1976.
137. Munson PL, Toverud SV, Boass A, et al: Calcitonin: Role during lactation. In Pecile A (ed): Calcitonin, 1980: Chemistry, Physiology, Pharmacology and Clinical Aspects. Amsterdam, Excerpta Medica, 1981, pp 110–122.
138. Gudmundsson TV, MacIntyre I, Soliman HA: The isolation of thyrocalcitonin and a study of its effects in the rat. Proc R Soc [Biol] 164:460–469, 1961.
139. Kenny AD, Heiskell CA: Effect of crude thyrocalcitonin on calcium and phosphorus metabolism in rats. Proc Soc Exp Biol Med 120:269–274, 1965.
140. Robinson CJ, Martin TJ, MacIntyre I: Phosphaturic effect of thyrocalcitonin. Lancet 2:83–85, 1966.
141. Martin TJ, Harris GS, Melick RA: Effect of calcitonin on serum inorganic sulphate and on the disappearance of injected radioactive sulphate in the rat. J Endocrinol 43:451, 1969.
142. Ardaillou R, Vuagnat P, Milhaud G, et al: Effects de la thyrocalcitonine sur l'excretion renale des phosphates, du calcium et des ions H chez l'homme. Nephron 4:298–305, 1967.
143. Bijvoet OLM, Van der Sluys Veer J, Jansen AP: Effects of calcitonin in patients with Paget's disease, thyrotoxicosis, or hypercalcaemia. Lancet 1:876–881, 1968.
144. Cochran M, Peacock M, Sachs G, et al: Renal effects of calcitonin. Br Med J 1:135–137, 1970.
145. Benabe JE, Martinez-Maldonaldo M: Hypercalcaemic nephropathy. Arch Intern Med 138:777–779, 1978.
146. Hosking DJ, Gilson D: Comparison of the renal and skeletal actions of calcitonin in the treatment of severe hypercalcaemia of malignancy. Q J Med New Series L111:359, 1984.
147. Bijvoet OLM, Van Der Sluys Veer J, Vries HR, et al: Natriuretic effect of calcitonin. N Engl J Med 284:681–688, 1971.
148. Williams CC, Mathews EW, Moseley JM, et al: The effects of synthetic human and salmon calcitonins on electrolyte excretion in the rat. Clin Sci 42:129–137, 1972.
149. Kawashima H, Torikai S, Kurokawa K: Calcitonin selectively stimulates 25-hydroxyvitamin D 3–1

alpha–hydroxylase in proximal straight tubule of rat kidney. Nature 291:327–329, 1981.

150. Chabades D, Gagnan-Brunette M, Imbert-Teboul M, et al: Adenylate cyclase responsiveness to hormone in various portions of the human nephron. J Clin Invest 65:439–448, 1980.

151. Dayer JM, Vassali J-D, Bobbitt JL, et al: Calcitonin stimulates plasminogen activator in porcine renal tubular cells: LLC–PK_1. J Cell Biol 91:195–200, 1981.

152. Nagamine Y, Sudol M, Reich E: Hormonal regulation of plasminogen activator mRNA production in porcine kidney cells. Cell 32:1181–1190, 1983.

153. Mahaffey JE, Dayer J-M, Krane SM, et al: Calcitonin stimulates urinary excretion of plasminogen activator activity. Calcif Tissue Int 31:59a (abstract), 1980.

154. Cooper CW, Schwesinger WH, Mahgoub AM, et al: Thyrocalcitonin: Stimulation of secretion by pentagastrin. Science 172:1238–1240, 1971.

155. Van Houten M, Rizzo AJ, Goltzman D, et al: Brain receptors for blood-borne calcitonin in rats: Circumventricular localization and vasopressin-resistant deficiency in hereditary diabetes insipidus. Endocrinology 111:1704–1710, 1982.

156. Fischer JA, Tobler PH, Henke H, et al: Salmon and human calcitonin-like peptides coexist in the human thyroid and brain. J Clin Endocrinol Metab 57:1314–1316, 1983.

157. Nakamuta H, Furukawa S, Koida M, et al: Specific binding of ^{125}I-salmon calcitonin to rat brain: Regional variation and calcitonin specificity. Jpn J Pharmacol 31:53–60, 1981.

158. Fischer JA, Sagar SM, Martin JB: Characterization and regional distribution of calcitonin binding sites in the rat brain. Life Sci 29:663–671, 1981.

159. Pecile A, Ferri S, Braga PC, et al: Effect of intracerebroventricular calcitonin in the conscious rabbit. Experientia 31:332–334, 1975.

160. Sexton PM, McKenzie JS, Mason RT, et al: Localization of binding sites for calcitonin gene-related peptide in rat brain by *in vitro* autoradiography. Neuroscience 19:12, 1986.

161. Gibson SJ, Polak JM, Bloom SR, et al: Calcitonin gene-related peptide immunoreactivity in the spinal cord of man and of eight other species. J Neurosci 4:3101–3111, 1984.

162. Lundberg JM, Franco-Cereda A, Hua X, et al: Coexistence of substance P and calcitonin gene-related peptide-like immunoreactivities in sensory nerves in relation to cardiovascular and bronchoconstrictor effects of capsaicin. Eur J Pharmacol 108:315–319, 1985.

163. Takami T, Kawai Y, Shiosaka S, et al: Immunohistochemical evidence for the coexistence of calcitonin gene-related peptide and choline acetyltransferase-like immunoreactivity in neurons of the rat hypoglossal, facial and ambiguous nuclei. Brain Res 328:386–389, 1985.

164. Mason RF, Peterfreund RA, Sawchenko PE, et al: Release of the predicted calcitonin gene-related peptide from cultured rat trigeminal ganglion cells. Nature 308:653–655, 1984.

165. Mulderry PK, Ghatei MA, Rodrigo J, et al: Calcitonin gene-related peptide in cardiovascular tissues of the rat. Neuroscience 14:947–954, 1985.

166. Brain SD, William TJ, Tippins JR, et al: Calcitonin gene-related peptide is a potent vasodilator. Nature 313:54–56, 1985.

167. Kubota M, Moseley JM, Butera L, et al: Calcitonin gene-related peptide increases cyclic AMP production in rat aortic smooth muscle cells. Biochem Biophys Res Comm 132: 88, 1985.

168. Goltzman D, Mitchell J: Interaction of calcitonin and calcitonin gene–related peptide at receptor site in target tissues. Science 227:1343–1345, 1985.

169. Heath H, Sizemore GW: Plasma calcitonin in normal man. Differences between men and women. J Clin Invest 60:1135–1140, 1977.

170. Hillyard CJ, Stevenson JC, MacIntyre I: Relative deficiency of plasma-calcitonin in normal women. Lancet 1:961–962, 1978.

171. Deftos LJ, Weisman MH, Williams GW, et al: Influence of age and sex on plasma calcitonin in human beings. N Engl J Med 302:1351–1353, 1980.

172. Milhaud G, Benezech-Le Fevre M, Moukhtar M: Deficiency of calcitonin in age-related osteoporosis. Biomedicine 29:272–276, 1978.

173. Chestnut CH, Baylink DJ, Sisom K, et al: Basal plasma immunoreactive calcitonin in postmenopausal osteoporosis. Metabolism 29:559–562, 1980.

174. Tiegs RD, Body J-J, Rolfe J, Heath H: Do calcitonin levels decrease with age? Reassessment with a new technique. Calcif Tissue Int 36:479 (abstract), 1984.

175. Taggart HM, Chestnut CH, Ivey JL, et al: Deficient calcitonin response to calcium stimulation in postmenopausal osteoporosis? Lancet 1:475–478, 1982.

176. Gruber HE, Ivey JL, Baylink DJ, et al: Long-term calcitonin therapy in postmenopausal osteoporosis. Metabolism 33:295–303, 1984.

MICHAEL F. HOLICK
JOHN S. ADAMS

5

Vitamin D Metabolism and Biological Function

The secosterol vitamin D has its origin dating back at least 0.5 billion years ago, when it was produced in ocean dwelling phytoplankton while they were being exposed to sunlight, possibly to act as a sunscreen.[1] With the evolution of the terrestrial vertebrates, vitamin D became important for the development and maintenance of the ossified skeleton. One of the principal physiologic functions of vitamin D is to maintain normal circulating concentrations of calcium and phosphorus for support of neuromuscular function and bone ossification. Vitamin D is able to accomplish this by enhancing the efficiency of the small intestine to absorb dietary calcium and phosphorus and increasing the mobilization of calcium stores from the bone.

During the past two decades, intense research has revealed that vitamin D is not a vitamin but a hormone. Once vitamin D is made in the skin or ingested in the diet it undergoes successive hydroxylations in the liver and kidney to be transformed to 1,25-dihydroxyvitamin D [1,25$(OH)_2$D].[2] 1,25$(OH)_2$D is the hormonally active form of vitamin D that leaves the kidney and travels in the circulation to its various target tissues and cells to carry out its physiologic functions. This knowledge has led to the development of assays for vitamin D metabolites, which have been invaluable in obtaining solid clinical evidence that acquired and inherited disorders of vitamin D metabolism are the cause of several hypo- and hypercalcemic disorders.

Although the major target tissues for 1,25$(OH)_2$D are the small intestine, bone, and kidney, recently it has been revealed that such diverse tissues and cells as the skin, pancreas, parathyroid gland, stomach, gonads, brain, monocytes, and activated T and B lymphocytes possess low-capacity, high-affinity nuclear receptors for this hormone. In a variety of experimental systems, both *in vivo* and *in vitro*, 1,25$(OH)_2$D has been shown to inhibit tumor cell proliferation and promote cellular differentiation; to stimulate insulin, thyroid-stimulating hormone, and interleukin-1 synthesis or release; to inhibit parathyroid hormone (PTH) and interleukin-2 synthesis and secretion; and to induce peripheral monocytes to mature into osteoclast-like cells. Although the physiologic relevance of these observations is unclear at present, these revelations have given rise to speculation that 1,25$(OH)_2$D is important for the recruitment of bone marrow stem cells to form new osteoblasts and osteoclast-like cells and to the novel use of 1,25$(OH)_2$D for the treatment of lymphomas and psoriasis.

The purpose of this chapter is to review the recent advances in the photobiology, biochemistry, and physiology of vitamin D and to recount how this fundamental knowledge has been useful for the diagnosis and treatment of a variety of disturbances in calcium and bone metabolism as well as diseases as diverse as psoriasis and cancer.

I. HISTORY OF VITAMIN D

A. Rickets and the Environment

There is firm evidence that most plants and animals that live on the Earth today have the capacity to produce vitamin D during exposure to sunlight.[1,3] In terms of human history, however, historians state that the disease rickets was reported to occur in humans as early as the second century AD, but the disease was not considered a significant health problem until people began to congregate into the cities of northern Europe just prior to its industrialization.[4] In the mid-17th century, Whistler, Glisson, and DeBoot each independently recognized that many of the children who lived in the sunless alleyways in the industrialized cities developed a severe disease of the bones. They noted that this disease was associated with deformities of the skeleton, particularly enlargement of the epiphyses of the joints of the long bones and the rib cage (commonly referred to as the rachitic rosary), bending of the spine, enlargement of the head, curvature of the thighs, and weak and toneless muscles, especially of the extremities (Fig. 5–1).[4,5] The incidence of this debilitating bone disease increased dramatically during the industrial revolution, especially in northern Europe and North America, and by the latter part of the 19th century, autopsy studies done in Leiden, the Netherlands, suggested that approximately 80% to 90% of children raised in the crowded cities of these areas had the disease.[6]

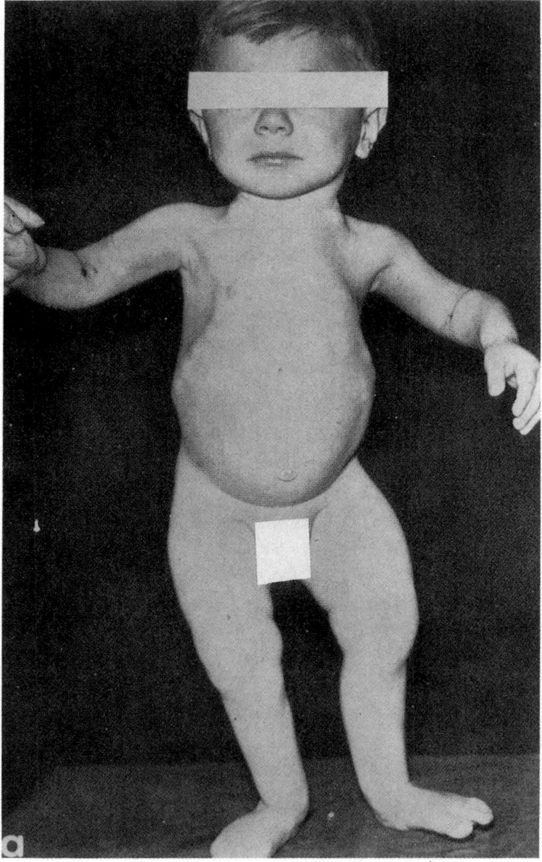

Figure 5–1. Child with rickets showing rachitic rosary of the rib cage, bowed legs, deformity of the long bones, and muscle weakness. (From Fraser D, Scriver CR: Hereditary disorders associated with vitamin-D resistance or defective phosphate metabolism. *In* DeGroot L, et al (eds): Endocrinology, vol 2. New York, Grune & Stratton, 1979, pp 797–807.)

As early as 1822, the Polish physician Sniadecki realized the importance of sun exposure for the prevention and cure of rickets.[7] He realized that children living in the inner city of Warsaw had a very high incidence of this bone disease, whereas children living in the rural areas outside of Warsaw were essentially free of this disorder. He advocated "if the parents' financial status permits, it is best to take the children out into the country and keep them as much as possible in the dry, open, and pure air. If not, at least they should be carried out in the open air, especially in the sun, direct action of which on our bodies must be regarded as one of the most efficient methods for the prevention and cure of this disease."[7] However, little attention was focused on the environment as a cause for this disorder until 1889 when an investigative committee of the British Medical Association reported that rickets was unknown in the rural districts of the British highlands but that it was prevalent in the large industrial towns.[8] A year later, Palm[9] reported his epidemiologic survey that included clinical observations from a number of physicians throughout the British Empire and the Orient. His information revealed that rickets was rare in children living in impoverished cities in China, Japan, and India where the people received poor nutrition and lived in squalor, whereas the children of the middle-class and poor who lived in the industrialized cities in the British Isles had a high incidence of rickets. Based on this survey he urged the following: "the establishment of a sunshine recorder in the heart of the city to record the chemical activity of the sun's rays rather than its heat; the removal of rachitic children, as early as possible, from the large towns to a locality where sunshine abounds and the air is dry and bracing; the systematic use of sunbaths as a preventative and therapeutic measure in rickets and other diseases; and the education of the public to the appreciation of sunshine as a means of health."

However, it was difficult at the time for people to believe that such a simple remedy as exposure to sunlight could have any significant effect on curing this crippling bone disease. At the turn of the 20th century, many theories had surfaced as to the cause of the debilitating disease, including infection, poor nutrition, lack of activity, and an inherited disorder. In 1905, Buchholz[6] exposed 16 rachitic children to a carbon-arc light source and suggested that there was a favorable response. However, in 1919 Huldschinsky demonstrated unequivocally for the first time that phototherapy alone was curative. He reported four patients with severe rickets who were cured (based on x-ray examination) after being treated with exposure to a mercury-vapor quartz lamp.[10] He speculated that the radiation responsible for this cure was the same radiation that causes melanization of the skin. He also showed that the effect of phototherapy was not local, inasmuch as exposure of one arm had equal and dramatic curative effects on both arms. Two years later, Hess and Unger[11] exposed seven rachitic children on the roof of a New York City hospital to varying periods of sunshine and reported that x-ray examinations showed marked improvement of the rickets of each child as evidenced by calcification of the epiphyses.

B. Vitamin D: The Nutrient

During the 19th century, cod-liver oil was frequently used for the prevention and cure of rickets. This knowledge prompted an intense investigation to determine what nutrient was responsible for preventing rickets. In 1919, Mellanby[12] reported that he could produce rickets in dogs by feeding them oatmeal and could cure the disease by adding cod-liver oil to their diet. In 1921, McCollum and colleagues[13] reported the profound influence of dietary phosphorus on the calcification of cartilage and ossification of bone in growing rats. They demonstrated that rats given a diet deficient in phosphorus and the antirachitic factor developed rickets, whereas rats given diets adequate in calcium and phosphorus but deficient in the antirachitic factor developed osteoporosis but not rickets. With this experimental model they examined the question of whether the antirachitic factor in cod-liver oil was identical to or distinct from vitamin A. In 1922, these workers oxidized cod-liver oil, destroying all vitamin A activity, and showed that the oxidized oil retained its antirachitic properties. Thus, it became clear that the antirachitic factor present in cod-liver oil was not vitamin A but a new fat-soluble vitamin that was to be called vitamin D. The fact that the antirachitic factor could be generated in the skin after exposure to sunlight or ultraviolet radiation or could be obtained from cod-liver oil caused some confusion as to whether there was more than one antirachitic factor. This issue was resolved when Powers et al.[14] reported that radiation from a mercury-vapor quartz lamp had similar if not identical healing effects on rachitic rats when compared with those brought about by the administration of cod-liver oil. Once it was known that exposure to sunlight could prevent and cure the disease, Steenbock and Black[15] and Hess and Weinstock[16] independently demonstrated that exposure of food and a variety of other substances to the vitamin D–producing radiation from the mercury-vapor quartz lamp could impart antirachitic properties to these substances. These investigators reported that exposure of rat liver, human serum, olive, cotton and linseed oils, lettuce, growing wheat, rat chow, and a variety of other substances endowed each with antirachitic properties. This concept was used to make milk antirachitic by adding the precursor of vitamin D to milk and exposing it to radiation from a mercury-arc lamp. Today, 400 IU (10 μg) of vitamin D_2 or vitamin D_3 is directly added to milk and other foods, resulting in almost complete elimination of rickets in the United States and in countries that use this practice.

Once it was established that the antirachitic factor could be produced *in vitro* by the ultraviolet (UV) irradiation of plant and animal tissues, several investigators began the quest to isolate and structurally identify the antirachitic factor. Originally, it was thought that the substance that was activated by UV radiation was cholesterol in animals and phytosterol in vegetable foods.[15,17] However, cholesterol lost the property of becoming antirachitic when it was purified by chemical means. It was concluded that the precursor of vitamin D (called provitamin D) was not cholesterol itself, but a substance associated with it.[18] The findings that ergosterol, a yeast sterol, had an intense ultraviolet absorption band at 280 nm (which was similar to the UV absorption maximum for the cholesterol-like sterol that had antirachitic properties) and that this yeast sterol could be rendered antirachitic by exposure to ultraviolet radiation suggested that the parent substance of vitamin D was either ergosterol or a highly unsaturated sterol similar to ergosterol. These observations prompted the quest of several laboratories to isolate and structurally identify the antirachitic factor. Reerink and van Wijk[19] and Askew et al.[20] purified vitamin D from irradiated ergosterol and reported almost identical UV absorption spectra with λ max at 265 and 262 nm, respectively. Initial characterization of vitamin D established that the structure retained the secondary hydroxyl group of the parent ergosterol, that ring B was opened between carbon 9 and 10, and that there were three double bonds in conjugation with each other (Fig. 5–2). Finally, in 1948 x-ray crystallographic analysis of a heavy atom derivative of vitamin D yielded the spacial orientation of vitamin D as a molecule that is quite different from its parent sterol (Fig. 5–2). The first vitamin D that was isolated from the irradiation of ergosterol was designated vitamin D_1. However, the product was found to be an impure mixture of vitamin D and lumisterol and the term was dropped. Vitamin D was finally purified from its irradiation products and was named ergocalciferol (vitamin D_2) (Fig. 5–2). Initially, it was thought that vitamin D_2 was identical to the vitamin D that was present in fish-liver oils and was produced in the skin by exposure to sunlight. However, in the 1930s it was reported that vitamin D obtained from the irradiation of ergosterol had little antirachitic activity in chickens, whereas the vitamin D that was isolated from the irradiation of cholesterol-like sterol yielded a very potent antirachitic substance.[21-23] The confusion as to whether vitamin D_2 was identical to the substance produced in skin was resolved when Windaus et al.[24] reported the synthesis of a new provitamin D analogue that was similar to ergosterol with the exception that the side chain was that of cholesterol (Fig. 5–2).

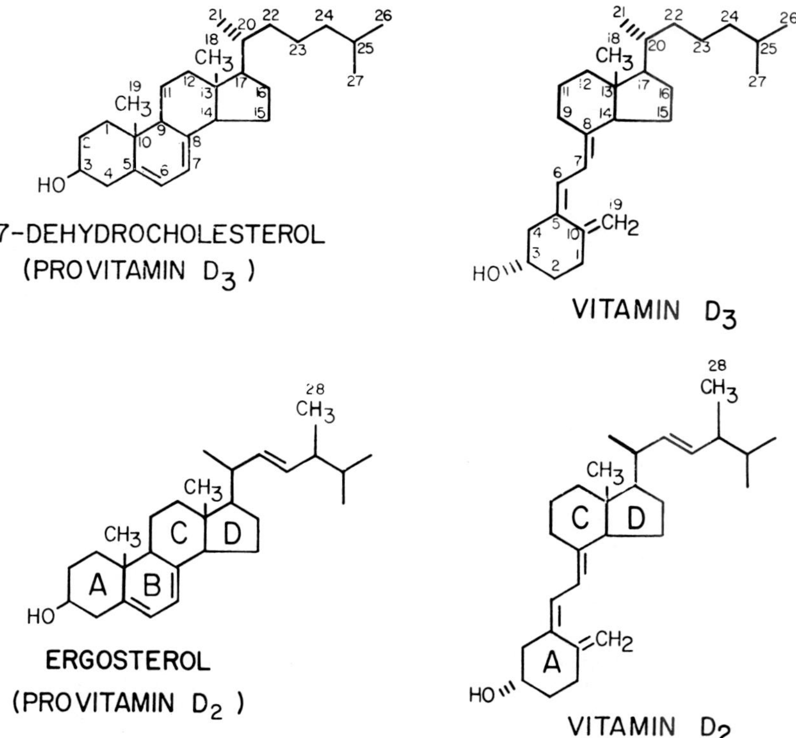

Figure 5–2. Structure of vitamins D_3 and D_2 and their respective precursors, 7-dehydrocholesterol and ergosterol. The only structural difference between vitamins D_2 and D_3 is their side chains; the side chain for vitamin D_2 contains a double bond between carbon-22 and carbon-23 and a carbon-24 methyl group. (From MacLaughlin JA, Holick MF: Photobiology of vitamin D_3 in the skin. *In* Goldsmith LA (ed): Biochemistry and Physiology of the Skin, vol 2. London, Oxford University Press, 1983, pp 734–754.)

This provitamin D was called provitamin D_3 or 7-dehydrocholesterol and upon irradiation gave rise to cholecalciferol (vitamin D_3) (Fig. 5–2). This new vitamin D had equal antirachitic activity in chick and rat to the vitamin D that was isolated from the cholesterol-like sterol and was identical to the vitamin D found in fish-liver oils and mammalian skin.[25] Therefore, it was concluded that 7-dehydrocholesterol rather than ergosterol was the parent compound present in the skin and that the resulting photoproduct was vitamin D_3.

II. PHOTOBIOLOGY OF VITAMIN D_3

A. Photosynthesis of Previtamin D_3 in Human Skin

The sun emits a broad spectrum of radiation. The high-energy photons that are most damaging to life on Earth (below 290 nm) are absorbed by the thin layer of ozone that envelops the Earth. When radiation between 290 and 315 nm (UV-B radiation) hits the skin, approximately 10% is reflected and the other 90% is absorbed or scattered.[26] During exposure to sunlight, UV-B photons are transmitted into the epidermis and dermis where cytoplasmic stores of provitamin D_3 are located. The 5,7-diene of provitamin D_3 absorbs this radiation, causing cleavage of ring B between carbons 9 and 10 and the formation of a 6,7-*cis*-conjugated triene to form a 9,10-seco (*seco* from the Greek term *split*) sterol known as previtamin D_3 (Fig. 5–3).[27] In adult skin, approximately 50% of the entire cutaneous stores of provitamin D_3 are found in the epidermis while the other 50% reside in the dermis.[27] When adult Caucasians and blacks are exposed to sunlight, approximately 70% to 80% and 95% to 98% of the UV-B photons are absorbed in the epidermis,

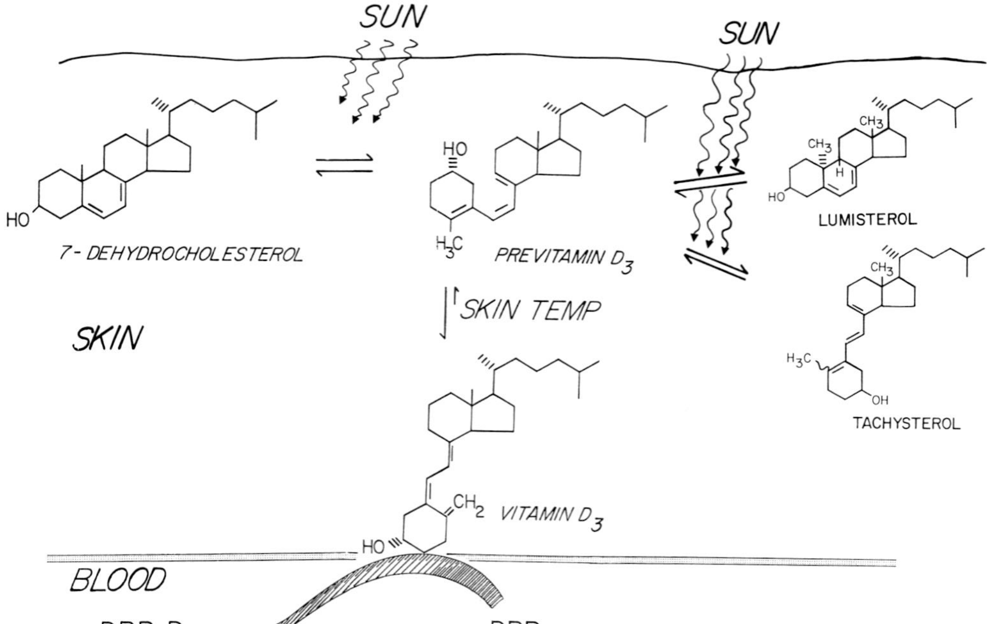

Figure 5–3. Schematic representation of the formation of previtamin D_3 in the skin during exposure to the sun and the thermal isomerization of preD_3, which is specifically translocated by the vitamin D–binding protein (DBP) into the circulation. During continual exposure to the sun, previtamin D_3 also photoisomerizes to lumisterol$_3$ and tachysterol$_3$, which are photoproducts that are biologically inert (i.e., they do not stimulate intestinal calcium absorption). Because the DBP has no affinity for lumisterol$_3$ but has minimal affinity for tachysterol$_3$, the translocation of these photoisomers into the circulation is negligible, and these photoproducts are sloughed off during the natural turnover of the skin. Because these photoisomers are in a state of quasiphotoequilibrium as soon as previtamin D_3 stores are depleted (owing to thermal isomerization to vitamin D_3), exposure of lumisterol and tachysterol to UV radiation will provoke these isomers to photoisomerize to preD_3. (From Holick MF, MacLaughlin JA, Doppelt SH: Science 211:590, 1981. Copyright by the American Association for the Advancement of Science.)

respectively. Therefore, approximately 80% to 90% of the previtamin D_3 that is formed occurs in the actively growing layers of the epidermis (stratum basale and stratum spinosum) while less than 20% occurs in the dermis.[27] In neonates, about 50% of the provitamin D_3 stores in the skin are present in the dermis, and because the epidermis transmits more UV-B photons into the dermis, the dermis is also a major site for previtamin D_3 synthesis.

Once previtamin D_3 is made in the skin, it immediately begins to thermally equilibrate to vitamin D_3 by a temperature-dependent process (Fig. 5–3).[27] This thermal equilibration takes approximately 1½ to 2 days to reach completion at body temperature (37° C) in humans.[27] Because most of the cutaneous previtamin D_3 synthesis in adults occurs in the actively growing layers of the epidermis, which is in close proximity to the dermal capillary bed, changes in the temperature of the surface of the skin resulting from exposure to very warm or cold climates do not significantly alter the rate of conversion of previtamin D_3 to vitamin D_3 in humans.[27] Although the exact mechanism for how vitamin D_3 exits the epidermal cells and journies to the dermal capillary bed is unknown, there is evidence that the vitamin D–binding protein, which has a relatively high affinity for vitamin D_3 in comparison to provitamin D_3 and previtamin D_3, helps translocate vitamin D_3 from the epidermis into the dermal circulation (Fig. 5–3).[27]

B. Regulation of Previtamin D_3 Synthesis in Human Skin

In 1967, Loomis[28] popularized a theory that skin pigmentation evolved for the purpose of regulating vitamin D_3 synthesis in the skin. He suggested that peoples living at or near the equator would have died of vitamin D intoxication as a result of daily exposure to intense solar radiation were it not for the evolution of more melanin pigmentation in the skin. Melanin is a natural sunscreen that is produced by the epidermis and acts as a neutral density filter absorbing wavelengths of sunlight that are responsible for producing previtamin D_3 in human skin.[29] Although it is clear that melanin can compete with 7-dehydrocholesterol for UV-B photons and therefore limit previtamin D_3 synthesis in the skin, this cannot be the only explanation for why Caucasians exposed to prolonged sunlight do not become vitamin D intoxicated.

It is now appreciated that there is a more fundamental process that regulates the photosynthesis of previtamin D_3 in human skin. Previtamin D_3 is sensitive to both thermal energy and ultraviolet radiation. Once previtamin D_3 is formed in the epidermis and dermis, it can either thermally isomerize to vitamin D_3 or during exposure to sunlight absorb a photon of UV-B radiation and isomerize to biologically inert isomers lumisterol and tachysterol (Fig. 5–3).[30] Thus, if a Caucasian is exposed to sunlight at the equator, during the initial few minutes of exposure provitamin D_3 is rapidly converted to previtamin D_3 (Fig. 5–4). Prolonged exposure to sunlight, however, does not increase previtamin D_3 production, but rather previtamin D_3 absorbs UV-B radiation and undergoes isomerization to form lumisterol and, to a small extent, tachysterol (Fig. 5–4).[30]

Thus, prolonged exposure to sunlight does not necessarily increase previtamin D_3 synthesis. In addition to the photolysis of previtamin D_3 in human skin that limits the amount of previtamin D_3 that is ultimately formed during a single exposure to sunlight, it is now appreciated that vitamin D_3 is exquisitely sensitive to exposure to sunlight. On a sunny day in Boston in June, vitamin D_3 is efficiently converted to 5,6-*trans*-vitamin D_3 and suprasterols 1 and 2 (Fig. 5–5).[31] The physiologic roles of the photoisomers of previtamin D_3 and vitamin D_3 are unknown at present.

C. Other Factors That Regulate the Cutaneous Production of Vitamin D_3

The photoproduction of previtamin D_3 in any layer of skin is dependent on the concentration of provitamin D_3, the presence of chromophores that compete with provitamin D_3 for UV-B photons, and the quantum of UV-B photons that are able to penetrate the skin and are absorbed by the provitamin D_3 chromophore. The average concentration of provitamin D_3 in a 6.25 cm^2 area of young adult human skin is approximately 5 μg for the epidermis and 1 to 3 μg for the dermis.[32] There is an inverse relation between the concentrations of provitamin D_3 in the epidermis with age (Fig. 5–6).[32] Compared with elderly

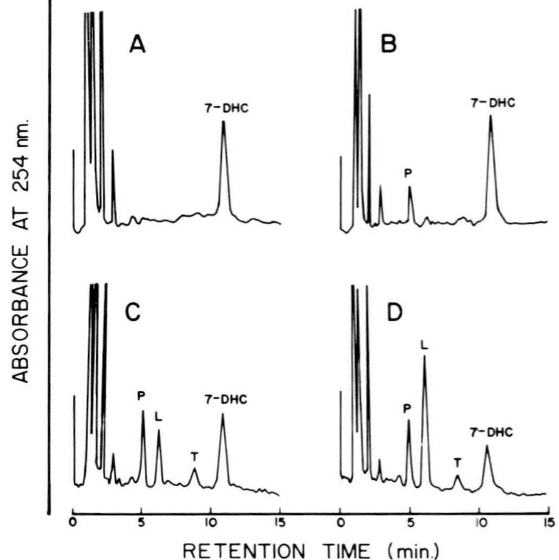

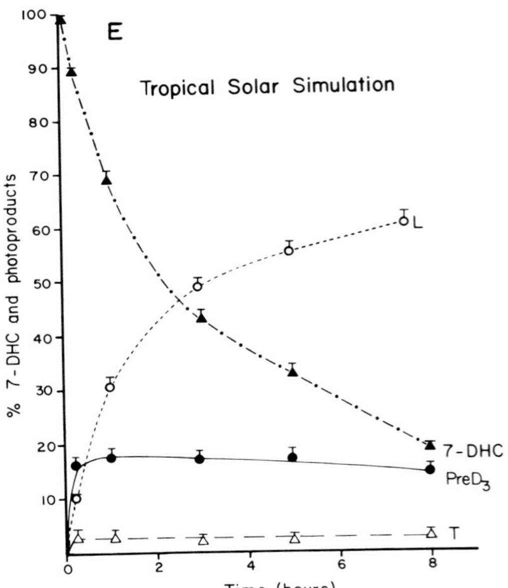

Figure 5–4. HPLC profiles of a lipid extract from the basal cells of surgically obtained hypopigmented skin that was previously shielded from (*A*) or exposed to (*B to D*) equatorial simulated solar ultraviolet radiation for 10 minutes (*B*), 1 hour (*C*), or 3 hours (*D*). *E*, An analysis of the photolysis of 7-dehydrocholesterol (7-DHC) in the basal cells and the appearance of the photoproducts previtamin D_3 (preD_3), lumisterol (L), and tachysterol (T) with increasing time of exposure to equatorial simulated sunlight. (From Holick MF, MacLaughlin JA, Doppelt SH: Science 211:590, 1981. Copyright 1981 by the American Association for the Advancement of Science.)

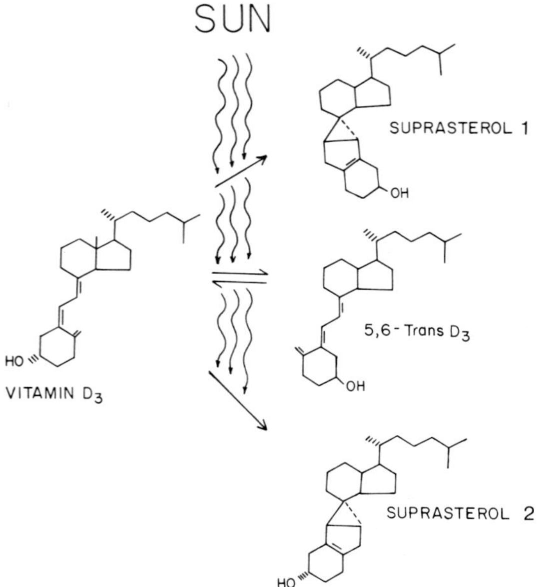

Figure 5–5. Photolysis of vitamin D_3 to 5,6-*trans*-vitamin D_3, suprasterol 1, and suprasterol 2. (From Holick MF, Smith E, Pincus S: Arch Dermatol 123:1677a, 1987.)

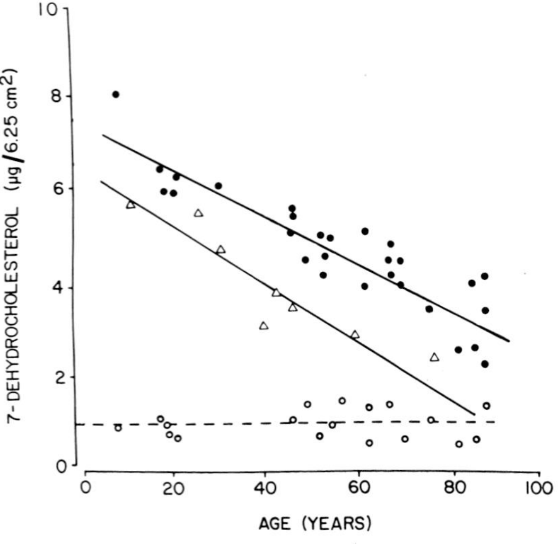

Figure 5–6. Effect of aging on 7-dehydrocholesterol concentrations in human epidermis and dermis. Concentrations of 7-dehydrocholesterol (provitamin D_3) per unit area of human epidermis (●), stratum basale (Δ), and dermis (O) obtained from surgical specimens from donors of various ages. A linear regression analysis revealed slopes of − 0.05, − 0.06, and − 0.0005 for the epidermis (r = − 0.89), stratum basale (r = 0.92), and dermis (r = 0.04), respectively. The slopes of the epidermis and the stratum basale are significantly different from the slope of the dermis ($p < 0.001$). (From MacLaughlin J, Holick MF: J Clin Invest 76:1536, 1985. By copyright permission of the American Society for Clinical Investigation.)

Table 5–1. Cutaneous Production of Vitamin D_3

	Epidermis		Dermis		Epidermis and Dermis	
Age	*7-DHC* *(ng/cm^2)*	*$preD_3$* *(ng/cm^2)*	*7-DHC* *(ng/cm^2)*	*$preD_3$* *(ng/cm^2)*	*$preD_3$* *(ng/cm^2)*	*% Formation pre D_3 Compared with 8-year-old*
8	1308	406	1800	36	442	100
18	1056	346	1125	22	368	80
77	605	144	1630	24	168	37
77	490	141	—	—	—	—
82	659	163	1040	20	183	40

7-Dehydrocholesterol (7-DHC) content before exposure to ultraviolet radiation and previtamin D_3 ($preD_3$) content after exposure to ultraviolet radiation in 1 cm^2 of human epidermis and dermis and the percentage (%) of $preD_3$ formed in the epidermis and dermis relative to the 8-year-old subject.

From MacLaughlin J, Holick MF: J Clin Invest 76:1536–1538, 1985.

adults, young adults can make two to three times more previtamin D_3 in their skin when they are exposed to the same amount of sunlight (Table 5–1).[32] Sunscreens, which are effective in preventing the damaging effects of sunlight, also prevent the beneficial effects of sunlight, the photosynthesis of previtamin D_3 in human skin.[29] It has been reported that the topical application of a sunscreen with a sun protection factor of 8 can completely block the photosynthesis of previtamin D_3 in human skin and prevent the elevation of the concentration of vitamin D_3 in the circulation after a whole-body exposure to a dose of ultraviolet radiation that is equivalent to a minimal erythemal dose.[29]

The percentage conversion of cutaneous provitamin D_3 to previtamin D_3 is also influenced by the solar zenith angle, which is inversely related to the amount of ultraviolet B photons in the solar spectrum, and by UV-B–absorbing chromophores that are present in the skin, such as melanin, urocanic acid, proteins, and RNA and DNA. An increase in the zenith angle either by the daily rotation of the Earth or by an increase in the distance north or south from the equator shifts the spectral distribution of sunlight toward longer wavelengths because of greater subtraction of shorter wavelengths (UV-B) by atmospheric absorption and scattering.[5] It is well known that in northern latitudes children are more prone to develop rickets during and immediately after the winter when compared with spring, summer, and fall. Originally it was thought that the principal cause for this was that children wore more clothing and were outdoors less. However, there is a more fundamental reason for this phenomenon. There is now evidence that exposure to sunlight between the months of November and March, in Boston (42° N), does not result in any cutaneous production of previtamin D_3.[31]

D. Effect of Whole-Body Ultraviolet Irradiation on Circulating Concentrations of Vitamin D and Its Metabolites

When young, healthy adult volunteers were exposed to a single whole-body dose of ultraviolet radiation that caused minimal erythema (1 minimal erythemal dose, or 1 MED), the circulating vitamin D concentrations increased from a baseline value of 2 ng/ml to 24 ng/ml within 24 hours and returned to a baseline value within 1 week after the exposure (Fig. 5–7).[33] The apparent half-life of vitamin D in the serum was determined to be about 48 hours.[33] Based on the assumption that the plasma volume is about 5% of the mean body weight, it was estimated that at least 30 μg of vitamin D_3 was released from each square meter of body surface area after exposure to 1 MED of ultraviolet radiation.[33] The role of skin pigment and ethnic background on limiting the cutaneous formation of vitamin D_3 was examined by exposing slightly pigmented Caucasians, moderately pigmented immigrants of Indian and Pakistani extraction, and heavily pigmented black volunteers to a single dose of ultraviolet radiation. Whole-body exposure of Caucasian subjects to 1.5 times their MED greatly increased the serum vitamin D concentrations by up to 60-fold 24 to 48 hours after exposure, whereas exposure to the same amount of radiation had no effect on serum vitamin D concentrations in the

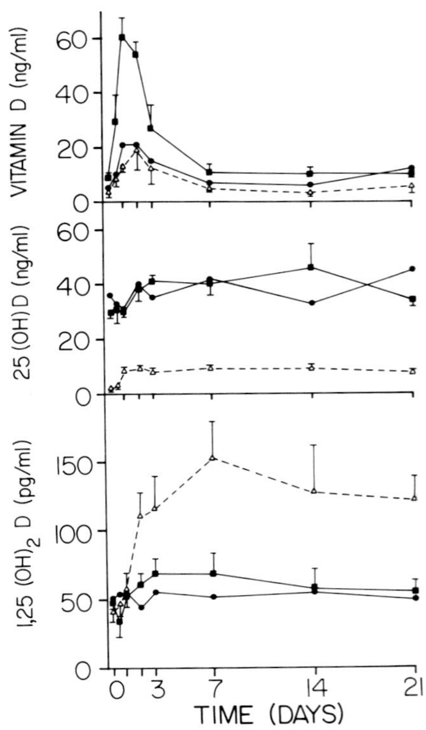

Figure 5–7. Changes in the serum concentrations of vitamin D and its metabolites after total-body exposure to ultraviolet radiation: concentrations of vitamin D, 25(OH)D, and 1,25$(OH)_2$D were measured in three normal subjects exposed to 3 minimal erythemal doses (MED) of ultraviolet radiation (UVR) (-■-), in a representative normal subject exposed to 1 MED of UVR (-●-), and in three vitamin D–deficient patients exposed to 1 MED of UVR (-Δ-). (From Adams JA, et al: N Engl J Med 306:722, 1982.)

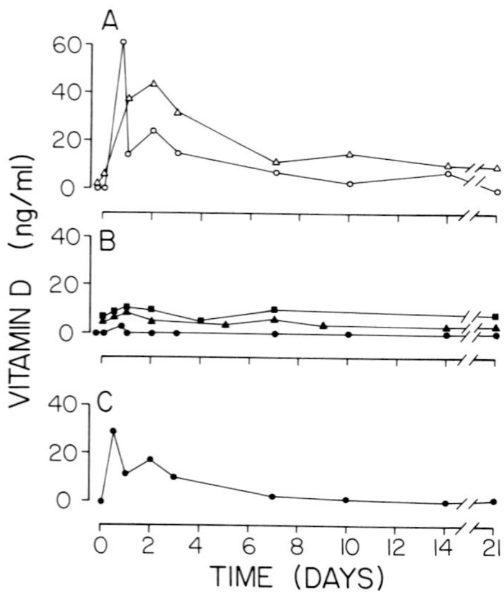

Figure 5–8. Serum vitamin D concentration in two lightly pigmented Caucasian (*A*) and three heavily pigmented black subjects (*B*) after total-body exposure to 0.054 J/cm^2 of UVR. *C*, Serial change in circulating vitamin D after reexposure of one black subject (● in panel B) to a 0.32 J/cm^2 dose of UVR. (From Clemens TL, et al: Lancet 1:74, 1982.)

black volunteers (Fig. 5–8).[34] The black subjects were then exposed to a dose of radiation that was equivalent to 6 times the MED for the Caucasian subjects (exposure of the Caucasian subjects to this amount of radiation would have caused severe second-degree sunburn), and circulating concentrations of vitamin D increased approximately 30-fold during the 24 hours after exposure (Fig. 5–8).[34] It is well recognized that Asians of Indian and Pakistani extraction living in Great Britain are more prone to develop rickets and osteomalacia. Although this may be due to the high phytate content in their diet, there has been some question as to whether these individuals have the same capacity as that of Caucasians and blacks to produce vitamin D_3. As can be seen in Figure 5–9, Indians and Pakistanis have the same capacity as that of Caucasians and blacks to produce vitamin D_3 in their skin as evidenced by increasing circulating concentrations of vitamin D that are comparable to those of Caucasian subjects exposed to 1 minimal erythemal dose (MED) of ultraviolet radiation.[35] Hence, blacks and Asians of Indian and Pakistani extraction have the same capacity as that of Caucasians to produce vitamin D_3 but require a much larger dose of ultraviolet radiation to do so because of the pigmentation that is present in their skin.

Although a single whole-body exposure to ultraviolet radiation has a dramatic effect on elevating the circulating concentration of vitamin D in a dose-dependent fashion, the effect on the circulating concentration of 25(OH)D and 1,25$(OH)_2$D is minimal. The serum 25(OH)D concentration increased only gradually, reaching a 50% increase in 7 to 14 days after exposure (Fig. 5–7).[33] There was no significant increase in circulating concentrations of 1,25$(OH)_2$D in the Caucasian subjects exposed to 1 and 3 MEDs of ultraviolet radiation (Fig. 5–7).[33] Vitamin D deficiency does not appear to alter provitamin D concentrations in the skin.[33] When vitamin D–deficient patients were exposed to 1 MED of whole-body ultraviolet radiation, their

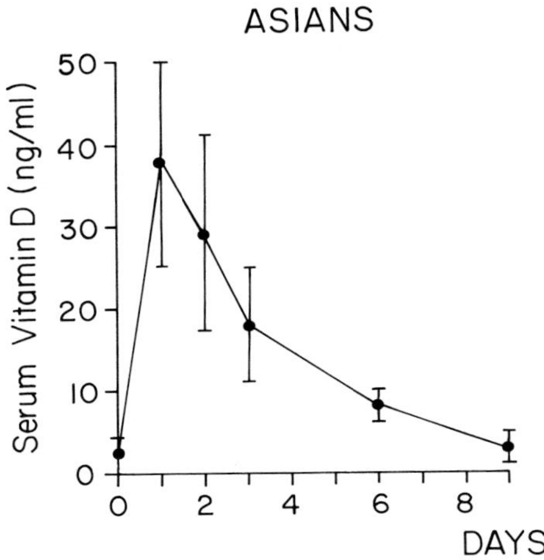

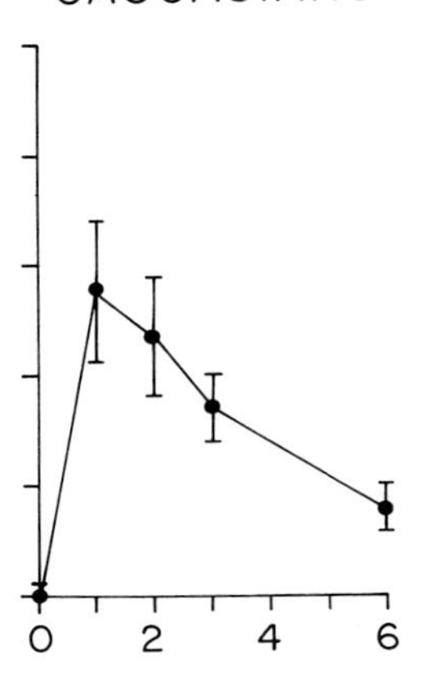

Figure 5–9. Serum vitamin D concentrations in Asians and Caucasians after 1.5 MED whole-body ultraviolet irradiation. Means ± standard deviations are shown at 0, 1, 2, 3, 6, and 9 days. There are no significant differences in serum vitamin D concentrations between Asians and Caucasians at any time point. (From Lo CW, Paris P, Holick MF: Am J Clin Nutr 44:683, 1986.)

circulating concentrations of vitamin D and 25(OH)D increased in a fashion almost identical to that seen for the vitamin D–sufficient volunteers (Fig. 5–7).[33] However, the serum $1,25(OH)_2D$ concentrations in the vitamin D–deficient patients increased by 3- to 4-fold within 7 days after the exposure and persisted at this concentration throughout the next 2 weeks (Fig. 5–7).[33] In these patients, the increase in circulating concentrations of $1,25(OH)_2D$ was most likely due to the fact that the high circulating concentrations of PTH enhanced the renal metabolism of 25(OH)D to $1,25(OH)_2D$ (see separate section on vitamin D metabolism and regulation for details).[33]

III. INTESTINAL ABSORPTION OF VITAMIN D

It is quite clear that for most of the population of the world cutaneous synthesis of vitamin D_3 is the principal source of this prohormone. The exceptions are probably peoples living in very northern and southern latitudes where the zenith angle of the sun does not permit sufficient vitamin D_3 production in skin. Very few foods contain vitamin D naturally; these include liver, egg yolks, and fish-liver oils. Several countries practice the fortification of some foods with vitamin D. In the United States, milk is the principal dietary component that is subject to vitamin D fortification with either vitamin D_2 or vitamin D_3. In other countries, some cereals, margarine, and breads also have small quantities of vitamin D added to them.

When vitamin D is ingested, this fat-soluble compound is incorporated into the chylomicron fraction and absorbed through the lymphatic system. Approximately 80% of the vitamin D enters the body via this mechanism. After the ingestion of a single dose of 50,000 IU of vitamin D_2, circulating concentrations of vitamin D are increased by as early as 4 hours, peak at 12 hours, and gradually decline to near baseline by 72 hours (Fig. 5–10).[36] Although aging significantly decreases the capacity of the skin to produce

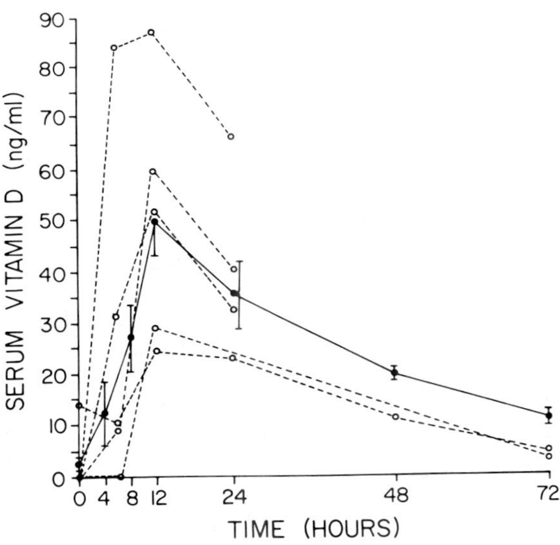

Figure 5–10. Vitamin D_2 absorption in young (•) and elderly (o) adults. Each subject received an oral dose of 50,000 IU of vitamin D_2, and at various times blood determinations were made for circulating concentrations of vitamin D. (From Holick MF: Clin Nutr 5:121, 1986.)

vitamin D_3, aging does not appear to significantly affect the intestinal absorption of vitamin D (Fig. 5–10).[37] On the other hand, intestinal malabsorption syndromes such as Crohn's disease, cystic fibrosis, and Whipple's disease can effectively prevent the intestinal absorption of vitamin D, whereas diseases that affect the more distal small intestine and large intestine appear to have little effect on the intestinal absorption of this fat-soluble vitamin (Fig. 5–11).[36] A simple method to determine whether an individual is capable of absorbing vitamin D is to conduct a provocative vitamin D absorption test. A blood sample is obtained before and 12 hours after a single oral administration of 50,000 IU of vitamin D_2 (Fig. 5–10).[36] If no elevation in the circulating concentration of vitamin D is observed, complete malabsorption of vitamin D should be suspected; however, an increase in the circulating concentration of vitamin D is reflective of vitamin D absorption, and the patient's dose of vitamin D can therefore be tailored accordingly.[36] Thus, patients who suffer from chronic liver disease or who have a disease of the small intestine are more prone to develop vitamin D deficiency owing to the inability to absorb this fat-soluble vitamin.

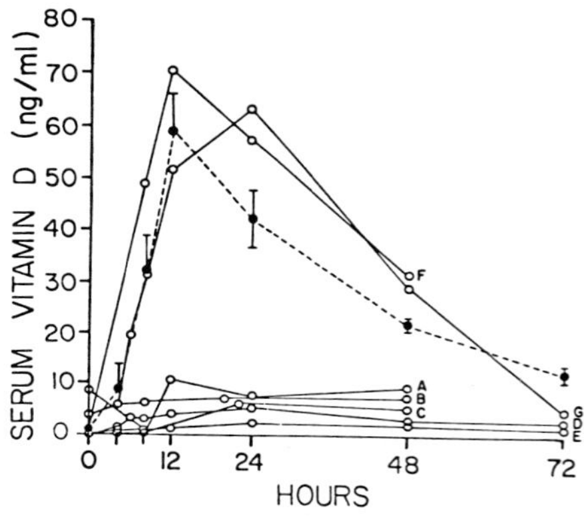

Figure 5–11. Serum vitamin D concentrations in seven patients with intestinal fat malabsorption syndromes after a single oral dose of 50,000 IU (1.25 mg) of vitamin D_2. For comparison, the means and standard errors of vitamin D concentrations measured in seven normal control subjects after a similar dose are indicated by the closed circles and dashed lines (—o—). Note that two patients, one with Crohn's ileocolitis (patient F) and one with ulcerative colitis (patient G), had essentially normal absorption curves. Five patients, however, showed a dramatic lack of response, with no values shown above 10 ng/ml. From Lo CW, et al: Am J Clin Nutr 42:644, 1985. Reproduced with permission from the American Society for Clinical Nutrition and The American Journal of Clinical Nutrition.)

IV. METABOLISM OF VITAMIN D TO 25-HYDROXYVITAMIN D

A. Hepatic Metabolism

Vitamin D_3 made in the skin or ingested in the diet along with dietary vitamin D_2 enters the circulation and is bound to a vitamin D–binding protein.[2] Vitamin D (the use of the term vitamin D without a subscript refers to either or both vitamin D_2 and vitamin D_3) is transported to the liver where it is hydroxylated on carbon 25 to generate the major circulating form of vitamin D, 25-hydroxyvitamin D [25(OH)D] (Fig. 5–12).[2,38] The vitamin D 25-hydroxylases are located in the mitochondria and microsomes of the parenchymal cells. The enzymatic reaction is supported by reduced NADP and molecular oxygen.[38] Although the mammalian liver has a large reserve of the vitamin D-25-hydroxylase, it is not the sole site for vitamin D 25-hydroxylation. In avian species, the kidney and intestine are capable of metabolizing vitamin D_3 to $25(OH)D_3$,[39] and hepatectomized rats metabolize vitamin D_3 to $25(OH)D_3$ to a small degree.[40] Vitamin D_2 and vitamin D_3 as well as vitamin D analogues, such as dihydrotachysterol and 1α-hydroxyvitamin D_3, are metabolized in the liver to their 25-hydroxy counterparts.[2] There is some evidence, however, that because the vitamin D–binding protein does not bind to vitamin D_2 as tightly as it does to vitamin D_3, vitamin D_2 is more available as a substrate for the hepatic enzyme and, therefore, is more efficiently converted to $25(OH)D_2$.[41] The half-life of 25(OH)D in the human circulation is about 2 to 3 weeks, and its concentration is a good reflection of the cumulative effects of dietary intake of vitamin D and exposure to sunlight.[2] It should be recognized, however, that the liver vitamin D-25-hydroxylase is relatively well regulated, inasmuch as the relative increase in circulating concentration of $25(OH)D_3$ in comparison to the cumulative intake of vitamin D_3 is relatively small (Fig. 5–13).[42] This may, in part, be due to negative feedback regulation of the hepatic vitamin D-25-hydroxylase by vitamin D, 25(OH)D, and/or $1,25(OH)_2D_3$.[43]

B. Clinical Disorders

Patients with severe parenchymal and cholestatic liver disease often have low circulating

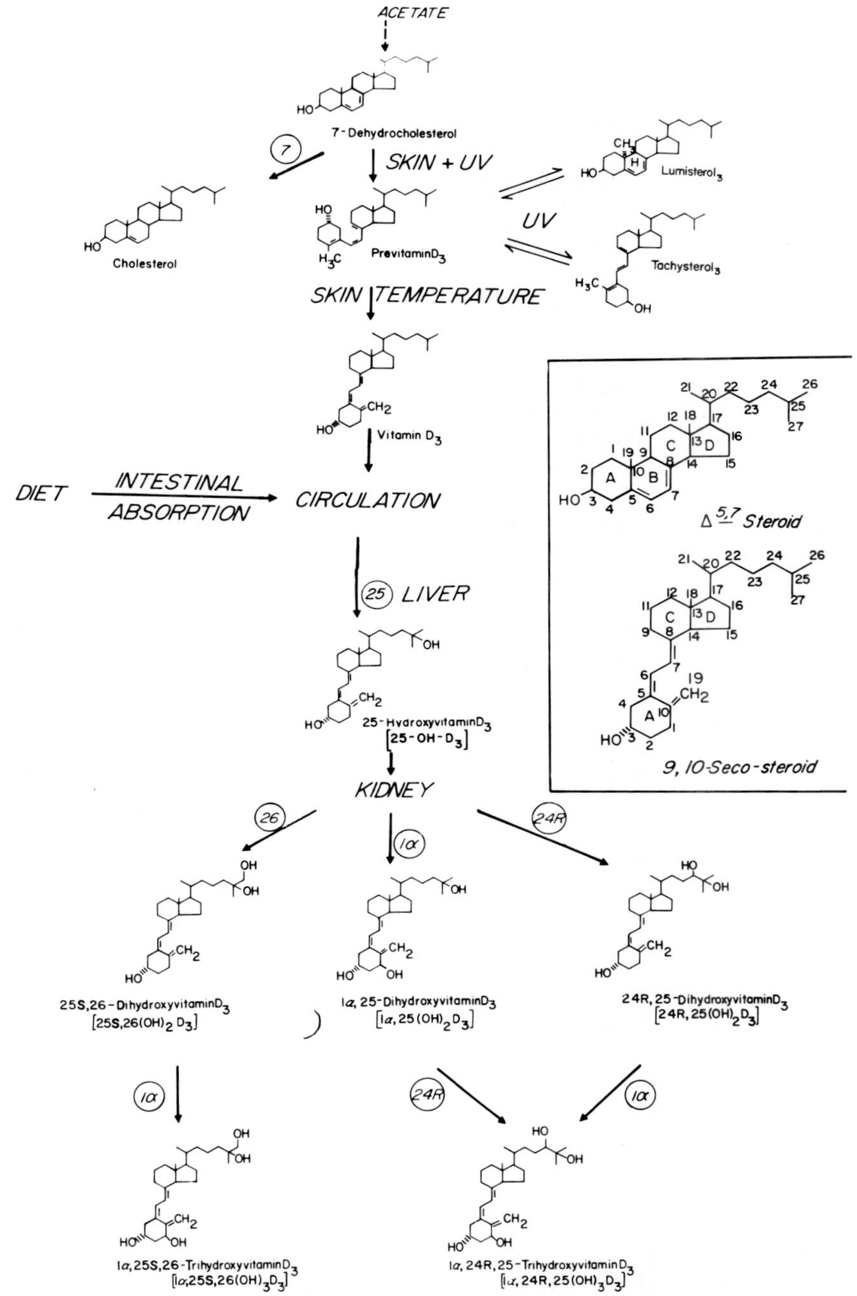

Figure 5–12. The photochemical, thermal, and metabolic pathways for vitamin D_3. Circled letters and numbers denote specific enzymes: (7) 7-dehydrocholesterol reductase; (25) vitamin D-25-hydroxylase; (1α) 25(OH)D-1α-hydroxylase; (24R) 25(OH)D-24R-hydroxylase; (26) 25(OH)D-26-hydroxylase. (From Holick MF, Potts JT Jr: Vitamin D. *In* Isselbacher KJ, et al (eds): Harrison's Principle of Internal Medicine, 10th ed. New York, McGraw-Hill, 1983, pp 1944–1949. Reproduced with permission.)

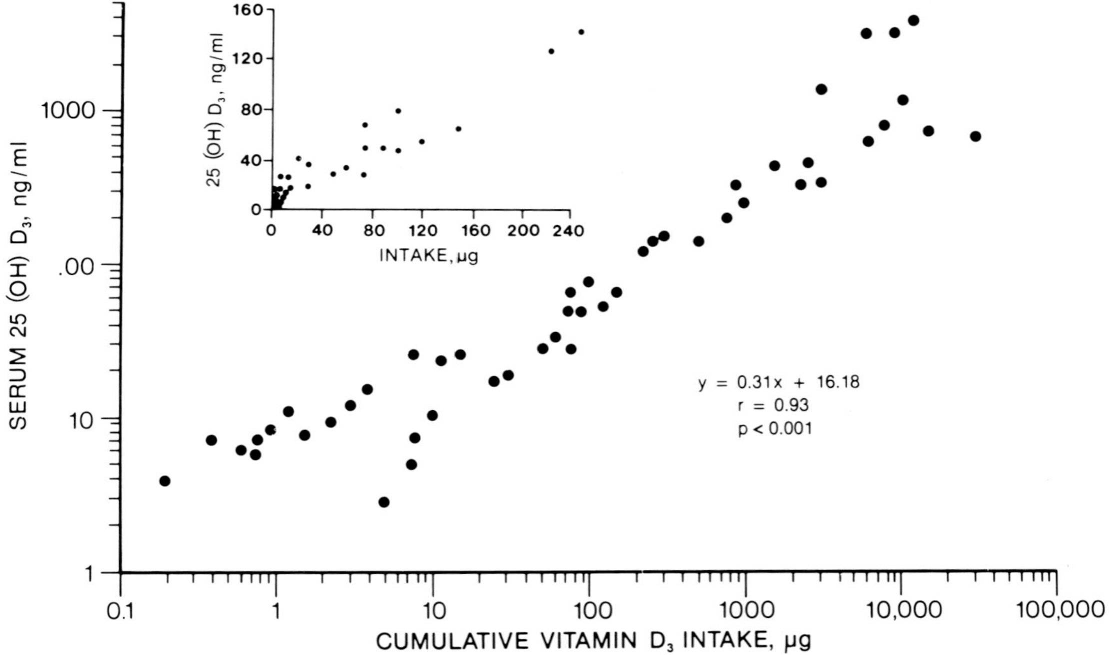

Figure 5–13. Serum levels of 25(OH)D_3 observed in response to various oral doses of vitamin D_3, given to vitamin D–deficient rats. There is a clear linear correlation that extends well into the pharmacologic range for both parameters. (Kindly supplied by the Nichols Institute.)

concentrations of 25(OH)D (Table 5–2).[44] This is partly due to the associated intestinal malabsorption of vitamin D as well as a decrease in the reservoir of the vitamin D-25-hydroxylase in the liver. Originally, it was believed that the low circulating concentration of 25(OH)D was responsible, in part, for the debilitating bone disease associated with severe liver failure. However, there is no correlation between the severity of the bone disease and circulating concentrations of 25(OH)D, and treatment of these patients with 25(OH)D or its metabolites provides no benefit.[44,45] However, because these patients are more prone to vitamin D deficiency due to associated fat malabsorption, it is wise to increase the vitamin D intake and monitor circulating concentrations of 25(OH)D (Chapter 11). The 25(OH)D concentrations in these patients should be maintained in the mid-normal range of approximately 25 to 45 ng/ml. Some patients will benefit by increasing the dose or frequency of oral administration of vitamin D once it has been determined, using the provocative oral vitamin D absorption test,[36] that the patient can absorb vitamin D. Otherwise, intravenous or intramuscular injections of vitamin D or increased exposure to sunlight will often provide adequate vitamin D nutrition for these patients. In disease states in which there is an increase in the metabolism of 25(OH)D to 1,25$(OH)_2$D, such as vitamin D–dependent rickets type II, sarcoidosis and other chronic granulomatous disorders, primary hyperparathyroidism, and hyperphosphatemic tumoral calcinosis, it has been reported that the circulating concentrations of 25(OH)D are often decreased, but usually not below the normal values.[43] Patients with nephrotic syndrome who have marked proteinuria (> 4 g/24 hr) may have decreased concentrations of 25(OH)D in the

Table 5–2. Serum Concentrations of 25(OH)D in Disorders of Calcium, Phosphorus, and Bone Metabolism

Disease State	Serum 25(OH)D
Vitamin D deficiency	↓
Intestinal malabsorption syndromes	↓
Liver disorders	↓
Nephrotic syndrome	↓
Osteopenia in the aged	N or ↓
Vitamin D intoxication	↑

circulation as a result of a loss in the urine of the vitamin D–binding protein (which is similar in molecular weight to albumin) with its tightly bound 25(OH)D. Thus, the turnover of 25(OH)D is markedly increased, and these patients will often benefit from additional vitamin D supplementation.[46] There is no need to treat these patients with either $25(OH)D_3$ or $1,25(OH)_2D_3$.

It is well documented that there is an association between osteomalacia or rickets and anticonvulsant drug therapy in epileptic patients.[47] Initially, it was thought that this resistance was because phenytoin and phenobarbital induced liver microsomal enzymes that rapidly metabolized and inactivated vitamin D and its metabolites. However, it now appears that these drugs also disrupt calcium homeostasis by additional mechanisms. Phenytoin inhibits vitamin D–dependent and vitamin D–independent intestinal calcium transport. Phenobarbital increases bile secretion (thereby increasing the turnover of vitamin D) and has a negative effect on the kinetics of the vitamin D-25-hydroxylase.[48] This problem appears to be more severe in children and adults who are institutionalized and who are taking several antiseizure medications. There does not appear to be a disruption in calcium or bone metabolism in otherwise healthy individuals who are taking a single anticonvulsant drug for prolonged periods of time. It has been reported that free-living cardiac patients free of known disorders of calcium metabolism have normal circulating concentrations of 25(OH)D despite 2 years of treatment with conventional doses of phenytoin.[49] The hallmark of this disorder is low circulating 25(OH)D. The associated disorders in calcium and bone metabolism are reversed when the oral intake of vitamin D is increased to raise 25(OH)D into the normal range.[50]

V. METABOLISM OF 25-HYDROXYVITAMIN D TO 1,25-HYDROXYVITAMIN D

A. Renal 25(OH)D-1α-Hydroxylase

Once 25(OH)D is formed in the liver, it is transported to the kidney on its vitamin D–binding protein and hydroxylated there on either carbon-1 or carbon-24 (Fig. 5–12).[2,38,50] In most mammalian species, including humans, the principal if not sole site for the metabolism of 25(OH)D to $1,25(OH)_2D$ is the kidney. However, during pregnancy the placenta plays a significant part in maintaining circulating concentrations of $1,25(OH)_2D$ by metabolizing 25(OH)D to $1,25(OH)_2D$.[51-53] Normal circulating concentrations of 1,25(OH)D in our laboratory are between 26 and 65 pg/ml, and the circulating half-life of the hormone is between 4 and 6 hours. There have been reports that there are extrarenal sites for the production of this hormone, but all of these have occurred in cultured cells originating from bone, skin, or peripheral monocytes.[54-56] Whether other tissues besides the kidney can produce 1,25(OH)D under normal circumstances in nonpregnant humans remains to be determined. It is known, however, that in patients who have had a bilateral nephrectomy or who have severe renal failure, the concentrations of $1,25(OH)_2D$ are usually very low or undetectable, suggesting that in humans the kidney is the principal, if not the sole, source of this hormone.[57]

The renal 25(OH)D-1α-hydroxylase is a mitochondrial cytochrome P-450 mixed-function oxidase that requires reduced NADP and molecular oxygen for its activity (Fig. 5–14).[38] In young vitamin D–deficient rats, this enzyme is located in the proximal convoluted tubules and pars recta of the proximal tubules.[58] *In vivo*, hypocalcemia enhances the renal mitochondrial 25(OH)D-1α-hydroxylase activity so that the rate of conversion of 25(OH)D to $1,25(OH)_2D$ increases. However, hypocalcemia, *per se*, does not appear to be directly responsible for enhancing this hydroxylation step *in vivo*. Any decrease in the serum calcium concentration below normal is a stimulus for increased secretion of parathyroid hormone. Parathyroid hormone, in addition to acting upon calcium and phosphorus metabolism in the kidney and bone, also acts physiologically as a tropic hormone to increase the renal synthesis of 1,25(OH)D from 25(OH)D.[59] The 25(OH)D-1α-hydroxylase in the proximal convoluted tubule in a neonatal rat is exclusively stimulated by parathyroid hormone, whereas the 1-hydroxylase in the pars recta is responsive only to calcitonin.[58] The mechanism by which these peptide hormones exert their influence on the renal metabolism of 25(OH)D has not been firmly established. It appears that PTH mediates its effect on the metabolism of 25(OH)D through cyclic AMP and on the renal handling of phosphate.

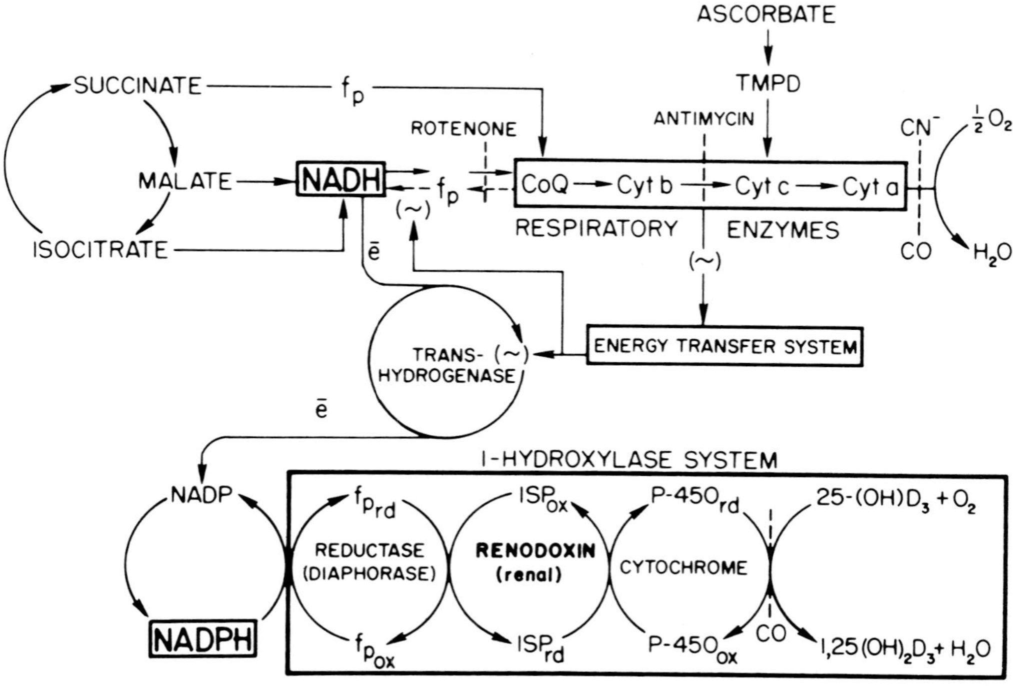

Figure 5–14. Mechanism of production of $1,25(OH)_2D_3$ by chick kidney mitochondria, illustrating the energy-dependent transhydrogenation reaction involved in electron supply for the hydroxylation reaction. (From DeLuca HF: The metabolism, physiology, and function of vitamin D. *In* Kumar R (ed): Vitamin D, Basic and Clinical Aspects. Boston, Martinus Nijhoff Publishing, 1984, pp 1–68. Reproduced with permission.)

B. Regulation of 25(OH)D Metabolism

When vitamin D–deficient rats are thyroparathyroidectomized, their ability to metabolize 25(OH)D to $1,25(OH)_2D$ is markedly diminished and then restored after parathyroid hormone is administered.[59] However, when vitamin D–deficient thyroparathyroidectomized rats were maintained on a high-calcium, low-phosphorus diet, the effects of thyroparathyroidectomy were reversed and the animals efficiently converted 25(OH)D to $1,25(OH)_2D$.[38] Furthermore, when another group of thyroparathyroidectomized rats were made hyperphosphatemic and hypocalcemic by dietary manipulation, the conversion of 25(OH)D to $1,25(OH)_2D$ was significantly reduced.[38] These data suggested that regulation of the serum phosphate was most important for 25(OH)D-1α-hydroxylase activity. In humans, this conclusion is further supported by the observation that in healthy men, phosphorus restriction caused an increase in circulating concentrations of $1,25(OH)_2D$ to 80% above control values. It was determined that this increase was due to an increase in the production rate without any change in the metabolic clearance of this hormone.[60] When similar male volunteers received phosphorus supplementation in their diets, the serum concentration of $1,25(OH)_2D$ decreased abruptly, reaching a nadir within 2 to 4 days. After 10 days of supplementation, the mean concentration of $1,25(OH)_2D$ was 29% lower than the value measured when the phosphorus was normal. Production rate decreased to 1.3 ± 0.2 μg/day, but the metabolic clearance rate did not change significantly (Fig. 5–15).[60] Therefore, although it has been demonstrated that hypocalcemia can induce the renal 25(OH)D-1α-hydroxylase, it appears that this is secondary to the effect of parathyroid hormone, which, in turn, stimulates adenylate cyclase activity in the renal proximal tubule, thus beginning a cascade of events that conclude with the enhancement of the renal tubular absorption of calcium, stimulation of secretion of phosphate into the urine, and

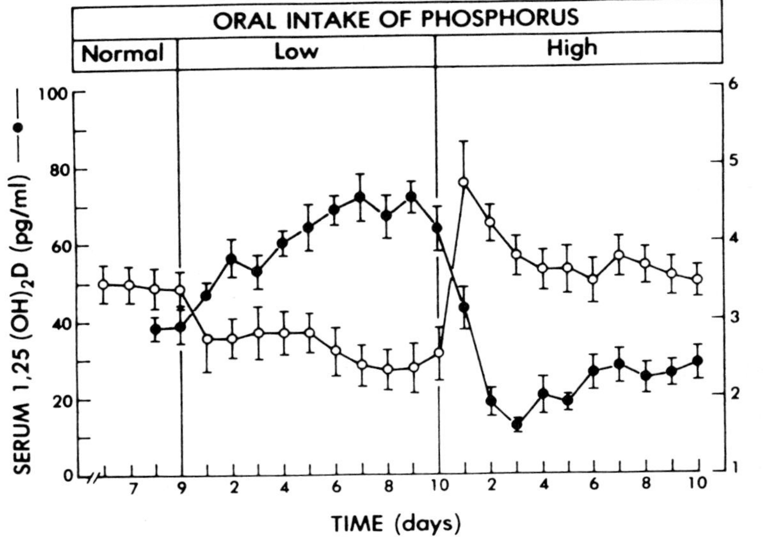

Figure 5–15. Effect of changes in the oral intake of phosphorus on the fasting serum concentrations of $1,25(OH)_2D$ and phosphorus in six healthy men. The bracketed points depict mean values + SEM. (From Portale AA, et al: J Clin Invest 77:7, 1986. By copyright permission of the American Society for Clinical Investigation.)

augmentation of the renal production of $1,25(OH)_2D$ (Fig. 5–16).[61] Although parathyroid hormone appears to be extremely important in the moment-to-moment regulation of the renal 25(OH)D-1α-hydroxylase, it should be appreciated that this enzyme is not absolutely dependent on this hormone for its activity. Patients with hypoparathyroidism often have low-normal circulating concentrations of $1,25(OH)_2D$ rather than low or undetectable concentrations of this hormone. Therefore, parathyroid hormone is not absolutely essential for the production of $1,25(OH)_2D$, but rather plays a role in modulating changes in the circulating concentration of this hormone at times of need.[38,50]

It is well known that during pregnancy, lactation, and skeletal growth, the body adapts to the increased need for calcium by enhancing the efficiency of the intestine to absorb dietary calcium. This adaptive response can be directly linked to the increased production of $1,25(OH)_2D$ during these physiologic stresses. There is evidence that estrogen, prolactin, and growth hormone either directly or indirectly enhance the renal production of $1,25(OH)_2D$ in various *in vitro* and *in vivo* animal models.[50,62] However, it should be noted that patients with hyperprolactinemia and acromegaly who have high circulating concentrations of prolactin and growth hormone, respectively, have no evidence of increased circulating concentrations of $1,25(OH)_2D$.[50,63,64] Thus, these hormones apparently, by themselves, cannot directly increase the production of $1,25(OH)_2D$ under normal circumstances and it is likely that other unidentified factors are also playing an important role as well.

The role of estrogen and progesterone on the renal production of $1,25(OH)_2D$ remains unclear. It is known, however, that in ovulating birds, the increased secretion of the sex hormones estrogen and progesterone markedly stimulates the renal production of this hormone. This compensatory increase in $1,25(OH)_2D$ synthesis is responsible for the utilization of calcium from the medullary bone and from the intestine for deposition into the developing egg shell. It is likely that the sex steroids have an indirect effect on the renal metabolism of 25(OH)D because it has been demonstrated *in vitro* that estrogen and progesterone do not stimulate the chick renal cells to produce $1,25(OH)_2D$.[65] In humans, the role of estrogen and progesterone on the renal metabolism of 25(OH)D to $1,25(OH)_2D$ is less clear. The circulating concentrations of $1,25(OH)_2D$ are not significantly altered in young women with estrogen deficiency caused by anorexia nervosa.[66] In sexually maturing boys, serum concentrations of testosterone increase at the onset of sexual maturation but do not significantly alter circulating concentrations of $1,25(OH)_2D$.[67] It has been strongly suggested, however, that the onset of menopause and decreased circulating concentrations of estrogen have a significant effect on the renal production of $1,25(OH)_2D$.[68] Although the circulating concentrations of this hormone have been re-

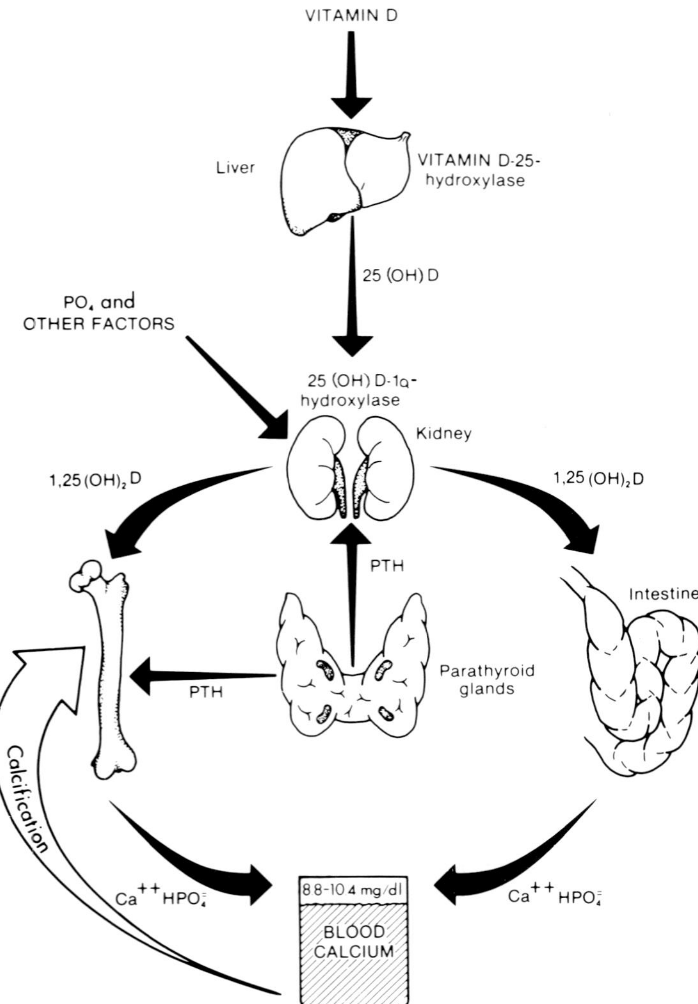

Figure 5–16. Schematic representation of the hormonal control loop for vitamin D metabolism and function. A reduction in the serum calcium below approximately 8.8 mg/100 ml serum prompts a proportional secretion of parathyroid hormone that acts to mobilize calcium stores from the bone. Parathyroid hormone also promotes the synthesis of $1,25(OH)_2D$ in kidney, which, in turn, stimulates the mobilization of calcium from bone and intestine. (Kindly provided by the Nichols Institute.)

ported to be slightly lower in osteoporotic women compared with aged-matched controls, estrogen replacement in postmenopausal women causes a slight, if significant, elevation in $1,25(OH)_2D$ in the serum. Aging may, however, decrease the influence of PTH on the renal metabolism of $25(OH)D_3$ to $1,25(OH)_2D_3$. As can be seen in Figure 5–17, when young volunteers were infused with the biologically active peptide fragment of PTH (1–34 PTH), there was a doubling of their circulating concentrations of $1,25(OH)_2D$ within 24 hours, whereas there was no significant change in $1,25(OH)_2D$ concentrations in elderly osteoporotics who received the same infusion of (1–34) PTH.[69] Therefore, aging may decrease the responsiveness of the kidney to produce $1,25(OH)_2D$ at critical times (such as when a person has little calcium in his or her diet) when the body needs to increase the efficiency of intestinal calcium absorption to maintain calcium homeostasis. When this system fails, the body calls upon the calcium stores in the bone by mobilizing mineral from the skeleton.[37] Thus, although the role of sex steroids in the regulation of $1,25(OH)_2D$ production in the laying hen is well established, less clear is the role of estrogen and androgens on $25(OH)D_3$ metabolism in humans.

C. Extrarenal Metabolism of 25(OH)D to $1,25(OH)_2D$

As early as 1940, it was first suggested that an abnormally high sensitivity of the intestine to vitamin D may be responsible for the

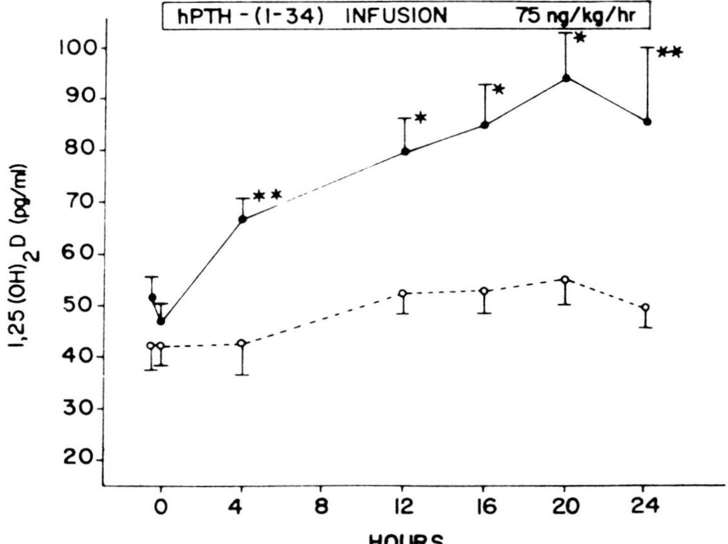

Figure 5–17. Effect of synthetic parathyroid hormone [hPTH-(1–34)] on concentrations of $1,25(OH)_2D$ in normal subjects (solid circles). All values are expressed as the mean ± SEM. The single asterisk denotes significant differences at $p < 0.01$, and the double asterisk at $p < 0.05$, between the level in the patients and that in the controls at corresponding time points. Asterisks also refer to significant differences between the preinfusion baseline levels and levels at particular time points. To convert values for $1,25(OH)_2D$ to picomoles per liter, multiply by 2.36. (From Slovik DM, et al: N Engl J Med 305:372, 1981.)

hypercalciuria and hypercalcemia that is associated in patients with sarcoidosis.[70] The revelation that vitamin D must be activated to $1,25(OH)_2D$ before it can carry out its biological function in the intestine was the impetus for investigators to speculate that the increased efficiency of intestinal calcium absorption in these patients was due to an abnormal production of $1,25(OH)_2D$. Indeed, it has now been clearly demonstrated that not only patients with sarcoidosis but patients who suffer from other chronic granulomatous disorders, including tuberculosis, silicosis, and fungal infections, have inappropriately high-normal or elevated circulating concentrations of $1,25(OH)_2D$.[50,71,72] Initially, it was thought that the elevated concentration of $1,25(OH)_2D$ was due to a defect in the regulation of the renal synthesis of this hormone. However, the observation that an anephric patient with sarcoidosis and hypercalcemia had elevated circulating concentrations of $1,25(OH)_2D$ led to the conclusion that 25(OH)D was metabolized to $1,25(OH)_2D$ at an extrarenal site (Fig. 5–18).[73] Based on the observations that $25(OH)D_3$ is metabolized to $1,25(OH)_2D_3$ *in vitro* by lymph node homogenates and cultured pulmonary alveolar macrophages from patients with sarcoidosis, it is believed that the granulomatous tissue of patients with chronic granulomatous disorders is responsible for this metabolism.[71,74] It does not appear that this extrarenal metabolism of 25(OH)D is regulated by either calcium, phosphorus, or parathyroid hormone. However, it has been recently demonstrated *in vitro* that resting macrophages that were activated by high concentrations of lipopolysaccharides from cell walls of gram-negative bacteria or gamma interferon had an enhanced metabolism of $25(OH)D_3$ to $1,25(OH)D_3$.[56,71]

Granulomas are not the only tissue that has the potential for metabolizing 25(OH)D to

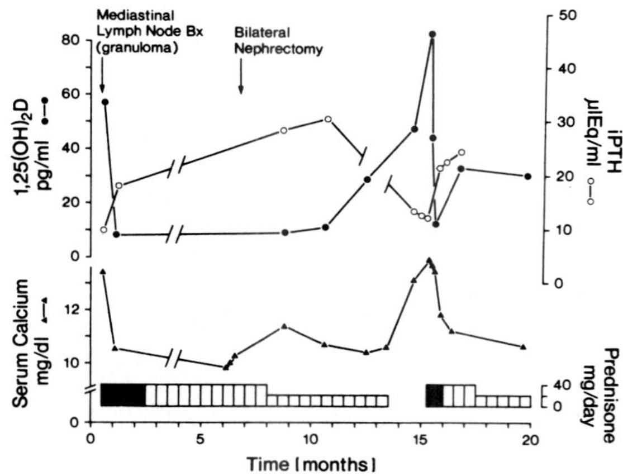

Figure 5–18. Relation of changes in serum levels of $1,25(OH)_2D$, iPTH, and calcium to doses of prednisone administered to control hypercalcemia. The solid portion of the bar representing the administration of prednisone indicates daily therapy, and the open portion indicates alternate-day therapy. Bx denotes biopsy. To convert values for $1,25(OH)_2D$ to picomoles per liter, multiply by 2.36. To convert values for calcium to millimoles per liter, multiply by 0.25. (From Barbour GL, et al: N Engl J Med 305:440, 1981.)

$1,25(OH)_2D$. It has been recently reported that unlike most patients with tumor-induced hypercalcemia, who have low circulating concentrations of $1,25(OH)_2D$, a few patients with Hodgkin's and non-Hodgkin's lymphoma with hypercalcemia have elevated circulating concentrations of this hormone.[75-78] Treatment with prednisone often suppresses $1,25(OH)_2D$ concentrations in these patients, similar to patients with chronic granulomatous disorders, and in turn resolves the hypercalcemia. In one patient, after the removal of the lymphoma, which was isolated in the spleen, the serum calcium and $1,25(OH)_2D$ concentrations returned to normal. Thus, it appears that certain types of lymphoma have the capacity to metabolize 25(OH)D to $1,25(OH)_2D$, similar to granulomas (see Chapter 22). Although the exact mechanism by which the 1-hydroxylase is stimulated in lymphomas is not clear, the recent observation that HTLV-1 infected cultured cord-blood lymphocytes induced the metabolism of $25(OH)D_3$ to a metabolite, which was unequivocally identified by mass spectroscopy as $1,25(OH)_2D_3$, provided strong evidence that these virus-infected cells have the necessary machinery to make this potent calciotropic hormone.[79] Since hypercalciuria and hypercalcemia in patients with either chronic granulomatous disorders or lymphoma are due to an abnormal production of $1,25(OH)_2D$, the treatment of these patients with prednisone, therefore, is reasonable (see Chapter 22).

VI. ALTERNATIVE METABOLISM OF 25-HYDROXYVITAMIN D AND 1,25-DIHYDROXYVITAMIN D

A. Metabolism of 25-Hydroxyvitamin D to 24,25-Dihydroxyvitamin D

The body possesses a variety of enzymes that have the capacity to transform 25(OH)D into innumerable dihydroxy, trihydroxy, and tetrahydroxy metabolites (Fig. 5–19).[38,50,80,81] In the early 1970s, it was appreciated that vitamin D–deficient rats, when provided radioactive vitamin D_3, efficiently converted the vitamin first to $25(OH)D_3$ and then to $1,25(OH)_2D_3$.[38,81] However, when these animals were given a diet that was high in calcium and contained vitamin D, $[^3H]25(OH)D_3$ was converted to a metabolite that was more polar[82] and was structurally identified as 24R,25-dihydroxyvitamin D_3 $[24,25(OH)_2D_3]$[83] (Fig. 5–12). Despite the fact that $25(OH)D_2$ has a methyl group in

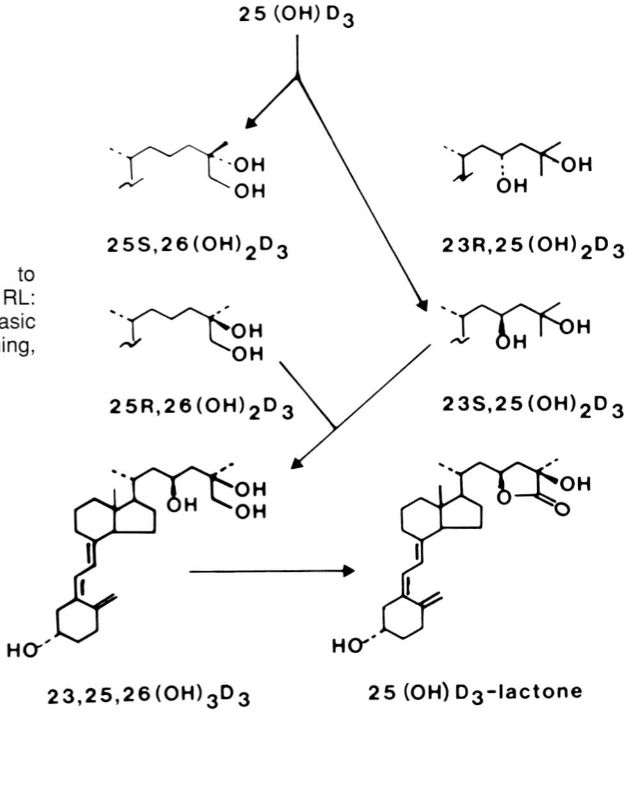

$25(OH)D_3$

$25S,26(OH)_2D_3$ $23R,25(OH)_2D_3$

$25R,26(OH)_2D_3$ $23S,25(OH)_2D_3$

$23,25,26(OH)_3D_3$ $25(OH)D_3$-lactone

Figure 5–19. Pathway of $25(OH)D_3$ metabolism to $25(OH)D_3$-26,23-lactone. (From Napoli JL, Horst RL: Vitamin D metabolism. *In* Kumar R (ed): Vitamin D, Basic and Clinical Aspects. Boston, Martinus Nijhoff Publishing, 1984. Reproduced with permission.)

the S configuration on carbon-24, it, too, is metabolized to $24,25(OH)_2D_2$. $24,25(OH)_2D$ is the major circulating metabolite of 25(OH)D, and its concentration, which is usually 2 to 4 ng/ml, is a reflection of the 25(OH)D concentration.[38,50,80] Although the kidney is the primary site for its production, most other tissues that possess nuclear receptors for $1,25(OH)_2D$ also have the enzymatic machinery to produce this metabolite (Fig. 5–20).[38,50,84] The renal 25(OH)D-24-hydroxylase is a mitochondrial enzyme requiring $NADPH^+$, molecular oxygen, and magnesium ions.[38,50] Originally, it was believed that parathyroid hormone, which enhanced the renal production of $1,25(OH)_2D$, was also responsible for decreasing the synthesis of $24,25(OH)_2D$. However, there is now firm evidence that parathyroid hormone does not influence the renal metabolism of 25(OH)D to $24,25(OH)_2D$. Parathyroid hormone stimulates the production of $1,25(OH)_2D$. This hormone, in turn, shuts off its own renal production and enhances the kidney's production of $24,25(OH)_2D$.[85-89]

The physiologic role of the 24-hydroxylation of 25(OH)D is unsettled at the present time. There are reports that $24,25(OH)_2D_3$ is capable of (1) promoting hatchability of chicken eggs,[90] (2) directly stimulating bone formation *in vitro* only in the presence of parathyroid hormone and $1,25(OH)_2D_3$,[91] (3) increasing the synthesis of proteoglycans in cultured chondrocytes,[92] (4) improving calcium retention in anephric patients,[93] and (5) more effectively promoting bone mineralization in humans when combined with $1,25(OH)_2D_3$ than $1,25(OH)_2D_3$ could by itself.[94] However, it is known that $24,25(OH)_2D_3$ at physiologic concentrations is biologically inert in anephric rats in inducing either intestinal transport or bone calcium mobilization.[95] Its biological activity is restored when it is hydroxylated on carbon-1 to act as an analogue of $1,25(OH)_2D_3$. This trihydroxy metabolite, 1,24,25-trihydroxyvitamin D_3, is less active than $1,25(OH)_2D_3$ in the stimulation of intestinal calcium transport and bone calcium mobilization.[95] Furthermore, this 1-hydroxylated metabolite does not have any specific function in enhancing bone mineralization. To further evaluate the role of the carbon-24 hydroxylation of $25(OH)D_3$, an analogue of $25(OH)D_3$ that had its hydrogens at carbon-24 replaced with fluorines (thus preventing this analogue from being hydroxylated

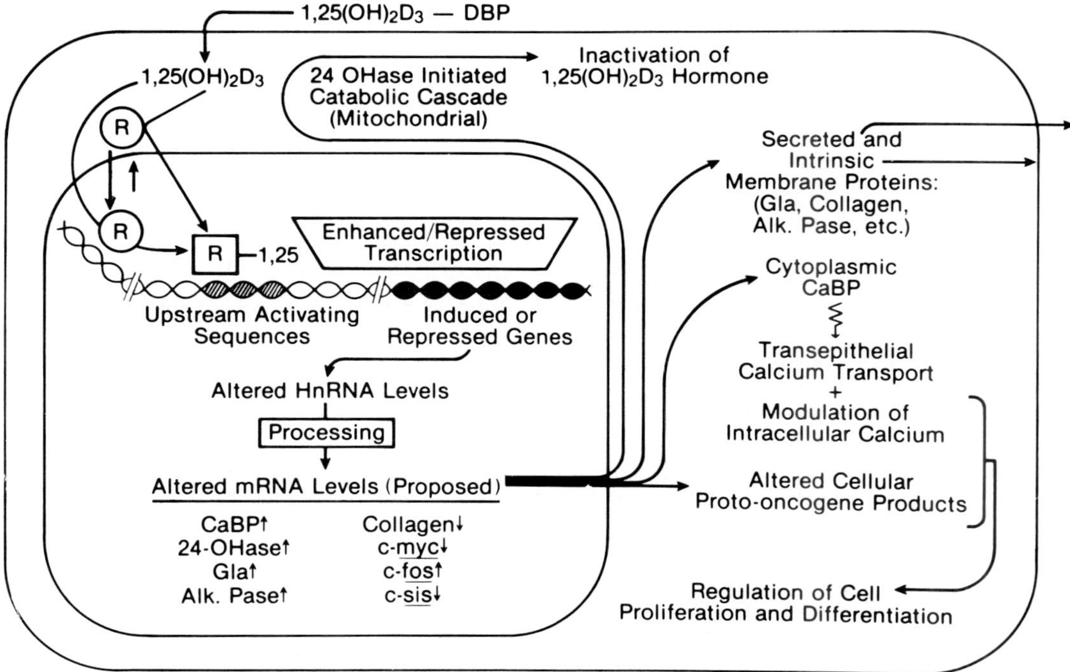

Figure 5–20. Proposed mechanism of action of $1,25(OH)_2D_3$ in target cells resulting in a variety of biological responses. (From Haussler MR, et al: Functions and mechanism of action of the 1,25-dihydroxyvitamin D_3 receptor. *In* Norman AW, et al (eds): Vitamin D. Berlin, de Gruyter, 1985, pp 83–92.)

on carbon-24), was synthesized and its biological activity evaluated. It was found that the 24,24′-difluoro-25-hydroxyvitamin D_3 has the same biological activity as 25(OH)D_3 in (1) enhancing intestinal calcium transport, (2) mobilizing calcium from bones, and (3) healing rachitic lesions in rats.[96] These results suggest that the carbon-24 hydroxylation of 25(OH)D_3 is not essential for the physiologic actions of vitamin D_3 in the rat. An alternative explanation for the presence of the 25(OH)D-24-hydroxylase in the kidney as well as other tissues that possess receptors for 1,25$(OH)_2D_3$ is that this enzyme acts as the initiator for the side-chain catabolism of 25(OH)D and 1,25$(OH)_2$D.[97]

B. Side-Chain and A-Ring Metabolism of 25(OH)D_3 and 1,25$(OH)_2D_3$

Under physiologic conditions, 25(OH)D is metabolized on carbon-26 to form 25S,26-dihydroxyvitamin D_3 [25,26$(OH)_2D_3$] (Fig. 5–12).[98] The circulating concentrations of 25,26$(OH)_2$D are also reflective of the vitamin D nutritional status of humans. Although 25,26$(OH)_2D_3$ does not have any special biological functions, it can mimic the biological actions of 1,25$(OH)_2D_3$ once it is hydroxylated in the kidney to 1,25S,26-trihydroxyvitamin D_3 (Fig. 5–12).[80,99] Although little is known about the regulation of this metabolic step, it appears that the kidney is the principal site for this metabolism.

The metabolism of 25(OH)D_3 on carbon-23 yields 23S,25-dihydroxyvitamin D_3 (Fig. 5–19).[80,99] This metabolite is apparently a precursor for an additional metabolic step that gives rise to a rather unusual metabolite that has been identified as 25-hydroxyvitamin D_3-23,26-lactone [25(OH)D_3-lactone] (Fig. 5–19).[80] This lactone is found in the circulation of humans and other animals that have received pharmacologic doses of vitamin D. Although there is no evidence that this lactone has vitamin D–like activity on either the intestine or bone, this compound is made in the kidney. It is curious that the vitamin D–binding protein recognizes this metabolite with a binding affinity that is about five to seven times greater than that for 25(OH)D_3.[38,80]

In addition to the multiple hydroxylations that can occur in the side chain, the hydroxyls can also be oxidized. 24,25$(OH)_2D_3$ and 23,25$(OH)_2D_3$ are oxidized to 24-keto-25(OH)D_3 and 23-keto-25(OH)D_3, respectively.[38,80] The multitude of hydroxylations and oxidations that 25(OH)D_3 can undergo are also seen for 1,25$(OH)_2D_3$. Therefore, the side chain of 1,25$(OH)_2D_3$ is recognized as a 25(OH)D_3 substrate and can undergo further oxidation and hydroxylation at carbon-23, carbon-24, and carbon-26 to form a number of metabolites including 1,24,25(OH)D_3; 1,25,26(OH)D_3; 24-keto-1,23,25$(OH)_3D_3$; 1,23,25$(OH)_3D_3$; and 1,25$(OH)_2D_3$-23,26-lactone.[38,50,80,100] It is believed that the metabolic importance of the side-chain modifications is for the deactivation and rapid clearance of 1,25$(OH)_2D_3$. This is particularly true for the carbon-23 oxidation, which ultimately gives rise to a biologically inactive water-soluble acid derivative known as 1α(OH)24,25,26,27-tetranor-23(COOH) vitamin D_3 (calcitroic acid).[38,50,80] To date, more than 22 metabolites of vitamin D have been structurally identified. All of these metabolites are less biologically active on a weight basis than 1,25$(OH)_2$D.

In addition to the multiple hydroxylations in the side chain, 25(OH)D_3 can have its A-ring oxidized whereby the carbon-19 is replaced with a keto group. This reaction occurs *in vivo* in ruminants and *in vitro* in chick kidney homogenates, resulting in the conversion of 25(OH)D_3 to the *cis* and *trans* isomers of 10-keto-19-nor-25-hydroxyvitamin D_3.[38,50,80]

VII. METABOLISM OF VITAMIN D_2

In the 1930s it was first appreciated that the vitamin D isolated from the irradiation of the sterol ergosterol yielded a vitamin D (vitamin D_2) that had minimum biological activity in the chicken when compared with the vitamin D (vitamin D_3) that was isolated from the irradiation of 7-dehydrocholesterol.[21-23] It is now recognized that vitamin D_2 is about 10 to 20 times less active than vitamin D_3 in the chicken. It has been assumed in mammals, including humans, that vitamin D_2 and vitamin D_3 have equal biological potency and are metabolized in identical fashion. However, it is known that in New World monkeys, as in chickens, the activities of vitamin D_2 and vitamin D_3 differ.[50] Originally, it was believed that vitamin D_2 is metabolized in a fashion identical to that of vitamin D_3. However, there are some exceptions. It is now recognized that the vitamin D–binding protein binds vitamin D_2 1.5 to 2 times less efficiently than vitamin D_3. This difference may be important because higher concentrations of the free form of vitamin D_2 can enter into the liver parenchyma and be more efficiently metabolized to $25(OH)D_2$.[50] Indeed, when a rat liver is perfused with an equal amount of vitamin D_2 and vitamin D_3, vitamin D_2 is preferentially metabolized to $25(OH)D_2$ when compared with vitamin D_3.[41] Similar to vitamin D_3, vitamin D_2 is metabolized to $25(OH)D_2$, which, in turn, is metabolized to 1,25-dihydroxyvitamin D_2, 24R,25-dihydroxyvitamin D_2, and 25S,26-dihydroxyvitamin D_2.[101] $1,25(OH)_2D_2$ is further metabolized to 1,24,25-trihydroxyvitamin D_2—a process believed to be important for the deactivation of $1,25(OH)_2D_2$.[50,102,103] Because vitamin D_2 has a methyl group at carbon-28, unlike vitamin D_3, this carbon is a target for a further hydroxylation to give rise to a variety of 28-hydroxylated metabolites, including 24,25,28-trihydroxyvitamin D_2 and 1,24,25,28-tetrahydroxyvitamin D_2.[104] The physiologic role of these metabolites remains uncertain; however, it is interesting to consider the possibility that $24,25,28(OH)_3D_2$ and $1,24,25,28(OH)_4D_2$ could be metabolized so that the carbon-28 methyl is oxidized and removed to yield a side chain that looks more like the side chain for vitamin D_3.[50]

VIII. BIOLOGICAL ACTIONS OF $1,25(OH)_2D$

A. Cellular Mechanism of Action in the Intestine

There is nearly unanimous agreement that the cellular actions of $1,25(OH)_2D$ are initiated by interaction of the hormone with a specific, high-affinity binding protein or receptor. The recent availability of anti-$1,25(OH)_2D_3$-receptor monoclonal antibodies that recognize avian[105] and mammalian receptor species[106] has added significantly to our knowledge of the $1,25(OH)_2D_3$-receptor interaction. Similar to other steroid hormones, the mammalian receptor for $1,25(OH)_2D_3$ is a rare intracellular protein. It has a molecular weight in the range of 52,000 to 56,000 daltons. It selectively binds the active metabolite of vitamin D, $1,25(OH)_2D$, with high affinity (equilibrium dissociation constant of 10^{-10} to 10^{-11} M) and binds avidly to nuclei and chromatin.[107] Although the receptor protein's hormone-binding domain is distinct and at some intramolecular distance from the DNA (nuclear)–binding domain,[108] it is apparent that these two separate regions of the protein are functionally linked; hormone binding induces a covalent modification (phosphorylation) of the receptor,[109] and increases the receptor's affinity for binding to nuclei and DNA.[110] The classic dogma for steroid hormones holds that the hormone traverses the cell membrane and binds to a receptor in the cytosol of the cell.[111] Binding of the steroid to its specific receptor "activates" the receptor and promotes binding of the receptor to acceptor sites (regulatory sequences) on nuclear DNA. Nuclear binding of the hormone-receptor complex regulates the transcription of hormone-specific mRNAs, which, in turn, govern the translation of protein. As has been recently suggested for the estrogens,[112-114] such a scenario may not be the case with $1,25(OH)_2D_3$. Autoradiographic studies employing radiolabeled $1,25(OH)_2D_3$,[115] as well as immunoperoxidase staining with anti-receptor monoclonal antibody,[116] demonstrate predominantly nuclear localization of both the hormone and the receptor in target cells. Furthermore, binding of the $1,25(OH)_2D_3$ to receptor, binding of receptor-hormone to specific DNA sequences, gene transcription, and new protein synthesis may not be a prerequisite for all of the cellular actions of $1,25(OH)_2D_3$. In the chick intestinal epithelial cell, for instance, there is evidence that receptor-bound $1,25(OH)_2D_3$ activates a unique gene sequence to stimulate transcription of a mRNA for calcium-binding protein (CaBP).[117] (See Chapter 6.) This protein is thought to be important in the transcellular transport of calcium in the intestine.[118] However, administration to animals of inhibitors of either transcription or translation, which terminate $1,25(OH)_2D_3$-directed CaBP production, will not block the $1,25(OH)_2D_3$-mediated uptake of calcium across the luminal membrane of the cell.[119,120] Time-course experiments indicate that calcium uptake by the enterocyte precedes or coincides with the synthesis of hormone-specific CaBP, further evidence that this $1,25(OH)_2D_3$ effect is not dependent on new protein synthesis. Workers have investigated the potential existence of a direct effect of $1,25(OH)_2D_3$ on the cell membrane.[121,122] They were able to demonstrate a $1,25(OH)_2D_3$-specific change in the lipid composition of the brush border membrane that either preceded or occurred simultaneously with the change in calcium transport rate across the membrane and was not affected by the administration of cycloheximide, an inhibitor of protein synthesis. Therefore, currently available evidence suggests that the interaction of $1,25(OH)_2D_3$ with a target cell may result in hormone-specific alterations in the cell at two levels, one of which is dependent on nuclear localization of the hormone-receptor complex and another that is independent of nuclear events. Recent work[123] may help provide a mechanistic explanation for the disparate modes of action of $1,25(OH)_2D_3$. Investigators have isolated two populations of $1,25(OH)_2D_3$ receptor from chick intestine, both of which possess a high binding affinity for $1,25(OH)_2D_3$. The most plentiful population of receptor (80% of the total cellular complement) is associated with the nucleus. When extracted from the nucleus, this species of receptor binds avidly to DNA cellulose. The second population is found in the cytosol of the cell. These receptors bind $1,25(OH)_2D_3$ avidly but do not bind to DNA cellulose. Therefore, although the cytosol receptor population has a high affinity for $1,25(OH)_2D_3$, it apparently lacks a DNA-binding domain. It is possible that $1,25(OH)_2D_3$ bound to the cytosol receptor may control the non–nuclear-mediated effects of the hormone, whereas interaction of the hormone with the more plentiful nuclear receptor population controls the effects of $1,25(OH)_2D_3$ that require gene transcription. Alternatively, the cytosol receptor population may represent receptor that was previously bound in nucleus and is in the process of being catabolized; the DNA-binding domain of the receptor is known to be exquisitely sensitive to proteolysis.[124]

B. Other Biological Actions of $1,25(OH)_2D_3$

In recent years there has been a considerable amount of effort directed toward identifying actions of $1,25(OH)_2D_3$ that are not directly related to maintenance of mineral ion homeostasis. The impetus for the search resulted from the identification and characterization of a specific, high-affinity receptor for $1,25(OH)_2D_3$ and from autoradiographic localization of radiolabeled $1,25(OH)_2D_3$ in a variety of tissues not previously thought to be a site for the action of the hormone (Table 5–3). It should be pointed out from the onset that most of the information on these "alternative" functions of $1,25(OH)_2D_3$ is derived from experiments performed *in vitro*. Hence, the physiologic significance, if any, of these effects of $1,25(OH)_2D_3$ in humans remains to be elucidated.

1. Differentiating and Antiproliferative Effects of $1,25(OH)_2D_3$

The first evidence that $1,25(OH)_2D_3$ possessed potent differentiating activity was provided by workers examining the effect of $1,25(OH)_2D_3$ on mouse (M-1) and human (HL–60) myeloblastic leukemia cell lines. They showed that M-1 cells and HL–60 cells could be induced to differentiate into monocyte-macrophages (Fig. 5–21).[125,126] The differentiating effect of $1,25(OH)_2D_3$ has recently been extended to normal human cells; investigators showed that under the influence of $1,25(OH)_2D_3$, mononuclear cells from human bone marrow will mature into monocytes or multinucleated macrophages *in vitro*.[127] $1,25(OH)_2D_3$ has also been shown to exert an antiproliferative effect on cultured cells. This effect of the hormone has been demonstrated in almost every animal or human cultured cell population, malignant or nonmalignant, in which it has been examined provided the cells harbor the specific receptor for $1,25(OH)_2D_3$.[50] In fact, inhibition of cell proliferation by $1,25(OH)_2D_3$ has been used as a bioassay of the $1,25(OH)_2D_3$ receptor interaction in cultured human dermal fibroblasts.[128] Preliminary, recent experimental results demonstrate that the antiproliferative effect of the hormone can be observed *in vivo*. The survival time of mice inoculated with M-1 (mouse myeloid leukemia) cells can be prolonged by administration of 1α-hydroxy-

Table 5–3. $1,25(OH)_2D_3$ Receptor Distribution Among Mammalian Tissues

Intestine	Thymus
Kidney	Lymphocytes
Bone	Monocytes-macrophages
Parathyroid	Testes
Brain	Ovary
Pituitary	Uterus
Parotid	Placenta
Pancreas	Breast
Stomach	Embryonic liver
Skin	Embryonic muscle

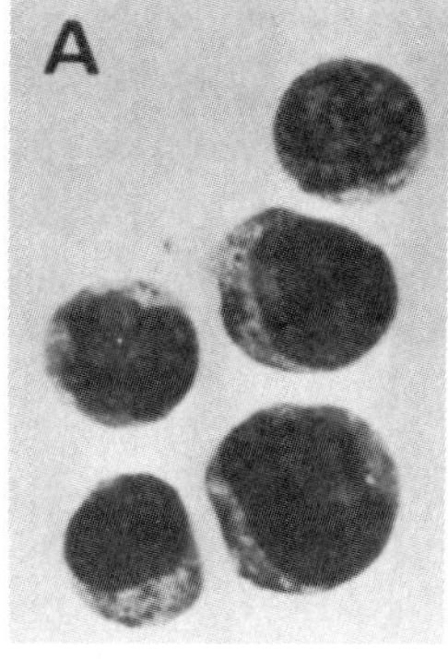

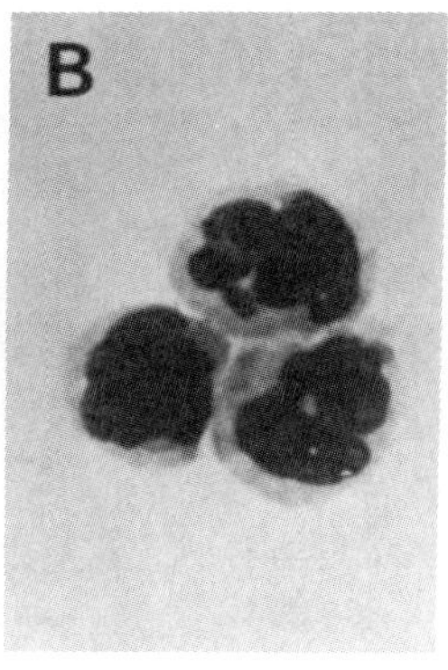

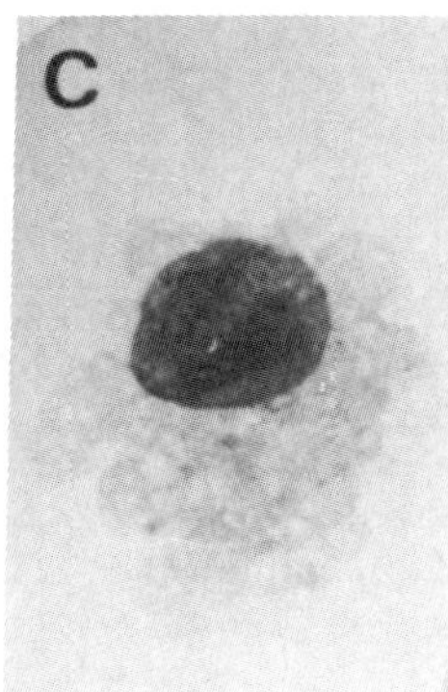

Figure 5–21. Morphologic changes in HL-60 cells, treated with vehicle (*A*), 1.2 x 10^{-8} M of $1\alpha,25(OH)_2D_3$ (*B*), or 1.0 x 10^{-9} M of TPA (*C*) for three days. Stained by the Wright-Giemsa procedures. (From Suda T, et al: Vitamin D in the differentiation of myeloid leukemia cells. *In* Kumar R (ed): Vitamin D, Basic and Clinical Aspects. Boston, Martinus Nijhoff Publishing, 1984, pp 343–363.)

vitamin D_3,[129] while growth of human $1,25(OH)_2D_3$ receptor-bearing tumor xenografts in immunoincompetent mice can be slowed by parenteral administration of $1,25(OH)_2D_3$.[130]

Inasmuch as osteoclasts, the active bone-resorbing cells in the human skeleton, are believed to originate from circulating cells of the monocyte- macrophage lineage,[131] the differentiating effects of $1,25(OH)_2D_3$ on these cells have recently received considerable attention. For instance, it is now known that $1,25(OH)_2D_3$-induced fusion of monocytes into multinucleated giant cells confers bone-resorbing potential on these cells *in vitro*.[132] Given the fact that mature chick osteoclasts lack the receptor for $1,25(OH)_2D_3$,[133] it is tempting to speculate that the action of $1,25(OH)_2D_3$ at the level of bone is to promote the maturation of monocyte-macrophage–like cells in bone into multinucleated osteoclasts (Fig. 5–22).[50,84]

2. *Immunoregulatory Effects of $1,25(OH)_2D_3$*

The presence of easily detectable numbers of receptors for $1,25(OH)_2D_3$ in mitogen- or antigen-activated human lymphocytes[134] and peripheral blood monocytes[135] suggests that

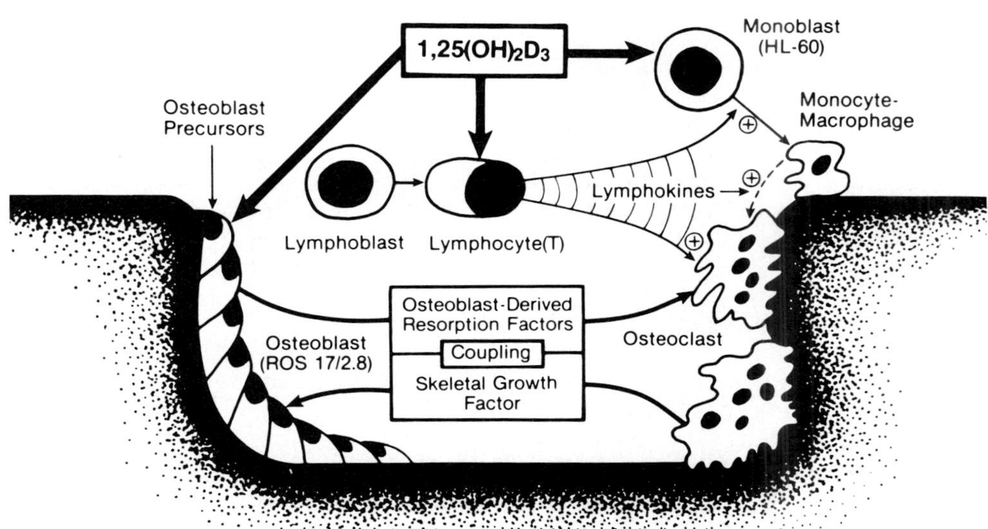

Figure 5–22. Proposed function of $1,25(OH)_2D_3$ and its receptor in bone remodeling and immunomodulation. (From Haussler MR, et al: Functions and mechanism of action of the 1,25-dihydroxyvitamin D_3 receptor. *In* Norman AW, et al (eds): Vitamin D. Berlin, de Gruyter, 1985, pp 83–92.)

that interaction of the active vitamin D metabolite with these cells may modulate the human immune response. Several laboratories[136-139] have demonstrated *in vitro* that physiologic concentrations of $1,25(OH)_2D_3$ inhibit the proliferation of activated, human peripheral blood mononuclear cells. This effect is specific for $1,25(OH)_2D_3$ [$25(OH)D_3$ and $24,25(OH)_2D_3$ are 500 to 1000 times less active], is mediated in part through inhibition of T-helper cell interleukin-2 (IL-2) production,[136,138] and results in suppression of immunoglobulin production *in vitro*.[138] Although not yet carefully examined, the immunoinhibitory effects of $1,25(OH)_2D$ in the peripheral blood of human subjects have not been detected *in vivo*. It is possible that the circulating concentration of $1,25(OH)_2D$ is quantitatively inadequate to modulate the peripheral immune response, but that the accumulation of the metabolite at certain tissue sites may be of immunologic importance in the cellular microenvironment of that tissue. For instance, workers[140] have suggested that the local production of $1,25(OH)_2D$ by resident alveolar macrophages in patients with sarcoidosis may be an important regulatory factor for lymphocyte proliferation and lymphokine production in the alveolar space of such patients. It is clear that more work in this area is required to determine whether $1,25(OH)_2D$ is an important immunoregulatory hormone in humans.

3. Effects of $1,25(OH)_2D_3$ on Skin Cells

In addition to being the source of vitamin D_3 synthesis,[27] mammalian skin also appears to be a target for the active form of the hormone. Receptors for $1,25(OH)_2D_3$ have been identified in rodent skin[141] and in cultured dermal fibroblasts and keratinocytes[128] from human hosts. Among the reported effects of $1,25(OH)_2D_3$ on cultured human cells are inhibition of proliferation of fibroblasts and keratinocytes,[128] stimulation of 7-dehydrocholesterol (provitamin D_3) synthesis,[142,143] cornification of keratinocytes,[144] and increased melanogenesis in melanoma cells.[145,146] The lack of bioeffective receptors for $1,25(OH)_2D_3$ in the developing skin of patients with vitamin D–dependent rickets type II has been suggested as a cause for the alopecia observed in some of these patients[147]; however, administration of large doses of $1,25(OH)_2D_3$ in such patients does not stimulate hair growth.[148] Most recently, oral (Fig. 5–23)[61] as well as topical administration of $1,25(OH)_2D_3$ to patients with psoriasis, a hyperproliferative disorder of the epidermis, has been shown to have remarkable therapeutic effect, suggesting that the hormone may be an effective pharmacologic agent in hyperproliferative skin disorders.[149-152]

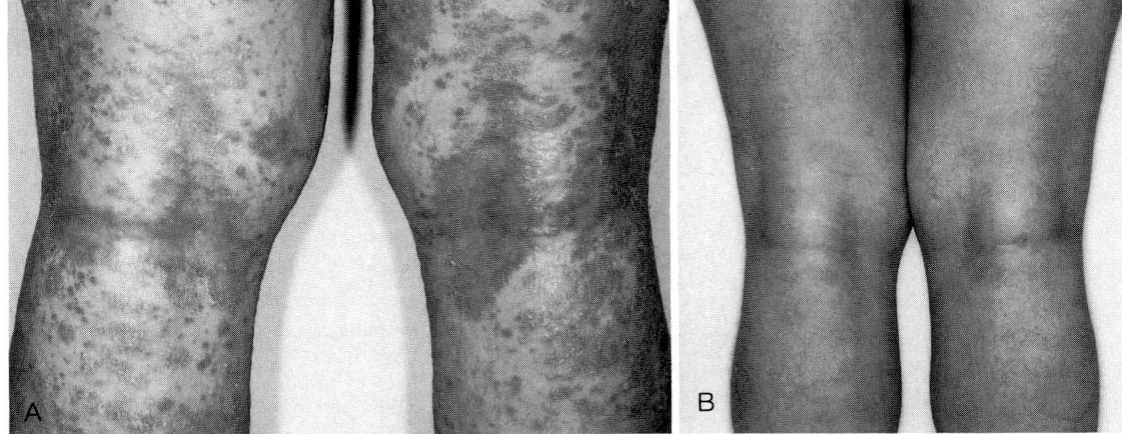

Figure 5–23. Views of the back of the legs of a female patient with erythrodermal psoriasis prior to treatment (*A*) and after 3 months of treatment with a daily oral dose of 2.0 μg of $1,25(OH)_2D_3$ (*B*). (From Holick MF: Kidney Int 32:912, 1987.)

IX. ASSAYS FOR VITAMIN D AND ITS METABOLITES

The ability to measure with precision vitamin D_2 and vitamin D_3 (collectively termed vitamin D) and their metabolites in the serum or plasma of human subjects has improved dramatically in the last 10 to 15 years. Before 1971, when the first competitive protein-binding assays for 25(OH)D were reported,[153,154] an estimate of the circulating concentration of active vitamin D metabolites was obtained solely by bioassay techniques. The "antirachitic" activity of human serum was determined by feeding a lipid extract of human serum to rats that were maintained on a high-calcium, low-phosphorus, vitamin D–deficient diet. One week later, the radii and ulnae were obtained, split, and stained with silver nitrate. The thickness of the line of new mineralization at the epiphyses "line test" was a measure of the effectiveness of the extract.[155] The ability of extracts of human serum to augment ^{45}Ca transport in the duodenum of vitamin D–deficient animals was another technique that was employed to measure vitamin D activity.[156,157] The advent of competitive protein-binding assays and the discovery that vitamin D was metabolized to more active compounds[158,159] ushered in the modern era of vitamin D metabolite assay technology. The introduction of high performance liquid chromatography (HPLC) for sample purification and the synthesis of radioligands of high specific activity are the two most important technological advances that have allowed the measurement of the less plentiful metabolites of 25(OH)D. For instance, it is now possible to detect $1,25(OH)_2D$, the active metabolite of the hormone, as low as 4.5 pg (10 fmol) in a single milliliter of serum.[160] Although the progress in assay technology has been rapid in terms of the vitamin D metabolites that have been measured, only measurements of the serum levels of 25(OH)D and $1,25(OH)_2D$ have been shown to be of clinical utility.

For that reason, particular attention will be paid to a description of the methods and significance of assaying these two metabolites and only brief mention will be made of the measurement of vitamin D and some of its other metabolites.

A. Assay Techniques

1. Measurement of Vitamin D_2 and Vitamin D_3

Quantitation of vitamin D_2 and vitamin D_3 in the serum is an arduous task and, at the present time, provides little useful information to the clinician. Because vitamin D_2 and vitamin D_3 are less polar than their hydroxylated metabolites, they cannot be purified or adequately resolved from one another on normal-phase HPLC. Therefore, if direct quantitation of vitamin D_2 and vitamin D_3 is desired, at least 2 ml of serum must be extracted and the lipid extract subjected to preparative open-column chromatography prior to purification on reverse-phase HPLC and quantitation on straight-phase HPLC (Table 5–4).[161-163] Although serial determinations of the vitamin D_3 concentrations may provide an index of the amount of vitamin D_3 synthesized in the skin after exposure to UV-B radiation (Fig. 5–7),[33] it is not an adequate measure of the vitamin D status of the individual. This is simplified in Figure 5–24, which shows the serum vitamin D concentrations in a group of normal subjects, all of whom had a normal serum concentration of 25(OH)D, who were sampled once during the summer and again in the winter. Because of the rapid disappearance of vitamin D from the serum,[33] the serum vitamin D concentration is variable and unpredictable. It may even be low in the summer if the person was not recently exposed to a significant amount of sunlight. However, there is now evidence suggesting that the serum vitamin D_2 level

Table 5–4. Indications for Assay

25(OH)D	Vitamin D deficiency Intoxication with exogenously administered vitamin D or $25(OH)D_3$ Following therapy with exogenously administered vitamin D or $25(OH)D_3$
$1,25(OH)_2D$	Vitamin D–dependent rickets, type I Vitamin D–dependent rickets, type II Hypercalcemia of sarcoidosis and other granulomatous diseases Humoral hypercalcemia associated with lymphoma Intoxication with exogenously administered $1\alpha(OH)D_3$ and $1,25(OH)_2D_3$ Absorptive hypercalciuria Idiopathic hypercalcemia of infancy (Williams syndrome) Renal failure

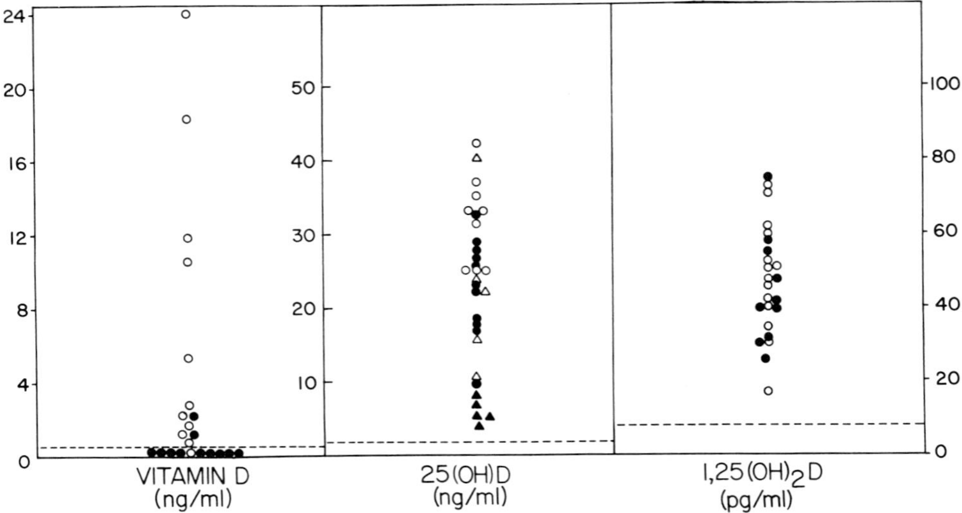

Figure 5–24. Distribution of circulating concentrations of vitamin D, 25(OH)D, and 1,25$(OH)_2$D in healthy subjects determined in the authors' laboratory. Vitamin D and 25(OH)D values determined in subjects during summer months (open symbols) were higher than those determined during winter months (closed symbols), whereas no seasonal variation was apparent for 1,25$(OH)_2$D concentration. Elderly adults (triangles) (aged 50 to 80 years) had significantly lower 25(OH)D concentrations than those in younger adults (circles). (From Clemens TL, Holick MF, Anast CS, Gray TK (eds): Perinatal Calcium and Phosphorus Metabolism. New York, Elsevier, 1983, pp 1–23.)

may be useful in judging the adequacy of absorption of an oral dose of 50,000 IU of vitamin D_2 (see Section III for details), thus providing a sensitive index of intestinal fat absorption and chylomicron formation.[36,164]

2. *Measurement of 25-Hydroxyvitamin D_2 and 25-Hydroxyvitamin D_3*

As shown in Table 5–4, the approach to determination of the 25(OH)D concentration may be varied, depending on the clinical situation and whether it is important to know the relative contributions of 25$(OH)D_3$ and 25$(OH)D_2$ to the overall circulating concentration of 25(OH)D. In assays not employing HPLC with direct UV absorbance for detection, a 25(OH)D concentration can be obtained easily from a few hundred microliters of serum. In all routine 25(OH)D assays, regardless of the method of detection, lipid extraction of the serum is necessary to dislodge the compound from the protein constituents of the serum that bind 25(OH)D. Lipid extraction for the 25(OH)D assay can be accomplished with a variety of solvents including chloroform and methanol,[165] methylene chloride and methanol,[166] diethyl ether,[167] acetonitrile,[168] or simply absolute ethanol.[169] The crude lipid extract may then be placed directly into a competitive protein-binding assay with some form of the serum vitamin D–binding protein (DBP) and [^{3}H]25$(OH)D_3$ as the displaceable ligand. Most 25(OH)D assays employ whole serum from vitamin D–deficient rats as a source of binding protein.[153,170] However, since only about 1% of the total binding sites on DBP are occupied by vitamin D or its metabolites, even in the vitamin D–sufficient state, serum from a vitamin D–replete animal can be used without significantly altering the sensitivity of the assay.

Obviously, whole lipid extracts will contain the total lipid complement of serum in addition to vitamin D, 25(OH)D, and other vitamin D metabolites. Therefore, it is not surprising that crude extracts containing 24,25$(OH)_2$D, 25,26$(OH)_2$D, and 25$(OH)D_3$-23,26-lactone, all of which are bound with high affinity by DBP,[171] as well as other non–vitamin D lipids that can bind to DBP yield values that are proportionately higher than values obtained after chromatography of the lipid extract.[172] Hence, a clearly low or undetectable value for 25(OH)D in a nonchromatographic assay is indicative of vitamin D deficiency; however, a value in the low-normal range in such an assay does not exclude vitamin D deficiency. Preparative chromatography of the lipid extract on silicic acid[154] or LH–20 Sephadex[173] to isolate a 25(OH)D-containing fraction of the extract prior to assay provides a more accurate estimate of the serum concentration of 25(OH)D. Further chromatography on normal-phase HPLC can be employed to separate $25(OH)D_2$ and $25(OH)D_3$ so that the two metabolites can be assayed independently.[174] It should be emphasized that the mammalian DBP does not significantly discriminate between $25(OH)D_3$ and $25(OH)D_2$, so $[^3H]25(OH)D_3$ may be the radioligand used in assaying either of the 25(OH)D metabolites. The truest possible estimate of the total $25(OH)D_2$ and $25(OH)D_3$ concentration is obtained by direct quantitation of the metabolites by a sensitive UV detector (coupled to an HPLC).[161,174,175] Inasmuch as the lower limits of detection by such an assay are in the range of 2 to 5 ng, direct quantitation of $25(OH)D_2$ and $25(OH)D_3$ requires the extraction of a larger volume of serum (2–5 ml), especially if the patient is thought to have vitamin D deficiency. Measurement of the $25(OH)D_2$ is of some clinical importance in the patient taking a multivitamin preparation containing vitamin D_2. Since the hepatic microsomal vitamin D-25-hydroxylase does not distinguish between vitamin D_2 and vitamin D_3 as substrates,[176] a low circulating concentration of $25(OH)D_3$ in such an individual may indicate that endogenous vitamin D_3 synthesis is deficient and that the patient is dependent on dietary or therapeutic supplements of vitamin D_2 to achieve an adequate vitamin D nutritional status. It should be noted, however, that in the United States foods are supplemented with either vitamin D_2 or vitamin D_3, and measurement of $25(OH)D_2$ and $25(OH)D_3$ cannot be used as a method for determining the source of vitamin D.

3. Measurement of 1,25-Dihydroxyvitamin D

The first serum assay for $1,25(OH)_2D$ was reported in 1974[177] just three years after the structural identification of $1,25(OH)D_3$ as the active metabolite of vitamin D_3.[178-180] The key to development of the assay was the detection of a high-affinity, low-capacity binding protein (receptor) in chick intestinal epithelium that could be employed as a specific binding protein in a radioligand binding assay.[181] The original assay required extraction of a large volume of serum (20 ml) and three separate chromatographic purification steps before assay and was sensitive to only 50 pg/tube. In recent years the availability of tracers of high specific activity, the application of sophisticated chromatography for sample purification, and the use of techniques to promote receptor stability have combined to greatly improve sample preparation and the analysis. The $1,25(OH)_2D$ assay is now available in most university hospitals and through several commercial laboratories. Although the assay for $1,25(OH)_2D$ in patients' serum or plasma is obtained with relative ease, there exists significant variability in its performance and there are caveats in its application to human health or disease (see section IX-B).

A purified lipid extract of human serum or plasma can be analyzed for its content of $1,25(OH)_2D$ in a variety of ways (Table 5–4). The classic binding protein in the competitive protein-binding assay for $1,25(OH)_2D$ is the hormone's own receptor protein isolated from intestinal epithelium of vitamin D–deficient chicks. Vitamin D–deficient birds are employed in order to improve the extraction of receptor that is not occupied by endogenously synthesized $1,25(OH)_2D$. A disadvantage in the use of the chick intestinal receptor in the binding assay is that it discriminates against $1,25(OH)_2D_2$ binding in favor of $1,25(OH)_2D_3$. Therefore, these two metabolites, which are biologically equipotent in humans, cannot be measured with comparable efficiency. This may account for the reports that the chick receptor assay underestimates the $1,25(OH)_2D_2$ concentration by 23% to 60%.[182-184] This failure is a significant liability when determining the serum concentration of $1,25(OH)_2D$ in patients relying on ingested vitamin D_2 for their vitamin D nutrition. These problems have been resolved with the increased use of the receptor derived from calf thymus, which binds $1,25(OH)_2D_3$ and $1,25(OH)_2D_2$ with equivalent affinity and capacity.[185] In fact, this assay can now be employed for the measurement of $1,25(OH)_2D$ in lipid extracts of small quantities of human serum (0.5–1.0 ml) after purification on a single silica cartridge.[186]

Several radioimmunoassays have been developed for detection of $1,25(OH)_2D$ in the serum.[187-191] Although potentially advantageous, radioimmunoassays suffer two major drawbacks. First, similar to the chick intestinal receptor, many antibodies raised against $1,25(OH)_2D_3$ analogues bind $1,25(OH)_2D_2$ less avidly than $1,25(OH)_2D_3$; therefore the radioimmunoassays suffer from an inability to determine accurately the $1,25(OH)_2D_2$ contribution to the overall $1,25(OH)_2D$ concentration. Second, antibodies raised against $1,25(OH)_2D_3$ exhibit cross reactivity with other vitamin D metabolites. Both of these deficiencies are related to the immunogen, which is usually a derivative of $1,25(OH)_2D_3$ conjugated to bovine serum albumin through the side chain of the molecule or in the A-ring at the carbon 3 position. The lack of good immunogen is undoubtedly the explanation for the failure of workers to develop a good antibody against the hormone.[187-191]

Stern et al.[192,193] have developed a very sensitive bioassay for $1,25(OH)_2D$ that measures the release of ^{45}Ca from prelabeled rat ulna and tibia maintained in organ culture. Although relatively labor-intensive by current standards, the bioassay does allow one to quantitate the biological effectiveness of a vitamin D metabolite or analogue. The cytoreceptor assay of Manolagas et al.[194,195] employs intact, receptor-possessing renal osteogenic sarcoma (ROS) cells and has the advantage of obviating the need for extensive chromatographic purification of the sample prior to assay. During the cytoreceptor assay, the ROS cells are incubated in an extracellular medium containing DBP, which binds $1,25(OH)_2D$ with less affinity than many of the contaminating vitamin D metabolites; this leaves relatively more $1,25(OH)_2D$ free to enter the ROS cells and to bind to its own high-affinity, intracellular receptor.

4. Measurement of 24,25-Dihydroxyvitamin D

Owing to the high affinity of DBP for $24,25(OH)_2D$,[196] this metabolite can be readily detected with ease in a competitive protein-binding assay (Table 5–4). However, $24,25(OH)_2D_2$ is bound two or three times less avidly than is $24,25(OH)_2D_3$,[197,198] making an estimation of the overall $24,25(OH)_2D$ concentration misleading in a person ingesting significant amounts of vitamin D_2. Accurate estimation of the total $24,25(OH)_2D$ concentration must, therefore, employ chromatographic techniques that resolve $24,25(OH)_2D_2$ and $24,25(OH)_2D_3$ and binding assays that use the appropriate radioinert metabolite in a standard curve. Recently, the use of a methylene chloride–isopropanol solvent system on a cyano-bonded μ-silica HPLC column has been shown to be capable of separating $24,25(OH)_2D_2$ and $25(OH)D_3$-23,26-lactone,[199] two metabolites of $25(OH)D_3$ that co-migrate with $24,25(OH)_2D$ on normal-phase HPLC μ-silica columns developed in hexane-isopropanol. It might be questioned whether determination of the circulating $24,25(OH)_2D$ concentration warrants the effort required. Although suggested by a number of investigators,[94,200] a physiologic role for $24,25(OH)_2D$ in human mineral metabolism has not been unequivocally demonstrated (see section VI-A). Until more convincing data are available, routine assay of $24,25(OH)_2D$ cannot be advocated.

5. Other Vitamin D Metabolites

In recent years the measurement of two additional metabolites, $25,26(OH)_2D$ and the $25(OH)D$-23,26-lactone, has been extensively investigated. For both, HPLC purification of the serum lipid extract is required prior to detection in a DBP-based competitive protein-binding assay (Table 5–4). Neither metabolite has been shown to be of physiologic significance in humans. In fact, the $25(OH)D_3$-23,26-lactone, a renal metabolite of $23,25(OH)_2D_3$,[201] is detected in human serum only in states of vitamin D excess. The significance of the extraordinarily high affinity of DBP for the lactone is not currently known. High circulating concentrations of this metabolite can theoretically displace $25(OH)D$ and $1,25(OH)_2D$ from the DBP, thereby facilitating the binding of these metabolites to the cellular receptor for $1,25(OH)_2D$ *in vivo*.[202]

B. Clinical Utility of the 25(OH)D and $1,25(OH)_2D$ Assays (Table 5–4)

1. 25(OH)D Assay

The 25(OH)D concentration is the test of choice for determining the adequacy of vitamin D nutrition from either endogenous or exogenous sources.[2,50] A very low or undetectable value in the competitive protein binding assay is indicative of (1) deficient substrate for the hepatic vitamin D-25-hydroxylase; (2) disease or hormone-related alteration in the activity of the hepatic vitamin D-25-hydroxylase; (3) failure to synthesize DBP or loss of DBP-bound 25(OH)D; or (4) accelerated catabolism of 25(OH)D. The first may result from diminished cutaneous sunlight exposure of the patient or from a combination of deficient sunlight exposure and intestinal malabsorption of vitamin D in persons consuming a diet supplemented with vitamin D. In either case, it is important to point out that deficient endogenous synthesis of vitamin D is required for vitamin D deficiency to occur. Clements et al.[203] recently reported that after oral or intravenous administration, neither vitamin D nor 25(OH)D undergoes significant enterohepatic circulation, precluding the possibility that one can become vitamin D– or 25(OH)D–deficient in the presence of adequate production of vitamin D_3 in the skin. A number of hepatocellular diseases can contribute to 25(OH)D deficiency in patients in whom the availability of substrate, vitamin D_2, or vitamin D_3 is compromised. However, it is unusual to encounter 25(OH)D deficiency in patients who are vitamin D–sufficient except for patients with severe liver disease,[44] because the "free" 25(OH)D concentration in such individuals is usually not altered.[204] Because human DBP is an alpha globulin with a relatively low molecular weight (58,000 daltons; albumin m.w. = 69,000), it is lost through the glomerular basement membrane in patients with nephrotic syndrome. The total serum concentration of 25(OH)D in such patients is directly correlated with the degree of proteinuria, and is expected to be low in patients with greater than 4 g of proteinuria per day.[46] Although patients with protein-losing enteropathies or severe burns may be subject to loss of DBP, 25(OH)D deficiency in such settings is rarely due to only a loss of DBP through the gastrointestinal tract or skin. Finally, in principle at least, the potential exists for accelerated 25(OH)D clearance from the serum as a cause for diminished circulating concentrations of the metabolite. It is known that administration of pharmacologic doses of $1,25(OH)_2D_3$ will accelerate $25(OH)D_3$ clearance in experimental animals[205] and ameliorate the increase in the serum 25(OH)D concentration in humans[43] given large daily doses of vitamin D_2 orally.

An assessment of the adequacy of therapy and patient compliance with therapy with vitamin D_3, vitamin D_2, or $25(OH)D_3$ in patients requiring vitamin D supplementation (i.e., hypoparathyroidism) can be made by following the serum concentrations of 25(OH)D. Therapy in most cases is aimed at maintaining the 25(OH)D level in the high-normal range, usually between 25 and 45 ng/ml.[2] Because 25(OH)D is bound with high affinity by the serum DBP, it has a long serum half-life with estimates ranging from 12 to 60 days.[2] Its prolonged half-life makes infrequent measurements of the serum 25(OH)D concentration (every 2 to 3 months) adequate for monitoring therapy in the noncompliant patient. Measurement of the 25(OH)D concentration is also the test of choice in establishing the diagnosis of vitamin D intoxication from ingestion or parenteral administration of vitamin D or $25(OH)D_3$. Ingestion of large quantities of vitamin D may result in 25-hydroxylation of vitamin D by hepatic mitochondria,[206-208] which possess a vitamin D-25-hydroxylase of lower affinity for vitamin D ($K_m = 10^{-6}$ M) than hepatic microsomes ($K_m = 10^{-8}$ M)[208,209] but a greater capacity for conversion of vitamin D to 25(OH)D.[210] The low-affinity, high-capacity mitochondrial system[211] does not appear to be product-inhibitable as is its microsomal counterpart[211] and is, therefore, capable of prolific 25(OH)D generation given enough substrate. Interestingly, in normal human subjects, excessive exposure to sunlight will not result in vitamin D_3 intoxication, because only a limited amount of vitamin D_3 will be formed in the skin (see section II-B); with continued photon bombardment of the skin, previtamin D_3 will be preferentially converted to two nonbiologically active photoisomers, tachysterol and lumisterol (Fig. 5–3) and vitamin D_3 is degraded to 5,6-*trans*-vitamin D_3 and suprasterols 1 and 2 (Fig. 5–5).

2. $1,25(OH)_2D$ Assay

In the authors' view there are few clinical circumstances in which a single determination of the serum concentration of $1,25(OH)_2D$, a metabolite with a circulating half-life of only 4 to 6 hours, will be of diagnostic value (Table 5–5). The finding of a very low or undetectable serum $1,25(OH)_2D$ concentration in a rachitic child with a normal or elevated serum concentration of 25(OH)D is indicative of vitamin D–dependent rickets type I, an inheritable defect, or

Table 5–5. Assay of Vitamin D and Vitamin D Metabolites

	Purification		Detection			
Sterol	*LPLC*	*HPLC*	*UV*	*CPBA*	*RIA*	*BIO*
Vitamin D	X	X	X			
	X	X		X		
25(OH)D				X		
	X			X		
	X	X	X			
	X	X		X		
$1,25(OH)_2D$	X			X		
	X	X		X		
	X	X			X	
	X	X				X
$24,25(OH)_2D$	X	X	X			
$25,26(OH)_2D$	X	X	X			
25(OH)D-23,26-lactone	X	X	X			

LPLC, open column (low pressure) liquid chromatography; HPLC, high performance liquid chromatography; UV, assay by ultraviolet light absorbance on HPLC; CPBA, competitive protein-binding assay; RIA, radioimmunoassay; BIO, bioassay.

absence of the renal 25(OH)D-1α-hydroxylase.[212] A very high circulating concentration of $1,25(OH)_2D$ in a rachitic child on vitamin D therapy is indicative of end-organ unresponsiveness to $1,25(OH)_2D$ and the diagnosis of vitamin D–dependent rickets type II.[213]

A high value for the $1,25(OH)_2D$ assay may occur in patients intoxicated with either dihydrotachysterol (DHT), 1α-hydroxyvitamin D_3 [$1a\alpha(OH)D_3$], or $1,25(OH)_2D_3$.[50] Intoxication with the former compounds is dependent to a great extent on hepatic 25-hydroxylation of DHT and of $1\alpha(OH)D_3$ to 25-hydroxydihydrotachysterol and $1,25(OH)_2D_3$, respectively, which cross-react with the $1,25(OH)_2D$ receptor. A frankly elevated or high-normal serum $1,25(OH)_2D$ concentration in a hypercalcemic patient with sarcoidosis,[72,214] tuberculosis,[215] silicone-induced granulomatous disease,[216] disseminated candidiasis,[217] or lymphoma[75-78] represents inappropriate endogenous production of the hormone in the presence of hypercalcemia (also see section V-C). The autonomous, extrarenal synthesis of $1,25(OH)_2D$ in sarcoidosis is almost always associated with extensive disease and high-intensity alveolitis.[218,219] The finding of an inappropriately high circulating $1,25(OH)_2D$ concentration in such a patient with granulomatous disease or lymphoma portends an excellent calcium-lowering effect with glucocorticoid therapy. In an older individual with suspected granulomatous disease or lymphoma, the failure of glucocorticoids to lower the serum $1,25(OH)_2D$ and calcium concentration within a few days strongly suggests the presence of a coexistent hypercalcemia-causing disease (i.e., primary hyperparathyroidism). Extrarenal $1,25(OH)_2D$ synthesis by the placenta will elevate the total and "free" concentration (that fraction of the total serum concentration not bound by a circulating binding protein) of $1,25(OH)_2D$ in the serum during the third trimester of pregnancy.[220,221]

A meaningful interpretation of the serum $1,25(OH)_2D$ concentration in states of vitamin D deficiency is difficult. It may be increased, decreased, or normal, depending on the circumstances in which the sample is obtained. This is illustrated in Figure 5–7. Shown are the serum concentrations of vitamin D, 25(OH)D, and $1,25(OH)_2D$ obtained in serial fashion from normal subjects and three hypocalcemic, vitamin D–deficient patients after exposure to UV-B radiation.[33] In the preirradiation period, the $1,25(OH)_2D$ concentration in the vitamin D–deficient subjects was normal; although normal, the level is inappropriately low in the presence of hypocalcemia. All three patients had secondary hyperparathyroidism, which accelerated their renal 25(OH)D-1α-hydroxylase in order to generate more active hormone from less substrate, 25(OH)D. In the absence of secondary hyperparathyroidism, their $1,25(OH)_2D$ levels would most certainly be lower. After synthesis of vitamin D in their skin in response to exposure to UV-B radiation, there was a small, gradual increase in the 25(OH)D concentration (30%), but a prompt and prolific increase in the $1,25(OH)_2D$ concentration (2- to 3-fold) into the supraphysiologic range. Therefore, in a patient with a low serum concentration of 25(OH)D, the serum concentration of 1,25$(OH)_2$D is dependent not only on the degree of stimulation of the renal 1α-hydroxylase by PTH, but also on the timing and amount of vitamin D entering the metabolic pathway.

Obtaining serial values for 1,25$(OH)_2$D in a single individual after a provocative stimulus to endogenous 1,25$(OH)_2$D synthesis is currently being investigated in various clinical settings (for example, postmenopausal osteoporosis).[69,222,223] However, at present, these techniques require frequent sampling and often prolonged stimulation of the renal 25(OH)D-1α-hydroxylase, such as a 6- to 12-hour infusion of hPTH(1–34), in order to measure a significant effect on the serum 1,25$(OH)_2$D concentration (Fig. 5–17). For the sake of practicality, the provocative tests are not yet a clinically useful tool, but they may become so in the future.

C. The Use of Vitamin D Assays in the Evaluation of the Hypocalcemic and Hypercalcemic/Hypercalciuric Patient

When confronted with a hypocalcemic patient, it is useful to consider whether the reduction in the serum ionized calcium concentration is due to deficiency in one or both of the calcemic hormones, 1,25$(OH)_2$D and PTH. In the case of the former hormone, measurement of the serum 25(OH)D concentration provides the most valuable information in the majority of cases. Owing to its long serum half-life, a 25(OH)D measurement provides an excellent index of the amount of vitamin D that is metabolized in the liver and the amount of substrate [25(OH)D] available for synthesis of the active metabolite, 1,25$(OH)_2$D. In the hypocalcemic patient, a frankly low 25(OH)D level almost always indicates deficient cutaneous synthesis and dietary intake of vitamin D. Patients with severe hepatocellular disease or nephrotic syndrome may have a low total serum calcium and 25(OH)D concentration due to either a decrease in hepatic synthesis or urinary loss of proteins that bind calcium (albumin, prealbumin) and 25(OH)D (DBP, albumin, lipoproteins) in the circulation. In such cases, a low serum concentration of ionized calcium and a compensatory elevation in the circulating PTH concentration may aid in establishing the presence of true ("free") 25(OH)D deficiency. Hypocalcemia with a normal or elevated 25(OH)D level points either to deficiency or decreased bioeffectiveness of PTH, an acquired abnormality in the metabolism of 25(OH)D to 1,25$(OH)_2$D (i.e., renal failure), an inherited defect in 1,25$(OH)_2$D synthesis, or a defect in the action of 1,25$(OH)_2$D at its target tissues. The last two situations, both rare, can usually be distinguished on biochemical grounds by the circulating 1,25$(OH)_2$D concentration, which will be low or nondetectable in patients with vitamin D–dependent rickets type I, and often dramatically increased in patients with vitamin D–dependent rickets type II.[2,50] In patients with hypocalcemia and diminished synthesis, release, or end-organ effectiveness of PTH (i.e., patients with hypoparathyroidism, magnesium deficiency, or pseudohypoparathyroidism), the 1,25$(OH)_2$D concentration will be inappropriately low. This is due to the lack of a stimulatory effect of PTH on the renal 25(OH)D-1α-hydroxylase and the inhibitory effect of hyperphosphatemia, a usual consequence of hypoparathyroidism, on the same enzyme. However, because of overlap of the serum 1,25$(OH)_2$D concentration into the normal range in such patients, measurement of this metabolite is not particularly helpful in establishing the diagnosis of hypoparathyroidism.

Whereas the 25(OH)D assay has a central role in the evaluation of the hypocalcemic patient, the utility of this assay in the workup of a hypercalcemic patient is limited. Only if 25(OH)D is present in high concentrations in the circulation and it (or its metabolites) binds to the high-affinity receptor for 1,25$(OH)_2$D is it capable of inducing hypercalcemia. Intoxication from an exogenous source may arise after ingestion of large amounts of vitamin D or 25$(OH)D_3$, whereas intoxication with endogenously synthesized 25(OH)D may be the etiologic explanation for the idiopathic hypercalcemia of infancy. The latter, referred to as the Williams syndrome when accompanied by the phenotypic markers of supravalvular aortic stenosis, elfin facies, and mental retardation, is a rare disorder that has been associated with an exaggerated increase in the serum concentration of 25(OH)D in response to a challenge with orally administered vitamin D_2.[223] These children have also been shown to possess inappropriately elevated serum concentrations of 1,25$(OH)_2$D.[224] In 25(OH)D intoxication, from either an exogenous or endogenous source, the serum 1,25$(OH)_2$D concentration may be normal or even reduced unless there is some additional abnormality in the regulation of the 1α-hydroxylation of 25(OH)D. As alluded to previously, normal individuals do not become vitamin D [25(OH)D] intoxicated from endogenously synthesized vitamin D. Lifeguards, for instance, may develop circulating 25(OH)D concentrations that are well above the normal range (> 100 ng/ml) but do not develop hypercalcemia or hypercalciuria.[203]

The usefulness of the 1,25$(OH)_2$D assay in evaluating a patient with hypercalcemia and/or hypercalciuria is, for the most part, restricted to patients with suppressed PTH secretion; an elevation in the serum 1,25$(OH)_2$D concentration is an expected accompaniment of primary hyperparathyroidism (unless renal failure is present), and there is little need for it to be measured when that diagnosis is certain or highly likely. (See Chapter 14.) Therefore, an inappropriate elevation in the serum 1,25$(OH)_2$D concentration and a suppressed plasma PTH concentration in a hypercalciuric/hypercalcemic patient is highly suggestive of (1) exogenous intoxication with 1α$(OH)D_3$, DHT, or 1,25$(OH)_2D_3$; (2) endogenous intoxication with 1,25$(OH)_2$D as may occur in sarcoidosis, other granulomatous diseases, and lymphoma; or (3) absorptive hypercalciuria[225] (see Chapter 22).

Determination of the serum 1,25$(OH)_2$D concentration may be of help in discerning the presence of primary hyperparathyroidism in patients who are suspected to harbor the disease but in whom confirmatory laboratory data are lacking. It should also be recognized that a frankly elevated serum 1,25$(OH)_2$D concentration may not be present in a hypercalcemic/hypercalciuric patient with concomitant hepatocellular disease or nephrotic proteinuria resulting in diminished production or loss of serum proteins that bind 1,25$(OH)_2$D. Although the "total" concentration of the hormone may be relatively low in such cases, the "free" concentration of 1,25$(OH)_2$D, which can adequately be determined from a knowledge of the serum albumin and DBP levels,[226] will be higher than normal.

X. CONCLUSION

As recently as 20 years ago, vitamin D was considered to be "just another one of those fat-soluble vitamins." The revelation that vitamin D must be hydroxylated in the liver and kidney to 1,25$(OH)_2$D before it is biologically active opened a new chapter for vitamin D research, and clinical medicine. The finding that the kidney was responsible for the final activation step for vitamin D metabolism provided a new insight into the cause of vitamin D resistance that was often associated with patients who suffered from chronic renal failure. The availability of reliable assays for the measurement of the circulating concentration of 25(OH)D and 1,25$(OH)_2$D has led to the identification of inborn and acquired disorders in 25(OH)D metabolism. These assays have provided new insights into the cause of a variety of hypo- and hypercalcemic disorders including vitamin D–dependent rickets types I and II,[233] primary hyperparathyroidism, and tumor-induced hypercalcemia associated with certain lymphomas and chronic granulomatous disorders. The knowledge of the crucial role of the kidney's metabolic conversion of 25(OH)D to 1,25$(OH)_2$D prompted the chemical synthesis of this kidney hormone and its 25-deoxy analogue, 1α-hydroxyvitamin D_3. These drugs have provided the clinician with an effective means for the treatment of a variety of hypocalcemic disorders that are caused by acquired and inborn errors in the metabolism of 25(OH)D to 1,25$(OH)_2$D.

The discovery of a rare intracellular protein (receptor) that binds 1,25$(OH)_2$D with high affinity and specificity has greatly advanced our understanding of the cellular mode of action of the hormone. In the 1970s the observation that a variety of tissues and cells (that are not classic target tissues for vitamin D) possessed nuclear receptors for 1,25$(OH)_2D_3$ opened up a new and exciting chapter in the evolving vitamin D story. It was found that such diverse tissues as the brain, parathyroid gland, gonad, thymus, pancreas, and skin had high-affinity, low-capacity nuclear receptors for 1,25$(OH)_2$D (Table 5–3). In addition, several circulating mononuclear cell populations including monocytes and activated B and T lymphocytes possessed receptors for this hormone. The initial reaction to these observations was that this was an epiphenomenon with little biological importance.

However, the observation that $1,25(OH)_2D$ could induce differentiation of $1,25(OH)_2D_3$ receptor-positive promyelocytic leukemic cells generated an enormous amount of interest regarding the potential biological effects of $1,25(OH)_2D$ on "nonclassical" target tissues. *In vivo* and *in vitro* studies have revealed that $1,25(OH)_2D$ can inhibit the proliferation and induce cellular differentiation of $1,25(OH)_2D_3$ receptor-positive cells and enhance or inhibit the synthesis and secretion of a variety of hormones, growth factors, and immunoglobulins. The physiologic importance of $1,25(OH)_2D$ on (1) regulating hormone secretion, (2) inducing maturation of a variety of tissues including the skin, (3) altering immune function, and (4) affecting myocardial activity is unknown. However, it is known that patients with vitamin D–dependent rickets type II or simple vitamin D deficiency do not have overt alterations in their immune systems, cardiac function, skin appearance, or hormone responsiveness to provocative stimulation.

Thus, although it is unlikely that $1,25(OH)_2D$ is essential for the normal functioning of these tissues, the observation that $1,25(OH)_2D$ can alter the biochemistry and physiology of receptor-positive tumor and normal cells has wide-ranging pharmacologic and physiologic applications. For example, the findings that parathyroid glands possess nuclear receptors for $1,25(OH)_2D_3$ and that *in vitro* $1,25(OH)_2D_3$ inhibits the expression of the parathyroid hormone gene[227] led to the intravenous use of $1,25(OH)_2D_3$ as a method to suppress parathyroid hormone secretion in chronic renal failure patients with marked secondary hyperparathyroidism (Fig. 5–25).[228] The observation that circulating monocytes possess receptors for $1,25(OH)_2D_3$ and differentiate into osteoclast-like cells when exposed to this hormone has prompted the concept that $1,25(OH)_2$ may be important for the mobilization of stem cells for the bone remodeling process (Fig. 5–22).

Initially it was thought that $1,25(OH)_2D$ would have great potential as an antitumor agent. However, it is now known that antimitogenic activity of $1,25(OH)_2D_3$ is reversible[229] and that tumor clones that have a decreased number of receptors for this hormone are resistant to its antimitogenic activity. Furthermore, when the hormone is given in pharmacologic doses, it causes severe hypercalcemia.[230] Despite these problems, $1,25(OH)_2D_3$ may be of great pharmacologic value, especially for dermatology. Unlike

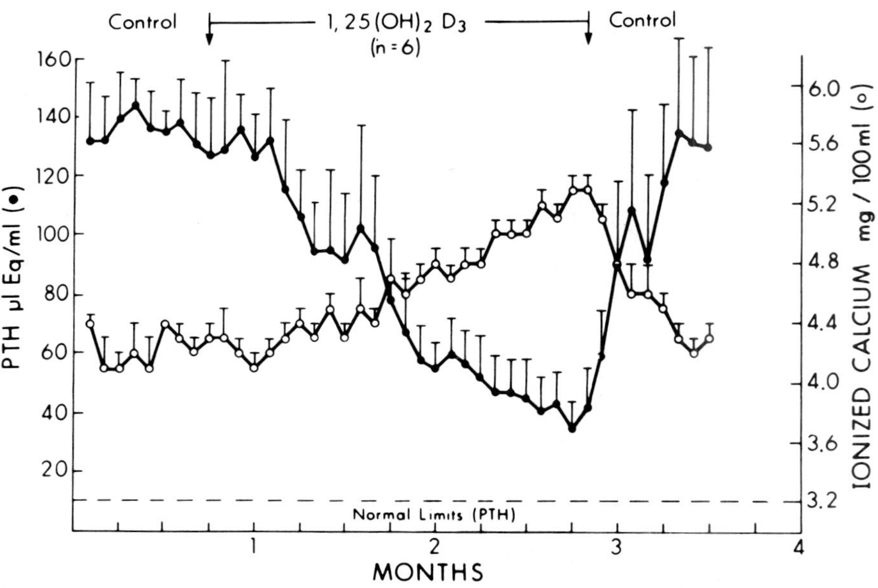

Figure 5–25. Temporal relationships between ionized calcium and serum iPTH, before, during, and after intravenous $1,25(OH)_2D_3$ administration in patients with moderate hyperparathyroidism. The maximum decrement in iPTH was 73.5%. In the first three weeks of treatment with $1,25(OH)_2D_3$ there was no change in ionized calcium; however, serum iPTH decreased from 132 ± 20 to 90 ± 20 µlEq/ml. (From Slatopolsky E, et al: J Clin Invest 74:2136, 1984. By copyright permission of the American Society for Clinical Investigation.)

tumor cells that can dedifferentiate when $1,25(OH)_2D_3$ is removed from their environment, when $1,25(OH)_2D_3$ induces human keratinocytes to differentiate, it does so in an irreversible manner. One practical application is the effective use of $1,25(OH)_2D_3$ for the treatment of hyperproliferative skin disorders such as psoriasis.

It is well documented that $1,25(OH)_2D_3$ causes many if not most of its biological effects by a nuclear-mediated mechanism. However, there is intriguing evidence that in some cells $1,25(OH)_2D$ may also increase intracellular calcium concentrations and alter phosphoinositol metabolism in both receptor-positive and -negative cells.[231,232] Thus, it may be possible to develop analogues of $1,25(OH)_2D_3$ that have selective effects on the plasma membrane and cytosolic calcium concentrations, while others could be developed that would interact with the nucleus to induce antimitogenic activity. The next decade holds great promise for the field of vitamin D research. $1,25(OH)_2D$ and its analogues offer great promise in areas of immunology, dermatology, cardiology, oncology, nephrology, and endocrinology. Thus, $1,25(OH)_2D_3$ is a hormone whose clinical and pharmacologic potential is yet to be realized.

References

1. Holick MF, Holick SA, Guillard RL: Photosynthesis of previtamin D in phytoplankton. *In* Loft B, Holmes WN (eds): Current Trends in Comparative Endocrinology, vol 2. Hong Kong, Hong Kong University Press, 1985, pp 1263–1266.
2. Holick MF, Krane SM, Potts JT Jr: Calcium, phosphorus, and bone metabolism: Calcium Regulating Hormones. *In* Braunwald E, Isselbacher KJ, Petersdorf RG, et al: Harrison's Principles of Internal Medicine, 11th ed. New York, McGraw-Hill, 1986, pp 1857–1870.
3. Horst RL, Reinhardt TA, Russell JR, Napoli JL: The isolation and identification of vitamin D_2 and vitamin D_3 from *Medicago sativa* (alfalfa plant). Arch Biochem Biophys 231:67–71, 1984.
4. Holick MF, MacLaughlin J, Parrish JA, Anderson RR: Photochemistry and photobiology of vitamin D. *In* Regan JD, Parrish JA (eds): Photomedicine. New York, Plenum Press, 1982, pp 195–218.
5. MacLaughlin JA, Holick MF: Mediation of cutaneous vitamin D_3 synthesis by uv radiation. *In* Goldsmith LA (ed): Biochemistry and Physiology of the Skin. North Carolina, Oxford University Press, 1983, pp 723–754.
6. Park EA: The etiology of rickets. Physiol Rev 3:106–159, 1923.
7. Sniadecki J (1822): Cited by W Mozolowski: Jedrzej Sniadecki (1768–1838) on the cure of rickets. Nature 143:121, 1939.
8. Owen I: Geographical distribution of rickets, acute and subacute rheumatism, chorea, cancer and urinary calculus in the British Islands. Br Med J 1:113–116, 1889.
9. Palm TA: The geographic distribution and etiology of rickets. Practitioner 45:270–279; 321–342, 1890.
10. Huldschinsky K: Heilung von Rachitis durch Kunstliche Hohensonne. Dtsch Med Wochenschr 45:712–713, 1919.
11. Hess AF, Unger LJ: Cure of infantile rickets by sunlight. JAMA 77:39–43, 1921.
12. Mellanby E: An experimental investigation on rickets. Lancet 1:407–412, 1919.
13. McCollum EV, Simmonds N, Becker JE, Shipley PG: Studies on experimental rickets. An experimental demonstration of the existence of a vitamin which promotes calcium deposition. J Biol Chem 53:293–312, 1922.
14. Powers GF, Park EA, Shipley PG, et al: The prevention of rickets in the rat by the means of radiation with the mercury vapor quartz lamp. Proc Soc Exp Biol Med 19:120–121, 1921.
15. Steenbock H, Black A: The induction of growth-promoting and calcifying properties in a ration by exposure to ultraviolet light. J Biol Chem 61:408–422, 1924.
16. Hess AF, Weinstock M: Antirachitic properties imparted to inert fluids and green vegetables by ultraviolet irradiation. J Biol Chem 62:301–313, 1924.
17. Hess AF, Weinstock M, Helman DF: The antirachitic value of irradiated phytosterol and cholesterol. J Biol Chem 63:305–308, 1925.
18. Rosenheim O, Webster TA: On the nature of the parent substance of vitamin D. Lancet 1:306–307, 1927.
19. Reerink EH, van Wijk A: The photochemical reactions of ergosterol. Biochem J 23:1294–1307, 1929.
20. Askew FA, Bourdillon RB, Bruce HM: The distillation of vitamin D. Proc R Soc Lond [Biol] 107:76–90, 1931.
21. Massengale ON, Nussmeier M: The action of activated ergosterol in the chicken. J Biol Chem 87:423–426, 1930.
22. Steenbock H, Kletzien SWF: The reaction of the chicken to irradiated ergosterol and irradiated yeast as contrasted with the natural vitamin D in fish liver oil. J Biol Chem 97:239–264, 1932.
23. Waddell J: The provitamin D of cholesterol. I. The antirachitic efficacy of irradiated cholesterol. J Biol Chem 105:711–739, 1934.
24. Windaus A, Schenck FR, von Werder F: Uber das antirachitisch wirksame Bestrahlungsprodukt aus 7-dehydrocholesterin. Z Physiol 241:100–103, 1936.
25. Brockmann H: Die Isolierung des antirachitischen Vitamins aus Tunfischleberol. Hoppe Seylers Z Physiol Chem 241:104–113, 1936.
26. Parrish J, Anderson RR, Urbach F, Pitts D (eds): Optical properties of the skin and eyes. *In* Biological Effects of Ultraviolet Radiation with Emphasis on Human Responses to Long-Wave Ultraviolet. New York, Plenum Press, 1978, pp 59–83.
27. Holick MF, MacLaughlin JA, Clark MB, et al: Photosynthesis of previtamin D_3 in human skin and the physiologic consequences. Science 210:203–205, 1980.

28. Loomis F: Skin-pigment regulation of vitamin D biosynthesis in man. Science 157:501–506, 1967.
29. Matsuoka LY, Ide L, Wortsman J, et al: Sunscreens suppress cutaneous vitamin D_3 synthesis. J Clin Endocrinol Metab 64:1165–1168, 1987.
30. Holick MF, MacLaughlin JA, Doppelt SH: Factors that influence the cutaneous photosynthesis of previtamin D_3. Science 211:590–593, 1981.
31. Webb AR, Kline L, Holick MF: Influence of season and latitude on the cutaneous synthesis of vitamin D_3. J Clin Endocrinol Metab 67:373–378, 1988.
32. MacLaughlin J, Holick MF: Aging decreases the capacity of human skin to produce vitamin D_3. J Clin Invest 76:1536–1538, 1985.
33. Adams JS, Clemens TL, Parrish JA, Holick MF: Vitamin-D synthesis and metabolism after ultraviolet radiation of normal and vitamin-D-deficient subjects. N Engl J Med 306:722–725, 1982.
34. Clemens TL, Adams JS, Henderson SL, Holick MF: Increased skin pigment reduces the capacity of the skin to synthesize vitamin D. Lancet 1:74–76, 1982.
35. Lo W, Paris P, Holick MF: Indian and Pakistani immigrants have the same capacity as Caucasians to produce vitamin D in response to ultraviolet irradiation. Am J Clin Nutr 44:683–685, 1986.
36. Lo CW, Paris PW, Clemens TL, et al: Vitamin D absorption in healthy subjects and in patients with intestinal malabsorption syndromes. Am J Clin Nutr 42:644–649, 1985.
37. Holick MF: Vitamin D requirements for the elderly. Clin Nutr 5:121–129, 1986.
38. DeLuca HF: The metabolism, physiology, and function of vitamin D. *In* Kumar R (ed): Vitamin D, Basic and Clinical Aspects. Boston/The Hague, Nijhoff, 1984, pp 1–68.
39. Tucker G III, Gagnon RE, Haussler MR: Vitamin D_3-25-hydroxylase: Tissue occurrence and apparent lack of regulation. Arch Biochem Biophys 155:47–51, 1973.
40. Olson EB Jr, Knutson JC, Bhattacharyya MH, DeLuca HF: The effect of hepatectomy on the synthesis of 25-hydroxyvitamin D_3. J Clin Invest 57:1213–1220, 1976.
41. Reddy GS, Napoli JL, Hollis BW: Differential 25-hydroxylation of vitamin D_2 versus vitamin D_3 in perfused rat liver. Calcif Tissue Int 36:524(abstract), 1984.
42. Holick MF, Clark MB: The photobiogenesis and metabolism of vitamin D. Fed Proc (FASEB) 37:2567–2574, 1978.
43. Bell NH: Vitamin D-endocrine system. J Clin Invest 76:1–6, 1985.
44. Long RG, Skinner RK, Meinhard E, et al: Serum 25-hydroxyvitamin D values in liver disease and hepatic osteomalacia. Gut 17:824–827, 1976.
45. Kaplan MM, Goldberg MJ, Matloff DS, et al: Effect of 25-hydroxyvitamin D_3 on vitamin D metabolites in primary biliary cirrhosis. Gastroenterology 81:681–685, 1981.
46. Pietrek J, Kokot F: Serum 25-hydroxyvitamin D in patients with chronic renal disease. Eur J Clin Invest 7:283–287, 1977.
47. Dent CE, Richens A, Rowe DJF, Stamp TCB: Osteomalacia with longterm anticonvulsant therapy in epilepsy. Br Med J 4:69–72, 1970.
48. Gascon-Barre M, Elbaz H, Hetu C, Joly J-G: Study on the liver microsomal incorporation and C-25 hydroxylation of [^{3}H]-vitamin D_3 in the rat. *In* Norman AW, Schaefer K, von Herrath D, Grigoleit H-G (eds): Vitamin D, Chemical, Biochemical and Clinical Endocrinology of Calcium Metabolism. Berlin, de Gruyter, 1982, pp 515–517.
49. Wark JD, Larkins RG, Perry-Keene D, et al: Chronic diphenylhydantoin therapy does not reduce plasma 25-hydroxyvitamin D. Clin Endocrinol 11:267–274, 1979.
50. Holick MF: Vitamin D: Biosynthesis, metabolism, and mode of action. *In* DeGroot LJ (ed): Endocrinology. 2nd ed. Philadelphia, WB Saunders, 1988, pp 902–926.
51. Weisman Y, Vargas A, Duckett G, et al: Synthesis of 1,25-dihydroxyvitamin D in the nephrectomized pregnant rat. Endocrinology 103:1992–1996, 1978.
52. Gray TK, Lester GE, Lorenc RS: Evidence for extrarenal 1-hydroxylation of 25-hydroxyvitamin D_3 in pregnancy. Science 204:1311–1313, 1979.
53. Tanaka Y, Halloran B, Schnoes HK, DeLuca HF: In vitro production of 1,25-dihydroxyvitamin D_3 by rat placental tissue. Proc Natl Acad Sci USA 76:5033–5035, 1979.
54. Howard GA, Turner RT, Sherrard DJ, Baylink DJ: Human bone cells in culture metabolize 25-hydroxyvitamin D_3 to 1,25-dihydroxyvitamin D_3 and 24,25-dihydroxyvitamin D_3. J Biol Chem 256:7738–7740, 1981.
55. Bikle DD, Nemanic MK, Whitney JO, Elias PW: Neonatal human foreskin keratinocytes produce 1,25-dihydroxyvitamin D_3. Biochemistry 25:1545–1548, 1986.
56. Reichel H, Koeffler HP, Barbers R, et al: 1,25-dihydroxyvitamin D_3 and the hematopoietic system. *In* Norman AW, Schaefer K, Grigoleit H-G, von Herrath D (eds): Vitamin D: Chemical, Biochemical and Clinical Update. Proceedings of the 6th Workshop on Vitamin D, Merano, Italy, March 1985. Berlin, de Gruyter, 1985, pp 167–176.
57. Shephard RM, Horst RL, Hamstra AJ, DeLuca HF: Determination of vitamin D and its metabolites in plasma from normal and anephric man. Biochem J 182:55–69, 1979.
58. Suda T, Kurukowa K: Characteristic localization of 25-hydroxyvitamin D_3-1α-hydroxylase along the fetal nephron. *In* Holick MF, Gray TK, Anast CS (eds): Perinatal Calcium and Phosphorus Metabolism. Amsterdam, Elsevier, 1983, pp 57–69.
59. Garabedian M, Holick MF, DeLuca HF, Boyle IT: Control of 25-hydroxycholecalciferol metabolism by parathyroid glands. Proc Natl Acad Sci USA 69:1973–1976, 1972.
60. Portale AA, Halloran BP, Murphy MM, Morris RC Jr: Oral intake of phosphorus can determine the serum concentration of 1,25-dihydroxyvitamin D by determining its production rate in humans. J Clin Invest 77:7–12, 1986.
61. Holick MF: Vitamin D and the kidney. Kidney Int 32:912–929, 1987.
62. Fraser D: Regulation of the metabolism of vitamin D. Physiol Rev 60:551–613, 1980.
63. Adams ND, Garthwaite TL, Gray RW, et al: The interrelationship among prolactin, 1,25-dihydroxyvitamin D and parathyroid hormone in humans. J Clin Endocrinol Metab 49:628–630, 1979.
64. Kumar R, Merimee TJ, Silva P, Epstein FH: The effect of chronic growth hormone excess or deficiency on plasma 1,25-dihydroxyvitamin D levels in man. *In* Norman AW, Schaefer K, von Herrath D, et al

(eds): Vitamin D, Basic Research and Its Clinical Application. Berlin, de Gruyter, 1979, pp 1005–1009.

65. Turner RT: Mammalian 25-hydroxyvitamin D-1α-hydroxylase, measurements and regulation. *In* Kumar R (ed): Vitamin D, Basic and Clinical Aspects. Boston/The Hague, Nijhoff, 1984, pp 175–196.
66. Rigotti NA, Nussbaum SR, Herzog DB, Neer RM: Osteoporosis in women with anorexia nervosa. N Engl J Med 311:1601–1606, 1984.
67. Krabbe S, Hummer L, Christiansen C: Serum levels of vitamin D metabolites and testosterone in male puberty. J Clin Endocrinol Metab 62:503–507, 1986.
68. Riggs BL, Gallagher JC, DeLuca HF, et al: A syndrome of osteoporosis, increased serum immunoreactive parathyroid hormone, and inappropriately low serum 1,25-dihydroxyvitamin D. Mayo Clin Proc 53:701–706, 1978.
69. Slovik DM, Adams JS, Neer RM, et al: Deficient production of 1,25-dihydroxyvitamin D in elderly osteoporotic patients. N Engl J Med 305:372–374, 1981.
70. Henneman PH, Dempsey EF, Carroll EL, Albright F: The cause of hypercalciuria in sarcoid and its treatment with cortisone and sodium phytate. J Clin Invest 35:1229–1242, 1956.
71. Mason RS: Extra-renal production of $1,25(OH)_2D_3$, the metabolism of vitamin D by non-traditional tissues. *In* Norman AW, Schaefer K, Grigoleit H-G, von Herrath D (eds): Vitamin D, Chemical, Biochemical and Clinical Update. Berlin, de Gruyter, 1985, pp 23–32.
72. Papapoulos SE, Clemens TL, Fraher LJ, et al: 1,25-Dihydroxycholecalciferol in the pathogenesis of the hypercalcemia of sarcoid. Lancet 1:627–630, 1979.
73. Barbour GL, Coburn JW, Slatopolsky E, et al: Hypercalcemia in an anephric patient with sarcoidosis, evidence for extrarenal generation of 1,25-dihydroxyvitamin D. N Engl J Med 305:440–443, 1981.
74. Adams JS, Singer FR, Gacad MA, et al: Isolation and structural identification of 1,25-dihydroxyvitamin D_3 produced by cultured alveolar macrophages in sarcoidosis. J Clin Endocrinol Metab 60:960–966, 1985.
75. Zaloga GP, Eil C, Medbery CA: Humoral hypercalcemia in Hodgkin's disease. Arch Intern Med 145:155–157, 1985.
76. Davies M, Mawer EB, Hayes ME, Lumb GA: Abnormal vitamin D metabolism in Hodgkin's lymphoma. Lancet 1:1186–1188, 1985.
77. Breslau NA, McGuire JL, Zerwekh JE, et al: Hypercalcemia associated with increased serum calcitriol levels in three patients with lymphoma. Ann Intern Med 100:1–7, 1984.
78. Rosenthal N, Insogna KL, Godsall JW, et al: Elevations in circulating 1,25-dihydroxyvitamin D_3 in three patients with lymphoma-associated hypercalcemia. J Clin Endocrinol Metab 60:29–33, 1985.
79. Fetchick DA, Bertolini DR, Sarin PS, et al: Production of 1,25-dihydroxyvitamin D_3 by human T cell lymphotrophic virus-I-transformed lymphocytes. J Clin Invest 78:592–596, 1986.
80. Napoli JL, Horst RL: Vitamin D metabolism. *In* Kumar R (ed): Vitamin D, Basic and Clinical Aspects. Boston/The Hague, Nijhoff, 1984, pp 91–123.
81. Mayer E, Kadowaki S, Williams G, Norman AW: Mode of action of 1,25-dihydroxyvitamin D. *In* Kumar R (ed): Vitamin D, Basic and Clinical Aspects. Boston/The Hague, Nijhoff, 1984, pp 259–301.
82. Boyle IT, Gray RW, DeLuca HF: Regulation by calcium of in vivo synthesis of 1,25-dihydroxycholecalciferol and 21,25-dihydroxycholecalciferol. Proc Natl Acad Sci USA 68:2131–2134, 1971.
83. Holick MF, Schnoes HK, DeLuca HF, et al: Isolation and identification of 24,25-dihydroxycholecalciferol: A metabolite of vitamin D_3 made in the kidney. Biochemistry 11:4251–4255, 1972.
84. Haussler MR, Donaldson CA, Kelly MA, et al: Functions and mechanism of action of the 1,25-dihydroxyvitamin D_3 receptor. *In* Norman AW, Schaefer K, Grigoleit H–G, von Herrath D (eds): Vitamin D, Chemical, Biochemical and Clinical Update. Berlin, de Gruyter, 1985, pp 83–92.
85. Henry H, Luntao EM: Further studies on the regulation of 25-OH-D metabolism in kidney cell culture. *In* Norman AW, Schaefer K, Grigoleit H-G, von Herrath D (eds): Vitamin D, Chemical, Biochemical and Clinical Update. Berlin, de Gruyter, 1985, pp 505–514.
86. Tanaka Y, Lorenc RS, DeLuca HF: The role of 1,25-dihydroxyvitamin D_3 and parathyroid hormone in the regulation of chick renal 25-hydroxyvitamin D_3-24-hydroxylase. Arch Bioichem Biophys 171:521–526, 1975.
87. Henry HL, Midgett RJ, Norman AW: Regulation of 25-hydroxyvitamin D_3-1-hydroxylase, *in vivo*. J Biol Chem 249:7584–7592, 1974.
88. Colston KW, Evans IMA, Spelsberg T, MacIntyre I: Feedback regulation of vitamin D metabolism by 1,25-dihydroxycholecalciferol. J Biol Chem 164:83–89, 1977.
89. Castillo L, Tanaka Y, DeLuca HF: Parathyroid hormone is not involved in 1,25-dihydroxyvitamin D regulation of 25-hydroxyvitamin D metabolism *in vivo*. Biochem Biophys Res Commun 100:1332–1336, 1981.
90. Henry HL, Norman AW: Vitamin D: Two dihydroxylated metabolites are required for normal chicken egg hatchability. Science 201:835–837, 1978.
91. Ornoy A, Goodwin D, Noff D, Edelstein S: 24,25-dihydroxyvitamin D is a metabolite of vitamin D essential for bone formation. Nature 276:517–519, 1978.
92. Corvol MT, Dumontier MF, Garabedian M, Rappaport R: Vitamin D and cartilage. II. Biological activity of 25-hydroxycholecalciferol and 24,25- and 1,25-dihydroxycholecalciferol on cultured growth plate chondrocytes. Endocrinology 102:1269–1273, 1978.
93. Kanis JA, Cundy T, Bartlett M, et al: Is 24,25-dihydroxycholecalciferol a calcium-regulating hormone in man? Br Med J 1:1382–1386, 1978.
94. Bordier P, Rasmussen H, Miravet L, et al: Vitamin D metabolites and bone mineralization in man. J Clin Endocrinol Metab 46:284–294, 1978.
95. Holick MF, Kleiner-Bossaller A, Schnoes HK, et al: 1,24,25-Trihydroxyvitamin D_3, a metabolite of vitamin D_3 effective on intestine. J Biol Chem 248:6691–6696, 1973.
96. Tanaka Y, DeLuca HF, Kobayashi Y, et al: Biological activity of 24,24-difluoro-25-hydroxylation on the functions of vitamin D. J Biol Chem 254:7163–7167, 1979.
97. Castillo L, Tanaka Y, DeLuca HF, Ikekawa N: On the physiological role of 1,24,25-trihydroxyvitamin D_3. Mineral Electrolyte Metab 1:198–207, 1978.

98. Suda T, DeLuca HF, Schnoes HK, et al: 25,26-Dihydroxycholecalciferol, a metabolite of vitamin D_3 with intestinal calcium transport activity. Biochemistry 9:4776–4780, 1970.
99. Reinhart TA, Napoli JL, Pramanik BC, et al: 1,25,26-Trihydroxyvitamin D_3: An *in vivo* metabolite of vitamin D_3. Biochemistry 21:6230–6235, 1981.
100. Mayer E, Kadowaki S, Williams G, Norman AW: Mode of action of 1,25-dihydroxyvitamin D. *In* Kumar R (ed): Vitamin D, Basic and Clinical Aspects. Boston/The Hague, Nijhoff, 1984, pp 259–302.
101. Jones G, Schnoes HK, DeLuca HF: Isolation and identification of 1,25-dihydroxyvitamin D_2. Biochemistry 14:1250–1256, 1975.
102. Horst RL, Reinhardt TA, Ramberg CF, et al: 24-Hydroxylation of 1,25-dihydroxyergocalciferol: An unambiguous deactivation process. J Biol Chem 261:9250–9256, 1986.
103. Reddy GS, Norman AW, Tserng K-Y: Isolation and identification of 1,23-dihydroxy-24,25,26,27-tetranor D_3: A new metabolite of 1,25-dihydroxyvitamin D_3 produced in the kidney. Biochemistry 26:324, 1987.
104. Reddy GS, Tserng Ky: Isolation and identification of 1,24,25-trihydroxyvitamin D_2, 1,24,25,28-tetrahydroxyvitamin D_3 and 1,24,25,26-tetrahydroxyvitamin D_2: New metabolites of 1,25-dihydroxyvitamin D_2 made in the kidney. Biochemistry 25:5328–5336, 1986.
105. Pike JW, Donaldson CA, Marion SL, Haussler MR: Development of hybridomas secreting monoclonal antibodies to the chicken intestinal 1α,25-dihydroxyvitamin D_3 receptor. Proc Natl Acad Sci USA 79:7719–7723, 1982.
106. Dame MC, Pierce EA, DeLuca HF: Identification of the porcine intestinal 1,25-dihydroxyvitamin D_3 receptor on sodium dodecyl sulfate/polyacrylamide gels by renaturation and immunoblotting. Proc Natl Acad Sci USA 82:7825–7829, 1985.
107. Pike JW: Interaction between 1,25-dihydroxyvitamin D_3 receptors and intestinal nuclei: Binding to nuclear constituents in vitro. J Biol Chem 257:6766–6775, 1982.
108. Allegretto EA, Pike JW: Trypsin cleavage of chick 1,25-dihydroxyvitamin D_3 receptors: Generation of discrete polypeptides which retain hormone but are unreactive to DNA and monoclonal antibody. J Biol Chem 260:10139–10145, 1985.
109. Pike JW, Sleator NM: Hormone-dependent phosphorylation of the 1,25-dihydroxyvitamin D_3 receptor in mouse fibroblasts. Biochem Biophys Res Commun 1131:378–385, 1985.
110. Hunziker W, Walters MR, Bishop JE, Norman AW: Unoccupied and in vitro and in vivo occupied 1,25-dihydroxyvitamin D_3 intestinal receptors. J Biol Chem 258:8642–8648, 1983.
111. Jensen EV, DeSombre ER: Estrogen-receptor interaction: Estrogenic hormones effect transformation of specific receptor proteins to a biochemically functional form. Science 182:126–134, 1973.
112. King WJ, Greene GL: Monoclonal antibodies localize oestrogen receptor in the nuclei of target cells. Nature 307:745–747, 1984.
113. Welshons WV, Lieberman ME, Gorski J: Nuclear localization of unoccupied estrogen receptors. Nature 307:747–749, 1984.
114. King RJB: Enlightenment and confusion over steroid hormone receptors. Nature 312:701–702, 1984.
115. Stumpf WE, Sar M, Reid FA, et al: Target cells for 1,25-dihydroxyvitamin D_3 in intestinal tract, stomach, kidney, skin, pituitary and parathyroid. Science 206:1188–1190, 1979.
116. Colston KW, Coombes RC, McClelland R, et al: Immunocytochemical localization of 1,25-dihydroxyvitamin D receptors in human breast cancer. J Bone Mineral Res 1:396 (abstract), 1986.
117. Thomasset M, Desplan C, Monktar M, Mathieu H: Intestinal calmodulin and calcium binding protein differ in their distribution and the effect of vitamin D steroid concentration. FEBS Lett 134:13–16, 1981.
118. Wasserman RH, Fullmer CS, Shimura F: Calcium absorption and the molecular effects of vitamin D_3. *In* Kumar R (ed): Vitamin D, Basic and Clinical Aspects. Boston/The Hague, Nijhoff, 1984, pp 233–257.
119. Bikle DD, Zolock DT, Morrissey RL, Herman RH: Independence of 1,25-dihydroxyvitamin D_3 mediated calcium transport from de novo RNA and protein synthesis. J Biol Chem 253:484–488, 1978.
120. Bikle DD, Morrissey RL, Zolock DT: The mechanism of action of vitamin D in the intestine. Am J Clin Nutr 32:2322–2338, 1979.
121. Goodman DBP, Haussler MR, Rassmussen H: Vitamin D_3-induced alteration of microvillar membrane lipid composition. Biochem Biophys Res Commun 46:80–85, 1972.
122. Rassmussen H, Matsumoto T, Fontaine D, Goodman DBP: Role of changes in membrane lipid structure in the action of 1,25-dihydroxyvitamin D_3. Fed Proc 41:72–77, 1982.
123. Nakada M, Simpson RU, DeLuca HF: Subcellular distribution of DNA-binding and non-DNA-binding 1,25-dihydroxyvitamin D receptors in chicken intestine. Proc Natl Acad Sci USA 81:6711–6713, 1984.
124. Pike JW: Intracellular receptors mediate the biologic action of 1,25-dihydroxyvitamin D_3. Nutr Rev 43:161–168, 1985.
125. Abe E, Miyaura C, Sakagami H, et al: Differentiation of rat myeloid leukemia cells induced by 1,25-dihydroxyvitamin D_3. Proc Natl Acad Sci USA 78:4990–4994, 1981.
126. Tanaka H, Abe E, Miyaura C, et al: 1,25-Dihydroxycholecalciferol and a human myeloid leukemia cell line (HL-60): The presence of cytosol receptor and induction of differentiation. Biochem J 204:713–719, 1982.
127. Miyaura C, Abe E, Kuribayashi T, et al: 1α,25-Dihydroxyvitamin D_3 induces differentiation of human myeloid leukemia cells. Biochem Biophys Res Comm 102:937–943, 1981.
128. Clemens TL, Adams JS, Horiuchi N, et al: Comparison of 1,25-dihydroxyvitamin-D_3-receptor binding in keratinocytes and fibroblasts from skin of normal subjects and a subject with vitamin-D-dependent rickets, type II: A model for study of the mode of action of 1,25-dihydroxyvitamin D_3. J Clin Endocrinol Metab 56:824–830, 1983.
129. Honma Y, Hozumi M, Abe E, et al: Prolongation of the survival time of mice inoculated with myeloid leukemia cells by 1,25-dihydroxyvitamin D_3. Proc Natl Acad Sci USA 80:201–204, 1983.
130. Eisman H, Barkla DH, Tutton PJM: 1,25-Dihydroxyvitamin D_3 suppresses the in vivo growth of human cancer cell solid tumor xenographs. J Bone Mineral Res 1:13 (abstract), 1986.
131. Bonucci E: New knowledge on the origin, function

and fate of osteoclasts. Clin Orthop 158:252–269, 1981.

132. Bar-Shavit Z, Teitelbaum SL, Reitsma P, et al: Induction of monocytic differentiation and bone resorption by 1,25-dihydrovitamin D_3. Proc Natl Acad Sci USA 80:5907–5910, 1983.
133. Merke J, Klaus G, Hugel U, et al: No 1,25-dihydroxyvitamin D_3 receptors on osteoclasts of calcium-deficient chicken despite demonstrable receptors on circulating monocytes. J Clin Invest 77:312–314, 1987.
134. Provvedini DM, Tsoukas CD, Deftos LJ, Manolagas SC: 1,25-dihydroxyvitamin D_3 receptors in human leukocytes. Science 221:1181–1182, 1983.
135. Bhalla AK, Amento EP, Clemens TL, et al: Specific high-affinity receptors for 1,25-dihydroxyvitamin D_3 in human peripheral blood mononuclear cells, presence in monocytes and induction in T lymphocytes following activation. J Clin Endocrinol Metab 57:1308–1310, 1983.
136. Tsoukas CD, Provvedini DM, Manolagas SC: 1,25-Dihydroxyvitamin D_3, a novel immunoregulatory hormone. Science 224:1438–1440, 1984.
137. Rigby WE, Stacy T, Fanger MW: Inhibition of T lymphocyte mitogenesis by 1,25-dihydroxyvitamin D_3 (calcitriol). J Clin Invest 74:1451–1455, 1984.
138. Lemire JM, Adams JS, Sakai R, Jordan SC: 1α,25-Dihydroxyvitamin D_3 suppresses proliferation and immunoglobulin production by normal human peripheral blood mononuclear cells. J Clin Invest 74:657–661, 1984.
139. Lemire JM, Adams JS, Bakke AC, et al: 1,25-Dihydroxyvitamin D_3 suppresses human T helper/inducer lymphocyte activity in vitro. J Immunol 134:23032–23035, 1985.
140. Adams JS, Gacad MA, Singer FR, Sharma OP: Production of 1,25-dihydroxyvitamin D_3 by pulmonary alveolar macrophages from patients with sarcoidosis. NY Acad Sci 465:587–594, 1986.
141. Horiuchi N, Clemens TL, Schiller AL, Holick MF: Detection and developmental changes of the 1,25$(OH)_2D_3$ receptor concentration in mouse skin and intestine. J Invest Dermatol 84:461–464, 1985.
142. Esvelt RP, DeLuca HF, Wichmann JK, et al: 1,25-Dihydroxyvitamin D_3 stimulated increase of 7,8-didehydrocholesterol levels in rat skin. Biochemistry 19:6158–6161, 1980.
143. Holick MF: Vitamin D photobiology: Recent advances in the biochemistry and some clinical applications. *In* Norman AW, Schaefer K, Grigoleit H-G, von Herrath D (eds): Vitamin D, Chemical, Biochemical and Clinical Update. Proc 6th Workshop, Vitamin D, Merano, Italy, 1985. Berlin, de Gruyter, 1985, pp 709–710.
144. Smith EL, Walworth NC, Holick MF: Effect of 1α,25-dihydroxyvitamin D_3 on the morphologic and biochemical differentiation of cultured human epidermal keratinocytes grown in serum-free conditions. J Invest Dermatol 86:704–714, 1986.
145. Colston K, Colston MJ, Feldman D: 1,25-Dihydroxyvitamin D_3 and malignant melanoma: The presence of receptors and inhibition of cell growth in culture. Endocrinology 108:1083–1086, 1981.
146. Hosoi J, Abe E, Suda T, Kuroki T: Regulation of melanin synthesis of B16 mouse melanoma cells by 1α,25-dihydroxyvitamin D_3 and retinoic acid. Cancer Res 45:1474–1478, 1985.
147. Marx SJ: Resistance to Vitamin D. *In* Kumar R (ed): Vitamin D: Basic and Clincal Aspects. Boston/The Hague, Nijhoff, 1984, pp 721–745.
148. Holick MF: Vitamin D resistance and alopecia, a causal or casual relationship? Arch Dermatol 121:601–603, (editorial), 1985.
149. Morimoto S, Onishi T, Imanaka S, et al: Topical administration of 1,25-dihydroxyvitamin D_3 for psoriasis; report of five cases. Calcif Tissue Int 38:119–122, 1986.
150. Kato T, Rokugo M, Terui T, Tagami H: Successful treatment of psoriasis with topical application of active vitamin D_3 analogue, 1,24-dihydroxycholecalciferol. Br J Dermatol 115:431–433, 1986.
151. Holick MF, Smith E, Pincus S: Skin as the site of vitamin D_3 synthesis and target tissue for (1,25-dihydroxyvitamin D_3): use of calcitriol (1,25-dihydroxyvitamin D_3) for treatment of psoriasis. Arch Dermatol 123:1677a–1683a, 1987.
152. Morimoto S, Yoshikawa K, Kozuka T, et al: An open study of vitamin D_3 treatment in psoriasis vulgaris. Br J Dermatol 115:421–429, 1986.
153. Belsey RE, DeLuca HF, Potts JT Jr: Competitive protein binding assay for vitamin D and 25-OH vitamin D. J Clin Endocrinol Metab 33:554–557, 1971.
154. Haddad JG, Chyu KJ: Competitive protein binding radioassay for 25-hydroxycholecalciferol. J Clin Endocrinol 33:992–995, 1971.
155. McCollum FG, Simmonds N, Shipley PG, Park EA: Studies on experimental rickets. XVI. A delicate biological test for calcium-depositing substances. J Biol Chem 54:41–50, 1922.
156. Schacter D, Rosen SM: Active transport of Ca^{45} by the small intestine and its dependence on vitamin D. Am J Physiol 196:357–365, 1959.
157. Schacter D, Dowdle EB, Schenker H: Active transport of calcium by small intestine of the rat. Am J Physiol 198:263–271, 1960.
158. Lund J, DeLuca HF: Biologically active metabolites of vitamin D_3 from bone, liver and blood serum. J Lipid Res 7:739–744, 1966.
159. Morii H, Lund J, Neville PF, DeLuca HF: Biological activity of a vitamin D metabolite. Arch Biochem Biophys 120:508–512, 1967.
160. Reinhardt TA, Horst RL, Orf JW, Hollis BW: A microassay for 1,25-dihydroxyvitamin D not requiring high performance liquid chromatography: Application to clinical studies. J Clin Endocrinol Metab 58:91–98, 1984.
161. Jones G: Assay of vitamins D_2 and D_3 and 25-hydroxyvitamins D_2 and D_3 in human plasma by high performance liquid chromatography. Clin Chem 24:287–298, 1978.
162. Horst RL, Littledike ET: Assay for vitamin D_2 and vitamin D_3 of dairy cows: Changes after massive dosing of vitamin D_3. J Dairy Sci 62:1746–1751, 1971.
163. Clemens TL, Adams JS, Nolan JM, Holick MF: Measurement of circulating vitamin D in man. Clin Chim Acta 121:301–308, 1982.
164. Clemens TL, Zhou XY, Myles M, et al: Serum vitamin D_2 and vitamin D_3 metabolite concentrations and absorption of vitamin D_2 in elderly subjects. J Clin Endocrinol Metab 63:656–660, 1986.
165. Bligh EG, Dyer WJ: A rapid method of total lipid extraction and purification. Can J Biochem Physiol 37:911–917, 1959.
166. Lambert PW, Syverson BJ, Arnaud CD, Spelsberg TC: Isolation and quantitation of endogenous vitamin

D and its physiologically important metabolites in human plasma by high performance liquid chromatography. J Steroid Biochem 8:929–937, 1977.

167. Caldas AE, Gray RW, Lemann J: The simultaneous measurement of vitamin D metabolites in plasma: Studies in healthy adults and in patients with calcium nephrolithiasis. J Lab Clin Med 91:840–849, 1978.

168. Turnbull H, Trafford DJH, Makin HLJ: A rapid and simple method for measurement of plasma 25-hydroxyvitamin D_2 and 25-hydroxyvitamin D_3 using Sep-Pak ^{18}C cartridges and a single high-performance liquid chromatographic step. Clin Chim Acta 120:65–76, 1982.

169. Preece MA, O'Riordan JLH, Lawson DEM, Kodicek E: A competitive protein binding assay for 25-hydroxycholecalciferol and 25-hydroxyergocalciferol in serum. Clin Chim Acta 54:235–242, 1974.

170. Horst RL, Littledike ET, Riley JL, Napoli JL: Quantitation of vitamin D and its metabolites and their plasma concentrations in five species of animals. Anal Biochem 116:189–203, 1981.

171. Horst RL: 25-OH-D_3-26,23 lactone: A metabolite of vitamin D_3 that is 5 times more potent than 25-OH-D_3 in the rat plasma competitive protein binding radioassay. Biochem Biophys Res Comm 89:286–293, 1979.

172. Dorantes LM, Arnaud SB, Arnaud CD: Importance of the isolation of 25-hydroxyvitamin D before assay. J Lab Clin Med 91:791–796, 1978.

173. Bouillon R, Van Kerkhove P, DeMoor P: Measurement of 25-hydroxyvitamin D_3 in serum. Clin Chem 22:364–368, 1976.

174. Horst RL, Shepard RM, Jorgensen NA, DeLuca HF: Assays for vitamin D and its metabolites. *In* Norman AW, Schaefer K, von Herrath D, et al (eds): Vitamin D: Basic Research and its Clinical Application. Berlin, de Gruyter, 1979, pp 213–221.

175. Kosky KT, VanDerSlik AL: High pressure liquid chromatographic method for determination of 25-hydroxycholecalciferol in cow plasma. Anal Biochem 74:282–291, 1976.

176. Jones G, Schnoes HK, DeLuca HF: An in vitro study of vitamin D_2 hydroxylases in the chick. J Biol Chem 251:24–28, 1976.

177. Brumbaugh PF, Haussler DH, Bursac KM, Haussler MR: Filter assay for 1α,25-dihydroxyvitamin D_3. Utilization on the hormones target tissue chromatin receptor. Biochemistry 13:4071–4097, 1974.

178. Lawson DEM, Fraser DR, Kodicek E, et al: Identification of 1,25-dihydroxycholecalciferol, a new kidney hormone controlling calcium metabolism. Nature (London) 230:228–230, 1971.

179. Holick MF, Schnoes HK, DeLuca HF, et al: Isolation and identification of 1,25-dihydroxycholecalciferol, a metabolite of vitamin D active in intestine. Biochemistry 10:2799–2804, 1971.

180. Norman AW, Myrtle JD, Midgett RJ, et al: 1,25-Dihydroxyvitamin D_3: Identification of the proposed active form of vitamin D_3 in the intestine. Science 173:51–55, 1971.

181. Brumbaugh PF, Haussler MR: 1α,25-Dihydroxycholecalciferol receptors in intestine. I. Association of 1α,25-dihydroxycholecalciferol with intestinal mucosa chromatin. J Biol Chem 249:1251–1257, 1974.

182. Dokoh S, Morita R, Fukunaga M, et al: Competitive protein binding assay for 1,25-dihydroxyvitamin D in human plasma. Endocrinology 25:431–436, 1978.

183. Hughes MF, Baylink DJ, Jones PG, Haussler MR: Radioligand receptor assay for 25-hydroxyvitamin D_2/D_3 and 1α,25-dihydroxyvitamin D_2/D_3. J Clin Invest 58:61–70, 1976.

184. Jones G, Byrnes B, Palna F, et al: Displacement potency of vitamin D_2 analogs in competitive protein-binding assays for 25-hydroxyvitamin D_3. J Clin Invest 50:773–775, 1980.

185. Reinhardt TA, Horst RL, Littledike ET, Beitz DC: 1,25-Dihydroxyvitamin D_3 receptor in bovine thymus gland. Biochem Biophys Res Comm 106:1012, 1982.

186. Hollis BW: Assay of circulating 1,25-dihydroxyvitamin D involving a novel single cartridge extraction and purification procedure. Clin Chem 32:2060–2063, 1986.

187. Clemens TL, Hendy GN, Graham RF, et al: A radioimmunoassay for 1,25-dihydroxycholecalciferol. Clin Sci Mol Med 54:329–332, 1978.

188. Bouillon R, DeMoor P, Baggiolini EG, Uskokovic MR: A radioimmunoassay for 1,25-dihydroxycholecalciferol. Clin Chem 26:562–567, 1980.

189. Gray TK, McAdoo T: A radioimmunoassay for 1,25-dihydroxyvitamin D_3. *In* Norman AW, Schaefer K, von Herrath D, et al (eds): Vitamin D: Basic Research and Its Clinical Application. Berlin, de Gruyter, 1979, pp 763–767.

190. Peacock M, Taylor GA, Brown W: Plasma 1,25-$(OH)_2$ vitamin D measured by radioimmunoassay and cytosol radioreceptor assay in normal subjects and patients with primary hyperparathyroidism and renal failure. Clin Chim Acta 101:93–101, 1980.

191. Perry HM, Clevinger BL, Haddad JG, Teitelbaum SL: Monoclonal antibody with high affinity for 1,25-dihydroxycholecalciferol. Biochem Biophys Res Commun 112:431–436, 1983.

192. Stern PH, Hamstra AJ, DeLuca HF, Bell NH: A bioassay capable of measuring 1 picogram of 1,25-dihydroxyvitamin D_3. J Clin Endocrinol Metab 46:891–896, 1978.

193. Stern PH, Phillips TE, Mavreas T: Bioassay of 1,25-dihydroxyvitamin D in human plasma purified by partition, alkaline extraction, and high-pressure chromatography. Anal Biochem 102:22–30, 1980.

194. Manolagas SC, Deftos LJ: Studies of the internalization of vitamin D_3 metabolites by cultured osteogenic sarcoma cells and their application to a non-chromatographic cytoreceptor assay for 1,25-dihydroxyvitamin D_3. Biochem Biophys Res Commun 95:562–602, 1980.

195. Manolagas SC, Culler FL, Howard JE, et al: The cytoreceptor assay for 1,25-dihydroxyvitamin D and its application to clinical studies. J Clin Endocrinol Metab 56:751–760, 1983.

196. Haddad JG, Min C, Mendelsohn M, et al: Competitive protein–binding radioassay of 24,25-dihydroxyvitamin D_3 in sera from normal and anephric subjects. Arch Biochem Biophys 182:390–395, 1978.

197. Horst RL, Littledike ET, Gray RW, Napoli JL: Impaired 24,25-dihydroxyvitamin D production in anephric man and pig. J Clin Invest 67:274–280, 1981.

198. Hay AWM, Jones G: The elution profits of vitamin D_2 metabolites from Sephadex LH20 columns. Clin Chem 25:473–475, 1979.

199. Jones G: Chromatographic separation of 24(R),25-dihydroxyvitamin D_3 and 25-hydroxyvitamin D_3-26,23-lactone using a cyano-bonded phase packing. J Chromatogr 276:69–74, 1983.

200. Hodsman AB, Wong EGC, Sherrard DJ, et al: Preliminary trials with 24,25-dihydroxyvitamin D_3 in dialysis osteomalacia. Am J Med 74:407–414, 1983.
201. Napoli JL, Pramanik BC, Partridge JJ, et al: 23S,25-Dihydroxyvitamin D_3 as a circulating metabolite of vitamin D_3: Its role in 25-hydroxyvitamin D_3-26,23-lactone biosynthesis. J Biol Chem 257:9634–9639, 1982.
202. Horst RL, Reinhardt TA, Napoli JL: 23-keto-25-hydroxyvitamin D_3 and 23-keto-1,25-dihydroxyvitamin D_3: Two new metabolites with high affinity for the 1,25-dihydroxyvitamin D_3 receptor. Biochem Biophys Res Commun 107:1319–1322, 1982.
203. Clements MR, Chalmers TM, Fraser DM: Enterohepatic circulation of vitamin D: A reappraisal of the hypothesis. Lancet 1:1376–1379, 1984.
204. Halloran BP, Bikle DD, Levens MJ, et al: Chronic 1,25-dihydroxyvitamin D_3 administration reduces the serum concentration of 25-dihydroxyvitamin D_3 by increasing the metabolic clearance rate. J Bone Mineral Res 1:18 (abstract), 1986.
205. Bell NH, Shaw S, Turner RT: Evidence that 1,25-dihydroxyvitamin D_3 inhibits the hepatic production of 25-hydroxyvitamin D in man. J Clin Invest 74:1540–1544, 1984.
206. Bjorkhem I, Holmberg I: Assay and properties of a mitochondrial 25-hydroxylase active on vitamin D_3. J Biol Chem 253:842–849, 1978.
207. Bjorkhem I, Holmberg I, Oftebro H, Pedersen JI: Properties of a reconstituted vitamin D_3-hydroxylase from rat liver mitochondria. J Biol Chem 255:5244–5249, 1980.
208. Yoon PS, DeLuca HF: Resolution and reconstitution of soluble components of rat liver microsomal vitamin D_3 25-hydroxylase. Arch Biochem Biophys 203:529–540, 1980.
209. Andersson S, Holmberg I, Wikvall K: 25-Hydroxylation of C_{27}-steroids and vitamin D_3 by a constitutive cytochrome P-450 from liver microsomes. J Biol Chem 258:6777–6781, 1983.
210. Pedersen JI, Bjorkhem I, Gustafsson J: 25-Hydroxylation of C_{27}-steroids by soluble liver mitochondrial cytochrome P-450. J Biol Chem 254:6464–6469, 1979.
211. Bhattacharyya MH, DeLuca HF: The regulation of rat liver calciferol-25-hydroxylase. J Biol Chem 248:2969–2973, 1973.
212. Fraser D, Kooh SW, Kind HP, et al: Pathogenesis of hereditary vitamin-D-dependent rickets: An inborn error of vitamin D metabolism involving defective conversion of 25-hydroxyvitamin D to 1α,25-dihydroxyvitamin D. N Engl J Med 289:817–822, 1973.
213. Brooks MH, Bell NH, Love L, et al: Vitamin-D-dependent rickets type II: Resistance of target organs to 1,25-dihydroxyvitamin D. N Engl J Med 298:996–999, 1978.
214. Bell NH, Stern PH, Pantzer E, et al: Evidence that increased circulating 1α,25-dihydroxyvitamin D is the probable cause for abnormal calcium metabolism in sarcoidosis. J Clin Invest 64:218–225, 1979.
215. Gkonos PJ, London R, Hendler ED: Hypercalcemia and elevated 1,25-dihydroxyvitamin D levels in a patient with end-stage renal disease and active tuberculosis. N Engl J Med 311:1683–1685, 1984.
216. Kozeny GA, Barbato AL, Bansal VK, et al: Hypercalcemia associated with silicon-induced granulomas. N Engl J Med 74:1103–1105, 1984.
217. Kantarjian HM, Saad MF, Estey EH, et al: Hypercalcemia in disseminated candidiasis. Am J Med 74:721–723, 1983.
218. Sandler LM, Winearls CG, Fraher LJ, et al: Studies of the hypercalcemia of sarcoidosis: Effect of steroids and exogenous vitamin D_3 on the circulating concentrations of 1,25-dihydroxyvitamin D_3. Q J Med 210:615–630, 1984.
219. Adams JS, Gacad MA, Endres DB, Sharma OP: Biochemical indicators of disordered vitamin D and calcium homeostasis in sarcoidosis. Sarcoidosis 3:1–6, 1986.
220. Bouillon R, Van Assche FA, Van Baelen H, et al: Influence of the vitamin D-binding aprotein on the serum concentration of 1,25-dihydroxyvitamin D_3. J Clin Invest 67:589–596, 1981.
221. Bikle DD, Gee E, Halloran B, Haddad JG: Free 1,25-dihydroxyvitamin D levels in serum from normal subjects, pregnant subjects, and subjects with liver disease. J Clin Invest 74:1966–1977, 1984.
222. Prince RL, Wark JD, Omond S, et al: A test of 1,25-dihydroxyvitamin D_3 secretory capacity in normal subjects and application in metabolic bone diseases. Clin Endocrinol 18:127–133, 1983.
223. Taylor AB, Stern PH, Bell NH: Abnormal regulation of circulating 25-hydroxyvitamin D in the Williams Syndrome. N Engl J Med 306:972–975, 1982.
224. Garabedian M, Jaeqz E, Guillozo H, et al: Elevated plasma 1,25-dihydroxyvitamin D concentrations in infants with hypercalcemia and elfin facies. N Engl J Med 312:948–952, 1985.
225. Broadus AE, Insogna KL, Lang R, et al: A consideration of the hormonal basis and phosphate leak hypothesis of absorptive hypercalciuria. J Clin Endocrinol Metab 58:161–169, 1984.
226. Bikle DD, Siiteri PK, Ryzen E: Serum protein binding of 1,25-dihydroxyvitamin D: A reevaluation by direct measurement of free metabolite levels. J Clin Endocrinol Metab 61:969–975, 1985.
227. Silver J, Russell J, Sherwood LM: Regulation of preproparathyroid hormone mRNA in bovine parathyroid cells in culture by vitamin D metabolites. *In* Norman AW, Schaefer K, Grigoleit H-G, von Herrath D (eds): Vitamin D, Chemical, Biochemical and Clinical Update. Proc 6th Workshop, Vitamin D, Merano, Italy, 1985. Berlin, de Gruyter, 1985, pp 24–33.
228. Slatopolsky E, Weerts C, Thielan HR, et al: Marked suppression of secondary hyperparathyroidism by intravenous administration of 1,25-dihydroxycholecalciferol in uremic patients. J Clin Invest 74:2136–2143, 1984.
229. Bar-Shavit Z, Kahn AJ, Stone KR, et al: Reversibility of vitamin D-induced human leukemia cell-line maturation. Endocrinology 118:679–686, 1986.
230. Koeffler HP, Hirjik S, Itri L, and the Southern California Leukemia Group: 1,25-Dihydroxyvitamin D_3: In vivo and in vitro effects on human preleukemic and leukemic cells. Cancer Treat Rep 69:1399–1407, 1985.
231. Baran DT, Moira ML: 1,25-Dihydroxyvitamin D increases hepatocyte cytosolic calcium levels: A potential regulator of vitamin D-hydroxylase. J Clin Invest 77:1622–1626, 1986.
232. Smith E, Holick MF: The skin: The site of vitamin D_3 synthesis and a target tissue for its metabolite 1,25-dihydroxyvitamin D_3. Steroids 49:103–131, 1987.
233. Fraser D, Scriver CR: Hereditary disorders associated with vitamin-D resistance or defective phosphate metabolism. *In* DeGroot L, et al (eds): Endocrinology, vol 2. New York, Grune & Stratton, 1979, pp 797–807.

6

STANLEY J. BIRGE
LOUIS V. AVIOLI

Pathophysiology of Calcium and Phosphate Absorptive Disorders

Calcium (Ca^{2+}) is the most abundant cation and fifth most common inorganic element of the human body. It not only serves as the principal component of the skeleton, imparting to it the structural integrity essential to support the increasing body size of the individual during growth, but also plays a vital role in a variety of essential physiologic and biochemical processes. Thus, maintenance of circulating Ca^{2+} within a narrow range is critical for the animal's survival. The homeostasis of Ca^{2+} in blood and extracellular fluid represents one of the most exquisite biological control systems in humans and is achieved by the interaction of a variety of hormones on the skeleton, kidneys, and intestine. It is evident that the availability of dietary Ca^{2+} is an important determinant of Ca^{2+} homeostasis. In this chapter we review the normal physiological regulation of Ca^{2+} absorption in humans and the alterations in intestinal Ca^{2+} absorption that characterize a variety of clinical disorders.

I. REGULATION OF INTESTINAL CALCIUM ABSORPTION

The average diet consumed daily by humans contains approximately 400 to 1000 mg Ca^{2+}. It and related alkaline earth cations, unlike Na^{+} and K^{+}, are only partially absorbed from the intestinal lumen. The net absorption of Ca^{2+} represents the summation of two unidirectional processes: the total transfer of Ca^{2+} from intestinal lumen to plasma; and the total transfer of Ca^{2+} from plasma to lumen, or endogenously secreted Ca^{2+}. Fecal Ca^{2+} consists not only of unabsorbed ingested Ca^{2+} but also of that Ca^{2+} endogenously secreted into the gastrointestinal tract that is not absorbed. Total intestinal Ca^{2+} excretion in humans averages 0.194 ± 0.073 g/day, whereas the secreted Ca^{2+} that is not absorbed, or endogenous fecal Ca^{2+}, averages 0.130 ± 0.047 g/cm per day.[1] Ca^{2+} excretion of the human jejunum is passive and approximates 0.008 mM/hr/20 cm.[2] Although endogenously secreted Ca^{2+} appears to play an insignificant role in maintaining circulating Ca^{2+} levels in humans, it may contribute to the adaptive response of lower mammals when subjected to varying levels of dietary Ca^{2+}.[3] Approximately 15% of the total intestinal Ca^{2+} secretion is assumed to be nonabsorbable, even under conditions when dietary Ca^{2+} is completely absorbed. These values are based on the assumption that dietary Ca^{2+} mixes homogeneously with endogenously secreted Ca^{2+}, that the absorptive efficiencies for both are identical, and that a portion of the endogenous Ca^{2+} is unabsorbed because it enters the gut distal to the absorptive site(s). Although in the past phosphate has been alleged to interfere with Ca^{2+} absorption as the result of the formation of poorly soluble calcium phosphates, high phosphate intakes have minimal effects on Ca^{2+} absorption.[3-5] The exception is undigestible organic phosphates (such as phytates or hexaphosphoinositol occurring in bran), which can form insoluble calcium salts. High concentrations of dietary Mg^{2+} can decrease Ca^{2+} absorption, presumably by competing for the Ca^{2+} transport site.[6] A variety of calcium salts have been used to supplement the diet including its lactate, chloride, gluconate, carbonate, citrate, or sulfate. There seems to be little difference in the intestinal utilization of Ca^{2+} from any of these salts.[7] However, there are a number of factors, such as oxalate,[7a] that when included in the diet can either influence the availability of Ca^{2+} to its site of transport or directly alter the transport process (Table 6–1). Certain

Table 6–1. Dietary Factors that Alter Intestinal Absorption of Calcium

Increased Absorption	Decreased Absorption
Amino acids	Oxalate
Tryptophan	Unabsorbed organic phosphates
Lysine	Tetracycline
Arginine	Unabsorbed fatty acids
Lactose and other complex sugars	Fiber
Dietary calcium deficiency	? Chronic magnesium deficiency
(short-term)	? Chronic iron deficiency

antibiotics and cationic amino acids such as lysine promote the absorption of calcium.[8] Similarly, lactose, other complex sugars, and glucose polymers significantly enhance calcium absorption.[9] Although it has been tacitly assumed that free acid alone is essential for calcium absorption, one must consider the other nutrients such as complex sugars in this regard.[10,11] Gastric acidity or achlorhydria appears to have limited, if any, effect on the intestinal absorption of certain oyster shell calcium supplements ingested as the carbonate salt.[12] In fact, in elderly populations high fiber intake significantly reduces calcium absorption irrespective of achlorhydria. Decreased acidity does not further reduce the bioavailability of calcium from food at high or low levels of fiber intake.[12a]

As an integral part of the Ca^{2+} homeostatic mechanism, the intestine has the ability to adapt to Ca^{2+} deprivation by increasing the absorption of dietary Ca^{2+}. This adaptation is achieved by the interplay of principally two hormones, parathyroid hormone (PTH) and $1,25(OH)_2D$. These two hormones modulate the rates of Ca^{2+} transfer across not only the intestine but also bone and kidney (Fig. 6–1). Under normal physiologic conditions, production and secretion of PTH are dependent on minute changes in the circulating concentration of Ca^{2+}. Thus, a reduction in dietary calcium results in increased levels of PTH secretion and an acute skeletal response designed to minimize alterations in serum Ca^{2+}. The increased intestinal absorption of Ca^{2+}, however, cannot be attributed to a direct effect of PTH on the intestine. Instead, the hormone, in conjunction with the reduced levels of Ca^{2+}, stimulates the renal production of $1,25(OH)_2D$ from its precursor 25(OH)D (see Chapter 5). The former sterol is approximately 500 times more potent than 25(OH)D in stimulating intestinal Ca^{2+} transport and is the effector hormone in the regulation of Ca^{2+} absorption. Estrogen also influences Ca^{2+} absorption, but again its effect is secondary to the induction of secondary hyperparathyroidism by decreasing the transfer of Ca^{2+} from bone into circulating fluids. In addition, there is some evidence suggesting that estrogen may have a direct or indirect effect on the renal production of $1,25(OH)_2D$.[13] In this instance, it is of interest that the placenta is also capable of contributing to the expanded production of $1,25(OH)_2D$.[14]

In humans, intestinal absorption of Ca^{2+} decreases with advancing age.[15-17] Similarly, the adaptation to low dietary Ca^{2+} is also blunted in the elderly.[2] These changes can be attributed to a progressive resistance to vitamin D that develops in the process of aging.[17,18] In addition, the renal production of $1,25(OH)_2D$ may also be impaired in the el-

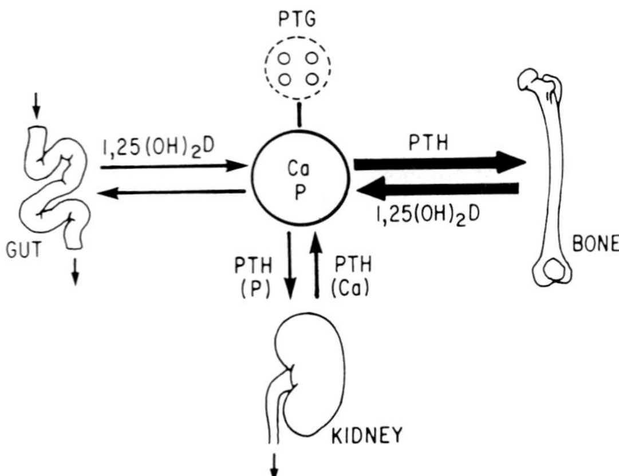

Figure 6–1. Schematic representation of calcium and phosphorus homeostasis. The major determinant of plasma calcium and phosphorus is the exchange of mineral between bone and plasma. The rate of exchange and net flux is dependent upon both parathyroid hormone (PTH) and $1,25(OH)_2D$. Calcium and phosphorus into plasma is accomplished by: (1) increased production of PTH, PTH stimulating bone turnover through a primary effect on osteoblasts and a secondary (osteoblast-mediated) effect on osteoclasts; and (2) increased production of $1,25(OH)_2D$ by the kidney, $1,25(OH)_2D$ stimulating increased intestinal absorption of calcium and phosphorus and increased osteoclastic activity and the mobilization of calcium and phosphorus from bone.

derly.[19] Consequently, the dietary intake of Ca^{2+} required to maintain positive Ca^{2+} balance progressively increases from 400 mg/day to 1200 to 1500 mg/day by the age of 65.[19]

There is considerable uncertainty as to whether the current United States Recommended Dietary Allowance (RDA) for calcium is adequate. The values listed in Table 6–2 are derived from balance studies in which the dietary calcium intake equals calcium losses in feces, urine, and sweat. They reflect the calcium intake required to achieve this balance in 95% of the population. What is at issue is whether these intakes provide a positive calcium balance and optimal bone mineralization. This is particularly relevant to the elderly, in whom intestinal calcium absorption is declining,[19a] as are their skeletal calcium reserves. Resolution of this issue is difficult, since it would require long-term assessment of bone mineral content in prospective clinical studies. The question is further complicated by the fact that the composition of the diet may significantly alter calcium absorption and retention. The majority of dietary calcium (i.e., 75%) is derived from dairy products alone, whereas approximately 12% is derived from fruits and vegetables. However, the addition of fruits and vegetables to a normal diet will often result in the development of a negative calcium balance.[20] The calcium contained in green leafy vegetables such as spinach is bound to oxalate and is not absorbed[7a,21] and, therefore, does not contribute to the absorbable calcium pool. Similarly, the presence of other elements in the diet (see Table 6–1) can significantly influence the amount of calcium absorbed and assimilated.

II. SITES OF CALCIUM ABSORPTION

The localization of the actual intestinal site(s) of Ca^{2+} absorption in humans and animals has preoccupied a host of investigators for a considerable time. It seems fairly well established that absorption occurs primarily in the upper portion of the small intestine of most species tested thus far and that the most efficient mechanism of absorption resides in the duodenum. *In vitro* experiments have demonstrated that the rate of Ca^{2+} absorption per unit segment (in terms of the amount of Ca^{2+} transferred per unit time) is maximal in the duodenum. However, when one also considers the transit time of Ca^{2+} through the intestinal tract, it becomes immediately obvious that more distal intestinal segments contain the major effective sites of Ca^{2+} absorption. Observations by Birge et al.[22] and Wensel et al.[23] suggest that similar but more sensitive mechanisms of Ca^{2+} absorption apply in humans. These studies demonstrated that although the calculated rate of Ca^{2+} absorption by the human duodenum was three times that of the rest of the gut, the intestinal segment distal to the duodenum was more sensitive to factors controlling Ca^{2+} absorption under normal physiologic conditions.[22] The studies also showed that flux from lumen to blood was independent of intraluminal Ca^{2+} concentration and was maximal in the more proximal intestinal segments.[23]

Recent studies have focused on the colon and cecum as sites for active Ca^{2+} transport. Both vitamin D and dietary Ca^{2+} restriction enhanced mucosal-to-serosal fluxes without changing secretory fluxes.[24] Some studies reveal that the secretory fluxes may be vitamin D–dependent and carrier-mediated,[25] whereas still others demonstrate a decrease in secretion fluxes with Ca^{2+} deprivation.[26] It is becoming increasingly evident that the large intestine must now also be considered as playing a potentially significant role in Ca^{2+} homeostasis, particularly during Ca^{2+} deprivation or as a consequence of the loss of ileal absorptive function.

Table 6–2. Recommended Dietary Allowances of Calcium (U.S.)*

Age	mg/day
0–0.5 yr	360
0.5–1.0 yr	540
1–10 yr	800
10–24 yr	1200
Adult	800
Pregnancy	1200–1400
Lactation	1200–1400
Elderly	1200–1600

*According to 10th Edition of RDA released October 24 1989.

III. MECHANISM OF CALCIUM ABSORPTION

A number of mechanisms that mediate the intestinal transport of Ca^{2+} have been identified. These include simple passive ionic diffusion, facilitated diffusion, and active transport. The primary driving force for "passive ionic diffusion" is the electrochemical gradient across the intestinal mucosa with the rate of diffusion linearly related to the magnitude of this gradient.

"Active transport" may be simply defined as a carrier-mediated process, directly coupled to energy-yielding reactions within the cell, which effects a net transport of a substance against an electrochemical gradient. It is generally believed that the so-called carrier proteins are either loosely bound to membranes or confined to a surface compartment located between the cell membrane and the cell wall. Despite the general acceptance that carrier proteins are involved in transport, most if not all of the evidence supporting this contention is still indirect.

Finally, "facilitated diffusion" may be defined as a passive process, with the driving force being that of the electrochemical gradient across the membrane. Since the transported ion is simply moving down its thermodynamic gradient, the mucosal flux ratio of facilitated diffusion is, like that of passive transport, identical to the theoretical flux ratio of Ussing.[27] However, the kinetics of ion movement that obtain when a substance is transported by facilitated diffusion are not those of the first-order relationship described for simple passive diffusion but instead are consistent with those features presently considered characteristic of a carrier-mediated transport system.

It seems well established that active transport contributes significantly to the intestinal absorption of Ca^{2+} in humans. A number of investigators have demonstrated that Ca^{2+} is transferred against a chemical gradient and that the "Ca^{2+} pump" can be saturated by increasing the concentration of Ca^{2+} in the precursor compartment and can be inhibited by hypothermia, anaerobiosis, and a variety of metabolic poisons.[23,28,29]

A role of phosphate in mediating active Ca^{2+} transport has been suggested, making the intestinal transport mechanism analogous to the phosphate-dependent Ca^{2+} transport in the kidney.[30] However, active transport of Ca^{2+} in the duodenum of experimental animals occurs in the absence of inorganic phosphate.[28,29] In the colon, stimulation of active transport of Ca^{2+} by vitamin D occurs in the absence of an effect of the vitamin on the active transport of inorganic phosphate, thus providing a clear dissociation between these two transport processes. The observed facilitation of Ca^{2+} transport by the addition of phosphate to the luminal compartment may be attributed to the restoration of depleted intracellular phosphate seen in the vitamin D–deficient experimental models used.[31]

In summary, the bulk of evidence accumulated to date supports the contention that in the duodenum, Ca^{2+} is transported by an active carrier-mediated, energy-dependent process. Passive transport or facilitated diffusion, or both, would appear to be the primary regulating mechanisms(s) for the absorption of Ca^{2+} in more distal intestinal segments. The higher pump efficiency of the more proximal intestinal segments may be due to intrinsic differences in the energy-generating systems or greater efficiencies of the intestinal cells in this location, a larger number of epithelial cells per unit length of intestine, and/or an increment in the amount of carrier essential to promote maximal active transport. The physiologic significance of the duodenal transport pump appears to have been well established in that its transport capacity is adaptive and decreases with age, is greater in pregnant than in nonpregnant states as well as during periods of low Ca^{2+} intake, and is stimulated by vitamin D and its biologically active metabolites. In general, the accumulated data are consistent with the fact that an active transport mechanism can increase the intestinal absorption of Ca^{2+} facultatively to meet the requirements of the organism. Despite repeated observations that the most rapid rate of Ca^{2+} transport per unit length of intestine is in the small intestine just beyond the pylorus, the transit time through the duodenum is normally so short that, in reality, the largest fraction of the total Ca^{2+} absorbed is probably from intestinal sites distal to the duodenum where passive and/or facilitated diffusion predominates.

IV. THE ROLE OF VITAMIN D

Vitamin D is the single most important factor regulating the intestinal absorption of Ca^{2+} in humans and animals. It had been well established that a 10- to 15-hour lag period obtained after vitamin D administration before stimulated intestinal Ca^{2+} transport was detectable. We now know that vitamin D, itself biologically inactive, is subsequently converted to a variety of metabolites with varying degrees of effectiveness in stimulating Ca^{2+} absorption by the intestine (see Chapter 5). It appears that the lag phase between administration and the biological response can be explained by (1) the prerequisite rate-limiting hepatic conversion of vitamin D to 25-hydroxycholecalciferol [25(OH)D_3]; (2) the subsequent transport of 25(OH)D in plasma to the kidney by a vitamin D–binding protein, immunologically identical to group-specific component (Gc) proteins; and (3) the renal conversion of 25(OH)D to either 1,25$(OH)_2D_3$, a metabolite that is approximately 500 times as active in stimulating intestinal transport as is the parent vitamin D substance, or 24,25$(OH)_2$, with a biological effectiveness on intestinal Ca^{2+} transport equal to that of 25(OH)D.

Although circulating levels of 25(OH)D and 24,25$(OH)_2D$ are much higher than those reported for 1,25$(OH)_2D$, the latter is primarily responsible for the increments in Ca^{2+} absorption observed following vitamin D_3 feeding to rachitic animals. The exact sequence of subcellular molecular events that characterize the intestinal response to 1,25$(OH)_2D$ (or other vitamin D_3 metabolites) continues to be an area of active investigation. Results of experiments with inhibitors of DNA-directed RNA synthesis are consistent with the interpretation that the stimulation of Ca^{2+} transport by 1,25$(OH)_2D$ is at least in part mediated by *de novo* protein synthesis and therefore analogous to the mechanism of steroid hormone action. A cytoplasmic receptor highly specific for 1,25$(OH)_2D$ has been demonstrated in intestine and with a sedimentation coefficient of 3.5 S. 1,25$(OH)_2D$ binding to this cytoplasmic receptor appears to represent an essential reaction prior to its subsequent binding to the nuclear chromatin of intestinal cells. The receptor protein has been identified in other target tissues of 1,25$(OH)_2D$ action, and clinical states of altered 1,25$(OH)_2D$ action have been associated with a variety of defects or absence of the 1,25$(OH)_2D$ receptor protein.

Pseudo–1-hydroxyl–containing analogs of 1α,25$(OH)_2D$ including isotachysterol$_3$, 5,6-*trans*-D_3, DHT_3, and 25(OH)DHT_3 are active in stimulating intestinal Ca^{2+} absorption; as such, these agents have been important therapeutic tools in treating patients with hypoparathyroidism, renal insufficiency, and other disorders characterized by impaired endogenous 1α-hydroxylation of vitamin D.

The molecular events resulting from the initiation of transcriptional processes that ultimately lead to an increase in Ca^{2+} transport across the intestinal epithelium have yet to be fully delineated. It has been demonstrated that vitamin D and its active metabolites stimulate the synthesis of a number of cell proteins. These include a Ca^{2+}-binding protein (CaBP),[32] alkaline phosphatase,[33] actin,[34] an intestinal membrane CaBP,[35] and a mitochondrial protein.[36] In addition, stimulation of cAMP,[37] alterations in membrane phospholipids,[38] and the phosphorylation of membrane proteins[39] have also been reported. These effects have all been alleged to contribute to the vitamin D–induced alterations in Ca^{2+} transport. In order to evaluate the potential role of these various molecular changes, it is necessary to appreciate which steps in the cellular translocation of Ca^{2+} are regulated by vitamin D.

Transport of Ca^{2+} across the intestinal epithelium can be considered to involve three steps: (1) transport across the brush border membrane; (2) transport across the cell cytosol to the basolateral membrane; and (3) transport across the basolateral membrane. The first step is along a downhill electrochemical gradient, whereas the third step is against a steep electrochemical gradient and is considered to be the rate-limiting step (Fig. 6–1). The early studies of Schachter and others[40,41] demonstrated that Ca^{2+} uptake by the mucosal surface of the intestinal epithelial cell is not an active process but one of facilitated diffusion that is carrier mediated. Unlike the Na^+ dependency of sugar and amino acid transport, movement of Ca^{2+} across the brush border is independent of Na^+.[42] That this uptake of Ca^{2+} across the brush border is stimulated by vitamin D has been amply demonstrated by numerous investigators. However, the mechanism of the vitamin's action at this site is still unknown. Some insight into this mechanism can be derived from the studies of Wong and Norman using the polyene antibiotic filipin, which interacts with membrane lipid.[43] In the intestine, filipin enhances the mucosal uptake of Ca^{2+} in both vitamin D–deficient and –replete chicks without altering overall net mucosal-serosal Ca^{2+} flux. These studies suggest that alterations in the brush border lipid membrane structure can lead to a specific increase in the permeability of the membrane to Ca^{2+} and the accessibility of a latent transport system for Ca^{2+}. Rasmussen and coworkers[38] have demonstrated that 1,25$(OH)_2D$ can alter phospholipid metabolism and composition of the brush border membrane. These changes in membrane lipid composition occur within a few hours and do not depend on new protein synthesis. Similarly, the vitamin-induced increase in Ca^{2+} permeability of brush border membrane vesicles also occurs within hours of $1,25(OH)_2D$ treatment and is not blocked by inhibitors of protein synthesis.[44] Vitamin D–dependent extrusion of Ca^{2+} across the basolateral membrane is not evident until 8 to 12 hours after treatment with the sterol and is blocked by inhibitors of both transcription and translation. Thus, there are at least two phases in the cellular response to $1,25(OH)_2D$. The first is an alteration in brush border membrane resulting in the facilitated diffusion of Ca^{2+} into the cell. This phase is followed by the stimulation of active extrusion of Ca^{2+} across the basolateral membrane. The delayed response of the second phase is attributed to the requirement for the *de novo* synthesis of protein(s) associated with the active transport of Ca^{2+} out of the cell.

Because of the potential toxicity of the Ca^{2+} entering the cell, a number of mechanisms have been proposed to transport the Ca^{2+} through the cell cytosol to the Ca^{2+} pump at the basolateral membrane. One such mechanism involves the mitochondria. These organelles have an impressive ability to concentrate Ca^{2+}, and indeed, following vitamin D administration, an increase in Ca^{2+} and phosphate granules can be demonstrated.[45] However, this increase in apparent uptake of Ca^{2+} is observed only during the initial phase of the cellular response to $1,25(OH)_2D$ and not during the second phase of active Ca^{2+} transport when intracellular levels of Ca^{2+} are restored, presumably to normal.[45] Thus, it is unlikely that mitochondria participate in the transcellular movement of Ca^{2+}. Instead they appear to serve as a "sump" in the prevention of Ca^{2+} toxic effects resulting from the increased accumulation of cell Ca^{2+} during the initial phase of $1,25(OH)_2D$ action. Another organelle that may serve as a shuttle for Ca^{2+} is the Golgi-derived membrane vesicle. One of the earliest responses of the intestine to $1,25(OH)_2D$ is the increased accumulation of Ca^{2+} by these vesicles[46] occurring within 30 minutes of the vitamin's administration. Pretreatment with cycloheximide inhibits both Golgi Ca^{2+} uptake and intestinal Ca^{2+} transport.[47] On the other hand, their capacity to accumulate Ca^{2+} in response to vitamin D may reflect the presence of newly synthesized Ca^{2+} transport protein(s) destined for the cell membrane.

At the basolateral membrane, two mechanisms are believed to be involved in the efflux of Ca^{2+} against the electrochemical gradient. One mechanism involves a Na^+-Ca^{2+} exchange based on a number of studies demonstrating the requirement of the Ca^{2+} pump for Na^+[41,48] and the analogy to Na^+-Ca^{2+} exchange pumps in other plasma systems. In addition, a second Ca^{2+} pumping mechanism has been identified in the enterocytes that is mediated by a Ca^{2+}-Mg^{2+}-ATPase.[49,50] This enzyme is localized exclusively to the basolateral membrane and is activated by 10^{-7} M Ca^{2+} similar to the Ca^{2+}-Mg^{2+}-ATPase in membranes of red blood cells or muscle. In contrast, the Ca^{2+}-Mg^{2+}-ATPase localized predominantly along the brush border is activated by 10^{-3} M Ca^{2+}. The Ca^{2+}-Mg^{2+}-ATPase of the enterocytes also forms a hydroxylamine-sensitive, phosphoenzyme intermediate that appears to be calmodulin regulated.[51,52] In addition, recent evidence suggests that the enzyme in the intestine is stimulated by vitamin D.[53]

Knowing the postulated sites for vitamin D action, it is still difficult to relate the known biochemical alterations induced by vitamin D in the enterocyte to the Ca^{2+} transport process.[54] One intriguing observation is the rapid rise in cAMP, which peaks between 30 and 90 minutes after the *in vitro* addition of $1,25(OH)_2D$.[55] A second rise in cAMP occurs coincident with the second phase in the stimulation of Ca^{2+} transport by the vitamin. The initial delay in the cAMP response to $1,25(OH)_2D$, however, is not typical of a cAMP-mediated hormone response. Considerable question remains as to whether the increase in cAMP is a primary event or secondary to other metabolic events such as an increase in intracellular phosphate and ATP induced by vitamin D.[56]

A number of CaBPs have been identified in the intestinal epithelial cell membrane and cytosol. The first CaBP described has proved to be a cytosolic protein with a molecular weight of 9000 to 13,000 in mammalian intestine and ranging up to 25,000 to 28,000 in avian intestine.[57] The protein has been identified in multiple animal species and a variety of tissues including kidney, pancreas, and brain. With the exception of brain, the protein is induced *de novo* by $1,25(OH)_2D$.[58] Its role in Ca^{2+} transport is suggested by the high affinity of the protein for the Ca^{2+} ($K_d \sim 10^{-5}$ M); the appearance of the protein parallels the increase in Ca^{2+} absorption of the second phase of the enterocyte response to $1,25(OH)_2D$ and the concentration of the protein in the various segments of the intestine correlates with the relative abilities of these segments to absorb Ca^{2+}. On the other hand, CaBP cannot be detected at a time when the initial increment in Ca^{2+} transport is demonstrated, and second, CaBP product can be blocked without inhibition of $1,25(OH)_2D$-stimulated Ca^{2+} transport. Although CaBP may not participate in membrane transport of Ca^{2+}, some role for the protein seems likely in the intestinal response to vitamin D. At present, it is postulated that the protein may serve as an intracellular carrier of Ca^{2+}, to facilitate the transfer of Ca^{2+} from mitochondria or Golgi to the Ca^{2+} pump of the basolateral membrane or as a buffer to protect the cell from the influx of Ca^{2+} induced by the vitamin. In addition to the well-characterized cytosolic CaBP, two CaBPs have been isolated from the brush border membrane with approximate molecular weights of 18,500 and 200,000, respectively.[58] The role of these proteins in the carrier-mediated entry of Ca^{2+} into the cell remains conjectural at this time.

Other proteins stimulated by vitamin D are brush border alkaline phosphatase and Ca^{2+}-ATPase, although there is considerable doubt whether these two enzymes are not in fact the same enzyme. Both enzyme activities are proportionally extracted from the membranes by butanol and inhibited equally by L-phenylalanine. The Ca^{2+}-Mg^{2+}-ATPase activity of the brush border that is stimulated by millimolar concentrations of Ca^{2+} is to be distinguished from the Ca^{2+} pump ATPase of the basolateral membrane stimulated by micromolar Ca^{2+} concentrations. The participation of either of these enzyme activities in either vitamin D–stimulated Ca^{2+} or phosphate transport is considered unlikely because L-phenylalanine, an inhibitor of alkaline phosphatase and the Ca^{2+}-ATPase, does not inhibit intestinal Ca^{2+} or phosphate transport. Second, the changes in alkaline phosphatase activity do not correlate well with the changes in Ca^{2+} transport induced by vitamin D. On the other hand, this ectoenzyme may play a role in increasing the availability of dietary organic phosphate to intestinal absorption. Other proteins not identified are also synthesized in response to vitamin D and are a part of generalized stimulation of RNA and protein synthesis.[112,146] This response of the intestinal epithelium reflects the generalized trophic effect of the vitamin characterized by an increase in DNA synthesis and mucosal proliferation.[59]

V. CLINICAL DISORDERS ASSOCIATED WITH ALTERATIONS IN CALCIUM ABSORPTION

A. Increased Absorption

As noted in Table 6–3, a variety of conditions can lead to an alteration in the absorption of Ca^{2+}. Regrettably, the techniques for measuring Ca^{2+} absorption remain cumbersome, time-consuming, and inaccurate. These various methods have been reviewed adequately elsewhere.[60,61] As a consequence of our inability to adequately assess Ca^{2+} absorption directly, one must rely for practical purposes on the clinical manifestations of increased or decreased availability of Ca^{2+}. Thus, it is appropriate to review in general

Table 6–3. Physiologic and Pathologic Factors that Alter Calcium Absorption

Increased Absorption
Physiologic states
Pregnancy
Lactation
Pathologic states
Sarcoidosis and granulomatous disorders
Primary hyperparathyroidism
Diabetes
Idiopathic hypercalciuric syndromes
Phosphorus depletion
Pharmacologically induced
Milk-alkali syndrome
Vitamin D intoxication
Estrogens
Nonabsorbable aluminum-containing antacids
Malabsorption
Physiologic states
Aging
Pathologic states
Intrinsic bowel disease
Hepatobiliary disease
Renal disease
Hyperthyroidism
Hypoparathyroidism
Pharmacologically induced
Anticonvulsants (Dilantin, phenobarbital)
Thiazides
Chemotherapeutic agents
Glucocorticoids
Antibiotics (tetracycline)

terms the clinical and biochemical expression of these states of altered Ca^{2+} homeostasis. First, with respect to states of intestinal hyperabsorption of Ca^{2+}, two basic mechanisms can be considered: physiologic and pathologic. Physiologic stimulation of Ca^{2+} absorption reflects the body's response to an increased requirement for Ca^{2+}. Under these conditions, urinary excretion of Ca^{2+} is either low or normal. On the other hand, pathologic states of increased Ca^{2+} absorption are in general associated with hypercalciuria (24-hr urine values) > 300 mg in men, > 250 mg in women, or > 4 mg/kg body weight. An exception to this rule occurs in early primary hyperparathyroidism (see Chapter 14). The effect of parathyroid hormone on the kidney is to stimulate the tubular reabsorption of Ca^{2+} resulting in the reduced renal excretion of Ca. Hypercalciuria prevails when the filtered load of Ca^{2+} exceeds the capacity of the tubules to reabsorb the Ca^{2+} presented. Urinary excretion of Ca^{2+} can be a very sensitive indicator of excessive assimilation of dietary Ca^{2+}, with changes being evident before increments in the serum Ca^{2+} can be appreciated. Its usefulness as a diagnostic tool requires a knowledge of the dietary Ca^{2+} content during and preceding the urine collection, since urinary excretion of Ca^{2+} is related to dietary Ca^{2+} intake in normal individuals. Similarly, sodium, protein, and carbohydrate intake must also be acknowledged, since each promotes calcium excretion. Urinary excretion of Ca^{2+} has not proved to be a reliable estimate of impaired Ca^{2+} transport at the level of the intestine. This is in part due to the fact that the kidney's capacity to conserve Ca^{2+} is limited in contrast to its ability, for example, to conserve Na^+ or phosphate. Serum Ca^{2+} levels are maintained within the normal range by the various homeostasis mechanisms described previously, so that the serum Ca^{2+} poorly reflects an altered state of Ca^{2+} homeostasis. Only under selected circumstances, specifically states of hypoparathyroidism or states of PTH resistance (Table 6–3), does this homeostatic mechanism fail. In these circumstances Ca^{2+} cannot be adequately mobilized from the skeleton, and the serum Ca^{2+} falls. In the absence of these clinical disorders, intestinal malabsorption of Ca^{2+} can result in the asymptomatic depletion of the skeleton of its mineral content. Regrettably, skeletal fracture may be the first and only manifestation of the malabsorption (see Chapter 11).

The cellular response of bone depends on numerous factors that are poorly understood. As a simplification, malabsorption associated with vitamin D deficiency is characteristically associated with a picture of osteomalacia—a disease of bone formation and a failure to mineralize the newly formed bone matrix (see Chapter 11). Malabsorption of Ca^{2+} without a deficiency of vitamin D results in a skeletal response characterized by osteoporosis with or without evidence of secondary hyperparathyroidism.[62] Growing children appear to be an exception, since they develop classic rickets with pure Ca^{2+} deficiency.[63]

Pregnancy and lactation are well recognized stimulants to intestinal Ca^{2+} absorption resulting in greater than a 2-fold increase in total Ca^{2+} absorbed. Despite this dramatic increase in response to the fetal and maternal Ca^{2+} requirements, the mechanism mediating this response is not understood. Heaney and Skillman[64] were able to demonstrate the increased absorption by the 20th week of pregnancy (the earliest time studied), at which time fetal Ca^{2+} storage is insignificant. One can postulate that the positive Ca^{2+} balance at this time will be utilized later in pregnancy for the fetus. Those factors that induce this intestinal adaptation to anticipate the needs of the mother later in her pregnancy are still ill-defined. A rise in maternal PTH does not occur until the last few weeks of pregnancy.[65] On the other hand, maternal serum concentrations of $1{,}25(OH)_2D$ rise progressively with pregnancy.[13,66] The origin of the apparent increased production of $1{,}25(OH)_2D$ has been attributed to the stimulation of the renal 1α-hydroxylase by prolactin or estrogens,[67] or to production by the fetal-placental unit.[68] These results must be interpreted with the understanding that the sex steroid hormones also produce elevations in vitamin D–binding protein.[69] Accordingly, estimates of "free" $1{,}25(OH)_2D$ do not increase in the maternal circulation until the last few weeks of pregnancy and again late in lactation. In addition, subsequent studies have failed to demonstrate increased concentrations of $1{,}25(OH)_2D$ in women with prolactinomas and elevated levels of prolactin in their serum.[70] Nor did these same investigators observe an increase in the intestinal absorption of Ca^{2+}, thus making it unlikely that prolactin is directly stimulating intestinal absorption of Ca^{2+}. Similarly, the role of estrogens in the enhanced absorption of Ca^{2+} is disputed. *In vitro* studies fail to demonstrate a direct effect of the hormone on renal production of $1,25(OH)_2D$, suggesting that its effects may be mediated through enhanced secretion of PTH. More recent data suggest that estrogen may induce an increase in the intestinal content of the $1,25(OH)_2D$ receptor protein[71] or perhaps an increase in mucosal villus height and number.[72]

Sarcoidosis is a disease of unknown origin characterized by a granulomatous infiltrate of multiple tissues (see Chapter 22). During the active phase of the disease, increased absorption of Ca^{2+} from the intestine occurs that results in hypercalciuria and occasionally hypercalcemia. These changes have been attributed to the finding of elevated levels of $1,25(OH)_2D$, which reflects an abnormal metabolism of the latter compound. Administration of a large dose of vitamin D suppresses $1,25(OH)_2D$ concentrations in normal patients, whereas as noted in Chapter 22, in patients with both active and inactive sarcoidosis, vitamin D feeding or sunlight exposure increases the levels of $1,25(OH)_2D$.[73] Of great interest is the origin of the $1,25(OH)_2D$, since the excess production persists following bilateral nephrectomy.[74] More recently, production of $1,25(OH)_2D$ by a variety of different tissues has been reported. One can speculate, therefore, that one of the cellular elements of the granulomatous reaction may be the origin of the excessive production of the sterol. Indeed, alveolar macrophages from sarcoid patients produce $1,25(OH)_2D$.[75] This phenomenon may not be restricted to sarcoidosis, since other granulomatous diseases have been associated with hypercalcemia, for example, coccidioidomycosis,[76] histoplasmosis,[77] berylliosis,[78] and tuberculosis.[79,80]

Although diabetes mellitus has been recognized as being associated with osteopenia,[81] the cause is still unknown (see Chapter 12). For the most part, animal studies have utilized the streptozotocin-induced chronic diabetic rat model and have revealed profound alterations in vitamin D metabolism and Ca^{2+} homeostasis. Biochemically, the chronic diabetic rat model displays an elevation in serum Ca^{2+} and depressed levels of PTH.[82] Serum concentrations of $1,25(OH)_2D$ are depressed, whereas those of $24,25(OH)_2D$ are increased.[83] Paradoxically, intestinal absorption of Ca^{2+} is increased and is associated with a marked hypercalciuria.[84] This increased absorption of Ca^{2+} can be attributed to (1) increased dietary intake, (2) hypertrophy of the intestine, and (3) a 5-fold increase in the intestinal mucosal receptors for $1,25(OH)_2D$.[84] Thus, the modest reduction in the circulating concentration of the sterol is more than compensated for by the increase in its tissue receptor protein. In diabetic children, a similar trend in the relative concentrations of the vitamin D metabolites is evident[85] as well as increased intestinal absorption of Ca^{2+}.[86]

Idiopathic hypercalciuria is a common finding in patients with recurrent renal calculi and in family members of such patients (see Chapter 23). An additional 5% of the population is estimated to have idiopathic hypercalciuria in the absence of renal lithiasis. The pathogenesis of these disorders is still in question, and, therefore, the diagnosis must be one of exclusion. Under the heading of idiopathic hypercalciuria, two major subgroups have been identified on the basis of the response to a low Ca^{2+} diet (< 400 mg/24 hr) or on the basis of the calcium/creatinine ratio in a 2-hour fasting morning urine collection followed by a 100 mg oral Ca^{2+} load and two additional urine collections over the next 4 hours.[87] The basic distinction between these two groups is that in "absorptive" hypercalciuria patients, the excessive excretion of Ca^{2+} is corrected with the reduction in dietary Ca^{2+}, whereas in "resorptive" hypercalciuria patients, the excessive excretion of Ca^{2+} persists after an overnight fast or on a low Ca^{2+} diet. The latter group can be further subdivided on the basis of their response to the Ca^{2+} load. The majority of patients in this subgroup apparently have a primary decrease in the renal tubular reabsorption of Ca^{2+} and are, therefore, classified as "renal hypercalciuria."[88] Their serum total calcium values tend to be low whereas their immunoreactive PTH levels are elevated as is the urinary excretion of cAMP; both suppress with calcium loading or thiazide therapy. The second subgroup includes those patients who appear to have a primary renal phosphate leak. Both the "absorptive" and the "resorptive" hypercalciuric syndromes have an increased intestinal absorption of Ca^{2+}.[87,88] In the resorptive group, the increased intestinal absorption of Ca^{2+} can be explained on the basis of the secondary hyperparathyroidism and the resultant increase in the production of $1,25(OH)_2D$. The bone biopsy lends additional credence to these physiologic changes, demonstrating increased osteoblastic and osteoclastic activity. Indeed, thiazide diuretic therapy, which stimulates renal tubular reabsorption Ca^{2+}, corrects the renal Ca^{2+} loss, restores the elevated serum concentrations of $1,25(OH)_2D$ to normal, and normalizes the intestinal absorption Ca^{2+}.[89] In the absorptive hypercalciurias, the pathogenesis of the increased intestinal Ca^{2+} absorption is not as clearly understood. PTH levels are probably suppressed in this disorder, which is reflected in the bone histologic features. Both osteoclastic and osteoblastic activity are reduced with an increase in the fraction of inactive osteoid (see Chapter 11). Although thiazide therapy corrects the renal excretion of Ca^{2+}, it does not normalize the increased intestinal absorption of the cation. This could be explained by the hypothesis that circulating levels of $1,25(OH)_2D$ are elevated in this disorder owing to a primary phosphate leak and hypophosphatemia.[90] Unfortunately, there is not general agreement as to whether patients with absorptive hypercalciuria have reduced concentrations of serum phosphate. Second, the role of phosphate depletion in the regulation of $1,25(OH)_2D$ synthesis can also be questioned. Finally, Zerwekh and Pak did observe that there was no change in the slightly elevated levels of blood $1,25(OH)_2D$ in their patients with absorptive hypercalciuria following thiazide treatment.[89] Perhaps another interpretation of the pathogenesis of this disorder is that the regulation of the renal 1α-hydroxylase by Ca^{2+} is impaired, resulting in the inappropriate elevation of the dihydroxy metabolite of vitamin D relative to the Ca^{2+} demands of the individual.

Phosphate depletion results in a recognized clinical entity characterized by a myopathy, hypercalciuria, accelerated bone resorption, osteomalacia, and increased intestinal absorption of Ca^{2+}. The pathophysiologic processes involved in the various features of this disorder are complex, and as yet the mechanism of the enhanced intestinal absorption of Ca^{2+} remains to be elucidated. The observed changes in the tubular reabsorption of Ca^{2+} and phosphate cannot be attributed to the reduction in circulating PTH. Thyroparathyroidectomy cannot abolish this adaptive response of the kidney. With the discovery of the renal conversion of 25(OH)D to $1,25(OH)_2D$ it was postulated that phosphate depletion resulted in the stimulation of $1,25(OH)_2D$ production. The increase in the vitamin D sterol resulted in turn in the increase in the intestinal absorption of Ca^{2+} and the rise in serum calcium. Indeed, increased production of $1,25(OH)_2D$ does occur as a result of phosphorus depletion. However, it soon became apparent that the changes in intestinal Ca^{2+} absorption and serum calcium did not require the renal metabolism of 25(OH)D and could be demonstrated in the vitamin D–deficient animal model.[91] Thus, the observed adaptations to phosphate depletion appear to be mediated by factors that are independent of the thyroid, the parathyroids, and vitamin D metabolism.

Pharmacologically induced states of increased Ca^{2+} absorption can be of major clinical significance. Before being adequately appreciated, the milk-alkali syndrome was a significant cause of irreversible renal failure. The syndrome is characterized by the excessive ingestion of Ca^{2+} and alkali, usually for the treatment of peptic symptoms, resulting in alkalosis and uremia; in its chronic form, hypercalcemia and calcinosis may be superimposed upon the renal impairment attributed to the alkalosis. The development of renal calcinosis leads to further reduction of glomerular filtration and increased retention of Ca^{2+}.[92] The increased intestinal absorption of Ca^{2+} is due only to the tremendous Ca^{2+} load presented to the intestine. Altering luminal pH over a wide range has no effect on Ca^{2+} transport, although normal gastric acidity is required to solubilize most $CaCO_3$ preparations. The systemic alkalosis, however, may contribute to a reduction in the glomerular filtration rate and thus the retention of Ca^{2+}, as would any underlying renal disease. However, alkalosis is usually associated with a rise rather than a fall in inulin and creatinine clearance. The rising serum calcium would reduce the glomerular filtration rate and thereby further exacerbate Ca^{2+} retention, hypercalcemia, and renal calcinosis. The advent of H_2-antagonist therapy for ulcer has reduced the incidence of this syndrome.

Vitamin D intoxication, although less common than previously reported, still presents a potentially serious problem in the use of vitamin D therapeutically.[93] With the advent of the more potent, faster acting analogues of vitamin D, $1\alpha(OH)D_3$ and $1\alpha,25(OH)_2D_3$, the incidence of vitamin D intoxication promises to increase. The mechanism of the increased intestinal absorption of Ca^{2+} in vitamin D intoxication is of interest in that it is mediated by 25(OH)D and its interaction with the

$1,25(OH)_2D$ receptor in the intestine, $1,25(OH)_2D$ production being suppressed by the hypercalcemia. Like vitamin D, 25(OH)D has a half-life of approximately 3 weeks because of its facility of being "stored" in adipose tissue and muscle. Consequently, following the withdrawal of the vitamin D, 2 to 6 months or more may be required before hypercalcemia and the enhanced absorption of Ca^{2+} is restored to normal.[94] The influence of estrogens on Ca^{2+} absorption in humans has been difficult to ascertain because the changes are not dramatic. However, calcium balance studies[95] and radioactive isotopic Ca^{2+} studies[96] suggest that estrogens induce a positive calcium balance in women that is associated with a reduction in fecal Ca^{2+} and increased intestinal absorption of Ca^{2+}. This effect of estrogens on intestinal Ca^{2+} absorption is probably secondary to a reduction in bone resorption and secondary hyperparathyroidism.[95] Recent studies indicate that estrogens can induce the intestinal receptor protein for $1,25(OH)_2D$.[71] Ovariectomy results in a prompt reduction in the rat intestinal $1,25(OH)_2D$ receptor protein content.[97] A direct stimulation of intestinal Ca^{2+} absorption by estrogens is unlikely, since the steroid probably inhibits the transport process.[98] Finally, the nonabsorbable antacids containing aluminum or magnesium hydroxide constitute a significant pharmacologic stimulation of intestinal Ca^{2+} absorption. In patients with normal renal function, these agents act by blocking the intestinal absorption of phosphate, leading to hypophosphatemia. As noted earlier, the hypophosphatemia leads to the stimulation of intestinal Ca^{2+} absorption by mechanisms that are poorly understood.

B. Decreased Absorption

Perhaps the most common cause of decreased intestinal absorption of Ca^{2+} is that which attends the normal aging process. Evidence has accumulated that in adults, intestinal absorption of Ca^{2+} decreases progressively with advancing age.[14,15] After the age of 65, absorption of Ca^{2+} is less than one third that measured in the third and fourth decades of life. The decrease in absorption occurs prior to menopause in females and, therefore, cannot be attributed entirely to the loss of sex steroids. A number of factors have been identified that contribute to this decline. First, the ability of the intestine to respond to the challenge of a low Ca^{2+} diet is impaired in the elderly.[2] This suggests that in the elderly the adaptive response is impaired either at the level of the production of the adaptive hormones [PTH and $1,25(OH)_2D$] or at the level of the intestinal response to the hormones. There is now evidence to suggest that aging impairs the adaptive response to calcium deprivation at both levels. In humans and in the laboratory animal model, aging results in decreased synthesis of $1,25(OH)_2D$. In osteoporotic women not only are the blood levels of $1,25(OH)_2D$ reduced, but there is no correlation between the levels of $1,25(OH)_2D_2$ and the measured absorption of Ca^{2+}[17] (see Chapter 12). These data can be interpreted by postulating a resistance of the intestine to the action of $1,25(OH)_2D$. It has also been recently demonstrated that the intestinal cytosolic receptor protein for $1,25(OH)_2D$ decreases in parallel with the reduction of Ca^{2+} transport associated with aging.

One of the major causes of osteomalacia is diseases of the bowel or surgical resection of the intestine (see Chapter 11). It is obvious that simple reduction of the absorptive surface area as in Crohn's disease, nontropical sprue, celiac disease, and intestinal bypass surgery will lead to the malabsorption of Ca^{2+}. However, other factors have been identified in these conditions that also contribute to the malabsorption. Of these factors, loss of bile salts and/or steatorrhea are clearly important. As noted earlier, increased concentrations of unabsorbed fatty acids within the intestinal lumen bind Ca^{2+} and limit the accessibility of the Ca^{2+} to its transport site. In addition, the increase in luminal fat concentrations impairs the absorption of vitamin D. Thus, the steatorrhea associated with pancreatic insufficiency has been shown to contribute to the malabsorption of vitamin D and osteomalacia. Like cholesterol, calciferol is a very nonpolar lipid with similar solubility characteristics. To permit absorption of these compounds by the intestinal mucosa, solubilization by micellar formation is essential. Thus, absorption of vitamin D and cholesterol is markedly impaired in experimental bile duct obstruction. Biliary cirrhosis and other chronic cholestatic syndromes with impairment of bile salt secretion result in marked reduction of serum 25(OH)D levels and osteomalacia,[99] whereas pure cirrhosis with

with loss of parenchymal function leads to only modest reductions of serum 25(OH)D levels. Although the liver is the primary site for hydroxylation of vitamin D, the enzymatic reserve is apparently sufficient to sustain marked losses of hepatic parenchymal tissue. In patients with severe forms of biliary cirrhosis, no impairment in the hydroxylation of vitamin D has been demonstrated. A third factor to be considered is the loss of vitamin D by interruption of its enterohepatic circulation. The sterol as 25(OH)D has been demonstrated to be secreted with the bile into the duodenum and reabsorbed in the ileum.[100] The significance of this enterohepatic circulation still remains controversial. Perhaps the most common gastrointestinal condition associated with Ca^{2+} malabsorption is gastric surgery and in particular subtotal gastrectomy and gastrojejunostomy.[101] An incidence of metabolic bone disease of up to 42% has been reported in patients with partial gastrectomy.[102] Vitamin D deficiency has been suggested to be one of the major causes of the bone disease of these patients owing to its impaired absorption or to poor intake. In the absence of vitamin D deficiency, the mechanism of the deranged mineral metabolism remains to be elucidated. Factors such as inadequate calcium intake, increased intestinal transit time, and inadequate acidification have been suggested as contributing factors.

Two endocrine disorders are associated with significant malabsorption of Ca^{2+}. In hypoparathyroidism, the loss of circulating PTH and the rise in serum phosphate result in the decreased renal production of $1,25(OH)_2D$ (see Chapter 14). The malabsorption of Ca^{2+} can, therefore, be attributed to the low levels of $1,25(OH)_2D$. Recent evidence suggests that PTH may also have a direct effect on intestinal Ca^{2+} transport[103] so that its absence may further contribute to the reduced intestinal absorption of Ca^{2+}. The second less obvious endocrine disorder leading to malabsorption of Ca^{2+} is that of hyperthyroidism (see Chapter 18). Increased concentrations of thyroid hormone stimulate bone resorption, resulting in the increased serum calcium and phosphate observed in this disorder. As a consequence of the hypercalcemia, PTH secretion is suppressed. Hence, as noted, the reduction in Ca^{2+} absorption observed in the hyperthyroid state can be attributed to the altered metabolism of vitamin D. Indeed, serum concentrations of $1,25(OH)_2D$ are reduced in patients with active hyperthyroidism.[104]

Chronic renal failure is characterized by a marked impairment in the intestinal absorption of Ca^{2+} (see Chapter 13). Patients with end-stage renal failure are also unable to adapt to alterations in dietary Ca^{2+} and, as a consequence, develop large fecal Ca^{2+} losses during periods of malnutrition or compromised Ca^{2+} intake, as may occur with low protein dietary regimens. Alterations in Ca^{2+} absorption usually are detectable when serum creatinine values are greater than 2.5 mg/100 ml,[105] although an inverse correlation between BUN level and Ca^{2+} absorption has been reported for patients with BUN levels between 25 and 250 mg/100 ml.[106] In patients with chronic renal disease, an intestinal defect in Ca^{2+} absorption has been demonstrated in the duodenum, jejunum, and ileum.[107,108] Distal non-vitamin D–dependent sites where Ca^{2+} absorption is primarily passive are apparently functionally intact. These findings are consistent with observations that uremic patients can absorb Ca^{2+} normally when dietary calcium intake is augmented to 4 to 10 g/day. The intestinal malabsorption of Ca^{2+} observed in patients with end-stage renal disease is resistant to vitamin D therapy [including $1\alpha(OH)D$ and $1,25(OH)_2D$], unaltered by chronic intermittent hemodialysis, and ultimately unrelated to the skeletal pathologic changes, since the progression of the osteodystrophic bone lesions is not attended by further deterioration of the intestinal absorption of Ca^{2+}.

The specific pathogenesis and exact nature of the intestinal Ca^{2+} transport defect in the chronic uremic state are still uncertain. There is mounting evidence obtained from experimental uremic animal models that renal insufficiency not only affects cellular Ca^{2+} transport parameters directly, but also results in derangements in vitamin D metabolism, with defective production of $1,25(OH)_2D$. Since $1,25(OH)_2D$ functions primarily to regulate intestinal absorption of Ca^{2+}, acquired alterations in its production by the diseased kidney obviously play a major role in initiating and perpetuating the intestinal malabsorption of Ca^{2+}. In addition, uremic toxins may alter cell metabolism directly, since a vitamin D–activated intestinal ATPase and mitochondrial activities, as well as intestinal cellular proliferation[109] and CaBP synthesis,[110] are all reportedly defective in the chronic uremic state. Moreover, reports of raised serum calcitonin levels in patients with chronic renal failure and calcitonin inhibition of vitamin D–induced intestinal Ca^{2+} absorption should also be considered.

Ca^{2+} malabsorption that is resistant to vitamin D therapy has also been observed in patients with either the nephrotic syndrome or classic forms of renal tubular acidosis. Since nitrogenous wastes and uremic toxins do not accumulate in either instance and functional renal mass is not severely impaired, the cause of the malabsorptive defect in these "tubular" forms of renal disease is most probably related to either the persistent hypoalbuminemia (nephrotic syndrome) or systemic acidosis (renal tubular acidosis). The relationship between the net intestinal absorption of Ca^{2+} and hypotonicity of circulating fluids in humans is still unknown, as is the effect of chronic acidosis on either the bioactivation of vitamin D or the intestinal response to vitamin D treatment. Since in animals Ca^{2+} absorption is dependent on circulating oncotic pressure and net lumen-plasma water movement, one might reasonably postulate that clinical disorders characterized by chronic hypotonicity of circulating fluids might, in fact, lead to an increase in plasma-lumen water flux and a subsequent decrease in the intestinal absorption of Ca^{2+}. The malabsorption of Ca^{2+} attending the course of patients with renal tubular acidosis may also be multifactorial. It can, however, be completely corrected by alkali therapy alone. However, although a systemic acidosis may directly impair the lumen-plasma transport of Ca^{2+}, the renal conversion of $25(OH)_2D_3$ to $1,25(OH)_2D_3$ is pH dependent, and an acidic pH is inhibitory for the reaction.[111] Isolated reports of calcium malabsorption induced by chronic anxiety and stress should also be mentioned, although the mechanisms involved are still conjectural at best.

Anticonvulsant drugs have become recognized as a significant cause of disordered mineral homeostasis and osteomalacia, with a reported incidence ranging from 4% to 40% in those receiving these drugs.[112,113] A number of factors have been identified that predispose the epileptic population to the development of osteopenia. Of these, the most prominent are the level of vitamin D intake and the exposure to sunlight. Thus, the incidence of disordered mineral metabolism is greatest in institutionalized epileptic patients who are confined indoors. Also of importance are the dose and duration of drug therapy and use of multiple anticonvulsant drugs. Use of acetazolamide or a ketogenic diet to produce a systemic acidosis further compromises the already disordered state of mineral homeostasis by accelerating the loss of mineral from bone and inhibiting the conversion of 25(OH)D to $1,25(OH)_2D$. The mechanism of the anticonvulsant drug action leading to osteomalacia appears to be basically 2-fold: first, an alteration of the metabolism of vitamin D; second, a direct inhibition of ion transport across the intestinal epithelium and an inhibition of osteoblastic activity. It is well recognized that the common anticonvulsants induce an increase in the hepatic P-450 mixed function oxidase enzyme activity. This results in the increased hydroxylation of vitamin D and 25(OH)D to biologically inactive, more polar metabolites that are eliminated in the bile and urine.[114] Hence, there is a marked decrease in the serum half-life of vitamin D and 25(OH)D. In an apparent response to hypocalcemia and increased levels of PTH, plasma levels of $1,25(OH)_2D$ are elevated in individuals receiving anticonvulsants, which suggests that other factors must be invoked to account for the breakdown in Ca^{2+} homeostasis. There is indeed good evidence that anticonvulsant drugs, particularly phenytoin, have a direct inhibitory effect on the intestinal transport of Ca^{2+}. Consequently, patients receiving combined drug therapy require above-normal circulating levels of vitamin D metabolites in order to maintain normal intestinal Ca^{2+} absorption.

Glucocorticoid steroids represent a second common drug-induced alteration in mineral homeostasis, which includes the malabsorption of Ca^{2+}[115] and the often profound loss of mineral from the skeleton. The pathophysiologic mechanisms of the events leading to steroid-induced osteoporosis are indeed complex. At the level of bone, the glucocorticoids have a number of actions that result in a relative increase in osteoclastic activity over osteoblastic activity. The inhibition of intestinal Ca^{2+} absorption has been a matter of some controversy. Originally, steroids were considered to impair the metabolism of vitamin D to its metabolically active derivatives. However, more recent studies in experimental animals have failed to demonstrate that cortisone alters the conversion of vitamin D to 25(OH)D and the conversion of 25(OH)D to

$1,25(OH)_2D$.[116] On the other hand, the clearance of $1,25(OH)_2D$ may be accelerated by its metabolism to more polar, biologically inactive metabolites to account for the reduction in $1,25(OH)_2D$ levels observed in patients with systemic lupus erythematosus or glomerulonephritis treated chronically with steroids.[117] The extent of this reduction, however, would not appear to be sufficient to explain the degree of malabsorption of Ca^{2+}. In short-term studies (2 weeks) in normal volunteers, moderate doses of prednisone produced significant increases in the circulating levels of $1,25(OH)_2D$.[118] These changes consistent with the interpretation that glucocorticoids have a direct effect on the intestinal epithelium, inhibiting the transport of Ca^{2+} at this site and thereby inducing a compensatory increase in PTH secretion must be reconciled with reports of a stimulatory action of glucocorticoids on epithelial calcium transport.[118a]

Chlorothiazide diuretic agents have a profound effect on the renal tubular reabsorption of Ca^{2+}, resulting in hypocalciuria. This mechanism of the diuretic action appears to be a direct stimulation of the distal nephron Ca^{2+} reabsorption and independent of PTH.[119] In addition, the thiazide diuretics inhibit the intestinal absorption of Ca^{2+} in patients with idiopathic hypercalciuria.[120] This inhibition of intestinal absorption of Ca^{2+} could be a direct effect of the diuretic on the intestine mediated through the prevention of secondary hyperparathyroidism through the action of the diuretic on the renal conservation of Ca^{2+}. In *in vitro* studies, thiazides have been shown to have no apparent effect on intestinal Ca^{2+} transport.[121] Thus, it would appear that the reduced intestinal absorption of Ca^{2+} observed in idiopathic hypercalciuria is the consequence of the suppression of PTH secretion and reduced synthesis of $1,25(OH)_2D$. Indeed, patients with increased bone turnover in association with idiopathic hypercalciuria experience a reduction in the cellular activity of bone consistent with reduced levels of PTH.[120]

Cytotoxic chemotherapeutic agents can induce profound malabsorption of Ca^{2+} by destroying the intestinal epithelium, which is uniquely sensitive to these agents because of the rapid turnover of the intestinal mucosal epithelium. However, the tetany associated with the drug *cis*-platinum results primarily from renal tubular cytotoxicity and hypomagnesemia.

In the last decade, the calcium channel blocking agents have become widely used in the effective treatment of hypertension and myocardial ischemia. Their mechanism of action is thought to be related to their inhibition of Ca transport through the slow channels of the cell membranes. Therapeutic concentrations of these drugs do not inhibit intestinal Ca^{2+} transport[122] and may even enhance absorption through increased production of $1,25(OH)_2D$.[123]

A number of nutritional factors have been identified that are required for the maintenance of normal intestinal Ca^{2+} absorption. The most obvious of these is vitamin D. Although vitamin D can be obtained from sunlight and a variety of dietary sources, the major dietary sources are limited to milk and certain cereals that have been supplemented with ergosterol (vitamin D_2). Even in those areas in which food products are supplemented with vitamin D, it would appear that requirements for vitamin D are met primarily by the endogenous production of calciferol (vitamin D_3) in skin, where 7-dehydrocholesterol is converted to calciferol under the influence of ultraviolet light.[124] Thus, the major circulating form of vitamin D is vitamin D_3, which is synthesized in skin.[125] This would suggest that a vitamin D deficiency state would require both deprivation of sunlight as well as a dietary deficiency of the vitamin. In addition to the simple nutritional deficiency of vitamin D, one must also be cognizant of a growing list of vitamin D–resistant states that are also characterized by a malabsorption of Ca^{2+} (see Chapters 11 and 24). Examples include the malabsorption of renal insufficiency, aging, and a number of rare familial disorders as discussed previously. Lead and other heavy metals will result in a clinical and biochemical characterization of osteomalacia due in part to their inhibition of 25-hydroxy-1α-hydroxylase as well as to their cytotoxic actions on the renal tubule.

Magnesium and iron deficiency probably constitutes yet another example of vitamin D resistance. The effects of magnesium deficiency on Ca^{2+} homeostasis are diverse and include an impaired secretion of PTH,[126] an inhibition of the skeletal response to PTH,[127] and an apparent resistance to the action of vitamin D on the intestine.[128] Thus an adequate dietary intake of magnesium is required for the normal absorption and assimilation of dietary Ca.[129] The influence of iron deficiency on Ca^{2+} homeostasis has not been adequately characterized. In the rat, chronic iron deficiency results in a significant decrease in intestinal Ca^{2+} absorption.[130] It has been the authors' experience that chronic iron deficiency in humans can lead to severe osteomalacia and intestinal malabsorption of Ca^{2+}, which is completely reversed by the replacement of the depleted iron stores. In this regard it should be emphasized that when calcium supplements are ingested together with foods containing iron or with iron supplements, the efficiency of iron absorption decreases.

Considerable attention has been focused recently on the calcium content of the American diet because of the growing appreciation of the relationship between calcium intake, the subsequent development of osteoporosis (see Chapter 12) later in life,[131] and the increased risk of hypertension and colon cancer.[132,133] The results of innumerable dietary surveys indicate that the majority of Caucasian women are consuming less than the recommended dietary allowances of calcium. Of note is the fact that after the age of 35 years, more than 75% of all females ingest less than the RDA in any given day. Second, these studies also revealed that the current recommended dietary allowances of calcium are more a statement of philosophy than sound criteria based on relevant scientific data. Third, these criteria do not take into consideration the bioavailability of the dietary calcium, the interactions between calcium and other dietary components, the effect of medications on calcium absorption and excretion, or the nutritional status of the individual, all of which may profoundly affect an individual's calcium requirements. These considerations have been reviewed by Allen in detail.[134] Clearly, further studies are needed to delineate the specific dietary requirement for calcium as individuals age. These studies will require a greater awareness of the physiologic role of Ca^{2+} in the development and maturation of the skeleton, in the pathogenesis of essential hypertension and eclampsias, and in as yet unrecognized pathologic processes that are the consequence of either dietary calcium deficiency or altered intestinal absorption of Ca^{2+}.

VI. PHOSPHATE

A. Homeostatic Mechanisms

Phosphorus is not only a major constituent of the skeleton in the form of hydroxyapatite, but it also is a mediator of energy transfer and participates in a wide variety of metabolic reactions in the cell. Because of the critical role of phosphorus as inorganic phosphate and phosphate esters in cell physiology, humans have developed elaborate mechanisms for extracting phosphate from the diet and for the conservation of the phosphate absorbed by the intestine. As a consequence, plasma phosphate and the extracellular fluid phosphate are maintained within a relatively narrow concentration range. Although the control of plasma phosphate concentration is not as finely regulated as that of calcium, we now recognize nonetheless that the plasma phosphate is indeed regulated through the interplay of a variety of homeostatic mechanisms. The intestine, which is involved in the extraction of phosphorus from dietary sources as inorganic phosphate, plays the principal role in the maintenance of an adequate supply of phosphate. The amount of phosphate excreted by the kidney is approximately equal to the amount of phosphate absorbed per day (see Chapter 7).

In adult humans, a dietary intake of approximately 800 mg of phosphate per day is required to maintain phosphate balance. During pregnancy and lactation this requirement is increased by 50%. Fortunately, phosphate is relatively abundant in a wide variety of foods so that nutritional phosphate deficiency is somewhat rare. Approximately four fifths of the dietary phosphorus in all age groups is contained in milk products, grains, and meat products. Dairy products constitute a major source of dietary phosphorus, with 1 cup of skim milk containing 247 mg and 1 oz of processed American cheese containing 210 mg. Food additives also contribute a considerable amount of phosphorus in the U.S. diet. These phosphorus-containing additives are used primarily in baked goods, cheeses, and other dairy products; phosphoric acid is also used in colas and carbonated beverages. In fact, food additives may contribute as much as 30% of the phosphorus of an average adult diet.[135] Dietary supplements of phosphorus are also readily available as mixed sodium and potassium mono- and dibasic salts. The laxative Fleet Phospho-Soda contains 129 mg/ml so that 1 teaspoon three times daily can provide over 1900 mg of phosphorus per day. Capsules and tablets are also available containing 250 mg or 500 mg of phosphorus as the sodium or potassium salt.

Consumption of phosphate in excess of 1800 mg will often be complicated by diarrhea. Approximately 60% of the dietary intake of phosphate is absorbed over a wide range of phosphorus intakes, with net absorption being proportional to intake. With increasing concentrations of phosphate in the diet, absorption occurs predominantly by a passive diffusion of phosphate across the intestine. Under these conditions, urinary excretion of phosphate parallels the dietary intake and is equal to the net phosphate absorbed. With reduced phosphate intakes, the intestinal absorption of phosphate occurs by active transport mechanisms. Urinary excretion of phosphate approaches zero as the tubular reabsorption of phosphate approaches 100% of the filtered load (see Chapter 7). Thus, both the intestine and the kidneys are able to respond to dietary phosphate restriction by enhancing the intestinal absorption and renal conservation of phosphate. Intestinal secretion of phosphate, which normally averages 3 mg/kg body weight/day, is also reduced. However, this adaptation occurs very slowly so that a net phosphate deficit may occur transiently.[136] In addition, humans are able to call upon endogenous stores of phosphate in order to maintain plasma phosphate concentrations. About 85% of the total body phosphorus is contained in the skeleton and is mobilized during phosphate depletion by increasing bone resorption. During an acute phase of phosphate depletion (i.e., 3–4 hr), the mobilization of phosphate from bone is not sufficiently rapid to maintain plasma phosphate. Under these conditions, skeletal muscle appears to play a dominant role in providing inorganic phosphate to the plasma.[137] During total starvation and pathologic states such as diabetic ketoacidosis, muscle catabolism may release sufficient quantities of intracellular phosphate to maintain normal or elevated levels of the anion. Since the released phosphate is lost in the urine, significant total body phosphate depletion can occur despite normal serum phosphate levels. During phosphate repletion, skeletal muscle, which comprises 40% of body weight, can rapidly deplete the smaller extracellular fluid (17% of body weight) of phosphate. During refeeding and the reversal of diabetic ketoacidosis, inorganic phosphate is sequestered in muscle hexose-phosphates and triose-phosphates of the glycolytic pathway; if not anticipated, profound hypophosphatemia may ensue. In normal individuals, these same mechanisms result in a postcibal fall in serum phosphate of about 0.25 mg/100 ml.[138] After sustained exercise or anaerobic muscle metabolism, plasma inorganic phosphate is rapidly taken up by muscle (5 mM/min) to replenish depleted phosphocreatine stores.[139,140] The decline in serum phosphate following myocardial infarction is perhaps yet another example of the shift in extracellular phosphate to intracellular sites in muscle.[141,142] Of the tissues involved in phosphate homeostasis, the renal handling of phosphate often represents the predominant determinant of the plasma phosphate (see Chapter 7). This is true in the chronic adaptation to both physiologic as well as pathologic disturbances of phosphate metabolism. Some of the factors that alter the renal handling of phosphate are listed in Table 6–4.

One of the humoral factors that plays the dominant role in the orchestration of the appropriate adaptation of the intestine, bone, and kidney to the challenge of phosphate depletion is the $1,25(OH)_2D$ metabolite of vitamin D_3. As detailed in Chapter 5, this metabolite is synthesized by a mitochondrial enzyme that hydroxylates the A-ring of 25-hydroxyvitamin D [25(OH)D] in the 1α-position.[143] As reviewed earlier, the enzyme is found predominantly in the kidney and its activity is governed primarily by parathyroid

Table 6–4. Factors that Decrease or Increase Renal Tubular Reabsorption of Phosphate

Factors that Decrease Phosphate Reabsorption
Parathyroid Hormone
Extracellular fluid volume expansion
Renal vasodilation
Diuretic agents
Alcohol ingestion
Parathyroid hormone
Calcitonin
Glucocorticoids
Antidiuretic hormone
Thyroid hormone
Calcitonin
High dietary intake of phosphate
Urinary alkalinization
Magnesium deficiency
Metabolic acidosis
Factors that Increase Phosphate Reabsorption
Glycosuria
Insulin
Growth hormone
Hypercalcemia
Hypermagnesemia
Dietary restriction of phosphate intake
Acute administration of vitamin D or $1,25(OH)_2D$

hormone[144,145] and circulating levels of inorganic phosphate.[146] Thus, when the plasma phosphate falls below the normal concentration, the production of $1,25(OH)_2D$ from its circulating precursor, 25(OH)D, is increased.

$1,25(OH)_2D$ stimulates the absorption of both calcium and phosphate by the intestine and the mobilization of calcium and phosphate from bone. The direct effect of $1,25(OH)_2D$ on renal phosphate conservation is relatively inconsequential (see Chapters 5 and 7). However, by increasing plasma calcium via its biological effects on the intestine and bone, $1,25(OH)_2D$ suppresses the production and secretion of parathyroid hormone. As noted in Chapter 13, $1,25(OH)_2D$ may also directly suppress PTH release. Parathyroid hormone is a major effector of renal phosphate clearance; it appears that in the presence of decreasing circulating levels of $1,25(OH)_2D$, PTH is able to enhance the renal tubular reabsorption of phosphate via cAMP and, hence, the conservation of phosphate. Unlike the renal proximal tubule, the adenylate cyclase system in jejunum is insensitive to PTH, and the P absorptive mechanism is resistant to cAMP.[149] It would appear that the renal metabolism of 25(OH)D also plays an important role in phosphate repletion when plasma phosphate concentration returns to normal or above. Under these conditions, the 25-hydroxycholecalciferol-1α-hydroxylase is suppressed and, in a reciprocal relationship, 24-hydroxylase activity is stimulated.[148] It has been postulated that the product, 24,25-dihydroxyvitamin D, is also essential for the maintenance of calcium and phosphate homeostasis, although other views have been expressed in this regard.[150] Although empirically attractive, hypotheses advanced to define the role of the vitamin D system on phosphate homeostasis are still controversial.[151,152] The phosphate-dependent metabolism of vitamin D is not the only factor regulating phosphate homeostasis. In the absence of vitamin D, the intestine, kidney, and bone respond to phosphate deprivation by enhancing the movements of phosphate into the circulation at each of the three anatomic sites.[91] This response also appears to be mediated by a humoral factor that is still unidentified.[137]

Other factors that influence phosphate homeostasis are conditions that cause a shift of phosphate between the extracellular and intracellular compartments. Extracellular inorganic phosphate shifts into cells when intracellular inorganic phosphate has been depleted by the phosphorylation of organic compounds. This occurs during glycolysis, glycogenolysis, and the synthesis of proteins and phosphocreatine. These processes are stimulated by the administration of carbohydrates, amino acids, or insulin and after sustained exercise as described previously. Respiratory alkalosis can also cause a rapid shift of phosphate into cells. Carbon dioxide diffuses rapidly across cell membranes and produces a fall in intracellular hydrogen ion concentration. The resulting increase in intracellular pH stimulates the glycolytic enzymes. Metabolic acidosis leads to a lowering of intracellular pH, inhibition of phosphorylation, and the release of phosphate from cells.[153]

During fasting, the concentration of phosphate in the lumen of the small intestine declines to about 2.0 mM/liter (6.2 mg/100 ml). The sources of endogenous phosphorus are saliva (4.0 mM/liter) and gastric, pancreatic, and intestinal secretion (1.0 mM/liter). Also, rapid turnover of enterocytes, which deliver approximately 250 mg of cellular debris into the intestinal lumen each day, contributes to the endogenous phosphate pool. Part of the endogenous phosphate pool is reabsorbed by the intestine, and the remainder (3.0–4.0 mM or 90–120 mg/day) is excreted in the feces.

Before considering the mechanism of phosphate transport across the intestine, it is necessary to first consider the structure and characteristics of the epithelial tissue involved in the transport process. The intestinal mucosa consists of villus structures lined with a columnar epithelium and a central core of lymphatics and capillaries that remove the substances transported by the columnar epithelium from the lumen of the intestine. The columnar epithelial cell is a highly differentiated cell that is asymmetric with respect to the structure and enzymatic composition of its cell membrane. That portion of the membrane facing the intestinal lumen is composed of a dense array of microvilli that extend into the lumen, thus greatly enhancing the absorptive surface area of the cell membrane. Accordingly, this surface of the cell is referred to as the "brush border." At the junction of the brush border and the lateral membrane, a dense structure connects the adjacent columnar cells and presumably serves to limit diffusion of substances between cells. The basal and lateral membranes are without convolutions or other distinguishing features microscopically. This membrane contains the Na^+-K^+-ATPase, whereas the brush border is relatively devoid of this enzyme. The exchange of Na^+ for K^+ is mediated by this enzyme, and this process creates an electrical potential difference across the cell membrane so that the cell is negative with respect to the outside of the cell.

This feature has two important implications with respect to the movement of the negatively charged phosphate ion across the intestine. First, because of the barrier imposed by the negative potential gradient, it can be assumed that passive intestinal absorption of phosphate would occur through channels between the lateral membranes of the columnar epithelium. Second, the negative potential gradient also implies that the rate-limiting and the site of active phosphate transport are located at the brush border. These assumptions are supported by the experimental observation that inhibitors of oxidative phosphorylation inhibit the rate of phosphate uptake by the mucosal epithelium.[154] Since the concentration of inorganic phosphate in the cytoplasm is of the order of 1 mM, efflux of phosphate across the basal lateral membrane would be passive along both a chemical and electrical potential gradient. The actual mechanisms of active phosphate transport remain to be delineated. The elucidation of this important transport process is made difficult by the fact that inorganic phosphate, unlike other "inert" ions, becomes rapidly organified once it enters the cell by a variety of metabolic reactions. Thus, the rate of phosphate uptake by the intestinal epithelial cell is not only a function of the transport process but also a function of the rate of esterification of the intracellular phosphate. In spite of these difficulties, a considerable amount of information has been accumulated that enables us to partially characterize the transport process in the intestine.

The available data indicate that phosphate absorption occurs through the cells of the intestinal mucosa and via the paracellular pathways in the duodenum, jejunum, and ileum, being greatest in the jejunum. The paracellular transport is mediated by diffusion and depends on a concentration gradient, whereas the transcellular transport is active, carrier-mediated and saturable, and independent of cAMP or PTH.[149]

There is now considerable evidence suggesting that there are at least two independent carrier-mediated processes for the transport of phosphate across the brush border of the intestinal epithelial cell.[155] In contrast to the high-affinity transport process (K_m = 0.08 mM), the low-affinity transport process displays a K_m for phosphate that is within the extracellular physiologic concentration of the anion. The two transport systems can be distinguished on the basis of a number of parameters. The high-affinity transport system is enhanced by acid pH, whereas the low-affinity system is stimulated by alkaline pH. Both processes are dependent on sodium and potassium; however, the low-affinity transport mechanism is stimulated by calcium. Much of the apparently conflicting data accumulated in the past can be attributed to the failure to recognize the existence of these two transport systems. Other factors that influence phosphate transport include arsenate, which competitively and irreversibly inhibits the transport at the brush border, providing additional support for the process as being carrier-mediated. As indicated, $1,25(OH)_2D$ and to a lesser extent other metabolites of vitamin D stimulate intestinal absorption of phosphate.

The molecular basis for the translocation of phosphate across the brush border is unknown. The membrane-bound enzyme alkaline phosphatase has been implicated by many investigators to be involved in the energy-dependent transport of phosphate into the cell. Indeed, phosphate deprivation results in the induction of synthesis of this enzyme, which parallels the increase in organic phosphate transport. This phenomenon has been documented in the mammalian renal tubule and intestine and in essentially every species examined including prokaryotic organisms.[156-158] In *Escherichia coli*, the enzyme has been studied extensively with selective gene mutations. From such studies it appears that the alkaline phosphatase enzyme is not required for inorganic phosphate transport but may influence the specificity of the transport system for phosphate relative to related anions.[159] Synthesis of the enzyme is co-regulated along with several other enzymes involved in cellular phosphate homeostasis in response to intracellular phosphate concentrations. The stimulation of intestinal alkaline phosphatase by vitamin D may be another expression of the genetic linkage between the alkaline phosphatase enzyme and the phosphate transport system.

B. Disorders of Intestinal Absorption of Phosphate

Disorders of phosphate absorption and the resulting phosphate depletion produce a clinical picture that is largely independent of the underlying cause.

The clinical manifestations of hypophosphatemia are summarized in Table 6–5. In general these changes can be attributed to two metabolic consequences of cellular phosphate depletion: (1) the reduction of ATP synthesis and thus the cell's source of energy; and (2) a shift in the oxyhemoglobin dissociation curve of the red blood cell.[160] Anaerobic metabolism of glucose is directly dependent on the serum phosphate level. Thus, the production of ATP by erythrocytes and other cells depends on the serum phosphate levels. The integrity and deformability of the erythrocyte membrane becomes less plastic when cell ATP levels fall, resulting in severe hemolytic anemias in patients with phosphate levels below 0.3 mg/100 ml.[161] Neurologic and muscular dysfunction associated with hypophosphatemia may also be attributed to the depletion of intracellular ATP. Symptoms of weakness, malaise, joint stiffness, and intention tremors occur in patients with serum phosphorus levels of 2 mg/100 ml.[162] More profound hypophosphatemia results in heart failure, rhabdomyolysis, paralysis, seizures, coma, and death.[163] An additional factor contributing to these neuromuscular symptoms may be tissue hypoxia resulting from the impaired delivery of oxygen.[160] Red cell phosphate depletion causes a decrease in the glycolytic intermediate 2,3-diphosphoglycerate, which is a major determinant of the binding avidity of oxygen to hemoglobin. Consequently, the oxyhemoglobin dissociation curve is shifted to the left with decreased delivery of oxygen to tissues. The skeletal effects of hypophosphatemia are osteomalacia and a clinical bone disease that resembles rickets (see Chapters 11 and 24). The mineralization defect and bone mineral loss appear to be independent of vitamin D and parathyroid hormone. Bone pain may be complicated with large-joint arthralgias and inflammatory arthritis.[164] Quantitative assessment of the role of the defective intestinal phosphate absorption in the phosphate depletion syndromes has been limited by the difficulties inherent in the measurement of intestinal phosphate absorption. Consequently, our knowledge of this aspect of phosphate homeostasis remains incomplete.

Table 6–5. Clinical Manifestations of Hypophosphatemia

Hematologic
Decreased release of O_2 from hemoglobin
Hemolytic anemia
Decreased polymorphonuclear chemotaxis and phagocytosis
Decreased clot retraction amd platelet survival
Hepatic
Hepatic coma ? to hypoxia
Skeletal
Osteomalacia and increased bone resorption
Neuromuscular
Muscle weakness
Paresthesias
Hyporeflexia
Rhabdomyolysis
Intention tremor
Ataxia
Paralysis
Convulsions
Heart failure
Coma

Through the years a number of approaches to the quantitation of phosphate absorption have been attempted. The most reliable has been the classic balance technique, which measures the net retention or loss of dietary phosphate over a period of 1 to 2 weeks. Not only is the technique tedious and impractical, it also does not measure intestinal phosphate transport specifically. A more simplified approach is the measurement of the rise in serum phosphate after an oral load of phosphate.[165] Although admittedly a crude estimation of the phosphate absorptive capacity of the intestine, the influence of the rate of phosphate utilization in cellular metabolism, the rate of deposition in bone, and intestinal secretion of phosphate on the observed response is less than the influence of these same factors on balance studies. Unfortunately, due to the high concentration of phosphate essential for studies of phosphate absorption, one is not able to assess the ability of the intestine to actively transport phosphate against a more physiologic concentration gradient. In an attempt to measure directly the intestinal transport of phosphate, peroral jejunal biopsies have been obtained from patients and the rate of [^{32}P]-phosphate accumulation of the mucosal tissue has been measured. This technique has been used to investigate a defect in the accumulation of [^{32}P]-phosphate in patients with vitamin D–resistant rickets.[166] Again, one must recognize that this technique measures the tissue accumulation of the isotope and not the actual transport of phosphate across the mucosa. All techniques including those in experimental animals have in common the problem of rapid organification of the phosphate upon entering the cell cytosol. As a result, it is difficult to ascertain the effective concentration gradient that limits the mucosal uptake of phosphate across the brush border.

The causes of impaired intestinal phosphate absorption may be divided into five functional categories (Table 6–6). Gastrointestinal disorders that result in steatorrhea such as pancreatic insufficiency and bile salt deficiency, intrinsic bowel disease (Crohn's disease and sprue), and short bowel syndromes (intestinal fistula, rapid transit states, ileal bypass procedures) can be associated with decreased intestinal absorption of phosphate and hypophosphatemia. The predominant mechanism leading to hypophosphatemia in these disorders is the renal wasting of phosphate secondary to overactive parathyroid glands induced by malabsorption of calcium and vitamin D.[167] As noted, vitamin D_3, and specifically the metabolite $1{,}25(OH)_2D_3$, is required for the normal intestinal absorption of phosphate. Malabsorption of the vitamin occurs in patients with steatorrhea resulting primarily from the absorption of the fat-soluble vitamin by the unabsorbed fats.[168] Absorption of the fat-soluble vitamin requires bile salts. Their defective synthesis in patients with severe liver disease and biliary cirrhosis accounts for the osteomalacia seen in these disorders. A failure to convert $25(OH)D_3$ to $1{,}25(OH)_2D_3$ by the renal tubule in chronic renal failure is a significant factor leading to defective absorption of phosphate.[169,170] Normal aging results also in decreased renal production of $1{,}25(OH)_2D_3$ in response to parathyroid hormone stimulation.[171] Thus, the elderly generate an inadequate response to dietary calcium restriction resulting in both negative calcium and phosphate balances. Other states resulting in impaired renal production of $1{,}25(OH)_2D_3$ and osteomalacia include heavy metal intoxication as with lead and strontium, diphosphonate therapy, and juvenile diabetes mellitus.

Table 6–6. Disorders of Intestinal Phosphate Absorption

Nonspecific Intestinal Malabsorption Syndromes
Vitamin D Deficiency States
- Nutritional vitamin D deficiency
- Liver disease
- Pancreatic insufficiency
- Gastric surgery

Disorders of Vitamin D Metabolism
- Advanced renal insufficiency
- Pseudo–vitamin D–resistant rickets
- Heavy metal intoxication
- ? Diphosphonate therapy
- Juvenile diabetes mellitus

Extrinsic Disorders of Intestinal Phosphate Absorption
- Nonabsorbable antacid therapy
- Phytates

Intrinsic Disorders of Intestinal Phosphate Absorption
- Familial hypophosphatemic vitamin D–resistant rickets
- ? Magnesium deficiency
- ? Aging
- Oncogenic hypophosphatemic osteomalacia

However, in humans there is no direct evidence that intestinal phosphate absorption is impaired in these states. The clinical importance of the dihydroxymetabolite of vitamin D is illustrated by the autosomal recessive disorder of pseudo–vitamin D–resistant rickets in which the 25-hydroxyvitamin D 1α-hydroxylase is defective.[172] By the first year of life these children develop hypophosphatemia and rickets resistant to vitamin D replacement but corrected completely by physiologic doses of $1{,}25(OH)_2D_3$ with restoration of normal growth and the return of biochemical abnormalities to normal.

In addition to vitamin D and its metabolites, there are a number of other factors that influence specifically the intestinal absorption of phosphate. Phosphate in the form of inositol hexaphosphoric acid or phytates, the major component of organic phosphate in cereals, forms insoluble salts with calcium and is, therefore, not available for absorption. Aluminum and magnesium ions, the principal elements of widely used antacids, also form insoluble salts with phosphate and are not absorbed. Inappropriate and continued use of aluminum-containing phosphate-binding antacids results in chronic hypophosphatemia, hypercalcemia, increased propensity toward renal calculi formation,[162] and osteomalacia (see Chapters 11 and 23). Increasing dietary calcium with the $CaCO_3$ salt to levels in excess of 1600 mg/day reduces the intestinal absorption of phosphate,[173] an effect that is utilized in the treatment of patients with chronic renal failure (see Chapter 13). Excessive use of antacids will complex with endogenously secreted phosphate and thereby rapidly deplete the body of inorganic phosphate. A number of factors directly influence the phosphate transport process. The least well understood is the influence of aging on intestinal transport functions. Both calcium and phosphate absorption are reduced by more than 50% with advancing age in humans. The intestinal response to vitamin D is similarly reduced, suggesting a state of vitamin D resistance.[18] In humans, intestinal absorption of phosphate has not been studied as a function of age. On the other hand, there is very good evidence that, in humans, intestinal calcium absorption is markedly limited after the sixth decade from its peak during the second decade of life.[15-17]

An interesting but complex disorder of phosphate absorption and homeostasis is that of magnesium deficiency. Severe magnesium deficiency in humans is associated with hypocalcemia due both to an inability of the parathyroid glands to secrete parathyroid hormone[174] and to a resistance of bone to the hormone's action[175] (Table 6–7). This disorder is further complicated by an apparent resistance to vitamin D. Despite the functional hypoparathyroidism, serum phosphate is often below normal. The hypophosphatemia can be attributed in part to an impairment in the intestinal absorption and renal tubular reabsorption of phosphate; magnesium supplementation of the deficient patient leads to an increase in phosphate balance. It is postulated that magnesium deficiency commonly associated with excessive ethanol ingestion may be one of the principal factors contributing to the severe hypophosphatemia of chronic alcoholism.[176]

Recent data suggest that oncogenic osteomalacia may result from the tumor production of a humoral factor that inhibits phosphate transport directly and blocks the renal production of $1,25(OH)_2D$ (see Chapter 11). The osteomalacia and renal wasting of phosphate may be profound but completely reversible by the excision of the typically small, often difficult-to-locate mesenchymal tumors. Their cell morphology is characterized by a mixture of mesenchymal elements including giant cells, vascular tissue, and hyaline cartilage.[177,178]

The most striking disorder of phosphate transport is the genetic defect that characterizes familial hypophosphatemic vitamin D–resistant rickets.[179] This disorder, which is inherited in an X-linked dominant fashion, is manifested by the early onset of growth failure and skeletal rickets (see Chapter 24). In contrast to pseudo–vitamin D–resistant rickets or nutritional rickets, vitamin D in even massive doses cannot correct the renal loss of phosphate and restore normal growth. Recently a strain of mice has been identified that develops hypophosphatemic rickets through a similar X-linked dominant mode of inheritance that phenotypically mimics the disorder in humans. In affected mice, impaired phosphate transport is apparent in both the intestine and the renal tubule. In humans, a similar pattern of involvement has emerged from investigations of the ability of peroral jejunal biopsies to accumulate [^{32}P] phosphate[166] and from oral phosphate tolerance tests.[165] Although phosphorus is an essential element in cell function and the regulation of cell metabolism, investigation of its role in clinical medicine has proved difficult. Consequently, our knowledge of the role of phosphate depletion and hypophosphatemia in the expression of disease still remains relatively limited. Too often, severe hypophosphatemia is not anticipated so that the catastrophic consequence becomes manifested before appropriate intervention is initiated. It is hoped that by increasing our familiarity with the factors contributing to hypophosphatemia and the clinical manifestations of the deficiency state, the life-threatening but reversible expressions of hypophosphatemia can be prevented.[180]

Table 6–7. Etiology of Hypoparathyroidism and Parathyroid Hormone–Resistant States

Hypoparathyroidism
Idiopathic
Surgical
Familial
Hypomagnesemia
Parathyroid Hormone–Resistant States
Uremia
Vitamin D deficiency (resistance)
Hypomagnesemia
Pseudohypoparathyroidism
? Aging

References

1. Heaney RP, Skillman TG: Secretion and excretion of calcium by the human gastrointestinal tract. J Lab Clin Med 64:19–35, 1964.

2. Ireland P, Fordtran JS: Effect of dietary calcium and age on jejunal calcium absorption in humans studied by intestinal perfusion. J Clin Invest 52:2672–2681, 1973.
3. Irving JR: Dynamics and function of phosphorus. *In* Comar CL, Bronner F (eds): Mineral Metabolism. New York, Academic Press, 1964, pp 249–313.
4. Spencer H, Menczel J, Lewin I, et al: Effect of high intake on calcium and phosphorus metabolism in man. J Nutr 86:125–132, 1965.
5. Cramer CF: Effect of Ca/P ratio and pH on calcium and phosphorus absorption from dog gut loops *in vivo*. Can J Physiol Pharmacol 46:171–173, 1968.
6. Brannan PG, Vergne-Marini P, Pak CYC, et al: Magnesium absorption in the human small intestine. J Clin Invest 57:1412–1418, 1976.
7. Patton MB, Sutton TS: The utilization of calcium from lactate, gluconate, sulfate and carbonate salts by young college women. J Nutr 48:443–452, 1952.
7a. Heaney RP, Weaver CM: Oxalale: Effect on calcium absorbability. Am J Clin Nutr 50:830–832, 1989.
8. Avioli LV: Intestinal absorption of calcium. Arch Intern Med 129:345–350, 1972.
9. Vaughan OW, Filer LJ: The enhancing action of certain carbohydrates on the intestinal absorption of calcium in the rat. J Nutr 71:10–14, 1960.
10. Kelly SE, Chawwla Singh K, Sellin JH, et al: Effect of meal composition on calcium absorption: Enhancing effect of carbohydrate polymers. Gastroenterology 87:596–600, 1984.
11. Recker RR: Calcium absorption and achlorhydria. N Engl J Med 313:70–73, 1985.
12. Bo-Linn GW, David GR, Buddrus DJ, et al: An evaluation of the importance of gastric acid secretion in the absorption of dietary calcium. J Clin Invest 73:640–647, 1984.
12a. Knox TA, Kassarjian Z, Dawson-Hughes B, et al: Effect of high fiber diet and gastric acidity on calcium absorption in the elderly by the whole-body counter method. J Am Coll Nutr 8:450, 1989.
13. Kumar R, Cohen WR, Silva P: Elevated 1,25-dihydroxyvitamin D plasma levels in normal human pregnancy and lactation. J Clin Invest 63:342–344, 1979.
14. Tanaka Y, Halloran B, Schnoes HF: *In vitro* production of 1,25-dihydroxyvitamin D_3 by rat placental tissue. Proc Natl Acad Sci USA 76:5033, 1979.
15. Bullamore JR, Wilkinson R, Gallagher JC: Effect of age on calcium absorption. Lancet 2:535–537, 1970.
16. Alevizaki CC, Ikkos DC, Singhelakis PJ: Progressive decrease of true intestinal calcium absorption with age in normal man. Nucl Med 14:760–762, 1973.
17. Gallagher JC, Riggs BL, Eisman J: Intestinal calcium absorption and serum vitamin D metabolites in normal subjects and osteoporotic patients. J Clin Invest 64:729–736, 1979.
18. Armbrecht HJ, Zenser TV, Davis BB: Effect of vitamin D metabolites on intestinal calcium absorption and calcium-binding proteins in young adult rats. Endocrinology 106:469–475, 1980.
19. Gray RW, Gambert SR: Effect of age on plasma $1,25(OH)_2D$ vitamin D in the rat. Age 5:54–56, 1982.
19a. Barrett-Comor E: The RDA for calcium in the elderly: too little, too late. Calcif Tissue Int 44:303–307, 1989.
20. Kelsay JL, Behall KM, Prather ES: Effect of fiber from fruits and vegetables on metabolic responses of human subjects. II. Calcium, magnesium, iron and silicon balances. Am J Clin Nutr 32:1836–1880, 1979.
21. Bonner P, Hummel FC, Bates MF: The influence of a daily serving of spinach or its equivalent oxalic acid upon the mineral utilization of children. J Pediatr 12:188–196, 1938.
22. Birge SJ, Peck WA, Berman M, Whedon GD: Study of calcium absorption in man: A kinetic analysis and physiologic model. J Clin Invest 48:1705–1713, 1969.
23. Wensel RH, Rich C, Brown AC, et al: Absorption of calcium measured by incubation and perfusion of the intact human small intestine. J Clin Invest 48:1768–1775, 1969.
24. Favus MJ, Kathpalia SC, Coe FL: Effects of diet calcium and 1,25-dihydroxyvitamin D_3 on colon calcium active transport. Am J Physiol 238:G75–G78, 1980.
25. Lee DBN, Walling MW, Gafter U, et al: Calcium and inorganic phosphate transport in rat colon. J Clin Invest 65:1326–1331, 1980.
26. Petith MM, Schedl HP: Intestinal adaptation to dietary calcium restriction: *In vivo* cecal and colonic calcium transport in the rat. Gastroenterology 71:1039–1042, 1976.
27. Ussing HH: The distinction by means of tracers between active transport and diffusion. Acta Physiol Scand 19:43–46, 1949.
28. Walling MW, Rothman SS: Phosphate-independent, carrier-mediated transport of calcium by rat intestine. Am J Physiol 217:1144–1148, 1969.
29. Martin DL, DeLuca H: Calcium transport and the role of vitamin D. Arch Biochem Biophys 134:139–149, 1960.
30. Bikle DD, Morrissey RL, Zolock DT: The mechanisms of action of vitamin D in the intestine. Am J Clin Nutr 32:2322–2338, 1979.
31. Bratbar N, Levine BS, Wading MW, et al: Intestinal absorption of calcium: Role of dietary phosphate and vitamin D. Am J Physiol 241:649–653, 1981.
32. Wasserman RH, Taylor AN: Vitamin D_3-induced calcium binding protein in chick intestinal mucosa. Science 152:791–793, 1966.
33. Birge SJ, Miller R: The role of phosphate in the action of vitamin D in the intestine. J Clin Invest 60:980–988, 1977.
34. Wilson PW, Lawson DEM: Incorporation of [^{3}H] leucine into an actin-like protein in response to 1,25 dihydroxycholecalciferol in chick intestine brush borders. Biochem J 173:627–631, 1978.
35. Kowarski S, Schachter D: Intestinal membrane calcium-binding protein. J Biol Chem 255:10834–10840, 1980.
36. Hobden AN, Harding M, Lawson DEM: 1,25-dihydroxycholecalciferol stimulation of a mitochondrial protein in chick intestinal cells. Nature (London) 288:718–720, 1980.
37. Corradino RA: Embryonic chick intestine in organ culture: Interaction of adenylate cyclase system and vitamin D_3-mediated calcium absorptive mechanism. Endocrinology 94:1607–1614, 1974.
38. Fontaine O, Matsumoto T, Goodman DBP, et al: Liponomic control of Ca transport: Relationship to mechanism of action of 1,25-dihydroxyvitamin D_3. Proc Natl Acad Sci USA 78:1751–1754, 1981.
39. Wilson PW, Larson DEM: Vitamin D dependent phosphorylation of an intestinal protein. Nature (London) 289:600–602, 1981.

40. Schachter DS, Kowarski JD, Finkelstein R-IW: Tissue concentration differences during active transport of calcium by intestine. Am J Physiol 211:1131–1136, 1966.
41. Urban E, Schedl HP: Comparison of *in vivo* and *in vitro* effects of vitamin D in calcium transport in the rat. Am J Physiol 217:126–130, 1969.
42. Martin DL, DeLuca HF: Influence of sodium on calcium transport by the rat small intestine. Am J Physiol 216:1352–1359, 1969.
43. Wong RG, Norman AW: Studies on the mechanism of action of calciferol. VIII. The effects of dietary vitamin D and the polyene antibiotic, filipin, *in vitro*, on the intestinal cellular uptake of calcium. J Biol Chem 250:2411–2419, 1975.
44. Bikle DD, Zobock DT, Morrissey R, et al: Independence of 1,25-dihydroxyvitamin D_3-mediated calcium transport from de novo RNA and protein synthesis. J Biol Chem 253:484–488, 1978.
45. Sampson HW, Matthews JL, Martin JH, et al: An electron microscopic localization of calcium in the small intestine of normal, rachitic and vitamin D-treated rats. Calcif Tissue Res 5:305–316, 1970.
46. MacLaughlin JA, Weiser MM, Freedman RA: Biphasic recovery of vitamin D-dependent Ca^{2+} uptake by rat intestinal Golgi membranes. Gastroenterology 78:325–331, 1980.
47. Weiser MM, Bloor JH, Dasmahapatia A: Intestinal calcium absorption and vitamin D metabolism. J Clin Gastroenterol 4:75–86, 1982.
48. Birge SJ, Switzer SC, Leonard DR: Influence of sodium and parathyroid hormone on calcium release from intestinal mucosal cells. J Clin Invest 54:702–709, 1974.
49. Birge SJ, Gilbert HR: Identification of an intestinal sodium and calcium-dependent phosphatase stimulated by parathyroid hormone. J Clin Invest 54:710–717, 1974.
50. Ghijsen WEJM, DeJong MD, Van Os CH: Dissociation between Ca^{2+}-ATPase and alkaline phosphatase activities in plasma membranes of rat duodenum. Biochim Biophys Acta 599: 538–545, 1980.
51. Nellans HN, Popovitch JE: Calmodulin-regulated ATP-driven calcium transport by basolateral membranes of rat small intestine. J Biol Chem 256:9932–9936, 1981.
52. DeJong HR, Ghijsen WEJM, Van Os CH: Phosphorylated intermediates of Ca-ATPase and alkaline phosphatase in plasma membranes from rat duodenal epithelium. Biochim Biophys Acta 647:140–149, 1981.
53. Schiffl H, Binswager U: Calcium ATPase and intestinal calcium transport in uremic rats. Am J Physiol 238:G424–G428, 1980.
54. van Corven JJM, De Jong MD, Van Os CH: The adenosine triphosphate–dependent calcium pump in rat small intestine: Effects of vitamin D deficiency and cell isolation methods. Endocrinology 120:868–873, 1987.
55. Corradino RA: Cyclic AMP regulation of $1,25(OH)_2D_3$-mediated intestinal calcium absorption mechanism. *In* Norman AW, Schaefer K, Coburn JW, et al (eds): Vitamin D: Biochemical, Chemical, and Clinical Aspects Related to Calcium Metabolism. Vitamin D: Biochemical, Chemical, and Clinical Aspects Related to Calcium Metabolism. de Gruyter, Berlin, 1977, pp 231–240.
56. Birge SJ, Miller RA: The role of phosphate in the action of vitamin D on the intestine. J Clin Invest 60:980–988, 1977.
57. Hitchman AJW, Harrison JE: Calcium binding proteins in the duodenal mucosa of the chick, rat, pig and human. Can J Biochem 50:758–765, 1972.
58. Kowarski S, Schachter D: Intestinal membrane calcium-binding protein: Vitamin D-dependent membrane component of the intestinal calcium transport mechanism. J Biol Chem 255:10834–10840, 1980.
59. Birge SJ, Alpers DH: Stimulation of intestinal mucosal proliferation by vitamin D. Gastroenterology 64:977–982, 1973.
60. Litwak L: Tracer studies of intestinal calcium absorption in man. Am J Clin Nutr 22:771–785, 1969.
61. Wootton R, Reeve J: The relative merits of various techniques for measuring radiocalcium absorption. Clin Sci 58:287–293, 1980.
62. Nordin BEC: Osteomalacia, osteoporosis and calcium deficiency. Clin Orthop Relat Res 17:235–258, 1960.
63. Mariel PJ, Pettifor JM, Ross FP, et al: Histological osteomalacia due to dietary Ca deficiency in children. N Engl J Med 307:584–588, 1982.
64. Heaney RP, Skillman TG: Calcium metabolism in normal human pregnancy. J Clin Endocrinol 33:661–669, 1971.
65. Pitkin RM: Calcium metabolism in pregnancy: A review. Am J Obstet Gynecol 12:724–737, 1975.
66. Wieland P, Fischer JA, Treschel U, et al: Perinatal parathyroid hormone, vitamin D metabolites, and calcitonin in man. Am J Physiol 239:E385–390, 1980.
67. Steichen JJ, Tsang RC, Gratton TL, et al: Vitamin D homeostasis in the perinatal period. N Engl J Med 302:315–319, 1978.
68. Weisman, T, Harrell A, Edelstein S, et al: 1α-25-dihydroxyvitamin D_3 and 24,25-dihydroxyvitamin D_3 *in vitro* synthesis by human decidua and placenta. Nature (London) 281:317, 1979.
69. Bouillon R, van Assche FA, van Baelen H, et al: Influence of the vitamin D-binding protein on the serum concentration of 1,25-dihydroxyvitamin D_3. J Clin Invest 67:589–596, 1981.
70. Kumar R, Abboud CF, Riggs BL: The effect of elevated prolactin levels in plasma 1,25-dihydroxyvitamin D and intestinal absorption of calcium. Mayo Clin Proc 55:51–53, 1980.
71. Miller RA, Russell JE, Birge SJ: Quantitation of the receptor proteins for $1,25(OH)_2D$ in the intestine of the aging rat. Calcif Tissue Int 35:697a, 1983.
72. Toraason M: Calcium flux in vivo in the rat duodenum and ileum during pregnancy and lactation. Am J Physiol 245:G624–G627, 1983.
73. Stern PH, DeOlazabal J, Bell NH: Evidence for abnormal regulation of circulating 1α,25-dihydroxyvitamin D in patients with sarcoidosis and normal calcium metabolism. J Clin Invest 66:852–855, 1980.
74. Barbour GL, Coburn JW, Slatopolsky E, et al: Hypercalcemia in a patient with sarcoidosis: Evidence for extrarenal generation of 1,25-dihydroxyvitamin D. N Engl J Med 305:440–443, 1981.
75. Adams JS, Singer FR, Garad MA, et al: Isolation and structural identification of 1,25-dihydroxyvitamin D_3 produced by cultured alveolar macrophages in sarcoidosis. J Clin Endocrinol Metab 60:960–966, 1985.

76. Lee JC, Catanzaro A, Parthemore JG, et al: Hypercalcemia in disseminated coccidiomycosis. N Engl J Med 297:431–433, 1977.
77. Walker JV, Baran D, Yakub YN, et al: Histoplasmosis with hypercalcemia, renal failure, and papillary necrosis: Confusion with sarcoidosis. JAMA 237:1350–1352, 1977.
78. Stoeckle JD, Hardy HL, Weber AL: Chronic beryllium disease: Long term follow-up of sixty cases and selective review of the literature. Am J Med 461:545–561, 1969.
79. Abbasi AD, Chemplavil JK, Farah BF, et al: Hypercalcemia in active preliminary tuberculosis. Ann Intern Med 90:324–328, 1979.
80. Gwinup G, Romdazzo G, Elias A: The influence of vitamin D intake on serum calcium in tuberculosis. Acta Endocrinol (Copenh) 97:114–117, 1981.
81. Levin ME, Boisseau VC, Avioli LV: Effects of diabetes mellitus on bone mass in juvenile and adult-onset diabetes. N Engl J Med 294:241–245, 1976.
82. Hough S, Avioli LV, Bergfeld MA, et al: Correction of abnormal bone and mineral metabolism in chronic streptozotocin-induced diabetes mellitus in the rat by insulin therapy. Endocrinology 108:2228–2234, 1981.
83. Seino Y, Seiena RI, Sonn YM, et al: The duodenal $1,25(OH)_2D_3$ receptor in rats with experimentally-induced diabetes. Endocrinology 113:1721–1725, 1983.
84. Hough S, Russell JE, Teitelbaum SL, et al: Calcium homeostasis in chronic streptozotocin-induced diabetes mellitus in the rat. Am J Physiol 242:E451–E456, 1982.
85. Fraser TE, White NH, Hough S, et al: Alterations in circulating vitamin metabolites in the young insulin-dependent diabetic. J Clin Endocrinol 53:1154–1159, 1981.
86. Witt MF, White NH, Santiago JV, et al: Increased calcium absorption in type I diabetic children. Pediatr Res 16:1129a, 1982.
87. Broadus AE, Dominguez M, Bartter FC: Pathophysiological studies in idiopathic hypercalciuria: Use of an oral calcium tolerance test to characterize distinctive hypercalciuric subgroups. J Clin Endocrinol Metab 47:751–760, 1978.
88. Pak CYC, Ohata M, Lawrence EC, et al: The hypercalciurias causes, parathyroid functions and diagnostic criteria. J Clin Invest 54:387–400, 1974.
88a. Pacifici R, Filipponi P, Mannarelli C, et al: Classification of idiopathic hypercalciuric patients by isotopic calcium absorption: A comparison with oral calcium tolerance test. Calcif Tissue Int 37:467–473, 1985.
89. Zerwekh JE, Pak CYC: Selective effects of thiazide therapy on serum 1α,25-dihydroxyvitamin D and intestinal calcium absorption in renal and absorptive hypercalciurias. Metabolism 29:13–17, 1980.
90. Gray RW, Wilz DR, Caldas AE, et al: The importance of phosphate in regulating plasma 1α,25-$(OH)_2$-vitamin D levels in humans. Studies in healthy subjects, in calcium stone-formers and in patients with primary hyperparathyroidism. J Clin Endocrinol Metab 45:299–306, 1977.
91. Brattbar N, Walling MW, Coburn JW: Interaction between vitamin D deficiency and deficiency and phosphorus depletion in the rat. J Clin Invest 63:335–341, 1979.
92. McMillan EE, Freeman RB: The milk alkali syndrome: A study of the acute disorder with comments on the development of the chronic condition. Medicine (Baltimore) 44:485–501, 1965.
93. Peterson CR: Vitamin D poisoning: Survey of causes in 21 patients with hypercalcemia. Lancet 1:1164–1165, 1980.
94. Shetty KR, Ajlouni K, Rosenfeld PS, et al: Protracted vitamin D intoxication. Arch Intern Med 135:986–988, 1975.
95. Recker RR, Saville PD, Heaney RP: Effect of estrogens and calcium carbonate on bone loss in postmenopausal women. Ann Intern Med 87:649–655, 1977.
96. Caniggia A, Gennari C, Bianchi V, et al: Intestinal absorption of ^{45}Ca in senile osteoporosis. Acta Med Scand 173:613–617, 1963.
97. Chan SDH, Chiu DRH, Atkins D: Oophorectomy leads to a selective disease in 1,25-dihydroxycholecalciferol receptors in rat jejunal villous cells. Clin Sci 66:745–748, 1984.
98. Finkelstein JD, Schachter D: Active transport of calcium by intestine: The effects of hypophysectomy and growth hormone. Am J Physiol 203:873–880, 1962.
99. Compston JE, Thompson RPH: Intestinal absorption of 25-hydroxyvitamin D and osteomalacia in primary biliary cirrhosis. Lancet 2:721–724, 1977.
100. Arnaud SB, Goldsmith RS, Lambert PW, et al: 25-hydroxyvitamin D_3: Evidence of an enterohepatic circulation in man. Proc Soc Exp Biol Med 149:570–572, 1975.
101. Imawari MK, Kozawa Y, Akamuma S, et al: 25-Hydroxyvitamin D and vitamin D-serum binding protein levels and mineral metabolism after partial and total gastrectomy. Gastroenterology 79:255–258, 1980.
102. Sitrin M, Meredith S, Rosenberg IH: Vitamin D deficiency and bone disease in gastrointestinal disorders. Arch Intern Med 138:886–888, 1978.
103. Nemere I, Szego CM: Early actions of parathyroid hormone and 1,25-dihydroxycholecalciferol on isolated epithelial cells from rat intestine I. Limited lysosomal enzyme release and calcium uptake. Endocrinology 108:1450–1462, 1981.
104. Bouillon R, Muls E, DeMoor P: Influence of thyroid function on the serum concentration of 1,25-dihydroxyvitamin D. J Clin Endocrinol Metab 51:793–797, 1980.
105. Coburn JW, Koppel MH, Brickman AS, et al: Study of intestinal absorption of calcium in patients with renal failure. Kidney Int 2:264–272, 1973.
106. Recker RR, Saville PD: Calcium absorption in renal failure: Its relation to blood urea nitrogen, dietary calcium intake, time on dialysis and other variables. J Lab Clin Med 78:380–388, 1971.
107. Brickman AS, Coburn JW, Rowe PH, et al: Impaired calcium absorption in uremic man: evidence for defective absorption in the proximal small intestine. J Lab Clin Med 84:791–801, 1974.
108. Vergne-Marini P, Parker TF, Pak CYC, et al: Jejunal and ileal calcium absorption in patients with chronic renal disease. J Clin Invest 57:861–866, 1976.
109. McDermott FR, Galbraith AJ, Dalton MK: Effects of acute renal failure on ileal epithelial cell kinetics: Autoradiographic studies in the mouse. Gastroenterology 66:235–239, 1974.
110. Piazolo P, Hotz H, Helmke K, et al: Calcium-bind-

ing protein in the duodenal mucosa of uremic patients and normal subject. Kidney Int 8:110–118, 1975.

111. Bikle D, Rasmussen H: The ionic control of 1,25-hydroxyvitamin D_3 production in isolated chick renal tubules. J Clin Invest 55:292–298, 1975.

112. Hahn TJ, Hendin BA, Scharp CR, et al: Effect of chronic anticonvulsant therapy on serum 25-hydroxycholecalciferol levels in adults. N Engl J Med 287:900–904, 1972.

113. Rodbor P, Christiansen C, Lund M: Development of anticonvulsant osteomalacia in epileptic patients on phenytoin treatment. Acta Neurol Scand 50:527–532, 1974.

114. Hahn TJ: Drug-induced disorders of vitamin D and mineral metabolism. Clin Endocrinol Metab 9:107–127, 1980.

115. Hahn TJ, Halstead LR, Teitelbaum S, et al: Altered mineral metabolism in glucocorticoid-induced osteopenia. J Clin Invest 64:655–665, 1979.

116. Carre M, Ayigebede O, Miravet L: The effect of prednisolone on the metabolism and action of 25-hydroxy- and 1,25-dihydroxyvitamin D_3. Proc Natl Acad Sci USA 71:2996–3000, 1974.

117. O'Regan S, Chesney RW, Hamstra A, et al: Reduced serum 1,25$(OH)_2$ vitamin D_3 levels in prednisone-treated adolescents with systemic lupus erythematosus. Acta Paediatr Scand 68:109–111, 1979.

118. Hahn TJ, Baran DT, Halstead LR: Alteration in mineral and vitamin D metabolism produced by subacute prednisone administration in man. Proceedings of the 61st Annual Meeting of The Endocrine Society, Baltimore, Williams & Wilkins, 1979, p 195.

118a. Lee DBN: Unanticipated stimulatory action of glucocorticoids on epithelial calcium transport. J Clin Invest 71:322–328, 1983.

119. Costanzo LS, Weiner IM: Relationship between clearances of Ca and Na: Effect of distal diuretics and PTH. Am J Physiol 230:67–73, 1976.

120. Ehrig U, Harrison JE, Wilson DR: Effect of long-term thiazide therapy on intestinal calcium absorption in patients with recurrent renal calculi. Metabolism 23:139–149, 1974.

121. Favus MJ, Coe FI, Kathpalia SC, et al: Effects of chlorothiazide on 1,25-dihydroxyvitamin D_3, parathyroid hormone, and intestinal calcium absorption in the rat. Am J Physiol 242:G575–G581, 1982.

122. Goligorsky MS, Chaimovitz C, Shany S: Verapamil improves defective intestinal calcium absorption in uremia. Adv Exp Med Biol 178:153–161, 1984.

123. Pinto JT, Johnson ME: The influence of verapamil in calcium-transport and uptake in segments of rat intestine. Pharmacology 27:343–349, 1983.

124. Holick MF, MacLaughlin JA, Clark MB, et al: Photosynthesis of previtamin D_3 in human skin and the physiologic consequences. Science 210:203–205, 1980.

125. Lawson DEM, Paul AA, Black AE: Relative contributions of diet and sunlight to vitamin D state in the elderly. Br Med J 2:303–305, 1979.

126. Muldowney FP, McKenna JS, Kyle LH, et al: Parathormone-like effect of magnesium replenishment in steatorrhea. N Engl J Med 282:61–68, 1970.

127. Freitag JJ, Martin KJ, Conrades MB, et al: Evidence for skeletal resistance to parathyroid hormone in magnesium deficiency. J Clin Invest 64:1238–1244, 1979.

128. Rosler A, Rabinowitz D: Magnesium-induced reversal of vitamin D resistance in hypoparathyroidism. Lancet 1:803–805, 1973.

129. Morgan KJ, Stampley GL, Zabik ME, Fischer DR: Magnesium and calcium dietary intakes of the U.S. population. J Am Coll Nutr 4:195–205, 1985.

130. Mahoney AW, Henricks DG: Utilization of dietary calcium by iron-deficient rats. Nutr Metab 18:6–15, 1975.

131. Heaney RP, Gallagher JC, Johnston CC, et al: Calcium nutrition and bone health in the elderly. Am J Clin Nutr 36:986–1013, 1982.

132. Ackley S, Barret-Conner E, Suarez L: Dairy products, calcium and blood pressure. Am J Clin Nutr 38:457–461, 1983.

133. Belizano JM, Villar J, Pineds O, et al: Reduction of blood pressure with calcium supplementation in young adults. JAMA 249:1161–1165, 1983.

134. Allen LH: Calcium bioavailability and absorption: A review. Am J Clin Nutr 35:783–808, 1982.

135. Greger JL, Krystofiak M: Phosphate intake of Americans. Food Technology, 36:78–84, 1982.

136. Stoff JS: Phosphate homeostasis and hypophosphatemia. Am J Med 72:489–495, 1982.

137. Birge SJ: Vitamin D muscle and phosphate homeostasis. Min Electrolyte Metab 1:57–64, 1978.

138. Annino JS, Relman AS: The effect of eating on some of the clinically important chemical constituents of the blood. Am J Clin Pathol 31:155–159, 1959.

139. Wilkie DR: The control of glycolysis in living muscle studied by nuclear magnetic resonance. J Physiol 267:703–735, 1977.

140. Danson MJ, Gadian DG, Wilkie DR: Contraction and recovery of living muscles studied by ^{31}P nuclear magnetic resonance. J Physiol 267:703–735, 1977.

141. Gould L: Decline in serum phosphorus in acute myocardial infarction. Angiology 30:219, 1979.

142. Yaroslavsky BM, Peer G, Bernhein J, Aviran A: Serum phosphate shift in acute myocardial infarction. Am Heart J 104:884–885, 1982.

143. Gray RW, Omdahl JL, Ghazarian JG, DeLuca HF: 25-hydroxycholecalciferol-1-hydroxylase. Subcellular location and properties. J Biol Chem 247:7528–7532, 1972.

144. Garabedian M, Holick MF, DeLuca HF, Boyle IT: Control of 25-hydroxycholecalciferol metabolism by parathyroid glands. Proc Natl Acad Sci USA 69:1673–1676, 1972.

145. Henry HL: Regulation of the hydroxylation of 25-hydroxyvitamin D_3 in vivo and in primary cultures of chick kidney cells. J Biol Chem 254:2722–2729, 1979.

146. Tanaka Y, DeLuca HF: The control of 25-hydroxyvitamin D metabolism by inorganic phosphorus. Arch Biochem Biophys 154:566–574, 1977.

147. Portale AA, Halloran BP, Murphy MM, Morris RC: Oral intake of phosphorus can determine the serum concentration of 1,25-dihydroxyvitamin D by determining its production rate in humans. J Clin Invest 77:7–12, 1986.

148. Tanaka Y, DeLuca HF: Rat renal 25-hydroxyvitamin D_3 1- and 24-hydroxylases: Their in vivo regulation. Am J Physiol 246:E168–E173, 1984.

149. Lee DBN, Walling MS, Palant CE et al: Jejunal phosphate transport is not regulated by the PTH-adenylate cyclase system. Mineral Electrolyte Metab 12:293–297, 1986.

150. Norman AW, Henry HL, Malluche HH: 24R, 25-dihydroxyvitamin D_3 and 1,25-dihydroxyvitamin D_3

are both indispensible for calcium and phosphorus homeostasis. Life Sci 27:229–237, 1980.
151. Miller SC, Halloran BP, DeLuca HF, et al: Studies on the role of 24-hydroxylation of vitamin D-deficient rats. Calcif Tissue Int 33:489–497, 1981.
152. Drezner MK: The role of abnormal vitamin D metabolism in x-linked hypophosphatemic rickets and osteomalacia. Adv Exp Med Biol 178:399–404, 1984.
153. Knochel JP: The pathophysiology and clinical characteristics of severe hypophosphatemia. Arch Intern Med 137:203–220, 1977.
154. Harrison HE, Harrison HC: Intestinal transport of phosphate: Action of vitamin D, calcium and potassium. Am J Physiol 201:1007–1012, 1961.
155. Avioli RC, Miller RA, Birge SJ: Characterization of phosphate uptake in isolated chick intestinal cells. Mineral Electrolyte Metab 5:287–295, 1981.
156. Kempson SA, Kim JK, Northrup TE, et al: Alkaline phosphatase in adaptation to low dietary phosphate intake. Am J Physiol 237:E465–E473, 1979.
157. McCraig LW, Motzok I: Regulation of intestinal phosphatase by dietary phosphate. Am J Physiol Pharmacol 50:1152–1156, 1972.
158. Lowendorf HS, Bazinet GF, Slayman CW: Phosphate transport in Neurospora. Depression of a high-affinity transport system during phosphorus starvation. Biochim Acta 389:541–549, 1975.
159. Willsby GR, Melaney MH: The loss of the phosperiplasmic protein leads to a change in the specificity of a constitutive inorganic phosphate transport system in Escherichia coli. Biochem Biophys Res Comm 60:226–233, 1974.
160. Lichtman MA, Miller DR, Cohen J, Waterhouse C: Reduced red cell glycolysis, 2,3-diphosphoglycerate and adenosine triphosphate concentration and increased hemoglobin-oxygen affinity caused by hypophosphatemia. Ann Intern Med 74:562–568, 1971.
161. Klock JC, Williams HE, Mentzer WC: Hemolytic anemias and somatic cell dysfunction in severe hypophosphatemia. Arch Int Med 114:360–364, 1974.
162. Lotz M, Zisman E, Bartter FC: Evidence for a phosphorus-depletion syndrome in man. N Engl J Med 278:409–415, 1968.
163. Fitzgerald F: Clinical hypophosphatemia. Ann Rev Med 29:177–189, 1978.
164. Moser CR, Fessel WJ: Rheumatic manifestations of hypophosphatemia. Arch Intern Med 134:674–678, 1974.
165. Condon JR, Nassins JR, Rutter A: Defective intestinal phosphate absorption in familial and non-familial hypophosphatemia. Br Med J 3:138–141, 1970.
166. Short EM, Binder HJ, Rosenberg LE: Familial hypophosphatemic rickets: Defective transport of inorganic phosphate by intestinal mucosa. Science 179:700–702, 1973.
167. Agus ZS, Goldfarb S, Wasserman A: Disorders of calcium and phosphorus balance. *In* Brenner BM, Rector FC (eds): The Kidney. 2nd ed. Philadelphia, WB Saunders, 1981, pp 940–1022.
168. Gertner JM, Lilburn M, Domenech M: 25-hydroxycholecalciferol absorption in steatorrhea and postgastrectomy osteomalacia. Br Med J 1:1310–1312, 1977.
169. Ahmed KY, Varghese Z, Wills MR, et al: Persistent hypophosphatemia and osteomalacia in dialysis patients not on oral phosphate-binders: Response to dihydrotachysterol therapy. Lancet 1:439–442, 1976.
170. Darrs FR, Zerwekh JE, Parker TF: Absorption of phosphate in the jejunum of patients with chronic renal failure before and after correction of vitamin D deficiency. Gastroenterology 85:908–916, 1983.
171. Ambrecht HJ, Wonsurawat N, Zenser TU: Differential effects of parathyroid hormone on the renal 1,25-dihydroxyvitamin D_3 and 24,25-dihydroxyvitamin D_3 production of young and adult rats. Endocrinology 11:1339–1344, 1982.
172. Fraser D, Kooh SW, Kind HP, et al: Pathogenesis of hereditary vitamin D dependent rickets. N Engl J Med 289:817–821, 1973.
173. Slatopolsky E, Weersts C, Lopez-Hilker S, et al: Calcium carbonate as a phosphate binder in patients with chronic renal failure undergoing dialysis. N Engl J Med 315:157–161, 1986.
174. Anast CS, Mohs JM, Kaplan SL, et al: Evidence for parathyroid failure in magnesium deficiency. Science 177:606–608, 1972.
175. Chase LR, Slatopolsky E: Secretion and metabolic efficacy of parathyroid hormone in patients with severe hypomagnesemia. J Clin Endocrinol Metab 38:363–371, 1979.
176. Adler AJ, Fillipone EJ, Berlyne GM: Effect of chronic alcohol intake on muscle composition and metabolic balance of calcium and phosphate in rats. Am J Physiol 249:E584–E588, 1985.
177. Reid IR, Teitelbaum SL, Dusso A, et al: Hypercalcemic hyperparathyroidism complicating oncogenic osteomalacia: Effect of successful tumor resection on mineral homeostasis. Am J Med 83:350–354, 1987.
178. Ryan EA, Reiss E: Oncogenous osteomalacia. Review of the world literature of 42 cases and report of two new cases. Am J Med 77:501, 1984.
179. Drezner MK, Lyles KW, Haussler MR: Evaluation of a role for 1,25-dihydroxyvitamin D_3 in the pathogenesis and treatment of X-linked hypophosphatemia rickets and osteomalacia. J Clin Invest 65:1020–1032, 1980.
180. Knochel JP: The clinical status of hypophosphatemia. An update. N Engl J Med 313:447–449, 1985.

7

KEITH A. HRUSKA
BRENDA R.C. KURNIK

Regulation of Renal Phosphate Transport

In 1844 Ludwig first proposed the theory of glomerular filtration and selective renal tubular reabsorption to explain the formation of urine. Cushney's theory, formulated in 1917, postulates that some substances are filtered in the renal glomeruli and actively reabsorbed through the walls of the renal tubules together with water at a rate required to produce an "optimal" concentration of substances reabsorbed into the extracellular fluid. In this manner, the concentration of solutes in the reabsorbed fluid characterizes renal function with respect to a given substance, and optimal concentrations of important solutes are maintained in the blood. With some modifications, this theory still describes renal handling of phosphate. In the steady state, variations in renal function are reflected by variations in plasma phosphate concentration. Variations in phosphate excretion, on the other hand, reflect corresponding variations in the net input of phosphate into the extracellular fluid from sites other than the kidney—for instance, bone or gut. Thus, the role of the kidney in extracellular phosphate homeostasis must be considered in relation to the physiology of other organs. To understand the function of the kidney as an organ of phosphate metabolism, one must understand the sites and nature of renal tubular phosphate transport mechanisms within the kidney.

I. THE ELEMENTS OF RENAL PHOSPHATE TRANSPORT

The glomeruli produce an ultrafiltrate of serum. As this ultrafiltrate passes along the renal tubules, its composition is altered because specific substances are subtracted by reabsorption and added by tubular secretion. Three processes, therefore, determine the final composition of urine: ultrafiltration, tubular reabsorption, and tubular secretion.

A. Glomerular Filtration

Micropuncture studies in amphibians and mammals provide a direct comparison of the simultaneous concentrations of phosphate in serum and in the glomerular filtrate. The results of many such studies indicate that these concentrations do not differ. Walser[1] has pointed out that the phosphate concentrations in glomerular filtrate and in serum can be equal only when about 13% of the serum phosphate is not filterable. One reason is that in measuring serum phosphate concentrations, the volume occupied by proteins is not taken into account. In addition, the presence of serum proteins on only one side of the ultrafiltering membrane will induce an electrochemical gradient across the membrane, and, as a result, the distribution of ions along the two sides of the membrane will be unequal (the Donnan equilibrium). Many earlier ultrafiltration studies of serum phosphate were unreliable because factors such as pH, pCO_2, or temperature had not been taken into account. The best available controlled studies and Walser's own studies in humans demonstrated that whatever the absolute value of the serum phosphate concentration, the ultrafiltrates of serum have approximately the same phosphate concentration as the serum itself. From this finding, Walser reasoned that on the average, 13% of the serum phosphate is protein-bound and nonfilterable[1] (Table 7–1). Therefore, it happens that despite considerable protein binding, the phosphate concentration in glomerular filtrate equals the serum phosphate concentration $[PO_4(w/v)]$. This is

Table 7–1. Concentrations of Phosphate in Normal Human Plasma

Phosphate	Concentration (mg/100 ml)	% Total
Free HPO_4^{2-}	1.55	43
Free $H_2PO_4^-$	0.34	10
Protein bound	0.43	12
$NaHPO_4$	1.02	29
$CaHPO_4$	0.12	3
$MgHPO_4$	0.10	3
Total	3.56	100

Reproduced from Walser M: J Clin Invest 40:723, 1961.

true for a wide range of serum phosphate concentrations. The filterable fraction of phosphate apparently does not change when phosphate is infused to raise its concentration in the blood to 10 mg/100 ml. However, rapid and marked elevations of calcium and phosphate levels can result in formation of nonfilterable colloidal complexes of calcium phosphate.[2] The filtration rate of phosphate in the kidney (filtered load, FL_{PO_4}, weight/time) can, therefore, be estimated as the product of serum phosphate concentration and glomerular filtration rate [GFR (volume/time)].

$$(1)\ FL_{PO_4} = [PO_4] \times GFR$$

This equation (1), which considers the Donnan equilibrium and the ultrafilterable phosphate concentration, closely approximates actuality.

Henceforth in this chapter, the amount of phosphate filtered per unit time will be designated as filtered load (FL_{PO_4}) and defined as $[PO_4] \times GFR$. Moreover, the serum phosphate concentration $[PO_4]$ can be considered as equal to the amount of phosphate filtered per unit volume of glomerular filtrate.

B. Tubular Transport—Reabsorption and Secretion

Renal tubular handling of phosphate is still not completely understood. In humans, tubular transport can only be defined as the difference between filtered load and excretion rate [$U_{PO_4}V$ (weight/time)], an indirect measurement (Eq. 2).

$$(2)\ T_{PO_4} = [PO_4] \times GFR - U_{PO_4}V$$

Such measurements demonstrate net phosphate reabsorption, but this does not preclude secretion of phosphate somewhere along the renal tubules, provided the reabsorption rate exceeds the secretion rate.

1. *Proximal Nephron*

The major site of phosphate reabsorption in the nephron is the proximal convoluted tubule. Micropuncture studies have shown that by the time glomerular filtrate has reached the late proximal tubules, 60% to 70% of the filtered phosphate has been reabsorbed.[3-5] This bulk reabsorption, however, is not achieved by a mechanism homogeneously distributed along the proximal tubule. In the first 25% of the proximal tubule, phosphate is reabsorbed avidly, exceeding the rate of fluid reabsorption.[6-8] In animals with intact parathyroid glands, phosphate reabsorption exceeds fluid reabsorption until the tubular phosphate concentration approximates 70% of the plasma level[3,4,9,10,11] (Fig. 7–1). At this point, the rate of phosphate reabsorption parallels that of fluid reabsorption and the tubular phosphate concentration remains relatively constant. In the absence of parathyroid hormone (PTH), the concentration of phosphate in the tubule does not stabilize, but continues to decline to values approximately 30% of that in plasma.[4,11-15] Recent studies of Na^+-dependent phosphate transport *in vitro* employing plasma membrane vesicles isolated from different nephron segments further indicate the presence of a "family" of phosphate transport proteins in the kidney.[16,17] This subject will be discussed in more detail in subsequent sections of this chapter.

2. *Distal Nephron Segments*

There is no phosphate reabsorption between the late accessible proximal tubule and early distal tubule in animals with intact parathyroid glands.[3,9,12,18-21] In the absence of PTH, phosphate is reabsorbed between the late proximal and early distal tubule, reflecting phosphate reabsorption in the pars recta.[12,15,22-25] Phosphate is not reabsorbed in other segments of the loop of Henle. Recent *in vivo* and *in vitro* microperfusion studies failed to detect reabsorption in the thin descending, thin ascending, and thick ascending limbs of the loop of Henle. Moreover, the phosphate permeability of these segments is very low.[25,26] The existence and significance of dis-

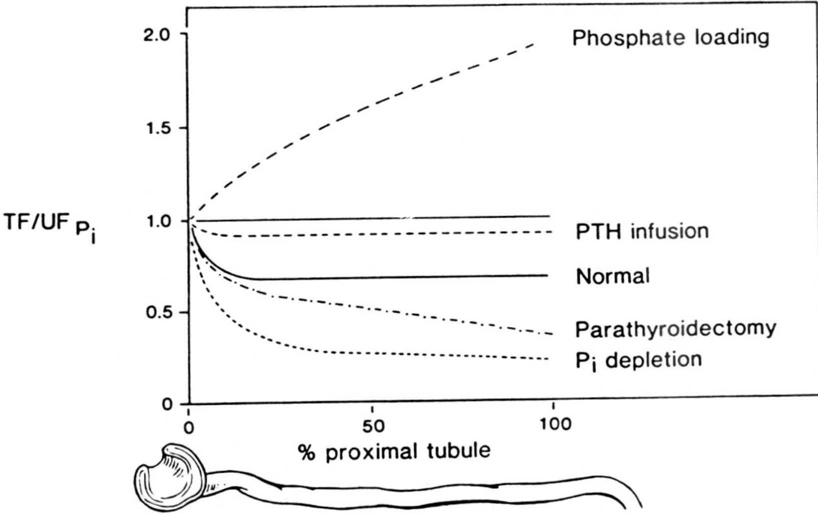

Figure 7–1. Generation of tubule fluid ultrafiltrate P_i ratio along the proximal convoluted tubule is attributable to more avid reabsorption of phosphate than isotonic fluid for most circumstances. P_i supply and PTH affect the avidity of phosphate transport.

tal phosphate reabsorption has been a topic of considerable interest in recent years. The answers remain unclear. Several studies have suggested that phosphate reabsorption occurs in the distal nephron, since fractional phosphate delivery is higher to the early superficial distal tubule than phosphate content in the urine.[9-12,15,18-20,27-31] This observation applies to animals with and without parathyroid glands. Direct micropuncture evidence localizes the reabsorption of up to 10% of the filtered phosphate load to the distal convoluted tubule in thyroparathyroidectomized rats, with the possibility of an additional 3% to 7% reabsorbed beyond the accessible late distal tubule.[29,30,32]

Unfortunately, other attempts at direct evaluation of phosphate handling by terminal nephron segments have not concurred with these results. The conflicts may relate to differences in species and methodology.[33] On the other hand, recent studies examining phosphate reabsorption in rats fed a low-phosphate diet demonstrate significant reabsorption by the time fluid enters the late distal tubule.[32,34,35] Nephron heterogeneity contributes to the discrepancy in the amount of distal phosphate delivered and phosphate excreted in the urine. Under conditions of phosphate retention induced by thyroparathyroidectomy, fractional phosphate delivery at the tip of the loop of Henle of juxtamedullary nephrons is significantly less than at the early distal tubule of superficial nephrons, but not different in amount from phosphate excreted in the urine.[28] Because, as pointed out later, no phosphate reabsorption is detectable along the superficial ascending limb of Henle, delivery of phosphate to the early distal site reflects the phosphate that escapes from reabsorption by the superficial proximal tubule and pars recta; it can be compared to the amount of phosphate delivered to the tip of the loop of Henle and juxtamedullary nephrons. Thus, the difference between superficial distal phosphate delivered and phosphate excreted in the urine may be largely accounted for by more avid phosphate reabsorption in deep nephron proximal tubules. Furthermore, there is evidence that a significant amount of phosphate is reabsorbed by juxtamedullary distal tubules and/or arcade segments connecting juxtamedullary distal tubules to the collecting ducts.[31]

3. Cellular Mechanisms of Renal Phosphate Transport—Luminal Membrane

Phosphate reabsorption in the proximal nephron is dependent on sodium in the lumen. In the presence of sodium, phosphate transport is inhibited by ouabain and other inhibitors of sodium-potassium ATPase. Thus, transcellular phosphate transport can be considered to be linked to the primary active transport of sodium. Co-transport of sodium and phosphorus has been demonstrated in isolated brush border membrane vesicles of kidneys of several mammalian species, including humans.[36-48] A typical experiment demonstrating sodium-dependent transport in brush border membrane vesicles isolated from dog kidneys is depicted in Figure 7–2. In the presence of a sodium gradient (Na^+ concentration out > Na^+ concentration in), phosphate is rapidly accumulated in the vesicles in concentrations that transiently exceed the equilibrium values several fold. In contrast, the imposition of an inwardly directed potassium gradient produces only a slow, equilibrating phosphate uptake. This type of experiment demonstrates that in the presence of a sodium gradient, phosphate is transiently accumulated in the vesicles against a concentration gradient and released back into the medium when the sodium gradient is dissipated. Similarly, the measurements of phosphate-dependent uptake of sodium have shown that sodium enters the vesicles together with phosphate.[42] Thus, there is firm evidence that the sodium-phosphate co-transport in the brush border membrane is energized by the electrochemical sodium gradient. The phosphate entry step into proximal tubular cells proceeds against an electrochemical gradient, and sodium-phosphate co-transport is commonly referred to as a secondary active transport mechanism.

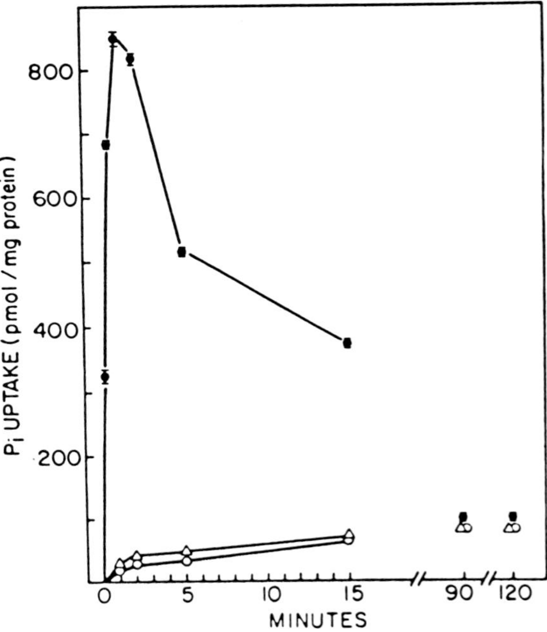

Figure 7–2 The time course of Na^+-dependent P_i uptake by canine renal brush border membrane vesicles (BBMV). BBMV were preloaded with 300 mM buffered mannitol •-100 mM NaCl extravesicular fluid; Δ-100 mM NaCl both inside and in the extravesicular fluid; ○-100 mM KCl in extravesicular fluid.

At pH 7.4, sodium-phosphate co-transport in rat brush border membrane vesicles is not sensitive to membrane potential. However, at acid extravesicular or tubular fluid pH, an electrogenic component of phosphate transport becomes apparent.[39,49] This is consistent with an electroneutral co-transport of two sodium ions and one divalent phosphate ion at physiologic pH and electrogenic transport of two sodium ions and a monovalent phosphate ion at acid pH (6.5). It is not known if the electroneutral and electrogenic components of sodium-phosphate co-transport are catalyzed by one transporter molecule in flexible specificity or by two different transporter molecules, one accepting divalent phosphate ($2Na^{++}HPO_4^{2-}$) and the other accepting monovalent phosphate ($2Na^{++}H_2PO_4^-$).

Data from several laboratories[16,50] suggest the existence of a heterogeneous population of sodium-phosphate co-transport systems within renal tubules. However, differing kinetics and stoichiometry of phosphate transport have been described, possibly depending on species, dietary regimen, and anatomic origin of the membranes, and a clear distinction between two or more transport systems with specified stoichiometries and kinetic characteristics has not yet been accomplished. The electroneutral, $2Na\text{-}HPO_4^{2-}$ co-transport system with a Km for phosphate of 0.2 to 0.4 mM/liter and a V_{max} of 130 to 170 pmol/mg/S seems to be dominant, at least in rat and canine proximal tubules. The electrogenic component can be demonstrated only at pH values lower than those normally encountered in the proximal tubule, under conditions of very low net P_i transport. Hence, it is not likely that this component plays a major role in the renal handling of P_i.

4. Phosphate Transport in Basolateral Membranes

Very little is known about phosphate transport from the cell to the peritubular fluid across the basolateral membrane. Participation of an anion exchanger in phosphate transport has been inferred from studies demonstrating inhibition of P_i influx from perfused capillaries into tubular cells by stilbene inhibitor, DIDS.[51] A contraluminal anion exchange mechanism accepting sulfate but not phosphate has been described, suggesting that separate pathways for sulfate and P_i transport are present in the basolateral membrane.[52]

The data on phosphate transport in basolateral membrane vesicles are few and conflicting. Hoffmann et al.[42] observed a rapid sodium-independent uptake of phosphate by basolateral membrane vesicles isolated from rat kidneys. Grinstein et al.[53] found that the sodium-independent efflux of phosphate from isolated basolateral membrane vesicles was inhibited by 4,4′diisothiocyanostilbene-2,2′-disulfonic acid (DIDS), which was in agreement with the *in vivo* data.[51] In dog kidney basolateral membrane vesicle preparations, a sodium gradient–dependent phosphate transport has been described.[54] The transport was electrogenic and carried a positive charge in the direction of phosphate movement, not unlike the electrogenic component of sodium-phosphate transport in the brush border membrane at acid pH. In contrast to brush border membranes, the sodium-dependent phosphate uptake in basolateral membranes was not stimulated when the pH was increased, nor could sodium-dependent glucose uptake be demonstrated. The K_m in the transport system was 14 μM and the V_{max} was 58 pmol/mg/min, approximately 1.4% of phosphate transport capacity of brush border membranes.[54] In the same basolateral membrane preparation, electrogenic sodium-independent phosphate transport with low affinity (K_m = 2.3 mM) and high V_{max} (74,000 pM/mg protein/min) was described.[54,55] Additional studies of rat basolateral membrane vesicles have demonstrated the existence of an anion exchanger with broad specificity on the basis of *trans* stimulation and *cis* inhibition of radioactive sulfate uptake by several anions, including P_i and phosphate.[56] However, Hagenbuch et al. were unable to demonstrate *trans* stimulation of phosphate uptake by intravesicular sulfate although phosphate-phosphate *trans* stimulation was apparent.[57]

From the available data, one can easily see that phosphate transport across the basolateral membrane remains incompletely elucidated. Investigations to date have been limited by technical difficulties associated with the basolateral membrane vesicle preparation. In contrast to brush border membranes, which are an almost uniform population of tightly sealed, right-side-out oriented vesicles, basolateral membrane vesicle preparations consist of a mixture of open sheets, inside-out and right-side-out vesicles, and only a small fraction of tightly sealed transport competent vesicles.[58] However, the available data suggest the existence of sodium-independent transport pathways, that is, an anion exchange sensitive to DIDS, and a low capacity for sodium-dependent phosphate transport.[54,56,57] The sodium-dependent phosphate transport system cannot be involved in phosphate exit from the cell because the driving forces of the sodium gradient and cell potential are always directed toward the cell interior, but it might provide for phosphate entry from the contraluminal side when phosphate entry from the lumen becomes restricted.[54,59] The specificity and stoichiometry of a sodium independent transport system that might be involved in phosphate exit from the cell are not known. Therefore, the driving forces for this system cannot be predicted. In addition to anion exchange, a rheogenic transport of phosphate, driven by cell potential, may be involved in phosphate exit from the cell.[54,55]

5. Relationship Between Phosphate Entry and Exit—Transcellular Movement

From available data one can surmise that functional coupling exists between the apical entry of phosphate and the basolateral exit. Intracellular phosphate is one of the factors determining the phosphorylation potential of the cell (ATP/ADP × phosphate), which in turn controls several metabolic pathways, including glycolysis, gluconeogenesis, and oxidative phosphorylation. One might expect that net phosphate transport across the cell occurs without large fluctuations of cytosolic free phosphate, $[P_i]_i$. This implies that P_i entry into the cell across the brush border membrane and its exit across the basolateral membrane must be coupled. The mechanisms involved in the maintenance of the constant $[P_i]_i$ are not clear, but useful information has been produced by studies of the metabolic effects of P_i in isolated perfused kidneys and isolated proximal tubules.[60-62] When isolated rat kidneys are perfused with phosphate-free medium, the total tissue phosphate decreases initially by 30% to 50% but then remains constant for several hours. The kidney is viable under these conditions, as indicated by near normal sodium reabsorption and oxygen uptake.[62] Thus, net phosphate efflux from the cell is completely inhibited after a certain amount of phosphate has been lost. The cytosolic phosphate concentration, measured by ^{31}P NMR, is 0.6 to 0.7 mM in this kidney preparation.[62]

6. Relationship of Phosphate Transport to Cell Metabolism

Since net phosphate efflux can be eliminated, either the transport systems in the basolateral membrane that catalyze phosphate efflux from the cell can be inhibited by some unknown regulatory process, or the uptake of phosphate into the cell becomes so efficient that it prevents a net loss of phosphate. Similar conclusions can be drawn from results of studies in isolated rabbit proximal tubules perfused with phosphate-free solution *in vitro*.[61] Omission of phosphate from the luminal perfusate in these experiments resulted in inhibition of net fluid absorption from the tubule, whereas omission of phosphate from the peritubular bath had no effect. Incubation of isolated tubule fragments in a phosphate-free medium, when phosphate was absent from both the luminal and contraluminal side of the cells, resulted in a considerable reduction of O_2 consumption. The inhibition of fluid absorption and respiration is dependent on the presence of glucose in the luminal solution and does not occur when glucose transport is inhibited with phloridzin or when glycolysis is inhibited by 2-deoxyglucose.[61] This is the so-called Crabtree effect, that is, hexose-induced inhibition of respiration and glycolysis, which occurs when intracellular phosphate is incorporated in the glycolytic intermediates and becomes a limiting factor in oxidative phosphorylation and glycolysis.[63] The occurrence of the Crabtree effect, when phosphate is removed from the lumen of rabbit proximal convoluted tubule but not when it is removed from the peritubular fluid, suggests several important points worth consideration. First, phosphate transport across the brush border membrane must be necessary for the maintenance of normal $[P_i]$ in the cell. Second, increased phosphate entry across the basolateral membrane must not be able to compensate fully for reduced phosphate transport across the brush border membrane. This may result from the low transport capacity of the basolateral membrane, the thermodynamic conditions for basolateral phosphate influx, which are unfavorable, or both. Finally, phosphate that enters the cell from the tubular lumen must come into equilibrium with the cytosolic phosphate pool that controls metabolism. This suggests that phosphate is not transported across the cell via discrete pathways such as vesicular transport.

II. REGULATION OF SODIUM-PHOSPHATE TRANSPORT

For the following discussion, several assumptions regarding sodium-phosphate transport are made. Although the sodium-phosphate symport has not been isolated, we are assuming that the system is an enzyme operating in a vectorial fashion catalyzing the transfer of phosphate from the extracellular fluid of the tubular lumen to the cell. Events that change the activity of the transport system fall into two broad categories, acute and chronic. Acute changes in enzyme activity (phosphate transport) may be produced by numerous factors including alterations in substrate, product, or co-enzyme concentrations or changes of pH. Two types of acute regulation of transport proteins are especially important. Allosteric regulation occurs when a regulating substance changes the enzyme activity by binding to the molecule at a regulatory site different from the substrate binding site, and activation-inactivation is the process of reversible covalent modification of the enzyme molecule by phosphorylation, ribosylation, methylation, and so on. These processes in turn are catalyzed by an additional set of regulatory enzymes such as protein kinases and protein phosphatases. The regulatory enzymes themselves may be subject to regulation, producing a regulatory cascade.

Chronic regulation may also be called adaptation. This process usually involves new synthesis of the transporter molecule and produces a sustained response in transport activity even when the intensity of the original stimulus has subsided. Since the phosphate transporter is most likely an intrinsic membrane protein, an additional process takes place between protein synthesis and the ultimate expression of phosphate transport. This is the transport and insertion of the protein into the target membrane. Transport and insertion may have different time courses and kinetics from those of protein synthesis, and these processes may also be subject to regulation. In recent years, a multitude of factors have been demonstrated to affect renal phosphate transport. They may be categorized within the broad framework of enzyme regulation discussed previously. However, information on sodium-phosphate co-transport is grossly insufficient. Since the transport protein has not been isolated, its molecular properties are completely unknown. The kinetics of the transport function have not been, as yet, investigated in full detail. Notably, the interaction of phosphate, sodium, and hydrogen with the cytoplasmic side can only be inferred from indirect evidence. The following sections, therefore, should be considered an attempt to organize available knowledge within the outline of regulation; no vital model of sodium-phosphate co-transport will be established.

A. Acute Regulation

1. Regulation of Phosphate Transport by Allosteric Modification Through Sodium and Protons

In most species, phosphate reabsorption in the proximal nephron is increased with increasing pH of the tubular fluid.[64] However, in isolated perfused tubules from the rabbit, the proximal nephron failed to demonstrate pH dependence,[24,65] although stimulation of sodium-phosphate co-transport by alkaline pH was demonstrated in brush border membrane vesicles isolated from rabbit kidneys.[40,46] The interaction of protons with the phosphate transport system is controversial. A complete discussion is beyond the scope of this chapter. The reader is referred to recent reviews for a complete discussion.[66,67]

Inorganic phosphate is present in physiologic pH values in two different anionic forms: HPO_4^{2-} and $H_2PO_4^-$. These two species are different in electrical charge and molecular size. At any given pH value, both phosphate forms are present. Most evidence reported to date suggests that both forms are transported by a single carrier. The divalent form, HPO_4^{2-}, has been thought by several investigators to be preferentially transported.[40,42,46,50,68-70] A different interpretation of the data has been provided by Murer et al.[36,71] These investigators have shown that brush border membrane vesicles prepared so that phosphate and sodium in the vesicular space were close to zero, expressed increasing phosphate transport as the external pH was raised from 6 to 8. Furthermore phosphate transport was stimulated at any pH by increasing sodium concentration. The sodium dependence of sodium-phosphate transport was sigmoidal at every pH, indicating interaction of more than one Na^+ with the transporter without a pH dependence on the number of Na^+ ions interacting. Kinetic analysis of the data indicated that pH had a strong effect on the affinity of sodium for the transport system, that phosphorus had no effect on the apparent affinity of sodium, and that the affinity for phosphorus was increased by sodium at both high and low pH. The investigators concluded that sodium activated the phosphate transport system and that at least two sodium ions are involved in the activation process. Another finding by these researchers was that hydrogen ion modulates the activity of sodium-phosphate co-transport by decreasing the affinity for sodium, and consequently for phosphate at saturating Na^+. However, hydrogen had little or no direct effect on phosphate affinity, and phosphate had no effect on the affinity of the transport system for sodium. Murer's group feels that both sodium and hydrogen are powerful allosteric modulators of brush border sodium-phosphate transport, that they interact at sites different from the phosphate binding site, and that by mutual interaction, they control the affinity for phosphate. The investigators are unable to explain the observation of Sacktor and Cheng[46] that intravesicular acidification stimulated sodium gradient–dependent phosphate transport. Sacktor and Cheng interpreted this as suggesting that at low pH values, phosphate may be trapped inside the vesicles as H_2PO_4, facilitating the uptake of HPO_4^{2-}. Thus, the allosteric effects of sodium, hydrogen, and phosphate, modifying the activity of the sodium-phosphate co-transport system, remain to be completely characterized.

2. Covalent Modification of Sodium-Phosphate Co-transport

Studies of the effects of parathyroid hormone (PTH) on renal phosphate transport, which are detailed in Chapters 3 and 14, have provided indications that cAMP-dependent phosphorylation of brush border membrane proteins may be involved in the regulation of sodium-phosphate transport,[72] that PTH-stimulated adenylate cyclase is localized in the basolateral membranes of proximal tubule cells,[73,74] and that cAMP-dependent protein kinase is present both in the cytosol and in the brush border.[75,76] Sodium-dependent phosphate transport is decreased in brush border membranes vesicles (BBMV) isolated from kidneys of animals treated with PTH.[43,68,77] The cAMP dependent phosphorylation of several protein bands has been demonstrated in BBMV *in vitro*.[72,78,81] These experiments have also demonstrated a correlation between cAMP-dependent phosphorylation and decreased sodium-phosphate co-transport in BBMV *in vitro*. Sodium-dependent uptake of 25 μM $^{32}P_i$ was inhibited[78,80] when dog BBMs were phosphorylated in the presence of 1 μM cAMP. Subsequently, other studies have demonstrated no effect on the kinetics of sodium-phosphate co-transport by cAMP-dependent phosphorylation, and the effect of cAMP-dependent protein phosphorylation on the regulation of sodium-phosphate co-transport has been disclaimed.[81,82] Methodologic difficulties associated with phosphorylation experiments *in vitro* complicate their interpretation. However, it would appear that cAMP-dependent phosphorylation is an important mechanism of regulation of sodium-dependent phosphate transport.

Several investigators have demonstrated that ADP-ribosylation of BBMV through membrane-bound ADP-ribosyltransferase produces an inhibition of sodium-phosphate co-transport.[79,83,84] Previous studies had demonstrated that $^{32}P_i$ uptake was inhibited when NAD was added to the suspension of BBMV.[85] However, the demonstration of NAD hydrolysis and rapid depletion of the added nucleotides leading to dilution of $^{32}P_i$[86,87] has cast a shroud upon these data. Other studies have demonstrated that nucleotides added to BBMV were rapidly hydrolyzed by alkaline phosphatase, 5′-nucleotidase, and nucleotide pyrophosphatase.[86-88] Additionally, sodium-dependent phosphate transport was not inhibited by NAD when hydrolysis of the nucleotide had been prevented.[87] In isolated perfused kidney[89] and in isolated perfused proximal tubules,[90,91] the oxidation and reduction of intracellular NAD with pyruvate and lactate, respectively, resulted in no appreciable changes in phosphate reabsorption. Thus, the role of ADP-ribosylation as a means of covalent modification of phosphate transport remains controversial.

B. Chronic (Long-Term)

Whereas the regulation of sodium-phosphate co-transport by allosteric or covalent modification of the transport protein may occur rapidly (within seconds), a longer term, slower regulation of transport activity is responsible for many forms of renal adaptation in phosphate transport. In a physiologic sense, adjustment of tubular phosphate reabsorption may be seen as a response to changing supply or demand for the ion. In a biochemical sense, adaptation of transport processes is usually associated with a change in the number of transport proteins in the membrane. Such adaptation would be reflected by an increase or decrease in the V_{max} of sodium-phosphate co-transport activity in the BBM. This has been shown to occur in response to variations in dietary supply but also as a secondary event when acute changes of phosphate reabsorption are produced by different cellular mechanisms. Numerous factors (Table 7–2) affect the activity of sodium-phosphate co-transport in renal BBMs. Characteristically, the adaptation is expressed as a change in V_{max} of the sodium-phosphate co-transport, whereas the K_m for phosphate

Table 7–2. Factors Producing Changes in Proximal Tubular Transport of Phosphate

Substance	Effect
Acute	
Parathyroid hormone	decrease
Acute P_i loading	decrease
Acute P_i deprivation	increase
Gluconeogenic stimuli	decrease
Insulin	increase
Chronic	
Chronic P_i deprivation	increase
Thyroxin	increase
Glucocorticoids	decrease
Metabolic acidosis	decrease
Growth hormone	increase
1,25 $(OH)_2D_3$	increase

remains unchanged.[16,43,50,92-97] These data suggest that chronic adaptation for phosphate transport is produced by changes in the number of cell membrane transport units. In addition, the increase in sodium-phosphate co-transport activity in phosphate depletion,[47] and a decrease in such activity in glucocorticoid-treated animals (Bertram Sacktor, personal communication) are both prevented by inhibitors of protein synthesis. The increase of sodium-phosphate co-transport activity in response to thyroxin is prevented by cytoskeletal inhibitors.[98] These data suggest that protein synthesis and membrane recycling may both be involved in the development of adaptation in phosphate transport rates. Recent studies performed in cell lines isolated from mammalian kidneys under culture conditions demonstrate that the adaptation to phosphate supply is biphasic.[99-103] These studies demonstrated that incubation of the cells in low-P_i medium results in a 2-fold increase of sodium-dependent phosphate transport. Two phases of adaptation were observed: a rapid, 30% increase in P_i transport that occurred within 10 minutes, and a slower phase that resulted in a doubling of phosphate transport rate after 15 hours. Both rapid and long-term adaptation was characterized by an increase in the V_{max} of sodium-dependent phosphate co-transport, demonstrated both in intact cells and in isolated brush border membrane vesicles isolated from the cultured cells.[101] The K_m for phosphate was not affected by adaptation. Only the longer term adaptation was inhibited by cycloheximide, suggesting that protein synthesis was involved in the slow adaptation only. Rapid changes in phosphate transport were produced by transfer of cells back and forth from media containing varying phosphate concentrations. These acute changes were resistant to cycloheximide. Apparently, two processes with different time courses are involved in the development of adaptation through phosphate transport: a slow one that requires protein synthesis and allows larger (greater than 100%) increases of phosphate transport rates, and a rapid one that is independent of protein synthesis and involves either activation or recruitment of preexisting transport units. The amplitude for rapid up and down regulation is low in cells grown in high-P_i medium, but it is dramatically increased in cells adapted to low-P_i medium that exhibit high rates of phosphate transport.

Exocytotic insertion of transport units from the intracellular pool into a target membrane has been proposed to be involved in adaptive regulation of proton ATPase in gastric mucosa[104] and turtle urinary bladder,[105] glucose transport in adipocytes,[106] and sodium-hydrogen exchange activity in rabbit proximal tubule.[107] Membrane recycling seems to be emerging as a general mechanism of adaptation of cellular transport systems. Results to date in studies of phosphate transport are at least consistent with the hypothesis that protein synthesis and membrane recycling are involved in the adaptation of the brush border sodium-phosphate co-transport system.

III. MECHANISMS OF REGULATION

In this section, regulation of phosphate transport in renal tubules is interpreted in terms of the membrane and cellular mechanisms described in section II. Sodium-phosphate co-transport in the brush border membrane is assumed to be the rate-limiting step in renal tubular transepithelial phosphate transport. The regulation of transport occurring in different situations is discussed as it is expressed at the level of the brush border membrane.

A. Parathyroid Hormone (PTH)

The effects of PTH on the proximal nephron are many. The hormone decreases fluid and sodium reabsorption, it inhibits phosphate bicarbonate and calcium reabsorption, and it stimulates proximal tubular gluconeogenesis.[108-116] The effects of PTH are initiated by an interaction of the hormone with receptors located on the basolateral membrane of proximal tubular cells. Some of these receptors couple to adenylate cyclase through the GTP-binding proteins G_s and G_i. Coupling of the receptor to adenylate cyclase stimulates cAMP production. Most of the cellular responses to PTH can be mimicked by exogenous cAMP or its analogues.[5,113,116,117] Recent data suggest additional pathways of cell activation by PTH.[118] PTH has been shown to stimulate the production of inositol trisphosphate and diacylglycerol in primary cultures of proximal tubular cells, basolateral membranes of proximal tubular cells, and opossum kidney cells.[118] It has also been shown to stimulate transient elevations of cytosolic calcium independent of stimulation of cAMP.[119-121] The relationship of this pathway of signal transduction related to PTH action remains to be fully elucidated. Recent results suggest that it may be important in stimulation of sodium-phosphate co-transport.[122] These data obtained from opossum kidney cells demonstrate that PTH stimulates phosphate transport at concentrations 1 log order less than required to stimulate adenylate cyclase activity. These results have essentially been confirmed by Malmström and Murer and by Caverzasio et al.[123,124] However, caution is advised in relating cAMP levels to activation of transport, since very small increases may be sufficient to fully activate protein kinase A.[124b]

Simultaneous inhibition of phosphate and bicarbonate reabsorption and the stimulation of gluconeogenesis by PTH suggest that these responses might be triggered by common cellular mechanisms. Inverse relationships between renal gluconeogenesis and phosphate transport as a general phenomenon have been reported.[85,125] The relationship between phosphate and bicarbonate reabsorption has been emphasized by several authors.[108,117,126] As a result, the suggestion has been made that the phosphaturic effect of PTH might be secondary to modification of cell pH, pH gradient, or cellular metabolism.[108] In a recent review,[67] stimulation of gluconeogenesis by PTH was proposed to be the mechanism of hormonally induced reductions in sodium-phosphate co-transport. Gluconeogenesis, by consuming protons and producing increased cytosolic phosphate, would produce allosteric inhibition of Na^+-P_i co-transport through alkalinization and inhibition of phosphate release from the transport protein (Fig. 7–3). The flaws in this reasoning are numerous. PTH produces cellular acidification,[127,128] not alkalinization, through inhibition of sodium-hydrogen exchange. Several authors suggest that the effect of PTH on sodium-hydrogen exchange is mediated through cAMP-dependent protein kinase.[129] In addition, transformed cell lines, which rely on glycolysis for metabolism and are not gluconeogeneic, that is, the opossum kidney cell line, retain exquisite sensitivity to PTH-mediated inhibition of sodium-phosphate co-transport.[122-124] Thus, as discussed before, the logical mechanism for

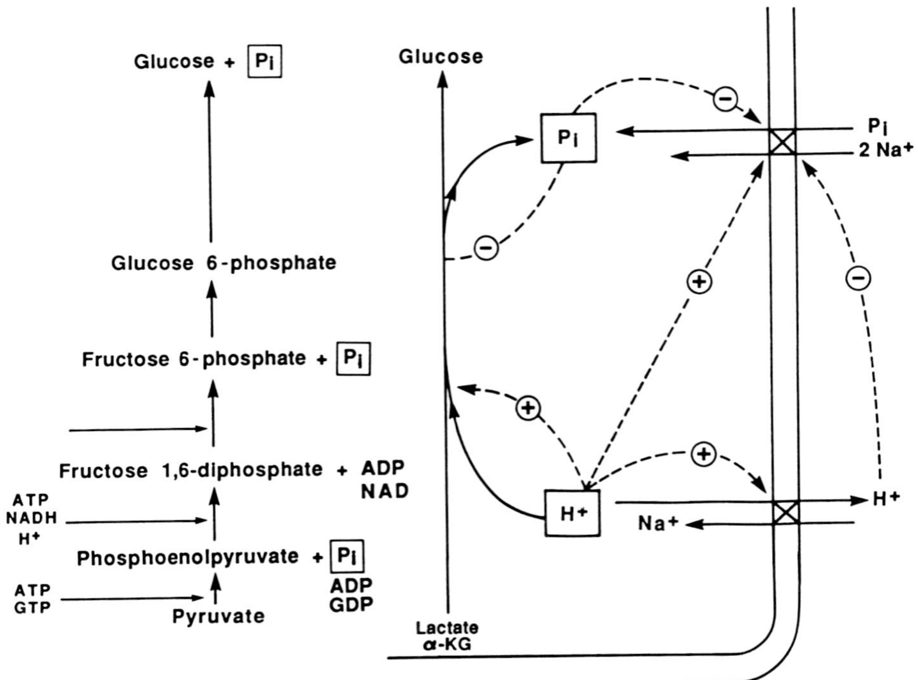

Figure 7–3 Relationship between gluconeogenesis and cytosolic P_i and protons. Gluconeogenesis releases P_i and consumes H^+. Cytosolic P_i has negative and H^+ positive effects on Na^+/P_i co-transport. Note that glycolysis would have effects opposite to those of gluconeogensis on P_i and proton supply in the cytosol.

PTH inhibition of sodium-phosphate co-transport appears to be membrane phosphorylation. Mediation of phosphorylation through cAMP-dependent protein kinase, diacylglycerol-stimulated protein kinase C, and calcium/calmodulin protein kinase and amplification of kinases by Ca^{2+} appear to be the logical mechanisms of covalent modification of Na^+-P_i co-transport as suggested by several authors.[80,118,122]

B. Dietary Intake—Phosphate Supply

Decreasing P_i availability in the diet stimulates P_i transport, and increasing the P_i supply decreases P_i transport.[8,34,35,43,45,47,50,93,94,130] The mechanism of signal transduction for changes in P_i availability is totally unknown. It is known that signal transduction emanates from the luminal membrane, since changes in luminal P_i affect energy metabolism of the cell but not changes in P_i on the basolateral side of the cell.[108] Numerous studies also demonstrate that the adaptation of Na^+-P_i co-transport on the basis of P_i supply appears to represent a totally independent mechanism of regulation from the control of P_i transport by PTH.[67,130] In most settings, the adaptation of P_i supply induced by P_i deprivation significantly impairs the adaptive response to changes in PTH, especially the response to increasing PTH levels.[131-134] Several maneuvers appear to act to restore the response to PTH. These include glucocorticoid and nicotinamide administration and induction of metabolic acidosis.[135-137] The mechanisms of regulation by these maneuvers must be elucidated before there can be clarification of the means by which they restore response to PTH-induced regulation in the face of P_i deprivation. As discussed in the section on chronic (long-term) regulation, recent studies performed in cell culture provide further elucidation of the mechanisms of adaptation to changes in P_i supply.[62,100-103] Thus, studies performed in several lines of cells derived from renal tubular cells demonstrate alterations in Na^+-P_i co-transport induced by changes in medium P_i concentration. These changes in P_i transport are expressed at the level of the luminal membrane Na^+-P_i co-transport system. The effects of lowering the medium P_i are time-dependent but occur relatively rapidly. Early effects can be seen within minutes after reducing medium P_i, but maximal effects require several hours (approximately 15) to develop. The early effects are independent of protein synthesis, whereas the later effects responsible for producing maximal adaptation are dependent upon protein synthesis. Biber and Murer and Caverzasio et al,[100,102] have envisioned that the acute effects represent an insertion of transport units from an available cytoplasmic pool into the membrane, whereas the late stages represent synthesis of new transport units and their traffic into the membrane. This concept of adaptation to P_i supply requires further study.

C. Acid-Base Status

A description of the effects of acute changes of acid-base balance on sodium-dependent phosphate transport, at the present time, is hampered by incomplete information regarding changes in intracellular pH and by controversy regarding the effects of changes in extracellular pH. Results obtained from micropuncture, microperfusion, and clearance experiments are divergent or even contradictory regarding the effect of external pH. Some investigators have found that phosphate reabsorption is stimulated by alkaline luminal perfusates.[138-141] The crux of these experiments appears to be luminal and intracellular phosphate concentration. At concentrations of phosphate that are not saturating, P_i transport is stimulated by increasing luminal pH.[139] However, at saturating or high phosphate concentrations, the dependency of P_i transport on luminal pH diminishes[140] and probably reverses.[65,142] These results agree well with those of recent studies of respiratory alkalosis and acidosis in rats *in vivo*.[70] In these studies, alkalosis stimulated and acidosis inhibited P_i reabsorption, but only at nonsaturating concentrations of P_i. Perhaps the apparently inconsistent results obtained in numerous studies[70,93,143-152] of acid-base effects on P_i transport in *in vivo* models can be understood by this finding, especially since many of the procedures involved were not controlled for phosphate and calcium supply.

Four major factors appear to control phosphate transport (Fig. 7–4), and their interactions determine the results of an experimental manipulation. Three of the factors, phosphate supply, protons (allosteric effects of hydrogen), and PTH, have been discussed in earlier

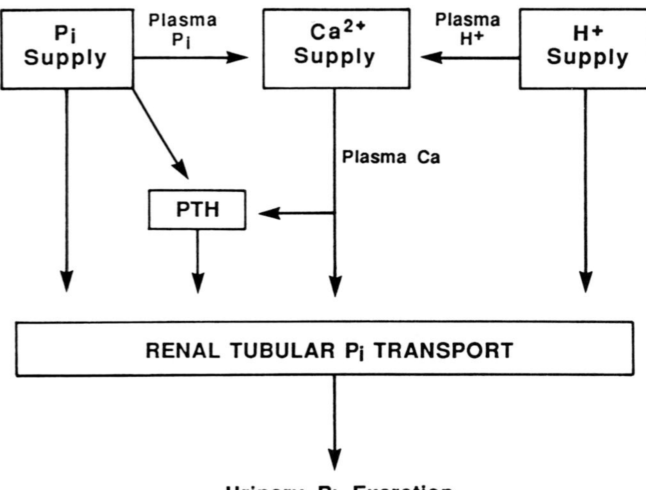

Figure 7–4 Interactions of plasma Ca^{2+}, PTH, and dietary phosphate and acid content in the regulation of phosphate transport. Supply may indicate electrolyte availability from exogenous (dietary) or endogenous (metabolic) sources.

sections of this chapter. The fourth, calcium, is poorly understood. Recent studies from Caverzasio and Bonjour[204] using the opossum kidney cell line in culture have demonstrated direct effects of extracellular calcium on sodium-P_i co-transport. Lowering $[Ca^{2+}]_e$ increases and elevating it decreases the rate of transport. The direct effects of cytosolic calcium on sodium-P_i co-transport remain to be determined. In this section, the interactions of P_i, sodium, calcium, and PTH with the sodium-P_i co-transport system(s) as discussed in section II-A (1a, allosteric modification), and the mechanisms of long-term adaptation as they are currently understood, will be used to interpret observations on the effects of acid-base status on renal P_i reabsorption.

The sodium-P_i co-transport of the brush border membrane was stimulated by alkaline pH at the luminal membrane but is inhibited by alkaline pH at the cytosolic membrane surface.[36] Studies by Ullrich[8] have demonstrated similar behavior of P_i reabsorption *in vivo*. The changes in pH at the luminal surface of the brush border membrane affect the affinities of the sodium-P_i co-transport system for sodium and P_i—an effect that would be expected to influence P_i transport only at nonsaturating P_i concentrations.[36] This behavior of P_i reabsorption has also been observed *in vivo*.[42-45,63,70,76,84,85,93,106,110-113,139,144-152] When P_i levels in the lumen are above carrier saturation, luminal pH no longer has an effect on the interaction of P_i with carrier. Cytosolic pH, however, may still influence the rate of P_i transport by affecting the rate of P_i dissociation from the carrier of the cytosolic surface of the membrane. This situation may occur during perfusions of proximal tubules with strongly buffered acid solutions containing a high phosphorus content.[65,139,142] Acidification of the cell, due to increased influx of hydrogen or product inhibition of sodium-hydrogen exchange, might have increased the rate of P_i dissociation from the carrier and stimulated the rate of P_i transport in these experiments.

Intracellular P_i concentration seems to be another important factor determining the rate of P_i dissociation into the cytosol. Experiments performed *in vivo* demonstrate that systemic P_i infusion reduces the rate of P_i reabsorption and reduces its sensitivity to luminal pH.[70,140] The effect of P_i infusion suggests that the rate of P_i unloading at the cytosolic surface of the brush border membrane is inhibited when cytosolic P_i is increased. This may become a rate-limiting factor in net P_i reabsorption. The interaction of P_i with a cytosolic aspect of the sodium-P_i co-transport system has not been investigated, and the kinetics of this reaction are unknown. If the kinetic properties of the sodium-P_i co-transport system are symmetric between the cytosolic and the luminal face of the membrane, data from *in vivo* experiments could easily be explained.

Disturbances of acid-base balance produce profound metabolic alterations that may indirectly affect renal reabsorption of P_i. Alkalosis is associated with inhibition of gluconeogenesis and stimulation of glycolysis.[113,115,145,153-158] Stimulation of glycolysis results in an increased incorporation of P_i into glycolytic intermediates, a shift of P_i from the extracellular fluid into the cells, and hypophosphatemia, which may in turn stimulate renal reabsorption of P_i.[145]

Acidosis and alkalosis affect bicarbonate reabsorption in the proximal tubule directly via stimulation and inhibition of sodium-hydrogen exchange in the brush border membrane.[107,159-162] These effects were mediated by direct allosteric control of sodium-hydrogen exchange activity by intracellular pH as well as by adaptive changes of sodium-hydrogen countertransport, at least in metabolic acidosis.[107,159,162] Stimulation of sodium-hydrogen exchange results in a decrease of luminal pH, which may result in inhibition of sodium-P_i co-transport.

Acidosis is associated with stimulation of renal gluconeogenesis, increased mitochondrial uptake of several anionic substrates (glutamine, glutamate, alpha-ketoglutarate, and citrate), and their oxidation to CO_2 and water.[154,157,163,164] Increased conversion of anionic substrates to either glucose or CO_2 involves increased intracellular consumption of hydrogen and may contribute to cell hydrogen homeostasis.[157] A relative alkaline shift of cell pH and P_i release from glycolytic intermediates may inhibit the dissociation of P_i on the cytosolic surface of the brush border membrane and may participate in the inhibition of P_i reabsorption observed in metabolic acidosis (Fig. 7–3).[143,148,149] In chronic metabolic acidosis, a large decrease of the V_{max} of sodium-P_i co-transport in isolated brush border membranes is observed, whereas the K_m for P_i is not changed.[93,95] However, in recent studies, Northrup et al.[165] have not observed this adaptation. Northrup's results suggest that the number of sodium-P_i co-transport systems in the membrane is decreased, an adaptive effect that must be distinguished from direct allosteric effects of hydrogen on P_i transport. Simultaneously, the V_{max} of sodium-hydrogen exchange and the rate of tubular acidification are increased,[107,161,162] which creates less favorable conditions for P_i reabsorption. Thus, in chronic metabolic acidosis, fewer sodium-P_i co-transport systems operate under less favorable kinetic conditions that together result in much slower P_i reabsorption in acidotic animals than in nonacidotic animals having the same plasma P_i.[93,95]

D. Steroid Hormones—1,25(OH)$_2$D$_3$ and Glucocorticoids

1. *Regulation of Phosphate Transport by 1,25(OH)$_2$D$_3$*

The effects of 1,25(OH)$_2$D$_3$ on the renal handling of P_i have recently been clarified and reviewed in Chapter 5. Controversy existed in the past owing to the animal models utilized to study P_i transport and the dosages employed. Clearance studies in human hypoparathyroid subjects[166] ingesting 1 to 2.5 μg per day of 1,25(OH)$_2$D$_3$ demonstrated a reduction in the fractional excretion of phosphorus but an increase in the amount of phosphorus appearing in the urine. In other words, the 1,25(OH)$_2$D$_3$ stimulated transport but P_i excretion increased related to an increase in the filtered load of P_i.

Animal clearance studies have shown both an inhibition of P_i transport[167,168] and a stimulation of P_i transport.[160,169-171] When mild vitamin D deficiency was produced in rats and secondary hyperparathyroidism was prevented,[169] the deficiency state was associated with an increase in P_i excretion. Sodium-dependent P_i transport in brush border membrane vesicles prepared from kidneys of vitamin D–deficient rats was also reduced. Repletion with physiologic doses of 1,25(OH)$_2$D$_3$ decreased P_i excretion and increased sodium-dependent P_i transport. These studies strongly support the stimulatory role of 1,25(OH)$_2$D$_3$ on the sodium-dependent P_i transport mechanism of the proximal tubule. They also support the earlier studies of the acute effects of vitamin D sterols on the renal handling of P_i.[170,171] These studies are discussed in the following section as they relate to the direct effects of the vitamin D sterols on membrane lipids.

Separation of acute and chronic effects of 1,25(OH)$_2$D$_3$ on P_i transport is important, since the chronic effects of the steroid may be affected by an increase in P_i availability due to stimulation of intestinal P_i absorption[172-174] (see Chapter 6). This could increase the filtered load of P_i and increase excretion despite stimulation of transport. Bonjour et al.[172,173] attempted to choose a physiologic dose of 1,25(OH)$_2$D$_3$ to study the chronic effects of the steroid on P_i transport in parathyroidectomized animals. They used sufficient 1,25(OH)$_2$D$_3$ to restore calcium absorption to normal and selected this as a physiologic dose. This dose increased P_i excretion and decreased the activity of the sodium-dependent P_i transport mechanism.[130] In vitamin D–deficient animals,[169] the dose was sufficient to produce hypercalcemia and an increase in plasma P_i. It increased P_i excretion at the same time that it increased the transport activity of isolated brush border membrane vesicles. In other studies,[175] small doses of $1,25(OH)_2D_3$ and PTH in thyroparathyroidectomized animals produced a decrease in P_i excretion over 6 hours. Results indicating an interaction between PTH and $1,25(OH)_2D_3$ were also observed in the state of P_i depletion.[176] In this setting, $1,25(OH)_2D_3$ increased the plasma P_i and restored the responsiveness to PTH measured in terms of P_i excretion.

The effects of $1,25(OH)_2D_3$ on P_i transport, determined by micropuncture of proximal and distal nephrons *in vivo,* remain controversial. An early report indicated stimulation of transport.[177] The most comprehensive analysis, performed in the Bonjour laboratory,[178] used a dose that may have been sufficient to increase the filtered load of P_i.

In the studies of Liang and Sacktor, $1,25(OH)_2D_3$ administered *in vivo* stimulated sodium-dependent phosphate uptake in cells isolated from chicken kidneys.[179-181] The effect was present at 3 hours following the administration of $1,25(OH)_2D_3$, but at 17 hours following an increase in the plasma P_i, the sodium-dependent phosphate uptake was decreased. These results suggest a stimulation of the transport process by $1,25(OH)_2D_3$, and a secondary inhibition related, again, to changes in the filtered phosphate load. The effect of $1,25(OH)_2D_3$ on phosphate transport in isolated chick renal cells was dose-dependent and very sensitive. The physiologic levels of $1,25(OH)_2D_3$ were maximally effective and stimulation was detectable at hormone levels of 10^{-14} M.[179-181]

The studies of Liang and Sacktor suggested that the effects of $1,25(OH)_2D_3$ were dependent on new protein synthesis since they were inhibited by cycloheximide. Earlier studies of the intestine had suggested that $1,25(OH)_2D_3$ produced specific effects on cell membrane phospholipid that stimulated calcium transport. Tsutsumi et al.[182] demonstrated that physiologic doses of $1,25(OH)_2D_3$ increased the phosphatidylcholine content and the fatty acid unsaturation of phosphatidylcholine in brush border membrane vesicles from the proximal tubular cells of the vitamin D–deficient rat kidney. Vitamin D depletion, itself, had decreased phosphatidylcholine content and increased the fatty acid saturation of phosphatidylcholine. The lipid dependency of phosphate transport was analyzed *in vitro* by the construction of Arrhenius plots.[183] These relate maximal rates of transport to temperature. Vitamin D deficiency significantly increased the activation energy for sodium-dependent phosphate transport. Physiologic repletion with $1,25(OH)_2D_3$ normalized the activation energy of the transport process.[183]

Recent studies from our laboratory have shown that $1,25(OH)_2D_3$ stimulates phospholipid exchange between plasma membrane vesicles and liposomes. The liposomes were either phospholipids that exhibit spontaneous transfer or physiologic forms of phosphatidylcholine.[183] We have also shown that the stimulation of phospholipid transfer from liposome to brush border membrane vesicle *in vitro* is associated with direct stimulation of phosphate transport.[184] These results strongly suggest a relationship between membrane lipid and the activity of sodium-dependent phosphate transport. They further suggest a relationship between $1,25(OH)_2D_3$, phosphatidylcholine biosynthesis, and the regulation of phosphate transport. Further studies are required to clarify the physiologic role of direct lipid effects of $1,25(OH)_2D_3$.

Recent studies have demonstrated that the brush border membrane of the proximal tubule isolated from HypY mice expresses a deficiency in phosphatidylcholine and phosphatidylethanolamine.[185] $1,25(OH)_2D_3$ stimuated phospholipid transfer from liposome to brush border membranes of the HypY mouse, but to the same extent that it stimulated transfer to normal brush border membranes. Stimulation of phosphate transport by lipid transfer was no greater in membranes from the HypY mouse than it was in membranes from normal mice. Thus, whereas the HypY mouse expresses an abnormality in phosphatidylcholine biosynthesis, this does not appear to be the genetic defect producing abnormal phosphate transport.[185]

Several lines of evidence suggest that glucocorticoids are important regulators of phosphate transport in the kidney.[186] In Cushing's disease and after glucocorticoid administration, lowered serum phosphate levels and enhanced phosphaturia have been reported. The site of action of glucocorticoids in decreasing P_i reabsorption is largely confined to the proximal tubule,[187,188] where glucocorticoid receptors but not mineralocorticoid receptors have been found.[189] Furthermore, it has been shown that dexamethasone but not aldosterone injected *in vivo* into rats results in decreased sodium-P_i co-transport in isolated brush border membrane vesicles.[97,190] Recent studies by Noronha-Blob and Sacktor[191] have investigated the mechanism of action of glucocorticoids on phosphate transport in primary culture of chick renal cells. Dexamethasone inhibited the sodium-dependent P_i uptake system. Sodium-independent P_i uptake and sodium-dependent uptakes of alpha-methylglucoside and proline were unaffected. Inhibition of sodium-dependent P_i co-transport by dexamethasone involved an induction period that was blocked by inhibitors of RNA and protein synthesis. The inhibitory effects of the glucocorticoids were rapidly reversed by removal of the steroid. Following reversal of P_i transport inhibition, cells responded again to glucocorticoids, however, with a much more rapid response time. The effects of glucocorticoids were inhibited by inhibitors of RNA and protein synthesis, actinomycin D, and cycloheximide. The authors suggest that glucocorticoids may mediate the renal adaptation of phosphate transport observed in chronic metabolic acidosis.

IV. CLINICAL DISEASE STATES ASSOCIATED WITH ABNORMAL P_i TRANSPORT

A. Chronic Renal Failure

Control of P_i reabsorption and maintenance of P_i balanced in the face of progressive loss of nephrons is observed during most of the course of chronic renal failure (see Chapter 13). Interactions of several factors (Fig. 7–4) probably account for the adaptation. The kidney is able to maintain normal plasma P_i levels until the glomerular filtration rate falls to approximately 25% of normal. Renal P_i reabsorption is depressed owing to separate, but associated, effects of PTH, P_i supply, and a metabolic acidosis. The effects of volume expansion and elevation of the filtered P_i load per functioning nephron appear also to play a role in the adaptation. Hyperphosphatemia ensues in advanced renal failure when the GFR falls to less than 25% of normal. This may be due to the maximal effects of the above factors on a small number of remaining nephrons so that further elevation of these influences is no longer effective in maintaining the phosphate balance of the body.

B. Vitamin D–Resistant Rickets—X-Linked Hypophosphatemic Rickets

Primary hypophosphatemic rickets or X-linked hypophosphatemic rickets is a well-described disorder, reviewed in Chapter 24, that is characterized by normocalcemia, hypophosphatemia, and inappropriate renal phosphate wasting. Evidence from an animal model, the X-linked hypophosphatemic mouse, in which the pathologic state appears to be very similar to the human disease, suggests that the primary basis for the hypophosphatemia is a defect in cellular phosphate absorption.[192,193] This may take the form of enhanced backflux from the cell into the tubule lumen or a decrease in uptake by the brush border membrane sodium-P_i co-transport system.[194] The biochemical defects include a relative decrease in PTH-responsive adenylate cyclase and alkaline phosphatase activities.[195] However, cAMP-dependent protein kinase and protein phosphatase activities appear not to be affected. Brush border membranes studied *in vitro* exhibit phosphorylation and dephosphorylation similar to normal controls even though sodium-dependent P_i transport is abnormally low.[197] These results suggest that the intrinsic abnormality of P_i transport is independent from mediation of the phosphaturic effect of PTH.[196-199] The role that these factors play in altering brush border membrane transport and the cellular events leading to this alteration are unknown. Because the renal cells respond appropriately to parathyroidectomy but abnormally to dietary phosphate restriction, it has been postulated that the underlying defect is a blunted response to the signal of intracellular P_i availability. This hypothesis requires testing.

Another group of hypophosphatemic patients who demonstrate renal tubular P_i wasting but no evidence of rickets has been described.[200] The renal wasting is not as severe as in patients with vitamin D–resistant rickets, and the P_i and cAMP excretion after response to PTH infusion is in marked contrast with the abnormal findings in X-linked hypophosphatemia subjects.[200] The pathogenesis in these subjects has not been well described since a suitable animal model is lacking.

C. Pseudohypoparathyroidism

Pseudohypoparathyroidism is a group of disorders in which there is a resistance to the action of PTH at the level of the renal proximal tubule.[201-203] Escape from the phosphaturic action of PTH due to secondary hyperparathyroidism and desensitization allows the renal cell to reabsorb inappropriate amounts of filtered phosphate and ultimately leads to hyperphosphatemia. Two forms of pseudohypoparathyroidism have been identified. In type I, patients demonstrate PTH resistance and absence of urinary cAMP response. In type II, patients have normal urinary cAMP excretion in response to PTH but fail to exhibit phosphaturia after PTH infusion. Calcium infusion restores the phosphaturic response in the type II form. These diseases appear to be due to a defect in PTH receptor, adenylate cyclase activation (type I), and post-cAMP defect or defective signaling through the calcium messenger system (type II) by the renal cell.[201-203]

References

1. Walser M: Ion association. VI. Interaction between calcium, magnesium, inorganic phosphate, citrate, and protein in normal human plasma. J Clin Invest 40:723, 1961.
2. McLean FC, Hinricks MA: Formation and behavior of colloidal calcium, phosphate in blood. Am J Physiol 121:580, 1938.
3. Strickler JC, Thompson DD, Klose RM, Giebisch G: Micropuncture study of inorganic phosphate excretion in the rat. J Clin Invest 43:1596–1607, 1964.
4. Agus ZS, Puschett JB, Senesky D, Goldberg M: Mode of action of parathyroid hormone and cyclic adenosine 3′-5′-monophosphate on renal tubular phosphate reabsorption in the dog. J Clin Invest 50:617–626, 1971.
5. Agus ZS, Gardner LB, Beck LH, Goldberg M: Effects of parathyroid hormone on renal tubular reabsorption of calcium, sodium and phosphate. Am J Physiol 224:1143–1148, 1973.
6. Baumann K, deRouffignac C, Roinel N, et al: Renal phosphate transport: Inhomogeneity of local proximal transport rates and sodium dependence. Pfluegers Arch 356:287–297, 1975.
7. McKeown JW, Brazy PC, Dennis VW: Intrarenal heterogeneity for fluid, phosphate, and glucose absorption in the rabbit. Am J Physiol 237:F312–F318, 1979.
8. Ullrich KJ, Rumrich G, Kloss S: Phosphate transport in the proximal convolution of the rat kidney. I. Tubular heterogeneity, effect of parathyroid hormone in acute and chronic parathyroidectomized animals and effect of phosphate diet. Pfluegers Arch 372:269–274, 1977.
9. Boudry JF, Troehler U, Toubai M, et al: Secretion of inorganic phosphate in the rat nephron. Clin Sci Mol Med 48:475–489, 1975 .
10. deRouffignac C, Morel F, Roinel N: Micropuncture study of water and electrolyte movement along the loop of Henle in psammomys with special reference to magnesium, calcium and phosphorus. Pfluegers Arch 344:309–326, 1973.
11. Greger R, Lang F, Marchand G, Knox FG: Site of renal phosphate reabsorption: Micropuncture and microinfusion study. Pfluegers Arch 369:111–118, 1977.
12. Amiel C, Kuntziger HE, Richet G: Micropuncture study of handling of phosphate by proximal and distal nephron in normal and parathyroidectomized rat. Evidence for distal reabsorption. Pfluegers Arch 317:92–109, 1970.
13. Beck LH, Goldberg M: Effects of acetazolamide and parathyroidectomy on renal transport of sodium, calcium and phosphate. Am J Physiol 224:1136–1142, 1973.
14. Frick A: Proximal tubular reabsorption of inorganic phosphate during saline infusion in the rat. Am J Physiol 223:1034–1040, 1972.
15. Kuntziger H, Amiel C, Roinel N, Morel F: Effects of parathyroidectomy and cyclic AMP on renal transport of phosphate, calcium and magnesium. Am J Physiol 227:905–911, 1974.
16. Brunette MG, Chan M, Muag U, Beliveau R: Phosphate uptake by superficial and deep nephron brush-border membranes. Effect of the dietary phosphate and parathyroid hormone. Pfluegers Arch 400:356–362, 1984.
17. Walker JJ, Yan TS, Quamme GA: Presence of multiple sodium-dependent phosphate transport processes in proximal brush-border membranes. Am J Physiol 252:F226–F231, 1987.
18. Kuntziger H, Amiel C, Gaudebout C: Phosphate handling by the rat nephron during saline diuresis. Kidney Int 2:318–323, 1972.
19. LeGrimellec C, Roinel N, Morel F: Simultaneous Mg, Ca, P, K, Na and Cl analysis in rat tubular fluid. I. During perfusion of either inulin or ferrocyanide. Pfluegers Arch 340:181–196, 1973.
20. Poujeol P, Chabardes D, Roinel M, deRouffignac C: Influence of extracellular fluid volume expansion on magnesium, calcium and phosphate handling along the rat nephron. Pfluegers Arch 365:203–211, 1976.
21. Staum BB, Hamburger RJ, Goldberg M: Tracer microinjection study of renal tubular phosphate reabsorption in the rat. J Clin Invest 51:2271–2276, 1972.
22. Brunette MG, Taleb L, Carriere S: Effect of parathyroid hormone on phosphate reabsorption along the nephron of the rat. Am J Physiol 225:1076–1081, 1973.
23. Dennis VW, Bello-Reuss E, Robinson R: Response of phosphate transport to parathyroid hormone in

segments of rabbit nephron. Am J Physiol 233:F29–F38, 1977.
24. Dennis VW, Woodhall PB, Robinson RR: Characteristics of phosphate transport in isolated proximal tubule. Am J Physiol 231:979–985, 1976.
25. Lang F, Greger R, Marchand GR, Knox FG: Stationary microperfusion study of phosphate reabsorption in proximal and distal nephron segments. Pfluegers Arch 368:45–48, 1977.
26. Rocha AS, Magaldi JB, Kokko JP: Calcium and phosphate transport in isolated segments of rabbit's Henle's loop. J Clin Invest 59:975–984, 1977.
27. Amiel C, Kuntziger H, Couette S, et al: Evidence for a parathyroid hormone-independent calcium modulation of phosphate transport along the nephron. J Clin Invest 57:256–263, 1976.
28. Haas J, Berndt T, Knox F: Nephron heterogeneity of phosphate reabsorption. Am J Physiol 234:F287–F300, 1978.
29. Harris CA, Sutton RAL, Dirks JH: Effects of hypercalcemia on calcium and phosphate ultrafilterability. Am J Physiol 233:F201–F206, 1977.
30. Pastoriza-Munoz E, Colindres RE, Lassiter WE, Lechene C: Effect of parathyroid hormone on phosphate reabsorption in rat distal convolution. Am J Physiol 235:321–330, 1978.
31. Poujeol P, Jamison RL, deRouffignac C: Phosphate reabsorption in juxtamedullary nephron terminal segments. Pfluegers Arch 387:27–31, 1980.
32. Haas JA, Berndt TJ, Haramati A, Knox FG: Nephron sites of action of nicotinamide on phosphate reabsorption. Am J Physiol 246:F27–F31, 1984.
33. Poujeol P, Corman B, Touvay C, deRouffignac C: Phosphate reabsorption in rat nephron terminal segments: Intrarenal heterogeneity and strain differences. Pfluegers Arch 371:39–44, 1977.
34. Haramati A, Haas JA, Knox FG: Adaptation of deep and superficial nephrons to changes in dietary phosphate intake. Am J Physiol 244:F265–F269, 1983.
35. Pastoriza-Munoz E, Mishler DR, Lechene C: Effect of phosphate deprivation on phosphate reabsorption in rat nephron: Role of PTH. Am J Physiol 244:F140–F149, 1983.
36. Amstutz M, Mohrmann M, Gmaj P, Murer H: The effect of pH on phosphate transport in rat renal brush border membrane vesicles. Am J Physiol 248:F705–F710, 1985.
37. Barrett PA, Gertner JM, Rasmussen H: Effect of dietary phosphate on transport properties of pig renal microvillous vesicles. Am J Physiol 239:F352–F359, 1980.
38. Beliveau R, Brunette MG: The renal brush border membrane in man. Protein pattern, inorganic phosphate binding and transport: comparison with other species. Renal Physiol 7:65–71, 1984.
39. Burckhardt G, Stern H, Murer H: The influence of pH on phosphate transport into rat renal brush border membrane vesicles. Pfluegers Arch 390:191–197, 1981.
40. Cheng L, Sacktor B: Sodium gradient-dependent phosphate transport in renal brush border membrane vesicles. J Biol Chem 256:1556–1564, 1981.
41. Dousa TP, Kempson SA, Shah SV: Adaptive changes in renal cortical brush border membrane. Adv Exp Med Biol 128:69–76, 1980.
42. Hoffmann N, Thees M, Kinne R: Phosphate transport by isolated renal brush border vesicles. Pfluegers Arch 362:147–156, 1976.
43. Hruska KA, Hammerman MR: Parathyroid hormone inhibition of phosphate transport in renal brush border vesicles from phosphate-depleted dogs. Biochim Biophys Acta 645:351–356, 1981.
44. Hruska KA, Klahr S, Hammerman MR: Decreased luminal membrane transport of phosphate in chronic renal failure. Am J Physiol 242:F17–F22, 1982.
45. Kempson SA, Dousa TP: Phosphate transport across renal cortical brush border membrane vesicles from rats stabilized on a normal, high or low phosphate diet. Life Sci 24:881–888, 1979.
46. Sacktor B, Cheng L: Sodium gradient-dependent phosphate transport in renal brush border membrane vesicles. Effect of an intravesicular greater than extravesicular proton gradient. J Biol Chem 256:8080–8084, 1981.
47. Shah SV, Kempson SA, Northrup TE, Dousa TP: Renal adaptation to low phosphate diet in rats. Blockade by actinomycin D. J Clin Invest 64:955–966, 1979.
48. Tenenhouse HS, Scriver CR: The defect in transcellular transport of phosphate in the nephron is located in brush border membranes in X-linked hypophosphatemia (Hyp mouse model). Can J Biochem 56:640–646, 1978.
49. Samarzija I, Molnar V, Froemter E: pH-dependence of phosphate absorption in rat renal proximal tubule. Proc Eur Dialysis Transplant Assoc 19:779–783, 1983.
50. Cheng L, Liang CT, Sacktor B: Phosphate uptake by renal membrane vesicles of rabbits adapted to high and low phosphorus diets. Am J Physiol 245:F175–F180, 1983.
51. Ullrich KJ, Murer H: Sulfate and phosphate transport in rat kidney proximal tubule. Philos Trans R Soc Lond [Biol] 299:549–558, 1982.
52. Brazy PC, Dennis VW: Sulfate transport in rabbit proximal convoluted tubules: Presence of anion exchange. Am J Physiol 241:F300–F307, 1981.
53. Grinstein S, Turner RJ, Silverman M, Rothstein A: Inorganic anion transport in kidney and intestinal brush border and basolateral membranes. Am J Physiol 238:F452–F460, 1980.
54. Schwab SJ, Klahr S, Hammerman MR: Na^+ gradient-dependent Pi uptake in basolateral membrane vesicles from dog kidney. Am J Physiol 246:F663–F669, 1984.
55. Hammerman MR, Schwab SJ: Phosphate transport in the kidney. Studies with isolated membrane vesicles. *In* Bonner F, Peterlik M (eds): Epithelial Calcium and Phosphate Transport: Molecular and Cellular Aspects. New York, Liss, 1984, pp 325–330.
56. Low I, Friedrich T, Burckhardt G: Properties of an anion exchanger in rat renal basolateral membrane vesicles. Am J Physiol 245:F334–F342, 1984.
57. Hagenbuch B, Stange G, Murer H: Transport of sulphate in rat jejunal and rat proximal tubular basolateral membrane vesicles. Pfluegers Arch 405:202–208, 1986.
58. Gmaj P, Ghijsen W, Murer H, Carafoli E: Calcium transport in isolated and reconstituted basal-lateral plasma membranes of rat kidney cortex. *In* Bonner F, Peterlik M (eds): Epithelial Calcium and Phosphate Transport: Molecular and Cellular Aspects. New York, Liss, 1984, pp 337–342.
59. Schwab SJ, Klahr S, Hammerman M: Uptake of Pi in basolateral vesicles after release of unilateral

ureteral obstruction. Am J Physiol 247:F543–F547, 1984.
60. Brazy PC, Balaban RS, Gulians SR, et al: Inhibition of renal metabolism. Relative effects of arsenate on sodium, phosphate and glucose transport by the rabbit proximal tubule. J Clin Invest 66:1211–1221, 1980.
61. Brazy PC, Gullans SR, Mandel LJ, Dennis VW: Metabolic requirement for inorganic phosphate by the rabbit proximal tubule. J Clin Invest 70:53–62, 1982.
62. Freeman D, Bartlett S, Radda G, Ross B: Energetics of sodium transport in the kidney. Saturation transfer ^{31}P-NMR. Biochim Biophys Acta 762:325–336, 1983.
63. Koobs DH: Phosphate mediation of the Crabtree and Pasteur effects. Science 178:127–133, 1972.
64. Murer H, Burckhardt G: Membrane transport of anions across epithelia of mammalian small intestine and kidney proximal tubule. Rev Physiol Biochem Pharmacol 96:1–53, 1983.
65. Ham LL, Kokko, JP, Jacobson HR: Effect of luminal pH and HCO_3^- on phosphate reabsorption in the rabbit proximal convoluted tubule. Am J Physiol 247:F25–F34, 1984.
66. Mizgala CL, Quamme GQ: Renal handling of phosphate. Physiol Rev 65:431–466, 1985.
67. Gmaj P, Murer H: Cellular mechanisms of inorganic phosphate transport in kidney. Physiolog Rev 66:36–70, 1986.
68. Brunette MG, Beliveau R, Chan M: Effect of temperature and pH on phosphate transport through brush border membrane vesicles in rats. Can J Physiol Pharmacol 62:229–234, 1984.
69. Braun-Werness JL, Jackson BA, Werness PG, Dousa TP: Binding of nicotinamide adenine dinucleotide by the renal brush border membrane fraction from rat kidney cortex. Biochim Biophys Acta 732:553–561, 1983.
70. Haramati A, Nienhuis D: Renal handling of phosphate during acute respiratory acidosis and alkalosis in the rat. Am J Physiol 147:F596–F601, 1984.
71. Murer H, Stern H, Burckhardt G, et al: Sodium-dependent transport of inorganic phosphate across the renal brush border membrane. Adv Exp Med Biol 128:11–23, 1980.
72. Hammerman MR, Hruska KA: Cyclic AMP-dependent protein phosphorylation in canine renal brush border membrane vesicles is associated with decreased phosphate transport. J Biol Chem 257:992–999, 1982.
73. Chabardes D, Imbert M, Clique A, et al: PTH sensitive adenyl cyclase activity in different segments of the rabbit nephron. Pfluegers Arch 354:229–239, 1975.
74. Shlatz LJ, Schwartz IL, Kinne-Safran E, Kinne R: Distribution of parathyroid hormone stimulated adenylate cyclase in plasma membranes of cell of the kidney cortex. J Membr Biol 24:131–144, 1975.
75. George ER, Balakir RA, Filburn CR, Sacktor B: Cyclic adenosine monophosphate dependent and independent protein kinase activity of renal brush border membranes. Arch Biochem Biophys 180:429–443, 1977.
76. Kinne R, Shlatz LJ, Kinne-Safran E, Schwartz IL: Distribution of membrane bound cyclic AMP-dependent protein kinase in the plasma membrane of cells of the kidney cortex. J Membr Biol 24:145–159, 1975.
77. Hammerman MR, Karl IE, Hruska KA: Regulation of canine renal vesicle P_i transport by growth hormone and parathyroid hormone. Biochim Biophys Acta 603:322–335, 1980.
78. Hammerman MR, Cohn DE, Tamayo J, Martin KJ: Effect of parathyroid hormone on Na+-dependent phosphate transport and cAMP-dependent ^{32}P phosphorylation in brush border vesicles from isolated perfused canine kidneys. Arch Biochem Biophys 227:91–97, 1983.
79. Hammerman MR, Hansen VA, Morrissey JJ: ADP ribosylation of canine renal brush border membrane vesicle proteins is associated with decreased phosphate transport. J Biol Chem 257:12380–12386, 1982.
80. Hammerman MR, Hruska KA: Cyclic AMP-dependent protein phosphorylation in canine renal brush border membrane vesicles is associated with decreaed phosphate transport. J Biol Chem 257:992–999, 1982.
81. Biber J, Malmström K, Scalera V, Murer H: Phosphorylation of rat kidney proximal tubular brush border membranes. Role of cAMP-dependent protein phosphorylation in the regulation of phosphate transport. Pfluegers Arch 398:221–226, 1983.
82. Malmström K, Biber J, Gmaj P, Murer H: Possible mechanisms for the regulation of the P_i transport in brush border membrane vesicles. *In* Bronner F, Peterlik M (eds): Epithelial Calcium and Phosphate Transport: Molecular and Cellular Aspects. New York, Liss, 1984, pp 331–336.
83. Hammerman MR, Corpus VM, Morrissey JJ: NAD^+-induced inhibition of phosphate transport in canine renal brush border membranes. Mediation through a process other than or in addition to NAD+ hydrolysis. Biochim Biophys Acta 732:110–116, 1983.
84. Kempson SA, Curthoys NP: NAD^+-dependent ADP-ribosyltransferase in renal brush-border membranes. Am J Physiol 245:C449–C456, 1983.
85. Kempson SA, Colon-Otero G, Ou SY, et al: Possible role of nicotinamide adenine dinucleotide as an intracellular regulator of renal transport of phosphate in the rat. J Clin Invest 67:1347–1360, 1981.
86. Angielski S, Zielkiewicz J, Dziezko G: Metabolism of NAD by isolated rat renal brush border membranes. Pfluegers Arch 395:159–161, 1982.
87. Tenenhouse HS, Chu YL: Hydrolysis of nicotinamide adenine dinucleotide by purified renal brush border membranes. Biochem J 204:635–638, 1982.
88. Lang RP, Yanagawa N, Nord EP, et al: Nucleotide inhibition of phosphate transport in the renal proximal tubule. Am J Physiol 245:F263–F271, 1983.
89. Baines AD, Ross BD: Gluconeogenesis and phosphate reabsorption in isolated lactate or pyruvate-perfused rat kidney. Mineral Electrolyte Metab 10:286–291, 1984.
90. Yanagawa N, Nagami G, Joe OK, et al: Dissociation of gluconeogenesis from fluid and phosphate reabsorption in isolated rabbit proximal tubules. Kidney Int 25:869–873, 1984.
91. Yanagawa N, Nagami GT, Kurokawa K: Cytosolic redox potential and phosphate transport in the proximal tubule of the rabbit. A study in the isolated perfused tubules. Mineral Electrolyte Metab 11:57–61, 1985.
92. Evers C, Murer H, Kinne R: Effect of parathyrin on the transport properties of isolated renal brush border vesicles. Biochem J 172:49–56, 1978.

93. Kempson SA: Effect of metabolic acidosis on renal brush border membrane adaptation to low phosphorus diet. Kidney Int 22:225–233, 1982.
94. Levine BS, Ho K, Hodsman A, et al: Early renal brush border membrane adaptation to dietary phosphorus. Mineral Electrolyte Metab 10:222–227, 1984.
95. Levine BS, Ho K, Kraut JA, et al: Effect of metabolic acidosis on phosphate transport by the renal brush border membrane. Biochim Biophys Acta 727:7–12, 1983.
96. Murer H, Stern H, Burckhardt G, et al: Sodium-dependent transport of inorganic phosphate across the renal brush border membrane. Adv Exp Med Biol 128:11–23, 1980.
97. Turner ST, Kiebzak GM, Dousa TP: Mechanism of glucocorticoid effect on renal transport of phosphate. Am J Physiol 243:C227–C236, 1982.
98. Yusufi ANK, Holets RJ, Dousa TP: Stimulation of renal brush border membranes (BBM) transport of phosphate (P_i) by thyroid hormones: Mechanisms of action. Fed Proc 43:663 (abstract), 1984.
99. Biber JC, Brown CD, Murer H: Sodium-dependent transport of phosphate in LLC-PK_1 cells. Biochim Biophys Acta 735:325–330, 1983.
100. Biber J, Murer H: Na-P_i cotransport in LLC-PK_1 cells: Fast adaptive response to P_i deprivation. Am J Physiol 249:C430–C434, 1985.
101. Brown CD, Bodmer M, Biber J, Murer H: Sodium-dependent phosphate transport by apical membrane vesicles from a cultured renal epithelial cell line (LLC-PK_1). Biochim Biophys Acta 769:471–478, 1984.
102. Caverzasio J, Brown CDA, Biber J, et al: Adaptation of phosphate transport in phosphate-deprived LLC-PK_1 cells. Am J Physiol 248:F122–F127, 1985.
103. Rabito CA: Phosphate uptake by a kidney cell line (LLC-PK_1). Am J Physiol 245:F22–F31, 1983.
104. Forte TM, Machen TE, Forte JG: Ultrastructural changes in oxyntic cells associated with secretory function: A membrane-recycling hypothesis. Gastroenterology 73:941–955, 1977.
105. Gluck S, Cannon C, Al-Awquati Q: Exocytosis regulates urinary acidification in the turtle bladder by rapid insertion of H^+ pumps into the luminal membrane. Proc Natl Acad Sci USA 79:4327–4331, 1982.
106. Kono T, Robinson FW, Blevins TL, Ezaki O: Evidence that translocation of the glucose transport activity is the major mechanism of insulin action on glucose transport in fat cells. J Biol Chem 257:10942–10947, 1982.
107. Tsai CJ, Ives HE, Alpern RJ, et al: Increased V_{max} for Na^+/H^+ antiporter activity in proximal tubule brush border vesicles from rabbits with metabolic acidosis. Am J Physiol 247:F339–F343, 1984.
108. Dennis VW, Brazy PC: Divalent anion transport in isolated renal tubules. Kidney Int 22:498–506, 1982.
109. Guder W: Regulation der Glukoneogenese der Niere. Munich, Dissertaionsdruck Schon, 1973.
110. Iino Y, Burg MB: Effect of parathyroid hormone on bicarbonate absorption by proximal tubules in vitro. Am J Physiol 236:F387–F391, 1979.
111. Karlinsky ML, Sagner DS, Kurtzman NA, Pillay VKG: Effect of parathormone and cyclic adenosine monophosphate on renal bicarbonate reabsorption. Am J Physiol 227:1226–1231, 1974.
112. Kurokawa K: Mechanism of renal action of parathyroid hormone. Adv Exp Med Biol 81:291–299, 1977.
113. Kurokawa K, Ohno T, Rasmussen H: Ionic control of renal gluconeogenesis. II. The effects of Ca^{2+} and H^+ upon the response to parathyroid hormone and cyclic AMP. Biochim Biophys Acta 313:32–41, 1973.
114. McKinney TD, Myers P: PTH inhibition of bicarbonate transport by proximal convoluted tubules. Am J Physiol 239:F127–F134, 1980.
115. Nagata N, Rasmussen H: Parathyroid hormone, 3′,5′-AMP, Ca^{++} and gluconeogenesis. Proc Natl Acad Sci USA 64:368–374, 1970.
116. Rasmussen H, Goodman DBP, Friedmann N, et al: Ionic control of metabolism. *In* Greep RO, Astwood EB (eds): Handbook of Physiology. Endocrinology, sect 7, vol VII. Washington, DC, American Physiological Society, 1976, pp 225–264.
117. Lau K, Goldfarb S, Goldberg M: The effects of parathyroid hormone on renal phosphate handling. *In* Massry SG, Fleisch H (eds): Renal Handling of Phosphate. New York, Plenum, 1980, pp 115–135.
118. Hruska KA, Moskowitz D, Esbrit P, et al: Stimulation of inositol trisphosphate and diacylglycerol production in renal tubular cells by parathyroid hormone. J Clin Invest 79:230–239, 1987.
119. Lowik CWGM, van Leeuwen JPTM, van der Meer JM, et al: A two-receptor model for the action of parathyroid hormone on osteoblasts: A role for intracellular free calcium and cAMP. Cell Calcium 6:311–326, 1985.
120. Hruska KA, Goligorsky M, Scoble J, et al: Effects of parathyroid hormone on cytosolic calcium in renal proximal tubular primary cultures. Am J Physiol 251:F188–F198, 1986.
121. Goligorsky MS, Loftus DJ, Hruska KA: Cytoplasmic calcium in individual proximal tubular cells in culture. Am J Physiol 251:F938–F944, 1986.
122. Cole JA, Eber SL, Poelling RE, et al: A dual mechanism for regulation of kidney phosphate transport by parathyroid hormone. Am J Physiol 253:E1–E7, 1987.
123. Malmström K, Murer H: Parathyroid hormone inhibits phosphate transport in OK cells but not in LLC-PK_1 abd JTC-12.P3 cells. Am J Physiol 251:C23–C31, 1986.
124. Caverzasio J, Brown CDA, Biber J, et al: Sodium-dependent phosphate transport inhibited by parathyroid hormone and cyclic AMP stimulation in an opossum kidney cell line. J Biol Chem 261:3233–3237, 1986.
125. Dousa TP, Kempson SA: Regulation of renal brush border membrane transport of phosphate. Mineral Electrolyte Metab 7:113–121, 1982.
126. Bank N, Malnic G: Effect of urinary alkalinization on renal phosphate reabsorption. *In* Massry SG, Fleisch H (eds): Renal Handling of Phosphate. New York, Plenum, 1980, pp 209–241.
127. Pollock AS, Warnock DG, Strewler GJ: Parathyroid hormone inhibition of Na^+/H^+ antiporter activity in a cultured renal cell line. Am J Physiol 250:F217–F255, 1986.
128. Reid IR, Civitelli R, Avioli LV, Hruska KA: Parathyroid hormone depresses cytosolic pH and DNA syntheses in osteoblast-like cells. Am J Physiol 255:E9–E15, 1988.
129. Weinman EJ, Shenolikar S, Kahm AM: cAMP-associated inhibition of Na^+/H^+ exchanger in rabbit kidney brush border membrane. Am J Physiol 252:F19–F25, 1987.
130. Stoll R, Kinne R, Murer H, et al: Phosphate transport

by rat renal brush border membrane vesicles: Influence of dietary phosphate, thyroparathyroidectomy, and 1,25-dihydroxyvitamin D_3. Pfluegers Arch 380:47–52, 1979.

131. Steele TH, Stromberg BA, Underwood JL, Larmore CA: Renal resistance to parathyroid hormone during phosphorus deprivation. J Clin Invest 58:1461–1464, 1976.
132. Steele TH: Renal response to phosphorus deprivation. Effect of the parathyroids and bicarbonate. Kidney Int 11:327–334, 1977.
133. Bonjour JP, Preston C, Fleisch H: Parathyroid hormone and renal handling of Pi effect of dietary Pi and diphosphonates. Am J Physiol 234:F497–F505, 1978.
134. Gloor HJ, Bonjour JP, Caverzusio J, Fleisch H: Resistance to the phosphaturic and calcemia actions of parathyroid hormone during phosphate deprivation: Prevention by 1,25-dihydroxyvitamin D_3. J Clin Invest 63:371–377, 1979.
135. Czekalski S, Knox FG, Dousa TP, et al: Restoration of phosphaturic response to parathyroid hormone by glucocorticoid treatment in phosphorus-deprived rats. J Lab Clin Med 100:858–865, 1982.
136. Haramati A, Knox FG: Tubular capacity of phosphate transport in phosphate-deprived rats: Effects of nicotinamide and PTH. Am J Physiol 244:F178–F184, 1983.
137. Guntupalli J, Eby B, Lau K: Mechanism for the phosphaturia of NH_4Cl: Dependence on acidemia but not on diet PO_4 or PTH. Am J Physiol 242:F552–F560, 1982.
138. Baumann K, Rumrich G, Papavassiliou F, Kloss S: pH dependence of phosphate reabsorption in the proximal tubule of rat kidney. Pfluegers Arch 360:183–187, 1975.
139. Lang F, Greger R, Knox FG, Oberteithner H: Factors modulating renal handling of phosphate. Renal Physiol 4:1–16, 1981.
140. Quamme GA, Wong NLM: Phosphate transport in the proximal convoluted tubule: Effect of intraluminal pH. Am J Physiol 246:F323–F333, 1984.
141. Ullrich KJ, Rumrich G, Kloess S: Phosphate transport in the proximal convolution of the rat kidney. III. Effect of extracellular and intracellular pH. Pfluegers Arch 377:33–42, 1978.
142. Cassola AC, Malnic G: Phosphate transfer and tubular pH during renal stopped flow microperfusion experiments in the rat. Pfluegers Arch 367:249–255, 1977 .
143. Quamme GA: Effects of dietary acid content on renal tubular changes to dietary phosphate intake. Proc Int Congr Nephrol, 9th, 1984, p 59A.
144. Hoppe A, Destro M, Knox FG: Effect of NH_4Cl on phosphaturic response to PTH in the hamster: Dissociation from acidemia. Am J Physiol 239:E328–E332, 1980.
145. Hoppe A, Metler M, Berndt TJ, et al: Effect of respiratory alkalosis on renal phosphate excretion. Am J Physiol 243:F471–F475, 1982.
146. Knox FG, Hoppe A, Kempson SA, et al: Cellular mechanisms of phosphate transport. *In* Massry SG, Fleisch H (eds): Renal Handling of Phosphate. New York, Plenum, 1980, pp 79–114.
147. Knox FG, Preiss J, Kim JK, Dousa TP: Mechanisms of resistance to the phosphaturic effect of the parathyroid hormone in the hamster. J Clin Invest 59:675–683, 1977.
148. Landberg H, Hartmann A, Kill F: Glomerular filtration rate and plasma pH as determinants of phosphate reabsorption. Kidney Int 26:128–136, 1984.
149. Steele TH, Challoner-Hue L, Gottstein JH, et al: Acid-base maneuvers and phosphate transport in the isolated rat kidney. Pfluegers Arch 392:178–182, 1981.
150. Webb RK, Woodhall PB, Tisher CC, et al: Relationship between phosphaturia and acute hypercapnia in the rat. J Clin Invest 60:829–837, 1977.
151. Wen SF: Indirect effect of hypercapnia on the phosphaturia of respiratory acidosis. Adv Exp Med Biol 128:113–115, 1980.
152. Wong NLM: The effect of bicarbonate on anion reabsorption along the dog nephron. Adv Exp Med Biol 128:135–143, 1980.
153. Hems DA, Gaja G: Carbohydrate metabolism in the isolated perfused rat kidney. Biochem J 128:412–426, 1972.
154. Kurokawa K, Rasmussen H: Ionic control of renal gluconeogenesis. I. The interrelated effects of calcium and hydrogen ions. Biochim Biophys Acta 313:17–31, 1973.
155. Kurokawa K, Rasmussen H: Ionic control of renal gluconeogenesis. III. The effects of changes in pH, pCO_2, and bicarbonate concentration. Biochim Biophys Acta 313:42–58, 1973.
156. Kurokawa K, Rasmussen H: Ionic control of renal gluconeogenesis. IV. Effect of extracellular phosphate concentration. Biochim Biophys Acta 313:59–71, 1973.
157. Dawson AG: Contribution of pH-sensitive metabolic process to pH homeostasis in isolated rat kidney tubules. Biochim Biophys Acta 499:85–98, 1977.
158. Relman AS: Metabolic consequences of acid-base disorders. Kidney Int 1:247–359, 1972.
159. Aronson PS, Shum MA, Nee J: Interaction of external H^+ with the Na^+-H^+ exchanger in renal microvillous membrane vesicles. J Biol Chem 258:6767–6771, 1983.
160. Murer H, Hopfer U, Kinne R: Sodium/proton antiport in brush border membrane vesicles isolated from rat small intestine and kidney. Biochem J 154:597–604, 1976.
161. Rector FC Jr: Sodium, bicarbonate, and chloride absorption by the proximal tubule. Am J Physiol 244:F461–F471, 1983.
162. Kinsella JL, Cujdik T, Sacktor B: Na^+-H^+ exchange in isolated brush border membrane vesicles in response to metabolic acidosis. Kinetic effects. J Biol Chem 259:13224–13227, 1984.
163. Simpson DP, Hager SR: pH and bicarbonate effects on mitochondrial anion accumulation. J Clin Invest 63:704–712, 1979.
164. Tannen RL, Sastrasinh S: Response of ammonia metabolism to acute acidosis. Kidney Int 25:1–10, 1984.
165. Northrup TE, Garella S, Cohen JJ: Na/H exchange in renal brush border (BBM) vesicles is not increased by acidemia. Clin Res 34:937A, 1986.
166. Neer RM, Holick MF, DeLuca HF, Potts JT Jr: Effects of 1α-hydroxy-vitamin D_3 and 1,25-dihydroxy-vitamin D_3 on calcium and phosphorus metabolism in hypoparathyroidism. Metabolism 24:1403–1413, 1975.
167. Ney RL, Kelly G, Bartter FC: Actions of vitamin D independent of the parathyroid glands. Endocrinology 82:760–766, 1968.

168. Crawford JD, Gribetz D, Talbot NB: Mechanism of renal tubular phosphate reabsorption and the influence thereon of vitamin D in completely parathyroidectomized rats. Am J Physiol 180:156–162, 1955.
169. Kurnik BRC, Hruska KA: Effects of 1,25-dihydroxycholecalciferol on phosphate transport in vitamin D-deprived rats. Am J Physiol 247:F177–F184, 1984.
170. Puschett JB, Moranz J, Kurnick WS: Evidence for a direct action of cholecalciferol and 25-hydroxycholecalciferol on the renal transport of phosphate, sodium, and calcium. J Clin Invest 51:373–385, 1972.
171. Popovtzer MM, Robinette JB, DeLuca HF, Holick MF: The acute effect of 25-hydroxycholecalciferol on renal handling of phosphorus. J Clin Invest 53:913–921, 1974.
172. Bonjour J-P, Caverzasio J, Muhlbauer R, et al: Acute and chronic effects of vitamin D metabolites on the renal handling of phosphate. *In* Norman AW, Schaefer K, Herrath DV, et al (eds): Vitamin D, Basic Research and Its Clinical Application. New York, de Gruyter, 1979, pp 307–314.
173. Bonjour J-P, Preston C, Fleisch H: Effect of 1,25-dihydroxy-vitamin D_3 on the renal handling of Pi in thyroparathyroidectomized rats. J Clin Invest 60:1419–1428, 1977.
174. Lee DBN, Walling MW, Brautbar N: Intestinal phosphate absorption: Influence of vitamin D and non-vitamin D factors. Am J Physiol 250:G369–G373, 1986.
175. Georgaki H, Puschett JB: Acute effects of a "physiological" dose of 1,25-dihydroxyvitamin D_3 on renal phosphate transport. Endocr Res Commun 9:135–143, 1982.
176. Brautbar N, Walling MW, Coburn JW: Interactions between vitamin D deficiency and phosphorus depletion in the rat. J Clin Invest 63:335–341, 1979.
177. Gekle D, Stroder J, Rostock D: The effect of vitamin D on renal inorganic phosphate reabsorption of normal rats, parathyroidectomized rats, and rats with rickets. Pediatr Res 5:40–52, 1971.
178. Muhlbauer RC, Bonjour J-P, Fleisch H: Tubular handling of P_i: Localization of effects of $1,25(OH)_2D_3$ and dietary P_i in TPXT rats. Am J Physiol 241:F123–F128, 1981.
179. Liang CT, Barnes J, Chenk L, et al: Effects of $1,25(OH)_2D_3$ administered in vivo on phosphate uptake by isolated chick renal cells. Am J Physiol 242:C312–C318, 1982.
180. Liang CT, Barnes J, Balakir R, et al: In vitro stimulation of phosphate uptake in isolated chick renal cells by 1,25-dihydroxycholecalciferol. Proc Natl Acad Sci USA 79:3532–3536, 1982.
181. Liang CT, Sacktor B: In vitro effect of $1,25(OH)_2D_3$ on the uptake of phosphate (P_i) by chick kidney cells. *In* Norman AW, Schaefer K, Herrath DV, Grigoleit HG (eds): Vitamin D, Chemical, Biochemical and Clinical Endocrinology of Calcium Metabolism. de Gruyter, New York, 1982, pp 437–439.
182. Tsutsumi M, Alvarez U, Avioli LV, Hruska KA: Effect of 1,25-dihydroxyvitamin D_3 on phospholipid composition of rat renal brush border membrane. Am J Physiol 249:F117–F123, 1985.
183. Kurnik BRC, Hruska KA: Mechanism of stimulation of renal phosphate transport by 1,25-dihydroxycholecalciferol. Biochim Biophys Acta 817:42–50, 1985.
183a. Kurnik BRC, Huskey M, Hagerty D, Hruska KA: Vitamin D metabolites stimulate phosphatidylcholine transfer to renal brush-border membranes. Biochim Biophys Acta 858:47–55, 1986.
184. Kurnik BRC, Huskey M, Hruska KA: 1,25-dihydroxycholecalciferol stimulates renal phosphate transport by directly altering membrane phosphatidylcholine composition. Biochim Biophys Acta 917:81–85, 1987.
185. Hruska KA, Roberts M, Avioli LV: Membrane phospholipid (PL) metabolism and phosphate transport in X-linked hypophosphatemia (Hyp-Y). Kidney Int 31:349, 1987.
186. Ritz E, Kreusser W, Bommer J: Effects of hormones other than parathyroid hormone on renal handling of phosphate. *In* Massry SG, Fleisch H (eds): Renal Handling of Phosphate. New York, Plenum Press, 1980, pp 137–195.
187. Frick A, Durasin I: Proximal tubular reabsorption of inorganic phosphate in adrenalectomized rats. Pflugers Arch 385:189–192, 1980.
188. Durasin I, Frick A, Neuweg M: Glucocorticoid-induced inhibition of the reabsorption of inorganic phosphate in the proximal tubule in the absence of parathyroid hormone. Renal Physiol 7:115–123, 1984.
189. Mishina T, Scholer DW, Edelman IS: Glucocorticoid receptors in rat kidney cortical tubules enriched in proximal and distal segments. Am J Physiol 240:F38–F45, 1981.
190. Freiberg JM, Kinsella J, Sacktor B: Glucocorticoids increase the Na^+/H^+ exchange and decrease the Na^+ gradient-dependent phosphate-uptake systems in renal brush border membrane vesicles. Proc Natl Acad Sci USA 79:4932–4936, 1982.
191. Noronha-Blob L, Sacktor B: Inhibition by glucocorticoids of phosphate transport in primary cultured renal cells. J Biol Chem 261:2164–2169, 1986.
192. Eicher EM, Southard JL, Scriver CR, Glorieux FH: Hypophosphatemia: Mouse model for human familial hypophosphatemia (vitamin D resistant) rickets. Proc Natl Acad Sci USA 73:4667–4671, 1976.
193. O'Doherty PJ, DeLuca HF: Intestinal calcium and phosphate transport in genetic hypophosphatemic mice. Biochem Biophys Res Commun 71:617–621, 1976.
194. Tenenhouse HS, Scriver CR, Melmes RR, Glorieux FH: Renal handling of phosphate in vivo and in vitro by the X-linked hypophosphatemic male mouse: Evidence for a defect in the brush border membrane. Kidney Int 14:236, 1978.
195. Brunette MG, Chan M, Lebrun M: Phosphatase activity along the nephron of mice with hypophosphatemic vitamin D-resistant rickets. Kidney Int 20:181–187, 1981.
196. Glorieux F, Scriver CR: Loss of a parathyroid hormone-sensitive component of phosphate transport in X-linked hypophosphatemia. Science 175:997–999, 1979.
197. Hammerman MR, Chase LR: Pi transport, phosphorylation, and dephosphorylation in renal membranes from HYP/Y mice. Am J Physiol 245:F701–F706, 1983.
198. Muhlbauer RC, Bonjour J-P, Fleisch H: Abnormal tubular adaptation to dietary Pi restriction in X-linked hypophosphatemic mice. Am J Physiol 242:F353–F359, 1982.
199. Tenenhouse HS, Scriver CR: Renal brush border membrane adaptation to phosphorous deprivation

in the HYP/Y mouse. Nature (London) 281:225–227, 1979.

200. Scriver CR, MacDonald W, Reade T, et al: Hypophosphatemic nonrachitic bone disease: An entity distinct from X-linked hypophosphatemia in the renal defect, bone involvement, and inheritance. Am J Med Genet 1:101–117, 1977.
201. Drezner MK, Neelon FA: Pseudohypoparathyroidism. *In* Stanbury JB, Wyngaarden JB, Fredrickson DS, et al (eds): The Metabolic Basis of Inherited Disease. New York, McGraw Hill, 1983, pp 1508–1527.
202. Chase LR, Melson GL, Aurbach GD: Pseudohypoparathyroidism: Defective excretion of 3'5'-AMP in response to parathyroid hormone. J Clin Invest 48:1832–1843, 1969.
203. Klahr S, Hruska KA: Effects of parathyroid hormone on the renal reabsorption of phosphorus and divalent cations. *In* Peck WA (ed): Bone and Mineral Research. Amsterdam, Elsevier Science, 1984, pp 65–124.
204. Caverzasio J, Bonjour J-P: Influence of calcium on phosphate transport in cultured kidney epithelium. Am J Physiol 254:F217–F222, 1988.

8

PAMELA GEHRON ROBEY
JOHN D. TERMINE

Biochemical Markers of Metabolic Bone Disease

Bone is an exquisite combination of cellular and noncellular constituents; the interactions and regulation of these constituents are critical to the maintenance of normal tissue function. During development, osteoprogenitor cells undergo differentiation into osteoblasts, the cells responsible for producing a mineralized extracellular bone matrix. As bone development continues, the initial mineralized matrix (calcified cartilage and woven bone) is remodeled by the sequential action of osteoclasts and osteoblasts, which eventually leads to the formation of true lamellar and osteonal bone. Bone modeling, which occurs during prenatal development and postnatal growth, results in the formation of marrow cavities and shape changes throughout the skeleton. However, focal remodeling (turnover) persists throughout life as a delicate balance between bone formation by osteoblasts and bone resorption by osteoclasts, composing the skeleton's physiologic response to the mechanical and metabolic needs of the body. Consequently, an understanding of normal osteoblast and osteoclast metabolism is of paramount importance to determine precisely the aberration(s) in metabolic bone disease that either result from or produce changes in bone turnover, that is, disrupt the balance of bone formation and resorption. Biochemical measurement of bone formation and resorption by noninvasive techniques is based on the identification of (1) synthetic products of osteoblasts released, at least partially, to circulation during their elaboration of a mineralized matrix, and (2) the subsequent degradation and release of the altered (degraded) products by osteoclasts. The list of bone constituents is increasing rapidly with ever more sensitive biochemical technology. Each one of these components, in either their native or degraded forms, provides a potential marker of bone metabolism. Careful estimates of their biochemical characteristics along with their correlation to histomorphometric analysis should in time prove the utility of each.

I. BONE MATRIX CONSTITUENTS

The identification of the molecular constituents in the extracellular matrix of bone has been facilitated by the development of techniques to chemically dissect both its organic and inorganic components.[1] The use of dissociative conditions (e.g., 4 M guanidine hydrochloride) as an initial step in the extraction of bone results in the removal of proteins not associated with the mineralized matrix (e.g., cellular and soft tissue proteins). Subsequent extraction under dissociative conditions in the presence of a demineralizing agent (normally, ethylenediamine tetraacetate) liberates proteins intimately associated with bone mineral.[2] However, it should be noted here that this procedure does not distinguish matrix components that are synthesized and deposited by osteoblasts from those that are exogenously derived.

A. Collagen

Collagen is the predominant secretory product of osteoblasts and composes 85% to 90% of the mineralized extracellular matrix.[3] Collagen is defined as a helical molecule composed of three polypeptides, termed α chains, that have a characteristic repeating amino acid sequence of Gly-X-Y throughout the molecule, where X and Y frequently are the amino acids proline and hydroxyproline, respectively. There are at least ten genetically distinct types of collagens (reviewed in ref. 4), but the mineralized matrix of bone contains only one of these, type I collagen, which is a heteropolymeric triple helical molecule composed of two α1(I) and one α2(I) chains. Type III and type V collagens have been purported to be present in trace amounts within bone; however, these collagen types are most likely blood vessel–associated.

As for all proteins, mRNA is transcribed from genes specific for collagen α chains in the nucleus of the cell (reviewed in ref. 5). The DNA encoding collagen α chains, like that of many other proteins, contains sequences that are not found in the final mRNA product that is translated. Collagen genes contain a large number of these intervening DNA sequences (50 in the case of the α1(I) chain of type I collagen). These intervening sequences are excised from the initial mRNA transcript (Hn mRNA) before or during transport of mRNA from the nucleus into the cytoplasm.

Collagen α chains are translated in a precursor form (prepro α) (reviewed in ref. 6). The initial sequence is the so-called signal peptide (pre) that allows the ribosome-mRNA complex to attach to the cytoplasmic side of the endoplasmic reticulum.[7] This portion is rapidly removed as translation continues and pro α chains are extruded into the lumen of the endoplasmic reticulum where specific enzymes hydroxylate certain of the prolyl and lysyl residues. The resultant amino acids, hydroxyproline and hydroxylysine, are for the most part unique to collagen, and are only rarely found in proteins that do not contain collagenous (Gly-X-Y) sequences. Pro α chains contain noncollagenous sequences at both the amino (termed pN) and carboxyl (termed pC) termini. After translation is completed, three pro α chains [two pro α1(I) and one pro α2(I) in the case of type I collagen] associate via their carboxyl propeptides, where inter- and intra-chain disulfide bonds are formed, and triple helix formation begins. Prolyl and lysyl hydroxlyation stops as triple helix formation proceeds, presumably owing to steric effects, that is, inaccessibility of the enzymes to the amino acid residues. During transport through the Golgi apparatus and to the cell surface, specific sugar transferase enzymes add galactose to certain collagen hydroxylysine residues, and in some cases glucose is added, resulting in the formation of either galactosyl-hydroxylysyl or glucosyl-galactosyl-hydroxylysyl residues on the collagen chain. Compared with the type I collagens found in nonmineralized tissues, the type I collagen of bone contains higher levels of hydroxylysyl residues, which usually are in the galactosylated form, whereas in skin there is more glucosyl-galactosyl-hydroxylysine.[8,9] In addition, N-linked oligosaccharides are often added to the propeptide extension of many collagen types. The completed procollagen molecule is then secreted from the cell.

The steps involved in the orderly deposition of collagen molecules to form collagen fibrils have not yet been definitively described. Several studies seem to indicate that collagen fibril formation can be initiated intracellularly.[10] In any event, the noncollagenous extension peptides (pN and pC) are removed by specific peptidases, which leave only small noncollagenous extensions at both the amino and carboxyl termini (telopeptides). However, it appears that at least one of these fragments, pN α1(I) (previously identified as a 24,000 M_r phosphoprotein[2]), persists in the extracellular matrix of bone.[11] This situation is similar to that found recently for the pC α1(II) fragment of type II collagen (chondrocalcin) in cartilage.[12] After removal of the propeptide extensions, collagen molecules associate both longitudinally (head to tail) and laterally in a one quarter–staggered fashion resulting in a periodicity of 640 Å noted at the electron microscopic level.[13] The factors that regulate fiber diameter are not well defined, but differences in the level of glycosylation of hydroxylysine residues[14] and proteins that bind to collagen, such as proteoglycans,[15,16] have been shown to influence fiber formation *in vitro*. In addition, some studies indicate that the persistence of amino-terminal extensions and incorporation of pN collagen molecules into a collagen fibril retards further growth in fiber diameter.[17] Consequently the types of posttranslational modifications particular to bone type I collagen and noncollagenous bone matrix proteins may dictate the ultimate molecular organization of the collagen scaffold upon which mineralization occurs.

Stabilization of the collagen scaffold is accomplished by the formation of covalent cross-links between α chains within the same triple helical molecule, and between chains of neighboring molecules (reviewed in ref. 18). Lysyl oxidase forms aldehydes from certain lysine and hydroxylysine residues (allysine and hydroxyallysine, respectively), particularly in telopeptide regions, which then condense either with each other, forming *intra*molecular crosslinks, or with other lysyl or hydroxylysyl residues (including the glycosylated forms), generally forming *inter*molecular crosslinks. As crosslinking continues, histidine or its aldehydic derivative may also become involved in complex organic structures in which as many as four α chains can be covalently crosslinked to each other. The types of crosslinks that are formed in bone are somewhat different from those in the soft tissues. Crosslinks in bone originate from hydroxyallysine and hydroxylysine (and glycosylated hydroxylysine), whereas in skin, the major crosslinks result from allysine and aldohistidine. Bone contains a higher level of borohydride-reducible crosslinks (an operational measurement) than does soft tissue. The reason behind this divergence in crosslink formation between bone and soft tissue is not yet understood, but may be a consequence of, or related to, the deposition of hydroxyapatite. One explanation is that mineral replaces the water surrounding collagen and immobilizes the molecule, which may prevent additional crosslink sites from chemically interacting.

B. Noncollagenous Bone Matrix Components

The noncollagenous portion of the bone matrix is composed of proteins synethesized by osteoblasts as well as those adsorbed from serum. Two-dimensional polypeptide maps of bone matrix extracts identified 40 major protein groups, with many more minor constituents; 14 of these were not present in maps of serum.[19] Based on these chemical data, and on biosynthetic experiments using osteoblasts *in vitro*, the number of major bone-specific gene products appears to be quite small. The content of noncollagenous proteins (ncp) in bone is dependent on the developmental stage and the age of the individual. In general, following puberty, the levels of noncollagenous proteins that remain intact decrease with increasing age.[20-23] The physiologic functions of either the endogenous or exogenous bone proteins remain largely undefined.

1. *Serum-Derived Bone Matrix Proteins*

On the average, approximately one third of the total noncollagenous bone matrix proteins are adsorbed from the circulatory system.[20,24] Since bone is a highly vascularized tissue, it is not surprising that serum proteins such as albumin, α_2-HS glycoprotein, immunoglobulins, transferrin, and apoA-I lipoprotein, for example, have been identified in the tissue, primarily in denaturing extracts.[19] However, in some cases, the amount of serum protein in demineralizing extracts of bone matrix may far exceed the level in circulation, presumably owing to their affinity for bone mineral. Serum albumin (M_r = 67,000) composes up to 3% of the total noncollagenous protein.[25] Another protein, α_2-HS glycoprotein, which in humans has a molecular weight of 50,000,[25] is synthesized by the liver and composes some 20% of the total bone noncollagenous protein.[26] However, this protein is found in the bone matrix at 50 to 100 times the concentration found in the circulation.[24,27] The reasons behind this enrichment of serum proteins in bone matrix are not yet known. In addition, exogenous growth factors (see later) also are entrapped in bone and retain their bioactivity. Thus, exogenous noncollagenous proteins can have at least potentially important roles in bone metabolism.

2. *Osteoblast-Derived Bone Matrix Proteins*

Osteocalcin. Of the noncollagenous osteoblast products, osteocalcin (also referred to as bone Gla protein, or BGP)[28,29] is the best characterized. The gene encoding osteocalcin has been cloned from both human[30] and rat[31] sources and contains three intervening sequences. The synthesis of osteocalcin has been shown to be stimulated by 1,25-dihydroxyvitamin D_3 *in vitro* in rat osteosarcoma cells,[32] in nontransformed human bone cells,[33] and *in vivo* in rats.[34] Osteocalcin mRNA codes for a 99–amino acid prepropeptide.[35] The first 23 amino acids are the hydrophobic signal peptide (pre), followed by a basically charged stretch of 26 amino acid residues (pro), and finally the 49–amino acid sequence of the mature molecule. Co-translationally, three specific glutamyl residues are modified by vitamin K–dependent enzymes to form γ-carboxyglutamyl (Gla) residues. Interestingly, osteocalcin shares a sequence homology in its propeptide region with other γ-carboxyglutamic acid–containing proteins (blood coagulation factors).[35] After γ-carboxylation, the propeptide is processed to the secreted form (49 amino acid residues). Osteocalcin, due to its Gla residues, binds both to ionic calcium (K_d ~10^{-3} M)[36] and to hydroxyapatite (K_d ~10^{-7} M).[37] If γ-carboxylation is blocked by inhibiting the vitamin K–dependent enzymes with warfarin, the rate of synthesis of osteocalcin does not appear to be affected; however, less than 2% of normal levels are retained in the bone matrix.[38] It should be noted here that in light of these experiments, the function of osteocalcin in bone remains nebulous, since no skeletal or mineral abnormalities were found in rats after 8 months of warfarin treatment. The sole change noted in these animals was a closing and mineralization of epiphyseal growth plates.[39] The amount of osteocalcin found in bone depends on the species[40] and differs during growth and development,[20,41-43] ranging from less than 1% to approximately 15% of the total noncollagenous protein, with human bone containing somewhat less than 1%.[24] In most species, embryonic and neonatal bone contains approximately 5% of the osteocalcin levels found in adult bone.[43]

Matrix Gla Protein. Bone matrix also contains another Gla-containing protein, which was identified in preparations of bone morphogenetic protein, to which it is tightly bound.[44] Matrix Gla protein (MGP), with a molecular weight of 10,000, contains five residues of Gla, although this posttranslational modification does not appear necessary for its accumulation in the extracellular matrix (unlike osteocalcin). Amino acid sequence analysis indicates that it shares a great deal of homology with osteocalcin, perhaps suggesting a common, precursor gene.[45] However, MGP appears to be present at an earlier stage of development than does osteocalcin, and the amount of MGP in rat bone remains relatively constant (approximately 2% of the noncollagenous proteins) during development and growth.[24,43]

Osteonectin. Phosphoproteins and glycoproteins are also major components of the extracellular matrix of bone. Of these, osteonectin is the most abundant.[11] Analysis of the bovine gene for osteonectin indicates that it contains at least eight intervening sequences (Findlay, unpublished results). Cell-free translation of osteonectin mRNA yields a preosteonectin molecule with a molecular weight of 47,000 by SDS gels. In cells, this signal peptide is co-translationally cleaved to yield the mature, secreted molecule with an apparent molecular weight of 38,000 on SDS gels.[46,47] Although this suggests the presence of an extremely long signal peptide, sequence analysis of the cDNA indicates that the signal peptide is only 30 amino acids in length, and thus, the large difference in molecular weight seen on SDS gels is due most likely to changes in protein conformation (Young, Bolander, Findlay, unpublished data). Osteonectin does not appear to have a pro form, since the size after removal of the signal peptide is not appreciably different from that of the protein extracted from the bone matrix.[48-50] Osteonectin contains phosphoserine, both N- and O-linked oligosaccharides,[11] and as many as seven disulfide bonds.[51] The amount of osteonectin found in bone is dependent on the species and developmental stage.[20,24] Rat bone contains relatively low levels,[52] whereas in human and bovine fetal and neonatal bone, osteonectin composes approximately 15% of the total noncollagenous protein.[11] With advancing age, the level of intact osteonectin in bone drops to low levels, as do all of the noncollagenous bone proteins, primarily due to proteolytic degradation.[21,22] Osteonectin binds to collagen, calcium, and hydroxyapatite *in vitro*[53,54] and may control mineralization *in vivo*. Although osteonectin has been shown to be synthesized by a wide variety of cell types *in vitro*[47,55-57] (Beresford and Gehron Robey, unpublished data), radioimmune assays[57] and immunocytochemistry[3,58] indicate that nonmineralized connective tissues generally contain less than 1% of the levels found in bone. Interestingly, platelets[59] and certain basement membranes that undergo frequent turnover[60,61] have recently been found to contain osteonectin; however, the function of the protein in these two sources is not yet known. The level of osteonectin found in serum is approximately 2 ng/ml and appears relatively constant with age in adults (Fisher, unpublished results).

Sialoproteins. Bone contains two sialoproteins, bone sialoprotein-I (which has recently been named osteopontin)[51,62-65] and bone sialoprotein-II,[51,62,63,66] both of which are phosphorylated. These proteins account for 5% to 10% of the noncollagenous proteins in developing bone.[20,24] To date, only sialoprotein-II has been identified in nonmineralized tissues. Bone sialoprotein-I (BSP-I) mRNA has been cloned and sequenced from a rat osteosarcoma cell line, and codes for a 20–amino acid signal peptide followed by a sequence encoding a protein with a molecular mass of approximately 33,000.[64] The fully processed (glycosylated and phosphorylated) protein that is extracted from bone matrix has an apparent molecular weight of 80,000 by SDS gels.[51,65] BSP-I also exhibits cell attachment activity for a variety of cell types *in vitro*.[64] Interestingly, the predicted amino acid sequence contains Arg-Gly-Asp, a cell-binding protein sequence identified in well-known cell attachment proteins such as fibronectin and vitronectin.[64]

BSP-II, a fragment of which was first described by Herring and coworkers,[67] has not yet been cloned at the molecular level, although the amino-terminal sequence of the matrix molecule has been determined.[51] The protein extracted from bone has an apparent molecular weight of 80,000 by SDS gels, contains 50% carbohydrate (both N- and O-linked oligosaccharides), and is more heavily sialylated (12% to 15% sialic acid)[66] than BSP-I (3% sialic acid).[51] Upon treatment of the intact protein with trypsin, a small fragment containing most of the carbohydrate is produced, similar to that which was first isolated by Herring. Thus, it is possible that some of this smaller fragment is produced by naturally occurring proteolysis *in vivo* and remains in adult bone matrix. mRNA for this protein has not yet been identified, but preliminary experiments utilizing bone cell cultures indicate that this protein may undergo several processing steps before the molecule is secreted into the medium.[68] To date, the function of this protein has not been determined.

Proteoglycans. Another class of extracellular matrix proteins, proteoglycans, constitute approximately 5% of the noncollagenous matrix of bone.[20] Proteoglycans are composed of a central protein core to which are attached glycosaminoglycans (chondroitin, dermatan, keratan, or heparan sulfate) and N- and/or O-linked oligosaccharides (reviewed in ref. 69). In bone, the two most abundant proteoglycans (PG-I and PG-II in the nomenclature of Rosenberg[70]) are relatively small, with apparent molecular weights between 100,000 and 200,000 by molecular sieve chromatography, and contain one or two attached chondroitin sulfate chains.[51,62,71-74] The concentrations of PG-I and PG-II are roughly equivalent in developing and neonatal human and bovine bone.[51,71] Although the protein cores (apparent molecular weight of approximately 46,000 or SDS gels) and the attached chondroitin sulfate (molecular weight of approximately 40,000) of PG-I and PG-II are similar, recent amino-terminal protein sequence data indicate that they are the product of different genes.[51] A large (M_r = 1,000,000) chondroitin sulfate proteoglycan composed of a 400,000 molecular weight core protein with chondroitin sulfate chains of 40,000 is also present at low levels in fetal bone matrix.[51] The functions of these proteoglycans during the initiation and continuation of mineralization events is not clear. However, the large chondroitin sulfate proteoglycan has been immunolocalized to the interstitial mesenchyme of developing subperiosteal bone and disappears as the mesenchyme is replaced by osteoid.[51,75] In development, the purpose of this loose interstitial mesenchyme may be to "capture" space destined to become bone. In bone remodeling, however, this mesenchyme is not needed, and consequently the large chondroitin sulfate proteoglycan is not synthesized.[75] The fate of PG-I and PG-II is less clear based on histochemical and biochemical data (reviewed in ref. 22). It has been suggested at least part of the newly synthesized proteoglycans (most likely PG-I) rapidly diffuses to the mineralization front,[75,76] whereas the remainder (PG-II) remains associated with the newly synthesized osteoid, directly adjacent to the osteoblasts. With time, PG-I appears to become relatively more degraded than PG-II, which may be maintained within a more protected mineralized bone compartment.[21,22,75]

Comparative studies of PG-I and PG-II isolated from different connective tissues indicate that they are immunologically and chemically similar in both mineralized and nonmineralized tissue (reviewed in ref. 77). However, in bone, PG-I and PG-II contain chondroitin sulfate, whereas in soft tissues they contain dermatan sulfate. In addition, bovine bone PG-II exhibits different sensitivities to enzymatic digestion than does PG-II from tendon.[78] These data suggest that the bone forms of these proteoglycans may be slightly different from those in soft tissues. PG-II mRNA has recently been cloned and sequenced from human placenta[79] and cloned from bovine bone-forming cells.[80] However, not enough information is currently available to determine if the chemical differences between bone and soft tissue PG-II are the result of slightly different backbone protein sequences, or from differing posttranslational modifications. Proteoglycans have been postulated to be regulators of collagen fibril formation,[15,16] and slight differences in proteoglycans from one tissue to another may reflect variable control by different cell types in the production and deposition of an extracellular matrix appropriate for the tissue in question.

Alkaline Phosphatase. Although not identified as a matrix protein, alkaline phosphatase is an important synthetic product of osteoblasts and has long been thought to be implicated in skeletal mineralization. The alkaline phosphatase of bone is similar to the liver and kidney isoenzymes, and distinct from the placental and intestinal forms, all of which have a molecular weight ranging from 100,000 to 200,000 (depending on the method of analysis), consisting of two identical disulfide-linked dimers.[81,82] The bone form of alkaline phosphatase may have slightly different internal sequences or posttranslational modifications from the liver and kidney forms as indicated by observed differences in thermal stability.[83] This difference provides yet another potential marker of bone metabolism. A cDNA clone coding for alkaline phosphatase has been isolated from a human osteosarcoma cell line, and the predicted sequence indicates that the unmodified protein has a molecular weight of 58,000.[84] Biosynthetic experiments using cells in culture show that (1) after glycosylation and reduction of disulfide bonds, alkaline phosphatase has a molecular weight of 76,000, and (2) it is not secreted by cells into the medium fraction, but is maintained within the cell layer, most probably associated with the plasma membrane.[85]

Several pieces of evidence suggest that alkaline phosphatase may be implicated in biomineralization. These are its presence in matrix vesicles in calcifying cartilage, its ability to hydrolyze pyrophosphate (a known inhibitor of hydroxyapatite deposition), and the increase in pyrophosphate found in the blood and urine of patients deficient in alkaline phosphatase (hypophosphatasia.)[86]

Low Abundance Matrix Proteins. Bone matrix also contains several less abundant proteins[19] and growth factors[87] that may or may not be unique to the tissue. Transforming growth factor-β has recently been identified in the bone matrix[88] and shown to be an osteoblastic cell product.[89,90] Other growth factors such as platelet-derived growth factor (PDGF),[87] skeletal[91] or bone-derived growth factor,[92] the different forms of fibroblast growth factor,[87] and others have been identified from denaturing and demineralizing extracts of bone, or from conditioned medium of bone organ and cell cultures. Most of these appear to originate from exogenous sources.

Lipids. Since hydroxyapatite deposition appears to be mediated, at least in part, by matrix vesicles in calcifying cartilage and woven bone, attention has been drawn to other membrane components that may be involved in biomineralization.[93,94] Proteolipids and Ca^{2+}-phospholipid-phosphate complexes have been isolated from the residual organic matrix of a variety of mineralized tissues and appear to be enriched in tissues undergoing mineralization. Both of these moieties appear to be capable of inducing hydroxyapatite precipitation *in vitro*. However, it is not yet clear whether these components are unique to calcifying tissue, or what role they play *in vivo*.

C. The Mineral Phase of Bone

The inorganic phase in bone is composed primarily of small crystals of a basic calcium phosphate mineral called hydroxyapatite. During mineralization (reviewed in ref. 95), the extracellular fluid surrounding the osteoblasts is supersaturated in calcium and phosphate. By processes that are not yet well defined, the initial mineral phases, transient precursors, such as amorphous calcium phosphate and/or octacalcium phosphate, are rapidly converted into hydroxyapatite. Moreover, the hydroxyapatite crystals in bone are not "pure" in the sense that they also contain carbonate and trace amounts of other elements. The bone mineral crystals are relatively small in size compared with the hydroxyapatite crystals formed in dental enamel. Proteins present in the surrounding environment most likely have a profound effect on the growth and replication of hydroxyapatite crystals.[96] Hydroxyapatite precipitation appears to occur via matrix vesicles in woven bone and by collagen fibril-mediated mineral nucleation in lamellar and osteonal bone (reviewed in ref. 93). The dissolution of bone hydroxyapatite crystals by osteoclasts is a significant source of inorganic ions during mineral homeostasis.

II. METHODS OF BIOCHEMICAL MEASUREMENT

The significance of noninvasive clinical analysis in determining the disease status of a patient is particularly dependent on the selection of appropriate biochemical parameters and the proper collection and storage of specimens. Three types of samples are available from patients: (1) blood-derived, (2) urine-derived, or (3) tissue biopsy. Although each type of sample can be used for a variety of assays to provide useful information, there are specific biochemical problems associated with each type of sample. As reviewed elsewhere, sequential tissue biopsies perhaps yield the most direct information. However, obtaining the biopsy is an invasive procedure and does not lend itself to frequent monitoring. In addition, the focal nature of bone turnover in normal tissue and in many metabolic bone diseases can make bone biopsy an inaccurate measure. The assay of body fluids, although noninvasive, is not without problems. Several variables have been identified that directly influence observed values for markers of bone metabolism, a few of which will be mentioned here. The overall nutritional and metabolic status of the patient at the time of sample collection is critically important. In many assays, it appears that a fasting or an altered diet is needed for accurate measurements. Circadian rhythms also affect circulating levels of certain bone markers. The renal clearance capacity of the patient greatly influences values for certain markers in both blood-derived and urine samples. Blood collection, appropriate separation of cellular from noncellular components, and proper storage are procedures that must be standardized and taken into account for each parameter to be assayed. A large amount of interpatient variability that has been noted in the literature for many bone markers may arise, at least in part, from differences in specimen procurement and handling.

A variety of biochemical assays are applicable to the measurement of a given parameter in plasma, serum, or urine samples. These assays involve (1) direct quantitation of a chemical substance such as measurement of calcium by atomic absorption spectrometry, or determinations of amino acid composition either before or after chemical separation methods; (2) measurement of enzymatic activity using color-generating substrates for the enzyme of interest; and (3) identification of molecules by immunologic assays such as RIA (radioimmune assay) or ELISA (enzyme-linked immunosorbent assay). Immunologic assays are perhaps the most sensitive and are quite useful in determining the levels of markers found in small amounts in the assay fluid (reviewed in ref. 97). The basic requirements for establishing a radioimmune assay are the availability of sufficient quantities of highly purified antigen and an antibody with a fairly high titer against that antigen. The specificity of the assay is highly dependent on the purity of the antigen, which is used both in "tagged" (most commonly with ^{125}I-iodine, although other markers can be used) and in the unmodified form as the specific competitor in the assay. Characterization of the antibody is also extremely important. In some cases, different animals injected with the same immunogen generate polyclonal antisera that recognize different sets of epitopes. Antisera may recognize epitopes from different regions of the molecule, called conformational-sensitive or sequence-discontinuous epitopes, found only in the native and not in a degraded molecule (or vice versa). Consequently, chemical characterization of the precise epitope(s) that each antisera actually measures is often useful in the interpretation of results. With the advent of automated peptide chemistry (both sequence analysis and synthesis of peptides with a known amino acid sequence), antibodies can be generated against specific sequence regions of a molecule and may be quite useful in establishing assays that measure specific domains of molecules that have specific chemical or biological functions.

The original method of RIA utilized soluble antigen and antibody, the complex of which was precipitated by the addition of a second antibody with resultant quantitation of the tracer in the precipitate. Now, solid phase assays are more commonly used, in which either the antigen or the antibody is immobilized onto a solid support, thereby allowing a more rapid and efficient separation of labeled from unlabeled antigen. Implicit in all RIA methods is the requirement that assay conditions be identical in all aspects for standards (controls) and unknown samples. For example, in comparing dilution curves generated by an unknown sample, it is important to note whether the slope is parallel to that of the standard curve. In a clinical setting, each sample may not always be assayed at multiple dilutions. When the standard or control curve is generated under one set of conditions, and the samples to be assayed differ significantly from these in some fashion, curves with different slopes are often obtained. Therefore, quantitation can be very tenuous. A variety of factors can lead to the generation of curves with different slopes, such as: total protein concentration; the presence of molecules in the unknown samples that share epitopes with the antigen; proteins in the unknown samples that interfere with the binding of the antigen to the antibody; and use of antibodies that recognize native forms, degraded forms, or both. Consequently, the chemical characterization of the immunoreactive substances with respect to their relationship to the original immunogen is often imperative to the proper interpretation of the results.

In some cases (frequently with connective tissue proteins), the development of an RIA is extremely difficult owing to poor solubility of the antigen in the buffers used for this assay. Maintaining solubility until the final precipitation step is critical for accurate determinations. Although generally not as sensitive as RIAs, ELISA assays are useful in quantitating certain proteins, such as proteoglycans, by either direct or indirect (competition) methods.[98] These ELISA assays are generally easy to conduct and have high reproducibility, particularly when sufficient serum levels warrant their use.

In spite of the difficulties noted, biochemical parameters have been and will continue to prove promising as useful measures of bone metabolism. Based on current progress in bone biology and biochemistry research, this area of clinical practice will continue to expand and improve in value. The reliability of such measurements will always be subject, however, to the caveats outlined previously. As long as these are taken properly into account, clinical applications of basic bone research findings should prove fruitful.

III. BIOCHEMICAL MARKERS OF BONE FORMATION

The noninvasive determination of bone formation by biochemical means is based on the assay and quantitation of biosynthetic products and by-products of osteoblasts. As mentioned previously, many of the extracellular matrix proteins of bone are synthesized in precursor forms and subsequently processed yielding free precursor fragment(s) that may, in turn, provide possible new parameters by which the biosynthesis of a particular protein can be measured. In addition, some proteins synthesized by osteoblasts and deposited in the extracellular matrix also escape into the circulation. It is generally desirable that the validity of any marker be established by comparison to histomorphometric analysis. However, histomorphometry also suffers its own inadequacies, since measurements are usually made in trabecular or endosteal samples and not in compact or cortical bone, and therefore may not be reflective of the entire skeleton.

A. Collagen

Because type I collagen is the predominant secretory product of osteoblasts, its precursor extension peptides (pN and pC), which are removed as fibers form the matrix and subsequently released into the circulation,[99,100] would appear to be good markers of bone formation. However, type I collagen is also the major matrix protein of several tissues, and consequently the assay of these peptides from serum would measure the rate of synthesis of type I collagen in all connective tissues. This, then, presents a "background" that must be taken into consideration in ascertaining specific changes contributed by bone. Currently, RIAs are available for measuring pN and pC peptide of type I collagen.[99,100] Very little information is available on serum pC levels at different stages of development and growth, but levels of approximately 100 ng/ml have been reported for normal adult human serum.[100,101] In one study, the level of pC was found to be elevated in Paget's disease, and those levels fell after treatment with calcitonin and dichloromethylene diphosphonate. The pC levels approached pretreatment values 7 hours following injection with calcitonin, but remained normal for several months after discontinuation of DCDP therapy.[101] Interestingly, levels of the pN peptide of another collagen type, type III, were also elevated in Paget's disease, and remained elevated after therapy. This is thought to reflect formation of fibrous lesions that contain type III collagen.[101] (See Chapter 15.)

Although not traditionally considered to be a parameter of bone formation, measurement of urinary hydroxyproline (uHYP), at least in part, may be reflective of new collagen synthesis.[102] Hydroxyproline is an amino acid that is fairly specific for collagen, and following collagen degradation, hydroxyproline is excreted (discussed later in more detail). Further analysis of total uHYP indicates that it is composed of 90% dialyzable HYP (D uHYP) and 10% nondialyzable HYP (ND uHYP).[103] It appears that D uHYP (fragments with molecular weights less than 4000) reflects the degradation of "old" collagen, collagen that had been incorporated into the matrix,[104] whereas ND uHYP (fragments between 5000 and 10,000 molecular weight) reflects the degradation of newly synthesized collagen that has not been incorporated into the matrix.[102,105,106] In several studies in which the amount of D versus ND uHYP were quantitated separately, increases in ND relative to D (reflecting new collagen synthesis) were found in Paget's disease,[105] various forms of rickets,[107] and Hodgkin's disease and prostate cancer with bone metastasis.[103] In addition, increases were found following treatment of postmenopausal osteoporosis with fluoride, and these increases were positively correlated with bone density and serum alkaline phosphatase.[108] Interestingly, the opposite effect (decreased ND uHYP) was noted in patients with skeletal fluorosis.[109]

The utility of estimating bone (collagen) formation by quantitating the amount of ND uHYP has not been verified by histomorphometric analysis. Further development of this assay may indicate that it is useful in assessment of collagen synthesis; however, as will be discussed later, it suffers from a lack of bone specificity, since it is a measurement of total collagen. In addition, there is considerable metabolism (reutilization of hydroxyproline), which may be variable in various disease states.[110]

B. Osteocalcin

Development of radioimmune assays specific for osteocalcin has led to the discovery that osteocalcin is present in serum[111] and that from 10% to 25% of total osteocalcin synthesized by bone cells escapes into the circulation and is not deposited in the bone matrix.[24] In one assay, it appears that circulating osteocalcin is a result of synthesis and not degradation, since this particular antiserum did not recognize at least the major forms of degraded osteocalcin.[112] A variety of RIAs have been developed using different antisera that crossreact with human osteocalcin,[113-128] including one using an antiserum raised against a synthetic peptide specific for the carboxyl-terminal region of the molecule.[129] In studies in which the serum levels were compared with histomorphometric analysis, there is general agreement that circulating osteocalcin is positively correlated with parameters of bone turnover, more specifically bone formation.[114,125,130,131] However, the correlation of circulating osteocalcin with more specific parameters of bone formation is somewhat controversial, with some studies indicating that it correlates with the rate of bone mineralization,[114] whereas others do not confirm these results.[120] In other studies, circulating levels were thought to reflect static parameters of bone formation,[130] whereas others found more positive correlations with dynamic parameters.[125] The biochemical basis for these discrepancies is not yet known, but may reflect differences in antisera used to measure circulating osteocalcin, different patient populations, and the focal nature of bone turnover.

Removal and degradation of circulating osteocalcin appears to be mediated primarily by the kidney.[132] After degradation, by a pathway that has yet to be elucidated, free Gla residues appear in the urine. The pattern of urinary Gla secretion, in general, is similar to the pattern of circulating osteocalcin levels in normal situations.[133] However, since other proteins (such as blood coagulation factors) contain Gla, the excretion of total Gla does not discriminate between bone and other sources.

The amount of osteocalcin in serum and plasma (values appear to be equivalent for both[24]) is age- and sex-dependent, and also exhibits a circadian rhythm, with low levels in the morning and nocturnal peak levels.[134] From the age of 1 year to puberty, the amount is found to be approximately 18 ng/ml, with a slight increase at puberty (more marked in males than in females) to approximately 25 to 39 ng/ml.[115,135] The levels then decline, although the exact amount is controversial, with several reports indicating levels between 5 and 7 ng/ml,[113,115,117,118,136] whereas others find between 12 and 16 ng/ml.[121,122,129] Correlation of circulating osteocalcin with advanced age has been controversial, with reports indicating that circulating osteocalcin decreases,[111] increases,[117,118] or remains unchanged.[129] It has been suggested that these differences are due to inadequate assessment of glomerular filtration rate (as measured by creatinine clearance).[137] Creatinine clearance declines with age, and changes in circulating osteocalcin could be affected by this decline in renal clearance. Again, the effect of renal status on osteocalcin levels is also contradictory, since in one study, mild renal impairment resulted in increases in circulating osteocalcin,[129] whereas in another study no change was noted except in chronic renal failure.[138] The variations noted with respect to age and renal status may also result from differences in the antibodies used in the radioimmune assay. Chemical characterization of all the immunoreactive substances present in serum and urine may well be critical for proper correlation of this parameter to the metabolic status of bone. For example, a recent study[130] indicated that several immunoreactive forms of osteocalcin that are lower in molecular weight than osteocalcin may exist in the serum of uremic patients. This suggests that circulating osteocalcin may be in both an intact and a degraded form in some situations, and in most cases, antibodies used for RIAs have not been characterized for their ability to bind to osteocalcin fragments.

Several histomorphometric studies have indicated that there is also a slight positive correlation between circulating osteocalcin and parameters of bone resorption,[120,125,130] and this correlation may arise from the measurement of degraded osteocalcin in the serum. In fact, several studies have indicated that osteocalcin, in either native or degraded form, is chemotactic for monocytes[139,140] and may induce differentiation of osteoclasts.[141] These findings raise the possibility, at least, of using assays specific for degraded osteocalcin that may reflect bone resorption.

Elevated levels of circulating osteocalcin have been reported in metabolic bone diseases that are characterized by an increase in bone turnover, such as in primary[126,142-144] and secondary[142] hyperparathyroidism, primary hyperthyroidism,[127,128,130] metastatic bone cancer,[142,143] and chronic renal failure.[138,143] Interestingly, in Paget's disease there is a marked increase in circulating osteocalcin,[113,133,142,143] whereas urinary Gla is not increased;[133] however, owing to the focal nature of Paget's disease, circulating osteocalcin that arises from the entire skeleton may not be a sensitive marker in this disease.[145] Less substantial or variable increases have been found in various forms of rickets[135,136,146] and X-linked hypophosphatasia. In postmenopausal osteoporotic women, the amount of circulating osteocalcin appears to vary from normal to elevated levels[113,116,133] and, interestingly, the urinary Gla is elevated.[133] By histomorphometry, at least three groups of osteoporotics can be identified with high, normal, and low rates of bone turnover.[119] It appears that in osteoporotics with increased rates of bone turnover, the levels of circulating osteocalcin are also increased.[119] (See Chapter 12.)

Decreases in circulating osteocalcin are generally found in situations of low bone turnover, such as in patients treated for long periods of time with corticosteroids,[128,131] and in situations of growth arrest, such as in growth hormone–deficient children.[147] Normal[123] to slightly depressed levels have been reported in hypothyroidism.[138]

Levels of circulating osteocalcin have also been used to evaluate the effect of various treatments of metabolic bone disease. Administration of 1,25-dihydroxyvitamin D_3 to patients with X-linked hypophosphatasia and autosomal recessive vitamin D–dependent rickets appears to increase levels of circulating osteocalcin.[146] In postmenopausal osteoporosis, circulating osteocalcin increased slightly with treatment with 1,25-dihydroxyvitamin D_3 and calcium supplementation, and with estrogen treatment.[148,149] In the treatment of Paget's disease and certain forms of metastatic bone cancer with salmon calcitonin, circulating osteocalcin levels were found to decrease.[143] Administration of parathyroid hormone to patients with X-linked hypophosphatasia caused only a transient drop in circulating osteocalcin (within 15 minutes), with a return to pretreatment levels by 75 minutes.[136] Parathyroidectomy in primary hyperparathyroidism was found to decrease osteocalcin in both males and females,[144] although in another study this decrease was found in women only.[143]

C. Serum Alkaline Phosphatase

The assay of serum alkaline phosphatase provides a useful marker for measurement of bone formation, although several factors qualify its significance in the absence of correlation to other parameters. Total serum alkaline phosphatase (TAP) is reflective of the enzyme activity contributed by liver, gastrointestinal tract, lung, and other sources as well as bone.[150] Consequently, metabolic disorders affecting these nonosseous tissues may have a profound effect on TAP. This is reflected in the less tight positive correlation of serum alkaline phosphatase levels with parameters of bone formation noted in many histomorphometric studies.[114,116,120,125,130] An inactivation-inhibition method is available for the determination of serum alkaline phosphatase arising from bone (BAP).[151] However, this assay is not used routinely in clinical situations. BAP levels were found to be higher in children than in adults, with a maximum level at puberty followed by a sharp decline to adult levels by the second decade.[152] BAP was positively correlated with plasma tartrate-resistant acid phosphatase and urinary hydroxyproline, two markers of bone resorption, although urinary hydroxyproline was proportionally higher before puberty. With advancing age, there is a gradual increase in TAP,[117,118] even when glomerular filtration rate is taken into account.[129]

In most cases, TAP is elevated in many of the same disorders that exhibit increases in circulating osteocalcin, that is, diseases with increased bone turnover, such as in Paget's disease,[142,143] primary and secondary hyperparathyroidism,[142] hyperthyroidism,[128] osteomalacia,[153] metastatic bone disease,[142] and renal osteodystrophy.[120,143,154] Patients with postmenopausal osteoporosis (PMO) have been reported to have increased TAP.[116] However, TAP did not distinguish between the three types of PMO (high, normal, and low turnover).[119] However, in certain cases, TAP does not correlate with circulating osteocalcin, such as in primary hyperparathyroidism.[113]

In monitoring the effect of treatment of metabolic bone disease, several dichotomies between circulating osteocalcin and TAP are noted. In metastatic bone cancer in remission following chemotherapy[142] and in post-dialysis renal osteodystrophy,[143] TAP remains elevated whereas osteocalcin is decreased. In primary hyperthyroidism treated by parathyroidectomy, TAP levels drop whereas osteocalcin levels remain elevated.[143] In PMO treated with 1,25-dihydroxyvitamin D_3, TAP does not change whereas osteocalcin increases.[124] In corticosteroid-induced bone degeneration, TAP levels are unchanged whereas osteocalcin is decreased. These dichotomies may be reflective of the inability to assay BAP rather than TAP in a clinical setting.

Serum Ca^{2+}. Since 99% of the total body calcium is in the skeleton, the skeleton plays a major role in the maintenance of plasma calcium homeostasis via bone turnover. Consequently, it would appear, in theory, that after injection of radioactive Ca^{2+}, measurement of radioactivity in plasma and urine or direct quantitation of total Ca^{2+} may be informative in metabolic bone disease.[155] Unfortunately, serum Ca^{2+} levels do not appear to correlate well with bone histomorphometric parameters. In addition, changes following administration of substances known to affect Ca^{2+} homeostasis are very small and difficult to measure with any statistical significance. However, because of the overall importance of maintaining calcium homeostasis in the treatment of metabolic bone disease, this parameter must necessarily be assessed, along with other biochemical markers.

IV. BIOCHEMICAL PARAMETERS OF BONE RESORPTION

Parameters that reflect bone resorption are the products generated by osteoclasts during the process of degradation of the mineralized extracellular matrix. These markers are either fragments of the molecular constituents of the matrix or products of the osteoclasts themselves. The processes by which proteins are removed from the matrix are not precisely known. As reviewed elsewhere, osteoclasts form in essence an extracellular lysosomal compartment with a lower pH than that in surrounding bone. This facilitates both hydroxyapatite dissolution or demineralization and the subsequent degradation of at least some of the matrix components. However, since osteoclasts do not always appear to degrade demineralized bone,[156] other cell types may participate in the removal of matrix.[156,157] In any event, the degraded components either are reutilized by the cell or are lost to the circulation and subsequently excreted.

A. Collagen Degradation Products

In soft tissues, a specific enzyme, mammalian collagenase, makes a single clip in collagen triple helical molecules at approximately three fourths of the distance from the amino terminus; after the initial cleavage, the remaining degradative pathway is not well defined, but it appears that certain cathepsins are involved in breaking down the collagen into smaller and smaller fragments (reviewed in ref. 158). Mammalian collagenase has not been detected in osteoclasts; however, osteoclasts appear to degrade collagen into approximately 10,000 M_r fragments via direct acid hydroxylysis.[159] Although collagenase has been isolated from bone, the cellular origin and its role in bone resorption are not well understood. In any event, collagen degradation results in the release of hydroxyproline and hydroxylysine, two amino acids that are somewhat unique to collagen, and measurement of collagen breakdown can be assessed by measuring the appearance of these two amino acids in urine specimens.[104,160,161] It must be remembered, however, that these two amino acids are present in all types of collagen (not just in type I collagen), and that the excretion of collagen degradation products is the total of both bone and soft tissue turnover.

1. *Urinary Hydroxyproline*

The measurement of urinary hydroxyproline (uHYP) is affected by dietary intake of gelatin and consequently requires a modified diet prior to sample collection.[102] The effect of this variable has been reduced by the development of a more sensitive assay that requires only an overnight fast and measurement of the uHYP with respect to creatinine levels.[162] Even with this improved assay, there are several drawbacks to its use. First of all, after collagen degradation, only 5% to 10% of the hydroxyproline is excreted; the remainder is metabolized and reutilized by the body.[110] In addition, there are two forms of hydroxyproline in the urine (as mentioned previously), dialyzable and nondialyzable.[110] The dialyzable fraction (D) of uHYP, which composes approximately 90% of the total uHYP,[103] appears to be reflective of degradation of "old" collagen, that is, collagen that was once incorporated in the extracellular matrix.[104] The nondialyzable (ND) uHYP (fragments between 5000 and 10,000), which composes the remainder, appears to reflect the degradation of newly synthesized collagen that was not incorporated into the extracellular matrix.[102,103,105,106] Consequently, the measurement of total uHYP without determination of D versus ND uHYP may not adequately reflect collagen metabolism. In addition, changes in renal function may greatly alter total uHYP and/or the ratio of ND versus D. In spite of all of these drawbacks, measurement of uHYP remains the single most used parameter for the measurement of bone resorption.

Total uHYP levels are higher in children than in adults and reach maximum levels at puberty followed by a sharp decline.[151,163] A direct relationship was found between total uHYP and height growth velocity.[163] In general, total uHYP appears to parallel BAP, indicating the coupling of bone formation and resorption, but before puberty, total uHYP is proportionally higher than BAP.[152] With advancing age, total uHYP increases slightly.[117]

Total uHYP is increased in a variety of bone disorders, such as Paget's disease,[105] hyperthyroidism,[123] and multiple myeloma with metastatic bone disease.[103,164] In studies in which the total uHYP was subfractionated (D versus ND), an increase in D uHYP (indicative of increased bone resorption) was found in multiple myeloma.[103,164] In postmenopausal osteoporosis, total uHYP levels have been reported to be normal[165] or increased.[116] In PMO treated with fluoride, total uHYP was unchanged, but there was an increase in ND HYP (concomitant with a decrease in D HYP), along with increases in TAP[108]; however, in individuals suffering from skeletal fluorosis, bone formation was found to be increased as measured by Ca^{2+} kinetics, but the levels of D uHYP were higher than normal.[109]

Since renal function has an effect on uHYP determinations, several studies have measured serum levels of HYP. Plasma contains free HYP, peptidyl HYP, and protein-bound HYP, all of which are elevated from normal levels in uremia[154] and renal osteodystrophy.[166] The protein-bound HYP is unaffected by dialysis and is probably indicative of proteins other than collagen, such as C1q. After kidney dialysis treatment, free and peptidyl HYP are decreased, but rise to predialysis levels after 24 hours. It should be noted, however, that the timing of this assay following dialysis is critical. Concurrent histomorphometric analysis indicates that free plus peptidyl HYP is positively correlated with the active resorption surface, indicating the utility of this parameter in measuring bone resorption in cases of renal failure.[154] If peptidyl HYP is the serum equivalent to ND uHYP, and free HYP the equivalent of D uHYP, it may be informative to correlate these two fractions to histomorphometric parameters of bone resorption and formation to determine their utility in assessing the synthesis and degradation of collagen.

2. *Urinary Glycosylated Hydroxylysine*

The advantage of measuring this modified amino acid in urine rises from the fact that glycosylated hydroxylysine generated by collagen breakdown is excreted.[160,161] Hydroxylysine residues are glycosylated during the processing of collagen α chains. The glycosylated forms produced are either glucosyl-galactosyl-hydroxylysine (GGHYL) or galactosyl-hydroxylysine (GHYL). The ratio of these two modified molecules (GGHYL/GHYL) is somewhat different depending on the tissue from which it is extracted. Bone has a ratio of 0.47 whereas skin is 2.06.[8,9] Consequently, measuring the ratio of these two modified amino acids in urine may be reflective of activity in one tissue as compared with another. In Paget's disease and hyperphosphatasia, an increase was found in the level of galactosyl-hydroxylysine compared with normal,[161] presumably due to increase in bone turnover, whereas burn patients were found to have increased levels of glycosyl-galactosyl-hydroxylysine, indicative of increased metabolism of the skin. After treatment of these two diseases with salmon calcitonin, the level of GHYL decreases to normal levels, that is, there is a decrease in bone collagen turnover.[161] However, this situation is complex, since the profile of GHYL and GGHYL excreted by normal patients treated with calcitonin is not reflective of skin or bone and must arise from other collagenous components such as C1q.[161] In addition, it has also been noted that in Paget's patients treated with calcitonin, there is also a decrease in GGHYL,[160] which suggests that some urinary GGHYL comes in part from the synthesis of bone-related collagen (perhaps type III collagen) that does not become incorporated into the extracellular matrix.

B. Tartrate-Resistant Acid Phosphatase

Although not used on a routine clinical basis, circulating tartrate-resistant acid phosphatase may be a direct method for the assay of osteoclast activity.[167] As reviewed elsewhere in this volume, there is a fair amount of controversy concerning the specificity of this marker for osteoclasts and their precursors; however, it remains one of the most used parameters for distinguishing osteoclasts from other cell types both histologically in tissue sections of bone and in cell cultures. Of the five acid phosphatases present in serum, only one is tartrate-resistant,[168] and in normal serum, the majority of the total circulating acid phosphatase is this particular acid phosphatase.[168,169] Recently, this marker was found to correlate positively with bone alkaline phosphatase and uHYP in primary hyperparathyroidism, again indicating the coupling between bone formation and resorption found in this disease.[170] Increased levels of this enzyme have been found in sera of patients with metastatic bone cancer.[171] Further evaluation of this parameter along with histomorphometric analysis is needed to ascertain the clinical value of this potentially specific osteoclastic marker.

V. OTHER BIOCHEMICAL MARKERS OF BONE TURNOVER

A number of assays have been developed to measure parameters that bear significance to certain specific processes in bone turnover, or to factors that are known to play a role in the causation of a certain disease. Although these assays are not commonly used, they may provide valuable information concerning the status of patients before and after therapy.

A. cAMP

The production of cAMP is mediated by the action of a variety of hormones on both osteoblasts and osteoclasts. Osteoblasts have been found to produce increased levels of cAMP in response to parathyroid hormone, prostaglandins, and factors that bind to beta-adrenergic receptors. On the other hand, calcitonin produces this increase in osteoclasts. After administration of calcitonin to normal individuals, a rapid increase was found in cAMP in serum and urine. Although cAMP could be produced by other tissues in response to calcitonin, studies indicate that it arises primarily from bone.[172,173] Calcitonin challenge of patients with Paget's disease and hyperparathyroidism produced a significantly higher response to calcitonin than in normal subjects, and interestingly, postmenopausal women were found to form higher levels than men.[174] It has been suggested that this parameter may be useful in determining the remodeling activity potential of a patient at risk for osteoporosis and to evaluate the effects of therapy.[174]

B. Alpha$_2$-HS Glycoprotein

Although α_2-HS glycoprotein is not a synthetic product of osteoblasts, the sequestering of this protein by bone may very well point to a role in bone metabolism. Different levels of α_2-HS are found during postnatal development, with children exhibiting higher levels than adults, and women exhibiting a more progressive decline than men. An increase in urinary α_2-HS was found with increasing age.[175] In spite of the fact that there are high levels of this protein in children, it appears that in Paget's disease, in which there is increased bone turnover, circulating levels are decreased,[25,177,178] and that it is negatively correlated with total serum alkaline phosphatase.[25] Following treatment of pagetic patients with calcitonin or diphosphonates, levels return to normal values.[176,177] Since production of this protein in the liver would presumably remain constant, reduction in circulating levels of α_2-HS may be reflective of the increased demand by newly formed bone matrix for this protein as a consequence of the mineralization process. However, it cannot be ruled out that α_2-HS may actually be required by osteoblasts during the turnover process and therefore may play a role in resorption rather than formation.[177] In fact, this protein displays chemotactic activity for monocytes.[139,140] Clearly, more study is needed to ascertain this intriguing protein's role in bone metabolism.

C. Urinary Glycosaminoglycan

Like virtually all of the bone matrix proteins described, proteoglycans are removed from the bone matrix during resorption, and degradation products are present in the urine, mainly as glycosaminoglycan chains attached to small remnants of the core proteins from which they arose. Little information is available concerning the contribution of bone-derived glycosaminoglycans to the total urinary pool. However, a recent study indicates that there is an increase in excreted chondroitin sulfate in patients suffering from spinal cord injury and mandatory immobilization. This increase in chondroitin sulfate excretion was found to be temporarily delayed from the increase in hydroxyprolinuria (which begins at 48 hours post injury) and calciuria (starting at 96 hours). However, the increases were sustained during the active phase of osteoporosis observed in these patients.[178] In view of the fact that there may be chemical differences in the immediate vicinity of the glycosaminoglycan attachment site on the core proteins of the small proteoglycan (PG-II) of bone and soft tissue (resulting from either amino acid sequence or posttranslational differences),[78] it may be possible to develop antibodies that recognize only the bone form of this molecule in urine.

VI. FUTURE DIRECTIONS

An honest evaluation of the present status of the value and/or potential of biochemical markers in monitoring metabolic bone disease is one of decidedly mixed accomplishments, but still of clear optimism. The addition of new bone markers (e.g., osteocalcin RIAs) has not yet afforded foolproof tools for the clinician, but the currently available data warrant extensive efforts to refine and extend our present armamentarium and technology in this area. Further, a simple perusal of the established bone constituents that can now be potentially used as markers of bone metabolism (Table 8–1) greatly increases the chances for success in this new field. No doubt, future progress will depend on and stem from recent advances in basic research in bone biology and biochemistry. The development and clinical application of sequence-specific polyclonal antibodies to individual bone proteins, as well as the utilization of monoclonal antibodies for which the reactive epitope (precise sequence of antigenic determinant) has been determined, will do much to clear up the ambiguities and contradictions confounding the present literature. Further, it is likely that tissue-specific sequence and/or posttranslational modifications will be described in detail over the next few years for those bone constitutents that also exist in nonbone tissues (e.g., alkaline phosphatase, osteonectin, bone proteoglycan). Assays using defined antisera capitalizing on these tissue-

Table 8–1. Potential Markers of Bone Metabolism

Constituent	Anabolic Potential	Catabolic Potential	Comments
Collagen, amino, and carboxyl propeptides	High; collagen is main osteoblast synthetic product	Unknown; degradation products unidentified	Widely distributed in other connective tissues; bone form may be phosphorylated
Osteocalcin	High; appears bone- and/or cartilage-specific	Unknown; however, degradation products may exist in circulation	Many assays presently in use; epitopes not defined
Osteonectin	High; major noncollagenous protein product of human osteoblasts	Unknown; however, its degradation products do exist in the bone matrix	Present in other, proliferative connective tissues; relative contributions of nonbone forms not yet established
Sialoproteins (BSP-I and BSP-II)	High; synthetic products of osteoblasts	Unknown; however, degradation products of BSP-II exist in adult bone	BSP-I may be a cell attachment protein
Proteoglycans (PG-I and PG-II)	High; synthetic products of osteoblasts	Unknown; degradation products unidentified	Tissue-specific modifications may exist for PG-II
Alkaline phosphatase	High; cell membrane constituent of osteoblasts and chondrocytes	Unknown; degradation pathway unidentified	Tissue-specific modifications may be identifiable with monoclonal antibodies
Urinary hydroxyproline or collagen glycopeptides	Nondialyzable HYP (see text)	Dialyzable HYP (see text)	Can come from multiple tissue sources
Tartrate-resistant acid-phosphatase	Unknown	Biosynthetic product of osteoclasts	Specificity of distribution not established

specific differences will then be capable of clearly delimiting the bone-related metabolic properties of these important proteins. Finally, the continuing development of better protein separative technologies (e.g., HPLC protein column, immunoaffinity procedures) should facilitate rapid separation and isolation of immunoreactive molecular species from biological fluids, thereby vastly improving immunoassay specificity. The advent of these new antibody and separative tools provides the exciting prospect of biochemical assay protocols that measure rates of bone formation and resorption simultaneously. For example, assays of serum levels for intact bone matrix proteins, or precursor segments removed during cellular processing and secretion, should be indicators of bone formation, whereas assays of levels for their defined internal degradation fragments may well be indicators of bone resorptive processes. It is easy to envision a series of crosscheck assays for several of the bone proteins to confirm such measurements in a clearly defined and concise fashion. The diagnostic and overall clinical import of such methodology is immediately apparent. Although at this writing, this goal only constitutes an investigator's dream, it seems only a matter of time for the full potential of present efforts to define the biochemical nature of bone cells and bone matrix constituents to become realized.

References

1. Termine JD, Belcourt AB, Miyamoto MS, et al: Properties of dissociatively extracted fetal tooth matrix proteins. J Biol Chem 255:9760, 1980.
2. Termine JD, Belcourt AB, Conn KM, et al: Mineral and collagen-binding proteins of fetal calf bone. J Biol Chem 256:10403, 1981.
3. Eyre DR: Collagen: Molecular diversity in the body's scaffold. Science 207:1315, 1980.
4. Martin GR, Timpl R, Miller PK, et al: The genetically distinct collagens. Trends Biochem Sci 10:285, 1985.
5. Cheah KSE: Collagen genes and inherited connective tissue diseases. Biochem J 229:287, 1985.
6. Fessler JH, Fessler LI: Biosynthesis of procollagen. Annu Rev Biochem 47:129, 1978.
7. Blobel G, Dobberstein:Transfer of proteins across membranes. J Cell Biol 67:835, 1975.
8. Pinnell SR, Fox R, Krane SM: Human collagens: Differences in glycosylated hydroxylysines in skin and bone. Biochim Biophys Acta 229:119, 1971.
9. Segrest JR, Cunningham LW: Variations in human urinary O-hydroxylysyl glycoside levels and their relationship to collagen metabolism. J Clin Invest 49:1497, 1970.
10. Weinstock M, Leblond CP: Synthesis, migration and release of precursor collagen by odontoblasts as visualized by autoradiography after ^{3}H-proline administration. J Cell Biol 60:92, 1974.
11. Fisher LW, Gehron Robey P, Tuross N, et al: The M_r 24,000 phosphoprotein from developing bone is the NH_2 terminal propeptide of the $\alpha 1$ chain of type I collagen. J Biol Chem 262:13457, 1987.
12. van der Rest M, Rosenberg LC, Olsen BR, et al: Chondrocalcin is identical with the C-propeptide of type II procollagen. Biochem J 237:923, 1986.
13. Piez KA: Structure and assembly of the native collagen fibril. Connect Tissue Res 10:25, 1982.
14. Valli M, Leonardi L, Strocchi R, et al: "In vitro" fibril

formation of type I collagen from different sources: Biochemical and morphological aspects. Connect Tissue Res 15:235, 1986.
15. Chandrasekhar S, Kleinman HK, Hassell JR: Regulation of type I collagen fibril assembly by link protein and proteoglycans. Coll Relat Res 4:323, 1984.
16. Scott JE: The periphery of the developing collagen fibril: Quantitative relationships with dermatan sulfate. *In* Chester MA, Heinegard D, Lundblad A, et al (eds): Proceedings of the Seventh International Symposium on Glycoconjugates. Lund, Sweden, Rahms Publishing Co, 1983, pp 830–853.
17. Fleischmajor R, Perlish JS: The role of the amino propeptide in collagen fibrillogenesis. Rheumatology 10:103, 1986.
18. Eyre DR, Paz MA, Gallop PM: Cross-linking in collagen and elastin. Annu Rev Biochem 53:717, 1984.
19. Delmas PD, Tracy RP, Riggs BL, et al: Identification of the noncollagenous proteins of bovine bone by two-dimensional gel electrophoresis. Calcif Tissue Int 36:308, 1984.
20. Conn KM, Termine JD: Matrix protein profiles in calf bone development. Bone 6:33, 1985.
21. Fisher LW, Termine JD: Purification of the noncollagenous proteins from bone: Technical pitfalls and how to avoid them. *In* Ornoy A, Harell A, Sela J (eds): Current Advances in Skeletogenesis. Amsterdam, Elsevier, 1985, pp 467–472.
22. Fisher LW, Termine JD: Noncollagenous proteins influencing the local mechanisms of calcification. Clin Orthop 200:362, 1985.
23. Dickson IR, Bagga MK: Changes with age in the noncollagenous proteins of human bone. Connect Tissue Res 14:77, 1985.
24. Triffitt JT: The special proteins of bone tissue. Clin Sci 72:399, 1987.
25. Ashton BA, Hohling HJ, Triffitt JT: Plasma proteins present in human cortical bone: Enrichment of the α_2-HS glycoprotein. Calcif Tissue Res 22:27, 1976.
26. Triffitt JT, Gebauer U, Ashton BA, et al: Origin of plasma α_2-HS glycoprotein and its accumulation in bone. Nature (London) 262:226, 1976.
27. Triffitt JT, Owen ME, Ashton BA, et al: Plasma disappearance of rabbit α_2-HS glycoprotein and its uptake by bone tissue. Calcif Tissue Res 26:155, 1978.
28. Hauschka PW, Lian JB, Gallop PM: Direct identification of the calcium-binding amino acid, γ-carboxyglutamate, in mineralized tissue. Proc Natl Acad Sci USA 72:3925, 1975.
29. Price PA, Otsuka AS, Poser JW, et al: Characterization of γ-carboxyglutamic acid containing protein from bone. Proc Natl Acad Sci USA 73:1447, 1976.
30. Celeste AJ, Rosen V, Buecker JL, et al: Isolation of the human gene for bone gla protein. EMBO J 5:1885, 1986.
31. Pan LC, Price PA: The propeptide of rat bone γ-carboxyglutamic acid protein shares homology with other vitamin K–dependent protein precursors. Proc Natl Acad Sci USA 82:6109, 1985.
32. Price PA, Baukol SA: 1,25-Dihydroxy vitamin D_3 increases synthesis of the vitamin K–dependent bone protein by osteosarcoma cells. J Biol Chem 255:11660, 1980.
33. Beresford JN, Gallagher JA, Poser JW, et al: Production of osteocalcin by human bone cells in vitro: Effects of 1,25-dihydroxy vitamin D_3, 24,25-dihydroxy vitamin D_3, parathyroid hormone and glucocorticoids. Metab Bone Dis Rel Res 5:229, 1984.
34. Price PA, Baukol SA: 1,25-Dihydroxy vitamin D_3 increases serum levels of the vitamin K–dependent bone protein. Biochem Biophys Res Commun 99:928, 1981.
35. Pan LC, Williamson MK, Price PA: Sequence of the precursor to rat bone γ-carboxyglutamic acid protein that accumulates in warfarin-related osteocarcoma cells. J Biol Chem 260:13398, 1985.
36. Hauschka PW, Gallop PM: Purification and calcium-binding properties of osteocalcin, the γ-carboxyglutamate-containing protein of bone. *In* Wasserman RH, Carrodino E, Carafoli RH, et al (eds): Calcium Binding Proteins and Calcium Function. North Holland, Elsevier, 1977, pp 338–347.
37. Poser JW, Price PA: A method for decarboxylation of γ-carboxyglutamic acid in proteins. J Biol Chem 254:431, 1979.
38. Price PA, Williamson MK: Effects of warfarin on the vitamin K–dependent protein in rat bone. J Biol Chem 256:12754, 1981.
39. Price PA, Williamson MK, Haba T, et al: Excessive mineralization with growth plate closure in rats on chronic warfarin treatment. Proc Natl Acad Sci USA 79:7734, 1982.
40. Price PA: Osteocalcin. *In* Peck WA (ed): Bone and Mineral Research, vol 1. Amsterdam, Excerpta Medica, 1983, pp 157–190.
41. Price PA, Lothringer JW, Nishimoto SK: Absence of the vitamin K–dependent bone protein in fetal rat mineral: Evidence for another γ-carboxyglutamic acid–containing component in bone. J Biol Chem 255:2938, 1980.
42. Price PA, Lothringer JW, Baukol SA, et al: Developmental appearance of the vitamin K–dependent protein of bone during calcification. J Biol Chem 256:3781.
43. Otawara Y, Price PA: Developmental appearance of matrix gla protein during calcification in the rat. J Biol Chem 261:10832, 1986.
44. Price PA, Urist MR, Otawara Y: Matrix gla protein, a new γ-carboxy-glutamic acid-containing protein which is associated with the organic matrix of bone. Biochem Biophys Res Commun 117:765, 1983.
45. Price PA, Williamson MK: Primary structure of bovine matrix gla protein, a new vitamin K–dependent bone protein. J Biol Chem 260:14971, 1985.
46. Kuwata F, Yao K-L, Sodek J, et al: Identification of pre-osteonectin produced by cell-free translation of fetal porcine calvarial mRNA. J Biol Chem 260:6993, 1985.
47. Young MF, Bolander ME, Day AA, et al: Osteonectin mRNA: Distribution in normal and transformed cells. Nucleic Acids Res 14:4483, 1986.
48. Otsuka K, Yao K-L, Wasi S, et al: Biosynthesis of osteonectin by fetal porcine calvarial cells in vitro. J Biol Chem 259:9805, 1984.
49. Gehron Robey P, Kirschner JA, Conn KM, et al: Biosynthesis of noncollagenous proteins by bone cells in vitro. *In* Ornoy A, Harell A, Sela J (eds): Current Advances in Skeletogenesis. Amsterdam, Elsevier, 1985, pp 461–466.
50. Gehron Robey P, Termine JD: Human bone cells in vitro. Calcif Tissue Int 37:453, 1985.
51. Fisher LW, Hawkins GR, Tuross N, et al: Purification and partial characterization of small proteoglycans I and II, and osteonectin from the mineral compartment of developing human bone. J Biol Chem 262:9702, 1987.

52. Zung P, Domenicucci C, Wasi S, et al: Osteonectin is a minor component of mineralized connective tissues in rat. Cell Biol Sci 64:356, 1985.
53. Termine JD, Kleinman HK, Whitson SW, et al: Osteonectin, a bone-specific protein linking mineral to collagen. Cell 26:99, 1981.
54. Romberg RW, Werness PG, Lollar P, et al: Isolation and characterization of native adult osteonectin. J Biol Chem 260:2728, 1985.
55. Wasi S, Otsuka K, Yao K-L, et al: An osteonectin-like protein in porcine periodontal ligament and its synthesis by periodontal ligament fibroblasts. Can J Biochem Cell Biol 62:470, 1984.
56. Gehron Robey P, Denholm LJ, Drum MA, et al: Biosynthesis of bone matrix proteins by osteogenesis imperfecta connective tissue cells. Am Soc Bone Mineral Res #126, 1985.
57. Gehron Robey P, Stubbs JC, Fisher LW, et al: Synthesis of osteonectin and a small proteoglycan (PG-II) by connective tissue cells in vitro. *In* Sen A, Thornhill T (eds): Development and Diseases of Cartilage and Bone Matrix. New York, Alan R Liss, 1987, pp 115–125.
58. Tung PS, Domenicucci C, Wasi S, et al: Specific immunohistochemical localization of osteonectin and collagen types I and III in fetal and adult porcine dental tissues. J Histochem Cytochem 33:531, 1985.
59. Stenner DD, Tracy RP, Riggs BL, et al: Human platelets contain and secrete osteonectin, a major protein of mineralized bone. Proc Natl Acad Sci USA 83:6892, 1986.
60. Dziadek M, Paulsson M, Aumailley M, et al: Purification and tissue distribution of a small protein (BM-40) extracted from a basement membrane tumor. Eur J Biochem 161:455, 1986.
61. Mason IJ, Taylor A, Williams JC, et al: Evidence from molecular cloning that SPARC, a major product of mouse embryo parietal endoderm, is related to an endothelial cell culture shock glycoprotein of M_r 43,000. EMBO J 5:1465, 1986.
62. Franzen A, Heinegard D: Proteoglycans and proteins of rat bone: Purification and biosynthesis of major noncollagenous molecules. *In* Butler WT (ed): The Chemistry and Biology of Mineralized Tissues. Birmingham, EBSCO Media, 1985, pp 132–141.
63. Franzen A, Heinegard D: Isolation and characterization of two sialoproteins present only in bone calcified matrix. Biochem J 232:715, 1986.
64. Oldberg A, Franzen A, Heinegard D: Cloning and sequence analysis of rat bone sialoprotein (osteopontin) cDNA reveals an Arg-Gly-Asp cell-binding sequence. Proc Natl Acad Sci USA 83:8819, 1986.
65. Prince CW, Oosawa T, Butler WT, et al: Isolation, characterization and biosynthesis of a phosphorylated glycoprotein form rat bone. J Biol Chem 262:2900, 1987.
66. Fisher LW, Whitson SW, Avioli LV, et al: Matrix sialoprotein of developing bone. J Biol Chem 258:12723, 1983.
67. Herring GM: The organic matrix of bone. *In* Bourne GH (ed): The Biochemistry and Physiology of Bone, vol 1. New York, Academic Press, 1972, pp 127–189.
68. Gehron Robey P, Fisher LW: Kinetics of noncollagenous bone matrix protein production by bone cells in vitro. *In* Cohn DV, Martin TJ, Meunier P (eds): Calcium Regulation and Bone Metabolism: Basic and Clinical Aspects. Amsterdam, Elsevier Sci Pub B.V., 1987, pp 438–443.
69. Hascall VC, Hascall GK: Proteoglycans. *In* Hay ED (ed): Cell Biology of Extracellullar Matrix. New York, Plenum, pp 3[illegible]–63.
70. Rosenberg LC, Cho HU, Tang L-H, et al: Isolation of dermatan sulfate proteoglycans from mature bovine articular cartilages. Biol Chem 260:6304, 1985.
71. Fisher LW, Termine JD, Dejter SW Jr, et al: Proteoglycans of developing bone. J Biol Chem 258:6588, 1983.
72. Franzen A, Heinegard D: Extraction and purification of proteoglycans from mature bovine bone. Biochem J 224:47, 1984.
73. Franzen A, Heinegard D: Characterization of proteoglycans from the calcified matrix of bovine bone. Biochem J 224:59, 1984.
74. Sato S, Rahemtula F, Prince CW, et al: Proteoglycans of adult bovine compact bone. Connect Tissue Res 14:65, 1985.
75. Fisher LW: The nature of the proteoglycans of bone. *In* Butler WT (ed): The Chemistry and Biology of Mineralized Tissues. Birmingham, EBSCO Media, 1985, pp 188–196.
76. Prince CW, Rahemtula F, Butler WT: Metabolism of rat bone proteoglycans in vivo. Biochem J 216:589, 1983.
77. Heinegard D, Björn-Persson A, Cöster L, et al: The core proteins of large and small interstitial proteoglycans from various connective tissues form distinct subgroups. Biochem J 230:181, 1985.
78. Vogel KG, Fisher LW: Comparisons of antibody reactivity and enzyme sensitivity between small proteoglycans from bovine tendon, bone and cartilage. J Biol Chem 26[illegible]:11334, 1986.
79. Krusius T, Ruoslahti E: Primary structure of an extracellular matrix proteoglycan core protein deduced from cloned cDNA. Proc Natl Acad Sci USA 83:7686, 1986.
80. Day AA, Ramis CI, Fisher LW, et al: Characterization of bone PG II cDNA and its relationship to PG II mRNA from other connective tissues. Nucleic Acids Res 14:9861, 198[illegible].
81. McKenna MJ, Hamilton TA, Sussman HH: Comparison of human alkaline phosphatase isoenzymes. Biochem J 181:67, 1979.
82. Stigbrand T, Fishman WH: Human alkaline phosphatases. *In* Stigbrand T, Fishman WH (eds): Progress in Clinical and Biological Research, vol 166. New York, Alan R Liss, 1983, pp 3–14.
83. Harris H: Multilocus enzyme systems and the evolution of gene expression: The alkaline phosphatases as a model example. *In* The Harvey Lectures: Series 76. New York, Academic Press, 1982, pp 85–123.
84. Weiss MJ, Henthorn PS, Lafferty MA, et al: Isolation and characterization of a cDNA encoding a human liver/bone/kidney-type alkaline phosphatase. Proc Natl Acad Sci USA 83:7[illegible]82, 1986.
85. Majeska RJ, Dean HW, Rodan GA: Alkaline phosphatase biosynthesis in ROS 17/2.8 rat osteosarcoma cells. J Bone Mineral Res 1[Suppl]:59, 1986.
86. Whyte MP: Alkaline phosphatase and the measurement of bone formation. *In* Potts JT, Frame B (eds): Clinical Disorders of Bone and Mineral Metabolism. Amsterdam, Excerpta Medica, 1983, pp 120–125.
87. Hauschka PV, Mavrakos AE, Iafrati MD, et al: Growth factors in bone matrix. J Biol Chem 261:12665, 1986.
88. Seyedin SM, Thompson AY, Bentz H, et al: Cartilage-inducing factor A. J Biol Chem 261:5693, 1986.

89. Centrella M, Canalis E: Transforming growth factor-β is a bifunctional regulator of replication and collagen synthesis in osteoblast-enriched cell cultures of fetal rat bone. J Biol Chem 262:2869, 1987.
90. Gehron Robey P, Young MF, Flanders KC, et al: Osteoblasts synthesize and respond to transforming growth factor-beta in vitro. J Cell Biol 150:457, 1987.
91. Farley JR, Baylink DJ: Purification of a skeletal growth factor from human bone. Biochemistry 21:3502, 1982.
92. Canalis E, Centrella J: Isolation of a nontransforming bone-derived growth factor from medium conditioned by fetal rat calvariae. Endocrinology 118:2002, 1986.
93. Boskey AL: Current concepts of the biochemistry and physiology of calcification. Clin Orthop Rel Res 157:165, 1981.
94. Boyan BD: Proteolipid-dependent calcification. *In* Butler WT (ed): The Chemistry and Biology of Mineralized Tissues. Birmingham, EBSCO Media, 1985, pp 125–131.
95. Posner AS, Betts F: Molecular control of tissue mineralization. *In* Veis A (ed): The Chemistry and Biology of Mineralized Connective Tissue. Amsterdam, Elsevier/North Holland, 1981, pp 257–266.
96. Eanes ED, Termine JD: Calcium in mineralized tissues. *In* Spiro TG (ed): Calcium in Biology. New York, John Wiley and Sons, 1983, pp 203–233.
97. Ristelli L, Ristelli J: Radioimmune assays for monitoring connective tissue metabolism. *In* Kühn K, Krieg T (eds): Connective Tissue: Biological and Clinical Aspects. Munich, Karger 1986, pp 216–245.
98. Rennard SI, Berg R, Martin GR, et al: Enzyme-linked immunoassays (ELISA) for connective tissue components. Anal Biochem 104:205, 1980.
99. Rohde H, Nowack H, Becker U, et al: Radioimmunoassay for the amino terminal peptide of procollagen pro α1(I) chain. J Immunol Methods 11:135, 1976.
100. Taubmann MB, Goldberg B, Sherr CJ: Radioimmunoassay for human procollagen. Science 186:1115, 1974.
101. Simon LS, Krane SM, Wortman PD, et al: Serum levels of type I and III procollagen fragments in Paget's disease of bone. J Clin Endocrinol Metab 58:110, 1984.
102. Laitinen O: Clinical applications of urinary hydroxyproline determination. Acta Med Scand 577[Suppl]:1, 1974.
103. Niell HB, Palmieri GM, Neely CL, et al: Total, dialyzable, and nondialyzable postabsorptive hydroxyproline: Values in patients with cancer. Arch Intern Med 143:1925, 1983.
104. Prockop DJ, Kivirikko KI: Relationship of hydroxyproline excretion in urine to collagen metabolism. Ann Intern Med 66:1234, 1967.
105. Krane SM, Munoz AJ, Harris ED Jr: Collagen-like fragments: Excretion in urine of patients with Paget's disease of bone. Science 157:713, 1967.
106. Krane SM, Munoz AJ, Harris ED Jr: Urinary polypeptides related to collagen synthesis. J Clin Invest 49:716, 1970.
107. Scriver CR: Glycyl-proline in urine of humans with bone disease. Can J Physiol Pharmacol 42:357, 1964.
108. Manzke E, Rawley R, Vose G, et al: Effect of fluoride therapy on nondialyzable urinary hydroxyproline, serum alkaline phosphatase, parathyroid hormone and 25-hydroxy vitamin D_3. Metabolism 2:1005, 1977.
109. Anasuya A, Rao Narasinger BS: Hydroxyproline peptides of urine in fluorosis. Clin Chim Acta 56:121, 1974.
110. Birkenhäger JC: The urinary excretion of hydroxyproline in metabolic disorders of connective tissue and bone. Folia Med Nederl 13:79, 1970.
111. Price PA, Nishimoto SK: Radioimmunoassay for the vitamin K–dependent protein of bone and its discovery in plasma. Proc Natl Acad Sci USA 77:2234, 1980.
112. Price PA, Williamson MK, Lothinger JW: Origin of the vitamin K–dependent bone protein found in plasma and its clearance by kidney and bone. J Biol Chem 256:12760, 1981.
113. Price PA, Parthemore JD, Deftos LJ: A new biochemical marker for bone metabolism. J Clin Invest 66:878, 1980.
114. Weinstein RS, Gundberg CM: Serum osteocalcin levels reflect bone mineralization in osteopenic patients. Clin Res 31:853A, 1983.
115. Gundberg CM, Lian JB, Gallop PM: Measurements of γ-carboxyglutamate and circulating osteocalcin in normal children and adults. Clin Chim Acta 128:1, 1983.
116. Delmas PD, Wahner HW, Mann KG, et al: Assessment of bone turnover in post-menopausal osteoporosis by measurement of serum bone gla-protein. J Lab Clin Med 102:470, 1983.
117. Delmas PD, Stenner D, Wahner HW, et al: Increase in serum bone γ-carboxyglutamic acid protein with aging women. J Clin Invest 71:1316, 1983.
118. Epstein S, McClintock R, Bryce G, et al: Differences in serum bone gla-protein with age and sex. Lancet 1:307, 1984.
119. Brown JP, Malaval L, Chapuy MC, et al: Serum bone gla-protein: A specific marker for bone formation in post-menopausal osteoporosis. Lancet 1:1091, 1984.
120. Malluche HM, Faugere M-C, Fanti P, et al: Plasma levels of bone gla-protein reflect bone formation in patients on chronic maintenance dialysis. Kidney Int 26:869, 1984.
121. Crouch M, Woods DA, Gallagher JA, et al: Serum osteocalcin in British subjects. Calcif Tissue Int 36:S3, 1984.
122. Melik RA, Farrugia W, Quelch KJ: Plasma osteocalcin in man. NZ Med J 15:410, 1985.
123. Martinez ME, Herranz L, dePedro C, et al: Osteocalcin levels in patients with hyper- and hypothyroidism. Horm Metab Res 18:212, 1985.
124. Zerwekh JE, Sakahee K, Pak CYC: Short-term 1,25-dihydroxy vitamin D_3 administration raises serum osteocalcin in patients with postmenopausal osteoporsis. J Clin Endocrinol Metab 63:615, 1985.
125. Charon SA, Delmas PD, Malaval L, et al: Serum bone gla-protein in renal osteodystrophy: Comparison with bone histomorphometry. J Clin Endocrinol Metab 63:892, 1986.
126. Yoneda M, Takatsuki K, Oiso Y, et al: Clinical significance of serum bone gla-protein and urinary γ-gla as biochemical markers in primary hyperparathyroidism. Endocrinol Jpn 83:89, 1986.
127. Garrel DR, Delmas PD, Malaval L, et al: Serum bone gla-protein: A marker of bone turnover in hyperthyroidism. J Clin Endocrinol Metab 62:1052, 1986.
128. Lukert BP, Huggins JC, Stoskopf MM: Serum osteocalcin is increased in patients with hyperthyroidism and decreased in patients receiving glucocorticoids. J Clin Endocrinol Metab 62:1056, 1986.

129. Catherwood BD, Marcus R, Madvig P, et al: Determinants of bone γ-carboxyglutamic acid-containing protein in plasma of healthy aging subjects. Bone 6:9, 1985.
130. Delmas PD, Malaval L, Arlot ME, et al: Serum bone gla-protein compared to bone histomorphometry in endocrine diseases. Bone 6:339, 1985.
131. Gundberg CM, Weinstein RS: Multiple immunoreactive forms of osteocalcin in uremic serum. J Clin Invest 77:1762, 1986.
132. Farrugia W, Melick RA: Metabolism of osteocalcin. Calcif Tissue Int 39:234, 1986.
133. Gundberg CM, Lian JB, Gallop PM, et al: Urinary γ-carboxyglutamic acid and serum osteocalcin as bone markers: Studies in osteoporosis and Paget's disease. J Clin Endocrinol Metab 57:1221, 1983.
134. Gundberg CM, Markowitz ME, Mizruchi M, et al: Osteocalcin in human serum: A circadian rhythm. J Clin Endocrinol Metab 60:736, 1985.
135. Cole DEC, Carpenter TO, Gundberg CM: Serum osteocalcin concentrations in children with metabolic bone disease. J Pediatr 106:770, 1985.
136. Cole DEC, Gundberg CM: Changes in serum osteocalcin associated with parathyroid hormone infusion in X-linked hypophosphatemic rickets. Clin Chim Acta 151:1, 1985.
137. Rowe JW, Andrus R, Tobin JD, et al: The effect of age on creatinine clearance in men: A cross-sectional and longitudinal study. J Gerontol 31:155, 1976.
138. Delmas PD, Wilson DM, Mann KG, et al: Effect of renal function on plasma levels of bone gla-protein. J Clin Endocrinol Metab 57:1028, 1983.
139. Malone JD, Teitelbaum SL, Griffin GL, et al: Recruitment of osteoblast precursors by purified bone matrix constituents. J Cell Biol 92:227, 1982.
140. Malone JD, Teitelbaum SL, Hauschka PV, et al: Presumed osteoclast precursors (monocytes) recognize two or more regions of osteocalcin. Calcif Tissue Int 34:511, 1982.
141. Mundy GR, Poser JW: Chemotactic activity of the γ-carboxyglutamic acid-containing protein in bone. Calcif Tissue Int 35:164, 1983.
142. Slovik DM, Gundberg CM, Neer RM, et al: Clinical evaluation of bone turnover by serum osteocalcin measurements in a hospital setting. J Clin Endocrinol Metab 59:228, 1984.
143. Deftos LJ, Parthemore JG, Price PA: Changes in bone gla-protein during treatment of bone disease. Calcif Tissue Int 34:121, 1982.
144. Delmas PD, Demiaux B, Malaval L, et al: Serum bone γ-carboxyglutamic acid-containing protein in primary hyperparathyroidism in malignant hypercalcemia. J Clin Invest 77:985, 1986.
145. Delmas PD, Demiaux B, Malaval L, et al: Serum bone gla-protein is not a sensitive marker of bone turnover in Paget's disease of bone. Calcif Tissue Int 38:60, 1986.
146. Gundberg CM, Cole DEC, Lian JB, et al: Serum osteocalcin in the treatment of inherited rickets with 1,25-dihydroxy vitamin D_3. J Clin Endocrinol Metab 56:1063, 1983.
147. Delmas PD, Chatelain P, Malaval L, et al: Serum bone gla-protein in growth hormone deficient children. J Bone Mineral Res 1:333, 1986.
148. Podenphant J, Christiansen C, Catherwood BD, et al: Serum bone gla-protein variations during estrogen and calcium prophylaxis of post-menopausal women. Calcif Tissue Int 36:536, 1984.
149. Podenphant J, Christiansen C, Catherwood BD, et al: Serum bone gla-protein and other biochemical estimates of bone turnover in early post-menopausal women during prophylactic treatment for osteoporosis. Acta Med Scand 218:329, 1985.
150. Posen S, Cornich C, Kleerekoper M: Alkaline phosphatase and metabolism bone disorders. *In* Avioli LV, Krane SM (eds) Metabolic Bone Disease. New York, Academic Press, 1977, pp 141–181.
151. Stepán JJ, Volek V, Kolár J: A modified inactivation-inhibition method for determining the serum activity of alkaline phosphatase isoenzymes. Clin Chim Acta 69:1, 1976.
152. Stepán JJ, Tesarová A, Havránek T, et al: Age and sex dependency of the biochemical indices of bone remodeling. Clin Chim Acta 151:273, 1985.
153. Peach H, Compston JE, Vedi S, et al: Value of plasma calcium phosphate and alkaline phosphatase measurements in the diagnosis of histological osteomalacia. J Clin Pathol 35:625, 1982.
154. Cundy T, Bartlett M, Bishop M, et al: Plasma hydroxyproline in uremia: Relationship with histologic and biochemical indices of bone turnover. Metab Bone Dis Rel Res 4:297, 1983.
155. Reeve J, Arlot M, Hesp R, et al: Tracer measurements of bone remodeling and their significance in involutional osteoporosis. *In* Potts JT, Frame B (eds): Clinical Disorders of Bone and Mineral Metabolism. Amsterdam, Excerpta Medica, 1983, pp 99–104.
156. Aaron JE: Histology and microanatomy of bone. *In* Nordin BEC (ed): Calcium, Phosphate and Magnesium Metabolism. London, Churchill Livingstone, 1976, pp 298–356.
157. Heersche JNM: The mechanism of osteoclastic bone resorption: An update of the helper cell hypothesis. *In* Silberman M, Slavkin HC (eds): Current Advances in Skeletogenesis. Amsterdam, Excerpta Medica, 1982, pp 232–237.
158. Weiss JB: Enzymic degradation of collagen. Int Rev Connect Tissue Res 7:1[illegible]2, 1976.
159. Blair HC, Kahn AJ, Crouch EC, et al: Isolated osteoclasts resorb the organic and inorganic components of bone. J Cell Biol 102:1164, 1986.
160. Askenasi R, DeBacker M, Devos A: The origin of urinary hydroxylysyl glycosides in Paget's disease of bone and in primary hyperparathyroidism. Calcif Tissue Res 22:35, 1976.
161. Krane SM, Kantrowitz FG, Byrne M, et al: Excretion of hydroxylysine and its glycosides as an index of collagen degradation. J Clin Invest 59:819, 1977.
162. Powles TJ, Rosset G, Leese CL, et al: Early morning hydroxyproline excretion in patients with breast cancer. Cancer 38:2564, 1976.
163. Clark S, Zorab PA: Hydroxyproline centiles for normal adolescent boys and girls. Clin Orthop Rel Res 137:217, 1978.
164. Stepán JJ, Neuwirtová R, Pacovský V, et al: Biochemical assessment of bone disease in multiple myeloma. Clin Chim Acta 142:203, 1984.
165. Moskowitz RW, Klein L, Katz D: Urinary hydroxyproline levels in an aged population: A study of nonosteoporotic and osteoporotic patients. Arthritis Rheum 8:61, 1965.
166. Varghese Z, Moorhead JF, Wills MR: Plasma hydroxyproline fractions in patients with dialysis osteodystrophy. Clin Chim Acta 110:105, 1981.
167. Minkin C: Bone acid phosphatase: Tartrate-resistant acid phosphatase as a marker of osteoclast function.

Calcif Tissue Int 34:285, 1982.

168. Lam WKW, Eastlund DT, Li CY, et al: Biochemical properties of tartrate-resistant acid phosphatase in serum of adults and children. Clin Chem 24:1105, 1978.
169. Lam WKW, Lee PF, Li CY, et al: Immunological and biochemical evidence for identity of tartrate-resistant isoenzymes of acid phosphatase from human serum and tissues. Clin Chem 26:420, 1980.
170. Stepán JJ, Silinková-Málková E, Havránek T, et al: Relationship of plasma tartrate-resistant acid phosphatase to the bone isoenzyme of serum alkaline phosphatase in hyperparathyroidism. Clin Chim Acta 133:189, 1983.
171. Tavassoli M, Rizo R, Yam LT: Elevation of serum acid phosphatase in cancers with bone metastasis. Cancer 45:2400, 1980.
172. Ardaillou R, Isaac R, Nivez MP, et al: Effect of salmon calcitonin on renal excretion of adenosine 3',5'-monophosphate. Horm Metab Res 8:136, 1976.
173. Caniggia A, Gennari C, Loré F, et al: Effects of parathyroid hormone and calcitonin on plasma and nephrogenous cyclic adenosine-3',5'-monophosphate in normal subjects and in pathological conditions. Eur J Clin Invest 10:99, 1986.
174. Minkhoff JR, Grant BF, Marcus R: Plasma cyclic AMP response to calcitonin: A potential clinical marker of bone turnover. Bone 6:285, 1985.
175. Dickson IR, Bagga M, Paterson CR: Variations in the serum concentration and urine excretion of α_2-HS glycoprotein, a bone-related protein, in normal individuals and patients with osteogenesis imperfecta. Calcif Tissue Int 35:16, 1983.
176. Ashton BA, Smith R: Plasma α_2-HS glycoprotein concentration in Paget's disease of bone: Its possible significance. Clin Sci 58:435, 1980.
177. Smith R, Vipond S, Ashton BA: Plasma α_2-HS glycoprotein and bone formation. *In* Potts JT, Frame B (eds): Disorders of Bone and Mineral Metabolism. Amsterdam, Excerpta Medica, 1983, pp 116–119.
178. Pilonchery G, Minaire P, Milan JJ, et al: Urinary elimination of glycosaminoglycans during the immobilization osteoporosis of spinal cord injury patients. Clin Orthop Rel Res 174:230, 1983.

9

S. H. COHN

Noninvasive Measurements of Bone Mass

Techniques for the evaluation of the skeletal system center on the measurement of bone mass. In the past decade, technological developments have made it possible to assess bone mass with noninvasive measurements. As a result, it is possible to quantify the slow demineralization process that accompanies the aging of all individuals, and thus to identify a population at risk of osteoporosis. The breakthrough in making this identification, in addition to the development of instrument systems with high sensitivity, is the concept of "normalization." In this procedure, the bone mass is expressed relative to the "normal" value for an individual, a predicted value based on the parameters of sex, age, body size, and habitus. Since, as detailed in Chapter 12, the rate of loss of bone in normal aging and in osteoporosis is very slow, methods for measuring these changes must be highly sensitive and precise.

Clinical symptoms of osteoporosis appear when the structural integrity of the bone, usually the vertebrae, is compromised through demineralization (see Chapter 12). The condition is generally manifested with the occurrence of one or more compression fractures in the vertebral bodies. All portions of the axial and appendicular skeleton, both cortical and trabecular bone, undergo demineralization. However, the vertebrae, because of their shape and size, are susceptible to spontaneous fracture due to compression, whereas other bones of the skeleton manifest their fragility chiefly in traumatic incidents. The compressive strength of the lumbar vertebral bodies has been correlated with the amount of bone quantified or the apparent density. Studies have also pointed out a close correlation between bone mineral mass and incidence of fracture. Two goals of the investigatory procedures in the study of osteoporosis are the accurate determination of the mass of bone relative to a "normal" value for a particular individual and the serial changes in bone mass resulting from therapy. The principles of the various techniques employed for the noninvasive measurement of bone mass have recently been reviewed, along with the clinical applications of the measurements.[1-5]

A variety of methods are presently available for the noninvasive measurement of bone mass of both normal individuals and patients with metabolic disorders. Chief among these methods are radiographic techniques such as radiogrammetry, photon absorptiometry, computed tomography, Compton scattering, and neutron activation analysis (Table 9–1). In this chapter, the salient features of the bone measurement techniques are discussed and their accuracy and precision noted. The most important developments in each of the various techniques for measuring bone mass are updated to the present state of the art, and their advantages and disadvantages are summarized. Where possible, intercomparisons are made. For greater detail, consult references 1 to 4.

I. RADIOGRAPHIC MORPHOMETRY (INDEXES)

Radiographic morphometry provides a useful tool for cross-sectional studies of bone mass in large populations. Radiographic indexes include vertebral biconcavity, femoral score, and femoral trabecular pattern. The first two indexes have been found to be related to the incidence of vertebral fractures. Additionally, the vertebral biconcavity index has been found to reflect extraskeletal factors that are pathogenic in spinal osteopenia, and

Table 9–1. Noninvasive Techniques for Quantitating Bone Mass

Technique	Site Measured	Cortical/ Trabecular %	Precision/ Accuracy	Discrimination	Response to Therapy	Radiation	Cost	Remarks
RG	Metacarpals							
	and/or	98/2	±2%/?	—	±*	10 mrem	$50–75	*estrogens
RD	Phalanges							
	Radius/ulna							
	(a) distal	80–95/ 20–5	±2–4% ±3–4%	—	±*			*estrogens
SPA								
	(b) ultradistal	25/75	±2–4%/?	?	?	10 mrem	$75–125	
	Os calcis	20/80	±2–4%/?	?	?			
	Spine: L1–L4*	35/65	±2–5%/ ±2–4%	±	+	10 mrem	$150–200	*total vertebral body including
DPA	Femur : neck :	75/25	±3–5%/?	—	?	10 mrem	$50–75	spinous
	trochanter	50/50	±3–5%/?	—	?	10 mrem		process
CT	Single-energy							
	spine: T12–L4*	5/95	±3–5%/ 6–30%†	±	+	500–750 mrem	$125–175	*area of interest within vertebral body
	Dual-energy							
	spine: T12–L4*	5/95	±5–10%/ ±5%	?	?	750 mrem	?	†Due to marrow fat?
TBC–NAA	Total skeleton	80/20	±2%/±5%	±	+	270–2000 mrem	$400–750	

From Chesnut CH: Bone imaging techniques. *In* Becker KL (ed): Principles and Practice of Endocrinology. Philadelphia, J.B. Lippincott, 1987.

the femoral score has been related to the degree of osteopenia. A reduced femoral trabecular pattern index may be associated with spinal osteopenia; however, the relation is not a direct proportionality, as the reduction also reflects the effects of stress.

Despite all of the above-mentioned relationships, none of these radiographic indexes is sufficiently sensitive and discriminating to identify those individuals in the early stages of osteopenia who are destined for the rapid and progressive loss of bone mass from the axial skeleton that culminates in vertebral collapse. Greater sensitivity is needed both to identify early osteopenia and to assess the response of skeletal mass to treatment.

II. RADIOGRAMMETRY

Radiogrammetry is the simplest and most widely used technique for the measurement of bone mass.[6] Conventional radiogrammetry is basically employed for the measurement of cortical bone. Since bone loss results primarily from endosteal resorption, cortical thickness reflects the loss quite well. Measurement of the cortical thickness of either the midshaft of the femur or metacarpal is utilized for estimation of the cortical bone mass. Correction for individual differences in bone size is effected by expressing cortical thickness as a percentage of the total width at midshaft.

The minimum level of cortical thinning that can be detected with this technique usually occurs in advanced stages of generalized osteoporosis.[6,7] Thus, the metacarpal index provides useful data in large-scale population surveys on the incidence of advanced osteoporosis. However, the technique is not adequate for the identification of the population at risk with respect to osteoporosis, since it is relatively insensitive to small decreases in bone mass. Moreover, measurements of cortical widths do not reflect bone resorption occurring within the cortex. The metacarpal index correlates with both regional and total osteopenia, and with the number of fractures of the dorsal spine. Since this measurement primarily reflects endosteal bone resorption rather than intracortical resorption, it appears to be somewhat less useful as an indicator of overall bone mass changes than are other techniques. Bone loss resulting from intracortical porosity can best be evaluated by magnification radiogrammetry; standard radiogrammetry is of limited value for this assessment. Changes in bone mass in patients with renal dysfunction, endocrine dysfunction, and other metabolic disorders have been widely measured by both standard and magnification radiogrammetry. Further work on the improvement of radiogrammetric measurements is required.

Studies are also needed to determine the degree of correlation among various peripheral bone measurements and total bone mass. Verification of the relationships is necessary in order that quantification of cortical bone mass in a particular appendicular portion of the skeleton may reliably form a basis for prediction of the fracture rate for other parts of the skeleton. Such studies can enhance the clinical usefulness of these techniques.

A. Clinical Applications

Radiogrammetry of cortical bone has provided normative data on both bone mass and remodeling rates as a function of age.[6,7] In addition, these data have been useful in quantifying remodeling in pathologic conditions and also for following the efficacy of various therapeutic programs such as estrogen therapy in osteoporosis (see Chapter 12).

The information obtained by radiogrammetry does not always correlate with that obtained by other noninvasive measurements of bone mass. However, the combination of radiogrammetry with data obtained by other techniques is useful for understanding bone changes in aging and in disease.

III. RADIOGRAPHIC DENSITOMETRY

Photodensitometric measurements with x-ray sources and radiographic films employing standardized aluminum wedges have proved to be quite reproducible. These measurements appear to be more sensitive than simple cortical measurements.[8] Certain technical problems inherent in this technique, however, reduce the accuracy of the measurement, and hence tend to limit its clinical usefulness. A basic problem is the present inability to correct the effects on the measurement of variation in the amount of soft tissue and fat overlying the bone. A second problem stems from the hardening of low-energy polychromatic x-ray beams; this hardening produces inaccuracies in the measurement. A third source of error derives from scattered radiation from the uncollimated x-ray beam, which affects the entire film. This effect is minimal in bones with a thin covering of soft tissues such as the carpals, metacarpals, and phalanges. Measurements of the metacarpals and phalanges have been more reliable than measurements made on bones in thicker areas of the body, although not as precise and sensitive as single-photon absorptiometry at the same location.[8-10]

Errors in density measurement of the order of 10% or more occur in both radiogrammetry and radiographic photodensitometry, and hence in the inferred bone mass measurement. The errors are inherent in x-ray measurement; they derive from variability in energy and film response. Errors that result from the use of the broad energy spectrum of x-rays, in addition to beam hardening, are nonuniformity of field intensity and energy, and radiation scattering. These problems can be reduced and some even eliminated by the use of monoenergetic photon sources such as those used in photon absorptiometry. Currently, the metacarpals can be measured in normal subjects with a precision of approximately 3%, and the phalanges with a precision of approximately 2%.[8]

Three basic problems remain to be solved for measurements made with radiographic densitometry and photon absorptiometry:

1. the need to convert a linear density measurement to an absolute measure of calcium,
2. the necessity for appropriately correcting for skeletal size, and
3. validation of the extrapolation of density from a very small sample of one type of bone to the bone mineral content of the entire skeleton.

IV. PHOTON ABSORPTIOMETRY

The present availability of monoenergetic radiation from radionuclide sources has led to the development of photon beam absorptiometric procedures. The principle of this technique is similar to that of roentgenography; the data obtained, however, are more precise. The bone mineral content is assumed to be directly proportional to the amount of photon energy absorbed by the bone.[11]

A. Single-Photon Absorptiometry (SPA)

Single-photon absorptiometric measurements are made on the appendicular skeleton rather than the axial skeleton, as the problems inherent in the interference of soft tissue are minimized at the former sites. To a lesser degree, these errors also occur, of course, in measuring the radius. Significant correction of this error may be made by the application of the dual-energy absorptiometric technique. There are also inherent errors resulting from the use of finite beam widths and from the nonuniformity of photon intensity across the beam width. Significant correction of these errors may be effected by numerical filtering methods.[12] Generally, cortical bone (diaphysis of the radius) is measured. In routine clinical scans of the shaft of the radius, the precision is reported to be 2% to 4%. The imprecision is largely the result of repositioning error. This error is minimized somewhat by utilizing the ratio of bone mineral content of the radius (BMC) to radius width as the index. The precision of the measurement made on the distal portion of the radius is less than that made on the diaphyseal portion. The sensitivity to changes in bone mass in the former is one half that of the latter. Thus, the metaphysis, although it contains proportionally more trabecular bone than the shaft, is nevertheless measured less frequently because of repositioning errors introduced by the irregularity of the bone architecture.[4]

In general, there is good correlation, in normal individuals, between the BMC of the radius shaft and the total body calcium. The correlation between SPA measurements of the appendicular and axial skeleton are, at best, moderate (0.6–0.7). The same correlations are not as good in osteoporotic patients. It should be emphasized that the BMC of the radius shaft is of limited value for predicting vertebral fractures.[13-15]

A number of technical advances in SPA have been made over the past four years.

1. A higher precision has been achieved in area measurements by the application of rectilinear scanning. Scanning over several centimeters has improved the precision from 2% to about 1.4% by reducing the error in scan repositioning.[11]
2. Several major advances over the last few years have resulted from the use of microprocessors in SPA instrumentation. With microprocessors, it has been possible to decrease errors by
   a. regulating the scan speed in proportion to counting statistics;
   b. improving the dead time correction;
   c. correcting for beam filtration ("hardening") due to overlying soft tissue;
   d. introducing algorithms for integration of bone attenuation and for edge detection to provide more accurate analysis of scan data.
3. Calibration and normalization have been improved. It is now possible to calibrate automatically against standards.

With the improvements achieved by the use of microprocessors and rectilinear scanners, it may be possible to make bone measurements in trabecular areas with SPA.[11] A precision of 1% has been reported for BMC in the distal forearm with the use of rectilinear scanning techniques.[16]

1. Clinical Applications

Single-photon absorptiometry is a useful technique for tracing normal changes in bone mass with aging and, in certain instances, changes resulting from therapeutic procedures. Considerable single-photon normative data are available from the wide clinical application of SPA.[10,11,16,17] Whereas the precision of the method is high, the accuracy of this technique, at the present time, is markedly reduced when it is applied to the measurement of the spinal column or any irregularly shaped bone surrounded by a large volume of tissue. If an absolute measurement is required, the data should be normalized for the size of the skeleton in each individual. A number of clinical studies performed with the use of SPA have been reported for the investigation of osteoporosis, renal osteodystrophy, and other metabolic bone diseases (see Chapters 12 and 13).

B. Dual-Photon Absorptiometry (DPA)

Dichromatic (dual-photon) absorptiometers with increased sophistication have recently been developed. These instruments employ two different photon energies in order to correct for overlying fat and tissue. Dual-photon absorptiometry (DPA) permits measurement of bone density to be made in areas such as the spine. These measurements are far less satisfactorily performed with single-photon techniques, as noted previously. With recent advances in DPA has come the application of the technique to the measurement of the bone mineral content of the lumbar spine, femoral neck, and total skeleton. The advances stem from the use of a dual-energy isotope, ^{153}Gd, which has optimal energies (44 and 100 keV) for resolving the two-component system of soft tissue and bone.[18,19]

The measurement of total body bone mass (TBBM) was also developed with the use of DPA.[18] The scan is performed with a modified rectilinear scanner and ^{153}Gd. It requires approximately 70 minutes. Actually, DPA is a linear density measurement, producing an integral of compact and cancellous bone in the scan path. The total body bone mass is expressed in grams, by validation against total body neutron activation measurement for calcium. A very good correlation (r = 0.99) was found between TBBM and TBCa measured by neutron activation.[20] The precision of TBBM measurements in young, healthy individuals is stated to be 2% to 3%.[18] The long-term precision of spinal measurements, femoral neck, and total skeleton is reported to be 2% to 3%.[21-25] An advantage of the DPA technique is the low radiation dose of 15 to 20 mrem.

The accuracy and precision of DPA are affected by a variety of physical and biological factors (Table 9–2). Corrections required for the factors influencing DPA measurements are as follows:

1. Since the inherent precision of DPA is not as high as that of SPA, radioactive sources of higher activity must be employed for DPA.

Table 9–2. Factors Affecting the Accuracy and Precision of Dual-Photon Absorptiometry

Geometry and collimation of the photon beam
Beam hardening and absorber thickness
Constancy of attenuation of coefficients of whole bone
Compton cross effect
Absorber thickness
Fat distribution
Localization of scanning area
Irregularities of bone shape
Scanning speed
Radionuclide source—count rate (dead time correction) and energy levels
Distance between scan paths
Scanning angle
Patient movement
Stability of electronics
Baseline determination

a. These sources require correction for dead time.

b. Gamma stripping is required to correct for the Compton contribution of higher energy peaks to lower energy peaks.

c. Correction is required for the effects of scattering of radiation of higher energy beams, which occurs particularly with large collimators.

2. Correction is required for the beam hardening with the lower energy radiation that occurs, since the 44 keV peak really consists of a number of different energies.

3. The beam energy is altered with changes in soft tissue thickness. If correction is not applied, the results are affected.

The fat composition of the soft tissue surrounding the spine affects DPA, but not to the degree that it affects CT scanning (described later). Since soft tissue is composed of variable amounts of fat and lean tissue, there is an inherent error in the attenuation correction that must be compensated. Correction is made for soft tissue composition with microprocessing algorithms. Soft tissue composition correction is more important for the total body calcium measurement than for local measurements by DPA.

The precision of DPA is also affected by

1. counting statistics;
2. sampling error due to the large step of the scan;
3. subject motion during the scan;
4. deviation from exponential attenuation (beam hardening), due to the polychromaticity of the lower energy photopeak;
5. inaccuracy introduced by nonuniformity of intensity across the finite beam profile (partial volume effect) at the edge of the bone (see section on SPA);
6. aortic calcification or vertebral osteophytosis, especially in the elderly, which results in false elevations of vertebral bone mass estimates.

The error introduced by factor 5 is a particular problem when deformed or crushed vertebrae are encountered in osteoporotic patients. All of these factors require correction for the appropriate application of the DPA technique.

1. Clinical Applications

The normal rate of loss of calcium from the spine appears to differ from that of compact bone in the appendicular skeleton. The loss also appears to begin at an earlier time.[11,23,26] Only moderate correlation exists between the appendicular mineral content and that of the spine. There is an even poorer correlation in patients with bone disorders.[15,23,24] DPA of the total skeleton gives a more representative indication of skeletal status than does the measurement of the appendicular skeleton.[18] Spinal DPA is useful in discriminating severe osteoporosis.[23,25] Hence, DPA may be useful for establishing a "fracture" threshold[2] in spinal osteoporosis and for monitoring therapeutic agents that preferentially affect trabecular bone in the spine. Total skeletal and femoral neck mineral content, however, may be less useful clinically than measurements of the spine.[11]

V. COMPUTED TOMOGRAPHY (CT)

The technique of CT scanning has the potential advantage of being able to separate cortical and cancellous bone by transaxial display. The basis for determining alterations in the skeleton by measuring cancellous bone resides in the high level of metabolic activity of this type of bone, which rapidly and sensitively reflects ongoing changes that affect bone mass (see Chapter 12).

For a three-dimensional reconstruction of a bone, a complete set of views is required. Relatively complex instrumentation and considerable data processing are also required. The attenuation coefficient of the bone is not measured directly, but rather is inferred from the measurements by the application of a series of line integrals.

The CT scanning technique for bone measurement has progressed considerably in the past several years.[27-34] With current equipment, precision of CT measurement for vertebral bone is 1% to 3% for single energy (80 kvp) and 3% to 5% for dual energy (80–120 kvp). Recent improvements in CT technology have further increased precision at a reduced exposure to 0.32% for single energy and 1.68% for dual-photon energy. The accuracy for CT (and DPA) can, however, be as low as 15% to 20% in elderly osteoporotic patients. The CT technique is open to a number of possible errors, and problems still exist. Among the sources of error are polychromatic distortion, changes in the size of the subject between measurements, and slight movements of the subject during the measuring process. Errors from these sources can significantly affect the measurements made.

Additionally, problems with the CT scanning instrumentation have been encountered, chiefly that of drift. Calibration is, therefore, required for each scan for a bone measurement. Another problem arises from the nonuniformity of the material scanned (the least resolvable picture element problem). Beam hardening errors are also inherent, as in any radiographic technique. The latter errors can be considerably reduced by employment of monoenergetic sources. However, as noted earlier, CT measurements made with a single energy source may have an error as high as 20% for vertebral mineral content. The error is produced by the effect of tissue and variable fat concentration in the vicinity of the spine.[28,32]

The primary source of error in the CT trabecular bone measurement technique derives from the effects of fatty marrow on the measurement.[28,32] The error is largely due to the presence of yellow marrow, the density of which is less than that of the red marrow. The result is a reduction of the spinal mineral equivalent. In spinal CT scans, uncertainties $> 10\%$ are reported to have been introduced by variance in the marrow;[32] in fact the error may be as high as 20%. The uncertainty is probably greater for spinal measurements in osteoporotic individuals, since the error due to fat increases as the bone volume decreases.[28,32] Thus, a large change in bone marrow composition may be associated with a high degree of bone loss, and results in a large error in the measurement of bone by this technique. Recent refinements in localization have shown that the error can be decreased to $\sim 3\%$.[34] In addition, as CT scans also reflect the collagen content, measurements in subjects with osteoid excess (see Chapter 11) may also have large errors.[32]

Several problems of CT measurement of trabecular bone in the appendicular skeleton with x-ray sources are minimized with the use of monoenergetic radionuclides.[35] A higher resolution capability may be achieved with the use of a monochromatic source such as ^{125}I, instead of x-rays, for the measurement of trabecular bone. With dual-energy capabilities, it is possible with CT (as with dual-photon absorptiometry) to correct for overlying tissue and fat, and thus to make a satisfactory determination of the bone mass of the spine.[32] With dual-energy CT scanning, the error attributable to fat can be reduced in elderly subjects to 2% to 4%.[28,29,32]

Since only partial correction can be made for the effect of scattered radiation, it still remains a problem. Another problem, arising from the calibration technique, is the difficulty of developing standards that are identical to the bone being measured. This problem can also be minimized by replacing x-ray sources with radionuclides.

A. Clinical Applications

Several different approaches are utilized for quantitative CT scanning for bone measurement (as discussed in the preceding). Whereas CT quantitative scanning is useful for the measurement of trabecular bone, care must be taken in interpreting the results in view of all the above-mentioned potential errors.

X-ray based CT scanning has a unique capability for accurate measurement of compact bone density. Cortical bone in the appendicular skeleton has been measured by CT scanning based on x-ray sources of a single energy.[31] Commercially available equipment is widely used for these measurements. With this technique, direct measurement of compact bone in the shaft of the radius may be made with a precision of <2%.[31,36,37] These measurements are easier to validate than those of trabecular bone.

Currently, the primary application of quantitative CT is the measurement of trabecular bone in the lumbar spine.[35-41] Another application is the measurement of trabecular bone in the limbs (distal radius) with the use of monoenergetic sources. The density measurement of the distal radius has been shown to correlate well with the density determined for the lumbar spine.[35] Measurement of the distal radius has been advocated as a means of differentiating osteoporotic women from their age-matched controls.[35] An advantage of this modification for appendicular skeletal measurements is the low radiation dose of approximately 10 mrem.

Age-related vertebral bone loss has been studied in a group of men and women ranging in age from 18 to 80 years.[28,33,42,43] The rate of change of spinal trabecular mineral with age in females averages 1.2% per year from age 20 to 80 years,[43] with accelerated loss occurring at the menopause.[42,43] Vertebral trabecular bone mass in men declines an average of 0.72% per year.[43] Vertebral fracture thresholds have also been defined using CT methods; in general, vertebral compression fractures or wedging occurs with vertebral mineral values below 110 mg/cm^3.[43] Vertebral strength and failure load have also been shown to correlate well with the measurement of trabecular bone density made by CT scanning.[44,45]

CT thus provides the clinician with still another tool for evaluating and monitoring therapeutic responses in the different forms of osteoporosis (see Chapter 12). Measurement of bone mass by the CT technique, however, is still limited by certain technical problems that require further experimental work for their resolution. Two areas requiring study for scanning accuracy are those of polychromatic errors and calibration problems (repositioning errors). Extraction of information from data obtained by the CT technique requires complex instrumentation and data processing. In addition to the need for sophisticated calibration and positioning techniques, careful technical monitoring is essential. With continued development, particularly with the dual-energy photon technique, CT scanning holds great promise both as an investigative and a clinical tool.

VI. COMPTON SCATTERING TECHNIQUE (CS)

The Compton scattering (CS) technique utilizes the scattering of a beam of gamma rays into a detector. Two orthogonal photon beams are employed. The level of activity detected is a function of the density of the bone target.[46] The measurement obtained is the average density of both the organic and the inorganic components of the volume of bone studied.

One advantage of the CS technique is that the scattering volume can be located entirely within weight-bearing trabecular bone. Another advantage of this technique is that, unlike other interactive processes that depend on both effective atomic number and mean density, the CS technique depends only on density. As repositioning of the scattering volume is relatively simple, the measurement is not a function of the thickness of the bone or of its possible rotation. Thus, the precision of the method is very high. The combined features of high Compton interaction probability and the ability to optimize the physical factors that determine the precision suggest that this technique has high potential for bone density measurement.

There are, however, several technical problems to be resolved before widespread use can be achieved.[47] The principal disadvantage of the Compton scattering technique results from the multiple scattering effects of a fixed point measurement. Thus, one of the technical problems is the evaluation of the contribution of those photons that are multiply scattered. Multiple scattering is a particular problem when the bone studied differs from the calibration standard. As mentioned, constituents of bone other than the mineral content are also reflected in the measurement. As in all partial body studies, patient or sample area positioning is very important. In this technique, the precision depends largely on the size of the volume measured. Density measurements of the os calcis have been considerably more reproducible than density measurements of the distal radius. Unfortunately, the density of the os calcis is influenced by body weight, as this bone reflects mechanical stress. It is possible that positioning problems may be encountered in the measurement of an area of cortical bone and that they may decrease the precision. Both development and application of the CS technique have advanced in recent years, and several different approaches for the application of this technique to bone measurement have been made.

In principle, the intensity of the photons scattered from bone depends on its electron density. The measured energy of the scattered radiation depends on the angle at which the scatter is measured. It is theoretically possible to detect scattered radiation from a very small volume (2–10 cm^3) of trabecular bone by the use of focused collimators. The effects of overlying soft tissue and compact bone can be minimized, so that only the trabecular bone is measured. Both the incident radiation and the emergent scattered radiation are, however, attenuated by overlying tissue. Initially, a second source having the same energy as that of the scatter radiation was used to correct for attenuation.[48,49] Presently, a single source with a high energy (100 keV) is used for both scattering and attenuation correction.[50]

Some of these problems are minimized by measuring the relative extent of both Compton and coherent scattering.[51-53] In all CS techniques for measuring bone, there are errors due principally to the multiple scattering and the uncertainty as to the scattering volume measured.[54,55] Results from studies employing ^{153}Gd and ^{153}Sm, a very small scattering angle, and GeLi solid state detectors indicate that the errors can be minimized.[56,57] A high correlation (r = 0.97) was obtained between coherent-Compton ratios and density of bone phantoms with the use of ^{241}Am and ^{153}Gd sources.[56] Filtered x-rays and ^{241}Am have also been used to measure trabecular bone by coherence scattering.[53,58] Whereas the marrow fat content produced a significant increase in the error, the attenuation by the surrounding tissue and compact bone was minimized. Since the CS techniques concentrate on measuring trabecular bone density, one must also be aware that the marrow fat affects the measurement. The precision of the technique has been established as 3% to 5%.

A. Clinical Applications

Changes with age of trabecular bone in the distal radius of normal subjects have been measured with CS scanning.[59] The trabecular density measurement was consistently higher than that reported with the use of other techniques.[11] This difference is possibly a result either of multiple scattering or of inappropriate correction for attenuation.[11] To date, it has not been possible to separate clearly osteoporotic individuals from normals on the basis of trabecular bone density measurements.

The coherent-Compton technique appears to provide a more accurate measurement of trabecular bone than CS scanning alone. Work is in progress to develop this technique and to resolve its inherent problems. The technique has considerable potential, and it is likely that with different sources, the use of microprocessors, and more sophisticated instrumentation, a clinically useful technique will emerge.

VII. STIMULATED POSITRON EMISSION (SPE)

Bone mass has also been quantified using stimulated positron emission (SPE) procedures.[60] A cross section of the body containing bone is excited by high-energy x-rays (hv > 1.022 MeV) to produce positron-electron pairs. The positron distribution is imaged by means of two detectors placed on opposite sides of the irradiated section, focused to receive annihilations produced inside the bone. Since the cross section for pair production in the bone tissue is proportional to the square of the atomic number of the absorber, demineralization of bone strongly affects the number of counts received from that region. This technique is unique among radiologic procedures for bone measurement in that it has direct three-dimensional imaging capability. Its precision is limited only by the allowable radiation dose and the volume of the bone target irradiated. Measurements can be confined to a specific bone site to maximize signal-to-noise ratio (i.e., ratio of surrounding tissue to bone tissue). High sensitivity to small changes (~5%) in density or amount of cortical bone can be obtained with a dose of < 0.5 rad. With the same dose, however, the method is less sensitive to changes in vertebral bone, as there is a lower amount of target mineral in this type of bone. A precision of 5% to 10% has been obtained with a 2 to 5 rad dose. The optimal energy for maximizing the sensitivity while minimizing the loss of spatial resolution due to the positron range lies between 2 and 3 MeV.

The unique features of the SPE technique are the direct three-dimensional imaging capability, high sensitivity to mineral content, well-defined signal, and relative immunity from the effects of changing body size. Unlike the CT scanning technique, SPE requires no mathematical algorithm for reconstruction of the image. The computational effort is considerably reduced, and errors associated with some types of transformation required in the process of reconstruction are eliminated. Thus the SPE technique appears to provide an attractive assessment of bone mass. Further work, however, is necessary to develop this technique before it can be advocated as clinically useful.

VIII. DUAL ENERGY RADIOGRAPHY (DER)

A new technique that uses dual-energy, pulsed x-ray technology provides quantification of bone mineral content in a shorter scan time and with lower dose to the subject than that used for CT or DPA.[61] The procedure, also known as quantitative digital radiography and x-ray absorptiometry, is similar to DPA in that total bone mineral of lumbar vertebrae L_1–L_4 is quantified. However, DER employs pulses of 70 and 140 kVp radiation alternating at 60 cycles/sec as the radiation source instead of ^{153}Gd. Preliminary results indicate a short-term precision for measurements of vertebral bone mass of 0.5% to 1.0%.[61]

IX. NEUTRON ACTIVATION

In all the techniques previously discussed, the precision or reproducibility is high for serial determinations in the same subject. Thus, even if absolute measurements are not accurate, relative measurements yield the data necessary for the study of time-related changes. For diagnostic determination, however, an accurate measure of bone mass is required for the evaluation of whole body or regional calcium deficits. Hence, for these studies, the bone mass must be measured absolutely. A technique that measures calcium directly, and hence bone mass, is neutron activation analysis. With the neutron activation technique, calcium may be measured either in a specified anatomic region (e.g., the hand, the torso) or in the entire body.

A. Partial Body

Determination of calcium and phosphorus in the hand is the simplest of the neutron activation measurements and requires the lowest radiation exposure to the individual.[62] The low radiation dose and the relative simplicity of the technique are its most attractive features. The measurement permits normalization for size by determination of hand volume. The results must, of course, be extrapolated to the whole skeleton, and the validity of the extrapolation verified. However, whereas there is a degree of uncertainty in extrapolating from the hand to the entire skeleton, it is less than that involved in extrapolating from the measurement of the linear density of a few millimeters of bone in the radius to the whole body, as is the procedure with absorptiometric measurements.

Partial body neutron activation analysis (PBNAA) of the torso is a compromise between hand activation and total body activation. The partial body neutron activation technique essentially measures the calcium in the trunk and upper thigh.[63-65] There are several advantages to irradiating the torso rather than a hand or the whole body. Since a large portion of the body is activated, the response is more representative of changes in the skeletal mass than is the response of an extremity such as the hand. Changes in the bone mass of osteoporotic patients may be more sensitively detected than with total body irradiation, as the spine is a larger fraction of the irradiated skeleton. Finally, the torso activation technique is somewhat simpler to apply than the total body neutron activation technique and as such has had considerable application in clinical studies.[63]

There are, however, some inherent disadvantages to the partial body neutron activation technique as compared with the total body neutron activation technique. As with all partial body measurement techniques, it is difficult to achieve an absolute measurement. In partial body activation techniques, the error introduced by repositioning alone can be substantial. In the torso activation technique, the size of the neutron irradiation field is fixed; hence, a variable portion of the skeleton of various individuals is irradiated and counted, depending on the body habitus of the subject. The portion that lies within the irradiated volume varies from 33% of the skeleton of large men to 50% of that of small women. The precision (reproducibility) of the system is ± 4% (1 SD) for the phantom used, and ± 5% for a human subject.[63]

The ^{238}Pu,Be sources used in this technique are relatively weak and have to be placed close to the body; thus, the geometry corrections for thickness of the irradiated subject are especially critical for this partial body activation technique. In addition, the proximity of the sources produces a radiation dose of 500 mrem. This is 1.8 times the dose to this critical body area received in the ^{238}Pu,Be total body neutron activation (270 mrem). An empirically derived factor has to be applied to the raw data to correct for the combined effects of nonuniformity of neutron fluence and gamma ray attenuation.

As for all the measurement techniques, it is highly important to normalize the data for skeletal size or analyze the data in terms of a reference standard to provide a rational uniform basis for the comparison of individuals of different sizes. For this purpose, the induced calcium counts have been normalized by the cube of the height of the individual.[63] The resulting value is termed the calcium bone index.[63] No correction is specifically provided for sex or age in the calculation of this particular normalization.

B. Total Body Neutron Activation

With the total body neutron activation analysis (TBNAA) technique, total body calcium is measured directly and absolutely.[66-70] The measurement reflects the total skeletal mass. With this technique, the patient is uniformly exposed to a beam of partially moderated fast neutrons. This exposure to neutrons provides a small skin dose (0.28–2.0 rem, for α,n sources and cyclotron neutrons, respectively) with the bone marrow dose less than one third the skin dose. As noted previously, the average dose equivalent to the skin in a total body activation is approximately one half of that delivered in the partial body activation of the torso.

The ^{49}Ca induced with this procedure is measured absolutely with an appropriate whole-body counter. From the data, not only the absolute values of total body calcium but also those of phosphorus, sodium, and chlorine can be determined.[66] The accuracy of this technique in a human subject is ± 5%, and the precision in an anthropomorphic phantom is ± 1.0% (1 SD). Total body calcium values are normalized for body size, sex, and age, so that the relative deficit in skeletal mass can be determined for each individual. Two sources of error in the TBNAA technique for calcium measurement derive directly from two primary requirements of the technique.[66] The first requirement is the necessity of achieving uniform neutron irradiation of the body calcium. The degree of uniformity of thermal neutron flux achieved by various investigators ranges from 5%, when the neutron source is a cyclotron, to 15% when portable α,n sources are utilized. The uniformity achieved by the various systems developed is generally satisfactory for measurement. Problems occur with grossly obese patients, and with patients who lose a large amount of weight during the course of therapy. The second requirement for TBNAA is the availability of a whole-body counter with an invariant counting response, or with a means of correcting for the attenuation of the induced ^{49}Ca. This correction is most accurate in the more advanced Brookhaven whole-body counter. In longitudinal studies, however, these two requirements do not significantly influence the precision, although they do affect the accuracy of the measurement.

The noninvasive nature of the technique and the low radiation dose to the subject allow the study of large normal populations as well as the study of osteopenic populations. The precision of the technique also makes it useful as a sensitive indicator of overall therapeutic efficacy. An obvious disadvantage of the TBNAA technique is that it is incapable of revealing a change confined to a small volume of the body. Small changes in bone mass at a particular site are masked by the large amount of calcium in the total body. Also, TBNAA cannot distinguish between skeletal and ectopic calcium.

Because TBNAA facilities are relatively complex and expensive, few are presently available. The limitations of the application of TBNAA are hence both technical and economic, in certain aspects.[70] However, both these limiting factors existed for the CT scanning technique, which now has wide acceptance and use in medical practice. The recent reduction in cost and increased availability of portable α,n neutron sources, as well as the recognition of the general usefulness of highly sensitive whole-body counters, should make this technique more readily available to medical research centers.[71] It is most likely that there will be a considerable growth in the application of this technique in medicine.[70,72,73]

The Brookhaven whole-body counter used in TBNAA studies to 1986 was updated with new detectors and electronics. These increased the sensitivity by a factor of approximately 4 and also enhanced the precision of the TBNAA technique for measuring total body calcium.

There are data to suggest that the ideal measure of demineralization that occurs with age or with certain diseases is the determination of calcium loss from the entire skeleton.[73-76] Thus, it is possible with TBNAA to infer skeletal mass with both high accuracy and high precision, since 99% of the total body calcium (TBCa) stored in the body is located in the skeleton.

C. Clinical Applications

The clinical utility of total body neutron activation was first demonstrated in 1972. Since that time, numerous studies employing measurement of both total and partial body calcium have been conducted[62-81] and changes in bone mass in normal subjects with respect to age, sex, and body size established.[76-78] The determinants of bone mass in postmenopausal women have also been reported.[79] Models describing the rate of loss of calcium from the body have been developed from TBNAA data[80] and both absolute and relative deficits in calcium in osteoporotic patients established.[77,78,81] A number of studies have used TBNAA and PBNAA to monitor the efficacy of therapy in osteoporosis.[66,73] Finally, logistic regression models have been developed from total body calcium (TBCa) data (and DPA and CT data as well) to identify women at risk for developing osteoporosis.[74,75]

X. METHODS OF EXPRESSING DATA; NORMALIZATION OF BONE MASS FOR BODY SIZE

In longitudinal studies, serial measurements of an individual are made in order to trace the time variation in bone mass. The individual, then, serves as his or her own reference control. The measurements made are relative and do not have to be expressed in absolute units. These measurements must, however, be reproducible within specific levels of precision. In a cross-sectional study, the bone mass of an individual is measured and compared with a reference standard or value. For these studies, an absolute measure of bone mass is generally required, or a reference must be available against which a particular measurement can be compared. However, the absolute amount of bone *per se* is not sufficient for evaluating the degree of calcification of an individual; body size, sex, age, and body habitus must be taken into account. The degrees of calcification of individuals differ markedly on the basis of these parameters. Total body calcium may vary from approximately 750 g in a 5 ft normal woman of small frame to 1250 g in a 6 ft normal man of large frame.

It is clear that bone mass measurement must be referred, or normalized, to skeletal size in order to determine the relative deficit or excess in bone calcium. This normalization is particularly important for those techniques that measure linear density (such as photon absorptiometry). Whereas normalization of bone mineral content values by the width of the radius, for example, decreases somewhat the variance of each sex-age group, the procedure does not satisfactorily normalize BMC for skeletal size. Such normalization is needed whenever the value of calcium deficit in an individual is desired. Comparison of individuals matched only for sex and age, or assessment of individuals with sex- and age-matched population, can lead to erroneous conclusions about the degree of mineralization, since the significant factor of body habitus is largely disregarded. (Some correction is introduced, of course, by the use of the parameter of sex.)

A technique developed for normalization of bone mineral content or, actually, total body calcium, employs a predicted normal value based on four parameters: height, lean body mass (based on the measurement of ^{40}K), age, and sex.[77,78] The variance of the ratio of the measured to predicted bone mass calculated with the use of these parameters is significantly less than the variance of the ratio of measured bone mass to that of age- and sex-matched normal individuals. Values of total body calcium predicted from height and weight are subject to larger errors than are values predicted from height and lean body mass, because of the effect of the highly variable fat content.[77] It is clearly important to interpret individual bone mass values in terms of a well-matched reference value. Some of the discrepancies in the bone mass measurements obtained by different investigators analyzing similar clinical situations can be explained by failure to normalize the bone mass data for skeletal size.

The large inherent variability in partial body measurements, particularly those involving density measurements, and the inability to normalize these data for skeletal size render these measurements rather unsatisfactory for the evaluation of the extent of osteopenia in a single individual. A highly important function which TBNAA fulfills is that it provides a reference value of total bone mass against which values obtained from various peripheral bone measurements may be compared. The technique of obtaining the total body calcium measurement, normalized for sex, age, skeletal size, and body habitus, provides an accurate method for evaluating the absolute as well as the relative loss of bone mass, and supplies an essential index for quantifying the degree of osteopenia in an individual.

Adequate normalization for bone and body size is required to minimize the intragroup biological variability and to maximize intergroup differences for measurements of bone mass.[81] Various attempts have been made to correct for bone mass variability in age-sex groups by the use of skeletal size parameters. For example, since the heterogeneity of skeletal size influences radiogrammetric measurements, Dequeker[83] related the absolute cortical bone mass index to an independent skeletal size parameter, namely, the metacarpal length. The effect of size of the metacarpal bone on cortical bone mass, however, was not uniform, and thus a correction for age was introduced as well. No consensus has been developed on how best to express the data from SPA, DPA, and CT scanning. Normalization of data for skeletal size appears to be applied only rarely to DPA or CT data.

For BMC of the radius,[82,84] it has been shown that it is possible to normalize for skeletal size with the use of height and lean body mass; the biological variation in a sex- and age-matched group was reduced.[82,84] The variability of lumbar BMC measured by DPA has also been related to skeletal size.[85] Because the effect of skeletal size correction was not uniform, it was necessary in addition to construct, for each decade, a cumulative percentage frequency distribution nomogram of the BMC data.[85] In some instances, normalizing bone mass against height, weight, and lean body mass did not reduce the biological variation in the BMC data.[86] In studies wherein attempts were made to separate normal individuals from osteoporotics, radial BMC data were adjusted by regression analysis with appropriate independent variables.[87]

No agreement has been reached on how best to express the BMC of the spine, whether measured by DPA or CT. DPA data are currently expressed as standard BMC per unit area in mg/cm^2; total integral bone mass (IBM) is expressed in grams or in a derived "corpus" measurement reflecting total integral bone density (IBD) in mg/cm^3. In a similar manner, the CT measurement is customarily expressed as vertebral body trabecular bone density in mg/cm^3, total integral bone mass (IBM) in grams, and total integral bone density (IBD) in mg/cm^3. There are few reports of attempts to normalize either DPA or CT spinal data for skeletal size directly, employing height or any parameter of bone size other than vertebral area, since the clinical interpretation of lumbar BMC data normalized to body height, weight, or vertebral size is considered by many to be of little use in discriminating between normal and osteoporotic patients.

XI. INTERCOMPARISON OF VARIOUS TECHNIQUES

The type of noninvasive measurement of bone mass selected for a study depends to a large extent on the nature and type of data required. Measurements of bone mass generally are employed in two basic types of studies, longitudinal and cross-sectional. Large-scale cross-sectional studies of osteopenia are easier and less expensive to conduct if bone mass can be ascertained by the relatively simple radiogrammetric or densitometric measurement of the metacarpals or the radius than by the more sophisticated photoabsorptiometric, CT, and neutron activation methods. Data accumulated by a number of laboratories indicate that measurements of the appendicular skeleton reflect total body calcium content reasonably well in most instances. The most interesting observation to be drawn from the reports of the results of the various bone measuring techniques is the considerable number of correlations that exist with respect to their clinical application. For example, the correlation coefficient of radial bone mineral content and total body calcium in crush-fracture osteoporotic patients has been reported to be as high as 0.826 ($p < 0.001$).[81] On the other hand, the correlation between the change in radial BMC and TBCa in osteopenic patients in response to therapy was very poor.

In a 1975 study, the correlation between TBCa (by TBNAA) and BMC (by SPA) at six different sites on the appendicular skeleton of osteoporotic females varied from 0.84 to 0.94 ($p < 0.001$).[88] By contrast, a 1984 study reported a correlation of 0.72 between radius BMC (by SPA) and total body bone mass (by DPA) in both normal and osteoporotic females.[89] The BMC of the radius, however, did not correlate well with spinal BMC (by DPA) in normal females ($r = 0.44$) and did not correlate at all in osteoporotic females.[89]

Currently, the three techniques that appear most useful for discriminating osteoporotic from normal individuals are dual-photon absorptiometry, computed tomography, and neutron activation analysis. Whereas the goal of each of these techniques is the same—to determine the degree of mineralization of the skeletal tissue—the measurements differ markedly. Neutron activation analysis (TBNAA and PBNAA) makes a direct measurement of the total or partial body calcium. Dual-photon absorptiometry (DPA) measures the trabecular and cortical bone in a section of vertebra, and computed tomography (CT) measures primarily trabecular bone in the spine. The results of the DPA and CT measurement of the spine are generally assumed to be a more critical index of bone change in osteoporotic patients than other whole-body or appendicular skeletal measurements of bone mineral content. TBCa, which measures the total trabecular and cortical bone in the body, has been shown to provide an effective method of monitoring the response to therapy and to discriminate between normal and osteoporotic patients.[73-75,90]

Few comparisons have been made, to date, in clinical studies, among absolute values of bone mineral, normalized values (values corrected for variation due to factors such as skeletal size), and percentage change over long periods of time as determined by means of the three techniques. Unnormalized data from neutron activation analysis for total body calcium and DPA data for localized areas are well correlated, since the values are a function of the size of the patient. However, the correlation is reduced when the data are normalized for body size.[85,91] It has been suggested that this weaker correlation may reflect an inappropriate application of the normalization procedure.[91] Normalization of only one of the sets of data also results in a lack of correlation.[91] It has to be emphasized that unnormalized values for total body calcium (or mineral content) yield little information on the adequacy of the mineralization of the individual. While there may be a lack of agreement on the appropriate normalization procedure, there cannot be any doubt that normalization for body size and habitus is essential for a meaningful interpretation of the data. Determination of the appropriate necessary normalization procedure presents considerable difficulty in all instances when extrapolation must be made from a measurement of a small localized area (or volume) to total body calcium or bone mineral content.

The assumption of uniformity may not hold; one may very well be sampling a volume that is not typical of the osseous system as a whole.

The most meaningful comparison between the results of the methods used to monitor the response to therapy examines the measurements of changes over a period of time. Most of these comparisons, however, have failed to demonstrate significant correlations. Reasonable agreement was found in one long-term study that compared the percentage change in bone mass measured by single-photon absorptiometry with that obtained by neutron activation at the same partial body site (the forearm).[91] The two techniques yielded data that were significantly correlated ($r = 0.61$, $p < 0.001$). Thus, these two techniques could be considered equally sensitive *in vivo* methods for monitoring changes in bone mineral content in the forearm.[91]

If an absolute measurement is required, the data must be normalized for the size of the skeleton in each individual, as previously discussed. The normalization process required with any partial body measurement is a very difficult one. When different areas or volumes of a bone are studied in various individuals and then intercompared, the common basis for comparison is often lost and an additional source of error is introduced. One problem encountered is that the fixed size of the photon beam results in measurement of different portions of a bone, in accordance with the size of the particular individual under study. Thus, varying percentages of bone contribute to the bone mineral content measurement. These errors can be reduced to some extent by careful repositioning of the photon beam centrally for each measurement of the vertebrae. The precision of the DPA technique for measuring bone mineral content in long-term studies is approximately the same as that of TBNAA, 2% to 3%.

The use of the CT and DPA techniques for osteoporotic patients is advantageous in several respects over the technique of TBNAA. Most of the patients identified as osteoporotic present with clinical symptoms of pain and disability associated with spontaneous crush fractures of one or more vertebrae. Hence, DPA measurements made on the spinal column are considered by most to be of prime importance, although not all investigators agree on this point.

An advantage of DPA is that the radiation dose to the individual is a small fraction of the dose required for TBNAA or CT scanning. Additionally, the apparatus of DPA is far less expensive than that required for TBNAA or CT. The cost of the source of radiation for DPA, ^{153}Gd, is lower than that of the multiple sources of ^{238}Pu,Be required for TBNAA. Further, no shielding is required. The cost of the DPA system is comparable to that of the partial body neutron activation system and far less than that of CT equipment.[66] CT has been widely used in recent years for measuring primarily the trabecular bone in the spine and also compact bone, peripherally. The potential advantage of the CT technique over that of DPA is its capability of precise three-dimensional anatomic localization, which provides a direct density measurement. It also has a capability for spatial separation of highly responsive cancellous bone from less responsive cortical bone.

The lumbar vertebral column has substantial amounts of compact bone in the dense vertebral plates and laminae, which are included in the DPA scan. DPA scan includes in the integral measurement vertebral compression and callous formation, angular and scoliotic deformity, hypertrophy of articular facets, and marginal osteophytosis as well as extraosseous calcification. The result is often an inaccurate and poorly reproducible measurement. Thus, in the DPA scan, the data represent an integral of compact and cancellous bone. Such an area projection may not be comparable to that obtained by CT because of the inclusion of low-turnover compact bone.

The most important criterion in the selection of a technique for measuring bone mass noninvasively would appear to be the ability to predict women at risk for development of osteoporosis, that is, the ability to discriminate between normal and osteoporotic patients prior to the appearance of a compression fracture. Another highly important criterion is the effectiveness of the technique for monitoring the response to therapy. Additional criteria are availability (commercial equipment is, of course, desirable), reasonable cost, low radiation exposure, and suitability for clinical application. The societal question of whether our finite medical resources should be allocated to mass screening of peri- and postmenopausal women in terms of cost and benefit has recently been addressed.[14,92,93]

A summary of the present characteristics of the various noninvasive techniques is presented in Table 9–1. The types of bone measured, sites of measurements, precision, discrimination ability, radiation dose, availability, cost, and patient acceptance are listed.

The correlations among the bone mass values obtained with six of the techniques in a group of 50 postmenopausal women have also been tabulated[90] (Table 9–3). Significant correlations were found between certain of the techniques as indicated. The average error in predicting bone mass at one site from measurement at a different location was 14%.[90]

The major conclusion from this study was the poor correlation between CT and the other techniques. It has been suggested, however, that when similar parameters of skeletal mineral content are measured by CT and DPA, no real discrepancy exists.[94] Some assume that the parameter that best correlates with fracture frequency is the vertebral trabecular density.[94] The data indicate, however, that residual fundamental differences in results do exist between those obtained by CT and those produced by other techniques. These differences may relate to the ability of the technique to define edges of the same volume for reproducibility; to inherent errors involved in CT-based measurements (such as the effect of bone marrow fat); or to the fact that CT measures primarily trabecular bone, whereas the other techniques also measure compact bone albeit in different amounts.

Table 9–3. Correlation Coefficients Between Techniques

	SPA-D	SPA-M	DPA	CT	X-ray
TBC	0.77 (49) ***	0.80 (49) ***	0.66 (40) ***	0.28 (33) ***	0.53 (48) ***
SPA-D	—	0.87 (50) ***	0.56 (36) ***	0.21 (32)	0.56 (48) ***
SPA-M		—	0.60 (36) ***	0.41 (32) *	0.53 (48) ***
DPA			—	0.07 (23)	0.48 (35)
CT				—	0.32 (32)

*p < 0.05; **p < 0.01; ***p < 0.001; ( ) = n.

TBC, Total body calcium by total body neutron activation analysis (g). *SPA-D,* Single-photon absorptiometry of diaphysis of radius (g/cm). *SPA-M,* Single-photon absorptiometry of metaphysis of radius (g/cm). *DPA,* Dual-photon absorptiometry of spine (L1–L4) g/scan line. *CT,* Computed tomography of spine (trabecular bone), (mg/cc) (T12–L3). *X-ray,* radiogrammography of third to fifth phalanges.

From Chesnut CH: Noninvasive techniques in the diagnosis of osteoporosis. *In* Osteoporosis Consensus Development Conference Statement, Clinical Center NIH, Apr. 2–4, 1984, Bethesda, MD, Vol. 5, No. 3, 1984.

XII. SUMMARY AND CONCLUSIONS

Each of the presently available noninvasive methods used to determine the degree of mineralization and the nature and degree of changes in skeletal tissue has significant advantages and limitations. Radiographic techniques are applicable to all parts of the entire skeleton, but lack the sensitivity required for quantifying levels of change associated with the development of pathologic conditions indicative of a patient at risk. Quantitative bone roentgenography or radiogrammetry, which measures cortical thickness of the appendicular skeleton, is relatively precise, but not necessarily indicative of the status of the axial skeleton. Single-photon absorptiometric techniques, although highly quantitative and precise, provide information on highly localized portions of the appendicular skeleton. Extrapolation of the findings to the axial skeleton have not proved to be valid for all individuals.

Large-scale cross-sectional studies of osteopenia are easier and less expensive to conduct if bone mass can be ascertained by the relatively simple radiogrammetric and densitometric measurement of the metacarpals or the radius than by the more sophisticated DPA, CT, or neutron activation methods. Data accumulated by a number of laboratories indicate that measurements of the appendicular skeleton reflect total body calcium content reasonably well, in most instances.

Comparison of the various noninvasive bone mass measuring techniques reveals a considerable number of correlations existing with respect to their clinical application. On the other hand, poor correlations were noted between CT and other techniques. Further, the correlation in osteopenic patients is, generally, not as high as that observed in a normal control population.

It was also noted that the rate of change of BMC at different sites varies when compared with the rate of change of TBCa. This finding is not surprising, in view of the differential rate of loss of bone in various parts of the skeletons of osteopenic patients. These differential rates are averaged in a total body calcium measurement.

The DPA and CT techniques appear to be the most useful for measurement of spinal bone density in the study of osteoporosis. Computed tomography offers significant potential advantages over other techniques, but still requires further work for the solution of inherent technical problems. Similarly, considerable additional work is required for Compton scattering techniques; the technical problems associated with these techniques are formidable. Neutron activation analysis permits the direct *in vivo* measurement of total calcium content of the body or parts of the body, and hence skeletal mass, with a high degree of precision. However, whereas there is a large clinical and research experience with partial body and total body neutron activation, the techniques are not yet routinely available. The development of commercial equipment along with some simplification of the elaborate research model could reduce the cost considerably.

Although all of these noninvasive techniques have been used for many years to estimate bone mass, the wide ranges of their precision and accuracy and their relative insensitivity to early small changes have precluded general applicability of any single technique for the early detection of osteopenic disorders that cause the individual to become fracture-prone.

The question has not been resolved as to whether bone mineral content measurement of the spine by DPA or CT or total body calcium measurement by neutron activation (the primary techniques) best reflects changes in bone mass after therapy. In particular, it has not been established that the contribution of trabecular bone to the strength of the human lumbar vertebrae is greater than that of cortical bone. The nondestructive compressive strength of excised human lumbar vertebrae indicates that 45% to 75% of the peak strength, regardless of percentage ash or physical density of the trabecular bone, is contributed by the cortex.[95] Further, studies of regional bone mineral "density" in osteoporotic women, performed with DPA, noted that ". . . there was not obvious preferential demineralization of the spine."[96,97] A unique advantage of the total body calcium measurement is that it can readily be normalized for body size, sex, and age, so that the relative deficiency in skeletal mass can be determined for each individual.[77,81] The usefulness of the normalization of the bone mass of osteoporotic patients obtained from localized measurements by means of the data obtained from normal young women is of questionable value.

A high degree of precision (reproducibility) is a necessity for meaningful relative bone measurements. Each of the primary techniques described is adequately precise (2% to 3%), although the accuracy is less (>5%). There is an inherent difficulty in measuring small bone mass changes in patients receiving therapy when the normal loss with age or disease is only about 1% to 2% per year in elderly women. It is necessary, therefore, to study large groups over long periods of time and/or increase the precision of the measuring techniques to obtain the data necessary for the appropriate evaluation of therapeutic regimens. TBNAA remains the only direct measure of bone (total body calcium) and thus serves as the ultimate standard for validation of indirect density measuring techniques such as DPA. With current technology, it is possible to increase the precision of the measurements. For example, some present neutron activation systems are at least 15 to 18 years old; updating the instrumentation would greatly enhance their sensitivity and precision and could also reduce the cost, so that the equipment could become more widely available.

Neither the CT nor DPA technique has yet been shown to discriminate as significantly between osteoporotic subjects and normals as the technique of total body neutron activation.[74] It is most useful to employ two or more measurements of bone mass for discriminating osteoporotics from normal individuals.[74] It is essential to obtain the measure of structural integrity by assessing total bone normalized for the individual in terms of sex, age, and body habitus. This normalization is most easily performed on TBNAA data. It is also desirable to have some measure of the change of the more metabolically active trabecular bone in the spine, as obtained by DPA and CT. Measurements of both these parameters are the most useful in therapeutic trials to determine the status of the disease and the efficacy of a therapeutic regimen.

It should be stressed that while the reduction in the bone mass is the single most important correlate with fracture incidence in osteoporosis, other factors are also involved. For example, trauma and structural changes in bone *per se* are also determinants of fracture incidence. Even if the precision of the systems were perfect, the biological characteristics of the bone remodeling system in humans are such that long-term extrapolation from rates of change of bone mass measured over relatively short periods of time is not always statistically possible.[98] The qualitative nature of bone also needs to be considered as well as the dynamics of the underlying cellular mechanisms (see Chapter 1).

It is important to continue the development of new methods for determining bone mass and to intercalibrate all the primary bone measuring techniques (such as CT and CS), along with the numerous secondary techniques, in large-scale, well-controlled clinical studies. Only in this way can one obtain information necessary to evaluate the efficacy of therapeutic agents in the treatment of demineralizing bone diseases. The information is also essential for a better understanding of the basic physiologic changes that occur in aging and in diseases that demineralize bone and leave the individual susceptible to both spontaneous and traumatic fracture.

References

1. Cohn SH (ed): Non-invasive Measurements of Bone Mass and Their Clinical Application. Boca Raton, CRC Press, 1981.
2. Mazess RB: Bone density in diagnosis of osteoporosis: Thresholds and breakpoints. Calcif Tissue Int 41:117–118, 1987.
3. Seldin DW, Esser PD, Alderson PO: Comparison of bone density measurements from different skeletal sites. J Nucl Med 29:168–173, 1988.
4. Wahner HW, Eastell R, Riggs BL: Bone mineral density of the radius: Where do we stand? J Nucl Med 26:1339–1341, 1985.
5. Mazess RB, Barden H, Ettinger M, Schultz E: Bone density of the radius, spine and proximal femur in osteoporosis. J Bone Mineral Res 3:13–18, 1988.
6. Meema HE, Meema S: Radiogrammetry. *In* Cohn SH (ed): Non-Invasive Measurements of Bone Mass and Their Clinical Application. Boca Raton, CRC Press, 1981, pp 6–50.
7. Fox KM, Tobin JD, Plato CC: Longitudinal study of bone loss in the second metacarpal. Calcif Tissue Int 39:218–225, 1986.
8. Colbert C, Bachtell RS: Radiographic absorptiometry (photo densitometry). *In* Cohn SH (ed): Non-invasive Measurements of Bone Mass and Their Clinical Application. Boca Raton, CRC Press, 1981, pp 51–84.
9. Shimmins J, Smith DA, Aitken M, et al: The accuracy and reproducibility of bone mineral measurements in vivo. Clin Radiol 23:47–51, 1972.
10. Goldsmith N, Johnston JO, Ury H, et al: Bone mineral estimation in normal and osteoporotic women. J Bone Joint Surg 53A:83–100, 1971.
11. Mazess RB: The noninvasive measurement of skeletal mass. *In* Peck WA (ed): Bone and Mineral Research, Annual I. Amsterdam, Excerpta Medica, 1983, pp 226–279.
12. Vartsky D, Ellis KJ, Pearlstein TB, et al: Numerical filtering method for elimination of errors in bone mineral measurements caused by finite photon beam size. Proceedings Fourth International Conference on Bone Measurement, NIH 80-1939, Toronto, 1980, pp 9–13.
13. Pocock NA, Eisman JA, Yeates MG, et al: Limitations of forearm bone densitometry as index of vertebral or femoral neck osteopenia. J Bone Mineral Res 1:369–375, 1986.
14. Ott SM, Kilcoyne RF, Chesnut III CH: Ability of four different techniques of measuring bone mass to diagnose vertebral fractures in postmenopausal women. J Bone Mineral Res 2:201–210, 1987.
15. Seeman E, Wahner HW, Offord KP, et al: Differential effects of endocrine dysfunction on the axial and the appendicular skeleton. J Clin Invest 69:1302–1309, 1982.
16. Christiansen C, Rodbro P: Long term reproducibility of bone mineral content measurements. Scand J Clin Lab Invest 37:321–323, 1977.
17. Grubb SA, Jacobson PC, Awbrey BJ: Bone density in osteopenic women: A modified distal radius density measurement procedure to develop an "at risk" value for use in screening women. J Orthop Res 2:322–327, 1984.
18. Peppler WW, Mazess RB: Total body bone mineral and lean body mass by dual-photon absorptiometry. I. Theory and measurement procedure. Calcif Tissue Int 33:353–359, 1981.
19. Bohr H, Schaadt O: Bone mineral content of femoral bone and the lumbar spine measured in women with fracture of the femoral neck by dual photon absorptiometry. Clin Orthop Rel Res 179:240–245, 1983.
20. Mazess RB, Peppler WW, Chesnut III CH, et al: Total body bone mineral and lean body mass by dual-photon absorptiometry. II. Comparison with total body calcium by neutron activation analysis. Calcif Tissue Int 33:361–363, 1981.
21. Krolner B, Pors Nielsen S: Measurement of bone mineral content (BMC) of the lumbar spine. I. Theory and application of a new two-dimensional dual-photon attenuation method. J Clin Lab Invest 40:653–663, 1980.
22. Dunn WL, Wahner H, Riggs BL: Measurement of bone mineral content in human vertebrae and hip by dual-photon absorptiometry. Radiology 136:485–487, 1980.
23. Riggs BL, Wahner HW, Dunn WL, et al: Differential changes in bone mineral density of appendicular and axial skeleton with aging: Relationship to spinal osteoporosis. J Clin Invest 67:328–335, 1981.
24. Krolner B, Pors Nielson S, Lund B, et al: Measurement of bone mineral content (BMC) of the lumbar spine. II. Correlation between forearm BMC and lumbar spine BMC. Scand J Clin Lab Invest 40:665–670, 1980.
25. Krolner B, Pors Nielson S: Bone mineral content of the lumbar spine in normal and osteoporotic women; cross sectional longitudinal studies. Clin Sci 62:329–336, 1982.
26. Stevenson JC, Banks LM, Spinks TJ, et al: Regional and total skeletal measurements in the early postmenopause. J Clin Invest 80:258–262, 1987.
27. Cann CE, Ettinger B, Gordon CS: Quantitative com-

puted tomography of vertebral spongiosa: A sensitive method for detecting early bone loss after oophorectomy. Ann Intern Med 97:699–705, 1982.

28. Pacifici R, Susman N, Carr PL, et al: Single and dual energy tomographic analysis of spinal trabecular bone: A comparative study in normal and osteoporotic women. J Clin Endocrinol Metab 64:209–214, 1987.
29. Cann CE, Genant HK: Single versus dual-energy CT for vertebral mineral quantification. J Comput Assist Tomogr 7:551–557, 1983.
30. Cann CE, Martin MC, Genant HK, et al: Decreased spinal mineral content in detection of pre-menopausal amenorrheic women. JAMA 251:626–633, 1984.
31. Revak CS: Mineral content of cortical bone measured by computed tomography. J Comput Assist Tomogr 4:342–350, 1980.
32. Mazess RB: Errors due to adipose tissue in measuring trabecular bone by computed tomography. Calcif Tissue Int 34:198–204, 1982.
33. Reinbold W-D, Genant HK, Reiser UJ, et al: Bone mineral content in early-postmenopausal and postmenopausal osteoporotic women: Comparison of measurement methods. Radiology 160:469–478, 1986.
34. Cann CE, Genant HK: Precise measurement of vertebral mineral content using computed tomography. J Comput Assist Tomogr 4:493–500, 1980.
35. Ruegsegger P, Anliker M, Dambacher M: Quantification of trabecular bone with low dose computed tomography. J Comput Assist Tomogr 5:384–390, 1981.
36. Pullan BR, Roberts TE: Bone mineral measurement using an EMI scanner and standard methods: A comparative study. Br J Radiol 51:24–28, 1978.
37. Jensen PS, Orphanoudakis SC, Rauschkolk EN, et al: Assessment of bone mass in the radius by computed tomography. Am J Radiol 134:238–292, 1980.
38. Orphanoudakis SC, Jensen PS, Rauschkolk EN, et al. Bone mineral analysis using single energy computed tomography. Invest Radiol 14:122–130, 1979.
39. Banzer D, Schneider U, Wegener O: Vertebral mineral by CT scanning. *In* Mazess RB (ed): Proceedings, Fourth International Conference on Bone Mineral Measurement. US Dept. of HEW, NIH Publ. 80-1938, Washington DC, 1980, pp 309–315.
40. McBroom RJ, Hayes WC, Edwards WT, et al: Prediction of vertebral body compressive fracture using quantitative computed tomography. J Bone Joint Surg 67A:1206–1214, 1985.
41. Cann CE, Genant HK, Ettinger K, et al: Spinal mineral loss in oophorectomized women. JAMA 244:2056–2059, 1980.
42. Firooznia H, Golimbu C, Rafii M, et al: Rate of spinal trabecular bone loss in normal perimenopausal women: CT measurement. Radiology 161:735–738, 1986.
43. Cann CE, Genant HK, Kolb FO, et al: Quantitative computed tomography for prediction of vertebral fracture risk. Bone 6:1–7, 1985.
44. McBroom RJ, Haues WC, Edwards WT, et al: Prediction of vertebral body compressive fracture using quantitative computed tomography (abstract). 30th Annual Meeting, Orthopaedic Research Society, Atlanta, GA, 1984.
45. Brassow F, Crone-Munzebrock W, Weh L, et al: Correlations between breaking load and CT absorption values of vertebral bodies. Eur J Radiol 2:99–101, 1982.
46. Webber CE: Compton scattering methods. *In* Cohn SH (ed): Non-invasive Measurements of Bone Mass and Their Clinical Application. Boca Raton, CRC Press, 1981, pp 101–120.
47. Kennett TJ, Webber CE: Bone density measured by photon scattering. II. Inherent sources of error. Phys Med Biol 21:770–780, 1976.
48. Clarke RL, Van Dyk G: A new method for measurement of bone mineral content using both transmitted and scattered beams of gamma-rays. Phys Med Biol 18:532–539, 1973.
49. Garnett ES, Kennett TJ, Kenyon DB, et al: A photon scattering technique for the measurement of absolute bone density in man. Radiology 106:209–212, 1973.
50. Huddleston AL, Bhaduri D: Compton scatter densitometry in cancellous bones. Phys Med Biol 24:310–318, 1979.
51. Olkkonen H, Karjalainen P: A 170-Tm gamma scattering technique for the determination of absolute bone density. Br J Radiol 48:594–597, 1975.
52. Puumalainen P, Uimarihuta A, Alhava EM, et al: A new photon scattering method for bone mineral density measurements. Radiology 120:723–724, 1976.
53. Ling S, Rustgi S, Karellas A, et al: The measurement of trabecular bone mineral density using coherent and Compton scattered photons in vitro. Med Phys 9:208–215, 1982.
54. Battista JJ, Bronskill MJ: Compton scattering tissue densitometry: Calculation of single and multiple scatter photon fluences. Phys Med Biol 23:1–23, 1979.
55. Huddleston AL, Bhaduri D, Weaver J: Geometrical considerations for Compton scatter densitometry. Med Phys 6:519–522, 1979.
56. Stalp JT, Mazess RB: Determination of bone density by coherent-Compton scattering. Med Phys 7:723–726, 1980.
57. Kerr SA, Kouris K, Webber CE, et al: Coherent scattering and the assessment of mineral concentration in trabecular bone. Phys Med Biol 25:1037–1047, 1980.
58. Puumalainen P, Uimarihuta A, Olkkonen H, et al: A coherent/Compton scattering method employing an x-ray tube for measurement of trabecular bone mineral content. Phys Med Biol 27:425–429, 1982.
59. Leichter I, Weinreb A, Hazan G, et al: The effect of age and sex on bone density, bone mineral content and cortical index. Clin Orthop Rel Res 156:232–235, 1981.
60. Benjamin M, Macovski A: On the potential use of stimulated positron emission (SPE) in the detection and monitoring of some bone diseases. Med Phys 7:112–119, 1980.
61. Kelley TL, Slovak DM, Schenfeld A, et al: Quantitative digital radiography *vs* dual photon absorptiometry of the lumbar spine. J Clin Endocrinol Metab 67:839–844, 1988.
62. Maziere B: Partial body neutron activation—Hand. *In* Cohn SH (ed): Non-invasive Measurements of Bone Mass and Their Clinical Application. Boca Raton, CRC Press, 1981, pp 151–164.
63. McNeill KG, Harrison JE: Partial body neutron activation—Truncal. *In* Cohn SH (ed): Non-invasive Measurements of Bone Mass and Their Clinical Application. Boca Raton, CRC Press, 1981, pp 165–190.
64. Smith MA, Tothill P: Development of an apparatus to measure calcium changes in the forearm and spine by neutron activation using ^{252}Cf. Phys Med Biol 24:317–326, 1979.
65. Boddy K, Robertson I, Glaros D: The development of

a facility for partial body in vivo activation analysis using Californium 252 neutron sources. Phys Med Biol 19:853–861, 1974.

66. Cohn SH: Total body neutron activation. *In* Cohn SH (ed): Non-invasive Measurements of Bone Mass and Their Clinical Application. Boca Raton, CRC Press, 1981, pp 191–214.
67. Chamberlain MJ, Fremlin JH, Holloway I, et al: In vivo use of the cyclotron for whole body neutron activation analysis: Theoretical and practical considerations. Int J Appl Radiat Isot 21:725–734, 1970.
68. Cohn SH, Dombrowski CS, Fairchild RG: In vivo neutron activation analysis of calcium in man. Int J Appl Radiat Isot 21:127–137, 1970.
69. Palmer HE, Nelp WB, Murano R, et al: The feasibility of in vivo neutron activation analysis of total body calcium and other elements of body composition. Phys Med Biol 13:269–279, 1968.
70. Cohn SH: In vivo neutron activation analysis: State-of-the-art and future prospects. Med Phys 8:145–154, 1981.
71. Cohn SH: Present status of in vivo neutron activation analysis in clinical diagnosis and therapy. Atomic Energy Review, IAEA, Vol. 18, No. 3, Vienna, 1980.
72. Nuclear based techniques for in vivo study of human body composition. Cohn SH, Parr R (eds): Report of IAEA Advisory Panel. Clin Phys Physiol Meas 6:275–301, 1985.
73. Cohn SH: Techniques for determining the efficacy of treatment of osteoporosis (editorial). Int J Calcif Tissue 34:433–438, 1982.
74. Cohn SH, Aloia JF, Vaswani AN, et al: Women at risk for developing osteoporosis: Determination by total body neutron activation analysis and photoabsorptiometry. Calcif Tissue 38:9–15, 1986.
75. Ott SM, Murano R, Lewellen TK, et al: Total body calcium by neutron activation analysis in normals and osteoporotic populations: A discriminator of significant bone mass loss. J Lab Clin Med 102:637–645, 1983.
76. Cohn SH, Aloia JF, Zanzi I, et al: The aging of the skeleton: U.S. experience. *In* Iio M, Wagner, HN (eds): Geriatric Nuclear Medicine. Tokyo, Igaku Shoin, Ltd, 1983, pp 319–328.
77. Cohn SH, Vaswani AN, Zanzi I, et al: Changes in body chemical composition with age measured by total body neutron activation. Metabolism 25:85–96, 1976.
78. Cohn SH, Vaswani AN, Zanzi I, et al: Effect of aging on bone mass in adult women. Am J Physiol 230:143–148, 1966.
79. Aloia JF, Vaswani AN, Yeh KJ, et al: Determinants of bone mass in postmenopausal women. Arch Intern Med 143:1700–1704, 1983.
80. Aloia JF, Ross P, Vaswani AN, et al: Rate of bone loss in postmenopausal and osteoporotic women. Am J Physiol 242:E82–E86, 1982.
81. Cohn SH, Ellis KJ, Wallach S, et al: Absolute and relative deficit in total body calcium and radial bone mineral content in osteoporosis. J Nucl Med 15:428–435, 1974.
82. Cohn SH, Aloia JF, Zanzi I, et al: Clinical applicability of bone mineral content measured by monoenergetic photon absorptiometry. Proceedings, Fourth International Conference on Bone Measurement, NIH 80-1938, Toronto, 1980, pp 1–5.
83. Dequeker J: Influence of sampling, sex, age and skeletal size on the variability of radiogrammetric bone mass values. *In* Dequeker J, Johnston CC (eds): Non-invasive Bone Measurements: Methodological Problems. Oxford, IRL Press, 1982, pp 107–113.
84. Cohn SH, Ellis KJ, Goldsmith NF: Validity of the absorptiometric measurement of bone mineral content of the radius. Am J Roentgenol 126:1286–1287, 1976.
85. Dequeker J, Geusens P, Wielandt L, et al: Lumbar BMC, skeletal size nomogram. *In* Christiansen C (ed): Osteoporosis. Proceedings, International Symposium on Osteoporosis, Copenhagen, June 1984, pp 341–344.
86. Christiansen C: Bone mineral measurement with special references to precision, accuracy, normal values and clinical relevance. *In* Dequeker J, Johnston CC (eds): Non-invasive Bone Measurements: Methodological Problems. Oxford, IRL Press, 1982, pp 95–105.
87. Johnston CC, Norton JA: Single energy photon absorptiometry: How to express the measurement. *In* Dequeker J, Johnston CC (eds): Non-invasive Bone Measurements: Methodological Problems. Oxford, IRL Press, 1982, pp 115–117.
88. Manzke E, Chesnut CH III, Wergedal JE, et al: Relationship between local and total bone mass in osteoporosis. Metabolism 24:605–610, 1975.
89. Mazess RB, Peppler WW, Chesney RW, et al: Does bone measurement of the radius indicate skeletal status? J Nucl Med 25:281–288, 1984.
90. Chesnut CH III: Non-invasive techniques in the diagnosis of osteoporosis. *In* Osteoporosis Consensus Development Conference Statement, Vol. 5, No. 3, Clinical Center, NIH, April 2–4, 1984, Bethesda, MD, pp 32–36.
91. Smith MA, Elton RA, Tothill P: The comparison of neutron activation and photon absorptiometry at the same part body site. Clin Phys Physiol Meas 2:1–7, 1981.
92. Cummings SR, Black D: Should perimenopausal women be screened for osteoporosis? Ann Intern Med 104:817–823, 1986.
93. Hall FM, Davis MA, Baran DT: Bone mineral screening for osteoporosis. N Engl J Med 316:212–214, 1987.
94. Genant HK, Powell MR, Cann CE, et al: Comparisons of methods for in vivo spinal bone mineral measurement. *In* Christiansen C (ed): Osteoporosis, Proceedings, International Symposium on Osteoporosis, Copenhagen, 1984, pp 97–102.
95. Rockoff SD, Sweet E, Bleustein J: The relative contribution of trabecular and cortical bone to the strength of human lumbar vertebrae. Calcif Tissue Res 3:163–175, 1969.
96. Mazess RB: Total body and regional bone mineral by dual-photon absorptiometry. Calcif Tissue Int 33:328 (abstract), 1981.
97. Cohn SH, Aloia JF, Yuen K, Vaswani AN: Comparison of cross sectional and longitudinal models of bone loss in women. XVIII European Symposium on Calcified Tissues, Angers, France, 1984.
98. Parfitt AM: Morphologic basis of bone mineral measurements: Transient and steady state effects of treatment in osteoporosis. Miner Electrolyte Metab 4:273–287, 1980.

HARTMUT H. MALLUCHE
MARIE-CLAUDE FAUGERE

10

Bone Biopsies: Histology and Histomorphometry of Bone

Improvements in diagnostic methods as well as in the effectiveness and availability of therapy have made metabolic bone diseases an essential part of medical practice. Clinicians and laboratory researchers now fully recognize the value of bone biopsies in the management of patients with metabolic bone disease. Moreover, these bone biopsies—for mineralized bone histology and the quantitative evaluation of histomorphometric parameters of bone structure, formation, and resorption—constitute a formidable research tool that continues to provide us with unique and indispensable information. For example, only bone histology can assess bone activity at the cellular, osteon, and tissue level, and even though bone histomorphometry is required for only a subset of special cases, it provides a useful and powerful method for understanding the pathophysiologic mechanisms of various metabolic bone diseases. This chapter represents a short review of the functional and structural organization of bone and explains in detail the indication, techniques, and rationale involved in performing bone biopsies for mineralized bone histology and histomorphometry.

I. THE FUNCTIONAL AND STRUCTURAL ORGANIZATION OF BONE

A. Axial and Appendicular Skeleton

The axial and appendicular skeleton can be distinguished functionally with the skull, spine, thorax, and pelvis composing the axial, and the extremities composing the appendicular skeleton. Pathologic processes may affect these skeletal sites in opposite directions,[1] and metabolic changes may be found predominantly in the axial or the appendicular skeleton[2,3] (C.C. Johnston, personal communication).

B. Compact and Cancellous Bone

Compact or cortical bone can be distinguished from cancellous or trabecular bone on the macroscopic level. Compact bone is mainly found in the diaphysis of long bones and on the surfaces of flat bones such as the ilium or vertebrae. Cancellous bone is limited to the metaphyseal region of long bones and is mainly found between the cortices of the smaller flat and short bones such as scapulae, vertebrae, and pelvis.

C. Lamellar and Woven Bone

Two different types of bone can be identified at the microscopic level: lamellar bone and woven bone (Figs. 10–1 and 10–2).

Lamellar bone is the main bone type of a mature skeleton and is characterized by an orderly arrangement of collagen bundles. The osteocytic lacunae in lamellar bone are uniform, are regularly distributed, and contain relatively monomorphic cells. Lamellar bone is typically formed in apposition to an existing surface as osteoblasts assume a distinct three-dimensional orientation in coordination with neighbor osteoblasts and form a continuous layer of unidirectional bone. This spatial orientation and polarized extrusion of protocollagen strands toward the bone matrix is a prerequisite for normal collagen production. The deposited collagen then exhibits an orderly lamellar pattern as circular layers of collagen alternate with longitudinal ones. This pattern is responsible for the birefringence under polarized light (Fig. 10–1).

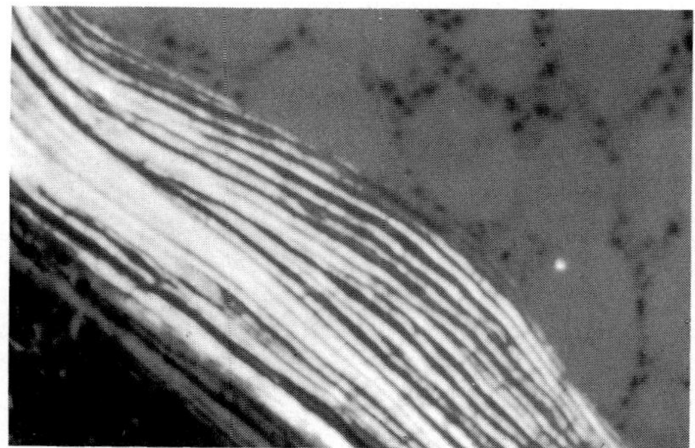

Figure 10–1. Lamellar osteoid and lamellar bone. Viewing under polarized light allows recognition of the orderly lamellar pattern of osteoid. Undecalcified, 3 μm thick section of human iliac bone (modified Masson-Goldner stain; ×125). (Figures 10–1 through 10–52 from Malluche HH, Faugere MC: Atlas of Mineralized Bone Histology. Basel, S. Karger AG, 1986) *See color plate I*

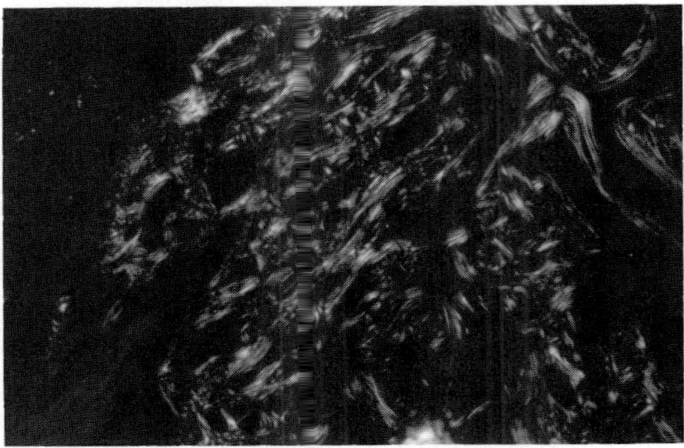

Figure 10–2. Woven osteoid and woven bone in predominant hyperparathyroid bone disease. Abundance of irregular woven osteoid in the center and presence of lamellar osteoid at the periphery of the trabecular bone. Undecalcified, 3 μm thick section of human iliac bone. Polarized light microscopy (modified Masson-Goldner stain; ×50). *See color plate I*

Contrasting with the regularity of lamellar bone, woven bone is composed of loosely and randomly arranged collagen bundles containing numerous osteocytes lying in lacunae of varying sizes and shapes. The walls of these lacunae are not well defined. Woven bone is formed by the irregular and unpolarized extrusion of protocollagen by osteoblasts, which bury themselves in the resulting matrix. This matrix consists of an orderless, crisscross texture that lacks the birefringence typical of lamellar bone under polarized light (Fig. 10–2).

Woven bone will be found in the embryonic skeleton and in both cortical and cancellous bone during stages of rapid bone growth, bone replacement, or high bone turnover. After the completion of bone growth, woven bone is replaced by lamellar bone in the normal skeleton. However, it will also be observed in certain pathologic conditions such as Paget's disease of bone (Chapter 15), callus formation at fracture sites, and osteitis fibrosa cystica resulting from primary or secondary hyperparathyroidism (Chapters 13 and 14). In adults, woven bone is indicative of rapid, uncontrolled bone formation and high bone turnover and is attributable to either local or systemic factors.

D. Bone Envelopes

Anatomically and functionally, there are three different bone surfaces. These bone surfaces undergo turnover in different ways and are affected differently by physiologic or pathologic stimuli. These surfaces include periosteal surfaces, haversian surfaces, and endosteal surfaces (Fig. 10–3). The three surfaces are referred to as "bone envelopes"[4]—a distinction valuable in describing and understanding histologic and functional abnormalities of bone.

E. The Osteon

Although bone structure does not normally change its microscopic appearance after closure of the epiphysis, it is, however, subject

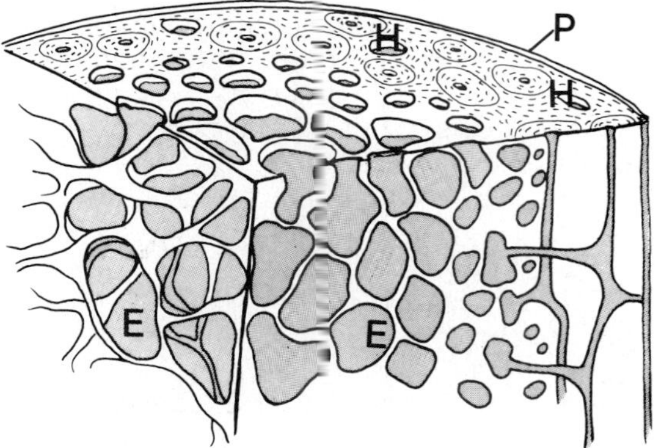

Figure 10–3. Bone envelopes. Periosteal surface (P), haversian surface (H), and endosteal surfaces (E). These surfaces are also referred to as different bone envelopes. On one side of the longitudinal cut of bone (left), the three-dimensional orientation of trabeculae is illustrated; on the other side (right), the histologic appearance of a bone section, that is, its two-dimensional image, is shown.

to continuous internal renewal by resorption and formation. Understanding this renewal process requires an understanding of the smallest, individually functioning unit of bone—the osteon (Fig. 10–4).

Each osteon contains a central "haversian" canal of blood vessels and connective tissue. Bone-resorbing and bone-forming cells, osteoclasts and osteoblasts, may be observed at the surface of these central canals (the haversian surfaces), thus indicating bone modeling or remodeling activity within the unit. Units undergoing modeling or remodeling are referred to as basic multicellular units (BMU).[4]

The central "haversian" canals are surrounded by concentric layers of osseous lamellae containing osteocytes arranged in a regular, coaxial order. These osteocytes are located within lacunae, and the bone matrix surrounding them may be completely or partially calcified. The osteocytes are joined together by cytoplasmic processes at all levels in osteons, and interstitial lamellae—the remains of incompletely resorbed osteons—are interspersed between histologically intact osteons (Fig. 10–4).

Cancellous or trabecular bone can be understood as longitudinally cut and unfolded osteons exhibiting, at their surface (endosteal surface), bone-forming and -resorbing cells and their product—the osteoid seams and resorption lacunae.

F. Bone Cells

1. The Osteoclasts

Osteoclasts are mono- or multinucleated cells characteristically seen in lacunae of resorbed bone and represent the main cells in the breakdown of the bone matrix and bone mineral. The cellular cytoplasm of the osteoclast reacts positively with specific stains for acid phosphatase[5] and displays a typical pink stain with the modified Masson-Goldner trichrome stain (Figs. 10–5*A*, *B*). Osteoclasts vary in size and usually display projections and lobes that give them an irregular appearance.

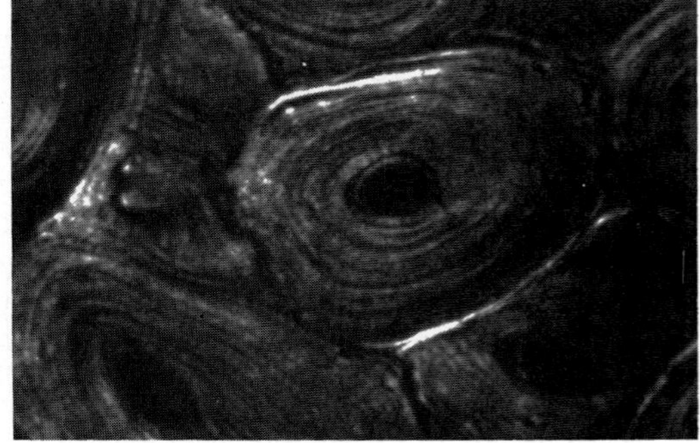

Figure 10–4. Osteons—smallest functioning units of bone. Concentric layers of osseous lamellae surrounding central canals. Interstitial lamellae interspersed between intact osteons. Undecalcified, unstained, 7 μm thick section of cortical human bone. Polarized light with red filter (×31). *See color plate I*

In a normal skeleton, osteoclasts are somewhat larger than macrophages and may have from one to three nuclei. *In vitro*, fusion of such smaller individual cells has been observed.[6] In pathologic states, the osteoclasts are large cells with a large number of nuclei (Fig. 10–5*B*). The nuclei are characteristically round or oval, most often with one or two prominent nucleoli.

The classic studies of Gaillard[7] revealed that osteoclasts are highly mobile and go through cycles of resorption and rest. Thus, it is not surprising that these cells vary in histologic appearance, depending on the point of the cycle at which they are observed. In routine preparations, however, osteoclastic cytoplasm is foamy and moderately acidophilic.

A criterion of osteoclastic activity is the histologic appearance of a "ruffled" border.[8] This is a special cytoplasmic differentiation seen at the surface of the osteoclast that is in contact with bone being resorbed. Bone mineral material and bone collagen within the ruffled border (evaluated by electron microscopy) indicate that this ruffled border plays a role in bone-resorbing activity.

Microcinephotography techniques[7,9] have revealed that bone is resorbed beneath osteoclasts that move from one place to another. The same techniques revealed a larger number of cytoplasmic vacuoles, and the energetically undulating ruffled borders have been shown to display vigorous pinocytosis.

The endosteum was postulated as the origination site for osteoclasts. Accordingly, the sequence of tissue events (i.e., resorption followed by new bone formation during remodeling of adult trabecular bone) was believed to correspond to the sequence of cellular events. Given this model, osteoclasts were postulated to form from precursor cells. The osteoclasts then shed nuclei that became osteoblasts. However, no direct cell-kinetic evidence has been provided to support this theory.

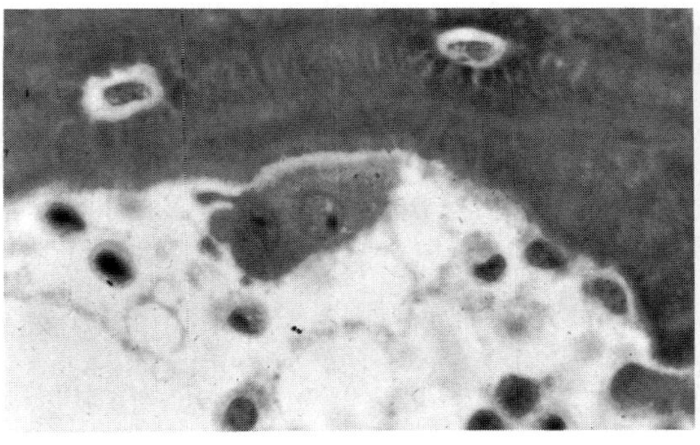
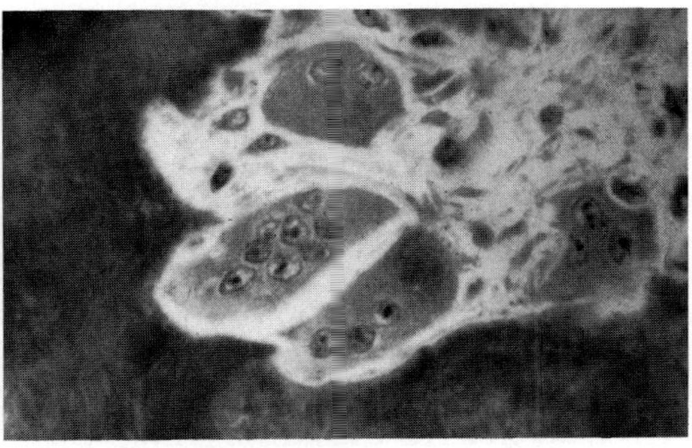

A B

Figure 10–5. Osteoclastic bone resorption. *A*, Shallow resorption of bone by an osteoclast with two nuclei and prominent nucleoli. Undecalcified, 3 μm thick section of human iliac bone (modified Masson-Goldner stain; ×125). *B*, Lacunar resorption. Osteoclasts resorbing mineralized bone in individual resorption zones forming a deep lacuna. Undecalcified, 3 μm thick section of human iliac bone (modified Masson-Goldner stain; ×125). *See color plate I*

Recent findings point to a different theory of the origin of osteoclasts. Kimmel and Jee[10] studied rat tibial bone at increasing distances from the growth cartilage and concluded that osteoblasts and osteoclasts derive from different cell sources and do not modulate from one cell type to another. Unfortunately, a definitive study of the endosteum is not available. Yet based on a series of studies using [^{3}H]-thymidine–labeled bone cells, Jee and Kimmel[11] were able to postulate the existence of preosteoclasts near sites of bone resorption—preosteoclasts similar or identical to mononuclear macrophages. These studies led to the hypothesis that osteoclast precursor cells (i.e., monocytes) are delivered to the bone surface through discontinuities in blood vessels. Subsequent studies supported the concept of phagocytes or monocytes as osteoclast precursors.[12,13] However, other experiments[14-16] suggest that a number of different cells can develop into osteoclasts. Thus, osteoclasts may have more than one osteoprogenitor cell line.

Just as the origin of osteoclasts is hypothetical, neither is it known in surety whether the osteoclasts or other indirect mechanisms are involved in the initiation and maintenance of bone resorption. In fact, there is little evidence that osteoclasts have receptors for parathyroid hormone or 1,25$(OH)_2D_3$ or respond to these hormones directly. Whereas circulating mononuclear cells, such as monocytes, have been shown to be osteoclast precursors and to resorb devitalized bone in culture, no effect of parathyroid hormone on chemotactic migration or resorbing activity could be demonstrated.[17,18] The normal osteoclastic activity observed in parathyroidectomized, newborn rats[19] and the lack of parathyroid hormone involvement in the osteoclastic defect associated with osteopetrosis[20] corroborate the notion that osteoclasts do not directly respond to parathyroid hormone.

Observations in our laboratories of marginal or negative correlations between circulating levels of parathyroid hormone and the number of osteoclasts, and a correspondingly good correlation between serum parathyroid hormone and the number of osteoblasts in bones of patients with end-stage renal failure,[21] support the hypothesis advanced by Rodan and Martin[22] that parathyroid hormone acts upon osteoblasts, which, in turn, allow osteoclasts to resorb bone (Chapter 1).

According to this hypothesis, osteoblasts, in the normal state, protect the bone matrix against osteoclastic resorption. Parathyroid hormone reverses or reduces this protective effect.

This hypothesis has far-reaching ramifications for the therapy of osteoporosis and other metabolic bone abnormalities. Whereas the response of osteoclasts to other bone-resorbing humoral factors such as prostaglandins or 1,25$(OH)_2D_3$ is uncertain, the response of osteoblasts grows increasingly clear. Just as it was found that osteoblasts, rather than osteoclasts, respond to parathyroid hormone, similarly, a growing body of evidence points to osteoblasts as target cells for prostaglandins and 1,25$(OH)_2D_3$.[21,23-32]

Lian et al.[33] observed that osteocalcin-deficient bone is poorly resorbed *in vivo* and *in vitro*, thus suggesting that osteocalcin might be an essential component of bone matrix for recruitment and/or differentiation of osteoclasts. The activity of osteoclasts was morphometrically assessed by Holtrop.[34] Shortly after the injection of parathyroid hormone, there was a rise in blood calcium levels (starting at 30 minutes, highest at 3 hours, and decreasing to normal at 6 hours). During this period a slight and continuous increase in the number of osteoclasts was noticeable. This increase was followed by a steeper increase after 6 hours, reaching values twice baseline at 12 hours. These data demonstrate that mechanisms other than the increasing number of osteoclasts are responsible for short-term mobilization of calcium from bone. Measuring cytoplasmic areas revealed that parathyroid hormone–treated osteoclasts were significantly larger than untreated osteoclasts 1.5 hours after injection of the hormone and that this increase returned to normal not before 12 to 24 hours after the injection of parathyroid hormone. In addition, the study showed that as early as 30 minutes after intravenous injection of parathyroid hormone, ruffled borders increased significantly in thyroparathyroidectomized rats. These changes were concurrent with changes in the plasma calcium level and were followed much later (i.e., after 12 hours) by significant increases in the number of osteoclasts.

These findings underscore an important concept describing the relationship between cell activity and cell number[35,36] wherein it has been demonstrated that an increase in the number of cells does not necessarily result in an increase in cell activity. In uremia, for example, an increase in the number of osteoclasts is seen concurrently with a decrease in activity at the cellular level.[31]

Histologically, there are three main types of osteoclastic resorption: (1) shallow and hook resorption (Fig. 10–5*A*); (2) lacunar resorption (Fig. 10–5*B*); and tunneling and dissective resorption.

1. This physiologic bone resorption respects lamellar boundaries, thus producing shallow or hook resorption cavities.
2. Lacunar resorption almost invariably reflects excessive pathologic bone resorption.
3. Tunneling resorption may occur when more than 60% of the trabecular surface is covered by osteoid—regardless of the type of disorder.[37]

It seems logical to conclude that in patients with tunneling resorption, osteoclastic activity is aimed at deeper layers of the trabeculae because of the low calcium content of the osteoid-covered surface. *In vivo*, osteoclasts are usually observed resorbing mineralized bone only. However, resorption of osteoid has been observed *in vitro*.[38,39] Studies in rachitic rats[40,42] indicate the existence of a factor inherent in bone that has never been mineralized. This factor seems to inhibit the appearance of osteoclasts as well as the initiation of bone resorption. Recent data from Bar-Shavit et al.[43] ascribe oligosaccharide-mediated binding mechanisms a role in facilitating osteoclast-bone attachment and, thus, bone degradation.

2. The Osteoblasts

Osteoblasts are mononucleated cells with basophilic cytoplasm, high nuclear ribonucleic acid content, and one to three nucleoli. They are the principal cells in bone formation.

Osteoblasts are usually arranged in a palisade-like configuration (Fig. 10–6*A*), and form bone in two successive stages: matrix or osteoid formation followed by mineralization. Matrix formation encompasses biosynthesis of both collagen and the ground substance of bone consisting of proteoglycans, glycoproteins, and other components. The mineralization stage denotes the deposition of hydroxyapatite crystals. Osteoblasts involved in the rapid deposition of bone are especially basophilic, plump, and polyhedral. They are called active osteoblasts (Fig. 10–6*A*). In contrast, resting osteoblasts are usually flat, their cytoplasm is less basophilic (Fig. 10–6*B*), and the juxtanuclear vacuoles cannot be seen.[8] With their epithelium-like organization, osteoblasts appear to form a barrier between the osteoid surface and the bone marrow. The mode of contact between osteoblasts is described as either "tight"[44] or "gap" junction.[45]

Approximately 10% to 20% of the trabecular surface exhibits osteoid. Thirty per cent to 40% of the osteoid surface is covered by active osteoblasts,[46,47] and 60% to 100% of the osteoid seams exhibit a zone called the mineralization or calcification front. This zone has characteristic staining properties that allow its identification with the toluidine blue stain or under fluorescent light after tetracycline administration.

Osteoid seam thickness decreases at sites of "maturing seams"[48] where osteoblasts are progressively less active. This reduced activity is preceded by a decrease in matrix synthesis and causes a depression of mineralization. At the tissue level, matrix and mineral apposition are considered to be balanced processes.

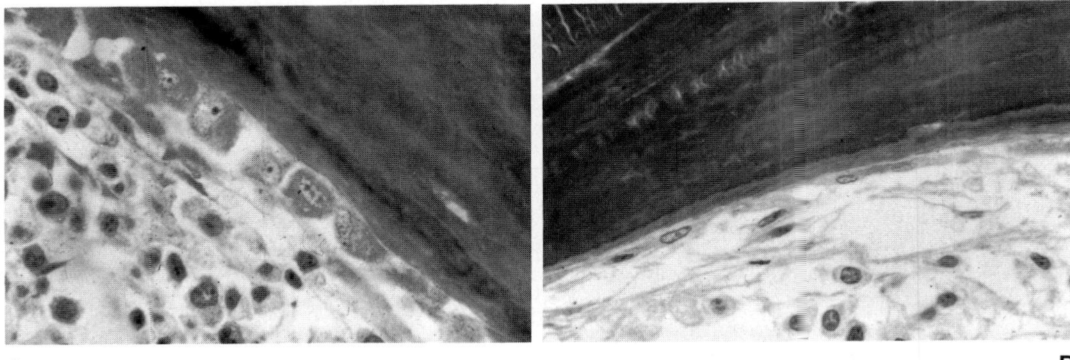

Figure 10–6. Osteoblasts. *A*, Active osteoblasts—epithelium-like layer of osteoblasts depositing newly formed bone. Regular arrangement of the mononucleated osteoblasts with one to three nucleoli. Undecalcified, 3 μm thick section of human iliac bone (modified Masson-Goldner stain; ×125). *B*, Resting osteoblasts—flat cells over a thin layer of osteoid, forming a barrier between the osteoid surface and the bone marrow space. Undecalcified, 3 μm thick section of human iliac bone (modified Masson-Goldner stain; ×125). *See color plate I*

Osteoblasts are thought to come from the osteoprogenitor cell population.[49-52] Yet even though it is possible to distinguish preosteoblasts from preosteoclasts of the osteoprogenitor pool through electron microscopy, no clear evidence is available supporting the previously advanced theory of interchange or modulation[53] between preosteoclasts and preosteoblasts.

3. The Osteocytes

After completing their bone matrix deposition, approximately 10% of the osteoblasts become trapped by the advancing edge of the bone and are surrounded, at first partly and then entirely, by the matrix. Thus, osteoblasts become osteocytes (Fig. 10–7*A*). Osteocytes are situated in lacunae and have cellular processes that traverse the matrix in canaliculi, connecting the osteocytes (Fig. 10–7*A*) and forming a syncytium including osteocytes and the osteoblasts of the trabecular surface.

Hypothetically, osteocytes (1) resorb bone, bone mineral, and bone matrix; (2) form new bone matrix (Fig. 10–7*B*); (3) mineralize newly formed matrix; and (4) play a role in non-osteoclast-mediated calcium release from bone.[53-63] Also, three different types of osteocytic lacunae have been distinguished: empty lacunae, large lacunae, and small lacunae.[64,65]

It was thought that osteocytes are involved in calcium homeostasis and possibly in the induction of bone remodeling.[66] However, that concept has been seriously challenged by Boyde,[67] whose data, although appealing, do

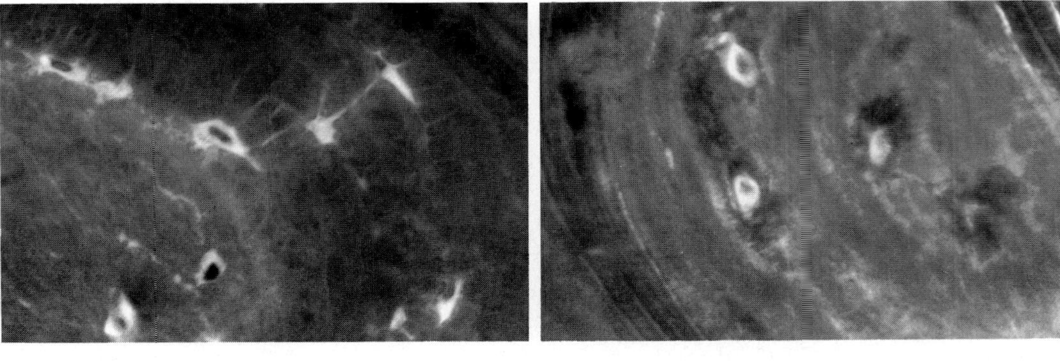

Figure 10–7. Osteocytes. *A*, Osteocytes situated in lacunae with processes traversing the matrix in canaliculi and connecting the osteocytes with each other. *B*, Osteocytes surrounded by osteoid, indicating either new bone formation by osteocytes or removal of mineral from the bone matrix. Undecalcified, 3 μm thick section of human iliac bone (modified Masson-Goldner stain; ×198). *See color plates I and II*

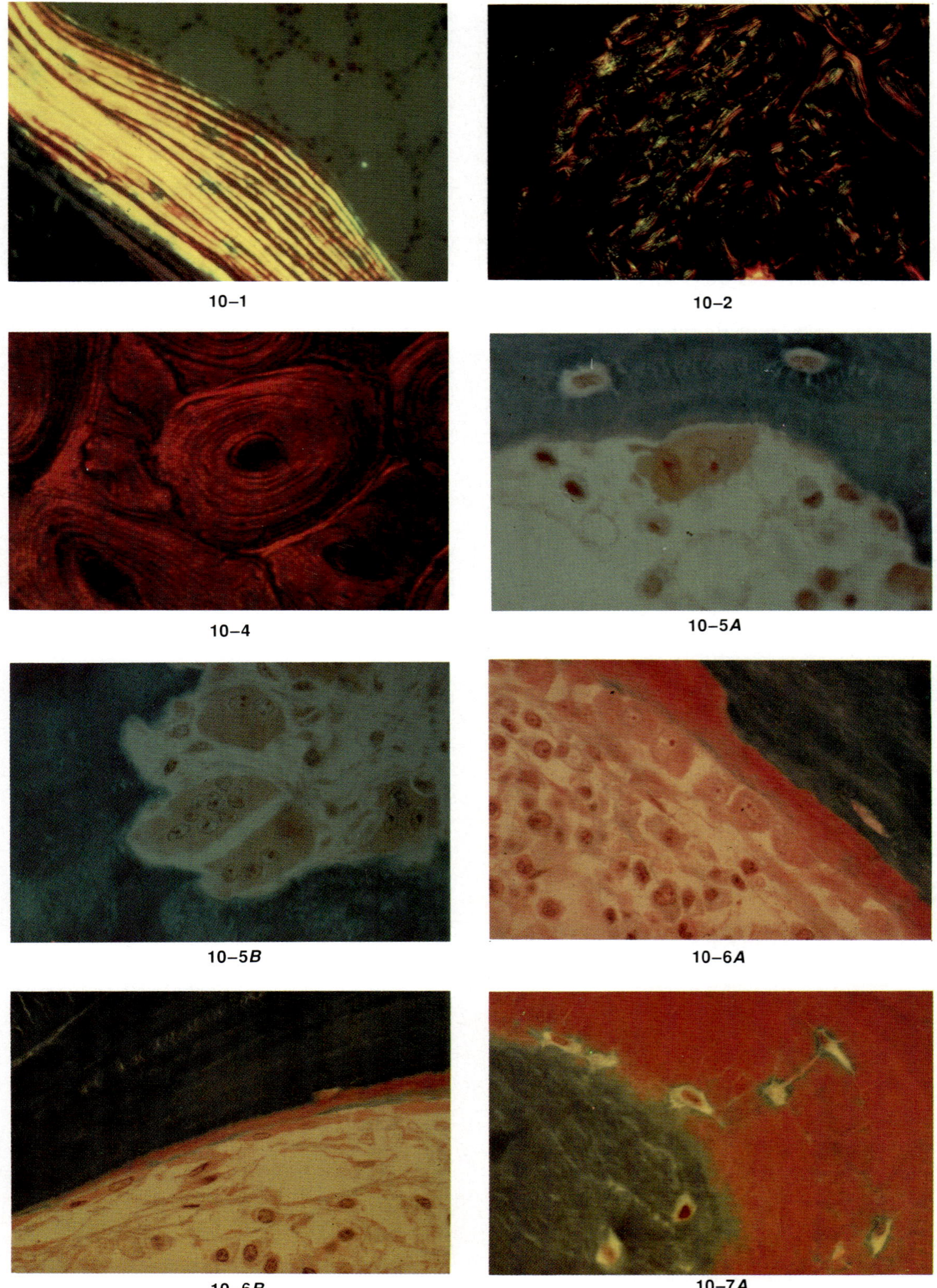
10–1

10–2

10–4

10–5*A*

10–5*B*

10–6*A*

10–6*B*

10–7*A*

PLATE I

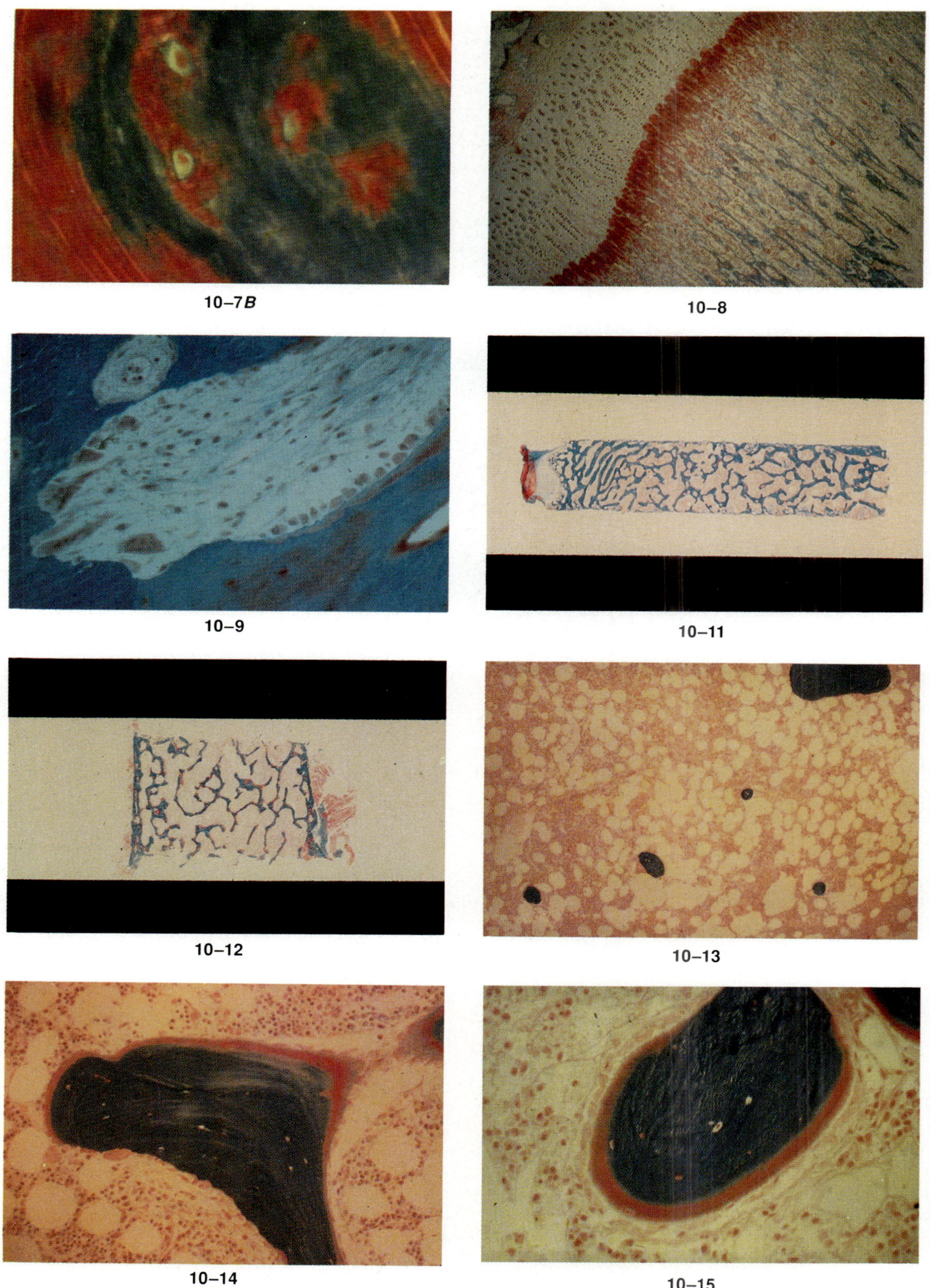

10–7*B*

10–8

10–9

10–11

10–12

10–13

10–14

10–15

PLATE II

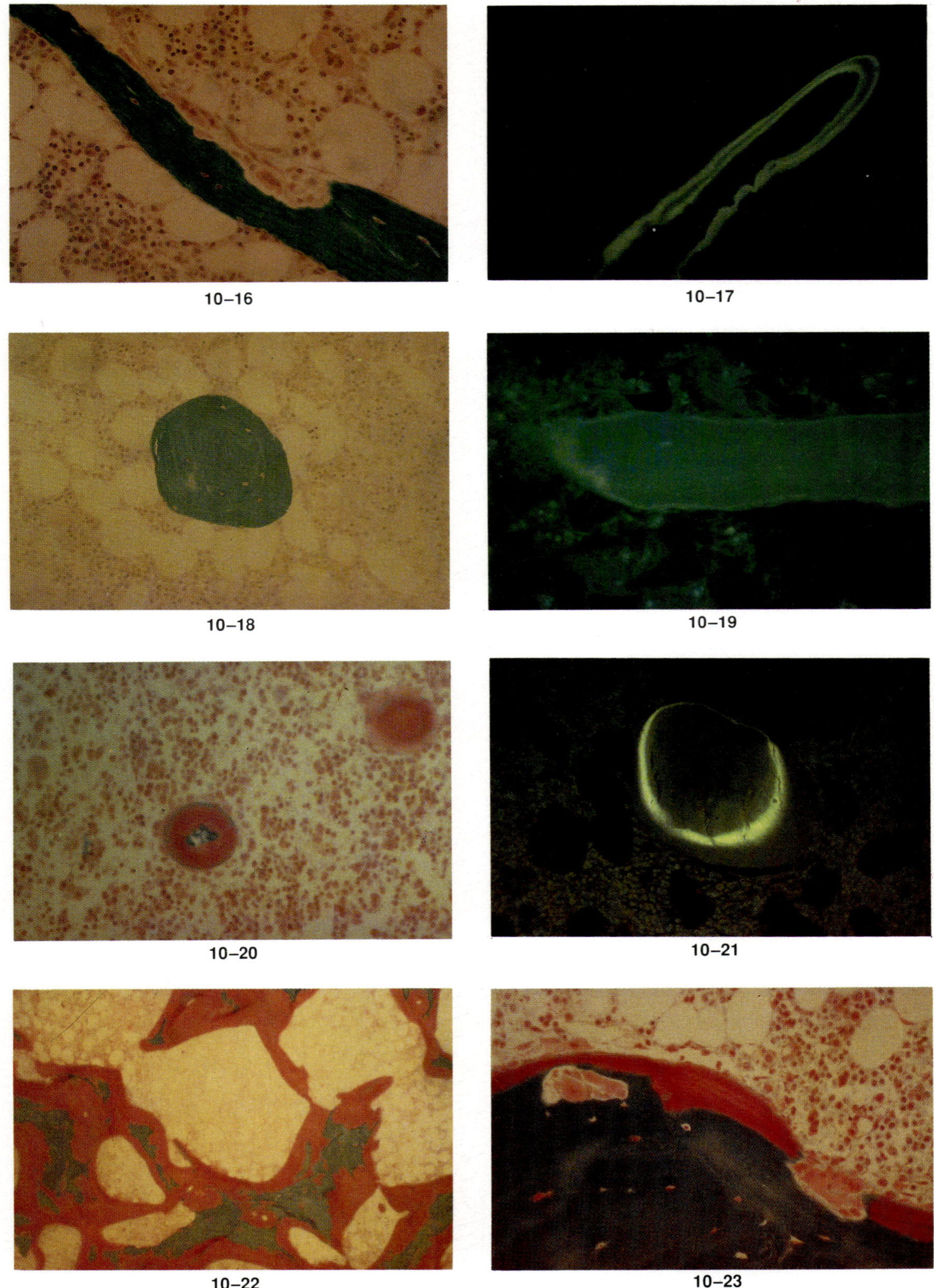

10–16

10–17

10–18

10–19

10–20

10–21

10–22

10–23

PLATE III

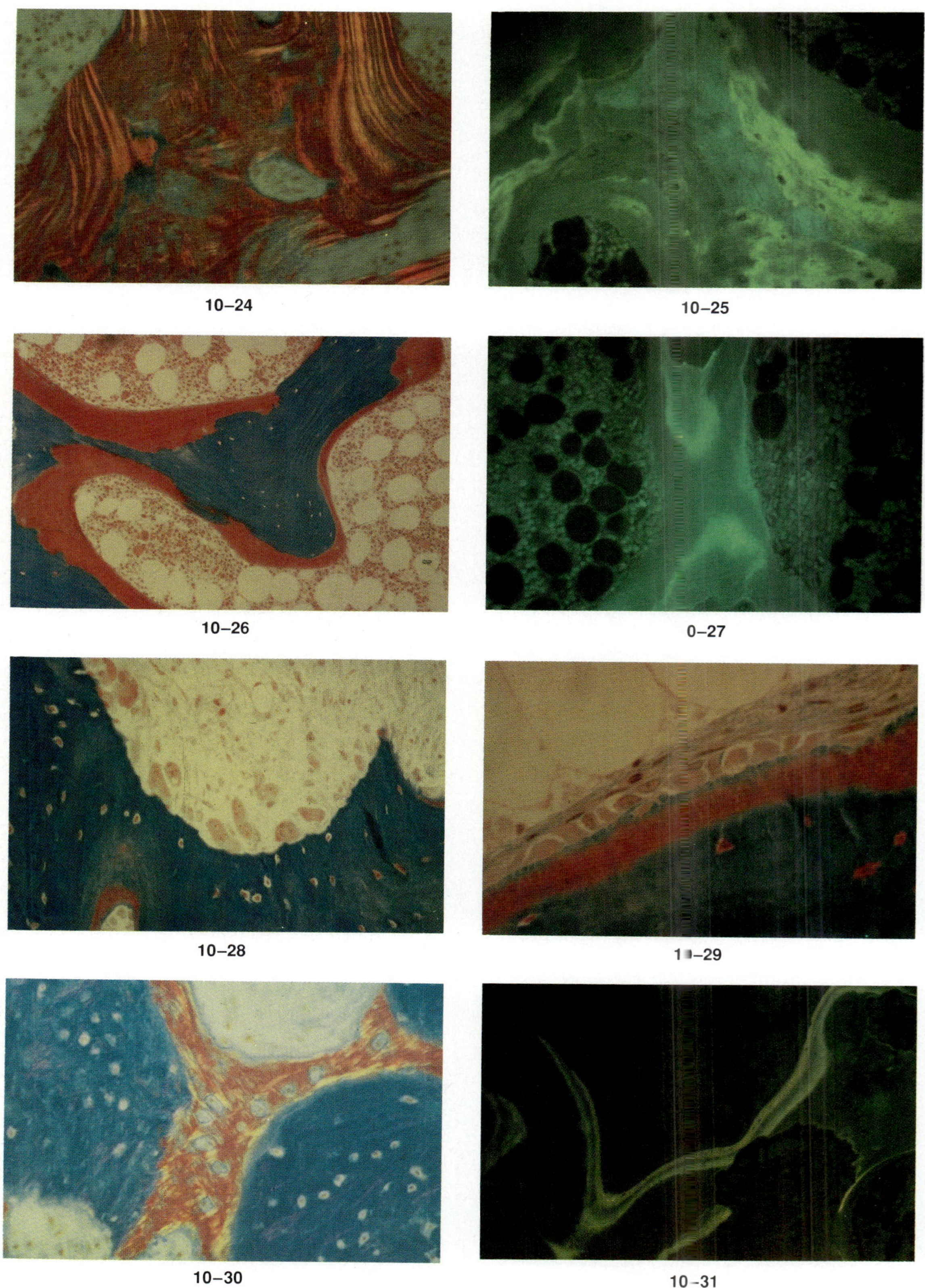

10–24 10–25

10–26 0–27

10–28 1–29

10–30 10–31

PLATE IV

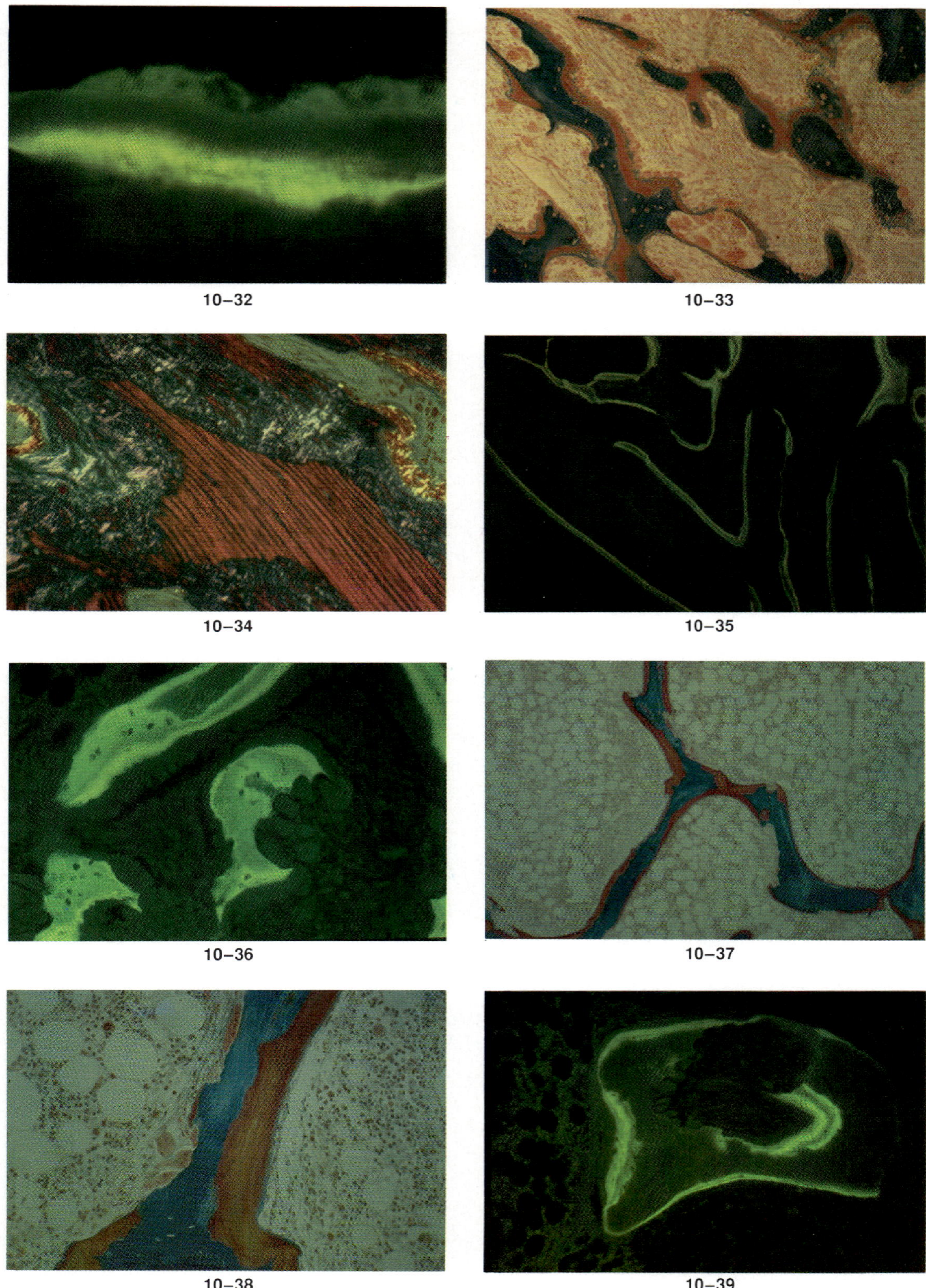
10–32
10–33
10–34
10–35
10–36
10–37
10–38
10–39

PLATE V

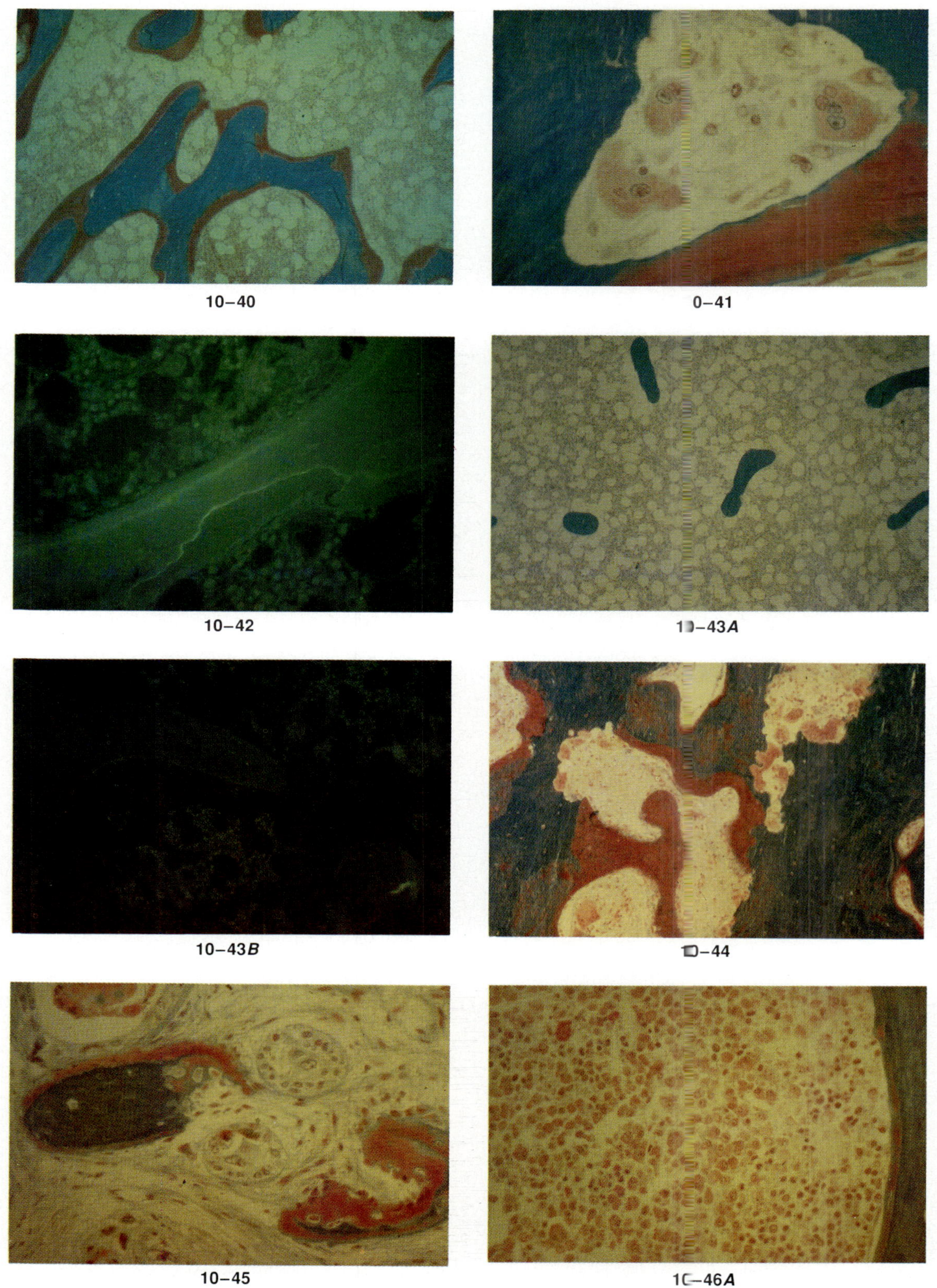

PLATE VI

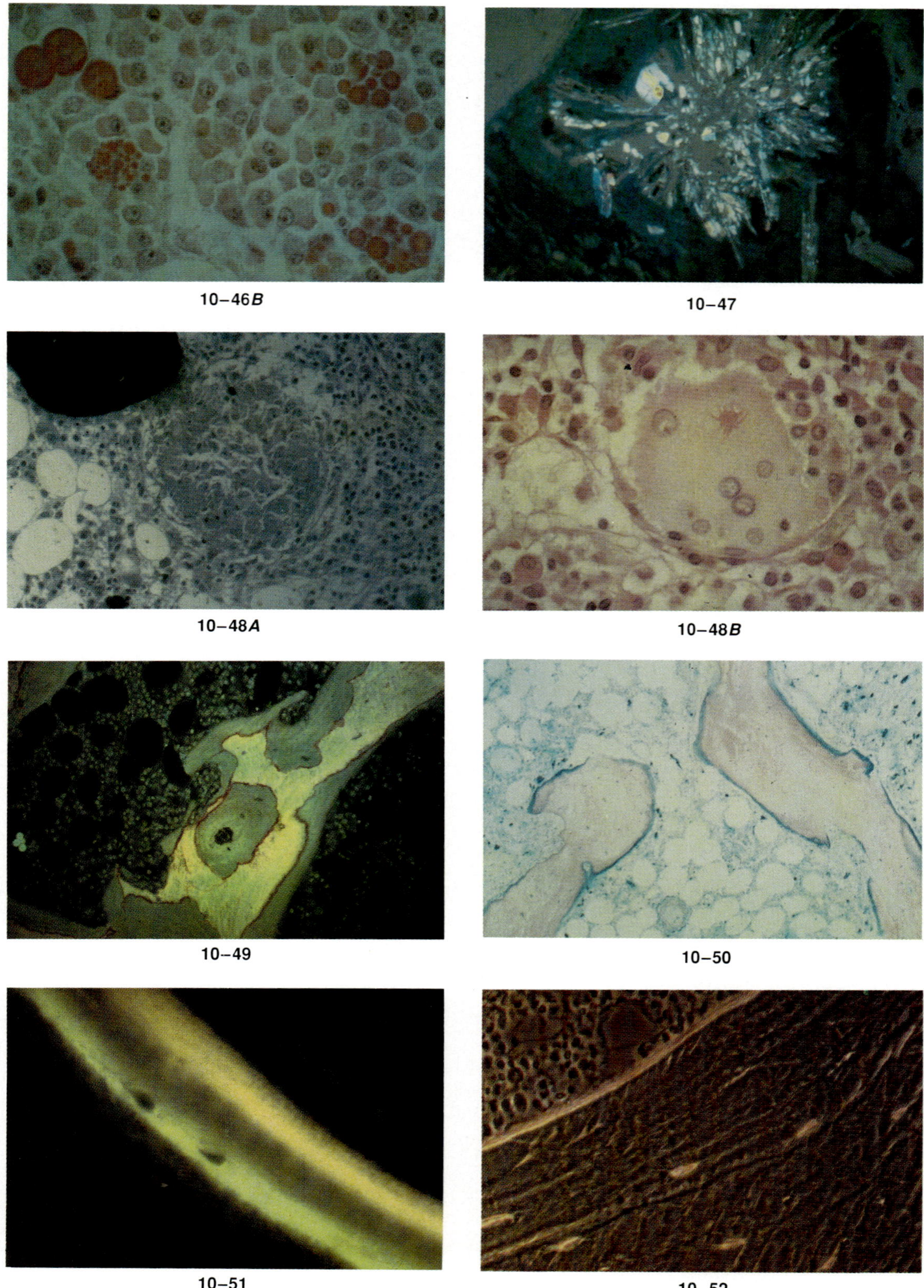

10–46*B*

10–47

10–48*A*

10–48*B*

10–49

10–50

10–51

10–52

PLATE VII

not offer an alternative model to replace the one it refutes. Further studies are obviously needed to determine the function of osteocytes in skeletal and/or calcium homeostasis.

G. Bone Modeling and Remodeling

The process of bone growth is called bone modeling, and there are two types of bone growth: longitudinal and appositional. Longitudinal growth (i.e., the growth of bone in length) occurs by enchondral ossification (Fig. 10–8), a process that creates new trabeculae until the epiphyseal growth plate fuses. Appositional growth (i.e., the growth of bone in width) proceeds by periosteal apposition of new bone and endosteal resorption of old bone. Appositional growth appears to occur without a coupling of the bone formation and bone resorption function, and thus represents one of the major differences between bone modeling and bone remodeling.

Bone remodeling describes the dynamic processes of the adult skeleton after closure of the epiphyseal growth plates. Basically, there is a continual renewal of bone tissue. A certain number of osteons enter a "remodeling cycle," which results in their partial or complete removal and replacement by new osteons. Systematic studies of bone remodeling activity in dogs[68,69] revealed that the removal of bone is followed by refilling and thus documented the sequential character of remodeling (Fig. 10–9).

The bone remodeling process is the physiologic basis of bone turnover and renewal in a mature skeleton. An osteon undergoing such remodeling is called an active bone remodeling unit,[4] and the formation of a new osteon is preceded by removal of old bone. Consequently, histologic cross sections of compact bone display osteoclastic activity near the center of a future osteon. The new osteon's diameter will be the composite result of both the activity and the duration of the resorptive phase.

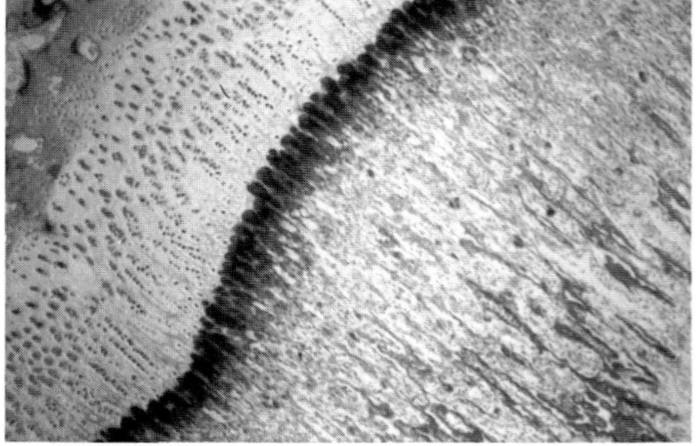

Figure 10–8. Growth plate. Longitudinal growth through enchondral ossification. Layers of proliferating and hypertrophic columnar cartilage followed by primary and secondary spongiosa. Undecalcified, 3 μm thick section of growing dog bone (modified Masson-Goldner stain; ×7.5). *See color plate II*

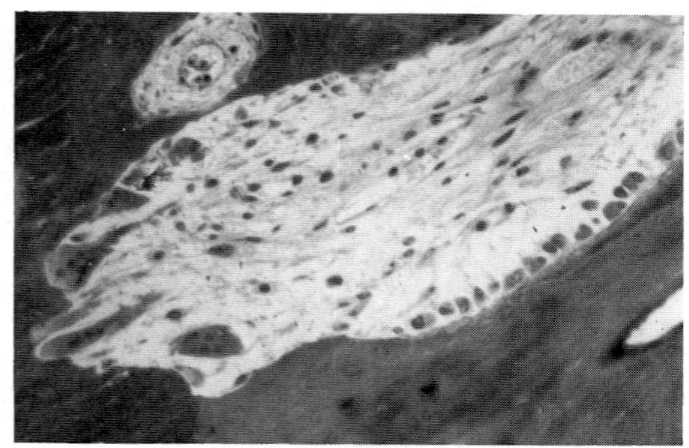

Figure 10–9. Bone remodeling. Cutting cone with several osteoclasts at its tip followed by peripheral deposition of new bone by osteoblasts. Between osteoblasts and osteoclasts, undifferentiated mesenchymal cells are seen. The sequential character of bone modeling is illustrated in this haversian remodeling site. Undecalcified, 3 μm thick section of human cortical bone (modified Masson-Goldner stain; ×50). *See color plate II*

"Mean wall thickness" is the composite result of the osteoclastic activity, the duration of osteoclastic resorption, and the activity and life span of osteoblasts in cancellous bone. Approximately 10 days after osteoblasts deposit bone matrix, mineralization begins at a distinct mineralization front. After the newly deposited bone has been completely mineralized, a remodeling cycle is completed. The time between the activation of resorbing cells and the completion of the sequence of events described earlier ("sigma"[4]) is 4 to 6 months in the adult skeleton.

Given the principles of bone remodeling, Frost advanced the concept of "the different levels of bone organization."[70] This distinction is important because a dissociation is possible between the different levels of bone organization. Activity on one level of organization may not necessarily parallel the activity at other levels. To account for dissociation at different levels of bone organization, the activity is broken down into (1) cell level activity, (2) osteon level activity, and (3) tissue level activity.

1. Cell level activity is determined by the amount of matrix resorbed and formed per cell and per unit time.
2. Osteon level activity is determined by the number and activity of cells per resorption and apposition site, and the lifetime of the individual resorption and apposition sites.
3. Tissue level activity is determined by the number and activity of resorption and apposition sites per unit volume of bone.

An example of the different levels of bone organization can be seen in uremia, in which overall bone resorption and formation (i.e., tissue level activity) may be increased, whereas cell level resorption and formation may be depressed (Malluche et al., unpublished observations). Therapy of uremic bone disease with the active vitamin D metabolite $1,25(OH)_2D_3$ may depress tissue level resorbing and forming activity while enhancing cell level activity.[71]

It should be noted that histologic changes in bone cell activity may prove transient, resulting from a past stimulus that triggered bone remodeling events. For instance, if the number of osteons entering a remodeling cycle (the "activation frequency") is temporarily increased, as seen with increased levels of thyroxin[72] or after administration of parathyroid hormone,[73] the first observation may reveal numerous osteoclasts and a negative bone balance. Subsequently, numerous osteoblasts and a positive bone balance may occur before surface cell density and bone balance return to baseline levels. Therefore, repeat bone biopsies are imperative in the evaluation of a particular therapy or regimen. These biopsies should always be performed after sufficient time has elapsed to allow the completion of a full remodeling cycle (sigma).

II. BONE BIOPSY

A. Prerequisites for Bone Biopsies

Bone biopsies provide qualitative information and quantitative results on the static and dynamic parameters of bone structure, formation, and resorption. *The major prerequisite for any technique employed is that the operator must obtain bone samples with adequate quantities of cortical and deep cancellous bone and without artifacts such as fractures of trabeculae or cortices, hemorrhage, compression of spongy bone, overlapping of trabeculae or cells, and/or cellular damage due to heat generated during the drilling procedure.*

Bone samples should be obtained from the sampling site without the application of major physical forces and without destructive instruments. (Even appropriate instruments become destructive when used without skill or understanding.) Typically, the more experienced the physician taking the biopsy, the better the quality of the specimen obtained. Several biopsy techniques are available that provide the skilled operator with adequate samples.

B. Bone Biopsy Instruments and Specimen Size

Available instruments for bone biopsies can be classified as manual trochars[74-82] or electric drills[83-85] (Fig. 10–10). Whereas the use of manual instruments requires special attention to avoid the overzealous application of physical force that may produce artifacts, the potential problem in the use of electric drills is the accumulation of bone powder in the periphery of the spongy bone if pressure is exerted during the drilling, or heat artifacts of bone cells if the speed of the instrument is too high.

The desired size of the bone sample mainly determines the degree of invasiveness of the bone biopsy. The optimal biopsy technique provides an appropriate-sized sample with minimal surgical invasion. Bone samples 0.5 cm

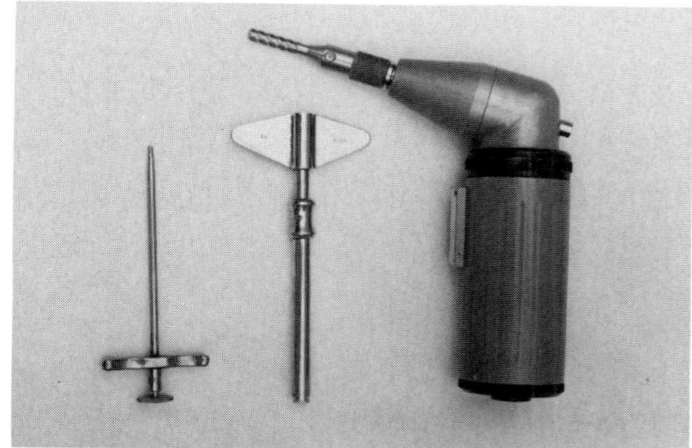

Figure 10–10. Bone biopsy instruments. Electric drill (right) for transiliac and vertical samples of 0.5 cm inner diameter and 3 to 4 cm length. Drilling bits of smaller diameter can be used for children. Manual trocar (center) for transiliac bone samples of 0.8 cm diameter. The 8-gauge Jamshidi needle (left) for vertical bone samples of 0.3 cm diameter and 2 to 3 cm length.

in diameter and 3.5 cm in length taken vertically from the anterior iliac crest (Fig. 10–11) have been established as sufficient for qualitative and quantitative bone histology.[47] Bone samples of 2 mm inner diameter and approximately 3.5 cm length obtained with a Jamshidi needle were claimed to provide useful qualitative results,[86] and since the Jamshidi technique is relatively noninvasive and inexpensive, its use was advocated for routine diagnostic bone biopsies. In a test of this advocacy, bone samples obtained with a new Jamshidi needle of 3 mm inner diameter and 3.5 length were compared with bone samples obtained with the previously described electric drill technique[47,84] providing samples of 5 mm inner diameter and 3 cm length. Both techniques were used during anterior iliac crest bone biopsies in 14 patients suffering from various metabolic bone disease.[87] The anterior and posterior samples were obtained using both instruments in alternation. Slides from samples with 3 mm and 5 mm diameter did not differ with respect to quality. Quantitative parameters of bone structure, such as cancellous bone mass and mean trabecular diameter, were not significantly different and correlated. Also, the volume and surface of osteoid and bone-osteoblast interface were the same and correlated. However, bone-osteoclast interface did not correlate, and mineral apposition rates were different. These findings question the advocacy of the Jamshidi technique, since bone samples of 3 mm inner diameter did not provide the same useful information as derived from the 5 mm samples. Only further studies will determine whether an increase in diameter from 3 to 4 mm (adding more than 30% additional area for examination) would give the same information that can be obtained from 5 mm bone samples.

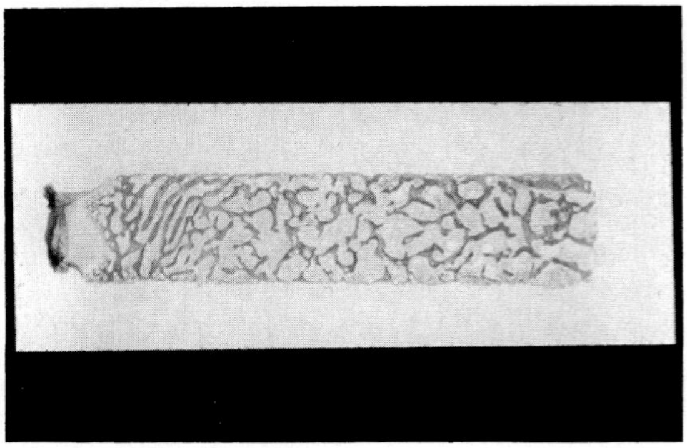

Figure 10–11. Bone slide of 3 μm thickness cut from samples of 5 mm diameter and 3 mm diameter. Photograph taken from original histologic slide. *See color plate II*

C. Skeletal Sites for Bone Biopsies

Metabolic bone diseases represent systemic diseases of the skeleton. Therefore, bone samples of adequate size obtained from any site on the skeleton should provide the useful information necessary for diagnosis. It is desirable to have both cortical and cancellous bone included in the specimen. Rib biopsies were routinely performed in the past.[88,89] This procedure is rarely used now, however, since cancellous bone is relatively scarce in rib samples and the iliac crest offers a more easily accessible site with fewer complications after the biopsy. Since most normative data were obtained from the iliac crest, this site is now considered to be optimal for bone biopsies. Certain local factors known to influence bone turnover (such as direct weight-bearing or tension, and forces exerted by muscle pull) are minimized at the anterior iliac crest. Studies comparing iliac crest bone samples with those from other skeletal sites showed differences in absolute values for bone volume or mineral apposition rate, but a good correlation between iliac crest and vertebrae[90] tibia, or femur.[91,92]

Bone samples can be obtained vertically from the anterior or posterior iliac crest, or horizontally from the anterior iliac crest (Fig. 10–12).

In choosing the mode of biopsy and the site of biopsy (i.e., left or right iliac crest, anterior

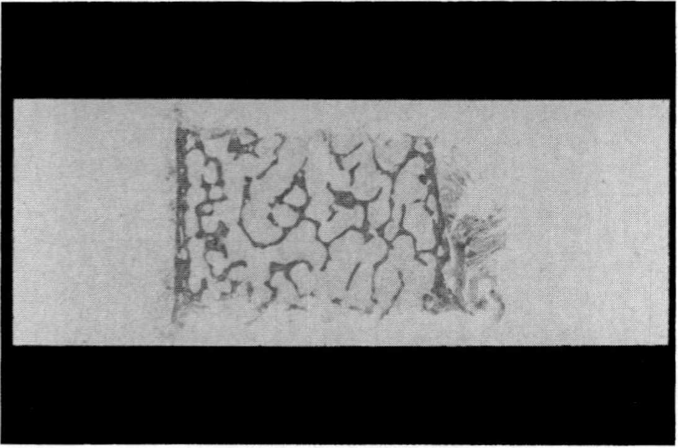

Figure 10–12. Bone slide of 3 μm thickness cut from a sample obtained horizontally using a trocar of 8 mm inner diameter. Inner and outer cortices are included in the sample. Undecalcified, 3 μm thick section of human iliac bone (modified Masson-Goldner stain). Photograph taken from original slide. *See color plate II*

or posterior iliac crest, horizontal or vertical, and superior or inferior), the variance of histomorphometric parameters within the iliac bone must be taken into consideration. There is no difference in cancellous bone mass between sections of vertical and horizontal bone biopsies. However, all other histomorphometric parameters are significantly higher in vertical biopsies—except the mean trabecular diameter. The superior-inferior variance must be taken into account when biopsy specimens are obtained horizontally, since the distance of the biopsy from the iliac crest may vary (i.e., one bone sample may be taken with a higher degree of superiority and the other with a higher degree of inferiority).

Quantitative bone parameters tend to be lower in sections from inferior biopsies than those from superior biopsies, but these differences are significant only for osteoid volume, mean osteoid seam thickness, bone-osteoblast interface, and osteoid surface ($p < 0.05$ to $p < 0.001$). Bone biopsy techniques obtaining samples vertically may provide bone samples from more anterior or more posterior sites; thus, the anterior-posterior variance along the iliac crest does not reveal significant differences in structural and cellular micromorphometric parameters of bone. Repeat biopsies are usually obtained from the contralateral site. Thus, the results are subjected to the right-left variance.

Studies in our laboratories on right-left variance reveal no difference in structural parameters of bone such as cancellous bone mass, mean trabecular diameter, volume of osteoid, osteoid surface, and mean osteoid seam thickness. However, the values for cellular parameters (such as osteoclastic index, bone-osteoblast interface, and trabecular surface exhibiting Howship's lacunae) are significantly higher ($p < 0.05$ to $p < 0.01$) in the right iliac crest bone.

These findings demonstrate that biopsies taken from contralateral sites of the iliac bone or obtained with different techniques can indeed be compared with each other if the ranges of variation are taken into account. (Note: Our data were obtained in 84 normal individuals.[47] These differences might be less if bone turnover is pathologically increased or more pronounced if bone turnover is suppressed.)

Ideally, one wants bone samples taken vertically and horizontally. This allows an assessment of subcortical cancellous bone and deep cancellous bone without restriction in size. The horizontally taken sample (again, ideally) would then provide information on the outer and inner cortices.

D. Indications for Bone Biopsies

In the past, bone biopsies were primarily performed for research purposes, and indications for diagnostic bone biopsies were restricted to the disabled or severely symptomatic patient. With the development and availability of histologic techniques allowing diagnosis of the various metabolic bone diseases, and with the advent of therapeutic modalities to reverse these abnormalities or slow their progression, performance of bone biopsies has been and should be considered more frequently. Bone biopsies performed in patients with end-stage or far-advanced diseases render little help to the patient and typically serve as mere documentation.

Given the time required for the development of severe or crippling bone diseases and their reversal by therapeutic regimens, bone biopsies should obviously be performed for early diagnosis rather than for late documentation of underlying bone disease. Note, however, that mineralized bone histology is a relatively new procedure not extensively employed in clinical diagnosis and research. Yet, as the frequency of bone biopsies and the clinical expertise in metabolic bone diseases increase, a deeper understanding of the underlying mechanisms of bone disease and novel therapeutic modalities will emerge. For example, novel noninvasive tests such as the recently introduced radioimmunoassay for bone Gla-protein[93-97] may become available for assessing metabolic bone diseases. As more of these tests become validated by bone histology, the indications for bone biopsies may be reduced. Conversely, knowledge derived from bone biopsies may well result in recognition of heretofore unknown pathologic features (such as the recently demonstrated accumulation of aluminum in bone of patients with renal failure or total parenteral nutrition), giving rise to new indications for bone biopsies.

Presently, bone biopsies are indicated for diagnosis and/or management of the following clinical problems

1. Osteoporosis (see Chapter 12)

Osteoporosis is not a homogeneous clinical entity, but rather a syndrome of bone loss associated with fractures. There is a wide range of etiologic factors for bone loss combined with heterogeneous histologic pictures. It seems logical to postulate that the different clinical syndromes of osteoporosis require different therapeutic approaches. Consequently, exact information on the histologic pattern of osteoporosis is desirable before an effective therapy can be instituted.

Histologically, a decrease in bone mass, that is, osteopenia, can be seen in cancellous and/or cortical bone. In cancellous bone, trabeculae appear thinner, that is, the trabecular diameter is reduced and there is increased separation between trabeculae. In histologic sections, a greater fraction of trabeculae are cut perpendicular to their long axis, producing the "button phenomenon," and there are fewer connections between trabeculae (Fig. 10–13).

Osteopenia can be histologically classified into two main groups based on cellular activities: active (or "high turnover") and inactive (or "low turnover") osteopenia. Active osteopenia (Figs. 10–14 to 10–16) is characterized by high-normal or increased number (and possibly activity) of osteoclasts with an increased number yet decreased activity of osteoblasts. Also, the fraction of trabecular surface exhibiting inactive resorption lacunae is increased in active osteopenia. It should be noted that inactive resorption lacunae reflect the composite activity of osteoclastic resorp-

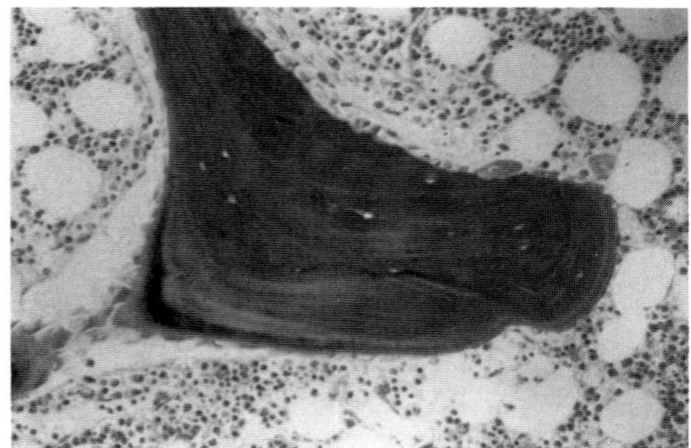

Figure 10–14. Active osteoporosis. High fraction of trabecular surface covered by osteoid and, on the opposite side of the trabecula, extended resorption zones. Undecalcified, 3 μm thick section of human iliac crest bone (modified Masson-Goldner stain; ×31). *See color plate II*

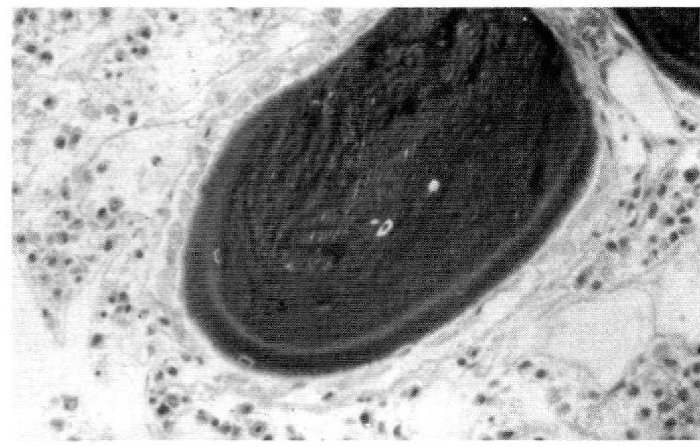

Figure 10–15. Active osteoporosis. High fraction of trabecular surface covered by osteoid, and presence of numerous osteoblasts covering the osteoid seam. Undecalcified, 7 μm thick section of human iliac bone (modified Masson-Goldner stain; ×40.) *See color plate II*

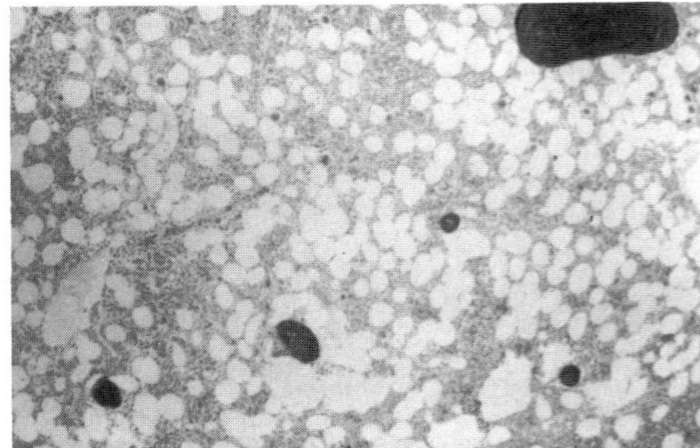

Figure 10–13. Osteopenia with "button phenomenon." Trabeculae cut perpendicularly to their long axis, producing the button phenomenon. Reduced connectivity between trabeculae. Undecalcified, 3 μm thick section of human iliac bone (modified Masson-Goldner trichrome stain; ×7.5). *See color plate II*

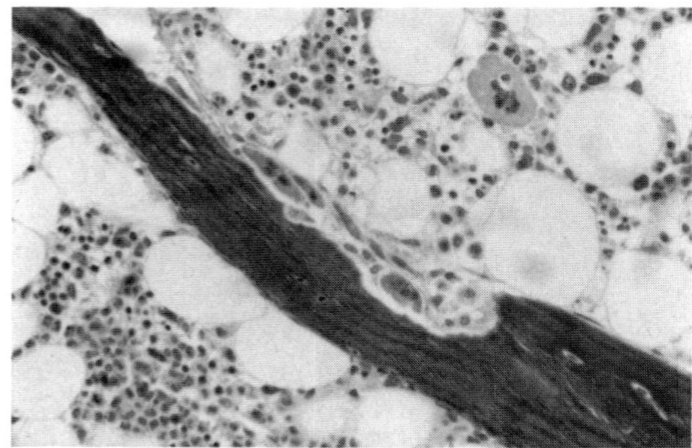

Figure 10–16. Active osteoporosis. Extended resorption lacunae with and without multinucleated osteoclasts. Undecalcified, 3 μm thick section of human iliac bone (modified Masson-Goldner stain; ×50). *See color plate III*

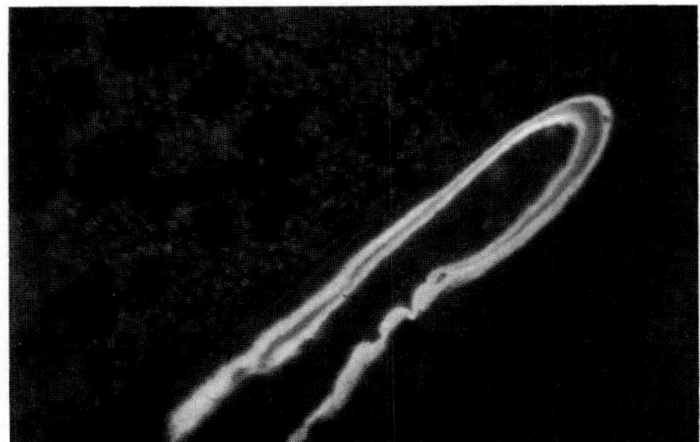

Figure 10–17. Active osteoporosis. High fraction of trabecular surface exhibiting tetracycline double labels. However, distance between labels varies from normal to low with appearance of merging of labels. Undecalcified, unstained, 7 μm thick section of human iliac bone. Fluorescent light microscopy (×25). *See color plate III*

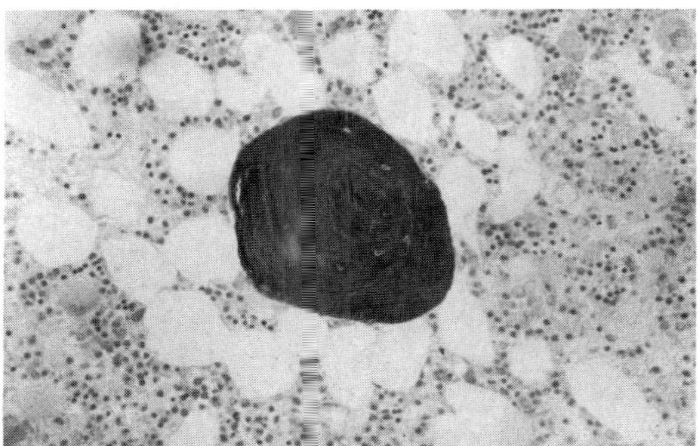

Figure 10–18. Inactive osteoporosis. Absence of osteoclasts and resorption zones. Absence of osteoid and osteoblasts. Undecalcified, 3 μm thick section of human iliac bone (modified Masson-Goldner stain; ×31). *See color plate III*

tion and osteoblastic refilling of the previously resorbed lacunae. Consequently, the fraction of trabecular surface exhibiting double labeling is normal or increased (Fig. 10–17).

Inactive osteopenia (Figs. 10–18 to 10–19) is characterized by few remodeling foci and a reduction in the number of osteoblasts and osteoclasts. Accordingly, the fraction of trabecular surface exhibiting resorption lacunae or tetracycline labels is usually less than normal (Fig. 10–19). In many instances, labels might merge, leading to an increased fraction of single labels. Moreover, the reduced number of foci may result in an increase in labeling escape and the appearance of more single labels.

Active and inactive osteopenia may appear in cortical as well as cancellous bone, and the histologic criteria are similar. In some patients, however, active osteopenia may appear in cancellous bone and inactive osteopenia in cortical bone, or vice versa. Whereas this phenomenon documents the functional identity of different envelopes in bone, only further studies will determine whether it has pathognomonic relevance or implications for therapy. Generally, however, osteoporotic patients with vertebral crush fractures have greater cancellous bone loss, whereas patients with hip fractures lose mainly cortical bone (C.C. Johnston, personal communication). It remains to be shown whether these differences are due to sequential bone loss in the two bone compartments or due to constant compartmental differences. In our experience, most patients experience bone loss in both cortical and cancellous bone, yet one compartment may be more severely affected than the other.[98]

Osteopenia in cortical bone is characterized by cortical thinning, increased porosity, and cancellization of cortex. The cortical thinning results primarily from resorption at the periosteal surface, increased porosity from resorption at the haversian surface, and cancellization from resorption at the endosteal surface.

A disturbance in the mineralization of bone may be associated with active and inactive osteopenia in cancellous or cortical bone. If this disturbance is not associated with a commensurate decrease in matrix production (as seen in inactive osteopenia), osteoid seam thickness increases and the combined histologic pattern of osteopenia and osteomalacia may be encountered (Figs. 10–20 and

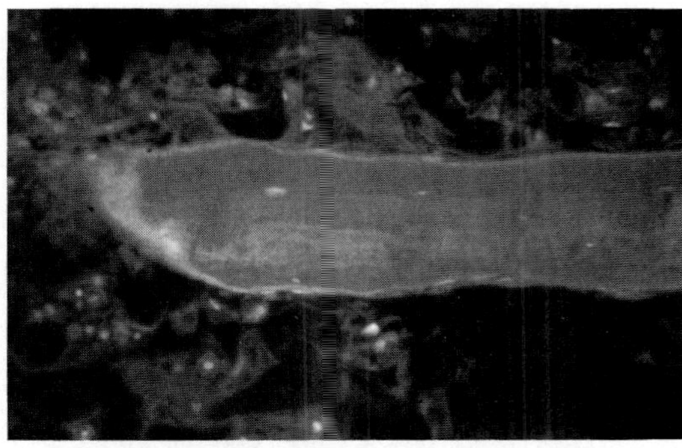

Figure 10–19. Inactive osteoporosis. Reduced tetracycline uptake. No double labels, only single labels of low intensity. Undecalcified, 7 μm thick section of human iliac bone. Fluorescent light microscopy (×31). *See color plate III*

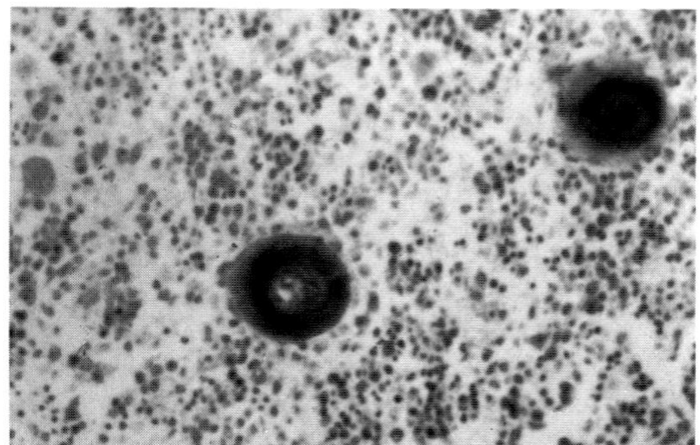

Figure 10–20. Osteopenia with osteomalacia. Reduced cancellous bone mass and increase in osteoid seam thickness. Undecalcified, 3 μm thick section from tibia of an oophorectomized and vitamin D–deficient rat (modified Masson-Goldner stain; ×20). *See color plate III*

10–21). Since osteoblastic dysfunction is frequent in osteopenia, the histologic pattern in patients with combined abnormalities may include low bone mass, increased fraction of trabecular surface covered by osteoid, low or normal osteoid seam thickness, decrease in the fraction of trabecular surface exhibiting tetracycline double labels with a relative increase in the fraction of trabecular surface exhibiting tetracycline single labels, and a decreased mineral apposition rate.

Repeat bone biopsies in patients with osteoporosis are performed to study mechanisms and to document success or to evaluate reasons for failure of the therapeutic regimen.

2. Defective Mineralization and Osteomalacia (see Chapter 11)

Osteomalacia was first described by Pommer[99] and defined as an abnormality in which

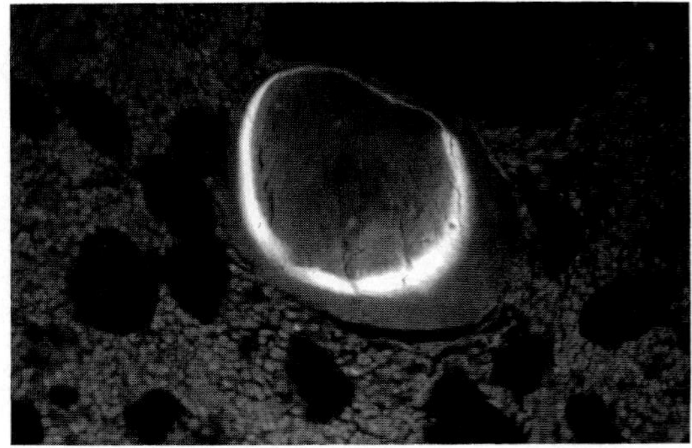

Figure 10–21. Osteopenia with osteomalacia. Presence of single tetracycline label with wide osteoid seam. Undecalcified, unstained, 7 μm thick section of human iliac bone (×31). *See color plate III*

newly formed bone matrix fails to mineralize in a normal or timely manner. The consequence of this condition is an accumulation of unmineralized matrix in bone. Clinically, the symptoms of osteomalacia include bone pain, muscle weakness, and spontaneous fractures or fractures occurring with minor trauma. X-ray techniques lack the sensitivity and specificity for diagnosing osteomalacia, since the reduction in mineral content of bone (in osteomalacia) cannot be differentiated roentgenologically from reduced bone mass without changes in the ratio between mineralized and unmineralized bone (i.e., osteopenia). Even the classic x-ray finding of Looser zones lacks the sensitivity and specificity to diagnose osteomalacia, as witnessed by the fact that Looser zones were not seen in most patients with histologically proven osteomalacia[100] whereas they were observed in patients with osteoporosis and not osteomalacia.[101] Bone biopsy is therefore essential for an unequivocal diagnosis of osteomalacia. The use of mineralized bone histology in diagnosing patients has revealed that the old concept of "soft bone resulting from too much osteoid" is insufficient for describing and classifying the changes observed in patients with osteomalacia (i.e., an abnormality in the ratio between bone formation and mineralization).

The introduction of tetracycline double labeling and the availability of routine biopsy techniques brought new insights into the different states of balance between bone matrix formation and mineral deposition. One such insight was that the number and extent of osteoid seams and the volume of osteoid represents the net result of the rate of appearance of new osteoid and the life span of the individual seams. This relationship was formulated by Frost[70,102] in the equation $O = \mu \times \text{sigma}$ (O = total osteoid; μ = birth rate of osteoid; and sigma = the life span of osteoid). This equation implies that the amount of osteoid present at any given time in the skeleton may be increased with enhanced formation of osteoid without an abnormality in mineralization being demonstrated. In other words, the amount of osteoid in the skeleton does not necessarily reflect the severity of the mineralization defect as was often implied in previous literature. Osteoid seams might increase in width or extent, thereby causing an increase in total osteoid volume. This increase in width or extent results from a lack of balance between the amount of osteoid formed and that mineralized per unit time. Consequently, "osteomalacia" describes the histologic finding of osteoid accumulation and wide osteoid seams, whereas "defective mineralization" describes commensurate abnormalities in bone formation and mineralization resulting in abnormal mineralization without an increase in osteoid seam width.

Histologically, three groups can be characterized: (1) active osteomalacia (Figs. 10–22 to 10–25); (2) inactive osteomalacia (Figs. 10–26 and 10–27); and (3) defective mineralization.

1. In active osteomalacia, there is an increase in osteoid volume resulting from an increase in the width of osteoid seams and an increase in the fraction of trabecular surface covered by osteoid (Fig. 10–22). A decrease in the mineral apposition rate and an increase in the fraction of single tetracycline labels of the broad diffuse type or the distinct single type documents that an abnormality in mineralization is contributing to the increase in osteoid volume (Fig. 10–25). Active osteomalacia is also characterized by numbers of osteoblasts and osteoclasts varying from low to low-normal or high-normal (Fig. 10–23); woven bone, woven osteoid (Fig. 10–24), and peritrabecular or marrow fibrosis is frequent.

2. Inactive osteomalacia with low bone turnover is characterized by an increase in osteoid volume associated with an increase in the thickness of osteoid seams and an increased fraction of trabecular surface covered by osteoid (Fig. 10–26). Abnormal mineralization is documented by a decrease in the fraction of trabecular surface exhibiting tetracycline labels. Not only are there fewer single labels, but there is a disproportionately greater reduction in double labels (Fig. 10–27).

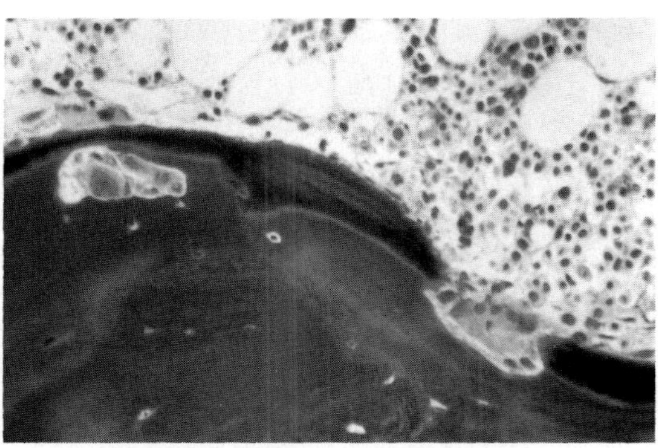

Figure 10–23. Active osteomalacia, moderate. Increase in fraction of trabecular surface covered by osteoid. Osteoid seam thickness high normal to increased. Trabecular surface without osteoid coating is being resorbed. Resorption cavities within mineralized trabecules under osteoid. Undecalcified, 3 μm thick section of human iliac bone (modified Masson-Goldner stain; ×50). *See color plate III*

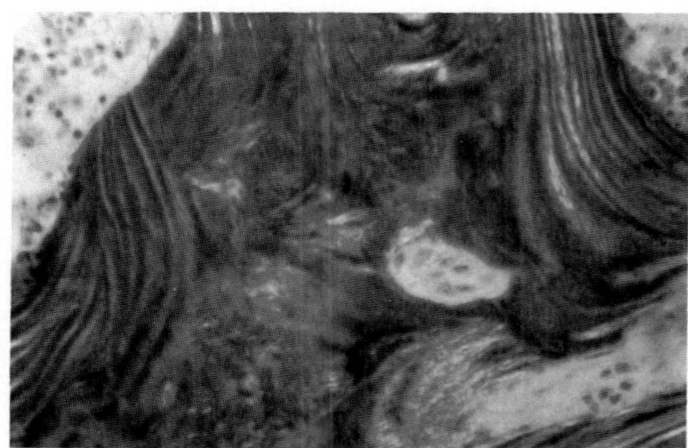

Figure 10–24. Active osteomalacia. Lamellar osteoid interspersed with woven osteoid and woven bone. Surface osteoid is mainly of the lamellar type. Undecalcified, 3 μm thick section of human iliac bone. Polarized light microscopy (modified Masson-Goldner stain; ×126). *See color plate IV*

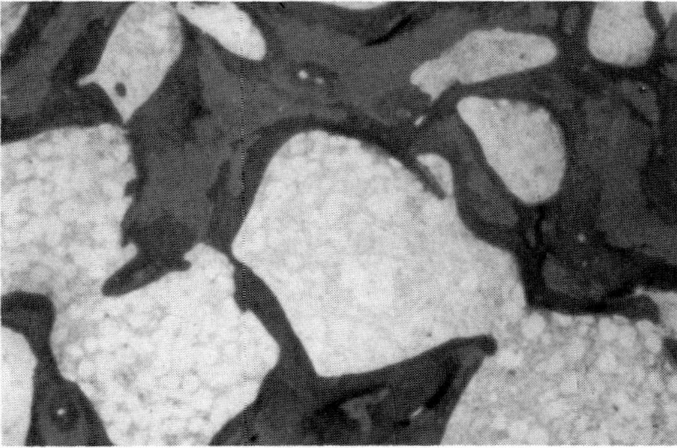

Figure 10–22. Active osteomalacia. Excessive accumulation of osteoid and increased width of osteoid seams. Undecalcified, 3 μm thick section of human iliac bone (modified Masson-Goldner stain; ×20). *See color plate III*

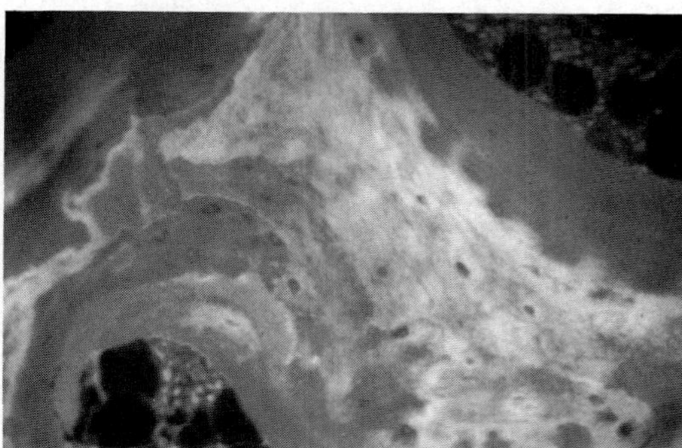

Figure 10–25. Active osteomalacia. Diffuse broad single labels of intense fluorescence. Undecalcified, unstained, 7 μm thick section of human iliac bone. Fluorescent light microscopy (×126). *See color plate IV*

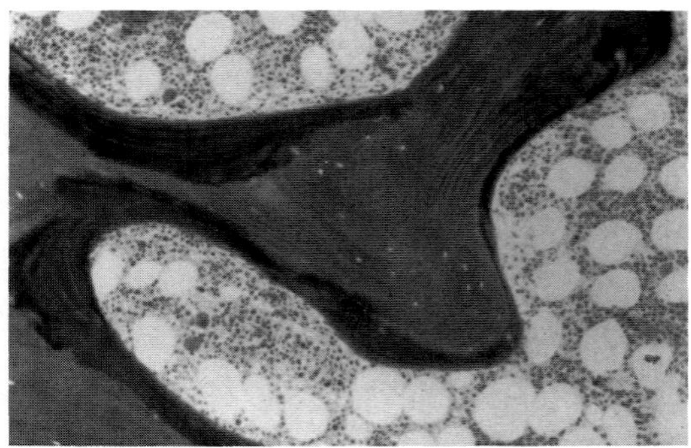

Figure 10–26. Inactive osteomalacia. Increased fraction of trabecular surface covered by osteoid. Osteoid seam thickness increased. Undecalcified, 3 μm thick section of human iliac bone (modified Masson-Goldner stain; ×31). *See color plate IV*

Inactive osteomalacia is usually associated with decreased mineral apposition rate, a decrease in bone-osteoblast interface, low bone-osteoclast interface, and absence of recent formation of woven osteoid or marrow fibrosis. The interface between mineralized bone and osteoid may be smooth or scalloped, reflecting low or high bone resorbing activity at the time osteoid was deposited.

3. Defective mineralization is characterized by a normal or increased volume of osteoid with normal osteoid seam thickness and an elevated fraction of trabecular surface covered by osteoid.

The mineralization defect is documented by the following dynamic parameters: a decrease in mineral apposition rate, normal or decreased fraction of tetracycline labeling with decreased fraction of double labels, and normal or increased fraction of single labels. The

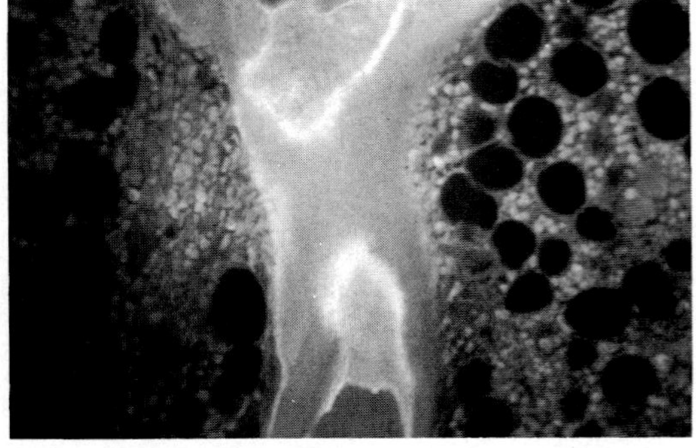

Figure 10–27. Inactive osteomalacia. Absence of tetracycline double labels, only a few thin or broad labels of low intensity. Undecalcified, unstained, 7 μm thick section of human iliac bone. Fluorescent light microscopy (×31). *See color plate IV*

single labels are usually thin. A state of low bone turnover is usually associated with the mineralization defect as evidenced by a reduced bone-osteoblast interface and low bone-osteoclast interface. If bone formation and bone resorption has become uncoupled, normal or high bone-osteoclast interfaces will result along with the other signs of low bone formation.

Teitelbaum[103] coined the term "appositional osteomalacia" to describe the histologic abnormality of reduced fractional labeling with decreased mineral apposition rate, and the term "maturational osteomalacia" for the histologic finding of broad single labels.

It is not clear whether high-turnover osteomalacia and low-turnover osteomalacia are distinct disease entities or whether they are merely phases of the same disease intercepted by bone biopsies at different times. It is conceivable that patients might initially develop high-turnover osteomalacia, wherein the higher bone turnover would serve as a compensatory mechanism to offset mineral losses from bone. As the disease progresses, bone turnover and cellular activities could conceivably decrease, thereby bringing on low-turnover osteomalacia.

3. Primary Hyperparathyroidism (see Chapter 14)

Positive clinical and laboratory tests for primary hyperparathyroidism do not represent an absolute indication for bone biopsies. However, normocalcemic patients with borderline or inconsistent elevations in parathyroid hormone levels and asymptomatic hypercalcemic patients with high-normal serum parathyroid hormone levels might well benefit from a bone biopsy. Mineralized bone histology will determine whether there are signs of severely increased parathyroid hormone activity on bone that warrants surgical intervention. A quantitative histology provides a level of information and objectivity for these sometimes difficult and equivocal clinical decisions. (It should be noted that serum parathyroid hormone levels fluctuate throughout the day, rendering interpretation of a single blood test difficult. Bone histology, however, reflects the integral of parathyroid hormone activity on bone over time.)

An overabundance of parathyroid hormone produces an increase in the number and size of all bone cells, including osteoclasts, osteoblasts, and osteocytes (Figs. 10–28 and 10–29).

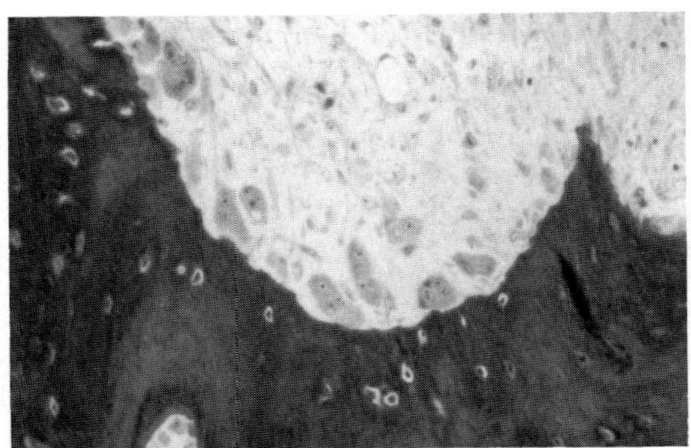

Figure 10–28. Primary hyperparathyroid bone disease. Increase in the number of osteoclasts and increased extent of trabecular surface exhibiting resorption lacunae. Increased density of osteocytes. Marrow fibrosis. Undecalcified, 3 μm thick section of human iliac bone (modified Masson-Goldner stain; ×50). *See color plate IV*

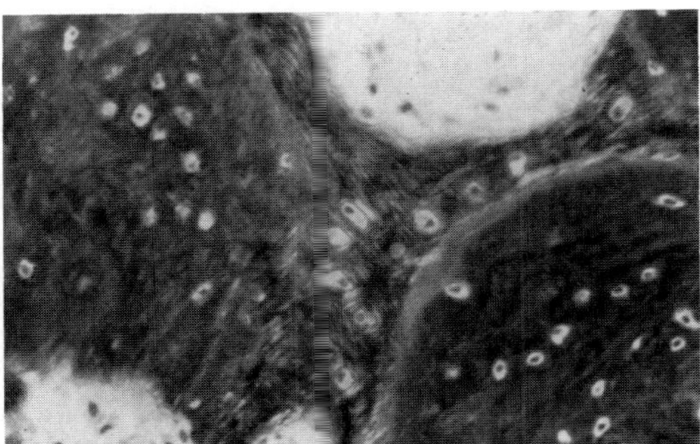

Figure 10–30. Primary hyperparathyroid bone disease. Appearance of woven osteoid. Undecalcified, 3 μm thick section of human iliac bone. Polarized light microscopy (modified Masson-Goldner stain; ×50). *See color plate IV*

Even though it is unclear whether there is increased activity at the cellular level, the increased number of cells may result in high activity at the tissue level—-as suggested by augmented osteoid volume, increased fraction of trabecular surface covered by osteoid, high bone-osteoclast interface with increased depth of resorption lacunae, increased number of osteocytes, and formation of woven osteoid (Fig. 10–30) and peritrabecular (Fig. 10–29) or marrow fibrosis. Bone mass may be normal, increased, or decreased depending on the prevailing bone balance.

If primary hyperparathyroidism occurs in postmenopausal women and patients with malnutrition or prolonged immobilization, osteopenia may ensue, whereas in patients with hyperphosphatemia, bone mass may be increased. (Note: Chronic continuous infusions of physiologic doses of parathyroid hormone in experimental dogs cause an increase in bone turnover without a significant effect on bone mass,[103] whereas chronic intermittent infusions of low-dose parathyroid hormone in osteoporotic patients are associated with an increase in bone mass.[104]) Dynamic parameters of bone, such as fractional tetracycline labeling and mineral apposition rate, are increased in cases of primary hyperparathyroidism (Fig. 10–31). The ratio, however, between double and single labels may decrease because of the increase in broad single labels resulting from an abnormal tetracycline uptake in woven bone (Fig. 10–32). We do not fully understand whether this phenomenon reflects a true mineralization defect or an abnormal mineral maturation in woven bone.

These changes in static and dynamic parameters of bone can be seen in various degrees in virtually all patients with hyperpara-

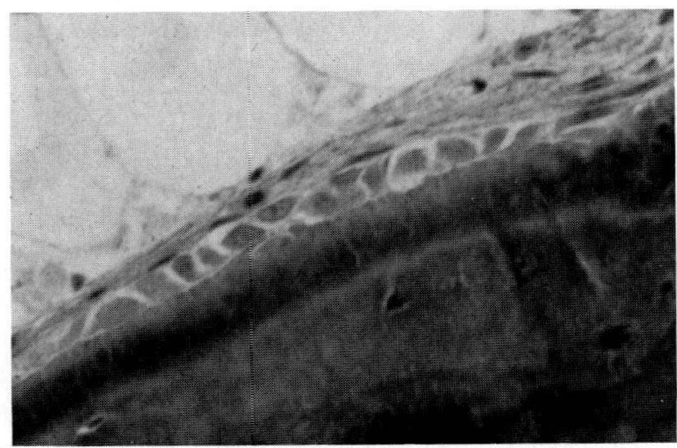

Figure 10–29. Primary hyperparathyroid bone disease. Increased number of osteoblasts. Peritrabecular fibrosis. Undecalcified, 3 μm thick section of human iliac bone (modified Masson-Goldner stain; ×126). *See color plate IV*

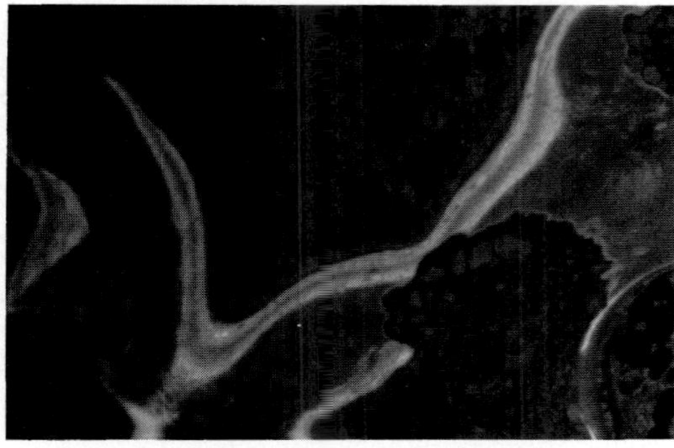

Figure 10–31. Primary hyperparathyroid bone disease. High fraction of trabecular surface exhibiting tetracycline uptake. Undecalcified, unstained, 7 μm section of human iliac bone. Fluorescent light microscopy (×31). *See color plate IV*

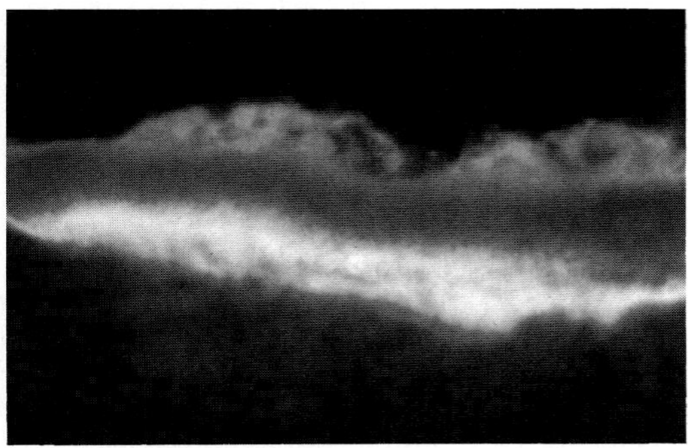

Figure 10–32. Primary hyperparathyroid bone disease. Appearance of bright and widespread labels reflecting tetracycline uptake in woven bone. Undecalcified, 7 μm thick section of human iliac bone. Fluorescent light microscopy (×126). *See color plate V*

thyroid bone disease. Bone histology may be more useful in some patients than x-rays or biochemical tests in the diagnosis of hyperparathyroid bone disease because x-ray imaging indicative of hyperparathyroid bone disease displays changes in cortical bone. Since turnover rates are lower in cortical than cancellous bone, the diagnostic information of x-ray imaging is restricted to late and pronounced stages of the disease. And since cancellous bone is well reflected in bone histology, this diagnostic tool is obviously superior to x-ray studies for early and sensitive diagnosis of hyperparathyroid bone disease. We have observed patients undergoing bone biopsies for osteoporosis whose serum parathyroid hormone levels and x-ray studies failed to reveal hyperparathyroid bone disease. Nevertheless, mineralized bone histology revealed clear signs of parathyroid hormone activity on the skeleton. Subsequent neck exploration showed diffuse parathyroid hyperplasia or microadenoma. As mentioned before, these observations could be explained in part by the fact that single measurements of serum parathyroid hormone concentrations do not necessarily reflect the integral of hormonal activity over time, whereas bone histology gives information on both the activity and the duration of parathyroid hormone effect on bone. Therefore, mineralized bone histology is a valuable tool for diagnosing and managing patients with mild or incipient hyperparathyroidism.

4. Renal Bone Disease (see Chapter 13)

A permanent reduction in glomerular filtration rate and abnormal bone metabolism are associated, not only in patients with end-stage renal failure but also in patients with creatinine clearances of 50 to 25 ml/minute. Patients requiring chronic maintenance dialysis display different groups of renal osteodystrophy. These groups include mixed uremic osteodystrophy (consisting of disturbed mineralization and signs of parathyroid hormone overactivity on bone), predominant hyperparathyroid bone disease, and predominant low-turnover osteomalacia, or adynamic bone disease. Since these subgroups require different therapeutic regimens, bone biopsies are essential for a rational approach. Also, there is aluminum accumulation in the bone of more than 95% of patients with low-turnover osteomalacia or adynamic bone disease, in 40% to 50% of dialyzed patients with mixed uremic osteodystrophy, and in 3% to 5% of those with predominant hyperparathyroid bone disease. Neither random determination of serum aluminum levels nor the change in serum aluminum levels after a single deferoxamine infusion is a reliable, noninvasive diagnostic test for aluminum-related bone disease. At the present, bone biopsies are the only available tool for diagnosing this disorder.

There are several bone abnormalities that develop after renal transplantation. The abnormality may be the result of persistent hyperparathyroidism, chronic steroid therapy, the administration of immunosuppressive drugs, or the prevalence of moderate renal failure.

Some patients with nephrotic syndrome experience urinary losses of vitamin D–binding protein resulting in bone abnormalities.[105] It remains unclear whether these patients develop more severe bone disease as their kidney function declines during the course of their underlying renal disease. However, bone biopsies in younger patients with nephrotic syndrome are particularly helpful in deciding whether to institute vitamin D therapy.

These bone abnormalities cannot be diagnosed by one or a combination of noninvasive tests. X-ray studies lack the sensitivity and specificity for diagnoses. In fact, x-ray images of subperiosteal resorption, endosteal erosion, longitudinal striations, acro-osteolysis, and rugger jersey spine are indicative of parathyroid overactivity on the skeleton and reflect changes in cortical bone. Yet, metabolic activity is much greater in cancellous bone.

Consequently, x-ray signs reflect advanced changes and cannot be used for early detection of bone abnormalities. If osteomalacic changes are superimposed upon previous hyperparathyroid bone disease, x-ray signs of hyperparathyroidism will persist and the osteomalacic abnormality cannot be recognized since osteoid is radiolucent. Oxalosis in bone may be a radiographic mimicry of renal osteodystrophy with predominant hyperparathyroid bone disease.[106] Thus, bone biopsies for mineralized bone histology are indicated if early and unequivocal diagnosis of renal bone diseases is desired and therapy is contemplated.

Histologic Pattern. Renal bone disease associated with the loss of kidney function (i.e., renal osteodystrophy) can be subdivided into three major histologic groups reflecting the pathogenetic factors known to contribute to the development of renal osteodystrophy: secondary hyperparathyroidism, defective renal production of 1,25(OH)$_2$D$_3$, and aluminum accumulation in bone. Accordingly, we make a distinction between predominant hyperparathyroid bone disease, mixed uremic osteodystrophy, and low-turnover osteomalacia. Yet, although these groups do not qualify as fully separate disease entities, distinguishing the three histologic patterns is necessary for the design and tailoring of therapeutic approaches to each group. Also, transformation from one group to another occurs, and the prevalence of a particular form varies, depending on geographic factors, aluminum exposure, therapy with vitamin D metabolites, dietary intake, and dialysis-related factors. Of unselected patients with end-stage renal failure, approximately 45% to 90% were found to have mixed uremic osteodystrophy, 5% to 20% predominant hyperparathyroid bone disease, and 5% to 35% low-turnover osteomalacia. And virtually all patients with mild to moderate renal failure have mixed uremic osteodystrophy.

Predominant Hyperparathyroid Bone Disease. Histologic changes in this subgroup of renal disease consist almost exclusively of signs of excess parathyroid hormone activity on the skeleton. In our unselected patients with end-stage renal failure, approximately 15% have predominant hyperparathyroid bone disease. Bone mass is significantly higher in this group than in patients with mixed uremic osteodystrophy or normal controls (Fig. 10–33). Whereas the mechanisms for this increase in bone mass remain unclear, possible factors are serum phosphorus, parathyroid hormone, calcium, 1,25(OH)$_2$D$_3$, or a combination of these factors. Also, patients with predominant hyperparathyroid bone disease may reveal excessive increases in trabecular bone mass alternating with hypercellular marrow—a finding illustrating the need for bone samples sufficient in size for the appropriate assessment of bone volume.

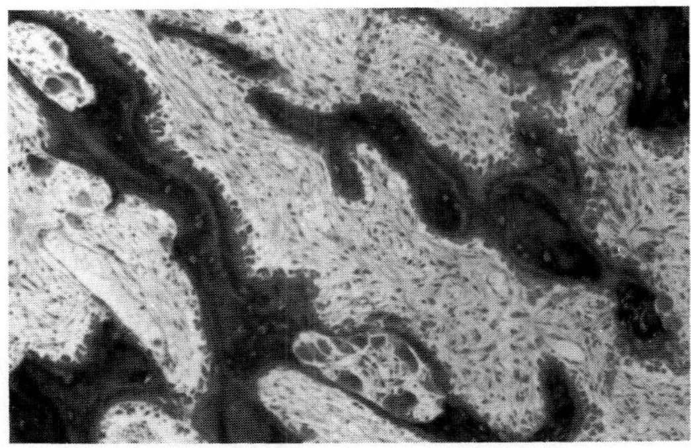

Figure 10–33. Renal osteodystrophy—predominant hyperparathyroid bone disease. High fraction of trabecular surface covered by osteoid seams. High osteoid-osteoblast interface. High bone-osteoclast interface with appearance of tunneling resorption. Marrow fibrosis. Undecalcified, 3 μm thick section of human iliac bone (modified Masson-Goldner stain; ×31). *See color plate V*

The term "osteosclerosis" is often used in describing bone mass increases observed in uremic patients with predominant hyperparathyroid bone disease. Yet, since osteosclerosis is also used to describe the radiologic finding of increased mineral density in bone, the term "increased bone mass" or "increased trabecular bone and/or cortical bone volume" is preferable.

When the high bone turnover associated with predominant hyperparathyroid bone disease develops in patients with preexisting negative bone balance (resulting from immobilization, malnutrition, heavy smoking, or other causes), an accelerated bone loss may occur that could cause severe osteopenia.

Osteoid volume and trabecular surface covered by osteoid are increased in predominant hyperparathyroid bone disease because of the enhanced production of woven osteoid (Fig. 10–34) and the high activation frequency of bone-remodeling sites as a result of parathyroid hormone overactivity. The augmented remodeling activity is reflected in the high fraction of trabecular surfaces exhibiting tetracycline labels (Fig. 10–35) and an increase

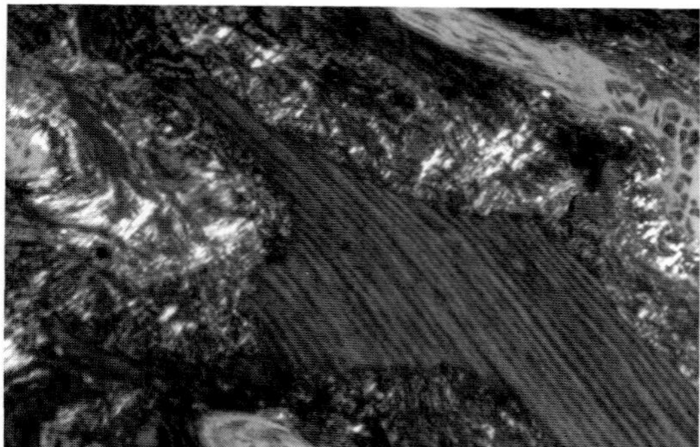

Figure 10–34. Woven osteoid and woven bone in predominant hyperparathyroid bone disease. Appearance of irregular crisscross pattern of mineralized bone (blueish-gray) and osteoid (golden-yellow-orange) surrounding an island of previously deposited normal lamellar bone exhibiting the typical birefringence (rust-brown). Undecalcified 3 μm thick section of human iliac bone. Polarized light microscopy (modified Masson-Goldner stain; ×50). *See color plate V*

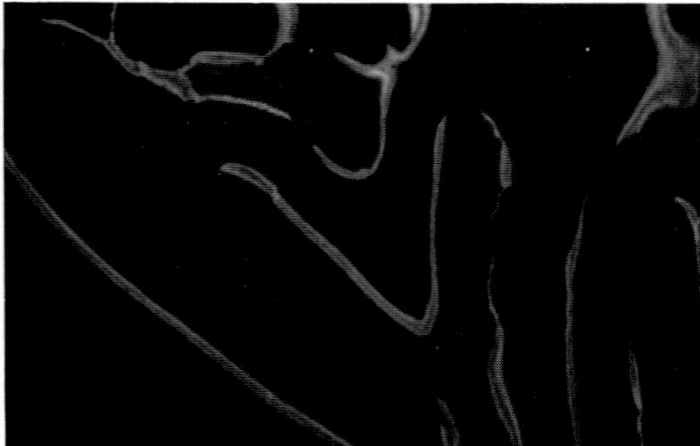

Figure 10–35. Mineralization in predominant hyperparathyroid bone disease. Increased fraction of trabecular surface exhibiting tetracycline uptake. The majority of the tetracycline labels exhibit regular double labels. Undecalcified, unstained, 7 μm thick section of human iliac bone. Fluorescent light microscopy (×22.5). *See color plate V*

in the mineral apposition rate. The diffuse uptake of tetracycline under fluorescent light demonstrates an abnormal mineralization of woven osteoid (Fig. 10–36). Mineralization proceeds rapidly and irregularly in predominant hyperparathyroid bone disease, an abnormality that may help explain the clinical paradox of patients being prone to fractures even though histologic findings reveal increased bone mass. Such a diagnostic difficulty merely underscores the need for bone histology, including an evaluation of bone texture and mineralization dynamics under polarized and fluorescent light.

Signs of stimulated bone activity at the tissue level in patients with predominant hyperparathyroid bone disease are paralleled by an increase in the number of bone cells and an abundance of osteocytes, osteoblasts, and osteoclasts (Fig. 10–33). As a result of excessive parathyroid hormone stimulation, the osteoblasts no longer deposit collagen exclusively toward the trabecular surface. Instead, collagen fibers are extruded into the marrow cavity, producing endosteal fibrosis. Advanced cases reveal hematopoietic or fat marrow entirely replaced by collagen fibers. Osteoblasts may vary in size and shape, losing their regular cuboidal form and appearing as very irregular polygonal or spindle-shaped osteoblasts. They may also present eccentric nuclei.

With the increased number of osteoblasts, an increased fraction is entrapped during bone formation, thus resulting in an increased number of osteocytes. Note that the increased number of osteoblasts does not necessarily reflect an increase in bone formation at the tissue level, since it might quite well represent a compensatory response to an insufficiency at the cellular level.[35]

Histologic signs of abnormal cell functions in predominant hyperparathyroid bone disease include osteocytic lacunae of irregular size and shape; the production of fibers and woven osteoid by osteoblasts; and the abundance and prominence of osteoclastic nuclei with increased cytoplasmic vacuolization. Osteoclasts appear as giant multinucleated cells with abundant cytoplasm breaking through lamellar boundaries and resorbing bone both from the trabecular surface and from within trabeculae. Consequently, lacunar resorption

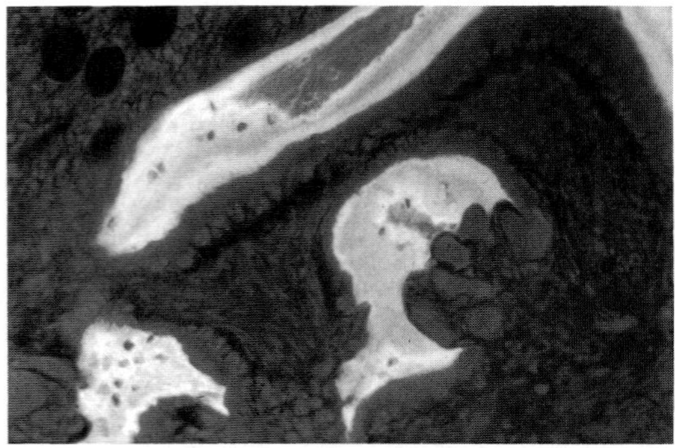

Figure 10–36. Mineralization in predominant hyperparathyroid bone disease. Presence of diffuse intense single labels in woven bone adjacent to double labels. Undecalcified, unstained, 7 μm thick section of human iliac bone. Fluorescent light microscopy (×31). *See color plate V*

or dissective excavating resorption may be seen, and since osteoclasts rarely resorb unmineralized bone, dissective or tunneling resorption is found in patients with excessive surface coverage of osteoid (Fig. 10–33). Finding osteoclasts over osteoid does not necessarily imply that osteoclasts resorb osteoid, but could result from an oblique cut through a nest of osteoclasts dwelling in an adjacent resorption cavity.

Early publications misinterpreted this hypercellularity in predominant hyperparathyroid bone disease as an indication of an inflammatory process; thus, the term "osteitis fibrosa" was coined to describe the hypercellularity and fibrosis.

Mixed Uremic Osteodystrophy. Mixed uremic osteodystrophy is found in the majority of patients with end-stage renal failure and consists of two major components, hyperparathyroid bone disease and defective mineralization. A spectrum of both histologic features may coexist at varying degrees in different patients. In our unselected patients undergoing 1 to 10 years of maintenance dialysis, approximately 80% revealed mixed uremic osteodystrophy.

Usually, patients with mixed uremic osteodystrophy have normal cancellous bone mass. Individual differences, however, are hardly surprising, since in cross-sectional studies, bone mass in any given patient must be the composite result of a net gain of bone occurring prior to the initiation of dialysis[107] and possible bone loss during maintenance hemodialysis.[108] These factors can only be unraveled in longitudinal prospective studies.

In our study of 20 patients on maintenance hemodialysis,[107] all patients were biopsied at the time of entry into the chronic dialysis program, and a second time 9 to 16 months later. Two bone samples were taken at each biopsy to provide an independent estimate of the sampling error. Mineralized bone histology and quantitative evaluation of volumetric density of bone were performed on all bone samples, and differences in bone mass were considered significant only when the changes between the first and second biopsy significantly exceeded the intraskeletal variance.

After 9 months of hemodialysis, 5% of patients showed a significant increase and 25% a significant decrease in volumetric density of bone. In four of the five patients with a significant decrease in bone mass, predisposing factors could easily be identified, including immobilization, catabolism with weight loss, and reversal of predialytic increase in bone mass. A determination of bone aluminum was not performed for this study. Our conclusions were that significant bone loss is not an invariable consequence of hemodialysis, even in the elderly and postmenopausal patient. Negative bone balance (i.e., a decrease in bone mass) results from an imbalance between the rate of bone deposition and the rate of bone resorption. The rate of bone loss increases with higher bone turnover. Consequently, in mixed uremic osteodystrophy with a marked component of hyperparathyroid bone disease, or in predominant hyperparathyroid bone disease, accelerated bone loss with severe skeletal destruction may ensue if the balance between bone deposition and bone resorption is not maintained.

The major structural abnormality in patients with mixed uremic osteodystrophy is the accumulation of osteoid (Fig. 10–37). Since both lamellar and woven osteoid can be distinguished under polarized light, an increase in the volume and surface of woven osteoid results in less lamellar osteoid. Even though total osteoid may not change, the ratio between woven and lamellar osteoid may be reversed. Consequently, routine polarized light microscopy is necessary for evaluating mixed uremic osteodystrophy.

Woven osteoid, then, provides a valuable criterion for distinguishing mixed uremic osteodystrophy from low-turnover osteomalacia

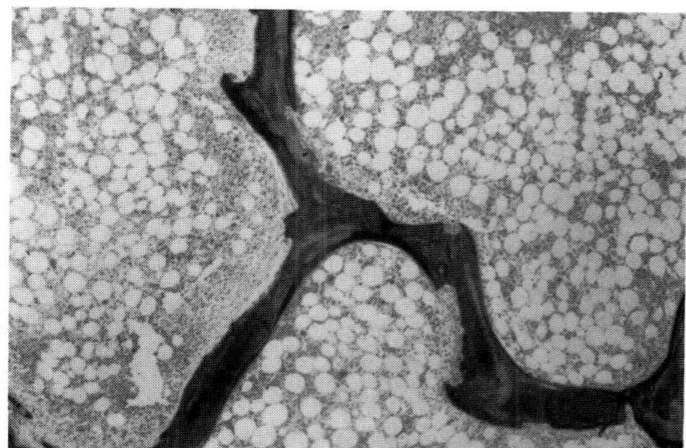

Figure 10–37. Mixed uremic osteodystrophy. Increased fraction of trabecular surface covered by osteoid. Mean thickness of osteoid seams is increased, resulting in high osteoid volume. Increased extent of trabecular surface exhibiting resorption lacunae filled with or void of osteoclast. Undecalcified, 3 μm thick section of human iliac bone (modified Masson-Goldner stain; ×7.5). *See color plate V*

or from hyperparathyroid bone disease. Lamellar osteoid accumulation is typical of low-turnover osteomalacia, and woven osteoid accumulation occurs mainly in predominant hyperparathyroid bone disease. Mixed uremic osteodystrophy, however, presents both types of osteoid.

The thickness of lamellar and woven osteoid is mildly to moderately increased in uremic osteodystrophy (Fig. 10–38), and cellular parameters such as the bone-osteoblast interface and bone-osteoclast interface are in the upper range of normal or elevated. There may be more or less cellularity and varying degrees of peritrabecular fibrosis, depending on whether the hyperparathyroid component or the defect in mineralization component predominates. Usually, not more than 30% of the trabecular surface is covered by collagen fibers.

Mixed uremic osteodystrophy also displays parameters of bone dynamics reflecting abnormal mineralization and bone formation (Fig. 10–39). This may result from either the impaired production of the active vitamin D metabolite or the accumulation of aluminum in bone. Our cross-sectional studies in patients revealed that 48% with mixed uremic osteodystrophy had aluminum deposition at the mineralization front—demonstrable by histochemical staining and energy-dispersive x-ray analysis.[109]

The fraction of lamellar osteoid seams exhibiting tetracycline double labeling is typically reduced and bone formation and resorption rates are decreased at both the osteon level and the cell level in mixed uremic osteo-

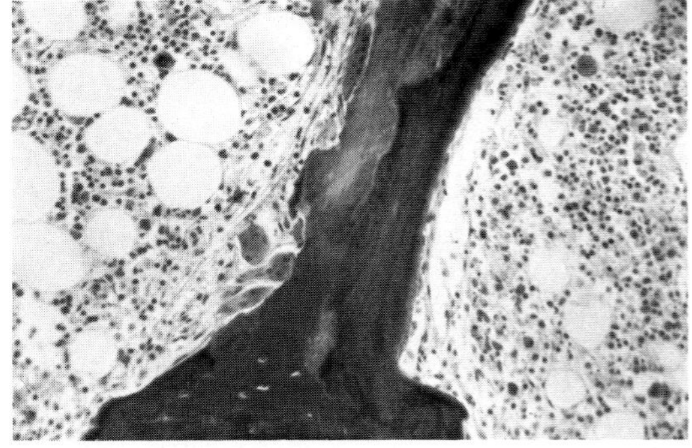

Figure 10–38. Mixed uremic osteodystrophy. Increased width of osteoid seams and resorption lacunae with multinucleated osteoclasts. Elevated osteoid-osteoblast interface. Mild peritrabecular fibrosis. Undecalcified, 3 μm thick section of human iliac bone (modified Masson-Goldner stain; ×31). *See color plate V*

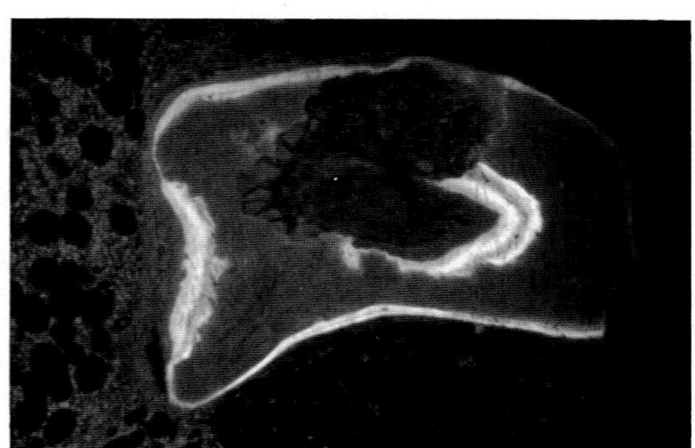

Figure 10–39. Mixed uremic osteodystrophy. Regular double uptake of tetracycline with increased distance between labels, single uptake and irregular diffuse uptake. Undecalcified, unstained, 7 μm thick section of human iliac bone. Fluorescent light microscopy (×20). *See color plate V*

dystrophy. Mineral apposition rate may be normal, mildly elevated, or decreased, dependent upon the relative presence of a hyperparathyroid component or a defect in mineralization (Fig. 10–39). The hyperparathyroid component is often mitigated in the presence of aluminum accumulation, that is, there are fewer osteoblasts and osteoclasts and signs of decreased activity of bone-forming and -resorbing cells.

Some patients with presumably recent aluminum exposure reveal a dissociation between osteoblastic and osteoclastic cell numbers—a decrease in osteoblasts with relatively large numbers of osteoclasts. This observation indicates that aluminum may initially affect osteoblasts and that the subsequent reduction in osteoclastic activity may be a result of the known coupling between bone formation and resorption. Whether mixed uremic osteodystrophy represents a distinct histopathologic group or whether there are subgroups included in this clinicopathologic entity awaits further study and clarification.

Low-Turnover Osteomalacia and Adynamic Uremic Bone Disease. Low-turnover or adynamic uremic bone disease occurs in a minority of patients with end-stage renal failure. These patients are prone to develop spontaneous fractures or fractures with minor trauma. They may present with normal or low levels of circulating parathyroid hormone, suffer from bone and muscle pain, and develop hypercalcemia after therapeutic trials using the available vitamin D metabolite.

Although there is considerable variation in the prevalence of low-turnover osteomalacia or adynamic uremic bone disease, there does seem to be an apparent geographic distribution. Centers in Great Britain,[110-112] the Federal Republic of Germany,[113] France,[114,115] and the United States[116,117] report that 20% to 30% of their patients undergoing hemodialysis reveal low-turnover osteomalacia or adynamic bone disease. Other dialysis centers in the United States[118] and the Federal Republic of Germany[119] report an incidence of low-turnover osteomalacia or adynamic uremic bone disease in 4% to 5% of their chronic dialysis patients, a finding in keeping with our present experience with unselected patients from various geographic areas. In individual dialysis centers, however, low-turnover osteomalacia or adynamic uremic bone disease occurs in more than 30% of the patients. (Note: Dialysis encephalopathy is also a relatively common occurrence in centers where low-turnover osteomalacia is frequent, pointing to a toxic and/or geographic factor in the development of uremic low-turnover osteomalacia.)

Recent claims that iron might also play a role in the pathogenesis of low-turnover osteomalacia[120] await clarification. Yet, in preliminary studies we applied a histochemical stain for iron (modified Gomori stain) and energy-dispersive x-ray analysis for the evaluation of patients with hemosiderosis with and without concomitant bone aluminum accumulation. Iron was discovered deposited at various sites, most commonly at the marrow-bone interface (including neutral surfaces), osteoid, and resorption zones. We also found iron distributed throughout osteoid or at the mineralization front. As yet, no clear-cut relationship has been established between iron deposition at the mineralization front and parameters of osteomalacia. Aluminum, however, was found localized at the mineralization front, and a clear correlation could be established between parameters of defective mineralization and aluminum deposition. These findings argue against the notion that iron represents another pathogenetic factor for low-turnover osteomalacia or adynamic uremic bone disease. However, the entire issue awaits further studies and clarification.

Low-turnover osteomalacia is histologically characterized by accumulation of lamellar osteoid occupying most of the trabecular surface (Fig. 10–40) and, not infrequently, 30% to 50% of trabecular bone volume. The excessive accumulation of lamellar osteoid may cause an increase in cancellous bone mass. There is low cellular activity and an absence or paucity of osteoclasts and osteoblasts. If osteoclasts are present, they are usually seen within trabecular bone (Fig. 10–41) or at the small fraction of trabecular surface left without osteoid coating.

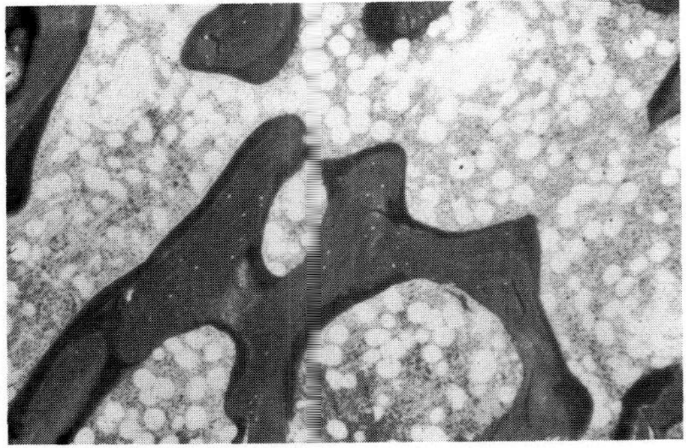

Figure 10–40. Renal osteodystrophy—low-turnover osteomalacia. Increase in osteoid volume. Absence of osteoblasts and surface resorption. Undecalcified, 3 μm thick section of human iliac bone (modified Masson-Goldner stain; ×8). *See color plate VI*

The irregular interface between osteoid and mineralized bone is in striking contrast to the smooth contour of the osteoid-marrow interface, perhaps reflecting previously enhanced resorbing activity. There is noticeable absence of peritrabecular and marrow fibrosis, and only a few fibers might be found associated with resorption (Fig. 10–41).

The decrease in osteoblast number is associated with low tetracycline uptake, and the osteoid seams lack fluorescent tetracycline labels or show thin single labels of low intensity at the bone-osteoid interface (Fig. 10–42). The number of remodeling sites with double labels as well as the distance between double labels is dramatically reduced, and bone for-

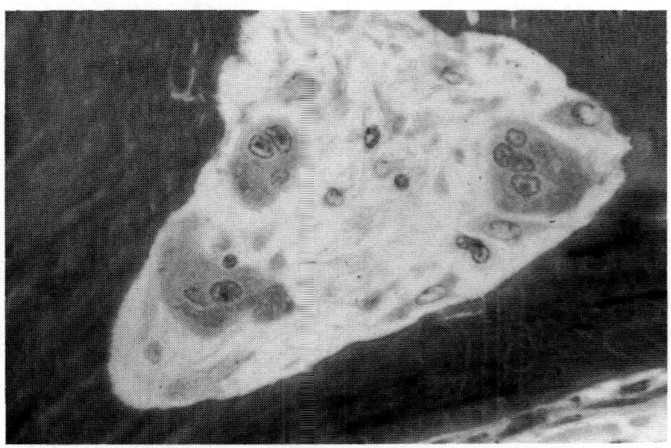

Figure 10–41. Renal osteodystrophy—low-turnover osteomalacia. Osteoclasts resorbing bone within trabecular bone and underneath osteoid. Fibers filling the resorption lacunae and thin layer of peritrabecular fibrosis (modified Masson-Goldner stain; ×126). *See color plate VI*

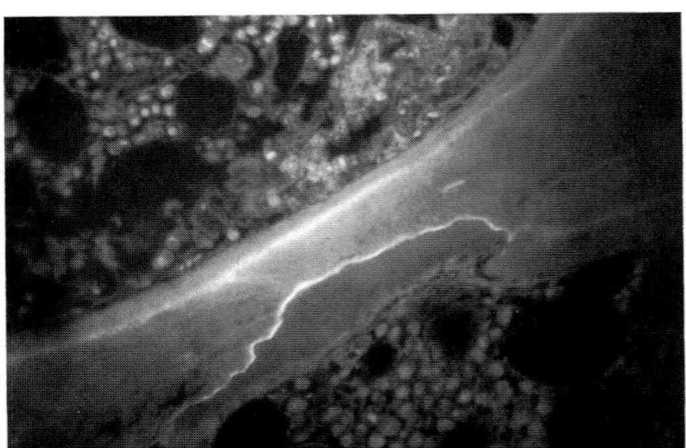

Figure 10–42. Mineralization defect in low-turnover osteomalacia. Absence of double labels. Thin single labels at the osteoid-bone interface of low intensity. Undecalcified, unstained, 7 μm thick section of human iliac bone. Fluorescent light microscopy (×31). *See color plate VI*

mation and resorption rates at the cellular and osteon level are extremely low.

Patients displaying all these histologic criteria, although without excessive osteoid seam thickness and increased osteoid volume, usually have a shorter history of uremia (Fig. 10–43). They may have been exposed to very high amounts of aluminum without long-standing prior hyperparathyroid bone disease, that is, without being subjected to the stimulatory effects of parathyroid hormone on bone formation. The terms "adynamic uremic bone disease" or "aplastic uremic bone disease" describe this entity.

Ninety-five per cent of the patients with low-turnover osteomalacia and adynamic uremic bone disease reveal aluminum accumulation. Although a cause-effect relationship between bone abnormalities and aluminum accumulation in bone is not yet fully established, clinical experience shows that the presence of stainable bone aluminum is associated statistically with a higher degree of disability.[121] This is partly due to increased fracture rate, delayed healing or nonhealing of fractures, and the poor success of orthopedic surgical interventions.

Renal Bone Disease Associated with Mild to Moderate Renal Failure. The serum biochemical derangements, intestinal malabsorption of calcium, and bone abnormalities associated with end-stage renal failure are also found in a milder form in patients with mild to moderate renal failure.[122-124] In 50 patients with mild to advanced renal failure (glomerular filtration rate: 30–50 ml/min), histologic studies found increased resorption cavities filled with loosely textured woven osteoid. This was observed without clearly increased bone-osteoclastic interface. Even though the number of osteoclasts is usually normal in patients with glomerular filtration rates over 50 ml/minute, the relatively wide normal range may conceal mild increments in the number of osteoclasts in individual patients with incipient renal failure.

Qualitatively, the osteoclasts appear larger and have more nuclei than in normal individuals. The histologic finding of increased trabecular surface covered by osteoclasts in some patients with incipient renal failure and normal parathyroid hormone level is of particular interest. Other than the possibility of methodologic problems in the parathyroid hormone radioimmunoassay, this finding could indicate that mechanisms other than parathyroid hormone regulate the number of osteoclasts, or that the mitotic response characteristic of osteoclast precursor cells to endogenous parathyroid hormone may be

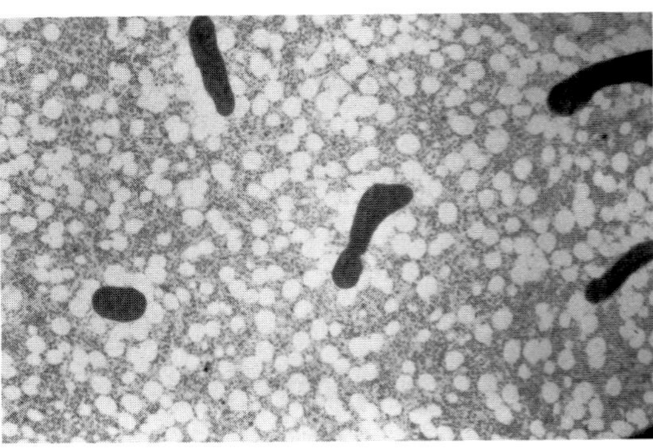

A

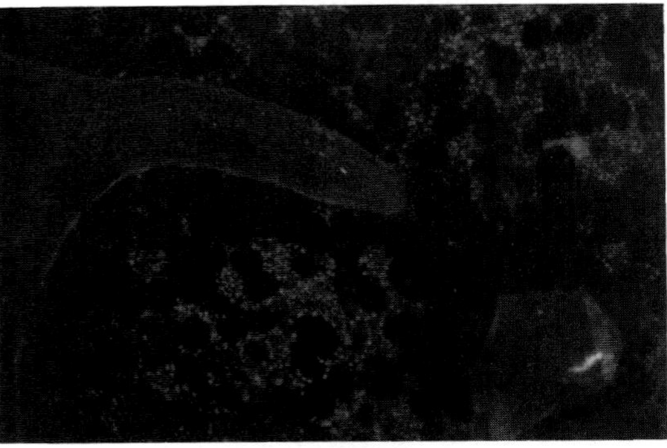

B

Figure 10–43. Adynamic uremic bone disease. *A*, No accumulation of osteoid. Absence of bone formation and resorption. Undecalcified, 3 μm thick section of human iliac bone (modified Masson-Goldner stain; ×20). *B*, Absence of tetracycline uptake documenting no mineralizing activity. Undecalcified, 7 μm thick section of human iliac bone. Fluorescent light microscopy (×31). *See color plate VI*

altered in incipient renal failure. Also, a single measurement of parathyroid hormone may not be at all representative for effects of parathyroid hormone on bone, since parathyroid hormone levels are known to fluctuate widely throughout the day.

Osteoid volume increases with falling glomerular filtration rate and is above normal in 50% of patients with a glomerular filtration rate between 50 and 60 ml/minute. Osteoid surface also increases with falling glomerular filtration rate and correlates with both the osteoclastic surface resorption and endosteal fibrosis, a finding indicating that the coupling between bone formation and resorption is maintained in mild to moderate renal failure. Woven osteoid, first appearing sporadically in resorption cavities, is seen in extended broad appositional fronts when the glomerular filtration rate falls below 40 ml/minute, and only after the glomerular filtration rate falls below 30 ml/minute does endosteal fibrosis occur.[123]

The exact threshold level of glomerular filtration rate at which a mineralization defect appears is difficult to define. Whereas there are patients with a glomerular filtration rate over 40 ml/minute who show an increased fraction of osteoid seams failing to incorporate tetracycline labels, most patients do not develop overt mineralization defect until the glomerular filtration rate falls below 40 ml/minute. In individual patients, however, even those in advanced renal failure, mineralization may be unremarkable.

The histopathologic findings in patients with mild to moderate renal failure are qualitatively identical to those seen in patients with end-stage renal failure and mixed uremic osteodystrophy. Felsenfeld et al.[125] report low-turnover osteomalacia in a patient with advanced renal failure before the onset of dialysis. Perhaps this resulted from aluminum accumulation in bone. But in a retrospective study of 100 patients with mild to moderate renal failure, we found stainable bone aluminum in 5%. The extent of trabecular surface with stainable bone aluminum was less than 30%, and the histologic diagnosis was mixed uremic osteodystrophy in all patients.[121]

5. Bone Abnormalities in Renal Stone Formers (see Chapter 23)

Tubular defects such as the adult Fanconi syndrome may cause mineral losses and associated severe bone abnormalities. Patients suffering from renal stone disease may have a bone abnormality contributing to their hypercalciuria and proclivity to form stones. In fact, the bone abnormality may prove to be the primary cause, as in the cases of patients with resorptive hypercalciuria;[126] the bone abnormality may be a secondary phenomenon resulting from renal calcium losses;[127] or the bone abnormality may represent an unexplained finding deserving further studies before we speculate on cause and effect.[128]

6. Pediatric Diseases (see Chapter 24)

Indications for bone biopsies in children are similar to those listed for adults. However, bone biopsies for mineralized bone histology are particularly helpful in the diagnosis and management of rickets, osteogenesis imperfecta, osteopetrosis, and other rare pediatric bone diseases. Note that the dosage required for diagnostic tetracycline labeling of bone neither discolors teeth nor affects skeletal growth. Also, growth is not affected by the biopsy even though the continuity of the growth plate may be temporarily disrupted by the biopsy.

7. Miscellaneous (see Chapters 15, 16, 17)

Bone biopsies are indicated in patients with unexplained bone pain, with unexplained elevation of serum alkaline phosphatase, with unexplained deviations from normal in serum calcium and phosphorus, and whenever the diagnosis of Paget's disease is not clearly established and malignancy has been ruled out.

Diphosphonates, which are used for treatment of patients with Paget's disease (Fig. 10–44), may induce a mineralization defect. Bone biopsies are therefore helpful in documenting normalcy of mineralization before the institution of therapy and to rule out abnormal mineralization after long-term therapy. Bone biopsies for mineralized bone histology are also indicated in patients with delayed fracture healing, pseudofractures, fractures after minimal trauma, and prolonged healing after bone and joint surgery, bone implants, or other orthopedic interventions.

In metastatic bone diseases, the biopsy may help to determine the origin of the primary tumor (Fig. 10–45). In sporadic cases, bone biopsies might reveal an unexpected mye-

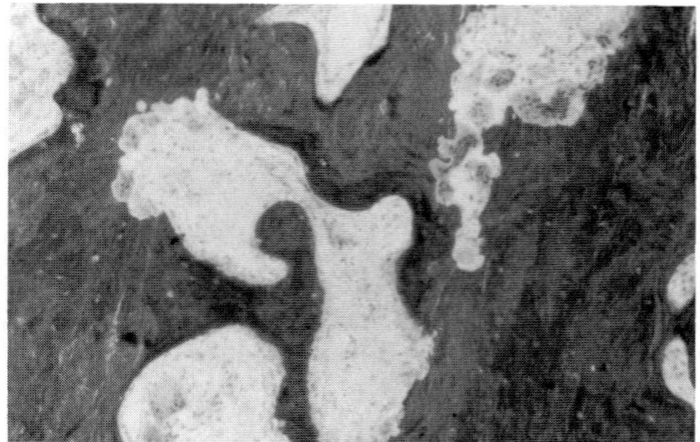

Figure 10–44. Paget's disease of bone. Increased trabecular surface covered by osteoid. Seam width increased. Lamellar osteoid and woven osteoid coexist. Undecalcified, 3 μm thick section of human iliac crest bone under polarized light (modified Masson-Goldner stain; ×31). *See color plate VI*

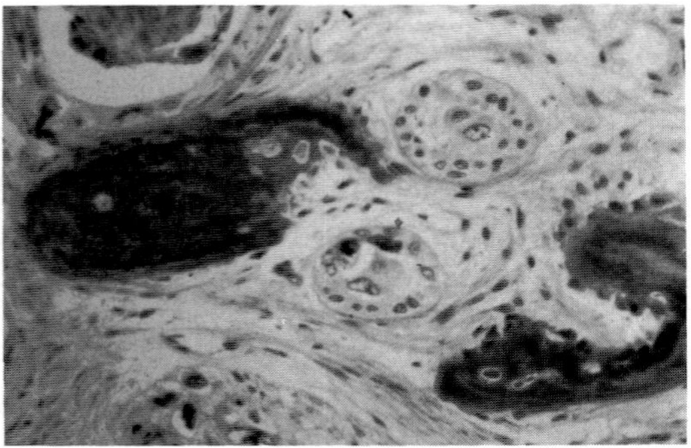

Figure 10–45. Bone abnormalities associated with malignancies. Metastatic epidermoid carcinoma. Presence of malignant cells in the bone marrow and stimulation of bone formation evidenced by high number of osteoblasts producing woven osteoid, woven bone, and fibers surrounding the trabecules and filling the marrow space. Undecalcified, 3 μm thick section of human iliac bone (modified Masson-Goldner stain; ×50). *See color plate VI*

loma, oxalosis, or sarcoidosis (Figs. 10–46*A*, *B* to 10–48*A*, *B*). The bone biopsy may also be helpful in understanding the radiologic finding of osteosclerosis through histologic findings consistent with fluorosis or Albers-Schönberg disease.

E. Complications of Bone Biopsies

Data concerning bone biopsy complications have been gathered and published by Duncan et al.[129] These authors sent a questionnaire to 18 different hospitals where bone biopsies are routinely performed. Of a total of 14,810 biopsies, 9030 were obtained from the iliac crest using the horizontal or transiliac approach, and 5780 were obtained by the superior or vertical approach. The overall frequency of complications was 0.52% (0.63% for the horizontal approach and 0.36% for the vertical).

Although many different types of instruments were used for these bone biopsies, generally, instruments providing smaller biopsies had fewer complications. These complications included hematoma, neuropathy, wound infection, and pain. Of those undergoing horizontal bone biopsy, one experienced fracture and one experienced osteomyelitis.

To assess the discomfort experienced during and subsequent to bone biopsy, a pain score was devised. The authors found that out of 37 patients, 21% reported no pain, 46% reported acceptable pain during or after the procedure, 30% experienced moderate pain, and 3% (one patient) reported severe pain.

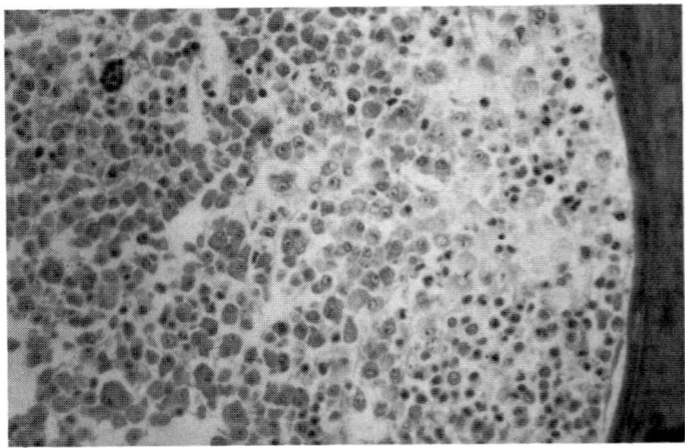

A

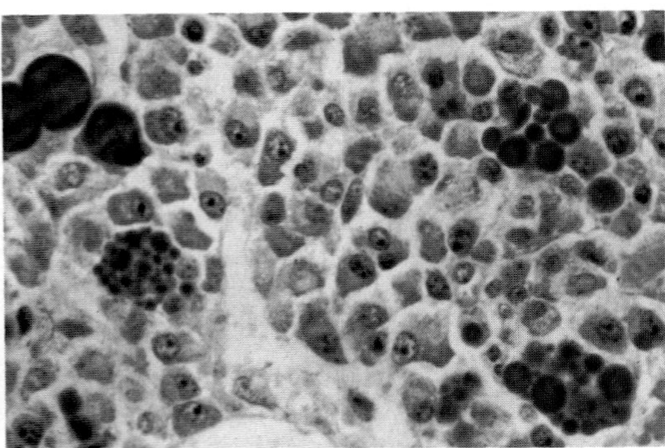

B

Figure 10–46. Bone abnormalities associated with malignancies. *A*, Multiple myeloma. Diffuse infiltration of the bone marrow by plasma cells without invasion of calcified bone. Undecalcified, 3 μm thick section of human iliac bone (modified Masson-Goldner stain; ×31). *B*, Multiple myeloma. High-power detail of plasma cells and Russell bodies. Undecalcified, 3 μm thick section of human iliac bone (modified Masson-Goldner stain; ×198). *See color plates VI and VII*

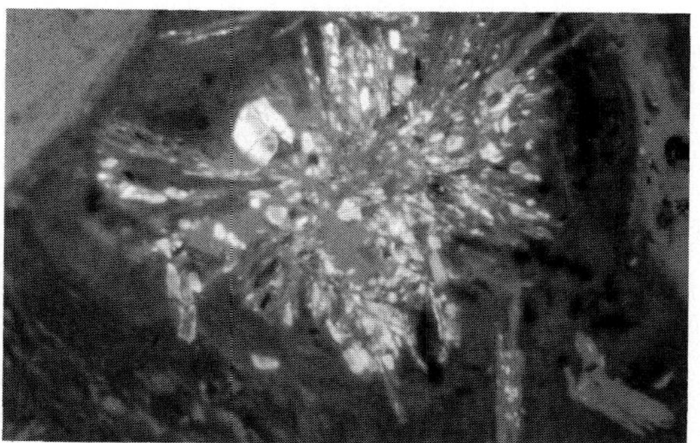

Figure 10–47. Oxalosis. Invasive crystal growth within trabecular bone and osteoid. Undecalcified, 3 μm thick section of human iliac bone. Partially polarized light microscopy (modified Masson-Goldner stain; ×50). *See color plate VII*

Similar observations were made at the Mayo Clinic,[85] where a power-driven transiliac trephine was used after local anesthesia application to the external and internal surfaces of the ilium. Of 48 subjects, 85% reported acceptable pain during or after the procedure, 10% experienced pain that was moderate, and 4% (two subjects) reported severe pain.

The experience of the operator remains the deciding factor in minimizing morbidity and maintaining the adequacy of the specimen.

In agreement with our earlier observations and recommendations, Duncan et al.[129] emphasize that the common mistake in bone biopsy procedure involves the use of heavy pressure on the trephine shaft. They too recommend a skilled and rotated cutting motion, allowing the teeth to cut the bone rather than being bent by the direct transmission of heavy pressure.

In summary, studies involving 9030 horizontal or transiliac bone biopsies and 5780 vertical or superior biopsies of the iliac crest revealed very little morbidity and no mortality in the bone biopsy procedure. Problems most commonly incurred included pain, hematoma, and, rarely, lateral femoral cutaneous neuropathy (observed mainly after transiliac bone biopsies). Such studies (along with personal experience and professional communications with colleagues) allow the conclusion that the iliac bone biopsy is a benign and safe procedure in the hands of a skilled operator.

III. TECHNIQUE OF MINERALIZED BONE HISTOLOGY

A. Fixation and Dehydration of Bone

Fixation should preserve bone tissue constituents and bone cells in a condition as lifelike as possible.[130] Consequently, the fixative must inhibit postmortem changes without removing the mineral from bone. This means that the tissue must be as fresh as possible and that the fixative must be potent enough to penetrate and inactivate acidic lysosomal enzymes without affecting mineral.

Fixatives can be divided into two major groups: precipitant fixatives that precipitate the cytosolic proteins as a coagulum (such as mercuric chloride, ethanol, picric and chromic acids), and nonprecipitant fixatives that fix protein by denaturing them. Examples of nonprecipitant fixatives include formalin, osmium tetroxide, and potassium dichromate.

Even though osmium tetroxide is a good fixative, we do not recommend its use for

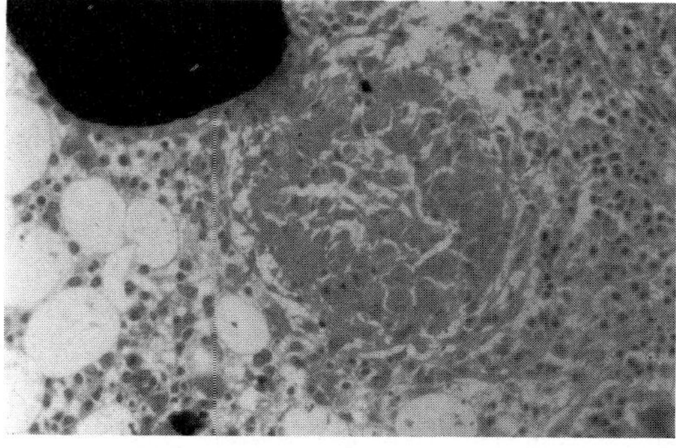

A

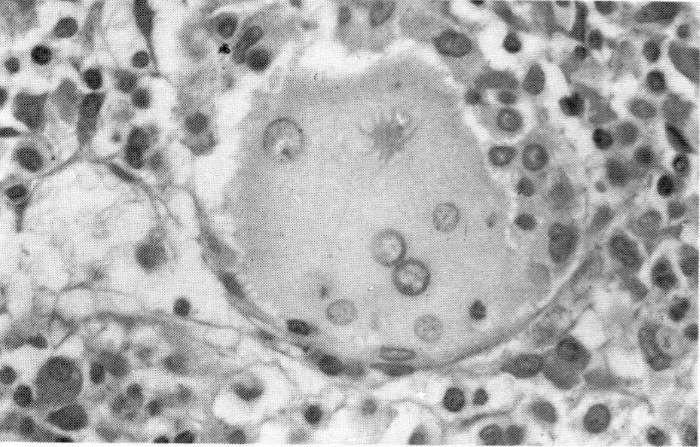

B

Figure 10–48. Sarcoidosis. *A*, Sarcoid noncaseating granuloma in bone marrow consisting of giant cells and histiocytic cells. Undecalcified, 3 μm thick section of human iliac bone (von Kossa's stain, counterstained with methylene blue; ×31). *B*, A characteristic asteroid body within a giant cell. Close-up view of bone marrow from the same patient shown in Figure 10–45 (hematoxylin-eosin stain; ×126). *See color plate VII*

mineralized bone histology because it reacts with and adds onto many cellular structures, promoting contrasts and, in a sense, "staining" tissue. Some fixatives—formalin in particular—may remove calcium, aluminum, and, thus, tetracycline from bone. Therefore, we do not recommend or use formalin. Our fixative of choice is ethanol—a relatively weak fixative that, according to our experience, does not remove calcium from bone within several weeks of exposure. Since the tissue penetration of alcohol is relatively weak, bigger pieces of bone must be divided before fixation.

The portion of the tissue placed into the fixing solution should be small enough to allow rapid fixation diffusion into the innermost part of the bone sample. The total volume of fixative should be at least 10 to 20 times that of the tissue. Usually, 24 hours of ethanol fixation are sufficient for bone biopsy samples of regular size.

It is necessary to dehydrate bone samples very thoroughly before embedding them in plastic, since all plastic monomers used for embedding bone are not miscible with water. To attain this dehydration, bone samples can be passed five times through pure ethanol, remaining in each ethanol container for 24 hours on a magnetic stirrer.

B. Embedding of Bone

The major challenge in doing bone histology without removing bone mineral is to find a suitable embedding medium. Its final degree of hardness should approximate the hardness of the bone; the substance should readily penetrate the bone specimen without causing artifacts such as bubbles; it should be safe, that is, nonflammable and nontoxic; it should be adjustable in hardness for final cutting; and solvents should be available for its dissolution after cutting.

After testing numerous substances, we found that methyl methacrylate, which was introduced by Arnold and Jee,[131] is among the most useful. Other plastic monomers such as bioplastic and glycol methacrylate can be employed for embedding. However, we encountered problems cutting bone samples embedded in bioplastic for longer periods of time, and we could find no suitable solvent for glycol methacrylate.

After the complete penetration of the liquid monomer, polymerization (hardening) is induced by heat or the addition of benzoyl peroxide. Vacuum application facilitates optimal penetration, and polymerization is promoted by keeping the samples at 48° C.

Note: Higher temperatures will prevent the gas from escaping because of rapid hardening, and gas bubbles will accumulate in the block. A slow, stepwise polymerization is required for optimally hardened plastic blocks.

C. Sectioning

Cutting mineralized bone requires special microtomes equipped with carbide edges or diamond knives. The most popular microtomes for large specimens are the older Jung microtome model K (Nussloch, FRG) and the newer Reichert-Jung polycut (Cambridge Instrument, Buffalo, NY).

For smaller bone samples, the universal microtome series (Model 1130–1150, Nussloch, FRG) and the newer Reichert-Jung universal rotary microtome Model 2050 (Cambridge Instruments, Buffalo, NY) are preferred. The cutting knife should advance at a slow speed, and the speed during the up and down or the to and fro motion should be the same. Various cutting fluids (water, ethanol) are used to keep the block and the sections moist.

Sections can be floated or directly transferred to glass slides, which should be precoated with gelatin to hold the relatively heavy bone specimen in place during the subsequent staining procedure. However, even the best microtomes need a skilled technician. The technician's level of training and experience determines whether marginal, satisfactory, or excellent sections of mineralized bone are cut.

D. Staining of Bone Sections

1. Staining Structural and Cellular Elements of Bone

The best bone staining results are obtained when the plastic embedding medium is first removed to allow optimal penetration of the stains. There are several staining techniques for discriminating calcified bone from uncalcified matrix.

The most valuable and most frequently used techniques include the Masson trichrome stain modified by Goldner[132] (and later in other laboratories), the solochrome cyanine stain,[133] and von Kossa's stain.[134] Calcified bone is stained green by the original Masson technique, blue by the modified Masson-Goldner technique, black by the von Kossa stain, and purplish-blue by solochrome cyanine.

Using these techniques, osteoid appears red (varying from orange-red to bright red) or blue. With the original and the modified Masson-Goldner technique, fibrin is stained red; connective tissue and mucus, green or blue; muscle tissue and red blood cells, pale red. Bone and bone marrow cells are also well stained. Cytoplasm of osteoclasts appears characteristically pink, and the cytoplasm of osteoblasts is reddish-blue (depending on ribonucleic acid content). Nuclei of osteoclasts and osteoblasts have brownish-blue membranes and chromatin with nucleoplasm appearing clear or light red and prominent red nucleoli. Osteocytes have similar staining characteristics with less prominent red nucleoli.

For differentiation or further classification, special stains are available. Osteoblasts can be differentiated from mononucleated osteoclasts by the pyronine green stain. Active osteoclasts are identified in some laboratories by histochemical staining of the lysosomal enzyme acid phosphatase.[5,135] However, note that precursor cells of lymphocytes and leukocytes are also stained by pyronine green, and all bone marrow cells with active lysosomes (i.e., granulocytes, monocytes, and macrophages) will react to the acid phosphatase stain. Also, acid phosphatase has been found in appreciable amounts in osteoblasts,[136] a finding that limits the value of histoenzymologic staining techniques for identification.

Villanueva[137,138] has described a special method for thick sections that stains the entire bone specimen. Calcified bone is usually stained yellowish-greenish-gray, and osteoid green or violet. Only further documentation will determine whether staining the entire specimen affects special stains—such as staining for aluminum, iron, and the like. We recommend referring to histology textbooks such as Pearse[139] for recipes of the various staining techniques.

2. *Staining Aluminum and Iron Deposits in Bone*

Several independent techniques can document the accumulation of aluminum in bone: atomic absorption spectrophotometry can be used to measure the aluminum content of bone; energy-dispersive x-ray analysis and histochemical staining for aluminum can identify aluminum at the mineralization front or at other sites. This latter technique identifies aluminum not only at the mineralization front (Fig. 10–49) and throughout osteoid and calcified bone, but at the cement lines as well. The different localizations of aluminum in bone may explain why direct measurements of aluminum content in bone using atomic absorption spectrophotometry do not always correlate with the extent of stainable bone aluminum at the bone-osteoid interface. Note, however, that the histopathologic changes associated with aluminum accumulation in bone correlate better with the extent of stainable bone aluminum at the mineralization front than with results of direct measurements of aluminum content in bone. The aurin-tricarboxylic acid method for stainable bone aluminum may well represent a more useful clinical tool than the measurement of bone aluminum content for assessing the patient's aluminum-related bone disease.[140]

Stainable bone aluminum may be found in patients treated with total parenteral nutrition[141] or in patients with reduced kidney function receiving large doses of aluminum-containing phosphate binders.[109,121,142-144] The aurin-tricarboxylic acid method is the most widely used technique for staining aluminum in bone.[145-147] We modify the procedure slightly in our laboratory in that we do not counterstain the slides. It is possible to assess the location and extent of aluminum deposits very well under fluorescent light, and this

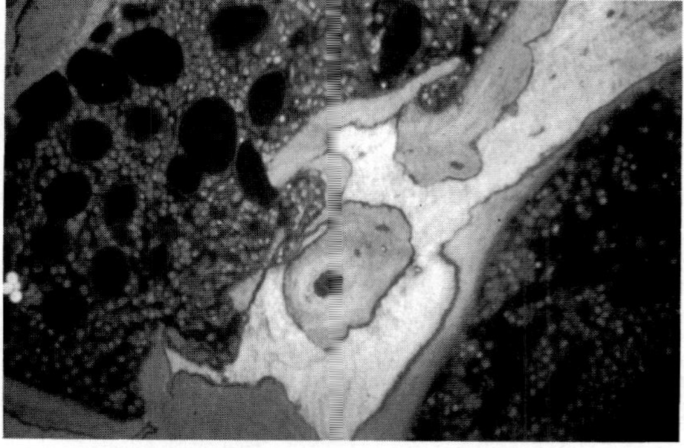

Figure 10–49. Aluminum deposits in bone. Stainable bone aluminum at the osteoid–mineralized bone interface, that is, the mineralization front. Undecalcified, 3 μm thick section of human iliac bone (aurin-tricarboxylic acid stain; ×31). *See color plate VII*

slight variation avoids the risk of masking some aluminum deposits with the counterstain.

Abnormal amounts of iron may also be found in bone, and there are four methods available for the demonstration of iron in microscopic slides: (1) the Berlin blue method of Perls;[148] (2) the iron sulfide reaction of Quincke;[149] (3) the Turnbull blue method of Schmeltzer;[150] and (4) the Gomori[151] technique that uses a mixture of equal parts 20% hydrochloric acid and a 10% solution of potassium ferrocyanide.

The Berlin blue method occasionally produces false-positive reactions, and both the Berlin blue and Turnbull blue preparations lose their color relatively soon. In fact, within a few months or even weeks, sections can become entirely unsuitable for comparison, a well-known phenomenon first described by Gans.[152] Consequently, we use a modified Gomori[151] method, primarily because of its major advantage of being specific for iron (Fig. 10–50).

The histochemical stain for aluminum and iron was validated in our laboratory by energy-dispersive x-ray microanalysis.[153] This technique involves processing small pieces of bone for transmission electron microscopy. The electron microscope sample is then exposed to an energy-active x-ray source and finally analyzed by an energy-dispersive x-ray detector. Throughout our years of validating the histochemical staining for aluminum by energy-dispersive x-ray analysis, we have invariably found a characteristic peak for aluminum (K = 1.485 eV) whenever the mineralization front revealed a positive histochemical staining for aluminum. And, importantly enough, those bone slides lacking stainable bone aluminum at the mineralization front did not exhibit the typical peak for aluminum by energy-dispersive x-ray analysis.

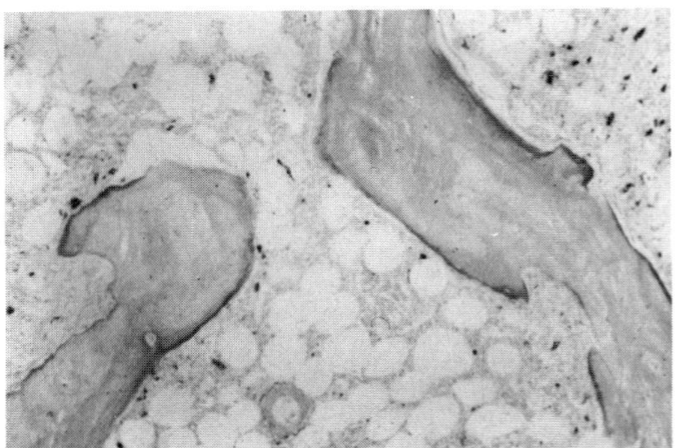

Figure 10–50. Histochemical staining of iron in bone. Iron can be demonstrated as blue linear deposits at the marrow-bone interface and in the bone marrow. Undecalcified, 7 μm thick section of human iliac bone (modified Gomori stain; ×31). *See color plate VII*

E. The Histologic Identification of the Mineralization Front

There are several methods available to identify the extent of the mineralization front. Toluidine blue is used to stain the mineralization front, whereas tetracycline or calcein is used for *in vivo* chelation of calcium deposited during mineralization. The spontaneous fluorescence of tetracycline or calcein makes it possible to identify the number of remodeling foci and the fraction of trabecular and haversian surface exhibiting an uptake of the fluorescent compound, thus indicating active mineralization.

We have found that toluidine blue sometimes fails to stain the mineralization front in a reproducible manner, and we advocate its use only for histologic identification of cement lines and mastocytes. Considering that tetracycline is relatively nontoxic to osteoblasts and other body cells, that there is only slow fading in appropriately stored blocks and slides, and given the reproducibility of tetracycline fluorescence, this labeling technique is the most useful marker for mineralization front activity in patients or experimental animals. Other markers such as calcein[154] or xylenol-orange[155] are helpful for repeat bone biopsies in experimental animals when a clear demarcation of the labels given at the first and second biopsy is needed.

F. Double Labeling Bone

Substances administered *in vivo* to identify the mineralization front can be time-spaced so as to be recognizable in cortical or cancellous bone under fluorescent light as rings or bands separated by a dark area—the dark area representing that period without administration. The first ring or band can be distinguished from the next by varying the durations of administration (which will provide different width) and/or by using two different substances (displaying different colors).

Principles of *in vivo* tetracycline labeling of bone were published by Frost in a series of papers and monographs[4,70,102,156-159] that extend the static histomorphometric evaluations to allow dynamic interpretation of bone turnover.

The tetracycline double labeling schedule routinely used in our laboratory is as follows: tetracycline hydrochloride (Tetracyn) is given at a dose of 7 mg/kg body weight three times daily for 2 days. The drug is then stopped for the following 10 days, and demeclocycline (Declomycin) is given at a dose of 4 mg/kg body weight three times daily during the 4 days thereafter.

Bone biopsies are performed within 4 to 5 days after administering the second label. The labeling-free interval following the second label is needed to allow bone to be deposited over the second label and, thus, to avoid leaching of tetracycline by organic solvents used for fixation or during the processing of slides.

The labeling-free interval between the first and second label may have to be prolonged to ascertain separation of labels in patients with bone abnormalities characterized by very low bone turnover. Conversely, patients with accelerated bone turnover and precipitous mineralization may be labeled using shorter labeling-free intervals.

Generally, the duration of the entire labeling protocol should not exceed the duration of a remodeling cycle, since the first labels may have been removed by the time of bone biopsy. Declomycin typically exhibits a golden-yellowish fluorescence; tetracycline hydrochloride fluoresces greenish-yellow (Fig. 10–51); and calcein fluoresces bright green. These differences allow the distinction of a single label from two merging labels in cases of low bone formation. In animal experiments and on those occasions when time constraints do not allow regular double administration of tetracycline, we inject tetracycline intravenously to ascertain administration, induce a faster rise and fall in serum levels, and get a sharper demarcation of the labels. In this technique, the dosage must be adjusted to kidney function.

We reduce the oral administration of tetracycline hydrochloride (from three times to twice per day) in patients with a glomerular filtration rate less than 25 ml/minute. Phosphate binders and other antacids also bind tetracycline. Therefore, these drugs should not be administered on days of tetracycline labeling. In our experience, patients with renal failure tolerate this short course of tetracycline administration relatively well, and children can be given tetracycline for labeling of bone at a dose adjusted to their body weight without immediate or long-term side effects. We observed no major side effects of tetracycline labeling using our dose regimen in over 1000 patients, many of whom had a reduction in kidney function.

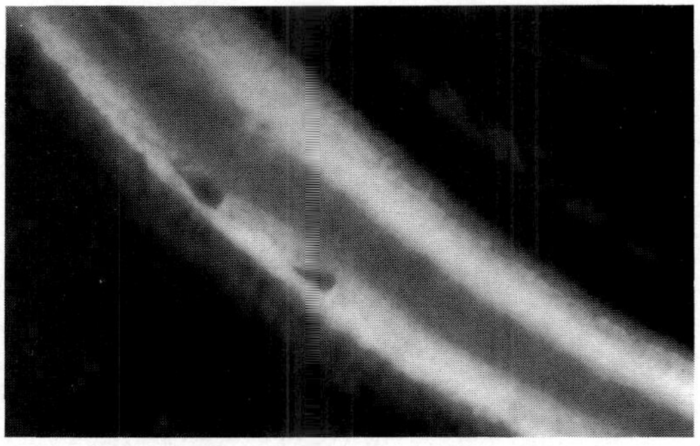

Figure 10–51. Labeling of bone. Tetracycline double labeling at the bone-osteoid interface. Two regular distinct labels. The outer golden-yellowish label represents administration of demeclocycline; the inner greenish-yellow label represents administration of tetracycline. Undecalcified, unstained, 7 μm thick section of human cancellous bone. Fluorescent light microscopy (×126). *See color plate VII*

There may be transient rises in blood urea nitrogen concentrations in individual patients undergoing chronic maintenance dialysis. This may be accompanied by nausea or vomiting. The symptoms, however, disappear with dialysis.

In rare cases, photosensitivity and allergic reactions may occur. The allergy may be against a particular or all tetracycline antibiotics. When a nonrenal patient receiving tetracycline antibiotics for an infection requires a bone biopsy, the "single continuous labeling technique" can be used. Note, however, that distinguishing the outer boundary of the broad single label will not always be easy, given the indistinct borders of tetracycline labels. Thus, for diagnostic purposes, tetracycline double labeling technique is preferred, since the individual labels are more easily identified.

There are six types of tetracycline labels that may be identified in bone under fluorescent light after a regular tetracycline double labeling protocol:

1. The regular, distinct "double labels" at the

bone-osteoid interface (Fig. 10–51);
2. Distinct single labels at the bone-osteoid interface;
3. Thin single labels at the bone-osteoid interface or at cement line;
4. Broad single labels at the bone-osteoid interface of lamellar bone;
5. Diffuse broad single labels of high intensity in woven bone; and
6. Thin single labels of low intensity at the trabecular or endosteal surface.

Formation sites that completed or started their mineralization during the labeling interval, thereby escaping either the second or the first label, may display distinct single labels. In addition, these labels may reflect the merging of two labels because of a low mineral apposition rate. Thin single labels may appear at the osteoid-bone interface or at cement lines as a result of passive uptake of tetracycline, thus indicating disturbed mineralization.

The broad single labels in lamellar bone and diffuse broad single labels of high intensity in woven bone reflect either abnormal irregular mineralization and/or diffuse passive uptake due to low diffusion impedance of unmineralized or incompletely mineralized osteoid or woven bone. Trabecular surfaces or endosteal surfaces with a thin low-intensity single label display the phenomenon of "surface fluorescence." This phenomenon is unrelated to normal bone mineralization and formation. It occurs mainly over neutral surfaces or less frequently over resorption zones. It is explained as unspecific ionic binding of calcium salts by tetracycline at sites of calcium exchange or release.

When double labels alone are evaluated for measurements of bone dynamics, bone formation rates will be underestimated owing to the "escape phenomenon" that produces distinct single labels. If all double and all single labels are included in calculations of bone formation rates, there will be an overestimation. This is because not all single labels are actively forming bone during the entire labeling period. Frost[160] addressed this problem by using a "ladder diagram" in calculating the correction factor for labeling escape. For practical purposes, however, including only 50% of the single labels in the calculation of bone formation rates provides an acceptable approximation.

Osteons cycle through "on" and "off" states and do not form bone continuously. Therefore, those osteons in the "off" state may passively accept a label and, after a rest period, may enter an "on" state. In this condition they actively begin mineralizing and take up the second label in a normal manner. This phenomenon produces a false and confusingly short distance between the two tetracycline labels. However, the intensities of the two labels should be significantly different. Documenting these theoretical considerations is difficult, and only future clarification will determine whether currently employed tetracycline labeling techniques are adequate or require further refinement.

Bone section thicknesses and tetracycline dosages may influence the fraction of trabecular surface exhibiting fluorescent labels (J.M. Harrelson, personal communication). Consequently, bone section thicknesses and tetracycline dosages should remain constant, and reference or comparison slides should be cut at the same thickness as slides under evaluation.

G. Staining the Bone Marrow

Those stains routinely used for structural and cellular elements of bone (such as Masson-Goldner) also stain bone marrow quite satisfactorily. If bone marrow abnormalities are observed, additional stains such as PAS and toluidine blue are desirable. They can also be used for sections of plastic-embedded mineralized bone. Refer to special texts for detailed descriptions of the process.[139,161]

H. Problems and Artifacts

Delaying the transfer of bone samples to fixative, deep-freezing bone, or use of hyper- or hypo-osmolar fixatives may cause cellular artifacts. Common fixatives such as formalin (particularly unbuffed formalin at room temperature) have been known to remove calcium, tetracycline, aluminum, and other substances from bone.

If kept in sufficient volumes of appropriate fixatives (10 to 20 times the volume of the sample), bone samples can be stored for longer periods, making deferred processing or mailing possible. However, insufficient exposure to the dehydrating agent will interfere with normal staining. This can be recognized by the intensely white appearance of mineralized bone on the cut surface of the block or on unstained slides. Note that insufficient vacuum application during plastic penetration traps air in the trabecular meshwork, resulting in small air bubbles within the hardened final block.

Excessive temperatures during the hardening process cause gas and irregular bubbles that might well render the bone specimen uninterpretable. If water drops fall into the liquid plastic monomer while it hardens, the plastic takes on a milky appearance. The benzoyl peroxide added to the plastic to start polymerization is explosive in its anhydrous form. Therefore, its hydrous form is used for storage and the water is reduced by heating shortly before it is added to the polymerization solution. Incomplete dehydration delays polymerization and the dissolution of benzoyl peroxide crystals, which might then explode within the plastic block during polymerization, thus damaging bone tissue.

These potential problems all point to the need of an experienced and skilled technician for artifact-free sectioning of bone. Indeed, most problems associated with mineralized bone histology result from incorrect cutting techniques and/or unskilled handling of the bone sections.

There are other potential problems that can arise. Organic cutting or stretching fluid use can remove tetracycline from the sections. Tears and overlaps of bone tissue can be, and usually are, caused by improperly balanced microtome, incorrect angle between cutting knife and plastic block, microtome knife in need of refiling, and unskilled transfer and stretching of sections onto slides. Outdated gelatin or incorrect mixtures may fail to hold the bone sections on the glass slide, resulting in partial or complete slide loss during staining.

Everyone in the discipline recognizes or should recognize the value of good technicians. The job requires excellent dexterity and an inordinate amount of patience. Mineralized bone histology, the processing, cutting, and staining of mineralized bone, requires continually meticulous attention to detail, accuracy, and exceptionally clean working habits. Even though mineralized bone histology became routine in an increasing number of laboratories, it is not a "cookbook" procedure and the skills do not come easily.

IV. BONE HISTOMORPHOMETRY

A. Qualitative Assessment of Bone Histology

Mineralized sections of bone can be evaluated qualitatively or quantitatively. Qualitative interpretation by an experienced bone pathologist is usually sufficient for routine diagnoses and classification of bone diseases (i.e., severe osteopenia, advanced osteomalacia, long-standing hyperparathyroid bone disease, Paget's disease, and bone abnormalities characterized by features such as oxalosis, sarcoidosis, metastatic infiltration of bone, malignancies of bone marrow, storage diseases, and accumulation of aluminum, iron, lead and other substances in bone).

Most metabolic bone diseases, however, are not characterized by qualitatively abnormal features. Instead, their diagnosis is based on the quantitative deviation from normal of one or several physiologic features. This fact, combined with the more widespread use of mineralized bone histology, particularly in patients with incipient or subtle disease states, may necessitate quantitative evaluation of bone for diagnostic purposes. Also, quantitative evaluation–histomorphometry is needed for reliable measurements of dynamic parameters of bone and objective documentation of histologic changes of bone after therapy.

B. Histomorphometry of Mineralized Bone Sections

Histomorphometric evaluation of bone provides objective data on the static and dynamic parameters of bone structure, formation, and resorption. Dynamic parameters obtained at the tissue, osteon, and cellular level provide an invaluable tool for research focusing on bone physiology and pathology.

Three major approaches are used in the histomorphometric evaluation of bone: manual or point counting techniques, semiautomatic computerized techniques, and fully automated computerized image analysis.

Manual techniques use integrating grids projected over the histologic structure under evaluation. Based on the principles of geometric probability,[162] three-dimensional structures are deduced from their two-dimensional images. The fraction of points overlying a structure is considered to represent an unbiased estimate of the volume fraction—the volumetric density of the structure. Therefore, volume fractions are obtained from point counting procedures.

Surface measurements in the point counting technique are obtained by counting random intersections between sampling lines and the histologic feature. The Merz and Schenk[163] method uses these principles and is the most widely used method in manual quantitative bone histology. The probability of sampling a given structure in a random plane (i.e., the plane of the section) depends on the position of the sampling plane relative to the position of the structure. If they are parallel, the probability is zero; if perpendicular, one.

According to Buffon's theorem,[164] the count must be corrected mathematically by multiplying the value for the surface density by the factor $4/\pi$. Iliac cancellous bone presents an isotropic nonrandom structure with preferential spatial orientation of trabeculae, which follow the strain pattern produced by mechanical forces. Therefore, according to Merz and Schenk, the integrating grid with its semicircular sampling lines is preferable to grids using straight lines.

The probability of an intersection between the semicircular sampling lines of the Merz and Schenk grid and the trabecular structure is largely independent of the trabecular orientation relative to the grid. When grids with straight parallel sampling lines are employed, the source of error has to be corrected by counting twice with the grid in two different positions perpendicular to each other. The number of random hits and boundary intersections are manually counted using blood cell calculators. Obviously, this approach is time-consuming.

The semiautomatic method of histomorphometry involves the use of a microscope equipped with a drawing tube. The image of a digitizing platen (positioned underneath the drawing tube) is drawn through the tube and projected over the optical field. Since the image is not projected outward, the optical resolution of the microscope is preserved for the observer. The digitizing platen is connected to a computer equipped with a black and white monitor, a double floppy disk drive, and a printer plotter—as designed and described by Malluche et al.[165] A more advanced version of this setup is now being commercially produced by Carl Zeiss, Thornwood, NY, under the tradename Osteoplan, and the design principle has been adopted by several other companies.

There is a cursor on the digitized platen, and the cursor is visible through the eyepiece of the microscope. The investigator selects and traces the histologic structures to be measured by moving the projection of the cursor over the histologic field under evaluation. Individual optical fields to be evaluated are determined by a square placed on the tablet. The size of this square can be adjusted by changing the position of the prism located within the drawing tube. As the individual microscopic structures are measured, values of perimeters and areas are transmitted to the computer, the printer, and the digitizer.

The measuring routine involves tracing and circuiting trabecular bone, osteoid, and endosteal fibrosis, counting osteoclasts and osteoblasts, and tracing those surface fractures exhibiting osteoblasts, osteoclasts, and resorption lacunae. Ideally, these routines are performed on 3 μm thick undecalcified bone sections, stained by the Masson-Goldner technique to allow optimal identification of structural and cellular parameters of bone in one section.

The measurements can be performed at any chosen magnification, and the quantitative static and dynamic parameters of bone structure, formation, and resorption measured by the Osteoplan are listed in Tables 10–1 to 10–3. An attempt to unify the nomenclature used for histomorphometric measurement has currently been made through the work of a committee appointed by the American Society of Bone and Mineral Research.

After the evaluation of a preselected number of fields, the parameters are printed along with standard deviations and ranges of individual results. The mean wall thickness is measured by tracing the endosteal surfaces and cement lines of completed osteons with phase-contrast microscopy (Fig. 10–52).

After these measurements have been completed, the incandescent light source is blocked and a fluorescent light (with the same cursor, illuminated by a fine red light in its center) traces the tetracycline double labels. Both measuring routines are performed on 7 μm thick unstained sections cut directly after the section used for bright field light microscopic evaluation.

Table 10–1. Static Parameters of Bone Structure, Formation, and Resorption

VV*	Volumetric density of bone (trabecular bone/total bone)	mm^3/cm^3
SV	Surface density of bone (trabecular bone/total bone)	mm^2/cm^3
D-TRAB	Mean trabecular diameter (mean trabecular width)	μm
VV-OS-l	Volumetric density of lamellar osteoid (volume of lamellar osteoid/total bone)	mm^3/cm^3
SV-OS-l	Surface density of lamellar osteoid (surface of lamellar osteoid/volume of total bone)	mm^2/cm^3
TH-OS-l	Thickness of lamellar osteoid (mean width of lamellar osteoid seams)	μm
OS-l	Percentage of trabecular surface covered by lamellar osteoid (surface of osteoid/total trabecular surface)	%
VV-OS-w	Volumetric density of woven osteoid (volume of woven osteoid/volume of total bone)	mm^3/cm^3
SV-OS-w	Surface density of woven osteoid (surface of woven osteoid/volume of total bone)	mm^2/cm^3
TH-OS-w	Thickness of woven osteoid (mean width of woven osteoid)	μm
OS-W	Percentage of trabecular surface covered by woven osteoid	%
SV-OSB	Surface density of osteoid covered by active osteoblasts (surface of osteoid covered by osteoblasts/total volume of bone)	mm^2/cm^3
VV-O-l	Relative volumetric density of lamellar osteoid (volume of lamellar osteoid/volume of trabecular bone)	mm^3/cm^3
SV-O-l	Relative surface density of lamellar osteoid (surface of lamellar osteoid/volume of trabecular bone)	mm^2/cm^3
VV-O-w	Relative volumetric density of woven osteoid (volume of woven osteoid/volume of trabecular bone)	mm^3/cm^3
SV-O-w	Relative surface density of woven osteoid (surface of woven osteoid/volume of trabecular bone)	mm^2/cm^3
SV-OB	Surface density of active osteoid covered by osteoblasts	mm^2/cm^3
OB/OS	Percentage of osteoid covered by osteoblasts (osteoid-osteoblast interface)	%
OB	Percentage of total trabecular surface covered by "active" osteoid (osteoblasts)	%
OBI	Osteoblastic index (number of osteoblasts/10 cm of trabecular boundary length)	
VV-FIB	Volumetric density of fibrosis (volume of fibrosis/total volume bone)	mm^3/cm^3
SV-FIB	Surface density of fibrosis (surface of peritrabecular fibrosis/total volume of bone)	mm^2/cm^3
TH-FIB	Thickness of peritrabecular fibrosis	μm
FIB-M	Percentage of bone marrow covered by fibrosis (area of fibrosis/area of bone marrow)	%
FIB	Percentage of trabecular surface covered by fibrosis	%
OCL	Percentage of trabecular surface covered by resorption lacunae filled with osteoclasts (bone-osteoclast interface)	%
HL	Percentage of trabecular surface exhibiting Howship's lacunae (surface of total resorption lacunae minus bone-osteoclast interface/total trabecular surface)	%
OCL-R	Percentage of mineralized trabecular surface covered by osteoclasts (bone-osteoclast interface/total trabecular surface minus osteoid surface)	%
L-TOT	Percentage of trabecular surface exhibiting total resorptive lacunae	%
SV-OCL	Surface density of osteoclastic lacunae (bone-osteoclast interface/total volume bone)	mm^2/cm^3
VV-LAC	Volume density of total resorption lacunae	mm^3/cm^3
SV-LAC	Surface density of total resorption lacunae	mm^2/cm^3
D-LAC	Mean depth of total resorption lacunae	μm
V-LAC	Relative volume density of total resorption lacunae	mm^3/cm^3
OCI	Osteoclastic index (number of osteoclasts/10 cm of boundary length)	

*See Table 10–2, footnote.

Table 10–2. Dynamic Parameters of Bone Remodeling

Md-d*	Mean distance between double labels	μm
LAB-OS-d	Fraction of osteoid seams exhibiting double labels (mean double label length/mean osteoid length)	
LAB-TS-d	Fraction of trabecular surface exhibiting double labels (mean double label length/mean trabecular length)	
MTH-s	Mean thickness of single labels	μm
LAB-OS-s	Fraction of osteoid seams exhibiting single labels (mean single label length/mean osteoid length)	
LAB-TS-s	Fraction of trabecular surface exhibiting single labels (mean single label length/mean trabecular length)	
MWTH	Mean wall thickness	μm
AR/D	Appositional rate per day (mean distance/labeling interval)	μm/day
AR/Y	Appositional rate per year (mean distance/labeling interval)	mm/year
BFR ts	Bone formation rate (tissue level–surface referent) (LAB-TS x AR/Y)	$[mm^3/(mm^2 \times yr)] \times 10^3$
BFR tv	Bone formation rate (tissue level–volume referent) (mean trabecular length x BFR ts/mean trabecular area)	$[mm^3/(mm^3 \times yr)] \times 10^3$
BFR bmu	Bone formation rate (BMU level–surface referent) (LAB-TS x AR/Y /OS)	$[mm^3/(mm^2 \times yr)] \times 10^3$
BFR cs	Bone formation rate (cell level–surface referent) (AR/Y)	$[mm^2/(cell \times yr)] \times 10^3$
BFR/OB	Bone formation rate/osteoblasts (BFR cs x length double labels)/#OB	$[mm^3/(mm^2 \times yr)] \times 10^3$
BRR ts	Bone resorption rate (tissue level–surface referent) (-BFR ts)	$[mm^3/(mm^2 \times yr)] \times 10^3$
BRR tv	Bone resorption rate (tissue level–volume referent) (-BFR tv)	$[mm^3/(mm^3 \times yr)] \times 10^3$
BRR bmu	Bone resorption rate (BMU level–surface referent) (-BRR ts/L-TOT)	$[mm^3/(mm^2 \times yr)] \times 10^3$
LRR	Linear rate of resorption (BRR bmu/L-TOT)	$[mm^3/(mm^2 \times yr)] \times 10^3$
BRR/ARS	Bone resorption rate/active resorptive surface (BRR ts/OCL%)	$[mm^2/(cell \times yr)] \times 10^3$
BRR-OC	Bone resorption rate/osteoclast (BRR/ARS x OCL% x mean trabecular length)#OC	$[mm^3/(mm^2 \times yr)] \times 10^3$
MIN LAG t	Mineralization lag time (mean osteoid seam width/apposition rate per day)	days
SIGMA f	Osteon formation time [MWT/(AR/Y)]	days
SIGMA r	Osteon resorption time [(L-TOT x SIGMA f)/OS%]	days
SIGMA	Osteon remodeling time (SIGMA f + SIGMA r)	days

*Symbols for histomorphometric parameters reflect those used in the authors' laboratory at the time of completion of the manuscript. During the time of typesetting, new abbreviations were published by the Committee on Nomenclature in Histomorphometry appointed by the American Society of Bone and Mineral Research.[166]

Table 10–3. Quantitative Parameters of Osteocytic Lacunae Obtained Under Light Microscopy

A-OCY f*	Mean area of osteocytic lacunae filled with cells	μ^2
ER-OCY f	Mean elliptical ratio of osteocytic lacunae filled with cells (short axis diameter/long axis diameter of filled osteocytic lacunae	
SS-OCY f	Mean specific surface of osteocytic lacunae filled with cells (surface of filled osteocytic lacunae/area of lacunae)	$1/\mu$
OI-OCY f	Index of osteocytic lacunae filled with cells (number of osteocytic lacunae filled with cells/unit area trabecular bone)	$\#/mm^2$
VV-OCY f	Volumetric density of osteocytic lacunae filled with cells (volume of osteocytic lacunae filled with cells/volume trabecular bone)	mm^3/cm^3
SV-OCY f	Surface density of osteocytic lacunae filled with cells (surface of filled osteocytic lacunae/volume trabecular bone)	mm^2/cm^3
A-OCY v	Mean area of void osteocytic lacunae	μ^2
ER-OCY v	Mean elliptical ratio of void osteocytic lacunae (short axis diameter/long axis diameter of void osteocytic lacunae)	
SS-OCY v	Mean specific surface of void osteocytic lacunae (surface of void osteocytic lacunae/area of lacunae)	$1/\mu$
OI-OCY v	Number of void osteocytic lacunae/unit area trabecular bone	$\#/mm^2$
VV-OCY v	Volumetric density of void osteocytic lacunae (volume of void osteocytic lacunae/volume trabecular bone)	mm^3/cm^3
SV-OCY v	Surface density of void osteocytic lacunae (surface of void osteocytic lacunae/trabecular bone volume)	mm^2/cm^3

*See Table 10–2, footnote.

By combining phase-contrast microscopy with fluorescent light microscopy, tetracycline uptake, status of mineralization, and mean wall thickness of the individual osteons within the same optic field can be evaluated. Dynamic histomorphometric data obtained are presented in Table 10–2. All static and dynamic parameters of cancellous bone or cortical bone can be obtained separately.

The method package consists of three main programs:

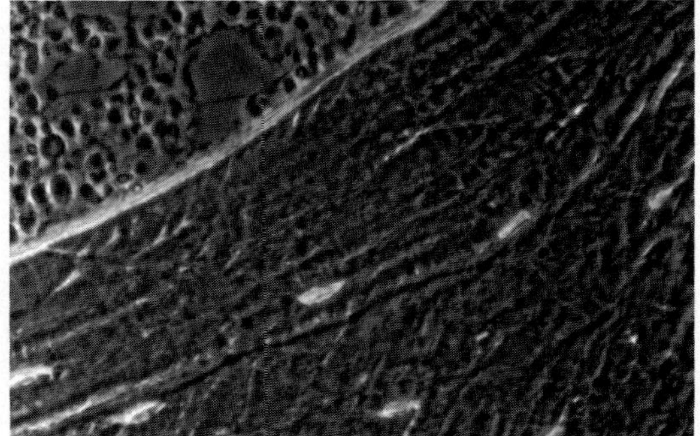

Figure 10–52. Trabecular osteon. The difference in orientation of lamellae allows identification of the boundaries of the osteon for measurement of mean wall thickness. Undecalcified, unstained, 7 μm thick section of human iliac bone. Phase-contrast microscopy (×80). *See color plate VII*

1. Micromorphometric parameters of bone evaluated under bright field light microscopy (LM);
2. Dynamic parameters of bone remodeling evaluated under fluorescent light and phase-contrast microscopy (FL); and
3. Qualitative analysis of osteocytes (OCY).

Quantitative parameters of osteocytes are obtained by tracing individual osteocytic lacunae. The evaluations of lacunae occupied by osteocytes and void lacunae are performed separately. (See Table 10–3 for quantitative osteocytic parameters calculated from measurements.) Histograms of areas and elliptical ratios of osteocytic lacunae are plotted.

This program makes it possible to evaluate the histologic field even when the bone matrix does not fully occupy the histologic field under consideration, thus permitting reliable calculations of the volumetric density and surface density of osteocytic lacunae. (Note: It is important to view the bone under polarized light before osteocytic lacunae are evaluated in order to ascertain that the osteocytic lacunae included in the evaluation are all measured in bone with identical orientation of collagen fibers.)

During the evaluation of each histologic slide, the investigator can graphically display all evaluated structural and cellular parameters on the printer. This immediate documentation is particularly helpful for teaching and for those occasions when permanent records of a slide are needed. If the investigator should have to stop, unexpectedly, before all the previously selected fields have been examined completely, the data can be stored without calculations or statistics. Then, as the remaining data are supplied in subsequent evaluations, the program can be run and the entire computational process completed. Importantly, a program overlay allows retrieval of any stored data from disks as required.

The third approach uses an image-analyzing computer to provide quantitative evaluations of histologic bone sections.[167] A video camera projects a microscopic image onto a black and white monitor, and the picture points are analyzed according to their "gray values." Using an image-analyzing computer drastically reduces the time required for quantitative evaluation of bone slides. At present, however, it is not feasible to analyze cellular and dynamic parameters of bone with this system because the computer is not yet capable of recognizing individual cells or distinguishing sectioning and staining artifacts from the histologic features under measurement. A newly developed automatic, image-analyzing system is currently undergoing tests in our laboratory. The price of this equipment, however, may prove prohibitive for widespread use.

C. Comparing Grid Technique and Semiautomatic Technique

The accuracy and precision of the manual and semiautomatic methods was determined by comparing the inter- and intraobserver errors involved in evaluating static, cellular, and dynamic parameters of bone histology. The two factors found to influence either method were the degree of bias and the level of precision.[168] The degree of bias refers to that human tendency of seeing or finding what we want or expect to find. Precision refers to the range or degree of spread among a series of observations. Thus, measurements may be unbiased but imprecise or precise but biased. The term "accuracy" refers to both the degree of bias and the level of precision. Accurate measurements are unbiased and precise.

We conducted a study of the accuracy of both the semiautomatic and the grid technique by analyzing intra- and interobserver errors. The only significant differences occurred in osteoid-osteoblast interface, bone-osteoblast interface, and mean trabecular diameter. The significant differences in the results for osteoblast interfaces between the two methods may be due to intraobserver variation or methodologic differences. The differences in mean trabecular diameter, however, probably arose because the semiautomatic method measures actual surfaces and areas, whereas the grid technique relies on random hits and intersections for area and surface measurements, respectively.

Structural parameters are obtained by both methods with the same variance when 50, 70, or 100 optical fields are evaluated at the same magnification. However, cellular parameters of bone resorption and formation are measured with a consistently lower coefficient of variation using the semiautomatic technique. Osteoclast parameters (which display the lowest degree of accuracy using the grid technique) were obtained by the semiautomatic method with coefficients of variance less than 50% of those inherent in the grid technique. Time requirements for the grid technique vastly exceed those of the semiautomatic technique, and the improved coefficients of variance for cellular parameters allowed a reduction in the number of fields evaluated by the semiautomatic technique. The coefficients of variance were such that the number of fields required to evaluate osteoclastic parameters could be reduced by 50% when the semiautomatic technique is used instead of the grid technique. Also, the substantially reduced level of interobserver error in the semiautomatic technique justified a further reduction in the number of evaluated fields without statistically jeopardizing the validity of the obtained results.

For practical purposes, evaluating 50 microscopic fields of a normal bone slide at a magnification of 200× will provide data with an overall coefficient of variance less than 20%, well within the acceptable standards for biological measurements. Obviously, the evaluation of more fields may be necessary for bone slides of pathologic states in which reduced activity prevails. Likewise, fewer fields may be required in states of very high bone activity.

An experienced investigator in our laboratory, using the grid technique, required from 4 to 5 hours to evaluate the minimum number of 250 optical fields. Only 50 to 60 minutes were required for comparable results using the semiautomatic method.

Few intraobserver errors occurred in measuring the structural parameters of bone (0.5%–3.1%), and noncellular parameters of bone resorption and formation revealed lower degrees of variation (2.6%–6.8%) than cellular parameters of resorption and formation (6.3%–10%).

There was remarkably little interobserver variation in structural parameters even when three different observers evaluated the slide at different times—a finding demonstrating the accuracy of the semiautomatic method. The mean deviation of structural parameters ranged from 4.5% to 6.8%. Parameters of bone resorption revealed a mean interobserver error of 6.2% to 9.8%. Quantitative parameters of bone formation were measured with a higher degree of interobserver difference than resorptive parameters, but even the largest mean difference did not exceed 11.6%. Finding that cellular parameters of osteoblasts reveal the widest range of variance may be a consequence of the known difficulties in defining distinct classification criteria for "active" osteoblasts, "inactive" osteoblasts, and "endosteal lining cells."

The difference between intra- and interobserver errors in structural parameters of bone and cellular parameters of osteoclasts was small, demonstrating that even in the hands of different investigators, histologic features of bone are measured with similar absolute results using the method. Therefore, it is possible to compare and/or pool data obtained in different laboratories using our semiautomatic method, and to do so with a degree of confidence.

Intraobserver errors involving two investigators evaluating dynamic parameters of bone remodeling were not statistically significant. (Note: Evaluating 50 fields at a magnification of 200× was sufficient to obtain a coefficient of variance of 7% and 6% respectively for mean distance between tetracycline labeling and for mean wall thickness in normal bone. Using additional fields yielded relatively small improvements in coefficients of variance. Consequently, 50 microscopic fields at 200× magnification proves sufficient for histomorphometric evaluation of these parameters in normal bone.)

Detailed dynamic parameters of bone formation and resorption could not be obtained in our laboratory using the manual or grid method because there was an extremely low degree of accuracy (coefficient of variance over 20%). The semiautomatic method, however, allowed quantitative parameters of bone formation and resorption with a coefficient of variance of 6% to 7% using not more than 50 optical fields and 200× magnification. The small variance of results from labeled appositional sites reveals a relatively constant rate at which bone is laid down and mineralized. The semiautomatic method also obtains dynamic parameters of bone formation and resorption at the cellular, osteon, and tissue level. This is particularly important for static quantitative bone parameters. For example, the total number of osteoclasts or osteoblasts may be increased at the tissue level because of decreased activity at the cellular level.

In addition to gathering and providing static and dynamic micromorphometric bone data, the semiautomatic method also provides a useful tool for quantitative evaluation of osteocytes. Previously, this was mainly done by mathematical approximations.[169-171] The semiautomatic technique allows a direct measurement of osteocytic lacunae with a coefficient of variance of 7% to 10%. A minimum of 170 individual osteocytic lacunae or 100 optical fields at a magnification of 787× should be evaluated in order to obtain an acceptable coefficient of variation—less than 20%.[165]

Introducing the "elliptical ratio" of osteocytes represents an objective approach to distinguishing small, inactive osteocytes[172] situated in flattened ellipsoid lacunae from enlarged active osteocytes seen in oval lacunae. The criterion of the irregularity of lacunar walls (which we have found rather subjective) is, thus, no longer an essential means of recognizing osteocytic activity. The routine plotting of histograms of data obtained for the area of osteocytic lacunae and the elliptical ratio of osteocytic lacunae allows differentiation between subpopulations of osteocytes. The usefulness of such quantitative data on osteocytic parameters was demonstrated in studies on bone response to physiologic and pharmacologic agents.[173,174]

D. Iliac Crest Histomorphometry in Normal Individuals

Histomorphometric results need to be compared with a reference scale of a proper control group. Geographic and methodologic differences should be taken into consideration in determining controls. In addition, interpreting histomorphometric bone data requires a knowledge of the variance of these data within the sites used for obtaining bone samples. This is of particular importance in evaluating the differences found in repeat bone biopsies performed after a treatment regimen or after certain experimental manipulations.

To establish a norm, we collected data on 149 subjects undergoing complete autopsy after suffering a violent or sudden death. Criteria for exclusion were history of prolonged bedrest, autopsy evidence of organ diseases, and information of clinical diseases from the family physician.

The criteria eliminated 28 subjects, leaving 121 individuals suitable for study. There were 88 males and 33 females, with ages ranging from 16 to 87 years. Dynamic parameters of bone remodeling were obtained from 28 volunteers who agreed to undergo bone biopsy after standard tetracycline labeling. This group included 14 males and 14 females whose ages ranged from 20 to 83 years.

Static micromorphometric parameters of bone structure, bone formation, and resorption were obtained from the subjects and are presented in Tables 10–4 to 10–9. The data on dynamic parameters of bone remodeling in normal individuals are given in Table 10–10. Notice that there is a tendency for volumetric density of bone (i.e., cancellous bone mass) to increase from the second to the fourth decade of life. After that, there is an obvious decline. Whether this decline is more pronounced in women than in men is still unknown and awaits further studies. Yet throughout all decades of life, bone mass is lower in women than in men (Chapter 12). The changes we observed in cancellous bone mass at various decades are, by and large, in agreement with European,[175-179] American,[180] and Australian[181] studies, despite the use of differing techniques.

The older age group displayed lower mean trabecular diameter. Whether this predisposes to a higher fracture rate is an interesting speculation, but awaits further clarification. All age groups presented similar static parameters of bone formation (i.e., volumetric density of osteoid and fraction of trabecular surface covered by osteoid). Similarly, the data concerning osteoid-osteoblast interface and mean thickness of osteoid seams do not reveal significant differences throughout adult life. While the osteoclastic index tended to fall from the second to the fifth decade, it increased subsequently. Whether this increase contributed to osteoporosis in the elderly remains unclear.

Howship's lacunae (i.e., the fraction of trabecular surface covered by resorption lacunae void of osteoclasts) declined from the second to the fifth decade, and thereafter increased. Since the extent of Howship's lacunae represents the composite result of bone resorbed by osteoclasts and refilled by osteoblastic activity, these observations may reflect an increase in osteoclastic resorption or a delayed filling by osteoblasts, that is, a decline in osteoblastic activity with age.

Table 10–4. Micromorphometric Parameters of Bone Structure in 33 Normal American Female Individuals

	Age:				
	11–20	21–30	31–40	41–60	>60
Cancellous bone mass %	20.9 ±4.9	21.4 ±6.1	20.3 ±6.1	17.4 ±7.4	14.8 ±7.1
Surface density of trabecular bone (mm^2/cm^3)	3055 ±542	3197 ±530	3596 ±705	3227 ±726	3014 ±408
Mean trabecular diameter (μm)	251 ±42.5	283 ±46	285 ±43	243 ±37	241 ±34
Mean wall thickness (μm)	*	62.4 ±1.0	58.4 ±8.7	45.5 ±9.5	*

Values are given as mean ± SD.

*Number of measurement does not allow statistical evaluation.

Table 10–5. Micromorphometric Parameters of Bone Structure in 88 Normal American Male Individuals

	Age:				
	11–20	**21–30**	**31–40**	**41–60**	**>60**
Cancellous bone mass %	21.8 ±2.0	21.9 ±3.7	22.9 ±1.7	19.0 ±1.6	17.8 ±1.3
Surface density of trabecular bone (mm^2/cm^3)	2862 ±392	3287 ±510	3025 ±430	2974 ±405	2916 ±370
Mean trabecular diameter (μm)	303 ±34	309 ±66	275 ±42	256 ±45	252 ±38
Mean wall thickness (μm)	62.1 ±13.7	60.9 ±7.4	64.0 ±11	65.0 ±19	62.0 ±14

Values are given as mean ± SD.

Table 10–6. Micromorphometric Parameters of Bone Formation in 33 Normal American Female Individuals

	Age:				
	11–20	**21–30**	**31–40**	**41–60**	**>60**
Absolute osteoid volume (mm^3/cm^3)	2.6 ±0.83	4.9 ±1.1	3.7 ±2.4	4.1 ±1.7	3.7 ±3.6
Relative osteoid volume (mm^3/cm^3)	14.3 ±6.1	24.7 ±2.1	11.9 ±6.5	25.8 ±16.2	21.0 ±18.0
Osteoid surface (%)	8.6 ±3.6	11.2 ±2.8	17.7 ±2.7	16.1 ±10.4	15.9 ±13.8
Mean osteoid seam thickness	9.2 ±2.5	11.5 ±0.7	9.0 ±2.1	10.1 ±3.6	8.7 ±1.8
Bone-osteoblast interface (%)	3.2 ±1.8	4.7 ±0.6	2.3 ±1.4	1.7 ±0.3	2.9 ±3.1
Osteoid-osteoblast interface	33.0 ±13.5	43.4 ±10.8	22.6 ±14.8	16.15 ±12.7	15.5 ±4.5

Values are given as mean ± SD.

Table 10–7. Micromorphometric Parameters of Bone Formation in 88 Normal American Male Individuals

	Age:				
	11–20	**21–30**	**31–40**	**41–60**	**>60**
Absolute osteoid volume (mm^3/cm^3)	5.57 ±2.0	4.21 ±1.8	3.96 ±3.4	4.5 ±2.4	4.6 ±1.6
Relative osteoid volume (mm^3/cm^3)	26.9 ±9.5	16.7 ±7.1	15.1 ±6.5	23.8 ±10.1	26.4 ±10.2
Osteoid surface (%)	16.1 ±4.8	12.2 ±4.5	10.8 ±4.6	13.8 ±4.3	18.5 ±9.0
Mean osteoid seam thickness	10.8 ±3.0	9.49 ±2.0	10.4 ±3.2	10.0 ±3.3	9.0 ±2.2
Bone-osteoblast surface (%)	6.37 ±3.90	4.74 ±2.57	3.8 ±2.25	3.1 ±2.26	4.1 ±2.11
Osteoid-osteoblast interface (%)	40.7 ±19.7	38.2 ±13.5	38.5 ±15.6	22.3 ±12.5	23.2 ±12.1

Values are given as mean ± SD.

Table 10–8. Micromorphometric Parameters of Bone Resorption in 33 Normal American Female Individuals

	Age:				
	11–20	21–30	31–40	41–60	>60
Total resorption lacunae	10.3 ±3.8	3.7 ±1.5	6.0 ±4.2	6.3 ±4.2	4.0 ±2.6
Bone-osteoclast interface (%)	1.33 ±0.34	0.75 ±0.32	0.77 ±0.46	0.53 ±0.27	0.61 ±0.17
Osteoclastic surface (%)	21.4 ±11.8	16.4 ±1.35	17.9 ±5.2	15.7 ±5.4	14.4 ±9.4

Values are given as mean ± SD.

Table 10–9. Micromorphometric Parameters of Bone Resorption in 88 Normal American Male Individuals

	Age:				
	11–20	21–30	31–40	41–60	>60
Total resorption lacunae	9.36 ±3.66	7.11 ±2.59	8.76 ±2.92	7.65 ±3.49	7.45 ±3.30
Bone-osteoclast interface (%)	1.33 ±0.80	1.29 ±0.54	1.08 ±0.79	0.97 ±0.48	1.04 ±0.45
Osteoclastic index	21.7 ±8.8	19.7 ±6.9	17.5 ±9.6	14.3 ±5.5	16.5 ±5.9

Values are given as mean ± SD.

Table 10–10. Dynamic Parameters of Bone Formation and Resorption in 28 Normal Individuals

	Females	Males
	Age: 20 to 80	
Mineral apposition rate (μm/d)	0.439 ±0.040	0.574 ±0.030
Doubly labeled osteoid seams (%)	47.5 ±5.1	54.2 ±4.1
Doubly labeled trabecular surface (%)	5.3 ±0.7	8.7 ±1.8
Singly labeled osteoid seams (%)	30.9 ±6.6	31.7 ±5.2
Singly labeled trabecular surface (%)	4.1 ±1.0	4.7 ±0.8
Bone formation rate—tissue level (volume referent) mm^3/cm^3 x yr x 10^3	184 ±35	201 ±37
Bone formation rate—BMU level mm^3/cm^3 x yr x 10^3	74 ±9	117 ±17
Bone formation rate/osteoblast mm^3/cm^3 x yr x 10^3	0.54 ±0.16	1.10 ±0.42
Bone resorption rate—BMU level mm^3/cm^3 x yr x 10^3	335 ±53	230 ±26
Bone resorption rate—osteoclast mm^3/cm^3 x yr x 10^3	71 ±13	68 ±12
Mineralization lag time (days)	21.8 ±1.5	17.5 ±1.5
Osteon remodeling time (days)	177 ±20	162 ±12

When histograms of micromorphometric parameters were plotted, osteoclastic index and bone-osteoclastic interface skewed left, whereas all other structural parameters of bone and all static parameters of bone formation and resorption revealed normal distribution. Finding normal distribution of all static morphometric parameters of bone except osteoclastic parameters demonstrated that the parametric tests are useful for statistical evaluations of all histomorphometric data of bone except the osteoclastic parameters.

The small variations documented in static and dynamic histomorphometric parameters of bone along with normal ranges of these quantitative bone parameters in normal individuals provides a solid and useful basis for distinguishing normal from abnormal bone. These control norm findings should help in the diagnosis and management of subtle and incipient pathologic conditions as histomorphometry takes its place in the clinical management of patients with metabolic bone disease.

References

1. Ritz E, Malluche HH, Bommer J, et al: Metabolic bone disease in patients on maintenance haemodialysis. Nephron 12:393–404, 1974.
2. Garn SM, Rohmann CG, Wagner B, et al: Population similarities in the onset and rate of adult endosteal bone loss. Clin Orthop Res 65:51–60, 1969.
3. Horsman A, Nordin BEC, Aaron J, Marshall DH: Cortical and trabecular osteoporosis and their relation to fractures in the elderly: *In* Deluca HG, Frost HM, Jee WSS, et al: Osteoporosis: Recent Advances in Pathogenesis and Treatment. Baltimore, University Park Press, 1981, pp 175–184.
4. Frost HM: Bone Remodeling Dynamics. Springfield, Charles C Thomas, 1963.
5. Evans RA, Dunstan CR, Baylink DJ: Histochemical identification of osteoclasts in undecalcified sections of human bone. Miner Electrolyte Metab 2:179–185, 1979.
6. Hancox NM: Motion picture studies of osteoclasts. *In* Rose GG: Cinematography in Cell Biology. New York, Academic Press, 1963, pp 141–190.
7. Gaillard PJ: Parathyroid gland and bone in vitro. Dev Biol 1:152–181, 1959.
8. Hancox NM: Osteoclastic bone resorption: *In* Harrison RJ, McMinn RMH: Biology of Bone. London, New York, Cambridge University Press, 1972, pp 113–135.
9. Goldhaber P: Bone resorption factors, cofactors and giant vacuole osteoclasts in tissue culture. *In* Gaillard PJ, Talmage RV, Budy AM: The Parathyroid Glands. Chicago, University of Chicago Press, 1965, pp 153–171.
10. Kimmel DB, Jee WSS: A quantitative histologic analysis of the growing long bone metaphysis. Calcif Tissue Int 32:113–122, 1980.
11. Jee WSS, Kimmel DB: Bone cell origin at the endosteal surface: *In* Meunier P: Bone Histomorphometry. Toulouse, Société de la Nouvelle Imprimerie Fournie, 1977, pp 113–131.
12. Tinkler SMB, Williams DM, Linden JE, Johnsson NW: Kinetics of osteoclast formation: The significance of blood monocytes as osteoclast precursors during 12-hydroxycholecalciferol-stimulated bone resorption in the mouse. J Anat 137:335–340, 1983.
13. Burger EH, van der Meer JWM: Precursor cell proliferation during osteoclast formation from bone marrow phagocytes. Calcif Tissue Int 36:454, 1984.
14. Heller M, McLean FC, Bloom W: Cellular transformations in mammalian bones induced by parathyroid extract. Am J Anat 87:315–339, 1950.
15. Tonna EA: Osteoclasts and the aging skeleton: A cytological, cytochemical and autoradiographic study. Anat Rec 37:251–269, 1960.
16. Altman AJ, Bandelin JG, Dominguez JH, Mundy GR: Differentiation of isolated calvarial cells into a mature heterogeneous population in culture. Metab Bone Dis Rel Res 1:25–79, 1978.
17. Walker DG: Bone resorption restored in osteopetrotic mice by transplants of normal bone marrow and spleen cells. Science 190:784–785, 1975.
18. Kahn AJ, Stewart CC, Teitelbaum SL: Contact-mediated bone resorption by human monocytes in vitro. Science 199:988–990, 1978.
19. Krukowski M, Kahn AJ: Normal osteoclast number and function in rat pups lacking parathyroid hormone. Experientia 25:871–872, 1980.
20. Rodan GA, Rodan SB, Marks SC: Parathyroid hormone stimulation of adenylate cyclase activity and lactic acid accumulation in calvaria of osteopetrotic rats. Endocrinology 102:1501–1505, 1978.
21. Faugere MC, Reitz R, Endress DB, Malluche HH: Serum parathyroid hormone levels reflect preferentially osteoblastic activity in patients with renal failure. Clin Res 32:753A, 1984.
22. Rodan GA, Martin TJ: Role of osteoblasts in hormonal control of bone resorption. Calcif Tissue Int 33:349–351, 1981.
23. Raisz LG, Koolemans-Beynen AR: Inhibition of bone collagen synthesis by Prostaglandin E2 in organ culture. Prostaglandins 8:377–385, 1974.
24. Wong GL, Luben RA, Cohn DV: 1,25-Dihydroxycholecalciferol and parathormone: Effects on isolated osteoclast-like and osteoblast-like cells. Science 197:663–665, 1977.
25. Malluche HH, Goldstein DA, Massry SG: Management of renal osteodystrophy with $1,25(OH)_2D_3$. II. Effects of histopathology of bone: Evidence for healing of osteomalacia. Mineral Electrolyte Metab 2:48–55, 1979.
26. Dietrich JW, Paddock DN: In vitro effects of ionophore A23187 on skeletal collagen and noncollagen protein synthesis. Endocrinology 104:493–499, 1979.
27. Manolagas SC, Haussler MR, Deftos LJ: 1,25-Dihydroxyvitamin D_3 receptor-like macromolecule in rat osteogenic sarcoma cell lines. J Biol Chem 255:4414–4417, 1980.
28. Partridge NC, Frampton RJ, Eisman JA, et al: Receptors for $1,25(OH)_2$ vitamin D_3 enriched in cloned osteoblast like rat osteogenic sarcoma cells. FEBS Lett 115:139–142, 1980.
29. Kream BE, Rowe DW, Gworek SC, Raisz LG: Parathyroid hormone alters collagen synthesis and

procollagen mRNA levels in fetal rat calvaria. Proc Natl Acad Sci USA 77:5654–5658, 1980.

30. Martin TJ, Partridge ND: Initial events in the activation of bone cells by parathyroid hormone, prostaglandins and calcitonin. *In* Cohn DV, Matthews JL, Talmage RV: Calcium Metabolism: Hormonal Control of Calcium Metabolism. New York, Elsevier/North Holland, 1981.
31. Malluche HH, Goldstein DA, Massry SG: Effect of $1,25(OH)_2D_3$ on activity of osteoblasts, osteoclasts and bone remodeling units in patients with renal osteodystrophy. Clin Res 29:563A, 1981.
32. Merke J, Klaus G, Hugel U, et al: 1,25-dihydroxyvitamin D_3 receptors on osteoclasts of calcium-deficient chicken despite demonstrable receptors on circulating monocytes. J Clin Invest 77:312–314, 1986.
33. Lian JB, Glowacki J, Key LL: Osteocalcin-deficient bone is poorly resorbed in vivo and in vitro. Calcif Tissue Int 36:464, 1984.
34. Holtrop ME: Quantitation of the ultrastructure of the osteoclast for the evaluation of cell function. *In* Meunier P: Bone Histomorphometry. Toulouse, Société de la Nouvelle Imprimerie Fournie, 1977, pp 133–145.
35. Malluche HH, Goldstein DA, Massry SG: $1,25(OH)_2$ Vitamin D modulates bone cell number and activity in uremia. Clin Res 30:754A, 1982.
36. Malluche HH, Matthews C, Faugere MC, et al: 1,25-Dihydroxyvitamin D maintains bone cell activity, and parathyroid hormone modulates bone cell number in dogs. Endocrinology 119:1298–1304, 1986.
37. Sato K, Byers PD: Quantitative study of tunneling and hook resorption in metabolic bone disease. Calcif Tissue Int 33:459–466, 1981.
38. Goldhaber P: Remodeling of bone in tissue culture. J Dent Res 34:490–499, 1966.
39. Melcher AH, Hodges GM: In vitro cultures of an organ containing mixed epithelial and connective tissues on a chemically defined medium. Nature (London) 219:301–302, 1968.
40. Weinman JP, Schour I: Experimental studies on calcification. II. The effect of rachitogenic diet on the alveolar bone of the white rat. Am J Pathol 12:833–855, 1943.
41. Weinman JP, Schour I: Experimental studies on calcification. V. The effect of phosphate on the alveolar bone and the dental tissue of the rachitic rat. Am J Pathol 21:1057–1067, 1945.
42. Young RW: Histophysical studies on bone cells and bone resorption. *In* Sognnaes RF: Mechanisms of Hard Tissue Destruction. Washington, DC, American Association for the Advancement of Science, 1973, pp 471–496.
43. Bar-Shavit Z, Teitelbaum SL, Kahn AJ: Saccharides mediate the attachment of rat macrophages to bone in vitro. J Clin Invest 72:516–525, 1983.
44. Whitson SW: Tight junction formation in the osteon. Clin Orthop 86:206–213, 1972.
45. Doty SB: Morphological evidence of gap junctions between bone cells. Calcif Tissue Int 33:509–512, 1981.
46. Schenk P: Basic symbolism for stereology. *In* Jaworski ZFG: Proceedings, 1st Workshop of Bone Morphometry, Ottawa, University of Ottawa, 1973, pp 360–362.
47. Malluche HH, Meyer W, Sherman D, Massry SG: Quantitative bone histology in 84 normal American subjects. Micromorphometric analysis and evaluation of variance of iliac crest bone. Calcif Tissue Int 34:449–455, 1982.
48. Parfitt AM, Villaneuva MM, Crouche MM, et al: Classification of osteoid seams by combined use of cell morphology and tetracycline labelling. Evidence for intermittency of mineralization. *In* Meunier P: Bone Histomorphometry. Toulouse, Société de la Nouvelle Imprimerie Fournie, 1977, pp 299–319.
49. Cooley LM, Goss RJ: The effects of transplantation and x-irradiation on the repair of fractured bones. Am J Anat 102:167–181, 1958.
50. Grillo HC: Origin of fibroblasts in wound healing: An autoradiographic study of inhibition of cellular proliferation by local x-irradiation. Ann Surg 157:45–457, 1963.
51. Urist MR: Osteogenesis by radioisotope labeled cell populations in implants of bone matrix under the influence of ionizing radiation. Clin Orthop Rel Res 76:231–243, 1971.
52. Kimmel DB: A light microscopic description of osteoprogenitor cells of remodeling bone in the adult. *In* Jee WSS, Parfitt AM: Bone Histomorphometry. Paris, Société Nouvelle de Publications Médicales et Dentaires, 1981, pp 181–188.
53. Rasmussen H, Bordier P: The Physiological and Cellular Basis of Metabolic Bone Disease. Baltimore, Williams and Wilkins, 1974.
54. Baud CA: Submicroscopic structure and functional aspects of the osteocyte. Clin Orthop Rel Res 46:227–236, 1968.
55. Vittali P: Osteocyte activity. Clin Orthop Rel Res 56:213–226, 1968.
56. Belanger LF: Osteocytic osteolysis. Calcif Tissue Res 4:1–12, 1969.
57. Meunier P, Bernard J, Vignon G: La mesure de l'elargissement périostéocytaire appliquée au diagnostic des hyperparathyroidies (a propos de 110 echantillons osseux). Pathol Biol (Paris) 9:371–378, 1971.
58. Tonna EA: Electron microscopic evidence of alternating osteocytic-osteoclastic and osteoblastic activity in the perilacunar walls of aging mice. Connect Tissue Res 1:221–230, 1972.
59. Whalen JP, Krook L, Nunez EA: A radiographic and histologic study of bone in the active and hibernating bat (Hyotis lucifungus). Anat Rec 172:97–108, 1972.
60. Krempien B, Geiger G, Ritz E, et al: Osteocytes in chronic uremia: Differential count of osteocytes in human femoral bone. Virchows Arch [A] 360:1–9, 1973.
61. Baylink D, Sipe J, Wergedal J: Vitamin D-enhanced osteocytic and osteoclastic bone resorption. Am J Path 244:1345–1357, 1973.
62. Bonucci E, Machio G, D'Angelo A, et al: Morphological aspects of bone tissue in chronic renal disease. A histological and electron microscopic study. *In* Norman AW, Schaefer K, Grigoleit HG, et al: Vitamin D and Problems Related to Uremic Bone Disease. New York, de Gruyter, 1975, pp 523–530.
63. Krempien B, Ritz E: Effects of parathyroid hormone on osteocytes. Ultrastructural evidence for anisotropic osteolysis and involvement of the cytoskeleton. Metab Bone Dis Rel Res 1:55–65, 1978.
64. Krempien B, Manegold C, Bommer J: The influence of immobilization on osteocyte morphology. Osteocyte differential counts and electron microscopical studies. Virchows Arch Abt A (Pathol Anat) 370:55, 1976.

65. Krempien B, Ritz E, Geiger G: Behavior of osteocytes in various ages and chronic uremia. Morphological studies in human cortical bone. *In* Jaworski ZFG: Proceedings, 1st Workshop on Bone Morphometry, Ottawa, University of Ottawa Press, 1976, pp 288–296.
66. Krempien B: Osteocyte activation, hormonal and mechanical factors. *In* Jee WSS, Parfitt AM: Bone Histomorphometry. Paris, Société Nouvelle de Publications Médicales et Dentaires, 1981, pp 257–268.
67. Boyde A: Evidence against "osteocytic osteolysis." *In* Jee WSS, Parfitt AM: Bone Histomorphometry. Paris, Société Nouvelle de Publications Médicales et Dentaires, 1981, pp 239–255.
68. Dhem A: Le forage des cannaux de Havers. Rev Chir Orthop 51:583–593, 1965.
69. Jaworski ZF, Lik E: The rate of osteoclastic bone erosion in Haversian remodeling sites of adult dog rib. Calcif Tissue Res 10:103–112, 1972.
70. Frost HM: Relation between bone-tissue and cell population dynamics, histology and tetracycline labelling. Clin Orthop 49:65–75, 1966.
71. Malluche HH, Fanti P, Friedler RM, Faugere MC: Decreased activity of bone cells contributes to the pathogenesis of early renal osteodystrophy—an abnormality reversed by $1{,}25(OH)_2D$. Kidney Int 31:353, 1987.
72. Meunier PJ, Bianchi GGS, Edouard CM, et al: Bony manifestations of thyrotoxicosis. Orthop Clin North Am 3:745–774, 1972.
73. Malluche HH, Sherman D, Meyer W, et al: Effects of long-term infusion of physiologic doses of 1–34 PTH on bone. Am J Physiol 242:F197 201, 1982.
74. Bordier P, Matrajt H, Miravet L, Hioco D: Mesure histologique de la masse et de la resorption des travées osseuses. Pathol Biol (Paris) 12:1238 1243, 1964.
75. Hocking DR: Bone marrow biopsy: A routine including marrow trephine. Med J Aust 2:915–917, 1964.
76. Ellis LD, Jensen WN, Westerman MP: Needle biopsy of bone and marrow. An experience with 1,445 biopsies. Arch Intern Med 114:213–221, 1964.
77. Byers P, Smith R: Trephine for full-thickness iliac-crest biopsy. Br Med J 1:682–683, 1967.
78. Duursma SA, Visser WJ, van Zoeren M, Korver MF: A bone biopsy procedure. Calcif Tissue Res 4:269–273, 1969.
79. Jamshidi K, Swaim WR: Bone marrow biopsy with unaltered architecture: A new biopsy device. J Lab Clin Med 77:335–342, 1971.
80. Fornasier VL, Vilaghy MI: The results of bone biopsy with a new instrument. Am J Clin Pathol 60:570–573, 1973.
81. Meunier PJ, Sellami S, Briancou D, Edouard C: Histological heterogeneity of apparently idiopathic osteoporosis. *In* DeLuca H, Frost HM, Jee WSS, Johnston CC, Parfitt AM (eds): Osteoporosis: Recent Advances in Pathogenesis and Treatment. Baltimore, University Park Press, 1981, pp 293–301.
82. Chappard D, Alexandre C, Bousquet G, Riffat G: Nouvelles modifications du trocart de Bordier pour la biopsie osseuse quantitative. Rev Rheum Mal Osteoartic 50:307–308, 1983.
83. Burkhardt R: Technische Verbesserungen und Ansendungsbereich der Histo-Biopsie von Knochenmark und Knochen. Klin Wochenschr 44:326–334, 1966.
84. Malluche HH: The value of bone biopsies for diagnosis of renal bone disease. *In* Moorhead JR, Baillod RA, Mion C: Dialysis, Transplantation, Nephrology. London, Pitman Medical, 1973, pp 111–115.
85. Johnson KA, Kelly PJ, Jowsey J: Percutaneous biopsy of the iliac crest. Clin Orthop 123:34–36, 1977.
86. Popplewell P, Philips PJ, Stehens M, et al: The Jamshidi needle—a simple instrument for bone biopsy. *In* Bone, Structure, Function and Disease. Adelaide, Australia, 2nd International Symposium, 1981, p 34.
87. Faugere MC, Malluche HH: Comparison of different bone biopsy techniques for qualitative and quantitative diagnosis of metabolic bone diseases. J Bone Joint Surg 65A: 1314–1319, 1983.
88. Frost HM, Villanueva AR: Human osteoblastic activity. I. A comparative method of measurement with some results. Henry Ford Hosp Med Bull 9:76–86, 1961.
89. Barer M, Jowsey J: Bone formation and resorption in osteoporosis. Clin Orthop 52:241–247, 1967.
90. Meunier PJ, Courpron P, Edouard CM: Physiological and comparative histological data. Clin Endocrinol Metab 2:239–259, 1973.
91. Faugere MC, Dorr LD, Malluche HH: Static and dynamic bone histology in primary and revision total knee arthroplasty. Orthop Trans 7:299–300, 1983.
92. Dorr L, Malluche HH, Faugere MC, et al: Bone structural and cellular characteristics in patients with total hip arthroplasty. 31st Annual Meeting, Orthopaedic Research Society, 1985.
93. Price PA, Nishimoto SK: Radioimmunoassay for the vitamin K–dependent protein of bone and its discovery in plasma. Proc Natl Acad Sci USA 77:2234–2238, 1980.
94. Deftos LS, Parthemore JG, Price PA: Changes in plasma bone Gla-protein during treatment of bone disease. Calcif Tissue Int 34:121–124, 1982.
95. Slovik DM, Gundberg OM, Lian JB, Neer RM: Clinical evaluation of bone turnover by serum osteocalcin measurements. Calcif Tissue Int 34:S15, 1982.
96. Delmas PD, Wahner HW, Mann KG, Riggs BL: Asessment of bone turnover in postmenopausal osteoporosis by measurement of serum bone GLA-protein. J Lab Clin Med 102:470–476, 1983.
97. Malluche HH, Faugere MC, Fanti P, Price PA: Plasma levels of bone Gla-protein reflect bone formation in patients on chronic maintenance dialysis. Kidney Int 26:85–90, 1984.
98. Dorr L, Arnala I, Faugere MC, Malluche HH: Bone histology in patients with osteoporosis and osteoarthritis undergoing total hip arthroplasty—histomorphometric studies of local and systemic changes. Clin Orthop, in press.
99. Pommer G: Rachitis and Osteomalacia. Leipzig, Vogel, 1885.
100. Ritz E, Krempien B, Bommer J, et al: Skeletal x-ray findings and bone histology in patients on hemodialysis. Kidney Int 13:316–326, 1978.
101. Perry HM, Weinstein RS, Teitelbaum SL, et al: Pseudofractures in the absence of osteomalacia. Skeletal Radiol 8:17–19, 1982.
102. Frost HM: The Bone Dynamics in Osteoporosis and Osteomalacia. Springfield, Charles C Thomas, 1966.
103. Teitelbaum SL: The histopathology of osteomalacia. *In* Jee WSS, Parfitt AM: Bone Histomorphometry. Paris, Société Nouvelle de Publications Médicales et Dentaires, 1981, pp 475–482.
104. Parsons JA, Meunier PJ, Neer RM, et al: Effects of synthetic human parathyroid hormone fragment (hPTH 1–24) on bone mass and bone mineral metabolism. *In* DeLuca HF, Frost HM, Jee WSS, et al: Os-

teoporosis. Baltimore, University Park Press, 1981, pp 457–465.

105. Malluche HH, Goldstein DA, Massry SG: Osteomalacia and hyperparathyroid bone disease in patients with nephrotic syndrome. J Clin Invest 63:494–500, 1979.

106. Julian BA, Faugere MC, Maluche HH: Oxalosis: A radiographic mimicry of renal bone disease. Am J Kidney Dis 9:436–440, 1987.

107. Malluche HH, Ritz E, Lange HP, et al: Bone mass in maintenance haemodialysis. Prospective study with seuqential biopsies. Eur J Clin Invest 6:265–271, 1976.

108. Faugere MC, Arnala IO, Ritz E, Malluche HH: Loss of bone resulting from accumulation of aluminum in bone of patients undergoing dialysis. J Lab Clin Med 107:481–487, 1986.

109. Faugere MC, Abreo K, Smith A, Malluche HH: Bone aluminum accumulation: Etiology, prevalence and its influence on vitamin D therapy in patients with mild to advanced renal failure. *In* Cohn DV, Potts JT Jr, Fujita T: Endocrine Control of Bone and Calcium Metabolism. Amsterdam, Excerpta Medica, 1984, pp 151–152.

110. Platts MD, Goode GC, Hislop JS: Composition of the domestic water supply and the incidence of fractures and encephalopathy in patients on home dialysis. Br Med J 2:657–660, 1977.

111. Ward MD, Feest TG, Ellis HA, et al: Osteomalacia dialysis osteodystrophy; evidence for a waterborne aetiological agent, probably aluminum. Lancet 1:841–844, 1978.

112. Parkinson IS, Ward MK, Feest TG, et al: Fracturing dialysis osteodystrophy and dialysis encephalopathy. Lancet 1:406–409, 1979.

113. Delling GR: Bone cells as well as bone remodelling surfaces in renal bone diseases and their changes after therapy: A quantitative analysis. *In* Norman AW, Schaefer K, Coburn JW, et al: Vitamin D: Biochemical, Chemical and Clinical Aspects Related to Calcium Metabolism. Berlin, de Gruyter, 1977, pp 165–174.

114. Vecchierini-Blineau MF, Thebaud HE, Brochard D, Coville P: Deux signes precurseurs de l'encephalopathie des hemodialyses: Osteodystrophie osteomalacique et alterations electroencephalographiques. Influence de la teneur en aluminium dans les bains de dialyse. Nephrologie 1:29–32, 1980.

115. Drueke T: Dialysis osteomalacia and aluminum intoxication. Nephron 26:207–310, 1980.

116. Pierides AM, Edwards WG, Cullum UX, et al: Hemodialysis encephalopathy with osteomalacic fractures and muscle weakness. Kidney Int 18:115–124, 1980.

117. Hodsman AB, Sherrard DJ, Wong EGC, et al: Vitamin D–resistant osteomalacia in hemodialysis patients lacking secondary hyperparathyroidism. Ann Intern Med 94:629–637, 1981.

118. Massry SG, Goldstein DA, Malluche HH: Current status of the use of $1,25(OH)_2D_3$ in the management of renal osteodystrophy. Kidney Int 18:409–418, 1980.

119. Ritz E, Malluche HH, Krempien B, Mehls O: Bone histology in renal insufficiency. *In* Davis DD: Perspectives in Nephrology and Hypertension. New York, Wiley, 1977, pp 197–233.

120. Pierce-Myli M, Pierides A: Iron and aluminum osteomalacia during hemodialysis. A new syndrome. Kidney Int 25:151, 1984.

121. Smith AJ, Faugere MC, Abreo K, et al: Aluminum associated bone disease in renal failure. A study on prevalence, histopathology, etiology and diagnosis in 197 patients. Am J Nephrol 6:275–283, 1986.

122. Massry SG, Llach F, Singer FR, et al: Homeostasis and action of parathyroid hormone in normal man and patients with mild renal failure. *In* Moorhead JR, Mion C, Baillod RA: Dialysis Transplantation Nephrology. London, Pitman Medical, 1975, pp 451–456.

123. Malluche HH, Ritz E, Lange HP, et al: Bone histology in incipient and advanced renal failure. Kidney Int 9:355–352, 1976.

124. Malluche HH, Werner E, Ritz E: Intestinal absorption of calcium and whole body calcium retention in incipient and advanced renal failure. Miner Electrolyte Metab 1:263–270, 1978.

125. Felsenfeld AJ, Gutman RA, Llach F, Harrelson JM: Osteomalacia in chronic renal failure: A syndrome previously reported only with maintenance dialysis. Am J Nephrol 2:147–154, 1982.

126. Bordier P, Ryckewaert A, Gjuens J, Rasmussen H: On the pathogenesis of so-called idiopathic hypercalciuria. Am J Med 63:398–409, 1977.

127. Coe FL, Canterbury JM, Firpo JJ, Reiss E: Evidence for secondary hyperparathyroidism in idiopathic hypercalciuria. J Clin Invest 52:134–142, 1973.

128. Malluche HH, Tschoepe W, Ritz E, et al: Abnormal bone histology in idiopathic hypercalciuria. J Clin Endocrinol Metab 50:656–658, 1980.

129. Duncan H, Rao SD, Parfitt AM: Complication of bone biopsy. *In* Jee WSS, Parfitt AM: Bone Histomorphometry. Paris, Société Nouvelle de Publications Médicales et Dentaires, 1981, pp 483–486.

130. Malluche HH, Faugere MC: Atlas of Mineralized Bone Histology. Basel, S. Karger, 1986.

131. Arnold JS, Jee WSS: Embedding and sectioning undecalcified bone and its application to radioautography. Stain Technol 29:225–239, 1954.

132. Goldner J: A modification of the Masson trichrome technique for routine laboratory purposes. Am J Pathol 14:237–243, 1938.

133. Matrajt M, Hioco D: Solochrome cyanin R as an indicator dye of bone morphology. Stain Technol 41:97–100, 1966.

134. Von Kossa G: Ueber die im Organismus kuenstlich erzeugbaren Verkalkungen. Beitr Pathol Anat 29:163–202, 1901.

135. Burstone MS: Histochemical demonstration of acid phosphatase activity in osteoclasts. J Histochem Cytochem 7:39–41, 1959.

136. Doty SB, Schofield BH: Enzyme histochemistry of bone and cartilage cells. Prog Histochem Cytochem 8:1–38, 1976.

137. Villanueva AR: An improved stain for fresh mineralized bone sections. Am J Clin Pathol 47:78–84, 1967.

138. Villanueva AR: Methods of preparing and interpreting mineralized sections of bone. *In* Jaworski ZF: Bone Histomorphometry. Ottawa, University of Ottawa Press, 1973, pp 341–353.

139. Pearse AGE: Histochemistry, Theoretical and Applied. 3rd ed, vol 2. Baltimore, Williams and Wilkins, 1972.

140. Faugere MC, Malluche HH: Stainable aluminum and not aluminum content reflect histologic changes in bone of dialyzed patients. Kidney Int 30:717–722, 1986.

141. Ott SM, Maloney NA, Klein GL, et al: Aluminum is

associated with low bone formation in patients receiving chronic parenteral nutrition. Ann Intern Med 98:910–914, 1983.

142. Ott SM, Maloney NA, Coburn JW, et al: The prevalence of bone aluminum deposition in renal osteodystrophy and its relation to the response to calcitriol therapy. N Engl J Med 307:709–713, 1982.
143. Andreoli SP, Bergstein JM, Sherrard DJ: Aluminum intoxication from aluminum-containing phosphate binders in children with azotemia not undergoing dialysis. N Engl J Med 310:1079–1084, 1984.
144. Freundlich M, Abitbol C, Zilleruelo G, et al: Infant formula as a cause of aluminum toxicity in neonatal uremia. Lancet 2:527–529, 1985.
145. Lillie PD, Fullmer HM: Histopathologic Technique and Practical Histochemistry. 4th ed. New York, McGraw-Hill, 1976, pp 534–535.
146. Ihle B, Buchanan MR, Plomley R, et al: Histology in dialysis osteomalacia secondary to aluminum toxicity. Kidney Int 19:149, 1981.
147. Maloney NA, Alfrey AC, Miller NL, et al: Histological quantitation of aluminum in iliac bone from patients with renal failure. J Lab Clin Med 99:206–216, 1982.
148. Perls M: Nachweis von Eisenoxyd in gewissen Pigmenten. Virchows Arch Pathol Anat 39:42–48, 1867.
149. Quincke H: Ueber directe Fe-Reaction in thierischen Geweben. Arch Exp Pathol Pharmkol 37:183–190, 1896.
150. Schmeltzer W: Der mikrochemische Nachweis von Eisen in Gewebselementen mittels Rhodan-Wasserstoffsaure und die Konservierung der Reaktion in Paroffinol. Z Wiss Mikrosk 50:99–102, 1933.
151. Gomori G: Microtechnical demonstration: A criticism of its methods. Am J Pathol 12:655–663, 1936.
152. Gans A: Das Abblassen des Turnbullblaues in mikroskopischen Schnitten. Z Wiss Mikrosk 40:310–313, 1923.
153. Russ JC: Resolution and sensitivity of x-ray microanalysis in biological sections by scanning and conventional transmission electron microscopy. Scan Electron Microsc 1:73–80, 1972.
154. Rahn BA, Perren SM: Calcein-blue as a fluorescent label in bone. Experientia 26:519–520, 1970.
155. Rahn BA, Perren SM: Xylenol-orange, a fluorochrome useful in poychrome sequential labeling of calcifying tissues. Stain Technol 46:125–129, 1971.
156. Frost HM: Measurement of human bone formation by means of tetracycline labeling. Can J Biochem Physiol 41:31–42, 1963.
157. Frost HM: Tetracycline-based analysis of bone remodeling. Calcif Tissue Res 3:211–317, 1969.
158. Frost HM: Bone Remodeling and Its Relationship to Metabolic Bone Diseases. Orthopaedic Lectures, vol III. Springfield, Charles C Thomas, 1973.
159. Frost HM: Bone Modeling and Skeletal Modeling Errors. Orthopaedic Lectures, vol IV. Springfield, Charles C Thomas, 1973.
160. Frost HM: Bone histomorphometry: Correction of the labelling "escape error." *In* Recker RR: Bone Histomorphometry: Technique and Interpretation. Boca Raton, CRC Press, 1983, pp 133–142.
161. Bartl R, Frisch B, Burkhardt R: Bone Marrow Biopsies Revisited. Basel, S. Karger, 1982.
162. Delesse MA: Procédé mécanique pour déterminer la composition des roches. C.r. Hebd Seanc Acad Sci (Paris) 25:544–552, 1847.
163. Merz WH, Schenk RK: Quantitative structural analysis of human cancellous bone. Acta Anat 75:54–66, 1970.
164. Buffon GLL: Essai d'arithmétique morale. Supplement à l'Histoire Naturelle (Paris), vol 4, 1777.
165. Malluche HH, Sherman D, Meyer R, Massry SG: A new semiautomatic method for quantitative static and dynamic bone histology. Calcif Tissue Int 34:439–448, 1982.
166. Parfitt AM, Drezner MK, Glorieux FH, et al: Bone histomorphometry: standardization of nomenclature, symbols and units. J Bone Min Res 6:595–610, 1987.
167. Meunier P: Use of an image-analyzing computer for bone morphometry. *In* Frame B, Parfitt AM, Duncan H: Clinical Aspects of Metabolic Bone Disease. Amsterdam, Excerpta Medica, 1973, pp 148–151.
168. Colton T: Statistics in Medicine. Boston, Little, Brown, 1974, pp 38–40.
169. Krempien B, Ritz E, Geiger G: Behavior of osteocytes in various ages and chronic uremia. Morphological studies in human cortical bone. *In* Jaworski ZF: Proceedings, 1st Workshop on Bone Morphometry. Ottawa, University of Ottawa Press, 1976, pp 288–296.
170. Meunier P, Bernard J: Morphometric analysis of periosteocytic osteolysis. *In* Jaworski ZF: Proceedings, 1st Workshop on Bone Morphometry. Ottawa, University of Ottawa Press, 1976, pp 279–287.
171. Baud CA: Histophysiology of the osteocyte: An introduction to morphometry of periosteocytic lacunae. *In* Jaworski ZF: Proceedings, 1st Workshop on Bone Morphometry. Ottawa, University of Ottawa Press, 1976, pp 267–272.
172. Baud CA, Auil E: Osteocyte differentiation count in normal human alveolar bone. Acta Anat 78:321–327, 1971.
173. Malluche HH, Henry H, Meyer-Sabellek W, et al: Effects and interactions of $24R25(OH)_2D_3$ on $1,25(OH)_2D_3$ on bone. Am J Physiol 238:E494–E498, 1980.
174. Malluche HH, Meyer-Sabellek W, Singer FR, Massry SG: Evidence for a direct effect of thiazides on bone. Miner Electrolyte Metab 4:89–96, 1980.
175. Bordier PJ, Tun-Chot S: Quantitative histology of metabolic bone disease. Clin Endocr Metab 1:197–215, 1972.
176. Schenk P: Standard values (histomorphometry) iliac crest cancellous bone. *In* Jaworski ZF: Proceedings, 1st Workshop of Bone Morphometry. Ottawa, University of Ottawa, 1973, pp 392–394.
177. Schultz A, Delling G: Histomorphometric preparation and technique: determination of trabecular bone volume. *In* Jaworski ZF: Proceedings, 1st Workshop of Bone Morphometry. Ottawa, University of Ottawa, 1973, pp 106–108.
178. Courpron P, Meunier P, Bressot C, Giroux JM: Amount of bone in iliac crest biopsy. Significance of the trabecular bone volume. Its values in normal and in pathological conditions. *In* Meunier P: Proceedings, 2nd International Workshop, Lyon, France, 1976, pp 39–53.
179. Melsen F, Melsen B, Mosekilde L, Bergman S: Histomorphometric analysis of normal bone from the iliac crest. Acta Pathol Microbiol Scand 86:70–80, 1978.
180. Whitehouse WJ: Cancellous bone in the anterior part of the iliac crest. Calcif Tissue Res 23:67–76, 1977.
181. Xipell JM, Brown DJ: Histology of normal bone—a computerized study in the iliac crest. Pathology 11:235–240, 1979.

A.M. PARFITT

11

Osteomalacia and Related Disorders

The term "osteomalacia" originally referred to generalized softening of bone leading to crippling deformities.[1,2] Histologic differentiation of osteomalacia from osteoporosis and osteitis fibrosa was first made by the German pathologist Pommer in the late 19th century,[3] but at that time bone was examined only in cadavers. A restatement of his observations in terms of current concepts of bone remodeling (Chapters 1 and 10) is that resorbed bone is replaced by the same volume of normal lamellar bone in young adults, by a lesser volume of normal lamellar bone in age-related bone loss and osteoporosis, by a complex mixture of woven bone and fibrous tissue in osteitis fibrosa, and by unmineralized bone matrix, or osteoid tissue, usually lamellar but occasionally woven, in osteomalacia.[4]

Soon after the discovery of vitamin D it became apparent that almost all cases of bone softening were the result of vitamin D deficiency, and osteomalacia came to be equated with the disease that could be cured by vitamin D administration.[1,2] Vitamin D deficiency can conveniently be classified as extrinsic, due to some combination of reduced dietary intake and reduced production in skin, and intrinsic, due to impaired intestinal absorption, with possible contributions from interruption of a putative enterohepatic circulation,[5] and altered metabolism due to malabsorption of calcium.[5a] Osteomalacia defined in this way has characteristic clinical, biochemical, radiographic, and histologic features, collectively referred to as the osteomalacic syndrome,[1] that have been described and illustrated many times. However, the deformed skeleton of advanced osteomalacia, with potentially catastrophic complications such as obstructed labor, is almost never seen except when and where extrinsic vitamin D deficiency is endemic, as in prerevolutionary China[6] and in some parts of present day India.[7]

Since it became feasible to examine bone microscopically during life, osteomalacia has usually been defined in histologic terms as the accumulation of osteoid tissue because of defective bone mineralization.[3,8] Unfortunately, because of erroneous notions of how defective mineralization should be identified histologically, some recent definitions of osteomalacia obscure the differences from other metabolic bone diseases to the extent that the term osteomalacia ceases to serve any useful purpose, thus effectively negating Pommer's pioneering work. One of the principal themes of this chapter is the formulation of a more rigorous histomorphometric definition of osteomalacia that restores many of its traditional connotations, allows more accurate evaluation of other diagnostic tests, clarifies the relationships to other forms of metabolic bone diseases, and elucidates pathogenesis.

Even with a more precise histologic definition, osteomalacia can result from a wide variety of causes other than vitamin D deficiency.[1,2,8,9] In children, in whom disordered mineralization is expressed as rickets, these other conditions, although individually rare, have in the developed countries become collectively more common than vitamin D deficiency. Diseases presenting in childhood include virtually all of the genetically determined forms of rickets and osteomalacia[2] and are described in detail in Chapter 24; they are considered here only to the extent that they raise issues of pathogenesis, diagnosis, or treatment that are relevant to adult medicine. One disadvantage of a histologic rather than a clinical definition of osteomalacia is that many of its rarer forms differ in one or more respects from the standard textbook description. Statements based on observations in one form of osteomalacia must never be assumed without evidence to apply to another. Even in vitamin D–related osteomalacia, with more widespread use of bone biopsy and consequent earlier diagnosis, some classic features such as Looser zones are now quite rare, and complete absence of symptoms, or the presence only of musculoskeletal symptoms unrelated to vitamin D, is much more common than in the past.

Although there are many nonhereditary causes of osteomalacia, intestinal malabsorption of vitamin D (intrinsic deficiency) still accounts for more than 75% of all current cases in U.S. adults without renal failure. This is so despite a lower prevalence than in the past of osteomalacia in some malabsorptive states, such as adult celiac disease, which are now earlier recognized and more effectively treated. An important difference from extrinsic vitamin D deficiency is that malabsorption of calcium is more severe, since it can occur also as a result of the primary intestinal disease, unrelated to lack of vitamin D. Patients with intestinal malabsorption are also at risk for nonosteomalacic osteopenia, associated sometimes with high bone turnover due to secondary hyperparathyroidism and sometimes with low bone turnover; the latter is likely related to malabsorption of other nutrients, some known and some unknown. A detailed characterization of the different forms of intestinal bone disease and their interrelationships is another major theme of this chapter.

Apart from problems resulting from incorrect histologic criteria for diagnosis, several other misconceptions about osteomalacia can be found in recent writings on the subject. Some authors have claimed that osteomalacia can frequently be present even when all the noninvasive diagnostic tests usually performed are normal,[10] but in the author's experience this is a rare occurrence. In some series, previously unsuspected osteomalacia has been found in up to 10% of patients with apparent age-related osteoporosis and compression fractures.[11] This probably reflects the referral bias that inevitably occurs at centers of tertiary care, since the prevalence of osteomalacia in unselected series of patients with postmenopausal osteoporosis in Detroit is less than 1%, although it may be higher in European countries that do not practice fortification of dairy products with vitamin D.[12]

But the most important misconception about osteomalacia is that all of its manifestations are curable. Although symptoms can readily be relieved, and biochemical and histologic abnormalities corrected, there has usually been irreversible damage to the skeleton by the time the diagnosis is made.[13] Symptomatic relief is gratifying to physicians, but its overemphasis can be counterproductive, because many patients have unrelated symptoms that are not relieved. This leads to poor compliance with treatment, the need for which is lifelong, regardless of symptoms. In many patients, osteomalacia is preceded for many years by clinically silent secondary hyperparathyroidism that accelerates the irreversible age-related loss of cortical and to a lesser extent cancellous bone.[14] Exposition of this concept is aided by using the term "hypovitaminosis D osteopathy" (HVO) to encompass the totality of osseous complications of deficiency or altered metabolism of vitamin D.[15,16] The possible role of HVO in the pathogenesis of age-related fractures, especially of the upper femur, represents a confusing but important borderland between osteoporosis and osteomalacia that is in need of clarification.

I. BONE MINERALIZATION AND THE MECHANISMS OF OSTEOID ACCUMULATION

A. Interpretation of Tetracycline Data

The use of *in vivo* double tetracycline labeling as a diagnostic and investigative tool is described in Chapter 10, but some additional details are important for the understanding of osteomalacia. Tetracycline chelates calcium, and when the blood level is raised, it binds reversibly to every bone surface accessible to the circulation, but is permanently incorporated into bone only at the mineralization fronts, which are the sites of currently active mineralization.[17] A few days after it has disappeared from the blood, tetracycline fluorescence is seen only in relation to these sites, which can also be identified by a band of granular structure and somewhat blurred outline that stains deeply with toluidine blue,[18] and by a wide variety of other histochemical features.[3,17] Tetracycline binds preferentially to the most recently formed mineral that is of small crystal size and high surface area (Chapter 2); there may also be a very small fraction of amorphous mineral with special affinity for tetracycline.[17] Because of the relatively low density and high water content of recently formed bone, tetracycline diffuses into it, away from the surface, to form the zone of instantaneous labeling, usually 2 to 3 μm in thickness.* As will be discussed later, in osteomalacia there can be an increase in the width of this band as well as a decrease in the distance between bands.

In all studies from the author's laboratory that form the basis of the conclusions to be presented later, by scheduling the biopsy before labeling is begun, the time interval between the end of the second labeling period and the biopsy has been kept constant at 4 days. Permanent tetracycline fixation occurs because during this time interval a layer of new mineral is deposited of sufficient thickness to prevent the escape of tetracycline when its blood level falls to zero, as occurs from all bone surfaces at which there is no mineral deposition. Depending on the particular tetracycline used and on the physical and chemical characteristics of the new mineral, there is some outward diffusion, so that the outermost border of the second fluorescent band may be quite close to the current location of the mineralization front, which has moved 2 to 3 μm away from its location at the time of administration of the second label.

There are several potential pitfalls in the interpretation of tetracycline measurements. A double band of fluorescence establishes unequivocally that bone formation occurred during the relevant time period, but only a single label can be deposited if formation begins or ends between the periods of label administration. Most single labels are evidence of bone formation, especially if they are in continuity with double labels, but in osteomalacia there are several mechanisms (described later) for the retention of a single label in the absence of any recent mineralization. Conversely, some mineralization can occur in the absence of tetracycline uptake, because if mineral apposition is very slow, too few tetracycline molecules may be retained to exceed the threshold for visible fluorescence. As a result, in some cases a higher proportion of the osteoid surface is unlabeled than can be accounted for by the delay in onset of mineralization, and the double tetracycline method underestimates the true bone formation rate by about 5% to 10%. It is also likely that some unlabeled osteoid results from a temporary cessation of mineralization to form a so-called resting seam[17] with subsequent resumption at a normal rate.[20]

*In the ilium, thickness (in three-dimensional space) = width (measured in two-dimensional sections) × 0.833, because of section obliquity.[19]

B. Life History of Individual Osteoid Seams

The formation of a new bone structural unit (B.St.U,* Chapter 10) begins at the cement surface, a thin layer of lowly mineralized collagen-poor but glycoprotein-rich connective tissue[20b] that is laid down on the floor of the resorption cavity at the end of the reversal phase of the remodeling cycle. In two-dimensional histologic sections stained with toluidine blue or gallocyanine, the three-dimensional cement surface is represented by the cement line, forming the boundary in the section of the new B.St.U.[21] The cement line, which remains in the same location, separating new bone from old, must be distinguished from the boundary between mineralized and unmineralized bone, referred to as the osteoid-bone interface, which normally moves away from the cement line during bone formation (Fig. 11–1). The mineralization front is always located at the osteoid-bone interface, but if mineralization fails to begin, or ceases temporarily or permanently, the mineralization front either never appears or disappears, but the interface remains.

Soon after deposition of the cement surface, a team of osteoblasts assembles and begins to deposit a layer of bone matrix referred to as an osteoid seam. Because of the local geometry, osteoid seams in cortical bone appear as rings, but in cancellous bone as crescents tapering at each end. Although their individuality is less apparent than in cortical bone and is obscured by the usual methods of histomorphometry (Chapter 10), osteoid seams in cancellous bone have a predictable range of dimensions and a measurable life span, during which characteristic changes occur in the morphologic features and function of the osteoblasts.[22,23] A provisional description of the life history of a typical osteoid seam in adult human cancellous bone, albeit simplified and incomplete, can be derived

*Terminology and symbols for bone histomorphometry are approved by the American Society of Bone and Mineral Research.[20a]

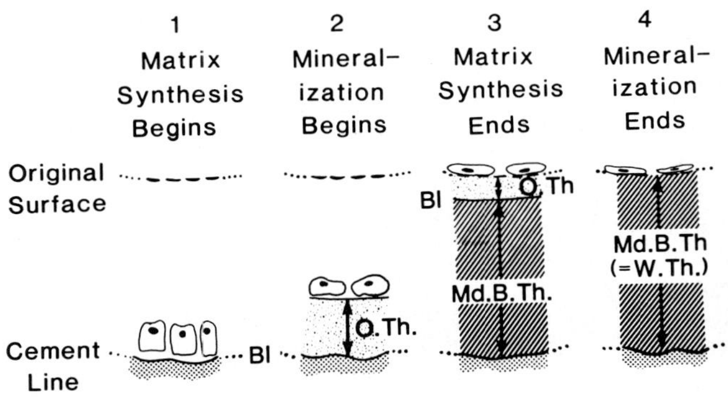

Figure 11–1. Stages in the completion of a new bone structural unit. O.Th, osteoid thickness; Md.B.Th, mineralized bone thickness; W.Th, wall thickness of completed bone structural unit. Note that bone interface (BI) moves away from the cement line during mineralization and that osteoblasts change progressively from cuboidal to flat.

from tetracycline-based kinetics (Figs. 11–1 and 11–2). Matrix apposition is most rapid (2.5–3.5 μm/day) at the outset and the seam reaches a maximum thickness of approximately 15 to 20 μm after about 10 days, just before mineralization begins. Mineral apposition is also most rapid at the outset (1.5-2.5 μm/day), and both matrix and mineral apposition progressively slow down with time, as the osteoblasts become flatter and more extended in shape and less basophilic in staining. About 50 days after the onset of mineralization, when the bone surface has returned to its previous location about 40 μm from the cement line, matrix synthesis stops. The osteoid seam thickness has by now fallen to about 6 μm, and mineral apposition continues at a progressively slower rate for a fur-

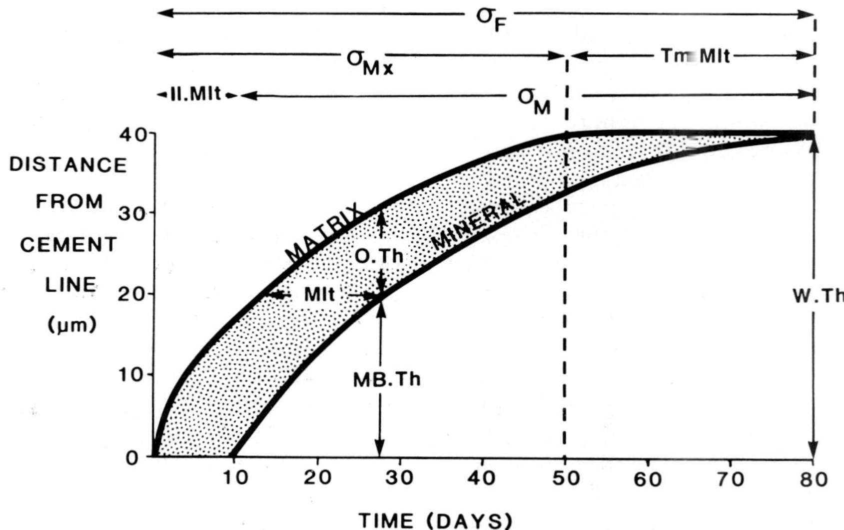

Figure 11–2. Relationship between matrix and mineral apposition during the life history of a single osteoid seam. The curved lines depict the distances of the edge of the matrix and of the bone interface from the cement line as functions of time from the onset of matrix synthesis: the slopes of the lines at any point correspond to the instantaneous rates of matrix and mineral apposition. σ_F, total duration of bone formation or formation period (80 days in this example); σ_{Mx}, total duration of matrix synthesis (50 days); Tm.Mlt, terminal mineralization lag time (30 days); Il.Mlt, initial mineralization lag time (10 days); σ_M, total duration of mineralization (70 days); W.Th, wall thickness (40 μm). The vertical distance between the two curved lines at any time represents the instantaneous osteoid seam thickness (O.Th) at that time. The horizontal distance between the curved lines at any distance from the cement line represents the instantaneous mineralization lag time at that distance. It follows that O.Th $*$ σ_F = Mlt $*$ W.Th. In the example shown, mean Mlt is 16 days, mean O.Th = 8 μm, and mean adjusted apposition rate = 0.5 μm/day. (Reprinted with permission from Parfitt AM: The physiologic and clinical significance of bone histomorphometric data. *In* Recker R (ed): Bone Histomorphometry. Techniques and Interpretations. Boca Raton, CRC Press, 1983. Copyright CRC Press, Inc.)

ther 30 days, until the osteoid seam disappears, because all the new matrix has become mineralized. The osteoblasts have now completed their histologic transformation into lining cells, and construction of the new B.St.U is finished.

According to this model, the durations of matrix synthesis and of mineralization overlap, but are neither co-extensive nor necessarily identical. Three separate stages can be recognized (Fig. 11–1). In the first stage, matrix synthesis occurs alone without mineralization, in the second stage matrix synthesis and mineralization occur together, and in the third stage mineralization occurs alone without matrix synthesis. In an alternative model,[23,24] the second and third stages are merged, matrix synthesis and mineralization terminating simultaneously. In either case, the third stage is probably when mineral apposition may sometimes be too slow for tetracycline fixation to occur. In considering the relationship between this model and the results of bone histomorphometry as ordinarily performed, it is important to distinguish between the mean values of various measured and derived quantities found in one individual and the instantaneous values that occur at different stages of the osteoid seam life history in that individual[23] (Fig. 11–2); where the context makes it necessary, a symbol that refers to such mean values will be identified by an upper horizontal bar.[17] For the mean value to be an accurate representation of the whole sequence of events, it is even more important that sampling is unbiased with respect to time than with respect to space. This is possible only if bone remodeling is in a steady state during the period of labeling and biopsy.

C. Mineralization Lag Time and Osteoid Maturation Time

A key quantity in understanding the mechanisms of osteoid accumulation and the pathogenesis and diagnosis of osteomalacia is the mineralization lag time, which is defined as the time interval between the deposition of an individual moiety of bone matrix and its mineralization.[25] During this time interval new matrix will be added (Fig. 11–3), so that the osteoid seam thickness (O.Th) is determined by the mineralization lag time (Mlt) and the osteoid apposition rate (OAR):

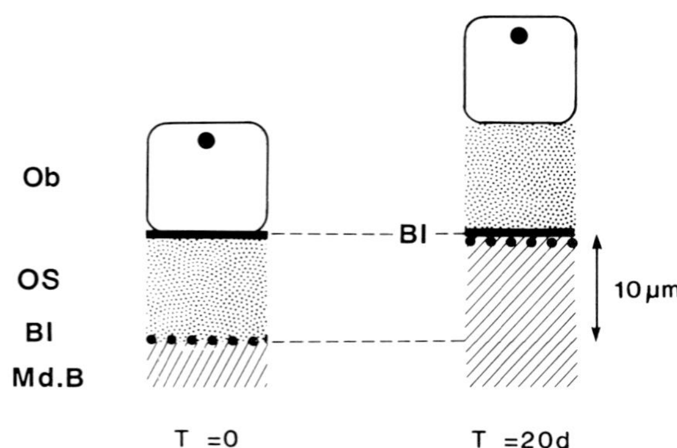

Figure 11–3. Calculation of mineralization lag time (Mlt). Ob, osteoblast; O, osteoid; BI, bone interface; Md.B, mineralized bone. At T = 0, the moiety of matrix immediately adjacent to the osteoblast (heavy solid line) has just been deposited. At T = 20 days, this moiety has just been reached by the advancing BI, which has traveled 10 µm (the thickness of the osteoid seam at T = 0) in 20 days for a mineral apposition rate of 0.5 µm/day. The thickness of the seam at T = 20 (the time of measurement) = 20 * matrix apposition rate (µm/day). In a steady state, mean thickness at T = 0 and at T = 20 are equal, and mean matrix and mineral apposition rates are equal. (Reprinted with permission from Parfitt AM: The physiologic and clinical significance of bone histomorphometric data. *In* Recker R (ed): Bone Histomorphometry. Techniques and Interpretations. Boca Raton, CRC Press, 1983. Copyright CRC Press, Inc.)

$$\mathrm{O.Th} = \mathrm{Mlt} * \mathrm{OAR},$$

which on rearrangement gives:

$$\mathrm{Mlt} = \mathrm{O.Th}/\mathrm{OAR} \qquad (1)$$

This concept was derived from studies of periosteal bone formation in rat tibia and cannot be applied without modification to adult human bone remodeling. In the growing rat, formation occurs over the entire periosteal surface and all the osteoid labels with tetracycline. Consequently, the osteoid apposition rate is virtually identical with the mineral apposition rate (MAR), so that:

$$\mathrm{Mlt} = \mathrm{O.Th}/\mathrm{MAR} \qquad (2)$$

In human bone, the fraction of osteoid surface that labels with tetracycline (MS/OS), whether based on the mean of the separately measured lengths of the first and second label or on the length of the second label alone,[17] is significantly less than unity. Since the total volumes of matrix and of mineralized bone formed are normally the same, the average rates of matrix and mineral apposition must also be the same. Consequently, the best estimate of the osteoid apposition rate is the mineral apposition rate averaged over the entire osteoid surface, referred to as the adjusted apposition rate:

$$Aj.AR = MAR * MS/OS$$

which in combination with equation (1) gives:

$$Mlt = O.Th/MAR * MS/OS \quad (3)$$

In the rat, bone formation is continuous, and the distinction between mean and instantaneous values is unimportant; but in humans, bone formation is cyclical. The instantaneous Mlt in young normal subjects increases progressively from about 10 days at the beginning of an osteoid seam life span (initial Mlt) to about 30 days at the end of the span (terminal Mlt), with a mean value of about 16 days (Fig. 11–4). The onset of mineralization is delayed because of a progressive increase in collagen crosslinking and other biochemical changes in the matrix that prepare it for mineralization[17,26,27]; the time needed for these changes to occur is the osteoid maturation time (Omt). If mineralization occurs as soon as maturation is complete, as is likely in the growing rat, then Mlt is the same as Omt. This probably also holds in humans at the onset (initial Mlt = Omt), but whether the subsequent increase in Mlt, which has no counterpart in the rat, results from slowing down of osteoid maturation is unknown. There could also be a decline in the supply of mineral, since the net inward calcium flux characteristic of osteoblasts must at some point change to the inward calcium gradient without net flux characteristic of lining cells.[28] To the extent that Mlt exceeds Omt, for whatever reason, Mlt is not an independent quantity but is the automatic consequence of the separately regulated rates of matrix and mineral apposition. But this does not detract from its usefulness in the understanding of histomorphometric data.

D. Mineral Accumulation and Fluorescent Label Width

The rate at which the bone interface advances ("horizontal" mineralization in Fig. 11–5) must be distinguished from the rate at which mineralization proceeds after it is initiated.[17]

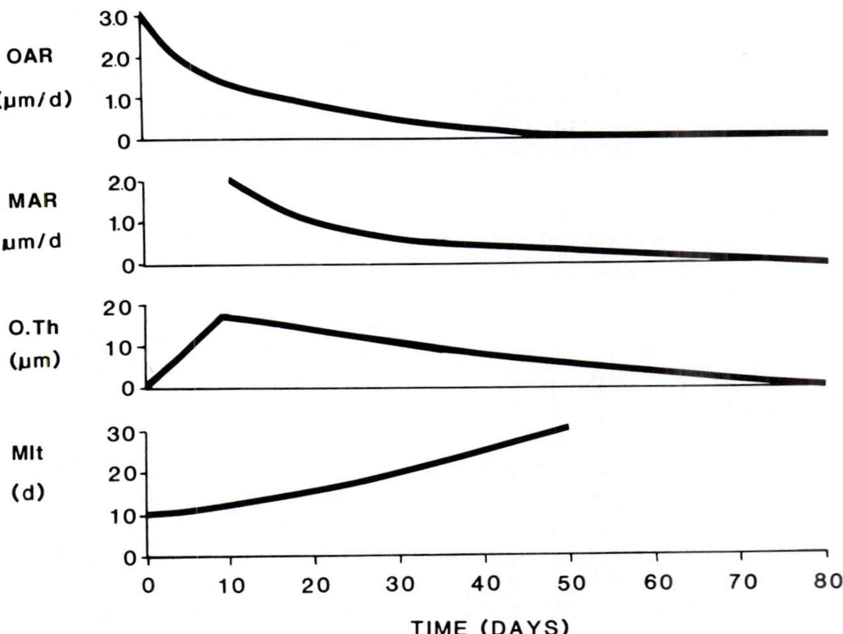

Figure 11–4. Changes in various indices of bone formation during the life history of an individual osteoid seam. Values correspond to the time course depicted in Figure 11–2. OAR, osteoid apposition rate; MAR, mineral apposition rate; O.Th, osteoid seam thickness; Mlt, mineralization lag time. (Reprinted with permission from Parfitt AM: The physiologic and clinical significance of bone histomorphometric data. *In* Recker R (ed): Bone Histomorphometry. Techniques and Interpretations. Boca Raton, CRC Press, 1983. Copyright CRC Press, Inc.)

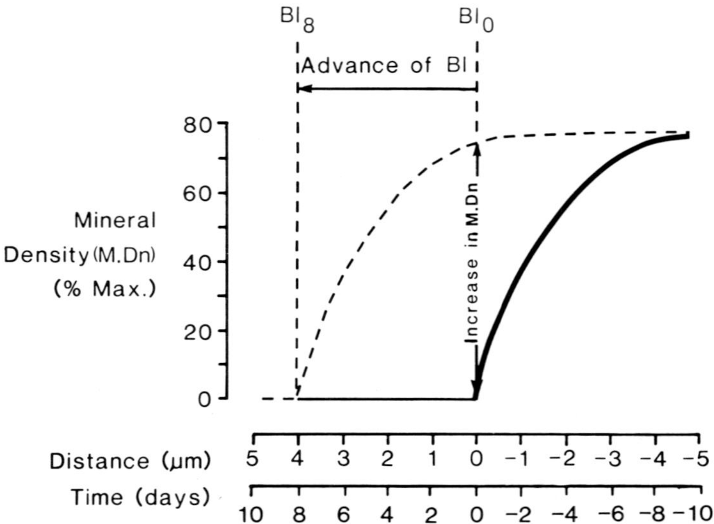

Figure 11–5. Distinction between two aspects of mineralization. In a plane perpendicular to a bone forming surface, mineral density (M.Dn) as percentage of maximum is plotted as a function of distance from the location of the bone interface (BI) at time zero (BI_0) and of time; osteoid is to the left and mineralized bone to the right. The correspondence between distance and time scales depends on movement of BI from right to left at a constant rate, assumed here to be 0.5 μm/day. The curved solid line shows M.Dn at different locations within mineralized bone at time zero. The curved dotted line shows M.Dn at different locations 8 days later, during which BI has advanced 4 μm to BI_8 and mineral density at BI_0 has increased to 75% of maximum. The distance from BD at which M.Dn has increased to the level that prevents diffusion of tetracycline molecules determines the width of the fluorescent band. The rate of advance of BI or mineral apposition rate ("horizontal mineralization") and the rate of mineral accumulation ("vertical mineralization") can vary independently, although they usually change in the same direction. (Reprinted with permission from Parfitt AM: The physiologic and clinical significance of bone histomorphometric data. *In* Recker R (ed): Bone Histomorphometry. Techniques and Interpretations. Boca Raton, CRC Press, 1983. Copyright CRC Press, Inc.)

In an individual moiety of bone matrix, mineral accumulation ("vertical" mineralization in Fig. 11–5) as a function of time is a continuous process that is conveniently subdivided into an early rapid increase usually completed in a few hours or days, referred to as primary mineralization, and a later slow increase that usually continues for several months, referred to as secondary mineralization.[17] As mineral density increases, a point is reached at which the bone is no longer permeable to tetracycline. For a given rate of mineral apposition, the time taken to reach this point determines the width of the fluorescent band.[29] In the rat, this relationship permits calculation of the rate of initial mineral accumulation, which is closely correlated with the rate of osteoid maturation.[25,26] In human subjects, this calculation cannot yet be formalized, but increased label width, presumably due to slower primary mineralization, is frequently observed in osteomalacia.

E. Osteoid Indices in Relation to Tetracycline-Based Kinetics

It is customary to ignore individual osteoid seam profiles and determine length, thickness, and volume for the entire section (Chapter 10). Thickness (width × 0.833) should be measured directly rather than calculated indirectly from volume and surface, both because of its intrinsic importance and because the frequency distribution of individual measurements sometimes gives more useful information than the mean value. The three osteoid indices are related as follows[30]:

$$\text{OV/BV (\%)} = \text{O.Th (mm)} * \text{OS/BS (\%)} * \text{BS/BV (mm}^2\text{/mm}^3\text{)} \quad (4)$$

where

$$\text{BS/BV (bone surface/volume)} = \text{(bone perimeter/area)/0.833}$$

A fall in trabecular thickness, as occurs to a modest extent in aging and in osteoporosis, will increase BS/BV and so increase OV/BV even if surface and thickness are unchanged, and for the most accurate interpretation, OV/BV should be corrected to the expected trabecular thickness for age and sex.[31]

The relationship between osteoid thickness and its kinetic determinants is given by rearrangement of equation 1, which applies to mean as well as to instantaneous values, or equation 3, which is difficult to apply to instantaneous values. Osteoid surface per unit of bone surface is determined entirely by the mean osteoid seam life span or formation period (FP) and by the average frequency with which new osteoid appears at any point on the bone surface, which in the steady state is the same as the frequency of remodeling activation (Ac.f):

$$\text{OS/BS}\ (\%) = \text{Ac.f}\ (/\text{y}) * \text{FP}\ (\text{y}) \times 100 \quad (5)$$

Osteoid volume is determined entirely by the fractional rate of bone turnover, which is the same as the volume-based bone formation rate (BFR/BV), and by the mean life span of an individual moiety of osteoid, which is the same as the mineralization lag time:

$$\text{OV/BV}\ (\%) = \text{BFR/BV}\ (\%/\text{y}) * \text{Mlt}\ (\text{y}) \quad (6)$$

Since in the steady state bone turnover is determined entirely by the frequency of remodeling activation and since FP is inversely proportional to the osteoid apposition rate,[17] the relationships between the static indices of osteoid accumulation and the kinetic indices can be summarized as in Figure 11–6. Note that each osteoid index is determined by different aspects of bone remodeling and bone cell function[30] and in particular that osteoid volume is independent of matrix (or mineral) apposition rate, which in the steady state affects surface and thickness in opposite directions.

F. Problems in the Definition of Impaired Mineralization

Although a reduction in mineral apposition rate is frequently taken to indicate defective mineralization, it is evident from Figure 11–2 that matrix and mineral apposition are closely coupled and that the mean mineral apposition rate can never exceed the mean matrix apposition rate. Consequently, a reduction in the mean rate of matrix apposition inevitably leads to, and is much the most common cause of, a reduction in the mean rate of mineral apposition. In postmenopausal osteoporosis, the adjusted apposition rate as previously defined averages about 65% of normal, with some values as low as 10%, reflecting different degrees of impairment of matrix synthesis by teams of osteoblasts.[32] Both in normal subjects and in every metabolic bone disease except osteomalacia, there is a significant positive correlation between mean osteoid thickness and mean adjusted apposition rate, with broadly similar slopes (b) and intercepts (a) of the regression lines.[30] Although such a relationship is to be expected, it has an unanticipated consequence for the interpretation of the mineralization lag time, since we can write:

$$\text{O.Th} = b(\text{OAR}) + a \quad (7)$$

If this is combined with equation 3, we obtain:

$$\text{Mlt} = b + a/\text{OAR} \quad (8)$$

Because of this relationship, which defines a rectangular hyperbola, when the adjusted apposition rate falls, the mineralization lag time increases (Fig. 11–7). This occurs in old normal subjects and in osteoporotic patients[32] and also in hypothyroidism.[33] Since prolongation of the lag time is an inevitable consequence of a fall in adjusted apposition rate, it does not by itself indicate defective min-

Rate of remodeling Activation ↑ → OS/BS↑
Rate of matrix apposition ↓ ↑
OV/BV↑
Mineralization Lag time ↑ → O.Th↑

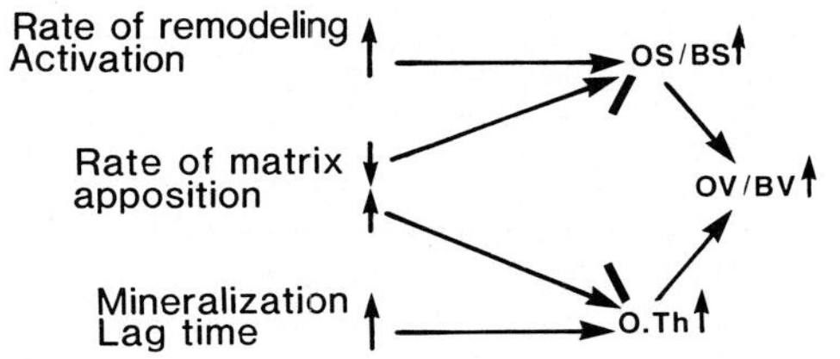

Figure 11–6. Mechanism of osteoid accumulation. Because a change in matrix apposition rate affects osteoid surface and thickness in opposite directions, in the steady state such changes have no influence on osteoid volume, which is determined only by the frequency of activation of remodeling and the mineralization lag time.

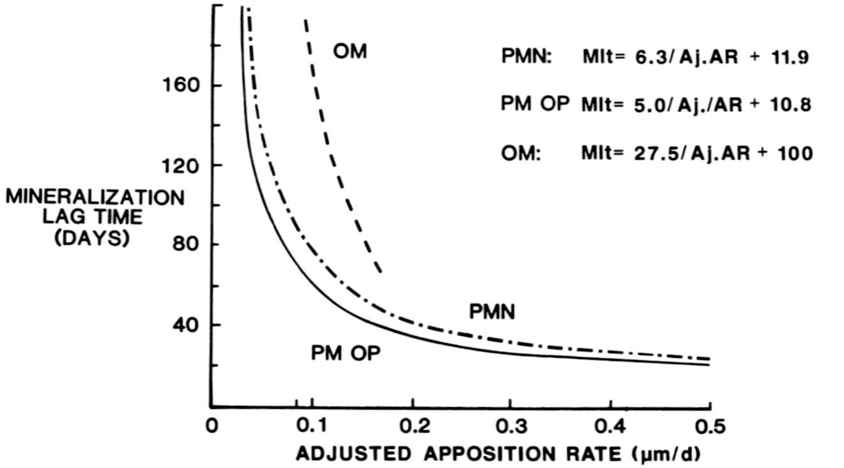

Figure 11–7. Hyperbolic relationship between mineralization lag time and adjusted apposition rate. PMN, postmenopausal normal; PMOP, postmenopausal osteoporosis; OM, osteomalacia due to hypovitaminosis D. Equations of the three lines given in inset based on published regression equations.[30] See also Table 11–1.

eralization.[30] Another way of arriving at the same conclusion is to consider the effect of prolongation of FP, which is also an inevitable consequence of a reduction in adjusted apposition rate. From Figure 11–2 it is clear that:

$$FP * \overline{O.Th} = W.Th * \overline{Mlt} \qquad (9)$$

Since O.Th has a minimum value (the intercept in equation 7) and W.Th (the mean thickness of a completed B.St.U) is constant at least in the short term, an increase in FP must be accompanied by an increase in Mlt.

An increase in surface extent but decrease in thickness of osteoid, a reduction in the proportion of labeled osteoid (or mineralization front), a fall in either mineral or adjusted apposition rate, and a prolongation of mineralization lag time can all be nonspecific consequences of impaired matrix synthesis by osteoblasts. Using any of these, alone or in combination, as a definition of osteomalacia serves only to obscure its distinction from osteoporosis. Although mineralization is a kinetic process, it turns out to be impossible to frame a rigorous and consistent definition of impaired mineralization *in vivo* using kinetic data alone without reference to osteoid thickness. To explain further why this is so, it is necessary to examine the evolution of hypovitaminosis D osteopathy as earlier defined.

G. Histologic Evolution of HVO and the Kinetic Definition of Osteomalacia

There is no relationship between osteoid thickness and osteoid surface either in normal subjects or in patients with postmenopausal osteoporosis, but in HVO, whether due to dietary deficiency or to intestinal malabsorption of vitamin D, there is a hyperbolic relationship between these variables[30,31] (Fig. 11–8*A*). This indicates that osteoid surface increases first and that osteoid thickness increases only slightly until OS/BS exceeds 70%, after which further increases in osteoid volume are due mainly to increasing thickness.[15,16] In the same patients, osteoid thickness shows a more complex relationship to adjusted apposition rate (Aj.AR; Fig. 11–8*B*). When this is above 0.1 μm/day, there is the usual positive relationship between these variables; below 0.1 μm/day, further decrements in Aj.AR are associated not with a fall in osteoid seam thickness as in all other situations, but with a progressive increase limited only by the normal thickness of new matrix or W.Th.[34] This reversal is the cardinal kinetic characteristic of defective mineralization, further illustrated in Figure 11–7, which shows that the mineralization lag time in osteoporosis, although prolonged in absolute value compared with normal subjects, is shortened relative to Aj.AR, whereas in osteomalacia the lag time is prolonged relatively,

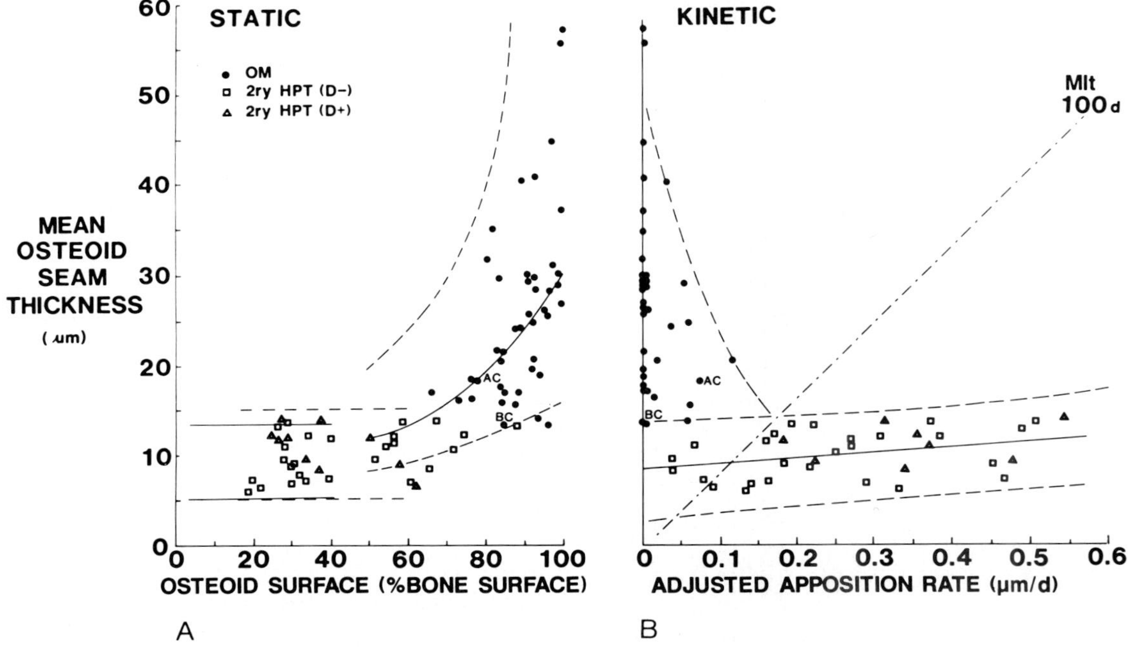

Figure 11–8. Osteoid thickness relationships in vitamin D deficiency, extrinsic or intrinsic. On left (Fig. 11–8*A*, static measurements), horizontal lines define mean and range for osteoid thickness and surface in normal subjects. The interrupted horizontal lines indicate the range for these variables in patients with secondary hyperparathyroidism with (D-; □) or without (D+; Δ) vitamin deficiency. The latter values represent patients with intestinal malabsorption of calcium alone. The curved solid line depicts the hyperbolic relationship found in osteomalacia (O.Th = 7.2/(1-0.0075) OS/BS) and the interrupted lines depict the 95% confidence limits. On the right (Fig. 11–8*B*, kinetic measurements), the straight solid line is the regression line of osteoid thickness on adjusted apposition rate (Aj.AR) in normal and hyperparathyroid subjects (OST = 7.2 Aj.AR + 7.8) and the 95% confidence limits for individual values. The oblique interrupted line represents mineralization lag time (Mlt) of 100 days. Note that in osteomalacia the osteoid thickness increases as adjusted apposition rate declines instead of decreasing as in all other situations. Patients with anticonvulsant bone disease (AC) and biliary cirrhosis (BC) individually identified because of the rarity of these causes of osteomalacia.

as well as absolutely; other differences are listed in Table 11–1.

Based on these relationships, the author defines osteomalacia by a combination of mean mineralization lag time more than 100 days and mean osteoid seam thickness above the upper 95% confidence limit predicted by the regression of osteoid thickness on Aj.AR in normal and osteoporotic subjects (Fig. 11–8), or more simply, above an absolute value of 12.5 µm (corrected for section obliquity). Patients with HVO who do not meet these criteria have increased volume and surface but not thickness of osteoid, increased bone formation rate, the normal positive relationship between O.Th and Aj.AR, and

Table 11–1. Kinetic Differences Between Osteoporosis and Osteomalacia

Feature	Osteoporosis	Osteomalacia
Mineralization lag time (Mlt)	Low for Aj.AR	High for Aj.AR
Osteoid maturation time	Normal	Increased
Adjusted apposition rate (Aj.AR)	Relative fall more than relative rise in Mlt	Relative fall less than relative rise in Mlt
	Never zero	Often zero
Osteoid thickness (O.Th)	Low	High
O.Th correlation with OS/BS	None	Positive
O.Th correlation with Aj.AR	Positive	Negative
Osteoblast defect	Matrix	Mineral

OS/BS, osteoid surface/bone surface.

increased osteoclast indices, resembling in every respect the histologic features of primary hyperparathyroidism[15,16] (Fig. 11–9). This analysis identifies the earliest stage of HVO (HVOi), when osteoid accumulation is due mainly to increased remodeling activation and bone turnover, before the emergence of a significant mineralization defect, as due to secondary hyperparathyroidism. For some purposes it is useful to refer to such patients as having preosteomalacia. Patients with HVO who meet the criteria for defective mineralization are further subdivided into those who retain some tetracycline double labels (HVOii) and those with no double labels (HVOiii).

A different perspective on the fundamental nature of osteomalacia can be gained from the model of osteoid seam life span (Fig. 11–10). In every other condition, all matrix formed eventually mineralizes; the slopes of the curves representing matrix and mineral apposition, although initially divergent, eventually converge, and the loop formed by these curves ultimately closes. By contrast, in osteomalacia some matrix remains permanently unmineralized, the slopes of matrix and mineral apposition remain divergent, and the loop never closes in the absence of treatment. The model also illuminates the difference between HVOii, in which the earliest formed matrix becomes mineralized but the later formed matrix does not, and HVOiii, in which none of the matrix formed becomes mineralized. Since all patients with HVOiii at the time of biopsy have likely been through the stage of HVOii, they show a mixture of the two types of osteoid seam depicted in Figure 11–10. Both thickness and volume of osteoid are significantly greater in HVOiii than in HVOii,[16,30] but even in the most severe cases, individual values for mean osteoid thickness fall within the reference range for mean wall thickness.[34]

A final point about the kinetic definition of osteomalacia is the identification of two variant forms. The definition does not explicitly refer to osteoid volume, which is the best index of the overall severity of osteoid accumulation. In cases that meet the kinetic criteria, OV/BV is almost always > 10% (twice the upper limit of normal), but occasionally it is normal. In these cases, contrary to the general rule, osteoid thickness increases earlier or to a relatively greater extent than osteoid surface, so that osteoid thickness is above the upper 95% confidence limit depicted in Figure 11–8*B*. This feature defines focal osteomalacia[35] as occurs in some drug-induced defects in mineralization, in which the initial increase in remodeling activation that characterizes HVO is absent for one or another reason. In mild cases, focal osteomalacia, although qualitatively evident on inspection, may be shown by measurement only as an abnormal frequency distribution of

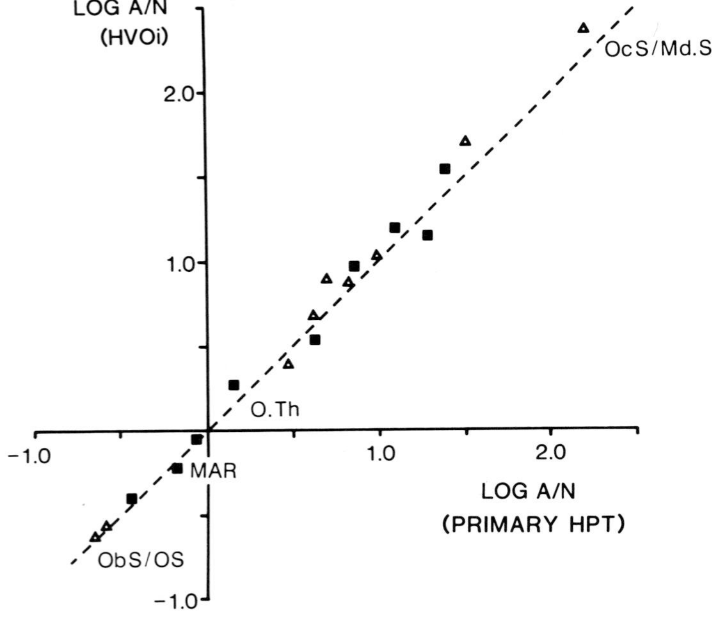

Figure 11–9. Comparison of histomorphometric data in primary hyperparathyroidism (HPT) and HVOi. ■, original measurements; Δ, calculated values. For each quantity, data are expressed as the natural logarithm of the ratio (mean value in patient group)/(mean value in normal controls). Four representative quantities are identified: ObS/OS, osteoblast surface/osteoid surface; MAR, mineral apposition rate; O.Th, mean osteoid thickness; Oc.S/Md.S, osteoclast surface/mineralized interface.

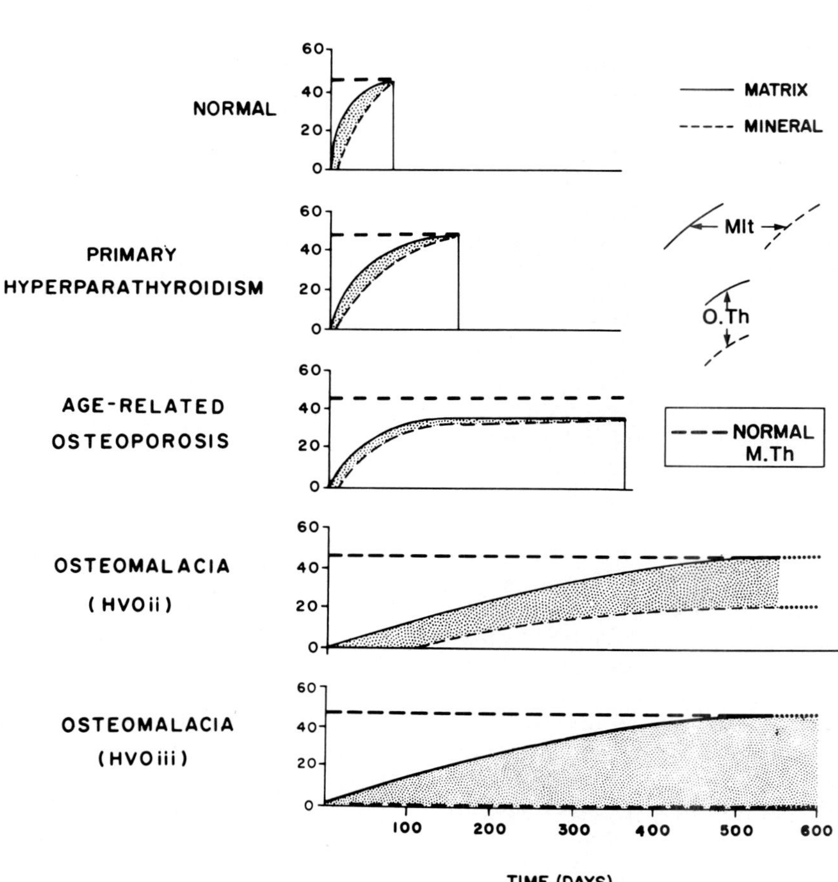

Figure 11–10. Kinetics of matrix and mineral apposition during evolution of a single bone remodeling unit in different forms of metabolic bone disease. Each panel is constructed in a manner similar to Figure 11–2. Mlt, mineralization lag time; O.Th, osteoid thickness. Note that in HVOii mineralization is delayed in onset, retarded in rate, and premature in termination, whereas in HVOiii no mineralization occurs at all.

individual osteoid seam thickness. A second and even rarer variant is the presence of substantial osteoid accumulation (OV/BV > 10%) in the absence of any increase in osteoid thickness, even when the frequency distribution of individual measurements is considered. This is referred to as atypical osteomalacia and may reflect a more severe impairment of matrix synthesis by osteoblasts than ordinarily occurs in osteomalacia.[31,36] The definitions of generalized, focal, and atypical osteomalacia and of HVO and its stages are summarized in Table 11–2; this classification will be used as a basis for describing the clinical, radiographic, and biochemical features of HVO and for comparing it with other forms of osteomalacia.

II. MANIFESTATIONS OF OSTEOMALACIA

Osteomalacia is accompanied by clinical, histopathologic, radiographic, biochemical, and radiokinetic features, the nature and frequency of which vary to some extent with the etiologic factor. The typical effects of vitamin D–related osteomalacia are described and the main exceptions, which will be covered in more detail in relation to specific types, are noted briefly. An important general principle is that the effects can differ markedly according to the age of onset. When defective mineralization begins in childhood, as well as rickets there is usually osteomalacia. If this persists untreated into adulthood, as charac-

Table 11–2. Criteria for Different Morphologic Forms of Osteomalacia and Different Stages of the Evolution of Hypovitaminosis D Osteopathy (HVO)

Form	Stage	O.Th[1](μm)	Mlt (d)	OV/BV[2](%)
Preosteomalacia	HVOi	<12.5[3]	<100	>5
Osteomalacia	HVOii	>12.5	>100	>10
Generalized	HVOiii	>12.5	∞[4]	>10
Focal	—	>12.5	>100	<5[5]
Atypical	—	<12.5	>50	>5[6]

O.Th, mean osteoid thickness (corrected for section obliquity); Mlt, mineralization lag time; OV/BV, osteoid volume per unit of bone volume.

[1]Corrected for regression on adjusted apposition rate in borderline cases.

[2]Corrected for trabecular thickness in borderline cases.

[3]Upper limit higher in renal osteodystrophy.

[4]No double label, so apposition rate zero.

[5]Cases with OV/BV between 5% and 10% are transitional between focal and generalized.

[6]In cases with OV/BV between 5% and 10% or with Mlt between 50 and 100, will need BFR to discriminate from HVOi or other forms of high-turnover osteoporosis.

teristically occurs in endemic vitamin D deficiency, severe deformity and gross radiographic abnormalities are common. When osteomalacia begins later in life without previous rickets, as is now the rule in the indigenous populations of developed countries, its manifestations are more subtle. The later the onset, the more the clinical features can resemble those of age-related osteoporosis and the more easily overlooked are the clues to osteomalacia, since its symptoms can easily be attributed to the locomotor or neurologic effects of aging. Except for Asian immigrants to Great Britain,[37] advanced endemic type osteomalacia is found only in an occasional patient with celiac disease[2,38] or vitamin D dependency.[2,39]

A. Clinical Features

The classic symptoms are bone pain and tenderness, muscle weakness, and difficulty in walking, often unremitting but lessening at the end of summer in mild cases. In the genetic forms of osteomalacia and in adult celiac disease there may be residual deformities of rickets[2] (Chapter 24), usually associated with short stature and possibly including subclinical basilar impression.[40] Deformities due to softening of the adult skeleton include kyphosis, coxa vara, and pigeon breast.[1,2,6,38,41,42] Protrusio acetabuli can ultimately compress the pelvic inlet to a triradiate shape and narrow the pubic arch, so that childbirth is only possible by cesarean section.[6] But in most patients there is no deformity other than the normal effects of aging on the spine. An unusual manner of presentation, most common in adult onset hypophosphatemic osteomalacia, is algodystrophy or reflex sympathetic dystrophy, probably as a result of increased load-bearing by the remaining mineralized bone.[42a,42b] The various types of fracture that occur in osteomalacia will be described after the radiographic changes. A few patients present with the effects of hypocalcemia, which are described in detail elsewhere in relation to hypoparathyroidism (Chapter 14). Some rarer symptoms, possibly due to hypocalcemia, that have been reported in osteomalacia but not in hypoparathyroidism are impaired function of the posterolateral columns of the spinal cord in the absence of vitamin B_{12} deficiency[43] and cochlear deafness.[44]

1. Bone Pain and Tenderness[2,4,45-47]

Like bone pain in general, pain in osteomalacia is dull and poorly localized but clearly felt in the bones rather than in the joints. It is often persistent, made worse by weight-bearing and contraction of locally attached muscles, rarely relieved completely by rest but sometimes by the adoption of a particular posture. The pain is usually symmetrical, beginning in the low back, later spreading to the pelvis and hips, upper thighs, upper back, and ribs. It is never of sciatic radiation and in the absence of fracture is rarely felt below the knees. The distribution of tenderness to percussion is similar, but usually includes the shins. Lateral compression of the ribs and posterior compression of the sternum are useful maneuvers to elicit pain. The anatomic localization to the axial rather than the appendicular skeleton has been attributed to its higher proportion of cancellous bone,[2] which accumulates relatively more osteoid than cortical bone and probably undergoes deformation more easily.

Although pain conforming to this description in every particular is easily recognized, usually it is less characteristic and is an uncertain basis for differential diagnosis. Some patients carry for many years one or more diagnoses that cover a broad spectrum of rheumatologic and orthopedic practice. Often these diagnoses are erroneous, but the patients commonly have other reasons for pain that do not respond to treatment of osteomalacia. A significant minority of patients are completely free of pain, especially those with severe hypocalcemia.[48,49] Others suffer excruciating pain with the least movement or the slightest touch. In X-linked hypophosphatemia (XLH) there is usually no bone pain until middle age despite lifelong osteomalacia in the absence of treatment, possibly because the cortices are thicker, so that even softened cancellous bone is less subject to strain. Although the general characteristics of bone pain as a form of deep somatic pain can be accounted for by the type and distribution of nerve fibers in bone,[4] its specific characteristics in different clinical circumstances are unexplained.

2. Muscle Weakness

Muscles of the proximal limb girdles, especially the lower, are often weak in osteomalacia, the severity varying from a slight abnormality detectable only on careful examination to severe disability verging on complete paralysis. In the only quantitative study, in 12 vitamin D–depleted patients, the force exerted during maximum voluntary isometric contraction of the quadriceps ranged from 14% to 67% of normal, with a mean of 37%.[50] Atrophy is mild in relation to the severity of weakness, tone is reduced, and fasciculation is absent, but deep tendon reflexes are increased.[51] In mild cases, true weakness must be distinguished from unwillingness to tense muscles because of pain. Specific symptoms include difficulty in rising from a chair or walking up or down stairs without using the arms[37] and a characteristic gait, described later. Electromyography usually shows motor unit potentials that are of short duration and reduced amplitude and often polyphasic.[51,52] Muscle biopsy shows no unequivocal features of primary muscle disease but mean fiber cross-sectional area is reduced to about the same extent as muscle strength,[50] with preferential loss of type II fibers.[53,54] The syndrome is commonly referred to as a myopathy, but the site of the lesion is unknown. There is variable evidence of a neurogenic component to the weakness,[53] but this could result from associated deficiencies of nutrients other than vitamin D.[52]

The syndrome can occur in every form of osteomalacia except XLH, but is more common in vitamin D–related cases. Among these, the frequency is only 10% to 30% when the diagnosis is made early by biopsy, but approaches 100% in endemic nutritional osteomalacia.[52] In gastrointestinal disorders with a high frequency of neurologic abnormality, "myopathy" is found only in patients with vitamin D malabsorption and osteomalacia,[55,56] and further evidence for specificity is induction of the muscle histologic changes by experimental vitamin D deficiency in the rat.[54] The similarity in clinical and laboratory findings between patients with "myopathy" associated with hypophosphatemia of various causes but variable severity[51] suggests that a common mechanism is depletion of phosphate at some critical intracellular location; this could be the result of severe phosphate deficiency, a specific transport defect in muscle under genetic control, or lack of some direct action of one or more vitamin D metabolites on muscle.[57] In patients with vitamin D depletion, muscle cell ATP and phosphoryl creatinine are reduced but do not correlate with the degree of weakness,[50] and preliminary NMR studies in one patient with hypophosphatemic osteomalacia were inconclusive.[58] Experimental phosphate depletion reduces muscle cell ATP and actomyosin content in the rat,[59] but several other mechanisms are possible. Severe proximal "myopathy" in the aluminum-related osteomalacia that occurs during hemodialysis[60] may be an exception to this generalization, reflecting instead the neurotoxicity of aluminum.[61]

3. Difficulty in Walking

Abnormal gait can be the result of either pain or weakness, but usually both contribute. A change in gait discriminates more reliably between young adults with and without osteomalacia than any other symptom.[62] Many patients feel pain only when walking, which they consequently undertake sparingly and gingerly. Because of weakness the legs may feel heavy and the patient tires easily, walks more slowly with a flat-footed, springless gait, and is more likely to stumble.[1] If the hip muscles can no longer keep the pelvis horizontal with asymmetrical support, the upper body bends laterally away from the outwardly swinging trailing leg, keeping the center of gravity over the leading leg. The combination of trunk oscillation, short steps, and wide track constitutes the classic penguin or ducklike waddling gait of advanced osteomalacia,[1,2,41] which is still common where vitamin D deficiency is endemic,[52] but is otherwise rare. A waddling gait must be differentiated from a broad-based gait resulting from outward bowing of the femora in the absence of muscle weakness.

B. Histopathology of HVO

The diagnostic criteria have already been discussed, but some additional histologic features are important for understanding the structural abnormalities in the skeleton and for the interpretation of noninvasive indices of bone remodeling.

Osteoid accumulation increases about 15-fold in both cancellous and cortical bone with a range of 5- to 30-fold, but the absolute increase in OV/BV is much greater in the former (10% to 60%) than in the latter (1% to 10%) because of the difference in their normal rate of turnover.[13,63] The corresponding decreases in mineralized bone volume are also much greater in cancellous bone, with values similar to those of patients with osteoporotic vertebral compression fractures.[12] Total cancellous bone volume, including osteoid, is usually normal or increased in extrinsic vitamin D deficiency but often reduced in intrinsic deficiency to levels intermediate between normality and established vertebral osteoporosis.[31] Because of increased bone turnover in HVOi, cortical bone porosity is increased about 2-fold, with little further change in HVOii and iii. Osteoid accumulation and porosity are reversible, but as a result of prolonged secondary hyperparathyroidism there is thinning of cortical bone due to increased net endocortical resorption that is irreversible and that forms the largest component of the total body bone mineral deficit.[14,63] With the increase in cancellous tissue space at the expense of the inner third of the cortex, the absolute amount of total cancellous bone may be normal even though its relative amount (analogous to concentration) is reduced.[63]

There are also qualitative changes in the bone. If completion of secondary mineralization is delayed, scattered areas of bone of subnormal mineral density may be revealed by quantitative microradiography[64] or by permeability to basic fuchsin.[17] Because of its high water content, such bone is more accessible than normal bone to exchange of mineral ions with the extracellular fluid. Low-density bone is seen especially around osteocyte lacunae,[65] which may also be lined by thin osteoid-like seams.[66] The asymmetrical perilacunar abnormality observed in XLH appears to be specific for that condition.[67] As well as being wider, tetracycline fluorescent bands are frequently blurred and indistinct.[3,36] The second label may still be visible at the zone of demarcation, even when mineralization is completely arrested, either because outward diffusion is retarded by thicker osteoid seams or because of binding to some constituent of the cement surface.[17] Woven osteoid, as in fracture callus, may mineralize even when adjacent lamellar osteoid does not.[68] Finally, scattered small foci of particulate mineral may be seen within the osteoid in toluidine blue-stained sections[3,69] and by electron microscopy.[70]

The interpretation of osteoclast indices, whether expressed as number of cells or nuclei or as extent of surface in contact with osteoclasts, rests on the observation that osteoclasts normally resorb only mineralized bone and avoid osteoid,[17,71] probably because their mechanism of attachment to the bone surface is impaired.[72] In HVOi the surface extent of osteoclasts is increased, whether related to the bone surface or the mineralized surface. As osteoid increases in extent, the osteoclast surface per unit of mineralized surface increases substantially, but in advanced osteomalacia the osteoclast surface per unit of bone surface may remain unchanged. For example, if the osteoid surface is 95% of bone surface and mineralized surface 5%, an osteoclast surface of 1% of bone surface is within the normal reference range for postmenopausal females but represents 20% of the mineralized surface. With the combination of reduced surface available for normal resorption and severe hyperparathyroidism, osteoclasts in typical Howship's lacunae are observed on osteoid, which appears to be undergoing resorption that is morphologically indistinguishable from the resorption of mineralized bone. Although the relative extent is small, osteoid resorption can account for more than half of the total osteoclast surface.[71] For a full description of bone remodeling in osteomalacia it is necessary to consider the formation, resorption, and balance of unmineralized bone and mineralized bone separately.

In a few patients with severe osteomalacia there are the typical findings of osteitis fibrosa—dissecting or tunneling intratrabecular resorption, giant subendocortical resorption cavities, increased fibrous tissue deposition adjacent to the cancellous and endocortical surfaces, within resorption cavities and within the marrow spaces, and formation of woven bone[4,73] (Chapter 10). In contrast to the osteitis fibrosa of hyperparathyroidism alone without a significant mineralization defect, in osteomalacia the osteoblasts cover a smaller than normal fraction of the osteoid surface[69,74] and when mineralization ceases altogether, the osteoid eventually becomes covered entirely by flat lining cells.[36] In vitamin D–related osteomalacia, the morphologic effects of hyperparathyroidism become more evident as mineralization becomes more defective, in contrast to the inverse relationship observed in the aluminum-related osteomalacia of hemodialysis[75,76] (Chapter 13). Osteoclast indices are also less increased in non–vitamin D–related hypophosphatemic osteomalacia, osteitis fibrosa is rare, and osteoid resorption does not occur.

C. Skeletal Radiology of HVO

Structural changes in bone detectable on x-ray examination result either from increased PTH secretion or from impaired mineralization. Secondary hyperparathyroidism accelerates net loss of bone from endocortical surfaces, leading to generalized thinning of cortical bone detected either by radiogrammetry or radial photon absorptiometry[14,63,77,78] (Chapter 9). If the loss is rapid, the endocortical surfaces may appear more irregularly scalloped than usual.[4,77] Increased bone turnover increases cortical porosity, recognizable as cortical striation in the metacarpals and phalanges on high-resolution films of the hands.[79] For a particular level of increase in turnover, the extent of cortical striation remains stable, but if mineralization becomes defective with the transition from HVOi to HVOii, cortical striations accumulate because refilling of resorption tunnels by osteoid does not alter their radiographic appearance[80,81]; by contrast, cortical thinning is probably retarded by osteoid insulation of the endocortical surface. Phalangeal subperiosteal erosion, the most specific sign of hyperparathyroidism, is not as common as in renal osteodystrophy[77,82] but in the absence of Looser zones (see later) may be the most tangible radiographic evidence of osteomalacia, since it is not seen in the usually less severe hyperparathyroidism of HVOi. Very rarely, patients with long-standing intestinal malabsorption develop generalized osteitis fibrosa cystica.[83,85] In no case has adequate bone histology been performed, so these patients could have undergone progression of HVOi without transition to osteomalacia, as occurs in renal osteodystrophy (Chapter 13).

The most common radiographic manifestation of impaired mineralization in cancellous bone is a nonspecific reduction in density,[4,9,82] usually referred to in the older literature as "demineralization" and in current literature as "osteopenia." Distinctive qualitative abnormalities in trabecular pattern occur only when severe osteomalacia began in childhood, as in celiac disease,[38,86,87] or in endemic vitamin D deficiency.[6,41] Many trabeculae were never formed and those present are more widely and irregularly spaced, and may become thicker and more clearly visible despite their lower mineral concentration. Horizontal lines of increased density in the metaphyses (Harris lines) resulting from resumption of growth after temporary arrest are also frequently seen in such patients.[38] Minor degrees of coarsening, blurring, and loss of detail have often been described but have not been validated by adequate bone histology and are of questionable value in differential diagnosis.[4] In most patients the appearances are indistinguishable from those of moderately severe age-related bone loss.

Of greater specificity are changes in bone shape. Minor degrees of protrusio acetabuli, detected by measuring the relationship between the acetabular and ilio-ischial lines, are much more common in osteomalacia than in osteoporosis[88] (see Chapter 12). More familiar, although rare in current practice, are changes in the spine, with biconcavity that is symmetrical about the horizontal axis of each vertebra and of similar degree in adjacent vertebrae, contrasting with the irregular distribution of altered vertebral shape in osteoporosis[2,4] (see Chapter 12). If anterior vertebral height is preserved there is no deformity, but a regular kyphosis with moderate height loss may result from generalized anterior wedging. In some patients with associated osteitis fibrosa, the abnormal vertebral shape is accompanied by irregular end-plate sclerosis as in renal osteodystrophy,[77] but osteosclerosis commonly occurs in osteomalacia only in XLH.[4,89] Bizarre spinal deformities can be seen in advanced endemic osteomalacia,[6,41,42] but substantial loss of trunk height with generalized vertebral compression is otherwise rare except in sporadic nonfamilial hypophosphatemia of adult onset, which in contrast to XLH is associated with severe cancellous osteopenia.[89] Osteomalacia in general has been claimed both to increase the risk of the osteoporotic type of vertebral compression fracture[12] and to protect against such fractures;[2] this issue will be discussed in section II-D.

The best known radiographic feature of osteomalacia is the Looser zone, a lucent band adjacent to the periosteum that represents an unhealed insufficiency type stress fracture.[2,4,27,38,77,82,87,89a] Stress fractures are incomplete fissures without displacement that occur as a result of repeated nonviolent subthreshold trauma; they are commonly divided into fatigue fractures in normal bone subjected to abnormal stress and insufficiency fractures in abnormal bone subjected to normal stress.[4] Looser zones occur most commonly in ribs, pubic rami, and outer borders of scapulae and less commonly in femoral necks, metatarsals, and shafts of long bones.[1,2] At some sites of predilection, localization may be determined by the proximity to arterial pulsation.[90] Although occasionally painless, they are more commonly associated with local tenderness and pain on activity.

If the lesions are multiple, symmetrical, and perpendicular to the periosteum with parallel margins and, in the absence of treatment, persist without callus or adjacent sclerosis, the diagnosis of osteomalacia is certain,[27,77,87] but exact conformity to this complete description (to which the term Looser zone should perhaps be restricted) is observed in fewer than 5% of patients with osteomalacia in current practice. More commonly the appearances are intermediate in one or more respects between classic Looser zones and typical stress fractures[91] (Table 11–3). Such lesions can occur in the absence of osteomalacia and so lack diagnostic specificity[27,89a] (Fig. 11–11). Indeed, in our recent experience, atypical lucent stress fractures are more often the result of osteoporosis than of osteomalacia,[89a] although the relative frequency remains much lower in the more common condition. Looser zones, like other types of stress fracture, show increased focal uptake on bone scan, which can lead to a mistaken diagnosis of metastatic disease[92] and to a fruitless and sometimes fatal search for a primary tumor.[93]

D. Fractures

Several types of fracture occur in patients with osteomalacia. Looser zones, like other types of stress fracture, can extend to produce a complete fracture with separation or displacement. This is common in the metatarsals[90] and is probably also the mechanism for

Table 11–3. Comparison of Classic Looser Zones and Typical Stress Fractures

	Looser Zones	Stress Fractures
Direction	Perpendicular	Can be oblique
Lucent band	Present	Usually absent
Margins	Parallel	Can diverge
Adjacent bone	Normal	Can be abnormal[1]
Number	Multiple	Usually single
Symmetry	Present	Absent
Sclerosis	Absent	Present
Visible callus	Absent	Present
Healing	Slow or absent	Rapid

[1]For example, in Paget's disease.

Modified from Parfitt AM: Bone fragility in osteomalacia: Mechanisms and consequences. *In* Uhthoff H (ed): Current Concepts of Bone Fragility. New York, Springer-Verlag, 1986.

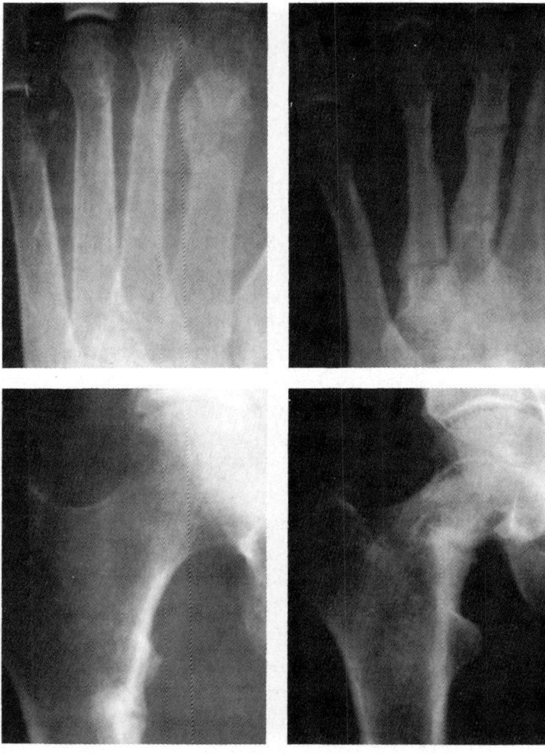

Figure 11–11. Atypical fractures in osteomalacia and osteoporosis. *Upper panel, left*: metatarsal fracture with central lucency and abundant callus formation in a patient with histologically verified osteomalacia; *right*: metatarsal fractures with more organized callus but persistent central lucency in a patient with histologically verified absence of osteomalacia. Resemblance to a classic Looser zone is somewhat greater in the latter case. *Lower panel, left*: incomplete fracture on medial aspect of upper femur in a patient with histologically verified osteomalacia; *right*: similar fracture in patient with histologically verified absence of osteomalacia. Although subtrochanteric location is more suggestive of osteomalacia, the other characteristics of the fractures do not differ significantly.

subtrochanteric fractures in the upper femoral shaft.[94] Multiple rib fractures in osteomalacia have caused death from hemothorax.[95] Occasionally a greenstick-type fracture can occur in severe osteomalacia, as in rickets.[96] When osteomalacia begins in childhood, the adult bones tend to be soft rather than brittle and fractures are rare.[6] Conversely, when osteomalacia begins in adult life, fractures are more common, occurring mainly in the extremities.[37,96] They differ from fractures in a normal skeleton only in needing a lesser degree of trauma, and from fractures in an osteoporotic skeleton only in a more varied anatomic distribution. An exception to this generalization is spontaneous fracture of the sternum, which is virtually confined to adult onset osteomalacia and myelomatosis (Fig. 11–12).

The major factor contributing to increased fracture risk is accelerated loss of cortical bone due to secondary hyperparathyroidism, so that repeated fractures are a common mode of presentation in HVOi.[14,16] The biomechanical significance of osteoid accumulation and cortical porosity is less clear. In an elderly population the ash content of a vertebral body is highly correlated with its compressive strength, which is equally reduced whether mineralized bone tissue is lost or replaced by unmineralized osteoid.[97] This effect is unlikely to be quantitatively important unless OV/BV exceeds 20%, but could increase vertebral fracture risk in those who have already lost cancellous bone.[12] Conversely, if bone matrix volume is normal, osteoid accumulation could decrease fracture risk by increasing elasticity.[1] Appendicular fractures are less common in HVOii and iii than in HVOi despite an equal or greater severity of cortical bone loss.[16] This is partly because activity is limited by pain and weakness—indeed, fracture risk increases when these symptoms are relieved by treatment. Another factor may be a shorter duration of greater risk because of more rapid progression and earlier diagnosis. The role of deficiency and altered metabolism of vitamin D in the pathogenesis of hip and vertebral fractures will be discussed in more detail in section V.

E. Noninvasive Indices of Bone Remodeling

A bone biopsy gives detailed information about cellular events in a small region but is

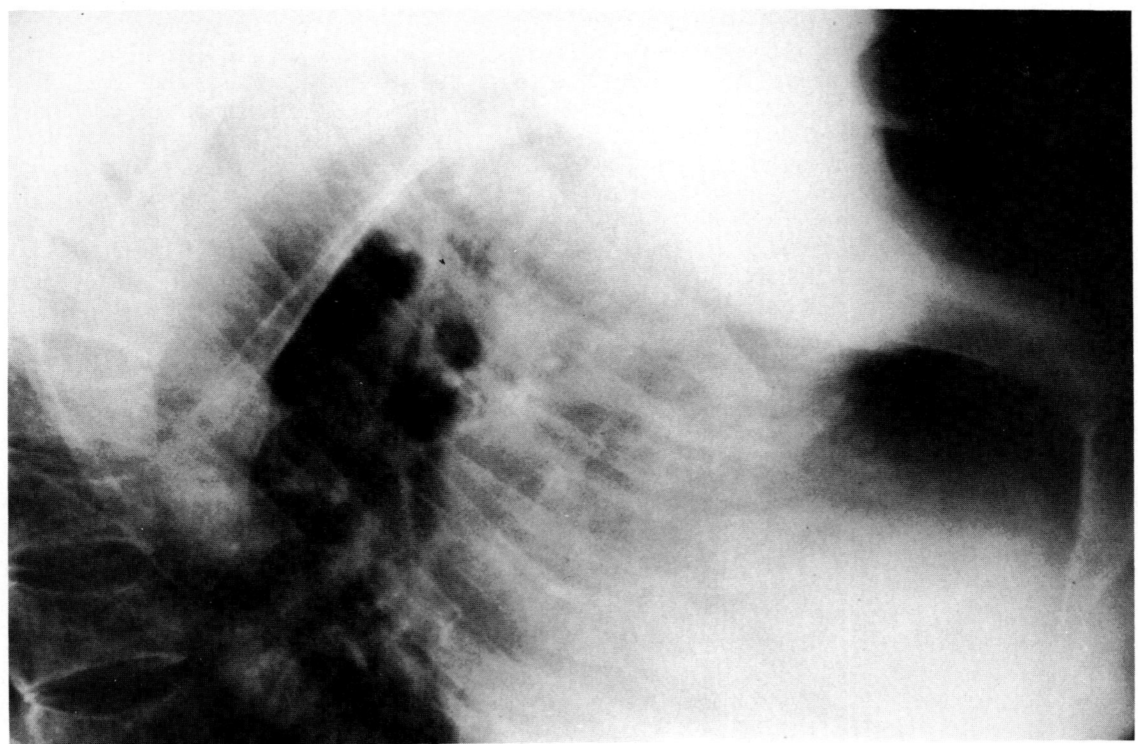

Figure 11–12. Combination of angulation of sternum due to spontaneous fracture and vertebral biconcavity in a patient with aluminum-related dialysis osteomalacia.

subject to appreciable sampling variation.[17] By contrast, radiokinetic and biochemical indices reflect the integrated activity of the entire skeleton (Chapter 8), but are governed mainly by the frequency of remodeling activation and give no information on individual cell function. In osteomalacia there are frequently increases in total urinary hydroxyproline, a marker of whole-body bone resorption,[98,99] and serum total alkaline phosphatase, a marker of whole-body bone formation.[1,2,37] In addition, radiocalcium kinetics often show an increase in accretion, an estimate of bone formation,[100,101] and there are also increases in skeletal uptake of various bone-seeking isotopes such as radiostrontium[102,103] and technetium-labeled diphosphonates[104-106] and in bone blood flow.[107] It is commonly inferred that bone turnover is high in osteomalacia,[37] but this interpretation is at variance with the histomorphometric evidence.

One explanation for the discrepancy is failure to differentiate between the different stages in the evolution of HVO. In HVOi, all methods of study are in agreement in showing increases in resorption, formation, and turnover, and it is likely that some patients included in previous reports did not have osteomalacia as rigorously defined, but rather preosteomalacia with the histologic, biochemical, and kinetic consequences of secondary hyperparathyroidism.[74] But other patients in the cited studies had undoubted osteomalacia despite lack of adequate histology. Another possibility is the local increase in cellular activity in relation to healing fractures, as mentioned in the previous section. There may also have been inadvertent inclusion of patients in the early stages of healing when histologically determined formation rates are very high, but this is unlikely in patients needing a pharmacologic rather than a physiologic dose of vitamin D. Furthermore, in patients studied by double tetracycline labeling, the level of serum alkaline phosphatase increases with the severity of the mineralization defect, and is highest when active mineralization has ceased[16] (Table 11–3).

Apparently increased kinetic accretion can probably be accounted for by the presence of significant amounts of bone of low mineral density and increased permeability, since this will enhance short- and medium-term exchange of radioactive calcium or strontium that may be impossible to differentiate from accretion without extended observation.[100] Increased uptake of labeled diphosphonate correlates with serum alkaline phosphatase but not with radiocalcium kinetics.[106] It has been proposed that the diphosphonate binds to some constituent of bone matrix and so is an index of osteoid accumulation with or without mineralization,[108] but in aluminum-related osteomalacia, diphosphonate uptake is low despite abundant osteoid.[109] Total hydroxyproline excretion is highest in patients with subperiosteal erosion,[98] and could reflect PTH-mediated resorption of unmineralized osteoid[71] even if the absolute level of resorption of mineralized bone was normal or even reduced. Utilization of newly synthesized collagen might be defective,[110,111] although the distribution of hydroxyproline-containing peptides between different chromatographic fractions is not altered.[98]

More difficult to explain is the increase in serum alkaline phosphatase. There is a high and significant correlation (r > 0.8) between log serum bone-specific alkaline phosphatase and log urinary hydroxyproline/creatinine in normal subjects and in several generalized disorders of bone. The regression slopes were similar, but in osteomalacia, alkaline phosphatase was higher relative to urinary hydroxyproline than in any other condition.[112] Alkaline phosphatase also correlates (r > 0.7) with radiostrontium uptake in osteomalacia due to vitamin D depletion[113] but not with bone blood flow.[107] Matrix apposition rate in osteomalacia is probably reduced, but total matrix synthesis could be increased, balancing the increase in unmineralized matrix resorption; this could account for the significant correlation between serum alkaline phosphatase and both osteoid surface and volume.[114] Inappropriate release of alkaline phosphatase might also reflect a disorder of osteoblast function induced by excess PTH, since aluminum-related osteomalacia in dialysis patients is usually accompanied by relatively low levels of both PTH and alkaline phosphatase.[60] Newer markers of osteoblast function, such as serum osteocalcin and procollagen type I carboxylterminal extension peptide (Chapter 8), have not yet been applied to the study of osteomalacia.

F. Abnormalities of Bone Mineral Metabolism in HVO

The cardinal metabolic abnormality is reduced net intestinal absorption of calcium[1,2,49] (Chapter 6). Fecal calcium excretion is close to and can even exceed dietary intake, but urinary calcium is low and calcium balance rarely more negative than −100 mg/day.[115] There is an equimolar deficit in net absorption of inorganic phosphate, but the relative change is much smaller.[1] According to the usual interpretation, calcium malabsorption leads in sequence to a fall in plasma calcium, secondary hyperparathyroidism, reduced renal tubular reabsorption of phosphate, hypophosphatemia, and reduction in calcium × phosphate product, which falls even further with the advent of more severe hypocalcemia. Eventually, deposition of mineral in osteoid is impaired because the supply of the relevant ions is reduced, and the alkaline phosphatase then rises. This traditional scheme requires considerable modification with regard to the order in which the changes occur, their pathophysiology, and their diagnostic significance.

In HVOi, the mean plasma calcium is slightly reduced, but the individual values are almost always normal (Table 11–4). There is

Table 11–4. Biochemical Evolution of HVO

	Normal	HVOi	HVOii	HVOiii
n	23	26	11	28
Age (years)	60.3 ± 1.3	57.2 ± 2.1	50.5 ± 6.3	58.1 ± 2.4
Plasma calcidiol (ng/ml)	23.7 ± 3.0	6.0 ± 0.5	6.8 ± 0.9([illegible]0)	4.1 ± 0.6(18)*
Plasma calcitriol (pg/ml)	40.8 ± 6.9	46.0 ± 4.7(11)	39.1 ± 3.7(8)	21.7 ± 3.2(10)†
Plasma calcium[1] (mg/dl)	9.64 ± 0.08	9.12 ± 0.11†	7.95 ± 0.39‡	8.02 ± 0.17
Plasma phosphate (mg/dl)	3.47 ± 0.08	3.36 ± 0.11	2.91 ± 0.23*	2.64 ± 0.13
Plasma Ca x P $(mg/dl)^2$	33.5 ± 0.7	30.7 ± 1.1*	23.3 ± 1.6	21.2 ± 1.2
Alkaline phosphatase (IU)	82.8 ± 3.9	132 ± 7.2‡	201 ± 31.[illegible]	284 ± 24.2*
NcAMP (nM/dlGF)	2.04 ± 0.26	4.01 ± 0.34‡	6.62 ± 0.79†	5.94 ± 0.61

Stages defined as in Table 11–1. Number of analyses shown in parentheses when less than number of subjects. Data shown as mean ± SE. Significance levels shown for difference in mean values from column immediately to the left. *$p < 0.05$, †$p < 0.01$, ‡ $p < 0.001$.

[1]Corrected for albumin.

no adult counterpart to the early hypocalcemia of infantile nutritional rickets,[116] which reflects difficulty in releasing calcium from the rapidly growing skeleton, and is only rarely observed in older children.[117] PTH secretion is increased as shown both by radioimmunoassay[118,119] and by excretion of nephrogenous cyclic AMP[16] (Table 11–4). Although mean TmP/GFR and plasma hosphate are both slightly reduced (see Chapter 7) individual values are usually normal. Twenty-four hour urinary calcium excretion and fasting urinary calcium/creatinine are often but not invariably reduced.[118] As already mentioned (section II-E), a moderate elevation of alkaline phosphatase is the most consistent abnormality, but can be absent in subjects without osteopenia.[119] Unlike the various types of osteomalacia with hypophosphatemia due to non–PTH-dependent defects in tubular phosphate reabsorption (referred to for convenience as primary), Albright and Reifenstein's first stage of "chemical osteomalacia with normal phosphatase"[120] does not occur during the evolution of HVO.

The vitamin D metabolite levels depend on the etiologic factor. In extrinsic vitamin D depletion, the plasma calcidiol level at which abnormal mineral metabolism can first be detected in an individual is usually below 5 ng/ml,[118,119] but in subjects with values between 5 and 10 ng/ml there is a slight but statistically significant depression of mean plasma calcium and phosphate and urinary calcium and elevation of iPTH,[118] and most patients with histologically verified HVOi have calcidiol values in this range[16] (Table 11–4). In patients with intrinsic vitamin D depletion, the complete biochemical, histologic, and bone densitometric syndrome of "HVOi" can occur at plasma calcidiol levels between 10 and 20 ng/ml,[16] presumably because there is an independent mechanism for calcium malabsorption and consequent secondary hyperparathyroidism that is unrelated to vitamin D. Increased PTH secretion accounts for normal or even increased levels of plasma calcitriol, as can also occur in anticonvulsant-treated patients,[121] but normal calcitriol levels in patients with extrinsic deficiency[118] are more puzzling. In such patients the malabsorption of calcium that is thought to be the initial event is without obvious explanation, a paradox that will be discussed later in relation to pathogenesis.

With progression to HVO stages ii and iii, in general all the biochemical abnormalities become more severe. Plasma and urinary calcium, TmP/GFR, and plasma phosphate levels become lower, and PTH, NcAMP, and alkaline phosphatase levels higher[16] (Table 11–4), but there are many individual exceptions. PTH hypersecretion and parathyroid gland hyperplasia occur in response not only to hypocalcemia but to the independent stimulus of calcitriol deficiency.[122,123] Patients with severe hyperparathyroidism may get impaired tubular reabsorption of bicarbonate and amino acids as well as phosphate, resembling proximal renal tubular acidosis or the Fanconi syndrome,[124] except for increased rather than decreased tubular reabsorption of calcium. Hypophosphatemia is adequately explained by increased PTH secretion without the need to postulate an additional effect of vitamin D metabolite deficiency.[57,125] Indeed, for the same increase in NcAMP, TmP/GFR is higher in secondary than in primary hyperparathyroidism because of the independent effect of plasma calcium on phosphate reabsorption.[48] Hypophosphatemia is of significantly lesser degree in HVO than in primary impairment of phosphate reabsorption, for both mean values and the frequency of individual low values.[1,47,126] Separation between the two groups is even clearer when the inverse relationship between TmP/GFR and NcAMP is considered.[48,57] Conversely, both individual and mean values for plasma calcium are almost always normal in patients with primary hypophosphatemia. The mean calcidiol level is significantly lower in HVOii than in HVOi, but does not fall further in HVOiii (Table 11–4). By contrast, the calcitriol levels can be normal in stage ii and do not become consistently subnormal until stage iii. Others have also found some normal but a majority of subnormal calcitriol levels in osteomalacia, although not classifying their cases in the same manner.[114,118]

In either HVOii or iii, a minority of patients present with hypocalcemic tetany, often with absence of bone pain and radiographically less severe bone disease.[48,49,113,127-130] Whether this is a pathogenetically distinct syndrome or simply one end of a spectrum is unclear, although probit analysis of plasma calcium values indicates two populations.[1] Because of lesser depression of phosphate reabsorption, higher than expected plasma phosphate, lower alkaline phosphatase, and lower incidence of phalangeal subperiosteal resorption, absence of the expected increase in PTH secretion was postulated.[113,120,127,129] This has been refuted, although PTH assays (greater increase in normocalcemic patients[130]) and NcAMP excretion (greater increase in hypocalcemic patients[48]) have given different results. Patients with severe hypocalcemia are resistant to the effects of PTH, both on calcium release from bone and on tubular phosphate reabsorption,[48,128-131] but maintain a normal cyclic AMP response to endogenous and sometimes exogenous PTH.[48,132] The biochemical resemblance to pseudohypoparathyroidism type II[48] (Chapter 14) is even closer in patients with absolute rather than relative hyperphosphatemia,[130-133] especially if the cyclic AMP response to exogenous PTH is impaired,[132,133] as may result from increased receptor occupancy.[134]

The syndrome has been attributed to magnesium depletion,[135] but this is only very rarely the explanation.[48] Although hypophosphatemia is not invariably absent, the effect of PTH on phosphate reabsorption is blunted by hypocalcemia and is restored by treatment that raises the plasma calcium.[48,129] The role of a relative failure to increase tubular reabsorption of calcium in response to PTH[136] is difficult to assess. In vitamin D–deficient monkeys, the syndrome can be reproduced by reducing dietary calcium intake to about 5% of normal,[137] but in osteomalacic patients no such clear relationship to dietary calcium intake is evident.[49] Neither insulation of bone surfaces by osteoid nor defective osteoclastic bone resorption accounts for severe hypocalcemia since no histologic difference was found between osteomalacic patients with low or with normal plasma calcium levels,[48] and some patients with the syndrome have radiographic as well as histologic evidence of osteitis fibrosa.[130,131] Furthermore, PTH-mediated resorption of cultured bone is unaffected by vitamin D deficiency.[138] There appears rather to be a failure of the calcium homeostatic system in bone, a system based not on osteoclastic bone resorption but on equilibration at quiescent bone surfaces.[28] The failure is unexplained, but the same mechanism operating with varying severity is probably the most important factor in all degrees of hypocalcemia in HVO.[1,57]

The rarest and least well understood biochemical abnormality in HVO is hypercalcemia.[130,139-141] Affected patients almost always have high PTH levels and osteitis fibrosa, and in an individual case it may be impossible to rule out coincidental primary hyperparathyroidism,[139] in which vitamin D deficiency reduces the plasma and urinary calcium levels, although frequently not to normal.[118] But it is well established that in chronic renal failure, hyperplastic glands may enlarge beyond the point needed to restore normocalcemia,[142] (Chapter 13) and there is much evidence that the same can occur in long-standing vitamin D deficiency;[130] in neither case is it known why cell proliferation (but not hormone secretion) becomes autonomous.[142] In such patients with hypercalcemia, the parathyroid secretory response to manipulation of the plasma calcium level resembles that of normocalcemic secondary rather than primary hyperparathyroidism,[130] as these terms have been defined elsewhere.[142] Even the finding of a single adenoma rather than generalized hyperplasia[139,141] does not establish that the hypercalcemia was independent of the vitamin D deficiency.[142] Rapid proliferation of a focus of cells abnormally responsive to mitotic stimulation could satisfy the increased demand for PTH, leading ultimately to a single adenoma without obvious hyperplasia of the other glands.[141] Alternatively, a diffuse increase in the rate of mitosis would make more likely a random mutation leading to adenoma formation.[143] It is to these cases, combining both primary and secondary factors in causation, that the term "tertiary hyperparathyroidism" should be restricted.[142] In hypercalcemic secondary hyperparathyroidism, as in primary hyperparathyroidism, vitamin D depletion may be intensified by increased hepatic catabolism of calcidiol[5a,143a] and also may mask the hypercalcemia, which becomes evident only after vitamin D administration.[144]

G. Summary of Temporal Evolution of HVO

In HVOi or preosteomalacia, there are characteristically no symptoms until a fracture occurs, which is one reason the existence of this intermediary stage was unrecognized for so long. The only biochemical abnormality that would be revealed by routine screening is a raised plasma alkaline phosphatase. Both fasting and 24-hour urinary calcium excretion are usually reduced. Skeletal radiographs are either normal or show only nonspecific osteopenia, but age-related loss of bone is accelerated, especially appendicular cortical bone but also axial trabecular bone, with a corresponding increase in fracture risk. Plasma calcidiol is usually, but not invariably low. There is both biochemical and histologic evidence of secondary hyperparathyroidism and of increased bone remodeling. Defective mineralization is either absent or no more severe than in primary hyperparathyroidism. Despite the lack of symptoms, treatment with some form of vitamin D is necessary to reduce PTH secretion to normal and prevent further irreversible bone loss. Whether some patients remain arrested at this stage or whether all eventually develop the complete clinical, biochemical, radiographic, and histologic syndrome of osteomalacia is unknown, but it may reasonably be assumed that all patients in stages ii or iii at the time of diagnosis traveled earlier through stage i.

H. Diagnostic Considerations

As in all fields of medicine, the most important step in diagnosis is to keep the condition in mind in the appropriate clinical settings, which will be described in section IV. In each setting the diagnostic value of a measurement must be independently validated and cannot be inferred from its importance in pathophysiology. But some aspects of diagnosis are logically considered here, because the existence of HVOi or preosteomalacia has an important bearing on the diagnostic process. Although crucial to understanding the disease, distinction between the different stages in the evolution of HVO is not essential for diagnosis, since it should not usually influence the decision to treat an individual patient with vitamin D. Consequently, the aim of diagnosis should be to identify HVO as early as possible in its evolution. Unfortunately, some diagnostic algorithms[62,126,145,146] have been based on the erroneous assumption that only osteomalacia, defined rather strictly, needs treatment and hence recognition.

The aim of preventing both occult bone loss and overt disease is best served by applying tests of high sensitivity (the probability of an abnormal result in a patient with disease) to the screening of populations at increased risk,[27,146] even if such tests are of low specificity (the probability of a normal result in a patient without disease). Most radioimmunoassays for PTH have been optimized for the diagnosis of primary rather than secondary hyperparathyroidism and frequently fail to detect a modest increase in individual PTH secretion (Chapter 14), but the immunoradiometric assay for intact PTH[146a] should be more useful. Other good screening tests are the plasma levels of total alkaline phosphatase and of calcidiol. For many tests, but especially alkaline phosphatase (and also urinary calcium), sensitivity is reduced by a large coefficient of variation, so that a biologically significant change could have occurred in an individual even though the result is still within the wide reference range. Sensitivity for alkaline phosphatase can be improved by more careful attention to sex and age differences, and both sensitivity and specificity can be improved by measurement of the bone-specific component (Chapter 8). A low plasma calcidiol level is a poor predictor of bone histology,[118,147-150] just as a low vitamin B_{12} level is a poor predictor of bone marrow histology. Nevertheless, it is the best available index of suboptimal vitamin D nutriture and consequent increased risk of HVO.

For the diagnosis of established osteomalacia without resort to an invasive procedure, test specificity is more important than sensitivity.[27] From this standpoint no test is very efficient when considered alone, especially in the very old in whom other causes for abnormal results are more prevalent.[151] Nevertheless, if the plasma calcium and phosphate levels (or calcium × phosphate product) are low and the alkaline phosphatase is high, osteomalacia is likely,[146] and if all three values are normal it is unlikely.[151] Between these extremes, the diagnostic value can be improved by various discriminant functions based on biochemical values alone[126,145] or combined with clinical and radiographic features.[146] But the validity of any particular discriminant function depends on the prevalence in a specific community and will not be the same in a young adult with suspected migrant osteomalacia, a nursing home resident with a hip fracture, or a patient with some form of intestinal malabsorption.

III. ETIOLOGIC CLASSIFICATION AND PATHOGENESIS OF OSTEOMALACIA

Osteomalacia can occur in diverse clinical settings, but in most types there is either a primary disorder of vitamin D metabolism or a primary (non–PTH-dependent) defect in the renal tubular reabsorption of phosphate.[2,9,57] In the former, hypocalcemia and secondary hyperparathyroidism are usual and hypophosphatemia is mild, whereas in the latter normocalcemia is the rule, secondary hyperparathyroidism is slight or absent, but hypophosphatemia is more severe (Table 11–5). In some forms of primary hypophosphatemia there are separate but interrelated disorders of both vitamin D and phosphate metabolism. Less common etiologic categories are the presence of a mineralization inhibitor, a primary abnormality of bone matrix, or a defect in alkaline phosphatase.[9]

A. Overview of Defects in Vitamin D Metabolism

Vitamin D metabolism can be affected at one of six levels (Table 11–6) (Chapter 5). Identification of the level is important in planning treatment, although the summation of independent factors at several levels may be needed to produce clinical effects, and some diseases affect more than one level. Each level is associated with a characteristic profile of vitamin D metabolite concentrations in blood (Table 11–6), but these must be interpreted with caution since changes in vitamin D–binding protein (DBP) can alter total concentrations without altering free concentrations.[152,153] Body stores of vitamin D, located mainly in fat and muscle, are derived either from the photochemical production in skin of cholecalciferol or from dietary intake and intestinal absorption of either chole- or ergocalciferol.[5,57,154] Although the former is more physiologic,[155] with current lifestyles the latter is equally important.[156] The distinction was made earlier between extrinsic vitamin D depletion, due to some combination of reduced skin synthesis and reduced intake, and intrinsic depletion, due to intestinal malabsorption of vitamin D, often augmented by some additional mechanism for increased fecal loss of vitamin D.[151a,157,158] One possibility is interruption of an enterohepatic circulation; this term refers to the excretion in bile of one or more metabolites of vitamin D with potential biological activity, which are reabsorbed at a more distal site in the intestine,[159] but the existence of such a conservative enterohepatic circulation has been denied.[160] Another possibility is increased hepatic catabolism of calcidiol to inactive metabolites as a result of increased PTH and/or calcitriol levels.[5a,151a]

The first step in vitamin D metabolism is hepatic 25-hydroxylation of calciferol to calcidiol, the principal transport form of vitamin D and an additional component of body stores, located mainly in muscle.[5,154] This process is impaired in cirrhosis of the liver,[161] but rarely to a level that causes osteomalacia (unless there is also malabsorption, as in biliary cirrhosis) because the liver has such a large reserve capacity.[154] Significant calcidiol deficiency that is not due to depletion of its precursor is most commonly the result of increased catabolism to biologically inactive metabolites from drug-induced enzyme induction,[162] or from stimulation of existing enzymes by calcitriol or PTH.[5a,151a] The possibility of increased fecal excretion of calcidiol was mentioned earlier. Loss of calcidiol

Table 11–5. Contrasting Features of Two Main Etiologic Categories of Osteomalacia

	Primary Disorder	
	Vitamin D	*Phosphate*
Plasma calcium	N or ↓	N
Plasma phosphate	N or ↓[1]	↓↓
PTH secretion	↑ or ↑↑	N or ↑
Alkaline phophatase	↑↑	↑
Osteoclast surface[2]	↑↑	↑
Osteitis fibrosa	Frequent	Rare
Cortical thickness	↓↓	↓
Cancellous volume	N or ↓	↑ or ↓[3]

[1]Occasionally increased.
[2]Difference clearer if referent is bone surface rather than mineralized surface.
[3]Varies with type. N, normal. ↑, ↓ change mild or slight. ↑↑, ↓↓ change severe or marked.

Table 11–6. Possible Levels of Disturbances of Vitamin D Metabolism

	Plasma Metabolite Concentration		
Level	*Calciferol*[1]	*Calcidiol*	*Calcitriol*[2]
Extrinsic depletion	↓	↓	N or ↓
Intrinsic depletion	↓	↓	N or ↓
Impaired 25-hydroxylation	N	↓	N or ↓
Increased catabolism	(↓)	↓	N or ↓
Impaired 1-hydroxylation	N	N	↓
Receptor defect	N	N	↑

[1]Inferential, few measurements available.
[2]May be increased if there is a vitamin D–independent mechanism for reduced intestinal calcium absorption and secondary hyperparathyroidism, leading to increased catabolism of calcidiol. [5a,151a]

bound to protein (both DBP and albumin) occurs in the nephrotic syndrome and leads to secondary hyperparathyroidism and osteoid accumulation in the absence of impaired renal function.[163-165] A similar mechanism operates during CAPD (Chapter 13), and urinary loss of calcidiol is also increased in patients with biliary cirrhosis.[154]

Calcitriol deficiency with normal body stores of vitamin D is most commonly the result of chronic renal failure (Chapter 13), but can also be due to a genetic defect in renal 1-α-hydroxylation, referred to as hereditary hypocalcemia[166] or vitamin D dependency type I[167] (Chapter 24). Plasma calcitriol levels are reduced by magnesium depletion,[154,168] but osteomalacia as a consequence has not been demonstrated. Calcitriol synthesis is impaired by deficiency of PTH (Chapter 5), but it is doubtful whether this causes osteomalacia, possibly because bone turnover is so low.[118] In a case believed initially to exemplify this relationship,[169] the patient was subsequently found to have concurrent XLH.[170] However, there is one adequately documented case of osteomalacia due to pseudohypoparathyroidism with secondary hyperparathyroidism.[171] Very low plasma calcitriol levels are found during prolonged total parenteral nutrition, but have not been clearly related to the presence or type of metabolic bone disease.[172] Finally, calcitriol may be ineffective because of one of several kinds of defect in its receptors, referred to as vitamin D dependency type II[166,173] (Chapter 24). Defects in calcitriol synthesis or receptor binding will not be considered further as causes of osteomalacia in this chapter. The role of such defects in the pathogenesis of age-related bone loss and fractures is discussed briefly in section V and in more detail in Chapter 12.

B. Overview of Defects in Phosphate Metabolism

The plasma phosphate level is regulated mainly by the tubular reabsorption of phosphate, best expressed as the mean renal threshold or TmP/GFR (Chapter 7). Intestinal absorption is much more efficient for phosphate than for calcium, net intestinal phosphate absorption remaining positive even with severe intestinal mucosal disease or with a large reduction in dietary intake.[57] Only if net absorption falls below 50 mg/day and the tubular transport mechanism is operating on the splay portion of the curve between the appearance and mean thresholds[174] can there be a sustained fall in plasma phosphate level below 2.5 mg/100 ml. Consequently, whole-body phosphate depletion sufficient to cause osteomalacia occurs only when net intestinal phosphate absorption becomes negative as a result of prolonged ingestion of large doses of phosphate-binding aluminum salts used as antacids.[175]

With this exception, chronic hypophosphatemia causing osteomalacia is invariably the result of a low renal phosphate threshold. When not due to hyperparathyroidism, primary or secondary, reduced phosphate reabsorption can be either a solitary or principal defect, with or without glucosuria and/or glycinuria, or one component of the Fanconi syndrome[57] (Table 11–7). This term refers to a global disorder of proximal tubular function with glucosuria, generalized amino aciduria, and impaired reabsorption of bicarbonate, urate, and less commonly, potassium, calcium, and sodium. Either type can be hereditary, usually presenting in infancy or early childhood, or non-hereditary, occurring at any age but most commonly during adolescence or adulthood. This simple ap-

Table 11–7. Classification of Primary (non–PTH-dependent) Defects in Tubular Reabsorption of Phosphate Causing Osteomalacia

Type			Plasma Calcitriol
Phosphate alone ± glucose	Hereditary	Classic	Normal[1]
		Hypercalciuric	High
	Nonhereditary	Tumor-induced[2]	Low
		Idiopathic	Low[3]
Multiple (Fanconi syndrome)	Hereditary	Primary[4]	Low[3]
		Secondary[5]	Low[3]
	Nonhereditary	Internal[6]	Variable
		External[7]	Unknown
		Idiopathic	Low[3]

[1]Low relative to plasma phosphate.
[2]Probably includes fibrous dysplasia and neurofibromatosis.
[3]Data inconclusive.
[4]Reduced reabsorption is a direct consequence of the genetic defect.
[5]Reduced reabsorption is an indirect consequence of the genetic defect, via accumulation of a nephrotoxic agent such as cystine or galactose.
[6]Resulting from extrarenal disease, such as light-chain nephropathy.
[7]Resulting from the harmful effect of a drug or environmental toxin; except for cadmium, such agents usually do not cause osteomalacia.

proach to classification breaks down in some causes of the Fanconi syndrome, such as galactosemia or cystinosis, in which proximal tubule function is affected, not directly but as an indirect consequence of a nephrotoxic substance that accumulates in abnormal amounts because of a genetically determined enzyme defect that is unrelated to renal tubular transport. These complexities are pursued in greater detail in Chapter 24.

The classic form of hereditary hypophosphatemia is familial hypophosphatemic vitamin D refractory rickets (or osteomalacia), often referred to as X-linked hypophosphatemia (XLH) because of the most common mode of inheritance.[89] Plasma calcitriol levels in the untreated state are normal for the rate of growth, but are lower than expected for the degree of hypophosphatemia[176] (Table 11–7). In a clinically similar disorder, hereditary hypercalciuric hypophosphatemia, the expected increase in plasma calcitriol levels occurs, leading to increased intestinal absorption of calcium.[177] In nonhereditary hypophosphatemia, most commonly due to a mesenchymal tumor, both symptoms and bone disease are more severe and there is an absolute, not just a relative, deficiency of calcitriol.[178] There are numerous causes of the Fanconi syndrome, but most cases in adults leading to osteomalacia are either idiopathic or the result of light-chain nephropathy.[179] Limited data suggest that in the Fanconi syndrome, whether hereditary or acquired, the plasma calcitriol level is usually low, either relatively or absolutely.[57,180] Renal tubular acidosis can be either a component of the Fanconi syndrome or unaccompanied by other primary defects in tubular reabsorption.[57] In the latter condition, the frequency and severity of hypophosphatemia are slightly greater than in vitamin D depletion, but less than in other types of hypophosphatemic osteomalacia.[1] There is no evidence for either absolute or relative calcitriol deficiency,[181] and it is possible that metabolic acidosis impairs mineralization directly as well as by reducing phosphate reabsorption. Finally, severe hypophosphatemia probably accounts for the rare occurrence of osteomalacia in primary hyperparathyroidism without vitamin D deficiency,[182] and after renal transplantation.[183]

C. Pathogenesis of Defective Mineralization

Despite much progress (Chapter 2), we still lack a detailed understanding of how and why biologic mineralization normally occurs only in some types of connective tissue and under close temporal and spatial control. Consequently, the pathophysiology of osteomalacia at the physicochemical, molecular, and cellular levels can be discussed only in a provisional and somewhat speculative manner. But several important general principles are known with reasonable certainty.[3,74,174,184] First, calcium, phosphate, and carbonate ions must be supplied and hydrogen ions removed for mineralization to occur. Second, the thermodynamic activities of the relevant ions in the fluid phase at sites of mineralization are influenced by, but are not the same as, those in the systemic extracellular fluid. Third, concentration gradients between mineralizing and nonmineralizing sites can be maintained either by cells (osteoblasts in bone or chondroblasts in cartilage), by structures derived from the cells, such as matrix vesicles, or by the ion-binding properties of macromolecules synthesized by the cells. Fourth, the exact chemical composition and three-dimensional structure of connective tissue matrices are major determinants of where and when mineralization can occur. Finally, rickets and osteomalacia can, under some circumstances, vary independently in severity and in response to treatment,[185] indicating that there are differences as well as similarities between the mineralization of growth plate cartilage and bone.

The role of vitamin D in sustaining normal mineralization has given rise to two related controversies[186,187] (Chapter 5). First, is the action of vitamin D mediated solely by changes in the calcium and phosphate concentrations in ECF,[26,101,188] or does it influence mineralization more directly?[8,189,190] Second, is calcitriol the only metabolite of physiologic importance, other than as a precursor,[118,188,191] or must some other metabolite also be considered?[26,190,192,193] In both cases the contestants have often failed to recognize the difference between an essential function that confers an absolute requirement and a contributory function that confers only a relative requirement. All the morphologic effects of vitamin D deficiency can be completely corrected by giving enough calcium and phosphate intravenously both in humans[194] and in the rat.[195] Clearly, vitamin D is not essential for mineralization, but nevertheless could have a direct action on bone cells that contributes to the process in normal circumstances.[192] Similarly, calcitriol alone can completely prevent or correct all the effects of vitamin D deficiency both in humans[196-200] and in the rat,[201,202] claims to the contrary[125,193] reflecting the inability of intermittent oral administration to sustain an adequate blood level.[201] Clearly, other metabolites are not essential, but it remains possible that one or more contribute to the evolution and reversal of defective mineralization. Alternatively, locally produced as well as systemic calcitriol could be involved.

1. *Evidence for Direct as Well as Indirect Effects of Vitamin D*

A plasma total Ca × P product [in $(mg/100ml)^2$] of less than 30 is a useful guide to the presence of infantile nutritional rickets,[101] but in older children and adults there is rarely such a consistent relationship between the plasma composition and the state of mineralization.[1,2,8,9,189,203] There are significant correlations between plasma phosphate and adjusted apposition rate and between plasma calcium and mean osteoid thickness,[204] but their magnitude is too low for useful prediction in individual patients. Calculation of an ion product more clearly related to the physical chemistry of bone mineral may remove some discrepancies,[101] but many remain. A more serious flaw in this line of reasoning is that single measurements in the fasting state, as in normal clinical practice, do not adequately represent body fluid composition because of the substantial circadian variation.[205,206] Nevertheless, it seems unlikely that such variation could account for the absence of osteomalacia in some patients with a degree of persistent hypophosphatemia that in other patients would be regarded as a sufficient explanation for their osteomalacia.[204,207] Even in the rat, a species in which mineralization probably depends more closely on plasma composition than in humans, healing of rickets can be detected radiographically in response to vitamin D administration while the Ca × P product is still subnormal.[202]

The persistence in early osteomalacia of some doubly labeled surfaces with normal or only moderately reduced rates of mineral apposition (section I-G) indicates that mineralization can proceed at the beginning of the osteoid seam life span, although it ceases prematurely. Mineralizing and nonmineralizing osteoid seams are often close together, sometimes even in direct continuity, and are exposed to the same microcirculation, so that the difference between them cannot be explained in terms of chemical changes alone. But at doubly labeled seams a higher proportion of the surface is lined by osteoblasts,[34,208] suggesting that these cells, possibly in conjunction with the osteocytes derived from them lying within the osteoid,[69,209] are able to promote mineralization in the face of a moderate reduction in plasma ion product, but do so for a shorter period of time than normal in vitamin D depletion. When this function is lost, mineralization ceases even though matrix apposition continues slowly and the osteoid seam gets progressively thicker. In more severe osteomalacia, osteoblasts are fewer or absent altogether, mineralization never begins, and double labels are not found. A similar relationship is observed during treatment—the recovery of mineralization in response to calcitriol administration, indicated by double labeling, occurs preferentially at surfaces where new osteoblasts have appeared.[210,211]

The bone histologic data in patients with osteomalacia strongly suggest that deficiency of calcitriol (and possibly also of other metabolites) impairs some function of the osteoblast that favors mineralization. This proposal is consistent with the presence in osteoblasts of calcitriol receptors,[212] the autoradiographic localization of labeled calcitriol in osteoblast nuclei,[213] the stimulation by calcitriol of the *in vitro* production by osteoblasts of alkaline phosphatase[214] and osteocalcin,[215] the *in vivo* enhancement by calcitriol of mineral apposition rate in young mice,[216] and the morphologic changes induced by calcitriol in the cells lining quiescent bone surfaces[217] that are of osteoblast lineage.[17,22] It is also consistent with the abnormalities in collagen crosslinking and other changes in bone matrix maturation and composition that have been found in vitamin D deficiency,[27,186] although it is less clear that these are the result of a direct rather than an indirect effect of vitamin D on osteoblast function. The proposal is also not in conflict with the evidence that unphysiologically large doses of calcitriol given to growing rats inhibit several aspects of osteoblast function[218] and in some circumstances can impair mineralization and lead to osteoid accumulation,[219,220] accounting for the paradoxical osteomalacia of prolonged hypervitaminosis D.[220a]

The concept that mineralization normally depends both on the availability of substrate ions via the circulation and on the activity of osteoblasts, although by no means rigorously established, enables all the apparently conflicting data, laboratory and clinical, to be reconciled. Which of the many functions of the osteoblast could be involved in mineralization is unknown. In addition to those previously mentioned, it seems likely that calcitriol could stimulate the inward transport of calcium and/or phosphate ions through or between cells at sites of mineralization,[57,118] consistent with its known effects on the cells of the intestinal mucosa and possibly the renal tubule (Chapter 5). The concept has the additional merit of providing a basis for unifying the pathogenesis of all major forms of osteomalacia, since hereditary or acquired defects in phosphate transport across the renal tubular epithelium could plausibly be accompanied by similar defects in transport across the quasi-epithelium that covers all bone surfaces.[57]

2. *Evidence that the Effects of Vitamin D Are Not Mediated Solely by Circulating Calcitriol*

In patients with histologically verified osteomalacia or with radiographically unambiguous rickets, plasma calcitriol concentrations can be within the appropriate reference ranges[114,118,197,221-225] (Table 11–4). The levels are indeed inappropriately low for the degrees of PTH hypersecretion and hypophosphatemia,[223] as is indicated by the very high levels attained during the early stages of treatment with vitamin D,[199,200,225] but the lack of target cell responses to an amount of calcitriol that is normally adequate requires explanation. In adults with osteomalacia, both biochemical and histologic indices of vitamin D depletion appear to correlate better with either the sum of calcidiol (in ng/ml) and calcitriol (in pg/ml) concentrations, or with calcidiol alone, than with calcitriol alone.[16,226] This suggests that calcidiol, or some other metabolite for which calcidiol is a precursor, such as 24-hydroxycalcidiol, might function as an agonist for calcitriol. In infants with untreated rickets, the plasma Ca × P product correlated with the plasma concentration of calcitriol and not calcidiol, although a higher than normal calcitriol level was needed to maintain a normal product.[225] This suggests that some other metabolite functions in a permissive manner, so that a fall in its concentration below a critical level would increase the need for calcitriol, but without dose-related effects above the critical level.[26]

Higher than normal calcitriol levels could be needed to correct hypocalcemia and to restore normal mineralization when the calcitriol-responsive cells are separated from the mineralized bone by a much wider than normal layer of uncalcified osteoid, through which the mineral ions must travel. But no similar reason is evident for the failure of intestinal mucosal cells to accomplish normal calcium transport, at least in patients who do not have an independent cause for impaired calcium absorption, such as intestinal disease or anticonvulsant administration.[227] Theories that ascribe all manifestations of osteomalacia to deficiency of circulating calcitriol alone may be able to account for its *persistence*, but have much greater difficulty accounting for its *initiation*. At the onset of HVO, what sustains calcium malabsorption and a small but significant fall in plasma calcium when plasma calcitriol is maintained at a normal level by secondary hyperparathyroidism? A similar argument applies to the increased vitamin D requirement of primary hyperparathyroidism, due to accelerated calcidiol catabolism in the presence of increased plasma calcitriol levels.[143a,151a]

During the evolution of HVO there is an early fall in plasma concentrations of both calcidiol[16,47,114,118] and 24-hydroxycalcidiol.[193,225] Calcium absorption and retention in bone are increased in humans by pharmacologic doses of 24-hydroxycalcidiol,[192] but there is no evidence for such effects at physiologic blood levels. Calcidiol binds to intestinal receptors for calcitriol, but with approximately 500- to 1000-fold lower affinity (Chapter 5), although calcidiol is only 100 times less effective than calcitriol in promoting bone resorption *in vitro*.[228] Seemingly, these differences in activity could be offset by the much higher total plasma concentration of calcidiol (Chapter 5), but there is only a 10-fold difference in free concentrations, based on current estimates of the association constants for binding to the same circulating protein.[152] Consequently, a fall in plasma calcidiol level below normal could not significantly modify total receptor occupancy in the target cells that respond to circulating calcitriol, although some more complex effect on receptor function remains possible.[229]

A more promising approach to the clinical paradox is the possibility that one or more dihydroxylated metabolites are produced locally in target tissues as is strongly suggested by studies with isolated bone and intestinal cells[230,231] and by the *in vivo* intestinal response to a pharmacologic oral dose of calcidiol.[232] If bone cell and intestinal cell 1α-hydroxylases were less influenced by PTH and phosphate than is the renal 1α-hydroxylase, local production of calcitriol would be more substrate-dependent than circulating calcitriol and would be impaired by a fall in plasma calcidiol concentration below normal. Similar considerations would apply to local production of 24-hydroxycalcidiol, if this compound could be shown to have a physiologically important function. But it is more consistent with the evidence that only calcitriol is essential[191] to postulate that circulating calcitriol is most important for the regulation of calcium homeostasis, locally produced calcitriol is most important for the regulation of bone remodeling, and both are important for the regulation of calcium absorption.

IV. OSTEOMALACIA RESULTING FROM ABNORMAL VITAMIN D METABOLISM

A. Extrinsic Vitamin D Depletion

Synthesis of vitamin D in the skin is reduced by residence at latitudes distant from the equator, atmospheric pollution, and increased skin pigmentation.[5] But the most important determinants are the duration of direct exposure to sunlight and the type and extent of protective clothing, which reflect cultural and social influences[9,233] as well as individual choice. Seasonal fluctuation is important in the U.K.; vitamin D status in the winter is largely dependent on the extent of body stores accumulated during the previous summer and in many persons is only marginally adequate, with a high prevalence of subclinical deficiency.[5,234,235] The same probably holds in many northern European countries.[156] Any chronic disease that impairs independence and mobility will inevitably reduce sun exposure or eliminate it altogether.[236]

Foods naturally abundant in vitamin D, such as swordfish, are consumed rarely if at all by most persons, so that dietary intake of vitamin D depends mainly on regional and national policy concerning fortification of food, for example, milk in the U.S. and margarine in the U.K. Differences in dietary intake of vitamin D contributed more than differences in latitude to the variation in mean plasma calcidiol level between countries, although both effects were significant.[156] Loss of dietary vitamin D, especially the contribution from less exotic fish and from eggs, is most likely to be important in those with an aversion to fatty foods or in strict vegetarians.[237,238] Vitamin D in multiple nutritional supplements is an unreliable source because most of the other constituents promote its chemical decomposition.[239] The dietary requirement of vitamin D is increased in the elderly,[5] who are more likely to be housebound or confined to nursing homes and are subject to age-related declines in the efficiency of vitamin D absorption and in the ability of the kidney to make calcitriol.

If the total supply of vitamin D, dermal and alimentary, is borderline, the occurrence of osteomalacia (and also of rickets) will be determined by other factors. Osteomalacia can occur locally in pagetic lesions[240,241] because bone of high turnover either needs more vitamin D or permits the more rapid development of the histologic expression of impaired mineralization; the opposite probably applies to bone of low turnover.[118] Pregnancy depletes vitamin D stores because calcidiol is transferred preferentially to the fetus,[242] which produces biochemical deterioration[243] and can precipitate overt osteomalacia.[49,244] The sacrifice of maternal vitamin D stores ceases at parturition,[242] but the calcium drain of lactation further weakens the bones, particularly if the dietary intake of calcium is low.[49] Calcium deficiency alone does not cause osteomalacia in adults but can do so in growing children.[245] The risk of osteomalacia is probably greater in populations that use breads made from whole meal or high extraction flour as a staple source of calories.[246-248] Such breads are rich in phytate, which binds dietary calcium and reduces its absorption, but the high fiber content is probably more important. Wheat fiber increases fecal excretion of bile acids,[247] which could impair the absorption of vitamin D, and a high-fiber diet reduces the plasma half-life of labeled calcidiol, an effect most likely due to increased fecal loss.[249]

In current practice in the developed countries, osteomalacia due to extrinsic (or privational) vitamin D depletion occurs mainly in two groups of persons—in young adults who have migrated from India or Pakistan, directly or via East Africa, to the U.K. and other European countries,[37,47] and in the elderly of every country.[5] Migrant osteomalacia has received the most attention. Although the roles of genetic susceptibility, skin pigmentation, and type of cereal consumption have been debated for many years, it is now clear that the major risk factor for the migrant population as a whole is a drastic reduction in solar exposure together with persistence of a very low dietary vitamin D intake.[37,47,235,250,250a] Although earlier studies were inconclusive,[248] it now seems clear that a higher intake of chapatti and a low intake of meat are additional risk factors.[250a] In one northern U.K. city there was a substantial improvement in various indices of vitamin D nutriture in the children of migrants over a 10-year period, probably reflecting adaptation to a Western lifestyle, but no improvement in the adults,[251] a public health problem that is still unsolved.[248,252]

It is generally agreed that osteomalacia in old people is much more common in the U.K. than in the U.S., although prevalence in a random community sample has not been determined in any country.[252] Reasons for increasing susceptibility with age were given earlier; why women remain more at risk than men long after cessation of childbearing is unknown. In the U.K., mean plasma calcidiol falls almost linearly with age in women from 30 to 90 years,[37,226] subclinical vitamin D depletion is especially common in the elderly,[156,234,235] and is the most important reason for impaired calcium absorption,[253] but similar data are not available for men. According to reasonable histologic criteria, osteomalacia is found in about 4% of unselected geriatric admissions in the U.K., a proportion that has remained stable for almost 20 years.[254-256] The prevalence is higher in nursing home residents and higher still in hip fracture patients[5]; whether the latter represents an etiologic relationship will be discussed later. No similar studies have been carried out in the U.S., although there are strong reasons for believing that the prevalence there would be lower in each of the four populations mentioned, but with the same rank order.[5] Nevertheless, some healthy free-living persons in the U.S. have subclinical vitamin D depletion.[257] Contrary to earlier belief,[120] privational osteomalacia does occur, especially with multiple risk factors,[257a] and being less common is more likely to be overlooked than in the U.K.[258]

B. Intrinsic Vitamin D Depletion

Although much less prevalent worldwide than extrinsic vitamin D depletion, in the U.S. and other countries that practice fortification of dairy products with vitamin D, intrinsic depletion is the commonest cause of osteomalacia, with the exception of dialysis osteodystrophy. In countries where it is common, extrinsic vitamin D depletion is a major determinant of the effect of intestinal disease on the skeleton[259]; this interaction is less evident in the U.S., although in Rochester (Minnesota) plasma calcidiol concentration in patients with adult celiac disease was significantly correlated with the duration of sun exposure.[260] Diverse other factors can influence the expression of vitamin D depletion in patients with gastrointestinal and hepatobiliary disease. Some have calcium malabsorption and consequent secondary hyperparathyroidism for reasons other than, or in addition to, vitamin D depletion.[16] Protein deficiency is common and could affect bone in many different ways.[261] Finally, other nutrients not normally thought of in the context of metabolic bone disease may turn out to have important influences on the function of bone cells.[31] Probably for this reason nonosteomalacic osteopenia with low bone turnover is especially common in patients with intestinal malabsorption, whether or not they have vitamin D depletion and secondary hyperparathyroidism.

Vitamin D needs intraluminal bile salts for absorption by a mechanism similar to other lipid-soluble substances, and enters the circulation via chylomicra in mesenteric lymph[174,262] (Chapter 5). In patients with both intestinal malabsorption and vitamin D depletion, a causal relationship is commonly assumed but difficult to prove. It is necessary to measure fecal excretion of radioactively labeled vitamin D after oral administration, since the rise in plasma vitamin D reflects also the rates of tissue uptake for storage or metabolism.[263] Calcidiol absorption is less dependent on bile and occurs directly into the portal circulation.[232,264] The increase in plasma calcidiol or the peak level after an oral load[265] is even less specific than the rise in plasma vitamin D, correlating neither with measured absorption nor with the degree of steatorrhea.[266] But a low value, although mainly indicative of reduced body stores of vitamin D, sometimes provides more information than the basal plasma level alone[266,267] and so may help to establish the *existence* of vitamin D depletion, although not necessarily establishing the *mechanism*.

Absorption of vitamin D is generally more depressed than absorption of calcidiol, but even with gross steatorrhea rarely falls below 40% of intake,[263] a level that would not cause vitamin D depletion in an adult ingesting the U.S. RDA of 10 μg/day.[262] Extrinsic factors that need to be considered even in relatively sunny regions are self-imposed avoidance of fatty foods to reduce fecal bulk, and limited sun exposure because of chronic illness or concern with body image.[31] But in many gastrointestinal disorders, the frequency and severity of vitamin D depletion are difficult to explain by these factors alone. For example, osteomalacia can occur after intestinal bypass surgery despite prescription of 1.25 mg/day of vitamin D,[268] from which absorption of only 1% would prevent depletion. Biliary excretion of vitamin D metabolites is increased by calcium malabsorption and secondary hyperparathyroidism[5a,151a] and possibly also by interruption of the enterohepatic circulation of bile salts[160].

Several authors have indicated the frequency of different absorptive and digestive disorders as causes of osteomalacia[208,262,267] (Table 11–8). Such lists reflect variation in surgical practice and individual physician interest as well as geographic differences in disease prevalence, and serve only to demonstrate the range of possibilities rather than to reveal epidemiologic truth. An increase in

Table 11–8. Frequency of Different Types of Intestinal Malabsorption as Causes of Osteomalacia at Henry Ford Hospital, 1976–1985

Type of Malabsorption	n	(%)
Postgastrectomy	14	(39)
Adult celiac disease	8	(22)
Bypass surgery	7	(19)
Chronic pancreatitis	4	(11)
Other short bowel	2	(6)
Biliary cirrhosis	1	(3)
Total	36	(100)

alkaline phosphatase can result from hepatobiliary disease or reflect the intestinal isoenzyme even in the absence of bone disease (Chapter 8) and so may be less useful in studies of prevalence than in extrinsic vitamin D depletion. But despite these possible drawbacks, alkaline phosphatase is a useful predictor of HVO in adult celiac disease.[269] Not surprisingly, there is much more information on the frequency and severity of vitamin D depletion (indicated by low plasma calcidiol levels) and of abnormal bone mineral metabolism than of histologically verified HVO. Currently unexplained is the high frequency of osteomalacia in the absence of vitamin D depletion after biliopancreatic bypass for obesity.[270]

Evidence for another form of bone disease in addition to HVO comes from several sources. Vertebral deformity and fractures are more common in patients who have had gastrectomy than in control subjects,[271,272] and 5% of patients referred for evaluation of vertebral fracture gave a history of gastrectomy compared with only 1% in control subjects.[273] Significant cortical and/or trabecular osteopenia without osteoid accumulation and in the absence of other etiologic factors such as corticosteroid therapy has been found after intestinal bypass surgery for obesity[31,268] and small bowel resection for Crohn's disease,[274] in primary biliary cirrhosis,[275-277] and in long-standing ethanol abuse.[278] In all these disorders a common bone histomorphometric profile can be discerned with thinner but more extensive osteoid seams, a low adjusted apposition rate indicating reduced collagen synthesis by teams of osteoblasts, and a low bone formation rate indicating reduced remodeling activation. A very similar disorder is also found in beagles with intestinal malabsorption.[279]

The state of decreased bone remodeling at the time of biopsy was probably preceded in many patients by high bone turnover typical of HVOi. Many of the patients still have vitamin D depletion and/or secondary hyperparathyroidism, to which their bone is not responding in the usual manner. In the non-osteomalacic osteopenia following intestinal shunt surgery, mean interstitial bone thickness is reduced, indicating a cumulative increase in resorption cavity depth in the past, even though resorption indices are no longer increased by the time of biopsy.[31] Finally, a few patients show atypical osteomalacia as previously defined, with similar kinetic defects to low-turnover osteopenia but with increased surface and volume but not thickness of osteoid.[31] This most likely represents a transition from HVOi, in which the usual morphologic expression of osteomalacia is blunted by an unusually severe defect in bone matrix synthesis by osteoblasts[36,268]; the same defect developing earlier in the course of the disease and accompanied by depression rather than stimulation of remodeling activation could prevent any osteoid accumulation in the patients with nonosteomalacic osteopenia (Fig. 11–13). Since these defects are similar to those found in patients with postmenopausal osteoporosis,[15,32] it is likely that in patients who have undergone accelerated bone loss, whether from secondary

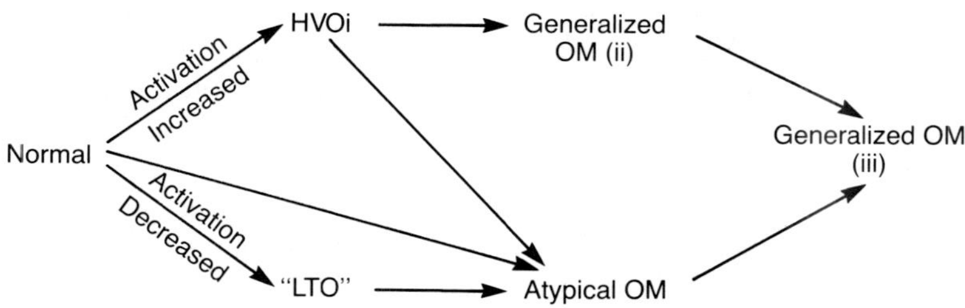

Figure 11–13. Possible deviations from normal development of HVO in intestinal bone disease. Transition from HVOi to atypical osteomalacia (OM) rather than to stage ii generalized OM reflects unusually severe depression of matrix synthesis, but if this continues very slowly, osteoid thickness will increase with eventual progression to stage iii generalized OM. If the initial increase in remodeling activation is blocked, the same defect in matrix synthesis with impaired mineralization will prolong FP and lead directly to atypical osteomalacia. If remodeling activation is depressed by some additional agent, there will be no osteoid accumulation, the disorder of cell function resembling low turnover osteoporosis ("LTO") but with normal instead of reduced osteoid seam thickness. If the mineralization defect persists, there will be gradual transition to atypical osteomalacia.

hyperparathyroidism or from menopausal estrogen deficiency, impaired recruitment and activity of osteoblasts limit bone repair and predispose to fracture.[31,32]

The previous discussion has emphasized the similarities between the various causes of intrinsic vitamin D deficiency, but there are also important differences. In postgastrectomy osteomalacia, extrinsic factors have been emphasized in the U.K.,[155,259,280] but hyperosteoidosis is common in countries where extrinsic vitamin D depletion is rare.[281,282] In most patients, steatorrhea is mild or absent and the mechanism of vitamin D depletion is unknown, although disruption of the normal digestive sequence could impair vitamin D absorption. In representative asymptomatic patients studied on average 9 years after operation, plasma calcidiol was reduced and calcitriol increased, but there was moderate impairment of calcium absorption and appendicular osteopenia.[283] In cystic fibrosis, mild vitamin D depletion and moderate osteopenia are common,[284,285] but rickets is very rare despite the severity of steatorrhea[286] and hyperosteoidosis has been verified histologically only in two adults, both with focal biliary cirrhosis and severe secondary hyperparathyroidism.[287,288] Osteomalacia is also rare in chronic pancreatitis and probably requires alcoholic liver disease as well as pancreatic enzyme deficiency.

Vitamin D depletion is common in Crohn's disease, but is severe enough to cause osteomalacia only in patients who have undergone small intestinal resection,[289,290] especially if treated with cholestyramine for bile acid–induced diarrhea.[291,292] After intestinal shunt surgery for obesity, serum calcidiol falls rapidly in the first 6 months and more slowly thereafter, and appendicular bone mass begins to fall after about 1 year despite little change in serum calcitriol.[293] Osteomalacia develops in about 12% of patients in Europe and in about 4% in the U.S., but for unknown reasons is less likely if hypomagnesemia is more severe.[31] The potential risk of osteomalacia is greatest in adult celiac disease[262,267,294-296] because the mucosal defect impairs absorption of vitamin D and calcium directly[103] and may also reduce local calcitriol synthesis.[232] In patients untreated for many years, osteomalacia develops in more than half, but can be forestalled by timely diagnosis.[296] Osteomalacia can occur even without steatorrhea and may be the presenting manifestation.[262,296] The distinctive features conferred by onset in childhood (even if subclinical) were emphasized previously.[38,83-87] Unlike postgastrectomy osteomalacia, there is no response to ultraviolet irradiation[297] or to moderate doses of vitamin D in the absence of a gluten-free diet.[298]

C. Impaired 25-Hydroxylation and Hepatobiliary Bone Disease

Despite the physiologic necessity of 25-hydroxylation, its impairment is of only minor importance in clinical medicine, unless the supply of vitamin D is low. If liver destruction is so extensive that too little calcidiol can be produced despite adequate substrate, the patient will usually die before developing HVO. Furthermore, no genetic defect in the 25-hydroxylase has yet been identified, except possibly in a single sporadic patient who also had target cell resistance to calcitriol.[299]

To understand what has been termed hepatic osteodystrophy,[300,300a] the separate effects of alcohol excess, loss of liver parenchyma, and cholestasis must be distinguished. Alcohol can cause osteopenia by a variety of adverse effects on bone mineral metabolism unrelated to vitamin D.[301,301a] Alcoholics are also especially prone to extrinsic vitamin D depletion,[302] which probably accounts for the coexistence of alcoholism and osteomalacia in a few patients with aseptic osteonecrosis.[303] Patients with cirrhosis of the liver, whether or not due to alcohol, often have mild steatorrhea[304] and impairment of vitamin D absorption.[305] Moderate reductions in plasma calcidiol in cirrhotic patients correlate with plasma albumin and other indices of liver function[306-308] probably because 25-hydroxylation is mildly impaired,[161,306,309] but plasma calcidiol can be raised above normal by oral vitamin D in the dose range 180 to 625 μg/day.[304] In hemochromatosis, venesection therapy increases plasma calcidiol, suggesting that iron accumulation can impair 25-hydroxylation independent of other effects on hepatocellular function.[310] In advanced cirrhosis, PTH secretion is slightly increased, but osteomalacia does not occur unless there is either cholestasis or extrinsic vitamin D depletion.[311]

In chronic cholestasis, whether in primary biliary cirrhosis or due to hepatitis or to extrahepatic biliary tract disease, intraluminal bile salt deficiency causes steatorrhea and impaired absorption of both vitamin D and calcidiol.[312-314] Also, some metabolite of vitamin D other than calcidiol is lost in the urine in proportion to the rise in serum bilirubin.[154,315] Consequently, plasma calcidiol levels are low and there is malabsorption of calcium that can be reversed by treatment with vitamin D or its metabolites,[316] but the frequency of osteomalacia due only to these abnormalities has been greatly exaggerated.[300a] Based on the kinetic criteria given earlier, or the osteoid measurements characteristic of these criteria, or on unequivocal clinical findings, the only acceptable published cases are four from the north of England, where extrinsic vitamin D depletion is common,[311,314] and three from London and one from the far north of Sweden,[317-320] of whom three were being treated for pruritus with cholestyramine, a drug that independently reduces vitamin D absorption.[321] In many other cases osteomalacia has been misdiagnosed because of one or more of the errors described in section I, failure to exclude HVOi,[322] or applying an unvalidated method to decalcified bone.[323,324] Data from the only definite case in the U.S. are shown in Figure 11–8.

By far the most important component of hepatic osteodystrophy is severe osteoporosis,[275,276,325] made worse in a few cases by corticosteroid therapy.[277] Bone pain and tenderness are frequently mentioned in clinical descriptions but they are the result of the multiple fractures to which these patients are especially prone, not of osteomalacia. Muscle weakness is also common, but can occur in primary biliary cirrhosis for several reasons unrelated to HVO. Even in asymptomatic patients there is significant vertebral osteopenia.[325] Two editorials mention increased bone turnover,[326,327] but careful attention to the actual data rather than to the authors' interpretations indicates that bone turnover is reduced, often markedly so, with low values for surface extent and volume of osteoid and extent and separation of tetracycline labeling.[275,276,325,328] The data indicate both depressed remodeling activation and impaired osteoblast function.[300a] Eroded surface without osteoclasts is increased,[329] but this reflects delayed formation rather than increased resorption. Furthermore, the indices of bone structure in transileal biopsies in primary biliary cirrhosis are very similar to those found in the nonosteomalacic osteopenia after intestinal shunt surgery, with cortical thinning and reduced thickness rather than density of trabecular plates.[328]

D. Increased Vitamin D Catabolism and Anticonvulsant Bone Disease

The metabolic pathways leading from calciferol to calcitriol have been extensively investigated, but are preferentially followed only when body stores are greatly depleted. Normally about 70% of the daily supply of both calciferol and calcidiol is converted to more polar metabolites of low or absent biological activity that undergo biliary and eventually fecal excretion, in part as glucuronide conjugates;[174] the proportions following these alternative pathways increase to 90% for calciferol and 99% for calcidiol in treated hypoparathyroidism.[330] Despite their quantitative importance in overall vitamin D economy, little is known about the metabolites formed, although by analogy with other steroid hormones, their production likely depends on hepatic microsomal mixed function oxidases.[331] These enzymes are inducible, with increased microsomal content of one of several types of cytochrome P-450, by a wide variety of drugs, including barbiturates, phenytoin and several other anticonvulsants, and the antituberculous drug rifampicin.[332] The degree of enzyme induction is roughly indicated by the increase in metabolic clearance of antipyrine or in urinary excretion of D-glucaric acid or 6 β hydroxycortisol, each marker showing a wide variation between different subjects taking the same drug, but correlating weakly with dose and blood level.[332]

Some patients on long-term anticonvulsant therapy develop a syndrome of low plasma calcidiol, intestinal malabsorption of calcium, slight fall in plasma calcium, secondary hyperparathyroidism, and cortical osteopenia.[162,333-338] Although commonly referred to as anticonvulsant osteomalacia, this term is misleading on several counts. Radiographic evidence of mild rickets has been found in 8% of children,[339] but systematic surveys of bone histology in adults have invariably failed to disclose osteomalacia,[340-343] except for a few doubtful cases in Scotland where privational vitamin D depletion is common.[344] With double tetracycline labeling, the bone formation rate is increased without defective mineralization,[341,343] and in this and every other respect the syndrome conforms exactly to the description of HVOi given earlier, with the exception of a higher incidence of acquired resistance to the phosphaturic effect of PTH[337,345] and disproportionate elevation of serum osteocalcin.[346] Osteomalacia, according to adequate clinical and radiographic and/or histologic criteria, has been found in a few cases, but is largely confined to patients with only marginally adequate vitamin D supply, prolonged treatment with multiple drugs, or other risk factors[347-356] (Fig. 11–8).

The term "anticonvulsant osteomalacia" is also misleading because the implication of uniform pathogenesis takes no account of significant differences between drugs.[357] Phenobarbital is a more potent enzyme inducer than phenytoin and has been convincingly shown to enhance the catabolism of calciferol and calcidiol in the liver[331,358,359] but does not usually by itself reduce plasma calcidiol levels[360] or cause rickets,[339] probably because the formation of calcidiol is increased as well as its destruction.[357,359,361] Phenytoin has not been shown to have any direct effect on vitamin D catabolism,[154,346] but is more commonly associated with abnormal bone mineral metabolism than phenobarbital because it can lead to hypocalcemia and secondary hyperparathyroidism by mechanisms unrelated to vitamin D,[337,343] such as impaired calcium release from bone and reduced calcium absorption.[227,335,346]

A further complexity is that in the only prospective study, the early effect of phenytoin in newly diagnosed epileptics was to increase plasma calcitriol at the expense of calcidiol, with a corresponding *increase* in calcium absorption but without change in parathyroid function,[362] consistent with the experimental demonstration of increased 1α-hydroxylase activity.[357,363] Multiple effects of phenytoin on vitamin D metabolism could account for differences in vitamin D metabolite profile[121,162,343,362,364,365] but make it more difficult to explain the production of osteomalacia, convincingly shown experimentally in the rat.[366] Paradoxically, the best evidence for the clinical importance of enzyme induction and enhanced vitamin D catabolism comes from studies not with anticonvulsants, but with rifampicin and isoniazid.[367,368]

Whatever the mechanism, anticonvulsant administration appears to increase vitamin D requirement by 10 to 15 μg/day in children[369,370] and possibly more in adults,[336,371] but whether this is clinically significant depends on the total dermal and dietary supply of vitamin D.[162,341,372] In otherwise healthy persons in sunny climates the effect is trivial,[373,374] although non–vitamin D–related effects of phenytoin may cause osteopenia.[343] By contrast, in mentally retarded institutional residents there is a substantial risk of clinically significant vitamin D depletion and its consequences.[371] At any level of supply, the amount by which requirement is increased depends on the dose and especially the number of drugs used, but also reflects individual susceptibility to enzyme induction. Consequently, both the frequency and the severity of the syndrome vary considerably between different populations. In some institutions, fractures due in part to anticonvulsant-induced osteopenia are a major health problem and overt rickets is common,[375-377] but in other institutions prolonged immobility appears a more important determinant of bone density than anticonvulsant therapy.[378]

As already emphasized, symptomatic bone disease is rare in noninstitutional settings, but the long-term effects of asymptomatic osteopenia are unknown. Although the clinical, biochemical, and histologic abnormalities respond well to treatment,[162,379] cortical bone loss is largely irreversible.[336] There is currently no consensus on whether all or only some anticonvulsant-treated patients should be given prophylactic vitamin D; if the latter, how they should be selected; and in either case whether ergo- or cholecalciferol is more effective.[336,338]

V. VITAMIN D AND AGE-RELATED OSTEOPOROSIS

Despite their obvious differences (Table 11–1), osteomalacia and osteoporosis have much in common. In both there is malabsorption of calcium, negative calcium balance, osteopenia, and increased fracture risk. In both, an initial state of high bone turnover, increased resorption, and accelerated bone loss is followed by a state of low bone turnover and impaired osteoblast function. These similarities suggest a possible role for vitamin D in the pathogenesis, differential diagnosis, and treatment of osteoporosis[380,381]; further information is given in Chapter 12.

A. Pathogenesis of Bone Loss and Fractures

In type I (postmenopausal) osteoporosis, low plasma calcitriol and impaired calcium absorption are secondary consequences of increased estrogen-dependent bone loss, and parathyroid function is normal or slightly depressed,[380-382] but in type II (senile) osteoporosis, a primary abnormality in vitamin D metabolism probably contributes to bone loss. Functioning renal tissue mass declines with age, and the aging kidney is less able to synthesize calcitriol in response to stimulation by PTH.[383] Because of this defect, augmented probably by other consequences of impaired renal function (Chapter 13) and possibly by an age-related decline in intestinal mucosal function,[384] PTH secretion increases with age to an extent that depends on the prevailing level of vitamin D nutriture.[253,385,386] Since all forms of secondary hyperparathyroidism that have been adequately studied accelerate the age-related loss of cortical and to a lesser extent trabecular bone,[14] it would be surprising if the same did not apply to the secondary hyperparathyroidism of aging.

In patients with vertebral compression fractures, HVOi is probably an important cause of high bone turnover, an abnormality that is common among such patients in France[12,387] where food is not fortified with vitamin D. In the U.S., high turnover is less common in compression fracture patients[11,15,32,388] except among those who have had a gastrectomy,[273] but even in the U.S. a few patients have clinically overt vitamin D depletion.[258] HVOi due to impaired 1α-hydroxylation probably accounts for the mild increase in OV/BV (3.5%–8%), reversible by administration of alfacalcidol, in patients with vertebral compression fractures, who because of their advanced age would be classified as type II rather than type I osteoporosis.[389] Muscle weakness and abnormal muscle histochemistry may also respond to alfacalcidol administration in these patients.[390]

As mentioned earlier, the prevalence of subclinical extrinsic vitamin D depletion, secondary hyperparathyroidism, and excess osteoid is frequently[5,391-393] but not invariably[5,393a] increased in patients with hip fracture. The available data are consistent with HVOi as an etiologic factor, but it remains possible that hypovitaminosis D is a nonspecific marker of ill health and inactivity, or that the muscle weakness of vitamin D deficiency increases the liability to fall. The former but not the latter possibility is consistent with the failure, in a controlled trial, of vitamin D supplements to increase the ability of elderly hospitalized patients with low plasma calcidiol levels to carry out activities of daily living.[394] But hip fracture patients with normal osteoid indices and low plasma calcidiol levels have increased surface extent of osteoclastic resorption and more severe cortical osteopenia than those with normal levels.[13] Also, increased osteoid accumulation and occasionally frank osteomalacia have been found in hip fracture patients with normal plasma levels of calcidiol but slightly reduced levels of calcitriol[395]; such an abnormality is less likely to be a nonspecific marker of ill health. These data increase the likelihood that HVOi, whether due to depletion or impaired metabolism of vitamin D, is a risk factor for hip fractures, but it is probably of etiologic importance in only a small proportion of patients.[393a]

B. Differential Diagnosis and Treatment of Osteoporosis

In all patients presenting with osteoporotic fractures of the spine or hip, especially after the age of 70, the physician should consider HVOi, which is both more common and easier to overlook than osteomalacia. If noninvasive indices of bone remodeling (Chapter 8) are increased, hyperparathyroidism (primary or secondary) and hyperthyroidism (endogenous or exogenous) must be excluded before resorting to estrogen replacement therapy. Serum osteocalcin correlates better with bone histology than alkaline phosphatase or urinary hydroxyproline[396] but has not yet been shown to be a better guide to the selection of treatment. Single photon absorptiometry of the radius, although an inaccurate predictor of vertebral bone status, is a good index of PTH-dependent bone loss.[63] Finally, although iliac bone histomorphometry after double tetracycline labeling is primarily a research tool, measurement of osteoid in a Jamshidi needle specimen is a simple and nontraumatic procedure with the potential for wide application.[397]

Vitamin D in a pharmacologic dose is commonly used in the management of osteoporosis, on the grounds that calcium alone would be inadequately absorbed and that subclinical osteomalacia would be corrected without the need for accurate diagnosis. It is doubtful whether in any other branch of medicine a treatment is so popular that combines such complete absence of supporting evidence with such potential for serious harm.[397a] Except in patients with vitamin D depletion (extrinsic or intrinsic), vitamin D has never been demonstrated to be beneficial in any form of osteoporosis. The only relevant data are that patients given vitamin D and calcium lose cortical bone faster than patients given only calcium, and that patients given vitamin D alone lose cortical bone faster than patients given no treatment at all.[398] In addition to its well-known toxic effects on the kidney,[5] vitamin D has an adverse effect on bone because one or more of its metabolites stimulates resorption[220a] and should not be given unless the plasma calcidiol level is low. Naturally, this proscription does not apply to the prophylactic administration of a physiologic amount (10–20 μg/day) to nursing home residents and others at increased risk of vitamin D depletion.[398b] The possible value of calcidiol, calcitriol, and alfacalcidol in correcting calcium malabsorption in patients with type I or type II osteoporosis[398a] is discussed in Chapter 12.

VI. OSTEOMALACIA RESULTING FROM ABNORMAL PHOSPHATE METABOLISM

Many of the similarities and differences between vitamin D–related and phosphate-related osteomalacia (Table 11–5) have already been referred to and can be readily accounted for, but one major question remains: What corresponds to HVOi in hypophosphatemic osteomalacia? In established cases, the relationships between osteoid seam thickness and both osteoid surface and adjusted apposition rate are the same as in HVO (Fig. 11–14), although seam thickness is greater and a higher proportion are in stage iii rather than stage ii. But there are almost no data on the mode of evolution at an earlier stage. The absence of focal osteomalacia indicates that, as in HVO, osteoid surface

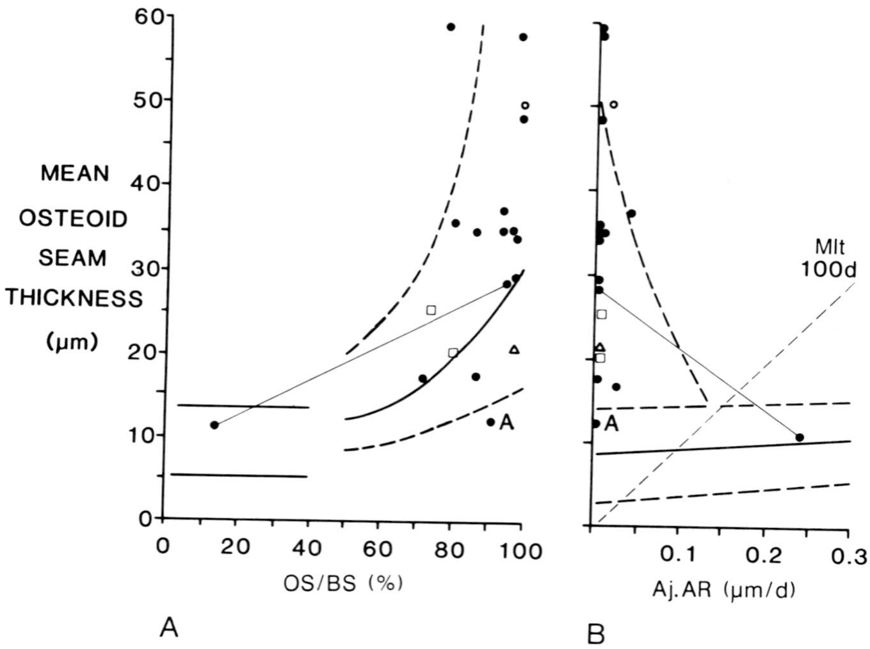

Figure 11–14. Osteoid thickness relationships in hypophosphatemic osteomalacia. Layout as in Figure 11–8 with static measurements on left (Fig. 11–14*A*) and kinetic measurements on right (Fig. 11–14*B*). Data are from 18 patients accumulated over 15 years, including six adults with XLH, seven with nonhereditary hypophosphatemia (five apparently without and two with a tumor, one cured by excision, with pre- and postoperative values joined), two with antacid-induced phosphate depletion (□), one with renal tubular acidosis secondary to Sjögren's syndrome (Δ), one adult with hereditary hypercalciuric hypophosphatemia (o), and one with atypical osteomalacia following renal transplantation (A).

increases before osteoid thickness, but without a stimulus to increased remodeling activation analogous to secondary hyperparathyroidism, osteoid surface can increase only as a result of prolongation of formation period, long known to be characteristic of hypophosphatemic osteomalacia.[10]

It can be inferred that all patients with impaired mineralization due to hypophosphatemia evolve through a stage of atypical osteomalacia, in which a reduction in the rate of mineral apposition is accompanied by a parallel reduction in the rate of matrix apposition or, looked at from a different viewpoint, by an inversely proportional prolongation of mineralization lag time. As osteoid surface increases, the surface available for initiation of remodeling would decrease, with a corresponding fall in bone formation rate, which would fall even further as mineralization became more defective. Except for one instance of atypical osteomalacia after renal transplantation (Fig. 11–14), data confirming this inference are lacking, most likely because the patients are not yet symptomatic and therefore not subjected to biopsy. Patients with hypophosphatemia, impaired osteoblast function, and reduced bone turnover but without osteomalacia[204,207] are presumably at an earlier stage at which disease progression is arrested because the fall in remodeling activation occurred sooner than would be dictated by the increase in osteoid surface, presumably from an independent cause. The situation is very similar to that in the nonosteomalacic low-turnover form of intestinal bone disease (Fig. 11–13), with the difference that in hypophosphatemia this is the usual manner of evolution, whereas in HVO it is an uncommon variant.

A. Phosphorus Depletion

Osteomalacia, according to reasonable criteria, has resulted from chronic phosphorus depletion in 10 cases[175,399,399a]; data on two more are shown in Figure 11–14. The patients have ranged in age from 26 to 69 years and included 10 women and 2 men, in keeping with the greater susceptibility of women to hypophosphatemia on a low-phosphate diet.[400] They had taken phosphate-binding antacids—aluminum hydroxide with or without magnesium hydroxide—in large quantities usually for at least 2 years. The clinical and radiographic features do not differ from those of osteomalacia in general, although symptoms of general debility may be more frequent and severe.[401] The plasma alkaline phosphatase is usually raised, but the abnormalities of bone mineral metabolism are unique. Plasma calcium is always normal and plasma phosphate usually but not invariably very low (0.9–3.2 mg/100 ml), but the most consistent and diagnostically reliable abnormality is that urine phosphorus excretion is always less than 50 mg/24 hours and often much lower. By contrast, urinary calcium excretion is increased, sometimes to very high levels[402]; in one case nephrolithiasis resulted and led to unnecessary parathyroid surgery.[403] The clinical and biochemical syndrome of phosphorus depletion, except for osteomalacia, can be induced experimentally within a few weeks in normal subjects by high-dose antacid administration.[400,401]

The osteomalacia is histologically typical, without evidence of aluminum deposition, and with increased osteoclast extent, less than in HVO but more than in other forms of primary hypophosphatemia.[175,399,403] Consequently, the hypercalciuria probably results from increased net bone resorption as well as from increased calcium absorption.[57,401,404] Since plasma calcidiol and PTH levels are normal, both sources of urinary calcium probably depend on an increased plasma calcitriol concentration, known to be induced by phosphate depletion[400] and demonstrated in the two most recent cases.[175,399] In retrospect, this abnormality was first observed more than 20 years ago in a patient with an increased plasma level of vitamin D activity, measurable at that time only by bioassay.[405] All manifestations are quickly reversed with cessation of antacid administration combined, if necessary, with supplemental phosphate. Looser zones have been observed to heal, but there is no histologic verification that osteomalacia can be completely cured. Other causes of osteomalacia with an increase in plasma calcitriol and/or hypercalciuria are shown in Table 11–9. In some of these conditions, calcitriol excess may paradoxically impair mineralization as it does in the rat.[219,220]

B. Hereditary Hypophosphatemia

Usually presenting in infancy, this condition is fully described in Chapter 24. The gene

Table 11–9. Unusual Causes of Osteomalacia with Increase in Plasma Calcitriol Concentration or Urinary Calcium Excretion or Both

	Plasma Calcitriol	Urinary Calcium ↑(Mixed)	Urinary Calcium ↑(Osseous)	Urinary Calcium ↓
Phosphate depletion	↑	+		
Hypercalciuric Hypophosphatemia[1]	↑	+		
Wilson's disease[2]	?	+		
Cadmium poisoning[2]	?	+		
Hypercalcemia HPT[3] with D-	↓		+	
Myeloma + LCN[2,4]	↓ or N		+	
Cystinosis[2]	↓		+	
Oculocerebrorenal syndrome[2]	?		+	
Renal tubular acidosis	N		+	
Bartter's syndrome[5]	?		+	
Vitamin D dependency type II[6]	↑			+
Calcium deficiency[7]	↑			+

Mixed hypercalciuria, increase in net intestinal absorption as well as net bone resorption. Osseous hypercalciuria, increase in net bone resorption alone.

[1]Ref. 177; previously referred to as Gentil-Dent syndrome.[404]

[2]Multiple renal tubular defects of Fanconi type.

[3]Hyperparathyroidism (primary or tertiary) and vitamin D deficiency.

[4]Light-chain nephropathy.

[5]Radiographic evidence of rickets; osteomalacia not verified.

[6]Defect in calcitriol receptor.

[7]Ref. 245.

Modified from Parfitt AM: Bone as a source of urinary calcium-osseous hypercalciuria. *In* Coe F (ed): Hypercalciuric States—Pathogenesis, Consequences and Treatment. New York, Grune & Stratton, 1984. (Additional references are given in this chapter for conditions not discussed in present text.)

has recently been localized, both in a murine model and in XLH, the most common form.[405a] In adults, the five separate but related components—hypophosphatemia, impaired mineralization, retarded growth, osteosclerosis, and ligamentous ossification—are of different relative importance and manner of expression than in children.[89,406] Impaired tubular reabsorption of phosphate is lifelong, but in other family members may be accompanied only by relative shortness of stature. After epiphyseal closure, treatment is often withdrawn but bone biopsy invariably shows osteomalacia and persistence of the asymmetrical perilacunar hypomineralization even in the absence of symptoms[407-409]; it is not known whether the same applies to hypophosphatemic relatives who never had rickets. Some patients experience recurrence of bone pain and difficulty in walking, appearance or reappearance of Looser zones, and progression of deformity after cessation of treatment. Others develop symptoms for the first time in late adult life. These differences cannot be related to the apparent histologic severity of the mineralization defect. In a unique family with X-linked recessive inheritance, the clinical features, mainly progressive lateral bowing of the femora, did not begin in any subject until adult life.[410]

The coarsened trabecular pattern often present in children may progress to a generalized increase in cancellous bone density, especially in the axial skeleton, producing a radiographic resemblance to osteopetrosis or renal osteodystrophy[89,406] (Chapters 13 and 16). Osteosclerosis may be especially severe in families with autosomal recessive rather than the more usual X-linked dominant inheritance.[411] Cancellous mineralized volume is normal or increased despite osteoid excess because cancellous bone volume is increased even more, both in the ilium (by histomorphometry; ref. 412 and unpublished data), in the distal radius (by computed tomography[413]), and in the spine (by neutron activation analysis[412]). The radiographic appearances reflect both the excess mineralized bone and the increased radiodensity of osteoid relative to other soft tissues because of its high sulphur content.[9] Cortical thickness is often increased in weight-bearing bones because of compensatory buttressing during growth,[89,412] but in non–weight-bearing bones is normal[413] or even decreased.

Osteosclerosis is asymptomatic, but ossification of ligaments, tendons, and joint capsules at their sites of attachment to bone, collectively known as entheses, is an important cause of disability in adults with hereditary hypophosphatemia.[406,414] The process begins as a roughening and irregularity of the periosteal surfaces, but progresses by extension of ossification beyond the original confines of the bone. Occasionally, ossicles due to ectopic ossification not continuous with the bone appear in the extremities and around the joints of the pelvis. There is usually pain, stiffness, and limitation of motion in relation to affected sites, and both x-ray appearances and clinical disability increase with age without relation to sex or treatment. Probably because of retarded growth and consequent shortness of the pedicles, the lumbar spinal canal is often narrow[415] with increased susceptibility to cord compression requiring surgical intervention.[89,416] Mild sensorineural hearing loss probably due to involvement of the cochlea by ligamentous ossification and bony expansion is also quite common.[417] The occurrence of similar lesions in a patient with cadmium-induced osteomalacia[406] suggests that they arise in response to prolonged tension on the surface of softened bones rather than representing an independent component of the genetic syndrome as previously suggested.[89]

C. Nonhereditary Hypophosphatemia, Idiopathic and Oncogenous

Hypophosphatemic osteomalacia sometimes appears for the first time in adolescence or adult life in the absence of rickets or retarded growth during childhood and with a negative family history.[89,418,419] In many cases the clinical, biochemical, and histologic abnormalities have been cured by removal of a mesenchymal tumor,[178] and several lines of evidence suggest that such a tumor is present in all cases. First, the characteristics that differ from hereditary hypophosphatemia (Table 11–10) are essentially identical in cases with and apparently without a tumor, including the frequency distribution of age of onset by decade. Second, with more widespread recognition of the need to search for a tumor in adult onset osteomalacia, reports of idiopathic cases have become notably less frequent.[420-423] Third, in many cases the tumors are so small that in an unfavorable location they could escape even the most sophisticated current methods of detection.[424] Finally, in at least one case initially reported as idiopathic, a tumor has been discovered during more extended observation.[425] But in one case encountered by the author, a tumor has still not been found nearly 40 years after the onset of symptoms, so that an occult tumor must not only be very small but very slowly growing. The longest interval between onset of symptoms and diagnosis in published cases is 14 years and has been 5 years or less in all cases reported since 1981.[178] The issue will likely not be settled until the pathophysiology is better understood.

The onset can be at any age but in most cases is between 20 and 50 years. In less than

Table 11–10. Differences Between Two Forms of Hypophosphatemic Osteomalacia

Feature	Hereditary	Nonhereditary[1]
Muscle weakness	No	Yes
Bone pain	No	Yes
Increased glycinuria	No	Yes
Osteopenia	No	Yes
Vertebral collapse	No	Yes
Loss of trunk height	No	Yes
Fractures[2]	No	Yes
Perilacunar low-density bone	Yes	No[3]
Osteosclerosis	Yes	No
Enthesopathy	Yes	No[4]
Deafness	Yes	No
Phosphate depletion[3]	No	Yes

Differences dependent only on age of onset are excluded.
[1]With or without a tumor.
[2]Looser zones occur in both.
[3]Evidence inconclusive.
[4]May depend on duration without treatment.
Modified from Parfitt AM, Kleerekoper M: Clinical disorders of calcium, phosphorus and magnesium metabolism. *In* Maxwell M, Kleeman CR (eds): Clinical Disorders of Fluid and Electrolyte Metabolism. 3rd ed. New York, McGraw-Hill, 1980.

10% of cases the symptoms begin before age 10 or after age 70, the former presenting as rickets rather than as osteomalacia.[426] Unlike adults with hereditary hypophosphatemia, most patients have bone pain, muscle weakness, and difficulty in walking and many have Looser zones. In contrast to hereditary hypophosphatemia, ligamentous ossification does not occur, and instead of axial osteosclerosis, there is often severe vertebral osteopenia with multiple compressions, loss of trunk height, and kyphosis, usually beginning 1 to 2 years after the other symptoms and progressing rapidly.[418,419] Osteopenia is often generalized, with pronounced cortical thinning; multiple fractures, especially of the femoral necks, are common. Due to the severity of the disease and the frequent delay in diagnosis, many of these patients in the past developed bizarre and crippling deformities including multiple angulations of the long bones, scoliosis as well as kyphosis, and pigeon chest due to fracture of the sternum.[89,427,428] Close to half of the patients, with or without tumor, have been bedridden before effective treatment was begun.[89,178]

The biochemical features are similar to those of hereditary hypophosphatemia, but malabsorption of calcium is more severe and the plasma phosphate level is lower. The mean value was 1.64 mg/100 ml in 27 nontumorous cases tabulated by Fanconi[419] and 1.52 mg/100 ml in 41 tumorous cases tabulated by Ryan and Reiss,[178] whereas in adults with hereditary hypophosphatemia, the plasma phosphate is usually above 2.0 mg/100 ml. Renal tubular responsiveness to exogenous PTH was blunted in one tumoral case[429] but exaggerated in one nontumoral case,[423] in keeping with the reported effect of parathyroidectomy,[430] but the data are too fragmentary to conclude that there is a difference in pathogenesis. Plasma calcitriol levels are uniformly low in the tumoral cases,[178,431] but have not been studied systematically in the nontumoral cases; in neither group does calcitriol administration consistently correct the defect in tubular reabsorption of phosphate,[178,421,422] probably because this requires maintenance of a supraphysiologic plasma level.[431] Urinary calcium excretion is either normal or sometimes increased, presumably owing to increased net bone resorption as a result of phosphate depletion.[418] Urinary excretion of glycine is often increased but other amino acids are normal, although a few cases manifest the Fanconi syndrome with generalized aminoaciduria and glucosuria with or without hyperchloremic acidosis.[178,431,432] Histologically, the bone is similar to that in severe vitamin D deficiency, but as in hereditary hypophosphatemia, osteoclastic resorption is usually less prominent[421,429,431,433,434] (Fig. 11–14). But in one case, resorption of osteoid was observed, indicating profound stimulation of osteoclast recruitment and activity.[434a]

Resection of a tumor when present is followed within a few days or weeks by a rise in low levels of plasma phosphate and calcitriol to normal, and by rapid improvement and eventual disappearance of symptoms and healing of Looser zones. Return of normal mineralization and healing of the osteomalacia has been confirmed histologically in a few cases[433] (Fig. 11–14). The tumors presumably secrete one or more humoral agents that impair both phosphate reabsorption and 1α-hydroxylation, but no such agent has yet been isolated, let alone identified. The tumors are mesenchymal but of variable origin in soft tissue or bone and with variable histologic features, often diagnosed as hemangiopericytoma. Almost all have the two main features of extreme vascularity and large numbers of spindle cells and multinucleated giant cells[178,435]; a recent, more detailed study suggested subdivision into four distinct groups.[435a] Osteomalacia (or rickets) that is clinically, biochemically, radiographically, and histologically very similar (except for earlier age of onset) occurs in some patients with fibrous dysplasia of bone (13 cases),[436-438] neurofibromatosis (9 cases, but only two recent),[439-442,442a] and linear sebaceous nevus syndrome (4 cases).[442b] In these disorders also, a humoral origin is likely, but is in most cases impossible to prove since the extent and multiplicity of lesions preclude surgical cure. However, partial excision of fibrous dysplasia in one case led to significant clinical and biochemical improvement.[436]

If a tumor is not found, treatment with some form of vitamin D in pharmacologic dose, together with supplemental phosphate and calcium, will lead to symptomatic relief and biochemical and radiographic improvement.[418] By analogy with hereditary hypophosphatemia (Chapter 24), calcitriol should be superior to calciferol and has been very effective in tumoral cases.[178] Only a moderate response was noted initially with short-term administration in nontumoral cases,[421,422] but an excellent long-term response was recently observed.[442b] Hypercalcemic hyperparathyroidism develops with unusual frequency during treatment,[420,443,443a] and is probably analogous to tertiary hyperparathyroidism with long-standing vitamin D depletion. These issues are discussed more fully in section VIII. A final peculiarity of idiopathic nonhereditary hypophosphatemia is that in at least two cases, spontaneous complete recovery has occurred, allowing treatment to be withdrawn.[433,444]

Osteomalacia has also been reported in a few patients with carcinoma of the prostate.[445-448] The plasma calcitriol level has been low in the three cases measured,[446,447] and the biochemical syndrome has been induced in nude mice transplanted with tumor tissue from affected patients,[449] but there are several differences from the usual form of oncogenous osteomalacia just described. First, with one exception,[445] osteomalacia has occurred in patients already known to have widespread osteoblastic metastases, with a total tumor burden that is much larger than in patients with a benign mesenchymal tumor. Second, hyperosteoidosis is due at least in part to stimulation of new woven bone by tumor cells[448] and is found also in patients with osteosclerosis for other reasons such as thorotrast toxicity[450] or myeloid metaplasia.[451] Third, affected patients are usually hypocalcemic as well as hypophosphatemic, the abnormalities being only slightly greater than in patients who have osteoblastic metastases without osteomalacia.[57] Finally, many patients with this form of osteomalacia lack clinical effects from it, with no proximal muscle weakness, bone pain no worse than can be accounted for by the osseous metastases, and no Looser zones or other radiographic features of osteomalacia. However, two patients treated with vitamin D[445] or calcitriol[447] derived substantial relief of bone pain.

D. Fanconi Syndrome

For the most part this is a childhood disorder[1,2,180] (Chapter 24), although Wilson's disease occasionally presents with osteomalacia without preceding rickets.[452] Onset in adult life does not rule out a genetic basis, probably always autosomal dominant,[453,454] but most cases are sporadic. Some are due to a known cause of renal tubular damage such as industrial or environmental cadmium intoxication[406,455-457] or light-chain proteinuria,[179] but Fanconi syndrome due to external toxicity rarely causes osteomalacia, presumably because the effects are usually reversible.[458] Some cases are tumor induced, as mentioned earlier, but many are diagnosed by exclusion as idiopathic.[459,460] There is usually a close clinical resemblance to nonhereditary hypophosphatemia without the Fanconi syndrome, although osteopenia is less prominent and the manifestations are less severe if bone biopsy is used to facilitate early diagnosis.[179]

Calcitriol levels when measured have usually been low,[180,461,462] except in one case of light-chain nephropathy,[179] probably because the defect in the proximal tubule occurs at a site of calcitriol synthesis; experimental induction of the Fanconi syndrome by administration of maleic acid also impairs 1α-hydroxylation.[463] Consistent with calcitriol deficiency, calcium absorption is impaired,[464] except in Wilson's disease[465] and cadmium poisoning,[404] where for unknown reasons it can be increased. Urinary calcium excretion is often high (Table 11–9); this sometimes results from associated proximal renal tubular acidosis and is correctable by alkali administration,[464] sometimes from phosphate depletion,[466,467] and sometimes from a separate defect in tubular reabsorption of calcium. Osteomalacia in the adult Fanconi syndrome responds well to treatment with oral phosphate either alone,[466,467] or combined with calcitriol if the plasma level is low.[179] In the autosomal dominant form there may be a greater need for alkali as well.[2,454]

E. Renal Tubular Acidosis and Ureteral Diversion

These two conditions have in common chronic metabolic acidosis in which the low plasma bicarbonate is balanced by an increase in chloride rather than in normally unmeasured anions such as lactate. Hyperchloremic acidosis also occurs with pharmacologic carbonic anhydrase inhibition and with congenital absence of carbonic anhydrase,[468] but these conditions have not been shown to cause osteomalacia. Renal tubular acidosis (RTA) is conveniently classified as proximal, in which bicarbonate reabsorption is reduced, and distal, in which the urine cannot be maximally acidified.[469] Proximal RTA is usually a component of the Fanconi syndrome (section

VII-D). Lone proximal RTA with rare exceptions[470] occurs only in infants, with spontaneous recovery after a few years,[471] and does not cause rickets. The concurrence of lone proximal RTA and osteomalacia[472] is usually a consequence of vitamin D depletion and secondary hyperparathyroidism.[124] In a possible exception to this rule,[473] the Fanconi syndrome was not adequately excluded.

Adult onset distal RTA in most cases is a complication of Sjögren's syndrome or other cause of hyperglobulinemia.[469,474] The major effects of RTA are potassium depletion, nephrolithiasis, and nephrocalcinosis,[1,2,180,469] their severity varying with the dietary acid load.[2] Osteomalacia was frequent in the past,[475] although rarely verified histologically.[404,474,476] Overt osteomalacia is now uncommon,[477,478] most likely because treatment is started earlier as a result of routine biochemical screening[469] and is more likely to require bone biopsy for diagnosis[473] (Fig. 11–14). It closely resembles vitamin D–related osteomalacia,[1,2] including the presence of proximal muscle weakness[479] and secondary hyperparathyroidism.[480,481] In one case the latter caused bone disease from osteitis fibrosa rather than from osteomalacia,[482] as sometimes happens in gluten enteropathy (section II-C), but in most cases is less severe than in HVO.[1] In the related condition of ureteral diversion, hyperchloremic acidosis is the result of preferential reabsorption of chloride and/or hydrogen ions from urine in contact with colonic or ileal epithelium. After ureterosigmoidostomy, histologically verified osteomalacia has developed in 5 to 18 years,[473,483-486] but with ileal replacement of ureters, osteomalacia has been manifest clinically in 2 years and histologically (in the absence of symptoms) in 6 months.[487] This form of osteomalacia is more common in the U.K. than in the U.S., and in several cases there has been marginal vitamin D deficiency.[485,486]

In both forms of hyperchloremic acidosis, the pathogenesis of osteomalacia is obscure. Despite the combined effects of hypokalemia, acidemia, and hyperparathyroidism, which all independently reduce tubular reabsorption of phosphate, mean plasma phosphate is only slightly lower than in vitamin D depletion[1] and plasma calcium is normal, so that the relevant formation product is probably not as low. Hypophosphatemia is significant only in an occasional patient with osteomalacia due to ureteral diversion.[484] Ammonium chloride administration increases urinary calcium excretion with little change in plasma calcium by simultaneously increasing net bone resorption and decreasing tubular reabsorption of calcium, but PTH secretion is unaffected so that this is an imperfect model for RTA.[488] Furthermore, absolute hypercalciuria is uncommon in RTA.[404]

Contrary to the predictions from animal experiments, metabolic acidemia does not impair calcitriol synthesis in humans,[488,489] and calcitriol levels are normal in both RTA[182] and ureteral diversion[473,486] unless there is significant renal insufficiency,[485] so that the usual malabsorption of calcium in RTA is unexplained. Acidemia probably impairs mineralization directly,[473] either by lowering trivalent PO_4^{2-} disproportionately,[490] or by compromising the removal of hydrogen ions from sites of mineral deposition. But several paradoxes remain; nonhyperchloremic acidosis, as in glycogen storage disease, does not impair bone mineralization, and in one family with isolated proximal RTA, hyperchloremic acidosis of similar severity to distal RTA was unaccompanied by any disorder of bone mineral metabolism.[470] Whatever the explanation, administration of alkali 1.5 to 2.5 mEq/kg body weight/day will usually raise plasma phosphate and heal the osteomalacia both in RTA[491-493] and in ureteral diversion[484,486,487] so that vitamin D is needed only in severe cases, or when delay in diagnosis has resulted in significant renal failure from nephrocalcinosis.[2]

VII. OSTEOMALACIA WITH NORMAL VITAMIN D AND PHOSPHATE METABOLISM

A. Inhibitors of Mineralization

Impaired mineralization and osteomalacia can be produced by sodium etidronate used in the treatment of Paget's disease (Chapter 15), sodium fluoride used in the treatment of osteoporosis (Chapter 12), and aluminum-containing phosphate-binding antacids used to control hyperphosphatemia in patients on maintenance hemodialysis (Chapter 13). Aluminum accumulation also contributes to bone disease in patients receiving total parenteral nutrition,[494] and a similar mechanism could be involved in thorium-related osteomalacia resulting from thorotrast exposure.[450]

In all varieties of toxic osteomalacia there is a high prevalence of both atypical and focal forms as defined in section I-G. Indeed, with the possible exceptions of pseudohypoparathyroidism[171] and hypophosphatasia,[495] focal osteomalacia is observed only with inhibitors of mineralization.

Sodium etidronate blocks mineralization *in vitro* and probably binds to the crystal surface of newly deposited mineral *in vivo*.[496] Osteoid accumulation and reduced tetracycline uptake were first observed with the use of etidronate in the treatment of osteoporosis,[497] but are now regularly seen in the treatment of Paget's disease in a dose of 10 mg/kg/day or more and are associated with increasing bone pain and increased fracture risk.[498,499] The mineralization defect develops earlier and is more severe in pagetic than in normal bone, presumably because of the difference in turnover.[74,499] In the largest series with individual data reported, osteomalacia was generalized in 11, focal in five, and atypical in four.[498] Although a dose of 5 mg/kg/day is generally considered to be safe,[499,500] focal osteomalacia is quite common after treatment with this dose for 6 months or longer[35] (Fig. 11–15), and in one case there was generalized osteomalacia presenting with a pathologic fracture.[501] The high frequency of focal osteomalacia probably results from the depression of remodeling activation by etidronate leading to reduced bone turnover before the emergence of a significant mineralization defect. Etidronate-induced osteomalacia is reversible, but the excess osteoid may not begin to mineralize for 3 to 6 months after the drug is discontinued.[74] Newer bisphosphonates such as clodronate are much less potent inhibitors of mineralization and do not cause osteomalacia, but may induce secondary hyperparathyroidism.[502]

In patients with osteoporosis treated with sodium fluoride, significant increases in the surface extent, thickness, and volume of unmineralized osteoid have usually been observed, but in most cases result from stimulation of matrix synthesis rather than from impaired mineralization.[503,504] Histologic evidence of osteomalacia was found in eight of 14 patients after 2 years' treatment but was clinically manifest only in one.[503] Symptomatic osteomalacia attributed to fluoride treatment has been reported only in a very few individual cases,[505,506] probably because osteoid is usually added to mineralized bone rather than replacing it, so that structural failure is less likely.[74] We have observed

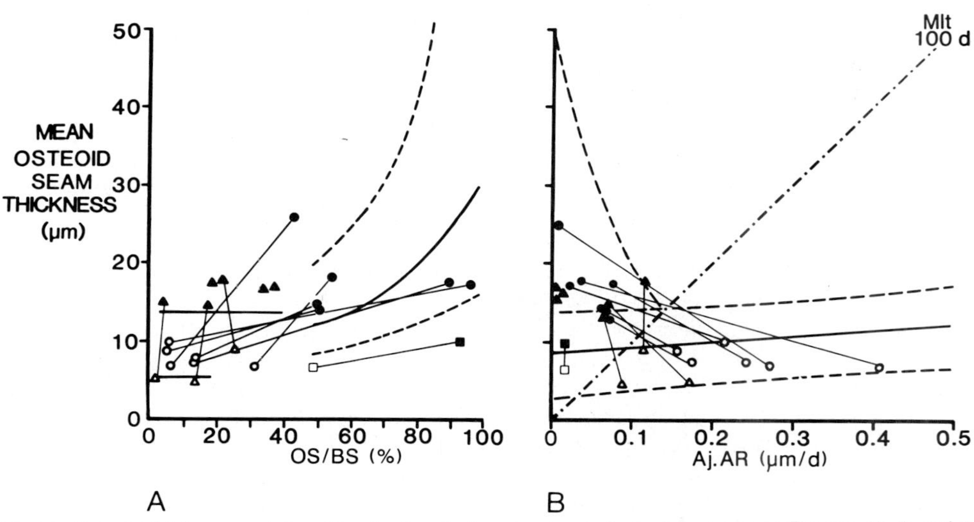

Figure 11–15. Osteoid thickness relationships in drug-induced osteomalacia. Layout as in Figures 11–8 and 11–14 with static measurements on left (Fig. 11–15*A*) and kinetic measurements on right (Fig. 11–15*B*). Data are from three patients with Paget's disease treated with EHDP 5 mg/kg body weight for 12 to 20 months giving rise to focal osteomalacia (single closed triangles), and 10 patients with osteoporosis treated with sodium fluoride in various regimens, with pretreatment values (open symbols) and posttreatment values (closed symbols) joined. Osteomalacia was focal in three cases (triangles), atypical in one case (squares) and generalized in six cases (circles). Note that complete arrest of mineralization was observed in all three EHDP-treated patients but in only one of 10 fluoride-treated patients.

osteomalacia in 10 cases, of which six were generalized, three focal, and one atypical (Fig. 11–15). Symptoms were present only in one patient with focal osteomalacia who had a painful stress fracture of a pubic ramus resembling a Looser zone.

The available data suggest that sodium fluoride in large doses significantly impairs mineralization in some patients, but the defect is not prevented by physiologic levels of vitamin D or related to abnormal vitamin D metabolism, is not caused by lack of substrate for mineralization, is not associated with secondary hyperparathyroidism, and probably reflects a direct toxic effect on osteoblasts. Osteomalacia is also found in some patients after prolonged treatment with niflumic acid, a fluorine-containing anti-inflammatory agent.[507] Since trabecular thickness increases more in patients who develop it than in those who do not (Kleerekoper and Parfitt, unpublished data), osteomalacia could be a stage in the evolution of a successful therapeutic response rather than a harmful side effect, but may contribute to the increased fracture rate in the first year of fluoride treatment especially if the dose is too high (Chapter 12).

Disabling osteomalacia with multiple spontaneous fractures, sometimes including the sternum (Fig. 11–12), is found with increasing frequency among patients on maintenance hemodialysis, especially after parathyroidectomy[60,75,76,508-511] (Chapter 13). Both atypical osteomalacia (referred to in this context as aplastic[508] or type II[509] and focal osteomalacia[511,512] are common, and some patients have low-turnover nonosteomalacic osteopenia.[512] The different histologic patterns reflect varying severity of prior hyperparathyroid bone disease, and of independent effects of aluminum to inhibit bone matrix synthesis and mineralization.[512a] In patients with generalized osteomalacia, the bone formation rate is no lower than in the osteomalacia of vitamin D depletion, but there is a closer resemblance to hypophosphatemic osteomalacia. The morphologic expression of hyperparathyroidism is less apparent and the mineralization defect is more severe, with osteoid seams that are relatively thicker (Fig. 11–16), and tetracycline uptake more often completely absent.[513]

Aluminum inhibits mineralization both *in vitro*[514] and *in vivo*[515] and dialysis osteomalacia is undoubtedly associated with

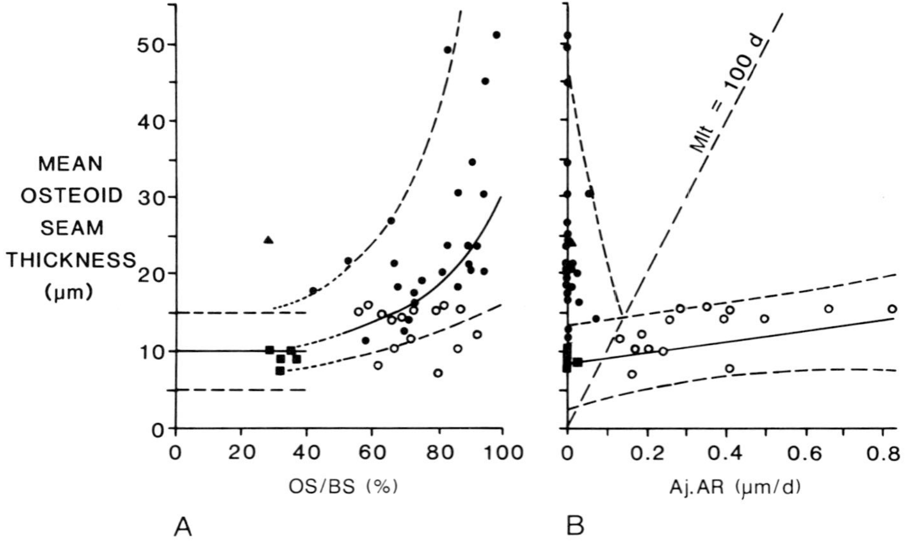

Figure 11–16. Osteoid thickness relationships in aluminum-related osteomalacia occurring during maintenance hemodialysis. Layout as in Figures 11–8, 11–14, and 11–15, with static measurements on left (Fig. 11–16*A*) and kinetic measurements on right (Fig. 11–16*B*). Data are from 46 patients, 15 with osteitis fibrosa (o), 25 with generalized osteomalacia (•), one with focal osteomalacia (▲), and five with aplastic bone disease (■); these represent an early stage of atypical osteomalacia with OV/BV between 5% and 10%. Note that there is considerable overlap in patients with and without osteomalacia by the static measurements, but clear demarcation by the kinetic measurements.

aluminum deposition at the bone interface.[75,76,508-513] But aluminum in the cement line, which is the initial location of the bone interface, frequently does not block mineralization in patients with osteitis fibrosa,[512a,516] and mineralization resumes after renal transplantation despite persistence of stainable aluminum.[517] Furthermore, nonuremic vitamin D–deficient animals given aluminum accumulate it in bone without impairing the healing response to vitamin D.[518,519] Clearly other factors must be involved in the pathogenesis of aluminum-related osteomalacia. One such factor could be the plasma level of citrate, which complexes aluminum to form a more potent inhibitor of mineralization than any other aluminum salt.[520] Another could be direct effects of aluminum on the function of osteoblasts, in which cells aluminum can be demonstrated within mitochondria.[512a]

B. Inability of Matrix to Mineralize

Although abnormal matrix maturation may contribute to osteomalacia in vitamin D depletion, osteomalacia due to defective bone matrix alone in the absence of any disorder of bone mineral or vitamin D metabolism has been established only in fibrogenesis imperfecta ossium.[521] In this rare condition, normal lamellar bone is replaced by matrix with no birefringence in polarized light and no fiber pattern detectable by light microscopy, but which by electron microscopy consists of a tangled mass of very thin, short, and irregularly curved fibers.[522] Mineralization of the abnormal matrix is delayed and retarded, but because the protein content of the matrix is reduced by as much as 75%, mineral density ultimately becomes higher than normal.[521] Nevertheless, bone surfaces are covered by thick and extensive layers of unmineralized matrix, the ultrastructural appearance of the mineralization front is abnormal,[523] and conformity to the kinetic criteria for generalized osteomalacia has been demonstrated by double tetracycline labeling.[524]

The condition most often presents in the fifth or sixth decade with intractable pain and multiple fractures, the patients often becoming unable to walk and dying within a few years.[525] The radiographic appearances are characteristic but can be confused with Paget's disease.[525,526] Since there is always some normal bone, the matrix defect must begin in adult life, probably only a few years before the onset of symptoms.[521] In one case, histologic and biochemical indices of bone resorption were increased, but there was no therapeutic response to calcitonin.[523] There is a high frequency of monoclonal gammopathy, and in one case with kappa light chains in serum and urine, complete clinical and histologic remission was achieved by combined treatment with cyclical melphalan and prednisolone,[527] an extraordinary observation with far-reaching implications for the cell biology of bone.

C. Disorders of Alkaline Phosphatase

The role of alkaline phosphatase in mineralization has been discussed for many years and is still unknown (Chapter 2), but osteomalacia occurs in hypophosphatasia, a genetic defect in the synthesis of alkaline phosphatase,[528] and in so-called axial osteomalacia, in which morphologically inactive osteoblasts stain with paradoxical intensity for alkaline phosphatase.[529]

Hypophosphatasia is usually an autosomal recessive disorder that presents in infancy with rickets, raised intracranial pressure, hypercalcemia, nephrocalcinosis, and early death; in mild cases the onset is in later childhood, and spontaneous radiographic improvement can occur[528] (Chapter 24). There is partial and variable deficiency (10%-30% of normal) of the bone/liver/kidney isoenzyme in cultured skin fibroblasts,[530] relatively greater reduction of the bone-specific than of other components of serum alkaline phosphatase,[531] and normal intestinal and placental isoenzymes. The plasma level and urinary excretion of phosphorylethanolamine and phosphorylserine are increased, most likely as a consequence of altered hepatic metabolism.[528,531] The plasma level and urinary excretion of inorganic pyrophosphate are even more increased[528,532]; alkaline phosphatase functions as a pyrophosphatase in bone, and failure to hydrolyze pyrophosphate in matrix vesicles could account for the mineralization defect that persists when epiphyseal cartilage from affected subjects is incubated *in vitro* in solutions that calcify normal cartilage.[528] There is no evidence for any abnormality in vitamin D metabolism.[533]

Adult hypophosphatasia is much commoner than previously suspected and is characterized by early loss of permanent teeth, osteopenia and increased fracture risk, and osteomalacia of variable severity, usually atypical, less commonly generalized, and occasionally focal.[495,534] Alkaline phosphatase staining in osteoblasts is of markedly reduced intensity, and its surface extent is inversely correlated with the amount of osteoid.[534] Most patients with abnormal bone histology are asymptomatic. The same biochemical abnormalities are found in blood and urine as in the childhood forms, except for one case similar in other respects but without increased phosphorylethanolamine excretion and with reduced intestinal alkaline phosphatase.[535] In some cases there is a history of rickets in childhood and the presence of deformities common in the childhood form such as prominent sternum and loss of normal curvature of the thoracic spine,[536] but in several large kindreds with autosomal dominant transmission the onset of clinical effects was clearly in adult life.[534,537,538] The expression of the biochemical defect varies considerably both within and between families.

The term "axial osteomalacia" is applied to a disorder in which cancellous bone of the axial skeleton is of increased radiodensity with an irregular, coarsened, and spongelike appearance[539] (Chapter 16). Pain in affected bone is mild or absent, and fractures do not occur. Histologically, the trabecular plates are irregularly thickened and closely packed, with increased surface extent and width of osteoid and reduced extent and separation of tetracycline uptake, but both mineralized and unmineralized bone is of lamellar structure with normal birefringence.[10,529,539-541] The appendicular skeleton is radiographically normal; in one case osteoid was abundant in the ilium and absent in a tibial malleolus, providing the first direct evidence that the mineralization defect is confined to the axial skeleton.[541a] The disorder is sometimes classified with fibrogenesis imperfecta ossium as a matrix defect, but supporting evidence is lacking. The serum alkaline phosphatase has been raised only in three of 13 published cases, two from one family, all other cases being sporadic.[529] The only clue to pathogenesis is the increased alkaline phosphatase content of osteoblasts, which is disproportionate to the increase in serum level and inconsistent with other indices of osteoblast activity. A defect either in the release of alkaline phosphatase at sites of bone formation or in its biological effectiveness could account for impaired mineralization, but would not explain the osteosclerosis.

VIII. THERAPEUTIC INTERVENTION IN OSTEOMALACIA

There is an important difference between the two main etiologic categories. Vitamin D–related osteomalacia occurs for the most part only in persons already known to be at risk and so in principle is largely preventable. By contrast, phosphate-related osteomalacia is usually less predictable, so that prevention is less often possible. Occasional measurement of urinary phosphate in patients on long-term antacid therapy would prevent phosphate depletion, and appropriate family surveillance might forestall symptoms in some genetic disorders. How best to manage familial hypophosphatemia after cessation of growth to minimize adult complications is unknown (Chapter 24). Routine multichannel biochemical screening probably leads to treatment of renal tubular acidosis before the onset of osteomalacia in most cases, but accidentally discovered hypophosphatemia is usually either transient or mild and of uncertain significance.[542,543] With these few exceptions, prevention can be usefully discussed only in relation to vitamin D.

A. Prevention of HVO

The prevention of intrinsic vitamin D depletion is primarily an issue of public health rather than of individual patient care, but many studies carried out with the object of influencing public policy have been poorly designed.[248] Attempts to eradicate migrant osteomalacia in the U.K. have included provision of free vitamin D tablets and various types of education, but neither measure has been convincingly demonstrated to improve health.[248] Any policy that requires ostensibly healthy Asian adults to permanently change their habits with respect to diet or sun exposure or to take daily medication indefinitely will inevitably fail. More realistic is to give a single oral dose of 2.5 mg of calciferol annually just before winter, an effective and safe method of maintaining adequate plasma calcidiol levels in Asians throughout the year.[544] Compliance with medical advice is likely to be better during pregnancy, and 25 µg of calciferol daily during the last trimester would improve fetal growth and ossification and minimize the occurrence of neonatal hypocalcemia as well as protect the mother.[545]

The same principles apply to prevention in the elderly. Very few will take a weekly serving of sardines or an annual vacation by the Mediterranean[546] because of medical advice. Therapeutic ultraviolet irradiation is both physiologic and effective, but it is also cumbersome, expensive, and potentially hazardous.[5,547] An oral vitamin D supplement of 20 µg/day given to old people at varying levels of risk in Ireland maintained satisfactory plasma levels of calcidiol, corrected any biochemical abnormalities indicative of subclinical HVO, and appeared to be entirely safe.[548] Unfortunately, the preparation used also supplied 60,000 IU/day of vitamin A, the long-term safety of which has not been rigorously established. Nevertheless, the observation supports the proposal that the RDA for vitamin D in the U.S. should be increased to 15 to 20 µg/day in the elderly[5] and should be heeded by those responsible for their nutritional needs.[398a] It should also encourage the governments of Northern European countries to adopt vitamin D fortification, at least to the level practiced in the U.S. and Canada and preferably extended to a wider range of foods. There is still no satisfactory pharmaceutical preparation for giving a physiologic daily dose of vitamin D to adults.[239]

Prevention of HVO in patients with gastrointestinal or hepatobiliary disease or receiving anticonvulsant therapy depends on medical awareness of the risk in these populations. The best policy has not yet been determined, but to be successful, it should be applied before serum alkaline phosphatase has increased or cortical osteopenia has developed. The degree of malabsorption of vitamin D varies widely between patients, and no single oral dose is uniformly safe and effective in prophylaxis. Absorption from intramuscular injections of vitamin D dissolved in oil is unpredictable,[549] and a water-soluble preparation that can be given intravenously is not generally available.[239] Individual monitoring is unavoidable and a reasonable policy is to give a capsule (not tablet) of 1.25 mg of ergocalciferol at a frequency that maintains plasma calcidiol between 20 and 40 ng/ml, although higher plasma levels will be needed in some patients with intestinal resection or refractory sprue. For most patients, the requisite frequency will lie somewhere between once a month and once a day. An amount of supplemental calcium should be added, such that the combination maintains urinary calcium excretion between 100 and 250 mg/24 hours (or calcium/creatinine ratio between 0.1 and 0.2 mg/mg) and plasma calcium, alkaline phosphatase, and the best available index of parathyroid function within normal limits. With these guidelines, some patients will be treated unnecessarily, in the sense that they would never have developed symptoms even if nothing was done, but many patients will benefit and none will be harmed.

B. Treatment of HVO

The aims of treatment are to relieve symptoms, restore bone strength by promoting mineralization of osteoid, and preserve mineralized bone by correcting secondary hyperparathyroidism. It is important that all three aims are explained to the patient and that the first is not permitted to overshadow the second and third. In extrinsic vitamin D depletion, these aims are best served by giving a modest dose of vitamin D (25-50 µg/day), together with adequate supplemental calcium. Urgent treatment of hypocalcemia, occasionally needed in patients with osteomalacia, is covered in Chapter 14. The responses to treatment and time course of healing will be described first, followed by some practical aspects of management and modifications of the regimen needed for other causes of HVO.

1. Response to Vitamin D

Giving a physiologic dose of vitamin D to a patient with extrinsic vitamin D depletion produces a characteristic series of changes.[1,2,37,47,49,200,239,550,551] The plasma calcitriol level begins to rise immediately and quickly reaches supranormal levels, intestinal calcium and phosphate absorption promptly increase, plasma calcium (if low) returns to normal in 1 to 4 weeks, PTH secretion falls rapidly but not to normal, and plasma phosphate rises to normal in 4 to 8 days and then to above normal for several months. Osteoclast function improves, and there is a rapid increase in urinary hydroxyproline.[99] Osteoblast function improves and mineralization resumes rapidly, probably within a week, plasma alkaline phosphatase increases further, calcium and phosphate are rapidly deposited in bone, and external balance becomes positive usually by the second 4-day period, with low fecal as well as urinary calcium excretion.[47,49] Symptoms improve soon after and a previously bedridden patient may become able to walk without pain in a few weeks, but restoration of normal bone structure,[63] normal muscle power,[50] and normal parathyroid function[118] can take up to 2 years or even longer, and it is important that the asymptomatic patient not default from follow-up. Some of these changes will now be described in more detail.

2. Effect on Bone Mineral Metabolism

When their substrate is depleted, both 25- and 1α-hydroxylase enzymes are maximally active and vitamin D is rapidly and almost quantitatively converted to calcitriol, so that the doses of calciferol and calcitriol needed for most rapid healing are almost the same, despite the 1000-fold difference in doses in other circumstances, such as the treatment of hypoparathyroidism.[550] Plasma calcidiol may not begin to rise for several weeks, but plasma calcitriol reaches three to five times the normal level and can remain elevated for many months,[199,200] sustained by continued hypersecretion of PTH despite restoration of normocalcemia[118,119] and probably also by continued low blood levels of calciferol and calcidiol. Plasma phosphate rises by about 1.0 mg/100 ml to reach a normal value in the first week with a transient fall in urinary phosphate indicating increased tubular reabsorption,[1,125,189] and continues to rise to a peak value about 1.0 mg/100 ml higher than normal by 3 to 4 weeks, and then falls slowly for the next 6 months.[47] Although both the rise in plasma calcium and the initial fall in PTH may contribute to the early rise in plasma phosphate, the later increase in tubular reabsorption of phosphate above normal is most likely the result of continued elevation of plasma calcitriol acting directly on the kidney.[550]

3. Effect on Bone Mineralization and Remodeling

Tetracycline-based histomorphometry during the healing of osteomalacia is limited, but serial measurement of the extent of toluidine blue–stainable mineralization front supports the inference from balance studies that substantial mineral deposition begins within a week of starting treatment.[69,125,209,551,552] However, it is unlikely that normal mineralization is immediately restored over the entire osteoid surface, since this would require calcium retention of 2.0 to 3.0 g/day rather than the 0.5 to 1.0 g/day usually found. Furthermore, even the thickest osteoid seam should mineralize completely within 3 months, but mean seam thickness can take much longer to return completely to normal. The most likely explanation for the delay is that mineralization can begin immediately only where osteoblasts are still present.[34,208-211] Elsewhere, the flat cells covering the osteoid surface must reacquire osteoblast function and morphologic features, and additional osteoblasts must be recruited to maintain coverage of the surface, processes that probably continue for several months and are responsible for the further increase in serum alkaline phosphatase that begins soon after starting treatment. At some of the thickest seams, mineralization may resume closer to the surface than the bone interface, leaving a layer of osteoid that remains permanently unmineralized as a residual "scar".[34]

In biopsies taken at varying times between 3 and 12 months after treatment was begun, mean values for mineral apposition rate were about 30% above normal and mean values for bone formation rate about five times greater than normal (Teotia and Parfitt, unpublished data). It is likely that osteomalacia heals by reversing its sequence of development, so that a patient in stage iii at the onset of treatment would pass successively through stage ii (return of double labels, but seam thickness still increased) and stage i (seam thickness normal, but formation rates still high) before returning completely to normal. This histologic evolution is accompanied by a gradual fall in alkaline phosphatase and, when remineralization is almost complete, by a rise in urinary calcium excretion. With the increase in mineralized bone surface and continued hyperparathyroidism there is an increase in absolute surface extent and number of osteoclasts, and a decline in total bone matrix volume, even though mineralized bone volume is increasing. Bone turnover probably remains elevated until the completion of parathyroid involution, which is a very slow process.[142]

4. Practical Aspects of Management

The ability of 1α-hydroxylated metabolites to cure the osteomalacia of extrinsic vitamin D depletion[196-198,553] is important to the understanding of physiology and pathogenesis, but it is simpler and safer to give the precursor and rely on the regulated endogenous production of calcitriol, which cannot lead to overtreatment and vitamin D intoxication.[198] Even in patients with age-related decline in renal function and 1α-hydroxylase activity, no advantage over calciferol has been demonstrated.[554] The dose of vitamin D is not critical; healing can be initiated with only 2 to 3 μg/day but will proceed more rapidly with a larger dose.[239,550] Calcium conservation is very efficient during the early stages of recovery,[49] but supplemental calcium 1.0 to 2.0 g/day will restore mineralized bone and suppress parathyroid hypersecretion more quickly[555] and make it less likely that replenishment of the axial skeleton will occur at the expense of the appendicular skeleton.[14] The most impressive calcium retention has been achieved with microcrystalline hydroxyapatite, which provides all the required minerals in the correct proportion,[47,550] but this preparation is not currently available in the U.S. and any form of calcium is satisfactory. Cortical bone that was lost during the development of the disease cannot be replaced,[63] and with the resumption of normal physical activity the risk of fracture increases, and the patient should be advised how to minimize the chance of falling.

The treatment of osteomalacia due to intrinsic vitamin D depletion follows the same general principles, but differs in several points of detail. First, as for prevention, the dose of vitamin D varies over a wide range and is unpredictable. Second, although vitamin D itself is the cheapest and safest compound for prevention, and for the correction of extrinsic depletion, calcidiol has several potential advantages in patients with intestinal or hepatobiliary disease. It is more precisely formulated,[330] is better absorbed,[263] bypasses any defect in 25-hydroxylation, leads to more predictable blood levels that can be monitored directly,[265,317,556] and is more rapid in onset and offset of its effects, so that the response to a change in dose can be detected more rapidly,[330,550] but retains physiologic regulation of 1-hydroxylation. Third, whatever compound is used, the dose requirement will be greatly affected by the response of the underlying disease to treatment,[27,262] and will (for example) show a larger and more rapid decline during the successful use of a gluten-free diet in celiac disease than during the attempted correction of pancreatic enzyme deficiency. Finally, because the dosage is both higher and varies more with time, more frequent and careful monitoring of the therapeutic response is required to avoid vitamin D intoxication[57,239] (Chapters 5 and 14). This should be on the same lines as previously recommended for prevention, but with particular attention to the approach of plasma alkaline phosphatase to normal and a rise in urinary calcium excretion, which may both give warning of a need to reduce the dose. A moderate increase in plasma creatinine during healing may reflect a change in muscle metabolism rather than a decline in renal function, and so is not by itself an indication for any change in treatment.[557]

C. Treatment of Hypophosphatemic Osteomalacia

X-linked hypophosphatemia (XLH), nonhereditary hypophosphatemia, and the Fanconi syndrome differ in many ways, but they have in common a primary (non–PTH-dependent) defect in tubular phosphate reabsorption and either relative or absolute impairment of calcitriol synthesis. In the absence of a tumor or of some reversible cause of renal tubular damage,[452] optimum treatment of all three conditions is based on some combination of supplemental phosphate and calcitriol.[27] The only other medications that may be needed are supplemental calcium in severe nonhereditary hypophosphatemia, and alkali in renal tubular acidosis, primary or secondary, as was previously indicated.

1. Phosphate Supplementation

Since phosphate is reasonably safe and sometimes effective by itself,[179,466,467] it is logical to use it initially as the only treatment (Chapter 24). With normal renal function, even a large phosphate supplement can produce only a modest increase in plasma phosphate, which depends much more on the renal threshold than on the phosphate load to be excreted (Chapter 7). Assuming 70% to 75% absorption and a GFR of 100 ml/minute, the mean plasma phosphate will rise by about 0.5 mg/100 ml for each 1.0 g/day increment in elemental phosphorus intake, with a smaller rise in fasting plasma phosphate. Even this theoretical maximum will be attained only if the phosphate is administered as the potassium rather than as the sodium salt, since expansion of the extracellular fluid volume by sodium may reduce tubular phosphate reabsorption and partly offset the rise in plasma phosphate.[558] Conversely, the effect of the supplement can be augmented by dietary salt restriction[57] or by diuretic therapy.[559]

The principal benefit of supplemental phosphate is direct enhancement of bone mineral deposition, but there can be additional benefits unrelated to a rise in plasma level. In patients with defective urinary acidification as well as impaired phosphate reabsorption, metabolic acidosis is improved by provision both of alkali and of additional urinary buffer to facilitate hydrogen ion excretion.[560] Also, phosphate supplements increase tubular reabsorption of calcium and reduce calcium excretion, even in the absence of metabolic acidosis.[57] When used in the treatment of hypercalcemia, supplemental phosphate may lead to hypocalcemia, soft tissue calcification, and impaired renal function,[57] but none of these effects are observed during the treatment of hypophosphatemic osteomalacia. Although diarrhea is troublesome in some patients, the only serious complication of long-term treatment is the emergence of hypercalcemic hyperparathyroidism needing surgical intervention. This has been reported after 2 to 14 years of treatment in 13 cases, eight with XLH and five with nonfamilial hypophosphatemia, three with and two without a tumor.[443a,561] The parathyroid pathology has been variable but with a predominance of multiple gland involvement. The pathogenesis is probably similar to the tertiary hyperparathyroidism of long-standing vitamin D depletion (section II-F).

2. Calcitriol

The effect of vitamin D in a pharmacologic dose in a nondepleted subject is quite different from its effect in a physiologic dose in a depleted subject.[239] First, the 25- and 1α-hydroxylase enzymes are relatively inactive and are suppressed further by excess of the substrate so that the response is much slower in onset. Second, even when maximum response has been achieved, less of the absorbed calcium and phosphate is retained in bone and much more is excreted in the urine. Finally, when treatment is stopped, the effect may persist for many months because of the large capacity of body storage sites for calciferol and calcidiol. There may be only a modest or even no increase in plasma calcitriol but a substantial rise in plasma calcidiol,[562] probably sufficient to increase the occupancy of calcitriol receptors despite its much lower affinity. Although with careful attention to detail satisfactory results can be achieved with calciferol,[89,239,418] and early results in nonhereditary hypophosphatemia showed little advantage for 1α-hydroxylated compounds,[421,422] it is likely that with increasing experience and better definition of optimum dose requirements calcitriol (or alfacalcidol, which produces calcitriol after hepatic 25-hydroxylation) will be the vitamin D metabolite of choice in all forms of hypophosphatemic osteomalacia[37,197,442b,562,563] (Chapter 24).

In vitamin D–replete patients, calcitriol increases intestinal absorption of calcium and phosphate more reliably than calciferol, but its most important therapeutic effect is to increase the renal tubular reabsorption of phosphate with a consequent rise in plasma phosphate.[562] Although commonly attributed to suppression of PTH secretion,[197,563] it is more likely a direct renal tubular effect of supraphysiologic plasma levels of calcitriol[562] as occurs during the treatment of extrinsic vitamin D depletion.[550] In children, the doses needed to achieve this effect are in the range of 50 to 80 ng/kg/day, which corresponds to 2.5 to 5 μg/day (or 4 to 8 μg/day of alfacalcidol) for most adults, preferably administered at frequent short intervals because of the short half-life. Even though the hypercalciuric and hypercalcemic effects are partly neutralized by concurrent administration of phosphate, this is very close to the intoxicating dose, particularly as the osteomalacia heals, and frequent and meticulous supervision is essential. Once healing has been achieved, the dose can be reduced to a safer and more manageable level.[197,562] The need for such large doses with their attendant hazards should be considered only after smaller doses have proved ineffective, since healing and symptomatic relief can often be accomplished by a dose that increases calcium absorption without increasing phosphate reabsorption, together with an adequate phosphate supplement[179] (Chapter 24). Concurrent calciferol does not prevent phosphate-induced tertiary hyperparathyroidism, but the likely greater effectiveness of calcitriol in this respect[561] remains to be demonstrated.

Acknowledgments. Many colleagues, present and former, contributed to the data and concepts presented in this chapter, but two were indispensable. D.S. Rao performed almost all of the transiliac bone biopsies, demonstrating that in expert hands it can be one of the safest and least unpleasant of all invasive procedures. A.R. Villanueva performed almost all the bone histomorphometry, with results that are a testament to his insight, skill, and experience.

References

1. Morgan DB: Osteomalacia, renal osteodystrophy and osteoporosis. Springfield, Charles C Thomas, 1973.
2. Dent CE, Stamp TCB: Vitamin D, rickets and osteomalacia. *In* Avioli LV, Krane SM (eds): Metabolic Bone Disease, vol 1. New York, Academic Press, 1977.
3. Aaron J: Histological aspects of the relationship between vitamin D and bone. *In* Lawson DEM (ed): Vitamin D. London, Academic Press, 1978.
4. Parfitt AM, Duncan, H: Metabolic bone disease affecting the spine. *In* Rothman R, Simeone F (eds): The Spine. 2nd ed. Philadelphia, W.B. Saunders, 1982, pp 775–905.
5. Parfitt AM, Gallagher JC, Heaney RP, et al: Vitamin D and bone health in the elderly. Am J Clin Nutr 36:1014–1031, 1982.
5a. Clements MR, Johnson L, Fraser DR: A new mechanism for induced vitamin D deficiency in calcium deprivation. Nature 325:62–65, 1987.
6. Maxwell JP, Miles LM: Osteomalacia in China. J Obstet Gynecol Br Empire 32:433–473, 1925.
7. Rizvi SNA, Vaishnava H: Occult osteomalacia in pregnant women in India. Lancet 1:1102, 1977.
8. Stanbury SW: Osteomalacia. Clin Endocrinol Metab 1:239–266, 1972.
9. Frame B, Parfitt AM: Osteomalacia: Current concepts. Ann Intern Med 89:966–982, 1978.
10. Arnstein AR, Frame B, Frost HM: Recent progress in osteomalacia and rickets. Ann Intern Med 67:1296–1330, 1967.
11. Avioli LV, Baran DT, Whyte MP, et al: The biochemical and skeletal heterogeneity of "post-menopausal osteoporosis." *In* Barzel US (ed): Osteoporosis II. New York, Grune & Stratton, 1978, pp 49–64.
12. Meunier PJ: Bone biopsy in diagnosis of metabolic bone disease. *In* Cohn DV, Talmage RV, Mathews JL (eds): Hormonal Control of Calcium Metabolism. Amsterdam, Excerpta Medica, 1981.
13. Parfitt AM: Bone fragility in osteomalacia: Mechanisms and consequences. *In* Uhthoff H (ed): Current Concepts of Bone Fragility. New York, Springer-Verlag, 1986, pp 265–270.
14. Parfitt AM: Accelerated cortical bone loss: Primary and secondary hyperparathyroidism. *In* Uhthoff H (ed): Current Concepts of Bone Fragility. New York, Springer-Verlag, 1986, pp 279–285.
15. Parfitt AM, Mathews C, Rao D, et al: Impaired osteoblast function in metabolic bone disease. *In* DeLuca HF, Frost H, Jee W, et al (eds): Osteoporosis: Recent Advances in Pathogenesis and Treatment. Baltimore, University Park Press, 1981, pp 321–330.
16. Rao DS, Villanueva A, Mathews M, et al: Histologic evolution of vitamin depletion in patients with intestinal malabsorption or dietary deficiency. *In* Frame B, Potts JT Jr (eds): Clinical Disorders of Bone and Mineral Metabolism. Amsterdam, Excerpta Medica, 1983, pp 224–226.
17. Parfitt AM: The physiologic and clinical significance of bone histomorphometric data. *In* Recker R (ed): Bone Histomorphometry. Techniques and Interpretations. Boca Raton, CRC Press, 1983, pp 143–223.
18. Villanueva AR, Kujawa M, Mathews CHE, Parfitt AM: Identification of the mineralization front: Comparison of a modified toluidine blue stain with tetracycline fluorescence. Metab Bone Dis Rel Res 5:41–45, 1983.
19. Schwartz MP, Recker RR: Comparison of surface density and volume of human iliac trabecular bone measured directly and by applied stereology. Calcif Tissue Int 33:561–565, 1981.
20. Hori M, Takahashi H, Konno T, et al: A classification of in vivo bone labels after double labeling in canine bones. Bone 6:147–154, 1985.
20a. Parfitt AM, Drezner MK, Glorieux FH, et al: Bone histomorphometry nomenclature, symbols and units. Report of the ASBMR Histomorphometry Nomenclature Committee. J Bone Mineral Res 2:595–610, 1987.
20b. Schaffler MB, Burr DB, Frederickson RG: Morphology of the osteonal cement line in human bone. Anat Rec 217:223–228, 1987.
21. Villanueva AR, Sypitkowski C, Parfitt AM: A new method for identification of cement lines in undecalcified, plastic embedded sections of bone. Stain Tech 81:83–88, 1986.
22. Parfitt AM: The cellular basis of bone remodeling. The quantum concept re-examined in light of recent advances in cell biology of bone. Calcif Tissue Int 36:S37–S45, 1984.
23. Parfitt AM, Villanueva AR, Mathews CHE, Aswani JA: Kinetics of matrix and mineral apposition in osteoporosis and renal osteodystrophy: Relationship to rate of turnover and to cell morphology. *In* Jee WSS, Parfitt AM (eds): Bone Histomorphometry: Third International Workshop. Paris, Armour-Montagu, 1981, pp 213–219.

24. Eriksen EF, Gundersen HJG, Melsen F, Mosekilde L: Reconstruction of the formative site in iliac trabecular bone in 20 normal individuals employing a kinetic model for matrix and mineral apposition. Metab Bone Dis Rel Res 5:243–252, 1984.
25. Baylink D, Stauffer M, Wergedal J, Rich C: Formation, mineralization and resorption of bone in vitamin D–deficient rats. J Clin Invest 49:1122–1134, 1970.
26. Baylink DJ, Morey EM, Ivey JL, Stauffer ME: Vitamin D and bone. *In* Norman AW (ed): Vitamin D. Molecular Biology and Clinical Nutrition. New York, Marcel Dekker, 1980.
27. Marel GM, McKenna MJ, Frame B: Osteomalacia. *In* Peck WA (ed): Bone and Mineral Research 4. Amsterdam, Elsevier, 1986, pp 335–412.
28. Parfitt AM: Bone and plasma calcium homeostasis. Bone 8:51–58, 1987.
29. Stauffer M, Baylink D, Wergedal J, Rich C: Decreased bone formation, mineralization, and enhanced resorption in calcium-deficient rats. Am J Physiol 225:269–276,1975.
30. Parfitt AM: The cellular mechanisms of osteoid accumulation in metabolic bone disease. *In* Mineral Metabolism Research in Italy, vol 4. Milano, Wichtig Editore, 1984, pp 3-9.
31. Parfitt AM, Podenphant J, Villanueva AR, Frame B: Metabolic bone disease with and without osteomalacia after intestinal bypass surgery: A bone histomorphometric study. Bone 6:211–220, 1985.
32. Parfitt AM, Mathews CHE, Villanueva AR, et al: Microstructural and cellular basis of age related bone loss and osteoporosis. *In* Frame B, Potts JT Jr (eds): Clinical Disorders of Bone and Mineral Metabolism. Amsterdam, Excerpta Medica, 1983, pp 328–332.
33. Melsen F, Mosekilde L: Trabecular bone mineralization lag time determined by tetracycline double-labeling in normal and certain pathological conditions. Acta Pathol Microbiol Scand [A], pp 88:83-88, 1980.
34. Meunier PJ, Van Linthoudt D, Edouard C, et al: Histological analysis of the mechanisms underlying pathogenesis and healing of osteomalacia. Proceedings, Sixteenth European Calcified Tissue Symposium, 1981, Abstracts 771–774.
35. Boyce BF, Smith L, Fogelman I, et al: Focal osteomalacia due to low-dose diphosphonate therapy in Paget's disease. Lancet 1:821–824, 1984.
36. Teitelbaum SL: Pathological manifestations of osteomalacia and rickets. Clin Endocrinol Metab 9:43–62, 1980.
37. Peacock M: Osteomalacia and rickets. *In* Nordin BEC (ed): Metabolic Bone and Stone Disease. Edinburgh, Churchill-Livingstone, 1984.
38. Hodson CJ: Metabolic and endocrine-induced bone disease. *In* Shanks SC, Kerley P (eds): A Text-book of X-ray Diagnosis by British Authors. 4th ed. Philadelphia, W.B. Saunders, 1971, pp 649-670.
39. Smith R: The pathophysiology and management of rickets. Orthop Clin North Am 3:601–621, 1972.
40. Hurwitz LJ, Banerji NK: Basilar impression of the skull in patients with adult coeliac disease and after gastric surgery. J Neurol Neurosurg Psychiatry 35:92–96, 1972.
41. Snapper I. Medical Clinics on Bone Diseases. 2nd ed. New York, Interscience, 1949.
42. Fairbank HAT: An Atlas of General Affections of the Skeleton. Edinburgh, E & S Livingstone, 1951.
42a. Huaux JP, Malghem J, Maldague B, et al: Reflex sympathetic dystrophy syndrome: An unusual mode of presentation of osteomalacia. Arthritis Rheum 29:918–925, 1986.
42b. Gerster JC, Jaeger P, Gobelet C, Boivin G: Adult sporadic hypophosphatemic osteomalacia presenting as regional migratory osteoporosis. Arthritis Rheum 29:688–692, 1986.
43. Knapp MS, Gough KR: An unusual neurological manifestation of hypocalcaemia. Lancet 1:475–477, 1967.
44. Brookes GB, Morrison AW: Vitamin D deficiency and deafness. Br Med J 283:273–274, 1981.
45. Rose GA, Lumb FH, Dent CE: Discussion on generalized aches and pain from metabolic bone diseases. Proc R Soc Med 50:371–380, 1957.
46. Dent CE, Watson L: Osteoporosis. Postgrad Med J 42[Suppl]:582–608, 1966.
47. Stamp TCB, Walker PG, Perry W, Jenkins MV: Nutritional osteomalacia and late rickets in greater London 1974–1979: Clinical and metabolic studies in 45 patients. Clin Endocrinol Metab 9:81–105, 1980.
48. Rao DS, Parfitt AM, Kleerekoper M, et al: Dissociation between the effects of endogenous parathyroid hormone on cAMP generation and on phosphate reabsorption in hypocalcemia due to vitamin D depletion: An acquired disorder resembling pseudohypoparathyroidism type II. J Clin Endocrinol Metab 61:285–290, 1985.
49. Parfitt AM: H.I. Chu: Pioneer clinical investigator of vitamin D deficiency and osteomalacia in China. A scientific and personal tribute (editorial). Calcif Tissue Int 37:335–339, 1985.
50. Young A, Edwards RHT, Jones DA, Brenton DP: Quadriceps muscle strength and fibre size during the treatment of osteomalacia. *In* Stokes IAF (ed): Mechanical Factors and the Skeleton. London, John Libbey, 1981, pp 137–145.
51. Schott GD, Wills MR: Muscle weakness in osteomalacia. Lancet 1:626–629, 1976.
52. Skaria J, Katiyar BC, Srivastava TP, Dube B: Myopathy and neuropathy associated with osteomalacia. Acta Neurol Scand 51:37–58, 1975.
53. Mallette LE, Patten BM, Engel WK: Neuromuscular disease in secondary hyperparathyroidism. Ann Intern Med 82:474–483, 1975.
54. Swash M, Schwartz MS, Sargeant MK: Osteomalacic myopathy: An experimental approach. Neuropathol Appl Neurobiol 5:295–302, 1979.
55. Banerji NK, Hurwitz LJ: Neurological manifestations in adult steatorrhoea (probable gluten enteropathy). J Neurol Sci 14:125–141, 1971.
56. Banerji NK, Hurwitz LJ: Nervous system manifestations after gastric surgery. Acta Neurol Scand 47:485–513, 1971.
57. Parfitt AM, Kleerekoper M: Clinical disorders of calcium, phosphorus and magnesium metabolism. *In* Maxwell M, Kleeman CR (eds): Clinical Disorders of Fluid and Electrolyte Metabolism. 3rd ed. New York, McGraw- Hill, 1980, pp 947-1152.
58. Smith R, Newman RJ, Radda GK, et al: Hypophosphataemic osteomalacia and myopathy: Studies with nuclear magnetic resonance spectroscopy. Clin Science 67:505–509, 1984.
59. Stroder J: The content of actomyosin in the skeletal muscle of rats with experimentally induced rickets. Helv Paediatr Acta 21:323–326, 1966.

60. Hodsman AB, Sherrard DJ, Wong EGC, et al: Vitamin-D-resistant osteomalacia in hemodialysis patients lacking secondary hyperparathyroidism. Ann Intern Med 94:629–637, 1981.
61. Wills MR, Savory J: Aluminium poisoning: Dialysis encephalopathy, osteomalacia and anaemia. Lancet 2:29–34, 1983.
62. Peach H, Compston JE, Vedi S: Value of the history in diagnosis of histological osteomalacia among Asians presenting to the NHS. Lancet 2:1347–1349, 1983.
63. Parfitt AM, Rao DS, Stanciu J, et al: Irreversible bone loss in osteomalacia: Comparison of radial photon absorptiometry with iliac bone histomorphometry during treatment. J Clin Invest 76:2403–2412, 1985.
64. Raina V: Rickets and osteomalacia—A morphological study. Indian J Med Res 61:190–194, 1973.
65. Frost HM: The dynamics of human osteoid tissue. *In* Hioco DJ (ed): L'Osteomalacie. Paris, Masson & Cie, 1967, pp 3–18.
66. Juster M, Oligo N, Laval-Jeantet M: Lisere preosseux et tissu osteoide. *In* Hioco DJ (ed): L'Osteomalacie. Paris, Masson & Cie, 1967, pp 39–63.
67. Steendijk R, Boyde A: Scanning electron microscopic observations on bone from patients with hypophosphatemic (vitamin D resistant) rickets. Calcif Tissue Res 11:242–250, 1973.
68. Ball J, Garner A: Mineralisation of woven bone in osteomalacia. J Pathol Bacteriol 91:563–567, 1966.
69. Rasmussen H, Bordier PJ: The Physiological and Cellular Basis of Metabolic Bone Disease. Baltimore, Williams and Wilkins, 1974.
70. Bonucci E, Matrajt H, Tunchot S, Hioco DJ: Bone structure in osteomalacia with special reference to ultrastructure. J Bone Joint Surg 51B:511–527, 1969.
71. Qiu M-C, Mathews C, Parfitt AM: Osteoclastic resorption of osteoid in secondary hyperparathyroidism. *In* Frame B, Potts JT Jr (eds): Clinical Disorders of Bone and Mineral Metabolism. Amsterdam, Exerpta Medica, 1983, pp 209–212.
72. Bar-Shavit Z, Kahn AJ, Teitelbaum SL: Defective binding of macrophages to bone in rodent osteomalacia and vitamin D deficiency. J Clin Invest 72:526–534, 1983.
73. Byers PD: The diagnostic value of bone biopsies in metabolic bone disease. *In* Avioli LV, Krane SM (eds): Metabolic Bone Disease, vol 1. New York, Academic Press, 1977.
74. Schenk RK, Olah AJ: What is osteomalacia? Adv Exp Biol Med 128:549–562, 1980.
75. Hodsman AB, Sherrard DJ, Alfrey AC, et al: Bone aluminum and histomorphometric features of renal osteodystrophy. J Clin Endocrinol Metab 54:539–546, 1982.
76. Ellis HA: Aluminum induced osteomalacia in patients with chronic renal failure and in animals. Nieren- und Hochdruckkrankheiten 12:S198–206, 1983.
77. Parfitt AM: The clinical and radiographic manifestations of renal osteodystrophy. *In* David DJ (ed): Perspectives in Hypertension and Nephrology: Calcium Metabolism in Renal Failure and Nephrolithiasis. New York, John Wiley, 1977, pp 145–195.
78. Anton HC: Width of clavicular cortex in osteoporosis. Br Med J 1:409–411, 1969.
79. Meema HE: Recognition of cortical bone resorption in metabolic bone disease in vivo. Skeletal Radiol 2:11–19, 1977.
80. Meema HE, Meema S: Improved roentgenologic diagnosis of osteomalacia by microradioscopy of hand bones. Radiology 125:925–935, 1975.
81. Wilson JS, Genant HK: In vivo assessment of bone metabolism using the cortical striation index. Invest Radiol 14:131–136, 1979.
82. Steinbach HL, Noetzli M: Roentgen appearance of the skeleton in osteomalacia and rickets. Am J Roentgenol 91:955–972, 1964.
83. Devlin JG, O'Donovan DK: Occult malabsorption causing osteitis fibrosa cystica. Acta Endocrinol 40:481–492, 1962.
84. Burkholder PK, DuBoff EA, Filmanowicz EV: Nontropical sprue with secondary hyperparathyroidism. A case report and review of the literature. Am J Dig Dis 10:75–85, 1965.
85. Ehrlich GW, Genant HK, Kolb FO: Secondary hyperparathyroidism and brown tumors in a patient with gluten enteropathy. Am J Roentgenol 141:381–383, 1983.
86. Bennett TI, Hunter D, Vaughan JM: Idiopathic steatorrhoea (Gee's disease). A nutritional disturbance associated with tetany, osteomalacia and anaemia. Q J Med 1:603–677, 1932.
87. Dent CE, Hodson CJ: Generalised softening of bone due to metabolic causes. II. Radiological changes associated with certain metabolic bone diseases. Br J Radiol 27:605–617, 1954.
88. Bible MW, Pinals RS, Palmieri GMA, Pitcock JA: Protrusio acetabuli in osteoporosis and osteomalacia. Clin Exp Rheumatol 1:323–326, 1983.
89. Parfitt AM: Hypophosphatemic vitamin D refractory rickets and osteomalacia. Orthop Clin North Amer 3:653–680, 1972.
89a. McKenna MJ, Kleerekoper M, Ellis BI, et al: Atypical insufficiency fractures confused with Looser zones of osteomalacia. Bone 8:71–78, 1987.
90. Steinbach HL, Kolb FO, Gilfillan R: A mechanism of the production of pseudofractures in osteomalacia (Milkman's syndrome). Radiology 62:388–394, 1964.
91. Simpson W, Young JR, Clark F: Pseudofractures resembling stress fractures in Punjabi immigrants with osteomalacia. Clin Radiol 24:83–89, 1973.
92. Macfarlane JD, Lutkin JE, Burwood RJ: The demonstration by scintigraphy of fractures in osteomalacia. Br J Radiol 50:369–371, 1977.
93. Parfitt AM, Oliver I, Villanueva AR: Bone histology in metabolic bone disease. The diagnostic value of bone biopsy. Orthop Clin North Am 10:329–346, 1979.
94. Chalmers J: Subtrochanteric fractures in osteomalacia. J Bone Joint Surg 52B:509–513, 1970.
95. Campbell AER: Haemothorax and osteomalacia. Lancet 2:542–543, 1965.
96. Chalmers J: Osteomalacia. J R Coll Surg Edinb 13:255–275, 1968.
97. Chalmers J, Barclay A, Davison AM, et al: Quantitative measurements of osteoid in health and disease. Clin Orthop 63:196–209, 1969.
98. Anderson J, Bannister DW, Parsons V, Tomlinson RWS: Total urinary hydroxyproline excretion in osteomalacia. Calcif Tissue Res 1:183–191, 1967.
99. Smith R, Dick M: Total urinary hydroxyproline in osteomalacia and the effect upon it of treatment with vitamin D. Clin Sci 34:43–56, 1968.
100. Heaney RP: Interpretation of kinetic studies in dis-

orders of mineralization. *In* Hioco DJ (ed): L'Osteomalacie. Paris, Masson & Cie, 1967, pp 239–247.

101. Nordin BEC, Smith DA: Pathogenesis and treatment of osteomalacia. *In* Hioco DJ (ed): L'Osteomalacie. Paris, Masson & Cie, 1967, pp 379–399.
102. Joplin GF, Robinson CJ, Melvin KEW, et al: Results of tracer studies in osteomalacia. *In* Hioco DJ (ed): L'Osteomalacie. Paris, Masson & Cie, 1967, pp 249–256.
103. Melvin KEW, Hepner GW, Bordier P, et al: Calcium metabolism and bone pathology in adult coeliac disease. Q J Med 3:83–113, 1970.
104. Fogelman I, Bessent RG, Turner JG, et al: The use of whole-body retention of Tc-99m diphosphonate in the diagnosis of metabolic bone disease. J Nucl Med 19:270–275, 1978.
105. MacFarlane JD, Khairi MRA, Ricciardone M, et al: Renal excretion of ^{99m}Tc-diphosphonate in osteomalacia. Ann Intern Med 90:350–351, 1979.
106. Knop J, Kröger E, Stritzke P, et al: Deconvolution analysis of ^{99m}Tc-methylene diphosphonate kinetics in metabolic bone disease. Eur J Nucl Med 6:63–67, 1981.
107. Tellez M, Wootton R, Reeve J: Skeletal blood flow measured with ^{18}F in patients with osteomalacia and hyperparathyroidism. Eur J Nucl Med 8:299–302, 1983.
108. Kaye M, Silverton S, Rosenthall L: Technetium-99m-pyrophosphate: Studies in vivo and in vitro. J Nucl Med 16:40–45, 1975.
109. Botella J, Gallego JL, Fernandez-Fernandez J, et al: The bone scan in patients with aluminium-associated bone disease. Proc EDTA-ERA 21:403–409, 1984.
110. Leading article: Vitamin-D deficiency, bone turnover, and urinary hydroxyproline. Lancet 1:1018–1019, 1968.
111. Saville PD, Alderman MH: Deficiency rickets in New York. Dissociation between urinary hydroxyproline and glycylproline with treatment. Arch Intern Med 125:341–343, 1970.
112. Stepan J, Pacovsky V, Horn V, et al: Relationship of the activity of the bone isoenzyme of serum alkaline phosphatase to urinary hydroxyproline excretion in metabolic and neoplastic bone disease. Eur J Clin Invest 8:373–377, 1978.
113. Thalassinos NC, Wicht S, Joplin GF: Secondary hyperparathyroidism in osteomalacia. Br Med J 1:76–79, 1970.
114. Compston JE, Vedi S, Merrett AL, et al: Privational and malabsorption metabolic bone disease: Plasma vitamin D metabolite concentrations and their relationship to quantitative bone histology. Metab Bone Dis Rel Res 3:165–170, 1981.
115. Stanbury SW: Vitamin D and calcium metabolism. *In* Norman AW (ed): Vitamin D. Molecular Biology and Clinical Nutrition. New York, Marcel Dekker, 1980.
116. Fraser D, Kooh SW, Scriver CR: Hyperparathyroidism as the cause of hyperaminoaciduria and phosphaturia in human vitamin D deficiency. Pediatr Res 1:425–435, 1967.
117. Vainsel M, Manderlier T, Corvilain J, Vis HL: Study of the secondary hyperparathyroidism in vitamin D deficiency rickets. I. Aspects of mineral metabolism. Biomedicine 21:368–371, 1974.
118. Stanbury SW: Vitamin D and hyperparathyroidism. J R Coll Physicians Lond 15:205–217, 1981.
119. Dandona P, Mohiuddin J, Weerakoon JW, et al: Persistence of parathyroid hypersecretion after vitamin D treatment in Asian vegetarians. J Clin Endocrinol Metab 59:535–537, 1984.
120. Albright F, Reifenstein EG: The parathyroid glands and metabolic bone disease. Selected studies. Baltimore, Williams and Wilkins, 1984.
121. Jubiz W, Haussler MR, McCain TA, Tolman KG: Plasma 1,25 dihydroxyvitamin D levels in patients receiving anticonvulsant drugs. J Clin Endocrinol Metab 44:617–621, 1977.
122. Madsen S, Olgaard K, Ladefoged J: Suppressive effect of 1,25-dihydroxyvitamin D_3 on circulating parathyroid hormone in acute renal failure. J Clin Endocrinol Metab 53:823–827, 1981.
123. Slatopolsky E, Weerts C, Thielan J, et al: Marked suppression of secondary hyperparathyroidism by intravenous administration of 1,25-dihydroxycholecalciferol in uremic patients. J Clin Invest 74:2136–2143, 1984.
124. Muldowney FP, Freaney R, McGeeney D: Renal tubular acidosis and aminoaciduria in osteomalacia of dietary or intestinal origin. Q J Med 37:517–539, 1968.
125. Bordier P, Rasmussen H, Marie P, et al: Vitamin D metabolites and bone mineralization in man. J Clin Endocrinol Metab 46:284–294, 1978.
126. Peach H, Compston JE, Vedi S, Horton LWL: Value of plasma calcium, phosphate, and alkaline phosphatase measurements in the diagnosis of histological osteomalacia. J Clin Pathol 35:625–630, 1982.
127. Salvesen HA, Boe J: Osteomalacia in sprue. Acta Med Scand 146;296–299, 1953.
128. Fourman P, Haapanen E: Parathyroid function in steatorrhoea with osteomalacia. Schweiz Med Wochenschr 94:886–891, 1964.
129. Bernstein D, Kleeman CR, Dowling JT, Maxwell MH: Steatorrhea, functional hypoparathyroidism, and metabolic bone defect. Arch Intern Med 109:43–49, 1962.
130. Stanbury SW, Lumb GA: Vitamin D. Clinical problems. Parathyroid function in chronic vitamin D deficiency in man: A model for comparison with chronic renal failure. Calcif Tissue Res 21[Suppl]:185–201, 1976.
131. Kanis JA, Walton RJ: Osteomalacia associated with increased renal tubular resorption of phosphate (hypohyperparathyroidism). Postgrad Med J 52: 295–297, 1976.
132. Dandona P, Freedman DB, Mohiuddin J, et al: Hyperphosphataemic rickets: A new variant. Br Med J 287:1765, 1983.
133. Sisson de Castro JA, Tucci JR: Extracellular cyclic AMP levels in osteomalacia. Acta Endocrinol 95:282–288, 1980.
134. Lewin IG, Papapoulos SE, Hendy GN, et al: Reversible resistance to the renal action of parathyroid hormone in human vitamin D deficiency. Clin Sci 62:381–387, 1982.
135. Muldowney FP, McKenna TJ, Kyle LH, et al: Parathormone-like effect of magnesium replenishment in steatorrhea. N Engl J Med 282:61–68, 1970.
136. Marshall DH: Calcium and phosphate kinetics. *In* Nordin BEC (ed): Calcium, Phosphate and Magnesium Metabolism. Edinburgh, Churchill-Livingstone, 1976.
137. Arnaud SB, Young DR, Berry P, Brown S: Nor-

mocalcemic and hypocalcemic vitamin D deficiency (-D) in the adult rhesus monkey. Abstracts of Annual Meeting of Endocrine Society, 1986.

138. Stern PH, Halloran BP, DeLuca HF, Hefley TJ: Responsiveness of vitamin D–deficient fetal rat limb bones to parathyroid hormone in culture. Am J Physiol 244 (Endocrinol Metab 7):E421–E424, 1983.

139. Vaishnava H, Rizvi SNA: Primary hyperparathyroidism associated with nutritional osteomalacia. Am J Med 46:640–644, 1969.

140. Teotia SPS, Teotia M: Hypercalcemic (tertiary) hyperparathyroidism in patients of longstanding vitamin D deficiency osteomalacia. *In* Teotia SPS, Teotia M (eds): Advances in Hormone, Bone and Mineral Metabolism. Proceedings of the Mid Term Conference of the Endocrine Society of India, Meerut, August 27-29, 1984, pp 111–118.

141. Smith JF: Parathyroid adenomas associated with the malabsorption syndrome and chronic renal disease. J Clin Pathol 23:362–369, 1970.

142. Parfitt AM: Hypercalcemic hyperparathyroidism following renal transplantation: Differential diagnosis, management, and implications for cell population control in the parathyroid gland. Mineral Electrolyte Metab 8:92–112, 1982.

143. Jackson CE: The two-hit theory of neoplasia: Implications for the pathogenesis of hyperparathyroidism. Cancer Genet and Cytogenet 14:175–178, 1985.

143a. Clements MR, Davies M, Fraser DR, et al: Metabolic inactivation of vitamin D is enhanced in primary hyperparathyroidism. Clin Sci 73:659–664, 1987.

144. Dent CE, Jones PE, Mullan DP: Masked primary (or tertiary) hyperparathyroidism. Lancet 1:1161–1164, 1975.

145. Hodkinson HM, Hodkinson I: A discriminant function for the biochemical diagnosis of osteomalacia in elderly subjects and its relevance to interpretation of borderline bone histological findings. J Clin Exp Gerontol 2:123–131, 1980.

146. McKenna MJ, Freaney R, Casey OM, et al: Osteomalacia and osteoporosis: Evaluation of a diagnostic index. J Clin Pathol 36:245–252, 1983.

146a. Nussbaum SR, Zahradnik RJ, Lavigne JR, et al: Highly sensitive two-site immunoradiometric assay of parathyrin, and its clinical utility in evaluating patients with hypercalcemia. Clin Chem 8:1364–1367, 1987.

147. Davie M, Lawson DEM, Jung RT: Low plasma-25-hydroxyvitamin D without osteomalacia. Lancet 1:820, 1978.

148. MacLennan WJ, Hamilton JC: Low plasma-25-hydroxyvitamin D without osteomalacia. Lancet 1:1210, 1978.

149. Kafetz K, Hodkinson HM: Osteomalacia in presence of "normal" serum 25-hydroxycholecalciferol concentration. Br Med J 283:1437–1438, 1981.

150. Hodkinson HM, Hodkinson I: Range for 25-hydroxy vitamin D in elderly subjects in whom osteomalacia has been excluded on histological and biochemical criteria. J Clin Exp Gerontol 2:133–139, 1980.

151. Hodkinson HM: Biochemical diagnosis of the elderly. London, Chapman and Hall, 1977, pp 53–66.

151a. Editorial. Acquired vitamin D deficiency and hyperparathyroidism. Lancet 1:451–452, 1988.

152. Bouillon R, Van Baelen H: Transport of vitamin D: Significance of free and total concentrations of the vitamin D metabolites. Calcif Tissue Int 33:451–453, 1981.

153. Bikle DD, Siiteri PK, Ryzen E, Haddad JG: Serum protein binding of 1,25-dihydroxyvitamin D: A reevaluation by direct measurement of free metabolite levels. J Clin Endocrinol Metab 61:969–975, 1985.

154. Mawer EB: Patterns of vitamin D metabolism in humans; relation to nutritional status. *In* Norman AW (ed): Vitamin D. Molecular Biology and Clinical Nutrition. New York, Marcel Dekker, 1980.

155. Fraser DR: The physiological economy of vitamin D. Lancet 1:969–972, 1983.

156. McKenna MJ, Freaney R, Meade A, Muldowney FP:Hypovitaminosis D and elevated serum alkaline phosphatase in elderly Irish people. Am J Clin Nutr 41:101–109, 1985.

157. Batchelor AJ, Watson G, Compston JE: Changes in plasma half-life and clearance of ^{3}H-25-hydroxyvitamin D, in patients with intestinal malabsorption. Gut 23:1068–1071, 1982.

158. Compston JE, Merrett AL, Ledger JE, Creamer B: Faecal tritium excretion after intravenous administration of ^{3}H-25-hydroxyvitamin D_3 in control subjects and in patients with malabsorption. Gut 23:310–315, 1982.

159. Rosenberg IH, Sitrin MD, Holt MJG: The enterohepatic circulation of vitamin D: Potential clinical implications. *In* Norman AW, Schaefer K, Herrath DV, et al (eds): Vitamin D, Basic Research and Its Clinical Application. Berlin, Walter de Gruyter, 1979, pp 487–492.

160. Clements MR, Chalmers TM, Fraser DR: Enterohepatic circulation of vitamin D: A reappraisal of the hypothesis. Lancet 1:1376–1379, 1984.

161. Jung RT, Davie M, Hunter JO, et al: Abnormal vitamin D metabolism in cirrhosis. Gut 19:290–293, 1978.

162. Hahn TJ: Drug-induced disorders of vitamin D and mineral metabolism. Clin Endocrinol Metab 9:107–129, 1980.

163. Malluche HH, Goldstein DA, Massry SG: Osteomalacia and hyperparathyroid bone disease in patients with nephrotic syndrome. J Clin Invest 63:494–500, 1979.

164. Goldstein DA, Haldimann B, Sherman D, et al: Vitamin D metabolites and calcium metabolism in patients with nephrotic syndrome and normal renal function. J Clin Endocrinol Metab 52:116–121, 1981.

165. Alon U, Chan JCM: Calcium and vitamin D homeostasis in the nephrotic syndrome: Current status (editorial). Nephron 36:1–4, 1984.

166. Liberman UA, Eil C, Marx SJ: Hereditary hypocalcemic vitamin D resistant rickets (HHDR). *In* Frame B, Potts JT Jr (eds): Clinical Disorders of Bone and Mineral Metabolism. Amsterdam, Excerpta Medica, 1983, pp 441–444.

167. Delvin EE, Glorieux FH, Marie PJ, Pettifor JM: Vitamin D dependency: Replacement therapy with calcitriol. J Pediatr 99:26–34. 1981.

168. Rude RK, Adams JS, Ryzen E, et al: Low serum concentrations of 1,25-dihydroxyvitamin D in human magnesium deficiency. J Clin Endocrinol Metab 61:933–940, 1985.

169. Drezner MK, Neelon FA, Jowsey J, Lebovitz HE: Hypoparathyroidism: A possible cause of osteomalacia. J Clin Endocrinol Metab 45:114–122, 1977.

170. Lyles KW, Burkes EJ Jr, McNamara CR, et al: The

concurrence of hypoparathyroidism provides new insights to the pathophysiology of X-linked hypophosphatemic rickets. J Clin Endocrinol Metab 60:711–717, 1985.

171. Epstein S, Meunier PJ, Lambert PW, et al: 1,25-dihydroxyvitamin D_3 corrects osteomalacia in hypoparathyroidism and pseudohypoparathyroidism. Acta Endocrinol 103:241–247, 1983.

172. Klein GL, Horst RL, Norman AW, et al: Reduced serum levels of 1,25-dihydroxyvitamin D during long-term total parenteral nutrition. Ann Intern Med 94:638–643, 1981.

173. Hirst MA, Hochman HI, Feldman D: Vitamin D resistance and alopecia: A kindred with normal 1,25-dihydroxyvitamin D binding, but decreased receptor affinity for deoxyribonucleic acid. J Clin Endocrinol Metab 60:490–495, 1985.

174. Parfitt AM, Kleerekoper M: The divalent ion homeostatic system: Physiology and metabolism of calcium, phosphorus, magnesium and bone. *In* Maxwell M, Kleeman CR (eds): Clinical Disorders of Fluid and Electrolyte Metabolism. 3rd ed. New York, McGraw-Hill, 1980, pp 269–398.

175. Godsall JW, Baron R, Insogna KL: Vitamin D metabolism and bone histomorphometry in a patient with antacid-induced osteomalacia. Am J Med 77:747–750, 1984.

176. Lyles KW, Clark AG, Drezner MK: Serum 1,25-dihydroxyvitamin D levels in subjects with X-linked hypophosphatemic rickets and osteomalacia. Calcif Tissue Int 34:125–130, 1982.

177. Tieder M, Samuel R, Liberman UA, et al: Hypercalciuric rickets: Metabolic studies and pathophysiological considerations. Nephron 39:194–200, 1985.

178. Ryan EA, Reiss E: Oncogenous osteomalacia. Review of the world literature of 42 cases and report of two new cases. Am J Med 77:501–512, 1984.

179. Rao DS, Parfitt AM, Villanueva AR, et al: Hypophosphatemic osteomalacia and adult Fanconi syndrome due to light-chain nephropathy: Another form of oncogenous osteomalacia. Am J Med 82:333–338, 1986.

180. Chesney RW: Etiology and pathogenesis of the Fanconi syndrome. Mineral Electrolyte Metab 4:303–316, 1980.

181. Chesney RW, Kaplan BS, Phelps M, DeLuca HF: Renal tubular acidosis does not alter circulating values of calcitriol. J Pediatr 104:51–55, 1984.

182. Woodhead JS, Ghose RR, Gupta SK: Severe hypophosphataemic osteomalacia with primary hyperparathyroidism. Br Med J 281:647–648, 1980.

183. Moorhead JF, Wills MR, Ahmed KY, et al: Hypophosphataemic osteomalacia after cadaveric renal transplantation. Lancet 1:694–697, 1974.

184. Boskey AL: Overview of cellular elements and macromolecules implicated in the initiation of mineralization. *In* Butler WT (ed): The Chemistry and Biology of Mineralized Tissues. Birmingham, AL, Ebsco Media, 1984, pp 335–343.

185. Glorieux FH, Marie PJ, Pettitfor JM, Delvin EE: Bone response to phosphate salts, ergocalciferol and calcitriol in hypophosphatemic vitamin D resistant rickets. N Engl J Med 303:1023–1031, 1980.

186. Stern PH: The D vitamins and bone. Pharmacol Rev 32:47–80, 1980.

187. Finkelman RD, Butler WT: Vitamin D and skeletal tissues. J Oral Pathol 14:191–215, 1985.

188. DeLuca HF, Schnoes HK: Vitamin D recent advances. Ann Rev Biochem 52:411–439, 1983.

189. Fourman P, Morgan DB: Effects of vitamin D in the human. *In* Nutritional Aspects of the Development of Bone and Connective Tissues. Nutritio et Dieta 13:30–43. Basel, Karger, 1969.

190. Rasmussen H: The role of $1{,}25(OH)_2D_3$ in the pathogenesis of osteomalacia. *In* Frame B, Potts JT Jr (eds): Clinical Disorders of Bone and Mineral Metabolism. Amsterdam, Excerpta Medica, 1983, pp 82–92.

191. Brommage R, DeLuca HF: Evidence that 1,25-dihydroxyvitamin D_3 is the physiologically active metabolite of vitamin D_3. Endocr Rev 6:491–511, 1985.

192. Kanis JA, Cundy T, Smith R, et al: Possible function of different renal metabolites of vitamin D in man. Contrib Nephrol 18:192–211, 1980.

193. Norman AW, Roth J, Orci L: The vitamin D endocrine system: Steroid metabolism, hormone receptors, and biological response (calcium binding proteins). Endocr Rev 3:331–366, 1982.

194. Popovtzer MM, Matthay R, Alfrey AC, et al: Vitamin D deficiency osteomalacia—Healing of the bone disease in the absence of vitamin D with intravenous calcium and phosphorus infusions. *In* Frame B, Parfitt AM, Duncan H (eds): Clinical Aspects of Metabolic Bone Disease. Amsterdam, Excerpta Medica, 1973, pp 382–387.

195. Weinstein RS, Underwood JL, Hutson MS, DeLuca HF: Bone histomorphometry in vitamin D–deficient rats infused with calcium and phosphorus. Am J Physiol 246:E499–E505, 1984.

196. Nagant de Deuxchaisnes C, Rombouts-Lindemans C, Huaux JP, et al: Healing of vitamin D–deficient osteomalacia by the administration of $1{,}25(OH)_2D_3$. *In* MacIntyre I, Szelke M (eds): Molecular Endocrinology. Amsterdam, Elsevier/North-Holland Biomedical Press, 1979, pp 375–404.

197. Peacock M, Heyburn PJ, Aaron JE, et al: Osteomalacia treated with 1α-hydroxyvitamin or 1,25 dihydroxy vitamin D. *In* Norman AW, Schaefer K, Herrath DV, et al (eds): Vitamin D. Basic Research and Its Clinical Application. Berlin, Walter de Gruyter, 1979, pp 1177–1183.

198. Stamp TCB, Perry W, MacArthur A, Jenkins MV: Treatment of privational late rickets and osteomalacia with the vitamin D. *In* Norman AW, Schaefer K, Herrath DV, et al (eds): Vitamin D. Basic Research and Its Clinical Applications. Berlin, Walter de Gruyter, 1979, pp 1153–1162.

199. Papapoulos SE, Clemens TL, Fraher LJ, et al: Metabolites of vitamin D in human vitamin D deficiency: Effect of vitamin D_3 or 1,25-dihydroxycholecalciferol. Lancet 2:612–615, 1980.

200. Stanbury SW, Taylor CM, Lumb GA, et al: Formation of vitamin D metabolites following correction of human vitamin D deficiency. Mineral Electrolyte Metab 5:212–227, 1981.

201. Parfitt AM, Mathews CHE, Brommage R, et al: Calcitriol but no other metabolite of vitamin D is essential for normal bone growth and development in the rat. J Clin Invest 73:576–586, 1984.

202. Lund B, Charles P, Egsmose C, et al: Changes in vitamin D metabolites and bone histology in rats during recovery from rickets. Calcif Tissue Int 37:478–483, 1985.

203. Rasmussen H, Baron R, Broadus A, et al:

$1,25(OH)_2D_3$ is not the only D metabolite involved in the pathogenesis of osteomalacia. Am J Med 69:360–368, 1980.

204. Parfitt AM, Villanueva AR: Hypophosphatemia and osteoblast function in human bone disease. *In* Massry SG, Letteri JM, Ritz E (eds): Proceedings, 5th International Workshop on Phosphate and Other Minerals. Regulation of Phosphate and Mineral Metabolism. Adv Exp Med Biol 151:209–216, 1982.
205. Markowitz ME, Rosen JF, Laxminarayan S, Mizruchi M: Circadian rhythms of blood minerals during adolescence. Pediatr Res 18:456–462, 1984.
206. Gundberg CM, Markowitz ME, Mizruchi M, Rosen JF: Osteocalcin in human serum: A circadian rhythm. J Clin Endocrinol Metab 60:736–739, 1985.
207. de Vernejoul MC, Marie PJ, Miravet L, Ryckewaert A: Chronic hypophosphatemia without osteomalacia. *In* Frame B, Potts JT Jr (eds): Clinical Disorders of Bone and Mineral Metabolism. Amsterdam, Excerpta Medica, 1983, pp 232–236.
208. Sebert JL, Meunier PJ: Role physiopathologique de la vitamine D et de ses metabolites dans l'osteomalacie. *In* Bouillon R, Boudailliez B, Marie A, et al (eds): Vitamine D et Maladies des Os et du Metabolisme Mineral. Paris, Masson, 1984, pp 109–145.
209. Bordier Ph J, Marie P, Miravet L, et al: Morphological and morphometrical characteristics of the mineralization front. A vitamin D regulated sequence of the bone remodeling. *In* Meunier PJ (ed): Bone Histomorphometry. Second International Workshop. Paris, Armour Montagu, 1976, pp 335–354.
210. Meunier PJ, Edouard C, Arlot M, et al: Effects of 1,25 dihydroxyvitamin D on bone mineralization. *In* MacIntyre I, Szelke M (eds): Molecular Endocrinology. Amsterdam, Elsevier/North-Holland Biomedical Press 1979, pp 283–292.
211. Marie PJ, Glorieux FH: Histomorphometric study of bone remodeling in hypophosphatemic vitamin D–resistant rickets. Metab Bone Dis Rel Res 3:31–38, 1981.
212. Manolagas SC, Haussler MR, Deftos LJ: 1,25-dihydroxyvitamin D_3 receptor-like macromolecule in rat osteogenic sarcoma cell lines. J Biol Chem 255:4414–4417, 1980.
213. Stumpf WE, Sar M, DeLuca HF: Sites of action of $1,25\ (OH)_2$ Vitamin D_3 identified by thaw-mount autoradiography. *In* Cohn DV, Talmage RV, Matthews JL: Hormonal Control of Calcium Metabolism. Amsterdam, Excerpta Medica, 1981, pp 222–229.
214. Manolagas SC, Burton DW, Deftos LJ: 1,25-Dihydroxyvitamin D_3 stimulates the alkaline phosphatase activity of osteoblast-like cells. J Biol Chem 256:7115–7117, 1981.
215. Lian JB, Coutts M, Canalis E: Studies of hormonal regulation of osteocalcin synthesis in cultured fetal rat calvariae. J Biol Chem 260:8706–8710, 1985.
216. Marie PJ, Hott M, Garba M-T: Contrasting effects of 1,25-dihydroxyvitamin D_3 on bone matrix and mineral appositional rates in the mouse. Metabolism 34:777–783, 1985.
217. Krempien B, Klimpel F: Action of 1,25-dihydroxycholecalciferol on cartilage mineralization and on endosteal lining cells of bone. Virchows Arch [A] 388:335–347, 1980.
218. Baylink D, Howard G, Ivey J, et al: Vitamin D and bone formation in mineralization. *In* Norman AW, Schaefer K, Herrath DV, Grigoleit H-G (eds): Vitamin D, Chemical, Biochemical and Clinical Endocrinology of Calcium Metabolism. Berlin, Walter de Gruyter, 1982, pp 363–368.
219. Hock JM, Gunness-Hey M, Poser J, et al: Stimulation of underminerlized matrix formation by pharmacologic doses of 1,25-dihydroxyvitamin D_3. Calcif Tissue Int 35:643(abstract), 1983.
220. Boyce RW, Weisbrode SE, Kindig O: Ultrastructural development of hyperosteoidosis in $1,25(OH)_2D_3$-treated rats fed high levels of dietary calcium. Bone 6:165–172, 1985.
220a. Davies M, Mawer EB, Freemont AJ: The osteodystrophy of hypervitaminosis D: A metabolic study. Q J Med, 234:911–919, 1986.
221. Eastwood JB, de Wardener HE, Gray RW, Lemann JL Jr: Normal plasma-$1,25\text{-}(OH)_2$-vitamin-D concentrations in nutritional osteomalacia. Lancet 1377–1378, 1979.
222. Kashiwa H, Nishi Y, Usui T, Seino Y: A case of rickets with normal serum level of $1,25\text{-}(OH)_2D$ and low 25-OHD. Hiroshima J Med Sci 30:61–63, 1981.
223. Chesney RW, Zimmerman J, Hamstra A, et al: Vitamin D metabolite concentrations in vitamin D deficiency. Are calcitriol levels normal? Am J Dis Child 135:1025–1028, 1981.
224. Adams JS, Clemens TL, Parrish JA, Holick MF: Vitamin-D synthesis and metabolism after ultraviolet irradiation of normal and vitamin D-deficient subjects. N Engl J Med 306:722–725, 1982.
225. Markestad T, Halvorsen S, Halvorsen KS, et al: Plasma concentrations of vitamin D metabolites before and during treatment of vitamin D deficiency rickets in children. Acta Paediatr Scand 73:225–231, 1984.
226. Nordin BEC, Heyburn PJ, Peacock M, et al: Osteoporosis and osteomalacia. Clin Endocrinol Metab 9:177–205, 1980.
227. Wahl TO, Gobuty AH, Lukert BP: Long-term anticonvulsant therapy and intestinal calcium absorption. Clin Pharmacol Ther 30:506–512, 1981.
228. Raisz LG, Trummel CL, Holick MF, DeLuca HF: 1,25-dihydroxycholecalciferol: A potent stimulator of bone resorption in tissue culture. Science 175:768–769, 1972.
229. Wilhelm F, Norman AW: Cooperativity in the binding of 1,25-dihydroxyvitamin D_3 to the chick intestinal receptor. FEBS 170:239–242, 1984.
230. Howard GA, Turner RT, Sherrard DJ, Baylink DJ: Human bone cells in culture metabolize 25-hydroxyvitamin D_3 to 1,25-dihydroxyvitamin D_3 and 24,25-dihydroxyvitamin D_3. J Biol Chem 256:7738–7740, 1981.
231. Puzas JE, Turner RT, Howard GA, Baylink DJ: Cells isolated from embryonic intestine sythesize 1,25-dihydroxyvitamin-D_3 and 24,25-dihydroxyvitamin-D_3 in culture. Endocrinology 112:378–380, 1983.
232. McDonald GB, Lau K-H W, Schy AL, et al: Intestinal metabolism and portal venous transport of $1,25(OH)_2D_3$, $25(OH)D_3$, and vitamin D_3 in the rat. Am J Physiol 248:G633–G638, 1985.
233. Groen JJ, Eshchar J, Ben-Ishay D, et al: Osteomalacia among the Bedouin of the Negev desert. Clinical and biochemical observations. Arch Intern Med 116:195–204, 1965.
234. Lawson DEM: Rickets and osteomalacia. Proc Nutr

Soc 43:249–256, 1984.

235. Preece MA, Tomlinson S, Ribot CA, et al: Studies of vitamin D deficiency in man. Q J Med 44:575–589, 1975.
236. O'Driscoll S, O'Driscoll M: Osteomalacia in rheumatoid arthritis. Ann Rheum Dis 39:1–6, 1980.
237. Dent CE, Smith R: Nutritional osteomalacia. Q J Med 38:195–209, 1969.
238. Elinson P, Neustadter LM, Moncman MG: Nutritional osteomalacia. Am J Dis Child 134:427, 1980.
239. Parfitt AM, Frame B: Drug treatment of rickets and osteomalacia. Semin Drug Treat 2:83–115, 1972.
240. Williams ED, Barr WT, Rajan KT, et al: Relative vitamin D deficiency in Paget's disease. Lancet 1:384–385, 1981.
241. Nagant de Deuxchaisnes C, Rombouts-Lindemans, Huaux JP, et al: Relative vitamin D deficiency in Paget's disease. Lancet 1:833–834, 1981.
242. Teotia M, Teotia SPS, Singh RK: Maternal hypovitaminosis and congenital rickets. Bull Inter Pediatr Assoc 3:39–46, 1979.
243. Howarth AT: Biochemical indices of osteomalacia in pregnant Asian immigrants in Britain. J Clin Pathol 29:981–983, 1976.
244. Parr JH, Ramsay I: The presentation of osteomalacia in pregnancy. Case report. Br J Obstet Gynaecol 91:816–818, 1984.
245. Marie PJ, Pettifor JM, Ross FP, Glorieux FH: Histological osteomalacia due to dietary calcium deficiency in children. N Engl J Med 307:584–588, 1982.
246. Berlyne GM, Ben Ari J, Nord E, Shainkin R: Bedouin osteomalacia due to calcium deprivation caused by high phytic acid content of unleavened bread. Am J Clin Nutr 26:910–911, 1973.
247. Robertson I, Ford JA, McIntosh WB, Dunnigan MG: The role of cereals in the aetiology of nutritional rickets: The lesson of the Irish Nutrition Survey 1943–8. Br J Nutr 45:17–22, 1981
248. Peach H: A review of aetiological and intervention studies on rickets and osteomalacia in the United Kingdom. Community Med 6:119–126, 1984.
249. Batchelor AJ, Compston JE: Reduced plasma half-life of radio-labelled 25-hydroxyvitamin D_3 in subjects receiving a high-fibre diet. Br J Nutr 49:213–216, 1983.
250. Marya RK, Saini AS, Rathee S, Arora SR: Osteomalacia in Hindu population of Haryana. Indian J Med Res 73:756–760, 1980.
250a. Henderson JB, Dunnigan MG, McIntosh WB, et al: The importance of limited exposure to ultraviolet radiation and dietary factors in the aetiology of asian rickets: A risk-factor model. Q J Med 241:413–425, 1987.
251. Stephens WP, Klimiuk PS, Warrington S, Taylor JL, et al: Observations on the natural history of vitamin D deficiency amongst Asian immigrants. Q J Med 51:171–188, 1982.
252. Peach H: A critique of survey methods used to measure the occurrence of osteomalacia and rickets in the United Kingdom. Community Med 6:20–28, 1984.
253. Francis RM, Peacock M, Storer JH, et al: Calcium malabsorption in the elderly: The effect of treatment with oral 25-hydroxyvitamin D_3. Eur J Clin Invest 13:391–396, 1983.
254. Anderson I, Campbell AER, Dunn A, Runciman JBM: Osteomalacia in elderly women. Scott Med J 11:429–435, 1966.
255. Hodkinson HM, Stanton BR, Round P, Morgan C: Sunlight, vitamin D, and osteomalacia in the elderly. Lancet 1:910–912, 1973.
256. Campbell GA, Kemm JR, Hosking DJ, Boyd RV: How common is osteomalacia in the elderly? Lancet 2:386–388, 1984.
257. Omdahl JL, Garry PJ, Hunsaker LA, et al: Nutritional status in a healthy elderly population: Vitamin D. Am J Clin Nutr 36:1225–1233, 1982.
257a. Kaplan FS, Soriano S, Fallon MD, Haddad JG: Osteomalacia in a night nurse. Clin Orthop Rel Res 205:216–221, 1986.
258. Barzel US: Vitamin D deficiency: A risk factor for osteomalacia in the aged. J Am Geriatr Soc 31:598–601, 1983.
259. Pittet PG, Davie M, Lawson DEM: Role of nutrition in the development of osteomalacia in the elderly. Nutr Metab 23:109–116, 1979.
260. Arnaud SB, Newcomer AD, Offord KP, Go VLW: 25-hydroxyvitamin D (25-OH-D) metabolism in nontropical sprue (NTS). *In* Norman AW, Schaefer K, Herrath DV, et al (eds): Vitamin D, Basic Research and Its Clinical Application. Berlin, Walter de Gruyter, 1979, pp 1023–1026.
261. Parfitt AM: Dietary risk factors for age-related bone loss and fractures. Lancet 2:1181–1184, 1983.
262. Meredith SC, Rosenberg IH: Gastrointestinal-hepatic disorders and osteomalacia. Clin Endocrinol Metab 9:131–150, 1980.
263. Davies M, Mawer EB, Krawitt EL: Comparative absorption of vitamin D_3, and 25-hydroxyvitamin D_3 in intestinal disease. Gut 21:287–292, 1980.
264. Maislos M, Silver J, Fainaru M: Intestinal absorption of vitamin D sterols: Differential absorption into lymph and portal blood in the rat. Gastroenterology 80:1528–1534, 1981.
265. Stamp TCB: Intestinal absorption of 25-hydroxycholecalciferol. Lancet 2:121–123, 1974.
266. Krawitt EL, Chastenay BF: 25-Hydroxy vitamin D absorption test in patients with gastrointestinal disorders. Calcif Tissue Int 32:183–187, 1980.
267. Rao DS: Bone and mineral metabolism. *In* Berk JE (ed): Bockus Gastroenterology, vol. 7. 4th ed. Philadelphia, W.B. Saunders, 1985, pp 4629-4638.
268. Parfitt AM, Miller MJ, Frame B, et al: Metabolic bone disease after intestinal bypass for treatment of obesity. Ann Intern Med 89:193–199, 1978.
269. Harris OD, Warner M, Cooke WT: Serum alkaline phosphatase in adult coeliac disease. Gut 10:655–658, 1969.
270. Compston JE, Vedi S, Gianetta E, et al: Bone histomorphometry and vitamin D status after biliopancreatic bypass for obesity. Gastroenterology 87:350–356, 1984.
271. Deller DJ, Begley MD: Calcium metabolism and the bones after partial gastrectomy. I. Clinical features and radiology of the bones. Australas Ann Med 12:282–294, 1983.
272. Nilsson BE, Westlin NE: The fracture incidence after gastrectomy. Acta Chir Scand 137:533–534, 1971.
273. Rao SD, Kleerekoper M, Rogers M, Frame B, Parfitt AM: Is gastrectomy a risk factor for osteoporosis? *In* Christiansen C, Arnaud CD, Nordin BEC, et al (eds): Osteoporosis. Proceedings of Copenhagen International Symposium on Osteoporosis, June 3–8, 1984, Aalborg Stiftsbortrykkeri, pp 775–777.
274. Hessov I, Mosekilde L, Melsen F, et al: Osteopenia with normal vitamin D metabolites after small-

bowel resection for Crohn's disease. Scand J Gastroenterol 19:691–696, 1984.
275. Matloff DS, Kaplan MM, Neer RM, et al: Osteoporosis in primary biliary cirrhosis: Effects of 25-hydroxyvitamin D_3 treatment. Gastroenterology 83:97–102, 1982.
276. Herlong HF, Recker RR, Maddrey WC: Bone disease in primary biliary cirrhosis: Histologic features and response to 25-hydroxyvitamin D. Gastroenterology 83:103–108, 1982.
277. Stellon AJ, Davies A, Compston J, Williams R: Osteoporosis in chronic cholestatic liver disease. Q J Med 223:783–790, 1985.
278. Bikle DD, Genant HK, Cann C, et al: Bone disease in alcohol abuse. Ann Intern Med 103:42–48, 1985.
279. Kunkle BN, Norrdin RW, Brooks RK, Thomassen RW: Osteopenia with decreased bone formation in beagles with malabsorption syndrome. Calcif Tissue Int 34:396–402, 1982.
280. Gertner JM, Lilburn M, Domenech M: 25-Hydroxycholecalciferol absorption in steatorrhoea and postgastrectomy osteomalacia. Br Med J 1:1310–1312, 1977.
281. Garrick R, Ireland AW, Posen S: Bone abnormalities after gastric surgery. Ann Intern Med 75:221–225, 1971.
282. Eddy RL: Metabolic bone disease after gastrectomy. Am J Med 50:442–449, 1971.
283. Nilas L, Christiansen C, Christiansen J: Regulation of vitamin D and calcium metabolism after gastrectomy. Gut 26,252–257, 1985.
284. Hahn TJ, Squires AE, Halstead LR, Strominger DB: Reduced serum 25-hydroxyvitamin D concentration and disordered mineral metabolism in patients with cystic fibrosis. J Pediatr 94:38–42, 1979.
285. Hanly JG, McKenna MJ, Quigley C, et al: Hypovitaminosis D and response to supplementation in older patients with cystic fibrosis. Q J Med 56:377–385, 1985.
286. Parfitt AM, Nassim JR, Collins J, Hilb A: Metabolic studies in a case of fibrocystic disease of the pancreas, in relation to treatment and to the incidence of bone disease. Arch Dis Child 37:25–33, 1962.
287. Scott J, Elias E, Moult PJA, et al: Rickets in adult cystic fibrosis with myopathy, pancreatic insufficiency and proximal renal tubular dysfunction. Am J Med 63:488–492, 1977.
288. Friedman HZ, Langman CB, Favus MJ: Vitamin D metabolism and osteomalacia in cystic fibrosis. Gastroenterology 88:808–813, 1985.
289. Compston JE, Horton LWL, Ayers AB, et al: Osteomalacia after small-intestinal resection. Lancet 1:9–12, 1978.
290. Driscoll RH Jr, Meredith SC, Sitrin MM, Rosenberg IH: Vitamin D deficiency and bone disease in patients with Crohn's disease. Gastroenterology 83:1252–1258, 1982.
291. Heaton KW, Lever JV, Barnard D: Osteomalacia associated with cholestyramine therapy for postileectomy diarrhea. Gastroenterology 2:642–646, 1972.
292. Compston JE, Horton LWL: Oral 25-hydroxyvitamin D_3 in treatment of osteomalacia associated with ileal resection and cholestyramine therapy. Gastroenterology 74:900–902, 1978.
293. Rickers H, Christiansen C, Balslev I, Rodbro P: Impairment of vitamin D metabolism and bone mineral content after intestinal bypass for obesity. A longitudinal study. Scand J Gastroenterol 19:184–189, 1984.
294. Rao DS, Marel G, Wong K, et al: Reversible and irreversible skeletal disease in adult coeliac disease. *In* Cohn DV, Potts JT Jr, Fujita T (eds): Endocrine Control of Bone and Calcium Metabolism. Amsterdam, Elsevier Science Publishers B.V., 1984, pp 279–280.
295. Mosekilde L, Melsen F, Hessov I, Bisballe S: Bone mass and bone remodeling in various gastro-intestinal disorders. *In* Cohn DV, Potts JT Jr, Fujita T (eds): Endocrine Control of Bone and Calcium Metabolism. Amsterdam, Elsevier Science Publishers B.V., 1984, pp 340–342.
296. Cooke WT, Holmes GKT: Coeliac disease. Edinburgh, Churchill Livingstone, 1984.
297. Rose GA: Some thoughts on osteoporosis and osteomalacia. Sc. Basis of Med Ann Rev 1967:252–275.
298. Nassim JR, Saville PD, Cook PB, Mulligan L: The effects of vitamin D and gluten-free diet in idiopathic steatorrhoea. Q J Med 28:141–162, 1959.
299. Zerwekh JE, Glass K, Jowsey J, Pak CYC: An unique form of osteomalacia associated with end organ refractoriness to 1,25-dihydroxyvitamin D and apparent defective synthesis of 25-hydroxyvitamin D. J Clin Endocrinol Metab 49:171–175, 1979.
300. Long RG: Hepatic osteodystrophy: Outlook good but some problems unsolved (editorial). Gastroenterology 78:644–647, 1980.
300a. Compston JE: Hepatic osteodystrophy: Vitamin D metabolism in patients with liver disease. Gut 27:1073–1090, 1986.
301. Saville PD: Alcohol and skeletal disease. *In* Lieber CS (ed): Metabolic Aspects of Alcoholism. Baltimore, University Park Press, 1977, pp 135–147.
301a. Feitelberg S, Epstein S, Ismail F, D'Amanda C: Deranged bone mineral metabolism in chronic alcoholism. Metabolism 36:322–326, 1987.
302. Bonjour JP: Vitamins and alcoholism. X. Vitamin D, XI. Vitamin E, XII. Vitamin K. Int J Vitam Nutr Res 51:307–318, 1981.
303. Arlot ME, Bonjean M, Chavassieux PM, Meunier PJ: Bone histology in adults with aseptic necrosis. J Bone Joint Surg 65A:1319–1327, 1983.
304. Posner DB, Russell RM, Absood S, et al: Effective 25-hydroxylation of vitamin D_2 in alcoholic cirrhosis. Gastroenterology 74:866–870, 1978.
305. Meyer M, Wechsler S, Shibolet S, et al: Malabsorption of vitamin D in man and rat with liver cirrhosis. J Mol Med 3:29–37, 1978.
306. Hepner GW, Roginsky M, Fai Moo H: Abnormal vitamin D metabolism in patients with cirrhosis. Dig Dis 21:527–532, 1976.
307. Imawari M, Akanuma Y, Itakura H, et al: The effects of diseases of the liver on serum 25-hydroxyvitamin D and on the serum binding protein for vitamin D and its metabolites. J Lab Clin Med 93:171–179, 1979.
308. Bouillon R, Auwerx J, Dekeyser L, et al: Serum vitamin D metabolites and their binding protein in patients with liver cirrhosis. J Clin Endocrinol Metab 59:86–89, 1984.
309. Lund B, Sorensen OH, Hilden M, Lund B: The hepatic conversion of vitamin D in alcoholics with varying degrees of liver affection. Acta Med Scand 202:221–224, 1977.
310. Chow LH, Frei JV, Hodsman AB, Valberg LS: Low serum 25-hydroxyvitamin D in hereditary hemo-

chromatosis: Relation to iron status. Gastroenterology 88:865–869, 1985.
311. Dibble JB, Sheridan P, Hampshire R, et al: Osteomalacia, vitamin D deficiency and cholestasis in chronic liver disease. Q J Med 51:89–103, 1982.
312. Compston JE, Thompson RPH: Intestinal absorption of 25-hydroxyvitamin D and osteomalacia in primary biliary cirrhosis. Lancet 1:721–724, 1977.
313. Barragry JM, Long RG, France MW, et al: Intestinal absorption of cholecalciferol in alcoholic liver disease and primary biliary cirrhosis. Gut 20:559–564, 1979.
314. Davies M, Mawer EB, Klass HJ, et al: Vitamin D deficiency, osteomalacia, and primary biliary cirrhosis. Response to orally administered vitamin D_3. Dig Dis Sci 28:145–153, 1983.
315. Jung RT, Davie M, Siklos P, et al: Vitamin D metabolism in acute and chronic cholestasis. Gut 20:840–847, 1979.
316. Bengoa JM, Sitrin MD, Meredith S, et al: Intestinal calcium absorption and vitamin D status in chronic cholestatic liver disease. Hepatology 4:261–265, 1984.
317. Compston JE, Horton LWL, Thompson RPH: Treatment of osteomalacia associated with primary biliary cirrhosis with parenteral vitamin D_2 or oral 25-hydroxyvitamin D_3. Gut 20:133–136, 1979.
318. Compston JE, Crowe JP, Horton LWL: Treatment of osteomalacia associated with primary biliary cirrhosis with oral 1-alpha-hydroxy vitamin D_3. Br Med J 2:309, 1979.
319. Compston JE, Crowe JP, Wells IP, et al: Vitamin D prophylaxis and osteomalacia in chronic cholestatic liver disease. Dig Dis Sci 25:28–32, 1980.
320. Danielson A, Lorentzon R, Larsson S-E: Normal hepatic vitamin-D metabolism in icteric primary biliary cirrhosis associated with pronounced vitamin-D deficiency symptoms. Hepatogastroenterology 29:6–8, 1982.
321. Thompson WG, Thompson GR: Effect of cholestyramine on the absorption of vitamin D_3 and calcium. Gut 10:717–722, 1969.
322. Reed JS, Meredith SC, Nemchausky BA, et al: Bone disease in primary biliary cirrhosis: Reversal of osteomalacia with oral 25-hydroxyvitamin D. Gastroenterology 78:512–517, 1980.
323. Long RG, Meinhard E, Skinner RK, et al: Clinical, biochemical, and histological studies of osteomalacia, osteoporosis, and parathyroid function in chronic liver disease. Gut 19:85–90, 1978.
324. Long RG, Varghese Z, Meinhard EA, et al: Parenteral 1,25-dihydroxycholecalciferol in hepatic osteomalacia. Br Med J 1:75–77, 1978.
325. Hodgson SF, Dickson ER, Wahner HW, et al: Bone loss and reduced osteoblast function in primary biliary cirrhosis. Ann Intern Med 103:855–860, 1985.
326. Arnaud SB: 25-Hydroxyvitamin D_3 treatment of bone disease in primary biliary cirrhosis (editorial). Gastroenterology 83:137–149, 1982.
327. Rosenberg IH: When is vitamin D–responsive bone disease not osteomalacia? Hepatology 4:157–158, 1984.
328. Stellon AJ, Webb A, Compston JE, Williams R: Low bone turnover state in primary biliary cirrhosis. Hepatology 7:137–142, 1987.
329. Cuthbert JA, Pak CYC, Zerwekh E, et al: Bone disease in primary biliary cirrhosis: Increased bone resorption and turnover in the absence of osteomalacia. Hepatology 4:1–8, 1984.
330. Parfitt AM: Adult hypoparathyroidism: Treatment with calcifediol. Arch Intern Med 138:874–881, 1978.
331. Hahn TJ, Scharp CR, Avioli LV: Effect of phenobarbital administration on the subcellular distribution of vitamin D_3-^3H in rat liver. Endocrinology 94:1489–1495, 1974.
332. Perucca E, Richens A: Biotransformation. *In* Woodbury DM, Penry JK, Pippenger CE (eds): Antiepileptic Drugs. 2nd ed. New York, Raven Press, 1982, pp 31–55.
333. Bouillon R, Reynaert J, Claes JH, et al: The effect of anticonvulsant therapy on serum levels of 25-hydroxy-vitamin D, calcium, and parathyroid hormone. J Clin Endocrinol Metab 41:1130–1135, 1975.
334. Hahn TJ: Bone complications of anticonvulsants. Drugs 12:201–211, 1976.
335. Stamp TCB, Flanagan RJ, Richens A, et al: Anticonvulsant osteomalacia. *In* Copp DH, Talmage RV (eds): Endocrinology of Calcium Metabolism. Amsterdam, Excerpta Medica, 1978, pp 16–22.
336. Hahn TJ, Halstead LR: Anticonvulsant drug-induced osteomalacia: Alterations in mineral metabolism and response to vitamin D_3 administration. Calcif Tissue Int 27:13–18, 1979.
337. Kruse K: On the pathogenesis of anticonvulsant-drug-induced alterations of calcium metabolism. Eur J Pediatr 138:202–205, 1982.
338. Tjellesen L, Gotfredsen A, Christiansen C: Different actions of vitamin D_2 and D_3 on bone metabolism in patients treated with phenobarbitone/phenytoin. Calcif Tissue Int 37:218–222, 1985.
339. Crosley CJ, Chee C, Berman PH: Rickets associated with long-term anticonvulsant therapy in a pediatric outpatient population. Pediatrics 56:52–57, 1975.
340. Jowsey J, Arnaud SB, Hodgson SF, et al: The frequency of bone abnormality in patients on anticonvulsant therapy. Electroencephalogr Clin Neurophysiol 45:341–347, 1978.
341. Mosekilde L, Melsen F: Dynamic differences in trabecular bone remodeling between patients after jejuno-ileal bypass for obesity and epileptic patients receiving anticonvulsant therapy. Metab Bone Dis Rel Res 2:77–82, 1980.
342. Fogelman I, Gray JMB, Gardner MD, et al: Do anticonvulsant drugs commonly induce osteomalacia? Scott Med J 27:136–142, 1982.
343. Weinstein RS, Bryce GF, Sappington LJ, et al: Decreased serum ionized calcium and normal vitamin D metabolite levels with anticonvulsant drug treatment. J Clin Endocrinol Metab 58:1003–1009, 1984.
344. Ashworth B, Horn DB: Evidence of osteomalacia in an outpatient group of adult epileptics. Epilepsia 18:37–43, 1977.
345. Kruse K, Kracht U, Göpfert G: Response of kidney and bone to parathyroid hormone in children receiving anticonvulsant drugs. Neuropediatrics 13:3–9, 1982.
346. Keith DA, Gundberg CM, Tassinari MS, et al: Phenytoin and bone metabolism. *In* Dixon AD, Sarnat BG (eds): Factors and Mechanisms Influencing Bone Growth. New York, Alan R. Liss, 1982, pp 517-526.
347. Dent CE, Richens A, Rowe DJF, Stamp TCB: Osteomalacia with long-term anticonvulsant therapy in epilepsy. Br Med J 4:69–72, 1970.
348. Genuth SM, Klein L, Rabinovich S, King KC: Os-

teomalacia accompanying chronic anticonvulsant therapy. J Clin Endocrinol Metab 35:378–386, 1972.
349. Greenwood RH, Prunty FTG, Silver J: Osteomalacia after prolonged glutethimide administration. Br Med J 1:643–645, 1973.
350. Marsden CD, Reynolds EH, Parsons V, et al: Myopathy associated with anticonvulsant osteomalacia. Br Med J 4:526–527, 1973.
351. Stamp TCB: Effects of long-term anticonvulsant therapy on calcium and vitamin D metabolism. Proc R Soc Med 67:64–68, 1974.
352. Pierides AM, Ellis HA, Ward M, et al: Barbiturate and anticonvulsant treatment in relation to osteomalacia with haemodialysis and renal transplantation. Br Med J 1:190–193, 1976.
353. Juttman JR, Barth JD, Birkenhäger JC: Treatment of anticonvulsant osteomalacia with 1α-hydroxycholecalciferol. Br Med J 1:551, 1977.
354. Broadus AE, Hanson TA, Bartter FC, Walton J: Primary hyperparathyroidism presenting as anticonvulsant-induced osteomalacia. Am J Med 63:298–305, 1977.
355. Mallette LE: Acetazolamide-accelerated anticonvulsant osteomalacia. Arch Intern Med 137:1013–1017, 1977.
356. Eastwood JB, Phillips ME, De Wardener HE: Effect of vitamin D_3 (cholecalciferol) in anticonvulsant osteomalacia. Metab Bone Dis Rel Res 2:83–86, 1980.
357. Mimaki T, Waison PD, Haussler MR: Anticonvulsant therapy and vitamin D metabolism: Evidence for different mechanisms for phenytoin and phenobarbital. Pediatr Pharmacol 1:105–112, 1980.
358. Hahn TJ, Birge SJ, Scharp CR, Avioli LV: Phenobarbital-induced alterations in vitamin D metabolism. J Clin Invest 51:741–748, 1972.
359. Silver J, Neale G, Thompson GR: Effect of phenobarbitone treatment on vitamin D metabolism in mammals. Clin Sci Mol Med 46:433–448, 1974.
360. Camfield CS, Delvin EE, Camfield PR, Glorieux FH: Normal serum 25-hydroxyvitamin D levels in phenobarbital-treated toddlers. Dev Pharmacol Ther 6:157–161, 1983.
361. Matheson RT, Herbst JJ, Jubiz W, et al: Absorption and biotransformation of cholecalciferol in drug-induced osteomalacia. J Clin Pharmacol 16:426–432, 1976.
362. Bell RD, Pak CYC, Zerwekh J, et al: Effect of phenytoin on bone and vitamin D metabolism. Ann Neurol 5:374–378, 1979.
363. Levison JC, Kent GN, Worth GK, Retallack RW: Anticonvulsant induced increase in 25-hydroxy-vitamin D_3-1α-hydroxylase. Endocrinology 101:1898–1901, 1977.
364. Christensen CK, Lund BI, Lund BJ, et al: Reduced 1,25-dihydroxyvitamin D and 24,25-dihydroxyvitamin D in epileptic patients receiving chronic combined anticonvulsant therapy. Metab Bone Dis Rel Res 3:17–22, 1981.
365. Keck E, Gollnick B, Reinhardt D, et al: Calcium metabolism and vitamin D metabolite levels in children receiving anticonvulsant drugs. Eur J Pediatr 139:52–55, 1982.
366. Harris M, Rowe DJF, Darby AJ: Anticonvulsant osteomalacia induced in the rat by diphenylhydantoin. Calcif Tiss Res 25:13–17, 1978.
367. Brodie MJ, Boobis AR, Hillyard CJ, et al: Effect of rifampicin and isoniazid on vitamin D metabolism. Clin Pharmacol Ther 32:525–530, 1982.
368. Shah SC, Sharma RK, Hemangini, Chitle AR: Rifampicin induced osteomalacia. Tubercle 62:207–209, 1981.
369. Silver J, Davies TJ, Kupersmitt E, et al: Prevalence and treatment of vitamin D deficiency in children on anticonvulsant drugs. Arch Dis Child 49:344–350, 1974.
370. Peterson P, Gray P, Tolman KG: Calcium balance in drug-induced osteomalacia: Response to vitamin D. Clin Pharmacol Ther 19:63–67, 1976.
371. Davie MWJ, Emberson CE, Lawson DEM, et al: Low plasma 25-hydroxyvitamin D and serum calcium levels in institutionalized epileptic subjects: Associated risk factors, consequences and response to treatment with vitamin D. Q J Med 52:79–91, 1983.
372. Mosekilde L, Melsen F: Anticonvulsant osteomalacia determined by quantitative analysis of bone changes. Acta Med Scand 199:349–355, 1976.
373. Wark JD, Larkins RG, Perry-Keene D, et al: Chronic diphenylhydantoin therapy does not reduce plasma 25-hydroxyvitamin D. Clin Endocrinol (Oxf) 11:267–274, 1979.
374. Weisman Y, Fattal A, Eisenberg Z, et al: Decreased serum 24,25-dihydroxyvitamin D concentrations in children receiving chronic anticonvulsant therapy. Br Med J 2:521–523, 1979.
375. Tolman KG, Jubiz W, Sannella JJ, et al: Osteomalacia associated with anticonvulsant drug therapy in mentally retarded children. Pediatrics 56:45–51, 1975.
376. Sherk HH, Cruz M, Stambaugh J: Vitamin D prophylaxis and the lowered incidence of fractures in anticonvulsant rickets and osteomalacia. Clin Orthop 129:251–257, 1977.
377. Wallöe A: Bone disease in epileptics. Thesis, The Department of Orthopaedic Surgery, Lund, Sweden, 1979.
378. Murchison LE, Bewsher PD, Chesters M, et al: Effects of anticonvulsants and inactivity on bone disease in epileptics. Postgrad Med J 51:18–21, 1975.
379. Mosekilde L, Melsen F, Christensen MS, et al: Effect of long-term vitamin D_2 treatment on bone morphometry and biochemical values in anticonvulsant osteomalacia. Acta Med Scand 201:303–307, 1977.
380. Slovik DM: The vitamin D endocrine system, calcium metabolism, and osteoporosis. Spec Top Endocrinol Metab 5:83–148, 1983.
381. Riggs BL: Vitamin D and involutional osteoporosis. *In* Kumar R (ed): Vitamin D. Boston, Martinus Nijhoff Publishing, 1984, pp 559–577.
382. Bouillon R, Guesens P, Dequeker J, De Moor P: Parathyroid function in primary osteoporosis. Clin Sci 57:167–171, 1979.
383. Tsai K-S, Heath H III, Kumar R, Riggs BL: Impaired vitamin D metabolism with aging in women: Possible role in pathogenesis of senile osteoporosis. J Clin Invest 73:1668–1672, 1984.
384. Francis RM, Peacock M, Taylor GA, et al: Calcium malabsorption in elderly women with vertebral fractures: Evidence for resistance to the action of vitamin D metabolites on the bowel. Clin Sci 66:103–107, 1984.
385. Chapuy M-C, Durr F, Chapuy P: Age-related changes in parathyroid hormone and 25-hydroxycholecalciferol levels. J Gerontol 38:19–22, 1983.
386. Marcus M, Madvig P, Young G: Age-related changes in parathyroid hormone action in normal

humans. J Clin Endocrinol Metab 58:223–230, 1984.

387. Joly R, Chapuy MC, Alexandre C, Meunier PJ: Osteoporoses a haut niveau de remodelage et fonction parathyroïdienne. Confrontations histobiologiques. Pathol Biol 28:417–424, 1980.
388. Whyte MP, Bergfeld MA, Murphy WA, et al: Postmenopausal osteoporosis: A heterogeneous disorder as assessed by histomorphometric analysis of iliac crest bone from untreated patients. Am J Med 72:193–202, 1982.
389. Sorensen OH, Anderson RB, Christensen MS, et al: Treatment of senile osteoporosis with 1α-hydroxyvitamin D_3. Clin Endocrinol 7:169S–175S, 1977.
390. Sorensen OH, Lund BI, Saltin B, et al: Myopathy in bone loss of ageing: Improvement by treatment with 1α-hydroxycholecalciferol and calcium. Clin Endocrinol 56:157–161, 1979.
391. Lips P, Netelenbos JC, Jongen MJM, et al: Histomorphometric profile and vitamin D status in patients with femoral neck fracture. Metab Bone Dis Rel Res 4:85–93, 1982.
392. Von Knorring J, Slätis P, Weber TH, Helenius T: Serum levels of 25-hydroxyvitamin D, 24,25-dihydroxyvitamin D and parathyroid hormone in patients with femoral neck fracture in Southern Finland. Clin Endocrinol 17:189–194, 1982.
393. Hoikka V, Alhava EM, Savolainen K, Parviainen M: Osteomalacia in fractures of the proximal femur. Acta Orthop Scand 53:255–260, 1982.
393a. Wilton TJ, Hosking DJ, Pawley E, et al: Osteomalacia and femoral neck fractures in the elderly patient. J Bone Joint Surg 69B:388–390, 1987.
394. Corless D, Dawson E, Fraser F, et al: Do vitamin D supplements improve the physical capabilities of elderly hospital patients? Age Ageing 14:76–84, 1985.
395. Lund BJ, Sorensen OH, Lund BI, et al: Vitamin D metabolism and osteomalacia in patients with fractures of the proximal femur. Acta Orthop Scand 53:251–254, 1982.
396. Brown JP, Delmas PD, Malaval L, et al: Serum bone Gla-protein: A specific marker for bone formation in postmenopausal women. Lancet 1:1091–1093, 1984.
397. Kemm JR, Campbell G, Cotton RE, et al: Osteoid in bones of elderly patients without bone disease. Age Ageing 13:144–151, 1984.
397a. Schwartzman MS, Franck WA: Vitamin D toxicity complicating the treatment of senile, postmenopausal, and glucocorticoid-induced osteoporosis. Am J Med 82:224–230, 1987.
398. Nordin BEC, Horsman A, Marshall DH, et al: The treatment of postmenopausal osteoporosis. *In* Barzel US (ed): Osteoporosis II. New York, Grune & Stratton, 1979.
398a. Editorial: Vitamin D supplementation in the elderly. Lancet i:306–307, 1987.
398b. Parfitt AM: Use of calciferol and its metabolites and analogs in osteoporosis; current status. Drugs 36:513–520, 1988.
399. Carmichael KA, Fallon MD, Dalinka M, et al: Osteomalacia and osteitis fibrosa in a man ingesting aluminum hydroxide antacid. Am J Med 76:1137–1143, 1984.
399a. Saadeh G, Bauer T, Licata A, Sheeler L: Antacid-induced osteomalacia. Cleve Clin J Med 54:214–216, 1987.
400. Dominguez JH, Gray RW, Lemann J Jr: Dietary phosphate deprivation in women and men. Effects on mineral and acid balances, parathyroid hormone and the metabolism of 25-OH-vitamin D. J Clin Endocrinol Metab 43:1056–1068, 1976.
401. Lotz M, Zisman E, Bartter FC: Evidence for a phosphorus-depletion syndrome in man. N Engl J Med 278:409–452, 1968.
402. Dent CE, Winter CS: Osteomalacia due to phosphate depletion from excessive aluminium hydroxide ingestion. Br Med J 1:551–552, 1974.
403. Cooke N, Teitelbaum S, Avioli LV: Antacid-induced osteomalacia and nephrolithiasis. Arch Intern Med 138:1007–1009, 1978.
404. Parfitt AM: Bone as a source of urinary calcium-osseous hypercalciuria. *In* Coe F (ed): Hypercalciuric States—Pathogenesis, Consequences and Treatment. New York, Grune and Stratton, 1984, pp 313–378.
405. Lotz M, Ney R, Bartter FC, Smith H: Osteomalacia and debility resulting from phosphorus depletion. Trans Assoc Am Physicians 77:281–295, 1964.
405a. Smith R, O'Riordan LH: Of mouse and man: The hypophosphataemic genes. Q J Med 245:705–707, 1987.
406. Davies M, Stanbury SW: The rheumatic manifestations of metabolic bone disease. Clin Rheum Dis 7:595–646,1981.
407. Drezner MK, Lyles KW, Haussler MR, Harrelson JM: Evaluation of a role for 1,25-dihydroxyvitamin D_3 in the pathogenesis and treatment of X-linked hypophosphatemic rickets and osteomalacia. J Clin Invest 66:1020–1032,1980.
408. Marie PJ, Glorieux FH: Histomorphometric study of bone remodeling in hypophosphatemic vitamin D–resistant rickets. Metab Bone Dis Rel Res 3:31–38, 1981.
409. Marie PJ, Glorieux FH: Relation between hypomineralized periosteocytic lesions and bone mineralization in vitamin D–resistant rickets. Calcif Tissue Int 35:443–448, 1983.
410. Frymoyer JW, Hodgkin W: Adult-onset vitamin D–resistant hypophosphatemic osteomalacia. J Bone Joint Surg 59A:101–106, 1977.
411. Perry W, Stamp TCB: Hereditary hypophosphataemic rickets with autosomal recessive inheritance and severe osteosclerosis. J Bone Joint Surg 60B:430–434, 1978.
412. Harrison JE, Cumming WA, Fornasier V, et al: Increased bone mineral content in young adults with familial hypophosphatemic vitamin D refractory rickets. Metabolism 25:33–40, 1976.
413. Exner GU, Prader A, Elsasser U, et al: Hypophosphatemic vitamin D resistant rickets (phosphate diabetes): Bone mineral problems studied by ^{125}I-computed tomography and microradiography. Helv Paediatr Acta 35:39–49, 1980.
414. Polisson RP, Martinez S, Khoury M, et al: Calcification of entheses associated with X-linked hypophosphatemic osteomalacia. N Engl J Med 313:1–6, 1985.
415. Cartwright DW, Masel JP, Latham SC: The lumbar spinal canal in hypophosphataemic vitamin D–resistant rickets. Aust NZ J Med 11:154–157, 1981.
416. Cartwright DW, Latham SC, Masel JP, Yelland JDN: Spinal canal stenosis in adult with hypophosphataemic vitamin D–resistant rickets. Aust NZ J Med 9:705–708, 1979.

417. Davies M, Kane R, Valentine J: Impaired hearing in X-linked hypophosphataemic (vitamin D-resistant) osteomalacia. Ann Intern Med 100:230–232, 1984.
418. Dent CE, Stamp TCB: Hypophosphataemic osteomalacia presenting in adults. Q J Med 40:303–329, 1971.
419. Fanconi A: Idiopathische hypophosphatämische Osteomalazie mit Beginn in der Adoleszenz. Helv Paediatr Acta 1971;26:535-549.
420. Kistler HJ, Bonetti A, Frey P, Fischer JA: Sporadische hypophosphatämische vitamin-D-resistente Osteomalazie (Phosphatdiabetes) im Erwachsenenalter und Hyperparathyreoidismus. Schweiz Med Wochenschr 106:1855–1862, 1976.
421. Offermann G, Delling G, Haussler MR: 1,25-dihydroxycholecalciferol in hypophosphataemic osteomalacia presenting in adults. Acta Endocrinol 88:408–416, 1978.
422. Ahmed KY, Varghese Z, Moorhead JF, Wills MR: The response to 1,25-dihydroxycholecalciferol and to dihydrotachysterol in adult-onset hypophosphataemic osteomalacia. Clin Chim Acta 97:33–37, 1979.
423. de Backer M, de Nutte N, Verbeelen D, et al: Renal responsiveness to parathyroid hormone in a case of nonfamilial hypophosphatemic osteomalacia. Klin Wochenschr 58:689–694, 1980.
424. Weiss D, Bar RS, Weidner N, et al: Oncogenic osteomalacia: Strange tumours in strange places. Postgrad Med J 61:349–355, 1985.
425. Renton P, Shaw DG: Hypophosphatemic osteomalacia secondary to vascular tumors of bone and soft tissue. Skeletal Radiol 1:21–24, 1976.
426. Prader VA, Illig R, Uehlinger E, Stalder G: Rachitis infolge Knochentumors. Helv Paediatr Acta 14:554–565, 1959.
427. Yoshikawa S, Kawabata M, Hatsuyama Y, et al: Atypical vitamin-D resistant osteomalacia. J Bone Joint Surg 46A:998–1007, 1969.
428. Boström H, Edgren B, Nilsonne U, Wester PO: Metabolic and orthopedic treatment of a case of adult nonfamilial hypophosphatemia with severe osteomalacia. Acta Orthop Scand 39:238–260, 1968.
429. Miller MJ, Marel G, Frame B, Neer R: Adult acquired vitamin D and PTH-resistant hypophosphatemic osteomalacia with multiple skeletal lesions. *In* Norman AW, Schaefer K, Herrath DV, Grigoleit HG (eds): Vitamin D. Chemical, Biochemical and Clinical Endocrinology of Calcium Metabolism. Fifth Workshop on Vitamin D. Berlin, Walter de Gruyter, 1982, pp 993-995.
430. Riggs BL, Sprague RG, Jowsey J, Maher FT: Adult-onset vitamin-D-resistant hypophosphatemic osteomalacia. Effect of total parathyroidectomy. N Engl J Med 281:762–766, 1969.
431. Drezner MK, Feinglos MN: Osteomalacia due to 1α-25,dihydroxycholecalciferol deficiency. Association with a giant cell tumor of bone. J Clin Invest 60:1046–1053, 1977.
432. Leehey DJ, Ing TS, Daugirdas JT: Fanconi syndrome associated with a nonossifying fibroma of bone. Am J Med 78:708–710,1985.
433. Yoshikawa S, Nakamura T, Takagi M, et al: Benign osteoblastoma as a cause of osteomalacia. A report of two cases. J Bone Joint Surg 59B:279–286, 1977.
434. Lejeune E, Bouvier M, Meunier P, et al: L'Osteomalacie des tumeurs mesenchymateuses. A propos d'une nouvelle observation. Rev Rhum 46:187–193, 1979.
434a. Siris ES, Clemens TL, Dempster DW, et al: Tumor-induced osteomalacia. Am J Med 82:307–312, 1987.
435. Weidner N, Bar RS, Weiss D, Strottmann MP: Neoplastic pathology of oncogenic osteomalacia/rickets. Cancer 55:1691–1705, 1985.
435a. Weidner N, Santa Cruz D: Phosphaturic mesenchymal tumors. Cancer 59:1442–1454, 1987.
436. Dent CE, Gertner JM: Hypophosphataemic osteomalacia in fibrous dysplasia. Q J Med 45:411–420, 1976.
437. McArthur RG, Hayles AB, Lambert PW: Albright's syndrome with rickets. Mayo Clin Proc 54:313–320, 1979.
438. Lever EG, Pettingale KW: Albright's syndrome associated with a soft-tissue myxoma and hypophosphataemic osteomalacia. Report of a case and review of the literature. J Bone Joint Surg 65B:621–626, 1983.
439. Swann GF: Generalised softening of bone due to metabolic causes. IV. Pathogenesis of bone lesions in neurofibromatosis. Br J Radiol 27:623–629, 1954.
440. Saville PD, Nassim JR, Stevenson FH, et al: Osteomalacia in von Recklinghausen's neurofibromatosis. Metabolic study of a case. Br Med J 2:1311–1313, 1955.
441. Balsan S, Guivarch J, Dartois A-M, Royer P: Rachitisme vitaminoresistant associe a une neurofibromatose probable chez un enfant. Arch Fr Ped 24:609–632, 1967.
442. Melick RA, Larkins RG, Greenberg PB, Wark JD: Osteomalacia due to unusual causes presenting in adults. Aust NZ J Med 9:253–257, 1979.
442a. Hogan DB, Anderson C, Mackenzie RA, Crilly RG: Hypophosphatemic osteomalacia complicating von Recklinghausen's neurofibromatosis: Increase in spinal density on treatment. Bone 7:9–12, 1986.
442b. Carey DE, Drezner MK, Hamdan JA, et al: Hypophosphatemic rickets/osteomalacia in linear sebaceous nevus syndrome: A variant of tumor-induced osteomalacia. J Pediatr 109:994–1000, 1986.
442c. Silverton SF, Haddad JG: Medical reversal of acquired hypophosphatemic osteomalacia. Am J Med 82:1077–1082, 1987.
443. Kleerekoper M, Coffey R, Greco T, et al: Hypercalcemic hyperparathyroidism in hypophosphatemic rickets. J Clin Endocrinol Metab 45:86–94, 1977.
443a. Reid IR, Teitelbaum SL, Dusso A, Whyte MP: Hypercalcemic hyperparathyroidism complicating oncogenic osteomalacia. Am J Med 83:350–354, 1987.
444. Dent CE, Friedman M: Hypophosphataemic osteomalacia with complete recovery. Br Med J 1:1676–1679, 1964.
445. Hosking DJ, Chamberlain MJ, Shortland-Webb WR: Osteomalacia and carcinoma of prostate with major redistribution of skeletal calcium. Br J Radiol 48:451–456, 1975.
446. Lyles KW, Berry WR, Haussler M, et al: Hypophosphatemic osteomalacia: Association with prostatic carcinoma. Ann Intern Med 93:275–278, 1980.
447. Kabadi UM: Osteomalacia associated with prostatic cancer and osteoblastic metastases. Urology 21:65–67, 1983.
448. Charhon SA, Chapuy MC, Delvin EE, et al: Histomorphometric analysis of sclerotic bone metastases from prostatic carcinoma with special reference to osteomalacia. Cancer 51:918–924, 1983.
449. Brazy PC, Lobaugh B, Lyles KW, Drezner MK: The pathogenesis of tumor-induced osteomalacia: A

new perspective. *In* Frame B, Potts JT Jr (eds): Clinical Disorders of Bone and Mineral Metabolism. Amsterdam, Excerpta Medica, 1983, pp 242-246.
450. Murphy WA, Seligman PA, Tillack T, et al: Osteosclerosis, osteomalacia, and bone marrow aplasia: A combined late complication of thorotrast administration. Skeletal Radiol 3:234–238, 1979.
451. Coindre JM, Reiffers J, Goussot JF, et al: Histomorphometric analysis of sclerotic bone from idiopathic myeloid metaplasia (nine cases). J Pathol 144:163–169, 1984.
452. Monro P: Effect of treatment on renal function in severe osteomalacia due to Wilson's disease. J Clin Pathol 23:487–491, 1970.
453. Smith R, Lindenbaum RH, Walton RJ: Hypophosphataemic osteomalacia and Fanconi syndrome of adult onset with dominant inheritance. Q J Med 45:387–400, 1976.
454. Brenton DP, Isenberg DA, Cusworth DC, et al: The adult presenting idiopathic Fanconi syndrome. J Inherited Metab Dis 4:211–215, 1981.
455. Adams RG, Harrison JF, Scott P: The development of cadmium-induced proteinuria, impaired renal function, and osteomalacia in alkaline battery workers. Q J Med 38:425–443, 1969.
456. Emmerson BT: "Ouch-Ouch" disease: The osteomalacia of cadmium nephropathy. Ann Intern Med 73:854–855, 1970.
457. Editorial: Cadmium pollution and Itai-itai disease. Lancet 1:382–383, 1971.
458. Ghozlan R, Dupuis M, Baviera E: Osteomalacia revelatrice d'un syndrome de Toni-Debre-Fanconi secondaire a la prise de methyl-3-chromone. Rev Rhum 52:61–62, 1985.
459. Mallette LE, Patten BM: Neurogenic muscle atrophy and osteomalacia in adult Fanconi syndrome. Ann Neurol 1:131–137, 1977.
460. Glassock RJ, Malluche HH, Tate M, et al: Recurrent fractures, hypophosphatemia, and renal insufficiency in elderly women. Am J Nephrol 4:329–335, 1984.
461. Baran DT, Marcy TW: Evidence for a defect in vitamin D metabolism in a patient with incomplete Fanconi syndrome. J Clin Endocrinol Metab 59:998–1001, 1984.
462. Colussi G, De Ferrari ME, Pontoriero G, et al: Vitamin D metabolites in the osteomalacia associated with the adult Fanconi syndrome in humans. *In* Mineral Metabolism Research in Italy, vol 4. Milano, Italy, Wichtig Editore, 1983, pp 197–200.
463. Brewer ED, Tsai HC, Szeto K-S, Morris RC: Maleic acid–induced impaired conversion of 25(OH)D_3 to 1,25$(OH)_2D_3$: Implications for Fanconi's syndrome. Kidney Int 12:244–252, 1977.
464. Saville PD, Nassim R, Stevenson FH, et al: The Fanconi syndrome. Metabolic studies on treatment. J Bone Joint Surg 37B:529–539, 1955.
465. Morgan HG, Stewart WK, Lowe KG, et al: Wilson's disease and the Fanconi syndrome. Q J Med 31:361–384, 1962.
466. Wilson DR, Yendt ER: Treatment of the adult Fanconi syndrome with oral phosphate supplements and alkali. Report of two cases associated with nephrolithiasis. Am J Med 35:487–511, 1963.
467. de Deuxchaisnes CN, Krane SM: The treatment of adult phosphate diabetes and Fanconi syndrome with neutral sodium phosphate. Am J Med 43:508–543, 1967.
468. Sly WS, Whyte MP, Sundaram V, et al: Carbonic anhydrase II deficiency in 12 families with the autosomal recessive syndrome of osteopetrosis with renal tubular acidosis and cerebral calcification. N Engl J Med 313:139–145, 1985.
469. Morris RC: Type 1 RTA ("classic" or "distal"). Physiologic characteristics. *In* Stanbury J, et al (eds): The Metabolic Basis of Inherited Diseases. 5th ed. New York, McGraw-Hill, 1983, pp 1812–1822.
470. Brenes LG, Brenes JN, Hernandez MM: Familial proximal renal tubular acidosis. A distinct clinical entity. Am J Med 63:244–249, 1977.
471. Nash MA, Torrado AD, Greifer I, et al: Renal tubular acidosis in infants and children. J Pediatr 80:738–748, 1972.
472. York SE, Yendt ER: Osteomalacia associated with renal bicarbonate loss. Can Med Assoc J 94:1329–1342, 1966.
473. Phelps KR, Einhorn TA, Vigorita VJ, et al: Acidosis-induced osteomalacia: Metabolic studies and skeletal histomorphometry. Bone 7:171–180, 1986.
474. Marquez-Julio A, Rapoport A, Wilansky DL, et al: Hyperglobulinemic purpura associated with renal tubular acidosis and osteomalacia: A report of two cases and review of the literature. Univ Mich Med Center J 42:26–32, 1976.
475. Courey WR, Pfister RC: The radiographic findings in renal tubular acidosis. Analysis of 21 cases. Radiology 105:497–503, 1972.
476. Heidbreder E, Hennemann H, Heidland A, Krempien B: Treatment of renal tubular acidosis and osteomalacia by salidiuretics. Lancet 1:52–53, 1973.
477. Brenner RJ, Spring DB, Sebastian A, et al: Incidence of radiographically evident bone disease, nephrocalcinosis, and nephrolithiasis in various types of renal tubular acidosis. N Engl J Med 307:217–221, 1982.
478. Harrington TM, Bunch TW, Van den Berg CJ: Renal tubular acidosis. A new look at treatment of musculoskeletal and renal disease. Mayo Clin Proc 58:354–360, 1983.
479. Vicale CT: The diagnostic features of a muscular syndrome resulting from hyperparathyroidism, osteomalacia owing to renal tubular acidosis, and perhaps to related disorders of calcium metabolism. Trans Am Neurol Assoc 74:143–147, 1949.
480. Coe FL, Firpo JJ Jr: Evidence for mild reversible hyperparathyroidism in distal renal tubular acidosis. Arch Intern Med 135:1485–1489, 1975.
481. Gonick HC, Lee DBN, Drinkard JP, Coulson WC: Interrelationship of acidosis, calcium balance, serum parathormone concentration, and bone morphology in type I renal tubular acidosis (RTA). *In* Frame B, Parfitt AM, Duncan H: Clinical Aspects of Metabolic Bone Disease. Amsterdam, Excerpta Medica, 1973, pp 403–406.
482. Wallach S, Baker RK, Nicastri A: Primary renal tubular acidosis and secondary hyperparathyroidism. Am J Med 52:809–816, 1972.
483. Leite CA, Frame B, Frost HM, Arnstein AR: Osteomalacia following ureterosigmoidostomy. With observations on bone morphology and remodeling rate. Clin Orthop 49:103–108, 1966.
484. Donohoe JF, Freaney R, Muldowney FP: Osteomalacia in ureterosigmoidostomy. Ir J Med Sci 2:523–530, 1969.
485. Perry W, Allen LN, Stamp TCB, Walker PG: Vitamin D resistance in osteomalacia after ureterosigmoidostomy. N Engl J Med 297:1110–1112, 1977.

486. Cunningham J, Fraher LJ, Clemens TL, et al: Chronic acidosis with metabolic bone disease. Effect of alkali on bone morphology and vitamin D metabolism. Am J Med 73:199–204, 1982.
487. Salahudeen AK, Elliott RW, Ellis HA: Osteomalacia due to ileal replacement of ureters: Report of 2 cases. J Urology 131:335–337, 1984.
488. Adams ND, Gray RW, Lemann J Jr: The calciuria of increased fixed acid production in humans: Evidence against a role for parathyroid hormone and 1,25$(OH)_2$-vitamin D. Calcif Tissue Int 28:233–238, 1979.
489. Kraut JE, Gordon EM, Ransom JC, et al: Effect of chronic metabolic acidosis on vitamin D metabolism in humans. Kidney Int 24:644–648, 1983.
490. Cochran M, Nordin BEC: Role of acidosis in renal osteomalacia. Br Med J 2:276–279, 1969.
491. Dundon S: Treatment of osteomalacia of renal tubular acidosis. Lancet 2:1204, 1972.
492. Richards P, Chamberlain MJ, Wrong OM: Treatment of osteomalacia of renal tubular acidosis by sodium bicarbonate alone. Lancet 2:994–997, 1972.
493. Mautalen C, Montoreano R, Labarrere C: Early skeletal effect of alkali therapy upon the osteomalacia of renal tubular acidosis. J Clin Endocrinol Metab 42:875–881, 1976.
494. Ott SM, Maloney NA, Klein GL, et al: Aluminum is associated with low bone formation in patients receiving chronic parenteral nutrition. Ann Intern Med 98:910–914, 1983.
495. Weinstein RS, Whyte MP: Heterogeneity of adult hypophosphatasia. Report of severe and mild cases. Arch Intern Med 141:727–731, 1981.
496. Russell RGG, Fleisch H: Pyrophosphate and diphosphonate in skeletal metabolism. Physiological, clinical and therapeutic aspects. Clin Orthop 108:241–263, 1975.
497. Jowsey J, Riggs BL, Kelly PJ, et al: The treatment of osteoporosis with disodium ethane-1-hydroxy-1,1-diphosphonate. J Lab Clin Med 78:574–584, 1971.
498. Khairi MRA, Altman RD, DeRosa GP, et al: Sodium etidronate in the treatment of Paget's disease of bone. A study of long-term results. Ann Intern Med 87:656–663, 1977.
499. Krane SM: Etidronate disodium in the treatment of Paget's disease of bone. Ann Intern Med 96:619–625, 1982.
500. Alexandre M, Chapuy MC, Vignon E, et al: Treatment of Paget's disease of bone with ethane-1, hydroxy-1,1 diphosphonate (EHDP) at a low dosage (5 mg/kg/day). Clin Orthop 174:193–205, 1983.
501. Evans RA, Dunstan CR, Hills E, Wong SYP: Pathologic fracture due to severe osteomalacia following low-dose diphosphonate treatment of Paget's disease of bone. Aust NZ J Med 13:277–279, 1983.
502. Delmas PD, Chapuy MC, Vignon E, et al: Long term effects of dichloromethylene diphosphonate in Paget's disease of bone. J Clin Endocrinol Metab 54:837–844, 1982.
503. Briancon D, Meunier PJ: Treatment of osteoporosis with fluoride, calcium, and vitamin D. Orthop Clin North Am 12:629–648, 1981.
504. Vigorita VJ, Suda MK: The microscopic morphology of fluoride-induced bone. Clin Orthop 177:274–282, 1983.
505. Grennan DM, Palmer DG, Malthus RS, et al: Iatrogenic fluorosis. Aust NZ J Med 8:528–531, 1978.
506. Compston JE, Chadha S, Merrett AL: Osteomalacia developing during treatment of osteoporosis with sodium fluoride and vitamin D. Br Med J 281:910–911, 1980.
507. Bonvoisin B, Bouvier M, Meunier PJ, Lejeune E: Osteomalacie histologique induite par l'administration prolongee d'acide niflumique. Nouv Presse Med 11:1636, 1982.
508. Sherrard DJ, Ott S, Maloney N, et al: Uremic osteodystrophy: Classification, cause and treatment. *In* Frame B, Potts J (eds): Clinical Disorders of Bone and Mineral Metabolism. Amsterdam, Excerpta Medica, 1983, pp 254–258.
509. Dunstan CR, Hills E, Norman AW, et al: The pathogenesis of renal osteodystrophy: Role of vitamin D, aluminium, parathyroid hormone, calcium and phosphorus. Q J Med 55:127–144, 1985.
510. Andress DL, Ott SM, Maloney NA, Sherrard DJ: Effect of parathyroidectomy on bone aluminum accumulation in chronic renal failure. N Engl J Med 312:468–473, 1985.
511. Boyce BF, Elder HY, Elliot HL, et al: Hypercalcaemic osteomalacia due to aluminium toxicity. Lancet 2:1009–1013, 1982.
512. Charhon SA, Chavassieux PM, Chapuy MC, et al: Low rate of bone formation with or without histologic appearance of osteomalacia in patients with aluminum intoxication. J Lab Clin Med 106:123–131, 1985.
512a. Parfitt AM: The localization of aluminum in bone: Implications for the mechanism of fixation and for the pathogenesis of aluminum-related bone disease (editorial). Int J Artif Organs 11:79–90, 1988.
513. Parfitt AM, Rao D, Stanciu J, Villanueva AR: Comparison of aluminum related with vitamin D related osteomalacia by tetracycline based bone histomorphometry. *In* Massry SG, Olmer M, Ritz E: Phosphate and Mineral Homeostasis. Adv Exp Biol Med 208:283–287, 1986.
514. Blumenthal NC, Posner AS: In vitro model of aluminum-induced osteomalacia: Inhibition of hydroxyapatite formation and growth. Calcif Tissue Int 36:439–441, 1984.
515. Goodman WG, Henry DA, Horst R, et al: Parenteral aluminum administration in the dog: II. Induction of osteomalacia and effect on vitamin D metabolism. Kidney Int 25:370–375, 1984.
516. Cournot-Witmer G, Zingraff J, Plachot JJ, et al: Aluminum localization in bone from hemodialyzed patients: Relationship to matrix mineralization. Kidney Int 20:375–385, 1981.
517. Podenphant J, Salem N, Sypitkowski C, et al: Reversal of aluminum related dialysis osteomalacia after transplantation. Proceedings, Fourth International Workshop on Bone Histomorphometry. Bone 6:405, 1985.
518. Hodsman AB, Anderson C, Leung FY: Accelerated accumulation of aluminum by osteoid matrix in vitamin D deficiency. Mineral Electrolyte Metab 10:309–315, 1984.
519. Quarles DL, Dennis VW, Gitelman HJ, et al: Aluminum deposition at the osteoid-bone interface: An epiphenomenon of the osteomalacic state in vitamin D deficient dogs. J Clin Invest 75:1441–1447, 1985.
520. Thomas WC, Meyer JL: Aluminum-induced osteomalacia: An explanation. Am J Nephrol 4:201–203, 1984.

521. Baker SL, Dent CE, Friedman M, Watson L: Fibrogenesis imperfecta ossium. J Bone Joint Surg 48B:804–825, 1966.
522. Swan CHJ, Shah K, Brewer DB, Cooke WT: Fibrogenesis imperfecta ossium. Q J Med 45:233–253, 1976.
523. Lang R, Vignery AMC, Jensen PS: Fibrogenesis imperfecta ossium with early onset: Observations after 20 years of illness. Bone 7:237–246, 1986.
524. Frame B, Frost HM, Pak CYC, et al: Fibrogenesis imperfecta ossium. A collagen defect causing osteomalacia. N Engl J Med 285:769–772, 1971.
525. Stoddart PGP, Wickremaratchi T, Hollingworth P, Watt I: Fibrogenesis imperfecta ossium. Br J Radiol 57:744–751, 1984.
526. Byers PD, Stamp TCB, Stoker DJ: Case report 296. Skeletal Radiol 13:72–76, 1985.
527. Stamp TCB, Byers PD, Ali SY, et al: Fibrogenesis imperfecta ossium: Remission with melphalan. Lancet 1:582–583, 1985.
528. Rasmussen H: Hypophosphatasia. *In* Stanbury J, et al (eds): The Metabolic Basis of Inherited Diseases. 5th ed. New York, McGraw-Hill, 1983, pp 1497–1507.
529. Whyte MP, Fallon MD, Murphy WA, Teitelbaum SL: Axial osteomalacia. Clinical, laboratory and genetic investigation of an affected mother and son. Am J Med 71:1041–1049, 1981.
530. Whyte MP, Vrabel LA, Schwartz TD: Alkaline phosphatase deficiency in cultured skin fibroblasts from patients with hypophosphatasia: Comparison of the infantile, childhood, and adult forms. J Clin Endocrinol Metab 57:831–837, 1983.
531. Millan JL, Whyte MP, Avioli LV, Fishman WH: Hypophosphatasia (adult form): Quantitation of serum alkaline phosphatase isoenzyme activity in a large kindred. Clin Chem 26:840–845, 1980.
532. Sorensen E, Flodgaard H: Adult hypophosphatasia. Report of a case with determination of inorganic pyrophosphate in plasma and urine during high phosphate intake. Acta Med Scand 197:357–360, 1975.
533. Whyte MP, Seino Y: Circulating vitamin D metabolite levels in hypophosphatasia. J Clin Endocrinol Metab 55:178–180, 1982.
534. Fallon MD, Teitelbaum SL, Weinstein RS, et al: Hypophosphatasia: Clinicopathologic comparison of the infantile, childhood, and adult forms. Medicine 63:12–24, 1984.
535. Paolaggi JB, Job Ch, Durigon M, et al: Hypophosphatasie de l'adulte a manifestations cliniques tardives. Nouv Presse Med 7:4285–4289, 1978.
536. Bethune JE, Dent CE: Hypophosphatasia in the adult. Am J Med 28:615–622, 1960.
537. Whyte MP, Teitelbaum SL, Murphy WA, et al: Adult hypophosphatasia. Clinical, laboratory, and genetic investigation of a large kindred with review of the literature. Medicine 58:329–347, 1979.
538. Whyte MP, Murphy WA, Fallon MD: Adult hypophosphatasia with chondrocalcinosis and arthropathy. Am J Med 72:631–641, 1982.
539. Frame B, Frost HM, Ormond RS, Hunter RB: Atypical osteomalacia involving the axial skeleton. Ann Intern Med 55:632–639, 1961.
540. Nelson AM, Riggs BL, Jowsey JO: Atypical axial osteomalacia. Report of four cases with two having features of ankylosing spondylitis. Arthritis Rheum 21:715–722, 1978.
541. Condon JR, Nassim JR: Axial osteomalacia. Postgrad Med J 47:817–820, 1971.
541a. VanErpecum KJ, Kroon HM, VanGroningen K, Harinck HIJ: Central and peripheral bone biopsy in a patient with axial osteomalacia. Neth J Med 28:505–508, 1985.
542. Betro MG, Pain RW: Hypophosphatemia and hyperphosphatemia in a hospital population. Br Med J 1:273–276, 1972.
543. Lundberg E, Bergengren H, Lindqvist B: Mild phosphate diabetes in adults. Acta Med Scand 204:93–96, 1978.
544. Stephens WP, Berry JL, Klimiuk PS, Mawer EB: Annual high-dose vitamin D prophylaxis in Asian immigrants. Lancet 2:1199–1201, 1981.
545. Brooke OG, Brown IRF, Bone CDM, et al: Vitamin D supplements in pregnant Asian women: Effects on calcium status and fetal growth. Br Med J 1:751–754, 1980.
546. Holdsworth MD, Dattani JT, Davies L, MacFarlane D: Factors contributing to vitamin D status near retirement age. Hum Nutr Clin Nutr 38C:139–149, 1984.
547. Toss G, Andersson R, Diffey BL, et al: Oral vitamin D and ultraviolet radiation for the prevention of vitamin D deficiency in the elderly. Acta Med Scand 212:157–161, 1982.
548. McKenna MJ, Freaney R, Meade A, Muldowney FP: Prevention of hypovitaminosis D in the elderly. Calcif Tissue Int 37:112–116, 1985.
549. Whyte MP, Haddad JG Jr, Walters DD, Stamp TCB: Vitamin D bioavailability: Serum 25-hydroxyvitamin D levels in man after oral, subcutaneous, intramuscular, and intravenous vitamin D administration. J Clin Endocrinol Metab 48:906–911, 1979.
550. Stamp TCB: Calcitriol dosage in osteomalacia, hypoparathyroidism and attempted treatment of myositis ossificans progressiva. Curr Med Res Opin 7:316–336, 1981.
551. Bordier Ph, Miravet L, Marie P, et al: Action des metabolites de la vitamine D sur la mineralisation du tissu osseux et les troubles du metabolisme phosphocalcique au cours de l'osteomalacie hypovitaminique D. Rev Rhum 45:241–248, 1978.
552. Bordier PH, Hioco D, Rouquier M, et al: Effects of intravenous vitamin D on bone and phosphate metabolism in osteomalacia. Calcif Tissue Res 4:78–83, 1969.
553. Bordier PH, Pechet MM, Hesse R, et al: Response of adult patients with osteomalacia to treatment with crystalline 1α-hydroxy vitamin D_3. N Engl J Med 291:866–871, 1974.
554. Hosking DJ, Campbell GA, Kemm JR, et al: Safety of treatment for subclinical osteomalacia in the elderly. Br Med J 289:785–787, 1984.
555. Cundy T, Kanis JA, Heynen G, et al: Failure to heal vitamin D–deficiency rickets and suppress secondary hyperparathyroidism with conventional doses of 1,25-dihydroxy vitamin D_3. Br Med J 284:883–885, 1982.
556. Haddad JG Jr, Rojanasathit S: Acute administration of 25-hydroxycholecalciferol in man. J Clin Endocrinol Metab 42:284–290, 1976.
557. Fonseca V, Weerakoon J, Mikhailidis DP, et al: Plasma creatinine and creatinine clearance in nutritional osteomalacia. Lancet 1:1093–1095, 1984.
558. Goldring SR, Krane SM: Cation effects on phos-

phate homeostasis in hypophosphatemic subjects. Adv Exp Med Biol 128:361–368, 1980.
559. Alon U, Chan JCM: Effects of hydrochlorothiazide and amiloride in renal hypophosphatemic rickets. Pediatrics 75:754–763, 1985.
560. Rose GA: Role of phosphate in treatment of renal tubular hypophosphataemic rickets and osteomalacias. Br Med J 2:857–861, 1964.
561. Firth RG, Grant CS, Riggs BL: Development of hypercalcemic hyperparathyroidism after long-term phosphate supplementation in hypophosphatemic osteomalacia. Report of two cases. Am J Med 78:669–673, 1985.
562. Harrell RM, Lyles KW, Harrelson JM, et al: Healing of bone disease in X-linked hypophosphatemic rickets/osteomalacia. Induction and maintenance with phosphorus and calcitriol. J Clin Invest 75:1858–1868, 1985.
563. Gertner JM, Brenton DB, Edwards RHT: 1α-hydroxyvitamin D_3 in the treatment of nutritional and metabolic rickets and osteomalacia. Clin Endocrinol 7[Suppl]:239–244, 1977.

LOUIS V. AVIOLI
ROBERT LINDSAY

12

The Female Osteoporotic Syndrome(s)

Osteoporosis is not unique to modern man, having been documented in prehistoric people living within the third millennium B.C.[1] "Osteoporosis" is a generic term used currently to define a specific form of generalized "osteopenia," a term initially introduced by Bauer as equal to "too little calcified bone."[2] According to classic histological criteria, osteoporosis is characterized by a reduction in trabecular bone mass in relation to the total area of the histologic section, and a ratio of mineral to organic matrix that approximates that of normal bone. Osteoporosis must be differentiated from osteomalacia (see Chapter 11) in which the ratio of mineral to organic matrix is by definition low, although total bone mass (i.e., osteoid plus mineral) may be normal, decreased, or even increased (Fig. 12–1). The distinction between osteoporosis and osteomalacia is established with certainty only by bone biopsy (usually of the rib or iliac crest) and inspection of appropriately stained, undemineralized, histologic sections. The distinguishing histologic features of osteomalacia observed on trabecular surfaces or newly forming haversian systems are wide osteoid seams and an increased number of surface seams per unit area of bone. In addition to these changes one classically finds a decreased rate of osteoid mineralization or so-called appositional rate at the calcification front, as shown by either special staining or tetracycline labeling techniques (see Chapters 10 and 11). These combined histologic criteria are essential to the diagnosis of osteomalacia *per se*, since other pathologic osteopenic disorders characterized by elevated appositional rates (i.e., hyperthyroidism, Paget's disease, or primary hyperparathyroidism) may also lead to an increase in the surface area occupied by osteoid seams despite ample evidence of osteoid mineralization. Not infrequently osteoporosis and some degrees of osteomalacia occur together without the so-called classic biochemical or radiologic "hallmarks" of osteomalacia (see Chapter 11). As detailed in Chapter 5, serum 25-hydroxycholecalciferol may be significantly lower in elderly females with symptomatic skeletal osteopenia. Variations in sunlight exposure, nutritional inadequacy, and acquired defects in the metabolism of 25-hydroxycholecalciferol and in the production of vitamin D_3 and $1,25(OH)_2D_3$ have been invoked as potential etiologic factors.[3-21] In fact, it has been estimated that 30% to 40% of elderly individuals in Great Britain and Boston, Massachusetts (U.S.A.), are vitamin D–deficient at the time of their first hip fracture.

To the radiologist, osteoporosis represents increased radiolucency of bones (particularly of the vertebrae), occasionally associated with biconcavity of vertebral bodies or ballooning of the intervertebral disks; with advanced rarefaction, some degree of vertebral collapse may occur (Figs. 12–2 and 12–3). Despite previous attempts to refine radiographic techniques, this definition is somewhat crude and misleading since a loss of over 30% of bone mineral is apparently necessary before the trained radiologist is certain of abnormal demineralization,[22,23] and radiologic criteria, such as ballooning of the vertebral disks, have been shown to be of little value in assessing the amount of bone loss.[24] Moreover, the amount of demineralization necessary for the radiologic diagnosis of osteopenia varies widely in different bones and in different parts of the same bone depending on the structural composition of the area in question. Decreased bone mass is more readily visible in bone characterized by an increased trabec-

OSTEOPENIA AND BONE MASS

(Schematic)

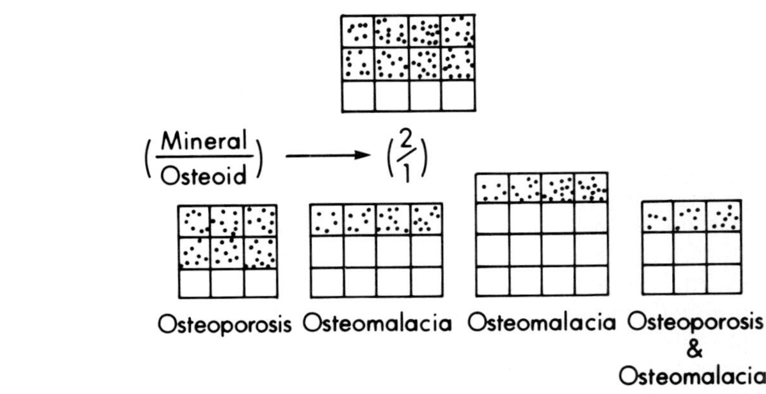

(Mineral / Osteoid) → (2/1) 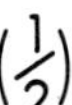 (1/2) (1/3) 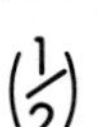 (1/2)

Figure 12–1. Schematic representation of bone mass and mineral-osteoid relationships in osteoporosis and osteomalacia. Each large block represents a hypothetical bone segment. The stippled areas denote mineralized osteoid; the clear areas, poorly mineralized or nonmineralized osteoid. The total number of small blocks in each hypothetical bone segment represents individual bone units. Note that bone mass is always decreased in osteoporosis, although the mineral-osteoid ratio is normal. Although bone mass may be normal, increased, or (when associated with osteoporosis) decreased in osteomalacia, the mineral-osteoid ratio is always decreased.

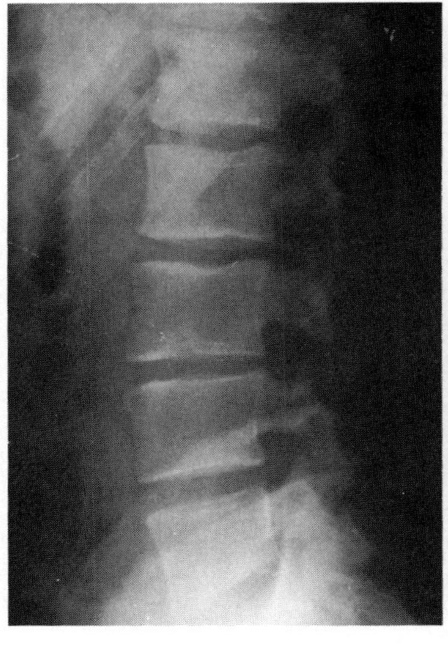

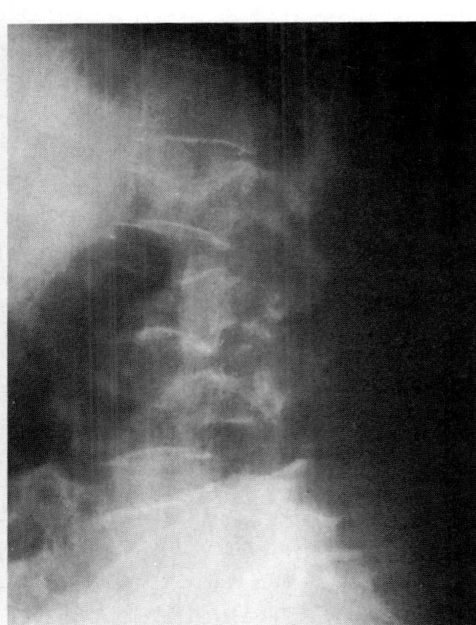

Figure 12–2. Lumbar vertebrae of a 29-year-old asymptomatic female on the left and that of a 55-year-old female with severe postmenopausal osteoporosis on the right.

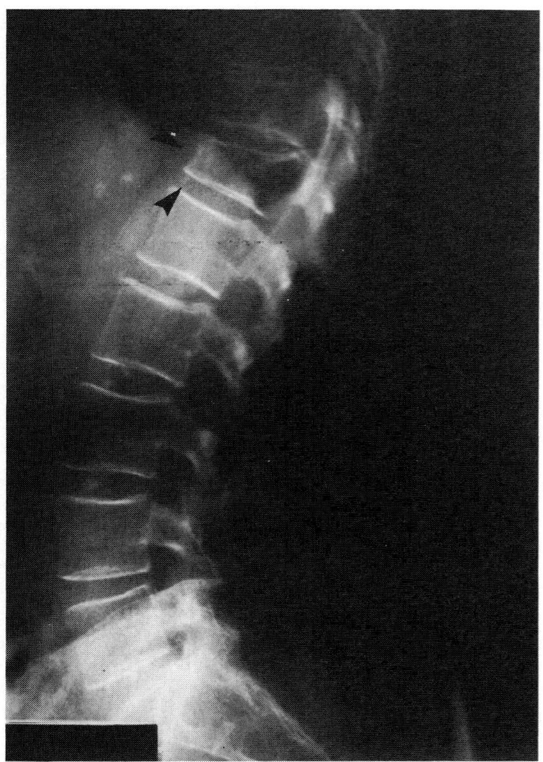

Figure 12–3. Anterior vertebral collapse (arrows) in an asymptomatic 58-year-old woman with postmenopausal osteoporosis.

ular content and relatively thin cortices. There are also individuals with excessive loss of vertebral trabecular bone without associated vertebral collapse as well as those with traumatic wedge fractures with a normal complement of trabecular bone. A lack of correlation also exists between bone mass in the axial (i.e., vertebral column and iliac crest) and appendicular (i.e., proximal ends of ulna and femur and small tubular bones of hands and feet) skeleton.[25-30] Obviously the propensity toward vertebral collapse and fracture in an osteoporotic individual depends not only on the mineral integrity of the skeletal site in question, but also on the quality of bone and the intensity of the mechanical forces applied to the area.[31]

I. PHYSIOLOGIC OSTEOPENIA

Bone affords an enormous depot of calcium that, when appropriately stimulated by a variety of hormones and metabolic agents, serves as the guardian of the circulating calcium pool. Unlike the mineral of tooth enamel that is relatively inert, the adult skeleton undergoes constant remodeling and turnover. The dynamic process of bone turnover normally results in the resorption and deposition of approximately 400 to 600 mg of calcium per day. Calcium is gradually deposited in the fetus during the early gestational period. During the final trimester, fetal accumulation of calcium is accelerated, and approximately two thirds of the calcium in the neonatal skeleton is deposited during this period. The total calcium content of a full-term child weighing 3500 g approaches 30 g or about 1% of the body weight. X-ray diffraction analysis of bones obtained from newborn infants reveals that both the apatite crystals and collagen are poorly oriented (see Chapter 2). This random pattern is converted to a highly oriented apatite-collagen relationship as the limbs are used and the skeleton is alternately stressed and relaxed.[32]

The turnover of skeletal calcium varies with age. It has been estimated to be 100% per year in infants up to 1 year, decreasing with age to a turnover rate of 10% in older children. The skeleton weighs approximately 100 g at birth and actually doubles in weight during the first year of life. Skeletal growth during childhood involves calcium retention of not more than 150 mg/day until after the first decade. During the peak adolescent growth "spurt," bone development is at its maximum. At this time calcium accumulation or "accretion" in bone may amount to between 275 and 500 mg/day, and bone mineral content increases by about 8.5% annually.[33] Thus, there are two periods of most rapid bone gain, that of infancy (through the second year) and that of adolescence (from ages 10 through 16 years, depending on sex and maturity rate). The adolescent spurt in subperiosteal new bone formation is earlier in females (from 10 through 16 years of age) than in males (from 12 through 16 years of age). The ratio of bone cortical area (i.e., second metacarpal) to total surface area is very similar to that of the 50th percentile curves of weight-for-age for all children aged 2 to 18 years.[34] By the age of 18, however, the ratio of cortical area to body weight is approximately 20% lower in females than in males. This relatively lower bone mass in females in early adult life may be one of the factors leading to a higher incidence of vertebral and hip fractures in postmenopausal women. Blacks have more bone and a heavier skeleton than do whites.[35] High bone density is not confined to black races, since bone mineral content of Polynesian women is also 20% greater than that of European women of similar ages.[36] These observations are also consistent with observations citing the important influence of genetic factors in control of bone development.[37] Alterations in the vitamin D–endocrine system[38,39] and blood calcitonin[40] that have been observed in blacks may also contribute to their propensity toward an increased bone mass. These acquired modifications include increased circulating levels of 1,25(OH)$_2$D as a result of secondary hyperparathyroidism (see Chapter 5), an enhanced renal tubular absorption of calcium, and increased circulating calcitonin levels (see Chapter 4). Children and young adults from impoverished areas or those suffering malnutrition characteristically exhibit a significant decrease in the amount of new bone formation during these periods.[41] Although ossification status (i.e., development of ossification centers) is not retarded by acute protein-calorie malnutrition, at a comparable "bone age" this acute insult leads to a dramatic decrease in compact cortical bone.[42] Subperiosteal growth in simple malabsorption states and in some disorders of oxygen transport is slower, but in addition endosteal bone resorption is accelerated. Bone "recovery" may also occur in adolescence in a variety of disorders, including osteogenesis imperfecta, vitamin D–resistant rickets, hypophosphatasia, and Down's syndrome.[43]

The rate of bone turnover is highest in cancellous or trabecular bones (i.e., vertebrae and ribs) than in compact bone, such as the long bones, skull, and mandible. The age-related remodeling processes of the skull probably differ from those of other skeletal parts, since skull bones are composed of two cortical layers, the outer and inner tables, separated by cancellous or "diploic" bone. As such, the bones in cross section from outside to within are characterized by two periosteum-lined surfaces, two compact layers of bone, and both endostei interspersed between diploic bone. This dual periosteal nature of the cranium leads to an increase in bone thickness. In contrast, the decreased thickness of "round" bones (i.e., rib, femur, and metacarpal) results from endosteal resorption exceeding periosteal apposition. It is still unclear whether either of the skull tables become thinner with age, a phenomenon that typifies the fate of comparable structural units (i.e., rib, femur, and metacarpal cortex). In adults, after epiphyseal closure and longitudinal growth have ceased, spinal (trabecular) bone density reaches its peak,[44] although skeletal turnover does not entirely cease, since there is both continuing subperiosteal cortical bone formation and a continuation of the later adolescent shift to endosteal bone formation or apposition, each of which contributes to increasing skeletal mass. At this time (25 to 30 years of age), the skeletal maintenance requires the deposition of approximately 180 g of calcium per year, or 15% of the total skeletal content. The skeleton is in a relatively steady state, since bone formation equals bone resorption with no net change in skeletal mass. Bone loss after skeletal maturity is a universal phenomenon. In men, bone loss tends to occur at the same rate as the loss of lean body mass[45] whereas in women there is an excessive loss of bone mass that exceeds the loss of lean body mass. In persons 35 to 50 years of age, there is a linear fall in the average amount of trabecular bone mass in women and men (Figs. 12–4 and 12–5). Using dual-photon densitometric measurements of *total* vertebral bone mineral, it has been shown that total bone mass in men and women declines 6% to 8% per decade, whereas the compact bone of the extremities decreases by 2% to 4% per decade after the age of 40 to 50 years.[46,47] More recent studies with computed tomographic techniques reveal that vertebral *trabecular* bone loss in women actually commences during or prior to the third decade.[48] The relationship between body size and skeletal mass may at least partly account for the racial differences in skeletal mass as well as the differences in bone mass between the sexes. It is, however, at the time of the menopause that the rate of bone loss increases significantly among women, and it is at this point that the true sexual dichotomy of bone loss becomes most obvious. Circulating estrogen levels play a major role in conditioning the rates of bone loss in women 42 to 58 years of age.[46,47,49,50] Estrogen deficiency following ovarian failure results in a 2-fold increase in bone turnover,[50] and an increased loss of vertebral trabecular bone that may be as great as 5% to 10% per year.[51] Cortical bone loss during this same period may be as much as 2% per year.[52] This loss is exponential, tends to decline after a

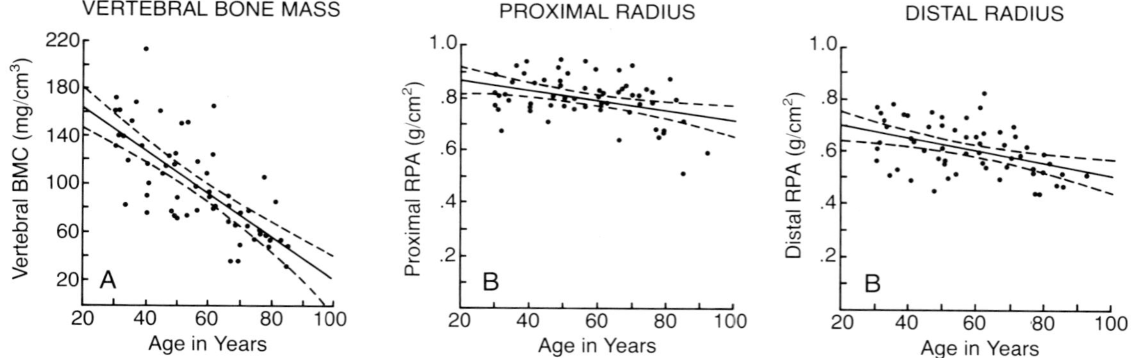

Figure 12–4. Regression of bone mineral content with age in healthy men (with 95% confidence interval of the estimates) for vertebrae. *A*, As measured by computer tomography. *B*, Both proximal and distal radius quantitated by radial photon absorptiometry (RPA). (From Meier DE, et al: Ann Intern Med 101:605–612, 1984.)

period of 4 to 8 years[53] (Fig. 12–6), and affects the entire skeleton, although it is far from uniform or homogeneous, proceeding at different rates in different parts.[54,55] Thus, the amount of cancellous trabecular bone of the vertebral bodies begins to decrease much earlier in life than does the cortical bone of the appendicular skeleton. Furthermore, the rates of bone resorption in various cancellous bones are also different, since vertebral bodies atrophy sooner than the calcaneum. Autopsy and *in vivo* noninvasive densitometric measurements of bone mass also demonstrate a positive correlation between bone size and bone density measurements.[35,56] Age-related decreases in mandibular alveolar bone also lead to diminution of tooth support, fenestration of the roots, and ultimate loss of teeth.[57,58]

General characteristics of the universal loss of skeletal mass with age can be summarized as follows: (1) in well-nourished individuals with calcium intakes greater than 700 to 800 mg/day, the decrease in bone mass is more rapid in females and is unrelated to calcium intake; (2) in females the trabecular bone loss begins during or prior to the third decade; (3) taller subjects of both sexes lose bone less rapidly; and (4) obese and black individuals during growth and modeling of bone develop greater skeletal mass for reasons yet unknown, although alterations in estrogen and calciotropic hormone production and/or metabolism have been implicated. Thus, since the maximum skeletal maturity is less for the white female than for the white male or the black male or female, and because the loss begins earlier in the female and proceeds at a more rapid rate after menopause, net skeletal mass is lowest in the slim postmenopausal white female.

Genetic and epidemiologic factors also appear to play important roles in determining the total bone mass of adult populations.

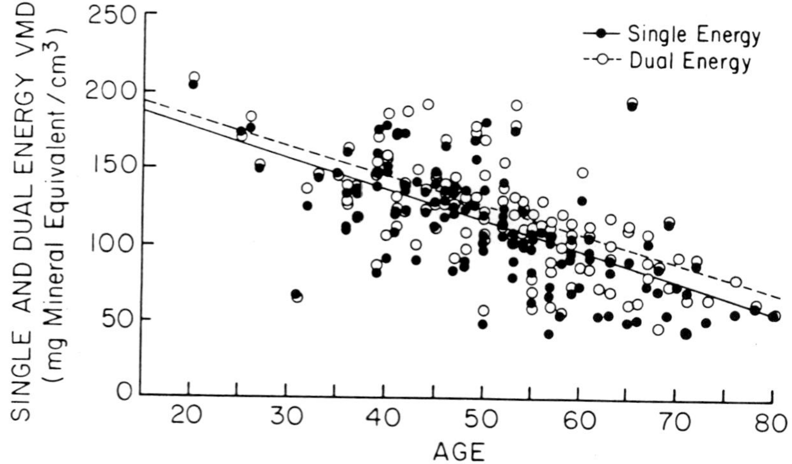

Figure 12–5. Regression of vertebral bone density with age in 133 normal women using computer tomography with either a single- or dual-energy source. (From Pacifici R, et al: J Clin Endocrinol Metab 64:209–214, 1987.)

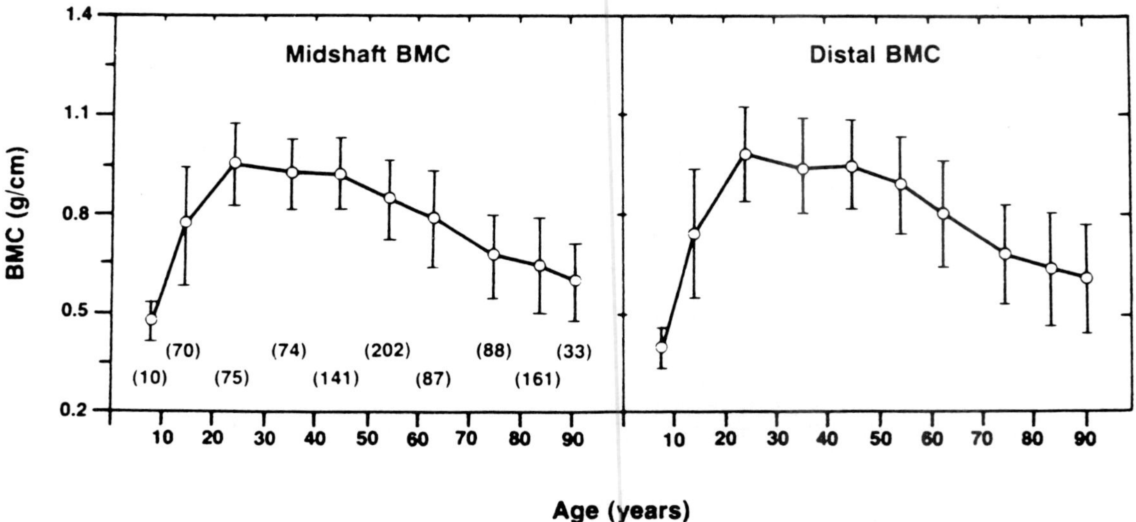

Figure 12–6. Photon absorption measurement of bone mineral content (BMC) of right radius in 941 white women. Number of subjects in each group is illustrated within the parentheses. (From Khairi MRA, Johnston CC: What we know — and don't know — about bone loss in the elderly. Geriatrics, Nov:67–70, 1978.)

Strikingly low levels of compact bone and vertebral density have been observed in prepubertal children with the XO variety of gonadal dysgenesis,[43] American-born and Asiatic-born Chinese and Japanese,[59] women of Anglo-Saxon origins,[60] and American Eskimos.[61] In this last group the demineralization has been associated with a decreased calcium intake and a "benign" systemic ketoacidosis that results from the Eskimo's high-protein acid-ash diet; high blood levels of $1,25(OH)_2D$ and very low levels of $24,25(OH)_2D$ have also been observed in the Eskimo and also attributed to a chronic low calcium intake.[62] Childhood osteopenia is seen in beta-thalassemia,[63] in patients with pseudo-pseudohypoparathyroidism,[64] and in subjects with chromosomal reduplications such as Klinefelter's syndrome (XXY).[43] Decreased bone mass also occurs in young XXXY and XXXXY individuals and in Down's syndrome.[43] In Down's syndrome, the osteopenia may be evident as early as the first year of life, but unlike in patients with XO Turner's syndrome, it is reversible with dramatic improvement observed during pubescence.[43] Studies of omnivores ingesting predominantly acid-ash diets with low calcium/phosphate ratios and of individuals with habitual excessive alcohol intakes also demonstrate significant losses in bone mass when compared with age- and sex-matched vegetarians[65] or nonalcoholics,[66] respectively. Moreover, since external mechanical forces, body weight, and skeletal muscle mass condition the structural integrity of bone,[67] the age-related loss of muscle mass combined with the gradual assumption of relatively sedentary lifestyles probably also contributes to the progressive decrease in skeletal mass that attends the aging process. One must also consider age-related changes in the intestinal absorption of calcium as another potential causative factor.[68] Although in early days no correlation between calcium intake and bone mass was demonstrated as reflected in either the thickness of the second metacarpal[69] or "spinal osteoporosis"[70] as estimated from routine radiographic analyses, more specific quantitative radiographic and photon absorptiometric measurements of bone mass demonstrate a significant negative correlation between calcium intake and bone mass.[71-76] Moreover, a negative linear correlation also exists between calcium absorption and age in both men and women,[77,78] and the adaptive efficiency of the intestine to a decreased calcium intake is impaired by the aging process[79] (Fig. 12–7). These factors together with the subtle alterations in renal function that characterize the aging process may lead to a chronic stimulated release of parathyroid hormone[80-84] (Fig. 12–8) and a failure to maximize the synthesis of the $1,25(OH)_2D_3$ vitamin D metabolite,[9,10,12] each of which perpetuates the accelerated rate of bone loss of aging individuals.

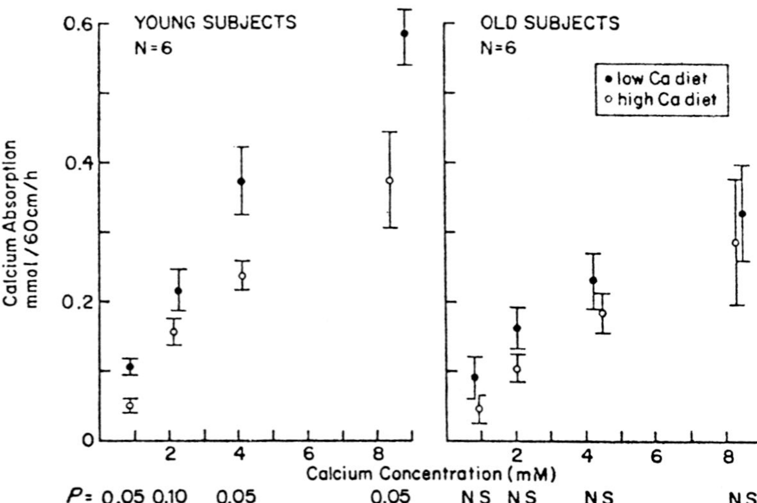

Figure 12–7. Effect of calcium intake on calcium absorption rates in young and old subjects. Each subject was studied twice, once on a low- and once on high-calcium diet. The rate of calcium absorption in the old subjects was significantly less than that observed in younger individuals, and the intestinal response of old individuals to calcium deprivation was blunted. NS, no significant difference. In this study, the urinary calcium was higher in the older subjects despite the fact that they absorbed less calcium. (From Ireland P, Fordtran JC: J Clin Invest 52:2672–2681, 1973.)

Other factors that may be implicated in the age-related bone loss phenomenon include defects in osteoblastic function,[85-90] changes in the quality[91] and quantity of the bone matrix,[31] an acquired impairment in calcitonin reserve and secretion,[92] and alterations in the immune system resulting in abnormal interleukin-1 activity.[93] Since subclinical cobalamin (vitamin B_{12}) deficiency is common in the elderly and since cobalamin deficiency is attended by defective osteoblastic activity,[94] it is conceivable that a chronic deficiency of this vitamin may also contribute to age-related bone loss in some individuals. The relationship between these age-dependent qualitative changes in bone matrix and skeletal mass and other changes in local and systemic factors that regulate bone cell function and metabolism[95] (see Chapter 1) is also consistent with the hypothesis that the progressive loss of bone mass that attends the aging process represents an acquired alteration in the orderly sequence of skeletal (mineral, cellular, and matrix) metabolism, which initially characterized the first two to three decades of life. Factors that also appear to play influential roles in this regard include race, weight, calcium intake, sex, ethnic origin, socioeconomic status, physical activity, and geographic area. The critical level of skeletal

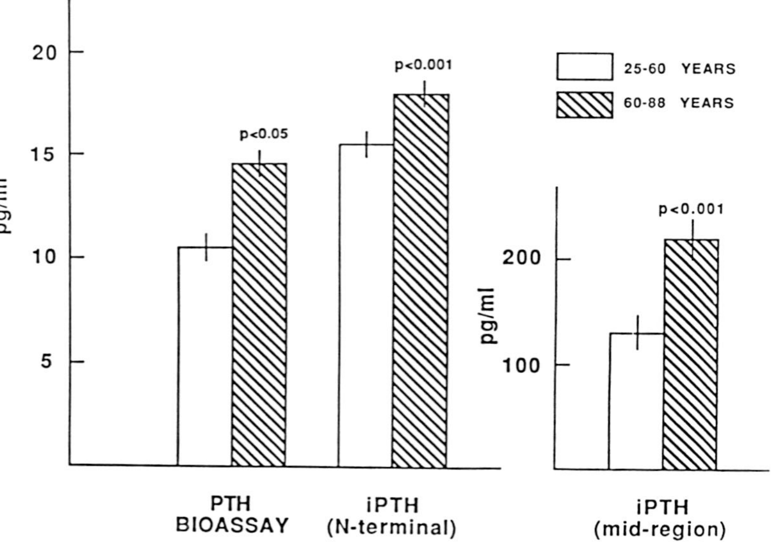

Figure 12–8: Circulating parathyroid hormone bioassay (PTH) and immunoassayable (iPTH) blood levels in young (25–60 years) and elderly (60–88 years) individuals. (Modified from Posillico JT, et al: Program and Abstracts of the 9th International Congress on Calcium-Regulating Hormones, Oct 25–Nov 1, 1986, Nice, France, p 143.)

mass at which osteopenia becomes radiologically or symptomatically manifest will be reached much earlier in the individual who failed to acquire the full complement of bone in adolescence. The individual with relatively lower skeletal mass at the time of maturity will be more susceptible not only to the complications of physiologic osteopenia at an earlier age but, as detailed later in this chapter, also to the skeletal insult imposed by drugs such as glucocorticoids, thyroid hormone, cytotoxic agents, or anticonvulsants, or any acquired disorder that results in a net loss of bone in excess of that attributable to the normal aging process.

II. DIAGNOSTIC AIDS

A. Radiology

Although bone mass normally decreases gradually with age in all adults, certain individuals with a variety of accumulated risk factors and/or inherited or acquired disorders of bone metabolism and others cited earlier will necessarily lose bone at a rate even greater than that imposed by senescence. It is often quite difficult to detect these individuals at greater risk for fracture since the amount of mineral that must be lost to be evident before the trained radiologic eye can suspect skeletal demineralization ranges from 20% to 60%. Furthermore, even when lack of mineral can be clearly visualized, it may be impossible to differentiate osteoporosis from osteomalacia,[96] malignant disorders with skeletal involvement such as multiple myeloma, or primary hyperparathyroidism.[97]

In the past, a number of "geographic" changes in bone roentgenograms have been used for the "diagnosis" of osteoporosis; these acquired alterations in vertebral structure become visually detectable only when bone loss is severe. In the vertebrae, one may see accentuation of end plate shadows and preservation and perhaps intensification of vertical trabeculae (Fig. 12–9) and biconcave compressions, localized to one or two vertebrae, usually with expansion of the intervertebral disks. In most forms of osteoporosis the vertebral cortex is thin and uninterrupted and gives the false impression of increased density because of the loss of trabeculae in the main body. Erosion of the cortex is rare in osteoporosis and should lead one to suspect malignant disease. The superior and inferior vertebral cortices are usually thickened or eburnated in patients with adrenal cortex overactivity (Fig. 12–10) or others on glucocorticoid therapy with osteoporosis.[98] As the bone loss progresses with advanced age, the trabecular pattern is accentuated because of the loss of horizontal trabecular structure and maintenance of vertebral trabeculae according to the structural lines of stress.[99] Further progression of the osteoporotic process may result in biconcave compression of the end plates by the pressure of the intervertebral disks on the hypomineralized vertebrae, resulting in "codfish" vertebrae and "ballooned" intervertebral disks

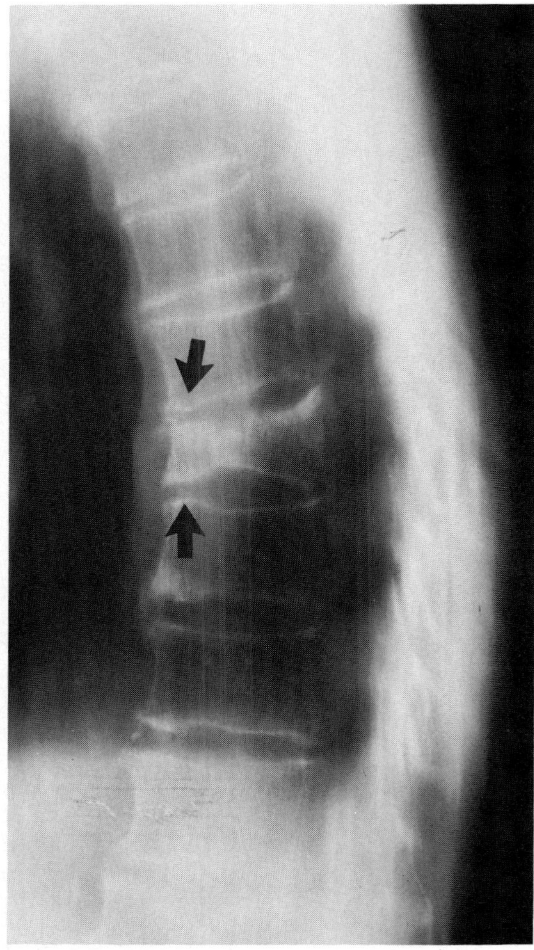

Figure 12–9. Laminogram of thoracic spine of a 60-year-old female with histologically confirmed osteoporosis. Note the accentuation of the vertical trabeculae and the areas of radiologic opacification (arrowheads) resulting from compression by the intervertebral disks and subcortical microfractures.

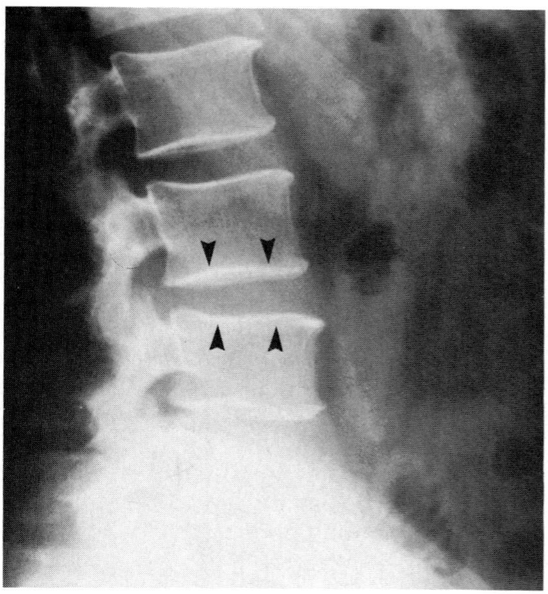

Figure 12–10. Vertebral osteoporosis in a patient with adrenal overactivity. Note thickened superior and inferior corticles (arrows).

(Fig. 12–11). Some advocate the use of a "spine" or "vertebral" index to document increased biconcavity of vertebral bodies. In this instance, if the ratio of the height of the central portion of the vertebral body to the height of the anterior or posterior cortex is less than 80%, significant bone loss is assumed. Localized herniations of the nucleus pulposus into the vertebral body, producing a concave mushroom-shaped defect in the upper or lower surface of the involved vertebrae or "Schmorl's nodes" (Fig. 12–11), may also be observed, although there is no association between Schmorl's nodes and the incidence of osteoporosis.[100] Isolated compression of the middle of the vertebral body must be evaluated carefully since this change in vertebral shape is rare and often an optical illusion.[101,102] Vertebral bodies demonstrating irregular end plates or multiple Schmorl's nodes may also reflect adolescent epiphysitis or Scheuermann's disease. Progressive vertebral demineralization leads subsequently to wedge or compression fracture. In osteopo-

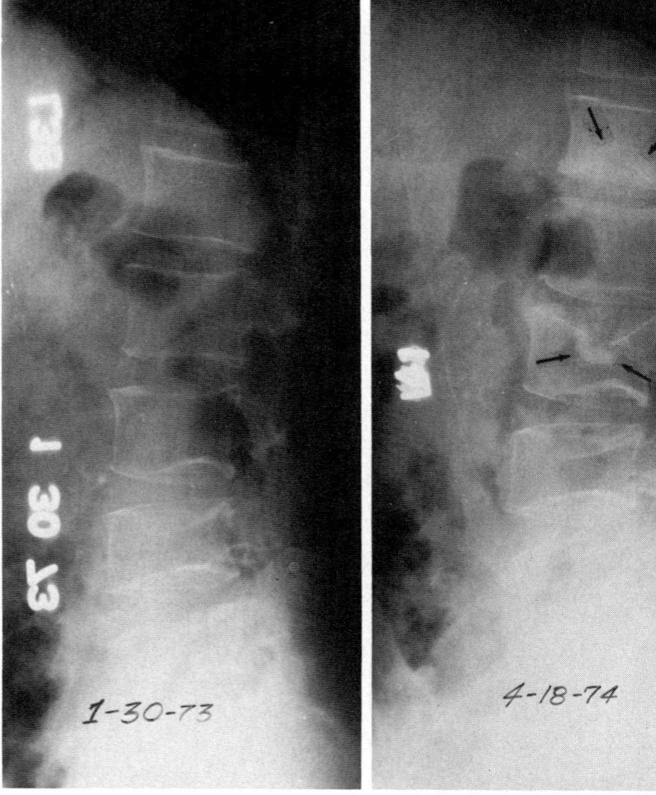

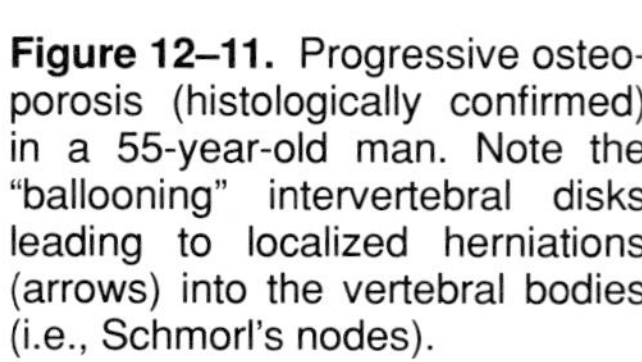

Figure 12–11. Progressive osteoporosis (histologically confirmed) in a 55-year-old man. Note the "ballooning" intervertebral disks leading to localized herniations (arrows) into the vertebral bodies (i.e., Schmorl's nodes).

rosis, the apex of a wedge fracture affecting mainly thoracic vertebrae is typically anterior (Fig. 12–3) and reflects advanced disuse when traumatic insults have not occurred.[101] Posterior wedging strongly suggests an underlying disease process distinct from osteoporosis, such as Paget's disease, trauma, or metastatic malignancy. Compression fractures that occur in osteoporotic patients may also result from vertebral osteomyelitis.[103] For patients with osteoporosis and acute vertebral compression fractures, occult osteomyelitis should always be considered, especially when there is severe back pain, persistent unexplained fever, elevated sedimentation rate, and bacteremia without an obvious extravertebral focus of infection.

The osteoporotic spine with irregularly spaced biconcave vertebral bodies containing Schmorl's nodes can often be distinguished from osteomalacia, which characteristically leads to biconcavity of the *majority* of vertebrae with expansion of the intravertebral spaces without Schmorl's nodes (see Chapter 11). These differences may be useful features for distinguishing the changes of osteoporosis and osteomalacia in the vertebral column with the following exceptions: (1) the vertebrae of osteoporotic children often reveal the regular shape changes described as characteristic for osteomalacia[104]; and (2) when osteoporosis and osteomalacia coexist in the same individual, the appearance of the spine may be classically that of osteoporosis. It should also be recognized that "pseudofractures" (Fig. 12–12)—"Looser zones," usually considered a hallmark of osteomalacia (see Chapter 11)—can also be observed in osteoporotic patients without histomorphometric evidence of osteomalacia.[96] This x-ray finding simply reflects the structural insufficiency of the skeleton. "Insufficiency fractures" of the pelvis that simulate metastatic disease are also seen in elderly individuals with severe bone loss.[105] Typical sites of involvement, such as the sacrum, the iliac bones, and the pubis, are often overlooked on initial radiographs and may require bone scanning and tomographs for identification (Fig. 12–13).

The presence of vertebral fractures in osteoporosis is highly correlated with the coexistence of other radiographic indications of osteoporosis, the association being particularly strong in the white female. Those individuals with a vertebral fracture in the midthoracic (T7–8) and thoracolumbar (T12–21) level of the spine have a 98% likelihood of having coexistent, generalized osteoporosis.[101,106] Fractures above the sixth thoracic vertebra with-

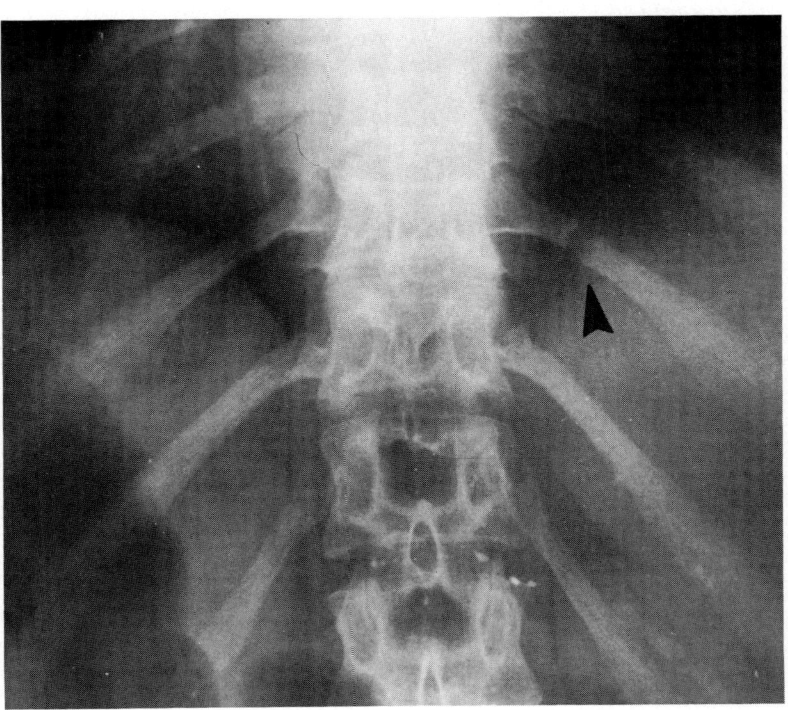

Figure 12–12. Pseudofracture of rib (arrow) in a postmenopausal woman with malabsorption and osteomalacia.

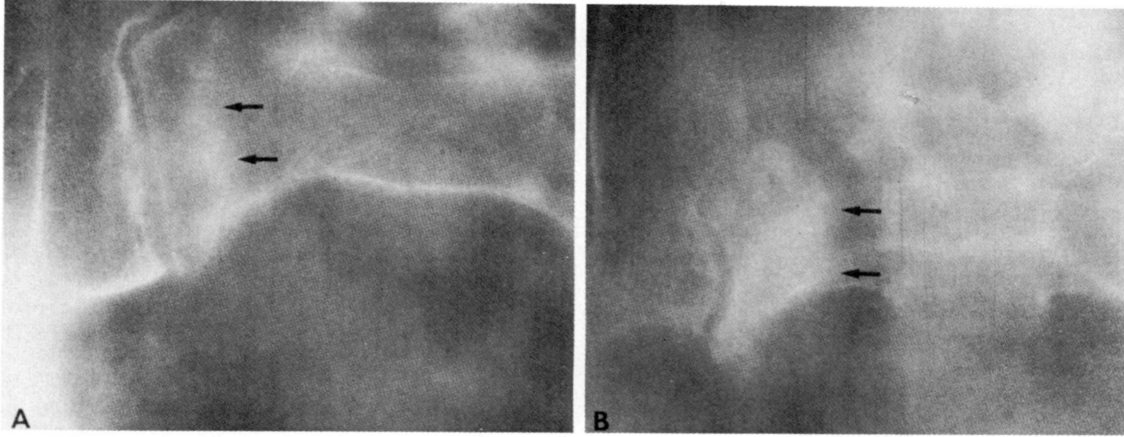

Figure 12–13. *A*, Tomogram of the sacrum and right sacroiliac joint, revealing vertebral band of sclerosis (arrows) in an osteoporotic patient with "insufficiency fractures" of the pelvis. *B*, Tomogram at a more posterior level demonstrating more pronounced sclerosis (arrows) adjacent to the right sacroiliac joint. (From Hauge MD, et al: Mayo Clin Proc 63:807–812, 1988.)

out concomitant disease below this level are rarely due to the loss of bone mass or "osteoporosis" that attends senescence. Spontaneous fractures above the fourth thoracic vertebrae should suggest metastatic cancer or septic spondylitis. Black individuals with vertebral fractures of the lower spine should always be considered to have generalized skeletal osteopenia until otherwise determined.

Radiographic changes, when apparent in peripheral skeletal sites, include cortical thinning of the long bones with irregularities of endosteal surfaces and diffuse demineralization (Fig. 12–14). Thinning of the tables of the calvarium is rare but when present is usually diffuse. Occasionally, the demineralization in the skull is spotty (Fig. 12–15), resembling multiple myeloma or metastatic carcinoma. These changes, seen usually only in advanced cases of osteoporosis, may be associated with decreased density of the floor and dorsum of the sella turcica. Pelvic and long bone involvement is characterized by a thin rim of well-mineralized cortex and a decreased amount of trabecular or cancellous bone (Fig. 12–14). The remaining trabecular pattern in the pelvis and femoral necks reflects the lines of stress applied to the skeleton and may actually appear more dense (Fig. 12–14). In this regard, some have advocated simple radiographic quantitation of trabecular content in the femoral heads (femoral neck or Singh "index") as a reliable method of categorizing various degrees of osteoporosis,[106,107] although this evaluation often proves unreliable.[108] A gross estimate of the severity of the osteoporotic process can also be obtained by measurements of cortical thickness of the femur, metatarsal, metacarpal, and phalangeal bones in relation to the total width of the shaft.[109] Combined thickness of the two cortices of less than 45% of the shaft width is considered to represent objective evidence of a significant decrease in bone mass. This technique often underestimates cortical bone loss since it fails to account for cortical porosity. Bone mineral in the phalangeal areas has also been quantitated by photodensitometric procedures,[110] although this technique is also of limited diagnostic value.[111] When the development of the osteoporotic process has been relatively rapid, as in severe forms of extreme immobilization, the earliest sign of demineralization may be a submetaphyseal band of rarefaction in the distal ends of the femora or tibiae. Only 1.5% to 2.5% of total body calcium loss (i.e., 20 to 30 g), when localized to specific areas in the long bones, is readily detected radiographically in cases of paralytic poliomyelitis[112] as early as 2 to 3 months after immobilization. Related roentgenographic features of limited diagnostic value are the absence of less than the usual amount of osteophytosis or spur formation along the vertebrae, a process that normally accompanies the aging process, and a relative increase in calcification of the aorta compared with that expected for the age of the pa-

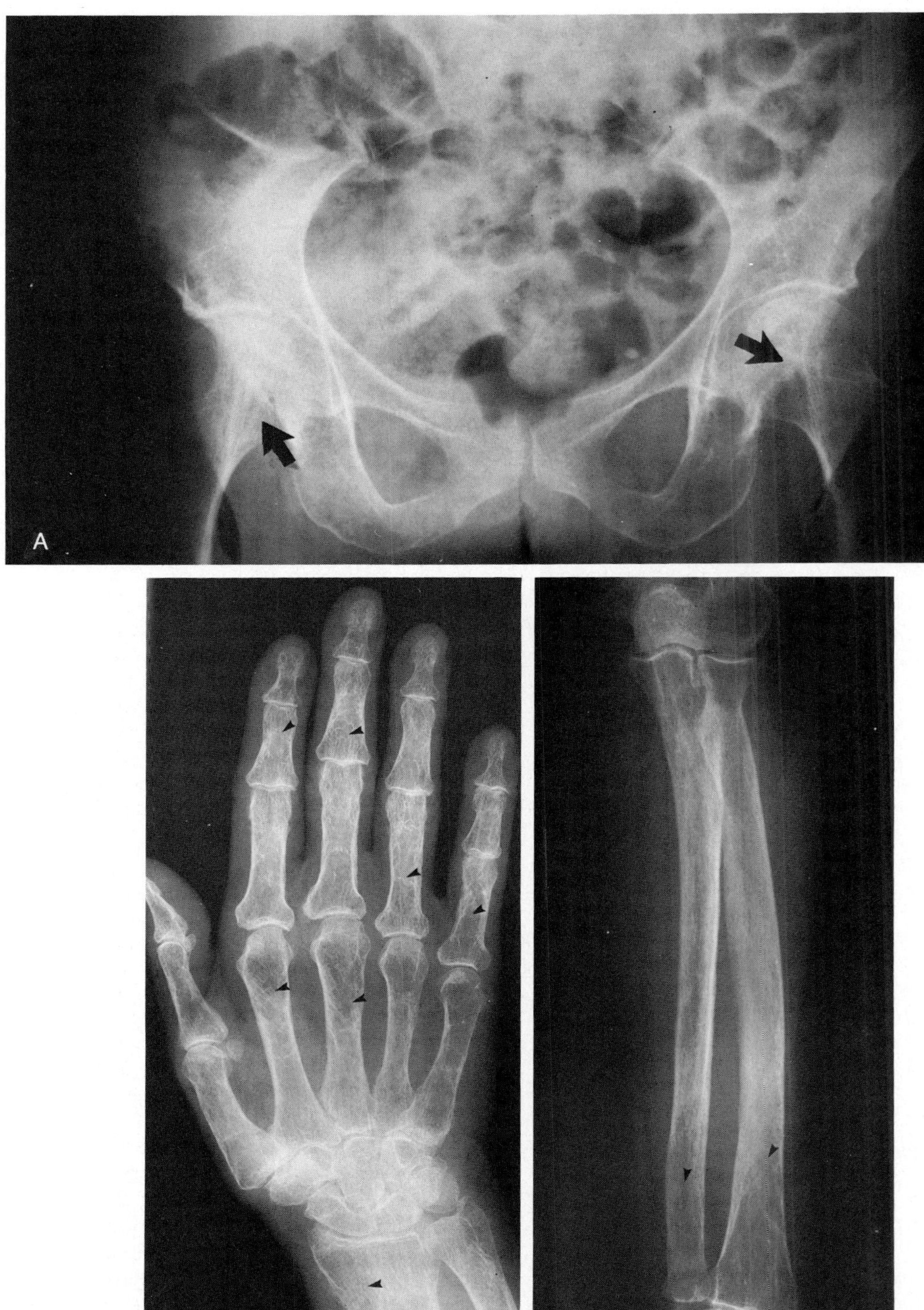

Figure 12–14. Radiographs of the pelvis (*A*), and (*B*), and right upper extremity (*C*) in a 65-year-old female with histologically documented osteoporosis. Cancellous bone of the right distal humerus, both femoral heads, and tubular bones of the hands have lost most of the trabeculae components (arrowheads). Remaining trabeculae in the femoral heads, representing those in the "line of stress," are increased in density and width.

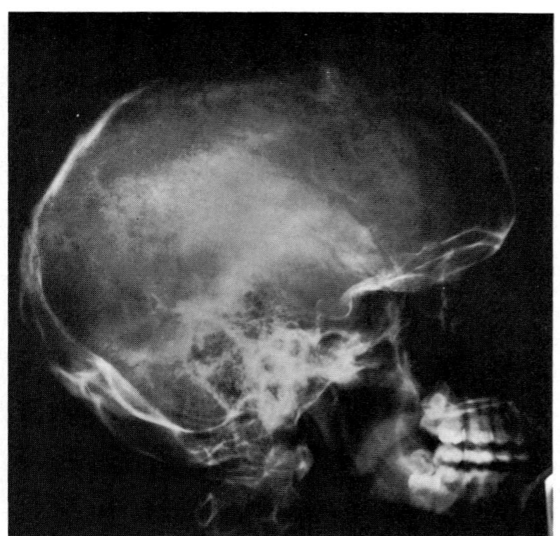

Figure 12–15. Spotty demineralization of the skull in a patient with bilateral adrenal cortical hyperplasia.

tient.[104] In severe cases, forward displacement of one vertebra over another (usually the fifth lumbar over the body of the sacrum or fourth lumbar over the fifth) mirrors the developmental defect in the pars interarticularis as seen in spondylolisthesis (Fig. 12–16).

Recently, a computer-derived spine deformity index (SDI) has been advocated as a simplified method for quantitating vertebral crush fractures on routine roentgenograms.[113] This technique, based on the observations (110 normal persons) that heights of all vertebral bodies are related to each other in a predictable and constant manner, it still is too premature for assessing its diagnostic specificity in individual patients.

B. Bone Mass Measurements

Over the past 15 to 20 years, a variety of noninvasive techniques have been developed for the estimation of bone mineral mass (see Chapter 9). It now seems possible that in the fairly near future, screening techniques for osteoporosis will include a routine bone mass measurement, perhaps at the time of the menopause and most assuredly in individuals with a preponderance of risk factors.[114-117] Currently, both dual- and single-beam photon absorptiometry (Fig. 12–6) and computer tomographic procedures (Figs. 12–4 and 12–5) are consistently used. The combination of these techniques allows measurement of peripheral bone, at the mid or distal radius site, and axial or central bone, usually the lumbar vertebrae or neck of the femur. The bone measured at the peripheral sites is primarily cortical bone, whereas the bulk of the bone measured at the vertebral site is trabecular bone. These combinations of measurements overcome the problem of possible diversities in behavior between different sites in the skeleton. Whether this is due to variations between cortical and trabecular bone behavior or to dissimilarities in behavior between axial and peripheral bone is not yet evident. Accumulating evidence suggests that changes occurring in the central or axial skeleton may differ significantly from changes occurring at the peripheral or appendicular skeleton.[26,28,29,118]

Although the peripheral measurement by single-photon absorptiometry is easy and may be performed in the average office setting, there is a high incidence of error in estimating central bone mass from peripheral measurements. The correlation coefficient between the two sites is low, usually about 0.4 to 0.6, and bone loss in the immediate postmenopausal phase of life is significantly greater at the vertebral site.[29,119] Also, it must be emphasized that there may be *no* relationship between the rate of change at either skeletal site.[26-29] A single measurement by both of these techniques results in a radiation exposure slightly less than that from a single chest roentgenogram, which under well-controlled techniques makes for an acceptable method of estimating and then following bone mass in individual patients. Recent software development allows dual-photon absorptiometry to be used to estimate total body calcium and femoral neck calcium with good precision and accuracy.[29]

Computed tomography (CT) provides, with any fourth-generation scanner and appropriate software, estimates of pure vertebral trabecular bone unobtainable by other techniques.[119-120] There is controversy about the accuracy of this technique, and there may also be arguments over its precision, particularly if a single-energy technique is used.[120] Precision and accuracy may also be reduced by the subjective decisions required to obtain the measurement site with this technique. The capability to measure pure trabecular bone within the vertebral body, eliminating interference from extraosseous

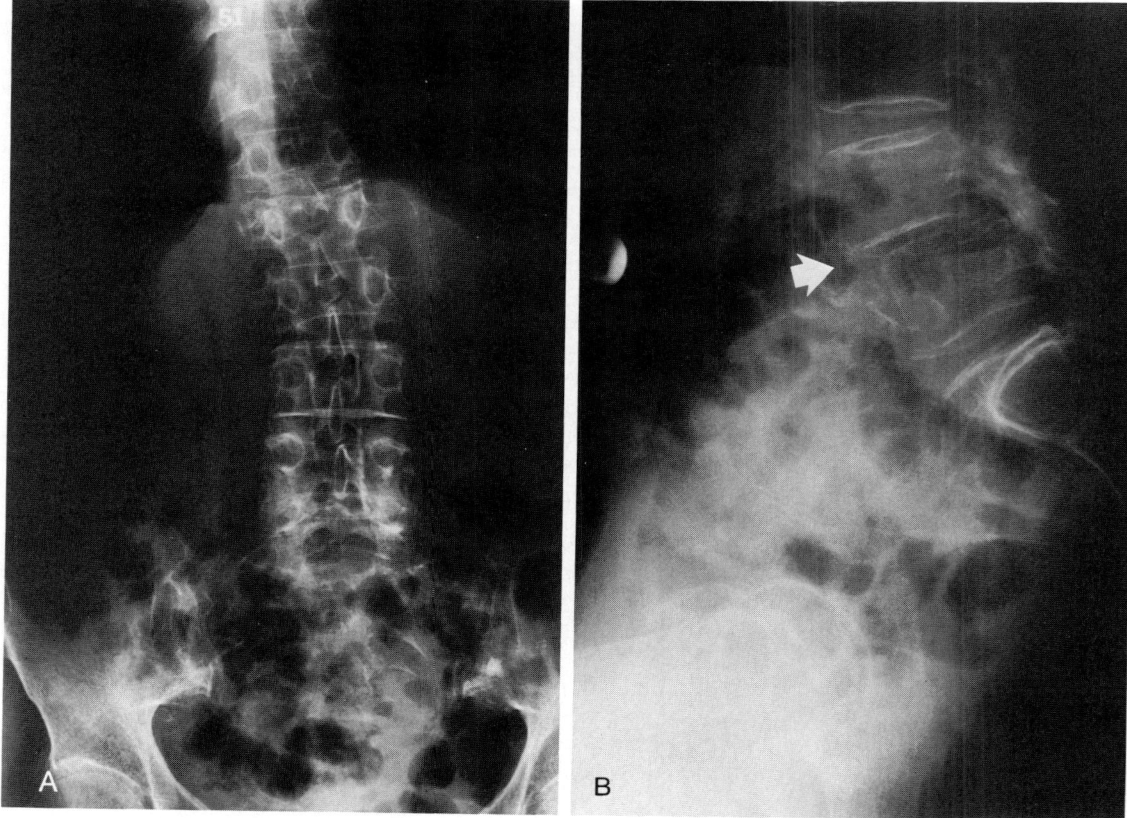

Figure 12–16. *A*, "Pseudospondylolisthesis" in a 79-year-old female with severe osteoporosis and scoliosis. *B*, Note the forward displacement of the fourth lumbar vertebra on the body of the fifth (arrow).

calcification such as osteophytes and aortic calcification (Fig. 12–17), makes this the method of choice (over techniques that are not restricted to the trabecular component of vertebral bone) in dealing with elderly patients with significant established osteoporosis.[120] However, the separation of patients with osteoporosis from the normal population tends to be better by dual-photon absorptiometry than by CT scanning.[15] The reason for this is not clear. In most CT settings, a phantom including a variety of concentrations of a bone mineral equivalent (usually K_2HPO_4) is scanned along with the patient (Fig. 12–17), allowing compensation for scanner drift over time and problems with beam hardening, but this does not compensate for the problems encountered with changes in marrow fat with age and decreased trabecular bone content. Particularly with the single-energy technique, these may result in significant errors in both accuracy and precision. To some extent this can be offset by dual-energy CT scanning. The cost is usually a larger radiation dose and longer scan time (see Chapter 9).

The most recent development in noninvasive bone mass measuring devices is "dual-energy radiography," also referred to as "quantitative digital radiography" (Fig. 12–18). Using dual-energy, pulsed x-ray technology, this technique can provide quantitation of bone mineral content in a shorter scan time with less radiation than either existing computed tomographic or dual-beam photon absorptiometric procedures. This new device is similar to dual-beam absorptiometry but differs in that an x-ray tube replaces the radioisotopic ^{153}gadolinium source. Although minimal experience is available for adequate assessment of its ultimate value in assessing bone mass, it has been demonstrated that the machine measures bone mass with higher resolution and greater speed than existing dual-photon absorptiometry equipment with precision values in the range of 0.3% to 0.4%.[121-122]

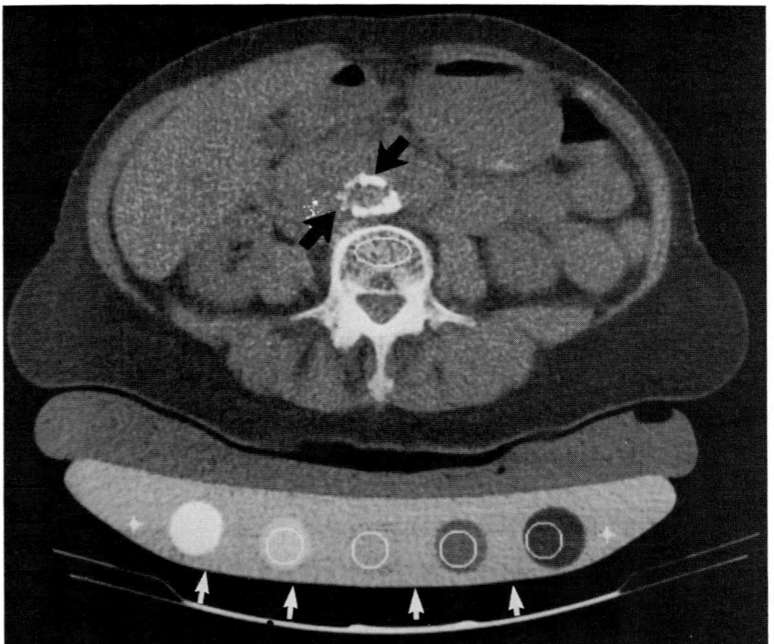

Figure 12–17. A computer tomographic representation of an osteoporotic patient with severe aortic calcification (two arrows). Note the elliptical area of measurement *within the vertebrae* and the K_2HPO_4 standard (four arrows).

None of these techniques measures bone turnover or gives any estimate of the metabolic activity within the skeleton. In order to determine rate of loss as well as mass at a single patient visit, a simplified method of quantitating skeletal turnover would be useful. A modification of the routine bone scanning technique, which has been found to be useful in determining skeletal metabolism, and which may add a predictive element to the bone mass measurement, has also been described.[123] This technique, which depends on the skeletal "retention" of a radioactive diphosphonate bolus, requires further investigation and validation before it could be put to general use. It does, however, help identify those patients with "high turnover" postmenopausal osteoporosis who, as detailed later, are excellent candidates for calcitonin therapy.[124] It seems likely that during the

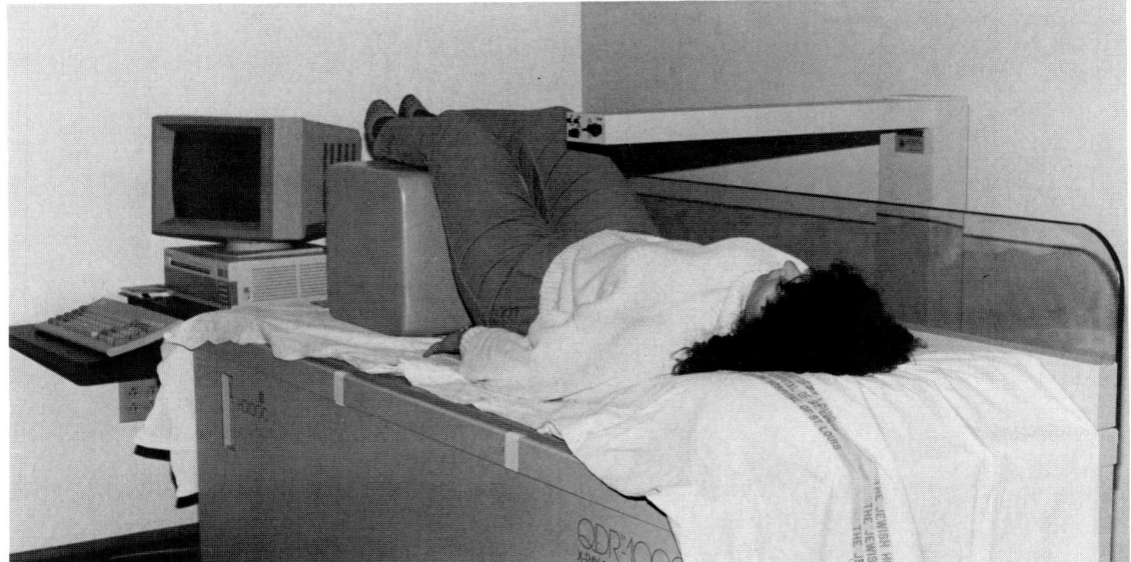

Figure 12–18. Patient in the process of vertebral bone mass measurement using the quantitative digital radiography technique.

coming decade, bone mass measurements will become more available to many clinicians, and it may be that bone mass values below a certain critical value[114-117] in patients with established risk factors will require the institution of preventive advice, if not pharmacologic treatment.

C. Clinical Characteristics

Most patients with osteoporosis are asymptomatic despite the presence of one or more vertebral fractures. When present, back pain is usually localized and of two types. Coincident with a vertebral fracture, the patient may experience sudden onset of sharp, severe pain aggravated by motion and located directly over a vertebral process. The pain may be spasmodic and characteristically radiates anteriorly around the flank into various portions of the abdomen, legs, or pelvis. In contrast to osteomalacia, generalized skeletal pain is uncommon, and between episodic bouts of vertebral fracture, the patient is usually completely free of pain. Nerve root and spinal cord compressions are also exceedingly rare complications of spinal osteoporosis, despite the presence of severe spinal deformities. With rest and with slight hyperextension of the back if necessary, the pain gradually subsides within 2 or 4 weeks regardless of any other treatment. The other more commonly observed pain is dull and aching, of long duration, and located several centimeters to one or both sides of the midline in the lower thoracic or lumbar region. These symptoms are often attributed to "rheumatism," "lumbago," or "sciatica."[125] Careful palpation usually detects associated spasm of the paravertebral muscles. The pain is apt to be exacerbated by sitting or standing for some time or by the Valsalva maneuver and is usually relieved by lying down.

The history may also reveal a gradual loss of height over a period of years or sometimes only months. The loss of height in osteoporosis is due to vertebral compression, most marked in the lumbar vertebrae and associated with lumbar scoliosis in over 45% of patients,[126] although it is also seen in the thoracic vertebrae. Clinically, the loss of height can be shown to be above the pubis by demonstrating that the distance from pubis to heel minus the distance from crown to pubis is greater than 2 inches, while the pubis-to-heel dimension is still one half the span from fingertip to fingertip. Stepwise decline in height and an associated lower dorsal kyphosis (commonly referred to as the "dowager's" or "widow's hump") are reliable clinical signs of progression of the osteoporotic process (Fig. 12–19). Progressive spinal deformity usually leads to downward angulation of the ribs and a narrowing of the normal gap between the lower ribs and the iliac crest, which may become so severe that patients complain of "rubbing together" of the iliac crest and lower ribs. At this point, measurable reduction in height usually ceases. For this reason, changes in linear height in the patient with severe dorsal kyphosis as a reflection of therapeutic responsiveness should be interpreted with caution. Abdominal distention (Fig. 12–19) and prominent horizontal skin creases are also seen across the abdomen resulting from an accordion-like folding of the torso (Fig. 12–19). In severe forms of the disease, the loss of the anterior lumbar curve may produce "pseudospondylolistheic" deformities (Fig. 12–16*B*), a forward pelvic tilt, hamstring contractures, permanent hip joint flexion, stiff ankles, and pronated feet; consequently patients may walk with a shuffling, unsteady gait and a broad stance and complain of chronic "lower back pain." Common sites of fracture other than vertebrae are the distal end of the radii (i.e., Colles' fracture) and the femoral neck.

D. Laboratory Testing

Calcium and inorganic phosphate in the plasma of patients with skeletal osteoporosis may be abnormal as a result of the underlying pathologic process. Occasionally, severe osteoporosis associated with multiple myeloma, occult malignant syndromes, hyperthyroidism, or acute immobilization may be present with a mild hypercalcemia and hyperphosphatemia, the former due to rapid resorption of skeletal mineral reservoirs and the latter possibly to parathyroid suppression induced by the hypercalcemia. Unrelated causes of hypercalcemia to be considered in patients with symptomatic or "crush fracture" osteoporotic syndromes include excessive vitamin A or vitamin D ingestion and chronic ingestion of diuretics, phosphate-binding "antacid" preparations, or subsali-

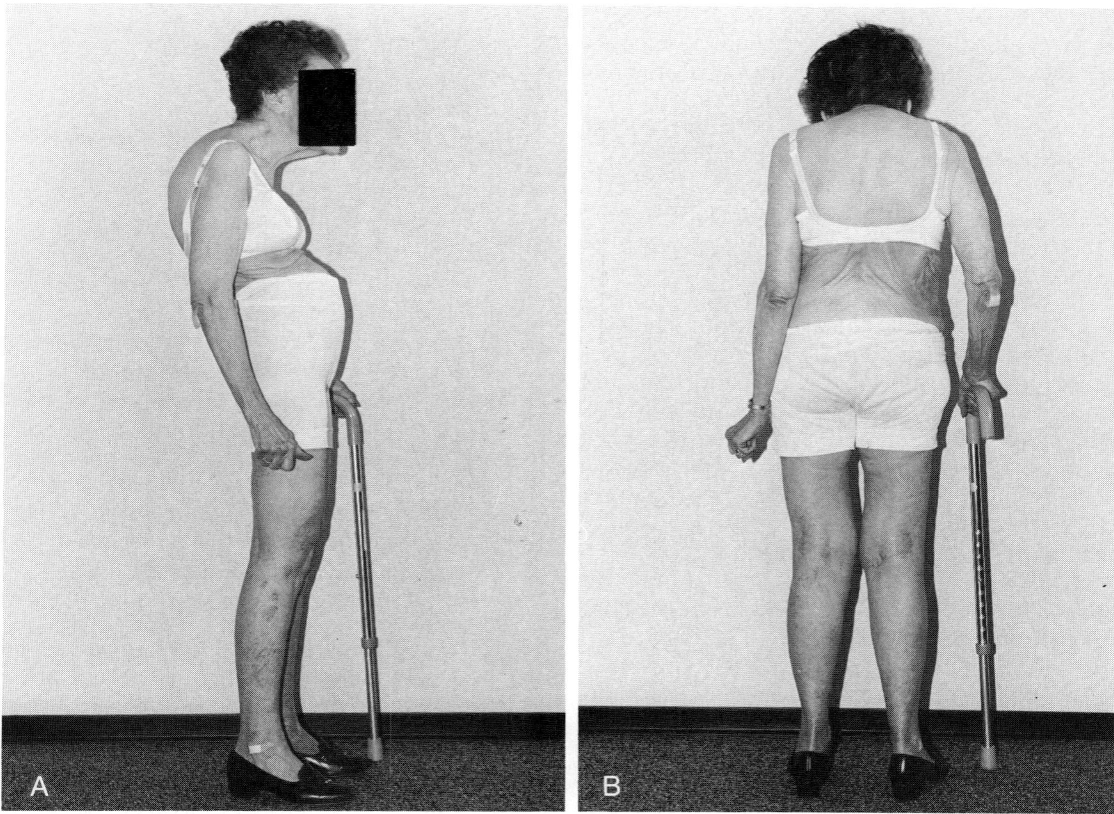

Figure 12–19. Severe thoracic kyphosis and abdominal distention (*A*) and scoliosis (*B*) in a 70-year-old osteoporotic woman.

cylate bismuth drugs such as Pepto-Bismol, which is often prescribed for the prevention of traveler's diarrhea (emporiatric enteritis). Unlike the liquid forms of Pepto-Bismol, the tablet forms contain 350 mg of calcium carbonate per tablet. Recommended doses of this agent to prevent diarrhea could deliver as much as 4.5 to 5.0 g/day of calcium and result in hypercalcemia. Although diagnostic significance has been attributed to the serum phosphate level in postmenopausal forms of osteoporosis, and a direct correlation has been observed between circulating phosphate values and bone-resorbing surfaces quantitated microradiographically in cross-sectional studies,[127] this sign is of little value in any one patient. Occasionally, states of adrenal corticoid excess may complicate postmenopausal osteoporotic state and result in hypocalcemia[128] and hypophosphatemia. Hypophosphatemia results from the phosphaturic effect observed in glucocorticoid-treated individuals (either indirectly because of elevations in circulating parathyroid hormone or as a direct effect of glucocorticoids on the kidney).

Although the chemical hallmark of primary hyperparathyroidism is hypercalcemia (see Chapter 14), total blood calcium is not infrequently in the "normal range" in elderly females with hyperparathyroidism who present with classic radiologic changes of "osteoporosis."[129] In these instances, ionized calcium values usually prove diagnostic.[129] Measurements of parathyroid hormone (PTH) levels must also be interpreted with caution since, although typically elevated in individuals with primary hyperparathyroidism (see Chapter 14), PTH levels not only *normally* increase with age[80-84] (Fig. 12–8) but may also be elevated in individuals with low-renin hypertension syndromes,[130] others on chronic glucocorticoid therapy,[131] and those with the benign hypercalcemic, hypocalciuric familial hyperparathyroid syndrome[132] (see Chapter 14). Elevated blood PTH levels in elderly individuals with progressive osteoporosis may also reflect an underlying "type II" form of osteoporosis (Table 12–1). Unlike the "type I" form, type II osteoporosis is characterized by the loss of both trabecular and cortical bone and presents with hip and pelvic fractures.[133-134] As reviewed in Chapter 3, the heterogeneity of the parathyroid hormone molecule and the development of a heterogeneous group of radioimmunoassays may also complicate the interpretation of results obtained. Moreover, it should also be stressed that estrogen and androgen treatment regimens for postmenopausal osteoporosis may mask the hypercalcemia of primary hyperparathyroidism,[135-136] the serum calcium rising whenever therapy is discontinued.[136] Mild hypocalcemia and hypocalciuria with radiologic signs indicative of osteoporosis suggest coexistent osteomalacia (see Chapter 11). Serum alkaline phosphatase is usually normal in osteoporosis, although vertebral osteoporosis in males is often attended by mild elevations.[106] Elevated values suggest either associated osteomalacia, Paget's disease of bone, healing fractures, primary hyperparathyroidism, or hypercortisolism. *Before attributing an elevated blood alkaline phosphatase to fracture healing, it should be recognized that the elevation is only detectable 7 to 10 days after the fracture occurs*[137] (Fig. 12–20). Occasionally, patients with osteogenesis imperfecta tarda and radiographic osteoporosis demonstrate elevations in serum alkaline phosphatase and acid phosphatase, although these changes are not characteristic for the disorder (see Chapter 17). Elevations in blood alkaline phosphatase can also be observed in individuals with occult osteomalacia on vitamin D "supplements," fibrous dysplasia, hyperthyroidism, hypernephroma, polymyalgia rheumatica, pregnancy, pulmonary embolization, thyroiditis, myocardial infarction, and certain forms of "benign" familial hyperphosphatasemia. Alkaline phosphatase can also be elevated following a normal meal and in

Table 12–1. Characteristics of Patients with Type I and Type II Osteoporosis

	Type I	Type II	p
Age (yr)	65.1 ± 5.4	83.6 ± 8.9	< 0.001
Calcium (mg/100ml)	9.5 ± 0.5	8.6 ± 1.0	< 0.001
PTH (pg/ml)	550 ± 398	852 ± 674	< 0.05
Radial bone mass (g/cm)	0.62 ± 0.12	0.62 ± 0.12	NS

Type I, vertebral fractures; type II, hip fractures.

Reproduced from Johnston CC, et al: J Clin Endocrinol Metab 61: 551–556, 1985.

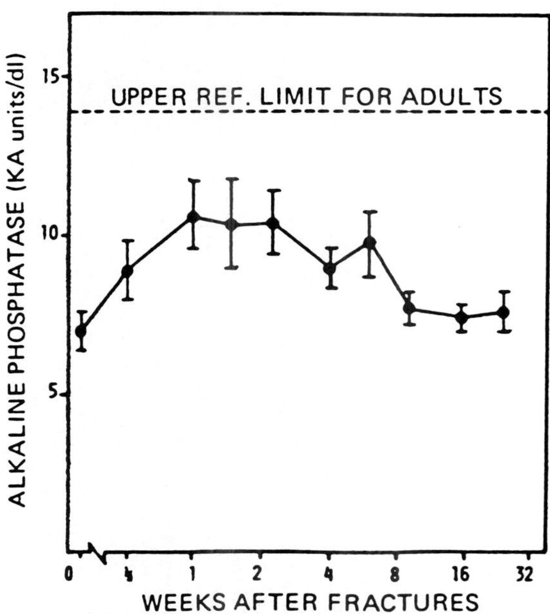

Figure 12–20. Means (●) and standard deviations (**I**) of serum alkaline phosphate activities of 63 patients with fracture of the femoral neck. (From Nilsson BE, Westlin NE: Acta Orthop Scand 43:564–567, 1972.)

patients with hepatobiliary disease, in those with lung cancer, or in others treated with a variety of unrelated drugs, that is, gold salts, nonsteroidal antiinflammatory agents, allopurinol, antibiotics, and oral hypoglycemic agents and following albumin infusions.[138-144] Tartrate-resistant acid phosphatase (TRAP) has also been proposed as a biochemical marker for bone resorption. Although accumulated data are still preliminary, circulating TRAP levels are abnormally high in osteoporotic women, and a negative correlation has been demonstrated between blood TRAP values and vertebral bone mass.[145]

Recent evidence suggests that there is a relationship between circulating bone gla-protein (BGP), a noncollagenous protein found only in bone and dentin, and bone turnover,[146-151] with elevated values observed whenever bone turnover is increased, that is, hyperthyroidism and hyperparathyroidism (see Chapter 8). The diagnostic significance of blood BGP in "osteoporotic" disorders has yet to be established with certainty, although individuals with the "high turnover" variety of postmenopausal osteoporosis are characterized by elevated values.[124,146] Postmenopausal osteoporotic patients on long-term glucocorticoid therapy and with low bone turnover may present with low BGP values.[124] Since circulating alkaline phosphatase and BGP do not possess equivalent specificity and sensitivity in differentiating osteoporotic disorders from normal, it has been suggested that both biochemical markers be assayed concurrently to ensure greater diagnostic efficiency.[152]

Androstenedione, an androgen secreted by the ovary and adrenal glands, is converted to estrogens in fat and muscle. Plasma androstenedione in postmenopausal women represents adrenal secretion only. Lower blood levels of androstenedione have been observed in some postmenopausal osteoporotic patients with "fracture-prone" loss of skeletal mass. This test, however, should not be presently considered diagnostic or helpful in establishing the severity of the osteoporotic state in any single patient. The major circulating adrenal androgen, dehydroepiandrosterone sulfate (DHEAS), has also been reported to be significantly lower in crush fracture-prone osteoporotic patients;[153] DHEAS is also positively correlated with vertebral bone density as qualitated by computed tomography.[154] These observations may be misleading since circulating levels of androstenedione and DHEAS are *elevated* in cigarette smoking females,[155,156] a select population of women with an *increased* propensity to develop osteoporosis.[58,157,158] Consequently, no diagnostic significance for blood values of either androstenedione or DHEAS can be established at this time.

Since vitamin D deficiency is common in elderly individuals,[3-21] especially those with poor sunlight exposure, blood levels of one of its active metabolites, 25-hydroxycholecalciferol (see Chapter 5), should prove helpful in establishing any occult "osteomalacic" contribution to the underlying osteoporotic disorder. Fasting blood levels below 10 to 11 ng/ml are consistent with underlying defects in bone mineralization and an underlying osteomalacic contribution to the osteoporotic syndrome. 25-Hydroxycholecalciferol levels may be decreased in patients with chronic malabsorptive or hepatic insufficiency syndromes and in others on long-term anticonvulsant regimens, situations that occasionally result in osteomalacia (Chapter 11) or premature bone loss and an "osteoporotic" radiographic presentation. Excessive sunlight exposure or the persistent use of vitamin D "supplements" in doses greater than 1000 to 1500 units per day may result in elevations in blood 25-hydroxycholecalciferol and urinary calcium much earlier than the hypercalcemia that ultimately occurs (see Chapter 5).

The majority of pathologic disorders that should be considered in any "osteoporotic" female are diagnosed by specific diagnostic testing procedures, that is, immunoelectrophoresis for multiple myeloma, bone marrow aspiration for systemic mastocytosis, blood thyroid hormone assays for hyperthyroidism, urinary cortisol for adrenal overactivity, and hepatic functional testing in patients with suspected hemochromatosis. One should be reminded of "osteoporotic" radiographs, which may occur in patients with "nonsecreting" forms of multiple myeloma, since in this form of the disease immunoelectrophoretic testing is characteristically nondiagnostic; bone marrow aspiration is essential to establish the diagnosis.

Urinary calcium is usually normal in individuals with osteoporosis unless it is attended by specific clinical disorders compromised by immobilization; malignancies such as multiple myeloma; oophorectomy; hyperthyroidism or during thyroid hormone replacement therapy; hyperparathyroidism; and glucocorticoid therapy. Hypercalciuria (i.e., 24-hour urinary calcium greater than 3.5 mg/kg body weight) may occur in patients during diuretic therapy, and when phosphate-binding antacids are taken indiscriminately. In selected instances, one of us (LVA) has noted hypercalciuria with histologic documentation of osteoporosis in the elderly female suggestive of an occult or senescent form of acquired distal renal tubular acidosis, although blood levels of serum bicarbonate and pH were normal. These patients, reminiscent of reports of decreases in acid excretion in the aged,[159,159a] can be identified with certainty by recording the urinary pH for 2 to 3 consecutive days and determining the response to NH_4Cl (0.1 g/kg body weight). Normally, the urine pH should rise after food intake ("alkaline tide") and also fall below 5.6 after NH_4Cl ingestion. Measurements of calcium and creatinine in a morning fasted urine specimen and the use of a calcium/creatinine ratio have been advocated as a "diagnostic index" of accelerated bone turnover.[124] A calcium/creatinine ratio greater than 0.16 is often consistent with accelerated bone breakdown.

Urinary hydroxyproline, an indirect measurement of bone collagen turnover (see Chapters 8 and 15), is also generally normal in osteoporotic subjects,[160] although it may be elevated in some patients with "high turnover" osteoporosis.[124] Fasting urinary hydroxyproline/creatinine ratios have been advocated for both diagnosis and following the response to therapy, with values greater than 0.012 suggesting rapid bone turnover. Increased hydroxyproline excretion usually attends the "osteoporotic-like" skeletal changes seen in patients with hyperthyroidism, hyperparathyroidism, metastatic malignancy, osteogenesis imperfecta tarda, acromegaly, Cushing's syndrome, and immobilization and in patients on thyroid replacement therapy.[161-163] Urinary hydroxyproline values are also markedly influenced by dietary sources of collagen-like peptides such as jellos, gelatin-containing products, and meat.

Recently, the urinary excretion of hydroxylysine glycosides has been introduced as a new index of collagen metabolism in bone, and the hydroxylysine glycosides are considered better tissue-specific markers of collagen turnover than is hydroxyproline[164] (see Chapter 15). β-1-Galactosyl-O-hydroxylysine (GH) appears to be more specific for bone collagen than is α-1,2-glucosyl-galactosyl-O-hydroxylysine (GGH), which is a marker for skin collagen. Vertebral mineral density measured by quantitative computed tomography and urinary GH are apparently inversely correlated, with high rates of bone mineral loss associated with increased urinary GH excretion.[164] Measurements of urinary GH should not be considered a "routine" laboratory test, since they require technical expertise with high-pressure liquid chromatographic techniques. As detailed in Chapter 15, other recent attempts to develop biochemical markers that reflect increased bone turnover and mineral loss include radioimmunoassays for the circulating type 1 procollagen carboxy-terminal extension peptide (pColl-I-C), the trimeric carboxy-terminal extension peptide of the procollagen molecule that is synthesized in the osteoblast.[165] However, no diagnostic value can yet be attributed to this test, since blood levels of pColl-I-C in patients with established osteoporosis do not consistently reflect bone turnover.[165]

III. EPIDEMIOLOGY AND INCIDENCE

The complication of the osteoporotic syndromes currently represents a major international public health problem and its prevalence is increasing. The disorder is only clinically relevant once a fracture (characteristically vertebral or hip) has occurred. However, prevention of bone loss may be a significantly more effective approach than treatment of the established disorder once the fracture has occurred. In the latter circumstance, it has proved difficult to document significant reduction in recurrence of fractures with some of the established pharmacologic approaches for a variety of reasons. Although the goal for preventive treatment remains the same as for treatment, that is, reduction in fracture incidence, the approach to the problem is generally simpler. Because it is assumed that fractures in osteoporosis result, at least partly, from a structurally unsound skeleton, most preventive measures in the younger individual can be devoted to maintenance of skeletal mass close to the maximum obtained at maturity. In addition to the prevention of skeletal deterioration, however, it must be recognized that particularly among the elderly, prevention of falls and acute stress on the axial skeleton, and avoidance of drugs and other precipitating factors that will predispose to falls, are important issues in the preventive aspects of fracture.[166-171]

When the reduction of bone tissue per unit volume of anatomic bone sufficiently compromises the skeleton, fractures may occur on minimal or trivial trauma. Many people with low bone mass will, however, not develop clinical fractures. We cannot as yet predict those individuals who will fracture, and indeed it may prove to be considerably easier to attempt to predict the greater number of individuals who will develop a significantly low bone mass as they age. Also, if clinicians are to recommend preventive measures aimed at reducing the incidence of bone loss among aging individuals, it seems more relevant and logical to consider the disorder in terms of bone mass rather than fracture. It is also noteworthy that the basic pathophysiologic mechanism of the disorder does not change following the chance occurrence of fracture.

A. Hip Fractures

Recent evidence from a variety of countries reveals that the prevalence of osteoporosis is increasing along with an increasing incidence of vertebral and hip fractures. In Belgium the incidence of hip fractures increased steadily and significantly between 1977 and 1982 by 28%[172]; from 1965 through 1983 the hip fracture rate in Sweden increased dramatically by 109%, with only 20% of the increment explained by age factors *per se*.[173-177] Similar trends of increasing hip fracture incidences during the second half of this century have been reported for Norway,[178] Spain,[179] Italy,[180] Canada,[181] The United Kingdom[182] (Fig. 12–21), and the United States[183-184] (Fig. 12–22), although age-adjusted fracture rates have been relatively stable in specific areas of the United States.[184] Results of studies performed in Australia predict an 83% increment in bed occupancy due to proximal femoral fracture between 1986 and 2011.[185]

In its 1981 annual report of the nation's health, the United States government announced that nearly 75% of Americans who reach the age of 65 years can now expect to live beyond the 75th year, a value that is 60% higher than that observed in 1940. Women aged 75 years and older represent only 18% of the 45-year and older female population, but 58% of the hospitalized "osteoporotic" population. Women aged 45 to 59 years presently represent 44% of the 45-year and older female population and 12% of the U.S. osteoporosis hospital population. For years it has been promulgated that the menopause represents a pivotal event in the development of osteoporosis contributing to the subsequent rise in vertebral and hip fracture rates in white women.[47,49,50,186] In fact, hip fracture rates for white women begin to rise abruptly between ages 40 and 44, 15 to 20 years earlier than generally assumed![187,188] Analysis of the U.S. National Hospital Discharge Survey from 1974 to 1979 revealed that the observed hip fracture incidence in white women rises from 3 fractures per 100,000 between ages 35 and 39 years, to 22 fractures per 100,000 between ages 40 and 44 years (Fig. 12–23). Using these accumulated data, it has been estimated that a postponement in the early rise in hip fracture increase in white women by 5 years would reduce overall hip fractures in this high-risk group by approximately 50%.[187] It appears justifiable to conclude that those risk factors that influence the onset and severity of bone loss that lead to hip fractures originate long before the clinical menopause occurs.[188a] The anticipated trends in the progressive increasing incidence of hip fracture may also

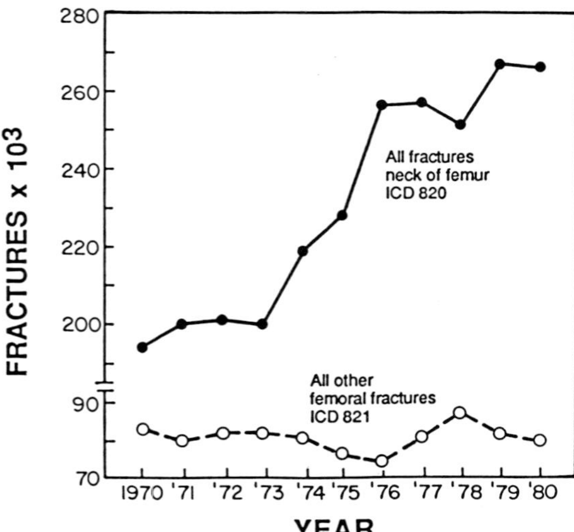

Figure 12–22. Changing occurrence of hip fracture (ICD 820) in the United States between 1970 and 1980. For comparison, there is no change in the number of traumatic fractures of the femur (ICD 821). (From Lindsay R: Clin Orthop Rel Res 222:44–59, 1987.)

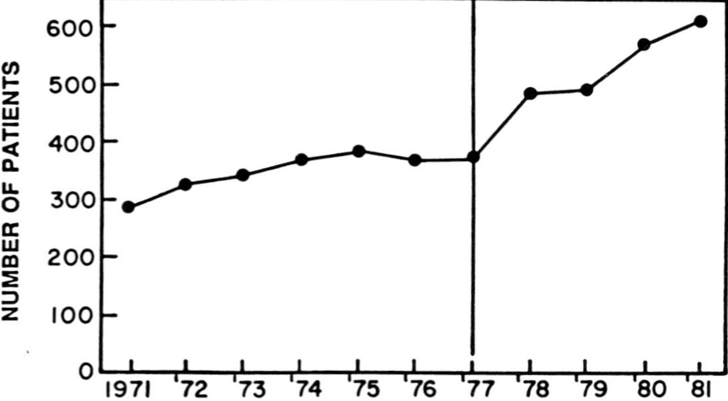

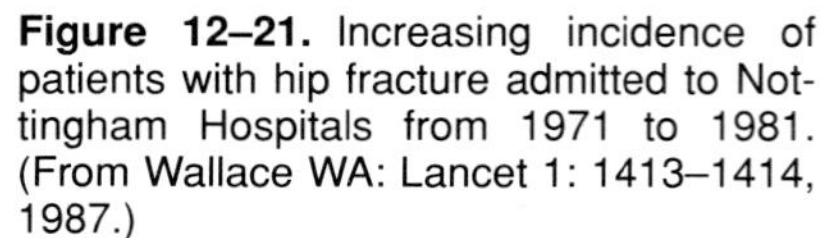
Figure 12–21. Increasing incidence of patients with hip fracture admitted to Nottingham Hospitals from 1971 to 1981. (From Wallace WA: Lancet 1: 1413–1414, 1987.)

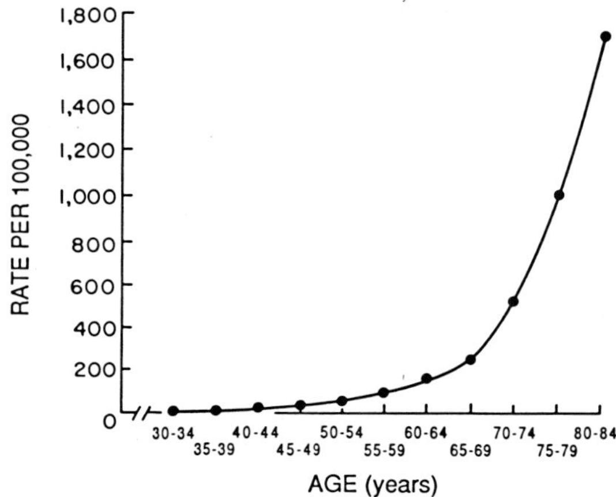

Figure 12–23. Age-specific hip fracture incidence rates for women by 5-year age intervals. U.S. National Hospital Discharge Survey 1974–1979. (From Brody JA, et al: Am J Public Health 74:1397–1398, 1984.)

prove to be low estimates, since the results of the National Center for Health Statistics Health and Nutritional Examination Survey (HANES I Survey) conducted in the United States between 1971 and 1975 revealed a surprising high prevalence (6% to 18%) of abnormally low cortical bone density in young individuals 25 to 34 years of age![189]

The incidence of femoral neck fracture in the United States, which can be used as one benchmark for the osteoporotic disorder, appears to be increasing by about 40% per decade (Fig. 12–23) with an increase in the age-dependent incidence among the at-risk population from 1.8% per annum to 2.05% per annum between the years 1970 and 1980.[184] In the United States, therefore, by the end of this decade some 5 to 10 million women will have a diagnosis of osteoporosis. Of the increase in femoral neck fractures documented in the United Kingdom, Sweden, and the United States, about 60% of this increment can be accounted for by the changing demography of the population; that is, an increase in the number of individuals at risk. If the current trend continues, there will be approximately 500,000 fractures of the hip per year in the United States by the end of the century. These estimates may prove to be conservative owing to progressive increments in the numbers of elderly, 70 years of age and older, in international communities who fall because of muscular degeneration, lower body disabilities with balance abnormalities, postural hypotension, and loss of cognitive function resulting from polypharmacy abuse of drugs. These statistics need not apply solely to the postmenopausal and more elderly females, since as noted earlier, fracture rates for U.S. white women climb steeply between the ages of 40 and 44 years.[187,188]

Hip fractures result in a considerable fiscal drain in terms of health care costs, and also in significant morbidity and mortality (Fig. 12–24).[188b] The National Osteoporosis Society of the United Kingdom reports that more women die from fractures caused by osteoporosis than of cancer of the cervix, uterus, and breast combined.[190] Current analyses of the complications of hip fractures reveal that there may be an associated mortality of as high as 50% one year following the hip fracture.[191] With such mortality figures, hip fracture (and presumably, indirectly, osteoporosis) would then become the 12th most common cause of death in the United States. Moreover, only 25% to 50% of patients with hip fractures maintain their level of function when daily living activities and walking ability are considered.[192] Although mean length of hospitalization for hip fracture varies considerably between countries and even within countries,[192-194] costs for hospitalization and subsequent care are becoming alarming on the international scene.[195] Changing patterns for hip fracture care, which includes extended use of acute hospital beds as well as rehabilitation and nursing home beds, are resulting in escalating annual costs in national budgets[184,196-197] that currently ap-

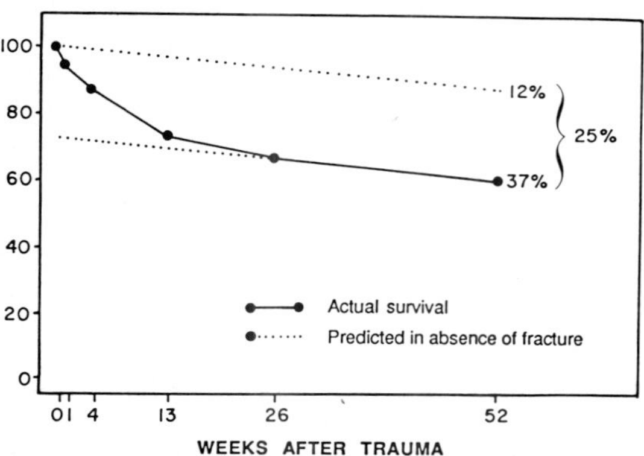

Figure 12–24. Relationship between survival and the passage of time since neck fracture occurred in 233 women. (From Aitken JM: Relationship between mortality after femoral neck fracture and osteoporosis. *In* Christiansen C, Johnsen JS, Riis BJ (eds): Osteoporosis 1987, vol 1. Viborg, Denmark, Norhaven Press, 1987, pp 45–48.)

proximate 10 billion dollars in the United States alone.[151,162,163] Moreover, although the implementation of the prospective payment system (PPS) for recipients of Medicare in the United States designed to decrease costs has decreased the average length of hospitalization for the hip fracture patient from 16.6 to 10.3 days, the quality of care of these patients appears to have deteriorated,[193] and the additional costs of nursing home care are now transferred to nongovernmental coffers.

B. Vertebral Fractures

Accurate data on the incidence of vertebral fractures (which are characteristically asymptomatic) and the costs to society are still unavailable for evaluation of the severity of this additional complication of postmenopausal and/or senile forms of osteoporosis. The incidence of vertebral fractures does increase with age, and as many as 20% to 35% of ambulatory females (compared with 5% to 47% of males) over the age of 60 years have one or more asymptomatic vertebral fractures on routine radiographs if anatomical changes such as vertebral "wedging" and "ballooning" as well as vertebral collapse are considered.[198-204] Using cross-sectional data from populations in the United States, it has been estimated that approximately 538,000 postmenopausal women will experience their first vertebral fracture each year.[200] Since there are approximately 32.5 million women over the age of 50 years, it has been estimated that the rate of first vertebral fractures in the United States is 17 per 1000 person-years. The prevalence of one or more vertebral fractures also increases with declining bone mass, approximating 42% in women with vertebral bone mineral density less than 0.6 g/cm^2 by dual-photon absorptiometry.[205] These statistics are startling when one considers that only half of the existing vertebral fractures are being diagnosed.[202] Age-related increments in vertebral fractures must also be reconciled with changing patterns (as noted earlier for hip fractures) in that both the incidence and prevalence of vertebral fractures appear to have increased dramatically with time.[202] A recent survey comparing vertebral fracture incidence in the 1950s to the 1980s in the same Scandinavian population revealed a 4-fold increment during the last 30 years[202] (Fig. 12–25).

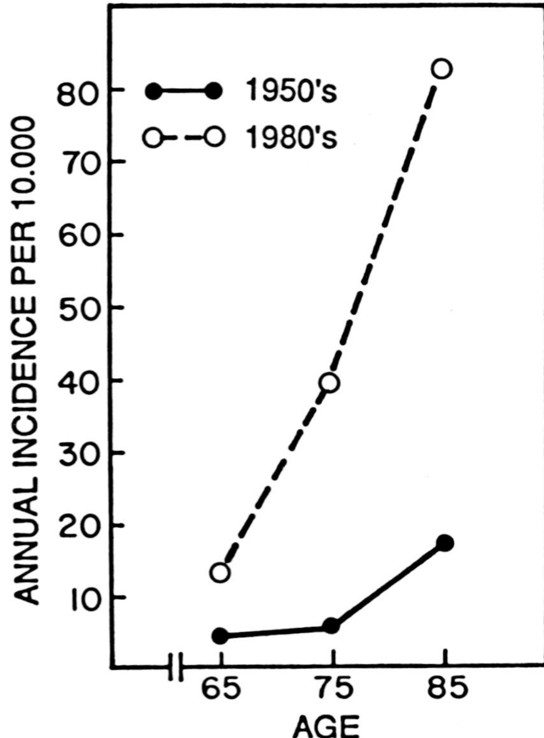

Figure 12–25. Age-specific annual incidence of vertebral fractures in Swedish women in 1950–1952 and 1982–1983. (From Bengnér U, et al: Calif Tissue Int 42:293–296, 1988.)

IV. IDENTIFICATION OF INDIVIDUALS AT RISK

A. Genetic and Lifestyle Factors

Factors that have been most closely associated with an increase in the risk of osteoporosis in the postmenopausal female are outlined in Table 12–2. It is obvious that any factor that increases the rate of bone loss in the premenopausal female results in a decrease in skeletal reserve at the time of the menopause. Vertebral fractures from osteoporosis are probably at least 10 times as common among women between 50 and 60 years of age as they are among men, and as summarized earlier, the true incidence of hip fracture is twice as common among women as among men. The sexual dimorphism in skeletal mass appears at the time of the completion of growth, and maximum skeletal mass in women occurs about the age of 25 to 30 years. This difference may result from a combination of higher calcium intakes in males[68]

Table 12–2. Factors Commonly Associated with the Female Osteoporotic Syndromes

Genetic
White or Asiatic ethnicity
Positive family history
Small body frame (less than 127 lb)
Lifestyle
Smoking
Inactivity
Nulliparity
Excessive exercise (producing amenorrhea)
Early natural menopause
Late menarche
Nutritional Factors
Milk intolerance
Lifelong low dietary calcium intake
Vegetarian dieting
Excessive alcohol intake
Consistently high protein intake
Medical Disorders
Anorexia nervosa
Acromegaly
Thyrotoxicosis
Parathyroid overactivity
Cushing's syndrome
Type I diabetes
Alterations in gastrointestinal and hepatobiliary function
Occult osteogenesis imperfecta
Mastocytosis
Rheumatoid arthritis
"Transient" osteoporosis
Prolonged parenteral nutrition
Prolactinoma
Endometriosis
*Partial hysterectomy
*Tubal ligations
Hemolytic anemia
Ankylosing spondylitis
Drugs
Thyroid replacement therapy
Glucocorticoid drugs
Anticoagulants
Chronic lithium therapy
Chemotherapy
GnRH agonist or antagonist therapy
Anticonvulsant drugs
†Extended tetracycline use
†Diuretics producing calciuria
†Phenothiazine derivatives
†Cyclosporine A

*Potential decrease in ovarian function due to vascular insufficiency.

†Not yet associated with decreased bone mass although identified as either toxic to bone in animals or inducing calciuria and/or calcium malabsorption in humans.

(Fig. 12–26), androgenic effects on the male skeleton during the growth spurt, and the increased vigorous exercise pursuits of the male population, even though the sex differences in exercise are declining somewhat.

Because of the accelerated phase of bone loss in the estrogen-deficient female during the immediate postmenopausal period,[50-53] and because of its relative ease of identification as a time marker, the menopause has been considered the most appropriate time to attempt to identify those women at risk. At this time bone mass is greater in those individuals with lifelong calcium intakes in excess of 800 mg/day[68,73,206-211] (Fig. 12–27), and in those who exercise routinely at least 45 to 60 minutes thrice weekly.[212-217] During the growth period and perhaps also during the period of skeletal consolidation that follows growth, routine exercise and adequate calcium intake may be of greater importance.[218]

Osteoporosis has been stated to be common among white and Asiatic populations.[59-61] Black individuals are less prone to develop either vertebral or hip fractures (Fig. 12–28). Recent circumstantial evidence, however, suggests that there may also be an increasing incidence of osteoporosis among blacks,[188] although this has not been documented in true epidemiologic fashion. When an adequate family history can be obtained, then a highly significant percentage of the individuals who suffer from osteoporosis will record the presence of kyphosis, height reduction, and perhaps also hip fracture in the female members of their family.[219,220] Whether it is genetic or the result of environmental influences occurring within families is debated. However, it is clear that bone mass at maturity is, to a significant extent, genetically related,[37,221] and because a significant component of the risk for osteoporosis is likely to be related to bone mass at maturity, it is clear there must at least be some genetic component in the risk of fractures from osteoporosis. In addition, it is known that families do tend to share environmental influences, particularly in diet and lifestyle, and these may also influence the incidence of osteoporosis within families.

Osteoporosis has also been regarded as a disorder of "thin" women.[35,222] This may be partly related to the loading of the skeleton, but may also be related to the reduced conversion of adrenal androgens, that is, androstenedione, to estrogens in the postmenopausal phase of life in women who have less than average body fat. The only source of estrogen of importance in postmenopausal women is this peripheral conversion of adrenal androgen. It has been established that bone mass is elevated in obese women,[35,223] and that even moderate obesity plays a protective role on postmenopausal bone loss.[223] In this regard, we should recognize

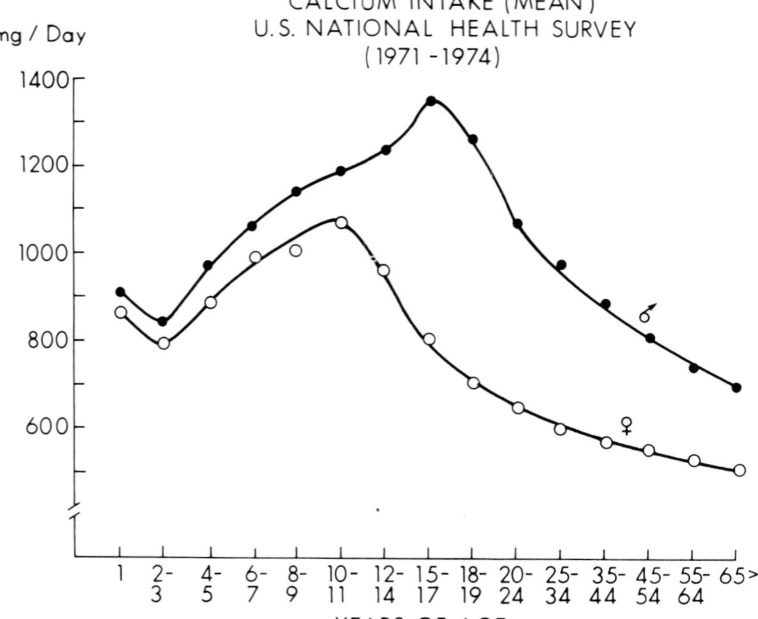

Figure 12–26: Mean calcium intakes of men (♂) and women (♀) in the United States from 1971 to 1974. (Adapted from DHEW Publication No. (HRA) 77–1647, July 1977.)

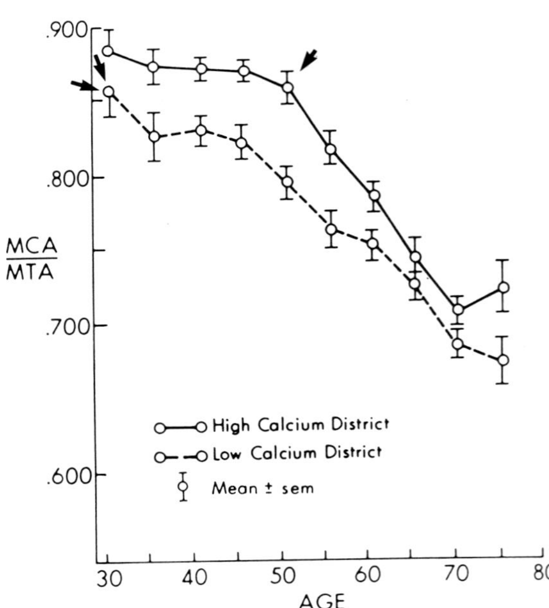

Figure 12–27: Relationship between cortical bone content (MCA/MTA) and age in individuals from either *high* (950 mg/day) or *low* (450 mg/day) calcium districts. Note that the bone density of those individuals of 50 years of age from the high-calcium district (single arrow) is comparable to that of 30-year-old individuals (double arrows) from the low-calcium district. (From Matkovic V, et al: Am J Clin Nutr 32:540–549, 1979.)

that the conversion of androstenedione to estrone increases with body weight,[224] resulting in higher circulating estrone levels in obese women. Albright et al., in their original description of osteoporosis,[85,86,225] demonstrated clearly the importance of ovarian failure and the postmenopausal state. It is now well recognized that premature ovarian failure and oophorectomy performed in the premenopausal phase of life are very important risk factors.[226] Moreover, acquired alterations in ovarian function that may result from anorexia nervosa,[227,228] excessive exercise,[229-232] and gonadotropin agonist or antagonist therapy[232-235] may result in premature accelerated rates of bone loss in the premenopausal female. It seems clear that the longer normal estrogen production is maintained, the less the risk of osteoporosis. We should recognize, in this regard, that there is a spectrum of ovarian function, even in postmenopausal women.[236] In these individuals, ovarian testosterone secretion is usually maintained but the secretion of estrone, estradiol, and androstenedione, although diminished, varies considerably.[236] Therefore, subtle changes in the production or metabolism of estrogen should be acknowledged, including the potential estrogen deficiency that may occur because of a late menarche,[237] following tubal ligation[238] or partial hysterectomy as a result of vascular insufficiency, and the increased fecal excretion

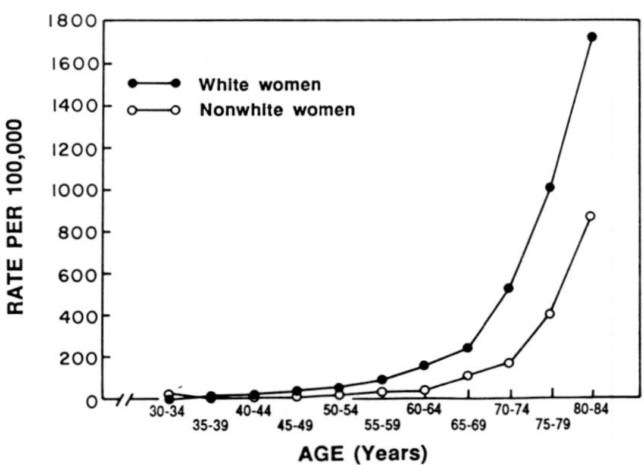

Figure 12–28: Age-specific hip fracture incidence rates for women by 5-year age intervals, U.S. National Hospital Discharge Survey 1974–1979. (From Farmer ME, et al: AM J Public Health 74:1374–1380, 1984.)

of estrogens resulting in lower blood levels in vegetarians who are at risk for low bone mass.[239]

The hepatic metabolism of estradiol results in either 2-hydroxy or 16-hydroxy metabolites. Whereas the 16-hydroxy metabolites possess potent estrogen effects, the 2-hydroxy metabolites are virtually biologically inert and cleared rapidly from the circulation. Factors that increase the hepatic formation of the inactive 2-hydroxy estrogen derivatives include cigarette smoking, anorexia, high-protein diets, and thyroid excess states.[240-241] Smoking does not, however, appear to influence the peripheral aromatization or metabolism of estradiol,[242] although it decreases the menopausal age by 1.74 years.[243] High-fat (low-protein, low-carbohydrate) diets and obese subjects are characterized by an increased production of the biologically active 16-hydroxy estrogen metabolites. Pregnancy and the use of oral contraceptives may increase exposure to sex hormones such that both of those may be associated with a higher bone mass at the time of the menopause. Breast feeding and lactation have been associated with either no alterations[244] or an actual increase[245] in bone mass. A sedentary lifestyle and the weightlessness that accompanies space flight must also be recognized as potent contributing factors to accelerated bone loss patterns.[214-217,246-249]

Increasing concerns with the difficulties in "weighting" the many and varied risk factors[250-253] have prompted attempts to identify those women who will lose bone rapidly within the immediate postmenopausal period. Some have identified 79% of "fast bone losers" (bone loss greater than 3% annually in the forearm) and 78% of "slow bone losers" utilizing a multiple regression analysis of single blood determination of alkaline phosphatase, a urinary calcium and hydroxyproline, and the measurement of body fat mass.[250] Although potentially significant for cross-sectional group analysis studies, these analytical "profiles" still offer limited diagnostic significance for detecting patients at risk for vertebral or hip fractures since, as noted earlier, forearm bone mass *cannot* and *should not* be used to predict the rate of change in vertebral or femoral bone mass. More recent (albeit still impractical) attempts to detect those early postmenopausal females at risk for rapid bone loss have been made in adult female monkeys utilizing short-term pituitary-ovarian suppression by a GnRH antagonist and measurements of urinary calcium/creatinine ratios.[254] Although promising, this approach needs further evaluation and confirmation before routine diagnostic testing in humans can be advocated. More detailed evaluation and confirmation of reports of elevated interleukin-1 (IL-1) blood levels in high turnover osteoporotic postmenopausal females,[93,255] and other reports of either elevations in circulating bone Gla-protein,[124] or an exaggerated blood cAMP response to intramuscular calcitonin in patients with accelerated bone turnover,[256] must be made before they can be considered appropriate diagnostic indices.

B. Nutritional Factors

The role of dietary indiscretion in either initiating or modulating the osteoporotic state has been a matter of debate and contention for decades. Although international controversy does exist,[257-260] there appears to be a consensus that (1) menopausal women are generally calcium-deficient; (2) osteoporotic women give histories of lower calcium intakes than do nonosteoporotic controls; and (3) the addition of calcium to calcium-deficient females can decrease the rate of bone loss and propensity to fracture.[68,70,71,73,74,76,209,210,214,252,261-270] Dietary factors other than calcium that have been proposed as contributing factors to the age-related and postmenopausal bone loss syndrome include caffeine, sodium, protein, and phosphate.[271-279] Increased consumption of frozen or "fast foods" with excessive amounts of phosphate-containing preservatives is of increasing concern since the combination of low calcium and high phosphate intakes may result in an acceleration of bone resorption.[273] In fact, recent studies reveal that parathyroid hormone secretion is elevated in individuals consuming high-phosphorus, low-calcium diets assembled from common household food supplies.[274] Excessive protein consumption does cause an increase in urinary calcium and in the amount of dietary calcium required to maintain calcium balance in humans.[275-277] The protein-induced alterations in calcium homeostasis (and bone mass?) have been attributed to increments in endogenous acid production and net acid excretion that is attributed entirely to the oxidation of the constituent sulfur-containing amino acids.[278] High caffeine intakes have been recorded in osteoporotic subjects,[157] and studies designed to analyze the effects of caffeine consumption in diets that included coffee, tea, and cola beverages reveal higher levels of urinary calcium and intestinal calcium secretion in caffeine users and a striking inverse correlation between dairy product intake and coffee-tea-cola intake.[279] The practical importance of these observations is still questionable, although one is led to the tentative conclusion that self-selected diets high in caffeine-containing beverages may mitigate the availability of dietary calcium. Obligatory calcium excretion does vary with sodium intake, and although the urinary calcium is in a sense more dependent on sodium intake,[280] the relationship between high sodium intake and bone mass is unknown. In a similar fashion, "significant correlations" have been observed between the degree of bone loss and dietary zinc, folate,[281] cobalamin,[98] boron,[282] and blood vitamin K[283] in both longitudinal and cross-sectional studies. The practical significance of these correlations is still ill-defined and conjectural at best. The abuse of alcohol is clearly an important risk factor for women as well as men.[66,284-286] In fact, studies in individuals consuming 100 g or more of ethanol daily show a significant decrease in osteoblastic activity and bone formation rates[286] (see Chapter 10). Although lactase deficiency has been equated with calcium malabsorption, there is apparently no significant difference in either vertebral or forearm bone mass content between normal and lactase-deficient subjects.[287]

C. Medical Disorders

Although a variety of seemingly unrelated disorders affect calcium homeostasis in an adverse fashion (see Table 12–2), some are more common than others and deserving of comment. Patients with hyperthyroidism lose both axial and appendicular bone, which can result in skeletal fractures.[288-293] Adverse effects of excessive thyroid hormone on calcium homeostasis include decreased calcium absorption and hypercalciuria. Thyroid hormone also conditions bone turnover, resulting in an inappropriately high degree of osteoclastic activity and increased bone resorption.[290-293] Significant restoration of the deficit in bone mass in hyperthyroid patients may not occur even following "cure" of the hyperthyroid state.[291]

Decreased calcium absorption, hypercalciuria, and alterations in the normal production and metabolism of parathyroid hormone and vitamin D that occur in Cushing's syndrome result in defective osteoblastic and accelerated osteoclastic activity, progressive osteoporosis, and fracture.[294-300] In fact, occult Cushing's syndrome may present with osteoporosis alone and the absence of the usual clinical features of hypercortisolism.[297-299] This "occult" osteopenic presentation of Cushing's syndrome should not be confused with those instances wherein "high turnover" forms of osteopenia are observed in oophorectomized women.[300] These individuals lose bone rapidly and have *high-normal* levels (more than 90 μg/24 hours) of urinary free cortisol with a paradoxically diminished cortisol response to corticotropin.[300] Occult renal insufficiency may also contribute to bone loss in aging women.[301] In this age group, loss of muscle mass may mask the underlying renal insufficiency since blood creatinine levels can be "normal" despite a fall in glomerular filtrate rate.[301]

Primary hyperparathyroidism, a frequent endocrinopathy in the postmenopausal female,[302-304] often presents only with "osteoporosis" and vertebral crush fractures (see Chapter 14). The diagnosis may prove difficult to establish in some instances, since elevated serum parathyroid hormone (PTH) levels in elderly patients must be interpreted with full recognition that mild alterations in renal function combined with subtle degrees of vitamin D deficiency may result in elevated levels of parathyroid hormone.[305,306] Moreover, as noted earlier in this chapter, PTH levels normally increase with age[80-84] (Fig. 12–8) and are also elevated in individuals with low-renin hypertension syndromes,[131] others on chronic glucocorticoid therapy,[130] and those with the benign hypercalcemic, hypocalciuric familial hyperparathyroid syndromes.[132]

Patients with rheumatoid arthritis (RA) are also prone to develop osteoporosis.[307-312] The osteoporosis is characterized by a juxta-articular bone loss, which occurs early in the disease, and an associated gradual, generalized progressive loss in bone mass. Although the specific cause of the osteoporotic process observed in RA has yet to be established with certainty, reduced physical activity, mast cell accumulation, prostaglandins, and cytokines such as interleukin-1 have all been considered contributory in this regard,[309,313] as well as therapeutic regimens that include glucocorticoids[307-310,314] and nonsteroidal antiinflammatory[310] drugs. The skeletal effects of prolonged treatment with either penicillamine or cytotoxic agents such as methotrexate[315] on bone mass in the RA patient are still unknown, although one should anticipate an adverse effect when the cytotoxic drugs are used indiscriminately (see later). Multiparity and increased physical activity appear to exert protective effects on vertebral bone mass in the patient with RA.

Decreased bone mineral content has been observed in a variety of studies of type I (insulin-dependent) diabetics in comparison with age- and sex-matched control subjects.[316] The decrease in bone mass in type I patients is most pronounced in those patients with childhood or adolescent onset of the disease and associated with the need for large insulin doses and poor glucose regulation.[316] Although preliminary studies on fracture incidence in diabetic patients did not reveal an increased fracture incidence between diabetics with 10 to 20 years' duration and a comparable number of nondiabetic controls,[317] the data are still ambiguous since, in these preliminary studies, diabetics and controls were selected from a "central diagnostic index" and neither diagnosis nor selection criteria of the nondiabetic control group were presented.[318] The derangements in calcium homeostasis in the type I diabetic patient include increased urinary excretion of calcium, phosphate, and magnesium, decreased plasma concentrations of magnesium and ionized calcium, normal to low blood levels of PTH and 1,25(OH)$_2$D, and a decreased bone formation rate.[317,319] Bone mineral density in women with type II (insulin-independent) diabetes is not decreased and may, in fact, be higher than normal.[320,321] This has been attributed to an associated obese state and elevated circulatory estrone levels.[321] In type II diabetic individuals, there is no relationship between bone mineral density, duration of diabetes, or hemoglobin A_{1c}.[320]

Other clinical disorders that can and often do accelerate either the physiologic bone loss in premenopausal women or the accelerated patterns of skeletal dissolutions in postmenopausal women include "transient regional" osteoporotic syndromes,[322] the osteoporosis associated with pregnancy and lactation,[323,324] occult forms of osteogenesis imperfecta that may become manifest only after the menopause,[325,326] systemic mastocytosis,[327,328] endometriosis,[234a] sarcoidosis,[329] hyperprolactinemia,[330-332] hemochromatosis,[333] gastrectomy,[334] chronic hemolytic states including porphyria,[335] hepatic,[336] and biliary[337] disease, "idiopathic" scoliotic syndromes,[338,339] during prolonged parenteral nutrition,[340,341] Turner's syndrome,[342] and acromegaly.[342a] Since vertebral bone mass reaches its peak at the time of cessation of longitudinal growth and epiphyseal closures,[343] and begins to decline during or prior to the third decade,[344] any acquired or inherited medical/surgical disorder that occurs early in life may result in an increased propensity toward fracture in the immediate postmenopausal period.

D. Drug Therapy

Drug therapy can and often does result in a variety of disturbances in mineral metabolism either indirectly by altering calcium absorption or excretion, and the release, metabolism, or skeletal response to the calciotropic hormones, or directly by inhibition of bone cell function as well as collagen production and mineralization. The resultant osteoporotic syndromes can be attended by normal or elevated values for blood parathyroid hormone; normal or low values for 25(OH)D; normal, low, or elevated circulating 1,25(OH)$_2$D; decreased or increased calcium absorption; and either hyper- or hypocalciuria. Thus, when considering either "type I" or "type II" osteoporotic syndromes (Table 12–1) and their respective classic biochemical profiles for blood calcium, phosphate, vitamin D metabolites, and parathyroid hormone[133,134] in patients on medications known to produce osteopenia (Table 12–2), the potential alterations in both histologic presentation and diagnostic tests by the drug-induced syndrome should be acknowledged.

Although there is uniform belief that chronic exposure to supraphysiologic levels of glucocorticoids leads almost inevitably to significant bone loss and an increased prevalence of rib and vertebral fractures,[345-347] there is still considerable contention regarding the effect of "low-dose glucocorticoid therapy" (LDGC) on bone.[348-351] In patients receiving prednisolone in doses ranging from 4 to 10 mg/day, there is a close negative correlation between total body calcium and steroid doses.[348] Moreover, the bone mass of the appendicular skeleton of premenopausal women is unaffected by the administration of LDGC (i.e., prednisone, 7.5 mg/day), whereas postmenopausal women on the same dose of glucocorticoids lose *twice as much bone* as age-matched postmenopausal women who are not taking glucocorticoids.[351] Glucocorticoid doses equivalent to less than 8 to 10 mg/day of prednisolone are usually considered safe,[350] although bone loss has been documented in individuals treated with as little as 5 mg/day of prednisone.[349] Although alternate-day glucocorticoid therapy can mitigate undesirable effects of daily glucocorticoid therapy on growth suppression, hypothalamic-pituitary-adrenal axis suppression, and infections, alternate day steroid regimens do not reduce the osteopenic effects recorded with daily steroid regimens.[352]

Disturbances in calcium and bone metabolism have also been recorded in patients on thyroid replacement therapy.[353-356] Despite a mild hyperthyroxinemia, serum triiodothyronine levels are characteristically normal and patients asymptomatic.[357,358] Studies in patients treated with contemporary L-thyroxine preparations reveal that 80% of patients ingesting 125 µg/day or more were "overdosed" as detected by thyrotropin response to thyrotropin-releasing hormone.[359] It is suggested that because of increased bioavailability of L-thyroxine thyroid hormone preparations, replacement doses should approximate 100 µg/day or 1.7 µg/kg body weight[359]; patients requiring thyroxine for suppression (i.e., goiter, cold nodules, thyroid cancer) will require more than 125 µg/day. It should also be recognized that especially in postmenopausal females, L-thyroxine dosage requirements decrease with age.[357] In order to minimize undesired skeletal effects of overly zealous thyroxine replacement therapy, doses of thyroid hormone administered to hypothyroid patients should be adjusted so that serum TSH, measured by the new sensitive assays, is within the normal range.[358]

Since initial reports of "anticonvulsant osteomalacia" appeared in the European literature in 1968, alterations in calcium and skeletal metabolism on anticonvulsant medications have been recorded worldwide.[345] Many drugs, including virtually all of the common anticonvulsants and many of the major and minor tranquilizers, are capable of inducing hepatic microsomal mixed oxidase enzyme activity. Some steroids share the hepatic microsomal degradation pathways with foreign substances; induction of these enzyme systems leads to an increased catabolism of a variety of steroid hormones,[360-362] resulting in accelerated production of polar, hydroxylated, biologically inactive products that are eliminated in the bile and urine. This has been demonstrated particularly well in the case of estrogens, progesterone, corticosteroids, and vitamin D. In the presence of an intact hypothalamic-pituitary axis, normal feedback control mechanisms increase the endogenous production of steroid hormones so that normal levels of biologically active hormones are usually maintained. This feedback control system explains why clinical evidence of drug-induced deficiencies of adrenal and gonad steroids is seldom observed, especially in individuals on low-dose regimens. On the other hand, chronic administration or large doses of hepatic microsomal-inducing agents, particularly phenobarbital (and anticonvulsant drugs that are metabolized to phenobarbital, such as primidone) and diphenylhydantoin, significantly reduces the biological effects of exogenously administered steroid hormones, most probably because of increased hepatic degradation.[360-362] Undesirable side-effects of anticonvulsant medications on calcium and skeletal metabolism include suppression of calcium absorption and direct inhibitory effects on basal, PTH, and 1,25$(OH)_2D_3$-induced bone turnover and inhibitory effects of collagen and noncollagen protein synthesis in bone.[345] The clinical severity of the bone disease observed in patients on anticonvulsant medications varies considerably, ranging from subclinical decreases in bone mass detectable only by the most sensitive noninvasive methods to marked hypocalcemia and severe osteopenia with multiple recurrent bone fractures. A trend toward increased skeletal demineralization has been associated with the length of anticonvulsant therapy,[345,363] although a "steady state" may be achieved in some adults.[363]

Glucocorticoids, thyroid supplements, and anticonvulsants presumably are well established as bone "toxins" when used indiscriminately or in inappropriately large doses. Heparin anticoagulants[364-366] can also decrease bone mass, whereas sodium warfarin drugs apparently do not adversely affect the skeleton,[367] despite reports of impaired carboxylation of osteocalcin in warfarin-treated patients[368] and decreased serum osteocalcin levels in patients treated with the vitamin K antagonist, phenprocoumon.[369] Lithium treatment results in elevations in circulating parathyroid hormone,[370] hypercalcemia (and hypermagnesemia), and a decrease in bone mineral content,[371] alterations that can occur as early as 3 months following treatment with oral lithium doses of 28 mEq/day.[372] Long-term lithium therapy is associated with an unusually high incidence of hyperparathyroidism, which may be mistaken for osteoporosis in older females.[373] Although "loop" diuretics, such as furosemide, result in hypercalciuria when used acutely,[374] prolonged use should not alter calcium homeostasis and bone content since the effect of the drug on calcium excretion is acute.[374]

Cytotoxic chemotherapy with drugs like vincristine and cyclophosphamide interfaces with the development of mineralized tissue,[375,376] and accelerated bone loss syndromes should also be anticipated in patients treated with methotrexate for malignant disorders,[377-379] rheumatoid arthritis,[315,380] or chronic inflammatory bowel disease.[381] Chemotherapy will result in a loss of skeletal mass either because of a direct toxic effect of the agent on calcifying tissue,[375,376] or because of the induction of gonadal damage and decreased levels of gonadal hormones.[377,378,382] "Medical gonadectomy," induced by GnRH or LHRH antagonist or agonist treatment for the premenstrual "tension" syndrome,[383] polycystic ovarian syndrome,[384] endometriosis,[234] and during breast feeding[384a] could,[233] and does,[385,386] result in bone loss, although the loss of bone appears to be reversible.[386] Finally, short-term studies in humans and in laboratory animals suggest that theophylline-like drugs,[387,388] phenothiazine derivatives,[389] and calcium channel blockers[390] may also interfere with calcium homeostasis if used chronically. Similarly, advocates for the use of cyclosporin A in psoriasis[391] or rheumatoid arthritis should proceed with caution, since this immunosuppressive agent is also toxic to bone in experimental animal models.[392-394] The increasing use of the nonsteroid "antiestrogen" tamoxifen in adjuvant therapeutic regimens for breast cancer in premenopausal women[395,396] does not result in progressive bone loss since tamoxifen is actually a potent estrogen *agonist* on trabecular and cortical bone.[397,398,398a]

Recognition of the potential adverse effects of a variety of seemingly unrelated medications on mineral and skeletal metabolism, and the appropriate use of either modified treatment regimens or drugs that protect the skeleton in situations in which potentially harmful medications cannot be changed or their doses altered, coupled with serial measurements of bone mass at predetermined intervals should help to minimize additional undesirable complications in osteoporotic individuals.

Despite the ready description of risk factors, it is difficult for the clinician to know what weight to attach to each genetic, medical, drug, or dietary risk factor when faced with a patient requesting advice for prevention of alterations in bone mass, or others requiring reasons to embark on a therapeutic program.[399] The relative prevalence of fracture should not be identified solely with a decrease in bone mass, since environmental factors, syncopal episodes, drugs, or other factors may have actually conditioned a fall or the traumatic insult that resulted in the fracture. It is clear, however, that recognition of the most prevalent risk factors will allow us to make some determination of risk for rapid losses in bone mass. Additionally, the presence of risk factors together with a low bone mass, or even the presence of a bone that is below the fifth percentile of maximum bone mass, may be considered in itself a risk factor justifying treatment. In the authors' clinics, if bone mass is low (that is, below one standard deviation of the young population), preventive measures are instituted. If bone mass is normal but repeated measurements suggest a loss of bone greater than the normal trend, then preventive steps are initiated at that point. If noninvasive bone mass measurements are not available, the presence of one of four major clinical associations is sufficient for the physician to consider preventive efforts. These are poor diet, poor lifestyle, a significantly early menopause (or other forms of acquired ovarian failure), and oophorectomy performed in the premenopausal phase of life. The first two are correctable by the patients themselves; the remainder requires physician intervention with appropriate therapeutic regimens.

V. PREVENTION AND THERAPY

A. Calcium

Although the need for calcium "supplementation" has achieved a "controversial status,"[257-267] there are dictums that appear to be well established and worthy of emphasis: (1) it is essential to guarantee adequate calcium nutrition during those formative years of bone and tooth growth and maturation; (2) adequate calcium intakes are required to maximize the effects of accepted therapeutic regimens, such as estrogens, exercise, and calcitonin[400]; (3) calcium supplementation *per se* is effective in suppressing bone loss in *some women* in the peri- or postmenopausal periods of life[208,210,211,263,264-270]; (4) calcium intakes of 1500 mg/day decrease the amount of estrogens necessary to suppress bone loss[401]; and (5) diets that contain adequate amounts of calcium are associated with a decrease in the incidence of hip fractures in later years.[263,264] In fact, *individuals with a calcium consumption of more than 765 mg/day are 60% less likely to experience a hip fracture!*[264] Given these clinical observations, the physician is then confronted with the pros and cons of recommending calcium "supplementation" for "all women." Dietary habits resulting in a deficiency in calcium intake usually develop early in life[402] and continue thereafter. Beyond the age of 35 years, more than 75% of apparently "healthy" females in the United States have calcium intakes much lower than detailed by the RDA.[170,403,404] A recent survey of calcium intake profiles of a postmenopausal U.S. population, 49 to 66 years of age, revealed 13% with an intake of 0 to 399 mg/day, 44% ingesting 400 to 699 mg/day, and 24% ingesting 700 to 899 mg/day. Only 19% had calcium intakes greater than 900 mg/day. Aging also produces a diverse heterogeneous population owing to differences in normal physiologic adaptations, various diseases, and a "potpourri" of drugs that can alter physiologic adaptations and calcium homeostasis.[271,405]

Supplementing diets of the elderly with calcium and calcium-rich foods can decrease the rate of cortical bone loss and should be considered an important health care issue.[211] Recommendations for calcium intake to ensure bone health and minimize bone loss rates should, therefore, be conditioned by individual requirements and adjusted accordingly if dietary habits reflect intake of foods with limited calcium content or bioavailability, consumption of excessive amounts of protein, sodium, and carbohydrate, or use of medications that either decrease the efficiency of calcium absorption or increase calcium excretion.[271] Emphasis should be placed on the need to "replete a relative calcium-depleted state" rather than to supplement an assumed "normal" calcium intake, as evident by the practice of repleting iron-deficient state. Although iron depletion can be documented by measurements of circulating iron and total iron binding capacity, the medical community has not yet been able to identify "calcium-deficient" females either by chemical testing or by the use of noninvasive measurements of bone mass. *Not all anemic patients are iron-deficient, although iron deficiency causes anemia. In a similar fashion, not all osteoporotic individuals are calcium-deficient, although calcium deficiency can accelerate the rate of bone loss.*[406-408] Of note is the fact that calcium deficiency of less than two thirds of the U.S. RDA is *four times* more frequent than iron deficiency of a similar magnitude. Given these observations, it seems prudent to accept the conclusion presented in 1984 in the United States at a National Institutes of Health (NIH) Consensus Conference:[409]

> Therefore, the RDA for calcium is evidently too low, particularly for postmenopausal women. . . . It seems likely that an increase in calcium intake to 1000–1500 mg/day, beginning well before the menopause, will reduce the incidence of osteoporosis in postmenopausal women.

Dairy products provide the source of most dietary calcium in the United States, although milk allergy or acquired distaste for milk as well as lactose intolerance often complicates the continued use of dairy sources.[410,411] Calcium may also be obtained from green vegetables, nuts, and certain canned fish. In some instances the "food" calcium is not readily biologically available[412]; in others, patients are resistant to changes in dietary habits and the physician must resort to calcium supplementation. As a rule of thumb, most patients who are normocalciuric are given a daily 1 g supplement of elemental calcium in divided doses, assuming a dietary calcium intake of 300 to 500 mg/day unless history reveals otherwise. Generally, the smallest number of tablets that provides the appropriate amounts of elemental calcium is preferred. For the most part, this entails the use of *bioavailable* forms of calcium carbonate that contain 40% elemental calcium. The elemental calcium content of calcium supplements varies widely (Table 12–3). Dolomite and bone meal should be considered poor sources of calcium since they may be contaminated with lead and other heavy metals. Recent convincing studies demonstrate that many generic (and some nongeneric) forms of calcium supplements have limited bioavailability,[413,414] and physicians should advise patients accordingly. Since in all preparations of calcium carbonate, calcium forms 40% of the total weight of the tablet, only two tablets of calcium carbonate may suffice to provide a daily supplement of 1 g of elemental calcium. Calcium citrate may provide an alternative source[415] with the potential benefits of improved calcium bioavailability, particularly when achlorhydria is present,[416] and reduction of the risk of urinary calculi; although on calcium intakes of 1000 to 1500 mg/day, this complication is theoretical at best.[417]

Finally, vitamin D insufficiency probably initially contributes to malabsorption of calcium and eventually osteomalacia in the elderly.[3-17] It is not entirely clear whether mild deficiency in the supply of vitamin D can contribute to the problems of bone loss and lead to osteoporosis. Severe forms of vitamin D deficiency can be easily documented by measurements of blood 25(OH)-cholecalciferol (see Chapters 5 and 11). When inadequate solar exposure and diet can combine to increase the risk of vitamin D deficiency, especially among elderly individuals, those living in northern latitudes,[418] and institutionalized populations,[17,419] vitamin D supplementation is required. This should be limited to 400 to 500 IU of vitamin D per day, which in most individuals with normal renal function will provide an adequate supply of the active metabolite 1,25-dihydroxyvitamin D. 25(OH)D_3, in doses of 20 μg three times weekly, can be used as a substitute for the vitamin D. The use of megadoses of vitamin D (50,000 units once or more weekly) is not recommended since hypercalciuria and hypercalcemia often result from this large dose.

Table 12–3. Calcium Content (%) of Commonly Used Calcium Supplements

Calcium carbonate	40%
Tribasic calcium phosphate	38%
Bone meal	31%
Calcium chloride	27%
Dibasic calcium phosphate	23%
Dolomite	22%
Calcium citrate	21%
Calcium lactate	13%
Calcium gluconate	9%
Calcium gluceptate	8%

B. Exercise

Undoubtedly one of the most important aspects of maintaining bone health is physical activity. Bone mass responds, at least in young patients, to skeletal stress, and is, for example, greater in the dominant forearm of tennis players than in the nondominant arm.[420] The level of physical activity in healthy premenopausal women also appears to be a determinant of peak total skeletal mass and vertebral bone density. Prospective studies do reveal that exercise may play a role in prevention of bone loss.[212-217] However, exercise is an ineffective stimulant of vertebral mass unless calcium intake is above 800 mg/day.[400] Additionally, the evidence that exercise-induced amenorrhea is detrimental to the skeletal health of competitive athletes,[230] especially in the presence of a reduced calcium intake, places physical activity in at least third place in importance among the preventive steps to be taken in order to minimize bone loss. Nonetheless, for a variety of health reasons, a moderate exercise program is recommended for both pre- and postmenopausal individuals.[421,422]

In general, the exercise pattern should follow the guidelines for exercise for good cardiovascular health.[423,424,424a] Thus, for the young healthy female a minimum of 30 minutes of vigorous aerobic exercise on alternate days or at least three times weekly is recommended.[424] This can easily be supplemented by increased walking and climbing stairs whenever possible. Because rate of change of force appears more important than absolute force, well-programmed competitive racquet sports are often useful for the young individual. For the older individual with vertebral fractures and severe loss of bone mass, walking may be the only relevant exercise.[421,422] Swimming, which is an excellent exercise for older individuals to condition muscle tone and strength, does not appear to influence skeletal homeostasis significantly. Bone mineral content in the spine may be increased somewhat by a modest exercise program and by more vigorous programs designed for individual heart target rate ranges, which depend on age and the maximum predicted pulse; maximum predicted pulse is 220 minus age in years. To determine the target pulse range, the maximum pulse is multiplied by 0.70 and 0.80. For example, a 70-year old individual would aim for a pulse between 105 and 120 during a vigorous exercise regimen. These aerobic conditioning exercise programs should be attempted with physician advice and should also include "warm-up" and "cool-down" intervals.[424,424a,425] In one such study of women 35 to 65 years of age subjected to an exercise regimen of 45 minutes/day, 3 days/week for 3 to 4 years, results were quite gratifying. Whereas nonexercising control groups of women lost bone at a rate of 2.44% per year, bone mass in the exercised women actually increased by 1.39% per 1 year. Beneficial skeletal effects of a supervised exercise program in women aged 53 to 74 years have also been recorded. In a program that included three weekly sessions of 45 to 50 minutes for 5 months, bone mass increased by 3.8% in the exercised group, whereas it decreased by 1.9% in the control nonexercised group.[426] When patients are subjected to exercise regimens characterized by 70% to 90% of maximum oxygen uptake capacity for 50 to 60 minutes three times per week, vertebral bone mineral increases by 4% in 9 months and by 6% after 21 months. Cessation of exercise results in a gradual but progressive loss of bone. When recommending exercise regimens for elderly women with established vertebral osteoporosis, adverse effects should also be anticipated and patients advised accordingly. Extension or isometric exercises are more appropriate for these individuals since vertebral compression fractures are more apt to occur during flexion-exercise programs.[425,427]

The mode of action of stress in the skeleton is still in doubt. It has been suggested that mechanical stimuli counter only the net hormonal influences driving resorption.[428] Presumably the mechanical stimulus is converted to a local electrical signal that stimulates osteoblast function, cAMP, or prostaglandin production.[429] However, remodeling processes at distant sites may be affected by mechanical loading and may be mediated through endocrine mechanisms. Growth hormone, which can be stimulated by exercise,[430] not only increases bone mass (in adult dogs) but also changes resorbing (endosteal) surfaces to sites of net bone formation.[431] Moreover, exercise results in a decrease in parathyroid hormone and increments in blood calcitonin,[432] a combination that should decrease bone resorption and bone loss (see Chapters 3 and 4).

C. Estrogens

Because ovarian failure is one of the most significant factors affecting bone mass loss in women, it is not surprising that treatment with ovarian steroids prevents bone loss[52,53,277-281,401,433-439] (Fig. 12–29, Table 12–4). In a recent retrospective cohort study of 2873 women in the U.S. Framingham Heart Study, estrogen use when initiated within 4 years of the clinical menopause decreased the incidence of hip fractures in later life,[433] an observation consistent with earlier retrospective epidemiologic studies.[435,436] However, the efficacy of estrogen therapy in preventing hip fractures when initiated over the age of 65

Table 12–4. Effect of Percutaneous 17β-Estradiol-Progesterone (E_2), Calcitonin (CT), and a Combination of Both Regimens (CT/E_2) on Vertebral Bone Loss in Postmenopausal Women

	N	Rates of Vertebral Bone Loss/Yr
Placebo	16	4.4%
CT	11	1.7%
E_2	15	1.2%
CT/E_2	16	1.1%

Adapted from MacIntyre I, et al: Bone 8:54, 1987.

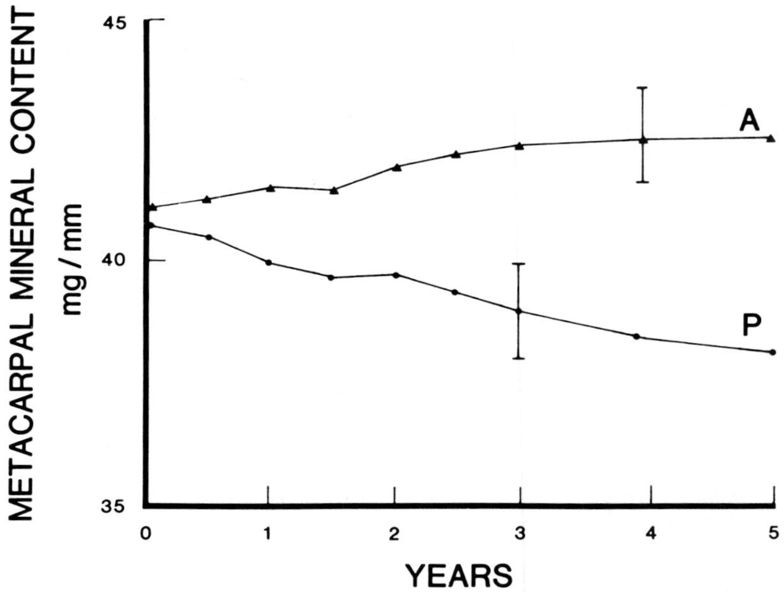

Figure 12–29: Preservation of bone mass measured by single-photon absorptiometry at the midpoint of the third right metacarpal bone. Group A is the estrogen-treated group; group P is treated with placebo.

was still unknown and conjectural at best, although some patients do respond with decreasing rates of bone loss.[438] The minimum effective estrogen dose essential to suppress bone loss is equivalent to 0.625 mg of oral conjugated equine estrogen (Fig. 12–30) or 1.0 to 2.0 mg of micronized 17 β-estradiol per day, 21 days each month.[274,282,430,437,438] Presently a transdermal therapeutic system (TTS) for estradiol is freely available in the United States, United Kingdom, and other European countries. The equivalent dose of the TTS for protection against osteoporosis is unknown at this time, although short-term studies (28 days) reveal that 50 μg of transdermal estradiol per 24 hours is as effective as 0.625 mg of oral estrogen in decreasing urinary calcium excretion.[440] Percutaneous estradiol applied daily as a cream is also effective in preventing bone loss.[266] Prolonged therapy with such cutaneous implants of estradiol (50 mg) combined with testosterone (100 mg) at 6-month intervals may prove as effective or even better than conventional oral estrogen progesterone regimens in

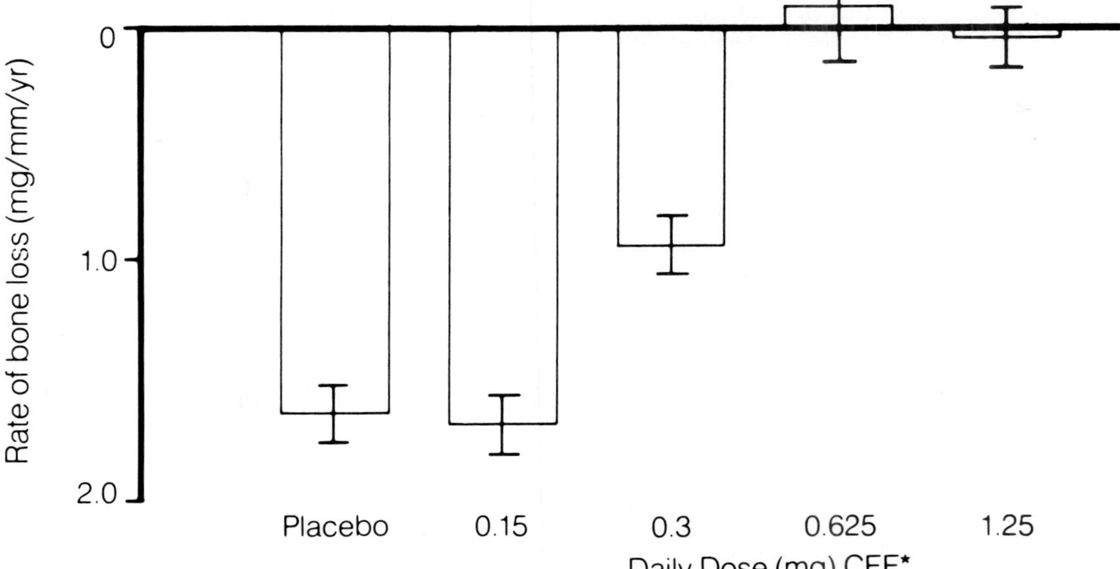

Figure 12–30: Dose response of bone mass changes with conjugated equine estrogens (CEE) in the early menopausal years.

preventing bone loss.[441] The effective oral estrogen dose can be decreased when calcium supplementation of 1200 to 1500 mg/day is also added to the regimen.[401] Withdrawal of estrogen treatment results in an acceleration of bone loss comparable to that seen in the immediate postmenopausal or postoophorectomy years.[53,442] The period of treatment required for fracture prevention is still debatable. It is at least 5 years if therapy is initiated immediately after the menopause,[439,443] and may be at least 10 years if a gap of several years intervenes between ovarian failure and onset of treatment.[439,443] The maximum effect that might be expected in compliant patients who initiate therapy within the first 5 years of menopause would be a 90% reduction in vertebral fracture frequency and a 50% reduction in hip fracture; that is, a reduction in fracture frequency among women to that which occurs among men[443] (Fig. 12–31). Since 20 to 30% of compliant patients may not respond to estrogens, serial measurements of bone mass at predetermined intervals of 6 months to 1 year should be made in order to document the required effect of therapy.

Despite preliminary evidence that estrogen receptors exist in active "osteoblast-like" cells,[444-446] it is entirely possible that the effects of sex steroids might also occur at the recruitment phase of bone remodeling. Although direct effects on osteoclast processes cannot be ruled out, the most popular theory of estrogen action depends more on the interaction of these steroids with the triad of hormones normally controlling calcium homeostasis: calcitonin, parathyroid hormone (PTH), and circulating vitamin D metabolites. The nature and manner of that interaction has yet to be completely elucidated. It has been suggested that part of the estrogen effect on bone is mediated via calcitonin since therapy with estrogen has been shown to increase circulating calcitonin levels (Fig. 12–32),[447] presumably as a result of a direct effect on calcitonin release by the thyroid gland.[448] The released calcitonin functions primarily to suppress osteoclastic bone resorption. As a consequence of the skeletal response to calcitonin, serum calcium would fall as the flow of calcium from bone to blood declines. In turn, PTH production would be stimulated either indirectly, because of the decrease in blood calcium, or directly as a response to estrogen, which is also a secretagogue for PTH,[449,450] resulting in an increase in the renal synthesis of 1,25-dihydroxyvitamin D.[448] Increments in this potent,

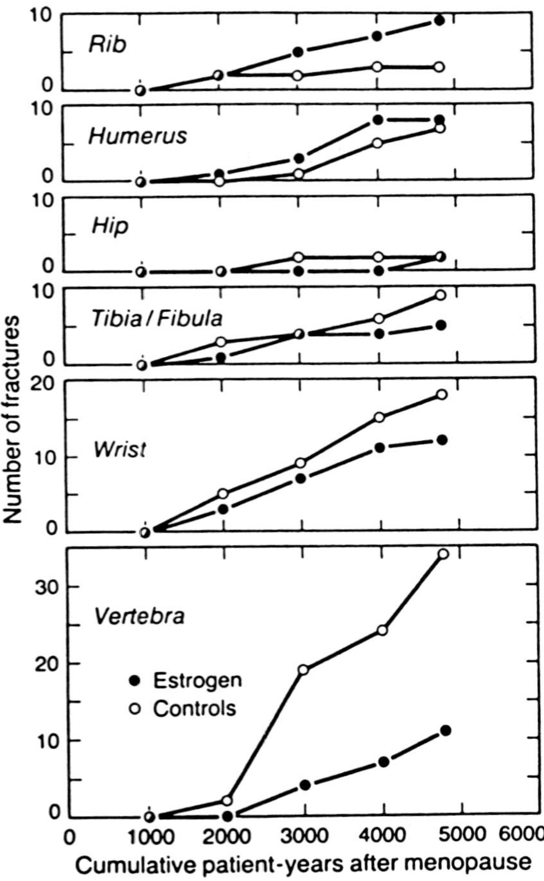

Figure 12–31: Effect of estrogen therapy on fracture incidence. The accumulated data reflect cumulative fractures according to type by postmenopausal patient-years at risk in 245 women and controls (From Ettinger B, et al: Ann Intern Med 102:319–324, 1985.)

biologically active vitamin D metabolite would account for improved calcium absorption from the gastrointestinal tract also observed during estrogen therapy.[447,451] The available data tend to support this complex mechanism of estrogen action, but a reconciliation of seemingly contrasting observations is required before the hypothesis can be accepted with certainty. For example, the theory must be reconciled with the observations that circulating PTH remains constant throughout the normal menstrual cycle despite wide fluctuations in estrogen levels,[452] and that estrogen-stimulated increments in circulating "free" $1,25(OH)_2D_3$ are not attended by elevations in blood PTH.[453] More recent studies describing markedly reduced urinary calcium excretion with associated elevations in blood 17β-estradiol and testosterone in postmenopausal women on boron supplements of 3 mg/day

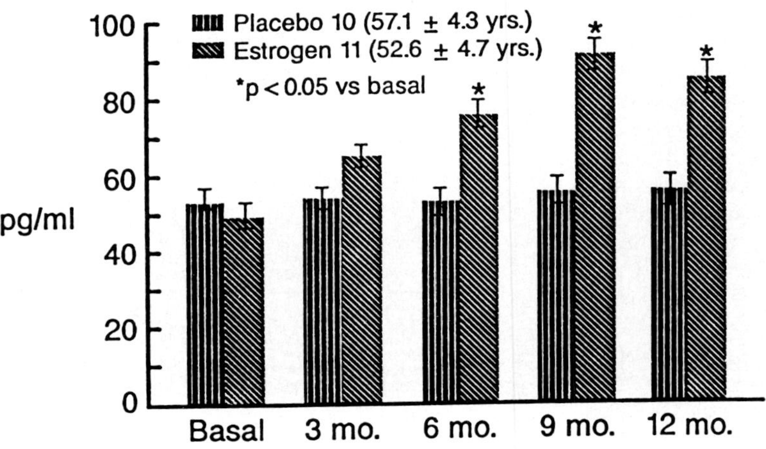

Figure 12–32: Effects of conjugated estrogen therapy (1.25 mg/day) on blood calcitonin levels in postmenopausal females. (Adapted from Civitelli R, et al: Calcif Tissue Int 42:77–86, 1988.)

should also be mentioned,[482] although the manner with which boron conditions estrogen metabolism is virtually unknown, as is the effect of this regimen on bone mass and fracture incidence.

Whereas a postmenopausal woman not taking estrogens has a 1 in 1000 chance each year of contracting endometrial carcinoma, a woman taking estrogens has 5 to 10 in 1000 chances each year. Other complications include alopecia, hirsutism, hypertension, weight gain and headaches, and thromboembolic phenomena. In order to minimize the incidence of endometrial carcinoma during estrogen therapy, progestational agents are also advocated in doses of 5 to 10 mg medroxyprogesterone daily for 10 to 13 days of each menstrual cycle. This time-dose relationship is essential to provide maximal maturation of the endometrium and to eliminate any hypoplastic changes. When estrogen-progesterone therapy is used to prevent bone loss in high-risk osteoporotic patients, one should also recognize reports of increased risk for developing breast carcinoma with long-term (>6 years) treatment regimens.[453a]

Preliminary observations suggest that the progestogens may have additional positive effects on stimulating bone formation,[454-457] although prolonged effects on bone mass and fracture frequency are unknown. Since androgenic progestogens of the 19-nortestosterone series reverse the beneficial effect of postmenopausal estrogen treatment on HDL cholesterol, and the hydroxyprogesterone derivative medroxyprogesterone acetate has no such effect,[458] medroxyprogesterone is recommended for estrogen-progesterone regimens as advocated for stabilizing bone mass. *Until other benefits* and risks that result from those doses of estrogen and progesterone essential to achieve this goal are more clearly defined, *we currently prescribe estrogen-progesterone therapy in the doses needed to retard bone loss only for women at greatest risk for osteoporosis and also recommend annual cervical cytologic studies and mammograms.*

D. Calcitonin

Due to its effect in suppressing bone resorption, which is presented in Chapter 4, calcitonin has proved effective in the treatment of hypercalcemia (Chapter 21) and in disorders of bone metabolism characterized by a dominance of osteoclastosis (or increased bone resorption) as cited in Chapter 15 for Paget's disease and immobilization (Fig. 12–33). It should ultimately prove to be exceptionally beneficial for the elderly osteoporotic female with a propensity toward hip fracture and high circulating PTH, which characterizes the type II osteoporotic syndrome (Table 12–1).[110,111]

Although calcitonin was approved in the United States in 1975 by the Food and Drug Administration (FDA) for treating Paget's disease, the experience with this drug for treating osteoporosis in the United States is still limited,[459,460] since FDA approval for its use in postmenopausal osteoporosis was announced only relatively recently in 1984. Reports of therapeutic response vary from those demonstrating acute anti-osteoclastic effects[461] and alterations in calcium metabolism consistent with suppression of bone turnover[462] to others showing dramatic clinical improvement with pain relief,[463] changes in

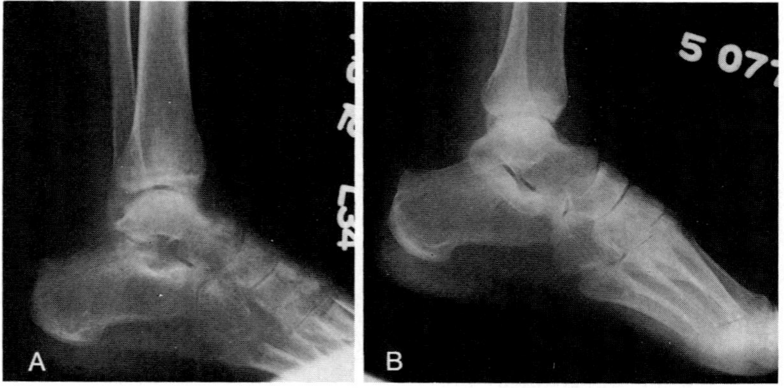

Figure 12–33: Effects of 24 months of treatment with salmon calcitonin (50 to 100 MRC units/day) on immobilization osteoporosis. *A*, Before therapy. *B*, After therapy. Note the radiologic evidence of increased bone mineral and increased definition of trabecular structure in *B*.

the skeletal coupling defects with a decrease in the rate of bone resorption, and quantitative increments in bone mass.[464-467,467a] An increase in intestinal calcium absorption has also been documented during calcitonin therapy.[465] More recent studies, designed to compare the effects of salmon calcitonin in patients with either "high" or "low" bone turnover, demonstrated a pronounced therapeutic effect in those with the high turnover form of the disorder[120] (Fig. 12–34). Studies also reveal that either parenteral[468] or nasal forms[469,470] of synthetic salmon calcitonin are effective in reversing bone loss in oophorectomized women and women in the immediate postmenopausal period[471] (Table 12–4). These observations should be considered when confronted with postmenopausal high-risk patients who are reluctant to follow estrogen-progesterone therapy because of a reportedly high incidence of breast carcinoma[453a] or ovarian-deficient states in previously menstruating, young females subjected to cytotoxic agents for breast cancer. As reviewed earlier in this chapter,[378,382] silent but accelerated bone loss should be anticipated in these women. Since estrogen replacement therapy to prevent progressive bone loss is obviously contraindicated in this population, calcitonin treatment should be considered. Similarly, since we can also anticipate progressive loss of vertebral bone during GnRH or LHRH agonist or antagonist treatment of certain gynecologic disorders because of decreased ovarian function,[384-386] calcitonin treatment offers a means to prevent bone loss if the treatment regimen cannot be discontinued.

As reviewed in Chapter 5, calcitonin has been widely employed in the treatment of

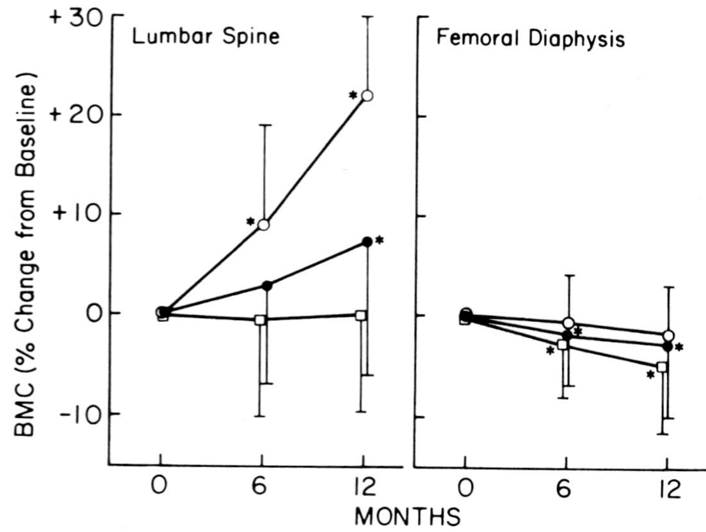

Figure 12–34: Effect of one year's treatment with salmon calcitonin on bone mineral content (BMC) of the lumbar spine and femoral diaphysis of postmenopausal osteoporotic patients: ○—○, "high turnover"; □—□, "normal turnover"; and ●—●, the pooled populations. (From Pacifici R, et al: J Clin Endocrinol Metab 64:209–214, 1987.)

Paget's disease of bone, in which the hormone exerts its beneficial effect by inhibiting bone resorption. Since the first therapeutic application in this disorder, it has been evident that calcitonin could be effective in relieving bone pain as well.[472] Relief of bone pain was first associated with a decrease in bone turnover. It soon became evident, however, that in many cases pain relief occurred prior to any modifications of the biochemical indices of bone disease.[472] Moreover, the analgesic effect induced by calcitonin administration in Paget's disease was maintained even when the skeletal response to calcitonin decreased,[472] observations that inferred that calcitonin could have an analgesic effect independent of its classic action on bone. The analgesic effect of calcitonin is now well documented not only in Paget's disease of bone but also in cancer patients with unbearable pain.[473] There is also mounting evidence that calcitonin significantly reduces bone pain in osteoporosis. Clinical trials in postmenopausal osteoporotic patients using calcitonin in doses ranging from 50 to 100 MRC units per day, and for periods spanning 1 to 19 months, have documented clinical improvement in pain and disability.[463,474,475] The analgesic effect can be evident as soon as the second week of treatment, and it increases with the length of treatment. These preliminary observations should be considered supportive of the potential symptomatic improvement to be offered by calcitonin treatment of the osteoporotic syndrome. The mechanism for the analgesic effect of calcitonin is yet to be clarified. Many hypotheses have been proposed, the most provocative of which include a stimulated release of beta-endorphin,[475] and a direct effect of calcitonin on central pain regulatory mechanisms with an enhancement of the "pain theshold."[475]

The expanding therapeutic use of calcitonin in a variety of bone diseases has also resulted in the recognition of its potential side-effects. At therapeutic doses, calcitonin is devoid of toxicity. Gastrointestinal (abdominal fullness and nausea) and vascular (flushing) side-effects have been observed and are usually mild and transient. Since calcitonin is a potent inhibitor of gastric free acid secretion, the gastrointestinal side-effects are mitigated if calcitonin is administered 3 to 4 hours following food ingestion. Pain at the site of injection, urinary frequency, and an unpleasant metallic taste have been described in isolated instances. The side-effects are much more severe when calcitonin is given intramuscularly, minimized with subcutaneous injections, and disappear with nasal spray forms of the hormone.[469,470] Finally, reactions to calcitonin, which characteristically occur at the initiation of therapy, tend to either decrease or disappear with continued administration of the drug.

E. Sodium Fluoride

Sodium fluoride has been prescribed for osteoporotic patients for decades,[476-490] although it is not yet approved by the FDA for use in osteoporosis in the United States. This substance should be restricted to formal protocols in study units with a research interest in the treatment of osteoporosis, as the frequency of significant gastrointestinal side-effects such as diarrhea, nausea, gastric pyrosis and bleeding, plantar fascial syndromes, arthralgia with synovitis, and increased fracture incidence may be quite high.[477,480,482,483,485,486,489] Despite testimonials to a favorable "risk/benefit" ratio and decreased incidence of vertebral fractures,[479,487,488] the enthusiasm should be tempered by other reports of increased incidence of nonvertebral fractures (including hip!) with frequencies *10 times* higher than anticipated.[480,489] Moreover, at least 30% of patients treated with fluoride may not respond to the drug, and many patients ultimately become intolerant of it.[489a] Limited experience with new "slow release" sodium reveals a decrease in the frequency of side-effects observed with ordinary sodium fluoride capsules,[481,490] although hip fracture rates are also 10 times higher than would be expected in a normal age-matched population.[489]

The results of a four-year randomized placebo-controlled, double-blind, clinical trial of continuous sodium fluoride therapy (75 mg/day) recently completed in the United States revealed no additional benefit on vertebral fracture rates than that observed from oral calcium carbonate supplements of 1500 mg/day.[490a] *In fact, a statistically significant increase in nonvertebral fracture rates was observed in the fluoride-treated patients.*

F. Coherence Therapy

Other therapeutic modalities for osteoporotic patients are also being explored. One popular approach is the modulation of the bone remodeling cycle to produce a positive bone balance at each remodeling site. The concept relies on the capacity to cyclically activate a large number of remodeling sites synchronously and to modulate their behavior in such a way that the osteoclast population will be inhibited and will resorb less bone; it is assumed that subsequently the osteoblast population will synthesize their normal quantity of osteoid.[491,492] Thus, a negative balance at each remodeling site will be converted to a positive balance, with an overall increase in bone mass. The "activation-inhibition" cycles would then be repeated, producing increments in bone mass for each repetition.[491,492] The concept is known by its acronym, ADFR (representing *A*ctivate-*D*epress-*F*ree-*R*epeat). However, there are still many unknowns, and there is a possible risk to this approach. First, it is not clear if bone cell activation that follows the administration of either of the agents normally used for this purpose is a coherent event. Second, the temporary inhibition of osteoclasts (for the period thought to be equivalent to their normal resorption period) may not be followed by replacement by osteoblasts and synthesis of new bone, but by further resorption as the inhibitory agent is removed. In addition, it is intrinsic to the ADFR hypothesis that continued osteoblastic function will overfill the smaller cavity produced by the osteoclast,[491,492] although there are no data to support that concept. Finally, the creation of a large number of resorption cavities by osteoclasts at the same time might temporarily prejudice the already weakened skeleton and increase the risk of fracture. A prospective, controlled study, designed to analyze the effect of the specific ADFR approach for a 2-year period in osteoporotic subjects using the PTH response to oral inorganic phosphate as the "activator" of bone turnover and diphosphonate as the osteoclastic "inhibitor," demonstrated no significant difference in bone loss when compared with a population receiving calcium supplements alone[493] (Fig. 12–35). The apparent failure of this combination of activator-depressor drugs may have resulted from a dose of phosphate that was insufficient to stimulate PTH[494] (Fig. 12–36) or the continued use of calcium supplements during the "free" period. Using a "pulse-dose" regimen of oral neutral phosphate (2.0 g/day for 7 days) and the etidronate disodium diphosphonate (20 mg/kg body weight for 5 days), and 8% gain in vertebral bone mass has been recorded after 12 months of therapy.[495] Pulse-doses of salmon calcitonin (50 IU × 5 days every third week) in patients treated with continuous oral phosphate increase trabecular bone volume by 30% or more after 12 months.[496,497] Other pulse-dose techniques have been advanced, albeit in a preliminary fashion,[498,499] which consist of concomitant or intermittent administration of antiresorptive agents such as the diphosphonates to osteoporotic subjects. Although encouraging, none of the currently

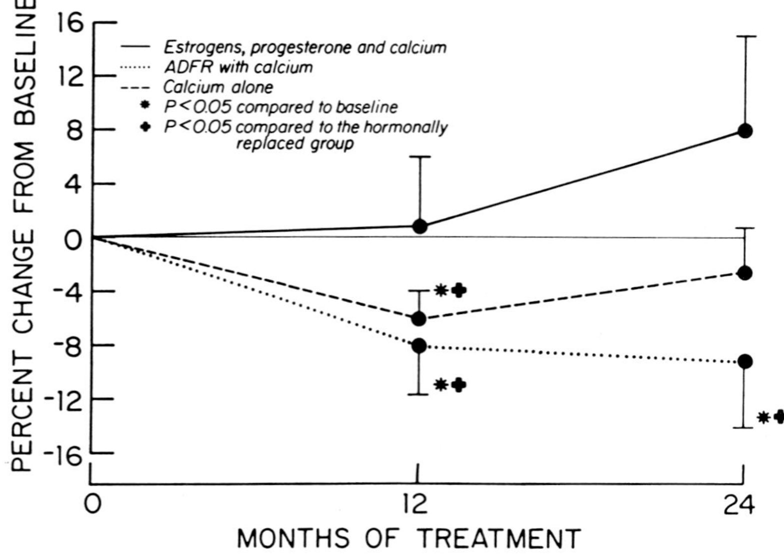

Figure 12–35: Comparative effects of therapeutic regimens in postmenopausal osteoporotic patients using the ADFR procedure. Bone cell activation was induced by oral phosphate, 1.5 g/day x 3 days. Depression was achieved by the diphosphate etidronate, 400 mg/day x 14 days; a free period of 8 weeks consisting of no drug therapy was followed by repetition of the cycle. Vertebral bone mass was quantitated by CT procedures (see Chapter 9). Note that after 24 months of treatment, bone mass had stabilized in patients treated with either estrogen, progesterone, and calcium, or calcium alone, whereas continued and progressive bone loss occurred with the ADFR-treated patients. (From Pacifici R, et al: J Clin Endocrinol Metab 66:747–753, 1988.)

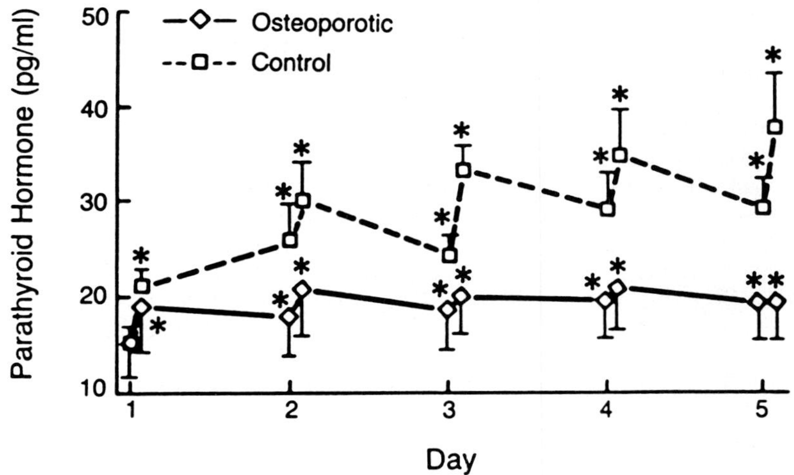

Figure 12–36: Response of parathyroid hormone to phosphate administration (2 g/day) in control and osteoporotic populations. Values are mean ±SEM for all subjects before and 2 hours after phosphate administration. An asterisk denotes a significant change from baseline. (From Silverberg SJ, et al: N Engl J Med 320:277–281, 1989.)

activated intermittent or "pulse-dose" regimens can be considered of proven therapeutic value until the appropriate long-term controlled study protocols are available for analyses. Recent studies with a relatively new diphosphonate, tiludronate (chloro-4-phenylthiomethylene bisphosphonate), are promising, since bone mineral density of the lumbar spine does stabilize following a 6-month course of a daily dose of 100 mg.[499a]

G. Parathyroid Hormone and Vitamin D Metabolites

The availability of a synthetic 1–34 amino-terminal fragment of human PTH (hPTH), and early observations that "small" PTH doses produced an anabolic effect by activating basic multicellular bone units with increasing bone mass in animals,[500] resulted in more sophisticated studies of hPTH in humans with osteoporosis.[501,502] Doses of 400 to 500 units of hPTH, 600 to 1200 mg of elemental calcium, and 0.25 to 0.50 μg of $1,25(OH)_2D_3$ for 12 months in eight males with "idiopathic osteoporosis" demonstrated an increase in trabecular bone density and an increase in calcium absorption.[502] Combination therapy using pulsatile doses of human PTH 1–38 fragments with sequential addition of nasal spray calcitonin has also resulted in increased bone mass in osteoporotic patients.[503] The sustained effect of these various treatment regimens and their potential benefit for chronic therapy in the postmenopausal osteoporotic syndrome have not yet been evaluated. Reports of transient hypoparathyroidism in patients treated with hPTH in doses of 100 μg/day must also be acknowledged.[504]

Alterations in circulating levels of vitamin D metabolites documented by some in postmenopausal and senile osteoporotic patients[9-19,339,340] have resulted in clinical trials of $1,25(OH)_2D_3$, its structurally related analogue $1\text{-}\alpha(OH)D_3$, $24,25(OH)_2D_3$, and $25(OH)D_3$ in osteoporotic patients. Isolated reports suggest that treatment with $1\text{-}\alpha(OH)D_3$ in doses of 1.0 μg/day results in an increase in bone mass[505] and a decrease in vertebral fractures.[506] Early studies with $1,25(OH)_2D_3$ were encouraging[507]; however, subsequent studies with $1,25(OH)_2D_3$ doses ranging from 0.25 to 1.0 μg/day for periods of 6 to 24 months have been less positive.[508-511] Although isolated reports of increased bone mass and decreased fracture incidence[509] are contrasted with other citations of decreased bone mass, decreased vertebral height,[508,510] and *increased* fracture incidence,[511] it is generally agreed that calcium absorption increases during $1,25(OH)_2D_3$ therapy.[507,512] Hypercalcemia and hypercalciuria appear to be recurrent problems during the administration of $1,25(OH)_2D_3$[509,511]; hypercalciuria necessitates significant decreases in calcium intake.[513]

The effects of $25(OH)_2D_3$ treatment for 12 to 18 months in doses of 50 μg/day reveal that some postmenopausal osteoporotic patients respond with an increase in calcium absorption and blood $1,25(OH)_2D_3$, whereas in others the response is negligible.[514] Finally, $24,25(OH)_2D_3$ doses of 10 μg/day for a 24-month period have no apparent effect on either appendicular or vertebral bone loss or calcium absorption.[515]

H. Miscellaneous

Androgens directly stimulate the proliferation of human osteoclast cells *in vitro*,[516] most probably by androgen receptor–mediated mechanisms.[517-519] Anabolic steroids increase whole-body calcium as well as forearm and vertebral bone density in postmenopausal osteoporotic individuals[517,520,521] with increments in vertebral bone density as high as 20% within 14 months.[520] However, undesirable side-effects such as voice changes and an increased growth rate of body hair usually mitigate the enthusiasm for this form of hormonal therapy. Moreover, changes in lipoprotein induced by certain oral 17α alkylated androgenic steroid preparations, such as a reduction in HDL cholesterol and LDL cholesterol, should also be considered undesirable in relation to the risk of coronary heart disease.[522,523] When used in combination with estrogens in osteoporotic females in the form of subcutaneous implants,[441] androgens are as effective as oral estrogen regimens in stabilizing vertebral bone mass.

Since thiazide therapy lowers urinary calcium excretion rate,[524] this family of diuretics has been advocated as relatively safe and effective in decreasing the rate of bone loss in the immediate postmenopausal period.[525-527] Retrospective analysis of fracture profiles of elderly hypertensive individuals on therapy for 6 or more years reveals an increase in bone mass and a decrease in fracture incidence,[528-530] with the fracture risk decreasing significantly with increased duration of thiazide usage.[530] The thiazide effects on bone are still ill-defined, although carbonic anhydrase inhibition may prove pivotal to its action.[531] Before advocating this form of therapeutic intervention on a routine basis, the overall benefit/risk ratio of prolonged thiazide use in the elderly must be considered, particularly with reference to hyperuricemic, hypercalcemic, and hypokalemic syndromes and other acquired central nervous system symptoms.[528]

VI. SUMMARY AND CONCLUSIONS

It is rational to provide advice about prevention to all at risk for early nontraumatic fracture syndromes. For practical purposes this currently means all slim white or Oriental women with either an early menopause, drug- or environment-induced changes in ovarian function, or oophorectomy. Recommendations to patients basically attempt to remove all risk factors amenable to such an approach. Until more experience is gained with androgens, ADFR procedures, sodium fluoride, and PTH analogues, preventive *therapy* requires intervention with calcium, exercise, estrogen, and calcitonin if estrogens are contraindicated, undesirable, or poorly tolerated in the immediate postmenopausal period. For more elderly women with painful crush fracture syndromes, calcitonin should be considered an effective deterrent to further bone loss and a good analgesic. Calcium supplementation, *using preparations with established bioavailability,* should be recommended when dietary sources are insufficient to provide a total intake of 1.0 to 1.5 g/day. Exercise prescription requires careful patient evaluation to avoid further insult to the skeleton and should include gravity-resistive exercises on a regular basis. Estrogen should be given in the minimum effective dose (0.625 mg conjugated equine estrogen or its equivalent per day for at least 21 days each month) or lower if calcium intake is increased; the use of a progestogen (and gynecologic supervision) is necessary if the patient has an intact uterus. The availability of nasal spray forms of salmon calcitonin with proven ability to prevent bone loss in the postmenopausal female represents a significant advance in therapy, especially for postmenopausal women who are not candidates for estrogen therapy and the elderly female who responds poorly to estrogens. Additionally, physicians must remind themselves of the "iatrogenic" problems that can be created by prolonged use of a variety of medications that can adversely affect the skeleton and the tendency toward polypharmacy in the elderly. Use of these medications must be scrutinized and carefully controlled, recognizing that pharmacokinetics are often altered in the elderly.

Finally, whereas it is commonly assumed that osteoporosis is a disorder of women, it is important to remember that the incidence of hip fracture is only twice as great among women as among men, and that chronic tobacco and alcohol use is significantly increased in men with osteoporosis. Hypogonadism increases risk in men, as in women; and obesity also has a protective effect in men. Preventive advice for men, therefore, follows a similar theme as that for women.

Detecting hypogonadism, removal of or minimizing dietary or habit-forming risks, and adhering to moderate exercise programs with adequate calcium nutrition are all relevant. Calcitonin should also be considered for those men with severe and debilitating forms of this disorder who are not candidates for androgen replacement therapy or who develop prostatic abnormalities during androgen treatment.[533]

References

1. Berg E: Paleopathology: Bone lesions in ancient peoples. Clin Orthop Rel Res 82:263–267, 1972.
2. Bauer GCH: Kinetics of calcium and strontium metabolism in man. *In* Rodahl K (ed): Bone As A Tissue. *In* Nicholson JI, Brown EM, Jr. New York, McGraw-Hill, 1960, pp 118–127.
3. Corless D: Vitamin D in the elderly. J Clin Exp Geront 6:113–144, 1984.
4. Parfitt AM, Gallagher JC, Heaney RP, et al: Vitamin D and bone health in the elderly. Am J Clin Nutr 36:1014–1031, 1982.
5. Francis RM, Peacock M, Taylor GA, et al: Calcium malabsorption in elderly women with vertebral fractures: Evidence for resistance to the action of vitamin D metabolites on the bowel. Clin Sci 66:103–107, 1984.
6. Lawson DEM, Paul AA, Black AE, et al: Relative contributions of diet and sunlight to vitamin D state in the elderly. Br Med J 2:303–305, 1979.
7. MacLaughlin J, Holick MF: Aging decreases the capacity of human skin to produce vitamin D_3. J Clin Invest 76:1536–1538, 1985.
8. Omdahl JL, Garry PJ, Hunsaker LA, et al: Nutritional status in a healthy elderly population: Vitamin D. Am J Clin Nutr 36:1125–1233, 1982.
9. Slovik DM, Adams JS, Neer RM, et al: Deficient production of 1,25-dihydroxyvitamin D in elderly osteoporotic patients. N Engl J Med 305:372–374, 1981.
10. Tsai K-S, Heath H, Kumar R, et al: Impaired vitamin D metabolism with aging in women. Possible role in pathogenesis of senile osteoporosis. J Clin Invest 73:1668–1672, 1984.
11. Lamberg-Allardt C: Vitamin D intake, sunlight exposure and 25-hydroxyvitamin D levels in the elderly during one year. Ann Nutr Metab 28:144–150, 1984.
12. Clemens TL, Zhou X-Y, Myles M, et al: Serum vitamin D_2 and vitamin D_3 metabolite concentrations and absorption of vitamin D_2 in elderly subjects. J Clin Endocrin Metab 63:656, 1986.
13. Lips P, van Ginkel F, Jongen M, et al: Determinants of vitamin D status in patients with hip fracture and in elderly control subjects. Am J Clin Nutr 46:1005–1010, 1987.
14. Bouillon RA, Auwerx JH, Lissens WD, et al: Vitamin D status in the elderly: Seasonal substrate deficiency causes 1,25-dihydroxycholecalciferol deficiency. Am J Clin Nutr 45:755–763, 1987.
15. Barzel US: Vitamin D deficiency: A risk factor for osteomalacia in the aged. J Am Geriat Soc 31:598–601, 1983.
16. Sharland DE: Osteomalacia in the elderly. J R Coll Physicians Lond 16:50–52, 1982.
17. McKenna M, Freaney R, Keating D, et al: The prevalence and management of vitamin D deficiency in an acute geriatric unit. Ir Med J 74:336–338, 1981.
18. Hordon LD, Peacock M: Vitamin D metabolism in women with femoral neck fracture. Bone and Mineral 2:413–426, 1987.
19. Knorring JV, Slätis P, Weber TH, et al: Serum levels of 25-hydroxyvitamin D, 24,25-dihydroxyvitamin D and parathyroid hormone in patients with femoral neck fracture in southern Finland. Clin Endocrinol 17:189–194, 1982.
20. Newton H, Sheltawy M, Hay A, et al: The relations between vitamin D_2 and D_3 in the diet and plasma $25OHD_2$ and $25OHD_3$ in elderly women in Great Britain. Am J Clin Nutr 41:760–764, 1985.
21. Gruber HE, Brautbar N: Metabolic bone disease and the elderly: Current approach to diagnosis and therapy. Nephron 38:76–86, 1984.
22. Lachman E: Osteoporosis: The potentialities and limitations of its roentgenologic diagnosis. Am J Roentgenol Radium Ther 74:712–715, 1955.
23. Wray JB, Sugarman ED, Schneider AJ: Bone composition in senile osteoporosis. JAMA 183:118–120, 1963.
24. Doyle FH, Gatteridge DH, Joplin GF, et al: An assessment of radiological criteria used in the study of osteoporosis. Br J Radiol 40:241–250, 1967.
25. Seeman E, Wahner HW, Offord KP, et al: Differential effects of endocrine dysfunction on the axial and the appendicular skeleton. J Clin Invest 69:1302–1309, 1982.
26. Pocock MA, Eisman JA, Yeates MG, et al: Limitations of forearm bone densitometry as an index of vertebral or femoral neck osteopenia. J Bone Mineral Res 1:369–375, 1986.
27. Ott SM, Kilcoyne RF, Chesnut CH II: Ability of four different techniques of measuring bone mass to diagnose vertebral fractures in postmenopausal women. J Bone Mineral Res 2:201–210, 1987.
28. Schaadt O, Bohr H: Different trends of age-related diminution of bone mineral content in the lumbar spine, femoral neck, and femoral shaft in women. Calcif Tissue Int 42:71–76, 1988.
29. Mazess RB, Barden H, Ettinger M, et al: Bone density of the radius, spine, and proximal femur in osteoporosis. J Bone Mineral Res 3:13–18, 1988.
30. Fox KM, Tobin JD, Plato CC: Longitudinal study of bone loss in the second metacarpal. Calcif Tissue Int 39:218–225, 1986.
31. Frost HM: The pathomechanics of osteoporoses. Clin Orthop Rel Res 200:198–225, 1986.
32. Chatterji S, Wall JC, Jeffrey JW: Changes in the degree of orientation of bone materials with age in the human femur. Experimentia 28:156–157, 1972.
33. Mazess RB, Cameron JB: Skeletal growth in school children: Maturation and bone mass. Am J Phys Anthropol 35:399–407, 1971.
34. Gryfe CI, Exton-Smith AW, Payne PR, et al: Pattern of development of bone in childhood and adolescence. Lancet 1:523–526, 1971.
35. Liel Y, Edwards J, Shary J, et al: Effects of race and body habitus on bone mineral density of the radius, hip, and spine in premenopausal women. J Clin Endocrinol Metab 66:1247–1250, 1988.
36. Reid IR, Mackie M, Ibbertson HK: Bone mineral content in Polynesian and white New Zealand

women. Br Med J 292:1547–1548, 1986.

37. Pocock NA, Eisman JA, Hopper JL, et al: Genetic determinants of bone mass in adults. A twin study. J Clin Invest 80:706–710, 1987.
38. Bell NH, Greene A, Epstein S, et al: Evidence for alteration of the vitamin D–endocrine system in blacks. J Clin Invest 76:470–473, 1985.
39. M'Buyamba-Kabangu JR, Fagard R, Lijnen P, et al: Calcium, vitamin D–endocrine system, and parathyroid hormone in black and white males. Calcif Tissue Int 41:70–74, 1987.
40. Stevenson JC, Myers CH, Ajdukiewicz AB: Racial differences in calcitonin and katacalcin. Calcif Tissue Int 36:725–728, 1984.
41. Garn SM: The course of bone gain and the phase of bone loss. Orthop Clin North Am 3:503–520, 1972.
42. Garn SM, Rohmann CG, Behar M, et al: Compact bone deficiency in protein-calorie malnutrition. Science 145:1444–1445, 1964.
43. Garn SM, Pozranski AK: Transient and irreversible bone losses. *In* Barzel US (ed): Osteoporosis. New York, Grune & Stratton, 1970, pp 114–123.
44. Gilsanz V, Gibbens DT, Carlson M, et al: Peak trabecular vertebral density. A comparison of adolescent and adult females. Calcif Tissue Int 43:260–262, 1988.
45. Meier DE, Orwoll ES, Jones JM: Marked disparity between trabecular and cortical bone loss with age in healthy men. Measurement by vertebral computed tomography and radial photon absorptiometry. Ann Intern Med 101:605–612, 1984.
46. Mazess RB, Barden HS, Ettinger M, et al: Spine and femur density using dual-photon absorptiometry in US white women. Bone and Mineral 2:211–219, 1987.
47. Stevenson JC, Banks LM, Spinks TJ, et al: Regional and total skeletal measurements in the early postmenopause. J Clin Invest 80:258–262, 1987.
48. Buchanan JR, Myers C, Lloyd T, et al: Early vertebral trabecular bone loss in normal premenopausal women. J Bone Mineral Res 3:583–587, 1988.
49. Nilas L, Christiansen C: Bone mass and its relationship to age and the menopause. J Clin Endocrinol Metab 65:697–701, 1987.
50. Heaney RP, Recker RR, Saville PD: Menopausal changes in bone remodeling. J Lab Clin Med 92:964–968, 1978.
51. Firooznia H, Golimbu C, Rafii M, et al: Rate of spinal trabecular bone loss in normal perimenopausal women: CT measurement. Radiology 161:735–738, 1986.
52. Lindsay R, Hart DM, Aiken JM, et al: Long-term prevention of postmenopausal osteoporosis by estrogen. Lancet 1:1038–1042, 1976.
53. Lindsay R, Hart DM, MacLean A, et al: Bone response to termination of estrogen treatment. Lancet 1:1325–1328, 1978.
54. Khairi MRA, Johnston CC: What we know—and don't know—about bone loss in the elderly. Geriatrics, Nov: 67–70, 1978.
55. Smith DM, Johnston CC, Yu PL: In vivo measurement of bone mass. JAMA 219:325–329, 1972.
56. Bell NH, Epstein S, Greene A, et al: Evidence for alteration of the vitamin D–endocrine system in obese subjects. J Clin Invest 76:370–373, 1985.
57. Israel H: Loss of bone and remodeling-redistribution in the craniofacial skeleton with age. Fed Proc Am Soc Exp Biol 26:1723–1728, 1967.
58. Daniell HW: Postmenopausal tooth loss. Contributions to edentulism by osteoporosis and cigarette smoking. Arch Intern Med 143:1678–1682, 1983.
59. Garn SM, Pao EM, Rihl ME: Compact bone in Chinese and Japanese. Science 143:1439–1440, 1964.
60. Smith RW Jr, Rizek J: Epidemiologic studies of osteoporosis in women of Puerto Rico and Southeastern Michigan with special reference to age, race, national origin, and to other related or associated findings. Clin Orthop Rel Res 45:31–48, 1966.
61. Thompson DD, Posner AS, Laughlin WS: Comparison of bone apatite in osteoporotic and normal Eskimos. Calcif Tissue Int 35:392–393, 1983.
62. Mazess RB, Barden HS, Christiansen C, et al: Bone mineral and vitamin D in Aleutian Islanders. Am J Clin Nutr 42:143–146, 1985.
63. de Vernejoul MC, Girot R, Gueris J, et al: Calcium phosphate metabolism and bone disease in patients with homozygous thalassemia. J Clin Endocrinol Metab 54:276–281, 1982.
64. Avioli LV: Hyperparathyroidism, hypoparathyroidism, pseudohypoparathyroidism and pseudopseudohypoparathyroidism. *In* Goldensohn ES, Appel SH (eds): Scientific Approaches to Clinical Neurology, Vol II. Philadelphia, Lea and Febiger, 1977, pp 1871–1883.
65. Ellis FR, Holish S, Ellis JW: Incidence of osteoporosis in vegetarians and omnivores. Am J Clin Nutr 25:555–558, 1972.
66. Nilsson BE, Westlin NE: Changes in bone mass in alcoholics. Clin Orthop Rel Res 90:229–232, 1973.
67. Meade JB, Cowen SC, Klawitter JJ, et al: Bone remodeling due to continuously applied loads. Calcif Tissue Int 36:S25–S30, 1984.
68. Avioli LV: Calcium and osteoporosis. Am Rev Nutr 4:471–491, 1984.
69. Garn SM: Calcium requirements for bone building and skeletal maintenance. Am J Clin Nutr 23:1149–1150, 1970.
70. Smith RW Jr, Frame B: Concurrent axial and appendicular osteoporosis: Its relation to calcium consumption. N Engl J Med 273:73–78, 1965.
71. Hurxthal LM, Vose GP: Relationship of dietary calcium intake to radiographic bone density in normal and osteoporotic persons. Calcif Tissue Res 4:245–256, 1969.
72. Sowers MFR, Wallace RB, Lemke JH: Correlates of mid-radius bone density among postmenopausal women: A community study. Am J Clin Nutr 41:1045–1053, 1985.
73. Sandler RB, Slemenda CW, LaPorte RE, et al: Postmenopausal bone density and milk consumption in childhood and adolescence. Am J Clin Nutr 42:270–274, 1985.
74. Freudenheim JL, Johnson NE, Smith EL: Relationships between usual nutrient intake and bone-mineral content of women 35–65 years of age: Longitudinal and cross-sectional analysis. Am J Clin Nutr 44:863–876, 1986.
75. Chan GM, McMurry M, Westover K, et al: Effects of increased dietary calcium intake upon the calcium and bone mineral status of lactating adolescent and adult women. Am J Clin Nutr 46:319–323, 1987.
76. Dawson-Hughes B, Jacques P, Shipp C: Dietary calcium intake and bone loss from the spine in healthy

postmenopausal women. Am J Clin Nutr 46:685–687, 1987.
77. Alevizaki CC, Ikkos DG, Singhelakis P: Progressive decrease of true intestinal calcium absorption with age in normal man. J Nucl Med 14:760–762, 1973.
78. Avioli LV, McDonald J, Lee SW: The influence of age in the intestinal absorption of Ca^{47} in women and its relation to Ca^{47} absorption in postmenopausal osteoporosis. J Clin Invest 44:1960–1965, 1965.
79. Ireland P, Fordtran JC: Effect of dietary calcium and age on jejunal calcium absorption in humans. J Clin Invest 52:2672–2681, 1973.
80. Epstein S, Bryce G, Hinman JW, et al: The influence of age on bone mineral regulating hormones. Bone 7:421–425, 1986.
81. Endres DB, Morgan CH, Garry PJ, et al: Age-related changes in serum immunoreactive parathyroid hormone and its biological action in healthy men and women. J Clin Endocrinol Metab 65:724–731, 1987.
82. Forero MS, Klein RF, Nissenson RA, et al: Effect of age on circulating immunoreactive and bioactive parathyroid hormone levels in women. J Bone Mineral Res 2:363–366, 1987.
83. Orwoll ES, Meier DE: Alterations in calcium vitamin D, and parathyroid hormone physiology in normal men with aging. Relationship to the development of senile osteopenia. J Clin Endocrinol Metab 63:1262–1269, 1986.
84. Young G, Marcus R, Minkoff JR: Age-related rise in parathyroid hormone in man: The use of intact and midmolecule antisera to distinguish hormone secretion from retention. J Bone Mineral Res 2:367–374, 1987.
85. Albright F, Smith PH, Richardson AM: Postmenopausal osteoporosis. JAMA 116:2465–2474, 1941.
86. Carasco MG, de Vernejoul MC, Sterkers Y, et al: Decreased bone formation in osteoporotic patients compared with age-matched controls. Calcif Tissue Int 44:173–175, 1989.
87. Reeve J, Arlot ME, Charassicut P, et al: Assessment of bone formation and bone resorption in osteoporosis: Comparison between tetracycline-based iliac histomorphometry and whole body ^{85}Sr kinets. J Bone Mineral Res 2:479–489, 1987.
88. Recker RR, Kimmel DB, Parfitt AM: Static and tetracycline-based bone histomorphometric data from 34 normal postmenopausal females. J Bone Mineral Res. 3:133–144, 1988.
89. Fiore CE, Falcidia E, Foti R, et al: Postoophorectomy bone loss is associated with reduced bone gla protein serum levels: A possible effect of osteoblastic insufficiency. Calcif Tissue Int 41:303–306, 1987.
90. Podenphant J, Johansen JS, Thomsen K, et al: Bone turnover in spinal osteoporosis. J Bone Mineral Res 2:497–503, 1987.
91. Ferris BD, Klenerman L, Dodds RA, et al: Altered organization of noncollagenous bone matrix in osteoporosis. Bone 8:285–288, 1987.
92. Reginster JY, Derasy R, Albert A, et al: Relationship between whole plasma calcitonin levels, calcitonin, secretory capacity and plasma levels of estrone in healthy women and postmenopausal osteoporosis. J Clin Invest 83:1073–1077, 1989.
93. Pacifici R, Rifas L, Teitelbaum S, et al: Spontaneous release of interleukin 1 from human blood monocytes reflects bone formation in idiopathic osteoporosis. Proc Natl Acad Sci 84:4616–4620, 1987.
94. Carmel R, Lau KH, Baylink DJ, et al: Cobalamin and osteoblast specific protein. N Engl J Med 319:70–75, 1988.
95. Raisz LG: Local and systemic factors in the pathogenesis of osteoporosis. N Engl J Med 318:818–828, 1988.
96. McKenna MJ, Kleerekoper M, Ellis BI, et al: Aytpical insufficiency fractures confused with Looser zones of osteomalacia. Bone 8:71–78, 1987.
97. Kochersberg G, Buckley NJ, Leight GS, et al: What is the clinical significance of bone loss in primary hyperparathyroidism? Arch Intern Med 147:1951–1953, 1987.
98. Murry RO: Radiologic bone changes in Cushing's syndrome and steroid therapy. Br J Radiol 33:1–19, 1960.
99. Atkinson PJ: Variation in trabecular structure of vertebrae with age. Calcif Tissue Res 1:24–32, 1967.
100. Boukhris R, Becker KL: Schmorl's nodes and osteoporosis. Clin Orthop Relat Res 104:275–280, 1974.
101. Hedlund LR, Gallagher JC, Meeger C, et al: Changes in vertebral shape in spinal osteoporosis. Calcif Tissue Int 44: 168–172, 1989.
102. Hurxthal LM: Measurements of anterior vertebral compressions and biconcave vertebrae. Am J Roentgen 103:635–644, 1968.
103. McHenry MC, Duchesneau PM, Keyes TF, et al: Vertebral osteomyelitis presenting as spinal compression fractures. Arch Intern Med 148:417–423, 1988.
104. Rose GA: The radiological diagnosis of osteoporosis, osteomalacia and hyperparathyroidism. Clin Radiol 15:75–83, 1964.
105. Hauge MD, Cooper KL, Litin SC: Insufficiency fractures of the pelvis that simulate metastatic disease. Mayo Clin Proc 63: 807–812, 1988.
106. Francis RM, Peacock M, Marshall DH, et al: Spinal osteoporosis in men. Bone and Mineral 5:347–357, 1989.
107. Singh M, Nagrath AR, Maini PS: Changes in trabecular pattern of the upper end of the femur as an index of osteoporosis. J Bone Joint Surg 52A:457–467, 1970.
108. Bohr H, Schaadt O: Bone mineral content of femoral bone and the lumbar spine measured in women with fracture of the femoral neck by dual photon absorptiometry. Clin Orthop Rel Res 179:240–245, 1983.
109. Barnett E, Nordin BEC: Radiological diagnosis of osteoporosis. Clin Radiol 11:166–174, 1960.
110. Colbert C, Bachtell RC: Radiographic absorptiometry. *In* Cohn SH (ed): Non-Invasive Measurements of Bone Mass and Their Clinical Application, Boca Raton, FL, CRC Press, 1981, pp 51–84.
111. Bachtell RS, Colbert C: Mineral computed from phalangeal x-rays compared with osteoporosis index assessed from spinal x-rays. *In* Menczel J, Robin GC, Makin M, Steinberg R (eds): Osteoporosis. New York, John Wiley and Sons, 1982, pp 98–108.
112. Whedon GD, Shorr E, et al: Metabolic studies in paralytic acute anterior poliomyelitis. II. Alterations in calcium and phosphorus metabolism. J Clin Invest 36:966–981, 1957.
113. Minne HW, Leidig G, Wüster C, Siromachkostov L, et al: A newly developed spine deformity index (SDI) to quantitate vertebral crush fractures in pa-

tients with osteoporosis. Bone and Mineral 3:335–349, 1988.
114. Avioli MD, Repa-Eschen L: Increasing osteoporosis screening referrals. Appl Radiol 17:25–35, 1988.
115. Ott S: Should women get screening bone mass measurements? Ann Intern Med 104:874–876, 1986.
116. Cummings SR, Black D: Should perimenopausal women be screened for osteoporosis? Ann Intern Med 104:817–823, 1986.
117. Riggs BL, Wahner HW: Bone densitometry and clinical decision-making in osteoporosis. Ann Intern Med 108:293–294, 1988.
118. Riggs BL, Wahner HW, Dunn WL, et al: Differential changes in bone and mineral density of the appendicular and axial skeleton with aging. J Clin Invest 67:328–334, 1981.
119. Genant HK, Cann CE, Ehinger B, et al: Quantitative computed tomography of vertebral spongiosa. A sensitive method for determining early bone loss after oophorectomy. Ann Intern Med 97:699–705, 1982.
120. Pacifici R, Susman N, Carr PL, et al: Single and dual energy tomographic analysis of spinal trabecular bone: A comparative study in normal and osteoporotic women. J Clin Endocrinol Metab 64:209–214, 1987.
121. Pacifici R, Rupich R, Vered I, et al: Dual energy radiography (DER). A preliminary comparative study. Calcif Tissue Int 43:189–191, 1988.
122. Kelley TL, Slovak DM, Schoenfeld A, et al: Quantitative digital radiography *versus* dual photon absorptiometry of the lumbar spine. J Clin Endocrinol Metab 67:839–844, 1988.
123. Fogelman I, Bessent RG, Cohen H, et al: Skeletal uptake of diphosphonates method for prediction of postmenopausal osteoporosis. Lancet 2:667–670, 1980.
124. Civitelli R, Gonnelli S, Zaccher F, et al: Bone turnover in postmenopausal osteoporosis. Effect of calcitonin treatment. J Clin Invest 82:1268–1274, 1988.
125. Frymoyer JW: Back pain and sciatica. N Engl J Med 318:291–300, 1988.
126. Healey JH, Lane JM: Structural scoliosis in osteoporotic women. Clin Orthop Rel Res 195:216–223, 1985.
127. Kelly PJ, Jowsey J, Riggs BL, et al: Relationship between serum phosphate concentration and bone resorption in osteoporosis. J Lab Clin Med 69: 110–115, 1967.
128. Hockaday TDR, Keynes WM: Low plasma calcium in adrenal overactivity. J Endocrinol 34:413–414, 1966.
129. Avioli LV: Preventing osteoporosis: The new significance of hyperparathyroidism. Geriatrics 41:30–37, 1986.
130. Resnick LM, Müller FB, Laragh JH: Calcium-regulating hormones in essential hypertension. Relation to plasma renin activity and sodium metabolism. Ann Intern Med 105:649–654, 1986.
131. Gennari C, Imbimbo B, Montagnani M, et al: Effects of prednisone and deflazacort on mineral metabolism and parathyroid hormone activity in humans. Calcif Tissue Int 36:245–252, 1984.
132. Marx SJ, Stock JL, Attie MF: Familial hypocalciuric hypercalcemia: Recognition among patients referred after unsuccessful parathyroid exploration. Ann Intern Med 92:351–356, 1980.
133. Riggs BL, Melton, LJ, III: Evidence for two distinct syndromes of involutional osteoporosis. Am J Med 75:899–901, 1983.
134. Johnston CC, Norton J, Khairi MRA, et al: Heterogeneity of fracture syndromes in postmenopausal women. J Clin Endocrinol Metab 61:551–556, 1985.
135. Horowitz M, Wishart J, Need, AG, et al: Treatment of postmenopausal hyperparathyroidism with norethindrone. Effects of biochemistry and forearm mineral density. Arch Intern Med 147:681–685, 1987.
136. Marcus R, Madvig P, Crim M, et al: Conjugated estrogens in the treatment of postmenopausal women with hyperparathyroidism. Ann Intern Med 100:633–640, 1984.
137. Nilsson BE, Westlin NE: The plasma concentration of alkaline phosphatase, phosphorus and calcium following femoral neck fracture. Acta Orthop Scand 43:504–510, 1972.
138. Christian DC: Drug-induced elevations in serum alkaline phosphatase. Am J Clin Pathol 54:118–142, 1970.
139. Fishman WH: Perspective in alkaline phosphatase isoenzymes. Am J Med 56:617–650, 1974.
140. Glick EN Raised serum alkaline phosphatase levels in polymyalgia rheumatica. Lancet 2:328, 1972.
141. Perez-Jimenez F, Jimenez Pereperez JA, Rivera J, et al: Thyroiditis and alkaline phosphatase. Ann Intern Med 91:500–501, 1979.
142. Stolback LL, Krant MJ, Fishman WH: Ectopic production of an alkaline phosphatase isoenzyme in patients with cancer. N Engl J Med 281:757–761, 1969.
143. Lum G, Gambino SR: Alkaline phosphatase after pulmonary infarction. N Engl J Med 287:361, 1972.
144. Leroux M, Perry WF: Serum heat stable alkaline phosphatase in pregnancy. Am J Obstet Gynecol 108:235–239, 1970.
145. de la Piedra C, Torres R, Rapado A, et al: Serum tartrate resistant acid phosphatase and bone mineral content in postmenopausal osteoporosis. Calcif Tissue Int 34:58–60, 1989.
146. Delmas PD, Malaval L, Arlot ME, et al: Serum bone gla-protein compared to bone histomorphometry in endocrine diseases. Bone 6:339–341, 1985.
147. Ismail F, Epstein S, Pacifici R, et al: Serum bone gla protein (BGP) and other markers of bone mineral metabolism in postmenopausal osteoporosis. Calcif Tissue Int 39:230–233, 1986.
148. Delmas PD, Stenner D, Wahner HW, et al: Increase in serum bone carboxyglutamic acid protein with aging in women. Implications for the mechanism of age-related bone loss. J Clin Invest 71:1316–1321, 1983.
149. Stepan JJ, Pospichal J, Presl J, et al: Bone loss and biochemical indices of bone remodeling in surgically induced postmenopausal women. Bone 8:279–284, 1987.
150. Lian JB, Gundberg CM: Osteocalcin. Biochemical considerations and clinical applications. Clin Orthop Relat Res 226:267–291, 1988.
151. Yasumura S, Aloia JF, Gundberg CM: Serum osteocalcin and total body calcium in normal pre- and postmenopausal women and postmenopausal osteoporotic patients. J Clin Endocrinol Metab 64:681, 1987.
152. Duda RJ, O'Brein JF, Katzmann JA, et al: Current assays of circulating bone-gla-protein and bone alkaline phosphatase: Effects of sex, age, and meta-

bolic bone disease. J Clin Endocrinol Metab 66:951–957, 1988.
153. Nordin BEC, Robertson A, Seamark RF, et al: The relation between calcium absorption, serum dehydroepiandrosterone, and vertebral mineral density in postmenopausal women. J Clin Endocrinol Metab 60:651–657, 1985.
154. Wild RA, Buchanan JR, Myers C, et al: Declining adrenal androgens: An association with bone loss in aging women. Proc Soc Exp Biol Med 186:355–360, 1987.
155. Khaw KT, Chir MBB, Tazake S, et al: Cigarette smoking and levels of adrenal androgens in postmenopausal women. N Engl J Med 318:1705–1709, 1988.
156. Longcope C, Johnston CC Jr: Androgen and estrogen dynamics in pre- and postmenopausal women: Comparison between smokers and nonsmokers. J Clin Endocrinol Metab 67:379–383, 1981.
157. Daniell HW: Osteoporosis of the slender smoker. Arch Intern Med 136:298–304, 1976.
158. Jensen J, Christiansen C, Rodbro P: Cigarette smoking, serum estrogens and bone loss during hormone replacement therapy early after menopause. N Engl J Med 313:973–975, 1988.
159. Adler S, Lindeman RD, Yiengst MJ, et al: Effect of acute acid loading on urinary acid excretion by the aging human kidney. J Lab Clin Med 72:278–289, 1968.
159a. Schuck O, Nadvornikova H, Teplan V: Acidification capacity of the kidneys and aging. Physiologia Bohemoslovaca 38:117–125, 1989.
160. Whyte MP, Bergfeld MA, Murphy WA, et al: Postmenopausal osteoporosis. A heterogenous disorder as assessed by histomorphometric analysis of the iliac crest bone from untreated patients. Am J Med 72:193–202, 1982.
161. Hyldstrup L, McNair P, Jensen GF, et al: Bone mass as a referent for urinary hydroxyproline excretion. Age and sex-related changes in 125 normals and in primary hyperparathyroidism. Calcif Tissue Int 36: 639–644, 1984.
162. Coindre JM, David J-P, Riviere L, et al: Bone loss in hypothyroidism with hormone replacement. Arch Intern Med. 146:48–53, 1986.
163. Yoneda M, Takatsuki K, Yamauchi K, et al: Influence of thyroid function on serum bone gla protein. Endocrinol Jpn 35:121–129, 1988.
164. Moro L, Mucelli RSP, Gazzarrini C, et al: Urinary β-1-galactosyl-0-hydroxylysine (GH) as a marker of collagen turnover of bone. Calcif Tissue Int 42:87–90, 1988.
165. Parfitt AM, Simon LS, Villanueva AR, et al: Procollagen Type I carboxy-terminal extension peptide in serum as a marker of collagen biosynthesis in bone: Correlation with iliac bone formation rates and comparison with total alkaline phosphatase. J Bone Mineral Res 2:427–436, 1987.
166. Ray WA, Griffin MR, Schaffner W, et al: Psychotropic drug use and the risk of hip fracture. N Engl J Med 316:363–369, 1987.
167. Kelsey JL, Hoffman S: Risk factors for hip fracture. N Engl J Med 316:404–406, 1987.
168. Udén G: Inpatient accidents in hospitals. J Am Geriatr Soc 33:833–841, 1985.
169. Prudham D, Evans JG: Factors associated with falls in the elderly: A community study. Age Ageing 10:141–146, 1981.
170. Aniansson A, Zetterberg C, Hedberg M, et al: Impaired muscle function with aging: A background factor in the incidence of fractures of the proximal end of the femur. Clin Orthop Rel Res 191:193–201, 1984.
171. Wootton R, Bryson E, Elsasser U, et al: Risk Factors for fractured neck of femur in the elderly. Age Ageing 11:160–168, 1982.
172. Nagant de Deuxchaisnes C, Devogelaer J-P: Increase in the incidence of hip fractures and of the ratio of trochanteric to cervical hip fractures in Belgium. Calcif Tissue Int 42:201–203, 1988.
173. Zetterberg C, Elmerson S, Andersson GBJ: Epidemiology of hip fractures in Göteborg, Sweden, 1940–1983. Clin Orth Rel Res 191:43–52, 1984.
174. Johnell O, Nilsson B, Obrant KJ, et al: Age and set patterns of hip fractures—changes in 30 years. Acta Orthop Scand 55:290–292, 1984.
175. Bengnér U, Johnell O, Redlund-Johnell I: Changes in the incidence of fracture of the upper end of the humerus during a 30-year period. A study of 2125 fractures. Clin Orthop Rel Res 231:179–182, 1988.
176. Hedlund R, Lindgren U, Ahlbom A: Age- and sex-specific incidence of femoral neck and trochanteric fractures. An analysis based on 20,538 fractures in Stockholm County, Sweden, 1972–1981. Clin Orthop Rel Res 222:132–139, 1987.
177. Obrant KJ, Bengnér U, Johnell O, et al: Increasing age-adjusted risk of fragility fractures: A sign of increasing osteoporosis in successive generations? Calcif Tissue Int 44:157–167, 1989.
178. Finsen V, Benum P: Changing incidence of hip fractures in rural and urban areas of Central Norway. Clin Orthop Rel Res 218:104–110, 1987.
179. Lizaur-Utrilla A, Puchades Orts A, Sanchez del Campo F: Epidemiology of trochanteric fractures of the femur in Alicante, Spain, 1974–1982. Clin Orthop Rel Res 218:24–31, 1987.
180. Gennari C: Epidemiology and financial aspects of osteoporosis. *In* Cohn DV, Martin TJ, Meunier PJ (eds): Calcium Regulation and Bone Metabolism, Vol. 9, Amsterdam, Elsevier, 1987, pp 897–899.
181. Martin AD, Silverthorn KG, Houston CS: Age specific increase in hip fractures in Canada. *In* Christiansen C, Johansen JS, Reis BJ (eds): Osteoporosis 1987, 1987, pp 111–112.
182. Wallace WA: The increasing incidence of fractures of the proximal femur: An orthopaedic epidemic. Lancet 1:1413–1414, 1983.
183. Lindsay R: Prevention of osteoporosis. Clin Orthop Rel Res 222:44–59, 1987.
184. Melton JL III, O'Fallon WM, Riggs BL: Secular trends in the incidence of hip fractures. Calcif Tissue Int 41:57–64, 1987.
185. Lord SR, Sinnett PF: Femoral neck fractures: Admissions, bed use, outcome and projections. Med J Aust 145:493–496, 1986.
186. Slemenda C, Hui SL, Longcope C, et al: Sex steroids and bone mass. A study of changes about the time of menopause. J Clin Invest 80:1261–1269, 1987.
187. Brody JA, Farmer ME, White LR: Absence of menopausal effect on hip fracture occurrence in white females. Am J Public Health 74:1397–1398, 1984.
188. Farmer ME, White LR, Brody JA, et al: Race and sex differences in hip fracture incidence. Am J Public Health 74:1374–1380, 1984.
188a. Steinberg KK, Freni-Titulau LW, DePuey EG, et al: Sex steroids and bone density in premenopausal

and perimenopausal women. J Clin Endocrinol Metab 69:533–539, 1989.
188b. Robert KA: Women with osteoporosis: The role of the family and service community. The Gerontologist 28:224–228, 1988.
189. Mangaroo J, Glasser JH, Roht LH, et al: Prevalence of bone demineralization in the United States. Bone 6:135–139, 1985.
190. From UK: 500 a day seek help on osteoporosis. Med News 4:8, 1987.
191. White BL, Fisher WD, Laurin CA: Rate of mortality for elderly patients after fracture of the hip in the 1980's. J Bone Joint Surg 69–A:1335–1340, 1987.
192. Jensen JS, Tondevold E, Sorensen PH: Costs of treatment of hip fractures. A calculation of the consumption of the resources of hospitals and rehabilitation institutions. Acta Orth Scand 51:289–296, 1980.
193. Fitzgerald JF, Fagan LF, Tierney WM: Changing patterns of hip fracture care before and after implementation of the prospective payment system. JAMA 258:218–221, 1987.
194. Pryor GA, Williams DRR, Myles JW, et al: Team management of the elderly patient with hip fracture. Lancet 1:401–403, 1988.
195. Melton JL, Riggs BL: Epidemiology and cost of osteoporotic fractures. *In* Vagenakis A, Soucacos P, Avramides A, et al (eds): 2nd International Conference on Osteoporosis. Social and Clinic Aspects. Milan, Masson Publishers, 1986, pp 23–27.
196. Aitken JM: Relationship between mortality after femoral neck fracture and osteoporosis. *In* Christiansen C, Johansen JS, Riis BJ (eds): Osteoporosis 1987, Vol 1. Viborg, Denmark, Norhaven Press, 1987, pp 45–48.
197. Owen RA, Melton LJ III, Gallagher JC: The national cost of acute care of hip fractures associated with osteoporosis. Clin Orthop Rel Res 150: 172–176, 1980.
198. Gershon-Cohen J, Rechtman AM, Schrarer H, et al: Asymptomatic fractures in osteoporotic spines of the aged. JAMA 153:625–627, 1953.
199. Jensen GF, Christiansen C, Boesen J, et al: Epidemiology of postmenopausal spinal and long bone fractures. Clin Orth 166:75–81, 1982.
200. Riggs BL, Melton LJ III: Involutional osteoporosis. N Engl J Med 314:1676–1686, 1986.
201. Iskant AP, Smith RW: Osteoporosis in women 45 years and over related to subsequent fractures. Public Health Reports 84:33–38, 1969.
202. Bengnér U, Johnell O, and Redlund-Johnell I: Changes in incidence and prevalence of vertebral fractures during 30 years. Calcif Tissue Int 42:293–296, 1988.
203. Harma M, Heliovaara M, Arpo A, et al: Thoracic spine compression fractures in Finland. Clin Orthop Rel Res 205:188–194, 1986.
204. Drinka PJ, Bauwens SF, DeSmet AA: Atraumatic vertebral deformities in elderly males. Calcif Tissue Int 41:299–302, 1987.
205. Melton LJ, Kan SH, Frye MA, et al: Epidemiology of vertebral fractures in women. Am J Epidemiol 129:1000–1011, 1989.
206. Sowers MFR, Wallace RB, Lemke JH: Correlates of mid-radius bone density among postmenopausal women: a community study. Am J Clin Nutr 41:1045–1053, 1985.
207. Matkovic V, Kostial K, Simonovic I, et al: Bone status and fracture rates in two regions of Yugoslavia. Am J Clin Nutr 32:540–549, 1979.
208. Hurxthal LM, Vose GP: The relationship of dietary calcium intake to radiographic bone density in normal and osteoporotic persons. Calc Tissue Res 4:245–256, 1969.
209. Buchanan JR, Myers CA, Greer RB: Determinants of atraumatic vertebral fracture rates in menopausal women: Biologic v mechanical factors. Metabolism 37:400–404, 1988.
210. Albanese AA: Calcium nutrition in the elderly. Maintaining bone health to minimize fracture risk. Postgrad Med 63:167–172, 1978.
211. Lee CJ, Lawler GS, Johnson GH: Effects of supplementation of the diets with calcium and calcium-rich foods on bone density of elderly females with osteoporosis. Am J Clin Nutr 34:819–823, 1981.
212. Aloia JF, Vaswani AN, Yeh JK, et al: Premenopausal bone mass is related to physical activity. Arch Intern Med 148:121–123, 1988.
213. Sandler RB, Cauley JA, Hom DL, et al: The effects of walking on the cross-sectional dimensions of the radius in postmenopausal women. Calcif Tissue Int 41:65–69, 1987.
214. Pocock NA, Eisman JA, Yeates MG: Physical fitness is a major determinant of femoral neck and lumbar spine bone mineral density. J Clin Invest 78:618–621, 1986.
215. Smith EL Jr, Smith PE, Ensign CJ, et al: Bone involution decrease in exercising middle-aged women. Calcif Tissue Int 36:S129–S138, 1984.
216. Dalsky GP, Stocke KS, Ehsani AA, et al: Weight-bearing exercise training and lumbar bone mineral content in postmenopausal women. Ann Intern Med 108:824–828, 1988.
217. Nelson ME, Meredith CN, Dawson-Hughes B, et al: Hormone and bone mineral status in endurance-trained and sedentary postmenopausal women. J Clin Endocrinol Metab 66:927–933, 1988.
218. Kanders B, Lindsay R, Dempster D, et al: Determinants of bone mass in young healthy women. *In* Christiansen C, Arnaud CD, Nordin BEC, et al (eds): Osteoporosis I. Copenhagen, Aalborg, Stifsbogtrykkeri, 1984, pp 337–340.
219. Evans R, Marel GM, Lancaster EK, et al: Bone mass is low in relatives of osteoporotic patients. Ann Intern Med 1:870–873, 1988.
220. Seeman E, Hopper JL, Bach LA, et al: Reduced bone mass in daughters of women with osteoporosis. N Engl J Med 320:554–558, 1989.
221. Smith DM, Nance WE, Kang K, et al: Genetic factors in determining bone mass. J Clin Invest 52:2800–2811, 1973.
222. Saville PD: Observations on 80 women with osteoporotic spine fractures. *In* Barzel U (ed): Osteoporosis. New York, Grune & Stratton, 1979, pp 38–46.
223. Ribot C, Tremollieres F, Pouilles J-M, et al: Obesity and postmenopausal bone loss: The influence of obesity on vertebral density and bone turnover in postmenopausal women. Bone 8:327–331, 1988.
224. MacDonald PC, Edman CD, Heansell DL, et al: Effect of obesity on conversion of plasma androstenedione to estrone in postmenopausal women with or without endometrial cancer. Am J Obstet Gynecol 130:448–453, 1978.
225. Albright F, Bloomberg E, Smith PH: Postmenopausal osteoporosis. Trans Assoc Am Phys 55:298–304, 1940.

226. Aiman J, Smentek C: Premature ovarian failure. Obstet Gynecol 66:9–14, 1985.
227. Rigotti NA, Nussbaum SR, Herzog DB, et al: Osteoporosis in women with anorexia nervosa. N Engl J Med 311:1601–1606, 1984.
228. Crosby LO, Kaplan FK, Portschak MJ: Effect of anorexia nervosa on bone morphometry in young women. Clin Orthop Rel Res 201:271–277, 1985.
229. Marcus R, Cann C, Madorg P, et al: Menstrual function and bone mass in elite women distance runners. Ann Intern Med 102:158–163, 1988.
230. Lindberg JS, Fears WB, Hunt MM, et al: Exercise-induced amenorrhea and bone density. Ann Intern Med 101:647–648, 1984.
231. Drinkwater BL, Nilson K, Chestnut CH III, et al: Bone mineral content of amenorrhea and eumenorrheic athletes. N Engl J Med 311:277–281, 1984.
232. Gudmundsson JA, Ljunghall S, Bergquist C, et al: Increased bone turnover during gonadotropin-releasing hormone superagonist-induced ovulation inhibition. J Clin Endocrinol Metab 65:159–163, 1987.
233. Henzl MR, Corson SL, Moghissi K, et al: Administration of nasal nafarelin as compared with oral danazol for endometriosis. A multicenter double-blind comparative clinical trial. N Engl J Med 318:485–489, 1988.
234. Steingold K, De Ziegler D, Cedars M, et al: Clinical and hormonal effects of chronic gonadotropin-releasing hormone agonist treatment in polycystic ovarian disease. J Clin Endocrinol Metab 65:773–777, 1987.
235. Frasen HM, Waxman J: Gonadotrophin releasing hormone analogues for gynaecological disorders and infertility. Br Med J 298:475–476, 1989.
236. Longcope C, Hunter R, Franz C: Steroid secretion by the postmenopausal ovary. Am J Obstet Gynecol 138:564–568, 1980.
237. Warren MP, Brooks-Gunn J, Hamilton LH, et al: Scoliosis and fractures in young ballet dancers. Relation to delayed menarche and secondary amenorrhea. N Engl J Med 314:1348–1353, 1986.
238. Cattanach J: Oestrogen deficiency after tubal ligation. Lancet 1:847–849, 1985.
239. Goldin BR, Adlercreutz H, Gorbach SL, et al: Estrogen excretion patterns and plasma levels in vegetarian and omnivorous women. N Engl J Med 307:1542–1547, 1982.
240. Michnovicz JJ, Hershcopf RJ, Naganuma H, et al: Increased 2-hydroxylation of estradiol as a possible mechanism for the anti-estrogenic effect of cigarette smoking. N Engl J Med 315:1305–1309, 1986.
241. Fishman J, Hellman L, Zumoff B, et al: Effect of thyroid on hydroxylation of estrogen in man. J Clin Endocrinol Metab 25:365–368,1964.
242. Longcope C, Johnston CC, Jr: Androgen and estrogen dynamics in pre- and postmenopausal women. A comparison between smokers and nonsmokers. J Clin Endocrinol Metab 67:379–383, 1988.
243. McKinlay SM, Bifano NL, McKinlay JB: Smoking and age at menopause in women. Ann Intern Med 103:350–356, 1985.
244. Koetting CA, Wardlaw GM: Wrist, spine and hip bone density in women with variable histories of lactation. Am J Clin Nutr 48:1479–1481, 1988.
245. Hreshchyshyn MM, Hopkins A, Zylstra S, et al: Association of parity, breast feeding and birth control pills with lumbar spine and femoral neck bone densities. Am J Obstet Gynecol 159:318–322, 1988.
246. Suominen H, Heikkinen E, Vainio P: Mineral density of calcaneus in men at different ages: A population study with special reference to life-style factors. Age Ageing 13:273–281, 1984.
247. Halioua L, Anderson JG: Lifetime calcium intake and physical activity habits: Independent and combined effects in the radial bone of healthy premenopausal Caucasian women. Am J Clin Nutr 49:534–541, 1989.
248. Whedon GD: Disuse osteoporosis: Physiological aspects. Calcif Tissue Int 36:S146–150, 1984.
249. Rambant PC, Goode AW: Skeletal changes during space flight. Lancet 2:1052, 1985.
250. Christiansen C, Riis BJ, Rodbro P: Prediction of rapid bone loss in postmenopausal women. Lancet 1:1105–1107, 1987.
251. Aloia JF, Cohn SH, Vaswani A, et al: Risk factors for postmenopausal osteoporosis. Am J Med 78:95–100, 1985.
252. Parfitt AM: Dietary risk factors for age-related bone loss and fractures. Lancet 2:1181–1185, 1983.
253. Editorial: Risk factors in postmenopausal osteoporosis. Lancet 1:1370–1372, 1985.
254. Abbasi R, Hodgen GD: Predicting the predisposition to osteoporosis. Gonadotropin-releasing hormone antagonist for acute estrogen deficiency test. JAMA 255:1600–1604, 1986.
255. Pacifici R, Rifas L, Vered I, et al: Interleukin-1 secretion from human blood monocytes in normal and osteoporotic women: Effect of menopause and estrogen/progesterone treatment. J Bone Mineral Res 3A:541, 1988.
256. Minkoff JR, Grant BF, Marcus R: Plasma cyclic AMP response to calcitonin: A potential clinical marker of bone turnover. Bone 6:285–290, 1985.
257. Hegstead DM: Calcium and osteoporosis. J Nutr 116:2316–2319, 1986.
258. Kanis JA, Passmore R: Calcium supplementation of the diet. I. Br Med J 298:137–140, 1989.
259. Kanis JA, Passmore R: Calcium supplementation of the diet. II. Br Med J 298:205–208, 1989.
260. Stevenson JC, Whitehead MI, Padwick M, et al: Dietary intake of calcium and postmenopausal bone loss. Br Med J 297:15–17, 1988.
261. Heaney RP, Recker RR, Saville PD: Calcium balance and calcium requirements in middle-aged women. Am J Clin Nutr 30:1603–1609, 1977.
262. Heaney RP, Recker RR, Saville PD: Menopausal changes in calcium balance performance. J Lab Clin Med 92:953–963, 1978.
263. Lau E, Donnan S, Barker DJP, et al: Physical activity and calcium intake in fracture of the proximal femur in Hong Kong. Br Med J 297:1441–1443, 1988.
264. Holbrook TL, Barrett-Connor E, Wingrau DL: Dietary calcium and risk of hip fracture: 14-year prospective study. Lancet 2:1046–1049, 1988.
265. Polley KJ, Nordin BEC, Baghurst PA: Effect of calcium supplementation on forearm bone mineral content in postmenopausal women: A prospective, sequential controlled trial. J Nutr 117:1929–1935, 1987.
266. Riis B, Thomsen K, Christiansen C: Does calcium supplementation prevent postmenopausal bone loss? A double-blind, controlled clinical study. N Engl J Med 316:173–177, 1987.
267. Lee CJ, Lawler GS, Johnson GH: Effects of supplementation of the diets with calcium and calcium-rich foods on bone density of elderly females with osteoporosis. Am J Clin Nutr 34:819–823, 1981.

268. Avioli LV: Adjunctive modes of therapy for postmenopausal osteoporosis. Pros and cons. Post Grad Med Sept:21–26, 1987.
269. Recker RR, Saville PD, Heaney RP: Effect of estrogens and calcium carbonate on bone loss in postmenopausal women. Ann Intern Med 87:649–655, 1977.
270. Heaney RP, Gallagher JC, Johnston CC, et al: Calcium nutrition and bone health in the elderly. Am J Clin Nutr 36:986–1013, 1982.
271. Spencer H, Kramer L, Osis D: Factors contributing to calcium loss in aging. Am J Clin Nutr 36:776–787, 1982.
272. Massey LK, Wise KJ: The effect of dietary caffeine on urinary excretion of calcium, magnesium, sodium and potassium in healthy young females. Nutr Res 4:43–50, 1984.
273. Greger JL, Krystofiak M: Phosphorus intake of Americans. Food Technology Jan:78–84, 1982.
274. Calvo MS, Kumar R, Heath H III. Elevated secretion and action of serum parathyroid hormone in young adults consuming high phosphorus, low calcium diets assembled from common foods. J Clin Endocrinol Metab 66:823–829, 1988.
275. Trilok G, Draper HH: Sources of protein-induced endogenous acid production and excretion by human adults. Calcif Tissue Int 45:335–338, 1989.
276. Yuen DE, Draper HH, Trilok G: Effect of dietary protein on calcium metabolism in man. Nutr Abst Rev Clin Nutr 54:447–459, 1984.
277. Anand CR, Linkwiler HM: Effect of protein intake on calcium balance of young men 500 mg calcium daily. J Nutr 104:695–700, 1974.
278. Trilok G, Draper HH: Effect of a high-protein intake on acid-base balance in adult rats. Calcif Tissue Int 44:335–388, 1989.
279. Heaney RP, Recker RR: Effects of nitrogen phosphorus and caffeine on calcium balance in women. J Lab Clin Med 99:46–55, 1982.
280. Nordin BEC: Calcium. J Food Nutr 42:67–82, 1986.
281. Freudenheim JL, Johnson NE, Smith EL: Relationships between usual nutrient intake and bone-mineral content of women 35–65 years of age. Longitudinal and cross-sectional analysis. Am J Clin Nutr 44:863–876, 1986.
282. Nielsen FH, Hunt CD, Mullen LM, et al: Effect of dietary boron on mineral estrogen and testosterone metabolism in postmenopausal women. FASEB J 1:394–397, 1987.
283. Hart JP, Shearer MJ, Klenerman L, et al: Electrochemical detection of decreased circulating levels of vitamin K, in osteoporosis. J Clin Endocrinol Metab 60:1268–1269, 1985.
284. Feitelborg S, Epstein S, Ismail F, et al: Deranged bone mineral metabolism in chronic alcoholism. Metabolism 36:322–326, 1987.
285. Spencer H, Rubio N, Rubin E, et al: Chronic alcoholism. Frequently overlooked cause of osteoporosis in men. Am J Med 80:393–397, 1986.
286. Diamond T, Stiel D, Lunzer M, et al: Ethanol reduces bone formation and may cause osteoporosis. Am J Med 86:282–288, 1989.
287. Horowitz M, Wishart J, Mundy L, et al: Lactase and calcium absorption in postmenopausal osteoporosis. Arch Intern Med 147:534–536, 1987.
288. Avioli LV: Osteoporosis: Pathogenesis and therapy. *In* Avioli LV, Krane SM (eds): Metabolic Bone Disease, vol. I. New York, Academic Press, 1977, pp 307–385.
289. Coindre JM, David JP, Riviera L, et al: Bone loss in hypothyroidism with hormone replacement. Arch Intern Med 146:48–53, 1986.
290. Adams PH, Jowsey J, Kelley PJ, et al: Effects of hyperthyroidism in bone and mineral metabolism in man. Q J Med 36:1–15, 1965.
291. Erikson EF, Mosekilde L, Melsen F: Trabecular bone remodeling and bone balance in hyperthyroidism. Bone 6:421–428, 1985.
292. Toh SH, Claunch BC, Brown PH: Effect of hyperthyroidism and its treatment on bone mineral content. Arch Intern Med 145:883–886, 1985.
293. Auwers J, Bouillon R: Mineral and bone metabolism in thyroid disease. A review. Q J Med 60:737–752, 1986.
294. Kugai N, Koide Y, Yamashita K, et al: Impaired mineral metabolism in Cushing's syndrome. Parathyroid function, vitamin D metabolites and osteocalcin. Endocrinol Jpn 33:345–352, 1986.
295. Aloia JF, Roginsky M, Ellis K, et al: Skeletal metabolism and body composition in Cushing's Syndrome. J Clin Endocrinol Metab 39:981–985, 1974.
296. Bressot C, Meunier PJ, Chapuy MC: Histomorphometric profile pathophysiology and reversibility of corticosteroid-induced osteoporosis. Metab Bone Dis Rel Res 1:303–311, 1979.
297. Ruder HJ, Loriaux DL, Lipsett MB: Severe osteopenia in young adults associated with Cushing's syndrome due to micronodular adrenal disease. J Clin Endocrinol Metab 39:1138–1147, 1974.
298. Hough S, Teitelbaum SL, Avioli LV, et al: Isolated skeletal involvement in Cushing's syndrome: response to therapy. J Clin Endocrinol Metab 52:1033–1038, 1981.
299. Kleerekoper M, Sudhaber DR, Frame B, et al: Occult Cushing's syndrome presenting with osteoporosis. Henry Ford Hosp Med J 28:132–137, 1980.
300. Manolagas SC, Anderson DC: Adrenal steroids and the development of osteoporosis in oophorectomized women. Lancet 2: 597–600, 1979.
301. Buchanan JR, Myers CA, Green RB III: Effect of declining renal function on bone density in aging women. Calcif Tissue Int 43:1–6, 1988.
302. Avioli LV: Preventing osteoporosis: The new significance of hyperparathyroidism. Geriatrics 41:30–37, 1986.
303. Dauphine RT, Riggs BL, Scholz DA: Back pain and vertebral crush fractures: an unemphasized mode of presentation for primary hyperparathyroidism. Ann Intern Med 83:365–367, 1975.
304. Kochersberger GG, Lyles KW: Osteoporosis followed by primary hyperparathyroidism. A reason for continued vigilance. J Am Ger Soc 35:61–65, 1987.
305. Petersen MM, Briggs RS, Ashby MA, et al: Parathyroid hormone and 25OHD concentrations in sick and normal elderly people. Br Med J 287:521–523, 1983.
306. Mori S, Shiraki M, Fujimaldi H, et al: Bone fracture in elderly female with primary hyperparathyroidism: Relationship among renal function, vitamin D studies and fracture risk. Horm Metab Res 19:183–185, 1987.
307. Sambrook PN, Reeve J: Bone disease in rheumatoid arthritis. Clin Sci 74:225–230, 1988.
308. Weisman MH, Orth RW, Catherwood BD, et al: Measures of bone loss in rheumatoid arthritis. Arch Intern Med 146:701–704, 1986.
309. Hahn TJ, Hahn BH: Osteopenia in patients with

rheumatic diseases. Principles of diagnosis and therapy. Semin Arthritis Rheum 6:165–188, 1976.

310. Reid DM, Kennedy NSJ, Smith MN: Total body calcium in rheumatoid arthritis effects of disease activity and corticosteroid treatment. Br Med J 285:330–332, 1982.
311. Sumbrook PN, Eisman JA, Champion D, et al: Sex hormone status and osteoporosis in postmenopausal women with rheumatoid arthritis. Arthritis Rheum 31:973–978, 1988.
312. Sumbrook PN, Eisman JA, Champion D, et al: Determinants of axial bone loss in rheumatoid arthritis. Arthritis Rheum 30:720–728, 1987.
313. Avioli LV: Osteoporosis in rheumatoid arthritis. Arthritis Rheum 30:830–832, 1987
314. Skibsted Als O, Gotfredsen A, Christiansen C: The effect ofglucocorticoids on bone mass in rheumatoid arthritis patients. Arthritis Rheum 28:369–375, 1985.
315. Tugwell P, Bennett K, Gent M: Methotrexate in rheumatoid arthritis. Ann Intern Med 107:358–366, 1987.
316. McNair P: Bone mineral metabolism in human type I (insulin-dependent) diabetes mellitus. Danish Med Bull 35:109–121, 1988.
317. Heath H, Melton LJ, Chu C-P: Diabetes mellitus and the risk of skeletal fracture. N Engl J Med 303:567–570, 1980.
318. Mazess RB: Diabetes mellitus and the risk of skeletal fractures. N Engl J Med 304:115, 1981.
319. Frost HM, Takahashi H: Decreased cortical bone resorption in ribs of patients with well-controlled diabetes. Diabetes 14:455–460, 1965.
320. Weinstock RS, Goland RS, Shane E, et al: Bone mineral density in women with type II diabetes mellitus. J Bone Mineral Res 4:97–101, 1989.
321. Johnston CC, Hui SL, Longcope C: Bone mass and sex steroid concentration in postmenopausal Caucasian diabetics. Metabolism 34:544–550, 1985.
322. Lakhanpal S, Ginsburg WW, Luthra HS, et al: Transient regional osteoporosis. A study of 56 cases and review of the literature. Ann Intern Med 106:444–450, 1987.
323. Gruber HE, Gutteridge DH, Baylink DJ: Osteoporosis associated with pregnancy and lactation: Bone biopsy and skeletal features in three patients. Metab Bone Dis Relat Res 5:159–165, 1984.
324. Smith R, Stevenson JC, Winearls CG, et al: Osteoporosis of pregnancy. Lancet 1:1178–1180, 1985.
325. Paterson CR, McAllion S, Stellman JL: Osteogenesis imperfecta after the menopause. N Engl J Med 310:1694–1740, 1984.
326. Paterson CR: Osteogenesis imperfecta in elderly women. Geriatr Med Today 4:29–34, 1985.
327. Fallon MD, Whyte MP, Teitelbaum SL: Systemic mastocytosis associated with generalized osteopenia. Human Pathology 12:813–820, 1981.
328. Cundy T, Beneton MNC, Darby AJ, et al: Osteopenia in systemic mastocytosis: Natural history and responses to treatment with inhibitors of bone resorption. Bone 8:149–155, 1987.
329. Fallon MD, Perry HM III, Teitelbaum SL: Skeletal sarcoidosis with osteopenia. Metab Bone Dis Relat Res 3:171–174, 1981.
330. Schlechte J, El-Khoury G, Kathol M, et al: Forearm and vertebral bone mineral in treated and untreated hyperprolactinemic amenorrhea. J Clin Endocrinol Metab 64:1021–1026, 1987.
331. Klibanski A, Greenspan SL: Increase in bone mass after treatment of hyperprolactinemic amenorrhea. N Engl J Med 315:542–546, 1986.
332. Klibanski A, Neer RM, Beitins IZ, et al: Decreased bone density in hyperprolactinemic women. N Engl J Med 303:1511–1514. 1980.
333. Diamond T, Stiel D, Posen S: Osteoporosis in hemochromatosis: Iron excess, gonadal deficiency, or other factors. Ann Intern Med 110:430–436, 1989.
334. Eddy RL: Metabolic bone disease after gastrectomy. Am J Med 50:442–447, 1971.
335. Pullon HWH, Cundy T, Bellingham AJ: "High turnover" osteoporosis in congenital erythropoietic porphyria. Clin Sci 76:18p, 1989.
336. Shih M-S, Anderson C: Does "hepatic osteodystrophy" differ from peri- and postmenopausal osteoporosis? A histomorphometric study. Calcif Tissue Int 41:187–191, 1987.
337. Hodgson SF, Dickson ER, Wahner HW, et al: Bone loss and reduced osteoblast function in primary biliary cirrhosis. Ann Intern Med 103: 855–860, 1985.
338. Velis KP, Healey JH, Schneider R: Osteoporosis in unstable adult scoliosis. Clin Orthop Rel Res 237:132–141, 1988.
339. Healey JH, Lane JM: Structural scoliosis in osteoporotic women. Clin Orthop Rel Res 195:216–223, 1985.
340. Vargas JH, Klein GL, Ament ME, et al: Metabolic bone disease of total parenteral nutrition: Course after changing from casein to amino acids in parenteral solutions with reduced aluminum content. Am J Clin Nutr 48:1070–1078, 1988.
341. Shike M, Shils ME, Heller A, et al: Bone disease in prolonged parenteral nutrition: Osteopenia without mineralization defect. Am J Clin Nutr 44:89–98, 1986.
342. Beals RK: Orthopedic aspects of the XO (Turner's) syndrome. Clin Orthop Rel Res 97:19–34, 1973.
342a. Diamond T, Nery MB, Posen S: Spinal and peripheral bone mineral densities in acromegaly: The effects of excess growth hormone and hypogonadism. Ann Int Med 111:567–573, 1989.
343. Gilsanz V, Gibbens DT, Carlson M, et al: Peak trabecular vertebral density. A comparison of adolescent and adult females. Calcif Tissue Int 43:260–262, 1988.
344. Buchanan JR, Myers C, Lloyd T, et al: Early vertebral trabecular bone loss in normal premenopausal women. J Bone Mineral Res 3:583–587, 1988.
345. Hahn TJ, Avioli LV: Acquired (non-inherited) disorders of vitamin D function. *In* DeGroot LJ (ed): Endocrinology, vol. 2. Philadelphia, W.B. Saunders, 1989, pp 1085–1110.
346. Adinoff AD, Hollister JR: Steroid-induced fractures and bone loss in patients with asthma. N Engl J Med 309:265–268, 1983.
347. Need AG: Corticosteroids and osteoporosis. Aust NZ J Med 17:267–272, 1987.
348. Reid DM, Kennedy NSJ, Smith MA, et al: Total body calcium in rheumatoid arthritis: effects of disease activity and corticosteroid treatment. Br Med J 285:330–332, 1982.
349. Sambrook PN, Eisman JA, Yeates MG, et al: Osteoporosis in rheumatoid arthritis: Safety of low dose corticosteroids. Ann Rheum Dis 45:950–953, 1986.

350. Sambrook PN, Eisman JA, Champion GD, et al: Determinants of axial bone loss in rheumatoid arthritis. Arth Rheum 30:721–728, 1987.
351. Nagant de Deuxchaisnes C, Devogelaer JP, Esselinckx W, et al: The effect of low dosage glucocorticoids on bone mass in rheumatoid arthritis: A cross-sectional and a longitudinal study using single photon absorptiometry. *In* Avioli LV, Gennari C, Imbimbo B (eds): Glucocorticoid Effects and Their Biological Consequences. New York, Plenum Press, 1984, pp 209–239.
352. Gluck OS, Murphy WA, Hahn TJ, et al: Bone loss in adults receiving alternate day glucocorticoid therapy. Arth Rheum 24:892–898, 1981.
353. Banovac K, Papic M, Bilsker MS, et al: Evidence of hyperthyroidism in apparently euthyroid patients treated with levothyroxine. Arch Intern Med 149:809–812, 1989.
354. Coindre J-M, David J-P, Riviere L, et al: Bone loss in hypothyroidism with hormone replacement. A histomorphometric study. Arch Intern Med 146:48–53, 1986.
355. Paul TL, Kerrigan J, Kelly AM, et al: Long-term L-thyroxine therapy is associated with decreased hip bone density in postmenopausal women. JAMA 259:3137–3141, 1988.
356. Fallon MD, Perry HM III, Bergfeld M, et al: Exogenous hyperthyroidism with osteoporosis. Arch Intern Med 143:442–444, 1983.
357. Wartofsky L: Osteoporosis: A growing concern for the thyroidologist. Thyroid Today 11:1–11, 1988.
358. Ross DS: Subclinical hyperthyroidism: Possible danger of overzealous thyroxine replacement therapy. Mayo Clin Pro 63:1223–1228, 1988.
359. Hennessey JV, Evaul JE, Tseng Y-C, et al: L-thyroxine dosage: A reevaluation of therapy with contemporary preparations. Ann Intern Med 105:11–15, 1986.
360. Conney AHL: Pharmacologic implications of microsomal enzyme induction. Pharmacol Rev 19:317–335, 1967.
361. Jubiz W, Meikle AW, Levinson RA: Effect of diphenylhydantoin on the metabolism of dexamethasone. Mechanism of the abnormal dexamethasone suppression in humans. N Engl J Med 283:11–15, 1970.
362. Levin W, Welsh RM, Conney AH: Effect of chronic phenobarbitol treatment on the liver microsomal metabolism and uterotropic action of 17 beta estradiol. Endocrinology 80:135–138, 1967.
363. Barden HS, Mazess RB, Chesney RW, et al: Bone status of children receiving anticonvulsant therapy. Metab Bone Dis Relat Res 4:43–47, 1982.
364. Griffith GC, Nichols G, Asher JD, et al: Heparin osteoporosis. JAMA 193:85–88, 1965.
365. Avioli LV: Heparin induced osteopenia. Adv Exp Med Biol 2:375–387, 1975.
366. Griffiths HT, Liu,DTY: Severe heparin osteoporosis in pregnancy. Postgrad Med J 60:424–425, 1984.
367. Piro LD, Whyte MP, Murphy WA, et al: Normal cortical bone mass in patients after long term coumadin therapy. J Clin Endocrinol Metab 54:470–473, 1982.
368. Menon RK, Gill DS, Thomas M, et al: Impaired carboxylation of osteocalcin in warfarin-treated patients. J Clin Endocrinol Metab 64:59–61, 1987.
369. Pietschmann P, Woloszczuk W, Panzer S, et al: Decreased serum osteocalcin levels in phenprocoumon-treated patients. J Clin Endocrinol Metab 66:1071–1074, 1988.
370. Mallette LE, Khouri K, Zengotita H, et al: Lithium treatment increases intact and midregion parathyroid hormone and parathyroid volume. J Clin Endocrinol Metab 68:654–660, 1989.
371. Christiansen C, Baastrup PC, Transbol I: Osteopenia and dysregulation of divalent cations in lithium-treated patients. Neuropsychobiology 1:344–354, 1975.
372. Christiansen C, Baastrup PC, Transbol I: Development of "primary" hyperparathyroidism during lithium therapy: Longitudinal study. Neuropsychobiology 6:280–283, 1980.
373. Stancer H, Forbath N: Hyperparathyroidism, hypothyroidism, and impaired renal function after 10 to 20 years of lithium treatment. Arch Intern Med 149:1042–1045, 1989.
374. Toft H, Roin J: Effect of furosemide administration on calcium excretion. Br Med J I:437–438, 1971.
375. Macleod RI, Welbury RR, Soames JV: Effects of cytotoxic chemotherapy on dental development. J R Soc Med 80:209, 1987.
376. Adatia AK: Effects of cytotoxic chemotherapy on dental development. J R Soc Med 80:784–785, 1987.
377. Redman JR, Bajorunas DR, Wong G, et al: Bone mineralization in women following successful treatment of Hodgkin's disease. Am J Med 85: 65–72, 1988.
378. Rivkees SA, Crawford JD: The relationship of gonadal activity and chemotherapy-induced gonadal damage. JAMA 259:2123–2125, 1988.
379. Ragab AH, Frech RS, Vieetti TJ: Osteoporotic fractures secondary to methotrexate therapy of acute leukemia in remission. Cancer 25:580–585, 1970.
380. Kremer JM: Long term methotrexate therapy in rheumatoid arthritis: A review. J Rheumatol 12[Suppl. 12]:25–28, 1985.
381. Kozarek RA, Patterson DJ, Gelfand MD, et al: Methotrexate induces clinical and histologic remission in patients with refractory inflammatory bowel disease. Ann Intern Med 110:353–356, 1989.
382. Henderson IC: Adjuvant therapy for breast cancer. N Engl J Med 318:443–444, 1988.
383. Muse KN, Cetel NS, Futterman LA, et al: The premenstrual syndrome. N Engl J Med 311:1345–1349, 1984.
384. McKenna TJ: Pathogenesis and treatment of polycystic ovary syndrome. N Engl J Med 318:558–562, 1988.
384a. Fraser HM, Dewart PJ, Smith SK, et al: Luteinizing hormone releasing agonist for contraception in breast feeding women. J Clin Endocrinol Metab 69:996–1002, 1989.
385. Henzl MR, Corson SL, Moghissi K, et al: Administration of nasal nafarelin as compared with oral danazol for endometriosis. N Engl J Med 318:485–489, 1988.
386. Cann CE, Henzl MR, Burrk K, et al: Reversible bone loss is produced by the GnRH agonist nafarelin. *In* Cohn DV, Martin TJ, Meunier PJ (eds): Calcium Regulation and Bone Metabolism: Basic and Clinical Aspects. Amsterdam, Elsevier, 1987, pp 123–127.
387. Prince RL, Monk KJ, Kent GN, et al: Effects of theophylline and salbutamol on phosphate and calcium metabolism in normal subjects. Mineral Electrolyte Metab 14:262–265, 1988.
388. Whiting SJ, Whitney HL: Effect of dietary caffeine and theophylline on urinary calcium excretion in the adult rat. J Nutr 117:1224–1228, 1987.

389. Komoda T, Nagata A, Kiyoki M, et al: Chlorpromazine alters bone metabolism of rats *in vivo*. Calcif Tissue Int 42:58–62, 1988.
390. Seely EW, LeBoff MS, Brown EM, et al: The calcium channel blocker diltiazem lowers serum parathyroid hormone levels *in vivo* and *in vitro*. J Clin Endocrinol Metab 68:1007–1012, 1989.
391. Ellis CN, Gorsulowsky DC, Hamilton TA, et al: Cyclosporine improves psoriasis in a double blind study. JAMA 256:3110–3116, 1986.
392. Movsowitz C, Epstein S, Ismail F, et al: Cyclosporin A in the oophorectomized rat: Unexpected severe bone resorption. J Bone Mineral Res 4:393–398, 1989.
393. Movsowitz C, Epstein S, Fallon M, et al: Cyclosporin-A *in vivo* produces severe osteopenia in the rat: Effect of dose and duration of administration. Endocrinology 123:2571–2577, 1988.
394. Schlosberg M, Movsowitz C, Epstein S, et al: The effect of cyclosporin A administration and its withdrawal on bone mineral metabolism in the rat. Endocrinology 124:2179–2184, 1989.
395. Legha SS: Tamoxifen in the treatment of breast cancer. Ann Intern Med 109:219–228, 1988.
396. The Ludwig Breast Cancer Study Group: Combination adjuvant chemotherapy for node-positive breast cancer. Inadequacy of a single perioperative cycle. N Engl J Med 319:677–683, 1988.
397. Turner RT, Wakley GK, Hannon KS, et al: Tamoxifen inhibits osteoclast-mediated resorption of trabecular bone in ovarian hormone-deficient rats. Endocrinology 122:1146–1150, 1988.
398. Turner RT, Wakley GK, Hannon KS, et al: Tamoxifen prevents the skeletal effects of ovarian hormone deficiency in rats. J Bone Mineral Res. 2:449–456, 1987.
398a. Fentiman IS, Caleffi M, Rodin A, et al: Bone mineral content of women receiving tamoxifen for mastalgia. Br J Cancer 60:262–264, 1989.
399. Johnson BE, Lucasey B, Robinson RG, et al: Contributing diagnoses in osteoporosis. Arch Intern Med 149:1069–1072, 1989.
400. Kanders B, Dempster DW, Lindsay R: Interaction of calcium nutritive and physical activity and bone mass in young women. J Bone Mineral Res 3:145–149, 1988.
401. Ettinger B, Genant HK, Cann CE: Postmenopausal bone loss is prevented by treatment with low-dosage estrogen with calcium. Ann Intern Med 106:40–45, 1987.
402. Mann P: Teenagers and the calcium crisis. Saturday Evening Post, April 1987, pp 68–71.
403. Carroll MD, Abraham S, Dressner R: Dietary intake source data: United States 1976–1980. Vital Health and Statistics. Series II. No. 23, DHHS, Pub. No. (PHS) 83–1681. National Center for Health Statistics, PHS, Washington, D.C., U.S. Gov. Printing Office, March, 1983.
404. Sandler RB, Slemenda CW, LaPorte RE, et al: Postmenopausal bone density and milk consumption in childhood and adolescence. Am J Clin Nutr 42:270–274, 1985.
405. Schneider EL, Vining EM, Hadley EC, et al: Recommended dietary allowances and the health of the elderly. N Engl J Med 314:157–160, 1986
406. Nordin, BEC, Polley KJ, Need AJ, et al: Calcium and osteoporosis. Ann Chir Gyn 77:212–218, 1988.
407. Need AG, Horowitz M, Philcox JC, et al: Biochemical effects of a calcium supplement in osteoporotic postmenopausal women with normal absorption and malabsorption of calcium. Mineral Electrolyte Metab 13:112–116, 1987.
408. Burnell JM, Baylink DJ, Chesnut CH III, et al: The role of skeletal calcium deficiency in postmenopausal osteoporosis. Calcif Tissue Int 38:187–192, 1986.
409. NIH Consensus Conference Statement. JAMA 252:799–802, 1984.
410. Fergus A: The potential deleterious effects of milk consumption in the elderly. Geriatric Med Today 4:122–128, 1988.
411. Nutritional implications of lactose and lactase activity. Dairy Council Digest 55:25–30, Sept-Oct, 1985.
412. Heaney RP, Weaver CM, Recker RR: Calcium absorbability from spinach. Am J Clin Nutr 47:707–709, 1988.
413. Barros M: Calcium tablets are not all created equal. New York Times, Wednesday, Jan 27, 1988, p C1.
414. Carr CJ, Shangraw RF: Nutritional and pharmaceutical aspects of calcium supplementation. Am Pharm NS27:149–157, 1987.
415. Harvey JA, Zobitz MM, Pak CYC: Dose dependency of calcium absorption: A comparison of calcium carbonate and calcium citrate. J Bone Mineral Res 3:253–258, 1988.
416. Recker RR: Calcium absorption and achlorhydria. N Engl J Med 333:70–74, 1985.
417. Licata AA, Gall DJ: Effect of supplemental calcium on serum and urinary calcium in osteoporotic patients. J Am Coll Nutr 7:419, 1988.
418. Webb AR, Kline L, Holick MF: Influence of season and latitude on the cutaneous synthesis of vitamin D_3: Exposure to winter sunlight in Boston and Edmonton will not promote vitamin D_3 synthesis in human skin. J Clin Endocrinol Metab 67:373–378, 1988.
419. Clemens TL, Myles M, Enders D, et al: Assessment of vitamin D_2 and D_3 status of institutionalized and ambulatory populations in New York. J Clin Endocrinol Metab 63:656–670, 1986.
420. Montoye HJ, Smith EL, Fardon DF, et al: Bone mineral in senior tennis players. Scand J Sports Sci 2:26–30, 1980.
421. Ettinger WH Jr, Evans WJ, Weindruch R, et al: Exercise for the elderly. Patient Care, Apr 15, 1989, pp 165–191.
422. Rippe JM, Ward A, Porcan JP, et al: Walking for health and fitness. JAMA 259:2720–2724, 1988.
423. Chow RK, Harrison JE, Brown CF, et al: Physical fitness effect in bone mass in postmenopausal women. Arch Phys Med Rehabil 671:231–235, 1986.
424. Morey MC, Cowper PA, Feussner JR, et al: Evaluation of a supervised exercise program in a geriatric population. J Am Geriatr Soc 37:348–354, 1989.
424a. Goodman CE: Osteoporosis: Protective measures of nutrition and exercise. Geriatrics 40:59–70, 1985.
425. Steinberg FU: Exercise in prevention and therapy of osteoporosis. *In* Avioli LV (ed): The Osteoporotic Syndrome. New York, Grune & Stratton, 1987, pp 109–119.
426. Simkin A, Ayalon J, Leichter I: Increased trabecular bone density due to bone-loading exercises in postmenopausal osteoporotic women. Calcif Tissue Int 40:59–63, 1987.
427. Sinaki M, Mikkelsen BA: Postmenopausal spinal os-

teoporosis: Flexion versus extension exercises. Arch Phys Med Rehabil 65: 593–596, 1984.
428. Lanyon LE: Functional strain as a determinant for bone remodeling. Calcif Tissue Int 36:556–561, 1984.
429. Farndale RW, Murray JC: Pulsed magnetic fields promote collagen production in bone marrow fibroblasts via athermal mechanism. Calcif Tissue Int 37:178–182, 1985.
430. Dawson-Hughes B, Stern D, Goldman J, et al: Regulation of growth hormone and somatomedin-C secretion in postmenopausal women: Effect of physiological estrogen replacement. J Clin Endocrinol Metab 63:424–432, 1986.
431. Harris WH, Heaney RP, Jowsey J, et al: Growth hormone: The effect on skeletal mineral in the dog. Calcif Tissue Res 10:1–8, 1972.
432. Aloia JF, Rasulo P, Deftos LJ, et al: Exercise-induced hypercalcemia and the calciotrophic hormones. J Lab Clin Med 106:229–232, 1985.
433. Kiel DP, Felson DT, Anderson JJ: Hip fracture and the use of estrogens in postmenopausal women. N Engl J Med 317:1169–1174, 1987.
434. Lindsay R, Hart DM, Purdle D, et al: Comparative effects of estrogen and a progestogen on bone loss in postmenopausal women. Clin Sci Mol Med 54:193–195, 1978.
435. Ettinger B, Genant HK, Cann CE: Long-term estrogen replacement therapy prevents bone loss and fractures. Ann Intern Med 102:319–324, 1985.
436. Kreiger N, Kelsey JL, Holford TR, et al: An epidemiologic study of hip fracture in postmenopausal women. Am J Epidemiol 116:141–148, 1982.
437. Lindsay R, Hart DM, Clark AC: The minimum effective dose of estrogen for prevention of postmenopausal bone loss. Obstet Gynecol 65:750–756, 1984.
438. Ted Quigley ME, Martin PL, Burnier AM, et al: Estrogen therapy arrests bone loss in elderly women. Am J Obstet Gynecol 156:1516–1523, 1987.
439. Weiss NS, Ure CL, Ballard JH, et al: Decreased risk of fractures of the hip and lower forearm with postmenopausal use of estrogen. N Engl J Med 303:1195–1198, 1980.
440. Chetkowski RJ, Meldrum DR, Steingold KA, et al: Biologic effects of transdermal estradiol. N Engl J Med 314:1615–1620, 1986.
441. Savvas M, Studd JWW, Fogelman I, et al: Skeletal effects of oral oestrogen compared with subcutaneous oestrogen and testosterone in postmenopausal women. Br Med J 297:331–333, 1988.
442. Horsman A, Nordin BEC, Crilly RG: Effect on bone of withdrawal of estrogen therapy. Lancet 2:33–35, 1979.
443. Lindsay R: Prevention and treatment of osteoporosis with ovarian hormones. Ann Chir Gynaecol 77:219–223, 1988.
444. Eriksen EF, Colvard DS, Berg NJ: Evidence of estrogen receptors in normal human osteoblast-like cells. Science 241:84–86, 1988.
445. Komm BS, Terpening CM, Benz DJ: Estrogen binding, receptor mRNA, and biologic response in osteoblast-like osteosarcoma cells. Science 241:81–84,1988.
446. Kaplan FS, Fallon MD, Boden SD, et al: Estrogen receptors in bone in a patient with polyostotic fibrous dysplasia (McCune-Albright syndrome). N Engl J Med 319:421–425, 1988.
447. Civitelli R, Agnusdei D, Nardi P, et al: Effects of one-year treatment with estrogens on bone mass, intestinal calcium absorption, and 25-hydroxyvitamin D-1-alpha-hydroxylase reserve in postmenopausal osteoporosis. Calcif Tissue Int 42:77–86, 1988.
448. Greenberg C, Kukreja SC, Bowser EN, et al: Effects of estradiol and progesterone on calcitonin secretion. Endocrinology 118:2594–2598, 1986.
449. Duarte B, Hargis GK, Kukreja SC: Effects of estradiol and progesterone on parathyroid hormone secretion from human parathyroid tissue. J Clin Endocrinol Metab 66:584–587, 1988.
450. Greenberg C, Kukreja SC, Bowser EN, et al: Parathyroid hormone secretion: Effect of estradiol and progesterone. Metabolism 36:151–154, 1987.
451. Gallagher JC, Riggs BL, DeLuca HF: Effect of estrogen on calcium absorption and serum vitamin D metabolites in postmenopausal osteoporosis. J Clin Endocrinol Metab 51:1359–1364, 1980.
452. Buchanan JR, Santen RJ, Cavaliere A, et al: Interaction between parathyroid hormone and endogenous estrogen in normal women. Metabolism 35:489–494, 1986.
453. Cheema C, Grant BF, Marcus R: Effects of estrogen on circulating "free" and total 1,25-dihydroxyvitamin D and on the parathyroid vitamin D axis in postmenopausal women. J Clin Invest 83: 537–542, 1989.
453a. Bergkvist L, Adami H-O, Persson I, et al: The risk of breast cancer after estrogen and estrogen-progestin replacement. N Engl J Med 321:293–297, 1989.
454. Christiansen C, Riis BJ, Nilas L, et al: Uncoupling of bone formation and resorption by combined oestrogen and progestagen therapy in postmenopausal osteoporosis. Lancet 2:800–801, 1985.
455. Lindsay R, Hart DM, Purdie D, et al: Comparative effects of oestrogen and a progestogen on bone loss in postmenopausal women. Clin Sci Mol Med 54:193–195, 1978.
456. Snow GR, Anderson C: The effects of continuous progestogen treatment on cortical bone remodeling activity in beagles. Calcif Tissue Int 37:282–286, 1985.
457. Snow GR, Anderson C: The effects of 17 beta-estradiol and progestogen on trabecular bone remodeling in oophorectomized dogs. Calcif Tissue Int 39:198–205, 1986.
458. Hirvonen E, Malkonen M, Manninen V: Effects of different progestogens on lipoproteins during postmenopausal replacement therapy. N Engl J Med 304:560–563, 1981.
459. Fatourechi V, Heath H III: Salmon calcitonin in the treatment of postmenopausal osteoporosis. Ann Intern Med 107:923–925, 1987.
460. McDermott MT, Kidd GS: The role of calcitonin in the development and treatment of osteoporosis. Endocr Rev 8:377–390, 1987.
461. Gonzalez D, Ghiringhelli G, Mautalen C: Acute antiosteoclastic effect of salmon calcitonin in osteoporotic women. Calcif Tissue Int 38:71–75, 1986.
462. Caniggia A, Gennari C, Bencini M, et al: Calcium metabolism and 47 calcium kinetics before and after long term thyrocalcitonin treatment in senile osteoporosis. Clin Sci 38:397–407, 1970.
463. Maresca V: Human calcitonin in the management of osteoporosis: a multicentre study. J Int Med Res 13:11–316, 1985.

464. Gennari C, Chierichetti SM, Bigazzi S, et al: Comparative effects on bone mineral content of calcium and calcium plus salmon calcitonin given in two different regimens in postmenopausal osteoporosis. Curr Ther Res 38:455–464, 1985.
465. Gruber HE, Ivey JL, Baylink DJ, et al: Long-term calcitonin therapy in postmenopausal osteoporosis. Metabolism 33:295–303, 1984.
466. Mazzuoli GF, Passeri M, Gennari C, et al: Effects of salmon calcitonin in postmenopausal osteoporosis: A controlled double-blind clinical study. Calcif Tissue Int 38:3–8, 1986.
467. Wallach S, Cohn SH, Ellis KJ, et al: Effect of salmon calcitonin on skeletal mass in osteoporosis. Curr Ther Res Clin Exp 22:556–572, 1977.
467a. Overgaard L, Riis BJ, Christiansen C, et al: Effect of salcalcitonin given intranasally on early postmenopausal bone loss. Br Med J 299:477–479, 1989.
468. Polatti F, Montrasio MG, Caprotti M, et al: Bone mineral content after oophorectomy: Effects of salmon calcitonin and oral calcium. Min Metab Res (Italy) 5:159–163, 1984.
469. Reginster JY, Albert A, Lecart MP, et al: 1-year controlled randomized trial of prevention of early postmenopausal bone loss by intranasal calcitonin. Lancet 2:1481–1483, 1987.
470. Christiansen C: Intranasal calcitonin for prevention and treatment of osteoporosis. Ann Chir Gynaecol 77:229–234, 1988.
471. MacIntyre I, Whitehead MI, Banks LM, et al: Calcitonin for prevention of postmenopausal bone loss. Lancet 1:900–901, 1988.
472. Nagant de Deuxchaisnes C: Calcitonin in the treatment of Paget's disease. Triangle 22:103–127, 1983.
473. Schiraldi GF, Scoccia S, Soresi E: Analgesic activity of high doses of salmon calcitonin in lung cancer. Curr Ther Res 38:592–598, 1985.
474. Franceschini R, Bottaro P, Panopoulos C, et al: Long-term treatment with salmon calcitonin in postmenopausal osteoporosis. Curr Ther Res 34:795–800, 1983.
475. Gennari C, Avioli LV: Calcitonin therapy in osteoporosis. *In* Avioli, L.V. (ed): The Osteoporotic Syndrome, 2nd ed. New York, Grune & Stratton, 1987, pp 121–143.
476. Kanis JA, Meunier PT: Should we use fluoride to treat osteoporosis? A review. Q J Med 210:145–164, 1984.
477. Farley SMG, Wergedal JE, Smith LC, et al: Fluoride therapy for osteoporosis: Characterization of the skeletal response by serial measurements of serum alkaline phosphatase activity. Metabolism 36:211–218, 1987.
478. Compston JE, Chadha S, Merrett AL: Osteomalacia developing during treatment of osteoporosis with sodium fluoride and vitamin D. Br Med J 281:910, 1980.
479. Hansson T, Roos B: Effect of fluoride and calcium on spinal bone mineral content: A controlled prospective (3 years) study. Calcif Tissue Int 40:315–317, 1987.
480. Dambacher MA, Ittner J, Ruegssegger P: Long-term fluoride therapy of postmenopausal osteoporosis. Bone 7:199–205, 1986.
481. Duursma SA, Glerum JH, Van Dihk A, et al: Responders and non-responders after fluoride therapy in osteoporosis. Bone 8:131–136, 1988.
482. Hasling C, Nielsen HE, Melsen F, et al: Safety of osteoporosis treatment with sodium fluoride, calcium phosphate and vitamin D. Mineral Electrolyte Metab 13:96–103, 1987.
483. Schnitzler CM, Solomon L: Trabecular stress fractures during fluoride therapy for osteoporosis. Skeletal Radiol 14:276–279, 1985.
484. Riggs BL, Baylink DJ, Kleerekoper M, et al: Incidence of hip fractures in osteoporotic women treated with sodium fluoride. J Bone Mineral Res 2:123–126, 1987.
485. Budden FH, Bayley TA, Harrison JE, et al: The effect of fluoride on histology in postmenopausal osteoporosis depends on adequate fluoride absorption and retention. J Bone Mineral Res 3:1227–1231, 1988.
486. Inkovaava J, Heikinheimo R, Marvinen K. et al: Prophylactic fluoride treatment and aged bones. Br Med J 3:730–734, 1975.
487. Mamelle N, Dusan R, Martin JL, et al: Risk-benefit ratio of sodium fluoride treatment in primary vertebral osteoporosis. Lancet 2: 361–365, 1988.
488. Pak CYC, Sakhaee K, Zerwekh JE, et al: Safe and effective treatment of osteoporosis with intermittent slow release sodium fluoride: Augmentation of vertebral bone mass and inhibition of fractures. J Clin Endocrinol Metab 68:150–159, 1989.
489. Hedlund LR, Gallagher JC: Increased incidence of hip fracture in osteoporotic women treated with sodium fluoride. J Bone Mineral Res 4:223–225, 1989.
489a. Hodsman AB, Drost DJ: The response of vertebral bone mineral density during the treatment of osteoporosis with sodium fluoride. J Clin Endocrinol Metab 69:932–938, 1989.
490. Pak CYC, Sakhaee K, Gallagher C, et al: Attainment of therapeutic fluoride levels in serum without major side effects using a slow-release preparation of sodium fluoride in postmenopausal osteoporosis. J Bone Mineral Res 1:563–571, 1986.
490a. Kleerekoper M, Peterson E, Phillips E, et al: Continuous sodium fluoride therapy does not reduce vertebral fracture rate in postmenopausal osteoporosis. J Bone Mineral Res 4 (Suppl. 1):S–376, 1989.
491. Frost HM: Treatment of osteoporosis by manipulation of coherent cell populations. Clin Orthop Rel Res 143:227–244, 1979.
492. Frost HM: Editorial. The ADFR concept revisited. Calcif Tissue Int 36:349–353, 1984.
493. Pacifici R, McMurtry C, Vered I, et al: Coherence therapy does not prevent axial bone loss in osteoporotic women. A preliminary comparative study. J Clin Endocrinol Metab 66:747–753. 1988.
494. Silverberg SJ, Shane E, de la Cruz L, et al: Abnormalities in parathyroid hormone secretion and 1,25-dihydroxyvitamin D_3 formation in women with osteoporosis. N Engl J Med 320:277–281, 1989.
495. Mallette LE, LeBlanc AD, Pool JL, et al: Cyclic therapy of osteoporosis with neutral phosphate and brief, high-dose pulses of etidronate. J Bone Mineral Res 4:143–148, 1989.
496. Marie PJ, Caulin F: Mechanisms underlying the effects of phosphate and calcitonin on bone histology in postmenopausal osteoporosis. Bone 7:17–22, 1986.
497. Alexandre C, Chappard D, Caulin F, et al: Effects of a one-year administration of phosphate and intermittent calcitonin on bone-forming and bone-resorbing cells in involutional osteoporosis: A histomor-

phometric study. Calcif Tissue Int 42:345–350, 1988.
498. Report. New treatments for osteoporosis add bone. Medical World News 28(21):33–34, 1987.
499. Conference Report. Br Med J 295:914, 1987.
499a. Reginster JY, Deroisy R, Collette J, et al: Prevention of postmenopausal bone loss by tiludronate. Lancet i:1469–1471, 1989.
500. Podbesek R, Edouard C, Meunier PJ, et al: Effects of two treatment regimes with synthetic human parathyroid hormone fragment on bone formation and the tissue balance of trabecular bone in greyhounds. Endocrinology 112:1000–1006, 1983.
501. Reeve J, Meunier PJ, Parsons JA, et al: Anabolic effect of human parathyroid hormone fragment in trabecular bone in involutional osteoporosis. A multicenter trial. Br Med J June 7:1340–1344, 1980.
502. Slovik DM, Rosenthal DI, Doppelt JH, et al: Restoration of spinal bone in osteoporotic men by treatment with human parathyroid hormone (1-34) and 1,25-dihydroxyvitamin D. J Bone Mineral Res 1:377–381, 1986.
503. Hesch RD, Busch U, Prokop M, et al: Increase of vertebral density by combination therapy with pulsatile 1-38hPTH and sequential addition of calcitonin nasal spray in osteoporotic patients. Calcif Tissue Int 44:176–180, 1989.
504. Audran M, Basle M-F, Defontaine A, et al: Transient hypoparathyroidism induced by synthetic human parathyroid hormone–(1-34) treatment. J Clin Endocrinol Metab 64:937, 1987.
505. Lindholm TS, Nilsson OS, Widhe T, et al: Preventive treatment of osteoporosis with 1-alpha-hydroxyvitamin D_3 and calcium. Evaluation of bone histomorphometry in osteoporotics and age matched controls. Acta Vitaminol Enzymol 4:179–184, 1982.
506. Orimo H, Shiraki M, Hayashi T, et al: Reduced occurrence of vertebral crush fractures in senile osteoporosis treated with 1-alpha(OH)-vitamin D_3. Bone and Mineral 3:47–52, 1987.
507. Gallagher JC, Jerpbak CM, Jee WSS, et al: 1,25-dihydroxyvitamin D_3: Short- and long-term effects on bone and calcium metabolism in patients with postmenopausal osteoporosis. Proc Natl Acad Sci USA 79:3325–3329,1982.
508. Finn GF, Christiansen C, Transbol I: Treatment of postmenopausal osteoporosis. A controlled therapeutic trial comparing oestrogen/gestagen, 1,25-dihydroxy-vitamin D, and calcium. Clin Endocrinol 16:515–524, 1982.
509. Aloia JF, Vaswani A, Yeh JK, et al: Calcitriol in the treatment of postmenopausal osteoporosis. Am J Med 84:401–408, 1988.
510. Brautbar N: Osteoporosis: Is 1,25-$(OH)_2D_3$ of value in treatment? Nephron 44:161–166, 1986.
511. Ott SM, Chesnut CH III: Calcitriol treatment is not effective in postmenopausal osteoporosis. Ann Intern Med 110:267–274, 1989.
512. Riggs BL, Nelson KI: Effect of long term treatment with calcitriol on calcium absorption and mineral metabolism in postmenopausal osteoporosis. J Clin Endocrinol Metab 61:457–461, 1985.
513. Smothers RL, Levine BS, Singer FR, et al: Relationship between urinary calcium and calcium intake during calcitriol administration. Kidney Int 29:578–583, 1986.
514. Zerwekh JE, Sakhaee K, Glass K, et al: Long term 25-hydroxyvitamin D_3 therapy in postmenopausal osteoporosis: Demonstration of responsive and nonresponsive subgroups. J Clin Endocrinol Metab 56:410–413, 1983.
515. Riis BJ, Thomsen K, Christiansen C: Does 24R,25$(OH)_2$-vitamin D_3 prevent postmenopausal bone loss? Calcif Tissue Int 39:128–132, 1986.
516. Gordan GS, Ricchi J, Roof BS: Antifracture efficacy of long-term estrogens for osteoporosis. Trans Assoc Am Phys 86:326–332, 1973.
517. Chesnut CH, Ivey JL, Gruber HE, et al: Stanozolol in postmenopausal osteoporosis. Therapeutic efficacy and possible mechanism of action. Metabolism 32:571–581, 1983.
518. Kasperk CH, Wergedal JE, Farley JR, et al: Androgens directly stimulate proliferation of bone cells in vitro. Endocrinology 124:1576–1578, 1989.
519. Colvard DS, Eriksen EF, Keeting PE, et al: Identification of androgen receptors in normal human osteoblast-like cells. Proc Natl Acad Sci USA 86:854–857, 1989.
520. Need AG, Horowitz M, Bridges A, et al: Effects of nandrolone decanoate and antiresorptive therapy on vertebral density in osteoporotic postmenopausal women. Arch Intern Med 149:57–60, 1989.
521. Johansen JS, Hassager C, Podenphant J, et al: Treatment of postmenopausal osteoporosis: Is the anabolic steroid nandrolone decanoate a candidate? Bone and Mineral 6:77–86, 1989.
522. Hassager C, Podenphant J, Riis BJ, et al: Changes in soft tissue body composition and plasma lipid metabolism during nandrolone decanoate therapy in postmenopausal osteoporotic women. Metabolism 38:238–242, 1989.
523. Thompson PD, Cullinane EM, Sady SP, et al: Contrasting effects of testosterone and stanozolol on serum lipoprotein levels. JAMA 261:1165–1168, 1989.
524. Brickman AS, Massary SG, Coburn JW: Changes in serum and urinary calcium during treatment with hydrochlorothiazide. Studies on mechanism. J Clin Invest 51:945–954, 1972.
525. Transbol I, Christensen MS, Jensen GF, et al: Thiazide for the postponement of postmenopausal bone loss. Metabolism 31:383–386, 1982.
526. Christiansen C, Christensen MS, McNair P, et al: Prevention of early postmenopausal bone loss: Controlled two-year study in 315 normal females. Eur J Clin Invest 10:273–279, 1980.
527. Wasnich RD, Benfante RJ, Yanko K, et al: Thiazide effect on the mineral content of bone. N Engl J Med 309:344–347, 1983.
528. Hale WE, Stewart RB, Marks RG: Central nervous system symptoms of elderly subjects using antihypertensive drugs. J Am Geriatr Soc 32:5–10, 1984.
529. Chesnut CH III: Editorial. Osteoporosis, fractures, and thiazides. J Am Geriatr Soc 32:3, 1984.
530. Ray WA, Downey W, Griffin MR, et al: Long-term use of thiazide diuretics and risk of hip fracture. Lancet 1: 687–689, 1989.
531. Boer WH, Koomans HA, Dorhout Mees EJ: Acute effects of thiazides, with and without carbonic anhydrase inhibiting activity, on lithium and free water clearance in man. Clin Sci 76:539–545, 1989.
532. Finkelstein JS, Klebanski A, Neer RM, et al: Increases in bone density during treatment of men with idiopathic hypogonadotropic hypogonadism. J Clin Endocrinol Metab 69:776–783, 1989.
533. Jackson JA, Watman J, Sprekerman AM: Prostatic complications of testosterone replacement therapy. Arch Intern Med 149:2365–2366, 1989.

13

EDUARDO SLATOPOLSKY
JACK W. COBURN

Renal Osteodystrophy

The term "renal osteodystrophy" is used in a generic sense to include all skeletal disorders that occur in patients with renal failure, including osteitis fibrosa, osteomalacia, osteosclerosis, growth retardation, and osteoporosis.

The association of renal failure with skeletal disease, hyperplasia of the parathyroid glands and abnormal vitamin D metabolism has been known for many years.[1,4] Now that the lives of patients with chronic renal failure can be prolonged through better conservative therapy, readily available dialysis, and successful renal transplantation, the morbidity associated with disordered divalent ion metabolism, soft tissue calcification, and renal bone disease has assumed greater clinical significance. The clinical features of renal osteodystrophy are better defined, and a rational approach to the prevention and treatment of renal osteodystrophy is possible.

I. OSTEITIS FIBROSA

Osteitis fibrosa represents the skeletal abnormalities secondary to high levels of circulating parathyroid hormone (PTH). Hyperplasia of the parathyroid glands and high levels of serum iPTH are among the most consistent pathogenetic factors affecting divalent ion metabolism in patients with chronic renal failure. Increased levels of serum iPTH have been reported in patients with only mildly abnormal renal function,[5,6] as shown in Figure 13–1.

The main factor leading to PTH secretion and causing parathyroid hyperplasia is hypocalcemia. The factors that contribute to hypocalcemia include (1) phosphate retention; (2) altered vitamin D metabolism; (3) skeletal resistance to the calcemic action of PTH; (4) an altered "set point" for calcium-regulated PTH secretion; and (5) impaired degradation of PTH secondary to reduced renal function (Fig. 13–2).

A. Phosphate Retention

The role of phosphate retention as a factor in the pathogenesis of secondary hyperparathyroidism has been emphasized by Slatopolsky and colleagues.[7-9] Considerable evidence supports an important role for phosphate retention in producing secondary hyperparathyroidism. Reiss et al.[10] demonstrated that an oral load of phosphorus, providing 1.0 gm of elemental phosphorus, led to an increase in serum phosphorus, a fall in ionized calcium level, and an increase in serum iPTH in normal subjects. Others have shown that long-term feeding of animals with a diet high in phosphate can produce parathyroid hyperplasia and increased levels of iPTH and can cause a mild reduction in serum calcium level.[11,12] Studies in experimental renal failure have shown that the restriction of dietary phosphate in proportion to the decrease in glomerular filtration rate (GRF) can prevent the development of secondary hyperparathyroidism in azotemic dogs followed for 2 months,[8] and subsequent studies[13] showed a substantial reduction of serum iPTH levels in animals with renal failure treated with proportional phosphate restriction for 2 years (Fig. 13–3). Llach et al.[14] indicated that a reduction in dietary phosphate intake in proportion to the decrease in GFR over a 2-month period in humans with creatinine clearances of 50 to 90 ml/minute was associated with a decrease in serum iPTH to normal levels. When phosphate intake was reduced in patients with more advanced renal insufficiency, serum iPTH fell substantially but remained above normal levels.[15] Other

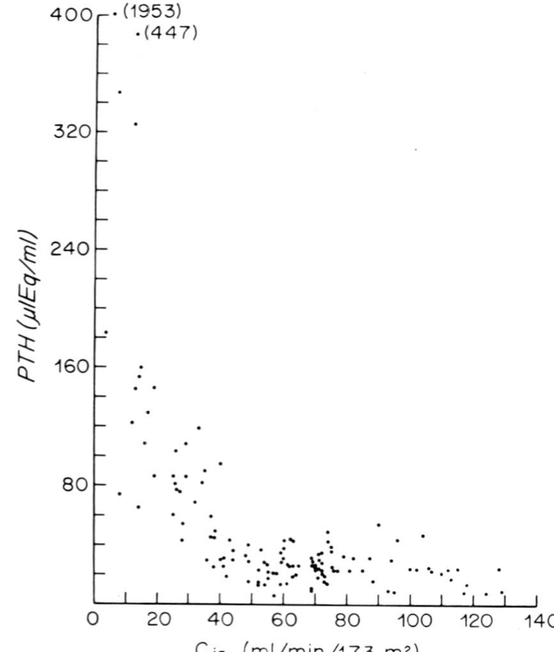

Figure 13–1. Relationship between serum iPTH and the renal clearance of inulin in patients with varying levels of renal function. (From Arnaud CD: Kidney Int 4:89, 1973.)

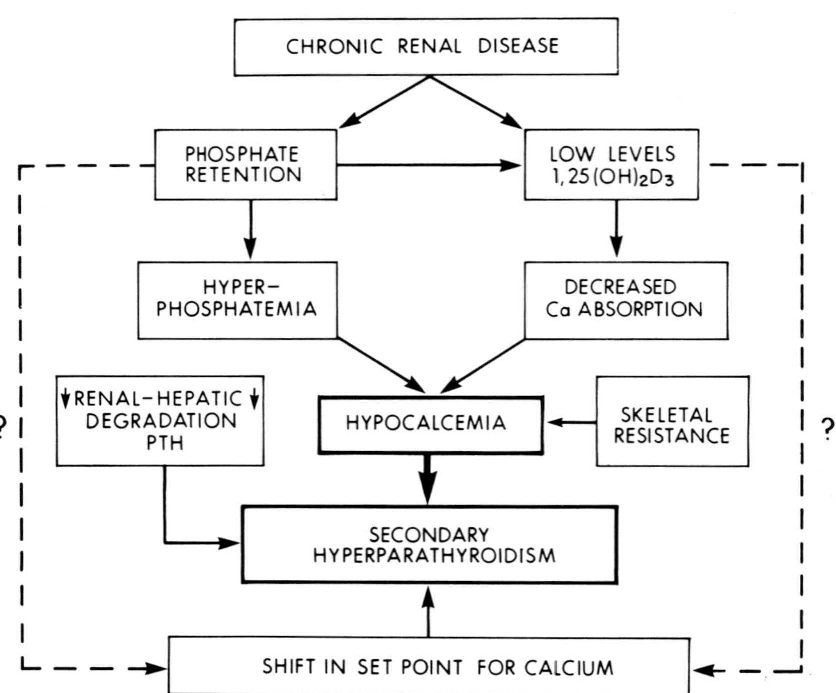

Figure 13–2. Schematic representation of the pathogenetic factors involved in the genesis of secondary hyperparathyroidism.

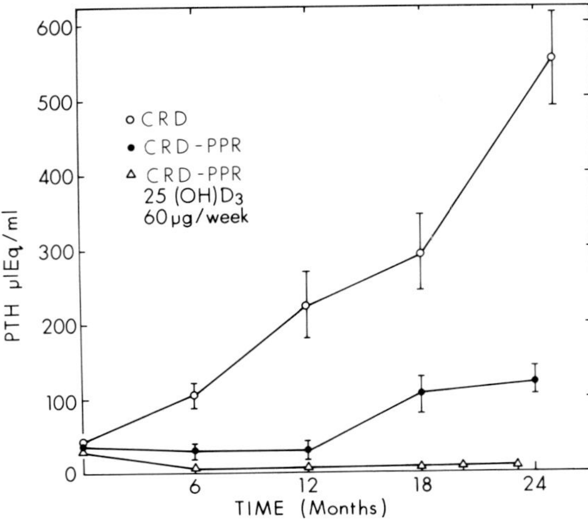

Figure 13–3. Serial values of iPTH in dogs with chronic renal insufficiency. The dogs received either a normal constant phosphate intake (o), a phosphate reduced in proportion to the decrease in glomerular filtration rate (•), or a proportional reduction in phosphate intake and $25(OH)D_3$, (Δ) for two years. (Modified from Rutherford WE, et al: J Clin Invest 60:332, 1977.)

studies have shown that serum iPTH levels correlate positively with the degree of hyperphosphatemia in patients undergoing dialysis,[16] an observation providing support for a role of hyperphosphatemia in causing parathyroid hypersecretion, particularly in patients with advanced uremia. Thus, phosphate loading could cause a small fall in the level of ionized calcium, or it may decrease the renal production of $1,25(OH)_2D_3$,[17] which may permit more secretion of PTH at any given level of serum calcium.[18] As renal disease advances and GFR falls below 25 ml/minute, hyperphosphatemia is usual;[19] under such circumstances, hypocalcemia is more directly related to a markedly increased level of serum phosphorus. Hyperphosphatemia *per se* does not increase PTH secretion. Although high concentrations of serum phosphate (7–9 mg/100 ml) precipitate calcium in soft tissues, the mechanism by which mild hyperphosphatemia affects the concentration of ionized calcium in serum is not known. It may decrease the release of calcium from bone[20] or affect the activity of the renal enzyme 1-α-hydroxylase responsible for the conversion of $25(OH)D_3$ to $1,25(OH)_2D_3$. Additional studies are necessary to define precisely the mechanism by which mild hyperphosphatemia affects the concentration of ionized calcium in serum. It is important to emphasize that correction of hyperphosphatemia alone will not reverse secondary hyperparathyroidism in patients with advanced renal failure (GFR less than 20 ml/minute), because many other factors are responsible for the increased PTH levels in blood.

B. Altered Vitamin D Metabolism

As reviewed in Chapter 5, the kidney is the major site for conversion of vitamin D to its active metabolite $1,25(OH)_2D_3$.[21] Thus, alterations in mineral homeostasis and skeletal disease can be expected in advanced renal failure. Because one of the main actions of vitamin D is to stimulate intestinal transport of calcium, it is easy to understand why the absorption of calcium from the intestine is decreased in patients with far-advanced renal insufficiency and low levels of $1,25(OH)_2D_3$. The evidence that altered vitamin D metabolism contributes to abnormal calcium metabolism in advanced renal failure is considerable. Metabolic balance studies usually show that fecal calcium losses are equal to or greater than dietary calcium intake in patients with advanced renal insufficiency,[22] and radioisotope techniques also show reduced intestinal absorption of calcium in most patients with advanced renal failure.[23] Currently, it is not known at what level of renal insufficiency vitamin D metabolism becomes abnormal. This information will be of considerable importance in elucidating the pathogenesis of secondary hyperparathyroidism of uremia. Slatopolsky et al.[24] compared the levels of $1,25(OH)_2D_3$ and iPTH in a group of adults with normal renal function, patients with mild decreases in GFR (GFR between 40 and 60 ml/minute) and patients with advanced renal failure (GFR between 5 and 20 ml/minute), and patients on dialysis. The plasma levels of $1,25(OH)_2D_3$ were normal or even slightly elevated in patients with creatinine clearance greater than 40 ml/minute. Cheung et al.[25] found similar results. As expected, patients with severe renal insufficiency had low levels of $1,25(OH)_2D_3$. If one assumes that a patient with a GFR of 50 ml/minute has lost roughly one half of the renal mass, and yet the levels of $1,25(OH)_2D_3$ are normal, one has to conclude that the production of $1,25(OH)_2D_3$ per unit of renal mass is greatly increased. This could be due to secondary hyperparathyroidism, which is usually present in patients with mild renal insufficiency. However, recent studies by Taylor et al.[26] in the dog showed that after unilateral nephrectomy, the remaining kidney increased the production of $1,25(OH)_2D_3$ even in the absence of PTH. Moreover, patients with a mild degree of renal insufficiency do not have calcium malabsorption. Coburn et al.[23] measured intestinal calcium absorption using ^{47}Ca isotope techniques in patients with different degrees of renal insufficiency. They found that patients with mild renal failure (serum creatinine less than 2.5 mg/100 ml) had calcium absorption values no different from those observed in normal volunteers. Malluche et al.[27] also studied calcium absorption in a large group of patients with renal disease. They found that as GFR decreased, there was a concomitant decrease in absorption of calcium. However, this abnormality became evident only at GFR values below 50 ml/minute. The results obtained in patients with GFRs greater than 60 ml/minute were not different from those obtained in patients with normal renal function. Thus, there is no good evidence for calcium malabsorption or low serum levels of $1,25(OH)_2D_3$ in patients with early renal insufficiency. Although the levels of $1,25(OH)_2D_3$ in most patients with advanced renal failure (GFR less than 20 ml/minute) are low, many patients lack histologic features of vitamin D deficiency. Thus, reduced synthesis of $1,25(OH)_2D_3$ may not be the only factor responsible for the development of osteomalacia in this group of patients.[28,29] Perhaps normal or elevated serum phosphorus levels may protect some uremic patients from osteomalacia. Abnormal generation of other vitamin D sterols, particularly 24,25 dihydroxy D_3, in the pathogenesis of renal osteodystrophy remains uncertain. The kidney is the organ primarily responsible for the formation of $24,25(OH)_2D$, but there is evidence that this metabolite may also be produced in the intestine and bone.[30] The role, if any, of $24,25(OH)_2D$ in the pathogenesis of renal osteodystrophy remains speculative. Recent studies by Olgaard et al.[31] in uremic dogs indicated that the administration of $24,25(OH)_2D_3$ did not have any beneficial effect.

C. Skeletal Resistance to the Calcemic Action of Parathyroid Hormone

Skeletal resistance to the calcemic action of PTH is another important cause of hypocalcemia in patients with renal insufficiency. The calcemic response to the infusion of parathyroid extract is significantly less in hypocalcemic patients with renal failure than in normal subjects or patients with hypoparathyroidism.[32] The finding of a delayed recovery from induced hypocalcemia in patients with mild renal insufficiency (creatinine clearances of 35 to 90 ml/minute) compared with results in normal subjects, despite a greater augmentation in serum iPTH levels, indicates that the skeletal resistance to endogenous PTH appears early in the course of renal insufficiency.[33] Such data suggest that the higher circulating level of PTH may be needed to maintain normal serum calcium levels in patients with renal failure.

The concept of skeletal resistance to PTH as an important factor in the development of secondary hyperparathyroidism has been challenged. Kaplan et al.[34] fed dogs with chronic renal failure a low-phosphate diet and prevented the development of secondary hyperparathyroidism. However, these animals developed skeletal resistance to the calcemic action of PTH. Thus, despite the presence of skeletal resistance to PTH, the dogs did not develop secondary hyperparathyroidism. Llach et al.[14] found that dietary phosphate restriction improved the calcemic response to a standardized infusion of PTH in patients with mild renal insufficiency. It is possible that alterations in vitamin D metabolism could be responsible for the resistance to the calcemic action of PTH seen in uremia. In dogs with acute renal failure,[35] treatment with $1,25(OH)_2D_3$ results in only partial correction of the blunted calcemic response to PTH, data supporting a possible role of altered vitamin D metabolism. Other observations suggest that hyperphosphatemia accounted for the skeletal resistance of parathyroid extract in rats with acute renal failure.[36] Results of studies of a bone-organ culture system indicate that the serum of uremic patients can inhibit PTH-stimulated release of calcium from the bone.[20]

D. Altered Calcium-Regulated PTH Secretion

A number of studies have suggested that most parathyroid hormone that is secreted in response to hypocalcemia is obtained from a recently synthesized pool of protein that is not in rapid equilibrium with most of the hormone stored in the cell.[37-41] Beta-agonist–stimulated hormone secretion, which is cAMP mediated, occurs from the pool of previously synthesized older protein.[42] Phenomenologically, the stimulation of hormone secretion by hypocalcemia, as opposed to stimulation by agents that operated through cAMP, appears to occur through different mechanisms[37, 43-44] (Fig. 13–4).

Calcium is an inhibitor of the adenylate cyclase activity of isolated parathyroid membranes.[45-49] Membranes prepared from hyperplastic glands are less susceptible to the inhibition of enzyme activity by calcium than are membranes prepared from normal human parathyroid tissue.[48] This suggests that the "set point for calcium" (the calcium ion concentration causing a 50% decrease in overall hormone secretion) to inhibit parathyroid adenylate cyclase may be elevated above normal in hyperfunctioning human parathyroid glands. Since calcium-mediated changes in cellular cAMP cannot account for all the calcium-induced changes in hormone secretion, it is suggested that the set point for calcium inhibition of adenylate cyclase is a general manifestation of the hyperplastic state.

In addition to the altered set point for the inhibition by calcium of parathyroid adenylate cyclase in membranes obtained from hyperfunctioning human glands, there is an altered set point for the inhibition of hormone secretion by calcium.[50-54] Accumulated data obtained for collagenase-dispersed human parathyroid cells indicates a set point in normal cells of 0.97 ± 0.04 mM calcium ion; whereas with cells from adenomas and both primary and secondary hyperplasia, the set point was increased to 1.26 ± 0.13 mM, 1.09 ± mM, and 1.17 ± 0.19 mM calcium ion respectively.[54] Not only was the set point for calcium elevated with respect to hormone secretion in cells obtained from hyperplastic parathyroid tissue, but the degree of responsiveness across the calcium-sensitive range was also altered. The degree of suppression of hormone secretion with increasing calcium is apparently less for cells obtained from all types of hyperplastic glands than for cells from normal glands.[54]

Several investigators[55-57] have provided evidence that vitamin D metabolites directly affect regulation of PTH secretion. In 1974, Oldham et al.[58] isolated a calcium-binding

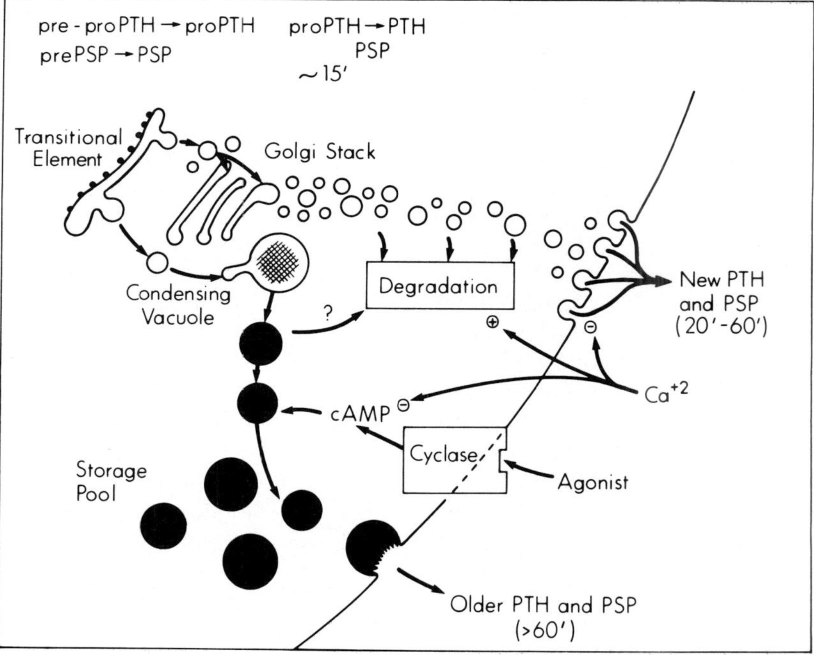

Figure 13–4. Cellular pathways in the parathyroid cell for the secretion of parathyroid hormone. Calcium primarily affects the secretion of newly synthesized PTH, whereas agents that influence cellular cyclic AMP levels affect the secretion of stored (older) hormone. (From Morrissey J, et al: Abnormalities in parathyroid hormone secretion in primay and secondary hyperparathyroidism. *In* Massry SG, Maschio G (eds): Phosphate and Other Minerals. New York, Plenum Press, 1983, pp 391.)

protein from porcine parathyroid glands with properties similar to those of the calcium-binding proteins found in mammalian intestinal mucosa. The administration of $25(OH)D_3$ to rachitic puppies increased the calcium-binding protein in the parathyroid glands. Subsequently, Brumbaugh et al.[59] demonstrated specific binding of $1,25(OH)_2D_3$ to cytosolic and nuclear receptors of the chick parathyroid glands *in vitro*. Chertow et al.[55] performed studies *in vivo* in the rat and *in vitro* with bovine parathyroid gland slices. These investigators clearly demonstrated an inhibitory effect of $1,25(OH)_2D_3$ on PTH release. After these initial publications, a series of papers appeared in the literature, suggesting that $1,25(OH)_2D_3$ did not have a direct effect on the secretion of parathyroid hormone.[60-61] Because of these controversial results, Golden et al.[62] studied in great detail the effect of $1,25(OH)_2D_3$ on parathyroid hormone secretion *in vitro*, using bovine parathyroid gland slices and isolated dispersed bovine parathyroid cells. The results failed to demonstrate an effect of $1,25(OH)_2D_3$ on PTH secretion by the isolated bovine parathyroid cells or by bovine parathyroid slices. It is critical to emphasize that the parathyroid glands used in these studies were obtained from normal cows that were not depleted of $1,25(OH)_2D_3$. Moreover, the studies were performed *in vitro* and the incubations were conducted over a 4 hour period. The fact that the animals were not depleted of $1,25(OH)_2D_3$ may have had an effect on the outcome of the results obtained in these studies. Studies by Oldham and collaborators[18] in vitamin D–deficient dogs clearly indicated that higher concentrations of calcium were necessary to suppress the release of parathyroid hormone in these animals. When similar studies were performed in the same animals after $1,25(OH)_2D_3$ was given to the dogs, the parathyroid glands appeared to be more sensitive to mild increments in serum calcium.

The low levels of $1,25(OH)_2D_3$ observed in patients with advanced renal insufficiency[24-25,63] could potentially play a role in the abnormal behavior of the parathyroid glands. Slatopolsky et al.[64] performed studies in dialysis patients using an intravenous form of $1,25(OH)_2D_3$. Twenty patients with hypocalcemia maintained on chronic hemodialysis were selected for the study. In the control part of the studies, blood was obtained before dialysis three times a week for a period of 3 weeks. In the treatment period, $1,25(OH)_2D_3$ was given intravenously at the end of each dialysis for a period of 8 weeks. The dose was 0.5 μg initially and gradually was increased to a maximum of 4.0 μg per treatment. Finally, a second posttreatment control period was continued for an additional 3 weeks.

The mean serum calcium increased from 8.5 to 9.4 mg/100 ml and with a peak response of 10.9 mg/100 ml during $1,25(OH)_2D_3$ administration. In the posttreatment period, serum calcium decreased to a mean of 9.0 mg/100 ml. In general, there was a tendency for serum phosphorus to increase during 1,25-dihydroxy D_3 administration. Magnesium, on the other hand, remained fairly constant during the entire study in all patients. Every single patient had a substantial decrease in the levels of PTH during $1,25(OH)_2D_3$ treatment. The mean decrement in PTH was 70.1% (Fig. 13–5). After 3 weeks of treatment, there was a gradual rise in the levels of ionized calcium. Concomitantly, there was a significant decrease in the levels of iPTH. After $1,25(OH)_2D_3$ was discontinued, PTH increased in every single patient. However, it would seem that early during the administration of $1,25(OH)_2D_3$ and before there was any significant increase in ionized calcium, there was a decrease in the levels of iPTH (Fig. 13–6).

Thus, the present studies demonstrate that $1,25(OH)_2D_3$ has remarkable suppressive effect on the release of PTH. Likely, the effects are mainly due to elevation in serum calcium to the upper limits of normal. However, it would seem that in addition to the calcemic effect, $1,25(OH)_2D_3$ *per se* modified the secretion of PTH. Recently, further evidence has been provided from *in vitro* studies indicating that $1,25(OH)_2D_3$ inhibits the synthesis[65] and secretion of PTH.[66] It is known that parathyroid glands obtained from uremic patients have a shift in the set point for calcium, requiring a higher concentration of ionized calcium than normal parathyroid glands for the suppression of PTH release. These studies raise the possibility that $1,25(OH)_2D_3$ may affect the regulation of PTH secretion by making the parathyroid gland more sensitive to calcium. Obviously, further studies are necessary to clarify this point.

E. Role of Reduced Degradation of PTH

An increased rate of PTH secretion is a major factor responsible for high plasma

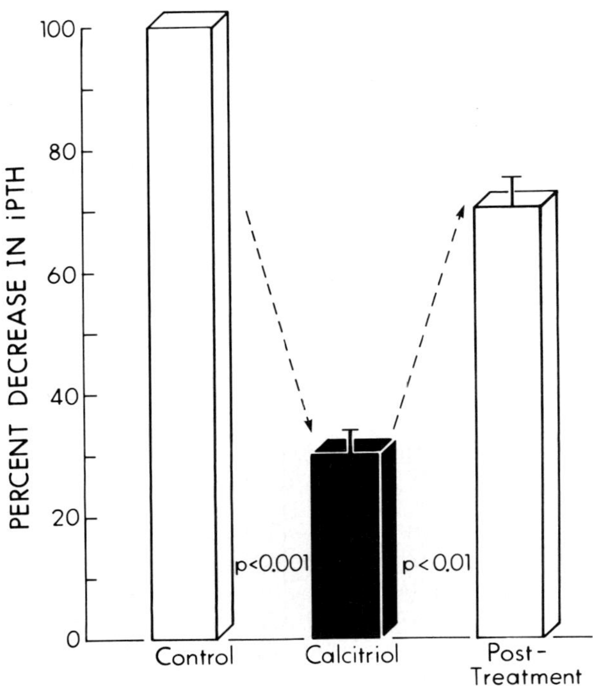

Figure 13–5. Changes in serum iPTH during and after the administration of intravenous 1,25$(OH)_2D_3$ expressed as percentage of pretreatment values. The mean decrement in serum iPTH was 70.1%. (Modified from Slatopolsky E, et al: J Clin Invest 74:2136, 1984.)

levels of iPTH in patients with renal insufficiency. Since the kidney plays an important role in the degradation of PTH and since the metabolic clearance of iPTH is slowed in renal failure, decreased degradation of PTH could be a factor contributing to the pathogenesis of hyperparathyroidism.[67] Because the kidney may be the only organ removing the carboxyl-terminal fragments of PTH from the circulation[68] (see Chapter 3), the level of C-terminal fragments is greatly increased in renal failure, and measurements of iPTH specific for the carboxyl fractions reveal values that are much higher in uremic patients than exist in patients with primary hyperparathyroidism.[69] However, the kidney also plays a role in the degradation of the intact 1–84 PTH molecule, and studies of the

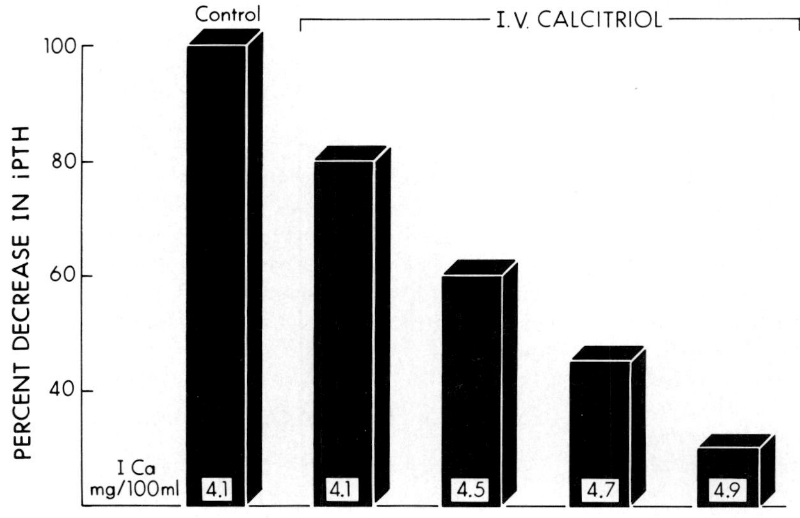

Figure 13–6. Temporal relationship between ionized calcium and serum iPTH before and during intravenous 1,25$(OH)_2D_3$ in all 20 patients. Serum iPTH decreased before there was any change in blood ionized calcium level. (Modified from Slatopolsky E, et al: J Clin Invest 74:2136, 1984.)

metabolic clearance of bovine PTH 1–84 suggest that its clearance rate is slowed in patients with renal failure.[70] If the uremic patient has a normal calcemic response to PTH and if the relationship that exists between ionized blood calcium and the secretion of PTH is normal, the effect of prolonged PTH degradation should be minimal. However, it is likely that a delayed degradation of PTH can result in higher levels of intact 1–84 PTH after any given rate of secretion of PTH than is the case in normal subjects.

II. OSTEOMALACIA

Osteomalacia, which is presented in detail in Chapter 11, is another important feature of the skeletal disease of some patients with advanced renal failure. In bone tissue, it is reflected by an increase in the osteoid seam width and an abnormal or decreased mineralization front. The pathogenesis of impaired skeletal mineralization in patients with chronic renal failure is not clear, and although alterations in vitamin D metabolism may play an important role, other factors undoubtedly contribute. The mechanism whereby altered vitamin D metabolism leads to impaired demineralization of bone is poorly understood. Whether vitamin D or $1,25(OH)_2D$ directly stimulates bone mineralization or leads to mineral deposition by increasing the levels of calcium and phosphate in the extracellular fluid surrounding bone is controversial. Although the plasma levels of $1,25(OH)_2D$ are reduced in patients with advanced renal insufficiency, overt osteomalacia is found in only a small fraction of patients.[28] Moreover, osteomalacia may be absent even in anephric patients.[29] Thus, other factors appear to participate in the pathogenesis of osteomalacia in uremic patients. One factor that may influence the development of osteomalacia is the plasma level of phosphorus, and hypophosphatemia *per se* can produce severe osteomalacia, even in patients with normal renal function. Alterations in collagen synthesis and maturation may also contribute to the development of osteomalacia. Experimental studies in uremic rats have shown a preponderance of immature soluble collagen that fails to mineralize normally. Treatment of such uremic animals with 25(OH)D can normalize collagen maturation.[71] Bone crystal formation also is affected in patients with renal insufficiency. Immature bone contains large quantities of amorphous calcium phosphate. Other alterations in the bone of uremic patients include an increase in magnesium, elevated levels of pyrophosphate, and diminished carbonate content. A combination of these factors may play a role in bone maturation and contribute to the development of uremic osteomalacia. Acidosis also may contribute to the pathogenesis of renal osteodystrophy. Administration of bicarbonate and correction of the acidosis in azotemic patients can reduce the fecal calcium[72] and, therefore, may be of therapeutic benefit.

It is now clear that the retention of aluminum plays an important role in the development of osteomalacia. In patients with advanced renal failure serum concentrations of aluminum above 100 to 200 μg/liter, the major source may be from the dialysate. In geographic areas with high aluminum content in tap water used for dialysate, the incidence of osteomalacia appears to decrease with deionization treatment.[73] However, recent evidence in the United States suggests that the main source of aluminum is due to the ingestion of phosphate binders containing aluminum, and the major cause of symptomatic vitamin D–resistant osteomalacia is the retention of aluminum, either from dialysate or from intestinal absorption of aluminum. In these patients, phosphate restriction in the diet is mandatory to allow decreased use of phosphate binders. Finally, recent evidence suggests that a lack of PTH, as has been seen in uremic patients after total parathyroidectomy, can precipitate the development of osteomalacia.[74,75]

III. CLINICAL AND BIOCHEMICAL FEATURES OF ALTERED DIVALENT-ION METABOLISM

Symptoms from altered divalent-ion metabolism usually appear only in patients with advanced renal failure. However, alterations in mineral homeostasis appear early in the course of renal insufficiency, and their identification may help the physician to introduce treatment early to prevent renal osteodystrophy. Numerous signs and symptoms can occur in association with altered divalent-ion metabolism in uremia. Bone pain can develop and progress slowly to the point that the patient becomes bedridden; moreover, this can occur whether the skeletal abnormality is osteitis fibrosa or osteomalacia. The bone pain is generally vague and commonly is located in the lower back, hips, knees, and legs. Low-back pain may arise from collapse of a vertebral body, and sharp chest pain may result from spontaneous rib fracture. However, physical findings frequently are lacking. Muscular weakness, when present, usually is proximal; it appears slowly and progresses. Plasma levels of muscle enzymes, creatinine phosphokinase and transaminase, usually are normal, and the electromyographic changes are nonspecific. The pathogenesis of such muscle weakness is uncertain. In patients with myopathy, electron micrographic studies have revealed localized disorganization of the myofibrils and dispersion of Z bands, changes that revert to normal following 25(OH)D.[76] The muscular weakness has also been attributed to secondary hyperparathyroidism on a neuropathic basis.[77] Finally, we have seen the resolution of muscle weakness following treatment of aluminum excess with chelating therapy. Pruritus, an especially common symptom in uremic patients with severe secondary hyperparathyroidism, has been attributed to increased levels of calcium in the skin. Moreover, pruritus can develop in uremic patients receiving pharmacologic doses of vitamin D and during the infusion of calcium. In patients with chronic renal failure, peripheral ischemic necrosis and vascular calcification have been reported. The lesions may involve the tips of the toes and fingers, when the skin becomes violaceous. Ulceration and scar formation may occur, with clear demarcation of the lesions from the surrounding skin. Most patients with such problems have concomitant severe secondary hyperparathyroidism, and some have benefited from subtotal parathyroidectomy.

Acute pain and swelling around one or more joints may develop in uremic patients. This syndrome of calcified periarthritis, which may be caused by the deposition of hydroxyapatite crystals, is associated with marked hyperphosphatemia.[78] Abnormal collagen metabolism, as is believed to exist in uremic bone, may also occur in tendon and may predispose to spontaneous tendon rupture.

Skeletal deformities are common in growing azotemic children. Bowing of the tibiae and femora and deformities from slipped epiphyses are not uncommon. Children with renal rickets sometimes exhibit typical radiographic findings of vitamin D deficiency. In adults with renal failure, particularly those with osteomalacia, marked skeletal deformities, with lumbar scoliosis, thoracic kyphosis, and deformities of the thoracic cage, may be observed. Growth retardation usually is seen in young children both before and during maintenance hemodialysis. Several factors, such as malnutrition, chronic acidosis, and severe osteomalacia, may contribute to the retarded growth. Caloric supplementation, correction of acidosis, and addition of $1,25(OH)_2D$ may improve the growth rate.

From the biochemical point of view, one of the early changes in patients with renal insufficiency (GFR between 60 and 80 ml/minute) is the presence of elevated levels of circulating iPTH. As the disease progresses (GFR less than 30 ml/minute), hypocalcemia may be present. Alterations in circulating ionized calcium are seen earlier than alterations in total calcium. This is because of an increase in the complexed fraction of blood calcium. However, the serum calcium may remain close to normal in patients with advanced renal insufficiency, and values below 7.5 mg/100 ml are infrequent. Usually, hypocalcemia is most marked in patients with severe osteomalacia or profound metabolic acidosis. Occasionally, hypercalcemia may be observed in uremic patients, particularly those undergoing long-term dialysis. This can arise from severe secondary hyperparathyroidism, ingestion of large amounts of calcium or vitamin D, unrelated diseases such as sarcoidosis or malignancy, or a "pure" mineralization defect that is believed to arise from aluminum accumulation.[79]

Hyperphosphatemia is common in patients with a GFR less than 25 ml/minute. The degree of hyperphosphatemia depends on the amount of phosphate ingested in the diet, the fraction absorbed by the intestine, and how much is excreted into the urine. Obviously, if the patient ingests phosphate binders, the serum phosphorus may remain normal despite advanced renal insufficiency. PTH can also influence the concentration of phosphate in serum. Although PTH decreases the reabsorption of phosphorus by the renal tubule, it mobilizes phosphate from bone. Thus, patients with severe hyperparathyroidism and advanced renal insufficiency usually have high concentrations of serum phosphate in plasma. Hypermagnesemia occurs in renal patients when the GFR falls below 15 ml/minute.

Intake of magnesium-containing antacids by patients with severe renal failure can lead to abrupt and marked hypermagnesemia. Increased serum magnesium usually is associated with increased content of magnesium in bone, a factor that may affect crystal formation. In patients receiving chronic hemodialysis, with a dialysate magnesium concentration of 1.5 mEq/liter, hypermagnesemia with blood levels of 2.5 to 3.5 mEq/liter is common. Serum alkaline phosphatase activity is often increased in uremic patients with osteitis fibrosa, osteomalacia, or mixed lesions. Although serum alkaline phosphatase activity is composed of isoenzyme activity arising from intestine, liver, kidney, and bone, routine alkaline phosphatase measurements, when increased in uremic patients, usually suggest increased osteoblastic activity. In dialysis patients, serum alkaline phosphatase activity correlates with the extent of bone osteoid surface covered with osteoblasts, resorbing surfaces, the number of osteoclasts, and the percentage of osteoid seams that take up tetracycline.[80,81] Coexistent liver disease, however, should be excluded as a cause of elevated alkaline phosphatase in uremic patients.

IV. BONE HISTOLOGY

Examination of bone is often important for the diagnosis and management of patients with renal osteodystrophy. As detailed in Chapter 10, the most common histologic finding is osteitis fibrosa secondary to high circulating levels of PTH. In these patients, the histologic findings are osteoclastosis and increased bone resorption surfaces (as reflected by many Howship's lacunae). They also show increased bone turnover as indicated from double tetracycline labeling, and increased quantities of woven osteoid, which differs from normal lamellar osteoid in that it exhibits a haphazard arrangement of collagen fibers. Woven osteoid can become mineralized; however, calcium may be deposited as amorphous calcium phosphate rather than as hydroxyapatite. The excess deposition of calcium phosphate in woven osteoid may explain the presence of osteosclerosis in some uremic patients. Osteoidosis, however, does not indicate the presence of osteomalacia or defective mineralization. The amount of osteoid present in bone depends on the rate and extent of its formation by osteoblasts and the rate and extent of calcification. Thus, in order to make the histologic diagnosis of osteomalacia, excess osteoid and an abnormal mineralization front must be present. The extent of bone surface undergoing calcification can be measured by techniques such as staining with toluidine blue *in vitro* or tetracycline labeling *in vivo*. Osteoidosis with a decreased calcification front has been taken to be evidence for osteomalacia. The use of double tetracycline labeling in conjunction with quantitative histomorphometric techniques can provide the best method for identification of defective mineralization. The bone turnover rate (measured with double tetracycline labeling) is normal or increased above normal in patients with osteitis fibrosa, whereas it is below normal in patients with osteomalacia (Fig. 13–7). Dialysis patients with pure osteomalacia usually show little or no evidence of secondary hyperparathyroidism.[79] This group fails to improve following 1-hydroxy D_3 or $1,25(OH)_2D$ therapy. Usually their bone biopsy stains positively for aluminum.

V. RADIOGRAPHIC FEATURES OF RENAL OSTEODYSTROPHY

Standard radiographic methods, as applied in clinical practice, often are inconsistent in identifying progression of renal osteodystrophy. Techniques to increase the sensitivity of x-ray studies (which are particularly applicable for views of the hands) include the use of fine-grain film (i.e., Kodak M industrial film or mammography film). The main radiographic feature of secondary hyperparathyroidism is increased bone resorption, most commonly seen on the subperiosteal surfaces of bone. Erosions that occur in conjunction with formation of new bone may appear as cysts or osteoclastomas (brown tumors). The presence of subperiosteal erosions correlates with serum iPTH and histomorphometric features of osteitis fibrosa on biopsy.[80,81] Subperiosteal erosions of the phalanges (detected by fine-grain hand radiographs) may be the most sensitive radiographic sign of secondary hyperparathyroidism (Fig. 13–8). The tuft of the terminal phalanx of the second or third digit commonly shows resorption, and there may be collapse of the overlying soft tissue, so that the finger appears clubbed. Bone erosions also may occur at the proximal end

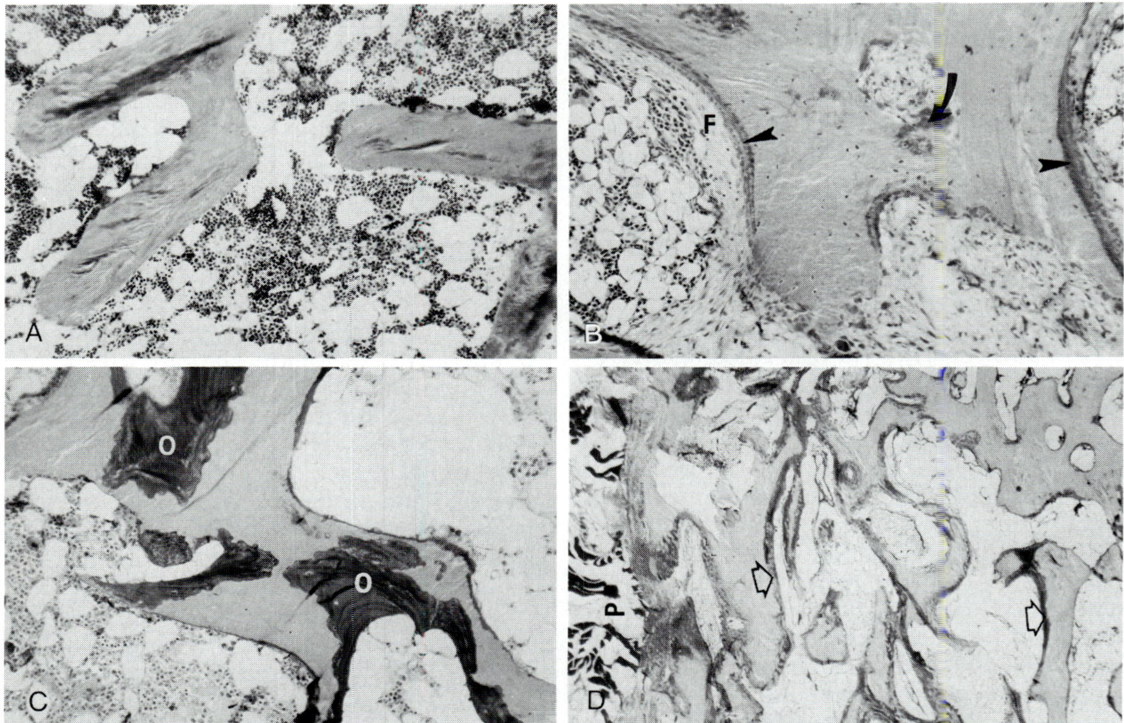

Figure 13–7. Photomicrographs showing representative features of renal osteodystrophy. *A*, Normal trabecular bone (undecalcified Goldner stain; magnification ×100). *B*, Osteitis fibrosa, with excess unmineralized osteoid covered by osteoblasts (arrows) and peritrabecular marrow fibrosis (F). *C*, Osteomalacia, showing wide osteoid seams (O). *D*, Lower power view of cortical and trabecular bone in a patient with chronic renal failure and osteosclerosis. The periosteum (P) is in the righthand corner. (Courtesy of Steven L. Teitelbaum, M.D.)

of the tibia, the neck of the femur or humerus, and the inferior surface of the distal end of the clavicle. In the skull, there is a mottled and granular appearance, with areas of resorption commonly associated with areas of osteosclerosis (Fig. 13–9). The lamina dura of the teeth often shows erosions in primary hyperparathyroidism, but is uncommonly affected by secondary hyperparathyroidism. Increased endosteal surface with widening of the central canal of long bones may also occur in secondary hyperparathyroidism. Osteosclerosis, another feature of osteitis fibrosa, is due to increases in the thickness and number of trabeculae in spongy bone and accounts for the typical "rugger jersey" appearance of the spine. Although the Looser zone or pseudofracture is considered pathognomonic of rickets in children or of osteomalacia in the adult, the x-ray features of osteomalacia often are less distinctive than those of secondary hyperparathyroidism. The typical x-ray feature of rickets, that is, widening of the epiphyseal growth plate, cannot develop after epiphyseal closure, and hence this radiographic sign of defective bone mineralization is limited to children. With mechanical stress on the skeleton affected by rickets or osteomalacia, a Looser zone may extend across a bone and produce a true fracture.[82] Features such as increased haziness or indistinctiveness of the trabeculae, biconcavity of the vertebral bodies (particularly in association with normal bone density), and deformities of long bones are said to be typical of osteomalacia, but these findings are uncommon and may not be easily recognized. Furthermore, uremic patients with osteomalacia commonly have secondary hyperparathyroidism with concomitant x-ray features of the latter. Thus, the definitive diagnosis of osteomalacia requires bone biopsy.

VI. EXTRASKELETAL CALCIFICATIONS

The factors that predispose to the appearance of soft tissue calcification include an increase in the circulating calcium × phosphate

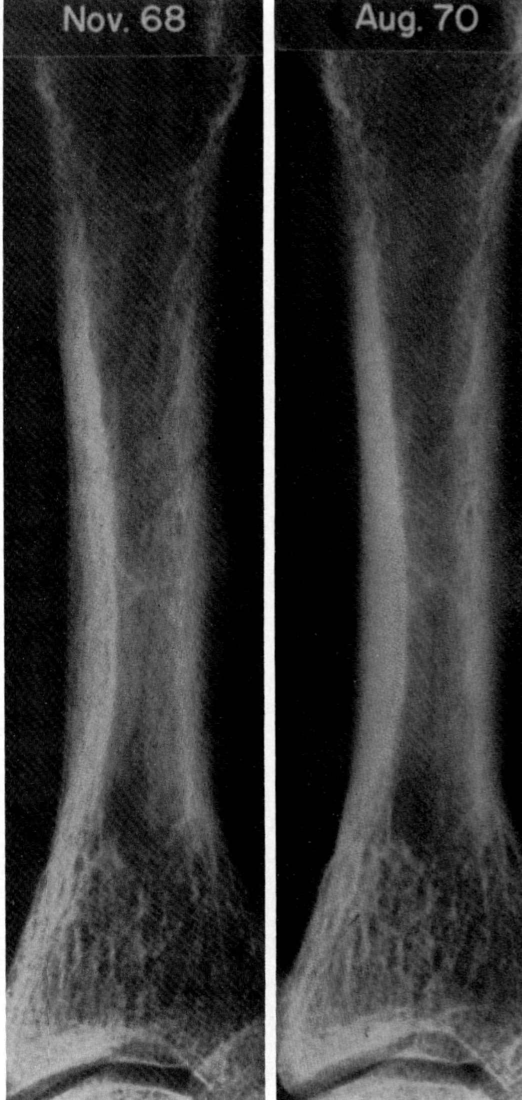

Figure 13–8. Magnification view of a digit obtained with fine-grain film, showing increased intracortical resorption (grade +3) in a 30-year-old uremic woman prior to her treatment with dialysis (left). Approximately two years later (right), the intracortical resorptive tunnels had disappeared, indicating that net bone formation exceeded net resorption. (From Meema HE, et al: Radiology 126:67, 1978.)

product in plasma, the degree of secondary hyperparathyroidism, the magnitude of alkalosis, and local tissue injury.[83] Three major varieties include: (1) calcification of medium-size arteries; (2) articular or tumoral calcification; and (3) visceral calcification affecting the heart, lung, and kidney. Arterial calcification often involves the media of the vessel. These calcifications are diffuse and continuous along the vessels, and their appearance contrasts to the regular discrete appearance of calcified intimal plaques. Such medial calcification of the vessels may be seen first in the dorsalis pedis artery, where it appears as a ring or tube as it descends between the first and second metatarsals. Other sites commonly involved are the ankles, abdominal aorta, feet, pelvis, hands, and wrists (Figs. 13–10 and 13–11).

VII. PREVENTION AND MANAGEMENT OF RENAL OSTEODYSTROPHY

A. Phosphate Retention

Hyperphosphatemia is a major factor accounting for the development and maintenance of secondary hyperparathyroidism in uremia. High serum phosphorus levels contribute to the development of soft tissue calcification in patients with advanced uremia; thus, the restriction of dietary phosphorus and the prevention of hyperphosphatemia are critical in the management of renal bone disease.

The dietary intake of phosphorus depends primarily on meat and dairy products in the diet; the usual phosphorus intake by normal adults in the United States is 1.0 to 1.6 g/day. One can lower the dietary intake of phosphate by restricting the intake of dairy products and by rigid adherence to a low-protein diet. However, there would be great difficulty in lowering phosphorus intake in proportion to the reduced GFR in patients with advanced renal failure by use of dietary manipulation. Moreover, low-phosphate diets are generally unpalatable to the tastes of most people living in the United States, and aluminum-containing compounds that reduce the intestinal absorption of phosphorus are usually given.[84] The aluminum-containing compounds employed to bind phosphorus in the intestinal tract include aluminum hydroxide and aluminum carbonate gels, which are available in liquid, tablet, and capsule form. The capsules are less effective than liquid gels in binding phosphorus,[85] but patient compliance is easier to achieve with capsules than with either the liquid or the tablets. The goal of such therapy is to reduce serum phosphorus to or near normal, and predialysis serum phosphorus levels are ideally main-

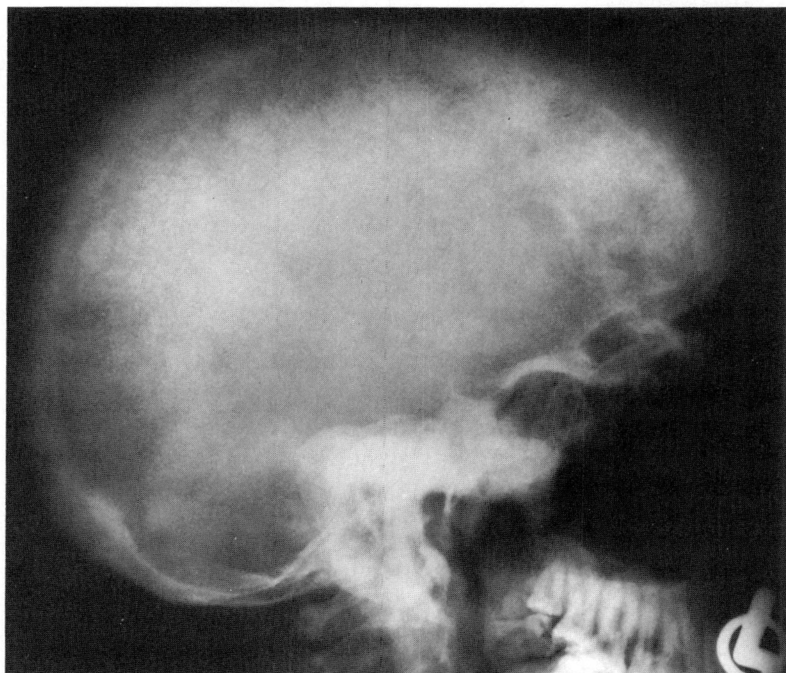

Figure 13–9. Abnormalities in the skull radiograph of a patient with a bone biopsy consistent with osteitis fibrosa. The skull has a diffuse granular appearance with focal areas of sclerosis.

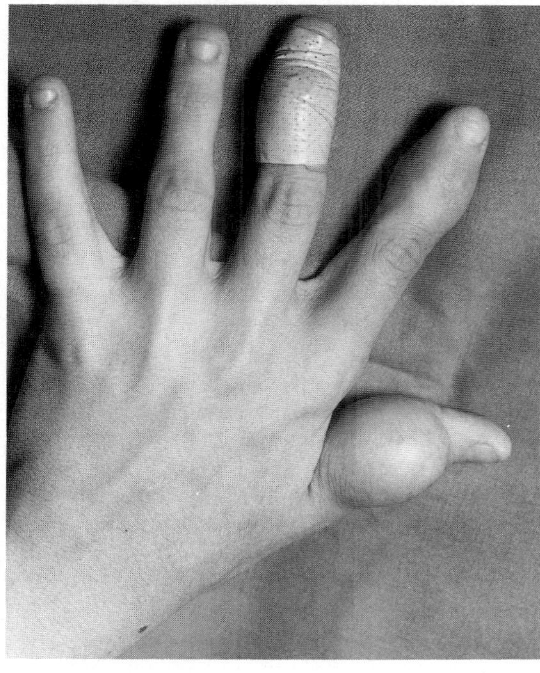

Figure 13–10. Hand of a patient with renal failure and high Ca-P product (Ca 8.5, P 14.2 mg/dl). Severe metastatic calcification of the left thumb.

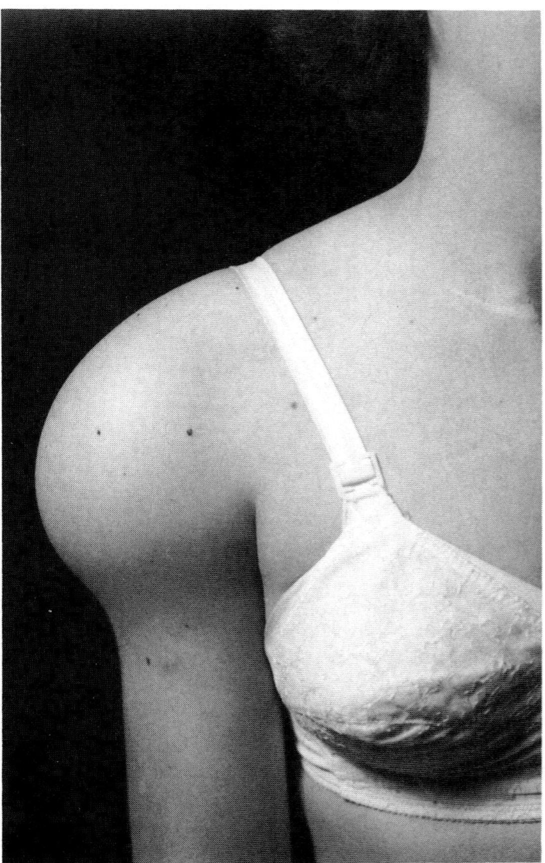

Figure 13–11. Advanced metastatic calcification of the right shoulder in a uremic patient with severe hyperphosphatemia.

tained at 5.0 to 5.5 mg/100 ml in dialysis patients (Fig. 13–12). In patients with creatinine clearances below 10 ml/minute and in those under treatment with dialysis, dietary phosphorus should be restricted to 800 to 900 mg/day, and two to four capsules of aluminum hydroxide or aluminum carbonate should be taken with each meal. Serum phosphorus should be monitored once or twice per month to permit appropriate dosage adjustment. If the serum phosphorus decreases below 4.5 mg/100 ml or remains above the desired range, the number of capsules should be decreased or increased by one or two per day. It is important to avoid reducing the serum phosphorus to subnormal levels to prevent phosphate depletion. Antacids containing magnesium should be avoided because of the risk of hypermagnesemia.

It is generally assumed that aluminum hydroxide and aluminum carbonate are nonabsorbable and safe; however, reported data suggest that orally administered aluminum may be absorbed in significant amounts in humans and in experimental animals, and such treatment can lead to increased plasma and tissue aluminum content.[86,87] Dialysis dementia[87] and some forms of renal osteodystrophy[88] may be related to tissue accumulation of aluminum. Recently, it has been shown[89-91] that calcium carbonate is an effective phosphate binder. Studies performed in 20 patients maintained on chronic dialysis have demonstrated that the administration of calcium carbonate 4 to 12 g daily in three to four doses per day is effective in controlling phosphorus in about 70% of the patients.[90] It is of utmost importance that patients ingest the calcium carbonate together with the meals, otherwise the drug will not be effective as a phosphate binder and the patient will develop hypercalcemia. Moreover, it is important to know the approximate amount of phosphorus ingested in each meal. For a small breakfast containing only 50 to 75 mg of phosphorus, 1 to 2 g of calcium carbonate may be sufficient. On the other hand, a large meal containing 600 mg of phosphorus may require 4 to 7 gm of calcium carbonate.

B. Calcium Supplements

Since impaired calcium absorption exists in patients with advanced renal failure, including those undergoing dialysis, and since their diets generally contain suboptimal quantities of calcium, oral calcium supplements are usually necessary in such patients. Studies of net intestinal calcium absorption suggest that a neutral or positive calcium balance can be achieved in uremic patients when calcium is added to increase the total calcium intake above 1.5 g/day.[92-93]

Long-term treatment with large doses of oral calcium supplements has been reported to reduce the incidence of bone resorption lesions, fractures, and episodes of pseudogout or extraskeletal calcification.[93] Another study showed lower plasma levels of alkaline phosphatase and iPTH in uremic patients receiving calcium supplements compared with those who did not receive them.[94]

Treatment with oral calcium supplements is not without risk. Calcium supplements should not be given to a patient with marked

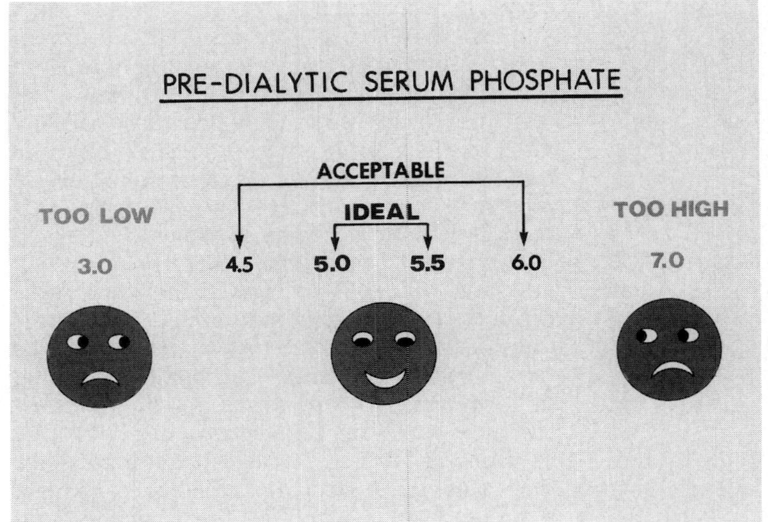

Figure 13–12. Schematic representation of the ideal predialytic serum phosphate. (From Slatopolsky E, Coburn JW: Bone and mineral disturbances in renal insufficiency. *In* Martinez-Maldonado M (ed): Handbook of Renal Therapeutics. New York, Plenum, 1983, p 397d.)

hyperphosphatemia because of the risk of increasing the Ca × P product and predisposing to extraskeletal calcification. Hypercalcemia clearly can develop in uremic patients during oral therapy with calcium salts.

Calcium carbonate is the first choice as a source of supplemental calcium, because it contains a high fraction of calcium, is inexpensive, tasteless, and relatively well tolerated. Calcium carbonate contains 40% elemental calcium. Calcium carbonate is available in several proprietary preparations, including Os-Cal, Titralac, and Tums (see Chapter 12).

A number of studies have been directed toward observing the effect of different dialysate calcium levels on the progress of renal bone disease. With the use of dialysate calcium levels lower than 6.0 mg/100 ml, evidence of progressive bone disease has been suggested by an increase in plasma alkaline phosphatase,[95] and bone deterioration on radiographs.[96-97] The ideal calcium in the dialysate should be 6.5 mg/100 ml.

C. Use of Vitamin D Sterols

Despite the dietary phosphate restriction, the use of phosphate binders, the choice of an appropriate level of calcium in dialysate, and the intake of adequate dietary calcium, a significant number of uremic patients still develop skeletal disease. Knowledge of the kidney's role in producing 1,25$(OH)_2D_3$ has created interest in the use of active vitamin D sterols in such patients.

When uremic patients have evidence of overt secondary hyperparathyroidism (e.g., bone erosions, high iPTH levels, and increased alkaline phosphatase), adequate treatment with a vitamin D sterol often leads to improvement. Thus, pharmacologic doses of D_2,[98] dihydrotachysterol,[99,100] 25-hydroxyvitamin D_3 (calcidiol),[101,102] 1α-hydroxyvitamin D_3,[103] and 1,25-dihydroxyvitamin D_3 (calcitriol)[104,105] can improve symptoms, the radiographic appearance of bone, and skeletal histology and can lower the serum levels of alkaline phosphatase and iPTH.

Vitamin D use is not without hazard; hypercalcemia can develop even in anephric patients and may require several weeks for resolution.[106] Such hypercalcemia develops as a consequence of high blood levels of 25(OH)D in the face of normal levels of 1,25$(OH)_2D_3$.[107] Vitamin D sterols should not be used when hyperphosphatemia is present because the increase in Ca × P product can predispose to the development of extraskeletal calcification.

Although there is an apparent block in the 1-hydroxylation of 25$(OH)D_3$, considerable data indicate that uremic patients can respond favorably to this sterol when it is given in doses of less than 100 mg/day. A reversal of symptoms of bone disease and improvement of histologic evidence of severe secondary hyperparathyroidism in bone cells have been observed in adults[108] and children[101] given 25$(OH)D_3$. Preliminary results from a six-center study indicate improvement in symptoms of bone pain and tenderness and fall in alkaline phosphatase during treatment of uremic patients with $25(OH)D_3$.[102] There was a decrease in the degree of osteitis fibrosa. Hypercalcemia developed in some patients and was associated with the increase in the plasma level of 25(OH)D to 200 to 300 ng/ml, which are supranormal levels.[102] However, another study showed improved bone mineralization during treatment with $25(OH)D_3$ in quantities that increased plasma levels of 25(OH)D only to normal.[109]

Such studies indicate that $25(OH)D_3$ may be effective in the treatment of symptomatic renal osteodystrophy; it was suggested from results of one study that bone formation was increased to a greater extent by $25(OH)D_3$ than $1\alpha(OH)D_3$,[110] and Bordier et al.[111] have reported that $25(OH)D_3$ was more effective than $1,25(OH)_2D_3$ or $1\alpha(OH)D_3$ in stimulating normal mineralization of bone in nonuremic patients with vitamin D deficiency. Further studies are necessary to verify whether $25(OH)D_3$ may have some specific effects on bone.

Results of several clinical trials indicate the efficacy of $1,25(OH)_2D_3$ in treating patients with symptomatic renal osteodystrophy. These clinical evaluations have shown a decrease in bone pain, improvement in muscle strength, and decrease in plasma alkaline phosphatase.[104-105,112] Studies of bone histology have revealed a prominent decrease in marrow fibrosis and other features of secondary hyperparathyroidism.[113,114] In addition, bone mineralization has improved in patients with osteomalacic lesions,[114,115] although these effects occurred more slowly. A decrease in serum phosphorus levels has been observed, particularly early in the course of treatment of patients who exhibited a favorable response. Increments in serum phosphorus levels have also been noted later in the course of treatment. Studies in uremic children indicate that treatment with $1,25(OH)_2D_3$ may increase the growth rate, particularly after plasma alkaline phosphatase and serum iPTH have decreased substantially toward normal.[116]

The quantities of $1,25(OH)_2D_3$ utilized in these trials have varied from 0.14 to 1.5 μg/day, and the major side effect of such treatment has been the appearance of hypercalcemia. From results in a small number of patients with symptomatic bone disease, it has been suggested that a smaller dose, 0.5 μg/day, may be efficacious and may result in a lower incidence of hypercalcemia.[117] Hypercalcemia may occur only after many weeks or months of treatment in patients who have a favorable response and may be heralded by a fall in plasma alkaline phosphatase to normal. Significant hypercalcemia may appear sooner in patients with aluminum-related bone disease or in those with severe secondary hyperparathyroidism (bone erosions and high serum iPTH) who have serum calcium levels that are slightly above normal before treatment;[118] such patients usually have massive parathyroid hyperplasia, and subtotal parathyroidectomy may be indicated.

The role of $1,25(OH)_2D_3$ treatment in the prophylaxis of skeletal disease for patients undergoing dialysis or those with mild renal failure has not yet been established; it has been suggested that renal function may decrease in patients during treatment with $1,25(OH)_2D_3$,[119] although this may be related to hypercalcemia or phosphate retention. Further studies are needed to establish the prophylactic role of $1,25(OH)_2D_3$ in renal failure. Whether a deficiency of $24,25(OH)_2D_3$ plays a role in the pathogenesis of renal osteodystrophy remains to be shown. Recent studies have indicated that $24,25(OH)_2D_3$ does not have beneficial effects in uremic dogs.[31]

D. Parathyroidectomy

The types of treatment just discussed often lead to improvement of calcium and phosphorus homeostasis, reversal of symptoms of bone disease, and suppression of parathyroid secretion. However, such measures may be unsuccessful, and certain features of secondary hyperparathyroidism may necessitate parathyroid surgery. When a problem leads to such a consideration, there should also be ample evidence for the presence of severe secondary hyperparathyroidism, for example, very high levels of serum iPTH with bone erosions or the presence of osteitis fibrosa on bone biopsy. Also, it is important that aluminum-related bone disease be excluded. The features that may indicate the need for parathyroid surgery include (1) persistent hypercalcemia, particularly when symptomatic; (2) intractable pruritus that does not respond to dialysis or other medical treatment; (3) progressive extraskeletal calcifications that occur in conjunction with a Ca × P product that is consistently greater than 75 to 80, despite appropriate phosphate restriction; (4) severe and progressive skeletal pain or fractures; and (5) the appearance of calciphylaxis (ischemic lesions of soft tissue and skin and vascular calcification).[120-122]

Persistent and significant hypercalcemia (serum calcium level greater than 11.0 mg/100 ml) that occurs in association with symptoms of nausea or vomiting or evidence of ulcer disease may indicate a need for subtotal parathyroidectomy. Hypercalcemia can develop in uremic patients who lack evidence of secondary hyperparathyroidism, and parathyroid surgery should not be undertaken unless bone erosions and elevated serum iPTH levels are seen.

The presence of marked hyperphosphatemia and overt secondary hyperparathyroidism in a noncompliant uremic patient presents a difficult therapeutic dilemma for the physician. Parathyroid surgery may lead to a transient lowering of blood phosphorus and even to the resolution of ectopic calcifications, but secondary hyperparathyroidism may recur, with all its manifestations, unless the patient follows the prescribed treatment with dietary phosphorus restriction and phosphate-binders, e.g., calcium carbonate.

The procedure for parathyroidectomy should be to identify four parathyroid glands, with the selection of one gland that is to be only partially resected. A part of this gland is removed, leaving 60 to 80 mg of viable tissue in place; after the frozen sections are available from the first gland, each of the other three glands can be removed. Alternatively, total parathyroidectomy should be done with transplantation of parathyroid tissue into the forearm.

After parathyroid surgery, the postoperative control of blood calcium levels may pose a problem, although this may be less serious when some parathyroid tissue is left in place. The preoperative presence of skeletal erosions is more often followed by severe hypocalcemia; the preoperative treatment of such patients with $1,25(OH)_2D_3$, the intravenous infusions of calcium gluconate, and treatment with oral calcium supplements may be needed. Tetany and even seizures can occur during the postoperative period; for reasons that are uncertain, tetanic seizures most often occur during the later period of hemodialysis or shortly after dialysis, when the degree of hypocalcemia is undoubtedly less marked than at other times. Such hypocalcemic tetany may occur 3 to 4 weeks postoperatively.[123] Serum levels of phosphorus and magnesium may decrease after parathyroid surgery, and phosphate-binders should be withheld if the serum phosphorus falls below 2.5 mg/100 ml. However, serum phosphorus should not be allowed to increase above 3.5 to 4.0 mg/100 ml because of the risk of aggravating hypocalcemia. Rapid remineralization of the skeleton is usually occurring during this period, and blood calcium will usually begin to rise after the "hungry" bones have been "repleted" with calcium. A fall in the elevated plasma alkaline phosphatase toward normal may be a clue that rapid skeletal remineralization is nearly completed and indicates that calcium supplements and vitamin D dosage may be reduced or discontinued.

The remnant parathyroid tissue may undergo hyperplasia and lead to the reappearance of overt secondary hyperparathyroidism, and the management of such a situation may be difficult. A second surgical procedure may be associated with greater technical difficulties and significant complications compared with the initial operation. Because of the difficulty and risk of a second surgical procedure, total parathyroidectomy with autotransplantation of some parathyroid tissue to the forearm has been recommended.[124] Such tissue transplanted to the forearm may be more accessible for subsequent surgical removal. Another risk of parathyroid surgery is the development of hypoparathyroidism. To avoid this, parathyroid tissue may be frozen and stored to be implanted later if persistent hypocalcemia appears. It would seem that total parathyroidectomy has little place in the management of renal bone disease, since it may predispose uremic patients to the development of an isolated mineralizing defect.

The availability of highly active forms of vitamin D has made the need for parathyroid surgery less urgent.[64] Whether one or more of the vitamin D analogues may be effective in leading to long-term suppression of the parathyroid glands must await further clinical evaluation.

E. Other Treatment Considerations: Aluminum Accumulation

The presence of excessive quantities of trace metals, particularly aluminum, in the water used to prepare dialysate can cause bone disease in uremic patients.[87] When a dialysis unit encounters an unusually high incidence of overt skeletal disease, the purity of the water supply should be tested and the methods of water treatment evaluated. Appropriate means of water purification are indicated in a center that encounters an excessively high incidence of bone disease, particularly osteomalacia. The amount of aluminum in the dialysate should not exceed 10 mμg/liter. Recently, however, it has become apparent that in the United States the main source of aluminum responsible for the development of bone disease is secondary to the ingestion of phosphate binders containing aluminum. Several reports have shown that desferrioxamine (Desferal), a chelating agent, is useful as a diagnostic tool as well as a therapeutic agent for patients with aluminum accumulation.[125-127] When Desferal is given intravenously in the dose of 40 to 60 mg/kg, it produces an increase in the levels of serum aluminum. When the increment in serum aluminum observed after the administration of Desferal is greater than 250 μg/liter, likely the patient is at risk to develop bone disease secondary to aluminum accumulation.[126] Aluminum can deposit in the mineralization front at the interface between bone and osteoid and impairs the normal mineralization of bone. Most of these patients also have low levels of circulating iPTH. Although the "Desferal test" (DFO test) is a useful noninvasive tool in the diagnosis of aluminum accumulation, bone histomorphometry with special staining for aluminum is the definitive test in the diagnosis of aluminum-induced osteomalacia. If a patient requires desferrioxamine treatment for aluminum-induced osteomalacia, the usual dose of Desferal is 1 to 3 g per week for 4 to 6 months. A second bone biopsy after 1 year can conclusively determine the effectiveness of the treatment (Table 13–1).

This work was supported by U.S. Public Health Service NIADDK grants AM–09976, AM–07126, and RR 00036.

The authors wish to express their appreciation to Mrs. Patricia Shy for her excellent assistance in the preparation of this manuscript.

Table 13–1. Guidelines for Management of Renal Osteodystrophy

Control of Serum Phosphorus (P) (5.0–5.5 mg/100 ml)

Restrict dietary phosphorus intake to 0.6 to 0.9 g/day
Individualize dosage of phosphate binders and ingest with meals: aluminum hydroxide, aluminum carbonate, or calcium carbonate; use minimum dose of aluminum-containing compounds
Avoid hypophosphatemia
Avoid aluminum excess

Adequate Calcium Intake

Give oral calcium supplements providing 1–2 g/day, when serum P is controlled
Dialysate Ca should be 6.0–6.5 mg/100 ml (3.0–3.25 mEq/liter)

Use of Vitamin D Sterols

Indications for treatment: Adequate control of serum P and:
- Hypocalcemia
- Overt secondary hyperparathyroidism (high iPTH and high alkaline phosphatase and bone erosions) with serum Ca < 11.0–11.5 mg/100ml
- Osteomalacia, particularly with secondary hyperparathyroidism
- Advanced renal failure in children
- Concomitant anticonvulsant therapy
- Proximal myopathy
- Prophylaxis in dialysis patients (cost-benefit ratio not established)
- Types and approximate daily doses:
  - Vitamin D_2 or D_3: 10,000–200,000 IU (0.25–5.0 mg/day)
  - Dihydrotachysterol: 0.25–2.0 mg/day
  - Calcidiol 25 (OH) D_3: 25–100 μg/day
  - Calcitriol 1,25 $(OH)_2D_3$: 0.25–1.0 μg/day; intravenous calcitriol more effective: 0.5–3.0 μg thrice weekly

Parathyroidectomy

Indications: Evidence of secondary hyperparathyroidism (x-ray erosions, biopsy, osteitis fibrosa, and adequately elevated iPTH), exclusion of Al-related bone disease, plus any of the following:
- Persistent hypercalcemia (serum Ca > 11.5–12.0 mg/100 ml)
- Progressive or symptomatic extraskeletal calcification (particularly with serum Ca x P product > 75 (both in mg/100 ml)
- Pruritis not responsive to other treatment
- Calciphylaxis (ischemic ulcers and necrosis)
- Symptomatic and persistent hypercalcemia after renal transplantation

Management of Aluminum Overload

Indications for treatment: Symptoms of osteomalacia, myopathy, or encephalopathy plus evidence of Al overload: bone biopsy, hyperaluminemia (200 μg/liter), or increment in plasma Al after desferrioxamine infusion (change 250μg/L after 30mg/kg)
- Substitute $CaCO_3$ for Al-containing PO_4 binders
- Desferrioxamine infusions for Al chelation (1.0–3.0 g, once weekly)

Other Treatment Considerations

Purification of water for dialysate preparation: aluminum conc. < 10 μg/liter; remove fluoride calcium, and magnesium
- Normalize acid-base status
- Appropriate dialysate magnesium: 0.6–1.0 mg/100 ml (0.5–0.8 mEq/liter)
- Avoid unnecessary treatment with phenytoin, barbiturates, or glutethimide

Modified from Coburn JW, et al: Altered divalent ion metabolism in renal disease and renal osteodystrophy. *In* Maxwell MH, Kleeman CR (eds): Clinical Disorders of Fluid and Electrolyte Metabolism. 3rd ed. New York, McGraw-Hill, 1980.

References

1. Albright F, Drake TG, Sulkowitch HW: Renal osteitis fibrosa cystica: Report of case with discussion of metabolic aspects. Johns Hopkins Med J 60:377–385, 1937.
2. Follis RH Jr, Jackson DA: Renal osteomalacia and osteitis fibrosa in adults. Johns Hopkins Med J 72:232–241, 1943.
3. Stanbury SW, Lumb GA: Metabolic studies of renal osteodystrophy. I. Calcium, phosphorus and nitrogen metabolism in rickets, osteomalacia, and hyperparathyroidism complicating chronic uremia and in the osteomalacia of the adult Fanconi syndrome. Medicine 41:1–31, 1962.
4. Dent CE, Harper CM, Philpot GR: Treatment of renal-glomerular osteodystrophy. Q J Med 30:1–31, 1961.
5. Reiss E, Canterbury JM, Egdahl RH: Measurement of serum parathyroid hormone in renal insufficiency. Trans Assoc Am Physicians 81:104–114, 1968.
6. Arnaud CD: Hyperparathyroidism and renal failure. Kidney Int 4:89–95, 1973.
7. Slatopolsky E, Caglar S, Pennell JP, et al: On the pathogenesis of hyperparathyroidism in chronic experimental insufficiency in the dog. J Clin Invest 50:492–499, 1971.
8. Slatopolsky E, Caglar S, Gradowska L, et al: On the prevention of secondary hyperparathyroidism in experimental chronic renal disease using "proportional reduction" of dietary phosphorus intake. Kidney Int 2:147–151, 1972.
9. Slatopolsky E, Bricker NS: The role of phosphorus restriction in the prevention of secondary hyperparathyroidism in chronic renal disease. Kidney Int 4:141–145, 1973.
10. Reiss E, Canterbury MJ, Bercovitz MA, et al: The role of phosphate in the secretion of parathyroid hormone in man. J Clin Invest 49:2146–2149, 1970.
11. LaFlame GH, Jowsey J: Bone and soft tissue changes with oral phosphate supplements. J Clin Invest 51:2834–2839, 1972.
12. Jowsey J, Reiss E, Canterbury JM: Long term effects of high phosphate intake on parathyroid hormone levels and bone metabolism. Acta Orthop Scand 45:801–806, 1974.
13. Rutherford WE, Bordier P, Marie P: Phosphate control and 25-hydroxycholecalciferol administration in preventing experimental renal osteodystrophy in the dog. J Clin Invest 60:332–341, 1977.
14. Llach F, Massry SG, Koffler A, et al: Secondary hyperparathyroidism in early renal failure: Role of phosphate retention. Kidney Int 12:459–463, 1977.
15. Fotino S: Phosphate excretion in chronic renal failure: Evidence for a mechanism other than circulating parathyroid hormone. Clin Nephrol 8:499–503, 1977.
16. Fournier AE, Arnaud CD, Johnson WJ, et al: Etiology of hyperparathyroidism and bone disease during chronic hemodialysis. II. Factors affecting serum immunoreactive parathyroid hormone. J Clin Invest 50:599–605, 1971.
17. Tanaka Y, DeLuca HF: The control of 25-dihydroxyvitamin D metabolism by inorganic phosphorus. Arch Biochem Biophys 159:566–570, 1973.
18. Oldham SB, Smith R, Hartenbower DL, et al: The acute effects of 1,25-dihydroxycholecalciferol on serum immunoreactive parathyroid hormone (iPTH) in the dog. Endocrinology 104:248–254, 1979.
19. Goldman R, Bassett SH: Phosphorus excretion in renal failure. J Clin Invest 33:1623–1628, 1954.
20. Raisz LG, Niemann I: Effect of phosphate, calcium and magnesium on bone resorption and hormonal responses in tissue culture. Endocrinology 85:446–452, 1969.
21. Fraser DR, Kodicek E: Unique biosynthesis by kidney of a biologically active vitamin D metabolite. Nature 228:764–766, 1970.
22. Liu SH, Chu HI: Studies of calcium and phosphorus metabolism with special reference to the pathogenesis and effect of dihydrotachysterol and iron. Medicine 22:103–161, 1943.
23. Coburn JW, Koppel MH, Brickman AS, et al: Study of intestinal absorption of calcium in patients with renal failure. Kidney Int 3:264–272, 1973.
24. Slatopolsky E, Gray R, Adams ND, et al: The pathogenesis of secondary hyperparathyroidism in early renal failure. *In* Norman A (ed): Fourth International Workshop in Vitamin D. Berlin, de Gruyter, 1979, p 1209.
25. Cheung AK, Manolagas SC, Cathewood BD, et al: Determination of serum $1,25(OH)_2D_3$ levels in renal disease. Kidney Int 24:104–109, 1983.
26. Taylor CM, Caverzacio J, Jung A, et al: Unilateral nephrectomy and 1,25-dihydroxyvitamin D_3. Kidney Int 24:37–42, 1984.
27. Malluche HH, Werner E, Ritz E: Intestinal absorption of calcium and whole body calcium retention in incipient and advanced renal failure. Mineral Electrolyte Metab 1:263–270, 1978.
28. Sherrard DJ, Baylink DJ, Wergedal JE, et al: Quantitative histological studies on the pathogenesis of uremic bone disease. J Clin Endocrinol 39:119–135, 1974.
29. Bordier PJ, Tun-chot S, Ewastwood JB, et al: Lack of histological evidence of vitamin D abnormality in the bones of anephric patients. Clin Sci 44:33–41, 1973.
30. Garabedian M, Pavlovitch H, Fellot L, et al: Metabolism of 25-hydroxyvitamin D_3 in anephric rats: A new active metabolite. Proc Natl Acad Sci USA 71:554–557, 1974.
31. Olgaard K, Finco D, Schwartz J, et al: Effect of $24,25(OH)_2D_3$ on PTH levels and bone histology in dogs with chronic uremia. Kidney Int 26:791–797, 1984.
32. Evanson JM: The response to the infusion of parathyroid extract in hypocalcemic states. Clin Sci 31:63–73, 1966.
33. Llach F, Massry SG, Singer FR, et al: Skeletal resistance of endogenous parathyroid hormone in patients with early renal failure: A possible cause for secondary hyperparathyroidism. J Clin Endocrinol Metab 41:339–345, 1975.
34. Kaplan MA, Canterbury JM, Gavellas GA, et al: The calcemic and phosphaturic effects of parathyroid hormone in the normal and uremic dog. Metabolism 27:1785–1792, 1978.
35. Massry SG, Stein R, Garty J, et al: Skeletal resistance to the calcemic action of parathyroid hormone in uremia: Role of $1,25(OH)_2D_3$. Kidney Int 1:467–474, 1975.
36. Somverville P, Kaye M: Evidence that resistance to the calcemic action of parathyroid hormone in rats with acute uremia is caused by phosphate retention. Kidney Int 16:552–560, 1979.

37. Morrissey J, Cohn DV: Regulation of secretion of parathormone and secretory protein-I from separate intracellular pools by calcium, dibutyryl cyclic AMP, and (1) isoproterenol. J Cell Biol 82:93–102, 1979.
38. Morrissey J, Cohn DV: Secretion and degradation of parathormone as a function of intracellular maturation of hormone pools. J Cell Biol 83:521–528, 1979.
39. MacGregor RR, Chu LLH, Hamilton JW, et al: Studies on the subcellular localization of parathyroid hormone in the bovine parathyroid gland: Separation of newly synthesized from mature forms. Endocrinology 93:1387–1397, 1973.
40. MacGregor RR, Hamilton JW, Cohn DV: The bypass of tissue hormone stores during the secretion of newly synthesized parathyroid hormone. Endocrinology 97:178–188, 1975.
41. Brown EM, Thatcher JC: Adenosine 3′,5′-monophosphate (cAMP)-dependent protein kinase and the regulation of parathyroid hormone release by divalent cations and agents elevating cellular cAMP in dispersed bovine parathyroid cells. Endocrinology 110:1374–1380, 1982.
42. Hanley DA, Takatsuki K, Birnbaumer ME, et al: In vitro perfusion for the study of parathyroid hormone secretion: Effects of extracellular calcium concentration and beta-adrenergic regulation on bovine parathyroid hormone secretion in vitro. Calcif Tissue Int 32:19–27, 1980.
43. Brown EM: Relationship of 3′,5′-adenosine monophosphate accumulation to parathyroid hormone release in dispersed cells from pathological human parathyroid tissue. J Clin Endocrinol Metab 52:961–968, 1981.
44. Blum JW, Fisher JA, Hunziker WH, et al: Parathyroid hormone response to catecholamines and to changes of extracellular calcium in cows. J Clin Invest 61:1113–1122, 1978.
45. Dufresne LR, Gitelman HJ: A possible role of adenyl cyclase in the regulation of parathyroid activity by calcium. *In* Talmage RV, Munson PL (eds): Calcium, Parathyroid Hormone and the Calcitonins. Amsterdam, Excerpta Medica Foundation, 1972, p 202.
46. Matsuzaki S, Dumont JE: Effect of calcium ion on horse parathyroid gland adenyl cyclase. Biochim Biophys Acta 284:227–234, 1972.
47. Rodriguez JH, Morrison A, Slatopolsky E, et al: Adenyl cyclase of human parathyroid glands. J Clin Endocrinol Metab 47:319–325, 1978.
48. Bellorin-Font E, Martin KJ, Freitag JJ, et al: Altered adenylate cyclase kinetics in hyperfunctioning human parathyroid glands. J Clin Endocrinol Metab 52:499–507, 1981.
49. Ontjes DA, Mahafdfee DD, Wells SA: Adenylate cyclase activity in human parathyroid tissues: Reduced sensitivity to suppression by calcium in parathyroid adenomas as compared with normal glands from normocalcemic-subjects or non-involved glands from hyperparathyroid subjects. Metabolism 30:406–411, 1981.
50. Habener JF: Responsiveness of neoplastic and hyperplastic parathyroid tissue to calcium *in vitro*. J Clin Invest 62:436–450, 1978.
51. Brown EM, Brennan MF, Hurwitz S, et al: Dispersed cells prepared from human parathyroid glands: Distinct calcium sensitivity of adenomas vs. primary hyperplasia. J Clin Endocrinol Metab 46:267–275, 1978.
52. Brown EM: Set-point for calcium: Its role in normal and abnormal parathyroid secretion. *In* Cohn DV, Talmage RV, Matthews JL (eds): Hormonal Control of Calcium Metabolism. Amsterdam, Excerpta Medica, 1981, p 35.
53. Brown EM, Wilson RE, Eastman RC, et al: Abnormal regulation of parathyroid hormone release by calcium in secondary hyperparathyroidism due to chronic renal failure. J Clin Endocrinol Metab 54:172–179, 1982.
54. Brown EM: Four-parameter model of the sigmoidal relationship between parathyroid hormone release and extracellular calcium concentration in normal and abnormal parathyroid tissue. J Clin Endocrinol Metab 56:572–581, 1983.
55. Chertow BS, Baylink DJ, Wergedal MH, et al: Decrease in serum immunoreactive parathyroid hormone in rats and in parathyroid hormone secretion *in vivo* by 1,25-dihydroxycholecalciferol. J Clin Invest 56:668–678, 1975.
56. Au WYW, Bukowsky A: Inhibition of PTH secretion by vitamin D metabolites in organ cultures of rat parathyroids. Fed Proc 35:530–531, 1976.
57. Dietel M, Dorn G, Montz R, et al: Influence of vitamin D_3, 1,25-dihydroxyvitamin D_3 and 24,25-dihydroxyvitamin D_3 on parathyroid hormone secretion, adenosine 3′,5′-monophosphate release, and ultrastructure of parathyroid glands in organ culture. Endocrinology 105:237–245, 1979.
58. Oldham SB, Fischer JA, Shen LH, et al: Isolation and properties of calcium-binding protein from porcine parathyroid glands. Biochemistry 13:4790–4796, 1974.
59. Brumbaugh PF, Hughes MR, Haussler MR: Cytoplasmic and nuclear binding components for 1α,25-dihydroxyvitamin D_3 in chick parathyroid glands. Proc Natl Acad Sci USA 72:4871–4875, 1975.
60. Llach F, Coburn JW, Brickman AD, et al: Acute actions of 1,25-dihydroxyvitamin D_3 in normal man, effect on calcium and parathyroid status. J Clin Endocrinol Metab 4:1054–1060, 1977.
61. Tanaka Y, DeLuca HF, Ghazarian JG, et al: Effect of vitamin D and its metabolites on serum parathyroid hormone levels in the rat. Mineral Electrolyte Metab 2:20–25, 1979.
62. Golden P, Greenwalt A, Martin K, et al: Lack of a direct effect of 1,25-dihydroxycholecalciferol on secretion of parathyroid hormone. Endocrinology 107:602–607, 1980.
63. Christiansen C, Christiansen MS, Melsen F, et al: Mineral metabolism in chronic renal failure with special reference to serum concentrations of $1,25(OH)_2D_3$ and $24,25(OH)_2D_3$. Clin Nephrol 15:18–22, 1981.
64. Slatopolsky E, Weerts C, Thielan J, et al: Marked suppression of secondary hyperparathyroidism by intravenous administration of 1,25-dihydroxycholecalciferol in uremic patients. J Clin Invest 74:2136–2143, 1984.
65. Silver J, Russell J, Lettieri D, et al: Vitamin D metabolites suppress cytoplasma in RNA coding for prepro-parathyroid hormone in isolated parathyroid cells. Clin Res 32:561A, 1984.
66. Chan YL, McKay C, Dye E, et al: The effect of 1,25-dihydroxycholecalciferol on parathyroid hormone secretion by monolayer cultures of bovine parathyroid cells. Clin Res 32:795A, 1984.
67. Hruska KA, Kopelman R, Rutherford WE, et al: Metabolism of immunoreactive parathyroid hormone

in the dog. The role of the kidney and the effects of chronic renal disease. J Clin Invest 56:39–46, 1975.

68. Martin KJ, Hruska KA, Lewis J, et al: The renal handling of parathyroid hormone. Role of peritubular uptake and glomerular filtration. J Clin Invest 60:808–814, 1977.

69. Freitag J, Martin KJ, Hruska KA, et al: Impaired parathyroid hormone metabolism in patients with chronic renal failure. N Engl J Med 298:29–32, 1978.

70. Hruska K, Korkor A, Martin K, et al: The peripheral metabolism of parathyroid hormone: Role of the liver and kidney and the effect of chronic renal failure. J Clin Invest 67:885–892, 1981.

71. Russell JE, Avioli LV: 25-hydroxycholecalciferol-enhanced bone maturation in the parathyroprivic state. J Clin Invest 56:792–798, 1975.

72. Litzow JR, Lemann J Jr, Lennon EJ: The effect of treatment of acidosis on calcium balance in patients with chronic azotemic renal disease. J Clin Invest 46:280–288, 1967.

73. Ward MK, Feest TG, Ellis HA, et al: Osteomalacic dialysis osteodystrophy: Evidence for a water borne aetiological agent, probably aluminum. Lancet 1:841–845, 1978.

74. Teitelbaum SL, Bergfeld MA, Freitag J, et al: Do parathyroid hormone and 1,25-dihydroxyvitamin D modulate bone formation in uremia? J Clin Endocrinol Metab 51:247–251, 1980.

75. Felsenfeld AJ, Harrelson JM, Gutman RA, et al: Osteomalacia after parathyroidectomy in patients with uremia. Ann Intern Med 96:34–39, 1982.

76. Schoenfeld PJ, Martin JA, Barnes B, et al: Amelioration of myopathy with 25-dihydroxyvitamin D_3 therapy 25(OH)D_3 in patients on chronic hemodialysis. Abstract Book. Third Workshop on Vitamin D. Asilomar, 1977, p 160.

77. Mallette LE, Patten BM, Engel WK: Neuromuscular disease in secondary hyperparathyroidism. Ann Intern Med 82:474–479, 1975.

78. Mirahmadi KS, Coburn JW, Bluestone R: Calcific periarthritis and hemodialysis. JAMA 223:548–552, 1973.

79. Coburn JW, Brickman AS, Sherrard DJ, et al: Defective skeletal mineralization in uremia without relation to vitamin D, serum Ca or P. Kidney Int 12:455–459, 1977.

80. Hruska KA, Teitelbaum SL, Kopelman R, et al: The predictability of the histologic features of uremic bone disease by non-invasive techniques. Metab Bone Dis Rel Res 1:39–44, 1978.

81. Ritz E, Malluche HH, Boimmer J, et al: Metabolic bone disease in patients on maintenance hemodialysis. Nephron 12:393–397, 1974.

82. Parfitt AM: Clinical and radiographic manifestations of renal osteodystrophy. *In* David DS (ed): Calcium Metabolism in Renal Failure and Nephrolithiasis. John Wiley and Sons, New York, 1977, p 150.

83. Parfitt AM: Soft tissue calcification in uremia. Arch Intern Med 124:544–552, 1969.

84. Fournier AE, Johnson WJ, Taves DR, et al: Etiology of hyperparathyroidism and bone disease during chronic hemodialysis. I. Association of bone disease with potentially etiologic factors. J Clin Invest 50:592–598, 1971.

85. Rutherford E, Mercado A, Hruska K, et al: An evaluation of a new and effective phosphorus binding agent. Trans Am Soc Artif Intern Organs 19:446–449, 1973.

86. Berlyne GM, Ben-Ari J, Pest D, et al: Hyperaluminaemia from aluminum resins in renal failure. Lancet 2:494–499, 1970.

87. Alfrey AC, LeGendre GR, Kaehny WD: Dialysis encephalopathy syndrome: Possible aluminum intoxication. N Engl J Med 294:184–187, 1976.

88. Ward MK, Feest TG, Ellis HA, et al: Osteomalacic dialysis osteodystrophy: Evidence for a water-borne aetiological agent, probably aluminum. Lancet 1:841–845, 1978.

89. Hercz G, Kraut JA, Andress DA, et al: Use of calcium carbonate as a phosphate binder in dialysis patients. Mineral Electrolyte Metab 12:314–319, 1986.

90. Slatopolsky E, Weerts C, Lopez-Hilker S, et al: Calcium carbonate as a phosphate binder in patients with chronic renal failure undergoing dialysis. N Engl J Med 315:157–161, 1986.

91. Salusky IB, Coburn JW, Foley J, et al: Calcium carbonate as a phosphate binder in children on dialysis. Kidney Int 27:185A, 1985.

92. Kopple JD, Coburn JW: Metabolic studies of low protein diets in uremia. II. Calcium, phosphorus and magnesium. Medicine 52:597–607, 1973.

93. Clarkson EM, Eastwood JB, Koutsaimanis KG, et al: Net intestinal absorption of calcium in patients with chronic renal failure. Kidney Int 3:258–263, 1973.

94. Meyrier A, Marsac J, Richet G: The influence of a high calcium carbonate intake on bone disease in patients undergoing hemodialysis. Kidney Int 4:146–153, 1973.

95. Curtis JR, De Wardener HE, Gower PE, et al: The use of calcium carbonate and calcium phosphate without vitamin D in the management of renal osteodystrophy. Proc Eur Dial Transplant Assoc 7:141–144, 1980.

96. Mirahmadi KS, Duff BS, Shinaberger JH, et al: A controlled evaluation of clinical and metabolic effects of dialysate calcium levels during regular hemodialysis. Trans Am Soc Artif Intern Organs 17:118–120, 1971.

97. Goldsmith RS, Johnson WJ: Role of phosphate depletion and high dialysate calcium in controlling dialytic renal osteodystrophy. Kidney Int 4:154–160, 1973.

98. Stanbury SW, Lumb GA: Parathyroid function in chronic renal failure: A statistical survey of the plasma biochemistry in azotemic renal osteodystrophy. Q J Med 35:1–26, 1966.

99. Kaye M, Chatterjee G, Cohen GF, et al: Arrest of hyperparathyroid bone disease with dihydrotachysterol in patients undergoing chronic hemodialysis. Ann Intern Med 73:225–231, 1970.

100. Kaye M, Sagar S: Effect of dihydrotachysterol on calcium absorption in uremia. Metabolism 21:815–820, 1972.

101. Witmer G, Margolis A, Fontaine O, et al: Effects of 25-hydroxycholecalciferol on bone lesions of children with terminal renal failure. Kidney Int 10:395–403, 1976.

102. Recker R, Schoenfeld P, Letteri J, et al: The efficacy of calcifediol in renal osteodystrophy. Arch Intern Med 138:857–861, 1978.

103. Papapoulos SE, Brownjohn AM, Goodwin FJ, et al: The effect of 1α-hydroxycholecalciferol on secondary hyperparathyroidism of chronic renal failure. *In* Norman AW, Schaefer K, Coburn JW, et al (eds): Vitamin D: Biochemical, Chemical and Clinical

Aspects Related to Calcium Metabolism. Berlin, de Gruyter, 1977, p 693.

104. Brickman AS, Sherrard DJ, Jowsey J, et al: 1,25-dihydroxycholecalciferol: Effect on skeletal lesions and plasma parathyroid hormone in uremic osteodystrophy. Arch Intern Med 134:883–889, 1974.

105. Silverberg DS, Bettcher KB, Dossetor JB, et al: Effect of 1,25-dihydroxycholecalciferol in renal osteodystrophy. Can Med Assoc J 112:190–194, 1975.

106. Counts SG, Baylink DJ, Shen FH, et al: Vitamin D intoxication in an anephric child. Ann Intern Med 82:196–203, 1975.

107. Hughes MR, Baylink DJ, Jones PG, et al: Radioligand receptor assay for 25-hydroxyvitamin D_2D_3. J Clin Invest 58:61–70, 1976.

108. Teitelbaum SL, Bone JM, Stein PM, et al: Calcifediol in chronic renal insufficiency: Skeletal response. JAMA 235:164–169, 1976.

109. Eastwood JB, Stamp TCB, De Wardener HE, et al: The effect of 25-hydroxyvitamin D_3 in osteomalacia of chronic renal failure. Clin Sci Mol Med 52:499–504, 1977.

110. Fournier AE, Bordier PJ, Gueris J, et al: 1α-hydroxycholecalciferol and 25-hydroxycholecalciferol in renal bone disease. Proc Eur Dial Transplant Assoc 12:227–232, 1976.

111. Bordier P, Rasmussen H, Marie P, et al: Vitamin D metabolites and bone mineralization in man. J Clin Endocrinol Metab 46:284–294, 1978.

112. Coburn JW, Brickman AS, Sherrard DJ, et al: Clinical efficacy of 1,25-dihydroxyvitamin D_3 in renal osteodystrophy. *In* Norman AW, Schaefer K, Coburn JW, et al (eds): Vitamin D: Biochemical, Chemical and Clinical Aspects Related to Calcium Metabolism. Berlin, de Gruyter, 1977, p 657.

113. Sherrard DJ, Coburn JW, Brickman AS, et al: A histologic comparison of $1,25(OH)_2$ vitamin D treatment with calcium supplementation in renal osteodystrophy. *In* Norman AW, Schaefer K, Coburn JW, et al: Vitamin D: Biochemical and Clinical Aspects Related to Calcium Metabolism. Berlin, de Gruyter, 1977, p 719.

114. Sherrard DJ, Brickman AS, Coburn JW, et al: Skeletal response to treatment with 1,25-dihydroxyvitamin D in renal failure. Contrib Nephrol 18:92–98, 1980.

115. Eastwood JB, Phillips ME, De Wardener HE, et al: Biochemical and histological effects of 1,25-dihydroxycholecalciferol in the osteomalacia of chronic renal failure. *In* Norman AW, Schaefer K, Grigoleit HG, et al (eds): Vitamin D and Problems Related to Uremic Bone Disease. Berlin, de Gruyter, 1975, p 595.

116. Chesney RW, Moorthy AW, Eisman JA, et al: Increased growth after long-term oral 1,25-vitamin D_3 in childhood renal osteodystrophy. N Engl J Med 298:238–241, 1978.

117. Ahmed KY, Wills MR, Varghese Z, et al: Long-term effects of small doses of 1,25-dihydroxycholecalciferol in renal osteodystrophy. Lancet 1:629–632, 1978.

118. Winkler SN, Brickman AS, Wong EGC, et al: Hypercalcemia during treatment of uremic patients with $1,25(OH)_2D_3$: Analysis of 43 cases. *In* Norman AW, Schaefer K, von Herrath D, et al: Vitamin D: Basic Research and Its Clinical Application. Berlin, de Gruyter, 1979, p 851.

119. Christiansen C, Rodbro P, Christiansen MS, et al: Deterioration of renal function during treatment of chronic renal failure with 1,25-dihydroxycholecalciferol. Lancet 2:700–708, 1978.

120. Wilson RE, Hampers CL, Bernstein DS, et al: Subtotal parathyroidectomy in chronic renal failure. Ann Surg 174:640–649, 1971.

121. Katz AD, Kaplan L: Parathyroidectomy for hyperplasia in renal disease. Arch Surg 107:51–59, 1973.

122. David SD: Calcium metabolism in renal failure. Am J Med 58:48–56, 1975.

123. Friedler RM, Rosenblatt MG, Corredor JW, et al: Seizures during hemodialysis, 2 to 20 months after parathyroidectomy, in patients with secondary hyperparathyroidism. Abstract Book, Clinical Dialysis and Transplant Forum, New Orleans, Louisiana, 1972, p 5.

124. Wells SA Jr, Gunnells JC, Shelburne JD, et al: Transplantation of the parathyroid glands in man: Clinical indications and results. Surgery 78:34–41, 1975.

125. Milliner DS, Nebeker HG, Ott SA, et al: Use of the desferrioxamine infusion test in the diagnosis of aluminum-related osteodystrophy. Ann Intern Med 101:775–780, 1984.

126. Ackrill P, Day JP, Gargstang FM, et al: Treatment of fracturing renal osteodystrophy by desferrioxamine. Proc Eur Dial Transplant Assoc 19:203–207, 1982.

127. Malluche HH, Smith AJ, Abreo K, et al: The use of desferrioxamine in the management of aluminum accumulation in bone in patients with renal failure. N Engl J Med 311:140–144, 1984.

JOEL F. HABENER
JOHN T. POTTS, JR.

14

Primary Hyperparathyroidism

Primary hyperparathyroidism is a disorder due to an excessive secretion of parathyroid hormone.[6] The abnormal concentration of circulating hormone usually leads to hypercalcemia and hypophosphatemia. Associated with these disturbances in mineral ion metabolism may be recurrent nephrolithiasis, peptic ulcers, mental changes, and excessive bone resorption. Recently it has been evident that the disease is more frequent than previously appreciated and is often asymptomatic.

This disorder was first recognized as a clinical entity over 50 years ago when it was discovered that surgical removal of parathyroid adenomas led to cure of the malady.[1-4,8] Albright and associates contributed considerably toward the understanding of the pathophysiology of this disease and described many of its protean manifestations.[5,6] An account of one of the first patients studied in depth was reported by Bauer and Federman.[7]

Primary hyperparathyroidism is diagnosed most commonly between the fifth and seventh decades,[9-12] but the disease is seen at earlier ages and occasionally in young children.[13,263,264] The incidence of the disease is two to five times higher in women than in men, and increases with age, particularly in women.[9,10] The prevalence of primary hyperparathyroidism is much higher than was recognized previously. As a consequence of the widespread introduction during the past decade of accurate and inexpensive measurement of serum calcium, the disease is diagnosed much more frequently than in earlier decades. Three decades ago the estimated prevalence was 1 case per 10,000.[11] At present in women over the age of 60 years, the annual incidence of primary hyperparathyroidism is reported to be 2 cases per 1000 persons per year. It is extremely difficult, therefore, to properly evaluate the frequency of occurrence of the various symptoms and complications of hyperparathyroidism; as many as 50% to 90% of patients seen at major medical referral centers present with no clearly identifiable symptoms.[9,12]

I. SIGNS AND SYMPTOMS

A. Renal Manifestations

Prior to the last decade, kidney involvement, particularly recurrent nephrolithiasis, was reported in 60% to 70% of patients.[14,15] The incidence of kidney involvement is less frequent today but is still an important manifestation of primary hyperparathyroidism in 5% to 20% of patients.[9,12,16-22]

The pathophysiologic effects of excessive parathyroid hormone on the kidney in patients with primary hyperparathyroidism can be considered in two broad categories: anatomic and functional. Under the category of anatomic defects is the occurrence of nephrolithiasis or nephrocalcinosis; under functional defects are included a spectrum of tubular and glomerular disorders that result from the deleterious effects of sustained hypercalcemia or excessive concentrations of parathyroid hormone, or both.

Although nephrolithiasis is not seen as frequently as in former years, the occurrence of this complication is frequent enough to deserve continued consideration. In patients with presumptive hyperparathyroidism but without symptoms at the time the diagnosis was established during the 1960s, the incidence of nephrolithiasis detectable radiographically was reported in 1971 to be as high as 32%[22] although much lower than the 60% to 70% of earlier decades. The incidence of nephrolithiasis is clearly falling still further as more and more asymptomatic patients with hyperparathyroidism are detected. In continuing long-term studies of primary hyperparathyroidism during the past decade at the Mayo Clinic and the Henry Ford Hospital (Detroit), nephrolithiasis was found in only 5% to 10% of patients.[9,20]

A variety of renal functional abnormalities occur in hyperparathyroidism, even in the absence of detectable nephrocalcinosis and/or nephrolithiasis.[14,23,24] These include elevation of blood urea nitrogen and serum creatinine, reflecting modest to marked reduction in glomerular filtration rate, and numerous renal tubular defects, particularly impairment of proximal tubular function. Parathyroid hormone has multiple direct effects on renal tubular function (Chapter 3). In severe hyperparathyroidism these effects cause a reduction in net acid secretion (renal tubular acidosis of the proximal, or type II, category, proximal RTA)[23] as well as aminoaciduria and glycosuria. Increased phosphate clearance with readily detectable abnormalities in measured parameters of renal tubular phosphate reabsorption leads to fasting hypophosphatemia, a classic laboratory indication of hyperparathyroidism (see Chapter 3 for details).

These overall defects occur in a continuous spectrum of severity and are influenced by anatomic changes in the kidney, such as diffuse calcium deposition (nephrocalcinosis) and the inflammation due to bacterial infection. Tubular defects involving compromise of proximal tubular function and urinary concentrating ability may be found in the absence of roentgenographically demonstrable renal calcification or evidence of infection.[10,23,25] A difficulty in attempting to assess the incidence and significance of more subtle tubular disorders is the lack of detailed evaluation of proximal and distal tubular function in most reported series of patients with hyperparathyroidism. With careful evaluation of renal function, it is found that (proximal) RTA is a rather common finding in primary hyperparathyroidism. This situation frequently results in mild hyperchloremic acidosis and reduction in serum bicarbonate. On the other hand,[25,26] hypercalcemia *per se* produced experimentally[27] or in disease states associated with hypercalcemia not due to hyperparathyroidism, such as carcinoma and acute vitamin D intoxication, is usually associated with mild alkalosis rather than acidosis.[28,29] Hyperchloremia and/or mild reduction in serum bicarbonate helps to distinguish hyperparathyroidism from other causes of hypercalcemia,[30,31] although the distinction is not always seen.[32] Similarities are noted in the abnormalities in renal function in patients with primary hyperparathyroidism and in patients with hereditary fructose intolerance; each disorder is characterized by a proximal type RTA.[23,33-36] A possible relationship between phosphate depletion and renal bicarbonate wasting has been suggested.[37] In studies in phosphate-depleted dogs, proximal renal tubular defects similar to those seen in hyperparathyroidism were noted, despite normal circulating levels of parathyroid hormone. Thus phosphate repletion *per se* might account in part for the restoration of normal proximal tubular bicarbonate and acid handling after successful parathyroid surgery.

Partial or complete reversibility of some or all of the defects in glomerular function and tubular function including acidification mechanisms and renal concentrating ability has been documented after surgical correction of hyperparathyroidism.[4,22,25,37-40] In one brief report, however, a more pessimistic view was presented with regard to the reversibility of renal functional abnormalities after surgical correction of hyperparathyroidism.[41]

The pathogenesis of nephrolithiasis in patients with hyperparathyroidism remains unclear. Although hypercalciuria is commonly present in the disease, there is no clear statistical relationship between hypercalciuria and the presence or absence of nephrolithiasis.[22,42,43] Some risk factors appear to be disturbances of urine acidification due to the influence of parathyroid hormone on bicarbonate transport in the proximal tubules with the ensuing acidosis leading to hypercalciuria,[40] an unexplained propensity for crystallization and crystal growth of stone-forming constituents in the urine,[44] and increased blood levels of 1,25-dihydroxyvitamin D.[45] A direct correlation with the occurrence of renal stones in patients with primary hyperparathyroidism has been reported if several, linked, variables are all increased—the circulating plasma concentration of 1,25-dihydroxyvitamin D, the gastrointestinal hyperabsorption of calcium, and the presence of hypercalciuria.[45] It seems reasonable to propose that excesses of vitamin D and/or calcium in the diet provide a positive risk factor for the development of renal stones in these patients.

B. Skeletal Manifestations

It is difficult to assess the cause, frequency, clinical significance, and prognosis of skeletal disease in hyperparathyroidism. These difficulties arise because of the clearly apparent reduction in frequency of symptomatic and overt manifestations of skeletal disease in hyperparathyroidism and because of the technical difficulties involved in the methods required to define pathophysiologic changes in the skeleton that may be serious but asymptomatic for long periods in milder forms of disease. Present information suggests that the pathognomonic form of skeletal disease in hyperparathyroidism, osteitis fibrosa cystica, is declining in relative frequency and that a subtle yet nonetheless clinically significant form of skeletal disease, simple diffuse osteopenia resembling osteoporosis, often without symptoms, is being seen more often. Certain reports have confirmed a continuing decline in osteitis fibrosa cystica and/or symptomatic bone disease. In an analysis of 138 cases of primary hyperparathyroidism it was noted that in the two decades 1930–1949, 53% of patients had symptomatic, generalized osteitis fibrosa cystica confirmed by radiologic examination,[14] whereas in the decade 1949–1960 only 21% were so afflicted[14] and, between 1965 and 1973 only 9% of 57 patients seen had skeletal pain or evidence of osteitis fibrosa cystica.[46] No skeletal symptoms at all were detected in 58 patients with primary hyperparathyroidism evaluated at the Henry Ford Hospital from 1980 to 1983.[20]

In one report it was emphasized that patients with primary hyperparathyroidism who have pain referable to the skeleton are most likely to present with findings of diffuse spinal rarefaction indistinguishable from that of senile or postmenopausal osteoporosis rather than the findings of osteitis fibrosa. The degree of osteopenia may be severe. Of 319 patients with surgically proved primary hyperparathyroidism seen at the Mayo Clinic over a 3-year period, 14 (4.4%) had diffuse osteopenia of the spine with evidence of vertebral crush fractures.[47] Nine of the 14 patients presented with a chief complaint of back pain. In none of these 319 patients, however, was there unequivocal roentgenographic evidence of osteitis fibrosa cystica. The patients with primary hyperparathyroidism demonstrated a statistically higher incidence of diffuse osteopenia of the spine and of vertebral crush fractures compared with a group of age- and sex-matched control patients with degenerative lumbar disk disease. In another report of 87 patients with primary hyperparathyroidism,[48] roentgenographic manifestations of osteopenia were found in 21% of the patients in the spine and in the hands of 36%. Evidence of fibrosa (subperiosteal resorption of the phalanges) was noted in only 8% of these same patients.[48]

Other groups have emphasized that hyperparathyroidism affects primarily cortical rather than trabecular bone and dispute the contention that vertebral crush fractures are more common in hyperparathyroidism than in the euparathyroid age-matched population.[48a,48b] Increased loss of cortical bone is confirmed by several methods and clearly affects the appendicular skeleton and pelvis but selective, parathyroid hormone-dependent vertebral osteopenia is not undisputably associated with mild hyperparathyroidism as distinct from the elderly population *per se*.[48a,48b]

Several histologic techniques including the older microradiography and histomorphometry[49,50] have confirmed increased bone turnover in patients with hyperparathyroidism. The percentages of total surfaces of trabecular bone involved by osteoclastic resorption and mean surface areas of osteocytic lacunae were significantly higher in hyperparathyroid than in normal subjects.[50] In addition to the microscopic evidence of increased bone turnover in many patients with primary hyperparathyroidism, evidence of decreased bone density has been found by various sensitive bone densitometric techniques: ^{125}I bone densitometry,[51] x-ray spectrophotometry,[52] and photon absorptiometric analyses.[53,56] For example, a study by single-photon absorptiometry of the bone mineral content of the radius in 30 patients with primary hyperparathyroidism revealed a decrease of more than one standard deviation in 23.[56]

The reason for the changing pattern of skeletal involvement (osteitis fibrosa vs. simple osteopenia) remains unclear. Milder forms of hyperparathyroidism may cause only increased bone turnover rather than extensive bone remodeling, or osteitis fibrosa cystica; the latter may occur only in severe hyperparathyroidism.[57] The present evidence for multiple effects of parathyroid hormone on the skeleton, including experimental data and clinical evidence of an anabolic effect of the hormone in experimental studies in osteoporosis, makes predictions difficult on a theoretical basis. It is possible that compensatory mechanisms or modifying influences in some way influence whether osteitis fibrosa cystica, osteoporosis, or a normal skeleton will be found in a given patient with hyperparathyroidism. These modifying influences may include production of calcitonin, in response to hypercalcemia; some factor relating to calcium absorption, either content[58] as originally thought but then doubted[59] or, more likely, efficiency of intestinal calcium absorption;[60] the levels of active metabolites of vitamin D; or phosphate balance and extracellular fluid concentrations of phosphate. Basically, the pathophysiologic causes of skeletal changes in this disease remain unclarified.

Clinically, however, a number of features of the bone disease, whether osteitis fibrosa cystica or simple osteopenia, are of importance in providing diagnostic clues to the presence of the disease or in helping to assess need for surgical treatment as well as the response of the patient after surgical correction. When severe osteitis fibrosa cystica develops,[63-66] radiologic examinations or, if performed, bone biopsy can directly establish the diagnosis. The most important roentgenograms for the diagnosis of generalized osteitis fibrosa cystica are those of the hands in the posteroanterior view.[61] In the majority of patients with roentgenographically demonstrable bone lesions, subperiosteal erosion of the radial aspect of the middle phalanges is seen (Fig. 14–1). The skull is the next most frequently involved area.[61] In advanced stages of the disease there is evidence of erosion of the outer cortical surfaces of bone throughout the skeleton, generalized demineralization of bones, and localized destructive lesions, often of cystic character (Figs. 14–2*A*, *B*).

Although the clinical manifestations of osteitis fibrosa cystica are often severe, with pain and fracture,[61] the involved bone undergoes extensive remineralization and healing post surgery (Fig. 14–3). Histologic examination of bone specimens from patients with severe osteitis fibrosa cystica reveals a number of changes that collectively define the presence of parathyroid overactivity. There is a reduction in the number of trabeculae, an increase in multinucleated osteoclasts seen in scalloped areas on the surface of the bone (Howship's lacunae), and a marked replacement of normal cellular and marrow elements by fibrovascular tissue (Fig. 14–3).

The major unsettled issue regarding skeletal manifestations is the frequency, specific relation to hyperparathyroidism, and reversibility (postparathyroidectomy) of the diffuse osteopenia attributed to many patients with the disease. A definite causal relation between hyperparathyroidism and diffuse osteopenia seems likely. With regard to reversibility of bone disease, one study found small but definite increases in mineralization of bone in the radius in 30 patients 1 year after removal of parathyroid adenomas.[56] However, bone mass did not return to normal. Further analysis of the patients for up to 3 years revealed that maximal recovery of bone mass is achieved at 1 year after cure of the hyperparathyroidism. It appears that loss of bone in primary hyperparathyroidism may be only partially reversible.[56,62] More study is needed using the more recently available, improved techniques for measuring bone mass. Longitudinal studies with multiple techniques are needed to document loss of bone over time, to establish the frequency of the problem and the reversibility of osteoporosis after parathyroidectomy.[56] If the osteopenia in such patients is not reversed after parathyroidectomy but its progression is simply halted or slowed,[56,62] it will become even more important to attempt early detection of progressive osteopenia in patients with hyperparathyroidism and to encourage surgical intervention to prevent further skeletal weakening to the point of pathologic fractures.

C. Neuromuscular and Neuropsychiatric Manifestations

Profound muscle weakness and atrophy were recognized in several of the earliest described cases of severe hyperparathyroidism.[1,7] The pathophysiologic features of neuromuscular involvement in hyperparathyroidism have been studied in some detail.[46,67] Symptoms include extreme weakness and fatigability, particularly involving proximal musculature (the lower more frequently than the upper extremities); often the symptoms disappear dramatically with surgery. There is, however, confusion in published reports concerning the frequency of these symptoms. Although most reports stress that many patients have no symptoms at all,[9,10,20] some recent studies have emphasized the frequency of neuromuscular symptoms.[11,46,67] In the specific syndrome that reverses with parathyroidectomy, the higher incidence in a few centers may reflect ascertainment bias from referral patterns or severity of disease at diagnosis; alternatively, some of the symptoms may reflect degenerative arthritis and not the specific syndrome seen with hyperparathyroidism.[46,67]

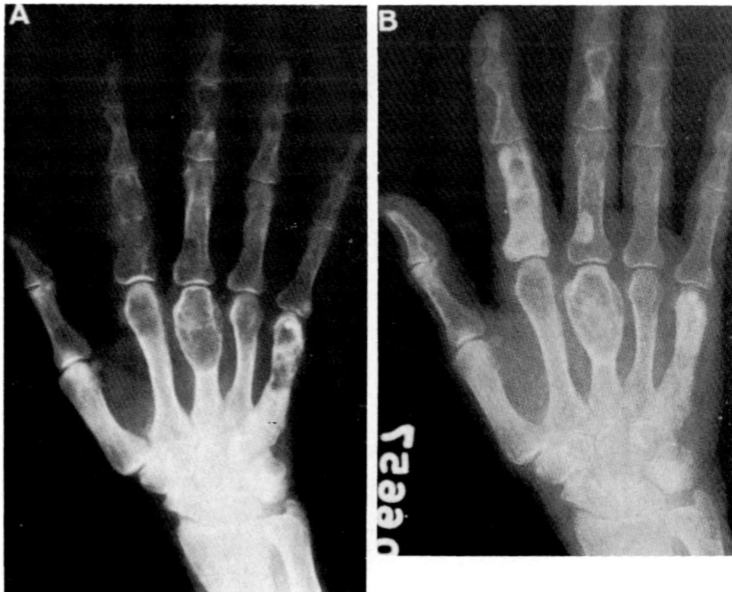

C

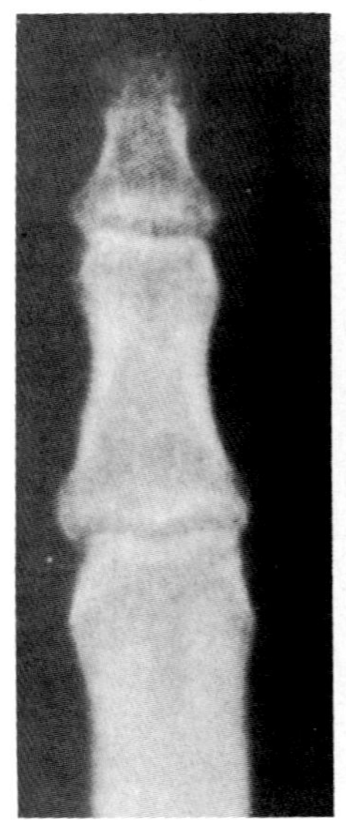

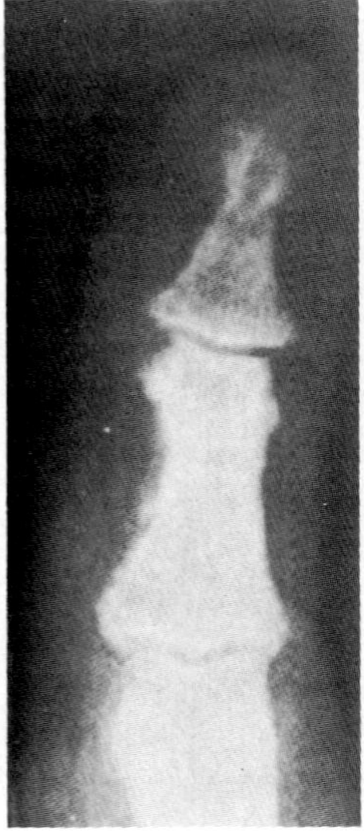

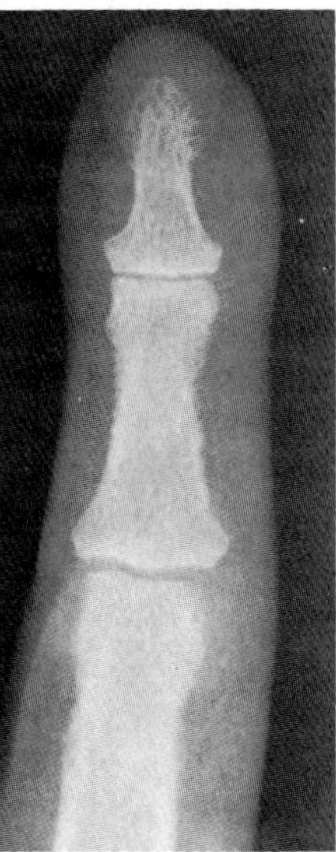

Figure 14–1. Hand films of patient with hyperparathyroidism and severe osteitis fibrosa cystica before (*A*) and after (*B*) removal of parathyroid adenoma. Cystic destruction of bone, subperiosteal resorption, and a pathologic fracture of the second proximal phalanx are evident. Some remineralization has occurred since the parathyroidectomy. (Courtesy of the Department of Radiology, Massachusetts General Hospital.) *C*, Magnification of x-ray film of normal finger (left) and finger from two patients with primary hyperparathyroidism (middle and right) to emphasize typical features. The abnormal fingers show decreased demineralization in the phalangeal tuft (middle) and subperiosteal bone resorption (middle and right). (Modified from Potts JT Jr, Deftos LJ: Parathyroid hormone, calcitonin, vitamin D, bone and bone mineral metabolism. *In* Bondy PK, Rosenberg LE (eds): Duncan's Diseases of Metabolism. Philadelphia, WB Saunders, 1974.)

The muscle weakness may be so profound that an initial diagnosis is entertained of amyotrophic lateral sclerosis, muscular dystrophy, or other serious neuromuscular disorders that are irreversible. Gross atrophy may be detectable in involved muscle groups. Striking reversal of muscle weakness and atrophy is noted in these patients after successful correction of the hyperparathyroidism. Electromyographic examinations reveal both short-duration/low-amplitude motor unit potentials and abnormally high-amplitude/long-duration polyphasic potentials, but motor nerve conduction velocities are normal.[67] Sensory abnormalities are absent. Patten et al.[67] emphasized that the overall findings including microscopic examination of affected tissue are consistent with a neuropathic rather than a myopathic origin of the neuromuscular disease.

In addition to the neuromyopathic manifestations of hyperparathyroidism, mental disturbances and impairment of higher central nervous system functions are reported in some patients.[68-72] Depression, personality changes, psychomotor retardation, memory impairment, and, occasionally, overt psychosis may occur. In severe hyperparathyroidism, mental obtundation and coma may be observed.[73]

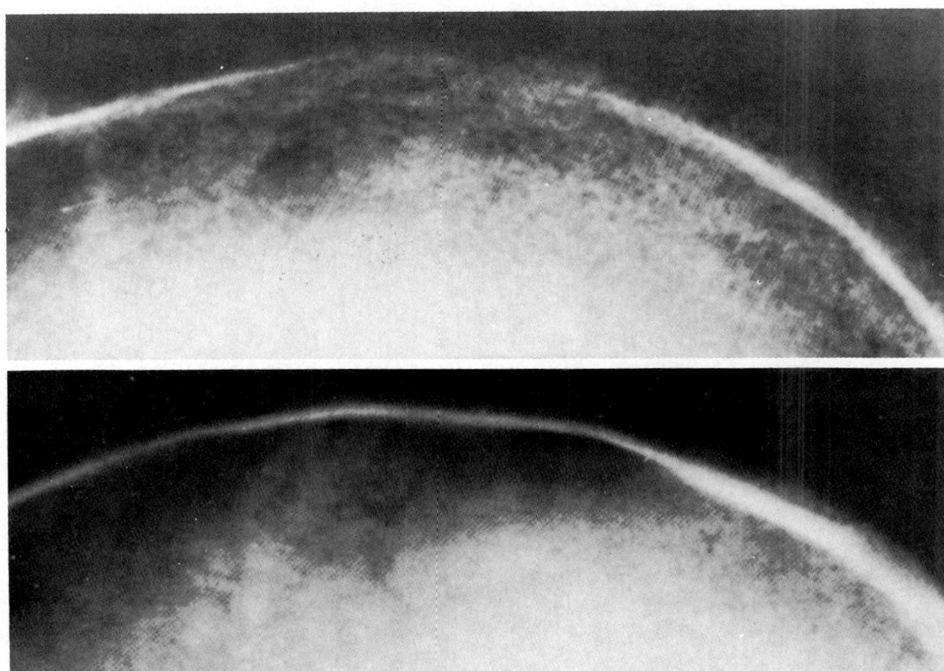

A

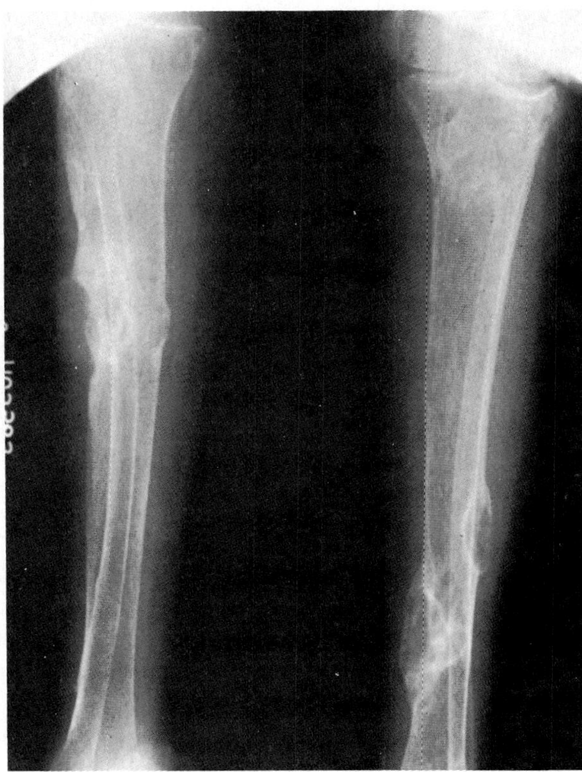

B

Figure 14–2. *A*, Magnification of skull x-ray film from a patient with primary hyperparathyroidism (top) and of a normal subject (bottom) to emphasize the appearance of localized resorption. (Courtesy of the Department of Radiology, Massachusetts General Hospital; from Potts JT Jr, Deftos LJ: Parathyroid hormone, calcitonin, vitamin D, bone and bone mineral metabolism. *In* Bondy PK, Rosenberg LE (eds): Duncan's Diseases of Metabolism. Philadelphia, WB Saunders, 1974.) *B*, Radii and ulnae of a patient with primary hyperparathyroidism. Severe osteopenia, increased trabeculation, and large areas of cystic degeneration are evident. (Courtesy of the Department of Radiology, Massachusetts General Hospital.)

These neuropsychiatric disturbances are thought to be due to the hypercalcemia *per se* rather than to any direct effects of parathyroid hormone[69]; characteristic electroencephalographic abnormalities have been described in hypercalcemia of many causes.[74,75]

On some occasions there is a striking improvement in a patient's sense of well being, including relief of fatigue and depression that may not have been noticeable prior to surgery.[72] It has been proposed that data obtained from a battery of psychological tests can serve as documentation of disruption of dominant hemispheric functions in patients with primary hyperparathyroidism and might be considered an indication for parathyroidectomy in the absence of other symptoms of hyperparathyroidism.[72] It should be emphasized, however, that mild depression and vague constitutional complaints alone are difficult to accept as an indication for surgery, because these symptoms are so common in the absence of hyperparathyroidism.

D. Gastrointestinal Manifestations

Peptic ulcer disease in patients with symptomatic primary hyperparathyroidism is seen with such high frequency that most investigators believe that the ulcer disease is causally related to the hyperparathyroidism. Some authors, on the other hand, have questioned this association.[76] Given the increased incidence of asymptomatic hyperparathyroidism in the elderly population,[9] it is clear that the earlier estimate of ulcer disease in 15% of patients is no longer valid.[9] It is useful, however, in establishing whether hyperparathyroidism and ulcer disease are causally related, to examine the frequency of association of the two diseases in symptomatic form. If the incidence of ulcer disease, based on appearance of symptoms, is greater in symptomatic hyperparathyroidism than in the general population, a causal relation is likely. This indeed seems to be true. In 10 reported series of peptic ulcer disease in patients with primary hyperparathyroidism, evidence of symptomatic and radiologically confirmed ulcer disease was present in 131 of 928 cases, an overall incidence of 14.2% (range 7.7% to 30.5%).[76,77] Inasmuch as the prevalence of peptic ulcer disease in the general adult population without hyperparathyroidism is reported to be much lower in the United States (estimates have ranged from a low of 2% to 3% [U.S.P.H.S. National Health Survey, 1960] to as high as 5% to 10%[76]), or in Great Britain (maximum estimate 7.8%[78]), it would appear that peptic ulcer disease is a true manifestation of primary hyperparathyroidism. On the other hand, the incidence of peptic ulcer disease in hyperparathyroidism in 1989 is much lower than 15%.[9] It is likely that in patients with asymptomatic disease, detected by blood calcium screening only, the disease is milder or the more effective counterregulatory mechanisms that minimize renal and osseous signs and symptoms may also minimize the frequency of peptic ulcer.

Some hyperparathyroid patients with peptic ulcer disease, particularly those with severe symptoms and multiple ulcers, are found to have Zollinger-Ellison syndrome[79] (multiple endocrine neoplasia syndrome, type I) with gastrin-producing tumors or diffuse hyperplasia of the pancreatic islet cells. These patients, however, constitute a small minority of patients with hyperparathyroidism and peptic ulcers; most patients have no recognized abnormalities of the endocrine pancreas.

The etiologic basis for the increased incidence of ulcer disease in most symptomatic hyperparathyroidism patients may be increased gastrin secretion, and resultant increased gastric acid production, induced by the hypercalcemia.[80] Levels of gastrin, although elevated, are considerably lower than in Zollinger-Ellison syndrome. In hyperparathyroidism, both basal acid secretion[81-85] and serum immunoreactive gastrin[81] are increased. Following parathyroidectomy, the excessive acid production, hypergastrinemia, and peptic ulcer symptoms usually return to normal[80,81,86] Evidence indicates that increased gastrin secretion and hyperacidity in hyperparathyroidism are due to the hypercalcemia and not to direct effects of the parathyroid hormone on gastrin production or on acid production *per se*. Even in the Zollinger-Ellison syndrome, the hyperacidity, elevated gastrin levels, and peptic ulcer symptoms may be reversed acutely by parathyroidectomy.[81] It has been argued persuasively that hyperparathyroidism always precedes the clinical expression of the Zollinger-Ellison syndrome.[82] Long-term follow-up of some of these patients has revealed ultimate recurrence of the Zollinger-Ellison syndrome despite the persistence of normal parathyroid function.

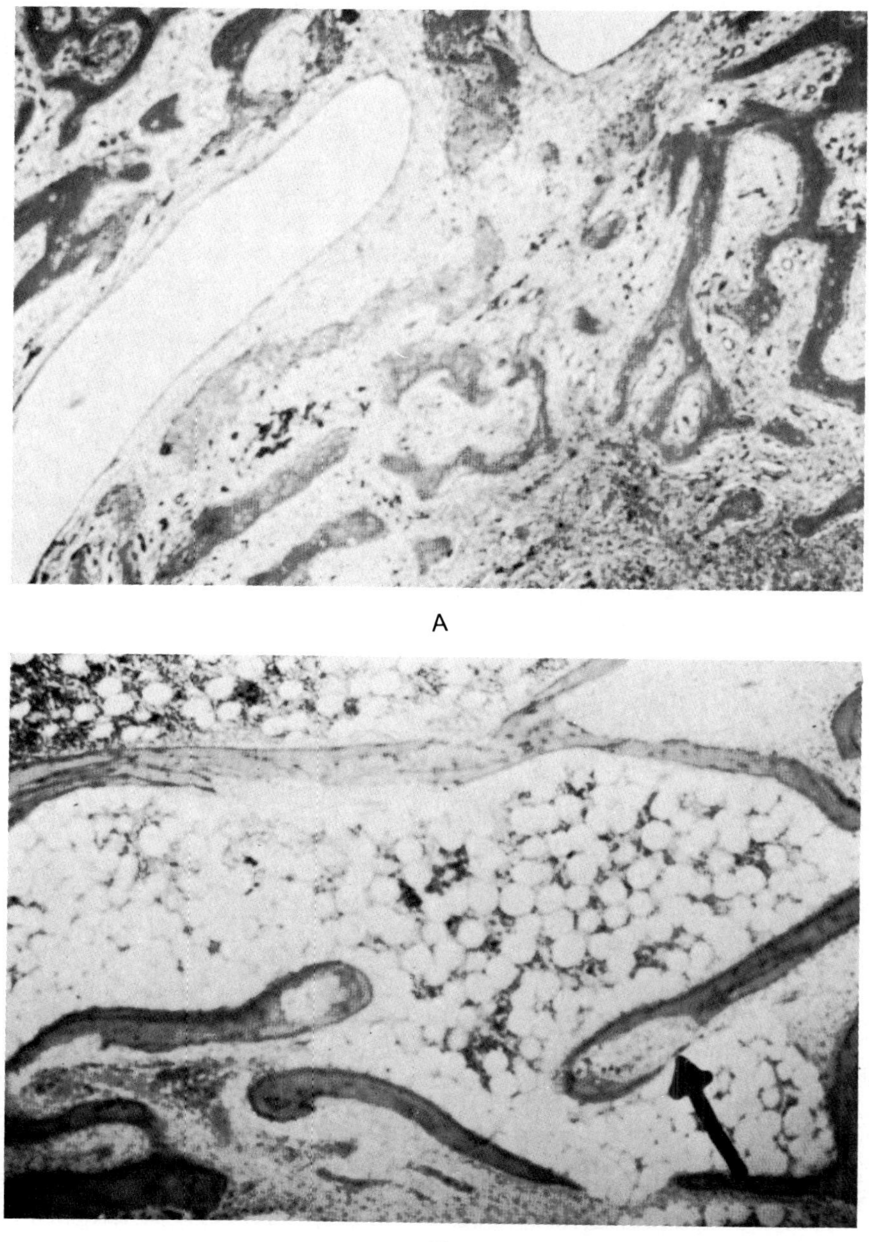

Figure 14–3. Microscopic appearance of osteitis fibrosa cystica in bone from an iliac crest bone. *A*, Extensive replacement of marrow with fibrovascular tissue; cystic cavities are evident. Osseous trabeculae showed evidence of both osteoclastic resorption and areas of osteoblastic bone formation. *B*, Classic appearance of dissecting osteitis within lamellar bone of trabeculae; several areas of fibrous replacement of marrow are evident.

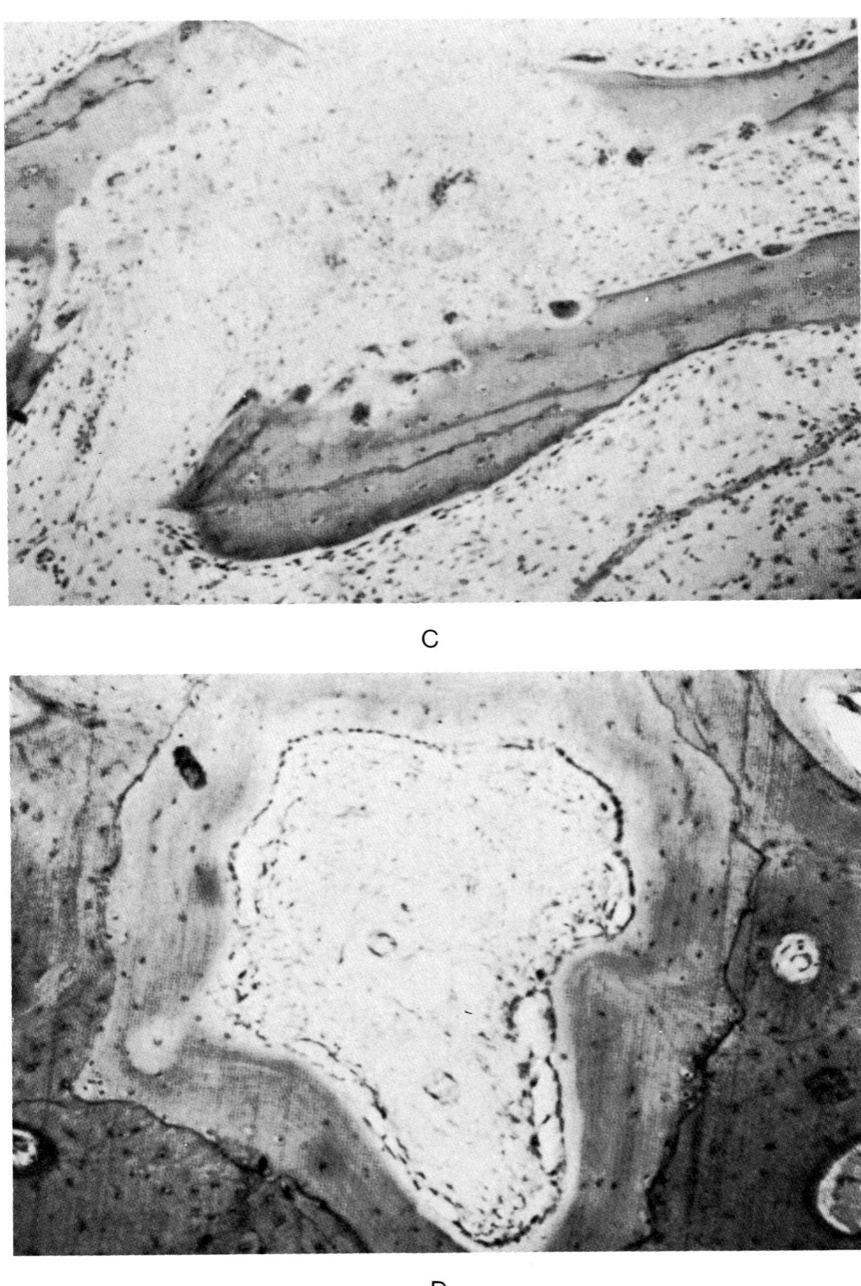

C

D

Figure 14–3 *Continued C,* Higher magnification of dissecting osteitis showing multinucleated osteoclasts resorbing bone. *D,* Osteone in cortical bone after parathyroidectomy, showing marked bone formation; innermost concentric circle of bone is unmineralized. Dark line represents calcification front; this osteomalacia is due to formation of matrix that is occurring faster than the process of mineralization. (Courtesy of the Department of Pathology, Massachusetts General Hospital.)

Pancreatitis was previously believed to be another gastrointestinal manifestation of hyperparathyroidism[87,88,92,94,95]; recent reports have called this contention into question.[89,90] Although an association of pancreatitis and hyperparathyroidism exists, the basis for it is unknown.[63,92-95] The long-standing, severe hypercalcemia *per se* associated with the hyperparathyroidism was felt to predispose to the development of pancreatitis.[92,94] One group even suggested that the hyperparathyroidism develops in response to pancreatitis.[93] In an early study, pancreatitis was reported to be the primary diagnostic clue to the presence of otherwise unrecognized hyperparathyroidism in 3% of 431 surgically proved cases.[87] More recent studies of patients with surgically proven hyperparathyroidism, however, have failed to show a high frequency of coexistent pancreatitis.[89-91] In a review of 1153 patients with primary hyperparathyroidism, one group found only 17 patients with coexisting pancreatitis for a prevalence of 1.5%.[90] In a study of 150 patients operated on for primary hyperparathyroidism between 1965 and 1975, another group[91] found associated pancreatitis in six (4%), whereas none of the 26 patients operated on from 1975 to 1981 had pancreatitis. In a recent study,[89] a survey of 1475 patients with pancreatitis between 1972 and 1982 found only five (0.4%) with hyperparathyroidism. It is notable that in these recent studies, the prevalence of hyperparathyroidism in patients with pancreati tis and the association of pancreatitis with primary hyperparathyroidism approximates the estimated prevalence of primary hyperparathyroidism in the population at large.[9,14-18] It has been suggested that the apparent association between hyperparathyroidism and pancreatitis may be a consequence of a subtle selection process that occurred mainly before the use of routine screening of serum calcium values.[90] Because of the understanding that pancreatitis can cause hypocalcemia, patients hospitalized for evaluation of pancreatitis were preferentially selected for testing of serum calcium and thus were preferentially evaluated for hyperparathyroidism.[90] These overall recent findings indicating a low frequency of coexistence of the two diseases bring into question whether there is indeed a causal pathophysiologic relationship between pancreatitis and hyperparathyroidism. However, in one report it is stated that in patients with pancreatitis and hyperparathyroidism, parathyroidectomy appears to ameliorate the pancreatitis, suggesting a cause and effect relationship.[89]

Although the nature of the pathogenetic interrelationships between pancreatitis and hyperparathyroidism is uncertain, awareness of this association does have several practical consequences. One should be aware still of the possible development of pancreatitis as a complication of severe hyperparathyroidism, particularly in acute parathyroid crisis, a condition in which an incidence of occurrence of 25% has been reported.[96] It is well documented also that both acute and chronic pancreatitis (the latter due to malabsorption) may cause a decrease in serum calcium concentration to deceptively normal or even low levels in hyperparathyroidism. Thus, the findings of even normal levels of serum calcium in the face of pancreatitis may be a clue to the concomitant existence of primary hyperparathyroidism.[92]

E. Articular Manifestations

A number of articular and periarticular disorders have been recognized in association with primary hyperparathyroidism, chondrocalcinosis with or without acute attacks of pseudogout, juxta-articular erosions, subchondral fractures, and traumatic synovitis, calcific periarthritis, and urate gout.[97-100]

Chondrocalcinosis is characterized by the deposition of calcium pyrophosphate dihydrate (CPPD) crystals in the articular cartilages and menisci (chondrocalcinosis)[101] and occasionally by the occurrence of acute attacks of arthritis (pseudogout), associated with CPPD in the synovial space, usually within polymorphonuclear leukocytes. The frequency of chondrocalcinosis in primary hyperparathyroidism was reported to be 7.5% to 18% in the 1960s.[102,103] In a recent study, chondrocalcinosis was detected in 10 of 32 patients with symptomatic hyperparathyroidism.[104] Those with chondrocalcinosis had greater parathyroid activity than those with no chondrocalcinosis. The patients were also older. These findings led to the suggestion that chondrocalcinosis is caused by the combined effects of sustained hypercalcemia and age-related changes in articular cartilage.[104] The diagnosis of chondrocalcinosis is suggested by the radiologic finding of characteristic calcium deposits in articular cartilages (Fig. 14–4); definite diagnosis is established by the

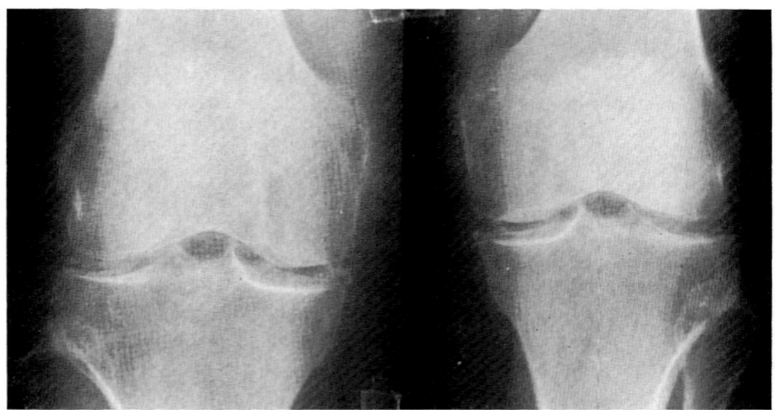

Figure 14–4. Radiographic appearance of chondrocalcinosis in articular cartilages of the knee. (Courtesy of Dr. S.M. Krane.)

finding of CPPD crystals in aspirates of joint fluid.[100] As with other disease manifestations, the frequency of chondrocalcinosis in hyperparathyroidism in 1989, if asymptomatic cases are included, is clearly much lower.[9]

In reviews published three decades ago, hyperuricemia was seen frequently in primary hyperparathyroidism[105] and was attributed to a decreased renal clearance of urates. Patients with chondrocalcinosis and hyperparathyroidism may also have hyperuricemia, a factor that may further confuse the diagnosis of the articular disorder.[100,106]

F. Hypertension

There have been numerous reports that hypertension occurs more frequently in hyperparathyroidism, particularly with elderly patients, than in the general population.[107-117] Estimates of the prevalence of hypertension in patients with primary hyperparathyroidism have ranged from 30% to over 60%.[108,110,115,116,118] In earlier studies, prevalences of the two diseases of 49% and 20% were reported.[107,118] Later studies[108,110,116] found an even higher correspondence. In a more recent study of 23 patients with surgically proven and cured primary hyperparathyroidism, 18 (78%) were found to be hypertensive, only five of whom had some degree of azotemia.[114] Another group[12] has reported finding a 4-fold increase in the prevalence of hypertension in hyperparathyroidism from 7% to 26% in patients studied before as compared with after 1975. The wide variation in the prevalence data is confusing; it may be partly due to varying criteria for the selection of patients and for the definition of hypertension. Inasmuch as the prevalence of hypertension in the general population is estimated to be 20% to 30%, depending on age and other factors,[119] it is difficult to conclude whether there exists a true association between hypertension and hyperparathyroidism based on statistical analysis of prevalence data and the ascertainment bias in hospitalized, surgically treated patients. At the present time there is no single factor or mechanism that can explain hypertension as a correlate of hyperparathyroidism.

In one review[114] several theories were discussed that have been proposed regarding the endocrine pressor mechanisms in primary hyperparathyroidism and consist of (1) peripheral vasoconstriction causing increased peripheral vascular constriction and increased cardiac contractility due to increased inotropism[120]; (2) renal tubular damage and increased renin production[121]; (3) renal damage secondary to nephrocalcinosis, renal calculi, obstructive nephropathy, and chronic pyelonephritis[107,118]; and (4) renal insufficiency and resultant increased sensitivity to the pressor effects of calcium.[122]

In this confusing situation it is important to determine whether parathyroidectomy leads to reversal of the hypertension; such would strengthen the supposed etiologic link. Obviously, in some patients, onset of renal damage and azotemia due to long-standing hypertension or nephrolithiasis could prevent return to a normotensive state whatever the original situation regarding cause and effect. In several recent studies, however, the majority of patients, free of overt renal damage, did not show a return to normal blood pressure but were still requiring treatment with antihypertensives[12,41,114] In one controlled study, no greater fall in blood pressure was detected in an age-matched set of 50 hypertensive patients after general surgical procedures compared with that seen in another 50 patients with hypertension and hyperparathyroidism after parathyroidectomy.[113] These observations suggest that hypertension *per se,* lacking presence of compounding factors such as multiple endocrine neoplasia syndromes, is not of itself an indication for parathyroid surgery on the expectation of benefit to the patient.

One aspect of the hypertension associated with hyperparathyroidism that has become clearly evident is that thiazide diuretics, often used as a first line of defense in the treatment of hypertension, aggravate the hypercalcemia.[112,123,124] Christensson et al.[123] screened approximately 16,000 "healthy" persons, 1000 of whom were taking thiazides. Twenty of 95 patients in the group who were found to be hypercalcemic were being treated with thiazides. Statistically, the prevalence of hypercalcemia in the thiazide-treated group was 1.9% compared with 0.6% in the entire population. Only five of the 20 patients with hypercalcemia became normocalcemic 1 year after discontinuation of the thiazides. Of the 15 patients who had persistent hypercalcemia, 14 underwent parathyroidectomy, and all had parathyroid adenomas. None of the patients had hyperplastic parathyroid glands characteristic of multiple endocrine neoplasia syndrome type II, in which pheochromocytomas are commonly present. Thiazides may need to be discontinued in hypertensive patients with hyperparathyroidism and replaced with furosemide or other agents that do not cause hypercalcemia if the patients are to be followed without surgery (as discussed below).

G. Other Clinical Manifestations

Skin necrosis, which may be found in patients with hypercalcemia of any cause, has also been found in hyperparathyroidism.[125] Calcification of the cornea (band keratopathy) is occasionally a manifestation of hypercalcemia of whatever cause[126]; however, it is not commonly found in primary hyperparathyroidism when serum phosphorus levels are low and renal glomerular function is maintained.

Certain distinctive clinical features are noted when hyperparathyroidism occurs in children. Primary hyperparathyroidism in patients under 16 years of age is rare. By 1980 there were reports of 85 proven cases of childhood primary hyperparathyroidism.[127-136] Two types of primary hyperparathyroidism are recognized, a severe hereditary form occurring in neonates and a milder, more typical form during childhood. Severe hypercalcemia is characteristically seen in the disease in neonates. Serum calcium levels are usually over 15 mg/100 ml and as high as 30.2 mg/100 ml in one reported case.[134] Neonatal hyperparathyroidism is often genetically transmitted as an autosomal dominant trait and is typically reported in families with the familial hypocalciuric hypercalcemia syndrome.[133-137] Twelve of 31 children with hyperparathyroidism reviewed by one group[133] were 3 months old or less and presented primarily with failure to thrive and skeletal abnormalities. The mortality rate in this group was 50%.[133-137] The characteristic pathologic change in neonatal primary hyperparathyroidism is chief cell hyperplasia of the parathyroid glands. Near total parathyroidectomy is required to control the disease. The prognosis following surgery is good provided a delay in diagnosis and treatment has not resulted in irreversible changes.

In children as distinct from neonates, hyperparathyroidism does not have known genetic inheritance, is caused by parathyroid adenomas, and should be considered merely an early onset of adult primary hyperparathyroidism. Rickets can occasionally occur in children with primary hyperparathyroidism.[138] Although rickets is usually not included in descriptions of the manifestations of hyperparathyroidism in childhood, 11 cases have been reported.[138] Eight of the 11 cases were due to parathyroid adenoma. Rickets is usually mild but may be severe in some. The pathogenesis of the rickets proposed is that parathyroid hormone enhances bone resorption and turnover, there is renal wasting of phosphate, and dietary calcium intake is limited owing to anorexia. The combination of these factors leads to a deficiency of bone mineralization in the rapidly growing skeleton of the child.

It is likely that with the increasing use of screening procedures, more instances will be found of hyperparathyroidism in children. The serum levels of calcium and phosphorus, however, should be interpreted with respect to the ranges of normal for that age. Data for normal children have been collected and used for this purpose.[131]

Primary hyperparathyroidism is a rare disease during pregnancy.[139-142] However, if the diagnosis is overlooked, the subsequent hypercalcemia often has deleterious effects upon both mother and fetus. The serious complications, of which neonatal tetany, stillbirth, and abortion are the most frequent ones, can usually be avoided if surgical treatment is instituted in time. The diagnosis of hyperparathyroidism during pregnancy depends on recognition of the usual symptoms and the finding of hypercalcemia. However, one should be aware that the total serum calcium levels in pregnant women are often reduced because of a decrease in the protein-bound fraction of calcium. Consequently, corrected and/or ionized serum calcium concentrations should be measured if hyperparathyroidism is suspected in a pregnant woman.

A common manifestation of untreated hyperparathyroidism in pregnancy is fetal tetany. Inasmuch as calcium readily crosses the placenta, maternal hypercalcemia inevitably results in fetal hypercalcemia and suppression of fetal parathyroid functions. Thus, infants are born with hypocalcemia due to functional hypoparathyroidism. In addition to having tetany, babies of mothers with hyperparathyroidism are usually small. Although some have indicated that surgery is not necessary during pregnancy when hyperparathyroidism is asymptomatic and mild,[142] some advocate surgery once the diagnosis is established.[139] Surgery is best carried out in the second trimester, at which time the fetus is fully developed and there is little chance of inducing premature labor. The risks of surgery and anesthesia appear to be no greater than they are in nonpregnant individuals.[139]

Parathyroid storm, or parathyroid crisis, is an acute medical and surgical emergency. Fortunately, the condition is rarely seen. In one review in 1980, 128 cases in the world literature were described.[144] Patients with this acute form of hyperparathyroidism present with very high serum levels (15 to 20 mg/100 ml, or higher) and marked mental disturbances.[144-146] The factors responsible for the development of the crisis state are unknown but likely involve contraction of the extracellular fluid volumes, stress from intercurrent illness, or hemorrhage within the parathyroid adenoma.[145] Definitive treatment is resection of the tumor. While the diagnosis is being sought, aggressive medical therapy should be instituted to control the hypercalcemia and the fluid and electrolyte balance. Failure of medical treatment, even in the presence of coma, is an indication for emergency parathyroidectomy.[146]

II. ETIOLOGY AND PATHOLOGY

Normally four parathyroid glands are present in the neck in tissue adjacent to the thyroid and/or thymus (Fig. 14–5). In a study of the distribution of normal glands in 160 autopsies of patients dying from causes unrelated to parathyroid disease, 156 subjects had four glands, three had five glands, and one had six glands.[8] The usual position occupied by the upper glands was posteriorly at the cricothyroid junction (77%) or behind the upper pole of the thyroid (22%). Of 312 parathyroid glands examined, only three upper

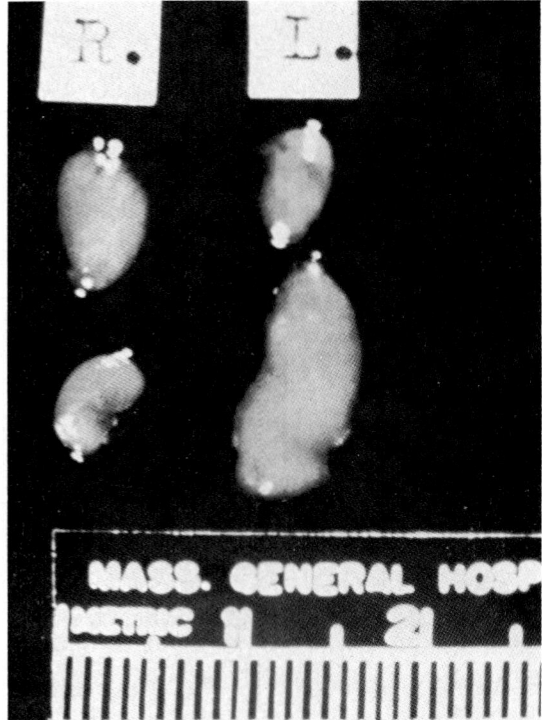

Figure 14–5. Gross appearance of four normal parathyroid glands removed at autopsy to illustrate relatively small size and variation in appearance. (Courtesy of the Department of Pathology, Massachusetts General Hospital.)

glands were found behind the upper esophagus.[8] The position of the normal lower glands varied more widely, from within the thymus to regions adjacent to the lower pole of the thyroid.[8] The lower glands were ectopically located more frequently than the upper glands. Several were at the carotid bifurcation, and the remainder were with thymic remnants near the carotid sheath at the thoracic inlet or within the mediastinum.

Enlargement of only a single gland is sufficient to cause excessive hormone secretion (Fig. 14–6). The enlarged gland is usually classified as a benign adenoma; only rarely is it a malignant carcinoma. Enlargement and diffuse hyperplasia of all four glands may be seen also (Fig. 14–7). Hyperplasia involving clear cells as a cause of primary hyperparathyroidism was described many years ago.[147] Later, appropriate emphasis was directed to the frequency of chief cell hyperplasia as a cause.[148] There are clearly familial cases of hyperparathyroidism (discussed below) in which inheritance follows an autosomal dominant pattern. Most cases of hyperparathyroidism are sporadic, without appearance in other generations. In the experience of most surgeons, a single abnormal gland, adenoma, is most often found in sporadic hyperparathyroidism, although enlargement of all four glands, hyperplasia, is reported in a few cases.[149-153] Hyperplasia is most commonly found in familial cases. Although an adenoma of a single gland was, and is still, regarded by many groups as the most common cause of primary hyperparathyroidism,[10-12,17,149-153] there continue to be adherents to the view that hyperplasia in multiple glands is a more frequent cause of primary hyperparathyroidism even in sporadic cases than is generally accepted.[152,153] (This controversy is examined in more detail in section VII dealing with surgical treatment.)

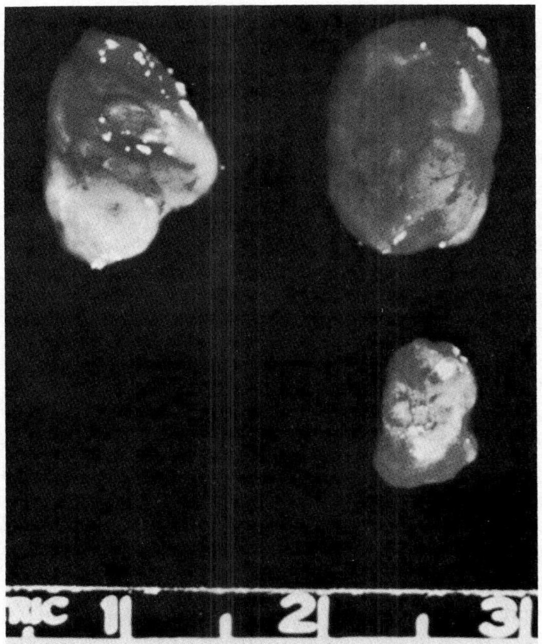

Figure 14–7. Gross appearance of primary chief cell hyperplasia of the parathyroids removed at surgery. Glands are irregular in outline and enlargement is variable. The fourth, a smaller gland, was left in the neck. (Courtesy of the Department of Pathology, Massachusetts General Hospital.)

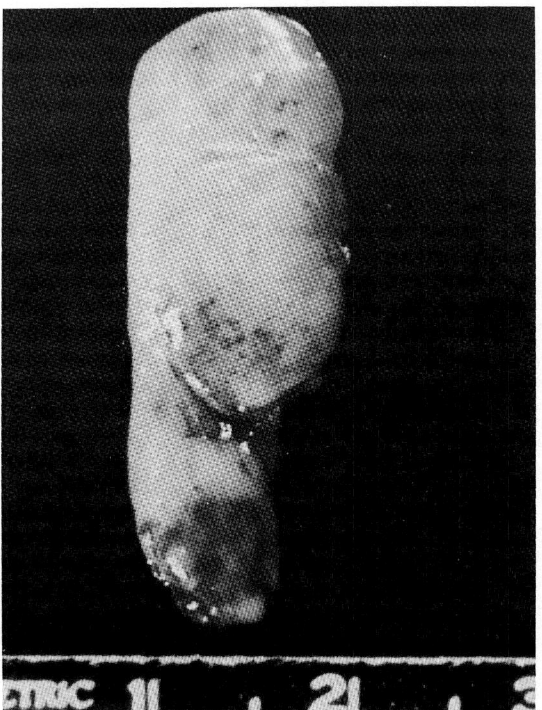

Figure 14–6. A 0.2 g parathyroid adenoma arising from a parathyroid gland to illustrate greater size than normal glands. Adenoma is at top and is compressing remaining normal parathyroid tissue below. (Courtesy of the Department of Pathology, Massachusetts General Hospital.)

Most surgeons and pathologists have continued to maintain that in over 80% of patients with primary hyperparathyroidism, a single abnormal gland or adenoma is the only abnormality, and that effective long-term cure can be obtained by the surgical removal of the single abnormal gland.[10-12,17,149-151,154,155]

The principal issues in pathologic classification have to do with etiology and prognosis. The etiologic factor is obscure for either adenoma or hyperplasia, although the earlier view that adenomas had a polyclonal origin[485,486] has been reevaluated by molecular biological studies that indicate a monoclonal origin.[487] In endocrine pathology generally, the concept of adenoma implies a neoplastic event in which a mature tumor results from a clonal expansion of a single transformed cell, whereas hyperplasia involves the response of multiple cells to an endogenous or exogenous stimulus.[482-487] Several techniques have been developed to study this problem, including analysis of X chromosome products in cells from tumors versus normal tissues in females. Advantage is taken of the random inactivation of the X chromosome in females during early fetal development. Polyclonality is shown by the presence of either chromosome in cells from the abnormal gland and in normal, nontumor cells; or monoclonality by exclusion of cells bearing one of the two X chromosomes, both of which are active in cells from normal tissues.[482-487]

Reports based on the use of the isometric forms of glucose-6-phosphate dehydrogenase, detectable in black patients, were used to examine the monoclonality or polyclonality of single parathyroid tumors or adenomas in black females undergoing parathyroid surgery. Surprisingly, the investigations pointed to a polyclonal origin of these solitary tumors, more consistent with the polyclonal origin of parathyroid tumors and strengthening the case for multiglandular origin of most cases of hyperparathyroidism.[485-486] The results seemed particularly impressive when the same techniques could be shown to confirm the monoclonal origin of adrenal adenomas and thyroid adenomas.[485-486] All such techniques have many potential methodologic and interpretative pitfalls, however. A more recent examination using techniques of molecular biology has permitted a more critical test of monoclonality versus polyclonality in abnormal parathyroid glands derived from patients with single-gland disease (adenoma) versus multiglandular disease (hyperplasia). In the majority of patients with adenomas, a monoclonal origin for the parathyroid tumor was confirmed.[487]

In the latter study more specific DNA testing was employed that permitted direct examination of X chromosome patterns in all female patients. Six of eight adenomas from women with sporadic parathyroid adenomas were shown to be monoclonal by testing of tumor versus nontumor DNA patterns.

A uniform pattern of X chromosome inactivation was found in the tumor versus the expected random pattern of X chromosome inactivation in peripheral cells. Also in all cells of the parathyroid tumors from two patients, a peculiar chromosome breakage of chromosome 11 with inversion of the chromosome between the two break points was determined. One break point in both patients was between exons 1 and 2 of the parathyroid gene; the other break point in one patient was on the long arm of chromosome 11 (11 q 13). The findings, in addition to confirming monoclonality, are intriguing with regard to potential genetic influences on cellular neoplasia. As then expected, there was no evidence for monoclonality in tumors from five patients with hereditary hyperparathyroidism and parathyroid hyperplasia.

Recent evidence based on genetic linkage studies in affected kindreds has pointed to the location of the genetic defect of the gene responsible for multiple endocrine neoplasia type-I (MEN-I), one of the forms of hereditary hyperparathyroidism, as being on chromosome 11 in the same region as the breakage point detected in the patient with a parathyroid adenoma.

This region of chromosome 11 is also near the region of the proto-oncogene INT 2, which is linked to the MEN-I gene locus.

Two recent studies have provided further surprising data concerning genetic abnormalities in hyperparathyroidism, both sporadic but also familial MEN-I kindreds.[487e,487f] Both groups have found in hyperplastic glands deletions of portions or even all of one parental copy of chromosome 11, in one study in ten of 16 tumors,[487e] and in the other study in three of six hyperplastic tumors.[487f] These findings, loss of heterozygosity in all cells from these 13 hyperplastic glands, unexpectedly established that these tumors are monoclonal, as found earlier only with parathyroid adenomas studied by the less informative technique of X chromosome inactivation patterns. These findings, which in the majority of cases could be shown to involve the loss of the MEN-I gene locus, could represent, in analogy with hereditary retinoblastoma[487d] and some other tumors,[487f] the loss of a genetic element that acts as an antioncogene or growth-controlling genetic element. In hereditary retinoblastoma, for example, one gene is inherited with a defect in the antioncogene locus; a somatically acquired deletion of the second allelic locus then presumably leads to unregulated cellular growth. The failure to detect loss of heterozygosity in all tumors from patients with hyperplastic parathyroid tumors might merely reflect the lack of suitable restriction fragment length polymorphisms in those patients to permit detection of small but significant chromosome deletions in the critical area, long arm chromosome 11 (11 q 13), the MEN-I gene region.

Speculation differed somewhat. One group[487e] found the tumors with chromosome 11 deletions to be larger than the tumors without detectable allelic loss. Hence one possibility offered was that hyperplasia of all glands results from a germ line defect in all glands; then chromosomal deletion leads to a monoclonal expansion and a larger tumor (an adenoma). In this respect they found that nine of 34 tumors from sporadic cases (a presumed single abnormal gland, an adenoma as based on both histologic and medical multiple criteria had detectable loss of chromosome 11 in the MEN-I gene locus. The other group[487f] seemed to favor the view that chromosome loss was essential for tumor development without postulating an intermediate stage of hyperplasia. Speculation about such details is all that is possible with the limited data; other potential growth-controlling genetic elements in the MEN-I locus, it was argued, could be involved. The overall results are unexpected in some respects and cannot yet be applied to change the clinical approach, which must be based on history, gland morphology, and histology (as discussed in Section VII, Surgical Management, below), but it seems likely that follow-up genetic studies ultimately may prove quite helpful both in understanding etiology and in planning surgery more rationally.

One reason for the continuing dispute about the pathologic etiology is that it is often difficult by either gross or histologic examination to distinguish between adenoma and hyperplasia or to decide by objective criteria whether abnormalities are present in only one or all four parathyroid glands. The older criterion used to distinguish between adenoma and hyperplasia, namely, finding a rim of normal tissue around the tumor nodule in an adenoma ("encapsulation," Fig. 14–8), may not always be found.[150] Moreover, compression of tissue around an area of hyperplasia may give also the appearance of a capsule ("pseudoencapsulation").[150]

Parathyroid carcinoma is estimated to be found in approximately 3% of patients (see Table 14–1).[10-12,17,149-152,155] Carcinoma of the parathyroid is characterized by the adherence of glandular tissue to surrounding structures (Fig. 14–9). Histologic criteria of malignancy[156] include the presence of nuclear mitotic figures (normally none are seen in an entire section), fibrosis, and capsular or blood vessel invasion (Fig. 14–10). Analysis of the data of Schantz and Castleman[156] and Wang[154] indicates that many carcinomas of the parathyroid are often slow-growing and relatively benign. If the involved parathyroid gland is removed without capsular rupture, long-term follow-up has generally shown no evidence of recurrence.[154] Clearly there is variation in aggressiveness of different tumors and there are reports of metastases before initial operation.[157]

When the parathyroid carcinoma does become metastatic, spread is usually to the lymphatics on the side of the neck where the original tumor developed.[154] Once hematogenous, parathyroid carcinoma localizes most frequently in the lung, but also in liver and bone.[157] Of 50 cases reviewed by Holmes et al.,[157] 46 of the carcinomas were hyperfunctioning and four carcinomas were not associated with excessive parathyroid hormone secretion. A feature often noted with these cases is the marked severity of hypercalcemia (greater than 14 mg/100 ml in 75% of cases.)

In the last several decades there has been increasing awareness of the hereditary aspects of hyperparathyroidism and the association of familial hyperparathyroidism with other well-defined, associated hereditable endocrine disorders.[158-171] Estimates of incidence in the United States suggest several thousand kindreds in which there is a genetic transmission of hyperparathyroidism, and/or other endocrine tumors.

There are two syndromes recognized of multiple hereditary endocrinopathy, which are genetically distinct from each other.[158] The first, now termed multiple endocrine neoplasia type I, consists primarily of tumors of

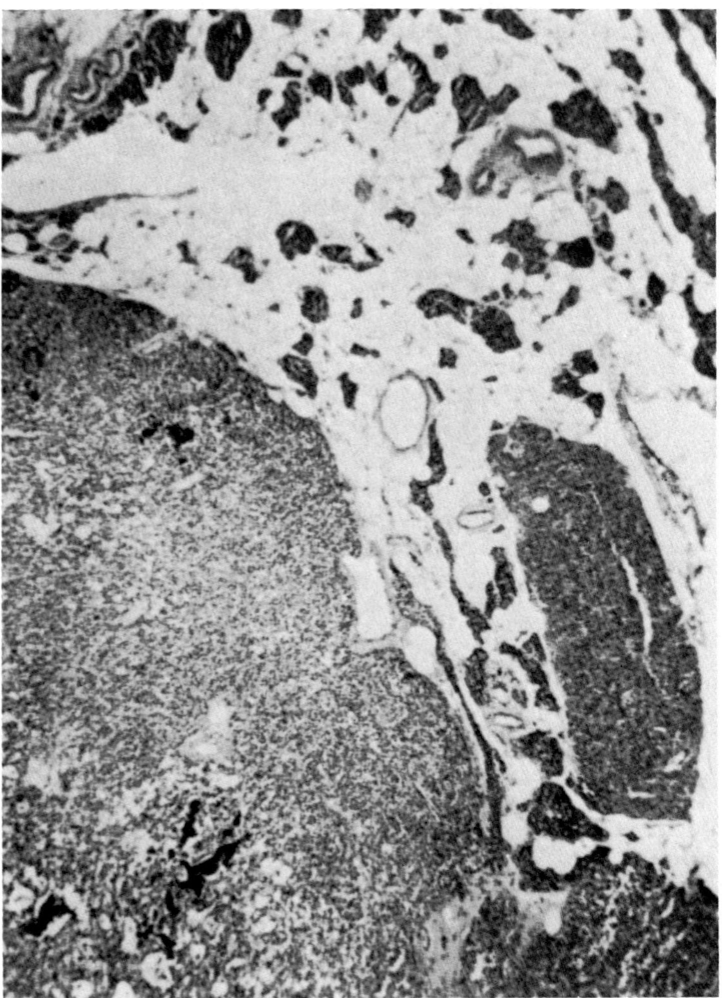

Figure 14–8. Microscopic appearance of a chief cell adenoma of the parathyroid gland. Adenoma is in lower left half of the field. Normal parathyroid tissue with characteristic fatty stroma and islands of chief cells and oxyphil cells is seen in lower left field. (Courtesy of the Department of Pathology, Massachusetts General Hospital.)

Table 14–1. Classification of Causes of Hypercalcemia

Parathyroid-Related	Vitamin D–Related
Primary hyperparathyroidism	Vitamin D intoxication
Solitary adenomas	1,25 $(OH)_2D$; sarcoidosis and other granulomatous diseases
Multiple endocrine neoplasia	Idiopathic hypercalcemia of infancy
Lithium therapy	
Familial hypocalciuric hypercalcemia	**Associated with High Bone Turnover**
Malignancy-Related	Hyperthyroidism
Solid tumor with metastases (breast)	Immobilization
Solid tumor with humoral mediation of hypercalcemia (lung, kidney)	Thiazides
Hematologic malignancies (multiple myeloma, lymphoma/leukemia)	Vitamin A intoxication
	Associated with Renal Failure
	Severe secondary hyperparathyroidism
	Aluminum intoxication
	Milk-alkali syndrome

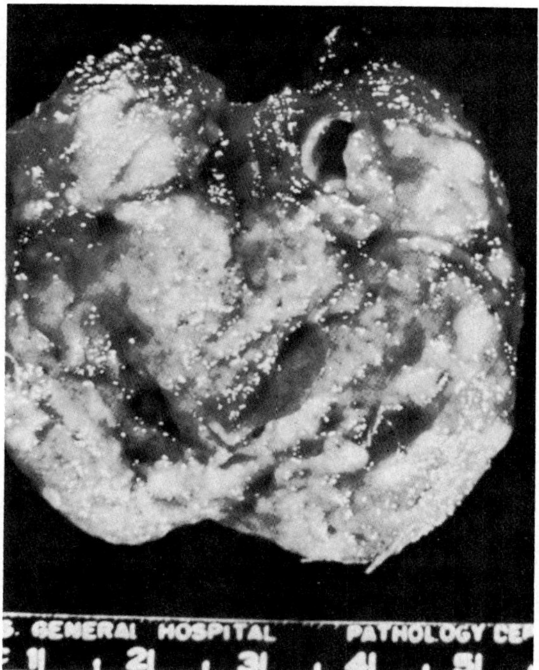

Figure 14–9. Cut section of a parathyroid carcinoma showing highly irregular, gritty surface due to extensive fibrosis. (Courtesy of the Department of Pathology, Massachusetts General Hospital.)

the parathyroid, pituitary, and pancreas. The second hereditary syndrome, termed multiple endocrine neoplasia type II, consists of medullary carcinoma of the thyroid, adrenal tumors (pheochromocytoma), and, again, tumors of the parathyroids. (See Chapter 18 for discussion of the latter syndrome).

Wermer[159] was the first to define the genetic aspects of the earliest recognized multiple endocrine syndrome, describing a pattern that featured pituitary, pancreatic, and parathyroid tumors (what is now termed MEN-I). Wermer correctly deduced that the high frequency with which one or more of these tumors were seen in family members from affected kindreds was compatible with an autosomal dominant inheritance.

The alternate syndrome, that of multiple endocrine neoplasia type II, was first reported, as a suspected separate clinical entity, by Sipple.[160] Schimke and Hartmann,[161] Schimke et al.,[162] and Steiner et al.[163] all noted the linkage between pheochromocytoma and medullary carcinoma of the thyroid as originally described by Sipple, plus the additional features of parathyroid tumors and mucosal neuromas. Steiner et al.[163] deduced an autosomal dominant pattern of inheritance in a total of 29 families who exhibited pheochromocytoma, medullary carcinoma of the thyroid, and hyperparathyroidism, and suggested the term multiple endocrine neoplasia type II (MEN-II) for the disorder involving the thyroid and adrenal medulla inasmuch as tumors of the pituitary and pancreas, common in the alternate endocrinopathy (which was then renamed multiple endocrine neoplasia type I syndrome or MEN-I), were absent from the kindreds with thyroid and adrenal tumors.

Several studies suggest that the Zollinger-Ellison syndrome,[164,165] familial medullary thyroid carcinoma,[166,167] familial pheochromocytoma,[163] and familial hyperparathyroidism[168] may occur as well as established hereditary syndromes in certain families without any evidence, despite careful screening, of any other endocrine disorder.[168] These

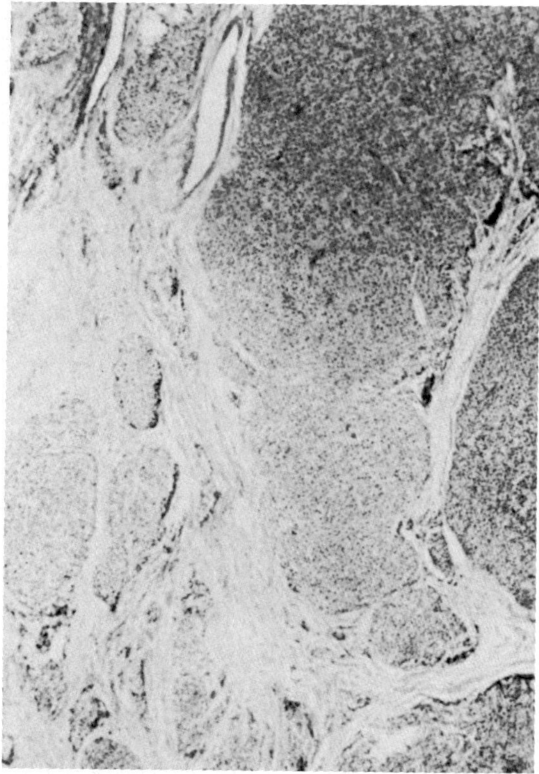

Figure 14–10. Microscopic appearance of a parathyroid carcinoma, showing large island of dense neoplastic chief cells separated by dense bands of connective tissue and occasional mitotic figures. (Courtesy of the Department of Pathology, Massachusetts General Hospital.)

findings of familial medullary carcinoma and pheochromocytoma as distinct from multiple endocrine neoplasia type II are discussed in Chapter 18.

Several explanations, none completely satisfactory, have been offered to explain the etiology of these multiple endocrine syndromes. There have been speculations based on the observations of Pearse[172] that the etiologic factor underlying multiple endocrine neoplasia syndromes involves a primary dysplasia of neuroectoderm.[173] Pearse[172] has discussed the hypothesis that cells originally of neural crest origin ultimately become the cells of origin of secretion of many of the hormones involved in the hereditary endocrine syndromes. These cells migrate widely during embryogenesis; the cells can be recognized by their histochemical characteristics (amine precursor uptake plus decarboxylation—hence the name APUD cells). Such a theory, however, does not account for the clustering of pituitary and pancreatic neoplasia only in kindreds with the MEN-I syndrome and a similar, apparent segregation of parafollicular cell and adrenal medullary tumors in the MEN-II syndrome; if a common cell type with ultimate dysplasia were the explanation, all endocrine tumors seen in the hereditary syndromes might be expected to appear in an affected kindred.

An alternative explanation offered for the syndrome is the occurrence of an initial overproduction of one hormone leading to a compensatory response of another endocrine organ resulting in hyperplasia and, eventually, neoplasia. One hypothesis is that nesidioblastosis or hypertrophy of pancreatic islet cells leads to overproduction of insulin and glucagon, which, in turn, stimulates excessive calcitonin release and, ultimately, parathyroid hyperplasia.[174] Similar speculations have involved a stimulus/response associated with regard to medullary carcinoma and parathyroid hyperplasia in MEN-II.

Against this view are several studies. Melvin et al.[175] established, by serial testing of asymptomatic members of a large kindred with MEN-II syndrome, that elevated blood levels of parathyroid hormone (indicating hyperplasia) with normal blood levels of calcitonin were seen in some patients, whereas, in others, elevated calcitonin levels (medullary carcinoma) were associated with normal parathyroid hormone levels. These results are consistent with an independent appearance of the discrete forms of endocrine neoplasia.

Thus, although a genetic pattern consistent with autosomal dominant inheritance of these syndromes has been demonstrated, a single, basic developmental defect explaining either the glandular disorder itself or the peculiar linkage or exclusion of endocrine gland tumors in the multiple endocrine syndromes has so far eluded detection.

As with other hereditary syndromes, the possibilities of direct genetic analysis (chromosomal abnormalities, restriction fragment length polymorphisms) offer the best hope for optimal yet efficient management by defining which kindred members carry the abnormal genetic constitution. The gene abnormalities responsible for hereditary retinoblastoma, for example, have shown that an autosomal dominant pattern is actually a homozygous recessive trait.[176] The linkage studies in families with MEN-I now permitting identification of the locus of an MEN-I gene may accelerate efforts for a gene marker[487b,487c]; the chromosome deletions found in parathyroid tumors may lead to the conclusion that, like hereditary retinoblastoma, the MEN syndromes are homozgous recessive.[487f]

III. DIAGNOSIS

A. General Considerations

Primary hyperparathyroidism is searched for in patients with symptoms or signs related to kidney stones, peptic ulcers, pancreatitis, chondrocalcinosis, osteitis fibrosa, or, with increasing frequency recently, asymptomatic and unexplained hypercalcemia.

Hypercalcemia is the most invariant manifestation of hyperparathyroidism. Repeated measurements of plasma calcium should be made in patients with suspected hypercalcemia (normal range in most centers is 8.6 to 10.4 mg/100 ml, with sometimes an even narrower range). It is important to eliminate errors or misinterpretations due to altered concentrations of blood proteins, venous stasis during collections of blood, or unsuspected variation in a given laboratory's range of normal. One may detect either a sustained hypercalcemia or a pattern of high-normal blood calcium values alternating with occasional slightly elevated values.

Patients with the pattern of intermittent hypercalcemia, suspected of having hyperparathyroidism, typically show all values to be at least in the upper 25% of the normal range, 10.0 mg/100 ml or greater, with some samples just above the upper limit of normal.

The serum inorganic phosphorus level in primary hyperparathyroidism is usually low but may be normal if patients had abnormal renal function. Hypophosphatemia can be a helpful clue, especially if blood calcium is equivocal. Detection of hypophosphatemia is less useful as an indicator of hyperparathyroidism, however, if blood calcium is markedly elevated, since severe hypercalcemia of any cause may lower serum phosphorus by altering renal tubular handling of phosphate.[177,178] To test for hypophosphatemia, blood samples should be obtained in the morning, under fasting conditions, since after eating there may be a sharp fall in blood phosphorus levels.

Hypercalciuria is also commonly seen in hyperparathyroidism with hypercalcemia. However, since parathyroid hormone reduces calcium clearance, the urinary excretion of calcium is lower in patients with hyperparathyroidism than in patients with equivalent degrees of hypercalcemia of nonparathyroid cause.[179] Blood alkaline phosphatase and urinary hydroxyproline excretion are elevated only when there is extensive bone involvement. Renal involvement can be reflected by a decreased concentrating ability, by specific tubular defects such as tubular acidosis, and by mild hyperchloremic acidosis.

A number of special tests based on responses in blood or urinary calcium and phosphate have been proposed to aid in establishing the diagnosis of hyperparathyroidism. These tests proved to be less useful than had been originally hoped. Most are now rarely performed, having been replaced by tests more specific for presence of excess parathyroid hormone; only a brief review of these older test procedures seems indicated.

Phosphate clearance is determined by standard techniques involving simultaneous measurements of urinary and blood phosphate and creatinine concentrations; usually urine samples are collected over a 1- to 4-hour period. Normal subjects have a phosphate clearance of 10.8 ± 2.7 ml/minute. Increases of 50% or greater above this figure have been detected in some patients with hyperparathyroidism. The ratio of phosphate clearance to creatinine clearance indicates the percentage of filtered phosphate excreted. The tubular resorption of phosphate can be calculated from the phosphate clearance and the glomerular filtration rate, the latter usually determined by creatinine clearance.

In normal subjects, the tubular resorption of phosphate exceeds 85%; in some patients with hyperparathyroidism, but unfortunately also in other subjects as well, tubular resorption of phosphate is lower. It is essential to control phosphate intake in such studies, as phosphate clearance and renal tubular phosphate transport, with or without excessive parathyroid effect, will vary with extremes of oral phosphate intake.[180] Variations in phosphate intake and numerous other confounding factors, including the practical difficulties encountered in collecting carefully timed urine and blood samples without special nursing and dietary assistance, have led to an abandonment of these tests in routine diagnostic use.

Thiazide diuretics in the usual doses of 1 to 2 g daily of chlorothiazide or its equivalent can produce sustained hypercalcemia in patients with hyperparathyroidism and borderline calcium values. Such a response is not seen in normal subjects. Although thiazide diuretics may produce transient elevations of blood calcium in normal subjects, normocalcemia returns in a few days despite continued administration. Thiazide administration, therefore, has been suggested as a provocative test for the presence of hyperparathyroidism (see discussion on differential diagnosis).[181]

Glucocorticoid administration was used for years to distinguish the hypercalcemia of hyperparathyroidism from that associated with sarcoidosis, multiple myeloma, vitamin D intoxication, and some malignant diseases with osseous metastases.[182,183] In these diseases, doses of hydrocortisone of 100 mg/day for 10 days result in a lowering of the serum calcium to normal levels, whereas calcium levels typically do not fall in primary hyperparathyroidism. This test also has been largely abandoned in routine use since it was defined as an in-patient[8] test, yet the length of stay required is prohibitive in modern hospital bed use. The test is sometimes used, however, in unusual patients with equivocal findings, since the false-positive rate in hyperparathyroidism is low.[182,183] When false-positive results in hyperparathyroidism are reported, it is when there is severe skeletal disease.[184,185]

B. Assays of Parathyroid Hormone

Clinically and physiologically useful assays for parathyroid hormone must be specific for detection of intact PTH or a defined fragment (immunoassays) or for a unique biological property of the hormone (bioassays). To be clinically practical and cost effective, the tests should be relatively simple to perform, be rapid in execution, and have high sensitivity and specificity. The assays should measure levels in all normal subjects, discriminate between normal subjects and those with hyperparathyroidism, and detect low levels in patients with hypercalcemia due to nonparathyroid causes who have suppressed gland function (hypercalcemia due to malignancy, hyperthyroidism, sarcoidosis, and other diseases with normal parathyroids).

Radioimmunoassays or immunoradiomimetic assays are widely available and are the most frequently used method for evaluating parathyroid gland function. These tests have improved considerably during the last decade and, particularly with double antibody methodology, have become highly useful in the evaluation of patients with disorders of calcium metabolism and hyperparathyroidism. Measurements of nephrogenous cAMP or urinary cAMP expressed as a function of glomerular filtrate are not widely used, although they show excellent discrimination among hyperparathyroidism, hypoparathyroidism, and normals. The tests are more inconvenient to perform and do not distinguish hypercalcemia related to malignancy from hyperparathyroidism. *In vitro* bioassays of blood samples based on PTH-dependent stimulation of renal glucose-6-phosphate dehydrogenase, a cytochemical bioassay, and PTH-dependent stimulation of adenylate cyclase have been developed principally as research tools. The details and relative efficacies of these assays are discussed in the following.

1. Radioimmunoassays

Subsequent to the initial description by Berson et al.[186] in 1963, immunoassays for circulating PTH have become an established diagnostic test in the evaluation of patients with hypercalcemia. Parathyroid hormone immunoassays have been troubled until recently by relatively severe problems with both false-negative and false-positive results.

Assays to measure plasma PTH have been difficult to develop and apply optimally because the circulating hormone concentrations are low and because there are multiple immunoreactive forms of the hormone, the secretion and clearance of which is modified by normal physiologic and pathologic changes[198,199] (see Chapter 3). Circulating concentrations of intact PTH are of the order of 10^{-11} M to 10^{-12} M when measured in the renal cytochemical bioassay[200] and by an amino-terminal specific radioimmunoassay,[191] the range predicted by studies *in vivo* using infused hormone.[201]

All investigators agree that intact PTH is the major form of secreted hormone, and that biologically inactive fragments of the parent molecule, composing the middle and carboxyl-terminal portions of the sequence, are the major forms of hormone found in the general circulation.[198]

The metabolic clearance rates of different immunoreactive forms of PTH differ (see Chapter 3). The half-time of intact PTH in blood is 5 minutes or less, whereas the half-time of middle carboxyl-terminal fragments is at least 5 to 15 times longer.[208] Endogenous amino-terminal fragments, if they circulate at all (Chapter 3), are likely to be cleared at rates comparable to that of intact hormone;[211] they do not appear to constitute a quantitatively significant fraction of total plasma immunoreactive PTH. Renal failure is associated with an increase in the concentrations of fragments relative to intact hormone;[221] glomerular filtration accounts for most, if not all, of the clearance of biologically inactive carboxyl-terminal fragments. Carboxyl-terminal fragments in humans with severe chronic renal failure may not decrease by even one half-time 24 hours after parathyroidectomy[212] (see Figures 3–3 through 3–11). Therefore, alterations in glomerular filtration greatly influence the concentration of circulating immunoreactive forms of PTH; the status of renal function, as well as the specificity characteristics of the PTH assay used, must be considered carefully when one reviews earlier published reports evaluating significance of radioimmunoassay results.

Amino-terminal fragments are detected by cytochemical bioassay[200] in patients with chronic renal failure but, as reviewed in Chapter 3, amino-terminal fragments are not released from peripheral sites of hormone cleavage in animal studies and it is possible that the material detected in the cytochemical assays is not PTH (or there is increased production or delayed clearance of amino fragments in renal failure). Further work is still necessary before firm conclusions can be made, but, as summarized in Chapter 3, there is no definite evidence that there are circulating amino-terminal fragments in humans with normal renal function.

In normal, young adult humans, concentrations of intact hormone are less than one third of the concentration of middle and carboxyl-terminal fragments; patients with surgically proven hyperparathyroidism have 3- to 20-fold higher concentrations of these inactive fragments than intact hormone.[193]

It is now clear that the desirable performance features in clinical diagnosis cited earlier in the introduction of this section are satisfied by the double-antibody assay technique, which provides high sensitivity and specificity, readily detecting all normal subjects and distinguishing patients with hyperparathyroidism from normals and those with malignancy and other nonparathyroid causes of hypercalcemia and hypoparathyroidism from normals. False-positive and false-negative findings are low in these diagnostic categories; the tests are very rapidly performed within hours or even, in special circumstances, minutes. The tests measure only intact hormone and are uninfluenced by any fragments of circulating hormone.

To understand, in contrast, the abundant literature concerning radioimmunoassay results in many earlier clinical reports, it is necessary to understand the limitations of the earlier techniques that used radioisotope displacement methodology and various types of antibodies and hormone-related ligands. Results with these tests are briefly reviewed as well. Several reports using radioimmunoassays with antisera recognizing epitopes in the middle third of the PTH molecule suggested that iPTH values increase as a function of age.[214-218] However, tests using an amino-terminal radioimmunoassay[219] and the cytochemical bioassay[220] suggest that this increase in PTH, at least in humans, can be attributed to age-related increased levels of biologically inactive middle and carboxyl-terminal fragments. Additional studies with subjects in whom dietary intake and vitamin D status are carefully controlled and the newer double antibody assays will be needed to definitely resolve this issue. Physiologic and pathologic decrease in glomerular filtration rate predictably will increase iPTH values in mid-region assays without necessarily influencing the concentrations of biologically active hormone in plasma. This contention is supported by the finding that radioimmunoassays that use amino-terminal specific antiserum are better predictors of severe hyperparathyroidism with osteitis fibrosa in patients undergoing maintenance hemodialysis than are mid-region assays.[222-227]

Most assays having sufficient sensitivity to measure plasma immunoreactive PTH[8] principally recognize determinants in the middle portion of the sequence, the sequence with greatest interspecies variability (see Chapter 3).[228-232] These assays measure both intact hormone and the middle and carboxyl-terminal fragments. The clinical utility of these middle and carboxyl region assays is due partly to the increased concentration of these fragments and certain favorable technical features of the methodology.[195]

PTH assays using antiserum specifically recognizing the amino-terminal portion of the PTH sequences should theoretically give the best correlation with the concentration of circulating intact, biologically active hormone (detected by its amino-terminus), since little, if any, amino-terminal fragments circulate. Amino-terminal assays with sufficient sensitivity to be clinically useful were difficult to develop because of the extraordinarily low concentrations of circulating intact hormone and because the amino-terminal portion of the PTH sequence appears to have low immunogenicity. Earliest reports concerning use of amino-terminal immunoassays suggested that normal circulating hormone levels were higher than predicted by the cytochemical bioassay; their clinical utility was not superior to other PTH radioimmunoassays.[198] A subsequently developed amino-terminal radioimmunoassay using a high affinity antiserum raised in chickens to human PTH[186-219] when applied to tests in humans indicated that circulating hormone concentrations in normal subjects are less than 100 pg/ml (expressed as equivalent of amino-terminal fragments less than 25 pg/ml), a level in good agreement with the cytochemical bioassay;[191] this assay has proved clinically useful.

Before considering the diagnostic uses of the parathyroid hormone immunoassay, it is useful to review the pathophysiology of parathyroid hormone secretion in hyperparathyroidism. In primary hyperparathyroidism, the mechanisms involved in the normal control of secretion of hormone must be abnormal, since patients have inappropriately high levels of the circulating hormone despite concomitant hypercalcemia.

The original hypothesis, that the abnormal pattern of secretion is due to autonomous secretion in dependent of blood calcium, was supported by one early report using radioimmunoassays.[326] The concept of autonomous secretion was challenged, however, by a subsequent study,[327] which showed, in patients with parathyroid adenomas, that hormone secretion was responsive to alterations in blood calcium caused by infusions of EDTA and/or calcium. These findings, subsequently confirmed by other studies *in vivo* and *in vitro* with parathyroid adenomas in tissue culture,[328-331] indicated that hormone production by parathyroid tumors was not autonomous. Because hormone secretion does respond to changes in serum calcium, one must conclude that the defect in control of hormone production is a mechanism more subtle than simple autonomy.

Two types of defect in secretion control or a combination of the two might theoretically explain PTH secretion in this disease. One possibility is that some fraction of hormone secretion is totally autonomous, that is, independent of the blood calcium concentration in both normals and those with hyperparathyroidism. The increased tissue mass in the latter leads to an inappropriately high hormone production despite hypercalcemia (Fig. 14–11*A*). The second defect implies that higher than normal levels of serum calcium are necessary to suppress hormone production, a "set point" error (Fig. 14–11*B*). In the latter instance, the secretion of hormone in patients with hyperparathyroidism would be suppressed, but at higher concentrations of serum calcium than in normal subjects (Fig. 14–11*B*). In the combination situation, the large mass of parathyroid tissue characteristic of hyperparathyroidism would result in an exaggeration of nonsuppressible secretion due to the increased number of cells *per se*; the requirement for higher calcium to suppress the fractional rate of secretion results in higher secretion per cell in adenoma despite hypercalcemia. The second defect combines with the first defect to cause excessive amounts of hormone to produce a state of hyperparathyroidism despite hypercalcemia, as is shown experimentally in humans (Fig. 14–11*C*).

Several lines of evidence had supported the possibility that nonsuppressible secretion plays a role in the abnormal secretion of parathyroid hormone.[332] (Chapter 3). Transplantation of several normal parathyroids into a single rat, thus considerably increasing the total mass of parathyroid tissue in the animal, produces hypercalcemia and a state of hyperparathyroidism.[332] Convincing evidence for incomplete suppression of hormone secretion in normal animals was obtained *in vivo*,[334,335] and considerable *in vitro* evidence, with gland tissue based on analyses of release of hormone at different calcium concentrations, indicated that a set point defect exists.[328-331]

Recently, as summarized in Figure 14–11C, reliable assays based on amino-terminal directed antisera have been applied to test the nature of the secretory defect in primary hyperparathyroidism directly in humans *in vivo*. The results of infusions of EDTA and calcium to lower and raise ionized calcium, respectively, have been coupled with hormone assays at various points during the calcium titration (see discussion and illustration of results in normals in Chapter 3). In the majority of patients with parathyroid adenomas there is responsiveness in hormone secretion as a function of blood calcium but the response is abnormal. There is an increased slope of secretory response and an increased level of calcium-independent, nonsuppressible hormone secretion as well as a "set point" defect, an increase in the degree of calcium elevation required to achieve 50% suppression of hormone production (Fig. 14–11*C*). All parathyroid carcinomas tested and a few adenomas had fixed elevated hormone output. The dynamic testing clearly distinguished all hyperparathyroid patients from euparathyroid individuals. Such testing may be useful in patients with equivocal clinical presentations or test results, such as patients with borderline calcium and PTH elevations and recurrent nephrolithiasis, for which parathyroid exploration might be useful.

Most of the radioimmunoassays used over the last two decades performed satisfactorily in distinguishing patients with primary hyperparathyroidism from normal subjects, regardless of the specificity of the antiserum. When evaluated against normal subjects without renal compromise, immunoreactive PTH levels were found to be elevated in 90% or more of patients with primary hyperparathyroidism.[191,196,211,229,231-234] Generally, there was a positive correlation between iPTH and the degree of hypercalcemia.

However, most of these radioimmunoassays for PTH failed to adequately distinguish patients with tumor-associated hypercalcemia from those with hyperparathyroidism. Results depended on the particular assay, generally

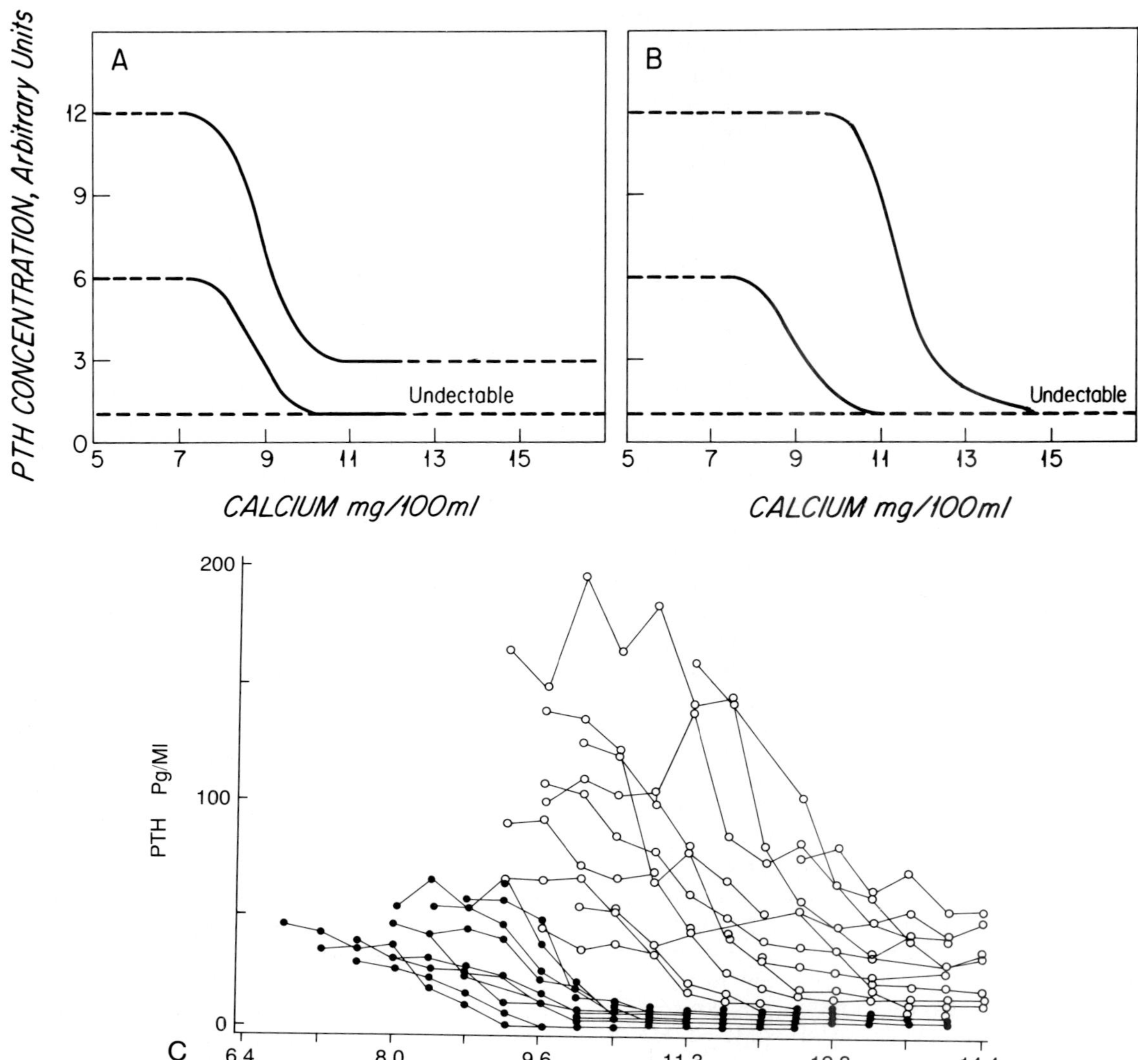

Figure 14–11. *A*, Diagram of one hypothesis (incomplete suppression) to explain secretory defect in primary hyperparathyroidism. Ordinate represents plasma parathyroid concentration; abscissa, plasma calcium. Dashed line at bottom of figure represents the lower limit of detectable PTH concentrations. Dashed extensions of curves describing changes in hormone concentration reflect extrapolations beyond the points where calcium concentrations could be safely varied. Hypothesis states that a small amount of hormone secretion persists despite elevated calcium. In the normal parathyroid, this quantity of secretion is small and insignificant. In hyperparathyroidism, greatly increased tissue mass leads to persistent secretion of hormone above detectable range (dashed line). Note slope describing secretion as a function of serum calcium for both normal and hyperparathyroid extrapolate to same calcium value (10.8 mg/100 ml) (no "set point defect"). *B*, Diagram depicting hypothesis of "set point" error to explain pathophysiologic mechanism of abnormality in hormone secretion in primary hyperparathyroidism. Hyperparathyroid individuals show steeper slopes of secretory response owing to large mass of tissue but, most critically, to explain persistent hypercalcemia; complete suppression of hormone output occurs only at abnormally high calcium level. *C*, Diagram illustrating the experimentally determined relationship between blood levels of Ca^{2+} and parathyroid hormone during Ca suppression and EDTA stimulation tests in normal adults (•) and patients with subsequently surgically confirmed primary hyperparathyroidism (o). Note that a complete separation of normal and abnormal subjects is possible if N-iPTH is measured while Ca^{2+} is systemically varied. Elements of both "set point" defect and persistent incomplete suppression are seen. (See also Figure 3–10, Chapter 3.)

giving normal rather than suppressed values in 15% to 50% of patients with tumor-associated hypercalcemia. Rarely apparent iPTH-levels were even elevated above normal, although in one assay, which shows excellent discrimination by levels of iPTH between normal subjects and those with primary hyperparathyroidism, elevated levels were detected in 27% of patients with tumor-associated hypercalcemia.[233] In contrast to primary hyperparathyroidism, "apparent" iPTH levels in hypercalcemic patients with cancer do not have a positive correlation with serum calcium levels.

Double antibody immunochemical methods have proved to eliminate most of the previous problems with radioimmunoassays. A "capture" antiserum, recognizing determinants in one portion of the molecule, is coupled to a solid-phase support and extracts hormone from a relatively large amount of plasma, which is then detected by a second, radioactive antibody that recognizes a second epitope on the molecule. One now extensively evaluated double antibody assay uses affinity-purified antibodies, an immobilized carboxyl-terminal antiserum, to "capture" intact hormone and carboxyl-fragments, and an amino-terminal radioiodinated second antiserum that selectively binds only intact hormone[494] (Fig. 14–12). Thus, the amount of radioiodinated antiserum bound to the solid phase varies as a function of intact hormone trapped or "sandwiched" between the two antisera.

The double antibody approach has been developed and applied by several laboratory groups[494a,494b] and is now offered by commercial laboratories. Extensive use of one immunoradiometric assay (IRMA)[494a] established a very sensitive standard curve, with detection of as little as 1 pg/ml (Fig. 14–12*A*). For the first time with any type of PTH assay, the sensitivity with double antibody assays is greater than needed to detect the lower limit of normal; also, hyperparathyroid patients are readily separated from those with the hypercalcemia of malignancy (Fig. 14–12*B*).

Such assays are highly useful to permit dynamic testing and to follow rapid changes in hormone concentration in blood after surgery.[494c,494d] The assay can be used to monitor the fall in hormone concentration after parathyroid surgery and to detect failure to remove sufficient parathyroid tissue when hormone concentration does not fall (Figs. 14–12*C*, 14–12*D*). It is possible to sacrifice sensitivity for speed when high levels of hormone are present as in hyperparathyroidism; a 15-minute assay applied to the same measurements of hormone level after surgery (Fig. 14–12*D*). The result suggests the eventual possibility of intraoperative monitoring in difficult cases (re-exploration, hyperplasia).

2. In Vivo *and* In Vitro *Urinary Cyclic AMP*

In normal subjects, total urinary cAMP excretion derives equally from filtered load and nephrogenous secretion of the nucleotide.[237] Plasma cAMP, which is normally maintained within narrow limits, increases with progressive renal impairment so that the nucleotide filtered load, when expressed as a function of glomerular filtration rate, remains relatively constant over creatinine clearance rates of 20 to 140 ml/minute.[237] Since filtered load remains constant over a wide range of renal functional status, nephrogenous cAMP becomes the major variable in urinary cAMP levels. Fortunately, although calcitonin, antidiuretic hormone, and PTH all stimulate renal adenylate cyclase *in vitro*, only the renal response to PTH results in urinary excretion of the nucleotide *in vivo*.[237]

To formally measure nephrogenous cAMP, the filtered load of plasma cAMP (nM/100 ml glomerular filtrate) is subtracted from the urinary cAMP (nM/100 ml glomerular filtrate).[238]

Measurement of the nephrogenous component was reported as unnecessary because the non-nephrogenous component is fairly constant although the test is not validated for severe renal failure (GFR below 20 to 30 ml/minute). Approximately 85% to 90% of patients with primary hyperparathyroidism will have elevated urinary cAMP levels when the volume is expressed parametrically as nM/100 ml GF.[237]

In vitro assays based on stimulation of adenylate cyclase or cyclic AMP accumulation in cells have been evaluated as assays to measure circulating elevated hormone concentrations but no normal levels can be detected.[229,240-242]

In general, with the advent of highly successful double antibody assays that measure intact hormone (since there is no evidence that intact hormone that is biologically inactive circulates) and that correlate well with physiologic or pathophysiologic states, assay based on cyclic AMP will probably be limited to research applications.

3. In Vitro *Cytochemical Bioassay*

Highly sensitive methods of measuring biologically active parathyroid hormone have been developed, based on cytochemical analysis of glucose-6-phosphate dehydro-

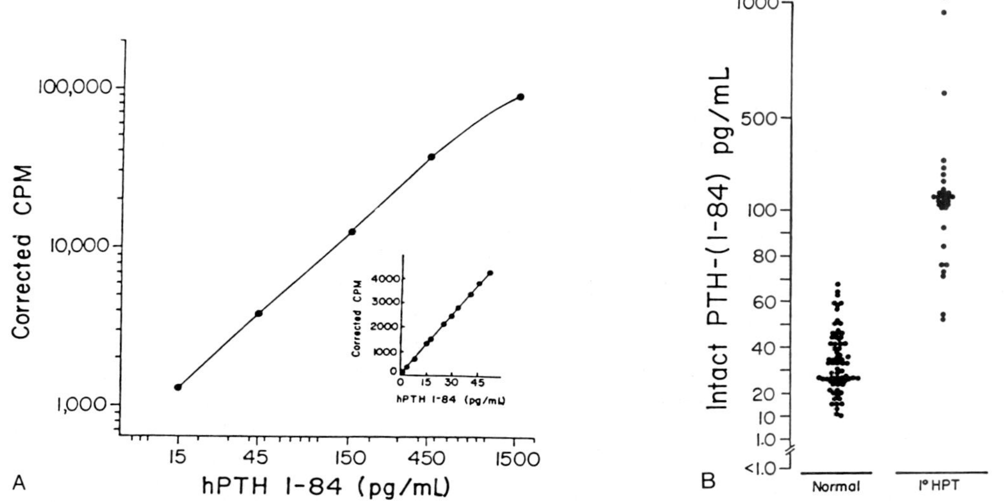

Figure 14–12. *A,* Dose-response plot for IRMA of PTH. Inset: linear plot for lower concentrations of PTH. Rest of plot is log–log. *B,* Intact PTH 1–84 measured by IRMA in sera from 72 normal individuals, 37 patients with surgically proven hyperparathyroidism (1° HPT), and 24 patients with hypercalcemia associated with malignancy. The normal reference interval is 12 to 65 pg/ml. Mean PTH in patients with hyperparathyroidism was 206 (± 43 SEM) pg/ml and 3.35 (± 0.8 SEM) pg/ml in individuals with hypercalcemia associated with malignancy. (*A* and *B* from Nussbaum SR, Zahradnik RJ, Lavigne Jr, et al: Highly sensitive two-site immunoradiometric assay of parathyrin and its clinical utility in evaluating patients with hypercalcemia. Clin Chem 33:1364–1367, 1987.)

genase activity in guinea pig–kidney distal convoluted tubules.[246,247] This method is at least 100 times more sensitive than available radioimmunoassays, allowing measurement of PTH in 1:1000 dilutions of plasma of normal individuals. Until recently, the assay was believed to be highly specific for PTH. Levels of hormone found in normal people, 2.9 to 29 pg/ml, were distinguished from values in hypoparathyroidism, less than 1 pg/ml, and from values in patients with primary or secondary hyperparathyroidism, 34 to 11,000 pg/ml.[200] Enthusiasm for the widespread clinical use of this assay has been dampened, however, because not only is the procedure technically difficult and time-consuming, but more important, further experience indicates that the assay fails to distinguish between hypercalcemic patients with hyperparathyroidism and those with cancer. Most hypercalcemic patients with hypercalcemia and elevated nephrogenous cAMP were found to have elevated circulating activity in the cytochemical bioassay. The remainder of these patients and most hypercalcemic cancer patients with suppressed nephrogenous cAMP were found to have normal levels of circulating activity. Less than 10% of the total of patients with hypercalcemia and malignancy had suppressed levels of activity.[248]

After gel filtration of plasma samples, cytochemical bioactivity was found in fractions of higher apparent molecular weight than that of PTH.[200] Tumor extracts enriched with these factors do not react with antisera to PTH, but the cytochemical bioactivity is inhibited by analogues of PTH that inhibit PTH binding and PTH-stimulated adenylate cyclase.[248-250] Testing of alternative enzymes has not yielded improved specificity.[250] Thus, PTH bioassays are important research tools with clinical utility limited by ambiguous results in hypercalcemia in association with cancers as well as by the technical complexities.

IV. DIFFERENTIAL DIAGNOSIS OF HYPERCALCEMIA

The various causes of hypercalcemia may be considered in terms of common pathophysiologic mechanisms (Table 14–1). The following discussion briefly reviews these en-

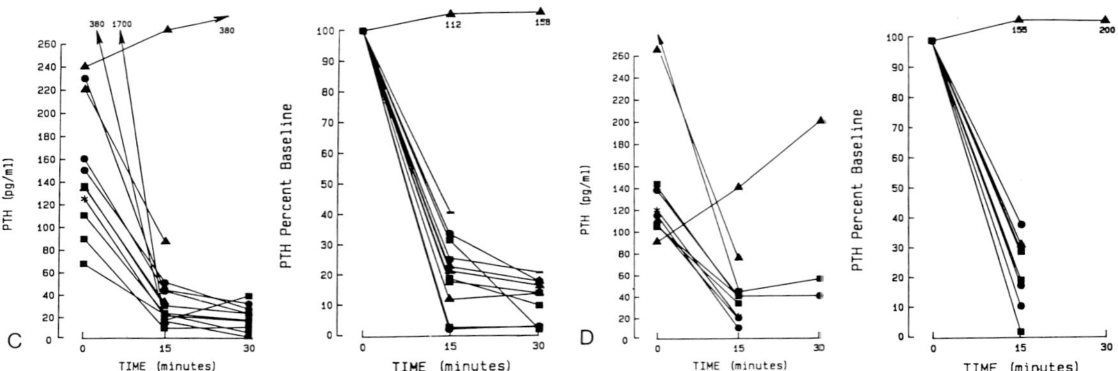

Figure 14–12 *Continued C,* Left, 24-hour IRMA for PTH serum PTH (1–84) concentrations, expressed as pg/ml, at baseline, 15 and 30 minutes after ligation of the vascular pedicle to the parathyroid adenoma. Right, Serum PTH concentrations expressed as a percentage of time zero value. In one patient with parathyroid carcinoma, PTH values did not fall. *D,* Left, 15-minute IRMA for PTH. Serum PTH-(1–84) concentrations at baseline, 15 and 30 minutes after ligation of the vascular pedicle to the PTH adenoma. Right, serum PTH-(1–84) expressed as a percentage of time zero value. In all patients cured of hyperparathyroidism by resection of an adenoma, PTH declined to 40% of basal values. In the patient with parathyroid carcinoma, PTH remained elevated. (*C* and *D* from Nussbaum SR, Thompson AR, Hutcheson KA, et al: Intraoperative measurement of parathyroid hormone in the surgical management of hyperparathyroidism. Surgery 104:1121–1127, 1988.)

tities except for tumor hypercalcemia, which is reviewed in Chapter 21. Although this consideration is a deliberate oversimplification, using only five categories of disease as potential causes of hypercalcemia, it seems useful as a logical approach in the differential diagnosis of hypercalcemia syndromes. Hyperparathyroidism is the most frequent cause of hypercalcemia. The disease is manifested as a chronic disorder in which symptoms develop over a period of months to years; alternatively, hyperparathyroidism can be entirely asymptomatic. Hypercalcemia can also be the earliest clue to the presence of a malignant tumor, the second most common cause of hypercalcemia in the adult population. Hyperparathyroidism and malignancy together account for greater than 90% of all cases of hypercalcemia. In most cases of tumor-associated hypercalcemia symptoms develop rapidly and are severe (see Chapter 21). Patients seek medical attention because of disabling symptoms arising from the underlying tumor, and the hypercalcemia is discovered during the evaluation. The interval between the first detection of hypercalcemia in patients with tumors and their death is often less than 1 year.

In the 10% or so of remaining cases of hypercalcemia not due to hyperparathyroidism or tumors, a variety of disorders are responsible. These other causes of hypercalcemia may be grouped into three categories (Table 14–1): (1) those associated with excessive vitamin D action, (2) those associated with high bone turnover from any of several causes, and (3) renal failure–related hypercalcemia, occurring either as a complication of the management of patients with primary renal failure or in which renal failure occurs secondarily, as in excessive ingestion of milk and alkali. Except in hypercalcemia associated with tumors, the hypercalcemia is usually easily corrected, allowing specific therapy of the underlying disease.

Malignancy-associated hypercalcemia is considered in Chapter 21. The following is a review of the clinical features of the causes of hypercalcemia other than primary hyperparathyroidism and cancer and suggests a general philosophy of approach to differential diagnosis of hypercalcemia.

A. Parathyroid-Related Causes of Hypercalcemia Distinct from Primary Hyperparathyroidism

1. Lithium Therapy

Lithium therapy, employed in the management of bipolar and other psychiatric disorders, causes hypercalcemia in approximately

10% of patients treated with customary doses for extended periods of time. The process seems to involve hypersecretion of the parathyroids with elevated PTH levels in mediation of the hypercalcemia, but one feature of the pathophysiologic mechanism is confusing. Generally, the hypercalcemia seems dependent on continued lithium treatment, remitting and recurring when lithium is stopped and restarted, yet when several patients were explored, parathyroid adenomas were found.

The presence of hypercalcemia does not correlate with plasma lithium level, but the frequency with which hypercalcemia occurs is sufficiently high to support a causal relationship between lithium and the hypercalcemia, particularly the dependence of the hypercalcemia on the continuation of the lithium.[255a] It is presumed that in most cases an adenoma is not present, merely hyperfunctioning glands; furthermore, the glands need not be postulated to be hyperplastic. Lithium, at the levels achieved in blood in treated patients, can be shown *in vitro* to shift the curve describing PTH secretion as a function of calcium level to the right, i.e., requiring higher calcium levels to lower PTH secretion.[257] It is logical to assume that this effect can cause elevated PTH and consequent hypercalcemia in otherwise normal individuals. If careful studies were done, elevated PTH levels might be found in many more lithium-treated patients than the 10% in whom frank hypercalcemia is detected. The adenomas reported in a few patients with lithium therapy and hypercalcemia may reflect the presence of an independently occurring parathyroid tumor; an effect of lithium on parathyroid gland growth need not be implicated (although it is not excluded), since clinically the majority of patients show complete reversal of hypercalcemia when lithium is stopped.[255a] Long-term follow-up studies have not been reported; many patients are continued on lithium because it is needed to treat psychiatric problems. These patients are presumably best managed according to the principles used in asymptomatic hypercalcemia, independent of lithium administration.[255a] If troubling symptoms or unfavorable signs develop, such as rising blood calcium levels, progressive bone demineralization, or kidney stones, it may be necessary to seek alternate psychotropic medication. Since it is unclear how often parathyroid adenomas will be found, it does not seem wise to recommend parathyroid surgery unless the hypercalcemia and elevated PTH persist after lithium is discontinued.

2. Familial Hypocalciuric Hypercalcemia

Familial hypocalciuric hypercalcemia (familial benign hypercalcemia, FHH) is transmitted as an autosomal dominant trait.[255a] Recognition of the disorder is important because affected individuals are frequently discovered owing to asymptomatic hypercalcemia; surgical exploration of the parathyroids is not indicated because it does not cure the disorder. It is therefore important to recognize such patients as differing from those with primary hyperparathyroidism.

The pathophysiology of FHH is not understood, and there is no single biochemical marker to distinguish these patients from patients with primary hyperparathyroidism. Nonetheless, the aggregate evidence serves to separate FHH clearly from primary hyperparathyroidism. The majority of patients with primary hyperparathyroidism have less than 99% renal calcium reabsorption,[262,262a] and most patients with FHH exceed 99% reabsorption. The hypercalcemia may be detectable in affected members of the kindreds in the first decade of life,[263-264] whereas hypercalcemia rarely occurs in primary hyperparathyroidism and the MEN syndrome in patients under the age of 10 years. The iPTH values may be elevated in FHH, but they are usually normal or lower than in patients with primary hyperparathyroidism.[262,262a] In patients who are inadvertently operated on, hypercalcemia and hypocalciuria persist without elevated PTH levels; the hypercalcemia and hypocalciuria, therefore, do not seem PTH-dependent.[262a] Serum magnesium levels are, on average, higher in FHH than in primary hyperparathyroidism.[260-262] The overall evidence favors some as yet uncharacterized nonparathyroid–dependent defect in calcium transport into or out of extracellular fluid.[262,262a]

Few clinical signs or symptoms are present in patients with FHH.[262] Unlike the MEN syndromes, other endocrine abnormalities are not present.[262] Most patients' disease is detected as a result of family screening after the diagnosis has been made in one member of the kindred. Unfortunately, the initial patient is frequently operated on without reversal of the hypercalcemia.[258-262a] At operation, the glands appear normal, or a moderate degree of hyperplasia of all parathyroid glands is seen.[262] No patient has had reversal of hypercalcemia by surgery unless all of the parathyroid tissue is inadvertently removed, rendering the patient hypoparathyroid, a most undesirable result.[262-262a] The high renal calcium reabsorption and the prompt recurrence of hypercalcemia as long as any parathyroid tissue remains make evident clinically that there is some abnormality in the regulation of the ratio of extracellular to intracellular calcium concentration or some abnormal mechanisms of calcium sensing in cell membranes in the kidney and/or elsewhere;[262a] independent of parathyroid hormone excess. The exact nature of this disorder and its natural history are not clear yet, but since the parathyroid glands are permissive rather than responsible for the syndrome, parathyroid surgery is not advocated; nor is medical treatment needed to lower the calcium levels, in view of the lack of symptoms.

B. Vitamin D–Related Hypercalcemia

Hypercalcemia related to excessive vitamin D action is due to either excessive ingestion or abnormal metabolism of the vitamin.[265,266] Abnormal metabolism of the vitamin is usually acquired in association with some widespread granulomatous disorder,[267-272] but there is one rare hereditary form of vitamin D sensitivity seen in infants in association with a variety of other developmental anomalies.[274] In certain disorders, defective regulation of the production of 1,25$(OH)_2D_3$ occurs; there is tight regulation of the renal 1-hydroxylase by several controlling factors (Chapter 5), but this normal feedback suppression by 1,25$(OH)_2D$ is less effective in infants than in adults and operates poorly, if at all, on 1-hydroxylase activity present in nonrenal ectopic sites, for example, in the granulomas of sarcoidosis.[268]

1. *Vitamin D Intoxication*

The chronic ingestion of large doses of vitamin D, usually at least 100 times the normal physiologic requirement (doses in excess of 50,000 to 100,000 units/day), is required to produce hypercalcemia in normal individuals (see Chapter 5). The excessive vitamin D action leads to an inappropriate increase in intestinal calcium absorption and probably also in bone resorption at least in humans.[266,273]

One obvious causative mechanism for the hypercalcemia is the excessive production of 25(OH)D that occurs as a consequence of a vast increase in the substrate, vitamin D. 25(OH)D production is much less tightly regulated than is the production of active metabolite, 1,25$(OH)_2D$. Hence, it is routine to detect concentrations of 25(OH)D 5 to 15 times or more above normal in patients who have been taking large doses of vitamin D, whether therapeutically, as in hypoparathyroidism, or accidentally, as in vitamin D intoxication.[265,266] 25(OH)D has a low but definite biological potency on the target cells for vitamin D action in intestine and bone. Hence, the excessive vitamin D action may be attributable to the high levels of 25(OH)D itself.[265] Disagreement exists in the few published reports concerning 1,25$(OH)_2D_3$ levels. An early report stressed excessive 25(OH)D levels but normal levels of 1,25$(OH)_2D_3$[265]; a more extensive report indicated elevated levels of 1,25(OH)D in seven of eight cases of vitamin D intoxication as well as massive increases in 25(OH)D levels.[266]

Clinically, the diagnosis is readily made in suspected patients by the detection of markedly elevated levels of 25(OH)D.[265,266] Hypercalcemia is usually well controlled by the discontinuation of the intake of vitamin D, a restriction of calcium in the diet, and increased fluid intake. Stores of vitamin D in fat are substantial, and vitamin D intoxication may persist for some weeks after vitamin D ingestion is terminated. Occasionally, treatment of these patients with glucocorticoid therapy is needed to ameliorate more persistent or severe hypercalcemia; the hypercalcemia is exquisitely sensitive to glucocorticoids. Normocalcemia is restored within several days by the administration of daily doses of 100 mg of hydrocortisone or its equivalent.

2. *Sarcoidosis and Other Granulomatous Diseases*

It has been recognized for a number of decades that patients with sarcoidosis have an abnormal sensitivity to ingested vitamin D (see Chapter 22). The pathophysiology of the hypercalcemia is now understood.[267-271,275] Similar pathophysiologic mechanisms are responsible for hypercalcemia seen in other granulomatous disease such as tuberculosis. Normal relations between 25(OH)D and the product, the active metabolite 1,25$(OH)_2D$ (Chapter 5), are not maintained in these patients; rather, there is excessive, unregulated production of $1,25(OH)_2D$.[267,268,276] A positive correlation exists between 25(OH)D levels (reflecting vitamin D intake) and the circulating levels of $1,25(OH)_2D$ (normally, there is no increase in the active metabolite despite increasing 25(OH)D levels). It is now understood that in patients with granulomatous diseases, synthesis of $1,25(OH)_2D$ occurs in macrophages of other cells contained within the granulomas. Studies of macrophages obtained from sarcoid granulomas reveal increased conversion of 25(OH)D to $1,25(OH)_2D$.[270] Hypercalcemia has occurred in an anephric patient with sarcoidosis in association with increased $1,25(OH)_2D$ levels.[271] The usual regulation of active metabolite production by calcium or PTH is not seen in these patients; high calcium intakes do not lead to a reduction in the level of $1,25(OH)_2D$ concentrations in the blood of patients with sarcoidosis as occurs in normal subjects.[267,268,272,276] Coexistent hypoparathyroidism and sarcoidosis in one patient led to normal production of $1,25(OH)_2D$ despite the absence of parathyroid hormone.[272] Based on these observations it seems certain that increased production of $1,25(OH)_2D$ by the granulomas rather than reduced metabolic clearance of the active metabolite is the mechanism responsible for the hypercalcemia. However, some evidence suggests there may be altered clearance of $1,25(OH)_2D$ from blood, as well.[267,268]

Patients with sarcoidosis, whether hypercalcemic or normocalcemic, have unregulated production of $1,25(OH)_2D$ in response to vitamin D loading.[267,268] Extensive exposure to sunlight, as in summer months,[277] or administration of small amounts of vitamin D is followed by demonstrably increased levels of the active metabolite and hypercalcemia.[267,268] Treatment with moderate doses of glucocorticoids reverses the hypercalcemia and the excessive rise in blood levels of $1,25(OH)_2D$ following oral ingestion of vitamin D.[267,268] The variation in the frequency of occurrence of hypercalcemia in sarcoidosis in earlier clinical reports over the preceding several decades (varying from less than 10% to as high as 60%) is probably explained by the moderating influence of steroids used often to control pulmonary complications and other manifestations of the granulomatous disease.[278] Presumably, multiple effects of the steroid administration occur in the disease, but both excessive production of the metabolite and responsiveness to it in target organs are blocked by steroids.[267]

In some patients with sarcoidosis, there are areas of lytic lesions in bone, but increased bone resorption does not appear to be a factor in most cases. The hypercalcemia is directly related to increased absorption of intestinal calcium.[278] Clinically, hypercalcemia is usually a manifestation of severe disseminated disease.[278] Hence, pulmonary involvement is usually always present. Chest films characteristically reveal a diffuse fibronodular infiltrate and/or prominent hilar adenopathy. An elevated blood gamma globulin may also occur. Definitive diagnosis relies on the demonstration of noncaseating granulomas in biopsies of liver or lymph nodes. Sarcoidosis may exist for several years with very few clinical signs.[278] In some patients, abnormal pulmonary function as tested by exercise-induced hypoxia or abnormal carbon monoxide diffusion time may be detected. Such findings in patients whose blood chemical indices are atypical for primary hyperparathyroidism (low PTH values, normal phosphate) may direct attention to a more detailed search for pulmonary sarcoidosis.

Management of the calcium metabolism in patients with sarcoidosis is best accomplished by avoiding excessive exposure to sunlight and by limiting intake of vitamin D and calcium. Glucocorticoids in the daily equivalent of 100 mg of hydrocortisone usually are sufficient to control persistent hypercalcemia.[278] Presumably, however, the abnormal sensitivity to vitamin D and abnormal regulation of $1,25(OH)_2D$ synthesis persist for as long as the granulomatous disease is active. Parathyroid hormone levels are suppressed and $1,25(OH)_2D$ levels are usually always elevated in patients with sarcoidosis.[279] There are, however, reports of the coexistence of primary hyperparathyroidism and sarcoidosis, but it is unclear whether this is more than a random association.

3. *Idiopathic Hypercalcemia of Infancy*

This unusual childhood syndrome, sometimes referred to as Williams syndrome, consists of multiple congenital developmental defects including three principal abnormalities—supravalvular aortic stenosis, mental retardation, and elfin facies—in association with hypercalcemia due to abnormal sensitivity to vitamin D.[274,280-283] The syndrome was first recognized in England in the post–World War II period following the vitamin D fortification of milk. Hypercalcemia develops during ingestion of as little as 2000 to 4000 units of vitamin D per day.[280,283] Recent studies have revealed marked increases in serum levels of $1,25(OH)_2D$, values ranging from 150 to 500 pg/ml.[274] The precise mechanism of the abnormal sensitivity to vitamin D and the increased circulating levels of $1,25(OH)_2D$ is as yet unclarified, but the hypercalcemia comes about by excessive intestinal calcium absorption.[274,280,282] After the first few years of life, the increased levels of $1,25(OH)_2D_3$ and increased sensitivity to vitamin D intake disappear.[274] One view concerning the pathophysiologic mechanism of the disease is that there is an abnormal clearance or inactivation of vitamin D or 25(OH)D.[280] The less precise regulation of the renal 1α-hydroxylase present in all infants leads to increased circulating $1,25(OH)_2D$ levels because of increased levels of substrate 25(OH)D. This view leads to the conclusion that the defect in these children involves the renal hydroxylase step indirectly and thus differs from the abnormality in sarcoidosis in which there is clearly an abnormal regulation of the 1-hydroxylase in granulomas.

The preferred treatment is restriction of calcium intake. Occasionally, the hypercalcemia can be quite severe before the presence of the syndrome is recognized. Calcium values above 16 mg/100 ml are recorded.[269] Treatment with glucocorticoids in the doses used for vitamin D intoxication or sarcoidosis, adjusted for body weight of the infant, rapidly reverses the hypercalcemia.

C. Hypercalcemia Associated with High Bone Turnover

1. *Hyperthyroidism*

Severe and symptomatic hypercalcemia is a rare complication of thyrotoxicosis (see Chapter 18). However, minimal elevations of serum calcium have been reported in as many as 23% of patients with hyperthyroidism.[284,285] The cause of hypercalcemia in hyperthyroidism appears to be secondary to increased bone resorption, probably due to direct effects of thyroxin and triiodothyronine on the skeleton.[286-291]

The turnover of calcium by the skeleton is increased by thyroid hormone.[288] One group reported that the serum calcium in hyperthyroid patients averaged 0.5 mg/100 ml higher than in a group of age-matched normal control subjects.[290] Serum inorganic phosphorus levels are more likely high or normal than low, and urinary phosphate clearance is decreased, suggesting that PTH secretion is suppressed. Low serum PTH levels have been reported in patients with hyperthyroidism and marked hypercalcemia.[292] Suppression of PTH secretion decreases tubular reabsorption of calcium and leads to hypercalciuria, which is frequently seen in patients with thyrotoxicosis.[286-294,296]

It has been emphasized that patients with thyrotoxicosis who develop severe hypercalcemia may have concomitant hyperparathyroidism, inasmuch as the hypercalcemia of uncomplicated thyrotoxicosis is usually mild.[295] One thyrotoxic patient with a serum calcium of 15 mg/100 ml later proved to have a parathyroid adenoma.[297] Another group described 17 patients with thyrotoxicosis and concomitant parathyroid adenomas.[298]

The diagnosis of hyperthyroidism usually offers no difficulties because, in most cases, it is the thyrotoxicosis rather than the hypercalcemia that brings the patient to the physician. However, particularly in the elderly, the signs of thyrotoxicosis may be minimal. During the treatment of a patient with thyrotoxicosis and hypercalcemia, repeated determinations of serum calcium should be made. If the serum calcium does not return toward normal as the thyrotoxicosis is brought under control, another cause for the hypercalcemia, such as hyperparathyroidism, should be suspected.

2. *Immobilization*

Immobilization is rarely associated with hypercalcemia in the absence of an associated disease in adults (Chapter 12), but may be associated with hypercalcemia in children and young adolescents, particularly after spinal cord injury and paraplegia or quadriplegia.[299,299a] If significant ambulation again becomes possible, the hypercalcemia in young patients usually returns to normal spontaneously.

The mechanism involves a change in bone turnover rates due to sudden loss of weight-bearing; resorption is favored over formation. In a young person with higher rates of bone turnover physiologically or in elderly patients with diseases that cause high bone turnover, absolute rates are high enough, when asynchronous, to cause hypercalcemia. The same phenomenon can be detected in normal volunteers subjected to extensive bed rest; hypercalciuria and marked skeletal calcium mobilization can be seen, although they do not usually become frankly hypercalcemic. In an adult patient, an underlying disease associated with high bone turnover, such as Paget's disease, may be discovered as the cause of hypercalcemia secondary to immobilization.

3. Thiazides

Administration of benzothiadiazides (thiazides)[304] can cause hypercalcemia in patients with high rates of bone turnover, such as patients with hyperparathyroidism,[305,306] hypoparathyroidism treated with large doses of vitamin D,[300] and juvenile, high-turnover osteoporosis.[306] Thiazides have been used as a provocative test to bring out borderline hypercalcemia in patients suspected of having hyperparathyroidism.[307] Thiazide administration to normal individuals causes a transient increase in blood calcium, usually within the normal range, which then reverts to preexisting levels after a week or more of continued thiazide administration.[302] The pharmacologic action of thiazides is complex. The drug appears to challenge calcium homeostasis by actions on renal calcium excretion, bone-calcium turnover, and intestinal calcium absorption (Chapter 23). The efficiency of PTH action *per se* is increased and may explain the observed effects in many patients.[300-303]

Several aspects of the actions of the thiazides, particularly in normal subjects and in patients with hypoparathyroidism, are not understood. Chronic administration of thiazide lowers urinary calcium excretion in normal subjects, which persists for the duration of the treatment. This hypocalciuric effect is not observed in some studies of hypoparathyroid patients[300,302,303] but is in others, at least when combined with sodium restriction.[308,309] The disparate observations are puzzling but probably indicate an action of thiazides on the renal tubule despite deficiency of PTH. Therefore, the actions of the drug are not merely an augmentation of the biological actions of PTH.[307] In fact, the substantial hypocalciuric effect of thiazides that can be elicited in hypoparathyroid patients on high-dose vitamin D and oral calcium replacement has been used successfully as an adjunct to therapy by achieving a satisfactory elevation of serum calcium without severe hypercalciuria.[309] A definite hypocalciuric effect of thiazides is seen in hypoparathyroid animals and some humans, the latter requiring sodium restriction.[309] The hypocalciuric effect in animals seems to involve reduced intestinal calcium absorption efficiency as well as increased renal calcium reabsorption, perhaps via compensatory reductions in levels of circulating $1,25(OH)_2D_3$ and ensuring intestinal calcium absorption.[307] The strong augmenting action of thiazides on the effectiveness of PTH in bone and kidney, however, is clearly a predominant action explaining the usual failure to see hypocalciuria in hypoparathyroidism. The potentiation of PTH has been shown experimentally with co-infusions of PTH and thiazides to patients with hypoparathyroidism.[306] The hypocalciuric effect of the drug involves, in part, the enhancement of proximal tubular resorption of sodium and calcium that results from chronic depletion of sodium and extracellular fluid volume. Hence, the hypocalciuric effect of thiazides involves both secondary effects of volume depletion and augmentation of PTH action.[302]

Two lines of evidence suggest that the skeleton is a locus of action of thiazides that involves potentiation of the actions of both PTH and vitamin D. Anephric patients, maintained on hemodialysis (see Chapter 13), show a hypercalcemic response to hydrochlorothiazide administration in dosages of 200 mg/day for 2 to 4 weeks.[301] The hypercalcemic response (both ionized and total calcium) to short-term chlorothiazide infusion is observed in normal subjects and patients with hyperparathyroidism even when urinary excretion of calcium (and sodium) was markedly increased.[303] The increased skeletal turnover and consequent hypercalcemia due to thiazides clearly requires a synergism with endogenous PTH or large doses of vitamin D. The serum calcium levels of hypoparathyroid patients do not rise during chlorothiazide infusion alone but do when PTH is infused along with the chlorothiazide.[303] On the other hand, a hypercalcemic response to thiazides independent of PTH is seen when the drug is administered chronically to patients with postoperative hypoparathyroidism treated with high dosages of vitamin D.[300,303] The overall results suggest that if normal hormonal function and calcium and bone metabolism are present, homeostatic controls can be reset to counteract the calcium elevating effect of thiazides. In the presence of hyperparathyroidism or increased bone turnover from another cause, such as with high-dose vitamin D therapy, homeostatic mechanisms cannot be reset.[300,302]

Clinically, it is important to recognize that the presence of hypercalcemia in association with thiazide administration points to an underlying disorder associated with calcium metabolism or bone turnover and is not a manifestation of iatrogenic disease in a normal subject. It is also important to remember the severity of hypercalcemia in hyperparathyroidism may be exaggerated if thiazides are being taken. The abnormal effects of the thiazide on calcium metabolism disappear within days of cessation of treatment with a drug. Treatment with thiazides should be stopped in hypercalcemic patients because it exaggerates the apparent degree of hypercalcemia, and it can confuse judgments about the need for surgery.

4. Vitamin A Intoxication

Hypercalcemia due to vitamin A intoxication is rare. Most examples of vitamin A intoxication result from accidental overdose from nutritional supplements.[310-312] Calcium levels have been reported to be elevated into the 12 to 14 mg/100 ml range in patients who have taken 50,000 to 100,000 units of vitamin A daily, 10 to 20 times the minimum daily requirement. The patients have typical features of severe hypercalcemia that include fatigue, anorexia, severe muscle pain, and sometimes diffuse bone pain.[310,311,312]

The mechanism of action of the excess vitamin A intake is presumed to be increased bone resorption; vitamin A causes increased bone resorption in large doses in bone cultures *in vitro*.

The diagnosis is established by history and by confirmatory measurements of vitamin A levels in serum, which are often increased several-fold above normal. Occasionally, characteristic skeletal x-ray features can be seen that reveal very distinctive periosteal calcifications, particularly in films of the hands.[311,312] Treatment consists of withdrawal of the vitamin, which is usually associated with the prompt disappearance of the hypercalcemia and reversal of the skeletal changes. If necessary, administration of 100 mg of cortisone or its equivalent per day leads to rapid normalization of the calcium.[242-244]

D. Hypercalcemia Associated with Renal Failure

1. Severe Secondary Hyperparathyroidism

Secondary hyperparathyroidism is the term used to apply to the state seen in certain diseases (vitamin D deficiency, renal failure) in which there is excessive production of PTH due to resistance to the metabolic actions of the hormone.[245] Parathyroid gland hyperplasia with resultant increased level of secretion of PTH occurs because of resistance to the effects of the normal circulating levels of the hormone; this resistance leads to chronic hypocalcemia, which, in turn, is a stimulus to enlargement of the parathyroid glands. As with any chronic adaptive state that represents an adjustment in normal homeostatic mechanisms, it is difficult to reconstruct precisely the sequential nature of events at any given point in the course of a patient's disease. Evidence that the sequence is resistance to PTH, hypocalcemia, parathyroid gland hyperplasia, and increased PTH secretion from enlarged glands,[313] is based on animal and human studies, the former involving experimental renal failure with phosphate retention,[314] and the latter occurring during the course of treatment of patients with diphosphonates that acutely block skeletal resorptive response.[315]

As noted in Chapter 13, secondary hyperparathyroidism occurs in patients with renal failure, but also in patients with osteomalacia (vitamin D deficiency) (Chapters 5 and 11) and pseudohypoparathyroidism (deficient receptor response to PTH). The clinical manifestations of secondary hyperparathyroidism vary greatly in these different disease states; hypercalcemia is usually detected only in renal failure where "overshoot" occurs.[315] It seems that primary and secondary hyperparathyroidism can be distinguished by the autonomous nature of the growth of the parathyroid glands in primary hyperparathyroidism (irreversible) and the merely adaptive increase in parathyroid gland size in secondary hyperparathyroidism (reversible).[313] In fact, reversal from an abnormal pattern of secretion accompanied by an involution of parathyroid gland mass to normal occurs in human subjects treated with diphosphonate after the drug is withdrawn and normal skeletal responsiveness recurs.[315]

In progressive kidney disease, the initial tendency to hypocalcemia is attributable to two causes: phosphate retention that develops because of the reduced renal capacity to excrete phosphate, and reduced concentrations of the enzyme 25(OH)D 1-hydroxylase concomitant with progressive renal damage (Chapter 13). The phosphate retention metabolically lowers the rate of $1,25(OH)_2D_3$ production, reduces skeletal responsiveness to PTH, and increases calcium outflow from extracellular fluid, while the reduced enzyme levels directly lower $1,25(OH)_2D_3$ synthesis.

2. Aluminum Intoxication

Aluminum intoxication occurs in patients on chronic dialysis, presumably owing to the aluminum present in dialysis fluids. Manifestations of the disorder include an acute dementia and a peculiar form of unresponsive severe osteomalacia.[316-319] The patients often develop severe bone pain, multiple nonhealing fractures, particularly of the ribs and pelvis, and a proximal myopathy.[318,320] Hypercalcemia is often encountered in these patients when they are treated by the administration of calcium and vitamin D or $1,25(OH)_2D$.[318,320] It is believed that acute hypercalcemia develops in response to the administration of vitamin D because of an impaired capacity of the skeleton to bind calcium due to the deposition of aluminum at mineralization sites.[318] Treatment with agents that chelate aluminum such as deferoxamine combined with $1,25(OH)_2D_3$ and $24,25(OH)_2D_3$ leads to improvement of the skeletal disorder and symptoms in some patients.[321]

3. Milk-Alkali Syndrome

The milk-alkali syndrome has been described in several distinctive clinical presentations—acute, subacute, and chronic—all of which feature the triad of hypercalcemia, alkalosis, and renal failure.[322-324] The syndrome is due to excessive ingestion of calcium and absorbable antacids such as milk or calcium carbonate.[322,324] The disorder is much less frequent since its widespread recognition and the availability of nonabsorbable antacids and H_2 receptor antagonists such as cimetidine and ranitidine for the treatment of gastric and duodenal ulcers.

In analysis of the factors responsible for development of the milk-alkali syndrome, it becomes apparent that individual susceptibility must be important in the pathogenesis because many patients have been treated with a high intake of calcium and alkali in the form of calcium carbonate without developing the syndrome.[322a] One known variation in susceptibility comes from analysis of variation in fractional intestinal calcium absorption as a function of calcium intake (as seen in patients with kidney stones, so-called dietary-dependent hypercalciuria). The small fraction of patients with a hereditary predisposition to excessive calcium absorption continue to absorb a high fraction of calcium despite intakes as high as 2 g or more of elemental calcium per day rather than reducing calcium absorption with high intake as is seen in the majority of normal subjects.[322a] Resultant mild hypercalcemia, which can be demonstrated after meals in such patients, is postulated to be the critical factor in the subsequent generation of alkalosis.[322a] Most individuals are quite resistant to the development of alkalosis after ingestion of even large quantities of non–calcium-containing alkali such as sodium bicarbonate. With the development of postprandial hypercalcemia, a mild increase occurs in sodium excretion and there is some depletion of total body water.[322a] These effects coupled with some suppression of endogenous PTH secretion would lead to increased bicarbonate reabsorption.[322a] This bicarbonate retention then leads to alkalosis in the face of continued calcium carbonate ingestion. It can be shown independently that alkalosis, *per se*, results in selective enhancement of calcium reabsorption in the distal nephron, thus aggravating the hypercalcemia.[323] The vicious cycle of mild hypercalcemia, bicarbonate retention, alkalosis, renal calcium retention, and severe hypercalcemia perpetuates and aggravates hypercalcemia and alkalosis as long as ingestion of large amounts of calcium and absorbable alkali continues. As renal failure develops, reduced capacity to excrete calcium due to loss of nephrons worsens the condition. On the other hand, normal individuals develop neither hypercalcemia nor alkalosis but rather absorb less calcium initially despite high intake and excrete the excess calcium and alkali in the urine.[324]

Acute development of hypercalcemia and alkalosis has been reported within days of beginning high rates of ingestion of calcium and alkali, a syndrome known as acute milk-alkali syndrome.[322a] Patients develop weakness, myalgia, irritability, and apathy. The impairment of renal function, including reduced renal concentrating ability and signs of tubular dysfunction as well as the hypercalcemia and alkalosis, reverses rapidly upon withdrawal of the excessive intake of calcium and alkali.[322a]

Patients with far-advanced milk-alkali syndrome, sometimes referred to as Burnett's syndrome,[322] represent the results of long-standing excessive calcium and alkali ingestion. Severe hypercalcemia, irreversible renal failure, and phosphate retention develop, often accompanied by ectopic calcification; the severity of the renal failure aggravates the hypercalcemia directly.[322a] There occasionally may be some improvement when calcium and alkali ingestion is reduced. However, in the original patients reported, prior to the availability of renal dialysis, renal failure progressed to death.[322a] There is an intermediate or subacute form of milk-alkali syndrome in which renal failure and ectopic calcium deposits are seen, but the renal failure is usually reversible over a period of weeks after withdrawal of excessive calcium and alkali intake.[325]

E. General Approach to Differential Diagnosis

Differential diagnosis in hypercalcemic disorders is still best achieved by using clinical criteria, but the radioimmunoassay for PTH, as now modified, is highly useful in distinguishing among major causes. The clinical points that deserve major emphasis in arriving at a correct diagnosis are the presence or absence of symptoms or signs of disease and evidence of chronicity. If one discounts fatigue or depression, which is common in this population, patients with *asymptomatic hypercalcemia* have primary hyperparathyroidism in well over 90% of the instances; symptoms of malignancy are usually present when hypercalcemia is caused by cancer (Table 14–1). Disorders other than hyperparathyroidism and malignancy are estimated to cause no more than 10% of all cases of hypercalcemia, and some of the nonparathyroid causes are associated with manifestations such as renal failure, the signs or symptoms of which are evident on initial routine laboratory test screening.

Chronicity is the second most important clinical point. If hypercalcemia has been manifest for more than 1 year, malignancy can usually (although not always) be excluded as the cause of hypercalcemia on clinical grounds alone. A striking feature of malignancy-associated hypercalcemia is the rapidity of the course, whereby signs and symptoms relatable to the underlying malignancy are evident within months of the first detection of hypercalcemia. Hyperparathyroidism is the likely diagnosis in patients with *chronic hypercalcemia*. Diseases other than hyperparathyroidism, such as sarcoidosis, are rare alternative causes of chronic hypercalcemia. A careful *history* of dietary supplements and drug use often readily reveals intoxication with vitamin D or A or the use of thiazides.

Although clinical considerations are helpful in arriving at the correct diagnosis of the cause of hypercalcemia, appropriate laboratory testing is essential for diagnosis. Theoretically, the radioimmunoassay for PTH should separate hyperparathyroidism from all other causes of hypercalcemia, those with hyperparathyroidism having elevated levels of iPTH despite hypercalcemia, and patients with malignancy and the other causes of hypercalcemia (except those related to primary hyperparathyroidism such as lithium-induced hypercalcemia) having levels of hormone below normal or undetectable. Assays in use over the last two decades sometimes give equivocal results, but the newer assays based on the double antibody method do separate hypercalcemic patients with malignancy from those with primary hyperparathyroidism, thus confirming the utility of the method as a test possessing the relevant specificity and sensitivity in the two disorders, which account for more than 90% of all cases of hypercalcemia. $1,25(OH)_2D$ levels are elevated in many patients (but not all) with primary hyperparathyroidism and are also increased in states of vitamin D intoxication, particularly sarcoidosis. In other disorders associated with hypercalcemia, concentrations of 1,25$(OH)_2$D would be expected to be low or, at the most, normal. However, since not all patients with hyperparathyroidism have elevated 1,25$(OH)_2D_3$ levels and not all non-parathyroid hypercalcemia patients have suppressed 1,25$(OH)_2D_3$, the test is of lower specificity and is not cost effective in differential diagnoses *per se*.

PTH levels are elevated in chronic renal failure; the elevation in older assays reflects, in part, accumulation of fragments secondary to renal failure rather than true parathyroid oversecretion. In general, with the older type single antibody assays, those based on middle or carboxyl-region epitopes, higher values were seen than in those based on amino-terminal recognition sites. The latter assays seemed to correlate better with other evidence of parathyroid overactivity, such as osteitis fibrosa. Results with the double antibody assay are similar to but overall superior to those seen with amino-terminal assays. Patients with sarcoidosis have low or undetectable levels of iPTH. No systematic surveys have been reported concerning PTH radioimmunoassay results with the double antibody technique in many of the other nonparathyroid-related causes of hypercalcemia, largely because of the infrequency with which the disorders are encountered, but it is predicted that they will be low or undetectable.

In summary, iPTH values are elevated in more than 90% of parathyroid-related causes of hypercalcemia, undetectable or low in malignancy-related hypercalcemia, and undetectable or normal in vitamin D–related and high bone turnover-related causes of hypercalcemia (although there are a paucity of data for these latter categories). The same general tendency to separate groups is seen with measurements of 1,25$(OH)_2$D.

Measurements of nephrogenous cyclic AMP are of limited value in distinguishing the two major causes of hypercalcemia, primary hyperparathyroidism and malignancy. Elevation of nephrogenous cyclic AMP occurs in some patients with malignancy and in essentially all patients with primary hyperparathyroidism. Specific laboratory tests are of utility in confirming the diagnosis of particular disorders (such as T4 with thyrotoxicosis); tests specific for tumor factors should be very helpful when developed.

Some general recommendations can be made as to the differential diagnosis of hypercalcemia. Two independent causes of hypercalcemia, although reported, are rare. If a specific disease traditionally associated with hypercalcemia is clinically evident, it is reasonable to assume that the disease is responsible for the hypercalcemia. It seems cost effective in view of the specificity and speed of the PTH radioimmunoassay and the high frequency of hyperparathyroidism in hypercalcemic patients to measure the iPTH level in all hypercalcemic patients unless malignancy is clinically evident or a specific diagnosis of a nonparathyroid disease is obvious. If hypercalcemia disappears in response to control of hyperthyroidism, for example, or after reduction of excessive intake of fat-soluble vitamins or alkali and calcium, as in the case of vitamin D intoxication or milk-alkali syndrome, there is no need to search for a second cause of hypercalcemia. If specific treatment does not lead to a reversal of the hypercalcemia, a search for an additional cause, by detailed laboratory testing, must be undertaken. Obviously, if signs suggestive of malignancy are evident, the management of the patient focuses on management of the malignancy.

When no clues are evident as to the diagnosis, either because the patient is asymptomatic or chronic illness obscures symptoms or signs that might provide a clue to the presence of malignancy, the following general approach can be used. If the patient is *asymptomatic* and if there is evidence by history of *chronicity* to the hypercalcemia, hyperparathyroidism is almost certainly the cause of the hypercalcemia. If iPTH levels (usually measured twice, at least) are elevated, little other evaluation is necessary. Hyperparathyroidism is never confirmed until abnormal parathyroid tissue is surgically removed, correcting the hypercalcemia, but patients with asymptomatic hypercalcemia who have the presumptive diagnosis on the basis of elevated concentration of iPTH can be followed without intervention but with careful monitoring, or recommended for surgery with reasonable confidence of cure. If in such patients there is a family history suggestive of other endocrine abnormality, more detailed screening for multiple endocrine neoplasia should be undertaken in the patient and family.

If the patient does not have clear-cut symptoms but there is only a short history or no clue to the duration of the hypercalcemia, *occult malignancy* must be considered with more care than if the hypercalcemia is known to be chronic. If the iPTH levels with the newer techniques in such an asymptomatic patient are increased convincingly, the diagnosis of asymptomatic hyperparathyroidism is established also, although the absence of clinical data favoring chronicity makes the laboratory data, increased iPTH, the only evidence against occult malignancy, and it is important to ensure that a clinically verified iPTH assay has been used.

If patients with only a short history of hypercalcemia have clear-cut systemic symptoms and/or the iPTH levels are not elevated, a thorough survey must be undertaken for malignancy, including chest x-ray, computerized tomography of chest and abdomen, and bone scan. Attention should also be paid to clues for underlying hematologic disorders such as anemia, increased plasma globulin, and abnormal serum immunoelectrophoresis; bone scans can be negative in patients with multiple myeloma.

Finally, if a patient is *asymptomatic* with *chronic hypercalcemia* but iPTH values are not elevated, malignancy seems unlikely on clinical grounds (*chronicity*) and it is useful to search for other chronic illnesses that cause hypercalcemia but may be atypical in presentation, such as occult sarcoidosis.

V. MEDICAL MANAGEMENT OF HYPERCALCEMIA

The measures available for the treatment of severe, life-threatening hypercalcemia are usually effective. In most patients with severe hypercalcemia, the serum calcium levels can be decreased by 3 to 9 mg/100 ml (0.75–2.25 mM/liter) over a period of 24 to 48 hours, a time that is sufficient to relieve the acute symptoms and prevent death. Once the severe hypercalcemia is corrected, however, the problem becomes one of the identification of the causative factors responsible for the hypercalcemia and the chronic management of hypercalcemia. Unless the underlying cause can be corrected, available therapies for the management of hypercalcemia are complicated by multiple ensuing side-effects.

In the management of hypercalcemia it is useful to focus on mechanisms whereby hypercalcemia is caused. There may be excessive release of calcium from the skeleton or absorption of calcium from the intestine; occasionally the extraction of calcium from the kidney may be impaired also. For example, hypercalcemia occurring in patients with metastatic cancer in the skeleton or in immobilized patients is likely primarily due to excessive release of calcium from the skeleton and would not be benefited by restriction of the patient's dietary calcium. On the other hand, patients with hypersensitivity to vitamin D (sarcoidosis) or vitamin D intoxication due to excessive ingestion of vitamin D have increased intestinal absorption of calcium. Severe restriction of dietary calcium in these patients is often beneficial, although it may not totally cure their hypercalcemia because high blood levels of vitamin D metabolites usually stimulate excessive skeletal calcium release. In all patients with increased bone dissolution, calcium entry into the circulation increases and hypercalcemia develops. The hypercalcemia interferes with renal concentrating mechanisms and may reduce thirst, leading to dehydration that worsens the hypercalcemia. In such a situation, measures of forced intakes of water should be instituted, thereby increasing urinary calcium excretion and thereby resulting in some amelioration of the hypercalcemia even though the other abnormalities of calcium turnover remain.

A. Hydration and Mild Diuresis

The first principle of the treatment of hypercalcemia is to increase the urinary excretion of calcium by maximizing the glomerular filtration of fluid and ions. Patients with hypercalcemia are often dehydrated as a result of frequent vomiting, inability to eat or drink, or hypercalcemia-induced defects in urinary concentrating ability. These factors lead to a decrease in both glomerular filtration of calcium and renal tubular clearance of calcium. Restoration of normal extracellular fluid volume will correct both of these abnormalities and can increase urinary calcium excretion by as much as 100 to 300 mg/day (2.5–7.5 mM/day). In a series of 16 patients with moderately severe hypercalcemia (mean 14.6 mg/100 ml, range 13.4–16.6), the intravenous infusion of isotonic saline (4 liters/day) alone lowered the serum total calcium concentration by an average of 2.16 mg/100 ml (corrected mathematically for initial concentration). By increasing the urinary sodium excretion to 400 to 500 mEq/day, the urinary calcium excretion will increase further than it will by simple rehydration because sodium and calcium clearance are closely linked.[336-340] Once adequate hydration has been achieved and hypercalcemia persists, the administration of moderate doses of furosemide or ethacrynic acid (twice daily) can be helpful; the diuretic will further depress the renal reabsorption of calcium.[338] The combined use of these three therapies—fluid, then saline, then diuretics—can produce an increase in urinary calcium excretion of as much as 400 to 800 mg/day in a hypercalcemic patient. Because this amount represents a substantial percentage of the daily exchangeable calcium pool, the serum calcium concentration may fall by as much as 3 mg/100 ml within 24 hours.

The therapeutic combination of high fluid intake and administration of sodium and furosemide or ethacrynic acid is also adaptable to long-term out-patient treatment. One must keep in mind the usual precautions regarding the potassium and magnesium depletion that occurs during chronic diuretic therapy. Diuretics must not be given before hydration is assured. Calcium-containing renal stones are a potential complication of the chronic therapy, but this risk is often acceptable in patients who are ill from hypercalcemia. Thiazide diuretics should be avoided in the treatment of hypercalcemic patients because they depress the renal clearance of calcium.

B. Forced Diuresis

In certain diseases, particularly cancer involving widespread destruction of bone, the high serum calcium levels can become life-threatening. Under such circumstances, therapy with diuretics should be pursued much more aggressively.[340] As much as 6 liters of isotonic saline (900 mEq sodium) daily plus furosemide in doses of 80 to 120 mg every 3 hours, or ethacrynic acid in doses of 20 to 40 mg every 1 to 2 hours, should be given to increase urinary calcium excretion to levels of 1000 mg/day or more. As a result of this therapy, serum calcium may decrease by 2 to 4 mg/100 ml within 24 hours. Because the decrease in serum calcium is dependent on the amount urinary calcium excretion exceeds the release of calcium from bone, patients with active lysis of bone require greater rates of calcium excretion to achieve reductions in serum calcium equivalent to those achieved in patients who are less severely ill. The occurrence of severe potassium and magnesium depletion is inevitable unless these minerals are replaced. Pulmonary edema may be precipitated by depletion of these minerals. These potential complications can be averted by continuous monitoring of central venous pressure and plasma or urine electrolytes. The demands, however, of these measures on the patient and medical staff are significant and should be considered before instituting this monitoring. It is important to remember that placement of a catheter in the bladder is helpful after the first 24 hours of institution of diuretics to alleviate inconvenient awakenings for the patient.

C. Phosphate

Patients who suffer from hypercalcemia frequently have hypophosphatemia. Hypophosphatemia decreases the rate of calcium uptake into bone,[341] increases intestinal calcium absorption[345,346] and both directly and indirectly stimulates the breakdown of bone.[341,346,347] Because these physiologic effects aggravate hypercalcemia, correction of the hypophosphatemia *per se* will help to lower the serum calcium concentration. The recommended treatment is the administration of 33 to 100 mM of phosphorus per day (1–3 g of phosphate phosphorus) to maintain the serum inorganic phosphate concentration above 3.1 mg/100 ml (1.0 mM/liter). Although phosphate therapy has been advocated periodically in the management of hypercalcemia,[349,350] there are grave concerns expressed about phosphate therapy, particularly ectopic calcification and even sudden fatality.[350,355-357] It remains uncertain whether toxic effects will occur if the increased phosphate intake restores serum inorganic phosphate levels only to normal. It is important to realize that the effects of oral supplements of phosphate on serum phosphate concentrations may be only transient. Serum inorganic phosphate levels should be monitored daily until it becomes clear that the doses of phosphate administered are adequate.

Raising the serum inorganic phosphate concentration above normal levels will predictably decrease serum calcium levels further[348] and has been proposed as a therapy for hypercalcemia.[349,350] Oral phosphate, beginning with a daily dose of 66 mM (2000 mg phosphate phosphorus), or intravenous phosphate, beginning with a dose of 45 mM (1500 mg phosphate phosphorus) over 6 to 8 hours, can be given. In response to this therapy with phosphate administration, serum calcium levels fell by 1.8 to 10.6 mg/100 ml (mean fall 5.6 mg/100 ml) in 15 patients with cancer. Hypercalcemia resulting from diseases other than cancer also responds to phosphate therapy; responses are reported in hyperparathyroidism,[348,349,351-353] sarcoidosis,[354] vitamin D intoxication,[349] and multiple myeloma.[355] Although oral or intravenous phosphate is one of the most effective treatments available to alleviate severe hypercalcemia, the potential toxicity is of concern. Severe, occasionally fatal hypocalcemia can be produced suddenly by excessive dosages of phosphate.[350,355-357] Serum calcium levels should be measured at frequent intervals when phosphate is being administered intravenously to detect the development of hypocalcemia before it becomes a life-threatening situation.[350]

Sodium phosphate does not eliminate calcium from the body. The amount of calcium in the urine generally declines after administration of oral or intravenous phosphate[348,349,351,352] and fecal calcium either declines or remains the same.[348,352,354] The decline in serum calcium levels therefore reflects a redistribution of calcium within the body. Studies of the kinetic distributions of strontium and calcium during intravenous phosphate therapy[358,359] indicate that calcium rapidly leaves the circulation. Similar rapid calcium efflux is observed in rats[359-361] with phosphate therapy. These observations suggest that acute precipitation of calcium-phosphate salts takes place, since the serum calcium concentrations begin to fall within minutes of the beginning of a phosphate infusion.[352]

Radiographics have demonstrated the precipitation of calcium salts in the walls of the vein receiving infusions of phosphate.[362] Decreases in serum calcium levels that occur during intravenous phosphate therapy are directly and linearly proportional to the mean ion product (calcium × phosphate) achieved during the phosphate infusion,[352] suggesting the precipitation of phosphate in soft tissues. The ultrafilterable factor of calcium multiplied by phosphate concentrations observed *in vivo* (solubility product) obtained from this linear relationship agrees closely with the solubility product for $CaHP0_4$ determined *in vitro* at physiologic temperature, pH, and ionic strength.[352]

Phosphate therapy can result in precipitates of calcium and phosphate in extraskeletal tissues that may cause problems. Metastatic calcification of phosphate salts has been reported in patients receiving oral or intravenous phosphate for treatment of hypercalcemia.[349,353,356,357,362] Such observations, however, are difficult to interpret because hypercalcemia by itself may lead to metastatic deposition of calcium-containing precipitates. Experimentally derived data in animals, where the effects of added phosphate could be compared at equivalent degrees of hypercalcemia, indicate that phosphates do aggravate the extent of deposits of calcium in the heart, kidneys, and other tissues.[363,364] Hyperphosphatemia also causes calcium phosphate deposits in multiple tissues of normocalcemic animals.[365,367] In patients with normal blood levels of calcium, phosphate administration has been reported to cause a marked deposition in the periarticular tissues.[368] The calcifications in the soft tissue of patients with uremia or renal failure are due in part to the accompanying hyperphosphatemia and may resolve when the serum phosphate is reduced.[369] It has long been recognized that hyperphosphatemia leads to intravascular precipitation of calcium phosphate, which is subsequently phagocytosed by the reticuloendothelial system and later slowly released into the circulation.[370,371]

Should phosphate be used acutely or chronically in the therapy of hypercalcemia? Although it seems likely that correction of hypercalcemia by administration of phosphate produces soft tissue calcification, it is not certain that this condition is permanent.[358,371] Furthermore, the few studies available do not demonstrate any definite functional toxicity of acute phosphate therapy in humans.[349,372] In view of this situation, particularly if mithramycin or forced diuresis is contraindicated and the hypercalcemia is severe and life-threatening, administration of oral or intravenous phosphate to hyperphosphatemic levels remains a justifiable treatment in an emergency. The use of phosphate for the treatment of chronic hypercalcemia is somewhat controversial. If long-term therapy with phosphate supplements is necessary, it should be prescribed in small doses, and the serum inorganic phosphate levels should be checked 1 or 2 hours after the administration of an oral dose. Serum phosphate levels should be maintained below 5.5 mg/100 ml to minimize the occurrence of calcium deposits in soft tissues.

The mechanism of the calcium-lowering effect of phosphate therapy is uncertain. As noted earlier, hypophosphatemia clearly aggravates hypercalcemia by effects on intestinal absorption of calcium and bone turnover.[341,345,346] It remains unsettled whether precipitation of calcium salts accounts entirely for the hypocalcemic effect of the administration of supplemental phosphate in the diet in individuals who are not hypophosphatemic prior to therapy. Small effects of phosphate on the release of calcium from stores in bone would have been missed by the kinetic studies cited previously. The application of sensitive morphologic techniques reveals an effect of hyperphosphatemia on skeletal resorption, opposite to that of hypophosphatemia;[341] high phosphate levels depress the release of calcium in bone culture.[373] Stimulation of parathyroid gland secretion can occur if phosphate levels lower calcium acutely. It should be noted that although serum inorganic phosphate levels return to baseline values within 18 hours after administration of intravenous phosphates, serum calcium levels take 2 to 4 days to return to normal.[352]

Preparations of inorganic phosphates are commercially available in liquid, powder, and capsule form for oral use and as a liquid for intravenous use. Preparations differ both in their content of phosphorus and their associated amounts of cations and pH, as shown in Table 14–2.

D. Mithramycin

In certain circumstances, mithramycin is a useful therapeutic agent for the acute management of hypercalcemia. Mithramycin is a cytotoxic substance derived from the microorganism *Streptomyces*. It is highly effective in its properties to inhibit bone resorption and to lower serum calcium levels and urinary calcium and hydroxyproline excretion.[374] Studies in mice show that mithramycin localizes in areas of active bone resorption.[375] These observations suggest that mithramycin exerts a direct skeletal effect. The direct effects of mithramycin on the skeleton are also evident during treatment of patients with Paget's disease of bone, because levels of urinary hydroxyproline and blood alkaline phosphatase fall markedly, and excessive skeletal turnover characteristic of the disease falls toward normal.[376]

In patients with hypercalcemia associated with the presence of cancer, one dose of mithramycin usually suffices to lower serum calcium levels into the range of normal within 48 hours;[377-379] the magnitude of response ranges widely from a decrement of 1.6 mg/100 ml to 11.0 mg/100 ml in the serum calcium. Occasionally, serum calcium levels fall more slowly after a single dose of mithramycin. If no response to mithramycin occurs during the first 24 to 48 hours, the initial dose is given every day until the serum calcium levels begin to fall.

The duration of action of mithramycin is variable but usually lasts several days. The serum inorganic phosphate often falls below 3.0 mg/100 ml after treatment with mithramycin, presumably as a result of the decrease in bone resorption.[378,379] The hypophosphatemia may be prevented by the administration of phosphate supplements as needed to maintain a normal serum con-

Table 14–2. Preparation of Inorganic Phosphate

	mM P	mg P	mEq Na	Eq K
Oral phosphate preparations				
Fleet Phospho-Soda (5 ml)	24	750	29	—
Neutra-Phos (1.25 g capsule)	8	250	7	7
Neutra-Phos-K (1.45 g capsule)	8	250	—	14
Intravenous phosphate preparations (1 ml)				
Sodium phosphate (Abbott)	3	93	4	—
Potassium phosphate (Abbott, McGaw)	3	93	—	4.5

Doses of phosphate are most clearly prescribed in millimoles, but are sometimes prescribed in milligrams of phosphate phosphorus since clinical laboratories still use such units to report serum and urine concentrations of inorganic phosphate. 1000 mg phosphate phosphorus = 33 mM. Milliequivalents are inappropriate units, since the valence is variable.

centration of inorganic phosphate, which may even augment the effectiveness of mithramycin in lowering levels of serum calcium. Mithramycin is usually effective in lowering serum calcium in patients with a wide variety of cancers regardless of whether they have skeletal metastases. Mithramycin is similarly effective in reversing the hypercalcemia of severe hyperparathyroidism through its effects on the skeleton rather than on parathyroid gland function.[380]

Mithramycin must be given intravenously. The usual dose for the treatment of hypercalcemia is 10 to 25 mg/kg body weight. One or two doses per week is usually sufficient; treatment should not be repeated until hypercalcemia recurs because the toxicity is strikingly dependent on the frequency of treatment and the total dose.[381,382]

Mithramycin is toxic and requires careful monitoring if continued doses are used. The major side-effects are thrombocytopenia (with normal bone marrow megakaryocytes), hepatocellular necrosis with increased LDH and AST levels and decreased clotting factors, and azotemia and proteinuria. Mild and reversible hepatic dysfunction occurred in 16% of patients receiving mithramycin for the treatment of hypercalcemia in one series of 67 patients, often after initial dosages.[383] Renal function should be monitored during therapy, because the hypercalcemia may have caused preexisting renal tubular or glomerular damage. Significant renal toxic effects can occur after a single dose of mithramycin in patients with preexisting azotemia.[384] Overdosage can lead to hypocalcemia.[374] The serum potassium should be monitored because mithramycin may lower serum potassium levels over several hours.[385] Hypercalcemic patients receiving the drug may already be potassium-depleted because of treatment earlier with diuretics or vomiting. Nausea, vomiting, stomatitis, and facial swelling can occur.[381,382] Severe toxicity is rare when only one or two doses are used and can be minimized by repeating single doses only when hypercalcemia recurs.[378] Toxic effects usually reverse after discontinuation of the drug.[375,382,386]

E. Glucocorticoids

Pharmacologic doses of glucocorticoids (e.g., 40–100 mg of prednisone or equivalent daily in divided doses) reverse the hypercalcemia of (1) vitamin D intoxication,[387] and (2) sarcoidosis, tuberculosis, and other granulomatous diseases,[388-390] and (3) the hypercalcemia caused by certain cancers.[391] Typically, the cancers causing hypercalcemia responsive to glucocorticoids are hematologic in origin, such as multiple myeloma, leukemias, Hodgkin's disease, and other lymphomas. Carcinoma of the breast also occasionally responds, at least early in the course of the disease; responses in the hypercalcemia caused by other cancers are unpredictable, and more reliable remedies are available for the treatment of hypercalcemia in such situations.[391]

Glucocorticoids alter serum calcium concentrations via multiple pathways. Given in large doses to normal volunteers or to patients with normal calcium metabolism, glucocorticoids increase renal calcium clearance and urinary calcium excretion,[392,393] decrease intestinal absorption of calcium,[394,395] and rapidly mobilize calcium from the skeleton.[395] The effects on the kidneys and intestines lower, whereas the effects on the skeleton raise, the serum calcium concentration. These counteracting effects, plus normal homeostatic mechanisms, maintain the serum calcium concentration unchanged when glucocorticoids are administered to normal volunteers[393,394] or to patients with normal calcium metabolism.[392] Similarly, the serum calcium concentration is usually unaffected when glucocorticoids are administered to patients with primary hyperparathyroidism.[388,396] The beneficial effects of glucocorticoids on the hypercalcemia of cancer are largely the result of their ability to reduce the size of the tumor,[437] to interfere with the mechanisms by which tumor cells mobilize calcium from bone,[397,398] and to increase renal calcium clearance even in well-hydrated hypercalcemic cancer patients.[399,400] The effects of glucocorticoids on intestinal calcium absorption are usually of secondary importance, because intestinal absorption of calcium is already less than normal in most patients.[401] The reduced intestinal absorption of calcium observed in these patients is consistent with the observation that serum levels of $1,25(OH)_2$ vitamin D are often suppressed.[399] Occasionally the hypercalcemia of cancer is associated with (and then may be partly or wholly caused by) elevated blood levels of $1,25(OH)_2$ vitamin D. In such patients, the effects of glucocorticoids on intestinal absorption of calcium may be an important aspect of their therapeutic effect.

In patients with granulomatous diseases, the hypercalcemia is caused by excessive production of 1,25$(OH)_2$ vitamin D by the granuloma cells.[402] Glucocorticoids lower the serum levels of 1,25$(OH)_2$ vitamin D to normal in patients with these illnesses,[390] either by decreasing production of the vitamin D metabolite or by accelerating its catabolism.[403] In addition, glucocorticoids may act directly on the intestinal epithelium to reduce the intestinal hyperabsorption of calcium that characterizes 1,25$(OH)_2$ vitamin D excess.[404]

F. Calcitonin

Calcitonin decreases the skeletal release of calcium, phosphorus, and hydroxyproline within minutes after intravenous injection.[405,406] The subsequent changes in serum calcium and phosphorus depend on the initial magnitude of skeletal resorption: subjects with the most rapid bone turnover show the greatest reduction in serum calcium concentration.[407] In the doses used clinically, calcitonin also increases the renal clearance of calcium and phosphorus (and sodium).[408,409] Increased skeletal uptake of phosphorus is also an initial effect of the drug in animals.[410]

Calcitonin is only moderately effective in lowering the serum calcium concentration in hypercalcemic patients (a 1–4 mg/100 ml or 0.25–1.0 mM/liter fall can be expected). There are published reports indicating greater effectiveness in some hypercalcemic states rather than others, but these distinctions may be more apparent than real given the multiple therapies used and the tachyphylaxis seen with calcitonin. Some reports suggest greater benefit in patients with hypercalcemia due to immobilization,[411] thyrotoxicosis,[412] or vitamin D intoxication.[413,414] Calcitonin is stated in other reports to be less effective than phosphate or mithramycin in patients with hypercalcemia due to cancer[415,416] or hyperparathyroidism.[411,414]

After several hours or days, escape from the hypocalcemic effects of calcitonin occurs in patients and animals.[417-419] An analogous phenomenon is seen in organ culture.[419] The effectiveness of calcitonin *in vivo* and *in vitro* can be restored by withholding the drug for several days.[419,420] Phosphate loading enhances and phosphate depletion inhibits the hypocalcemic effect of the hormone.[421] However, calcitonin-induced hypophosphatemia does not account for the tachyphylaxis.[417] The co-administration of glucocorticoids prolongs the effects of calcitonin in organ culture, delaying or preventing the "escape" phenomenon;[419] a similar synergism is reported to occur *in vivo*.[422] Calcitonin is effective by intravenous, intramuscular, or subcutaneous injection, but it is inert when taken by mouth or sublingually. It is also effective when administered intranasally, but mucosal absorption is relatively poor, requiring doses that are prohibitively expensive. Salmon calcitonin is more potent than porcine or human calcitonin and can be given in doses of 25 to 50 units every 6 to 8 hours. Human calcitonin must be given in greater dose by weight but has the advantage of reduced incidence of antibody formation (neutralizing antibodies are rare, however, even with salmon calcitonin). In dilute solutions, calcitonin adheres to glass; if it is given by continuous infusion of dilute solutions, heat-inactivated human albumin (1 mg/ml) or some other protein must be added to the solution.

Although calcitonin is expensive, it is largely free from toxic effects. Used in combination with other drugs, especially in the first day or two of therapy prior to onset of refractoriness, it may allow a reduction in dose of the more potent, but more toxic, alternative therapies; further efforts to achieve prolongation of effect might increase the utility of calcitonin.

G. Indomethacin/Aspirin

Prostaglandins, particularly PGE_2, stimulate the resorption of bone in organ culture,[423] and a large body of experimental evidence suggests they may be involved in the production of bony metastases and/or hypercalcemia by malignant cells.[424,425] Many patients with hypercalcemia of malignancy have biochemical evidence of increased prostaglandin synthesis, which can be restored to normal by aspirin in doses sufficient to produce a serum salicylate level of 20 to 30 mg/100 ml, or indomethacin in doses of 25 mg every 6 hours. In only a minority of patients, 20% or less, however, has there been convincing control of hypercalcemia, although earlier reports were encouraging.[426-429] Blood levels of prostaglandins may not predict accurately whether prostaglandins are involved in the mediation of the hypercalcemia. Bone-resorbing factors distinct from prostaglandins may be more important in local stimulation of bone breakdown. Prostaglandins are inactivated by passage through the lung. Hence, measurement of overall prostaglandin synthesis, rather than merely blood levels, is necessary before and after attempts at blockade of prostaglandin synthesis to make valid correlations among the variables: (1) pretreatment levels of prostaglandin production, (2) responses of blood calcium levels to treatment with aspirin or indomethacin, and (3) posttreatment changes in indices of prostaglandin production. Such correlations have not been made. Unfortunately, it is not presently possible to offer predictions as to which tumors might best respond. Because methods necessary to define excessive prostaglandin production are not widely available, a therapeutic trial may be the only way to assess the value of treatment with inhibitors of prostaglandin synthesis in individual patients. Drugs that inhibit prostaglandin synthesis also decrease the glomerular filtration rate. Such changes in renal function can interfere with the renal excretion of calcium, especially in patients who are dehydrated or have impaired renal function, findings common among hypercalcemic patients;[430] this side-effect can limit the calcium-lowering effect. Sulindac inhibits prostaglandin synthesis in extrarenal tissues without decreasing the glomerular filtration rate in such patients, probably because the active form of the drug is inactivated in the kidneys.[431,432] The effectiveness of prostaglandin inhibitors as a treatment for the hypercalcemia of cancer is receiving further evaluation.

H. Bisphosphonates (Diphosphonates)

Bisphosphonates are hydrocarbons with two inorganic phosphate groups bonded to a connecting carbon. They are analogues of inorganic pyrophosphate (in which two inorganic phosphate groups are bonded to a connecting oxygen). In contrast to the P-O-P bond, the P-C-P bond is not hydrolyzed, so bisphosphonates, when used in medical applications, persist in tissues and eventually are excreted unchanged in the urine. Bisphosphonates are potent inhibitors of bone resorption and hence are extremely effective in reversing and controlling the hypercalcemia of cancer and hyperparathyroidism, but anxieties about their possible toxicity have so far inhibited their chronic use and their commercial development. The only bisphosphonate approved for clinical use in the United States is ethane-1-hydroxy-1,1-bisphosphonate (etidronate). Given by daily intravenous infusion over several hours, etidronate usually reduces the serum calcium concentration to normal over 2 to 10 days in patients with hypercalcemia caused by cancer or hyperparathyroidism.[433] Intravenous formulations of the drug are, however, not commercially available. Intestinal absorption of the drug is low when given in usual doses (designed for chronic therapy of Paget's disease). Therefore, etidronate must be given for several weeks before it effectively blocks bone resorption.[434] In addition, there is a narrow range between drug concentrations that block bone resorption and those that block bone mineralization, the latter leading to osteomalacia and possible risk of fracture. This limits the effectiveness of etidronate for the chronic management of hypercalcemia, but it can be very useful to control the symptoms of hypercalcemia for several months in patients with a limited life expectancy.[433]

The bisphosphonates APD (3-amino-1-hydroxypropylidene-1,1-bisphosphate) and clodronate (dichloromethylene-bisphosphate) block bone resorption as effectively as etidronate and somewhat faster,[433,435,439a] but block bone mineralization only at high dosages. Consequently, they not only lower serum calcium levels and urine calcium and hydroxyproline excretion[436,437] but they also produce a positive calcium balance when administered to hypercalcemic patients.[437,438] Usual doses do not cause osteomalacia; in fact they allow skeletal mineral to increase. The greatest effectiveness of APD and clodronate as agents for the treatment of hypercalcemia has been demonstrated in patients with osteolytic metastases,[433,437,439,440] multiple myeloma,[439,441] humoral hypercalcemia of cancer,[439,442] primary hyperparathyroidism[434,435,442] parathyroid carcinoma,[436] and immobilization. Despite their efficacy, APD and clodronate have not been marketed because of potential toxicity (febrile reactions with APD in high dosage and several cases of leukemia among recipients of clodronate). Recently, APD is being more widely introduced in the U.S. and has been shown to be effective in the management of hypercalcemia of malignancy.[439a]

I. Dialysis

Hypercalcemia complicated by severe renal failure is difficult to manage; if treatment is appropriate, dialysis is the first choice. Peritoneal dialysis can remove 500 to 2000 mg of calcium in 24 to 48 hours and lower the serum calcium concentration by 3 to 12 mg/100 ml (0.75–3.0 mM/liter), if calcium-free dialysis fluid is used.[443] Standard commercial peritoneal dialysis fluids generally contain 5 to 8 mg Ca/100 ml, which is higher than the normal serum ionized calcium concentration. Dialysis with these standard fluids cannot be used to relieve hypercalcemia. With calcium-free fluids and 30-minute exchanges of 2 liters each, ultrafilterable calcium clearances exceed the urea clearances.[443] Equilibration of plasma and peritoneal fluid calcium concentrations takes 90 to 120 minutes.[444,445]

Hemodialysis is equally effective.[446] The membranes of artificial kidneys are quite permeable to calcium; large calcium transfers can occur over relatively short intervals if the dialysate is calcium-free.[447,448] In addition to special salt mixtures, this may require the use of deionized water if the local tap water contains much calcium.[449]

Because commercial dialysis solutions contain little or no inorganic phosphate, phosphate clearances are high during peritoneal dialysis[484] and hemodialysis.[448] Large quantities of phosphate are therefore lost during conventional dialysis, and serum inorganic phosphate concentrations usually fall. Since hypophosphatemia will aggravate hypercalcemia, the postdialysis serum inorganic phosphate concentration should be measured if dialysis has been used to treat hypercalcemia, and phosphate supplements added to the diet or to subsequent dialysis fluids if necessary to maintain a normal serum inorganic phosphate concentration.

J. Summary

The various therapies are listed in Table 14–3 with their particular indications and principal toxicities. The choice of therapy depends on the basic disease, the severity of the hypercalcemia, the serum inorganic phosphate level, and the patient's renal, hepatic, and bone marrow function. The treatment of hypercalcemia must be approached in the context of overall patient care. If the underlying disease is unknown or is thought likely to be a candidate for successful treatment, treatment should be aggressive. If, on the other hand, the patient suffers from a cancer for which all definitive or effective ameliorative measures have been exhausted, aggressive therapy of the hypercalcemia is not indicated.

Mild hypercalcemia (less than 12 mg/100 ml or 3 mM/liter) can usually be managed with good hydration. Intravenous sodium chloride and small doses of furosemide or ethacrynic acid may be useful for more severe hypercalcemia not responsive to hydration alone. Severe hypercalcemia (greater than 15 mg/100 ml or 3.75 mM/liter) requires rapid correction. Vigorous sodium/calcium diuresis with large doses of furosemide and ethacrynic acid works rapidly, but can be attempted only if renal and cardiac function are adequate and if appropriate monitoring is available. Mithramycin is an important drug in this situation, since it has the advantage of great effectiveness and simplicity of use; the principal contraindication is its toxicity.[434] Renal, hepatic, or bone marrow disease may preclude its use, however. These two approaches, diuretic therapy to increase urinary calcium excretion and mithramycin to block bone resorption, are the most effective and widely applied treatments for hypercalcemia; they can be used well in combination. APD may now prove to be an effective alternative approach to mithramycin to achieve rapid blockade of bone resorption.[439a]

Other measures have value in special circumstances. Phosphate therapy can be useful when hypophosphatemia is present; intravenous phosphate therapy, although effective, has serious toxic potential, and should be reserved for special circumstances in which mithramycin and/or saline/furosemide therapy cannot be used because of underlying hematologic, hepatic, or renal disease. Glucocorticoids and prostaglandin synthesis inhibitors work only over several days and are unpredictable in many applications; these agents should not be relied upon as the initial treatment for severe hypercalcemia. Dialysis should be reserved for hypercalcemia complicating acute or chronic renal failure.

Table 14–3. Therapeutic Strategy in Treating Hypercalcemia

Therapy	Therapeutic Details	Indications	Complications	Precautions
		Most Generally Useful Therapies		
Hydration	2 liters or more	Universal	—	—
High salt intake	Achieve urine Na of 300 mEq/day or more	Universal	Edema	—
Furosemide or ethacrynic acid	40–160 mg/day 50–200 mg/day	Universal	K and Mg	Measure serum K and Mg
Forced diuresis	4–6 liters fluid IV/day containing 600–900 mEq Na plus furosemide every 1–2 hr, plus at least 60 mEq K/day, plus at least 60 mEq Mg/day	Universal	Pulmonary edema; K and Mg	Intensive monitoring, including venous pressure and serum Mg and K
Mithramycin	10–25 μg/kg IV, repeat prn	Increased bone resorption	Liver, kidney, marrow toxicity	Monitor platelets, CBC, BUN, AST
Oral phosphate	250 mg P every 6 hr PO	Universal if serum P 3 mg/100 ml	Ectopic calcification	Keep serum P below 5–6 mg/100 ml
		Special Therapies for Particular Uses		
Prednisone or equivalent	5–15 mg every 6 hr	Breast cancer, lymphomas, leukemias, multiple myeloma, vitamin D poisoning, sarcoidosis	Cushing's syndrome if chronic prescription	Alternate-day prescription for chronic use
IV phosphate	1500 mg P every 12 hr until P 5 mg/100 ml	Severe hypercalcemia, diuresis, or mithramycin contraindicated	Ectopic calcification, severe hypocalcemia	Monitor serum Ca and P closely
Calcitonin	2 units/kg every 4 hr subcutaneously	Adjunct when bone reabsoption; paralysis, immobilization	—	—
Indomethacin	25 μg every 6 hr PO	Certain types of cancer	Na retention, GI bleeding; headache	Careful clinical monitoring
Dialysis	Low-Ca bath	Acute renal failure	Multiple	Monitor serum P after dialysis

VI. MEDICAL TREATMENT OF HYPERPARATHYROIDISM

A. Management of Asymptomatic Hyperparathyroidism

The extensive use of routine measurements of serum calcium as a medical screening device and wider studies of families of patients with hyperparathyroidism are bringing to medical attention considerable numbers of asymptomatic hypercalcemic patients.[9,12] If the hypercalcemia is discovered accidentally, and the patient is asymptomatic, the need for parathyroid surgery is often not clear. It is not difficult to recommend surgery when symptomatic bone, renal, or gastrointestinal disease is present, but balancing the risks and benefits of prophylactic parathyroid surgery is often done intuitively since it is difficult to predict which patients may have silent complications; the natural history of asymptomatic hyperparathyroidism has not been systematically studied. Efforts to study the natural history of the disease and derive predictive indices regarding the need for surgery are currently being undertaken.

Information on the natural history of this disease is provided by a report from the Mayo Clinic of 147 surgically untreated or incompletely treated patients with primary hyperparathyroidism, 134 of whom had mild asymptomatic disease.[470] Over a 10-year period, 20% of these patients required surgery (which was unsuccessful in 5 of 29 patients). Most of the surgery was necessary during the first 5 years of follow-up, most often because of renal calculi or anxiety. About 62% of the patients escaped surgery (4% because they died of related causes). The remaining 18% were lost to follow-up. There is a need for parallel follow-up studies in surgically treated patients, since renal deterioration has been reported in some patients despite successful surgery,[450] possibly related to renal infection, prior nephrocalcinosis, or persistent renal calculi.

When faced with an asymptomatic patient with hyperparathyroidism, it is first important to confirm the diagnosis, define the symptoms or lack thereof concerning the variable symptoms of primary hyperparathyroidism, measure the creatinine clearance and renal tubular function, and search for urinary tract calculi or infection. If renal function is significantly impaired, or renal calculi are present, surgery is probably warranted. It is important to recall that hypercalcemia causes a functional defect in urinary concentrating capacity that is reversible and so not, *per se*, an indication for surgery.

The skeletal mass should be evaluated simultaneously, including quantitative measurements of cortical bone density if possible. Single-photon bone densitometry or cortical bone in the shaft of the radius is particularly sensitive and useful for detecting early bone loss in such patients.[448,451,452] If bone mass is already low (for whatever reason), parathyroid surgery may be advisable to prevent further bone loss for the hyperparathyroidism. Lastly, if the hypercalcemia is severe (above 13 mg/100 ml or 3.25 mM/liter), the risks of more severe life-threatening hypercalcemia (for example, with dehydration secondary to acute illness) are great enough to warrant surgery. Other considerations are the age and general health of the patient and the skill of the available parathyroid surgeons. The difficulties of lifelong follow-up for an asymptomatic illness are considerable. Some young patients will therefore warrant surgery simply because of their unwillingness or inability to maintain a regular follow-up. A final consideration should be the patient's anxieties, either about surgery and anesthesia or about having an uncorrected abnormality. These anxieties may influence therapy significantly if consideration of the preceding factors produces only equivocal arguments for or against parathyroid surgery.

Such a thorough review of medical and practical issues dictates surgery for many of these patients, but a significant residue of truly asymptomatic patients without complications will remain. In these patients, serial quantitative measurements of renal glomerular and tubular function and bone mass at 6-month and later at 12-month intervals are extremely helpful. Such serial follow-up measurements will allow developing complications to be detected early, before significant permanent damage occurs. Asymptomatic patients will accept parathyroid surgery more readily if told that serial tests reveal developing deterioration of renal function or skeletal mass. Many patients with mild hyperparathyroidism will show no deterioration or symptoms during prolonged follow-up and can be confidently reassured after such periodic reevaluations. Until it is possible to predict which patients will deteriorate and which will not, this empiric approach is the only alternative to recommending universal prophylactic surgery for asymptomatic primary hyperparathyroidism. At the present time, it is probably wise to resist any temptation to treat asymptomatic patients with specific medical therapies.

Recently, attention has been directed to the beneficial effects of estrogen and/or norethindrone in the management of primary hyperparathyroidism.[461,462] Treatment with ethinyl estradiol (30 mg daily) or, in patients deemed unsatisfactory for estrogen, norethindrone (5 mg daily) led to improvements in serum calcium and indices of bone turnover without an apparent increase in PTH concentrations despite significant calcium lowering (hormone measured as basal levels with a carboxyl-terminal based immunoassay). Estrogen was more effective than norethindrone. The effects were observed for 3 to 6 months; results were similar to those reported earlier.[462] A critical review of the issue concluded that it was difficult, based on the data available, to recommend estrogen therapy as a viable alternative to surgery or simple medical surveillance. The risk/benefit of estrogen therapy is still under evaluation. There is insufficient knowledge on the long-term skeletal benefits to accept the risks, but a long-term study is indicated.[462]

B. Active Medical Treatment of Primary Hyperparathyroidism

Lowering serum calcium with phosphate leads to increased PTH excretion, which may aggravate rather than ameliorate renal and osseous deterioration.[453] If treatment is necessary, the patient is no longer asymptomatic, and the primary therapeutic approach should still be surgery.

Occasionally, however, patients with primary hyperparathyroidism must be treated medically because of complications such as symptomatic hypercalcemia, because repeated surgery is unsuccessful, coincidental illness makes surgery inadvisable, or the patient refuses surgery. Since remedies that decrease the serum calcium concentration may increase the serum PTH concentration, it is advisable to lower the serum calcium concentration only enough to eliminate symptoms, minimize the dangers of hypercalcemic crises, and keep the urinary calcium excretion below 300 mg/day (7.5 mM/day). Maintaining a serum calcium below 11 to 12 mg/100 ml (2.75-3.0 mM/liter) will usually accomplish all this. Although it is generally assumed that the risk of ectopic calcification in the kidneys, blood vessels, joint cartilages, heart, and elsewhere is directly proportional to the serum calcium concentration, there are no controlled clinical observations to support this. In fact, many patients never develop significant ectopic calcification despite many years of untreated illness. Animal experiments have even indicated that lowering calcium by increasing phosphate may aggravate ectopic calcifications.[454]

Many patients with primary hyperparathyroidism are, however, significantly phosphate-depleted because of the increased renal phosphate clearance induced by the PTH excess. In these patients, if medical treatment of hypercalcemia seems necessary, it may be possible to decrease the serum calcium concentration, without harming the skeleton, by correcting the phosphate deficiency. The correction of severe phosphate depletion can produce a positive skeletal calcium and phosphorus balance and an improvement in bone mass despite a secondary increase in the serum parathyroid hormone concentration. Albright et al. demonstrated such a sequence in two of four patients with primary hyperparathyroidism treated with supplemental oral phosphate to correct severe phosphate depletion.[455] Whether the skeletal benefits of phosphate repletion and the general benefits of the resultant decrease in the serum calcium concentration outweigh the risks of increased PTH secretion in every patient with surgically untreatable primary hyperparathyroidism is unclear.[456] At present, it seems reasonable to recommend dietary phosphate supplements in patients in whom it is necessary to treat hypercalcemia and in whom hypophosphatemia is present.

Patients with primary hyperparathyroidism are sometimes vitamin D–deficient, as revealed by low serum concentrations of 25-hydroxyvitamin D, or 1,25$(OH)_2$ vitamin D.[456-460] Vitamin D deficiency may aggravate the skeletal disease by superimposing osteomalacia upon the already present hyperparathyroid bone disease or by simply increasing demands on skeletal calcium reabsorption to maintain serum calcium. On the other hand, vitamin D deficiency will moderate the hypercalcemia by limiting intestinal calcium absorption and skeletal calcium release. Correcting vitamin D deficiency in such patients will, therefore, aggravate the hypercalcemia, even though it may improve the bone disease. The desirable balance between these two effects can be established only by a cautious therapeutic trial. In patients who are not ideal or willing operative candidates, the benefits of improving skeletal mass often outweigh the risks of some increase in blood calcium, particularly if there is only mild hypercalcemia and severe reduction in bone mass or osteitis fibrosa cystica is present.[362,363]

VII. SURGICAL MANAGEMENT OF PRIMARY HYPERPARATHYROIDISM

The surgical management of hyperparathyroidism, involving the removal of one or more hyperfunctioning parathyroid glands, restores normal calcium and parathyroid function in 92% to 96% of patients, based on analyses of reports from major medical centers summarizing results from large series of patients in each institution.[463-471] Controversies persist, however, about surgical strategies owing to persistent disagreements concerning surgical findings. Satisfactory results are most often encountered in all series when a single enlarged gland or parathyroid adenoma is found. All groups agree that surgical outcomes are more often unsatisfactory when multiple gland disease, typically seen in chief cell hyperplasia, is found[463-471]; risks of persistent hypercalcemia or permanent hypoparathyroidism are considerably higher in hyperparathyroidism due to multiple gland hyperplasia.[472,473]

The experience of the surgeon is generally regarded as the most important factor in determining the success of the surgical exploration.[469,471] Although there has been considerable interest in a variety of techniques for preoperative localization of hyperfunctioning hyperparathyroid glands and some techniques have been extensively evaluated, recent reviews suggest that the techniques be used only when the initial operation has been unsuccessful in locating the abnormal parathyroid tissue.[471]

The postoperative management of patients generally is accomplished without great difficulty unless complicating factors such as extensive bone disease, renal failure, or the need to remove a substantial fraction of the four parathyroid glands increases the risk of more serious postoperative hypocalcemia.[471-473]

A. Surgical Strategies and Results: Persistent Controversies

The majority view is that disease in a single gland, a parathyroid adenoma, is responsible for the hyperparathyroidism in approximately 80% of patients.[463-472] Hyperplasia of the parathyroids accounts for 10% to 15%, carcinoma 2% to 4%, and in a small percentage of patients, abnormal parathyroid tissue is not found.[463-471] Most experienced surgeons advocate limited removal of parathyroid tissue; there are differences in approach, however, even among those favoring a conservative approach. Some advocate unilateral exploration if an abnormal parathyroid gland is found and a second gland is identified and biopsy suggests it is normal.[469,486] The reasoning behind this approach is that double adenoma is extremely rare, its existence even disputed, and hyperplasia involving all glands is excluded by the biopsy results indicating one normal gland.[469] Most of the groups, however, that advocate the conservative approach favor a bilateral exploration of the neck with identification, if possible, of at least four parathyroid glands.[463-466,471] If only one gland is grossly enlarged, that gland is removed and it is assumed that single gland disease is responsible for the hyperparathyroidism and that its removal will lead to a restoration of normocalcemia. Most of the reports do not indicate whether all glands are biopsied, but one group[471] advocates the biopsy of all glands to assure that tissue which was identified as parathyroid is indeed a parathyroid gland. Biopsy proof, confirming the location of all four glands, is felt to be important if a reexploration is indicated because of failure to reverse the hypercalcemia.[471]

Several groups disagree with the majority opinion, feeling that multiple gland disease is more common than the 10% to 20% quoted by the majority. One group advocated removal of three parathyroid glands and approximately 50% of the fourth as routine procedure in all cases, with the view that a higher rate of initial cure would be achieved without incurring an excessive incidence of hypoparathyroidism.[475] The Paloyan group reports multiglandular disease in 40% of patients and single gland disease in 60%. Abnormalities limited to two glands, what might be termed by others "double adenoma," was found in 30% of those considered as having multiple abnormal glands. Two other groups have provided evidence supporting a higher incidence of multigland disease,[476,477] but the surgical strategies differed. One group advocated biopsy of all four glands with the extent of surgery based on biopsy results. A single abnormal gland was found in 56% of cases and multiglandular disease in 42%.[477] Yet another group, relying on gross examination of the parathyroids rather than biopsy results, reported 68% to have single gland enlargement, 22% either two or three gland enlargement, and 10% four gland enlargement in a series of a total of 350 patients; only glands seen grossly to be abnormal were removed.[476]

It is difficult to reconcile these differing opinions from centers in which large numbers of patients are operated on by experienced surgeons with extensive histopathologic examination of removed tissue. It is clear that a single preferred surgical approach cannot be deduced on the basis of results so far reported with respect to such issues as reversal of hyperparathyroidism at the initial exploration, rate of recurrent disease, frequency of transient but symptomatic hypoparathyroidism, or permanent hypoparathyroidism.

What are some of the problems encountered in parathyroid surgery that account for these unresolved controversies, and what approaches might assist in their resolution? Anatomic variation in the apparent number and location of parathyroid glands, as well as their small size, representing a few hundred milligrams in total, explains the difficulties encountered by all surgeons in finding the abnormal glands and in determining the functional status of individual glands. In all reported series, for example, in a small percentage of patients, an abnormal gland is not located on the initial exploration or even with reexploration despite strong laboratory and clinical evidence of presumptive hyperparathyroidism.[463-471] In two reported extensive autopsy series in patients dying from diseases not involving known abnormalities of the parathyroids, although four parathyroid glands were found in 90% of subjects, five glands and three glands, respectively, were found in approximately 5% of patients.[478,479] Although sometimes only three glands are found, despite the opportunity to perform careful examination during an autopsy, four glands may actually be present in all patients, at least as based on two other studies[480,481] in which at least four parathyroids were found when serial sectioning was performed in human embryos. These results merely serve to underscore the inherent difficulty in locating an abnormal parathyroid gland that can be quite metabolically active with a tissue weight of a few hundred milligrams.

There is general agreement that hyperplasia of the parathyroids can be asymmetric, with one or two glands much larger than the other two even though histologic examination reveals hyperplastic changes in all glands, that is, reduction in normal fat content and increased numbers of chief cells or water clear cells. Hence, distinction between adenoma and hyperplasia by gross appearances is sometimes difficult[463-469]; there is also intrinsic difficulty, confusion, and disagreement over histopathologic criteria for adenoma and hyperplasia.[473-475,477,478,485-487]

What are the actual details of the published reports in which disagreements persist, and what can be concluded, at present, about the best surgical strategy? Review of the published reports from groups practicing a more conservative approach versus those who favor more extensive resection does not reveal convincing differences in stated outcomes, despite the striking differences in technique. Presumably, if clear-cut differences in results were evident, greater uniformity in surgical approach would be practiced at present. A Swedish group reports, in a series of 441 patients, adenoma in 77% and hyperplasia in 18%. The remaining percentage either could not be satisfactorily classified or had no abnormal tissue found. As defined by most surgical groups, persistent hypercalcemia was defined as patients not rendered normocalcemic at surgery or "relapsing" within 6 months of surgery. Recurrent hypercalcemia was defined as the appearance of hypercalcemia after a normocalcemic period of at least 6 months. Persistent hypercalcemia was found in 8% of the patients overall, in half of whom a second operation led to normocalcemia. Recurrent hypercalcemia occurred in 16% of the patients with hyperplasia compared with 3% of patients diagnosed as having parathyroid adenomas at initial exploration. Approximately 5% of the patients experienced hypocalcemia in the preoperative period, requiring supplemental calcium and vitamin D therapy. Overall, the results showed normal parathyroid function and normal calcium level in 88% (including successful reoperations in those who required them), persistent hypercalcemia in 5%, and permanent hypocalcemia in 3%.[463] These authors concluded that the conservative approach was justified in the majority of patients. In another report[464] summarizing results in 273 patients, single gland enlargement classified as adenoma was found in 83%, and hyperplasia of all identified parathyroid glands was found in 15%. The authors reported an overall cure rate, referring to results of initial surgery, of 96%; long-term follow-up results were not provided. In a third report, from the Mayo Clinic, the results in 500 patients were summarized.[465] This group, as with several others favoring the conservative approach, nevertheless identified all four parathyroid glands whenever possible. Grossly enlarged glands were removed, usually only one being found. Both enlarged glands were removed when double adenoma was found (3% of patients). If more than two glands were enlarged, the patients were regarded as having hyperplasia and had a subtotal parathyroidectomy involving all four glands. Single enlarged gland or adenoma was found in 76% overall, double adenoma 2.3%, hyperplasia 15%, carcinoma 0.4%, and the remaining percentage unclassified or having no discernible abnormal parathyroid tissue. The acute cure rate was 92%; 10% of patients had symptomatic hypocalcemia requiring calcium supplementation in the immediate postoperative period. Permanent hypoparathyroidism was noted in only 2% of the entire group, disproportionately, as in the experience of others, resulting from patients with parathyroid hyperplasia and multiple gland disease. In another interesting report, a group of surgeons attempted to compare conservative versus liberal approaches with respect to surgical technique and extent of tissue removed.[466] Fifty patients were in each of three groups. One surgeon used the conservative approach, removing enlarged glands only, with or without biopsy of one additional gland. A second surgeon did 50 consecutive cases with a more liberal approach defined as routine removal of at least two glands, or removal of 3½ glands when more than one gland was enlarged, and liberal use of biopsy identification. This same surgeon who used the liberal approach then switched to the conservative approach with another group of 50 patients. Clinical outcomes and pathologic diagnoses were compared and contrasted. The incidence of multiple gland disease was designated at 14% with the conservative approach of the first surgeon; in the liberal approach used by the second surgeon, multiple gland disease was estimated to be present in 46%, including such diagnoses as chief cell hyperplasia, nodular chief cell hyperplasia, multiple adenomas, and increased cellularity with abnormal increase in the ratio of parenchyma over fat affecting more than one gland. When the second surgeon adopted the conservative approach, removing only enlarged glands, the frequency with which normal glands were biopsied is not stated. Not surprisingly, however, the incidence of multiple gland disease when the second surgeon used a conservative approach fell to 10%. Clearly, if fewer glands were available for histologic examination, there was less opportunity to designate multiple gland disease. The important issue to these investigators was, of course, the surgical outcome: 96% of patients operated on by the first surgeon with a conservative approach attained normocalcemia; the same took place when the second surgeon used his conservative approach. If anything, a lower incidence of normocalcemia was detected when the liberal approach was used; the details of the patients with persistent hypercalcemia are not given, but at least one had a mediastinal adenoma.

Temporary hypocalcemia requiring treatment occurred in 4% of the patients by the first surgeon with a conservative approach, and 2% by the second surgeon with a conservative approach. On the other hand, 20% of the patients operated on with the liberal approach by the second surgeon had temporary hypocalcemia requiring treatment. Permanent hypocalcemia did not occur in this small series of 50 patients in either of the two conservative groups, but was found in 4% of those with the more extensive resection. Long-term follow-up was not provided in this report, so the frequency of recurrent hypercalcemia (a problem with limited resection, it is argued by those who favor more extensive resection) was not addressed by the approach used by these surgeons. On the other hand, it was impressive as an internally consistent study performed entirely by one group that the frequency of successful surgical outcomes (normal parathyroid function at least over the several years of the study) was equally favorable, if not superior, with the conservative approach, and that problems with temporary or permanent hypocalcemia were much improved. The authors did attempt to deal with the issue of long-term recurrent hypercalcemia by turning to historical evidence, citing the extensive report by Clark and associates[488] that surveyed a series of 3200 patients treated by selective removal of only abnormally enlarged parathyroid glands where recurrent hyperparathyroidism was reported in less than 1% of these patients; 80% single gland disease was reported in 11 of the 16 extensive reports of several hundred or more patients in each of the reported series that was summarized by Clark and colleagues. The length of follow-up period, however, did vary among many of the reported series so that there is still legitimate uncertainty about late recurrence (beyond a decade).[488]

The conservative approach, advocated by the majority of medical centers with large experience in hyperparathyroidism, appears to have impressive results, with high rates of restoration of normocalcemia that persists for at least several years after surgery and a low incidence of hypoparathyroidism. The minority of surgeons who favor more extensive exploration offer as their principal criticism of clinical results achieved by conservative approach the lack of long-term follow-up. It was noted, for example, by the Swedish group advocating a conservative approach that recurrent hypercalcemia did occur in 3% of the patients in whom there was resection of a single gland and the presumptive diagnosis of adenoma at the time of initial surgery. None of the recurrences occurred earlier than 9 years after surgery, leaving that group to suggest that the surgeon may be occasionally misled as to single versus multiple gland disease at initial operation. The majority argument appears to be that since most patients are permanently cured, at least over the time period of several decades, with the more limited procedure, it is not warranted to remove more tissue with a higher risk of permanent hypoparathyroidism in order to eliminate a low frequency of recurrence.

Paloyan and colleagues are the principal proponents of the more extensive surgical resection. In their initial report,[474] they advocated removal of all but a portion of one parathyroid gland, independent of the gross appearance of any of the four parathyroid glands. Detailed histologic examination of the removed tissue indicated to these authors that true single gland disease occurred in only 33% of patients with a much higher incidence of multiple gland disease of varying pathologic character, including nodular hyperplasia and diffuse hyperplasia. In a subsequent report,[475] Paloyan and colleagues modified their approach to meet criticism of those who argue that routine 3½ gland resection is excessive. In their more recent strategy, half of two parathyroid glands, for a total of 75 to 100 mg of parathyroid tissue, are left after the remainder of the parathyroid tissue is resected. In the more recent report,[475] the earlier results of the 3½ gland resection and the more recent, modified, less extensive subtotal parathyroidectomy were reviewed together as a total group of approximately 300 patients. An overall cure rate of 98% is reported, with persistent hyperparathyroidism in 7%, and no recurrent hyperparathyroidism in the time period over which the patients are followed. Of those with persistent hyperparathyroidism, the majority were subsequently cured by a second procedure and successful removal of an ectopic parathyroid gland. Symptomatic postoperative hypocalcemia requiring treatment was reported by these authors to be only 10% and permanent hypoparathyroidism only 1%. This latter result is surprising in view of the higher incidence of hypoparathyroidism reported by other groups when extensive surgery is performed.[463-473] It is especially puzzling that the stated incidence of hypoparathyroidism is lower even than that reported with more conservative surgery; criteria for defining hypoparathyroidism may differ. The claim that multiple abnormalities in the parathyroid glands exist, however, when extensive resections and/or biopsies are performed, is supported by two other recent reports. One careful surgical study indicates that multiple gland disease can be found in as high as 42% of patients;[488] the functional significance of the abnormalities is unclear, however, in view of the apparent success of limited resections.[463-467,488] Another report claims the rather astonishing figure of 75% as the incidence of multiple gland disease; however, the criteria used for pathologic classification of many of the patients operated on in the series[153] as indicative of hyperplasia would not be accepted by most centers. Rather, these authors used unusual criteria for an adenoma, which, if not found, led them to classify the pathologic process as multiple gland hyperplasia.[153] This report does not seem interpretable or applicable to the general controversy in view of the criteria used and the lack of clinical correlation.

In any event, the critical issues are those involving long-term evaluation of surgical results, particularly to compare the incidence of recurrent hyperparathyroidism and postoperative hypoparathyroidism with conservative surgery versus that seen with more extensive resection. Follow-up over decades, a length of observation greater than that evident in a survey of the current reports from most centers, is required to provide assurance about persistence of the euparathyroid state. Dynamic testing of residual parathyroid function with the new, more reliable immunoassays recently developed may help to detect earlier, and define by more objective criteria, the frequency of recurrence of hyperparathyroidism that follows the use of the conservative strategy and whether the more radical surgical procedures tend to limit parathyroid reserves significantly and cause a higher frequency of frank hypoparathyroidism. Such continued long-term clinical analysis and/or provocative testing may eventually be useful in making a firm conclusion as to optimal surgical approach. Also, modern techniques of molecular biology may prove helpful by permitting further examination of the polyclonality versus monoclonality of cell types associated with enlarged glands, particularly the confusing issue of whether monoclonality is typical of most cases of familial hyperplasia (as discussed above in Section II, Etiology and Pathology). At the present time, the bulk of evidence seems to favor a conservative approach with removal of only visibly enlarged parathyroid glands;

cure rates seem satisfactory and the suspicion persists[463-466] that more radical surgery[474,475] may cause more hypoparathyroidism. Further clinical and laboratory work is clearly required, however, to satisfactorily resolve the controversies that are still evident in surveys of surgical strategies and results.

B. Preoperative Localization Techniques

In view of the vagaries of parathyroid surgery discussed, it is not surprising that there has been considerable interest in techniques for preoperative localization of the parathyroid glands. Many reports have appeared on a variety of techniques over the past decade. The NIH group has recently undertaken a critical review of the various methods.[471] Unfortunately, there is a paucity of reviews in which cost-effectiveness, sensitivity and specificity, risk and benefit, and morbidity and inconvenience are critically analyzed and compared among techniques. Noninvasive techniques have received much wider attention recently and now are more often used than invasive techniques, or at least precede, in most cases, the use of invasive procedures such as arteriography.[471] Almost all of the techniques are based on the principle of detecting a suspicious mass lesion, presumed to be an abnormal parathyroid gland, in the neck or mediastinum, rather than representing a functional test of parathyroid gland activity. This indirect character of most localization techniques leads to a higher than desirable frequency of false-positive results.[471,512-519] The overall success of the techniques such as ultrasound, computer tomography, and thallium/technetium scans in preoperative localization prior to any surgery ranges from 60% to 70%.[471,512-522] Since, as noted previously, the success reported at the initial operation in correcting the hyperparathyroidism is greater than 90% for experienced surgeons without the benefit of any preoperative localization techniques, the NIH group, among others, strongly recommends that localization techniques be used only in patients who are reexplored because of failure to find the abnormal parathyroid gland at the initial exploration.[471] There seems general agreement that the invasive techniques should be reserved for patients requiring reexploration.[507]

Ultrasound techniques have several advantages, including the avoidance of radiation, lower cost, and good results for lesions found in the neck in the vicinity of the thyroid. The disadvantage of the technique is that the overall success rate[512-515] in accurate preoperative localization prior to the initial surgical exploration is only 60% to 70%. Furthermore, it is generally agreed that results are poor for lesions located in the mediastinum. Computer tomography is also noninvasive, has a minimum radiation exposure, and is helpful in localization of ectopic glands present in the anterior or posterior superior mediastinum, the last feature being a clear advantage over ultrasound. Nonetheless, the overall success rate is estimated at 60%.[517-519] In addition, some of the lesions identified as potential parathyroid glands prove to be mass lesions that are benign but not of parathyroid origin.[471]

Radiothallium/technetium scanning is based on subtracting the uptake of radiotechnetium by the thyroid from the combined uptake of radiothallium of both the thyroid and the parathyroid.[520,522] Thallium tends to detect thyroid and parathyroid tissue by virtue of their hypervascularity. The technique seems most effective for lesions within the neck and is sometimes particularly helpful for glands located at the cervicothoracic inlet. The technique is not, as with ultrasound, very helpful for mediastinal lesions because of interference by thallium activity in the heart and thoracic vascular structures. There is some disagreement about the value of the technique with reports claiming sensitivity as high as 70% to 80%,[520-522] whereas the NIH group claims the success rate is closer to 50% to 60%.[471]

In all of the techniques, it is clear that even the advocates indicate a localization success below that of the experienced surgeon without the assistance of any of the techniques. Furthermore, many surgeons advocate, as discussed previously, identifying all four parathyroid glands even when an abnormal gland is discovered early in the exploration; this strategy argues further against the routine use of localization techniques, even of the noninvasive character, prior to the initial exploration.[471]

There is a clear consensus, on the other hand, that in patients with persistent or recurrent hyperparathyroidism, there should be extensive use made of these techniques—ultrasound, computer tomography, and thallium/technetium scanning—as well as, in most cases, arteriography. The NIH group, which has extensive experience with reexploration because of cases referred with failure at initial operation, states that the noninvasive techniques, in their experience, if applied collectively, provide an accurate localization preoperatively of the abnormal gland in about 50% of patients. When arteriography, the usual invasive technique now used, is added, the successful preoperative localization rises to 75% to 80%.[471] It is stated that ultrasound by itself achieves preoperative localization in reexplored cases in about 40% to 50%.[523,524] Again, the success of the technique is best for lesions in the neck, particularly intrathyroidal parathyroid adenomas. Computer tomography seems particularly helpful for the more difficult problem of mediastinal lesions, being successful, it is reported, in 50% to 60% of cases.[526,527] The NIH group states that in their experience,[471] computed tomography is not successful in patients under the age of 30 years because of less distinction in tissue density between the thymus and the parathyroid; with increasing age, the thymus is replaced with fat, which provides a more ready discrimination between the parathyroid gland mass and the thymus. It has been reported that thallium/technetium scanning has been successful in 42% of patients at the time of reexploration.[525]

The NIH group has suggested that there is value to performing needle biopsy of suspicious mass lesions detected by the noninvasive techniques to confirm that the tissue is parathyroid in character. Aspiration is performed with a narrow-gauge needle, guided by computer tomography or ultrasound. Determination of parathyroid hormone in the aspirate has led to preoperative positive localization of a mass as parathyroid tissue in 17 of 20 cases.[471] Other groups have also been using the technique of needle aspiration with success.[528,529]

The technique of venous catheterization of the superior, middle, and inferior thyroid veins, the veins closest to the parathyroid effluent vessels, combined with selective radioimmunoassay, was practiced with considerable success in several centers for several years.[507,510,511] Detection of a localized increase in immunoassayable hormone often led to the correct prediction that the parathyroid adenoma was located in the side of the neck where the gradient was detected. The technique was basically a lateralization rather than a localization procedure, in that the gland itself was not directly visualized. This is a critical deficiency in the technique; at the same time, the procedure is based on a functional test, namely, the output of parathyroid hormone. For the most part, selective venous catheterization has been replaced by arteriography. The initial procedure used was selective arteriography with injections into the inferior or superior thyroid or internal mammary arteries.[508,509] The success rate was 90% to 95%;[507-509] unfortunately, the technique required great skill to avoid injection into vessels feeding the spinal cord and brain stem. Complications related to damage to the central nervous system were reported in 1% to 5% of cases, even with skilled angiographers.[507] Fortunately, this procedure has now been replaced by intra-arterial digital angiography. Dilute contrast media is injected into the ascending aorta. All the potential arterial supply is filled; the application of the digital subtraction techniques then allows high resolution analysis leading to detection of the abnormal parathyroid gland in a high percentage of cases. Success as high as 90% is reported by the NIH group.[471,530]

The NIH group has also popularized the procedure of treating parathyroid adenomas in selected patients by nonsurgical techniques. When a gland is identified by digital arteriography, lesions, particularly those located within the mediastinum, can often be approached by selective catheterization of small feeding arteries. With the catheter so positioned, an injection of an excess of dye normally used to produce a radiopaque image of the parathyroid gland results in a protracted staining of the tumor with apparent intraglandular extravasation of dye and destruction of the tumor.[531,532] Results indicate destruction of the gland in a majority of a series of approximately 20 patients;[532] the follow-up for intermediate periods of up to several years has not yet shown recurrence.

The NIH surgeons have also demonstrated the utility of intraoperative, rapid measurements of urinary cAMP as a guide to the adequacy of the parathyroid surgery. Urinary cAMP may fall to normal values within 1/2 hour to 1 hour after an adequate amount of parathyroid tissue is removed.[471] There have not yet been reports of the use of this specialized method at other centers, but the general approach of looking for rapidly available information relating to the abnormal function of the parathyroid tissue is a promising approach for the future for both cAMP measurements and the recent, more rapid and sensitive radioimmunoassays. It is unclear whether the latter will ever be made sufficiently rapid to be of value intraoperatively.

C. Postoperative Management

Many issues arise in the management of patients in the immediate perioperative and postoperative period of parathyroid surgery. Adequacy of the surgery as well as the function of residual normal tissue is most effectively evaluated by serial determination of plasma calcium and phosphate values on successive days after neck exploration. The rate of change in serum calcium levels after successful parathyroid surgery, such as removal of a single adenoma, has been carefully documented.[489] Serum calcium usually falls by several milligrams per 100 ml within the first 24 hours after surgery. Thereafter, calcium values fall typically to low-normal or subnormal values in the range of 8 to 9 mg/100 ml over a period of 3 to 4 days. The nadir of the serum calcium is usually reached in about 2 to 5 days, and then there is return to normal or to the lower level of normal. In earlier studies, patients with high serum alkaline phosphatase levels and other evidence of osteitis fibrosa showed a more profound fall to values often less than 7 mg/100 ml; the nadir in serum calcium was not reached for as long as 5 to 50 days after operation, presumably reflecting continued uptake of calcium and phosphate by bone in excess of that released, "hungry bones."[489] The abrupt reduction in levels of parathyroid hormone in the circulation results in a cessation of excessive bone resorption, whereas stimulation of new bone formation persists. Serial bone biopsies examined after parathyroidectomy have shown a marked osteoblastic response manifested by the deposition of large amounts of osteoid in areas previously involved by osteoclastic resorption (Fig. 14–13). Osteoid is apparently laid down much faster than it is mineralized, resulting in a histologic picture resembling that seen in osteomalacia. Hence, for several weeks to months after operation, in patients with osteitis fibrosa cystica, reparative processes in the skeleton may be limited by the availability of calcium and phosphorus from the circulation. The persistent uptake of calcium and phosphate, even though inadequate to heal bone rapidly, nonetheless causes severe hypocalcemia and hypophosphatemia requiring treatment. Accelerated uptake of calcium and phosphate by the skeleton in many patients, even without frank osteitis, is a major factor contributing to the hypocalcemia and hypophosphatemia that may be seen for weeks in the postoperative period.

A critical analysis of the relative importance of various factors controlling the extent and time course of the fall in serum calcium after successful parathyroid surgery has never been performed. This comes about largely because of the lack of effective means, such as repetitive analyses by parathyroid hormone immunoassays, to accurately measure the rate of secretion of hormone from the residual parathyroid tissue, particularly biologically active hormone (as distinct from inactive fragments). It seems likely that the hypocalcemia seen in the first few days postoperatively in all patients reflects lack of hormone secretion from the normal glands, increased losses of calcium to bone and urine, and possibly other factors, such as a reduced number of hormone receptors that results from "down-regulation" of receptor number during the period of excessive hormone secretion.

Data that bear on the issue of the secretory activity, if any, of the normal glands as a function of long-standing hypercalcemia are minimal. There are two types of evidence. One group[490] showed that in the normal animal, induction of sustained hypercalcemia for periods of as long as 40 hours is associated with continued secretion of hormone, although at a low level. These findings are consistent with observations[491] of continued cellular activity in remaining normal glands in patients with parathyroid adenomas. A contradictory line of evidence derives from studies with samples taken from the venous drainage of normal glands at the time of localization studies.[492] No increase over immunoassayable hormone levels in peripheral blood is seen in the parathyroid effluent, in contrast to the high gradients detected in the effluent from the affected, hyperfunctioning gland.[492,493] The lack of detection of hormone output from the normal glands indicates that their functional activity in long-standing hyperparathyroidism with persistent hypercalcemia must be low or absent. The persistent hormone production despite hypercalcemia in cows may have reflected the short-term nature of the hypercalcemia, hours rather than months.[490]

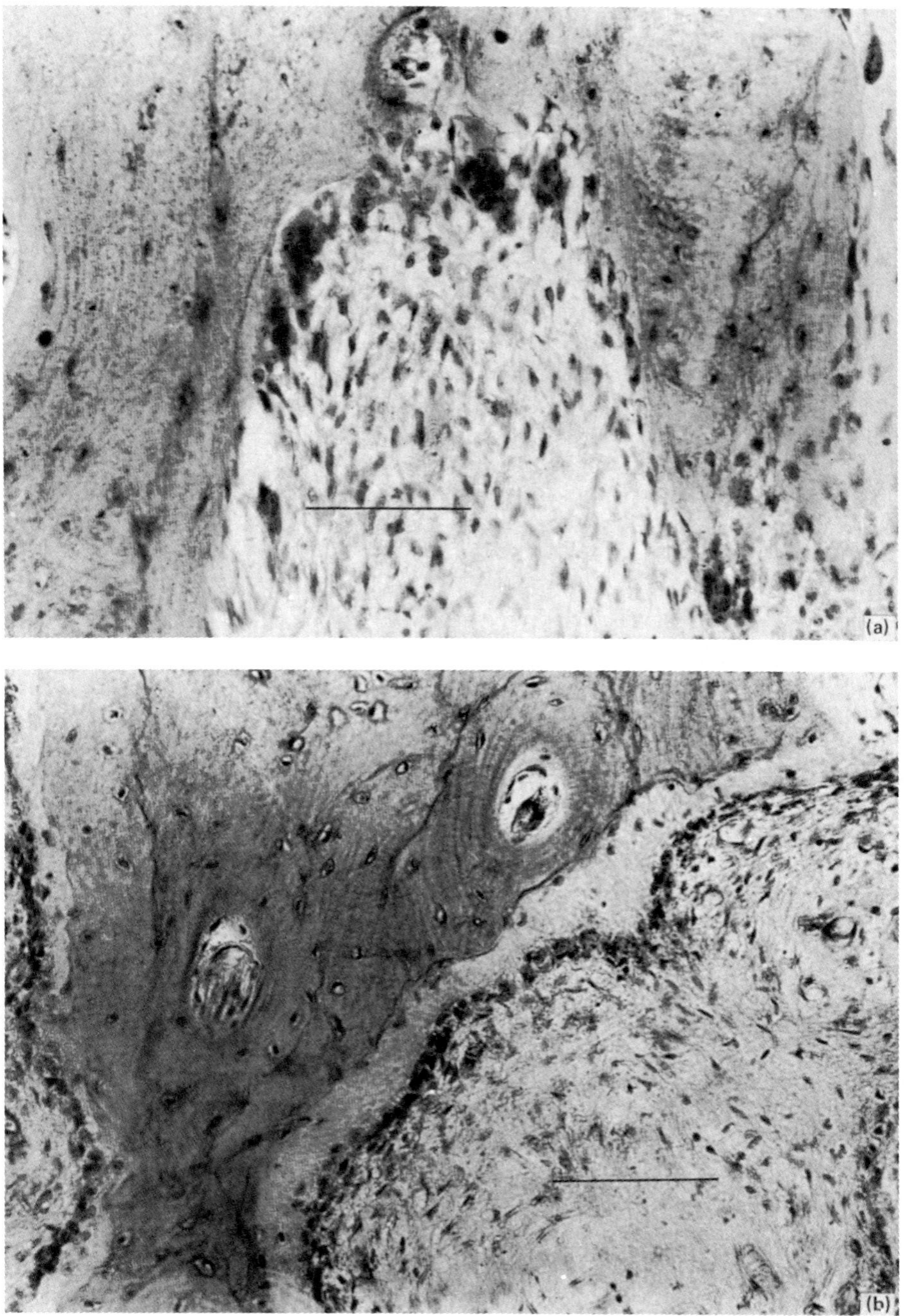

Figure 14–13. (Illustration continued on following page.)

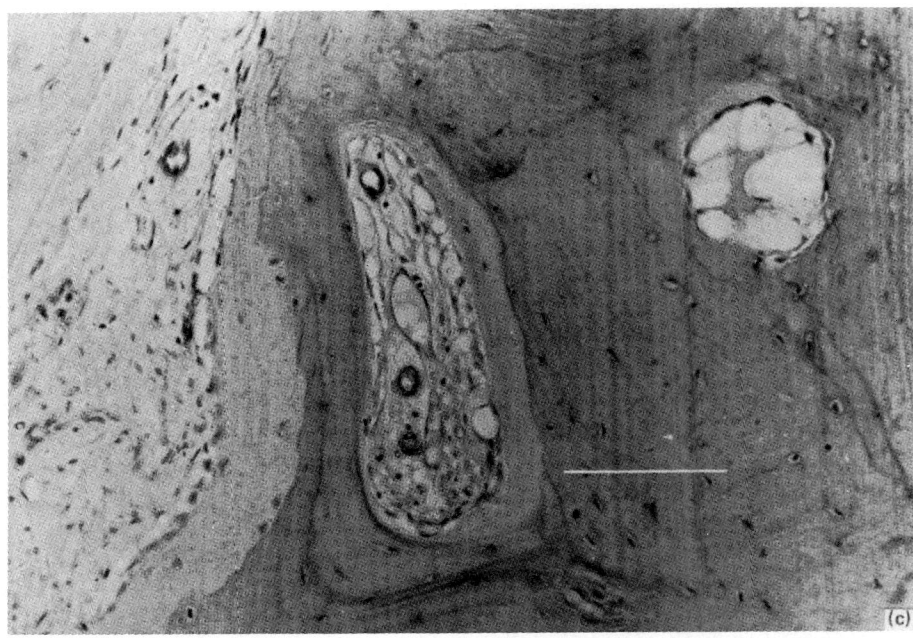

Figure 14–13. Serial photomicrographs of bone biopsies of the tibia taken during and after removal of a parathyroid adenoma. *A*, Day of parathyroidectomy; *B*, 7 days, and *C*, 35 days after surgery. At time of surgery (*A*), typical histologic findings of osteitis fibrosa cystica are evident. There is marked fibroblastic proliferation with several large, multinucleotoid osteoclasts adjacent to the surface of laminar bone. These findings are indicative of active bone resorption. By 7 days after parathyroidectomy (*B*), the histologic findings have changed completely. A large seam of unmineralized osteoid has appeared adjacent to the mineralized bone, which, in turn, is lined by a continuous row of osteoblasts. These findings indicate the rapid formation of new bone. Osteoid is being laid down faster than the process of mineralization, resulting in a histologic picture similar to that seen in osteomalacia. Considerable poorly mineralized osteoid is still evident by 35 days after surgery (*C*). The patient was severely hypocalcemic (serum calcium values of 5.1–5.5) during this time, requiring the intermittent intravenous administration of calcium chloride with ingestion of large amounts of calcium glycerol phosphate to prevent tetany. The photomicrographs, provided by Dr. S.M. Krane, were retaken by the Department of Pathology, Massachusetts General Hospital, from the original histologic preparations from case No. 8 described by Albright and Reifenstein (1948). H and E stain of partially decalcified tissues. Magnification × 300 (horizontal bar = 300 μm).

The interpretation that seems most reasonable from these data is that the normal parathyroid glands in the presence of a functioning adenoma have a negligible rate of hormone secretion. Presumably, the rapid fall in serum calcium after the removal of the abnormal, hyperactive gland reflects in part the delay required for resumption of normal rates of secretory activity by the residual, suppressed parathyroid glands. Eventually, it should become possible to obtain frequent measurements of plasma parathyroid hormone using techniques that measure reliably and exclusively the biologically active intact hormonal molecule. The newer assays have already been used to obtain preliminary data concerning the time course of recovery of parathyroid secretory rate to normal levels after operation.[494] Such studies could be used to decide to what extent and how often normal glands are suppressed prior to correction of the hyperparathyroidism. Whether the normal glands are completely suppressed has not been answered by these studies, but subnormal levels of parathyroid hormone are seen for approximately 24 hours followed by return of immunoassayable hormone levels to normal values, confirming full function of the normal parathyroids.[494] Such studies could be useful in predicting in individual patients whether the hypocalcemia is merely transient or whether more permanent hypoparathyroidism requiring vitamin D therapy is likely.

Failure of the serum calcium level to fall below 10 mg/100 ml in the first 2 or 3 postoperative days is usually a sign of inadequate surgery.[495,496] When multiple glands are hyperplastic and at least one hyperfunctioning gland has eluded detection by the surgeon, the usual fall in blood calcium to subnormal levels does not occur, owing to the continued secretion of a greater than normal level of parathyroid hormone.

Regardless of whether the failure to correct hyperparathyroidism surgically is due to failure to remove either any or all of the involved abnormal parathyroid tissue, it is recommended[155] that reexploration be deferred for several months because of the technical difficulties encountered in examining the recently explored tissues of the neck. As discussed earlier, special localization techniques may be of use in localization of the remaining abnormal tissue if reexploration is required. It has been reported that when reexploration is performed, the residual abnormal tissue is still found within the neck in at least 75% of cases.[155] In one report dealing with 71 reexplored cases, the missing gland was found within the neck in 82% of the patients; in only 18% was a sternotomy required to reach an abnormal gland.[155]

The occurrence of protracted postoperative hypocalcemia varies greatly in frequency depending on the presence or absence of associated medical complications and to some extent, as discussed before, the type of surgical approach used. In patients in whom all four glands are biopsied or subtotally resected, there is a greater risk of temporary or permanent hypoparathyroidism.[463-466,472,473] Persistent hypocalcemia may be due to inadequate residual parathyroid tissue, that is, true hypoparathyroidism, either temporary or permanent. Hypocalcemia may also be caused by failure of systemic tissue to respond to adequate levels of circulating parathyroid hormone, for example, severe hypomagnesemia, chronic renal failure, severe bone disease with large mineral deficits in the skeleton, malabsorption or other causes of vitamin D lack, and, rarely, intraoperative pancreatitis.[497,500-502]

A clue to the onset of permanent hypoparathyroidism is often provided by serial determinations of blood phosphate as well as calcium. Normally, after correction of hyperparathyroidism, persistent hypophosphatemia due to rapid repair of bone mineral deficits occurs. When hypoparathyroidism is present, hyperphosphatemia occurs as a consequence of the loss of parathyroid action on renal phosphate clearance, an effect that predominates over skeletal uptake of phosphate.

Oral calcium supplementation may suffice as treatment for mild symptomatic hypocalcemia in the postoperative period. Because intestinal absorption of calcium is reasonably efficient for several days after parathyroidectomy,[489] addition to the diet of several grams of elemental calcium per 24 hours (given as any of several preparations, plus liberal use of milk as tolerated) will often lead to a lessening of the symptoms of increased neuromuscular irritability. Chvostek's sign may be useful to monitor the success of oral therapy. If hypocalcemia is severe and/or continues, intravenous calcium is necessary to avoid serious consequences such as tetany, laryngospasm, and convulsions. Solutions of calcium (gluconate or chloride) at a concentration of 1 mg/ml may be administered in 5% dextrose/water. The rate and duration of intravenous calcium therapy are determined by the severity of symptoms and the response to therapy detected by monitoring both blood calcium levels and signs of neuromuscular irritability. A rate of infusion of 0.5 to 2 mg/kg/hour or 30 to 100 ml/hour of the 1 mg/ml solution will usually suffice to relieve symptoms. In most instances, parenteral therapy will be required for only a few days. If the requirement for parenteral calcium continues for more than 4 or 5 days, replacement therapy with 1,25-dihydroxycholecalciferol and/or oral calcium should be initiated.

If true hypoparathyroidism is present, 10 days or longer may be required for the calcium-raising action of large doses of vitamin D plus oral calcium to take effect;[489] 1,25-dihydroxycholecalciferol can raise serum calcium to normal within 24 hours after initiation of treatment, hence use of this rapidly acting derivative of vitamin D is preferred regardless of whether the hypocalcemia is permanent or transient.[498]

Postoperative hypocalcemia is frequent in patients who have primary hyperparathyroidism and coexistent chronic renal failure and/or vitamin D deficiency or malabsorption. Significant magnesium depletion and resulting severe hypomagnesemia occasionally appear in patients with primary hyperparathyroidism.[500-502] The magnesium deficiency *per se* may be responsible for persistent and refractory hypocalcemia, and unless magnesium levels are restored to normal, it may be difficult if not impossible to correct postoperative hypocalcemia. The hypocalcemia associated with magnesium depletion arises principally from impairment of the secretion of parathyroid hormone from the residual parathyroid gland.[504,505] As discussed, repletion of magnesium leads to a prompt restoration of the normal secretory activity of the parathyroids.

Detection of hypomagnesemia may provide a clue to a readily reversible cause of protracted hypocalcemia that is not due to hypoparathyroidism. Magnesium deficiency should therefore be promptly corrected whenever detected. $MgCl_2$ is sufficiently soluble to be effective by mouth, but preparations of this compound are not widely available, and oral repletion is slower. Accordingly, repletion should usually be parenteral. The extent of total-body magnesium deficiency may well be as great as 150 to 200 mEq. Inasmuch as the depressant effect of magnesium on central and peripheral neural function is not seen below 4 mEq/liter (normal range is 1.5–2.0 mEq/liter), magnesium replacement can be accomplished rapidly. A dose as great as 100 mEq/kg can be given over 8 to 12 hours if severe hypomagnesemia is detected, provided renal function is not impaired.[506] The magnesium is given either as an intravenous infusion over 8 to 12 hours or in divided doses intramuscularly. If hypocalcemia is due to hypomagnesemia, blood calcium usually returns to normal within 24 to 48 hours.[504,505] If in doubt, a guide to the correction of the magnesium deficit is the restoration of normal rates of excretion of Mg, that is, excretion of 70% to 90% of the administered dose[506] when the intracellular deficit is corrected.

References

1. Mandl F: Klinisches und experimentelles zur frage der lokalisierten ostitis fibrosa: B. Die generalisierte form der ostitis fibrosa. Arch Klin Chir 143:1, 1926.
2. Gold E: Mitt Grenzgeb Med Chir 41:63, 1928.
3. Barr DP, Bulger HA: The clinical syndrome of hyperparathyroidism. Am J Med Sci 179:449–476, 1930.
4. Wilder RM: Hyperparathyroidism: Tumor of the parathyroid glands associated with osteitis fibrosa. Endocrinology 13:231, 1929.
5. Albright F, Aub JC, Bauer W: Hyperparathyroidism. A common and polymorphic condition as illustrated by seventeen proved cases from one clinic. JAMA 102:1276–1287 (April 21), 1934.
6. Albright F, Reifenstein EC Jr: The Parathyroid Glands and Metabolic Bone Disease: Selected Studies. Baltimore, Williams and Wilkins, 1948.
7. Bauer W, Federman DD: Metab Clin Exp 11:21, 1962.

7a. Erdheim J: Zur normalen und pathologischen histologie der glandula thyreoidea, parathyreoidea, und hypophysis. Beitr Pathol Anat 33:158, 1903.

7b. Cushing H, Davidoff LM: *In* The Pathological Findings in Four Autopsied Cases of Acromegaly, with a Discussion of Their Significance. New York, Rockefeller Inst. Med. Res., Monogr. No. 22, 1927.

7c. Rossier PH, Dressler M: Schweiz Med Wochenschr 69:985, 1939.

8. Wang CA: Ann Surg 183:271, 1976.
9. Heath H, Hodgson SF, Kennedy MA: Primary hyperparathyroidism: Incidence, morbidity, and potential economic impact in a community. N Engl J Med 302:189–193, 1980.
10. Bainbridge ET, Barney AD: Some changing aspects of primary hyperparathyroidism. Ann R Coll Surg Engl 65:67–70, 1983.
11. Diamond TH, Botha JR, Shires R: Primary hyperparathyroidism. S Afr J Med 69:94–97, 1986.
12. Browder W, Rakinic J, Schlecter R, Krementz ET: Primary hyperparathyroidism in the seventies: A decade of change. Am J Surg 146:360–365, 1983.
13. Chaves-Carballo E, Hayles AB: Parathyroid adenoma in children: Report of three cases, with unusual articular manifestations in one case. Am J Dis Child 112:553–557, 1966.
14. Hellstrom J, Ivemark BI: Primary hyperparathyroidism: Clinical and structural findings in 138 cases. Acta Chir Scand [Suppl] 294:1–112, 1962.
15. Riddick FA Jr: Primary hyperparathyroidism. Med Clin North Am 81:871–881, 1967.
16. Watson L: Primary hyperparathyroidism. Clin Endocrinol Metab 3:215–235, 1974.
17. Brennan MF: Primary hyperparathyroidism. Annu Rev Surg 25–47, 1983.
18. Boonstra CE, Jackson CE: Serum calcium: Surgery for hyperparathyroidism: Results in 50,000 clinic patients. Am J Clin Pathol 55:523–534, 1971.
19. Wang CA: Surgery of the parathyroid glands. Adv Surg 5:109–127, 1971.
20. Rao DS: Primary hyperparathyroidism: Changing patterns in presentation and treatment decisions in the eighties. Henry Ford Hosp Med J 33:194–197, 1985.
21. Mundy GR, Cove DH, Fisken R: Primary hyperparathyroidism: Changes in the pattern of clinical presentations. Lancet 1:1317–1320, 1980.
22. Purnell DC, Smith LH, Scholz DA, et al: Primary hyperparathyroidism: A prospective clinical study. Am J Med 50:670–680, 1971.
23. Morris RC Jr, Sebastian A, McSherry E: Renal acidosis. Kidney Int 1:322–340, 1972.
24. Thoren L, Werner I: Hyperparathyroidism: Clinical observations in a series of 85 patients. Acta Chir Scand 135:395–401, 1969.
25. Epstein FH: Calcium and the kidney. Am J Med 45:700–714, 1968.
26. Epstein FH: Bone and mineral metabolism in hyperthyroidism. Ann Int Med 68:490–491, 1986.
27. Richet G, Ardaillou R, Amiel C, et al: Acidification de l'urine par injection intraveineuse de sels de calcium. J Urol Nephrol 69:373–398, 1963.
28. Heinemann HO: Metabolic alkalosis in patients with hypercalcemia. Metabolism 14:1137–1152, 1965.
29. Verbanck M: Le fonctionnement du rein dans les etats d'hypercalcemie: Etude clinique et experimentale. Acta Clin Belg [Suppl]1:1–130, 1965.
30. Wills MR, McGowan GK: Plasma-chloride levels in

hyperparathyroidism and other hypercalcemic states. Br Med J 1:1153–1155, 1964.
31. Palmer FJ, Nelson JC, Bacchus H: The chloride-phosphate ratio in hypercalcemia. Ann Intern Med 80:200–204, 1974.
32. Coe FL: Magnitude of metabolic acidosis in primary hyperparathyroidism. Arch Intern Med 134:262–265, 1974.
33. Morris RC Jr: An experimental renal acidification defect in patients with hereditary fructose intolerance. I. Its resemblance to renal tubular acidosis. J Clin Invest 47:1389–1398, 1968.
34. Morris RC Jr: An experimental acidification defect in patients with hereditary fructose intolerance. II. Its distinction from classic renal tubular acidosis; its resemblance to the renal acidification defect associated with the Fanconi syndrome of children with cystinosis. J Clin Invest 47:1648–1663, 1968.
35. Morris RC Jr: Renal tubular acidosis: Mechanisms, classification and implications. N Engl J Med 281:1405–1413, 1969.
36. Morris RC Jr, McSherry E, Sebastian A: Modulation of experimental renal dysfunction of hereditary fructose intolerance by circulating parathyroid hormone. Proc Natl Acad Sci 68:132–135, 1971.
37. Gold LW, Massry SG, Arieff AI, et al: Renal bicarbonate wasting during phosphate depletion: A possible cause of altered acid-base homeostasis in hyperparathyroidism. J Clin Invest 52:2556–2562, 1973.
38. Edvall CA: Renal function in hyperparathyroidism. A clinical study of 30 cases with special reference to selective renal clearance and renal vein catheterization. Acta Chir Scand[Suppl 229], 1958.
39. Purnell DC, Scholz DA, Smith LH, et al: Treatment of primary hyperparathyroidism. Am J Med 56:800–809, 1974.
40. Muldowney FP, Carroll DV, Donahoe IF, et al: Correction of renal bicarbonate wastage by parathyroidectomy: Implications in acid-base homeostasis. Q J Med 40:487–498, 1971.
41. Britton DC, Thompson MH, Johnston IDA, et al: Renal function following parathyroid surgery in primary hyperparthyroidism. Lancet 2:74–75, 1971.
42. Lloyd HM: Primary hyperparathyroidism: An analysis of the role of the parathyroid tumor. Medicine (Baltimore) 47:53–71, 1968.
43. Mallette LE, Bilezikian JP, Heath DA, et al: Primary hyperparathyroidism: Clinical and biochemical features. Medicine (Baltimore) 53:127–146, 1974.
44. Pak CYC, Holt K: Nucleation and growth of brushite and calcium oxylate in urine of stone-formers. Metabolism 25:665–673, 1976.
45. Broadus AE, Horst RL, Lang R, et al: The importance of circulating 1,25-dihydroxyvitamin D in the pathogenesis of hypercalciuria and renal-stone formation in primary hyperparathyroidism. N Engl J Med 302:421–426, 1980.
46. Aurbach GD, Mallette LE, Patten BM, et al: Hyperparathyroidism: Recent studies. Ann Intern Med 79:566–581, 1973.
47. Dauphine RT, Riggs BL, Scholz DA: Back pain and vertebral crush fractures: An unemphasized mode of presentation for primary hyperparathyroidism. Ann Intern Med 83:365–367, 1975.
48. Genant HK, Baron JM, Straus FH II, et al: Osteosclerosis in primary hyperparathyroidism. Am J Med 59:104–113, 1975.
48a. Kleerekoper M, Villanueva AR, Mathews CHE, et al: PTH mediated bone loss in primary and secondary hyperparathyroidism. *In* Frame B, Potts JT Jr (eds): Clinical Disorders of Bone and Mineral Metabolism. Amsterdam, Excerpta Medica, 1983, pp 200–203.
48b. Wilson R, Rao SD, Kleerekoper M, Parfitt AM: Is asymptomatic primary hyperparathyroidism (PHPT) a risk factor for vertebral crush fractures (VCF)? J Bone Mineral Res 2 [Suppl 1]: abstract 109, 1987.
49. Jowsey J: Quantitative microradiography: A new approach in the evaluation of metabolic bone disease (editorial). Am J Med 40:485–491, 1966.
50. Meunier P, Vignon G, Bernard J, et al: Clinical Aspects of Metabolic Bone Disease. *In* Frame B, Parfitt AM, Duncan H (eds): Clinical Aspects of Metabolic Bone Disease. Amsterdam, Excerpta Medica, 1973, p 215.
51. Forland M, Strandjord NM, Paloyan E, et al: Bone density studies in primary hyperparathyroidism. Arch Intern Med 122:236–240, 1968.
52. Balen N, Hjern B: Bone mineral content in patients with primary hyperparathyroidism without radiological evidence of skeletal changes. Acta Endocrinol 75:297–304, 1974.
53. Pak CYC, Stewart A, Kaplan R, et al: Photon absorptiometric analysis of bone density in primary hyperparathyroidism. Lancet 2:7–8, 1975.
54. DeVogelaer JP, Huaux P, Nagant de Deuxchaisnes C: Does mild, asymptomatic, primary hyperparathyroidism require surgery to avoid bone loss in post-menopausal females? *In* Christiansen C, Arnaud CD, Nordin BEC, et al (eds): Osteoporosis. Copenhagen, Aalborg Stiftsbogtrykkeri, 1984, pp 365–367.
55. Seeman E, Wakman HW, Offord KP, et al: Differentiational effects of endocrine dysfunction in the axial and the appendicular skeleton. J Clin Invest 69:1302–1309, 1982.
56. Martin P, Bergmann P, Gillet C, et al: Partially reversible osteopenia after surgery for primary hyperparathyroidism. Arch Intern Med 146:689–691, 1986.
57. Bordier PJ, Arnaud CD, Hawker C, et al: Relationship between serum immunoreactive parathyroid hormone, osteoclastic and osteocytic bone resorptions and serum calcium in primary hyperparathyroidism and osteomalacia. *In* Frame B, Parfitt AM, Duncan H (eds): Clinical Aspects of Metabolic Bone Disease. Amsterdam, Excerpta Medica, 1973, p 222.
58. Albright F, Reifenstein EC Jr: The Parathyroid Glands and Metabolic Bone Disease: Selected Studies. Baltimore, Williams and Wilkins, 1948.
59. Dent CE: Some problems of hyperparathyroidism. Br Med J 2:1419–1425, 1962.
60. Peacock M: Renal stone disease and bone disease in primary hyperparathyroidism and their relationship to the action of parathyroid hormone on calcium absorption. *In* Talmage RV, Owen M, Parsons JA (eds): Calcium-Regulating Hormones, Proceedings of the Fifth Parathyroid Conference. Amsterdam, Excerpta Medica, 1975, p 78.
61. Steinbach HL, Gordan GS, Eisenberg E, et al: Primary hyperparathyroidisms: A correlation of roentgen, clinical, and pathologic features. Am J Roentgenol Radium Ther Nucl Med 86:329–343, 1961.
62. Parfitt AM: The actions of parathyroid hormone on bone: Relation to bone remodeling and tumors, cal-

cium homeostasis and metabolic bone disease. Metabolism 25:1033–1069, 1976.
63. Potts JT Jr, Deftos LJ: Parathyroid hormone, calcitonin, vitamin D, bone and bone mineral metabolism. *In* Bondy PK, Rosenberg LE (eds): Duncan's Diseases of Metabolism. Philadelphia, WB Saunders, 1974, p 1225.
64. Recklinghausen F von: Die fibrose oder deformirende Ostitis, die Osteomalacie und die osteoplastiche Carcinose in ihren gegenseitigen Beziehungen. *In* Festschrift Rudolf Virchow zu seinem 71 Geburtstage. Berlin, G Reimer, 1891, p 1.
65. Hirschberg K: Zur Kenntniss der Osteomalacie und Ostitis malacissans. Bietr Pathol Anat 6:513–524, 1889.
66. Mandl F: Klinisches und Experimentelles zur Frage der lokalisierten und generalisierten Ostitis fibrosa. (Unter besonderer Berucksichtigung der Therapie der letzteren.) Arch Klin Chir 143:1–26, 245–284, 1926.
67. Patten BM, Bilezikian JP, Mallette LE, et al: Neuromuscular disease in primary hyperparathyroidism. Ann Intern Med 80:182–193, 1974.
68. Henson RA: The neurological aspects of hypercalcemia: With special reference to primary hyperparathyroidism. J R Coll Physicians Lond 1:41–49, 1966.
69. Petersen P: Psychiatric disorders in primary hyperparathyroidism. J Clin Endocrinol 28:1491–1495, 1968.
70. Lehrer GM, Levitt MF: Neuropsychiatric presentation of hypercalcemia. J Mt Sinai Hosp 27:10–18, 1960.
71. Hockaday TDR, Keynes WM, McKenzie JK: Catatonic stupor in elderly women with hyperparathyroidism. Br Med J 1:85, 1966.
72. Neumann PJ, Torppa AJ, Blumetti AE: Neuropsychologic deficits associated with primary hyperparathyroidism. Surgery 96:1119–1123, 1984.
73. Wilson RE, Bernhard WF, Polet H, et al: Hyperparathyroidism: The problem of acute parathyroid intoxication. Ann Surg 159:79–93, 1964.
74. Moure JMB: The electroencephalogram in hypercalcemia. Arch Neurol 17:34–51, 1967.
75. Allen EM, Singer FR, Melomed D: Electroencephalographic abnormalities in hypercalcemia. Neurology 20:15–22, 1970.
76. Ostrow JD, Blanshard G, Gray SJ: Peptic ulcer in primary hyperparathyroidism. Am J Med 29:769–779, 1960.
77. Barreras RF: Calcium and gastric secretion. Gastroenterology 64:1168–1184, 1973.
78. Doll R, Jones FA, Buckatzsch MM: Occupational factors in the aetiology of gastric and duodenal ulcers. Medical Research Council Special Report Ser No. 276. London, His Majesty's Stationery Office, 1950.
79. Zollinger RM, Ellison EH: Primary peptic ulcerations of the jejunum associated with islet cell tumors of the pancreas. Ann Surg 142:709–728, 1955.
80. Barreras RF, Donaldson RM Jr: Role of calcium in gastric hypersecretion, parathyroid adenoma and peptic ulcer. N Engl J Med 276:1122–1124, 1967.
81. Dent RI, James JH, Wang CA, et al: Hyperparathyroidism: Gastric acid secretion and gastrin. Ann Surg 176:360–369, 1972.
82. Betts JB, O'Malley BP, Rosenthal FD: Hyperparathyroidism: A prerequisite for Zollinger-Ellison syndrome in multiple endocrine adenomatosis Type I—report of a further family and a review of the literature. Q J Med New Series XLIX, 193:69–76, 1980.
83. Patterson M, Wolma F, Drake A, et al: Gastric secretion and chronic hyperparathyroidism. Arch Surg 99:9–14, 1969.
84. Ward JT, Adesola AO, Welbourn RB: The parathyroids, calcium and gastric secretion in man and the dog. Gut 5:173–183, 1964.
85. McGuigan JE, Colwell JA, Franklin J: Effect of parathyroidectomy on hypercalcemic hypersecretory peptic ulcer disease. Gastroenterology 66:269–272, 1974.
86. Wilder WT, Frame B, Haubrich WS: Peptic ulcer in primary hyperparathyroidism: An analysis of fifty-two cases. Ann Intern Med 55:885–893, 1961.
87. Cope O, Culver PJ, Mixter CG Jr, et al: Pancreatitis, a diagnositc clue to hyperparathyroidism. Ann Surg 145:857–863, 1957.
88. Wang C-A: Surgery of the parathyroid glands. Adv Surg 5:109–127, 1971.
89. Prinz RA, Gerard AV: The association of primary hyperparathyroidism and pancreatitis. Am Surg 51:325–329, 1985.
90. Bess AM, Edis AJ, von Heerdon JA: Hyperparathyroidism and pancreatitis: Chance or counsel association. JAMA 243:246–247, 1980.
91. Paloyan D, Simonowitz D, Paloyan E, et al: Pancreatitis associated with primary hyperparathyroidism. Am Surg 48:366–368, 1984.
92. Mixter CG Jr, Keynes WM, Cope O: Further experience with pancreatitis as a diagnostic clue to hyperparathyroidism. N Engl J Med 266:265–272, 1962.
93. Paloyan E, Lawrence AM, Straus FH II, et al: Alpha cell hyperplasia in calcific pancreatitis associated with hyperparathyroidism. JAMA 200:757–761, 1967.
94. Edmondson HA, Berne CJ, Homann RE Jr, et al: Calcium, potassium, magnesium and amylase disturbances in acute pancreatitis. Am J Med 12:34, 1952.
95. Snodgrass PJ: Diseases of the pancreas. *In* Wintrobe MM, Thorn GW, Isselbacher KJ, et al (eds): Harrison's Principles of Internal Medicine. 7th ed. New York, McGraw-Hill, 1974, pp 1568–1579.
96. Kelly TR: Relationship of hyperparathyroidism to pancreatitis. Arch Surg 97:267–274, 1968.
97. Bywaters EGL, Dixon AStJ, Scott JT: Joint lesions of hyperparathyroidism. Ann Rheum Dis 22:171–187, 1963.
98. Wang C-A, Miller LM, Weber AL, et al: Pseudogout: A diagnostic clue to hyperparathyroidism. Am J Surg 117:558–565, 1969.
99. Grahame R, Sutor DJ, Mitchener MB: Crystal deposition in hyperparathyroidism. Ann Rheum Dis 30:597–604, 1971.
100. McCarty DJ Jr: Diagnostic mimicry in arthritis—patterns of joint involvement associated with calcium pyrophosphate dihydrate crystal deposits. Bull Rheum Dis 25:804–809, 1975.
101. McCarty DJ Jr, Haskin ME: The roentgenographic aspects of pseudogout (articular chrondrocalcinosis): An analysis of 20 cases. Am J Roentgenol 90:1248–1257, 1963.
102. McCarty DJ Jr: Mod Trends Rheumatol 1:287, 1966.
103. Dodds WJ, Steinbach HL: Primary hyperparathyroidism and articular cartilage calcification. Am J Roentgenol 104:884–892, 1968.

104. McGill PE, Grange AT, Royston CS: Chondrocalcinosis in primary hyperparathyroidism: Influence of parathyroid activity and age. Scand J Rheumatol 13:56–89, 1984.
105. Mintz DH, Canary JJ, Carreon G, et al: Hyperuricemia in hyperparathyroidism. N Engl J Med 265:112–119, 1961.
106. Scott JT, Dixon AStJ, Bywaters EGL: Association of hyperuricaemia and gout with hyperparathyroidism. Br Med J 1:1070–1073, 1964.
107. Hellstrom J, Birke G, Edvall CA: Hypertension in hyperparathyroidism. Br J Urol 30:13–24, 1958.
108. Rosenthal FD, Roy S: Hypertension and hyperparathyroidism. Br Med J 4:396–397, 1972.
109. Christensson T, Hellstrom K, Wengle B: Hypercalcemia and primary hyperparathyroidism. Arch Intern Med 137:1138–1142, 1977.
110. Blum M, Kerstein M, Worth MH Jr: Reversible hypertension caused by the hypercalcemia of hyperparathyroidism. JAMA 237:262–263, 1977.
111. Christensson T, Hellstrom K, Wengle B: Blood pressure in subjects with hypercalcemia and primary hyperparathyroidism detected in a health screening program. Eur J Clin Invest 7:109–113, 1977.
112. Kleerekoper M, Rao DS, Frame B: Cardiovasc Med 6:1283–1288, 1978.
113. Bradley EL III, Wells JO: Primary hyperparathyroidism and hypertension. Am Surg 49:569–570, 1983.
114. Lueg MC: Hypertension and primary hyperparathyroidism: A five-year case review. S Med J 75:1371–1374, 1982.
115. Brinton GS, Jubiz W, Lagerquist LD: Hypertension in primary hyperparathyroidism: The role of the renin angiotensin system. J Clin Endocrinol Metab 41:1025–1029, 1975.
116. Pyrah LN, Hodgkinson A, Anderson CK: Primary hyperparathyroidism. Br J Surg 53:245–316, 1966.
117. Madhaven T, Frame B, Block MA: Influence of surgical correction of primary hyperparathyroidism on associated hypertension. Arch Surg 100:212–214, 1970.
118. George JM, Robson A, Ketchum A, et al: Calcareous renal disease and hyperparathyroidism. Q J Med 34:291–301, 1965.
119. Blood pressure of persons 6–74 years of age in the United States. U.S. Dept. of Health, Education, and Welfare publication (PHS–HSA) No. 1. Washington, DC, U.S. Government Printing Office, 1976.
120. Haddy FJ: Local control of vascular resistance as related to hypertension. Arch Intern Med 133:916–931, 1974.
121. Oparil S, Haber E: The renin-angiotensin system. N Engl J Med 291:446–457, 1974.
122. Rubin RP: The role of calcium in the release of neurotransmitter substances and hormones. Pharmacol Rev 22:389–428, 1970.
123. Christensson T, Hellstrom K, Wengle B: Arch Intern Med 137:1138–1142, 1977.
124. Jorgensen FS: Effect of thiazide diuretics upon calcium metabolism. Dan Med Bull 23:223–230, 1976.
125. Anderson DC, Steward WK, Piercy DM: Calcifying panniculitis with fat and skin necrosis in a case of uraemia with autonomous hyperparathyroidism. Lancet 2:323–325, 1968.
126. Cogan DG, Albright F, Bartter FC: Hypercalcemia and band keratopathy: Report of nineteen cases. Arch Ophthalmol 40:624–638, 1948.
127. Nolan RB, Hayles AB, Woolner LB: Adenoma of the parathyroid gland in children: Report of case and brief review of the literature. Am J Dis Child 99:622–627, 1960.
128. Reinfrank RF, Edwards TL Jr: Parathyroid crisis in a child. JAMA 178:468–471, 1961.
129. Rajasuriy AK, Peiris OA, Ratnaike VT, et al: Parathyroid adenomas in childhood: A case report and a review of the current literature. Am J Dis Child 107:442–449, 1964.
130. Lloyd HM, Aitken RE, Ferrier TM: Primary hyperparathyroidism resembling rickets of late onset. Br Med J 2:853–856, 1965.
131. Steendijk R: Metabolic bone disease in children. Clin Orthop 77:247–275, 1971.
132. Girard RM, Belanger A, Hazel B: Primary hyperparathyroidism in children. Can J Surg 25:11–13, 1982.
133. Norwood S, Andrassy RJ: Milit Med 148:812–814, 1983.
134. Lillquist K, Illum N, Jacobsen BB, Lockwood K: Primary hyperparathyroidism in infancy associated with familial hypocalciuric hypercalcemia. Acta Paediatr Scand 72:625–629, 1983.
135. Matsuo M, Okita K, Takemine H, Fujita T: Neonatal primary hyperparathyroidism in familial hypocalciuric hypercalcemia. Am J Dis Child 136:728–731, 1982.
136. Spiegel AM, Harrison HE, Marx SJ, et al: Neonatal primary hyperparathyroidism with autosomal dominant inheritance. J Pediatr 90:269–272, 1977.
137. Rhone DP: Primary neonatal hyperparathyroidism: Report of a case and review. Am J Clin Pathol 64:488–499, 1975.
138. Heintz GE, Sizonenho PC, Pounier L: Primary hyperparathyroidism and rickets: A case report and review of the literature. Helv Paediatr Act 39:509–516, 1984.
139. Kristoffersson A, Dahlgren S, Lithner F, Jarhult J: Primary hyperparathyroidism in pregnancy. Surgery 97:326–330, 1985.
140. Delmonico FL, Neer RM, Cosmi AB, et al: Hyperparathyroidism during pregnancy. Am J Surg 131:328–332, 1976.
141. Goehe RK, Kaplan EL, Lindheimer MD, et al: Maternal primary hyperparathyroidism of pregnancy. JAMA 238:508–511, 1977.
142. Lowe DK, Orwall ES, McClung MR, et al: Hyperparathyroidism and pregnancy. Am J Surg 145:611–619, 1983.
143. Chow S, Williams C, Cole E: Parathyroid storm: Rare manifestation of primary hyperparathyroidism. Can Med Assoc J 134:503–504, 1986.
144. Bayat-Mokhtari R, Palmieri GMA, Moinuddin M, et al: Parathyroid storm. Arch Intern Med 140:1092–1095, 1980.
145. Wang CA, Guyton SW: Hyperparathyroid crisis: Clinical and pathologic study of 14 patients. Ann Surg 190:782–790, 1979.
146. Maselly MJ, Lawrence AM, Brooks M, et al: Hyperparathyroid crisis: Successful treatment of ten comatose patients. Surgery 90:741–746, 1981.
147. Albright F, Bloomberg E, Castleman B, Churchill ED: Hyperparathyroidism due to diffuse hyperplasia of all parathyroid glands rather than adenoma of one. Arch Intern Med 54:315–329, 1934.
148. Cope O, Barnes BA, Castleman B, et al: Vicissitudes of parathyroid surgery: Trials of diagnosis and

management in 51 patients with a variety of disorders. Ann Surg 154:491–508, 1961.
149. Roth SI: Pathology of the parathyroids in hyperparathyroidism: Discussion of recent advances in the anatomy and pathology of the parathyroid glands. Arch Pathol 73:495–510, 1962.
150. Roth SI: Recent advances in parathyroid gland pathology. Am J Med 50:612–622, 1971.
151. Thompson NW, Eckhauser FE, Harness JK: The anatomy of primary hyperparathyroidism. Surgery 92:814–824, 1982.
152. Paloyan E, Paloyan D, Pickelman JR: Hyperparathyroidism today. Surg Clin North Am 53:211–220, 1973.
153. Ghandur-Mnaymneh L, Kimura N: The parathyroid adenoma: A histopathologic definition with a study of 172 cases of primary hyperparathyroidism. Am J Pathol 115:70–83, 1984.
154. Wang CA: Parathyroid re-exploration. Ann Surg 186:140–148, 1977.
155. Wang CA, Cope O: Reoperation for hyperparathyroidism. *In* Hardy JD (ed): Rhoad's Textbook of Surgery: Principles and Practice. Philadelphia, JB Lippincott, 1977.
156. Schantz A, Castleman B: Parathyroid carcinoma: A study of 70 cases. Cancer 31:600–605, 1973.
157. Holmes EC, Morton DL, Ketcham AS: Parathyroid carcinoma: A collective review. Ann Surg 169:631–640, 1969.
158. Habener JF, Potts JT Jr: Parathyroid physiology and primary hyperparathyroidism. *In* Avioli LV, Krane SM (eds): Metabolic Bone Disease. New York, Academic Press, 1978.
159. Wermer P: Genetic aspects of adenomatosis of endocrine glands. Am J Med 16:363–371, 1954.
160. Sipple JH: The association of pheochromocytoma with carcinoma of the thyroid gland. Am J Med 31:163–166, 1961.
161. Schimke RN, Hartmann WH: Familial amyloid-producing medullary thyroid carcinoma and pheochromocytoma: A distinct genetic entity. Ann Intern Med 63:1027–1039, 1965.
162. Schimke RN, Hartmann WH, Prout TE, et al: Syndrome of bilateral pheochromocytoma, medullary thyroid carcinoma and multiple neuromas: A possible regulatory defect in the differentiation of chromaffin tissue. N Engl J Med 279:1–8, 1968.
163. Steiner AL, Goodman AD, Powers SR: Study of a kindred with pheochromocytoma, medullary thyroid carcinoma, hyperparathyroidism and Cushing's disease. Multiple endocrine neoplasia, Type 2. Medicine 47:371–409, 1968.
164. Ellison EH, Wilson SD: The Zollinger-Ellison syndrome: Re-appraisal and evaluation of 260 registered cases. Ann Surg 160:512–530, 1964.
165. Fox PS, Hofmann JW, Decosse JJ, et al: The influence of total gastrectomy on survival in malignant Zollinger-Ellison tumors. Ann Surg 180:558–566, 1974.
166. Williams ED: Histogenesis of medullary carcinoma of the thyroid. J Clin Pathol 19:114–118, 1966.
167. Block MA, Horn RC Jr, Miller JM, et al: Familial medullary carcinoma of the thyroid. Trans Am Surg Assoc 85:101–110, 1967.
168. Marx SJ, Powell D, Shimkin PM, et al: Familial hyperparathyroidism: Mild hypercalcemia in at least nine members of a kindred. Ann Intern Med 78:371–377, 1973.
169. Scholz DA, Purnell DC, Edis AJ, et al: Primary hyperparathyroidism with multiple parathyroid gland enlargement. A review of 53 cases. Mayo Clin Proc 53:792–797, 1978.
170. Von Heerden JA, Kent RB III, Sizemore GW, et al: Primary hyperparathyroidism in patients with multiple endocrine neoplasia syndromes. Arch Surg 118:533–536, 1983.
171. Rizzoli R, Green J III, Marx SJ: Am J Med 78:467–474, 1985.
172. Pearse AGE: Evolutionary and developmental relationships among the cells producing peptide hormones. *In* Parsons JA (ed): Peptide Hormones. London, MacMillan, 1976, pp 33–46.
173. Weichert RF III: The neural ectodermal origin of the peptide-secreting glands: A unifying concept for the etiology of multiple endocrine adenomatosis and the inappropriate secretion of peptide hormones by nonendocrine tumors. Am J Med 49:232–241, 1970.
174. Vance JE, Stoll RW, Kitabchi AE, et al: Nesidioblastosis in familial endocrine adenomatosis. JAMA 207:1679–1682, 1969.
175. Melvin KEW, Miller HH, Tashjian AH Jr: Early diagnosis of medullary carcinoma of the thyroid gland by means of calcitonin assay. N Engl J Med 285:1115–1120, 1971.
176. Knudson AG: Hereditary cancer, oncogenes, and antioncogenes. Cancer Res 45:1437–1443, 1985.
177. Eisenberg E: J Clin Invest 44:942, 1965.
178. Schussler GC, Verso MA, Memoto T: J Clin Endocrinol Metab 35:497, 1972.
179. Nordin BEC, Peacock M: Lancet 2:1280, 1969.
180. Neer RM, Potts JT Jr: Medical management of hyperparathyroidism and hypercalcemia. *In* DeGroot LJ et al (eds): Endocrinology, 2nd ed. Philadelphia, WB Saunders, 1989, vol. 2, chapter 61.
181. Duarte CG, Winnacker JL, Becker KL, Pace A: N Engl J Med 284:828, 1971.
182. Dent CE: Br Med J 2:1419, 1962.
183. Dent CE, Watson L: Br Med J 1:646, 1966.
184. Gwinup G, Sayle B: Ann Intern Med 55:1001, 1961.
185. Boonstra CE, Jackson CE: Ann Intern Med 63:468, 1965.
186. Berson SA, Yalow RS, Aurbach GD, Potts JT Jr: Immunoassay of bovine and human parathyroid hormone. Proc Natl Acad Sci USA 49:613–617, 1963.
187. Raisz LG, Yajnik CH, Bockman RS, Bower BB: Comparison of commercially available parathyroid hormone immunoassay in the differential diagnosis of hypercalcemia due to primary hyperparathyroidism or malignancy. Ann Intern Med 91:739–740, 1979.
188. Zanelli JM, Gaines Das RE: The first international reference preparation of human parathyroid hormone for immunoassay: Characterization and calibration by international collaborative study. J Clin Endocrinol Metab 57:462–469, 1983.
189. Minne HW: Quality control in parathyroid hormone radioimmunoassays: A multicenter study performed by the European Parathyroid Hormone Study Group. Eur J Clin Invest 14:16–23, 1984.
190. Fischer JA, Binswanger U, Dietrich FM: Human parathyroid hormone: Immunological characterization of antibodies against a glandular extract and the synthetic amino-terminal fragments 1–22 and 1–34 and their use in the determination of immunoreactive hormone in human sera. J Clin Invest 54:1382–1394, 1974.

191. Segre GV: Amino-terminal radioimmunoassays for human parathyroid hormone. *In* Frame B, Potts JT Jr (eds): Clinical Disorders of Bone and Mineral Metabolism. Amsterdam, Excerpta Medica, 1983, pp 14–17.
192. Segre GV, Tregear GW, Potts JT Jr: Development and application of sequence-specific radioimmunoassays for analysis of the metabolism of parathyroid hormone. Methods Enzymol 37:38–66, 1975.
193. Segre GV, Habener JF, Powell D, et al: Parathyroid hormone in human plasma: Immunochemical characterization and biological implications. J Clin Invest 5:3163–3172, 1972.
194. D'Amour P, Labelle F, Lazure C: Comparison of four different carboxyl-terminal tracers in a radioimmunoassay specific to the 68–84 region of human parathyroid hormone. J Immunoassay 5:183–204, 1984.
195. Marx SJ, Sharp ME, Krudy A, Rosenblatt M: Radioimmunoassay for the middle region of human parathyroid hormone: Studies with a radioiodinated synthetic peptide. J Clin Endocrinol Metab 53:76–84, 1981.
196. Mallette LE, Tuma SN, Berger RE, Kirkland JL: Radioimmunoassay for the middle region of human parathyroid hormone using an homologous antiserum with a carboxy-terminal fragment of bovine parathyroid hormone as radioligand. J Clin Endocrinol Metab 54:1017–1024, 1982.
197. Papapoulos SE, Manning RM, Hendy GN, et al: Studies of circulating parathyroid hormone in man using a homologous amino-terminal specific immunoradiometric assay. Clin Endocrinol (Oxf) 13:57–67, 1980.
198. Martin KJ, Hruska KA, Freitag JJ, et al: The peripheral metabolism of parathyroid hormone. N Engl J Med 301:1092–1098, 1979.
199. Mayer GP, Keaton JA, Hurst JG, Habener JF: Effects of plasma calcium concentration on the relative proportion of hormones and carboxyl fragments in parathyroid venous blood. Endocrinology 104:1778–1784, 1979.
200. Goltzman D, Henderson B, Loveridge N: Cytochemical bioassay of parathyroid hormone: Characteristics of the assay and analysis of circulating hormonal forms. J Clin Invest 65:1309–1317, 1980.
201. Parsons JA, Rafferty B, Gray D, et al: Pharmacology of parathyroid hormone and some of its fragments and analogues. *In* Talmage RV, Owens M, Parsons JA (eds): Calcium-Regulating Hormones. Amsterdam, Excerpta Medica, 1975, pp 33–39.
202. Morrissey JJ, Hamilton JW, MacGregor RR, Cohn DV: The secretion of parathormone fragments 34–84 and 37–84 by dispersed porcine parathyroid cells. Endocrinology 107:164–171, 1980.
203. Flueck JA, DiBella FP, Edis AJ, et al: Immunoheterogeneity of parathyroid hormone in venous effluent serum from hyperfunctioning parathyroid glands. J Clin Invest 60:1367–1375, 1977.
204. Habener JF, Kemper B, Potts JT Jr: Calcium-dependent intracellular degradation of parathyroid hormone: A possible mechanism for the regulation of hormone stores. Endocrinology 97:431–444, 1975.
205. Segre GV, D'Amour P, Potts JT Jr: Metabolism of parathyroid radioiodinated hormone in the rat. Endocrinology 99:1645–1652, 1976.
206. Segre GV, Niall HD, Sauer RT, Potts JT Jr: Edman degradation of radioiodinated hormones: Application to sequence analysis and hormone metabolism *in vivo*. Biochemistry 16:2417–2427, 1977.
207. Hruska KA, Korkor A, Martin K, Slatopolsky E: Peripheral metabolism of intact parathyroid hormone: Role of liver and kidney and the effect of chronic renal failure. J Clin Invest 67:885–892, 1981.
208. Segre GV, D'Amour P, Hultman A, Potts JT Jr: Effects of hepatectomy, nephrectomy and nephrectomy/uremia on the metabolism of parathyroid hormone in the rat. J Clin Invest 67:439–448, 1981.
209. Segre GV, Perkins AS, Witters LA, Potts JT Jr: Metabolism of parathyroid hormone by isolated rat Kupffer cells and hepatocytes. J Clin Invest 67:449–457, 1981.
210. D'Amour P, Huet P-M, Segre GV, Rosenblatt M: Characteristics of bovine parathyroid hormone extraction by bone liver *in vivo*. Am J Physiol 241 (Endocrinol Metab 4):E208–214, 1981.
211. Silverman R, Yalow RS: Heterogeneity of parathyroid hormone: Clinical and physiologic implications. J Clin Invest 52:1958–1971, 1973.
212. Berson SA, Yalow RS: Immunochemical heterogeneity of parathyroid hormone in plasma. J Clin Endocrinol Metab 28:1037–1047, 1968.
213. Martin KJ, Freitag JJ, Conrades MB, et al: Selected uptake of the synthetic amino-terminal fragment of bovine parathyroid hormone by isolated perfused bone. J Clin Invest 62:256–261, 1978.
214. Marcus R, Madvig P, Young G: Age-related changes in parathyroid hormone action in normal humans. J Clin Endocrinol Metab 58:223–230, 1984.
215. Wiske PS, Epstein S, Bell NH, et al: Increases in immunoreactive parathyroid hormone with age. N Engl J Med 300:1419–1421, 1979.
216. Gallagher JC, Riggs BL, Jerpbak CM, Arnaud CD: The effect of age on serum immunoreactive parathyroid hormone in normal and osteoporotic women. J Lab Clin Med 95:373–385, 1980.
217. Insogna KL, Lewis AN, Lipinski BA, et al: Effect of age on serum immunoreactive parathyroid hormone and its biological effects. J Clin Endocrinol Metab 53:1072–1075, 1981.
218. Chapuy MC, Durr F, Chapuy P: Age-related changes in parathyroid hormone and 25 hydroxycholecalciferol levels. J Gerontol 38:19–22, 1983.
219. Marcus R, Minkoff J, Young G, et al: Age-related rise in parathyroid hormone: Comparison of NH_2-terminal and mid-molecule assays. J Bone Mineral Res 1 [Suppl 1]:abstract 343, 1986.
220. Loveridge N, Stamp TCB, Saphier PW: PTH bioactivity in elderly normal subjects and in osteoporotic patients. IX International Conference on Calcium-Regulating Hormones and Bone Metabolism, Nice, France, abstract 858, 1987.
221. Freitag J, Martin KJ, Hruska KA, et al: Impaired parathyroid hormone metabolism in patients with chronic renal failure. N Engl J Med 298:29–32, 1978.
222. Voigts A, Felsenfeld AJ, Andress D, Llach F: Parathyroid hormone and bone histology: Response to hypocalcemia in osteitis fibrosa. Kidney Int 25:445–452, 1984.
223. Piraino BM, Rault R, Greenberg A, et al: Spontaneous hypercalcemia in dialysis patients: Etiology and therapeutic considerations. Am J Med 80:607–615, 1986.
224. Andress DL, Endres DB, Maloney NA, et al: Comparison of parathyroid hormone assays with bone histomorphometry in renal osteodystrophy. J Clin Endocrinol Metab 63:1163–1169, 1986.

225. Hruska K, Teitelbaum SL, Kopelman R, et al: The predictability of the histological features of uremic bone disease by non-invasive techniques. Metab Bone Dis Rel Res 1:39–44, 1978.
226. Dunstan CR, Hills E, Norman AW, et al: The pathogenesis of renal osteodystrophy: Role of vitamin D, aluminum, parathyroid hormone, calcium and phosphorus. Q J Med 55:127–144, 1985.
227. Chan YL, Furlong TJ, Cornish CJ, Rosen S: Dialysis osteodystrophy. Medicine 64:296–309, 1985.
228. Juppner H, Rosenblatt M, Segre GV, Hesch RD: Discrimination between intact and mid-C-region PTH using selective radioimmunoassay systems. Acta Endocrinol 102:543–548, 1983.
229. Lindall AW, Elting J, Ells J, Roos BA: Estimation of biologically active intact parathyroid hormone in normal and hyperparathyroid sera by sequential N-terminal immunoextraction and midregion radioimmunoassay. J Clin Endocrinol Metab 57:1007–1014, 1983.
230. Hackeng WHL, Lips P, Netenlenbos JC, Lips CJM: Clinical implications of estimation of intact parathyroid hormone (PTH) versus total immunoreactive PTH in normal subjects and hyperparathyroid patients. J Clin Endocrinol Metab 63:447–453, 1986.
231. Reiss E, Canterbury JM: The radioimmunoassay for parathyroid hormone in man. Proc Soc Exp Biol Med 128:501–504, 1968.
232. Arnaud CD, Goldsmith RS, Bordier PJ, Sizemore GW: Influence of immunoheterogeneity of circulating parathyroid hormone on results of radioimmunoassays of sera in man. Am J Med 56:785–793, 1974.
233. Slatopolsky E, Hruska K, Martin K, Freitag J: Physiological and metabolic effects of parathyroid hormone. *In* Brenner B, Stein J (eds): Contemporary Issues in Nephrology, vol 4. New York, Churchill Livingstone, 1979, pp 169–193.
234. Conaway HH, Anast CS: Double-antibody radioimmunoassay for parathyroid hormone. J Lab Clin Med 83:129–138, 1974.
235. DiBella FP, Haroker CD: Use of an "intact" parathyroid hormone assay increases "step-up" gradients in samples obtained by selective venous catheterization. Calcif Tissue Int 33:320, 1981.
236. Harris ST, Segre GV, Meng X-W, Potts JT Jr, Ner RM: unpublished observations.
237. Broadus AE, Mahaffey JE, Bartter FC, Neer RM: Nephrogenous cyclic adenosine monophosphate as a parathyroid function test. J Clin Invest 60:771–783, 1977.
238. Broadus AE: Nephrogenous cyclic AMP. Recent Prog Horm Res 37:667–701, 1981.
239. Steward AF, Horst R, Deftos LJ, et al: Biochemical evaluation of patients with cancer-associated hypercalcemia: Evidence for humoral and non-humoral groups. N Engl J Med 303:1377–1383, 1980.
240. Nissenson RA, Nyiredy KD, Arnaud CD: Guanyl nucleotide potentiation of parathyroid hormone–stimulated adenylate cyclase in chicken renal plasma membranes: A receptor-independent effect. Endocrinology 108:1949–1953, 1981.
241. Nissenson RA, Abbott SR, Teitelbaum AP, et al: Endogenous biologically active human parathyroid hormone: Measurement by a guanyl nucleotide-amplified renal adenylate cyclase assay. J Clin Endocrinol Metab 52:840–846, 1981.
242. Seshadri MS, Chan YL, Wilkinson MR, et al: An adenylate cyclase bioassay for parathyroid hormone: Some clinical experiences. Clin Sci 3:321–326, 1985.
243. Seshadri MS, Chan YL, Wilkinson MR, et al: Some problems associated with adenylate cyclase bioassays for parathyroid hormone. Clin Sci 3:331–319, 1985.
244. Nissenson RA, Strewler GJ, Hsu F, et al: Utility of a parathyroid hormone bioassay in the differential diagnosis of hypercalcemia. Program of the 1984 Annual Meeting, Am Soc Bone Mineral Res A-57, 1984.
245. Hsu FS, Clark OH, Serata TY, Nissenson RA: Rapid localization of parathyroid tumors by selective venous catheterization and parathyroid hormone bioassay. Surgery 94:873–876, 1983.
246. Chambers DJ, Dunham J, Zanelli JM, et al: A sensitive bioassay of parathyroid hormone in plasma. Clin Endocrinol [illegible]:375–379, 1978.
247. Fenton S, Somers S, Heath DA: Preliminary studies with the sensitive cytochemical bioassay for parathyroid hormone. Clin Endocrinol 9:381–384, 1978.
248. Goltzman D, Stewart AF, Broadus AE: Malignancy-associated hypercalcemia: Evaluation with a cytochemical bioassay for parathyroid hormone. J Clin Endocrinol Metab 53:899–904, 1981.
249. Stewart AF, Insogna KL, Goltzman D, Broadus AE: Identification of adenylate cyclase and cytochemical glucose 6-phosphate dehydrogenase stimulating activity in extracts of tumors from patients with humoral hypercalcemia of malignancy. Proc Natl Acad Sci USA 80:1454–1458, 1983.
250. Loveridge N, Kent GN, Heath DA, Jones EL: Parathyroid hormone-like bioactivity in a patient with severe osteitis fibrosa cystica due to malignancy: Renotropic actions of a tumour extract as assessed by cytochemical bioassay. Clin Endocrinol 22:135–146, 1985.
251. Colt EWD, Kimbell D, Fieve RR: Renal impairment, hypercalcemia, and lithium therapy. Am J Psychiatry 138:1, 106–108, 1981.
252. Christiansen C, Baastrup PC, Landgreen P: Endocrine effects of lithium. II. "Primary" hyperparathyroidism. Acta Endocrinol 88:528–534, 1978.
253. Christensson TAT: Lithium, hypercalcemia, and hyperparathyroidism. Lancet 2:144, 1976.
254. Graze KK: Hyperparathyroidism in association with lithium therapy. J Clin Psychiatry 42:1, 38–39, 1981.
255. Herman SP: Lithium, hypercalcemia, and hyperparathyroidism. Biol Psychiatry 16:593–595, 1981.
255a. Mallette LE, Eichorn E: Effects of lithium carbonate on human calcium metabolism. Arch Intern Med 146:770, 1986.
256. Lau K, Goldfarb S, Grabie M, et al: Mechanism of lithium-induced hypercalciuria in rats. Am J Physiol 234:E294–E300, 1978.
257. Brown EM: Lithium induces abnormal calcium-regulated PTH release in dispersed bovine parathyroid cell. J Clin Endocrinol Metab 52:1046–1048, 1981.
258. Foley TP Jr, Harrison HC, Arnaud CD, Harrison HE: Familial benign hypercalcemia. J Pediatr 81:1060–1067, 1972.
259. Marx SJ, Powell D, Shimkin PM, et al: Familial hyperparathyroidism: Mild hypercalcemia in at least nine members of a kindred. Ann Intern Med 78:371–377, 1973.

260. Marx SJ, Spiegel AM, Brown EM, Aurbach GD: Family studies in patients with primary parathyroid hyperplasia. Am J Med 62:698–705, 1977.
261. Marx SJ, Spiegel AM, Brown EM, et al: Divalent cation metabolism: Familial hypocalciuric hypercalcemia versus typical primary hyperparathyroidism. Am J Med 65:235, 1978.
262. Marx SJ, Attie MF, Levine MA, et al: The hypocalciuric or benign variant of familial hypercalcemia: Clinical and biochemical features in fifteen kindreds. Medicine 60:397–409, 1981.
262a. Stuckey BGA, et al: Fasting calcium excretion and parathyroid hormone together distinguish familial hypocalciuric hypercalcaemia from primary hyperparathyroidism. Clin Endocrinol 27:525, 1987.
263. Lillquist K, Illum N, Jacobsen BB, Lockwood K: Primary hyperparathyroidism in infancy associated with familial hypocalciuric hypercalcemia. Acta Paediatr Scand 72:625–629, 1983.
264. Spiegel AM, Harrison HE, Marx SJ, et al: Neonatal primary hyperparathyroidism with autosomal dominant inheritance. J Pediatr 90:269–272, 1977.
265. Hughes MR, Baylink DJ, Jones PG, Haussler MR: Radioligand receptor assay for 25-hydroxyvitamin D_2/D_3 and 1α,25-dihydroxyvitamin D_2/D_3: Application to hypervitaminosis D. J Clin Invest 58:61–70, 1976.
266. Davies M, Mawer EB: The pathogenesis of hypercalcaemia in vitamin D poisoning. *In* Norman AW, et al (eds): Vitamin D: A Chemical, Biochemical and Clinical Update. Proceedings of the Sixth Workshop on Vitamin D, Merano, Italy. Berlin, Walter de Gruyter, 1985, pp 57–58.
267. Bell NH, Stern PH, Pantzer E, et al: Evidence that increased circulating 1α,25-dihydroxyvitamin D is the probable cause of abnormal calcium metabolism in sarcoidosis. J Clin Invest 64:218–225, 1979.
268. Bell NH: Vitamin D–endocrine system. J Clin Invest 76:1–6, 1985.
269. Barbour Gl, Coburn JW, Slatopolsky E, et al: Hypercalcemia in an anephric patient with sarcoidosis: Evidence for extrarenal genesis of 1,25-dihydroxyvitamin D. N Engl J Med 305:440–443, 1981.
270. Adams JS, Singer FR, Gacad MA, et al: Isolation and structural identification of 1,25-dihydroxyvitamin D_3 produced by cultured alveolar macrophages in sarcoidosis. J Clin Endocrinol Metab 60:960–966, 1985.
271. Lambert PW, Stern PH, Avioli RC, et al: Evidence for extrarenal production of 1α,25-dihydroxyvitamin D in man. J Clin Invest 69:722–725, 1982.
272. Zimmerman J, Holick MF, Silver J: Normocalcemia in a hypoparathyroid patient with sarcoidosis: Evidence for parathyroid-hormone-independent synthesis of 1,25 dihydroxyvitamin D. Ann Intern Med 98:338, 1983.
273. Habener JF, Potts JT Jr: Parathyroid physiology and primary hyperparathyroidism. *In* Avioli LV, Krane SM (eds): Metabolic Bone Disease, vol 2. New York, Academic Press, 1978, pp 1–147.
274. Garabedian M, Jacqz E, Guillozo H, et al: Elevated plasma 1,25-dihydroxyvitamin D concentrations in infants with hypercalcemia and an elfin facies. N Engl J Med 312:948–952, 1985.
275. Shai F, Baker RK, Addrizzo JR, Wallach S: Hypercalcemia in mycobacterial infection. J Clin Endocrinol 34:251, 1972.
276. Stanbury SW: Vitamin D and hyperparathyroidism: The Lumleian lecture 1981. J R Coll Physicians Lond 15:205–217, 1981.
277. Papapoulos SE, Clemens TL, Fraher LJ, et al: 1,25-dihydroxycholecalciferol in the pathogenesis of the hypercalcaemia of sarcoidosis. Lancet 1:627, 1979.
278. Winnacker JL, Becker KL, Katz S: Endocrine aspects of sarcoidosis. N Engl J Med 278:427–434, 1968.
279. Cushard WG Jr, Simon AB, Canterbury JM, Reiss E: Parathyroid function in sarcoidosis. N Engl J Med 286:395–398, 1972.
280. Goodyer PR, Frank A, Kaplan BS: Observations on the evolution and treatment of idiopathic infantile hypercalcemia. J Pediatr 105:771–773, 1984.
281. Williams JCP, Barratt-Boyes BF, Lowe JB: Supravalvular aortic stenosis. Circulation 24:1311–1318, 1961.
282. Veldhuis JF, Kulin HE, Demers LM, Lambert PW: Infantile hypercalcemia with subcutaneous fat necrosis: Endocrine studies. J Pediatr 95:460–462, 1979.
283. Aarskog O, Aksnes L, Markestad T: Vitamin D metabolism in idiopathic infantile hypercalcemia. Am J Dis Child 135:1021–1024, 1981.
284. Rose E, Boles RS Jr: Hypercalcemia in thyrotoxicosis. Med Clin North Am 37:1715, 1953.
285. Bryant LR, Wulsin JH, Altemeier WA: Hyperparathyroidism and hyperthyroidism. Ann Surg 159:411, 1964.
286. Aub JC, Bauer W, Heath C, et al: Studies of calcium and phosphorus metabolism. III. Effects of thyroid hormone and thyroid disease. J Clin Invest 7:97, 1929.
287. Laake H: Osteoporosis in association with thyrotoxicosis. Acta Med Scand 151:229, 1955.
288. Krane SM, Brownell GL, Stanbury JB, et al: The effect of thyroid disease on calcium metabolism in man. J Clin Invest 35:874, 1956.
289. Adams PH, Jowsey J, Kelly PJ, et al: Effects of hyperthyroidism on bone and mineral metabolism in man. Q J Med 36:1, 1967.
290. Adams P[H], Jowsey J: Bone and mineral metabolism in hyperthyroidism: An experimental study. Endocrinology 81:735, 1967.
291. Krane SM, Goldring SR: Hyperthyroidism: skeletal system; hypothyroidism: skeletal system. *In* Werner SC, Ingbar SH (eds): The Thyroid. New York, Harper and Row, 1976.
292. Castro JH, Genuth SM, Klein L: Comparative response to parathyroid hormone in hyperthyroidism and hypothyroidism. Metabolism 24:839, 1975.
293. Harrison MT, Harden R McG, Alexander WD: Some effects of parathyroid hormone in thyrotoxicosis. J Clin Endocrinol 24:214, 1964.
294. Bouillon R, DeMoor P: Parathyroid function in patients with hyper- or hypothyroidism. J Clin Endocrinol Metab 38:999, 1974.
295. Epstein FH, Freedman LR, Levitin H: Hyercalcemia, nephrocalcinosis and reversible renal insufficiency associated with hyperthyroidism. N Engl J Med 258:782, 1958.
296. Epstein FH: Bone and mineral metabolism in hyperthyroidism. Ann Intern Med 68:490, 1968.
297. Baxter JD, Bondy PK: Hypercalcemia of thyrotoxicosis. Ann Intern Med 65:429, 1966.
298. Breuer RI, McPherson HT: Hypercalcemia in concurrent hyperthyroidism and hyperparathyroidism. Arch Intern Med 118:310, 1966.

299. Winters JL, Kleinschmidt AG Jr, Frensilli JJ, et al: Hypercalcemia complicating immobilization in the treatment of fractures: A case report. J Bone Joint Surg 48A:1182, 1966.
299a. Maynard FM: Immobilization hypercalcemia following spinal cord injury. Arch Phys Med Rehabil 67:41, 1986.
300. Parfitt AM: The interactions of thiazide diuretics with parathyroid hormone and vitamin D: Studies in patients with hypoparathyroidism. J Clin Invest 51:1879–1888, 1972.
301. Koppel MH, Massry SG, Shinaberger JH, et al: Thiazide-induced rise in serum calcium and magnesium in patients on maintenance hemodialysis. Ann Intern Med 72:895–901, 1970.
302. Brickman AS, Massry SG, Coburn JW: Changes in serum and urinary calcium during treatment with hydrochlorothiazide: Studies on mechanisms. J Clin Invest 51:945–954, 1972.
303. Popovtzer MM, Subryan VL, Alfrey AC, et al: The acute effect of chlorothiazide on serum-ionized calcium: Evidence for a parathyroid hormone–dependent mechanism. J Clin Invest 55:1295–1302, 1975.
304. Goodman LS, Gilman A: The Pharmacological Basis of Therapeutics. 4th ed. New York, Macmillan, 1970.
305. Duarte DG, Winnacker JL, Becker KL, et al: Thiazide-induced hypercalcemia. N Engl J Med 284:828, 1971.
306. Parfitt AM: Chlorothiazide-induced hypercalcemia in juvenile osteoporosis and hyperparathyroidism. N Engl J Med 281:55, 1969.
307. van der Sluys VJ, Birkenhager JC, Smeenk D: De invloed van oraal toegediende diuretica op de calcium-en fosfaatstofwisseling. Ned Tijdschr Geneeskd 109:1795, 1965.
308. Rizzoli R, Hugi K, Fleisch H, Bonjour JP: Effect of hydrochlorothiazide on 1,25-dihydroxyvitam D_3 induced changes in calcium metabolism in experimental hypoparathyroidism in rats. Clin Sci 60:101–107, 1981.
309. Porter RH, Cox BG, Heaney P, et al: Treatment of hypoparathyroid patients with chlorthalidone. N Engl J Med 298:577–581, 1978.
310. Katz CM, Tzagouronis M: Chronic adult hypervitaminosis A with hypercalcemia. Metabolism 21:1171, 1972.
311. Frame B, Jackson CE, Reynolds WA, et al: Hypercalcemia and skeletal effects in chronic hypervitaminosis A. Ann Intern Med 80:44, 1974.
312. Caffey J: Chronic poisoning due to excess of vitamin A: Description of clinical and roentgen manifestations in 7 infants and young children. Am J Roentgenol Radium Ther Nucl Med 65:12, 1951.
313. Mahaffey JE, Potts JT Jr: Secondary hyperparathyroidism: Pathophysiology and etiology. *In* DeGroot LJ, et al (eds): Endocrinology, vol 2. New York, Grune & Stratton, 1979, pp 725–734.
314. Slatopolsky E, Caglar S, Gradowska L, et al: On the prevention of secondary hyperparathyroidism in experimental chronic renal disease using "proportional reduction" of dietary phosphorus intake. Kidney Int 2:147, 1972.
315. Harris ST, Neer RM, Segre GV, et al: Secondary hyperparathyroidism associated with dichloromethane diphosphonate treatment of Paget's disease. J Clin Endocrinol Metab 55:1100–1117, 1982.
316. Ott SM, Maloney NA, Coburn JW, et al: The prevalence of bone aluminum deposition in renal osteodystrophy and its relation to the response to calcitriol therapy. N Engl J Med 307:709–713, 1982.
317. Ellis HA, McCarthy JH, Herrington J: Bone aluminum in haemodialysed patients and in rats injected with aluminium chloride: Relationship to impaired bone mineralisation. J Clin Pathol 32:832–844, 1979.
318. Llach F, Felsenfeld AJ, Coleman MD, et al: The natural course of dialysis osteomalacia. Kidney Int 29 [Suppl 18]:S74–S79, 1986.
319. Hodsman AB, Wong EGC, Sherrard DJ, et al: Preliminary trials with 24,25-dihydroxyvitamin D_3 in dialysis osteomalacia. Am J Med 74:407–414, 1983.
320. Orwoll ES: The milk-alkali syndrome: Current concepts. Ann Intern Med 97:242–248, 1982.
321. Sutton RAL, Wong NLM, Dirks JH: Effects of metabolic acidosis and alkalosis on sodium and calcium transport in the dog kidney. Kidney Int 15:520–533, 1979.
322. Burnett CH, Commons RR, Albright F, et al: Hypercalcemia without hypercalciuria or hypophosphatemia, calcinosis and renal insufficiency: A syndrome following prolonged intake of milk and alkali. N Engl J Med 240:787, 1949.
322a. Orwoll ES: The milk-alkali syndrome: current concepts. Ann Intern Med 97:242, 1982.
323. McMillan DE, Freeman RB: The milk alkali syndrome: A study of the acute disorder with comments on the development of chronic condition. Medicine 44:485, 1965.
324. Henneman PH, Benedict PH, Forbes AP, et al: Idiopathic hypercalciuria. N Engl J Med 259:802–807, 1958.
325. Vincent PC, Radcliff FJ: The effect of large doses of calcium carbonate on serum and urinary calcium. Am J Dig Dis 2:286–295, 1966.
326. Reiss E, Canterbury JM: N Engl J Med 280:1381, 1969.
327. Murray TM, Peacock M, Powell D, et al: Clin Endocrinol 1:235, 1972.
328. Targovnik JH, Rodman JS, Sherwood LM: Regulation of parathyroid hormone secretion *in vitro*: Quantitative aspects of calcium and magnesium ion control. Endocrinology 88:1477–1482, 1971.
329. Habener JF: Responsiveness of neoplastic and hyperplastic parathyroid tissues to calcium *in vitro*. J Clin Invest 62:436–450, 1978.
330. Brown EM, Gardner DG, Brennan MF, et al: Calcium-regulated parathyroid hormone release in primary hyperparathyroidism. Am J Med 66:923–931, 1979.
331. Wagner PK, Krause U, Rothmund M: Effect of calcium and magnesium on parathyroid hormone release from human adenomatous and secondary hyperplastic parathyroid tissue *in vitro*. Res Exp Med 181:205–210, 1982.
332. Gittes RF, Radde IC: Endocrinology 78:1015, 1966.
333. Targovnik JH, Rodman JS, Sherwood LM: Endocrinology 88:1477, 1971.
334. Mayer GP: Program, 55th Annual Meeting, American Endocrine Society, 1973, p A-160.
335. Mayer GP, Habener JF, Potts JT Jr: J Clin Invest 57:678, 1976.
336. Hosking DJ, Cowley A, Bucknall CA: Rehydration in the treatment of severe hypercalcemia. Q J Med 200:473–481, 1981.

337. Walser M: Calcium clearance as a function of sodium clearance in the dog. Am J Physiol 200:1099, 1961.
338. Walser M: Treatment of hypercalcemia. Mod Treatment 7:662, 1970.
339. Tori JA, Hill LL: Hypercalcemia in children with spinal cord injury. Arch Phys Med Rehabil 59:443–446, 1978.
340. Suki WN, et al: Acute treatment of hypercalcemia with furosemide. N Engl J Med 283:836, 1970.
341. Baylink D, et al: Formation, mineralization, and resorption of bone in hypophosphatemic rats. J Clin Invest 50:2519, 1971.
342. Lotz M, et al: Osteomalacia and debility resulting from phosphorus depletion. Trans Assoc Am Physicians 77:281, 1964.
343. Freeman S, McLean F: Experimental rickets: Blood and tissue changes in puppies receiving diets very low in phosphorus with and without vitamin D. Arch Pathol 32:387, 1941.
344. Nagant C, Krane S: The treatment of adult phosphate diabetes and Fanconi syndrome with neutral sodium phosphate. Am J Med 43:508, 1967.
345. Lotz M, et al: Evidence for a phosphorus-depletion syndrome in man. N Engl J Med 278:409–415, 1968.
346. Tanaka Y, Deluca H: The control of 25 hydroxyvitamin D metabolism by inorganic phosphorus. Acta Biochem Biophys 154:566, 1973.
347. Day HG, McCollum EV: Mineral metabolism, growth, and symptomatology of rats on diet extremely deficient in phosphorus. J Biol Chem 130:269, 1939.
348. Albright F, et al: Studies in parathyroid physiology: Effect of phosphate ingestion in clinical hyperparathyroidism. J Clin Invest 11:411, 1932.
349. Goldsmith RS, Ingbar SH: Inorganic phosphate treatment of hypercalcemia of diverse etiologies. N Engl J Med 274:1, 1966.
350. Goldsmith RS, Ingbar SH: Phosphate, sulfate, and hypercalcemia. Ann Intern Med 67:463, 1967.
351. Eisenberg E: Effects of varying phosphate intake in primary hyperparathyroidism. J Clin Endocrinol Metab 28:651, 1968.
352. Hebert LA, et al: Studies of the mechanism by which phosphate infusion lowers serum calcium concentration. J Clin Invest 45:1886, 1966.
353. Dent CE: Some problems of hyperparathyroidism. Br Med J 2:1495, 1962.
354. Pak CY, et al: Control of hypercalcemia with cellulose phosphate. J Clin Endocrinol Metab 28:1828, 1968.
355. Goldsmith RS, et al: Phosphate supplementation as adjunct in the therapy of multiple myeloma. Arch Intern Med 122:128, 1968.
356. Shackney S, Hasson J: Precipitous fall in serum calcium, hypotension, and acute renal failure after intravenous phosphate therapy for hypercalcemia. Report of two cases. Ann Intern Med 66:906, 1967.
357. Breuer PI, LeBauer J: Caution in the use of phosphates in the treatment of severe hypercalcemia. J Clin Endocrinol Metab 27:695, 1967.
358. Eisenberg E: Effect of intravenous phosphate on serum strontium and calcium. N Engl J Med 282:889, 1970.
359. Milhaud CR, et al: Etude du mecanisme de l'effet hypocalcemiant du phosphate mineral et de l'interaction eventuelle avec la thyrocalcitonine. C R Acad Sci (Paris) 266:1;169, 1968.
360. Pechet MM, et al: Regulation of bone resorption and formation. Influences of thyrocalcitonin, parathyroid hormone, neutral phosphate, and vitamin D_3. Am J Med 43:696, 1967.
361. Feinblatt J, et al: Effect of phosphate infusion on bone metabolism and parathyroid hormone action. Am J Physiol 218:1624, 1970.
362. Carey RW, et al: Massive extraskeletal calcification during phosphate treatment of hypercalcemia. Arch Intern Med 122:150, 1968.
363. Schneeberger EE, Morrison AB: Increased susceptibility of magnesium-deficient rats to a phosphate-induced nephropathy. Am J Pathol 50:549, 1967.
364. Spaulding SW, Walser M: Treatment of experimental hypercalcemia with oral phosphate. J Clin Endocrinol Metab 31:531, 1970.
365. Hamuro Y, et al: Acute induction of soft tissue calcification with transient hyperphosphatemia in the KK mouse by modification in dietary contents of calcium, phosphorus and magnesium. J Nutr 100:404, 1970.
366. Jowsey J, Balasubramanian P: Effect of phosphate supplements on soft-tissue calcification and bone turnover. Clin Sci 42:289, 1972.
367. Craig JM: Observations on the kidney after phosphate loading in the rat. Arch Pathol 68:306, 1959.
368. Wilber JF, Slatopolsky E: Hyperphosphatemia and tumoral calcinosis. Ann Intern Med 68:1043, 1968.
369. Parfitt AM: Soft tissue calcification in uremia. Arch Intern Med 124:544, 1969.
370. Grollman A: Condition of inorganic phosphorus of blood with special reference to calcium concentration. J Biol Chem 72:565, 1927.
371. Gersh I: Improved histochemical methods for chloride, phosphate-carbonate and potassium applied to skeletal muscle. Anat Rec 70:331, 1938.
372. Stamp TCB: The hypocalcaemic effect of intravenous phosphate administration. Clin Sci 40:55, 1971.
373. Raisz C, Nilmann I: Effect of phosphate, calcium and magnesium on bone resorption and hormonal responses in tissue culture. Endocrinology 85:446, 1969.
374. Parsons V, et al: Effects of mithramycin on calcium and hydroxyproline metabolism in patients with malignant disease. Br Med J 1:474, 1967.
375. Kennedy BJ, et al: Studies with tritiated mithramycin in C_3H mice. Cancer Res 27:1534, 1967.
376. Ryan WG, et al: Effects of mithramycin on Paget's disease. Ann Intern Med 70:549, 1969.
377. Perlia CP, et al: Mithramycin treatment of hypercalcemia. Cancer 25:389, 1970.
378. Elias E, et al: Control of hypercalcemia with mithramycin. Ann Surg 175:431, 1972.
379. Elias E, et al: Hypercalcemic crisis in neoplastic diseases: Management with mithramycin. Surgery 71:631, 1972.
380. Singer F, et al: Mithramycin treatment of intractable hypercalcemia due to parathyroid carcinoma. N Engl J Med 283:634, 1970.
381. Brown JH, Kennedy BJ: Mithramycin in the treatment of disseminated testicular neoplasms. N Engl J Med 272:111–118, 1965.
382. Ream NW, et al: Mithramycin therapy in disseminated germinal, testicular cancer. JAMA 204:1030, 1968.
383. Green L, Donehower RC: Hepatic toxicity of low

doses of mithramycin in hypercalcemia. Cancer Treat Rep 68:1379–1381, 1984.

384. Benedetti RG, Heilman KJ, Gabow PA: Nephrotoxicity following single dose mithramycin therapy. Am J Nephrol 3:277–278, 1983.
385. Fillastre JP, Maitrot J, Canonne MA, et al: Renal function and alterations in plasma electrolyte levels in normocalcemic and hypercalcemic patients with malignant diseases given an intravenous infusion of mithramycin. Chemotherapy 20:280–295, 1974.
386. Kofman S, et al: Mithramycin in the treatment of embryonal cancer. Cancer 17:938, 1964.
387. Verner JV Jr, et al: Vitamin D intoxication: Report of two cases treated with cortisone. Ann Intern Med 48:765, 1958.
388. Dent CE, Watson L: The hydrocortisone test in primary and tertiary hyperparathyroidism. Lancet 2:662, 1968.
389. Henneman PH, et al: Cause of hypercalciuria in sarcoid and its treatment with cortisone and sodium phytate. J Clin Invest 35:1229, 1956.
390. Bell NH, Stern P, Pantzer E, et al: Evidence that increased circulating 1-alpha-25-dihydroxy vitamin D is the probable cause for abnormal calcium metabolism in sarcoidosis. J Clin Invest 64:218–225, 1979.
391. Fulmer DH, et al: Treatment of hypercalcemia. Comparison of intravenously administered phosphate, sulfate and hydrocortisone. Arch Intern Med 129:923, 1972.
392. Laake H: The action of corticosteroids in the renal reabsorption of calcium. Acta Endocrinol (Kbh) 34:60, 1960.
393. Zerwekh JE, Pak CYC, Kaplan RA, et al: Pathogenic role of 1-alpha,25-dihydroxy vitamin D in sarcoidosis and absorptive hypercalciuria: Different response to prednisone therapy. J Clin Endocrinol Metab 51:381–386, 1980.
394. Pechet MM, et al: Metabolic studies with a new series of 1,4-diene steroids. II. Effects in normal subjects of prednisone, prednisolone, and 9-alpha-fluoroprednisolone. J Clin Invest 38:691, 1959.
395. Caniggia A, Nuti R, Lore F, Vattimo A: Pathophysiology of the adverse effects of glucoactive corticosteroids on calcium metabolism in man. J Steroid Biochem 15:153–161, 1981.
396. Watson L, Moxham J, Fraser P: Hydrocortisone suppression test and discriminant analysis in differential diagnosis of hypercalcemia. Lancet 1:1320–1325, 1980.
397. Tashjian AH Jr, Voelkel EF, Levine L: Effects of hydrocortisone on the hypercalcemia and plasma 13,14 dihydro-15-keto PEG_2 in mice bearing the $HSDM_1$ fibrosarcoma. Biochem Biophys Res Commun 74:199–206, 1977.
398. Mundy GR, Rick ME, Turcotte R, et al: Pathogenesis of hypercalcemia in lymphosarcoma cell leukemia. Role of an osteoclast activating factor-like substance and mechanism of action for glucocorticoid therapy. Am J Med 65:600–606, 1978.
399. Stewart AF, Horst R, Deftos LF, et al: Biochemical evaluation of patients with malignancy-associated hypercalcemia; evidence for humoral and nonhumoral groups. N Engl J Med 303:1377–1383, 1980.
400. Ralston SH, Fogelman I, Gardiner MD, Boyle IT: Relative contribution of humoral hypercalcemia and metastatic factors to the pathogenesis of hypercalcemia in malignancy. Br Med J 1:1405–1408, 1984.
401. Coombes RC, Ward MK, Greenberg PB, et al: Calcium metabolism in cancer: Studies using calcium isotopes and immunoassay for parathyroid hormone. Cancer 38:2111–2120, 1976.
402. Adams JS, Singer FR, Gacad MA, et al: Isolation and structural identification of 1,25-dihydroxy vitamin D_3 produced by cultured alveolar macrophages in sarcoidosis. J Clin Endocrinol Metab 60:960–966, 1985.
403. Carre M, Ayigbede O, Miravet L, Rasmussen H: The effect of prednisolone upon the metabolism and action of 25-hydroxy and 1,25-dihydroxyvitamin D_3. Proc Natl Acad Sci USA 71:2996–3000, 1974.
404. Favus MJ, Walling MW, Kimberg DV: Effects of 1,25-dihydroxycholecalciferol on intestinal calcium transport in cortisone-treated rats. J Clin Invest 52:1680–1685, 1973.
405. Milhaud G, et al: Etude du mecanisme de l'action hypocalcemiante de la thyrocalcitonine. C R Acad Sci (Paris) 261:813, 1965.
406. Deftos LJ, First BP: Calcitonin as a drug. Ann Intern Med 95:192–197, 1981.
407. Milhaud G, et al: *In* Talmage RV, Belanger LF (eds): Parathyroid Hormone and Thyrocalcitonin (Calcitonin). Amsterdam, Excerpta Medica, 1968, p 86ff.
408. Haas HG, et al: Renal effects of calcitonin and parathyroid extract in man. Studies in hypoparathyroidism. J Clin Invest 50:2689, 1971.
409. Bijvoet O, et al: Natriuretic effect of calcitonin in man. N Engl J Med 284:681, 1971.
410. Talmage RV, et al: The influence of calcitonins on the disappearance of radiocalcium and radiophosphorus from plasma. Endocrinology 90:1185, 1972.
411. Neer RM, et al: Pharmacology of calcitonin: Human studies. *In* Taylor S, Foster G (eds): Calcitonin 1969. London, Heinemann, 1970, pp 547–554.
412. Bijvoet O, et al: Effects of calcitonin on patients with Paget's disease, thyrotoxicosis, or hypercalcemia. Lancet 1:876, 1968.
413. Buckle R, et al: Vitamin D intoxication treated with porcine calcitonin. Br Med J 3:205, 1972.
414. West TET, et al: Treatment of hypercalcemia with calcitonin. Lancet 1:657, 1971.
415. Kammerman S, Canfield R: Effect of porcine calcitonin on hypercalcemia in man. J Clin Endocrinol Metab 31:70, 1970.
416. Foster GV, et al: Effect of thyrocalcitonin in man. Lancet 1:107, 1966.
417. Neer RM, et al: Escape from calcitonin (CT) during therapy of hypercalcemia. Clin Res 18:676, 1970.
418. Sorensen OH, Hindberg I: Calcitonin and bone. Lancet 1:1061, 1970.
419. Raisz L, et al: Induction, inhibition and escape as phenomena of bone resorption. *In* Talmage RV, Munson PC (eds): Calcium, Parathyroid Hormone, and Calcitonin. Amsterdam, Excerpta Medica, 1972, p 446.
420. Au WYW: Calcitonin treatment of hypercalcemia due to parathyroid carcinoma. Arch Intern Med 135:1594–1597, 1975.
421. Kennedy JW, Talmage RV: *In* Talmage RV, Belanger L (eds): Parathyroid Hormone and Thyrocalcitonin (Calcitonin). Amsterdam, Excerpta Medica, 1968, p 407ff.
422. Binstock ML, Mundy GR: Effect of calcitonin and glucocorticoids in combination on the hypercalcemia of malignancy. Ann Intern Med 93:269–272, 1980.
423. Klein DC, Raisz L: Prostaglandins: Stimulation of

bone resorption in tissue culture. Endocrinology 85:657–661, 1970.
424. Greaves M, Ibbotson KJ, Atkins D, et al: Prostaglandins as mediators of bone resorption in renal and breast tumors. Clin Sci 58:201–210, 1980.
425. Mundy GR, Martin TJ: The hypercalcemia of malignancy: Pathogenesis and management. Metabolism 31:1247–1277, 1982.
426. Seyberth HW, et al: Prostaglandins as mediators of hypercalcemia associated with certain types of cancer. N Engl J Med 293:1278, 1975.
427. Seyberth HW, et al: Characterization of the groups of patients with hypercalcemia of cancer who respond to treatment with prostaglandin synthesis inhibitors. Trans Assoc Am Physician 89:92, 1976.
428. Coombes RC, Neville AM, Bondy PK: Failure of indomethacin to reduce hyproxyproline excretion or hypercalcemia in patients with breast cancer. Prostaglandins 12:1027–1035, 1976.
429. Brenner DE, Harvey HA, Lipton A, Demers L: A study of prostaglandin E_2, parathormone, and response to indomethacin in patients with hypercalcemia of malignancy. Cancer 49:556–561, 1982.
430. Clive DM, Stoff JS: Renal syndrome associated with nonsteroidal antiinflammatory drugs. N Engl J Med 310:563–572, 1984.
431. Ciabattoni G, Cinotti GA, Pierucci A, et al: Effects of sulindac and ibuprofen in patients with chronic glomerular disease. N Engl J Med 310:279–283, 1984.
432. Zambraski EJ, Chremos AN, Dunn MJ: Comparison of the effects of sulindac with other cyclooxygenase inhibitors on prostaglandin excretion and renal function in normal and chronic bile duct–ligated dogs and swine. J Pharmacol Exp Ther 28:560–566, 1984.
433. Jung A: Comparison of two parenteral diphosphonates in hypercalcemia of malignancy. Am J Med 72:221–226, 1982.
434. Mundy GR, Wilkinson R, Heath DA: Comparative study of available medical therapy for hypercalcemia of malignancy. Am J Med 74:421–432, 1983.
435. Sleeboom HP, Bijvoet OL, van Oosterom AT, et al: Comparison of intravenous (3-amino-1-hydroxypropylidene)-1,1-bisphosphonate and volume repletion in tumour-induced hypercalcemia. Lancet 2:239–243, 1983.
436. Shane E, Jacobs TP, Siris ES, et al: Therapy of hypercalcemia due to parathyroid carcinoma with intravenous dichloromethylene diphosphonate. Am J Med 72:939–944, 1982.
437. Jacobs TP, Siris ES, Bilezikian JP, et al: Hypercalcemia of malignancy: Treatment with intravenous dichloromethylene diphosphonate. Ann Intern Med 94:312–316, 1981.
438. Jung A, Chantraine A, Donath A, et al: Use of dichloromethylene diphosphonate in metastatic bone disease. N Engl J Med 308:1499–1501, 1983.
439. van Breukelen FJ, Bijvoet OL, Frijlink WB, et al: Efficacy of amino-hydroxypropylidene bisphosphonate in hypercalcemia: Observations on regulation of serum calcium. Calcif Tissue Int 34:321–327, 1982.
439a. Theibaud D, et al: Oral versus intravenous AHPrBP (APD) in the treatment of hypercalcemia of malignancy. Bone 7:247, 1986.
440. Chapuy MC, Meunier PJ, Alexandre CM, Vignon EP: Effects of disodium dichloromethylene diphosphonate on hypercalcemia produced by bone metastases. J Clin Invest 65:1243–1247, 1980.
441. Paterson AD, Kanis JA, Cameron EC, et al: The use of dichloromethylene diphosphonate for the management of hypercalcemia in multiple myeloma. Br J Haematol 54:121–132, 1983.
442. Douglas DL, Duckworth T, Russell RG, et al: Effect of dichloromethylene diphosphonate in Paget's disease of bone and in hypercalcaemia due to primary hyperparathyroidism or malignant disease. Lancet 1:1043–1047, 1980.
443. Nolph KD, Stoltz M, Maher JF: Calcium-free peritoneal dialysis. Treatment of vitamin D intoxication. Arch Intern Med 128:809, 1971.
444. Stoltz ML, et al: Factors affecting calcium removal with calcium-free peritoneal dialysis. J Lab Clin Med 78:389, 1971.
445. Garrett JJ, Cuddihee RE: Calcium absorption during peritoneal dialysis. Trans Am Soc Artif Intern Organs 14:372, 1968.
446. Cardella CJ, Birkin BL, Rapoport A: Role of dialysis in the treatment of severe hypercalcemia: Report of two cases successfully treated with hemodialysis and review of the literature. Clin Nephrol 12:285–290, 1979.
447. Schreiner G: Dialysis of poisons and drugs—annual review. Trans Am Soc Artif Intern Organs 18:563, 1972.
448. Wolf AV, et al: Artificial kidney function: Kinetics of hemodialysis. J Clin Invest 30:1062, 1951.
449. Free RM, et al: Hard-water syndrome. N Engl J Med 276:1113, 1967.
450. Britton DC, et al: Renal function following parathyroid surgery in primary hyperparathyroidism. Lancet 2:74, 1971.
451. Forland M, et al: Bone density studies in primary hyperparathyroidism. Arch Intern Med 122:236, 1968.
452. Pak CYC, et al: The hypercalciurias. Causes, parathyroid function, and diagnostic criteria. J Clin Invest 54:387, 1974.
453. Murray TM, et al: Non-autonomy of hormone secretion in primary hyperparathyroidism. Clin Endocrinol 1:235, 1972.
454. Jowsey J, et al: Effect of phosphate supplements on soft tissue calcification and bone turnover. Clin Sci 42:289, 1972.
455. Albright F, et al: Studies in parathyroid physiology: Effect of phosphate ingestion in clinical hyperparathyroidism. J Clin Invest 11:411, 1932.
456. Dudley FJ, Blackburn CRB: Extraskeletal calcification complicating oral neutral-phosphate therapy. Lancet 2:628, 1970.
457. Woodhouse NJY, Dagle FH, Joplin GH: Vitamin D deficiency and primary hyperparathyroidism. Lancet 2:283, 1971.
458. Lumb GA, Stanbury SW: Parathyroid function in human vitamin D deficiency, and vitamin D deficiency in primary hyperparathyroidism. Am J Med 56:833, 1974.
459. Albright F, Reifenstein EC Jr: The Parathyroid Glands and Metabolic Bone Disease: Selected Studies. Baltimore, Williams and Wilkins, 1948.
460. Habener J, Potts JT Jr: Parathyroid physiology in primary hyperparathyroidism. *In* Avioli LV, Krane SM (eds): Metabolic Bone Disease, vol 2. New York, Academic Press, 1978.
461. Selby PL, Peacock M: Ethinyl estradiol and

norethindrone in the treatment of primary hyperparathyroidism in postmenopausal women. N Engl J Med 314:1481, 1986.

462. Coe FL, Favus MJ, Parks JH: Is estrogen preferable to surgery for postmenopausal women with primary hyperparathyroidism? N Engl J Med 314:1508, 1986.

463. Rudberg C, Akerstrom G, Palmer M, et al: Late results of operation for primary hyperparathyroidism in 441 patients. Surgery 99:643–651, 1986.

464. Thompson NW, Eckhauser FE, Harness JK: The anatomy of primary hyperparathyroidism. Surgery 92:814–821, 1982.

465. Russell CF, Edis AJ: Surgery for primary hyperparathyroidism: Experience with 500 consecutive cases and evaluation of the role of surgery in the asymptomatic patient. Br J Surg 69:244–247, 1982.

466. Edis AJ, Beahrs OH, van Heerden JA, Akwari OE: "Conservative" versus "liberal" approach to parathyroid neck exploration. Surgery 82:466–473, 1977.

467. Taylor GW: Surgery of hyperparathyroid disease. Br J Surg 67:732–735, 1980.

468. Cope O: Am J Surg 99:394, 1960.

469. Wang CA: Surgical management of primary hyperparathyroidism. *In* DeGroot LJ, et al (eds): Endocrinology, vol 2. New York, Grune & Stratton, 1979.

470. Purnell DC, Scholz DA, Smith LH, et al: Am J Med 56:800, 1974.

471. Norton J, Aurbach GD, Marx SJ, Doppman JL: Surgical management of hyperparathyroidism. *In* DeGroot LJ, et al (eds): Endocrinology, vol 2. Philadelphia, WB Saunders, 1988.

472. Edis AJ, van Heerden JA, Scholz DA: Results of subtotal parathyroidectomy for primary chief cell hyperplasia. Surgery 86:462, 1979.

473. Castleman B, Schantz A, Roth SI: Parathyroid hyperplasia in primary hyperparathyroidism. Cancer 38:1668, 1976.

474. Paloyan E, Lawrence AM, Baker WH, Strauss FH: Near total parathyroidectomy. Surg Clin North Am 49:43, 1968.

475. Paloyan E, Lawrence AM, Oslapas R, et al: Subtotal parathyroidectomy for primary hyperparathyroidism: Long-term results in 292 patients. Arch Surg 118:421–431, 1983.

476. Wells SA Jr, Leight GS: The surgical management of patients with primary hyperparathyroidism. *In* Frame B, Potts JT Jr (eds): Clinical Disorders of Calcium and Bone Metabolism. Amsterdam, Excerpta Medica, 1983.

477. McGarity WC, McKeown PP, Sewell CS: The role of routine biopsy of all parathyroid glands in primary hyperparathyroidism. Am Surg 51:8–15, 1985.

478. Wang CA: The anatomic basis of parathyroid surgery. Ann Surg 183:271, 1975.

479. Alveryd A: Parathyroid glands in thyroid surgery. Acta Chir Scand 389:[Suppl 1], 1968.

480. Boyd JD: Development of thyroid and parathyroid glands and thymus. Ann R Coll Surg Engl 7:455, 1950.

481. Norris EH: The parathyroid glands and the lateral thyroid in man: The morphogenesis, histogenesis, topographic anatomy, and prenatal growth. Contrib Embryol 26:247, 1937.

482. Knudson AG, Strong LC, Anderson DE: Heredity and cancer in man. Prog Med Genet 9:113–158, 1973.

483. Knudson AG: Hereditary cancer, oncogenes, and antioncogenes. Cancer Res 45:1437–1443, 1985.

484. Linder D, Gartler SM: Glucose 6-phosphate dehydrogenase mosaicism: Utilization as a cell marker in the study of leiomyomas. Science 150:67–69, 1965.

485. Fialkow PJ, Jackson CE, Block MA, Greenawald KA: Multicellular origin of parathyroid "adenomas." N Engl J Med 297:696–698, 1977.

486. Jackson CE, Cerny JC, Block MA, Fialkow PJ: Probable clonal origin of aldosteronomas versus multicellular origins of parathyroid "adenomas." Surgery 92:875–879, 1982.

487. Arnold A, Staunton CE, Kim HG, et al: Monoclonality of parathyroid adenomas: Clonally abnormal parathyroid hormone genes and clonal patterns of X chromosome inactivation. N Engl J Med 318:658–662, 1988.

487a. Arnold A, Staunton CE, Kim HG, Gaz RD: Cloning and characterization of the rearranged PTH gene in a parathyroid adenoma. J Bone Mineral Res 3:Suppl:S–210, abstract, 1988.

487b. Larsson C, Skogseid B, Oberg K, Nakamura Y, Nordenskjold M: Multiple endocrine neoplasia type I gene maps to chromosome 11 and is lost in insulinoma. Nature 332:85–187, 1988.

487c. Bale SJ, Bale AE, Stewart K, et al: Linkage analysis of multiple endocrine neoplasia type 1 with Int2 and other markers on chromosome 11. Genomics 4:320–322, 1989.

487d. Cavenee WK, Murphree AL, Shull MM, et al: Prediction of familial predisposition to retinoblastoma. N Engl J Med 314:1201–1207, 1986.

487e. Friedman E, Sakaguchi K, Bale AE, et al: Clonality of parathyroid tumors in familial multiple endocrine neoplasia type 1. N Engl J Med 321:213–218, 1989.

487f. Thakker RV, Bouloux P, Wooding C, et al: Association of parathyroid tumors in multiple endocrine neoplasia type 1 with loss of alleles on chromosome 11. N Engl J Med 321:218–224, 1989.

488. Clark OH, Way LW, Hunt TK: Recurrent hyperparathyroidism. Ann Surg 184:391, 1976.

489. Albright F, Reifenstein EC Jr: The Parathyroid Glands and Metabolic Bone Disease: Selected Studies. Baltimore, Williams and Wilkins, 1948.

490. Mayer GP, Habener JF, Potts JT Jr: J Clin Invest 57:678, 1976.

491. Roth SI: Am J Med 50:612, 1971.

492. Bilezikian JP, Doppman JL, Shimkin PM, et al: Am J Med 55:505, 1973.

493. Powell D, Murray TM, Pollard JJ, et al: Arch Intern Med 131:645, 1973.

494. Nussbaum SR, Potts JT Jr, Wang CA, et al: Development of a highly sensitive 2 site immunoradiometric assay for parathyroid hormone and its clinical utility in the evaluation of patients with hypercalcemia. Endocrine Society 69th Annual Meeting (abstract), 1987.

494a. Nussbaum SR, Zahradnik RJ, Lavigne JR, et al: Highly sensitive two-site immunoradiometric assay of parathyrin, and its clinical utility in evaluating patients with hypercalcemia. Clin Chem 33:8, 1364–1367, 1987.

494b. Brown RC, Aston JP, Weeks I and Woodhead JS: Circulating intact parathyroid hormone measured by a two-site immunochemiluminometric assay. J Clin Endocrinol Metab 65:407–414, 1987.

494c. Brasier AR, Wang CA, Nussbaus SR: Recovery of parathyroid hormone secretion after parathyroid adenomectomy. J Clin Endocrinol Metab 66:495–500, 1988.

494d. Nussbaum SR, Thompson AR, Kelly A, et al: Intraoperative measurement of parathyroid hormone in the surgical management of hyperparathyroidism. Surgery 104:1121–1127, 1988.

495. Cope O, Barnes BA, Castleman B, et al: Ann Surg 154:491, 1961.
496. Cope O: N Engl J Med 274:1174, 1966.
497. Potts JT Jr: Diseases of the parathyroid gland and other hyper- and hypocalcemic disorders. *In* Braunwald E, et al (eds): Harrison's Principles of Internal Medicine. 11th ed. New York, McGraw-Hill, 1986, pp 1870–1889.
498. Kooh SW, Fraser D, DeLuca HF, et al: N Engl J Med 293:840, 1975.
499. Neer RM, Holick MF, DeLuca HF, Potts JT Jr: Metab Clin Exp 24:1403, 1975.
500. Barnes BA, Krane SM, Cope O: J Clin Endocrinol Metab 17:1407, 1957.
501. Agna JW, Goldsmith RE: N Engl J Med 258:222, 1958.
502. Potts JT Jr, Roberts B: Am J Med Sci 235:206, 1958.
503. Sutton RAL: Br Med J 1:529, 1970.
504. Anast CS, Winnacke JC, Forte LR, Burns TR: Proceedings, 57th Annual Meeting, American Endocrine Society A-47:74, 1975.
505. Singer FR, Segre GV, Habener JF, Potts JT Jr: Metab Clin Exp 24:139, 1975.
506. Shils ME: Medicine (Baltimore) 48:61, 1969.
507. Eisenberg H, Pallotta JA: Special localizing techniques for parathyroid disease. *In* DeGroot LJ, et al (eds): Endocrinology, vol 2. New York, Grune & Stratton, 1979, pp 717–724.
508. Eisenberg H, Pallotta JA, Sherwood L: Selective arteriography, venography, and venous hormone assay in diagnosis and localization of parathyroid lesions. Am J Med 56:810–820, 1974.
509. Doppman JL, Wells SA, Shimkin PM: Parathyroid localization by angiographic techniques in patients with previous neck surgery. Br J Radiol 46:403–418, 1973.
510. Doppman JL, Hammond WG: Localization of parathyroid adenoma. N Engl J Med 281:1248, 1969.
511. Shimkin P, Powell D, Doppman JL: Parathyroid venous sampling. Radiology 194:571, 1972.
512. Simeone JF, Mueller PR, Feriucci JT, et al: High resolution real time sonography with a parathyroid. Radiology 141:745–751, 1981.
513. Van Heerden JA, James EM, Caselle PR, et al: Small part ultrasonography in primary hyperparathyroidism. Ann Surg 195:774–780, 1982.
514. Scheible W, Deutsch Al, Leopold GP: Parathyroid adenoma: Accuracy of preoperative localization by high resolution real time sonography. J Clin Ultrasound 9:325–330, 1981.
515. Reading CC, Charboneau JW, James EM, et al: High resolution parathyroid sonography. AJR 139:325–330, 1982.
516. Brewer WH, Walsh JW, Newsome HH Jr: Impact of sonography on surgery for primary hyperparathyroidism. Am J Surg 145:270, 1983.
517. Sommer B, Welter HF, Spelsberg F, et al: Computed tomography for localizing enlarged parathyroid glands in primary hyperparathyroidism. J Comput Assist Tomogr 6:521–526, 1982.
518. Stark DD, Moss AA, Gooding GAW, et al: Parathyroid scanning by computer tomography. Radiology 148:297, 1983.
519. Stark DD, Gooding JW, Moss AA, et al: Parathyroid imaging; comparison of high resolution CT and high resolution sonography. AJR 141:633–638, 1983.
520. Young AB, Gaunt JI, Croft DN, et al: Location of parathyroid adenoma by thallium 201 and technetium-99m subtraction scanning. Br J Med 286:1384–1386, 1983.
521. Okerlund MD, Sheldon K, Corpuz S, et al: A new method with high sensitivity and specificity for localization of abnormal parathyroid glands. Ann Surg 200:381, 1984.
522. Ferlin G, Camerani M, Conte N, et al: New perspectives in localizing enlarged parathyroids by technetium/thallium subtraction scan. J Nucl Med 24:438, 1983.
523. Krudy AG, Shaawker TH, Doppman JL, et al: Ultrasonic parathyroid localization in previously operated patients. Clin Radiol 35:113–118, 1984.
524. Reading CC, Charboneau JW, James EM, et al: Postoperative parathyroid high-frequency sonography: Evaluation of persistent or recurrent hyperparathyroidism. AJR 144:399–400, 1985.
525. Skibber JM, Reynolds JC, Spiegel AM, et al: Computerized thallium/technetium scans and reoperative parathyroid surgery. Am Assoc Endocrine Surgeons (abstract), 1985.
526. Doppman JL, Brennan MF, Kohler JO, et al: CT scanning for parathyroid localization. J Comput Assist Tomogr 1:30–36, 1977.
527. Doppman JL, Krudy AG, Brennan MR, et al: CT appearance of enlarged parathyroid glands in the posterior-superior mediastinum. J Comput Assist Tomogr 6:1099–1102, 1982.
528. Gooding GAW, Clark OH, Stark DD, et al: Parathyroid aspiration biopsy under ultrasound guidance in the postoperative hyperparathyroid patient. Radiology 155:193–196, 1985.
529. Solbiati L, Montali G, Croce F, et al: Parathyroid tumors detected by fine needle aspiration biopsy under ultrasonic guidance. Radiology 148:793–797, 1983.
530. Krudy AG, Doppman JL, Miller DL, et al: Detection of mediastinal parathyroid glands by nonselective digital arteriography. AJR 142:693–695, 1984.
531. Doppman JL, Popovsky M, Girton M: The use of iodinated contrast agents to ablate organs; experimental studies and histopathology. Radiology 138:333–340, 1981.
532. Geelhoed GW, Krudy AG: Long term followup of hyperparathyroid patients treated by transcatheter staining with contrast agent. Surgery 94:849–862, 1983.

15

FREDERICK R. SINGER
STEPHEN M. KRANE

Paget's Disease of Bone

Paget's disease of bone is a focal disorder of unknown etiology characterized initially by excessive resorption and subsequently by excessive formation of bone, culminating in a "mosaic" pattern of lamellar bone associated with extensive local vascularity and increased fibrous tissue in adjacent marrow. In the strict sense this is not a metabolic bone disease, since some portion of the skeleton is spared, no matter how widespread the disease process may be. It is the extraordinary extent of the abnormal remodeling seen in some cases and its metabolic consequences that make necessary a detailed consideration of the disorder in this volume.

I. HISTORICAL ASPECTS

Sir James Paget in 1876 described the clinical and pathologic aspects of a disease resulting in focal enlargement and deformity of the skeleton[1] (Fig. 15–1). His subsequent papers provided further details.[2,3] It was his opinion that the pathologic basis for the disease was a chronic inflammation of bone, hence the term "osteitis deformans."

Descriptions of the disorder had been published earlier: Rullier,[4] Wrany,[5] Wilks[6] and Czerny[7] all reported single cases that resembled those of Paget. Nagant de Deuxchaisnes and Krane[8] have summarized evidence that the disease may have existed in prehistoric times. A detailed historical review of Paget's disease can be found in *Paget's Disease of Bone* by Barry.[9]

II. INCIDENCE AND EPIDEMIOLOGY

The incidence of Paget's disease in a given population is difficult to estimate since the great majority of affected individuals are asymptomatic.[10] The types of studies that have been undertaken to obtain data are autopsies of unselected persons, review of roentgenograms, and review of hospital admissions. The first major study was that of Schmorl[11] in Dresden who found at autopsy that 3% of 4614 patients over 40 years of age had Paget's disease. Collins[12] in England found an incidence of 3.7% in 650 autopsies. These figures were confirmed by the radiologic survey of Pygott,[13] who found an incidence of 3.5% in London in 9775 patients over 45 years of age. The incidence in hospitalized patients, however, is less than 1%. Newman[14] reported 82 cases out of 127,000 admissions at the Hospital of the University of Pennsylvania. Rosenkrantz and colleagues[15] found 111 cases out of 94,112 patients admitted to the New York Veterans Administration Hospital. Barry[9] reviewed admissions to the main teaching hospitals of Australia and found 2630 cases out of 1,769,664 admissions (1 in 673).

The most striking aspect of the epidemiology of Paget's disease is the great variation in prevalence throughout the world.[16] By roentgenographic survey it occurs most frequently in England,[17] but it is also commonly found in Australia,[18] New Zealand,[19] North America,[20,21] and France.[22] Although the autopsy study of Schmorl indicated a common occurrence in Dresden,[11] a roentgenographic survey comparing Europe to Great Britain indicated a low prevalence in Essen, West Germany.[22] Great variability of prevalence may be found even within one country as evidenced by the strikingly high prevalence of Paget's disease in Lancashire[17] compared with the rest of England and by the much lower prevalence in the southern compared with the northern United States.[20,21]

Surprisingly, in Ireland few affected individuals have been identified.[23] The disease is very rare in Scandinavia,[22] Japan,[24] and China. A recent epidemiologic study examined the past exposure of pagetic patients to household pets.[25] Dog ownership was more common in pagetic patients than in control subjects with diabetes mellitus. A follow-up study failed to confirm these results, however.[25a]

Paget's disease is usually first identified in individuals over the age of 40 years, although the disorder has been detected in younger persons, almost none of whom have been under 20 years of age. The incidence then rises with increasing age so that by the ninth decade it has been reported to range from 5% to 11%. In the large series that have been reported, men are affected somewhat more frequently than are women. In Barry's series of 2630 patients,[9] 1420 were men, a ratio of seven men to six women. There is a rare syndrome in children of congenital hyperphosphatasia characterized by fragile and deformed bones, which has also been called juvenile Paget's disease. The involved bones do not have the morphologic characteristics of Paget's disease and this disorder should therefore be considered as a separate entity.[26]

Paget's disease may occur in more than one member of a family. Evens and Bartter have described a kindred with definite Paget's disease in seven members and probable disease in two others.[27] The results of an analysis of 407 family history questionnaires completed by patients with Paget's disease indicated that 14% had at least one family member also affected by the disease.[28] In another study, 25% of 75 patients had a family history of Paget's disease.[29] In 56 families affected by Paget's disease, 31 exhibited a pattern of distribution consistent with autosomal dominant inheritance of the disease.[28] In 25 other families, the disease was identified only in siblings but not in their parents, consistent with autosomal recessive inheritance. Although the pattern of autosomal recessive inheritance was suggestive, it could not be established in this series since bone scans and/or roentgenographic surveys of the parents were not conducted to rule out subclinical disease. Despite the evidence of Paget's disease in families, Martin and Melick were able to find only five recorded cases in identical twins.[30]

In an attempt to identify possible genetic markers for the disease, the frequencies of HLA antigens in patients with Paget's disease were determined by several investigators.[31-34] The phenotypic frequencies of the HLA-A and HLA-B antigens were found not to differ significantly from those of control populations. In five kindreds with a pattern of inheritance consistent with autosomal dominant transmission, however, typing of the HLA-A, B, C (class I) antigens and linkage analysis revealed an association between the haplotype and clinical demonstration of the disease.[35,36] In a preliminary study of class II HLA antigens in patients with Paget's disease, an increased frequency of DQW1 and its associated DR antigens was found.[37] If con-

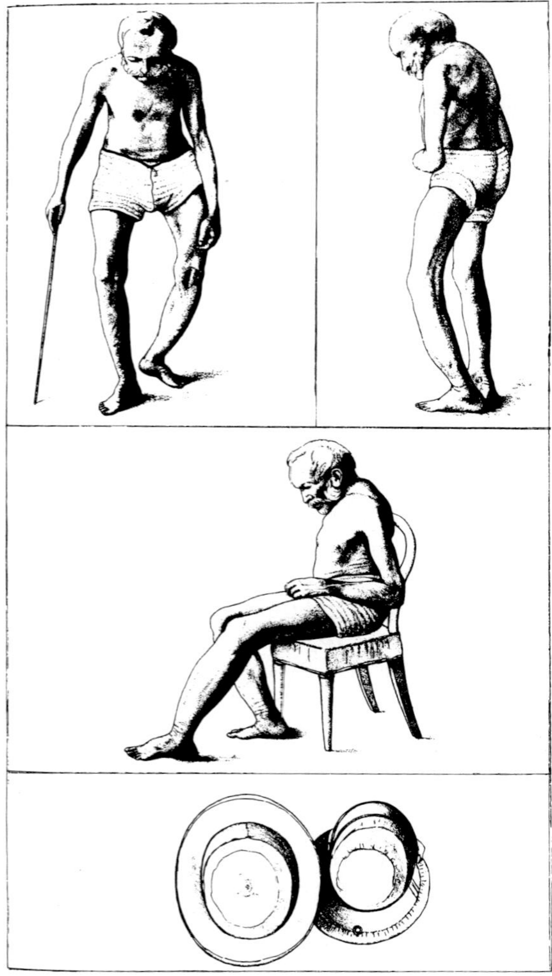

Figure 15–1. A drawing of the original patient of Sir James Paget showing marked skeletal deformities including enlargement of the skull, represented here by change in hat size.

firmed, the latter findings are consistent with an immunoregulatory abnormality linked to the class II histocompatibility genes in patients with Paget's disease.

III. HISTOPATHOLOGY (see also Chapter 10)

There is a general agreement that the pathologic process of Paget's disease of bone may be divided into three phases.[11,38-40] In the first, the osteolytic or "hot" phase, there is intense resorption of existing bone. This is soon accompanied by accelerated deposition of spicules of lamellar bone in a disorganized fashion (the mixed phase). In the final phase, the osteoblastic or "cold" phase, bone formation is dominant, and the irregularly shaped trabeculae are characterized by the "mosaic" pattern of cement lines, which appear haphazardly between fragments of lamellar bone. Any single bone may have separate foci, each of a different phase of the disease process, or various bones may be in different phases. It is possible for all three phases of the disorder to be found in the same focus in a single bone.

The diagnostic feature of Paget's disease is the abnormal architecture of lamellar bone. The osteons in normal compact bone are cylindrical, whereas they form regular arches or packets in spongy bone. The lamellar arrangement of normal bone results from the parallel arrangement of collagen fibers in a regular orientation and is best visualized by polarized light. There are relatively few osteocytes per unit area of matrix, and there is uniformity in size and shape of the osteocytes, which generally appear as small cells with dark nuclei. There are a number of types of lamellar bone in the normal cortex. The outer and inner circumferential lamellae are those on the periosteal and endosteal surfaces, respectively. These surround the osteons or haversian systems, which are composed of concentric lamellae. The interstitial lamellae found between osteons are the remnants of previously formed and partially resorbed circumferential lamellae. The trabeculae of the medulla are also normally composed of lamellar bone but do not contain osteons. There are few, if any, complete osteons composed of lamellar bone in Paget's disease.

Woven bone, which is almost never found under normal conditions after the epiphyses close except in areas of rapid remodeling, is the type of bone most frequently seen in response to a stress, for example, fracture or tumor. In woven bone there is a seemingly chaotic, unorganized pattern of deposition of collagen fibers, large numbers of osteocytes per unit area of matrix, and large variations in size and shape of the osteocytes. This type of bone is frequently seen in "tissue patches" of Paget's disease, which have scalloped contours and prominent cement lines where there is interaction with other patches.[11] This pattern of deposition of woven bone should be distinguished from the diagnostic "mosaic" pattern of pagetic lamellar bone. Although woven bone may occasionally be the predominant finding in an active phase of Paget's disease, it is not a diagnostic feature, and the percentages of woven and lamellar bone vary from patient to patient and lesion to lesion.[38]

The major changes seen in the osteolytic phase of the disease are due to the activity of osteoclasts. These large multinucleated cells are often found in great profusion adjacent to any bone surface and are presumably derived from similar hematopoietic precursor cells as are normal osteoclasts (Fig. 15–2). In Paget's disease, however, the osteoclasts may assume bizarre shapes, and often contain more than 8 to 12 or as many as 100 nuclei.[39,41-43] Osteoclasts of this type are rarely seen in other forms of nonneoplastic bone disorders characterized by increased remodeling, such as hyperparathyroidism.

The osteoclastic resorption occurs prior to the fibrous tissue replacement of adjacent normal fatty or hematopoietic bone marrow by a fibrous stroma. Noteworthy at this stage of the disease is the early development of vascular hypertrophy, hyperplasia, and venous ectasia in the marrow spaces and the influx of undifferentiated mesenchymal cells adjacent to the osteoclastic foci. As resorption continues, there is an increase in the deposition of this fibrous stroma, and the vascularity becomes more prominent. There is evidence consistent with increased vascular perfusion in this bone but not for the existence of arteriovenous shunts, as will be discussed subsequently. In the cortex, the osteoclasts widen the osteons centrifugally until they become confluent with other osteons or Volkmann's canals. This process may continue until resorption extends to the endosteal and periosteal surfaces (Fig. 15–3). In some cases the outer circumferential lamellae will remain in-

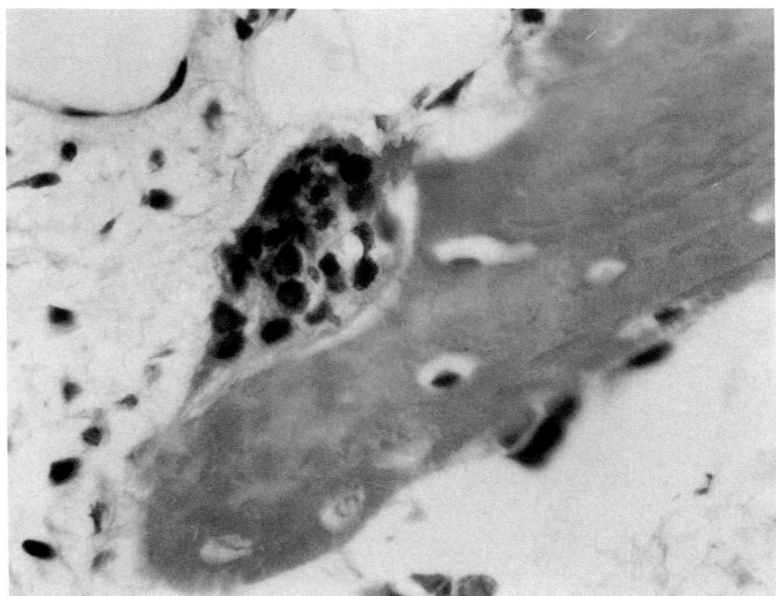

Figure 15–2. A large multinucleated pagetic osteoclast in a resorption lacuna in a spicule of lamellar bone. This cell contains at least 30 nuclei (H and E; ×790).

tact. If there is penetration of the outer circumferential lamellae, formation of periosteal new bone takes place; often woven bone is deposited in these areas in a manner similar to that observed in fracture callus. If the disease continues, this new bone will also be resorbed and eventually replaced by pagetic lamellar bone with its characteristic "mosaic" pattern.

Despite the fact that osteoclasts are the principal cells of interest in the lytic phase, foci of intense osteoblastic activity may also be seen at this stage. These osteoblasts are responsible for the deposition of lamellar bone, often adjacent to areas of irregular resorption (Fig. 15–4), although woven bone is also occasionally seen in these areas. The newly formed woven bone may be resorbed

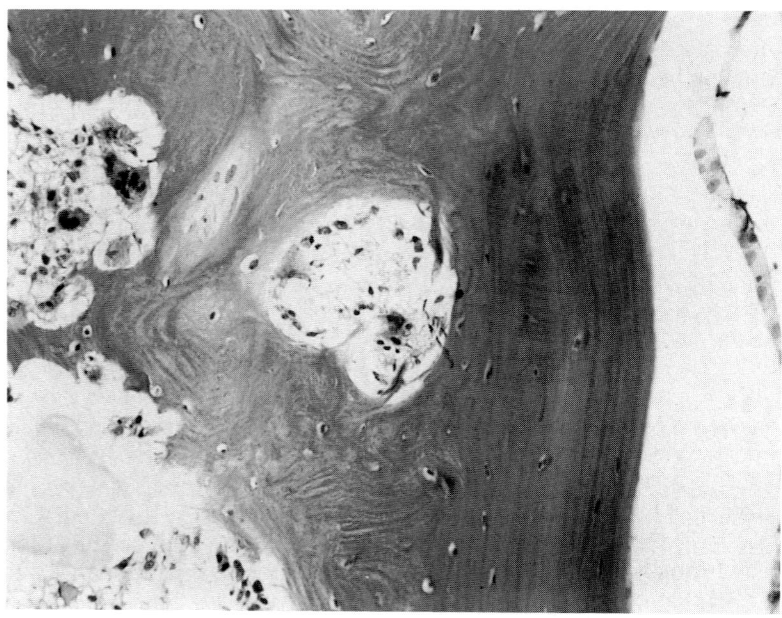

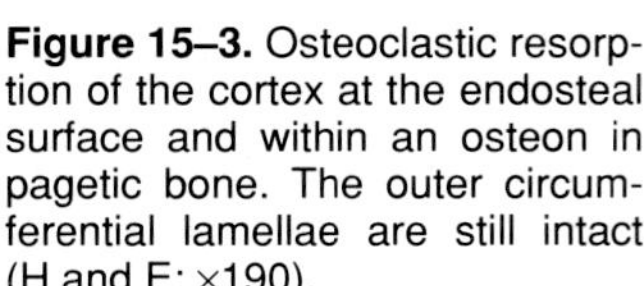

Figure 15–3. Osteoclastic resorption of the cortex at the endosteal surface and within an osteon in pagetic bone. The outer circumferential lamellae are still intact (H and E; ×190).

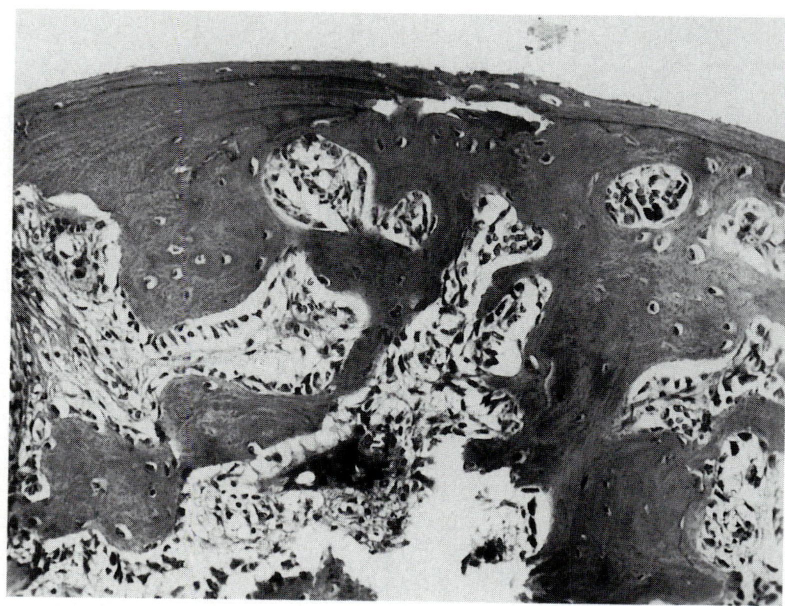

Figure 15–4. Resorption of the cortex is almost complete, although a thin rim of outer circumferential lamellae is still intact. Note the prominent bone formation surfaces lined by osteoblasts. Much of the new bone in this section is woven bone (H and E; ×190).

soon after deposition based on the pattern of tetracycline labeling.[44]

Similar changes are seen in the cancellous bone of the medulla, where the trabecular bone may be rapidly resorbed by numerous osteoclasts. Thin bands of new bone of either lamellar or woven type may also be found in the marrow cavity adjacent to areas of resorption. Occasionally, hemorrhagic cysts surrounded by fibrous marrow containing hemosiderin-laden macrophages are found in the medulla. Such cysts may persist into the third phase of the disease. These defects develop from microinfarcts of trabecular bone and marrow secondary to rupture of numerous thin-walled dilated vessels.[38]

In most patients with Paget's disease there is abundant evidence for abnormal bone resorption. The large osteoclasts (which contain the inclusions consistent with viral nucleocapsids, as will be discussed subsequently) are deeply embedded in the resorption lacunae. Meunier et al.[41] have observed that a few normal-sized osteoclasts may be found adjacent to the giant osteoclasts, which they interpret as evidence for the survival of the normal bone remodeling process adjacent to the pagetic lesion. In their series of 72 patients, Meunier et al.[41] have attempted to quantitate the abnormal resorption in Paget's disease. The mean value for the total resorption surface as compared with total surface was found to be 23.1% ± 8.3%, approximately 6-fold that of the mean in the 130 normal controls (3.6% ± 1.1%). The number of osteoclasts was found to be 3.18 ± 2.3/mm^2 in pagetic bone compared with 0.33 ± 0.23/mm^2 in nonpagetic bone.

The "mixed" phase of Paget's disease occurs at that stage when osteoclasts become less numerous and their activity begins to wane, and osteoblasts become more numerous. New lamellar bone formation occurs with lines of easily recognized plump osteoblasts closely applied to bone. The appearance of classic pagetic bone with the "mosaic" arrangement of the cement lines then follows. This diagnostic histologic feature of Paget's disease is characterized by irregular, jigsaw-shaped pieces of lamellar bone with an erratic arrangement of cement lines (Fig 15–5). The scalloped appearance of these cement lines represents sites of prior osteoclastic resorption. As mentioned earlier, it is unusual to find completely intact osteons and/or to be able to trace a single unit of lamellar bone for any distance (Fig. 15–6). Bone lamellae haphazardly faceted together are readily observed using polarized light microscopy (Fig. 15–7). The interfaces between these units or patches of pagetic bone are represented by the cement lines observed using light microscopy. Each new wave of osteolysis will leave a resorption line, which subsequently remains as a cement line when new lamellar bone is deposited. Thus, pagetic bone reflects the repeated pattern of resorption and deposition of lamellar bone waxing

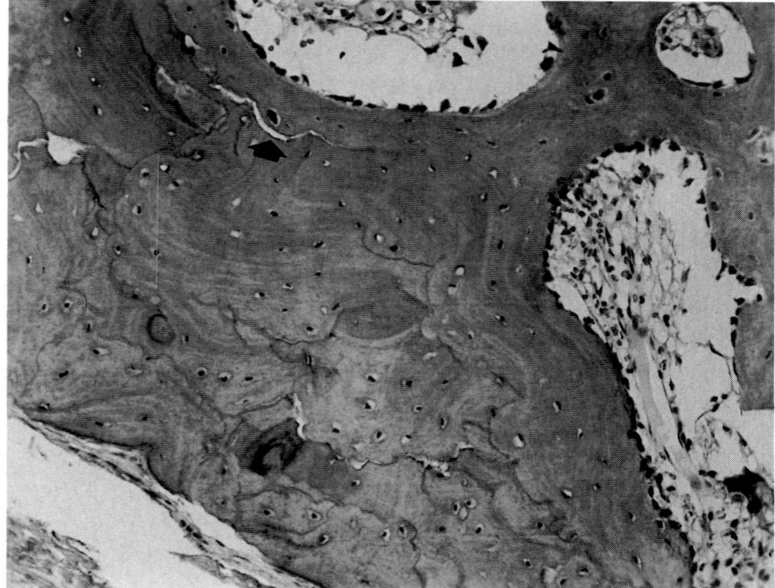

Figure 15–5. The mixed phase of Paget's disease with prominent rows of osteoclasts lining lamellar bone, which is arranged in the typical "mosaic" pattern. Note the replacement of fatty marrow by loose fibrovascular stroma. The crack (arrow), which is an artifact, separates two units of lamellar bone and is usually seen as a blue cement line (H and E; ×190).

and waning in the same area. The marrow contiguous with areas of osteoblastic and osteoclastic activity is replaced by the fibrovascular stroma (Fig. 15–8).

Although most attention has been directed toward the abnormal osteoclasts and their role in initiating the increased bone resorption that characterizes Paget's disease, osteoblastic function is also abnormal. Numerous, plump osteoblasts can readily be found lining formation surfaces, which are considerably increased in pagetic bone. It is the increased number and activity of the osteoblasts that accounts for elevations of serum alkaline phosphatase levels. There is no conclusive evidence, however, whether the abnormalities in osteoblastic number and function originate in the osteoblasts themselves or are induced by factors produced by osteoclasts or the proliferating stromal cells that replace the

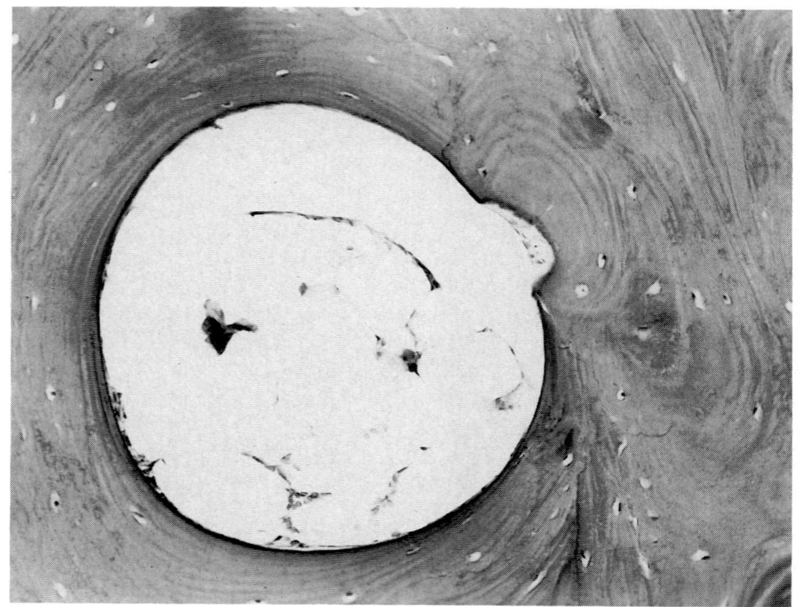

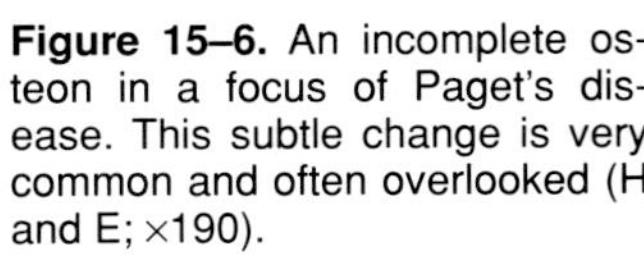

Figure 15–6. An incomplete osteon in a focus of Paget's disease. This subtle change is very common and often overlooked (H and E; ×190).

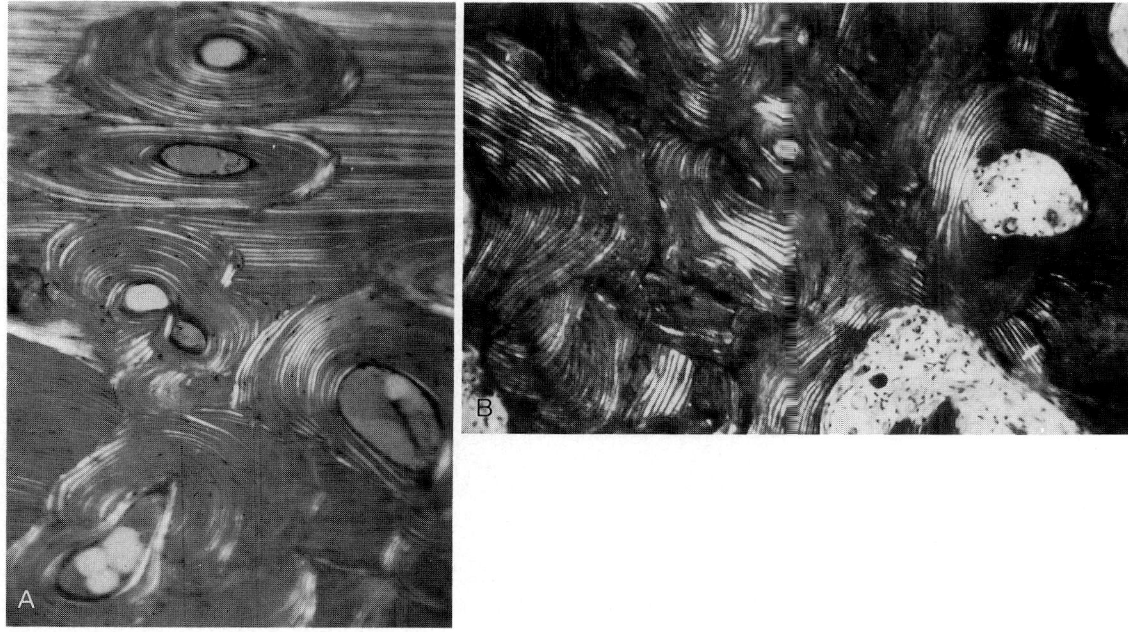

Figure 15–7. Polarized views of lamellar bone. *A*, Normal cortex with circumferential and concentric lamellar bone (H and E; ×150). *B*, Lamellar bone in Paget's disease with the typical "mosaic" pattern (H and E; ×190).

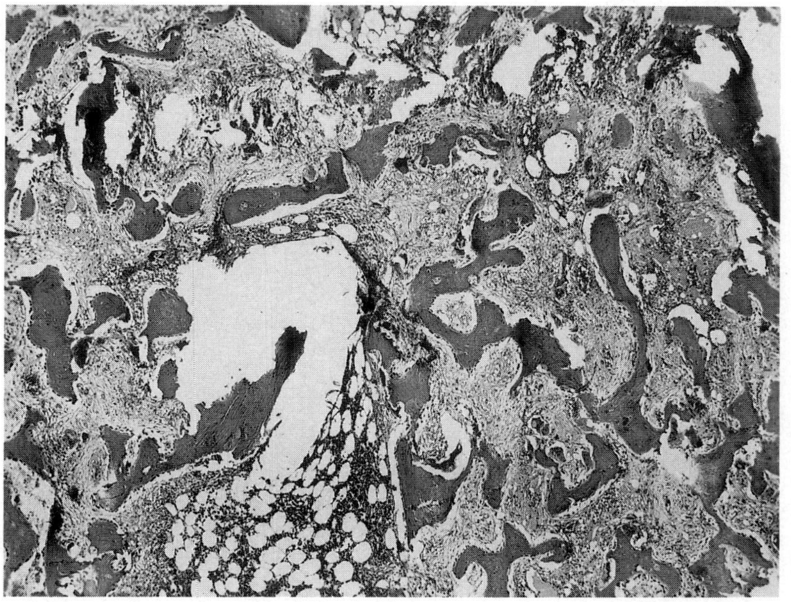

Figure 15–8. A cross-sectional view of a rib showing the mixed phase of Paget's disease. Most of the cortex has been replaced by irregular spicules of pagetic bone and loose fibrovascular stroma instead of normal marrow. The remnants of medulla and hematopoietic marrow are seen in the lower center of the photomicrograph (H and E; ×44).

normal hematopoietic bone marrow within or adjacent to the pagetic lesions. The "hyperosteoblastosis" is associated with marked changes in the amount and distribution of osteoid tissue. Meunier et al.[41] found osteoid volume to be increased in pagetic bone (2.5-fold in males; 4.2-fold in females) as well as osteoid surfaces (3.4-fold in males; 5.0-fold in females). On the other hand they found that the thickness index of pagetic osteoid borders was slightly decreased compared with controls. These results were interpreted as indicating that the calcification rate is slightly faster than the osteoblastic appositional rate in Paget's disease, the reverse of what is found in osteomalacia. The calcification rate was calculated to be 1.36 ± 0.27 μm/day in pagetic subjects compared with 0.72 ± 0.12 in controls. Meunier et al.[41] considered that the nonpagetic bone in the patients with Paget's disease was also abnormal with significant increases in trabecular resorption and osteoid surfaces.

In later stages that constitute the so-called osteoblastic or sclerotic phase of the disease, dense, irregular masses of pagetic bone are found with relatively little cellular activity (Fig. 15–9). The normal marrow is almost entirely replaced with fibrous tissue containing scattered telangiectatic vessels, and osteoblasts line bone surfaces. There may be scattered chronic inflammatory cells present as well. Periodic acid–Schiff positive droplets are found in the marrow adjacent to some osteoblasts. The pagetic bone in the sclerotic phase has no tendency to orient around vascular canals or to form osteons and is therefore relatively avascular and grossly hard to cut. Belanger,[43] using microradiography, found that the thin metachromatic cement lines of the early phases formed into high-density bands of calcification in the late sclerotic phase.

It was proposed by Belanger et al.[45] that the first morphologic event in Paget's disease is the resorption of surrounding lamellar bone by osteocytes (osteocytic osteolysis). Microradiographs of lamellar bone in a focus of Paget's disease close to the junction of normal bone do show widened osteocyte lacunae with irregularly bosselated or etched borders. Belanger et al.[45] suggested that these lacunae are continuously enlarged by osteocytes until they communicate with the haversian system or Volkmann's canal. Occasional osteocyte lacunae also may appear scalloped and enlarged even by random light microscopy (Fig. 15–10). Evidence has been presented indicating, however, that the increased size of the periosteocytic lacunae does not represent "osteolysis" but is a feature of the woven bone *per se*, which characteristically contains relatively large osteoblasts (osteocytes).[41,46]

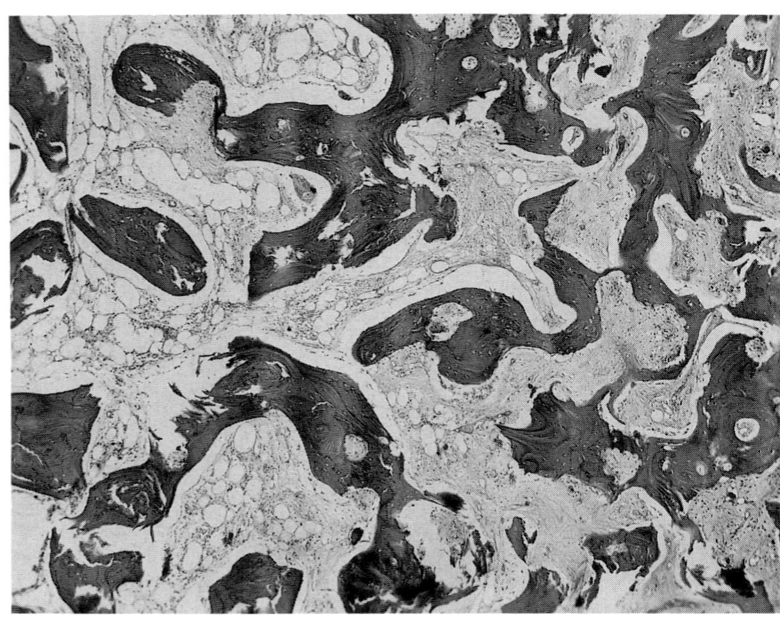

Figure 15–9. The osteoblastic phase of Paget's disease with thickened irregular spicules of pagetic bone and a loose fibrous stroma. There is very little cellular activity in this section even at higher magnification (H and E; ×44).

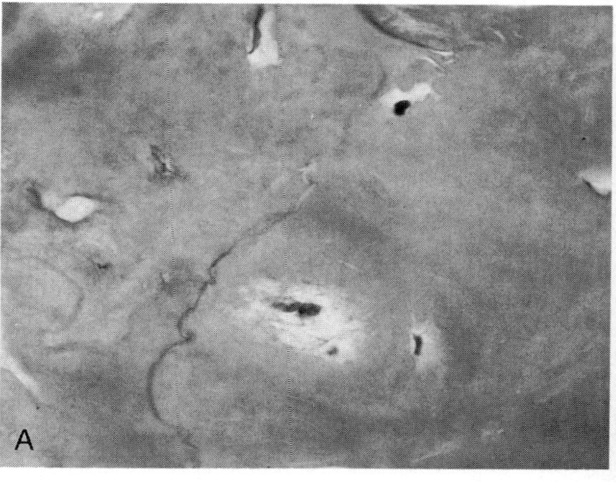

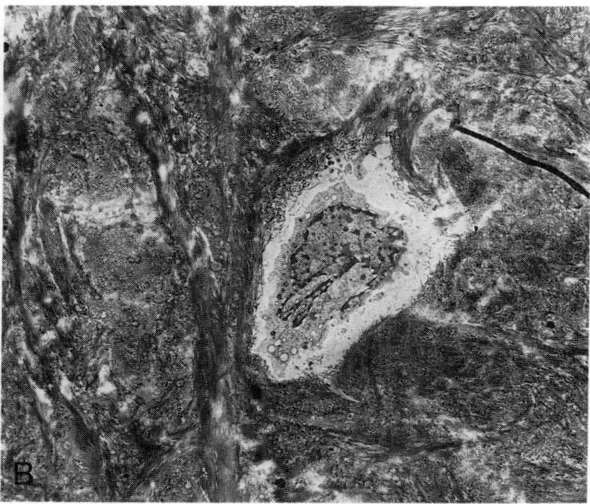

Figure 15–10. Enlarged osteocytic lacunae in a section of pagetic bone. *A*, An enlarged scalloped osteocyte lacuna that may represent osteocytic osteolysis (H and E; ×790). *B*, Electron micrograph of demineralized bone from a different patient with Paget's disease illustrating an osteocyte surrounded by a large zone in which mineralized bone is absent. The osteocyte has a large lobulated nucleus and clumped chromatin. Note the large number of peripherally located dense bodies in the cytoplasm with the appearance of lysosomes. There are also vacuoles and dilated cisternae of the rough endoplasmic reticulum. The edge of the cell has numerous filapodia extending into the lacunar space, which contains amorphous material and loose collagen fibrils. The perilacunar wall is frayed and the osmiophilic lamina is lost. The collagenous structure of the bone is disorganized and there are no distinct lamellae (×6840). (Courtesy of Dr. Barbara Mills).

The cement lines, seen with hematoxylin and eosin staining as blue lines at the interfaces between circumferential lamellae and osteons, between interstitial lamellae and osteons, or in trabecular bone, appear when a new unit of bone is added to preexisting bone. Cement lines, therefore, are at the interface between units of bone, even between woven and lamellar bone. The later accumulation of these cement lines in lamellar bone creates the diagnostic "mosaic" pattern seen in Paget's disease.

Although there may be more than normal bone per unit volume in Paget's disease, it is architecturally unsound. Grossly, the bone in the osteolytic phase may be soft enough to be cut with a knife without prior demineralization if resorption and the decrease in the mass of mineralized bone are severe enough. In the osteoblastic phase, the macerated bone often crumbles like a pumice stone. This is presumably due to the improper alignment along stress lines of the collagen fibers in each spicule of plate or bone. Although each spicule of bone is arranged according to stress lines, each is weaker than a comparable normal spicule of lamellar bone and will readily break.

The characteristic biological abnormalities of Paget's disease are obvious in all phases of bone remodeling even though it is likely that the initial event is focal osteoclastic bone resorption. Although it has been generally assumed that the formation of pagetic bone is a coupled response to the increased resorption, there is evidence that all of the pagetic bone is abnormal: osteoblast number, osteoblastic surface, and osteoblastic activity are all increased. These altered remodeling events can be interpreted as consistent with an increased "birth rate" of all of the bone cell populations. Meunier et al.[41] have also pointed out that their quantitative data also indicate that there is an increased occurrence of new "bone cell differentiation foci" and a decrease in the ratio of appositional to resorption surfaces. These findings are consistent with a shortened phase of formation or a prolonged phase of resorption or both.

A. Pertinent Aspects of Histologic Differential Diagnosis

From the point of view of diagnostic histopathology, there are a few entities that may mimic the pattern of pagetic bone, although none has the striking "mosaic" pattern of Paget's disease. In *hyperparathyroidism*, irregular fragments of lamellar bone surrounded by a fibrous marrow adjacent to brown tumors or cysts are seen. However, there is no great profusion of cement lines, and dissecting osteitis, not seen in Paget's disease, is frequently present. Similarly, periosteal reactions in *syphilis* or *fracture callus* may include spicules of lamellar bone with many cement lines, but complete osteons can still be identified, and the irregular cement lines are rarely as evident as in Paget's disease. Slowly formed reactive lamellar bone, such as that about a *Schmorl's nodule* in the spine, a *Brodie's abscess* in a long bone, or *endosteal callus*, may also be confused with Paget's disease. These lesions often contain large, irregularly shaped trabeculae of lamellar bone, but cement lines are not very numerous. *Accessory scaphoid bones*, especially those subjected to constant pressure, also have a confusing histologic picture, but again cement lines are not numerous.[38] *Osteoblastic metastases* may stimulate formation of lamellar bone spicules, which are embedded in a sea of fibrous tissue. However, numerous cement lines are lacking in this new bone, and metastatic tumor cells should be identified in adjacent marrow.

In *fibrous dysplasia*, the trabeculae are irregularly shaped and consist of woven bone with numerous cement lines surrounded by dense fibrovascular connective tissue. However, prominent osteoblasts on the surface of bone trabeculae, a characteristic feature of Paget's disease, are not seen in fibrous dysplasia. Moreover, abnormal lamellar bone, diagnostic of Paget's disease, is absent in fibrous dysplasia.

In the few reported cases of so-called *congenital hyperphosphatasia* or *hyperphosphatasemia* studied microscopically,[47-51] the bone contains irregular trabeculae of woven bone instead of compact normal cortex with osteon formation. This rare, autosomal recessive disease, which occurs in children and has also been called juvenile Paget's disease, osteoclasia, osteochalasia, and hyperostosis corticalis deformans juvenilis, is characterized by rapid turnover of subperiosteal bone and may share certain clinical and biochemical features of Paget's disease, for example, multiple bone involvement, skull deformities, elevated total urinary hydroxyproline excretion and serum alkaline phosphatase activity, and even the presence of angioid streaks. Histologically, however, the skeletal lesions can be readily differentiated from those of Paget's disease, since hyperphosphatasemia represents a lack of normal cortical remodeling; hence, the classic "mosaic" pattern of faceted units of lamellar bone is absent. We have had the opportunity to review the tumorous left radius in one of the three cases reported by Thompson et al.[48] The mass had numerous misshapen spicules of mineralized woven bone surrounded by a dense fibrovascular marrow, similar to a focus of fibrous dysplasia. The pattern of Paget's disease was not present, and we feel that the term "juvenile Paget's disease" is not warranted.

IV. FOCAL MANIFESTATIONS

The clinical presentation of patients with Paget's disease depends on the extent and site of skeletal involvement.[51a] The disease may be monostotic or polyostotic, with or without symptoms. When polyostotic, the disease may lead to crippling deformities. Symptoms arise from fractures, enlargement, and excessive vascularity of bone as well as from compression of neural structures. Joints may undergo so-called degenerative changes due to abnormal mechanical stress on the articular cartilage resulting from structurally altered, deformed bones. It is our impression that some patients with very severe, extensive disease may be withdrawn or somnolent, or complain of fatigue and weakness, even in the absence of specific involvement as described later. This is especially true in those with severe skull involvement. On the basis of angiographic studies it has been postulated that in some of these individuals there may be a shunting of blood through the external carotid system to the detriment of the brain, a so-called pagetic steal (vol pagetique).[52]

A. Pain

Although the majority of pagetic lesions encountered are not painful,[53] pain may be prominent in patients with Paget's disease. Pain may result from the primary pagetic process or from complications that arise because of the abnormal bone. The pain associated with an uncomplicated pagetic lesion is usually dull and boring but may occasionally be sharp and radiating. Weight-bearing may increase the severity of pain in lesions in the vertebrae, pelvis, and lower extremities, but nocturnal pain is also common in these areas. Khairi et al. found that pagetic lesions detected by $Na^{18}F$ bone scan but not seen on roentgenograms are generally painful.[54] An evaluation by Vellenga and colleagues of 45 roentgenographically normal lesions detected by ^{99m}Tc-EHDP scanning, however, indicated that only 11% were associated with typical pain of Paget's disease.[55] Fogelman and Carr also found that symptoms were not associated with any of 33 roentgenographically normal lesions in 23 patients.[56]

It is uncertain how the abnormal structure of the bone accounts for the development of pain. Steindler postulated that stretching of the periosteum as the bone enlarges in addition to associated hyperemia of the marrow cavity stimulates somatic sensory nerve endings in these areas.[57] It is likely, however, that microfractures are a significant cause of pain in weight-bearing areas. The overgrowth of bone encroaching on nervous tissue may also result in severe pain syndromes; since associated neurologic signs are frequently absent, it is nevertheless difficult to ascribe the pain to the lesions detected roentgenographically or on bone scan.

Frequently pain may be due to joint involvement by other disease processes distinct from Paget's disease, such as degenerative arthritis, gouty arthritis, calcific periarthritis, or rheumatoid arthritis and its variants.[58] It is of great importance to appreciate the variety of factors that can account for such pain in order to be able to institute the appropriate mode of therapy.

B. The Skull

Paget's disease involves the skull in two major patterns, although both may be present at the same time or one may develop into the other. Presumably the earliest lesion and one of the patterns seen in the skull that is usually asymptomatic has been termed osteoporosis circumscripta[59,60] (Fig. 15–11). Histologically the inner and outer tables are resorbed and replaced by fibrovascular tissue.[38] Therefore, the involved area is grossly red-violet because of the vascular marrow unobscured by the bone tables. These circumscribed radiolucent areas in the calvarium may persist for years before new bone deposited in a patchy fashion is appreciated radiologically (Fig. 15–12). A second pattern, which probably develops decades after the stage of osteoporosis circumscripta (or possibly independently), is enlargement of the cranium, usually greatest in the occipital and frontal regions. In extreme instances, the circumference of the skull may increase by as much as 15 cm. This increase results from cortical thickening, primarily the result of deposition of pagetic bone on the outer table. As the process continues, however, the diploe is also replaced, resulting in a calvarium that is coarsely thickened yet still vascular. Roentgenograms at this stage may show the classic "cotton wool" appearance (Fig. 15–13).

The patient with an enlarged cranium may be asymptomatic or have a variety of problems. Rarely, the increased weight of the skull can make it difficult for the patient to hold the head erect, leading to spasm in the muscles

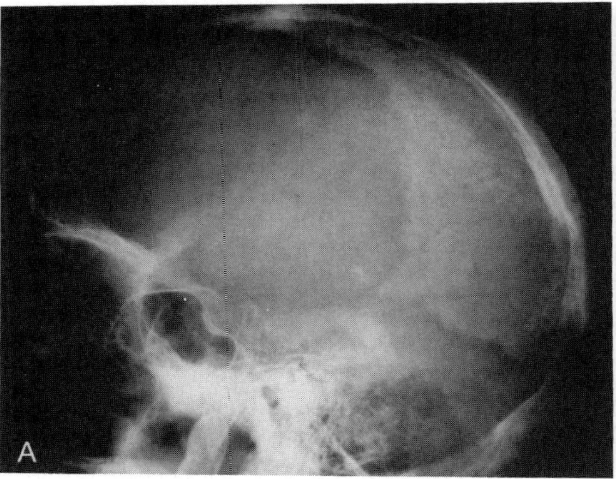

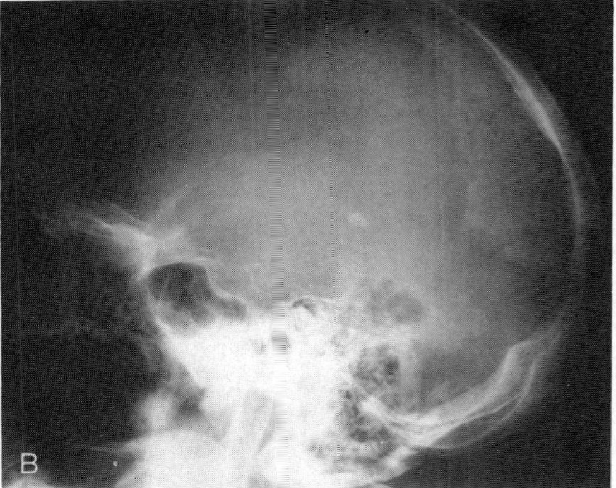

Figure 15–11. Progression of osteoporosis circumscripta in Paget's disease. *A*, The skull of a 52-year-old man, which shows a focal irregular osteoporotic area. *B*, The same patient, one year later, now with almost total skull involvement.

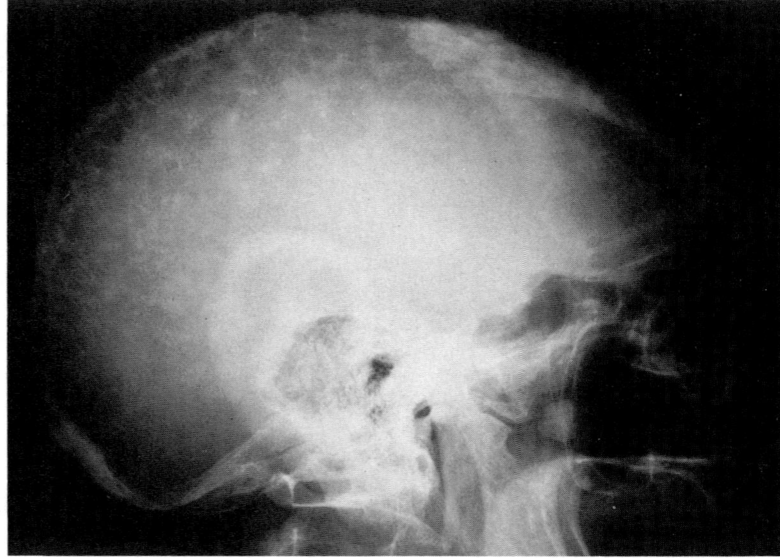

Figure 15–12. An 83-year-old woman with a "honeycomb" skull produced by patchy deposition of new bone in a focus of osteoporosis circumscripta.

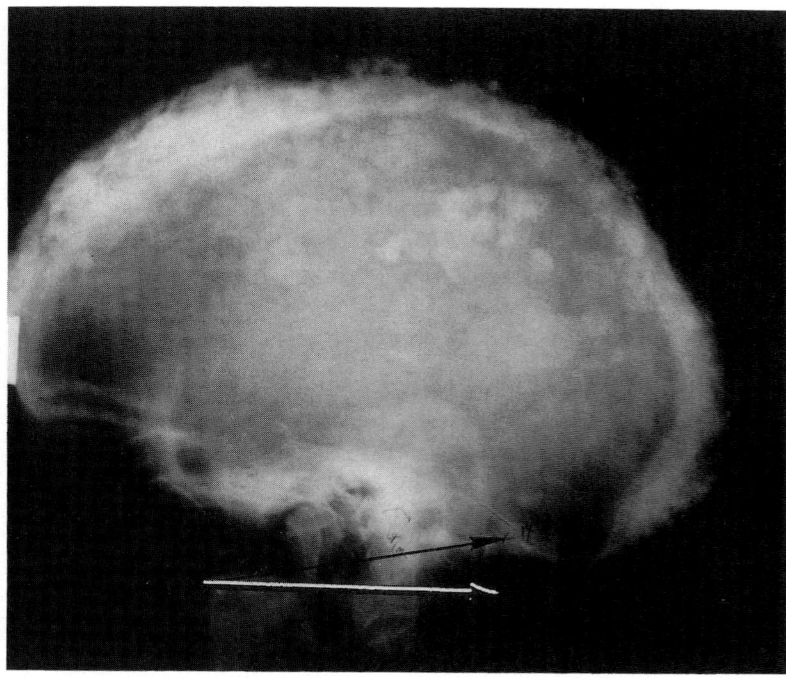

Figure 15–13. An enlarged skull with the "cotton wool" pattern of diffuse cortical thickening and platybasia. Chamberlain's line (black arrow), which extends from the posterior end of the hard palate to the dorsal rim of the foramen magnum, is well below the tip of the dens. McGregor's line (white arrow), which extends from the posterior surface of the hard palate to the most caudal point of the occipital curve, is below the dens by more than 4 mm. Both of these measurements aid in defining platybasia.

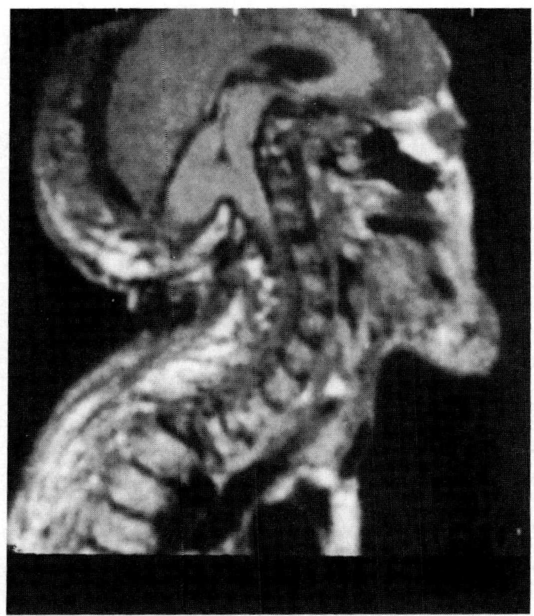

Figure 15–14. Magnetic resonance imaging of the skull and spine of a 74-year-old woman with polyostotic Paget's disease who developed weakness of the lower extremities and loss of bladder control. Note the markedly thickened calvaria, basilar invagination, low lying cerebellar tonsils and dilated ventricles. Anterior offset of T2 on T3 secondary to pagetic deformity and thickening of facial bones are also present. (Courtesy of Dr. Patrick Colletti.)

of the neck. A potentially more serious complication caused by pagetic remodeling of the base of the skull is protrusion of bone through the foramen magnum. The degree of such basilar invagination or platybasia may be measured radiographically as an increase in the angle between the basisphenoid and the basilar portion of the occiput (Fig. 15–13). Although basilar invagination is not uncommon in Paget's disease, neurologic abnormalities resulting from compression of structures in the posterior fossa[61] or less commonly from cerebellar tonsillar herniation[62] are rare. When there is such neural compression, laminectomy of the upper cervical vertebrae and suboccipital craniectomy have been successfully performed to relieve pressure on the structures of the posterior fossa.[61] Hydrocephalus may also develop in patients with Paget's disease, which produces disturbances in gait, urinary incontinence, and varying degrees of dementia[63] (Fig. 15–14). Ventricular shunts may reverse these abnormalities.[63]

Difficulties in hearing and maintaining balance result from Paget's disease of the temporal bone. These complications can be ascribed to direct involvement of the ossicles, the labyrinth, or the external auditory canal by the pagetic process. Sensorineural loss from cochlear involvement or from impingement on the eighth cranial nerve by pagetic bone narrowing the auditory foramen may also produce decreased hearing.[64-66]

Although disturbances of function of other cranial nerves are unusual, optic atrophy has been reported as a complication of Paget's disease and may be more common than is generally thought.[67] Direct bony compression of the optic nerve appears to account for only a minority of the cases of optic atrophy, however. An example of pagetic bone overgrowth causing compression of the optic nerve is shown in Figure 15–15.

C. The Jaws

The jaws and bones of the face are uncommonly involved with Paget's disease. The maxilla is most often affected.[68] Leontiasis ossea, which occurs when all the facial bones are involved, and is more typically a feature of fibrous dysplasia, is a rare complication of Paget's disease.

Paget's disease involving the bone of the alveolar socket may produce serious dental

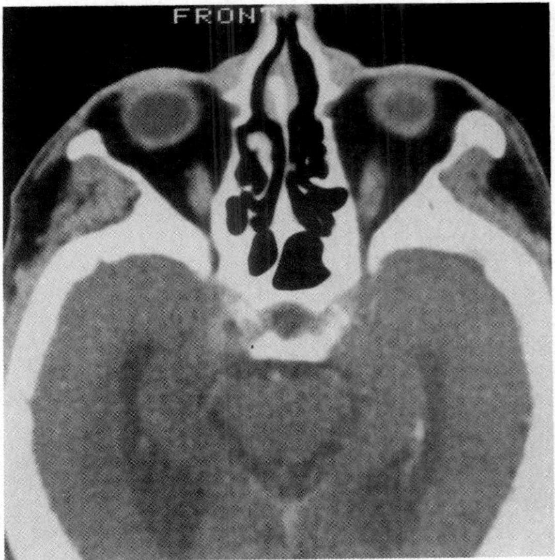

Figure 15–15. Computed tomographic scan of the head of a 79-year-old man with extensive Paget's disease who presented with six months of blurring of vision in his right temporal field. There is narrowing of the structures at the orbital apex and optic foramina bilaterally.

problems.[68] The bone adjacent to the teeth can be involved in all phases of the disease, but the enamel and dentin are spared. Particularly prominent is hyperplasia of the cementum surrounding the teeth, partial loss of the lamina dura, and displacement of the teeth (Figs. 15–16 and 15–17).

D. The Spine

The spine, particularly in the lumbar and sacral regions, is one of the commonest sites in which Paget's disease is found. Although Paget's disease of the spine is most often asymptomatic, pain may be ascribable to the pagetic lesions. The early vertebral lesion may resemble osteoporosis, especially when the entire body is involved. More commonly the vertebral bodies appear enlarged radiologically with thickening at the margins and central coarse vertical striations producing a characteristic framed pattern (Fig. 15–18). Although multiple adjacent vertebrae may be affected, the disease process frequently skips vertebrae. The vertical height of a vertebral body may be decreased owing to inadequate mechanical strength and the development of micro- and/or macrocompression fractures. In extreme instances a vertebral body may nearly completely resorb, take on the appearance of a thin transverse osseous rod, and perhaps be mistakenly identified as a calcified intervertebral disk.

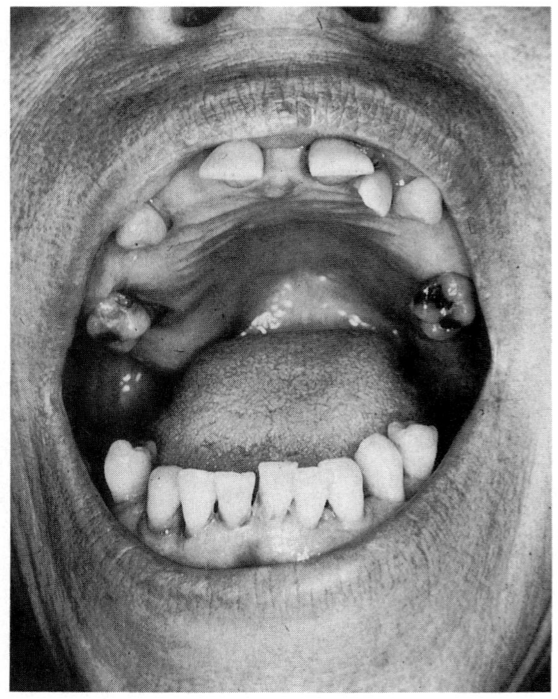

Figure 15–16. Severe displacement of the maxillary teeth in a patient with Paget's disease.

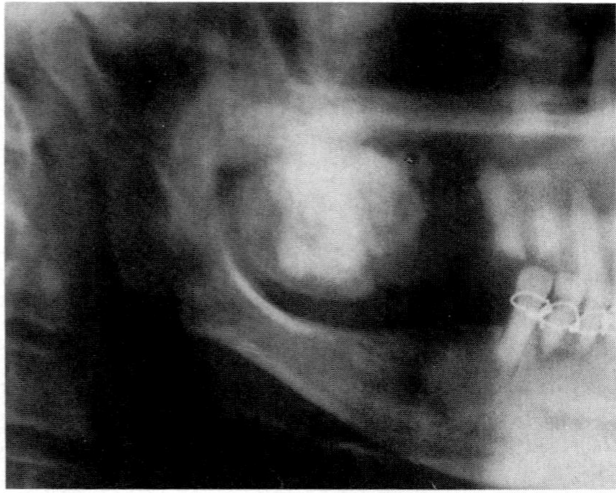

Figure 15–17. A Panovex view of the mouth showing a marked hypercementosis appearing as a bosselated radiodense mass. Such a lesion could easily be confused with a dental tumor were it not for the associated pagetic changes in the adjacent bone. (Courtesy of Dr. W. Guralnick.)

Compression of the spinal cord or nerve roots may result from enlarging vertebral bodies, pedicles, and laminae involved by Paget's disease.[69,70,70a] Neurologic compression of this sort is most common in the thoracic area. The symptoms resulting from these lesions include back pain, numbness and paresthesias of the feet, difficulty in walking, and progressive paresis of the legs. If untreated, the patient may develop spastic paraparesis with abnormal bladder and bowel function and an upper thoracic sensory loss. Myelography performed in the lumbar and suboccipital regions reveals the inferior and superior limits of the compression, which often extends over multiple adjacent thoracic segments.[71] The noninvasive techniques of computed tomography (Fig. 15–19) and magnetic resonance imaging are excellent methods of determining anatomic abnormalities of the spine, particularly in the neural arch, where routine roentgenograms are least helpful.

In the presence of neural compression of this sort, the treatment of choice is decompressive laminectomy if recovery cannot be

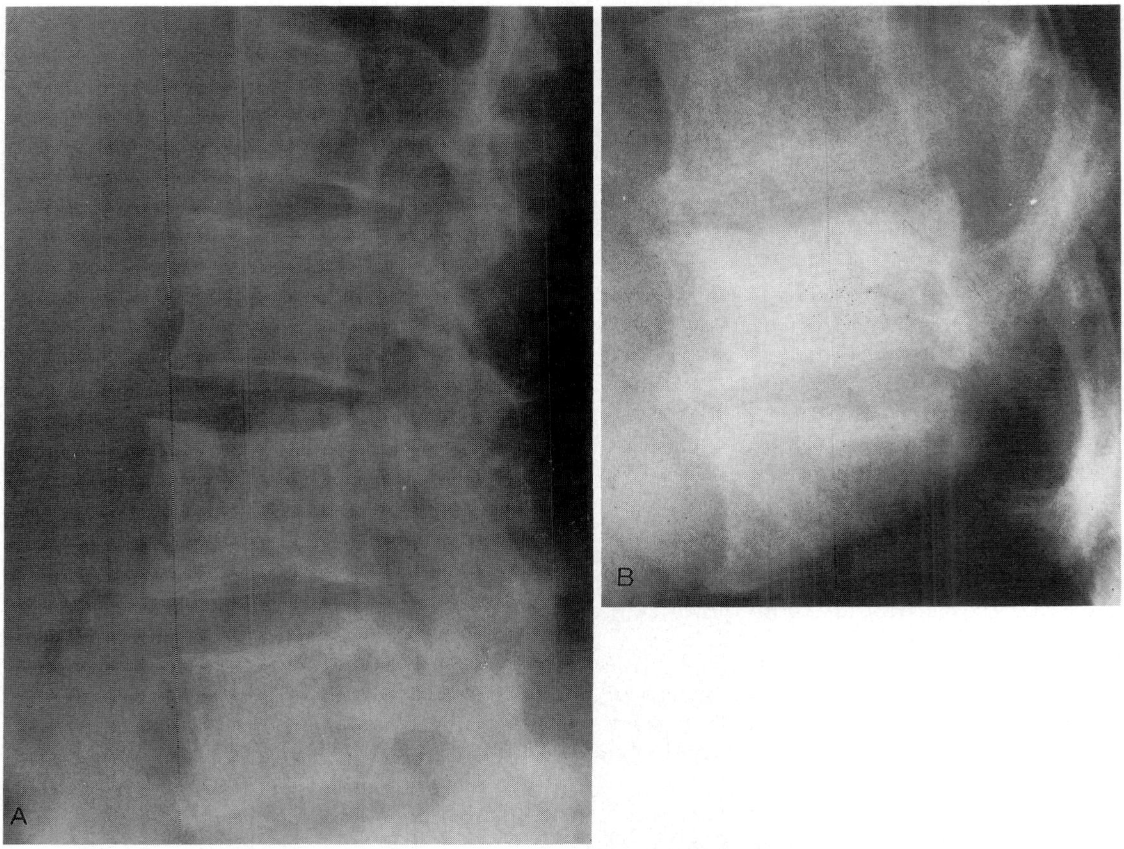

Figure 15–18. Paget's disease of the spine in a 60-year-old man. *A*, Enlarged vertebral bodies with thickened margins and coarse central vertical striations producing the appearance of the so-called framed vertebrae. *B*, A higher power view.

induced by medical therapy (to be discussed). An uncommon feature found in some patients is the development of a discrete paraspinal mass, which consists of partially calcified osteoid tissue that infiltrates the epidural region by direct extension from the vertebral periosteum and paraosseous connective tissue.[71] We observed yet another lesion in a 61-year-old man with extremely severe, generalized Paget's disease (urinary hydroxyproline 1200 mg/24 hours), which appeared, over a period of months, on roentgenograms of the chest as a rapidly enlarging mass (Fig. 15–20). An exploratory thoracotomy performed to rule out a pleural tumor or malignant transformation revealed a large oval mass arising from several thoracic vertebrae, which was composed of a central marrow cavity and a peripheral capsule of pagetic bone. This case and four others have been described in greater detail,[72,73] particularly with respect to the occurrence of myelopathy.

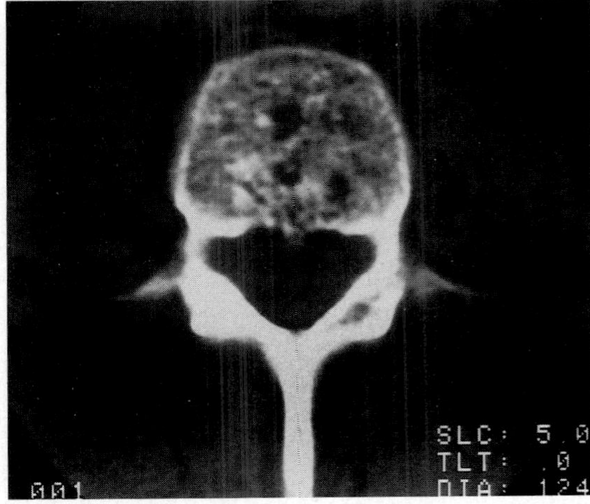

Figure 15–19. Computed tomographic scan of the third lumbar vertebra of a 71-year-old man with Paget's disease. Typical changes of Paget's disease are seen in the vertebral body.

Although severe clinical problems that are the consequence of neural compression are most often seen with thoracic involvement, lumbar spine pain associated with lumbosacral involvement is more common. For example, in the series of Altman and Collins,[74] significant lumbar spine pain was present in 106 patients compared with only six patients with dorsal spine pain. In the latter, compression of vertebral bodies due to associated osteoporosis was thought to be the underlying pathologic process. Indeed, it is important to consider that intervertebral disk disease or arthritis unrelated to Paget's disease may be the cause of lumbar pain as well.

An association of ankylosing spondylitis and Paget's disease was reported by Bitar[75] and Layani and colleagues[76] in a total of six patients. We evaluated an additional six patients with Paget's disease who also had physical findings that suggested ankylosing spondylitis.[58] Limitation of chest expansion was present in each. Spinal flexion was impaired in four, and four had peripheral joint disease. Apparent ossification of spinal ligaments was present in two patients, and extensive osteophytosis in the other four. Sacroiliac joint obliteration was found in four patients, and squaring of the vertebral bodies in two. Syndesmophytes were not seen, however. Paget's disease was present in the pelvis of five patients and in the lumbosacral spine of four. Fatigue, stiffness, and back pain were common complaints. Although the clinical findings in this group of patients were strongly suggestive of ankylosing spondylitis, it is conceivable that pagetic involvement adjacent to certain joints might mimic spondylitis. Our approach to understanding the nature of spinal symptoms in Paget's disease is to consider the results of HLA typing. From 88% to 96% of patients with ankylosing spondylitis have the HLA antigen B27 as compared with approximately 8% of control Caucasian populations.[77,78] In four of our six patients with Paget's disease associated with the features of spondylitis, none had the B27 HLA antigen. It is thus likely that small joints of the spine and the costovertebral joints are affected secondarily by Paget's disease in adjacent bone, and that the resultant clinical syndrome mimics that produced by ankylosing spondylitis. In the two cases described by Altman and Collins,[74] syndesmophytes were present consistent with true Marie-Strümpell's spondylitis coexisting with Paget's disease.

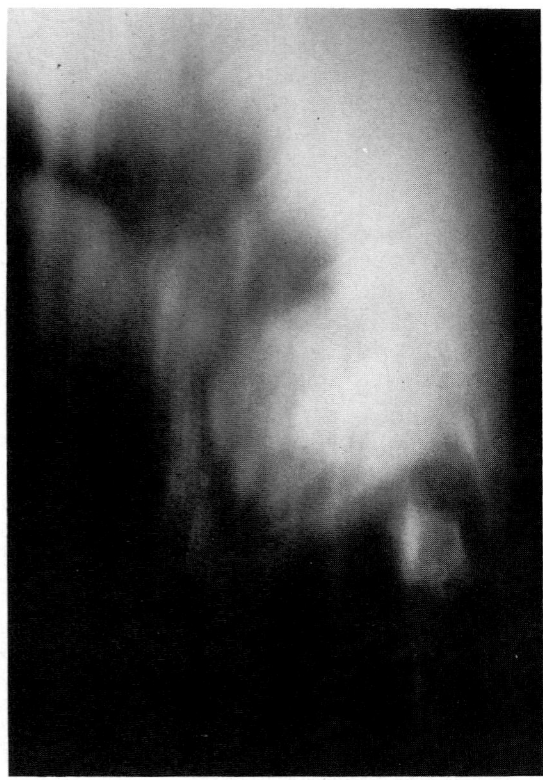

Figure 15–20. A tomogram of a 61-year-old man with severe generalized Paget's disease and a rapidly growing paraspinal mass arising from several thoracic vertebrae.

E. The Pelvis and Extremities

In the extremities, the femur and tibia are most commonly involved with Paget's disease. It is not unusual to find a monostotic focus in either of these bones (Fig. 15–21). When these bones are involved, clinical manifestations such as pain, deformity, and increase in skin temperature are frequently present. The deformity associated with Paget's disease of the femur is an outward bowing combined with a coxa vara deformity causing external rotation of the lower leg. The tibia is usually bowed anteriorly and laterally (Fig. 15–22); on the other hand, the fibula is almost never affected. The upper extremities are less frequently affected by Paget's disease and are often asymptomatic (Figs. 15–23 and 15–24). However, involvement of the humerus and ulna does occur. Rarely the disease

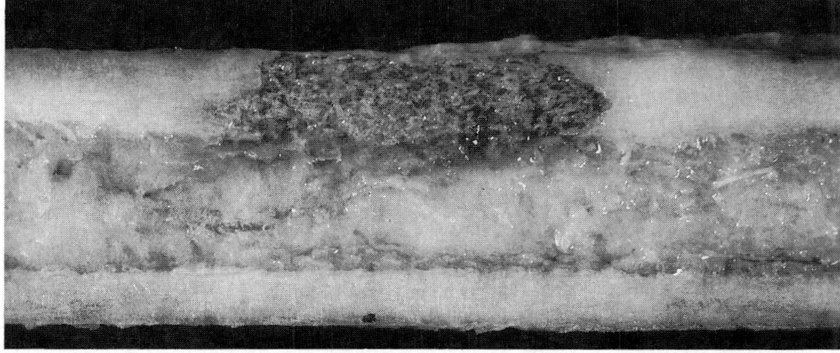

Figure 15–21. An osteolytic focus of Paget's disease in the cortex of the tibia. Note the coarsely trabeculated pattern of bone spicules and the rich vascular marrow within this focus. (From Taylor GW, Castleman B: Clinicopathological conferences of the Massachusetts General Hospital. N Engl J Med 269:808–813, 1963.)

appears in the hands and feet; it is usually in a single bone and is almost always asymptomatic (Figs. 15–25 and 15–26).

The major clinical problem that may develop after years of involvement of the pelvis and upper femur is so-called pagetic coxopathy, a form of degenerative joint disease of the hip, which may cause considerable morbidity from pain and decreased mobility.[79] Although Barry[9] feels that the incidence of this problem is low, we[58] and Altman and Collins[74] have found pagetic coxopathy to be a common source of discomfort in Paget's disease. Involvement of the hip joint could result from pagetic changes in the subchondral bone or from altered mechanics at the hip due to deformity of the entire bone. Roper[80] suggested that if the narrowing of the hip joint space in patients with Paget's disease is predominantly superior in the zone of

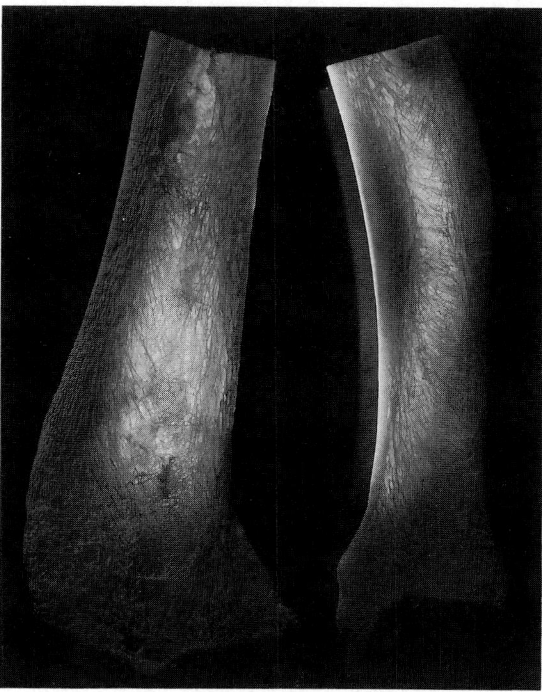

Figure 15–22. A transillumination of a macerated hemisected tibia with Paget's disease showing the thickened cortex and densely packed, coarsely thickened trabeculae, as well as typical bowing deformity.

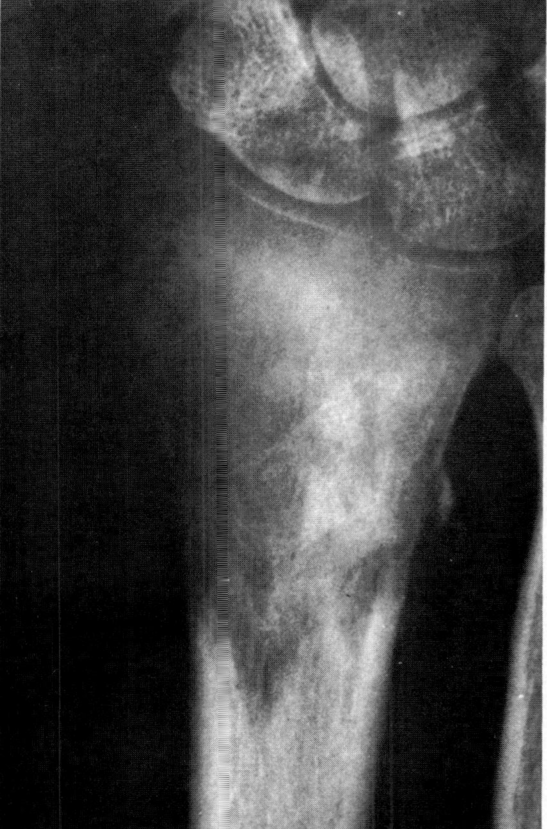

Figure 15–23. An osteolytic monostotic focus of Paget's disease in the radius of a patient who presented with wrist pain. Note the flame shape or sawtooth pattern produced by the advancing edge of osteoclastic activity which distinguishes this lesion from a malignant tumor.

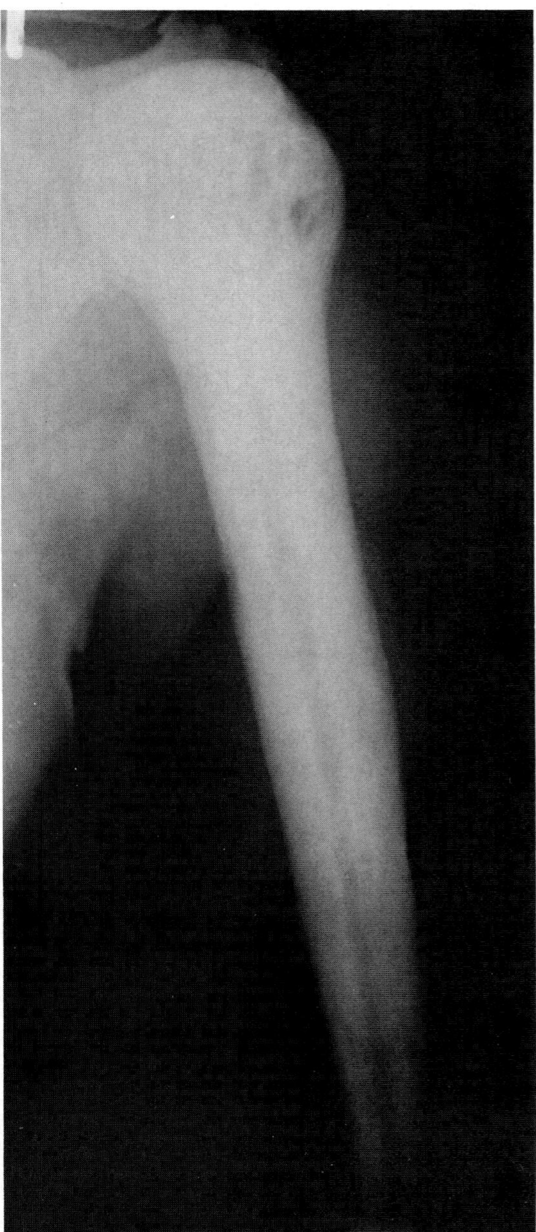

Figure 15–24. Paget's disease of the humerus. Note the cyst in the humoral head representing cystic degeneration, which may occur in a focus of Paget's disease. The cortices are markedly thickened by coarse trabeculae.

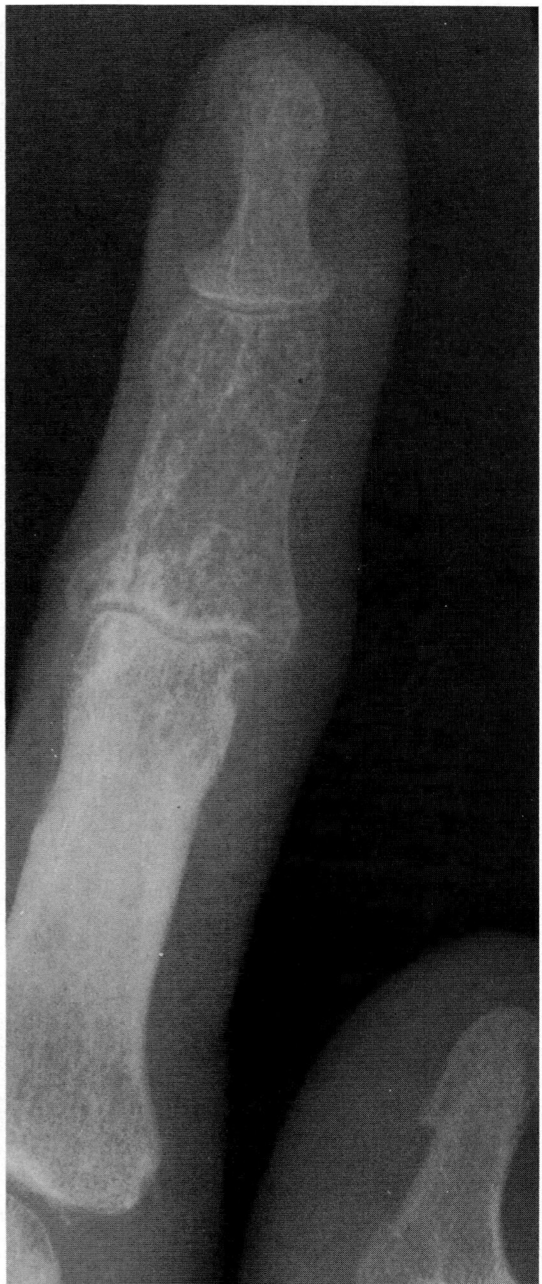

Figure 15–25. Involvement of two phalanges in a 78-year-old man with severe generalized Paget's disease. Note the thickened cortex of the proximal phalanx and the coarsely thickened trabeculae of the middle phalanx. These lesions were not symptomatic.

maximal weight-bearing, coincidental, unrelated degenerative joint disease is probably the cause. He concluded that if the joint space narrowing is medial and accompanied by protrusio acetabuli, the Paget's disease is the cause. In our study of 41 patients with disease involving 76 hips, we have found that pagetic involvement of the proximal femur in the absence of acetabular involvement is rare, whereas acetabular disease without femoral involvement is common[58] (Fig. 15–27). The latter is associated with narrowing of the superior joint margin, usually without protrusio acetabuli, and relatively few symptoms. The most severe disease occurs in patients with both acetabular and proximal femoral disease (Fig. 15–28). Protrusio acetabuli is usually associated with both superior and medial joint space narrowing (Fig. 15–29). In these patients the abnormal remodeling of pagetic bone permits the forces of weight-bearing to drive the femoral head in a superior and medial direction. Some symptomatic relief from the pain of hip disease is obtained by the use of orthopedic devices, salicylates, or indomethacin (or related anti-inflammatory drugs), but in others total hip replacement is required for adequate relief of pain and definitive treatment.[81,82]

Knee pain is common in patients with Paget's disease of the distal femur and proximal tibia[58] and is more likely to be present if the disease is adjacent to the joint. Severe joint space narrowing is observed in these patients and is almost always accompanied by pain, although the severity of the pain and impaired mobility are usually less than in patients with pagetic hip disease. Osteophytes may also be found. When synovial effusions occur, they usually have the characteristics of noninflammatory (type I) fluids.[74] Excellent resolution of the pain and impaired mobility in patients with tibial disease can be achieved by tibial osteotomy and realignment of the distorted anatomy of the distal lower extremity.[83] Paget's disease may also involve the patella, which may become enlarged and warm to the touch. The focal nature of the disease is illustrated by the fact that a pagetic patella may be present in the absence of any

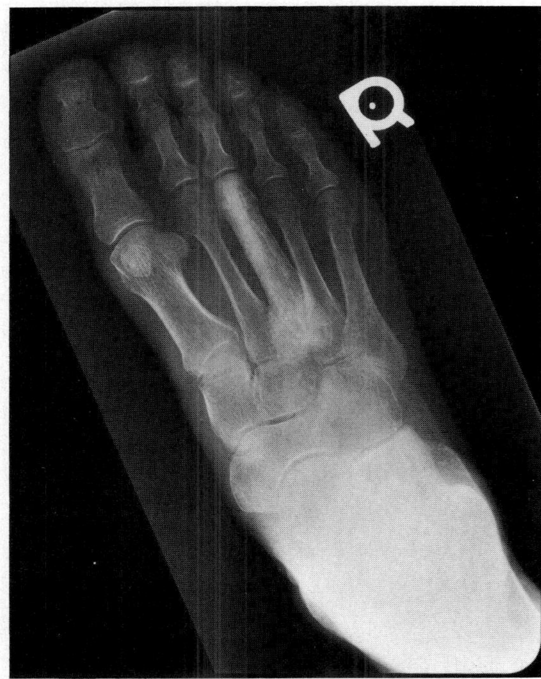

Figure 15–26. Paget's disease of the third metatarsal. Note the increased trabeculation and dimensions of the bone.

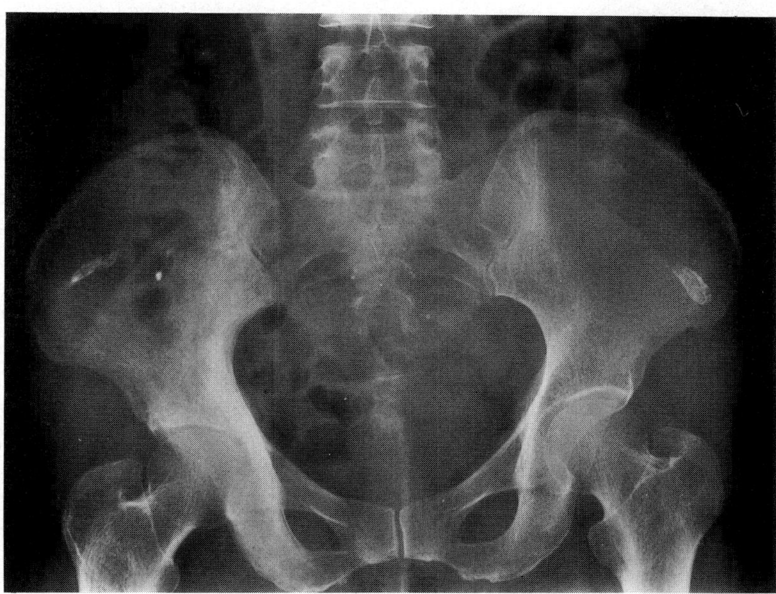

Figure 15–27. Early involvement of the right half of the pelvis characterized by a dense rim of pagetic bone surrounding the acetabulum, the "brim" sign. This is a frequent early finding in the pelvis.

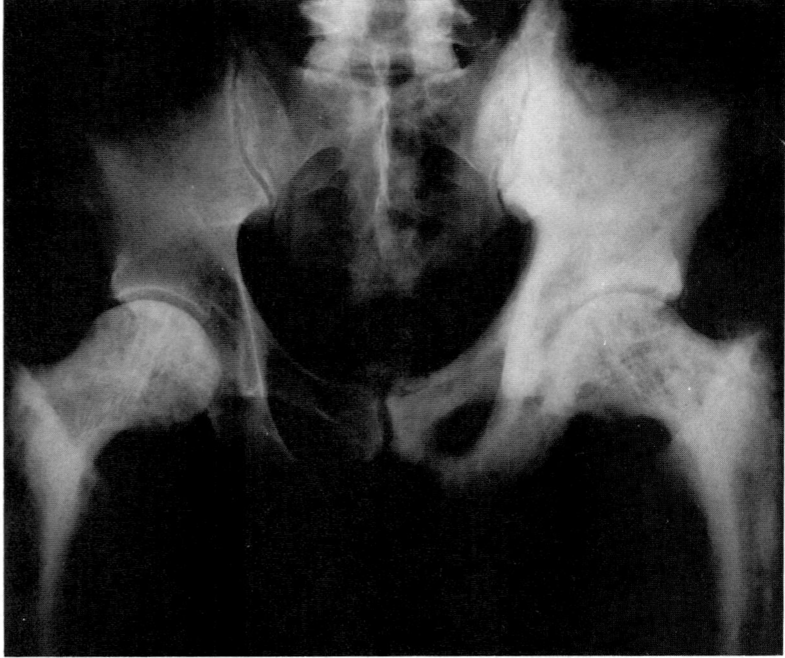

Figure 15–28. More severe involvement of the left pelvis and femur by Paget's disease. Note that the left portion of the sacrum is also involved.

other involvement of the particular extremity and is not necessarily associated with Paget's disease of the femur or tibia (Fig. 15–30).

V. LOCAL COMPLICATIONS

A. Fractures

Fractures are the most common complication of Paget's disease.[84] They are character-

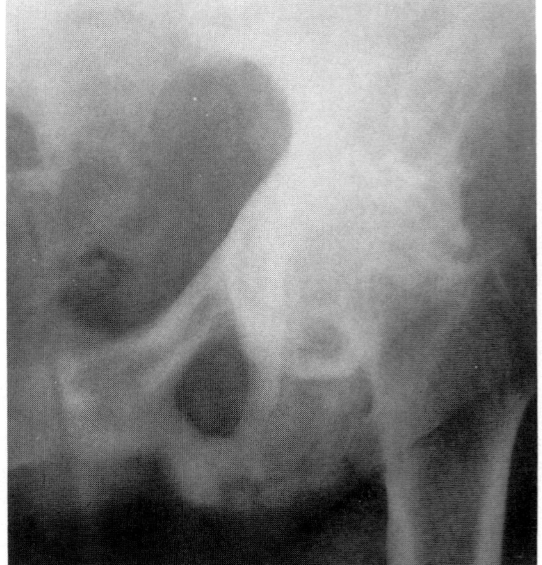

Figure 15–29. Protrusio acetabuli in Paget's disease involving the proximal femur and acetabulum.

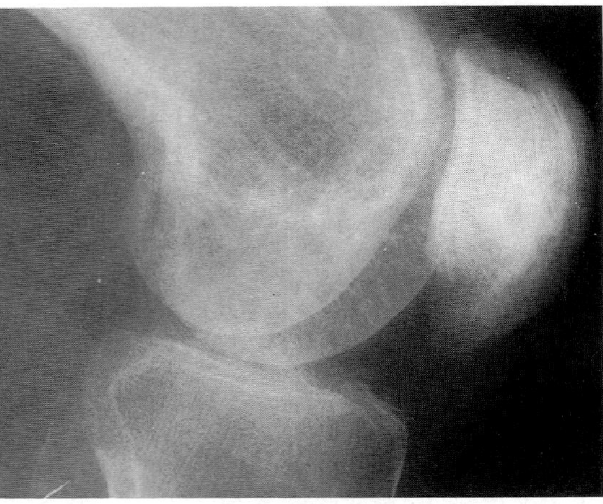

Figure 15–30. Paget's disease of the patella. There is marked exaggeration of the cortical and medullary bone produced by the pagetic bone, following normal stress lines.

istically transverse whether complete or incomplete, and lie perpendicular to the cortex. The incomplete fissure fracture, or infraction, seen in the long bones is infrequently a precursor to complete transverse fractures[85] and need not result from external trauma. Femoral fractures are twice as common as fractures of the tibia;[38] the main femoral site is just below the lesser trochanter, whereas the main tibial site is at the upper third of the shaft.[86] The small cortical incomplete fractures often occur at multiple sites on a single long bone, primarily along the periosteal edge of the convex surface of the curved bone, and penetrate to various depths through the cortex. These lesions are seen on roentgenograms as narrow slitlike radiolucent transverse lines (Fig. 15–31). Repeated occurrence and remodeling of incomplete fractures is partly responsible for the increase in total degree of curvature in diseased tubular bone. The majority of incomplete fractures occur during the osteolytic phase, whereas complete fractures tend to be more

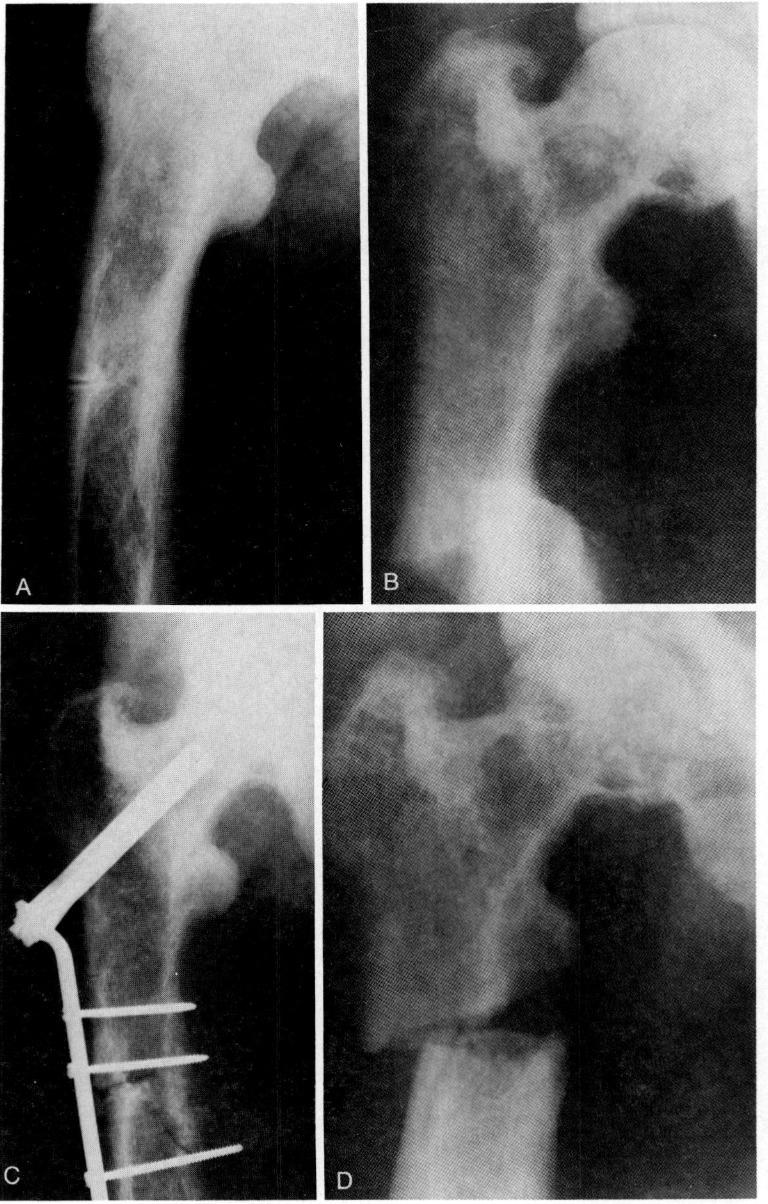

Figure 15–31. Fractures in Paget's disease. *A*, Two fissure fractures of a femur involved by Paget's disease. *B*, One month later, a complete "chalk stick" fracture occurred at the site of the distal fissure fracture. Note that the proximal fissure fracture is still present. *C*, A month after the fracture was pinned, it began to heal. *D*, Two years later, a complete "chalk stick" fracture occurred at the site of the proximal fissure fracture.

common in the osteoblastic phase. This would be anticipated, since the energy required for the propagation of the fracture is dissipated by the numerous separate trabeculae of the bone of the lytic phase.

Fractures in pagetic bone can heal as efficiently as in normal bone while the callus underlying the break itself undergoes the bony changes of Paget's disease. In the largest reported series of 182 complete femoral fractures, however, the incidence of nonunion was high, that is, 40%.[87] In complete fractures, which are usually transverse as if the bone were snapped like a piece of chalk, the periosteum will be torn with a wide separation of fragments (Fig. 15–31*D*). There is a bias (over 30%) for the occurrence of complete shaft fractures at a site just below the lesser trochanter, with resultant flexion abduction deformity of the proximal fragment. The frequency of this subtrochanteric site of fracture in Paget's disease should be contrasted with the frequency of femoral neck site of fracture in older persons without Paget's disease. Since incomplete fractures are most common at the subtrochanteric level, this area would be expected to be the site of the most extensive femoral remodeling and proliferation of abnormal bone in Paget's disease. Accordingly, a combination of internal expansion and remote compression trauma might be sufficient to elicit complete fracture. Tibial fractures follow the femoral pattern. At times the fibula, which is almost never involved with Paget's disease, may nevertheless be fractured as a consequence of the tibial fracture. Pelvic fracture is usually through one or both pubic or ischial rami. It is often difficult to determine whether vertebral body deformity results from pagetic resorption *per se* or superimposed authentic fracture.

It has been noted that spontaneous fracture may occur through an osteolytic lesion of Paget's disease and result in rapid local spread of the pagetic osteolytic process.[9,88] These events may be confused radiographically with malignant transformation.

B. Associated Neoplasia

The precise incidence of malignant change in Paget's disease is unknown. Although there have been estimates as high as 10% in generalized, severe disease,[38] an incidence of approximately 1% probably reflects a more accurate picture if all cases are taken into account.[9,84,89] Rarely osteosarcomas may develop in multiple members of families with Paget's disease.[9,90,91]

In all patients with bone sarcoma over the age of 60 years, over half will have Paget's disease.[91] In Barry's series[9] of 116 sarcomas arising in Paget's disease, men were affected twice as often as were women. Malignant change is rare below the age of 50 years. The most common symptoms are pain and swelling, which in some instances predate radiographic findings by a period of months. Pain may be absent in malignancies involving the skull. In some cases the neoplasm itself, as a soft tissue tumor, may be the presenting sign. A postulated correlation of fractures in pagetic bone and the site of sarcomatous change has never been substantiated, since histologic demonstration of neoplasms arising at a fracture site has rarely been reported even though Paget's disease and neoplasms may be found in the same bone.[9] Furthermore, in one survey no predisposition to malignancy was found following fracture.[93] Therefore, local injury or excessive trauma, so often invoked as causally related to malignant transformation, is more likely to be the event that draws attention to the previously undetected tumor.

Sarcomas in Paget's disease are found most frequently in the pelvis, femur, humerus, skull, and facial bones, but are uncommon in vertebrae.[9,89,94-96] The distribution of sarcomas can be contrasted with the distribution of Paget's disease itself, which affects the vertebrae, skull, pelvis, femur, tibia, and humerus in that order. The reasons why sarcomatous change favors the humerus are obscure.[9] The malignant changes always take place within a focus of Paget's disease. Therefore, only in cases of advanced and extensive polyostotic disease are multifocal sarcomas found,[38,94] and when they do occur, the skull is the most common site.[9] Jaffe[38] described cases in which sarcoma developed in the only bone involved with Paget's disease. In the studies of Collins, Paget's disease was polyostotic in two thirds of the patients with sarcoma.[84] Autopsy data suggest that when multiple sarcomas are present, each is of independent origin and not metastatic. Multiple scalp tumors were seen in 24 cases in Barry's series of 116 sarcomas.[9] Such lesions were often associated with lysis of the underlying calvarium and invasion directly into the brain. Death ensued within 6 months after diagnosis.

The sarcomas vary widely in cell composition,[9,38,89,92-96] reflecting the pluripotentiality of the mesenchymal elements of the bone marrow. Sarcomatous tumors have a spectrum of histologic patterns, which include the following: (1) cell-poor, collagen-rich fibrosarcomas (Fig. 15–32); (2) poorly differentiated fibrosarcomas with abundant giant cells; (3) anaplastic sarcomas with giant cells, spindle cells with plump nuclei, and osteoclast-like giant cells resembling so-called malignant giant cell tumors of bone; (4) rare chondrosarcomas, nine of which were reviewed by Barry;[9] (5) conventional giant cell tumors found mostly in the skull, but with occasional spinal, innominate, or femoral involvement; (6) sarcomatous stroma that may contain osteoid and may be classified as osteosarcoma; (7) reticulum cell sarcoma;[97] and (8) multiple myeloma.[98] This histologic spectrum appears to be a continuum from benign to malignant, since benign but bizarre cellular changes in fibrous bone marrow remote from the tumor site may be seen.[38,99] Thus, there is a danger in interpreting a biopsy taken from one portion of a tumor, since different histologic patterns may be found in different parts of the neoplasm, and for this reason we prefer the broadly descriptive term "sarcoma." As Jaffe[38] concluded: "It would seem that the connective tissue from which they [sarcomas] arise may reveal, even within the same tumor, manifold potentialities for differentiation and dedifferentiation along mesenchymal lines."

Radiographically sarcomas usually appear as small, irregular radiolucent foci with mottled or speckled areas of calcification superimposed on the background of Paget's disease (Fig. 15–33). The dense areas of tumor bone and the sunburst pattern (periosteal reaction) characteristic of osteosarcoma of the young are not usually seen in sarcomas associated with Paget's disease. In addition, the tumors associated with Paget's disease are not confined to the ends of the bones but occur anywhere along the shaft. For example, in Barry's series[9] of 24 tumors involving the femur, 10 were in the proximal third of the shaft, 5 in the mid-third, and 9 in the distal third. Most tibial tumors were in the proximal portion of the shaft. Sarcomas appear to originate in the medulla,[9,38] as manifested by the radiographic signs of early subcortical medullary bone lysis. This progresses to cortical bone loss and the eventual development of a soft tissue mass. Computed tomography is now essential in delineating the soft tissue extension. A pathologic fracture may be seen as a terminal event of this biological sequence.[9] Although many patients with Paget's disease who develop osteosarcomas have increased levels of serum alkaline phosphatase activity compared with previous levels, so-called explosive rises of serum enzyme activity are not seen.

The prognosis for sarcomas arising in Paget's disease is dismal.[9,38,89,92-96] The 5-year survival in pagetic patients with sarcomas in one study was 7.5% as compared with a survival of 37% in elderly patients in whom the tumor arose *de novo*.[92] Most patients die

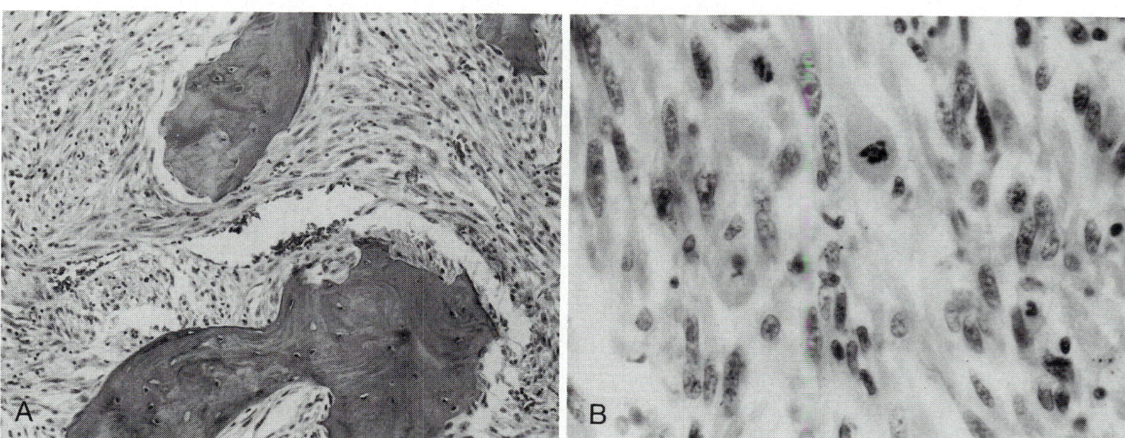

Figure 15–32. A spindle cell sarcoma. *A*, Abnormal fibroblasts mainly compose the tumor, which surrounds fragments of pagetic bone (H and E; ×190). *B*, Atypical mitoses are seen in several of the spindle sarcoma cells (H and E; ×750).

within 2 years after the diagnosis is established. In Barry's series of 116 tumors,[9] no patient survived longer than 5 years, with the average duration of survival being 12 months from diagnosis. Those patients with multiple sarcomas died within 6 months with pulmonary metastases.[38] At present, radiotherapy is only palliative, and the treatment of choice appears to be amputation if the tumor is painful or disfiguring. In contrast to the remarkable increase in efficacy of several chemotherapeutic programs used to treat osteosarcomas in children,[100] adjuvant chemotherapy has not yet proved effective in prolonging survival when the osteosarcomas arise in patients with Paget's disease.[92]

A peculiar neoplasm deserving special mention here is the giant cell tumor associated with Paget's disease. These are uncommon tumors that most often involve some portion of the calvarium or facial bones. They have rarely been reported to occur in familial Paget's disease.[101] In Barry's review[9] of 15 such tumors (five in the calvarium, two each in the maxilla, mandible, and tibia, and one each in the humerus, ilium, sacrum and ethmoid), a spectrum ranging from classic benign giant cell tumors to malignant sarcomas with giant cells was seen. Similar cases have been reported under the broad term of giant cell tumor. Although the prognosis varies with each case, survival rates appear to be more favorable than for other neoplasms associated with Paget's disease. Jaffe[38] has described an astounding case in which, over an 8-year period, 12 such tumors appeared successively in the frontal, parietal, temporal, occipital, and facial bones. We have also observed these tumors to occur in multiple bones (all pagetic) in the same individual.[102] We had under our care a man with extensive polyostotic Paget's disease known since age 35 (serum alkaline phosphatase levels as high as 114 Bodansky units) who at age 46 was discovered to have a tumor containing giant cells in the mandible. He was treated with curettage and radiation but the tumor recurred on several occasions over several years. Eleven years after the mandibular lesion was identified, he developed a right iliac bone tumor with iliac vein obstruction, which was identical histologically to the lesion in the jaw (Fig. 15–34). The pelvic lesion did not respond to radiation therapy but became smaller with the administration of calcitonin. At the time of this patient's death from

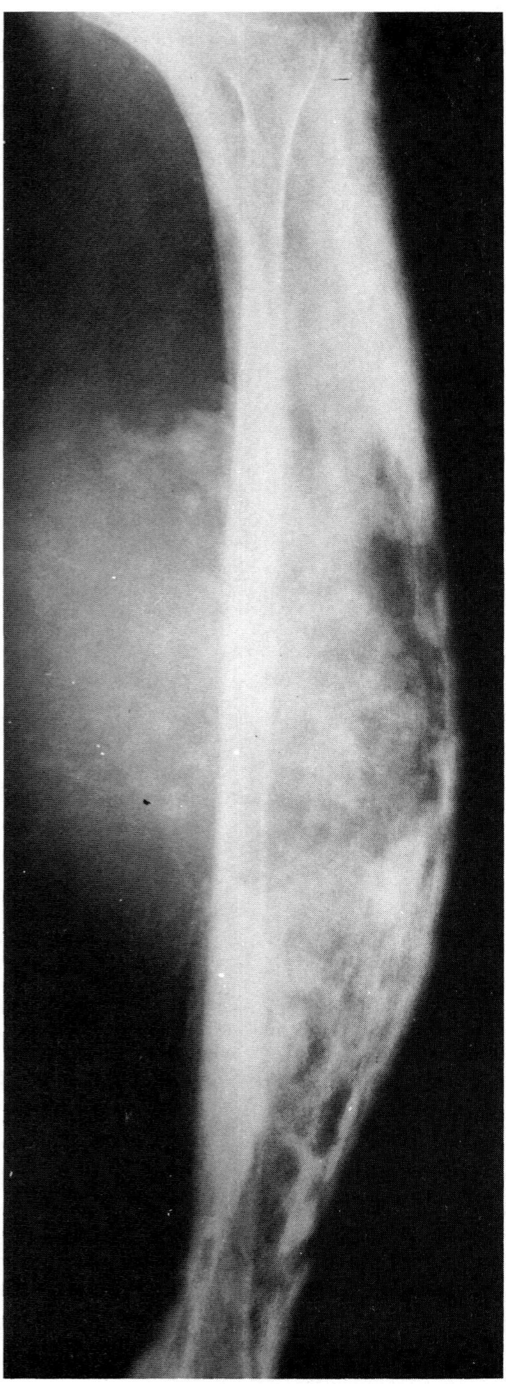

Figure 15–33. An 82-year-old man with osteosarcoma arising in a tibia involved with Paget's disease. The tumor has extended into the soft tissue and has multiple radiodense areas, some of which have the trabecular pattern of bone formation. Note the underlying changes of Paget's disease in the tibia.

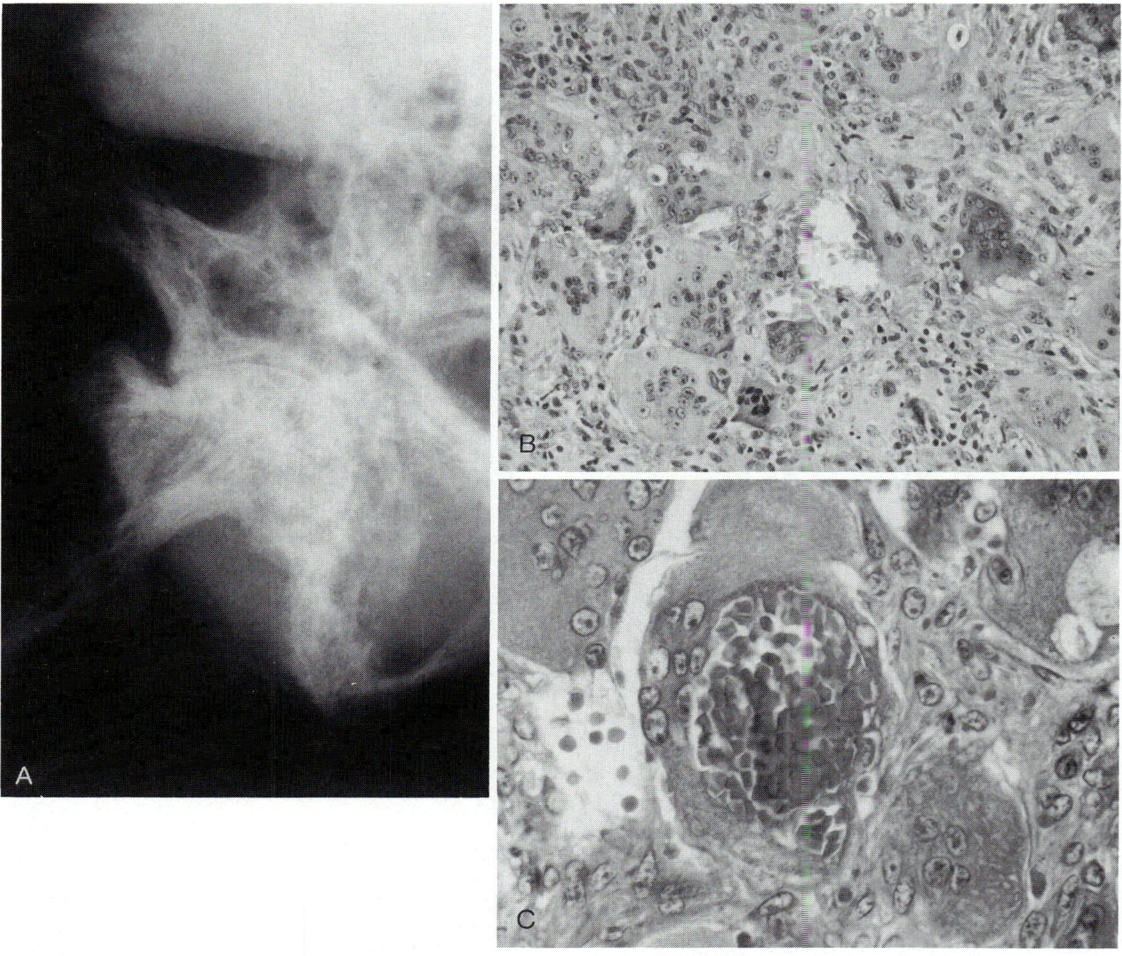

Figure 15–34. A giant cell reparative granuloma in the right iliac bone of a 57-year-old man with extensive Paget's disease of most bones. *A*, The lesion is seen as a large cystic defect in the ilium. There is severe Paget's disease of the pelvis and femur. This lesion was histologically indistinguishable from a giant cell reparative granuloma of the jaw in the same individual. *B*, The jaw and iliac lesions were composed of benign-appearing spindle cells with plump fusiform nuclei and prominent nucleoli. The many osteoclast-type giant cells were generally arranged about areas of hemorrhage (H and E; ×270). *C*, Such giant cells often contained large aggregates of erythrocytes (H and E; ×700).

coronary heart disease, 19 years after the jaw lesion was discovered, there was no evidence of metastases.

Microscopically these tumors consist of benign spindle cells with plump fusiform nuclei and clumped chromatin or nucleoli (Fig. 15–34). Mitoses are rare. Scattered among these cells are osteoclast-type giant cells not randomly dispersed, but congregated about foci of hemorrhage or scar and often associated with hemosiderin-laden macrophages. Some of the giant cells have phagocytized erythrocytes. Small scattered fragments of pagetic bone were found adjacent to some tumor cells in addition to reactive woven bone spicules, which are generally peripherally disposed. Fibrous marrow adjacent to these tumors has similar gradations of cellular atypicality such that the tumors merge subtly with the nearby fibrous marrow.

We feel that these lesions represent an atypical proliferative process similar to the giant cell reparative granulomas of the jaw. This conclusion was reached after review of four additional cases at the Massachusetts General Hospital as well as 35 others in the literature.[102] The reasons for considering the lesions distinct from true giant cell tumors are as follows: Histologically the giant cell lesions of Paget's disease differ from true giant cell tumors in the number and distribution of giant cells, the benign appearance of the stromal cells, and the increased production of collagenous matrix. Clinically the true giant cell tumors occur predominantly in the ends of the long bones, whereas the pagetic tumors are usually found in facial bones. A small percentage of true giant cell tumors may be malignant as documented by occurrence of distant metastases, whereas reparative granulomas do not metastasize. The cases reported by Jacobs et al.[101] also resemble ours clinically and histologically. What is of particular interest in that series[101] is that three of five patients were related and all patients traced their ancestral roots to Avellino, Italy (three of the five patients in our series were also of Italian ancestry, at least one of whom had relatives from Avellino). It is possible that all or most of the previously reported cases are reparative granulomas, although not all pathologists agree with the interpretation that these lesions are not true giant cell tumors.[103] Whether or not the giant cell lesions found in association with Paget's disease are neoplasms, they are frequently very aggressive and locally destructive and attain large dimensions. The soft tissue mass in one of our patients extended at least 28 to 30 cm, estimated by computed tomography (Fig. 15–35). Although the lesions may respond to radiation therapy, they do recur, and chemotherapy with agents such as doxorubicin may be required.[103] Dexamethasone may be of limited value as reported in the series of Jacobs et al.[101]

Attempts have been made to correlate the skeletal distribution of Paget's disease with that of metastatic cancer, but the correlation would hold only for the axial skeleton, which is among the most favored sites for metastases of many types of cancer. The ribs are a preferential site for metastases, but rib involvement in Paget's disease is unusual. On the other hand, the tibia, which is among the most favored sites of Paget's disease, is an infrequent location for metastatic cancer.[9] A correlation would seem to depend on the degree of abnormal bone vascularization. The few examples of the coexistence of multiple myeloma and Paget's disease, two diseases that commonly affect the axial skeleton of the elderly, appear to be coincidental.[98] Paget's disease is also occasionally the site of skeletal metastases of carcinomas. We have encountered a few such instances that included a metastasis from prostatic carcinoma and lung carcinoma. In view of the high vascularity of pagetic bone, it is surprising that metastases to such bone are not encountered more frequently.

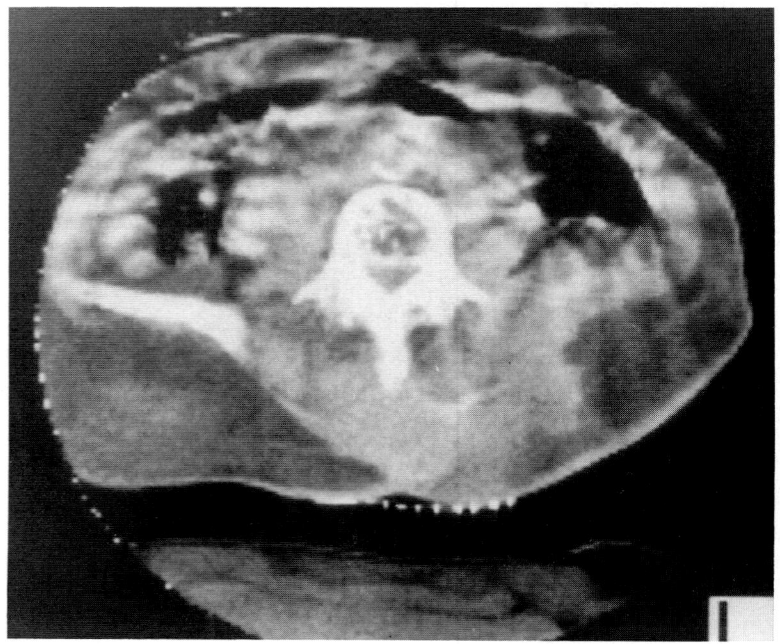

Figure 15–35. Computed tomographic scan of the lumbar spine of a 71-year-old woman with extensive Paget's disease and a paraspinal mass consistent with giant cell reparative granuloma. This scan was similar to that previously reported as Patient 1.[101]

VI. METABOLIC ASPECTS OF PAGET'S DISEASE

A. Mineral Metabolism

Clinical and histopathologic evidence suggests that the primary defect in Paget's disease is excessive resorption of bone in a focal area. Characteristically this excessive resorption is soon accompanied by an increase in bone formation, which may continue even after the resorption has slowed. Despite the focal nature of the disorder and its limited extent in some patients, the increased remodeling is readily detected by overall assessment of the turnover of the mineral and organic phases of bone.

As bone is resorbed, mineral ions are released into the extracellular fluid. If excessive resorption occurs in one part of the skeleton, the increased concentration of mineral ions in the extracellular fluid would, because of the resultant hypercalcemia, decrease secretion of parathyroid hormone and increase renal clearance of calcium. In patients with Paget's disease, however, concentrations of calcium and phosphorus in plasma are usually normal, concentrations of parathyroid hormone measured by radioimmunoassay are usually normal,[104-107] and urinary calcium excretion is not characteristically increased in the absence of fractures of bone or immobilization of patients in bed.[8] These observations imply that the increased release of mineral ions that results from increased bone resorption must be accompanied by closely geared local reutilization of such ions for the formation of the new mineral phase. Therefore, the external calcium balance in Paget's disease, which reflects differences in bone formation and resorption, does not usually give any indication of the *rates* of these processes. It should be pointed out, however, that calcium balances in pagetic subjects are rarely more than 200 mg/day positive or negative. Analysis of the disappearance from the plasma of tracer doses of mineral ions does indicate how greatly accelerated the turnover of these ions may be, even though the process may be confined to a limited region of the skeleton.

The results of studies of several authors utilizing kinetic analysis of plasma disappearance rates and/or skeletal uptake of ^{47}Ca, ^{45}Ca, ^{85}Sr,[8,108,109] and Mg[110] or ^{99m}Tc-diphosphonate,[111,112] although not strictly comparable quantitatively, have all shown that the rates of both bone formation and resorption can be greatly increased in patients with Paget's disease. As an example, the pattern of disappearance of injected ^{47}Ca from the serum of a patient with extensive Paget's disease is shown in Figure 15–36. From data of this sort it is possible to calculate the size of the exchangeable calcium pool and rates of entrance into (V_{o+}) and exit from (V_{o-}) this pool.[113,114] Although there is disagreement as to the significance of such calculations and their physiologic meaning and what corrections need to be applied to take into account factors such as long-term isotope exchange, it is possible to use the numbers derived to compare different subjects with each other and with normals. The increased values for V_{o+} and V_{o-} calculated in patients with Paget's disease are mean rates for the whole skeleton. It should be emphasized that some areas of bone would be remodeling at a rate manyfold that of others. Calculations of the kinetic parameters in patients such as those listed in Table 15–1 probably overestimate rates of calcium resorption, V_{o-} (as well as calcium deposition, V_{o+}). However, in comparison with the rates calculated for normal subjects, both formation and resorption may be increased occasionally more than 20-fold. Although the physical properties of ^{32}P have precluded its widespread use to study phosphorus kinetics in humans except in individuals who are terminally ill, it is likely that an abnormality similar to that observed with the tracer cations would be seen. Fluoride ions can be incorporated into the hydroxyapatite crystal lattice, and evidence of increased retention of absorbed fluoride has also been found in patients with Paget's disease.[8]

Although the whole-body turnover of mineral ions is increased in pagetic subjects, results obtained by external scanning following administration of the radioactive isotopes ^{47}Ca, ^{85}Sr, ^{18}F, and bisphosphonate coupled to ^{99m}Tc[111,112,115-117] indicate that the tracer is localized mainly to diseased areas of the skeleton. This phenomenon has led to the use of bone-seeking isotopes in defining the extent and activity of the disease in clinical practice. The pattern of uptake of ^{99m}Tc-labeled bisphosphonate in monostotic and polyostotic Paget's disease is illustrated in Figure 15–37.

It was found earlier that pagetic bone initially takes up more ^{47}Ca than normal bone

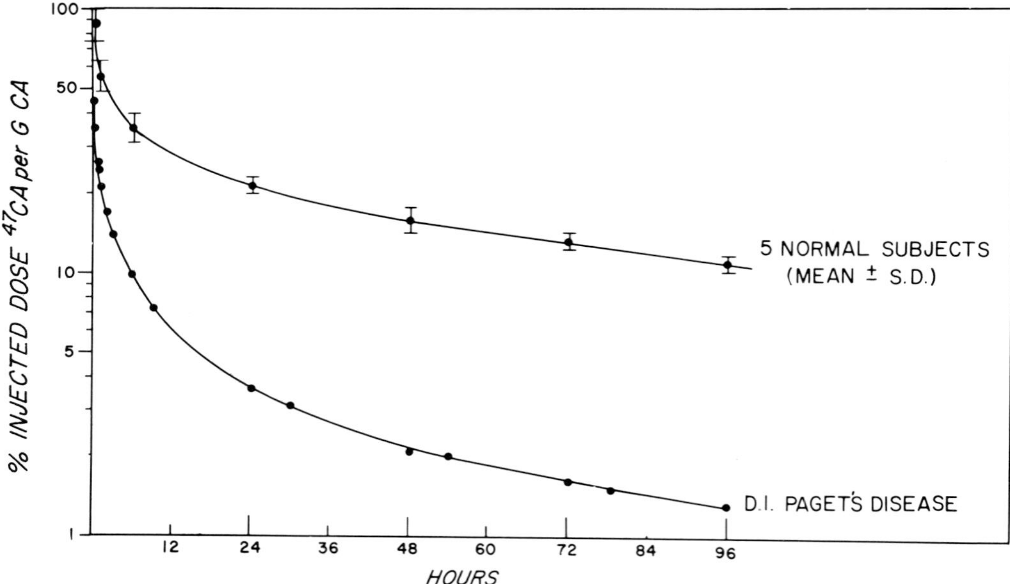

Figure 15–36. The pattern of egress of ^{47}Ca from the serum of a patient with extensive Paget's disease as compared to that from five normal subjects. (From Nagant de Deuxchaisnes C, Krane SM: Paget's disease of bone: Clinical and metabolic observations. Medicine 43:233–266, 1964. By permission from the publisher, the Williams and Wilkins Co.)

and retains the isotope for longer times.[8] This increased uptake is not due entirely to rapid exchange processes, since the high level of activity persists in the involved bones even when the specific activity of ^{47}Ca in plasma has fallen to low levels. Whether such retention is the result of the formation of a new mineral phase or some long-term exchange process[118,119] is not yet known. On the basis of the uptake of ^{47}Ca and the subsequent decay of this isotope to its daughter isotope ^{47}Sc, we concluded that the calcium that enters pagetic bone becomes "fixed" and no longer available for short-term exchange processes.[8] Thus a model can be proposed in which there is rapid formation of new bone with the calcium-phosphate mineral phase of the older bone "insulated" by newly deposited mineral phase. Skeletal uptake of agents such as ^{99m}Tc-diphosphonate would be proportional to the surface of newly formed calcium-phosphate mineral phase as well as to the magnitude of the blood flow to the pagetic bone.[112] As discussed previously, although there is increased blood flow through dilated superficial vessels overlying a pagetic bone, there is convincing evidence using ^{18}F clearance techniques that blood flow is in-

Table 15–1. Calcium Resorption and Hydroxyproline Excretion in Paget's Disease

Patient	Calcium Resorption Rate (V_{o-}) (1) (g/24 hr)	Hydroxyproline Excretion (2) (g/24 hr)	Bone Resorption (g/24 hr) Based on (1)	(2)
1	14.2	0.590	50.7	17.5
2	6.9	0.497	24.6	14.8
3	4.9	0.238	17.5	7.1
4	4.1	0.114	14.6	3.4
5	3.6	0.147	12.9	4.4
6	3.5	0.223	12.5	6.6
7	2.3	0.078	8.2	2.3
Normal values	<0.670	<0.040	<2.4	<1.2

Calculated from Nagant de Deuxchaisnes C, Krane SM: Medicine (Baltimore) 43:233, 1964.

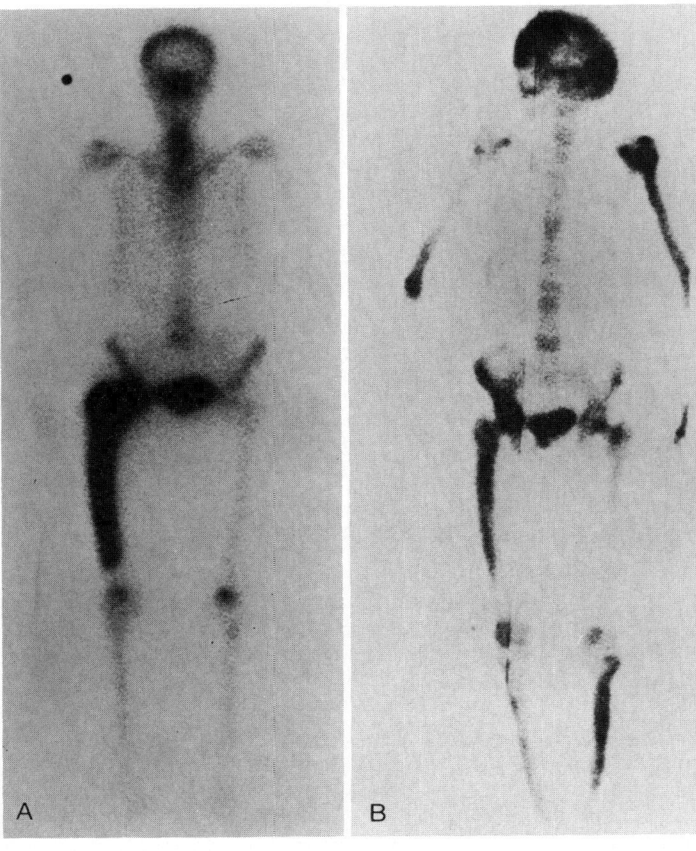

Figure 15–37. Bone scans in two patients with Paget's disease. *A*, An example of monostotic disease in which nearly the entire right femur shows increased uptake of ^{99m}Tc-bisphosphonate. *B*, Polyostotic Paget's disease involving the skull, multiple vertebrae, the right hemipelvis and multiple long bones.

creased to pagetic bone. The intensity of the remodeling in diseased bone may also result in the rapid clearance of tracer ions from the blood, leaving little tracer available for uptake by normal bone. Thus, uptake over an uninvolved tibia at an arbitrary interval following injection of ^{47}Ca is less in patients with Paget's disease than in normal subjects.[8]

The kinetic data obtained in patients with Paget's disease imply that despite enormous increases in both bone resorption and formation, the rates of the two processes are very similar. We have speculated[8] that the increase in bone formation is the homeostatic response of the organism to maintain the concentration of calcium in the plasma constant despite the great egress of calcium from bone to extracellular fluid. It is possible that it is this homeostatic requirement for bone formation that accounts for the irregular deposition of new bone that characterizes Paget's disease. The delicate equilibrium between formation and resorption is easily upset by such events as fractures or immobilization of the patients and would be reflected in alterations in calcium balance or in elevation of serum calcium levels.

Serum magnesium concentrations were found to be low in 25% of 64 patients in Liverpool.[120] Metabolic balance studies in 19 patients indicated that the hypomagnesemic individuals had a significantly more positive balance and a higher net absorption of magnesium than normomagnesemic individuals. It was suggested that the hypomagnesemia probably resulted from increased uptake by bone.

In the only study assessing the level of vitamin D metabolites in the circulation, serum 25(OH)D and 1,25$(OH)_2D_3$ levels were within the normal range, but serum 24,25$(OH)_2D_3$ levels were more than 50% lower than those of an age-matched control group.[121] The degree of disease activity was higher in the patients with the lower levels of 24,25$(OH)_2D_3$. The significance of these findings remains to be established.

B. Metabolism of Bone Matrix

1. Pagetic Bone Matrix

When bone is resorbed, not only is there release of mineral ions from the inorganic phase, but there is resorption of the organic phase as well. As discussed in Chapters 1 and 2, the organic phase of bone consists mainly of collagen in addition to several noncollagenous proteins.

The major, if not the exclusive, type of collagen in normal bone is type I collagen.[122] Small amounts of type III collagen may also be found, usually in the walls of blood vessels. The amino acid composition of pagetic bone analyzed after demineralization in EDTA is indistinguishable from normal bone. Furthermore, the few samples of pagetic bone that have been examined by cyanogen bromide digestion and chromatography showed a pattern also indistinguishable from that of normal bone and do not show the presence of detectable amounts of type III collagen peptides.[123] Moreover, pagetic bone fragments in organ culture synthesize only type I collagen, whereas skin fibroblasts synthesize both types I and III collagens.[124] It has not been proved by microdissection techniques that all of the collagen in lamellar as well as woven pagetic bone is type I. Histologic examination of specimens of pagetic bone, however, characteristically shows a loose, fibrous stroma replacing normal marrow elements. This fibrous stroma probably includes types III and V collagens. It is possible that the inability to detect type III collagen chemically in bone is accounted for by the relatively low percentage of stroma in the samples examined.[125]

Normal bone and skin both contain the same heterotrimeric type I collagen. Only one gene has been identified for each component alpha$_1$(I) and alpha$_2$(I) chains.[126] Unless there is some alternative pathway of processing the primary gene transcript of these type I collagen chains, then the amino acid sequence of the type I collagen chains in skin and bone should be identical. Skin and bone collagens are not identical from the point of view of posttranslational modifications, however. For example, the pattern of glycosylation of the hydroxylysine residues is clearly different in human skin and bone.[127-129] The ratio of glucosyl-galactosyl hydroxylysine [Hyl(Glc-Gal)] to galactosyl-hydroxylysine [Hyl(Gal)] is 0.47 ± 0.01 in normal human bone and 2.06 ± 0.47 in normal human skin, whereas the total glycosylated hydroxylysine is similar in the collagens from these tissues.[128] In five pagetic bone samples the ratio of Hyl(Glc-Gal)/Hyl(Gal) ranged from 0.40 to 0.74, not significantly different from normal.[130] The reducible crosslinks of normal bone can also be distinguished from those of normal skin.[131] In normal bone the predominant compound is hydroxylysino-hydroxynorleucine, the reduced Schiff base of hydroxylysine and hydroxylysine aldehydes.[131] A minor crosslink, hydroxylysinonorleucine, has been found to be relatively increased in pagetic bone compared with normal bone,[132] although the significance of this finding remains to be established. Other major crosslinks in mature skeletal collagens are the 3-hydroxpyridinium residues.[131,133] The major compound, hydroxylysyl pyridinolone (HP), is derived from three residues of hydroxylysine, whereas the less abundant lysyl pyridinolone (LP) is derived from two hydroxylysine residues and one lysine residue. Measurements of these compounds in blood or urine should provide other useful markers in the evaluation of Paget's disease.

It is probable that there is no major abnormality of the type, primary structure, and/or distribution of collagen in pagetic bone proper. There may be minor differences in posttranslational modifications of bone collagens that could reflect the "maturity" of the bone sampled and the turnover, that is, the rates of formation and resorption. If the sample is from the more loosely structured cancellous bone, then there might be a greater relative contribution of stromal collagens that would include types III and V collagens. A systematic study of all of the noncollagenous proteins in pagetic bone compared with normal bone has yet to be reported. The concentrations of alpha$_2$HS-glycoprotein, albumin, and sialic acid (for bone sialoprotein) have been measured in a small number of samples and found to be significantly increased in pagetic bone.[134] This has been attributed to the increased rate of bone turnover.

2. Collagenolysis

In order for bone to be resorbed, it is essential to remove the mineral phase so that the matrix can be attacked by proteolytic enzymes. Current evidence suggests that these processes occur in the uniquely acidic environment of the extracellular compartment adjacent to the ruffled border of the osteoclast.[135,136] At the low pH in this compartment, dissolution of the calcium-phosphate of bone is presumably the initial event. It was first proposed by Vaes[137] and subsequently elaborated upon further[138] that acid hydrolases, which would function optimally at the low pH in this compartment, would be involved in the resorption of the organic matrix. Although there are data[139-141] indicating that a neutral metalloproteinase, a collagenase,[142] is produced in bone, it has been suggested that the source of this enzyme is osteoblast-like cells rather than osteoclasts[143] and the collagen-resorbing activity of osteoclasts is an acid hydrolase distinct from collagenase. Whatever the mechanism, since the rate of bone resorption in Paget's disease is characteristically increased, it follows that the rate of collagenolysis is also increased, which is reflected in the urinary excretion of peptides derived from collagen. It has been found that biopsy specimens of pagetic bone release significantly more labeled amino acids from collagen gels than do normal bones.[144] Whether this enhanced collagenolysis is due to increased numbers of cells (and which cells) or enhanced collagenolytic activity per cell is not known.

3. *Hydroxyproline and Hydroxylysine Excretion (see Chapter 8)*

In normal animals and humans, the free hydroxylysine[145] and hydroxyproline[146] released from collagen-derived peptides are not reutilized for collagen synthesis and are degraded to small carbon fragments.[147,148] However, oligopeptide-bound hydroxyproline[148,149] and hydroxylysine[8,128,130] and glycosylated hydroxylysine[128,130,150-152] are excreted in the urine, the rate of excretion roughly reflecting the rate of collagen degradation.[123,153] The presence of increased urinary excretion of peptides containing hydroxyproline and other collagen markers in patients with Paget's disease provides a useful tool for the study of collagen turnover in humans and for assessing responses to therapy.

The excretion of hydroxyproline-containing peptides is greater than normal in almost all patients with Paget's disease, even in those with monostotic involvement.[148,154] In general, the amount of hydroxyproline excreted is directly correlated with the extent of the Paget's disease[58,155,156] as well as with the degree of disease activity as determined, for example, by ^{47}Ca kinetics.[8] The fact that the concentrations of oligopeptide hydroxyproline in the plasma are also increased,[157,158] despite rapid clearance by the kidney,[159] indicates that the increased urinary excretion is not due simply to increased renal clearance. Although the evidence is indirect, it is likely that the excessive urinary excretion of hydroxyproline in pagetic subjects has its source in bone. The evidence is as follows: (1) The level of excretion of hydroxyproline is directly related to the extent and the degree of the activity of the Paget's disease. (2) As will be discussed in detail later in this chapter (section VIII-B), treatment of Paget's disease with agents that have their major effects on bone (e.g., calcitonin) results in decreased hydroxyproline excretion. (3) There is no histopathologic evidence that collagens in tissues other than bone, such as the dermis, are involved to a degree sufficient to explain the increased collagen degradation, although minor morphologic changes in appearance of the dermis in pagetic subjects have been observed. (4) The total urinary excretion of hydroxylysine as well as hydroxyproline is increased in Paget's disease, and the pattern of glycosylated hydroxylysines excreted in the urine of several patients studied resembles that of bone collagen.[126,150-152,156] The ratio of Hyl(Glc-Gal)/Hyl(Gal) in five patients with extensive Paget's disease ranged from 0.40 to 0.74, closer to that of bone collagen (0.47) than to that of skin (2.06) or other collagens (> 2.0).[127] The urinary ratios are distinctly lower than the mean in nonpagetic subjects of 1.49.[150]

4. *Other Collagen Peptides*

Dialyzable oligopeptides containing hydroxyproline compose over 90% of the total urinary hydroxyproline.[148,160] These consist primarily of the dipeptide prolylhydroxyproline and its diketopiperazine and the tripeptide glycylprolylhydroxyproline. The sequence of the peptide components is consistent with that in mammalian collagens in which glycine occurs every third residue and 4-hydroxyproline only in the residue preceding glycine, never in the position following glycine.

One might expect that other peptides of the collagen sequence, such as glycylproline, would be excreted in the urine in excess when collagen degradation is increased. Scriver[161] identified glycylproline in the urine of patients with rickets and found that the rate of its excretion diminished with healing of the rickets. Alderman et al.[162] observed marked increases in urinary excretion of glycylproline in patients with a familial skeletal disorder characterized by thickened cortices of long bones, bow deformities, and fractures. They were also able to detect glycylproline in the urine of some subjects with rickets and osteogenesis imperfecta but were unable to find the peptide in the urine of patients with other bone diseases including Paget's disease, although data on hydroxyproline excretion in these patients were not given. In unpublished studies, S.R. Pinnell and S.M. Krane found the excretion of glycylproline to range from 1.04 to 1.47 μmoles per milligram creatinine in four samples of urine from a patient with severe Paget's disease and total urinary hydroxyproline excretion averaging 1300 μg per milligram creatinine (normal adults usually excrete < 40 μg hydroxyproline per milligram creatinine). The level of excretion of glycylproline in this subject was in the range of that reported by Alderman et al.[162] for their patients. However, the hydroxyproline excretion in the pagetic subject was six times greater and is consistent with the observations of Alderman et al.[162] that the excretions of glycylproline and hydroxyproline are not directly proportional.

5. Nondialyzable Urinary Hydroxyproline

The nondialyzable fraction of urinary hydroxyproline consists of a number of heterogenous polypeptides of approximately similar molecular weight, averaging about 5 K_d, estimated by sedimentation equilibrium.[163-165] These polypeptides obtained from the urine of patients with Paget's disease share several characteristics with the collagen chains including the typical amino acid composition, susceptibility to proteolytic cleavage with purified clostridial collagenase, and a negative optical rotation in solution that increases on cooling. Some features distinguishing several of these peptides from bone collagens on the basis of amino acid composition are the high ratio of 4-hydroxyproline to proline, the absence of 3-hydroxyproline, and the high ratio of lysine relative to arginine. It seems likely, however, that these polypeptides are derived from bone for reasons similar to those considered previously, which suggest that the major source of total urinary hydroxyproline in Paget's disease is bone. However, the pattern of distribution of the glycosylated hydroxylysines in the urinary polypeptide fraction is different from that of whole bone or whole urine from pagetic subjects, with a ratio of Hyl(Glc-Gal)/Hyl(Gal) of approximately 1.7 (S.M. Krane and M. Byrne, unpublished).

The results of studies using tracer doses of [^{14}C]-proline in three patients with Paget's disease were similar and suggested that these nondialyzable urinary polypeptides are related to collagen synthesis. Within hours following oral administration of the [^{14}C]-proline, [^{14}C]-hydroxyproline was detected in the urinary polypeptide fraction. At the peak of labeling, the specific activity in the polypeptide fraction was several-fold greater than that in the oligopeptide fraction (Fig. 15–38). After chromatography on phosphocellulose of one of these polypeptide peaks, the specific activity of the [^{14}C]-hydroxyproline was higher in every fraction isolated than in the total dialyzable small peptide fraction.

Polypeptides similar to these were also found in the urine of patients with other skeletal disorders including severe fibrous dysplasia of bone, hyperphosphatasia, and hyperparathyroidism with osteitis fibrosa, all conditions characterized by high skeletal turnover.[164] A similar portion of the hydroxyproline in the urine of normal subjects is also nondialyzable, although the chemical composition of the normal polypeptides has not been determined.

It is likely that the collagen-like polypeptides excreted in the urine in large amounts by patients with Paget's disease, representing about 10% of the total hydroxyproline, are at least in part related to collagen synthesis. The component chains of type I collagen are synthesized by the osteoblasts in bone as precursor procollagen molecules that contain both amino-terminal and carboxyl-terminal globular (i.e., noncollagen triple helical) extensions. The amino-terminal extension peptide contains a small collagen triple helical repeat near its carboxyl-terminal end. Prior to formation of the collagen fibrils and fibers of bone, these extensions are cleaved by specific en-

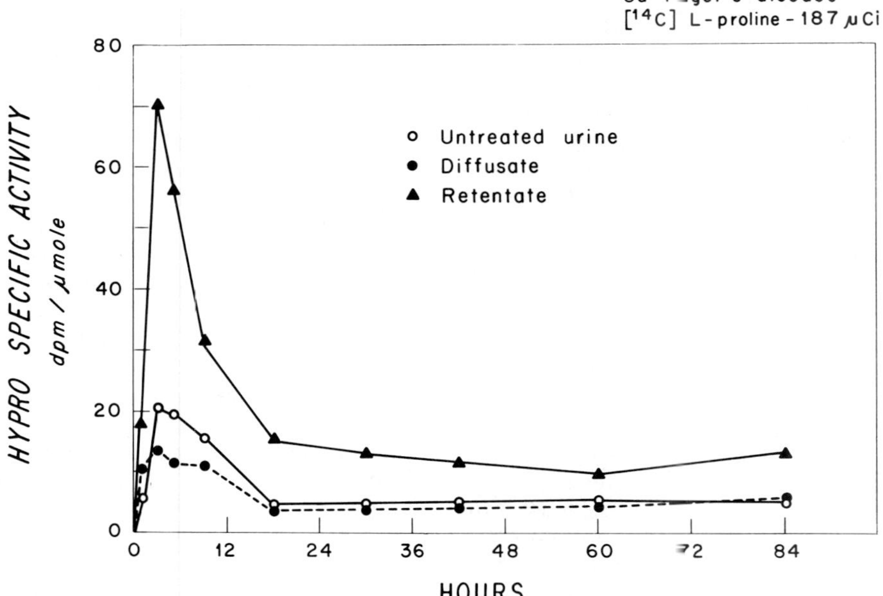

Figure 15–38. Multiple specific activities of ^{14}C-hydroxyproline (hypro) in urine and its fractions after dialysis as a function of time after administration of ^{14}C-proline to a patient with Paget's disease. (From Krane SM, et al: Science 157:713, 1967. Copyright 1967 by the American Association for the Advancement of Science.)

dopeptidases to yield the helical trimers.[122,126,166] One of the urinary peptides analyzed by Szymanowicz[167] contained one third glycine (Gly) and approximately equal amounts of proline (Pro) and hydroxyproline (Hyp) and could thus be composed of at least five -Gly-Pro-Hyp triplets and arise from the minor collagen helix of the amino-terminal propeptide of either the pro alpha$_1$(I) or pro alpha$_2$(I) chain. In preliminary findings using chromatofocusing and high-performance liquid chromatography, we have purified a similar peptide from pagetic urine as well as other peptides whose sequences match those in regions of the pro alpha$_1$(I) chain (M. van der Rest, L.S. Simon, M. Byrne, and S.M. Krane, unpublished).

On the basis of the sequences, the molecular weight of at least some of these peptides is lower than we originally estimated. Depending on their position on the collagen chains of each of these nondialyzable urinary polypeptides, the evidence is most consistent with their origin in newly synthesized chains or portions of chains in bone, which are then selectively removed soon after synthesis or in the amino-terminal peptides of type I collagen.

The pattern of alteration in the metabolism of mineral ions and the matrix components considered up to this point in patients with Paget's disease is thus consistent with the high rate of skeletal turnover inferred from radiologic and histologic observations of the course of the disorder. We noted that the mineral ion kinetics probably overestimate the mean rate of bone calcium deposition and resorption and that the total urinary hydroxyproline excretion reflects both (bone) collagen synthesis and degradation. The urinary hydroxyproline contained in low molecular weight fractions largely reflects collagen breakdown. An unknown portion of these peptides, however, is cleaved to yield free hydroxyproline, which in turn is further degraded in the liver.[148] Therefore, the calculation of collagen degradation based on the excretion of hydroxyproline peptides alone gives too low an estimate. Determination of the glycosylated hydroxylysines[127,128,130,150-152,156] provides a more accurate index of collagen degradation, since their further metabolism is relatively limited. Despite these caveats, we have estimated the amount of bone resorbed in a number of pagetic patients based on ^{47}Ca kinetics compared with that based on total urinary hydroxyproline excretion as shown in Table 15–1. Since the level of hydroxyproline excretion was high in these subjects, sources of collagen other than bone would be expected to contribute little to total excretion, and the figure based on matrix resorption would be a minimum one. Therefore, the magnitude of the turnover determined by ^{47}Ca kinetics is not unreasonable.

6. Serum Procollagen Peptides

The potential value of assays of procollagen peptides as markers of collagen synthesis was first explored by Goldberg et al.[168,169] and Taubman et al.,[170] who developed antibodies to carboxyl-terminal fragments of type I collagen purified from human fibroblast–conditioned medium. Since the procollagen peptide extensions of type I collagen are cleaved prior to fibril formation, measurements of these peptides would theoretically be of considerable value if they were not extensively degraded by proteases before release into the circulation. The carboxyl-terminal propeptide of type I procollagen is a heterotrimer of approximately 110 K_d that is stabilized by interchain disulfide bonds. Taubman et al.[170] described elevated levels of these peptides (which we termed pColl-I-C[125]) in the serum of patients with Paget's disease compared with normal subjects, and the levels of these peptides correlated with the extent and activity of the disease, determined by the activity of serum alkaline phosphatase.

We corroborated these findings in a more recent report[125] in which we also observed a decrease in the levels of pColl-I-C in pagetic subjects who received dichloromethylene bisphosphonate for 4 to 7 months. Furthermore, we observed an acute fall in the levels of p-Coll-I-C in patients given single subcutaneous injections of salmon calcitonin. There are several explanations for these results, including the possibilities that these fragments are released when bone is resorbed or that these therapies alter the metabolism of the procollagen peptides. We interpreted these results, however, as indicating that the fall in pColl-I-C following administration of calcitonin or bisphosphonates reflects a decrease in bone formation coupled to the decrease in resorption, similar to that observed using measurements of nondialyzable urinary hydroxyproline.[171]

We also found that levels of the amino-terminal propeptide of type III procollagen (pColl-III-N), determined by radioimmunoassay,[172] were elevated in serum from patients with Paget's disease and that the levels correlated in most individuals with the extent and/or activity of the disease.[125] We presume that the elevated serum levels of pColl-III-N in Paget's disease result from synthesis of type III procollagen by the stromal fibroblasts in close proximity to the pagetic bone spicules.

Unfortunately, the levels of the procollagen peptides may be modulated by alterations in metabolic clearance, and we have no data pertinent to metabolism of these peptides with the exception that no pColl-I-C immunoreactivity can be detected in urine.[125] The pColl-I-C is released before collagen fibers are formed, however, and there is no evidence that this peptide is entrapped in mineralized bone. The situation is different with respect to pColl-III-N, which is probably retained within the collagen matrix in normal skin. It has been proposed by Fleischmajer et al.[173,174] that pColl-III-N cleaved from type III procollagen can fit into the holes formed by the staggered packing of collagen molecules but that the more cumbersome carboxyl-terminal peptide of either type I or III procollagen cannot. Thus, it is unlikely that resorption of bone collagen results in the release of the carboxyl-terminal peptides of type I procollagen, although resorption of the fibrous stroma could result in the release of amino-terminal peptides of type III procollagen. Since the levels of type III procollagen peptides remain elevated above normal while the levels of serum alkaline phosphatase and p-Coll-I-C fall to within the normal range after treatment of the Paget's disease with dichloromethylene bisphosphonate, stromal fibroblasts synthesizing the loose fibrous stroma containing type III collagen may be less sensitive to the drug than the osteoblasts synthesizing type I procollagen. Similar findings were reported in a recent study of calcitonin treatment.[174a]

It should also be pointed out that the amino-terminal peptides of both types I and III procollagens have a potential functional role in bone remodeling. The amino-terminal propeptides have been proposed as negative feedback regulators of collagen synthesis that inhibit translation of procollagen mRNAs.[175,176]

7. Metabolism of Noncollagenous Bone Proteins in Paget's Disease of Bone (see Chapter 8)

Circulating levels of alpha$_2$HS-glycoprotein have been measured in patients with Paget's disease of bone and found on the average to be lower than those in normal adults.[177] The levels are inversely related to the activity of plasma alkaline phosphatase. These decreases of the concentration of alpha$_2$HS-glycoprotein in pagetic *serum* are to be contrasted with increases in pagetic *bone*,[134] and are consistent with the idea that alpha$_2$HS-glycoprotein is synthesized in the liver, circulates in plasma, and is taken up into newly synthesized bone matrix.[178] When the pagetic subjects were treated either with a bisphosphonate or calcitonin, the serum levels of alpha$_2$HS-glycoprotein tended to increase toward normal.[177] The changes observed after calcitonin therapy were considered to be too rapid and too large to be accounted for on the basis of decrease in bone formation alone, and the possibility of increased hepatic synthesis was raised.

Levels of bone Gla-protein have also been found to be increased on the average in individuals with Paget's disease compared with normal subjects.[179-185a] Although in some series very high levels of alkaline phosphatase activity have been associated with only slight increases in bone Gla-protein levels, there has been on the average a significant positive correlation between serum levels of bone Gla-protein and activity of alkaline phosphatase in untreated patients with Paget's disease.[182] The serum levels of bone Gla-protein, however, have not always fallen when the Paget's disease has been treated with bisphosphonates to the extent predicted based on changes in total urinary hydroxyproline excretion and serum activity of alkaline phosphatase. We have actually noted marked increases during long-term calcitonin therapy in most patients (Table 15–2). Thus, in Paget's disease, levels of bone Gla-protein are not sensitive markers of pagetic bone turnover and may not reflect the same aspects of bone metabolism or even the same cellular source (e.g., osteoblasts versus bone

Table 15–2. Serum Alkaline Phosphatase, Urinary Hydroxyproline, and Serum Bone Gla-Protein (Osteocalcin) Levels Before and During Long-term Human Calcitonin (HCT) Treatment

Patient	Therapy and Duration	Serum Alkaline Phosphatase B-L-B U/ml (normal 1–3)	Urinary Hydroxyproline mg/24 hr (normal <40)	Serum Bone Gla-Protein pM/ml
1	Control	30	178	26
	HCT 0.5 mg/day 1.7 years	6.3	77	46
2	Control	43.1	362	33
	HCT 0.5 mg/day 7 years	9.9	130	314
3	Control	44.4	493	45
	HCT 0.5 mg/day 4.5 years	12.4	188	110
4	Control	71.7	1952	126
	HCT 0.5 mg/day 8.5 years	28.2	961	>314
5	Control	39	551	21
	HCT 0.5 mg/day 4.75 years	21.3	289	>314
6	Control	15.1	95	23
	HCT 0.5 mg/day 4 years	1.2	20	116
7	Control	9.5	173	80
	HCT 0.5 mg/day	1.3	47	38

Serum bone Gla-protein measurements provided by Dr. Bayard Catherwood.

stromal fibroblasts). Observations that urinary excretion of total Gla (*not* bone Gla-protein) is not different in pagetic subjects compared with normals[186] simply reflect the fact that there are many sources of Gla (such as several clotting factors) other than bone Gla-proteins. Total urinary Gla is therefore not a useful discriminant in Paget's disease.

Radioimmunoassays have also been developed that permit measurement of circulating osteonectin. In a preliminary report,[187] levels were found to be increased in patients with Paget's disease but not to the extent observed even using immunoassays for bone Gla-protein. Indeed, no correlation was found between serum levels of osteonectin and those of bone Gla-protein in Paget's disease or other forms of metabolic bone disease.

C. Acute Effects of Calcitonin

The use of the calcitonins in treatment of Paget's disease will be discussed subsequently. The acute effects of calcitonin are so striking in pagetic subjects, however, that it is appropriate to discuss them as they relate to bone turnover. Bijvoet et al.[157] were the first to demonstrate that a decrease in serum calcium and phosphorus concentrations was readily produced by injection of porcine calcitonin in pagetic patients, whereas no such response was detected in normal subjects. The fall in serum calcium was accompanied by a marked decrease in plasma levels and urinary excretion of hydroxyproline peptides. These results were confirmed and extended to include the effects of salmon calcitonin by Singer et al.[105] and Krane et al.[171] The major decrease in hydroxyproline excretion occurs in the oligopeptide fraction. Observations that in response to calcitonin administration, the ratio of Hyl(Glc-Gal)/Hyl(Gal) rises (from the low values of bone) as the total hydroxylysine and hydroxyproline fall are consistent with a calcitonin-induced decrease in degradation of bone collagen rather than collagen from some other source.[130]

The acute decrease in bone resorption induced by calcitonin appears to be due to an inhibition of osteoclastic activity. Within 30 minutes after administration of calcitonin to pagetic patients, the osteoclasts become less adherent to bone, lose their ruffled borders, and begin to fragment (Fig. 15–39). It thus seems reasonable to conclude, since the calcitonins have been shown to have their major action on decreasing bone resorption, that the pagetic subjects in whom bone turnover is markedly accelerated would show the greatest serum calcium response to a decrease in bone resorption. This conclusion is based in part on the demonstration that normal subjects respond to calcitonin by decreasing total urinary hydroxyproline excretion without significantly changing serum calcium levels.[130] The fall in total urinary hydroxyproline excretion in normal subjects is similar in percentage to that seen in patients with Paget's disease, although the absolute decrease is orders of magnitude less. In the normal subjects, as in the patients with Paget's disease, the decrease in excretion of polypeptide hydroxyproline and the increase in the ratio of polypeptide/oligopeptide excreted occur at the nadir of the calcitonin response. As an explanation of these observations, we proposed that the decrease in plasma and urinary hydroxyproline is greater than the decrease in plasma calcium because the size of the exchangeable calcium pool is large relative to rates of entry into this pool, even in Paget's disease in which the amount of calcium entering and leaving the pool is much greater than normal. In contrast, the size of the pool of small peptides containing hydroxyproline is small relative to rates of entry into this pool from degradation of collagen. Therefore, a given decrease in resorption would more profoundly affect the size of the oligopeptide hydroxyproline pool than that of the calcium pool. The results of this study further suggest that an acute decrease in bone matrix formation (as shown by decrease in excretion of polypeptide hydroxyproline) accompanies the fall in bone resorption. Other evidence for a decrease in bone matrix formation is provided by observations that there is a corresponding acute fall in circulating levels of the carboxyl-terminal procollagen peptide pColl-I-C within hours after administration of calcitonin.[125] Whether this response is mediated by parathyroid hormone, which can acutely decrease collagen synthesis, or by a fall in the level of plasma phosphorus is not known.

D. Citrate Metabolism

A large fraction of total body citrate is present in bone, where it is bound to calcium

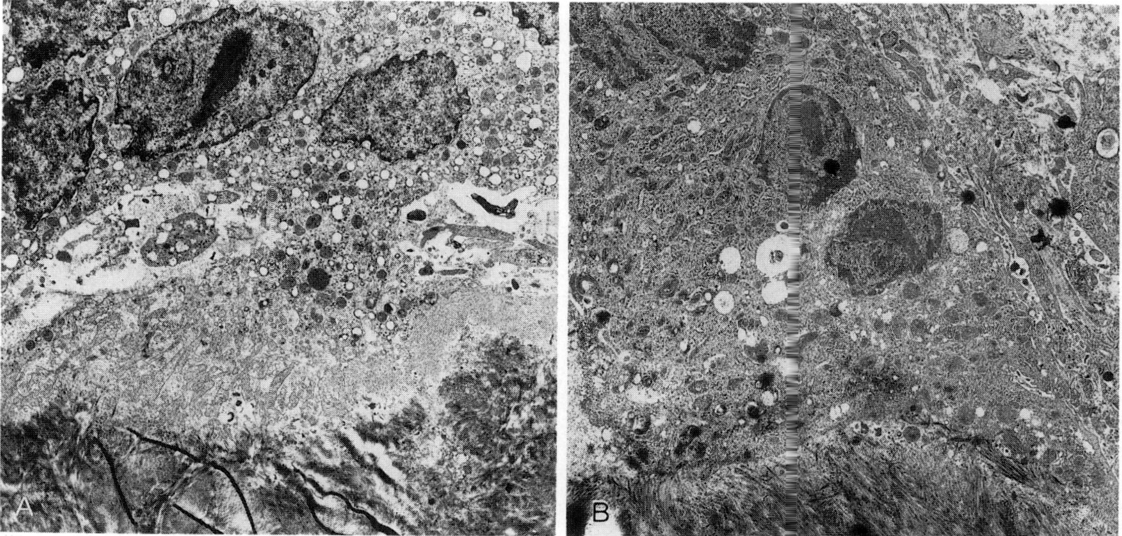

Figure 15–39. Electron micrographs of iliac crest biopsies taken from a 60-year-old woman with Paget's disease prior to *A* and 30 minutes following 20 μg salmon calcitonin IV *B*. *A*, Edge of active osteoclast showing wide ruffled border containing collagen fibrils and bone mineral. Note numerous as well as large vacuoles immediately adjacent to the ruffled border (×4200). *B*, Osteoclast displaying reduction in activity shown by the loss of the ruffled border and relatively smooth appearance of the cytoplasmic membrane bordering bone. Note the reduction in numbers of vacuoles but an increase in autophagic vacuoles compared with the initial biopsy (×7800). (Courtesy of Dr. Barbara G. Mills.)

ions on the surface of the calcium-phosphorus mineral phase. When bone is resorbed, the release of calcium ions is accompanied in many systems by release of citrate.[188,189] Parathyroid hormone inhibits citrate oxidation and release in bone and other tissues[190,191] and increases plasma citrate levels. Hypocitremia follows parathyroidectomy and the citrate levels can be restored by administration of parathyroid hormone.[191] Calcitonin decreases the effects of parathyroid hormone on citrate accumulation by bone in culture[190] and decreases plasma citrate when administered to rats.[191]

In human diseases associated with decreased bone resorption, such as hypoparathyroidism, reduced concentrations of serum citrate are found, whereas in hypercalcemic states such as hyperparathyroidism with osteitis fibrosa,[192] citrate levels are usually increased.[193] Urinary citrate levels parallel those of calcium in patients with renal stone disease, with and without hyperparathyroidism[194] and the administration of parathyroid extract increases the urinary citrate excretion in hypoparathyroidism.[195]

In Paget's disease, the serum citrate levels may be elevated in patients with high alkaline phosphatase levels even though the serum calcium levels are normal.[196] This is consistent with other evidence of increased bone resorption. We have measured urinary citrate excretion by the method of Natelson et al.[197] in a few patients with extensive Paget's disease. Basal levels of excretion in two patients with severe disease were 600 and 1390 μg per milligram creatinine, and total hydroxyproline excretion was 61■ and 1300 μg per milligram creatinine, respectively. Although the range of citrate excretion in normal subjects is broad[198] and there is some diurnal variation in the excretion pattern, it is probable that the citrate excretion in the more severely affected subject was increased. However, in both patients, citrate excretion increased strikingly following calcitonin injection. In the subject whose data are shown in Figure 15–40, serum citrate levels prior to calcitonin infusion were elevated to 4.9 mg/100 ml, well above the upper limit of normal of 3.6 mg/100 ml.[192] At the peak of the response to calcitonin, citrate levels fell to 4.1 mg/100 ml and citrate clearance increased from 13.9 to 37.0 ml/minute. It is probable that the initial fall in serum citrate resulted from calcitonin suppression of bone resorption but that the increased urinary citrate excretion and clearance was due to an increase in secretion of parathyroid hormone.

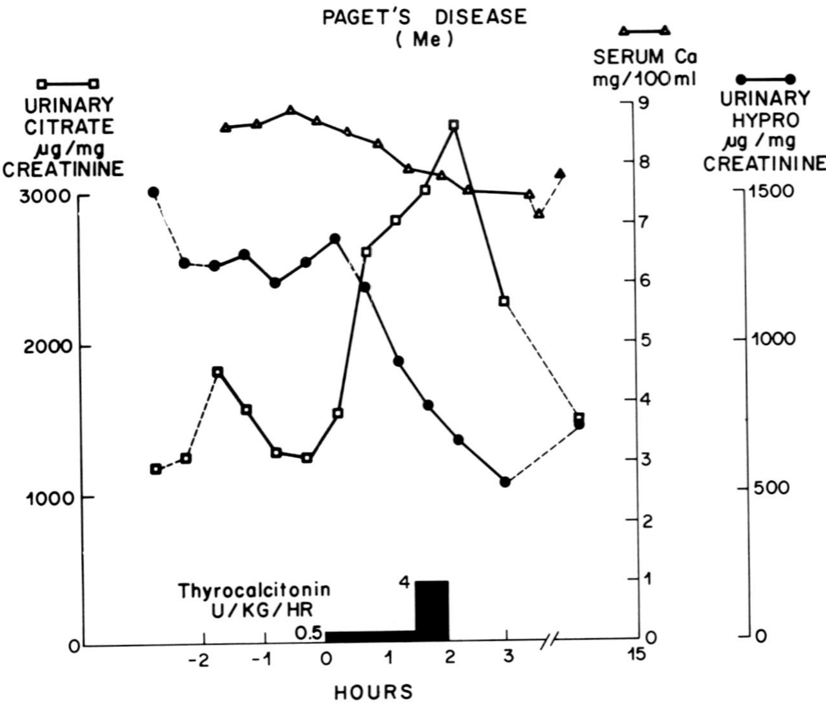

Figure 15–40. Acute effect of porcine calcitonin on serum calcium and urinary hydroxyproline and citrate excretion in a 69-year-old woman with Paget's disease.

E. Serum Alkaline Phosphatase

The role of alkaline phosphatase in bone and its pattern of variation in disease in general has been discussed in detail in Chapters 1 and 8. A few comments are pertinent here, however. Alkaline phosphatase in bone is localized in osteoblasts. Although the role of this enzyme is still not clear, there is a strong correlation between biological mineralization and high alkaline phosphatase levels in bone-derived cells such as cultured osteosarcoma cells. This alkaline phosphatase has the properties of the "bone-liver-kidney" enzyme, one of the three members of the alkaline phosphatase gene family.[199,200] Differences in chemical properties of the enzymes from bone, liver, and kidney are accounted for by posttranslational modifications including sialylation.[200] Elevation of the level of alkaline phosphatase in serum is characteristically seen in patients with Paget's disease, an observation made first by Kay.[201] Indeed, the highest recorded values for alkaline phosphatase are found in patients with Paget's disease. The level correlates with the extent as well as the activity of the disease, as does the level of urinary hydroxyproline excretion. Serum alkaline phosphatase and urinary hydroxyproline excretion also correlate with each other[58,155,156] (Fig. 15–41). In almost all studies, the circulating alkaline phosphatase in Paget's disease is indistinguishable from that normally present in bone or in plasma in other bone diseases. Recently, alkaline phosphatase purified from pagetic serum was found to behave differently from the enzymes purified to homogeneity from several other human tissues, that is, liver, kidney, intestine, and placenta.[202] When the native pagetic enzyme was desialylated, however, it behaved identically with respect to electrophoretic and isoelectric focusing properties with the desialylated forms from liver and kidney, but could be distinguished from the desialylated enzyme from placenta or intestine. In two pagetic subjects who were plasmaphoresed and the plasma replaced with albumin, the alkaline phosphatase activity that fell immediately to one third the initial levels returned to baseline within 10 to 15 days. The biological half-life of the enzyme in these subjects was therefore approximately 1 to 2 days.[203]

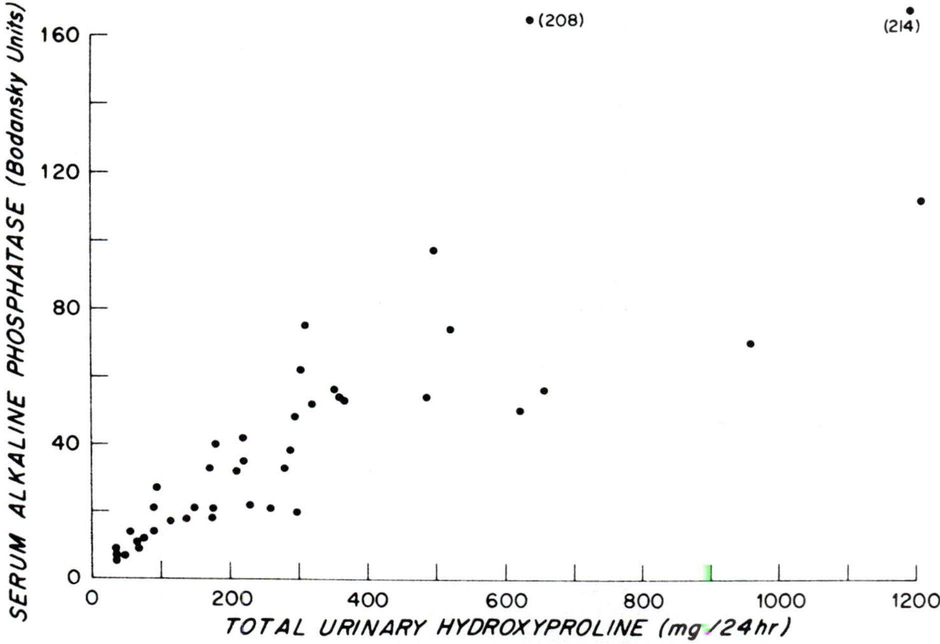

Figure 15–41. The relationship between serum alkaline phosphatase and urinary hydroxyproline excretion in 42 patients with Paget's disease. (Data calculated from Franck et al.[58])

It is distinctly unusual to see markedly elevated levels of alkaline phosphatase in subjects with Paget's disease who have isolated involvement of a small bone such as a vertebral body, and, indeed, the levels may be normal in 15% of patients with only one or two lesions determined by ^{99m}Tc-diphosphonate imaging.[199] Isolated involvement of larger bones, however, is associated with a broad range of phosphatase levels. In our experience, involvement of the skull alone is often associated with levels of phosphatase higher in proportion to the percentage of skeleton involved; the converse is true for pelvic involvement.[58] In general, with increasing numbers of pagetic lesions there is an approximately linear correlation of number with alkaline phosphatase levels.[204] When the disorder enters the sclerotic or osteoblastic phase and cellular activity decreases, even extensive involvement may be associated with limited elevations.

In patients followed over years, the levels of alkaline phosphatase tend to show a long-term upward trend with a tendency to plateau in a range characteristic for that individual.[205] Some patients show cyclic fluctuations about this more or less constant baseline. Although "explosive" elevations in serum alkaline phosphatase have been observed in individuals in whom osteosarcoma develops on the background of Paget's disease, this is an unusual occurrence and is not discussed at all in most large series.[206]

F. Other Phosphatases

In patients with Paget's disease and moderately elevated alkaline phosphatase levels, the activity of 5′-nucleotidase is usually normal. Modest elevations in 5′-nucleotidase may be seen, however, in serum from patients with very high alkaline phosphatase levels.[207] The level of acid phosphatase is usually normal in patients with Paget's disease, although in subjects with widespread, advanced lesions and very high alkaline phosphatase levels, mild elevations of acid phosphatase levels may also be encountered.[208] Using monophenyl phosphate as substrate, it was found that 18% of 96 patients with Paget's disease had levels between 3.0 and 4.9 units and only 3% between 5.0 and 9.9 units (normal value < 3.0 units). When beta-glycerophosphate was the substrate, however, in only one pagetic patient out of more than 100 was an elevation of acid phosphatase noted.[205,209] Recently, a spectrophotometric assay for tartrate-resistant acid phosphatase activity was proposed as a marker of osteoclastic activity.[209a] High levels were found in the serum of patients with Paget's disease.

VII. SYSTEMIC COMPLICATIONS AND ASSOCIATED DISEASES

A. Hypercalciuria, Renal Calculi, and Hypercalcemia

Urinary calcium excretion in patients with Paget's disease may be high, low, or normal[210] since the amount excreted appears to be dependent on the rates of bone resorption and formation relative to each other,[8] as well as on homeostatic influences such as variations in the secretion of parathyroid hormone in response to changes in plasma calcium concentrations. In the majority of patients with Paget's disease, however, rates of resorption and formation are similar and therefore urinary calcium excretion is usually normal. In those patients in whom bone resorption is greater than formation, hypercalciuria is more likely to occur. Hypercalciuria may also occur when this equilibrium is disturbed, for example, following fractures or in association with extended immobilization.[211]

In an individual patient, hypercalciuria may predispose to the formation of renal calculi. This is not a common complication of Paget's disease, although in one series 15.6% of patients had urinary calculi.[212] Nagant de Deuxchaisnes and Krane,[8] after reviewing the literature on this subject, found an overall incidence of 5% among 1382 pagetic patients. Two factors other than the Paget's disease probably account for such an association. First, since patients with urinary calculi frequently have roentgenograms of the abdomen and pelvis, asymptomatic and presumably incidental Paget's disease in these areas would be detected more readily. Second, prostatic hypertrophy, which is common in elderly males, often leads to urinary tract obstruction, infection, and calculi. Ridlon[213] found that more than half of 22 pagetic patients with urinary calculi had prostatic hypertrophy.

Hypercalcemia is distinctly uncommon in patients with Paget's disease. Nagant de Deuxchaisnes and Krane[8] were able to find in the literature only 17 patients with a serum calcium greater than 12 mg/100 ml after excluding those patients with coincidental hyperparathyroidism and multiple myeloma. In several of these reported instances it was uncertain that analysis of serum calcium levels was performed with sufficient accuracy to be confident about its interpretation. Reifenstein and Albright[211] reported originally that hypercalcemia developed in immobilized patients with Paget's disease, and it is difficult to separate the general effects of immobilization from the local effects of fractures.

Hypercalcemia in patients with Paget's disease may also develop as a result of coincidental hyperparathyroidism[214-216] or malignancy.[217] Rarely hyperparathyroidism may be misdiagnosed as Paget's disease because of radiologic similarities in pelvic lesions.[216] A complete skeletal survey and, if necessary, measurement of serum parathyroid hormone concentration should distinguish the two disorders. Secondary hyperparathyroidism with or without mild hypocalcemia has been reported in some patients with Paget's disease and normal renal function.[218,218a] This has been attributed to an increased rate of bone formation compared with that of resorption that may occasionally be observed. It was pointed out earlier that histomorphometric findings consistent with secondary hyperparathyroidism have been found in nonpagetic bone from patients with Paget's disease.[41]

B. Hyperuricemia and Gout

The association of Paget's disease and gout is commented upon in some of the early descriptions of Paget's disease.[212] Despite further reports of such an association between these two diseases,[219-222] there had been little evidence to indicate that patients with Paget's disease have an increased incidence of hyperuricemia or gout until we reported our studies of the concentration of serum uric acid and the incidence of gout in 47 patients with Paget's disease.[58] The results suggested that the pagetic process could be an etiologic factor in the development of gout. In this study of 28 men and 18 women, 19 patients (40.4%), 16 of whom were men, were found to be hyperuricemic. Serum uric acid concentrations in the group correlated with both the extent and the activity of the bone disease as defined by the percentage of bone involved radiologically, the serum alkaline phosphatase, and the total urinary hydroxyproline excretion. Seven of the males had clinical episodes of gouty arthritis. Urinary uric acid excretion was measured in six patients. Three were hyperuricosuric and three were hypouricosuric. The one patient who had a family history of gout had the most severe form of the disease (Fig. 15–42). It seemed reasonable to speculate that the turnover of nucleic acids in the active cells of pagetic bone might increase the urate pool and result in secondary hyperuricemia.[223] In a second large series, a history of gouty arthritis was present in only 11 of 149 patients and hyperuricemia was present in 20% of 118 patients not on allopurinol.[74] These findings were interpreted as indicating no increase in the levels of serum urate or the incidence of gout above that expected in the general population. It is probable that our series[58] included individuals with more severe disease and greater skeletal turnover, which may explain the different results. In a recent study of radionuclide imaging in patients with gout, 23% of the patients were found to have Paget's disease compared with 2.1% of a reference population who had had bone scans ordered for other reasons.[223a]

C. Calcific Periarthritis and Chondrocalcinosis

Franck et al.[58] reviewed the roentgenograms of multiple joints from 55 patients with Paget's disease and found a 36% incidence of periarticular calcifications. The association, although striking, could still be coincidental. The shoulders were most commonly involved but the elbow, wrist, hip, knee, metacarpophalangeal, and interphalangeal joints were also affected. Acute inflammatory episodes occurred in relation to these deposits. In general the calcifications were not adjacent to areas of Paget's disease and there was no correlation between the extent of the Paget's disease and the calcifications.

Radi et al.[224] have reported that six of 14 patients with Paget's disease had chondrocalcinosis on roentgenograms of wrists and knees. In contrast, Franck et al.[58] found only two instances of chondrocalcinosis in 54 patients who had wrist and knee films. The main difference between the two series was that the patients without chondrocalcinosis had a mean serum alkaline phosphatase level seven times greater than the mean in the patients with chondrocalcinosis. It is conceivable that the high concentrations of alkaline

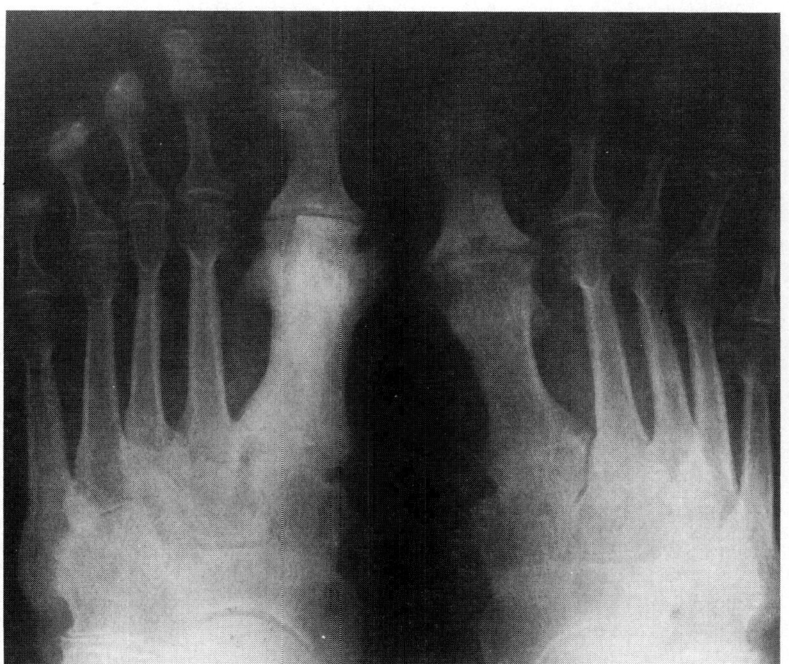

Figure 15–42. A 59-year-old man with gout and generalized Paget's disease who has both diseases involving the left first metatarsal. The pagetic bone is radiodense and widened. The associated scalloped destruction of the metatarsal head is due to gouty arthritis. (From Franck et al: Rheumatic manifestations of Paget's disease of bone. Am J Med 56:592–603, 1974.)

phosphatase, which acts as an organic pyrophosphate at neutral pH, by decreasing ambient concentrations of inorganic pyrophosphate would protect against the deposition of calcium pyrophosphate dihydrate crystals that characterize chondrocalcinosis.

D. Cardiovascular Complications

In the osteolytic and mixed phases of Paget's disease there is a marked increase in blood flow through involved extremities, manifested often by elevated skin temperature over the affected bone.[225] That this increased blood flow is not due to anatomic arteriovenous anastomoses but rather to increased perfusion of pagetic bone was shown by Rutishauser et al.,[226] who injected the vessels of such bone at autopsy, and by Rhodes et al.,[227] who showed, using injections of microspheres, that there are no such channels greater than 15 μm in diameter. Others have concluded that there is associated vascular hyperplasia and ectasia in pagetic bone.[228]

It has been found that most, if not all, of the increased blood flow to pagetic extremities can be accounted for by increased cutaneous flow, as measured with water plethysmographs and by demonstrating that epinephrine iontophoresis reduces blood flow of an affected extremity almost to normal.[229] In addition, local heating of the pagetic extremity fails to increase blood flow in the pagetic limb as it does in the normal limb. Thus, reflex cutaneous dilation is the likely explanation for the cutaneous hyperthermia and the elevated pO_2 in the venous blood of an involved limb. The extent to which increased vascularity of the bone proper contributes has been demonstrated using methods such as ^{18}F clearance,[230] which show increased flow in pagetic bone and reduction following treatment.[231,232]

Increased cardiac output secondary to increased blood flow to skeletal and nonskeletal tissue may be found in patients with generalized disease of at least 15% of the skeleton involved,[225,233-235] although we have observed increased cardiac output in patients with Paget's disease limited to the skull. This increased cardiac output in elderly individuals with Paget's disease may contribute to congestive heart failure, but particularly in the presence of other coexistent heart disease. It is generally responsive to the usual modes of treatment.

Intracardiac calcification has been reported in association with Paget's disease. Harrison and Lennox[236] concluded that such calcification of the cardiac tissues was five times more common in patients with generalized Paget's disease than in control subjects. Since the calcification may involve the interventricular septum and the aortic and mitral valves, heart block may develop as a result of septal calcifications. Usually, however, the valvular calcifications are not of clinical significance, although in one report a patient with Paget's disease and calcification of the interventricular septum and aortic and mitral valves developed complete heart block and required a permanent transvenous pacemaker.[237] Recently Strickberger et al.[237a] reported a correlation of calcific aortic valve disease with the severity of Paget's disease.

Arterial calcifications are also common in patients with Paget's disease. For example, O'Reilly and Race[210] found an incidence of 43% in their series. The calcifications are particularly common in limb arteries and may be detected by radiographic examination in as many as 50% of patients.[238] Such calcifications are generally of the Mönckeberg type (medial involvement and preservation of the lumen) and are usually of no clinical importance.

E. Pseudoxanthoma Elasticum, Angioid Streaks, and Skin Changes

The association of pseudoxanthoma elasticum and Paget's disease[239-241] has provoked speculation that Paget's disease may be a widespread disorder of connective tissue rather than a disease limited to the skeleton. Characteristics common to these two diseases include angioid streaks, vascular calcification, and skin calcification.[242] Although this concept is interesting, it is incompatible with the fact that the vast majority of patients with Paget's disease have normal skin and no excessive mobility of the joints.

We have examined skin biopsies from six patients with Paget's disease. Abnormal patterns of elastic fibers seen in four of these biopsies included a decrease in the number of the superficial fine elastic fibers with fragmentation and clumping of fibers as seen with elastic tissue stains. In the reticular layer, the coarse fibers were sparse and the few remaining ones greatly fragmented so that few interconnecting bundles were present. Such changes were also noted by Paton,[242] but he felt that after treatment with various connective tissue stains and digestion with beta-glucuronidase there was no evidence of any abnormality in the collagen or elastic fibers. Paton[242] explained his findings on the basis of the great variation of the cutaneous elastic fibers found normally in various portions of the body. We have not been able to refute this valid point, since the normal variations of cutaneous elastic fibers have not been well documented. Therefore, although the changes in the skin may be purely specious, we have recorded our findings so that future investigators may deal with this problem.

Although angioid streaks are found in 8% to 15% of advanced cases of Paget's disease,[242,243] comparatively little has been written about such lesions in Paget's disease (Fig. 15–43). The changes described for the angioid streaks seen in Paget's disease are histologically identical to those of pseudoxanthoma elasticum and include basophilia and cracking of Bruch's membrane and proliferation of fibrovascular tissue through the defects. It was suggested that since calcification may occur at the site of elastic fibers in the skin of patients with Paget's disease, the same event may occur in Bruch's membrane.[242] Bruch's membrane is a composite extracellular matrix resembling that of basement membranes and although it contains a thin elastin-bearing lamina, it does not contain the large elastic fibers found in the dermis.[244] There are no elastic fibers in bone except those found in the walls of large arteries.

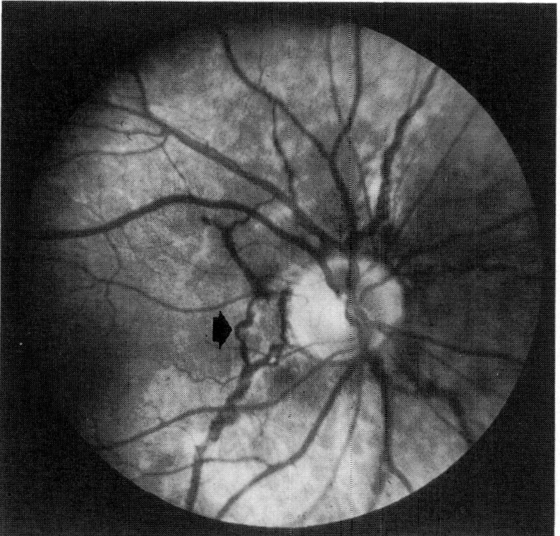

Figure 15–43. Multiple angioid streaks in Paget's disease (arrow indicates most extensive one).

Some evidence that supports the concept of a generalized connective tissue abnormality in Paget's disease was reported by Francis and Smith,[245] who examined the nature of skin collagen in 11 patients with Paget's disease and control subjects. They found a decreased amount and stability of the polymeric collagen fraction in the pagetic patients and speculated that a progressive failure of glycoprotein and collagen crosslinking reactions could account for the observed abnormalities. As previously discussed, however, there are no other indications of a major structural abnormality of bone collagen specific for Paget's disease.

F. Malabsorption Syndrome

Somayaji[246] described eight patients with Paget's disease who had a variable pattern of gastrointestinal malabsorption. Diarrhea, steatorrhea, xylose malabsorption, and folate deficiency were prominent features. It was postulated that secondary folate deficiency or relative ischemia of the bowel secondary to increased bone blood flow might be responsible for the observations. No confirmatory reports have been published.

VIII. DRUG TREATMENT

A. Indications

Most patients with Paget's disease require no treatment, since the disorder is usually asymptomatic and produces little or no morbidity. The advanced age of many affected individuals would also preclude the use of potentially toxic drugs. There are several criteria, however, that we propose for considering patients with Paget's disease as potential candidates for specific therapy. These have been grouped under definite and possible indications in Table 15–3.

Various modes of treatment affect certain manifestations of Paget's disease. Bone pain is decreased by a variety of drugs, and elevated cardiac output is diminished as a result of suppression of the activity of the disease. Numerous examples of improvement of neurologic deficits have been reported. Sup-

Table 15–3. Indications for Drug Treatment of Paget's Disease

Definite

Severe bone pain corresponding to areas of pagetic involvement as demonstrated by roentgenograms and/or isotope scanning procedures
Cardiac failure associated with a high output state
Hypercalcemia due to the Paget's disease
Recurrent renal calculi due to hypercalciuria
Neurologic deficit arising from vertebral disease
Elective orthopedic surgery involving pagetic bone or associated with prolonged immobilization

Possible

Multiple fractures in pagetic bone
Early onset of Paget's disease in an area where disabling deformity or hearing loss is to be anticipated
Prevention of osteogenic sarcoma
Otherwise unexplained disabling weakness and fatigue in a patient with severe, extensive Paget's disease

pression of disease activity and vascularity prior to elective surgery on affected bones appears to reduce the risk of excessive blood loss, although this has not been examined in controlled trials. There have been no formal studies on the use of drugs in the control of hypercalcemia, hypercalciuria, or gout in pagetic patients, although on theoretical grounds there is a strong likelihood that suppression of the disease would help correct these complications. Much more careful investigation will be required to determine the effect of treatment in prevention of pathologic fractures or osteogenic sarcoma. If it can be shown that drug treatment not only can suppress existing disease over prolonged periods of time but also can prevent the appearance of lesions in other bones, it would be important to treat younger patients with mild Paget's disease in order to avoid future major disabilities. There are some patients with widespread Paget's disease who have disabling weakness and lassitude. If such clinical problems cannot be explained by other disease mechanisms, then treatment of the Paget's disease may be considered.

Effective therapeutic agents such as the calcitonins and the bisphosphonates appear to act primarily by decreasing bone resorption through effects on osteoclasts and the generation of osteoclasts. Thus, a temporary state results in which bone formation rate exceeds bone resorption rate. With time, however, the bone formation rate also falls and coupling is restored. Effective therapy therefore converts a high bone turnover state to a lower turnover state in which the new bone formed appears structurally normal.

B. Calcitonin

Calcitonin is a peptide hormone, the main pharmacologic property of which is to decrease bone resorption. This effect results from the inhibition of the function of osteoclasts present in bone (an acute response) and a decrease in the number of osteoclasts, which probably results from a decreased generation of osteoclasts from the hematopoietic precursors (chronic response).

Milhaud and colleagues[247] suggested and Bijvoet and colleagues[157,248] and Canniggia and Gennari[249] first demonstrated that calcitonin produces an early, dramatic hypocalcemic effect in patients with Paget's disease. Bijvoet et al.[157] noted a striking, acute decrease in urinary hydroxyproline excretion in such patients, a response subsequently confirmed by Singer et al.[105(b2)]

Porcine calcitonin was used in the initial studies of the chronic effects of calcitonin in patients with Paget's disease.[250] When it was shown that salmon calcitonin was more potent in acutely lowering plasma calcium in humans, this form of the hormone was introduced into clinical trials.[105,250] Human calcitonin has been used to a lesser extent than the salmon hormone[250-252] and has only recently been approved for use in the United States.

The clinical experience in Paget's disease with all three forms of calcitonin has, in general, been similar. Calcitonins are administered by subcutaneous or intramuscular injection, usually on a daily basis. With few exceptions, affected individuals have responded with a fall in urinary hydroxyproline excretion within days and a fall in serum alkaline phosphatase levels within weeks. Calcium balance usually becomes more positive during the initial 1 to 4 months of treatment,[253-255] and continued treatment (9–19 months) is not associated with any change in calcium balance.[256] In one series of 38 patients treated up to 5 years, mean total of body calcium as assessed by neutron activation actually fell by 4%.[257] Histological examination of sequential bone biopsies in patients treated with calcitonin shows a reduction in osteoclast number as well as a reduction in woven bone and the extent of fibrosis of the bone marrow.[255,258]

The reported clinical benefits associated with chronic calcitonin therapy include relief of bone pain,[259,260] reduction of increased cardiac output,[261] reversal of central and peripheral neurologic deficits,[262] stabilization of hearing deficits,[263] healing of osteolytic lesions,[264,265] reduction of skeletal blood flow,[266] and prevention of excessive hemorrhage associated with orthopedic surgery.[267] Of particular interest is the radiologic improvement of osteolytic lesions, which is readily demonstrable during long-term therapy. An example of the efficacy of salmon calcitonin on healing of bone lesions is shown in Figure 15–44. In some patients the formation of a more normal cortex in long bones, the restoration of the corticomedullary junction, and a reduction in the total diameter of the shaft of expanded bones is observed. Beneficial effects on the skeletal lesions observed radiologically may, however, require larger doses of calcitonin than are needed to produce maximal biochemical suppression.[264] As would be expected, improvement in bone scans during long-term calcitonin therapy is also observed.[268] Gallium scans appear to be a more sensitive means of detecting responses to calcitonin therapy, perhaps because gallium uptake is a better index of bone cell activity.[269] This concept is supported by the recent finding that gallium localizes in the nuclei of osteoclasts in Paget's disease.[269]

Several patterns of response to calcitonin are apparent during long term treatment of Paget's disease. In one pattern, there are complete biochemical and clinical remissions[105,255] (Fig. 15–45). A more common pattern (the "plateau response") is that in which there is an initial decrease in indices of bone remodeling, but normalization of bone remodeling does not take place with continued treatment[105] (Fig. 15–46). Patients who show this pattern usually maintain clinical improvement associated with biochemical evidence of decreased bone turnover. On the average, the biochemical indices in these

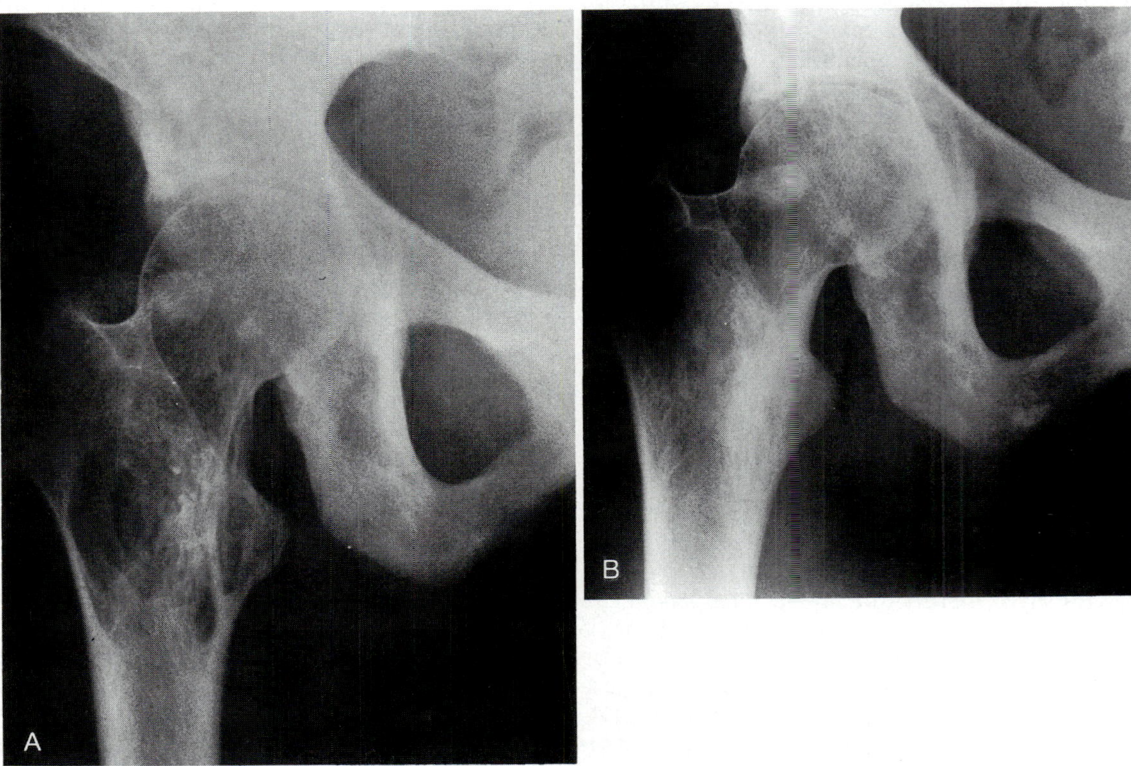

Figure 15–44. Osteolytic lesion in right proximal femur. *A*, Before treatment. *B*, Two years after treatment with salmon calcitonin. (Courtesy of Dr. Jane Mahaffey.)

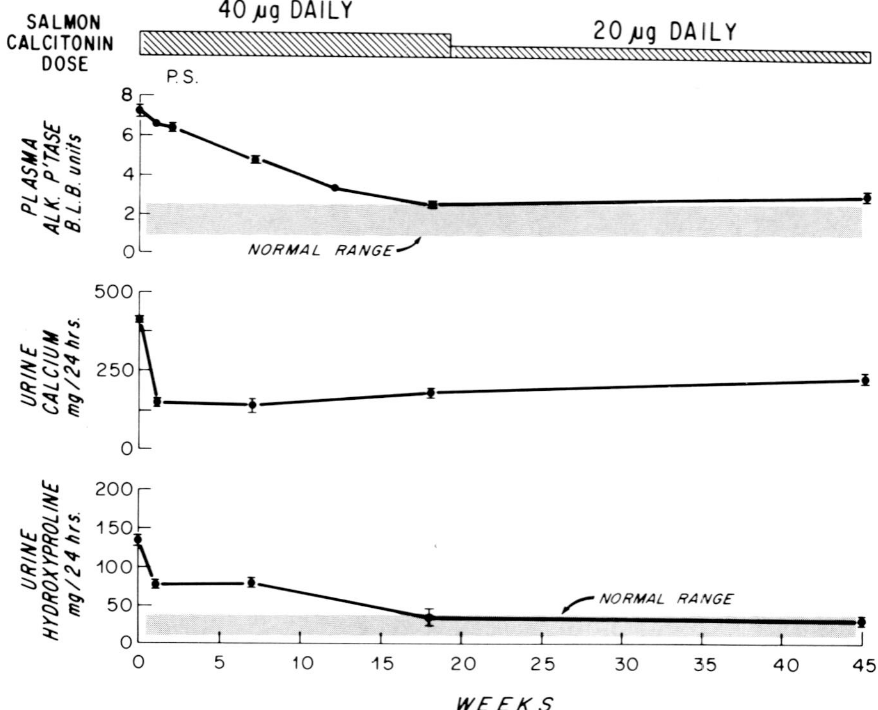

Figure 15–45. Result of a 45-week period of daily administration of salmon calcitonin to a 78-year-old man with Paget's disease. Data are expressed as mean ± SE of multiple determinations made during a one-week period before and during treatment. (From Singer FR, et al: Pharmacological effects of salmon calcitonin in man. *In* Talmage RV, Munson PL [eds]: Calcium, Parathyroid Hormone and the Calcitonins. Amsterdam, Excerpta Medica, 1972.)

patients are stabilized at approximately 50% of pretreatment levels. A third pattern is characterized by an initial response comparable to that in the other groups, but as treatment is continued, biochemical and clinical abnormalities recur[270-274] (Fig. 15–47).

The plateau response has been observed in patients treated with each type of calcitonin. In an attempt to exclude inadequate dosage of hormone as a factor in the plateau response, Singer and colleagues[105] increased the dose of salmon calcitonin up to 10-fold in four patients but found no significant further decreases in the biochemical indices of disease activity.

The third pattern of acquired resistance to the effects of calcitonin has been found in some patients treated with porcine,[274] salmon,[270,271,273,275,275a] or human calcitonin.[272] In the great majority of patients treated with the nonhuman calcitonins who become resistant to metabolic effects, high titers of antibodies to these species of calcitonin have been demonstrated in the circulation. Resistance to porcine,[274] salmon,[273-275] and human calcitonin,[272] however, may also rarely develop in the absence of detectable circulating antibodies. With the exception of a single individual treated with human calcitonin who developed clinically insignificant antibody titers,[276] antibodies to human calcitonin in treated patients have not been detected. It is not certain whether antibody-associated calcitonin resistance is a rare or common event. Martin and colleagues[275,277,278] found that only one individual out of 36 who were treated with salmon calcitonin became resistant owing to high antibody titers. Results of our own experience[270,273] suggest that resistance due to the formation of salmon calcitonin antibodies is a common event in the United States. Resistance to salmon calcitonin developed during long-term treatment in 22 of our 85 patients (26%).[272] Antibodies to salmon calcitonin were detected in 56 of the 85 patients (66%), and in 19 of the 19 patients whose antibody titer was 1:1500 or greater, calcitonin resistance was evident. Antibodies,

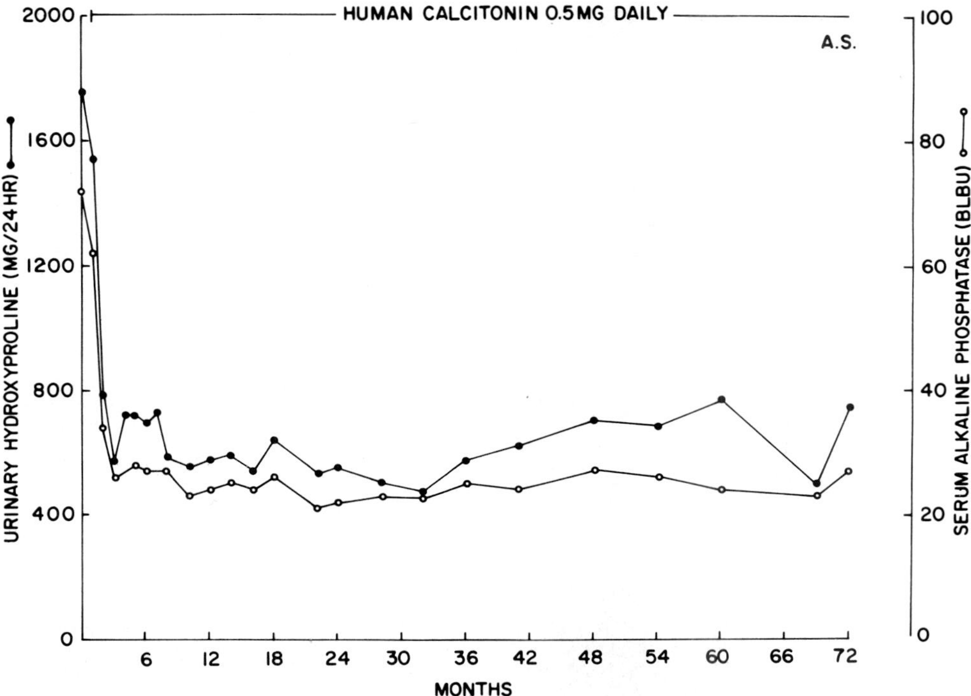

Figure 15–46. Result of a 72-month period of daily subcutaneous administration of human calcitonin to a 68-year-old man with Paget's disease. The upper limit of normal for urinary hydroxyproline is 40 mg/24 hr and for serum alkaline phosphatase activity is 3 Bessey-Lowrey-Brock units.

in titer < 1:1500, did not interfere with the efficacy of long-term therapy. In the three patients who became resistant to calcitonin in the absence of antibodies, no other explanation could be established for the mechanism of resistance. Further evidence for the clinical significance of high antibody titers is established by the observation that 15 of 15 resistant patients (including five unpublished cases) have responded to treatment with human calcitonin.[273,279] These results are consistent with those studies *in vitro* in which it has been demonstrated that antibodies to salmon calcitonin do not bind human calcitonin. An example of successful response to human calcitonin of a patient who was resistant to salmon calcitonin is illustrated in Figures 15–48 and 15–49.

Another factor that might alter the clinical response of patients treated with calcitonin is the stimulation of parathyroid hormone secretion secondary to calcitonin-induced hypocalcemia.[105] Dube and colleagues[280] observed a slight elevation of the levels of serum immunoreactive parathyroid hormone in five patients treated with porcine calcitonin and proposed that the development of secondary hyperparathyroidism could account for resistance to calcitonin. Burckhardt and colleagues[106] studied the parathyroid hormone response to calcitonin-induced hypocalcemia in 12 patients with Paget's disease before and during treatment with salmon calcitonin and also observed increases in serum levels of parathyroid hormone. *Hyper*secretion after prolonged treatment, however, was not observed. Other investigators also found no evidence of hyperparathyroidism in their patients.[256,274,281-283] The possibility remains, however, that the persistent stimulation of parathyroid hormone secretion may interfere with the clinical response. Conclusive evidence for this response would be provided only if the histologic changes of hyperparathyroidism were to be documented in bone uninvolved with Paget's disease. There is suggestive evidence of hyperparathyroidism in nonpagetic bone of individuals treated with human calcitonin,[281] although a similar appearance has also been described in untreated patients.[41]

Attempts have also been made to suppress the activity of Paget's disease by stimulating

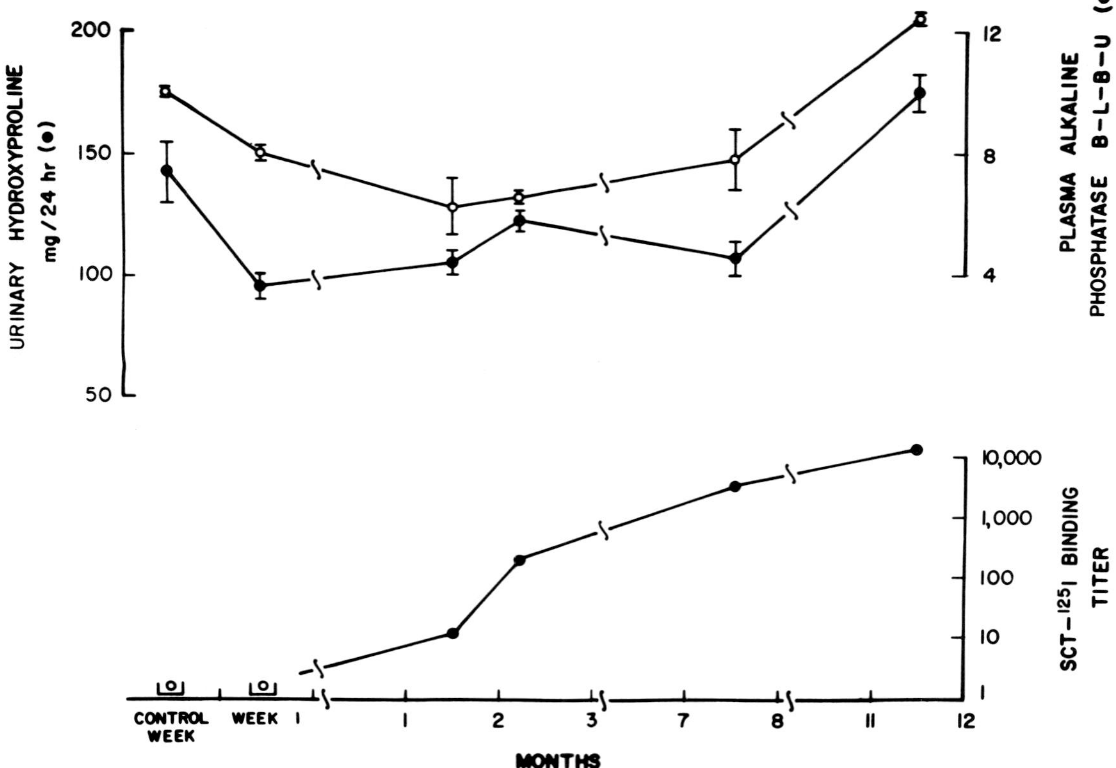

Figure 15–47. The control and treatment levels of urinary hydroxyproline, plasma alkaline phosphatase and salmon calcitonin-^{125}I binding titer during an 11.5-month period when a 51-year-old male received 100 MRC units of salmon calcitonin daily. The hydroxyproline data points represent the mean SE of at least five 24-hr urine collections during a one-week period. The upper limit of normal is 40 mg/24 hr. The alkaline phosphatase data points represent the mean SE of at least three blood samples taken during the week. The upper limit of normal is 2.6 Bessey-Lowrey-Brock units. The binding titer is plotted on a log scale. (From Singer FR, et al: J Clin Invest 51:2331, 1972.)

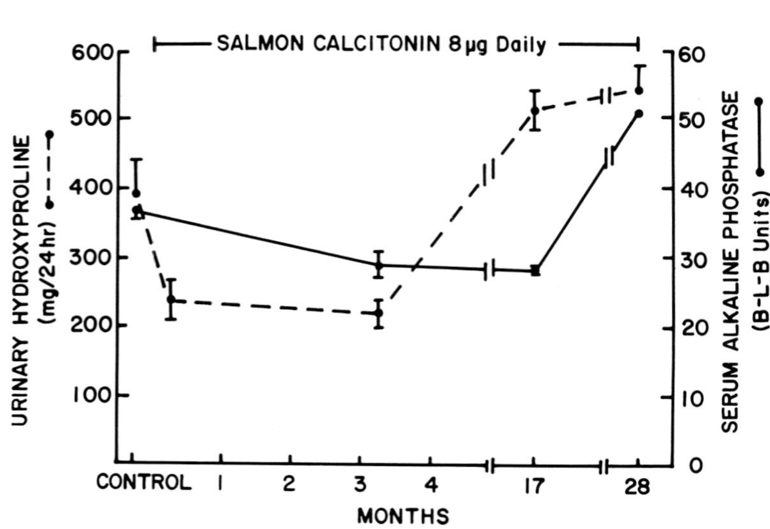

Figure 15–48. Response of a 62-year-old woman treated for 28 months with subcutaneous salmon calcitonin. After an initial decrease of bone turnover, she became resistant to continuing treatment. Antibodies to salmon calcitonin were present in her serum at a titer of 1:8000 at 28 months. (From Singer FR, Rude RK, Mills BG: Studies of the treatment and aetiology of Paget's disease of bone. *In* MacIntyre I (ed): Human Calcitonin and Paget's Disease. Bern, H. Huber, 1977, pp. 93–110.)

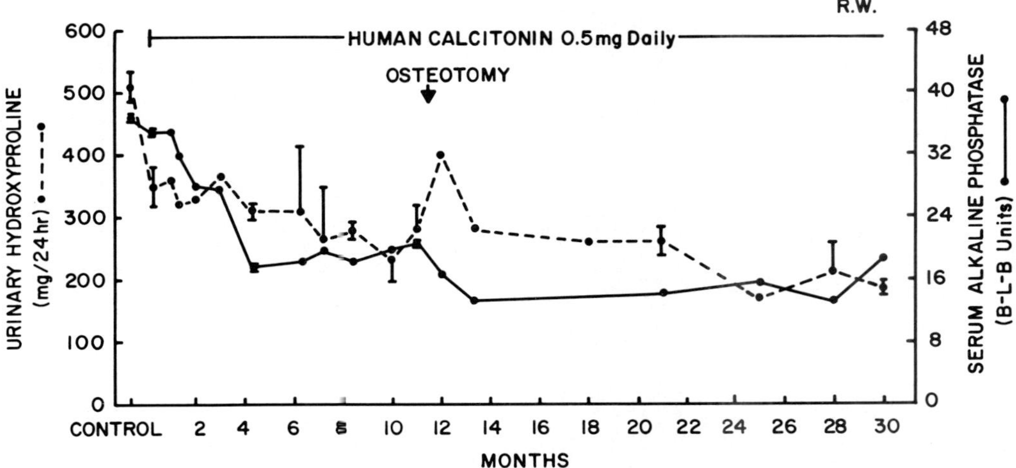

Figure 15–49. Results of human calcitonin treatment of the patient with resistance to salmon calcitonin illustrated in Figure 15–48. Note the continuing response after 30 months. (From Singer FR, Rude RK, Mills BG: Studies of the treatment and aetiology of Paget's disease of bone. *In* MacIntyre I (ed): Human Calcitonin and Paget's Disease. Bern, H. Huber, 1977, pp 93–110.)

endogenous calcitonin secretion by means of oral calcium supplementation in combination with the diuretic chlorthalidone.[284] This regimen has been shown to significantly lower serum alkaline phosphatase activity and urinary hydroxyproline excretion as well as improve symptoms in most patients, although no direct evidence of increased calcitonin secretion has been presented. It is unlikely that this program is as effective as treatment with exogenous calcitonin, since the abnormal biochemical indices are not suppressed to the same degree and healing of osteolytic lesions has not been reported. Nevertheless, a trial of 1500 mg of supplemental calcium with 25 mg of chlorthalidone or equivalent of another thiazide diuretic may be worth considering in selected patients who have bone pain and mainly sclerotic lesions who are unable (e.g., for financial reasons) to embark on a course of calcitonin therapy.

On the basis of more than 15 years of successful clinical use of the calcitonins in Paget's disease it can be concluded that these hormones can effectively and safely suppress abnormal bone remodeling as well as induce a variety of beneficial clinical responses. Although side-effects of nausea and facial flushing may be troublesome in some individuals, rarely has significant toxicity been reported.[259] It should be stressed that joint pain, a common complication, will probably not respond to calcitonin therapy.

The optimum dose of the salmon calcitonin is in the range of 50 to 100 MRC units administered daily or three times weekly by subcutaneous self-injection. Human calcitonin is usually administered in a dose of 0.5 mg daily, although 1 mg daily may be necessary to induce optimal radiologic improvement.[264] If treatment is continued for at least 1 year and then discontinued, there is considerable variation in the time period when manifestations of the disease reappear.[285] It may therefore be worthwhile to wait until symptoms reappear or the alkaline phosphatase increases. In those individuals in whom neurologic deficits are improved, the hormone may have to be administered indefinitely. The elucidation of the mechanism of calcitonin resistance in those individuals who do not develop significant titers of neutralizing antibodies will probably require studies of calcitonin receptors in the plasma membrane of the osteoclasts, a formidable task. The pathogenesis of nausea and facial flushing after calcitonin injection is not understood.

The mode of administration of calcitonin by self-injection or even by a nurse or relative is not accepted by some patients. Preliminary results obtained with nasal spray and suppository formulations of salmon calcitonin suggest that in the future these modes of administration could replace parenteral therapy.[275a,286,286a]

C. Bisphosphonates

Bisphosphonates (formerly diphosphonates) are synthetic analogues of inorganic pyrophosphate in which -P-C-P- bonds are substituted for -P-O-P- bonds. The bisphosphonates bind to the surface of calcium phosphate mineral. This property is responsible in part for localization of the bisphosphonates coupled to a radionuclide, in regions of active bone formation. *In vitro*, the bisphosphonates retard precipitation of calcium phosphate from solution and slow the growth and dissolution of hydroxyapatite crystals. Extensive studies in experimental animals and humans indicate that they inhibit bone resorption and formation, but their precise mode of action is still uncertain.[287] One such compound that has been extensively studied since 1971 is disodium etidronate (disodium ethane-1-hydroxyl-1,1-bisphosphonate). This drug can be administered orally, although gastrointestinal absorption is variable.

Disodium etidronate is usually administered to patients with Paget's disease in doses ranging from 5 to 20 mg/kg body weight daily for 1- to 6-month periods.[232,265,288-332d] The minimum effective dose appears to be 2.5 mg/kg body weight daily; but 5 mg/kg daily over a 6-month period has become the standard initial dose. Treatment with 5 mg/kg daily results in a slow decrease in serum alkaline phosphatase activity and urinary hydroxyproline excretion, which reach a nadir between 3 to 6 months after beginning treatment. The decrease in urinary hydroxyproline excretion usually occurs prior to the decrease in serum alkaline phosphatase activity. After a 6-month period of treatment, their biochemical abnormalities may remain suppressed for one year or more[300,303,315] in many patients (Fig. 15–50). As has been found with calcitonin therapy, there are several patterns of biochemical response to disodium etidronate.[328] Approximately 40% of patients have a prolonged response after a single course of therapy. These individuals are often those with modest initial elevation of biochemical indices of disease, although this was not observed in all patients with long-term remissions such as those illustrated in Figure 15–50. A second group of patients[328] (approximately 45%) experience a good response to the initial course of therapy but require retreatment with disodium etidronate 3 to 63 months after the initial therapy, and then respond similarly to 20 mg/kg/day but not as well to 5 mg/kg/day. The final group of patients[328] (approximately 15%) do not respond to retreatment during an average follow-up of 6 years. Resistance is best predicted by an initial urinary hydroxyproline level of more than 10 times normal.

Following high-dose disodium etidronate therapy, a reduction in cardiac output is observed coincident with reduction of biochemical activity.[305] The mean reduction of approximately 27% is probably explained by a proportionate reduction in skeletal blood flow.[232] Other features of the clinical response to disodium etidronate are not identical to those produced by calcitonin, however. Bone pain may be relieved in 50% or more of patients[320] over a period of several months, but in 10% to 38% of patients a dramatic increase in bone pain develops in the site of pagetic lesions.[295,301,302,307] This is more likely to occur with 20 mg/kg/day, but we have noted a paradoxical increase in pain even in patients treated with 5 mg/kg/day. After treatment is stopped, the pain usually resolves within several weeks to months. The pathogenesis of disodium etidronate–induced bone pain is not known but is likely related to inhibition of bone mineralization, which will be discussed subsequently.

Another puzzling aspect of the response to disodium etidronate is that despite considerable suppression of biochemical indices of disease, the extent of osteolytic lesions may increase during treatment.[265,295,300,301,304,306] An example is illustrated in Figure 15–51. The increase in radiolucent lesions associated with disodium etidronate therapy is most likely to occur with a dose of 10 or 20 mg/kg/day. We have also observed worsening of osteolytic lesions in several patients treated with 5 mg/kg/day, although this is observed only in a minority of treated patients. Little evidence for healing of osteolytic lesions has been presented. In one report, two of three lesions healed during multiple courses of therapy.[308] In another report, radiologic healing was evident in three patients with multiple osteolytic lesions but the results were not consistent.[265] A minority of the lesions improved, but the majority deteriorated. After treatment is

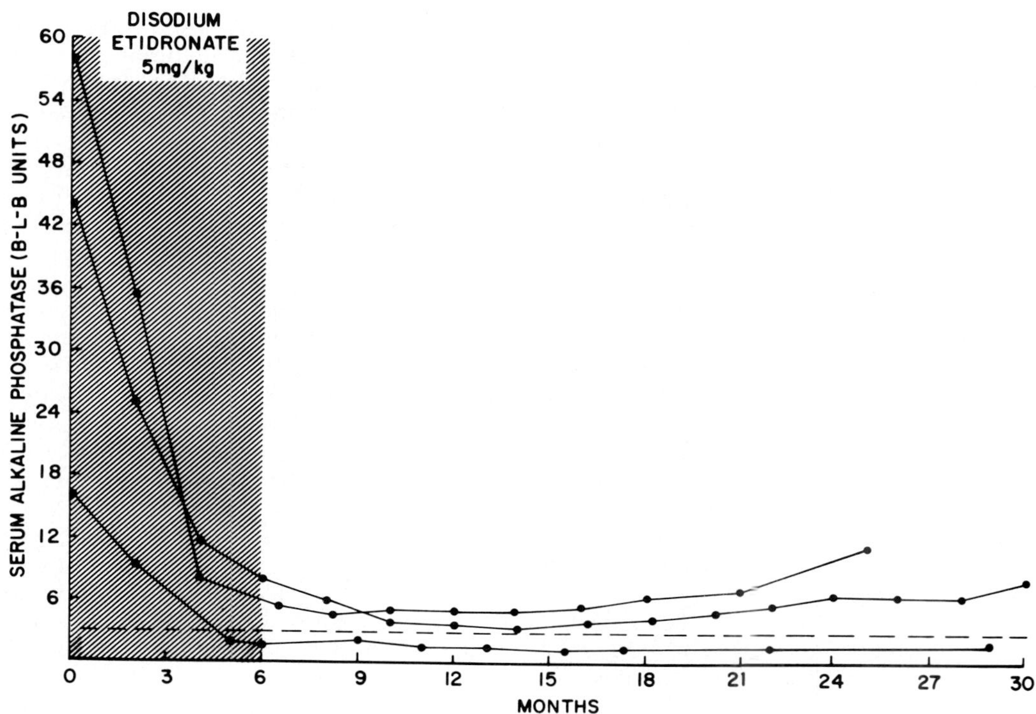

Figure 15–50. Results of disodium etidronate therapy in three patients with Paget's disease. Note the prolonged suppression of serum alkaline phosphatase activity after stopping the treatment. The interrupted line indicates the upper limit of normal of serum alkaline phosphatase activity.

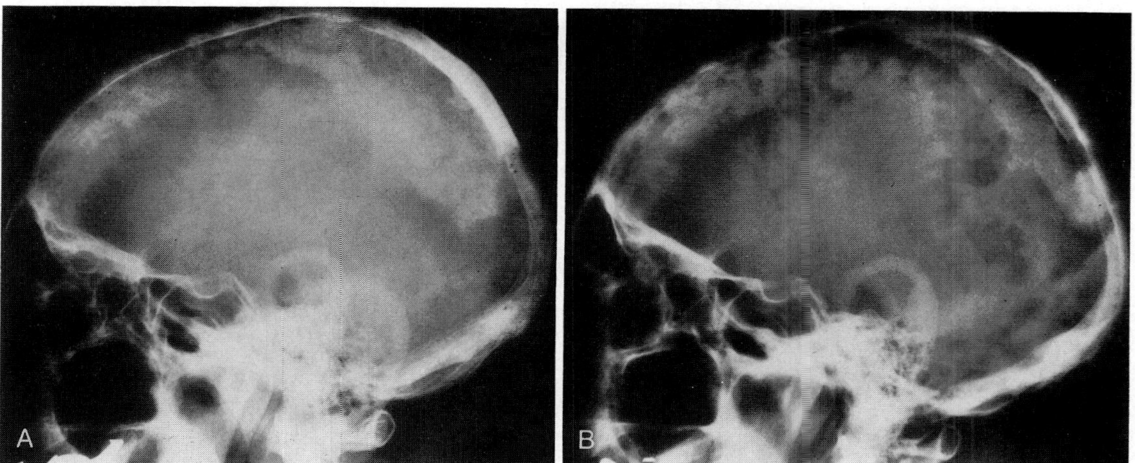

Figure 15–51. The evolution of osteolytic skull lesions in a 60-year-old man treated with disodium etidronate, 5 mg/kg/day, for seven months. *A*, Osteolytic lesion of the skull at the time treatment was started. *B*, New osteolytic lesions have appeared six months after treatment was discontinued despite the observation that serum alkaline phosphatase activity had decreased by 66% at this time.

stopped, healing may occur spontaneously[318] and may be accelerated if calcitonin therapy is instituted.[265]

The explanation for the paradoxical increase in bone pain experienced by some patients and the worsening of osteolytic lesions may be found in an examination of bone biopsies from treated patients. A characteristic finding in patients treated with 20 mg/kg/day is an increase in osteoid surface and osteoid seam thickness, which develops as a consequence of impaired mineralization.[318] This mineralization defect is probably dose-related, since in several series patients treated with 5 mg/kg/day infrequently accumulated excess osteoid.[293,302,311,320] Boyce et al.,[326] however, noted osteomalacia in 9 of 13 transiliac biopsy specimens in patients treated for 6 months with 5 to 8 mg/kg/day. An unusual feature observed in this study was that thickened osteoid seams with absent mineralization were found in a focal distribution along the trabecular surfaces. This finding contrasts with the diffuse distribution of the thickened osteoid seams of vitamin D deficiency. It has also been reported that 1 month of treatment with 20 mg/kg/day of disodium etidronate results in a clinical response superior to that of 5 mg/kg/day for 6 months.[330] Although bone histomorphometry revealed transient impaired mineralization in these subjects, a sustained decrease in bone resorption was produced. These observations led to the proposal that short-term high-dose therapy may maximize suppression of disease activity but decrease the likelihood of clinically significant osteomalacia. These conclusions were disputed as a result of similar studies by another group of investigators who nevertheless reported similar histologic changes.[331] Long-term studies of a large number of patients would be necessary to demonstrate the safety of these short-term high-dose regimens. Impairment of mineralization in disodium etidronate–treated patients is probably not ascribable to inhibition of vitamin D metabolism, since in one study of this problem, intestinal calcium absorption actually increased and serum $1,25(OH)_2D$ levels remained within the normal range.[312]

A desirable therapeutic effect observed histologically in disodium etidronate–treated patients is a reduction in osteoclastic bone resorption, which is more profound in patients treated with 20 mg/kg/day.[293,296,311,320,326] Ultrastructural analysis of osteoclasts reveals considerable evidence of cell degeneration, although the characteristic nuclear and cytoplasmic inclusions are unaltered.[325] Bone marrow fibrosis is reduced, and areas of woven bone may be replaced by lamellar bone.

Side-effects of disodium etidronate therapy, in addition to increased bone pain, include nausea and diarrhea, both of which are uncommon except at higher dosages. Hyperphosphatemia is a common occurrence at high dosages and is a consequence of increased renal tubular reabsorption of phosphate.[287] Mild hyperphosphatemia may develop even following treatment with low dosages[326] and may indicate that greater than the average amount of drug has been absorbed. There is some controversy whether the incidence of fractures is increased by disodium etidronate therapy. After a multicenter review of 737 patients treated for varying periods with 2.5 to 20 mg/kg/day, it was concluded that treatment was not associated with an increased fracture incidence.[319] Nevertheless, it is likely that high-dose therapy, and, in some instances, low-dose therapy, can contribute to the development of fissure fractures[326] and completed pathologic fractures.[295,300-302,304,321,332] This is likely to result from the decreased strength of active pagetic bone when the resorptive phase is dominant and when the new bone formed is inadequately mineralized. Because of this, we feel that disodium etidronate therapy should be avoided, if possible, in patients with osteolytic lesions in weight-bearing regions of the skeleton.

Two second-generation bisphosphonates have shown considerable promise in clinical trials primarily undertaken in Europe and South America. Dichloromethylene bisphosphonate (Cl_2MDP)[333-342a] and (3-amino-1-hydroxypropylidene)-1,1-bisphosphonate (APD)[343-353e] are potent inhibitors of bone resorption in patients with Paget's disease and in the doses used have produced no defect in mineralization[332,337,338,342] with a normally mineralized bone matrix. Thus, APD can induce healing of osteolytic lesions[345,350] with a normally mineralized bone matrix. These agents would therefore not have the undesirable property of inducing a form of osteomalacia that may predispose to pathologic fractures. These agents act rapidly, particularly when given intravenously, with evidence of significant decreases in bone resorption in a matter of days. After weeks of intravenous administration or months of oral drug, the indices of bone turnover may be brought into normal range and remain there for months or years. Thus, long-term remissions may be induced. Preliminary studies suggest that one-to-seven day courses of oral or intravenous APD can also produce prolonged remissions.[353b,353c,353e]

Transient hypocalcemia and secondary hyperparathyroidism occur during the early phase of treatment with Cl_2MDP[333,337] and APD,[339,341,342] but these biochemical consequences of inhibition of bone resorption do not interfere significantly with the therapeutic response. With return of bone turnover to the normal range (a common event), normocalcemia and a euparathyroid state follow and formation/resorptive coupling is restored.

Side-effects and toxic effects due to Cl_2MDP therapy have been few and generally mild. An increase in bone pain does not occur, and hyperphosphatemia is not observed. Minor intestinal disturbances have not led to discontinuation of therapy. One patient was reported to have developed leukemia,[338] but he had also been exposed to benzene, and the possible role of Cl_2MDP in the development of this malignancy was not established. APD use has been associated with transient fever, transient leukopenia, gastric distress, oral ulcers, and skin rashes.

It is likely that one or more of the new bisphosphonates will replace calcitonin and disodium etidronate as the most commonly used drugs in treating Paget's disease if the incidence of toxic effects continues to remain low in clinical trials. Other agents such as the aminobutane[353f] or aminohexane bisphosphonates[353g,353h] are also effective and may be commercially successful. The oral route of administration, the absence of osteomalacia, and the great potency of these agents provide significant advantages to their use.

D. Mithramycin

Mithramycin is an antibiotic that has proved to be an effective antitumor drug in the treatment of embryonal tumors of the testis. The drug also has a potent cytotoxic effect on bone cells, particularly osteoclasts, possibly through inhibition of RNA synthesis. This has made it an effective agent in the acute control of severe hypercalcemia. Ryan and colleagues have pioneered the use of mithramycin in the treatment of patients with Paget's disease.[354-359] They and subsequent investigators[360-370] have demonstrated occasionally dramatic effects of this drug in patients with high skeletal turnover (Fig. 15–52). In a manner analogous to the effects of calcitonin or intravenous bisphosphonates, acute hypocalcemia and hypophosphatemia, a reduction in urinary hydroxyproline excretion, and a rise in serum parathyroid hormone levels result from a single infusion of mithramycin.[364,367,371] In contrast to calcitonin, however, daily infusions produce persistent mild hypocalcemia, which resolves after treatment is discontinued. These effects are consistent with a potent inhibition of osteoclastic bone resorption. It is less certain whether osteoblastic function is affected acutely, although serum alkaline phosphatase activity may be decreased within as short a period as 12 hours of mithramycin infusion.[371] These observations are particularly significant since the half-life of circulating skeletal alkaline phosphatase has been estimated to be 1 to 2 days.[372]

After 10 daily infusions of mithramycin at 10 to 25 μg/kg body weight, urinary hydroxyproline excretion and serum alkaline phosphatase activity may decrease into the normal range in many patients. These decreases are maintained for a variable period ranging from several months to as long as 12 years (rare). Weekly infusions of 15 to 25 μg/kg body weight also have been reported to produce prolonged biochemical remissions.[356] Bone scans may revert toward a normal pattern[365] and roentgenograms also, although the latter have not been extensively evaluated.

A reduction in bone pain (frequently rapid) has been noted in the great majority of treated patients, although no double blind trials have been undertaken. There is a good correlation between pain relief and biochemical remission as well as recurrence of pain and worsening of biochemical parameters.

There are significant problems encountered in using mithramycin. The drug can be administered only by intravenous infusion and must be infused carefully, since extravasation can lead to painful soft tissue injury. Side-effects may be troublesome. Nausea and vomiting may occur but are less likely to develop if the drug is infused over 4 hours or more rather than as a bolus. Toxic effects from

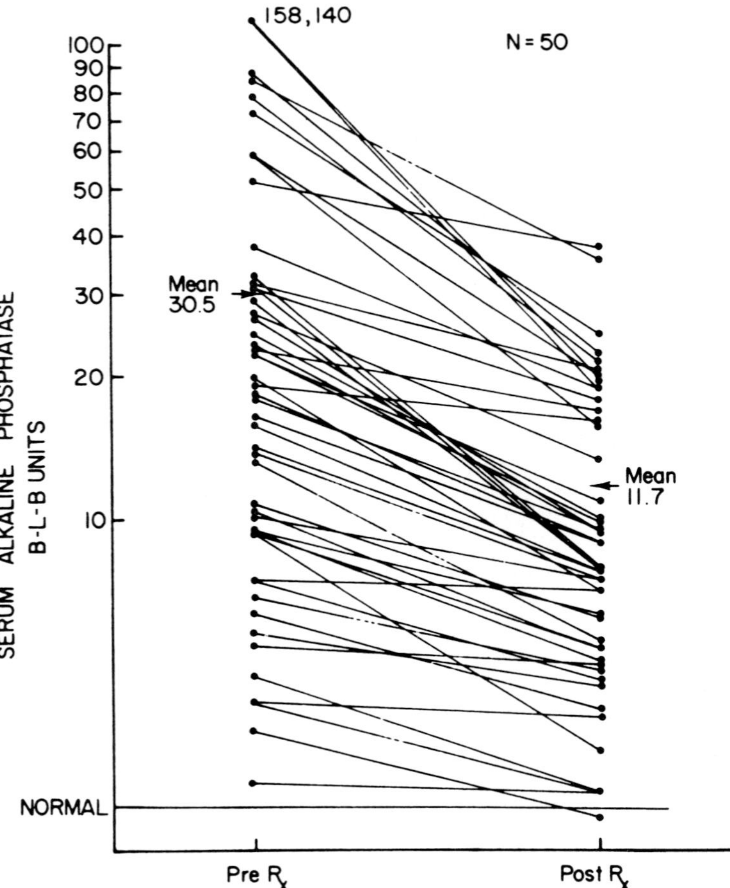

Figure 15–52. The effect of mithramycin therapy on serum alkaline phosphatase activity (Bessey-Lowrey-Brock units) in 50 patients with Paget's disease. (From Ryan WG, et al: Treatment of Paget's disease with mithramycin—further experiences. Semin Drug Treatment 2:57, 1972.)

mithramycin therapy include abnormal bleeding ascribable to impaired platelet function and decreased production, hepatitis as manifested by increased levels of circulating hepatic enzymes, and renal failure. In most patients, the toxic effect is transient, although persistence of reduced glomerular filtration rate has been reported.[359] If smaller doses or weekly therapy is utilized, the incidence of toxic effects is considerably reduced.

Although mithramycin and another cytotoxic drug, actinomycin D,[373-375] have been shown to suppress the activity of Paget's disease, these agents should not be considered first-line agents in therapy of the disease. The use of potentially lethal drugs in a benign disorder seems unwarranted in the majority of patients. Their primary use should be reserved for patients who have not responded to the other available agents or others who cannot tolerate such therapies. Mithramycin may possibly be the drug of choice in the unusual patient in whom rapid suppression of disease activity is imperative. Careful monitoring of platelet number, liver enzymes, and renal function is critical during the treatment course if toxicity is to be minimized. Reduction of dosage is recommended in patients with liver or renal disease.

E. Miscellaneous Drugs

Many other drugs have been used to treat Paget's disease, including arsenic,[210] magnesium carbonate,[376] aluminum acetate,[377,378] anabolic steroids,[379,380] folic acid,[381] phenylbutazone,[8] acetylsalicylic acid,[8,382-384] adrenocorticoid-steroids or ACTH,[383,385-390] sodium fluoride,[8,110,391-395] phosphate,[396] glucagon,[397-400] and colchicine.[401] Some of these drugs were evaluated at a time when only subjective criteria were available to assess efficacy. Others, particularly acetylsalicylic acid and glucocorticoids, have produced significant although transient suppression of the disease, although relatively large doses were required and their use was accompanied by intolerable side-effects. Drugs such as sodium fluoride, phosphate, glucagon, and colchicine have either produced variable results or have been studied in only a few subjects. At present none of these drugs is widely used. We have found, however, that anti-inflammatory drugs such as acetylsalicylic acid and indomethacin are of use in controlling symptoms, particularly those associated with the joint involvement of the hips and knees secondary to Paget's disease in adjacent bones.

F. Combination Therapy

Combinations of calcitonin and disodium etidronate,[265,306,402-404,404a,404b] calcitonin and mithramycin,[368] mithramycin and glucagon,[368] and mithramycin and disodium etidronate[359] have been utilized in a relatively small number of patients to attempt to obtain additive suppressive effects on the disease and perhaps reduce toxicity. The results suggest that combination therapy may produce greater suppression of biochemical indices, but no compelling clinical evidence has been presented that patients will therefore benefit to greater extent than from single-agent therapy. On the contrary, the calcitonin–disodium etidronate combination is not as useful in inducing healing of osteolytic lesions as is calcitonin alone.[265,306]

IX. SURGERY

Surgery in patients with Paget's disease is often deferred or withheld for a variety of reasons. Some feel that the advanced age of many patients is a relative contraindication. The technical problems associated with operations on sclerotic bone, the fear of excessive hemorrhage from bone or adjacent soft tissue, the possibility of delayed union or nonunion, and the unproven speculation that surgery may predispose to induction of osteosarcomas have all contributed to a reluctance to operate on patients in whom these are otherwise appropriate indications for surgery. The problem of excessive hemorrhage has been considerably reduced by treatment with one of the available agents prior to surgery. In our experience, the benefits of appropriate surgery considerably outweigh any of the other potential problems.

In patients with basilar impression, suboccipital craniectomy and laminectomy of upper cervical vertebrae may be necessary to decompress the posterior fossa and thereby relieve neurologic impairment.[61] Ventricular shunts have been proposed as a means of preventing progressive dementia arising from progressive communicating hydrocephalus.[63] The more common problem of hearing loss in patients with skull involvement has been treated with equivocal results utilizing stapes mobilization or stapedectomy. Spinal stenosis or nerve root compression as a consequence of intervertebral foraminal encroachment may require laminectomy or foraminotomy. Results of surgery on the spine are generally quite good.[69,70,70a]

The complication of arthropathy involving joints adjacent to pagetic bone disease provides the most frequent indication for surgery. Total hip replacement is highly effective in patients with intractable hip pain and impaired mobility[81,82] (Fig. 15–53). Heterotopic ossification may develop postoperatively (Fig. 15–54) but fortunately does not often produce symptoms or disability. It is our impression that this complication may be more common in Paget's disease than in the general population of patients undergoing hip replacement. Involvement of the knee joint is a common problem in patients with distal femoral disease or severe bowing of the tibia. Correction of the varus deformity by tibial and fibular osteotomy may relieve knee pain and improve mobility[83] (Fig. 15–55). It is occasionally necessary to carry out total knee replacement in these patients.

Open reduction and fixation of fractures in Paget's disease is usually reserved for fractures of the femur.[87] Because of the high incidence of nonunion of femoral fractures, various forms of fixation are required to produce optimum healing. Fractures of the tibia and other long bones generally heal with immobilization by casting alone.

In patients in whom elective surgery is scheduled, suppression of disease activity should be accomplished over a 3- to 4-month period utilizing one of the available drugs. If serum alkaline phosphatase activity is reduced by approximately 50% prior to surgery, hemorrhage should be minimized. The optimum length of postoperative treatment has not been established but it seems reasonable to continue treatment at least until healing is considered complete.

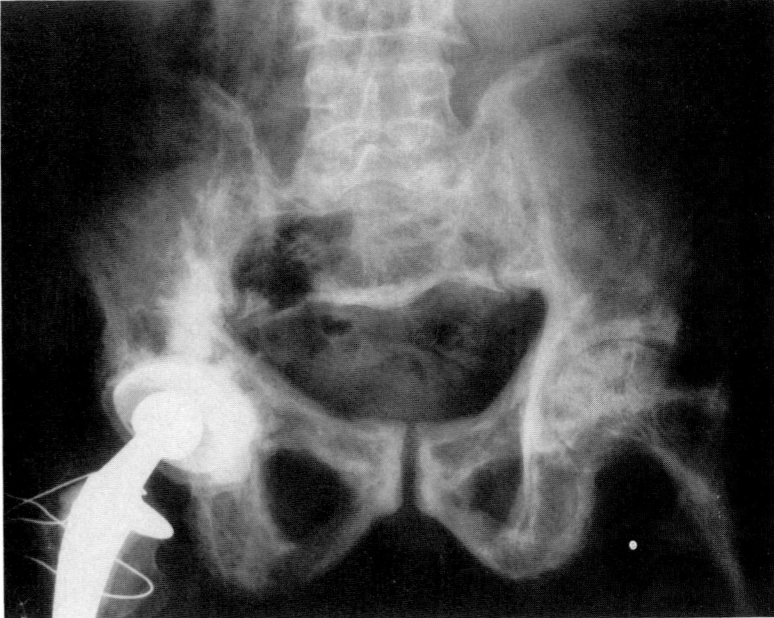

Figure 15–53. Total hip joint replacement in a 68-year-old patient with severe pagetic coxopathy. Note the joint space narrowing of the left hip which may be an indication for a future second hip joint replacement.

X. ETIOLOGY

Speculation as to the cause of Paget's disease began with the initial paper of Paget.[1] His concept of the disease as a chronic inflammatory disorder did not gain widespread acceptance, in large part because there are few inflammatory cells in pagetic lesions. Interest in this idea was revived by the reports of Albright and Henneman[389] and Maurice and colleagues,[382] in which the anti-inflammatory drugs ACTH, cortisone, and aspirin were shown to suppress Paget's disease. However, since the glucocorticoids affect many different cell functions, their effects in Paget's disease may represent interference with the function and/or differentiation of osteoclasts and osteoblasts rather than an "anti-inflammatory effect." For example, effects of acetylsalicylic acid and glucocorticoids on Paget's disease could be due to decreasing prostaglandin synthesis by bone cells rather than to "suppressing inflammation."

Since Paget proposed an inflammatory etiology of Paget's disease, a variety of other theories of etiology and pathogenesis have been proposed.[405] These include considerations of Paget's disease as a disorder of secretion of growth hormone, parathyroid hormone or calcitonin, a benign neoplastic

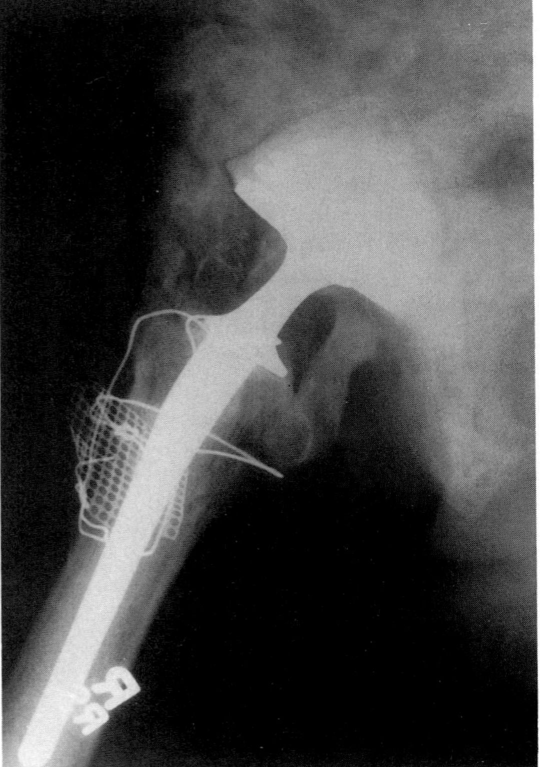

Figure 15–54. Heterotopic ossification surrounding a hip joint replacement in a 72-year-old patient 3 months postoperatively.

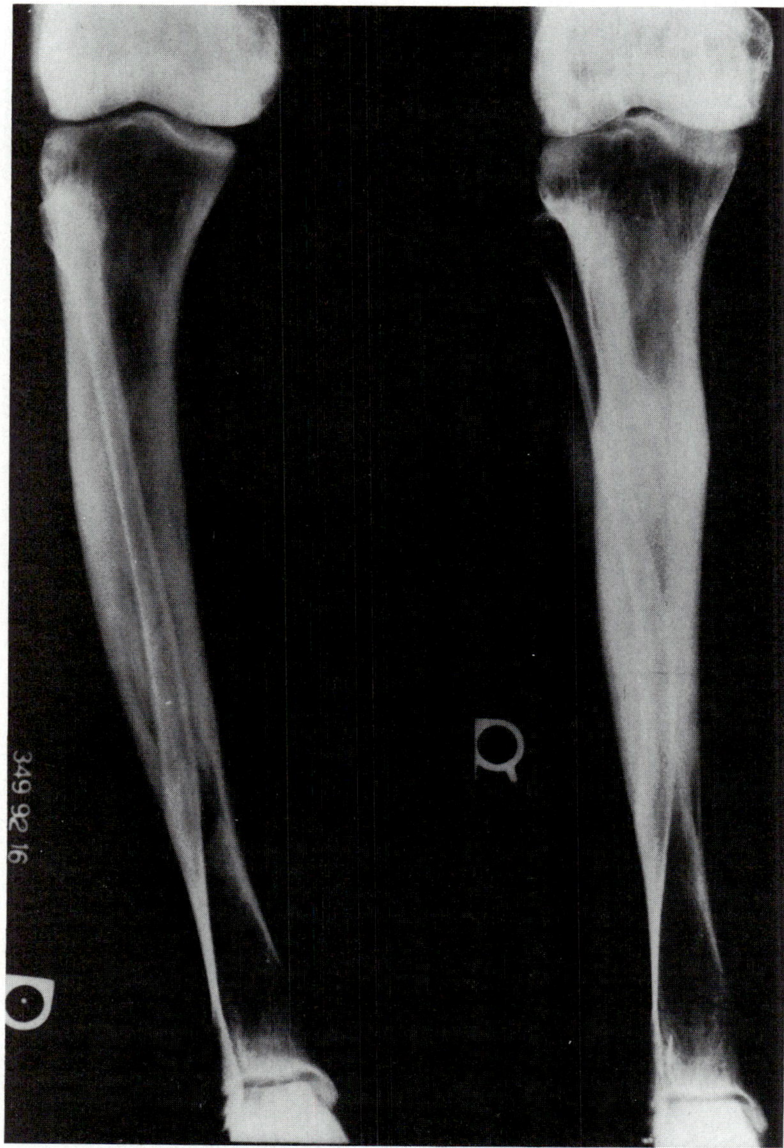

Figure 15–55. The results of a right tibial osteotomy to correct bowing and recurrent knee effusions in a patient with Paget's disease. On the left is the tibia prior to surgery. (From Singer FR: Paget's Disease of Bone. New York, Plenum, 1977.)

process, a primary vascular disorder, and an inborn error of connective tissue. No significant evidence to support any of these hypotheses has been reported. The role of calcitonin perhaps deserves closest scrutiny, since this hormone has such a potent effect upon osteoclasts and does improve many manifestations of the disease. However, athyroidal subjects with low levels of circulating calcitonin do not develop pagetic lesions with increased frequency, and calcitonin levels in patients with Paget's disease are within the normal range.[406]

In 1974, the first study of the ultrastructure of bone cells in Paget's disease appeared.[407] Rebel and colleagues observed intranuclear inclusions that resembled nucleocapsids of the Paramyxoviridae virus family in the osteoclasts of four French patients (Fig. 15–56). These results led to the concept that Paget's disease might be considered a slow virus infection of bone, analogous to the post-measles virus infection of the brain, subacute sclerosing panencephalitis.[408] Subsequently, investigators in the United States,[409] Germany,[410] Italy,[411] Canada,[412] England,[413] and Japan[413a] found identical inclusions in the nuclei and, at times, the cytoplasm of pagetic osteoclasts in each patient from whom adequate bone specimens were obtained. These nucleocapsid-like structures have not been observed in any other bone or marrow cells and have not been found in osteoclasts from normal subjects or from patients with a variety of metabolic disorders such as primary and secondary hyperparathyroidism. Similar structures have, however, been described in a small percentage of giant cells in some patients with giant cell tumors of bone[414] and in the osteoclasts of several patients with pyknodysostosis[415] and osteopetrosis.[416]

In addition to the morphologic evidence of virus-related structures in pagetic osteoclasts, immunohistologic studies have shown the presence of viral antigens. Initially Rebel and colleagues reported the presence of measles virus antigens in pagetic osteoclasts,[417] whereas Mills and colleagues found respiratory syncytial virus antigens in osteoclasts (Fig. 15–57) and cultured mononuclear cells from pagetic bone specimens.[418] Subsequently, in a later study, measles virus and respiratory syncytial virus antigens were both identified in serial sections of the same osteoclasts.[419] Basle and colleagues have also described the presence of SV5 and parainfluenza 3 viral antigens in some pagetic specimens but could not detect respiratory syncytial virus antigens.[420] Utilizing the technique of *in situ* hybridization, Basle and colleagues have detected measles virus nucleocapsid mRNA in bone specimens from four patients.[421] Unexpectedly the mRNA was found not only in osteoclasts but in osteoblasts, osteocytes, fibroblasts, and other marrow elements. The lack of discernible inclusions and immunohistologic evidence of viral antigens in any cells other than osteoclasts suggests that the measles virus mRNA may not be translated in the mononuclear cells of bone and bone marrow. Perfect controls to validate *in situ* hybridization techniques are frequently difficult to obtain.

There is no entirely satisfactory explanation for the presence of several different Paramyxoviridae viral antigens in the osteoclasts of Paget's disease. A reasonable possibility is that the high spontaneous mutation rate of these RNA viruses[422] accounts for the confusing antigenic pattern found in the studies reported. Based on morphology alone, the inclusions most closely resemble nucleocapsids of respiratory syncytial virus.[411,412] The presence of both nuclear and cytoplasmic inclusions, however, is more consistent with the intracellular distribution of measles virus;

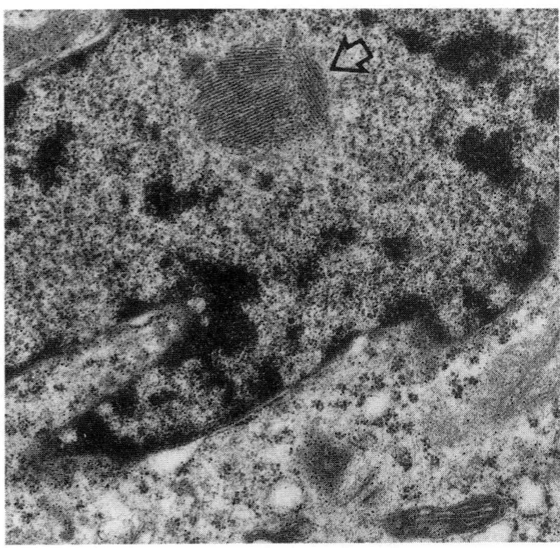

Figure 15–56. Nucleus of an osteoclast from a patient with Paget's disease. The arrow indicates the characteristic nuclear inclusion in longitudinal section. Each microfilament measures approximately 1 nm in diameter (decalcified; ×20,250). (From Singer FR, et al: Acute effects of calcitonin on osteoclasts in man. Clin Endocrinol 5[Suppl]: 333s–340s, 1976. Permission from Blackwell Scientific Publications, Ltd.)

respiratory syncytial virus has seldom been observed within the nucleus by electron microscopy. Unfortunately, efforts to rescue an infectious virus from bone cell cultures derived from pagetic bone have not been successful,[423,424] and budding of viruses from osteoclasts has not been observed by electron microscopy. If the putative viral agent is sufficiently defective, an infectious virus may never be isolated. Identification of the exact nature of the viral structures in pagetic osteoclasts will require the use of multiple cDNA probes for components of numerous Paramyxoviridae viruses as well as continuing attempts to rescue an infectious agent from cell cultures. If more definitive identification of the agent is obtained, a number of critical questions will still remain. Is Paget's disease a slow virus infection of bone, or do the nuclear inclusions result simply from infections of susceptible cells with a virus that has no significant effects on the function of those cells? Can the racial and familial patterns of the prevalence of Paget's disease be explained by subtle immunologic abnormalities linked to the HLA system? Elevated serum IgM levels have been reported in five of 26 patients, but the relevance of this observation is unknown.[425] Finally, if Paget's

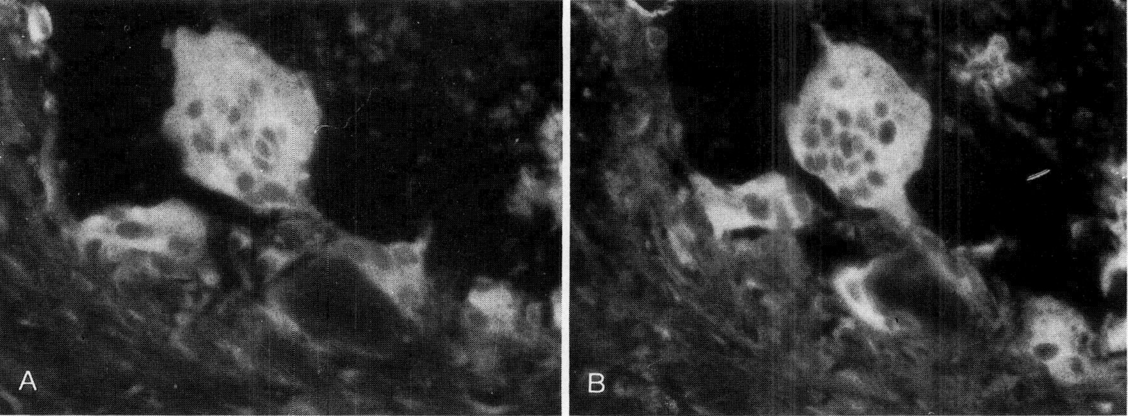

Figure 15–57. *A*, A group of osteoclasts in a pagetic lesion. The multinucleated cells exhibit strong immunofluorescence when treated by an indirect immunofluorescent technique utilizing an antibody to respiratory syncytial virus. The cytoplasm but not the nuclei is stained. *B*, Serial section showing the same group of osteoclasts as in *A*. The cells exhibit a similar degree and localization of fluorescence when treated with an antibody to measles virus (From Mills BG, et al: Proc Natl Acad Sci USA 78:1209, 1981. Original magnification ×320.)

disease is proved to be a slow virus infection, will immunization prevent and antiviral therapy reverse the disease process? Preliminary attempts to treat one patient with measles vaccine[426] and four patients with inosiplex,[342] an antiviral drug effective in subacute sclerosing panencephalitis, have produced negative results. These data do not, however, disprove the slow virus hypothesis of Paget's disease. Considerably more time and effort will be required before the etiology of Paget's disease is resolved.

References

1. Paget J: On a form of chronic inflammation of bones (osteitis deformans). Med-Chir Trans 60:37–64, 1877.
2. Paget J: The Bradshaw lecture on some rare and new diseases. Br Med J 2:1189–1193, 1882.
3. Paget J: Additional cases of osteitis deformans. Med-Chir Trans 65:225–236, 1882.
4. Rullier PR: Sur un accroissement extraordinaire de os plats. Bull Fac Med Paris 2:94, 1812.
5. Wrany: Spongiose Hyperostose des Schadels, des Beckens und des linken Oberschenkels. Vierteijahresschr Prakt Heilkd 93:79, 1867.
6. Wilks S: Case of osteoporosis, or spongy hypertrophy of the bones (calvaria, clavicle, os femoris and rib, exhibited at the Society). Trans Pathol Soc Lond 20:273–277, 1869.
7. Czerny V: Eine lokale Malacie des Unterschenkels. Wien Med Wochenschr 23:985, 1873.
8. Nagant de Deuxchaisnes CN, Krane SM: Paget's disease of bone: Clinical and metabolic observations. Medicine 43:233–266, 1964.
9. Barry HC: Paget's Disease of Bone. Edinburgh, E and S Livingstone, 1965, p 3.
10. Ziegler R, Holz G, Rotzler B, Minne H: Paget's disease of bone in West Germany. Prevalence and distribution. Clin Orthop Rel Res 194:199–204, 1985.
11. Schmorl G: Uber Ostitis deformans Paget. Virchows Arch Pathol Anat Physiol 283:694–751, 1932.
12. Collins DH: Paget's disease of bone–incidence and subclinical forms. Lancet 2:51–57, 1956.
13. Pygott F: Paget's disease of bone. The radiological incidence. Lancet 1:1170–1171, 1957.
14. Newman FW: Paget's disease. J Bone Joint Surg 28:798–804, 1946
15. Rosenkrantz J, Wolf J, Kaicher J: Paget's disease—review of 111 cases. Arch Intern Med 90:610–633, 1952.
16. Barker DJP: The epidemiology of Paget's disease. Metab Bone Dis Rel Res 4, 5:231–234, 1981.
17. Barker DJP, Chamberlain AT, Guyer PB, Gardner MJ: Paget's disease of bone: The Lancashire focus. Br Med J 1:1105–1107, 1980.
18. Gardner MJ, Guyer PB, Barker DJB: Radiological prevalence of Paget's disease of bone in British migrants to Australia. Br Med J 1:1655–1657, 1978.
19. Reasbeck JC, Goulding A, Campbell DR, et al: Radiological prevalence of Paget's disease in Dunedin, New Zealand. Br Med J 286:1937, 1983.
20. Rosenbaum HD, Hanson DJ: Geographic variation in the prevalence of Paget's disease of bone. Radiology 92:959–963, 1969.
21. Guyer PB, Chamberlain AT: Paget's disease of bone in two American cities. Br Med J 280:985, 1980.
22. Detheridge FM, Guyer PB, Barker DJP: European distribution of Paget's disease of bone. Br Med J 285:1005–1008, 1982.
23. Detheridge FM, Barker DJP, Guyer PB: Paget's disease of bone in Ireland. Br Med J 287:1345–1346, 1983.
24. Tohgo O, Ito K, Takeda H, et al: Paget's disease of bone. Orthop Traum Surg (Jpn) 27:525–530, 1984.
25. O'Driscoll JB, Anderson DC: Past pets and Paget's disease. Lancet 2:919–921, 1986.

25a. Barker DJP, Detheridge FM: Dogs and Paget's disease. Lancet 2:1245, 1985.

26. Woodhouse NJY, Fisher MT, Sigurdsson G, et al: Paget's disease in a 5-year old: Acute response to human calcitonin. Br Med J 4:267–269, 1972.
27. Evens RG, Bartter FC: The hereditary aspects of Paget's disease. JAMA 205:900–902, 1968.
28. Sofaer JA, Holloway SM, Emery AEH: A family study of Paget's disease of bone. J Epidemiol Community Health 37:226–231, 1983.
29. Canfield R, Rosner W, Skinner J, et al: Diphosphonate therapy of Paget's disease of bone. J Clin Endocrinol Metab 44:96–106, 1977.
30. Melick RA, Martin TJ: Paget's disease in identical twins. Aust NZ J Med 5:564–565, 1975.
31. Simon L, Blotman F, Seignalet J, Claustre J: Etiologie de la maladie osseuse de Paget. Rev Rhum Mal Osteoartic 42:535–544, 1975.
32. Seignalet J, Simon L, Blotman F: Repartition des antigenes HL-A dans la maladie de Paget. Nouv Presse Med 4:2204, 1975.
33. Cullen P, Russell RGG, Walton RJ, Whiteley J: Frequencies of HLA-A and HLA-B histocompatibility antigens in Paget's disease of bone. Tissue Antigens 7:55–56, 1976.
34. Singer FR, Schiller AL, Pyle EB, Krane SM: Paget's disease of bone. *In* Avioli LV, Krane SM (eds): Metabolic Bone Disease, vol II. New York, Academic Press, 1978, p 493.
35. Fotino W, Haymovits A, Falk CT: Evidence for linkage between HLA and Paget's disease. Transplant Proc 9:1867–1868, 1977.
36. Tilyard MW, Gardner RJM, Milligan L, et al: A probable linkage between familial Paget's disease and the HLA loci. Aust NZ J Med 12:498–500, 1982.
37. Singer FR, Mills BG, Park MS, et al: Increased HLA-DQW1 antigen pattern in Paget's disease of bone. Clin Res 33:574A, 1985.
38. Jaffe HL: Metabolic, Degenerative and Inflammatory Diseases of Bones and Joints. Philadelphia, Lea and Febiger, 1972.
39. Rasmussen H, Bordier P: The Physiologic and Cellular Basis of Metabolic Bone Disease. Baltimore, Williams and Wilkins, 1974, pp 292–303.
40. Jaffe HL: The classic Paget's disease of bone. Clin Orthop Rel Res 127:4–42, 1977.
41. Meunier PJ, Coindre JM, Edouard CM, Arlot ME: Bone histomorphometry in Paget's disease. Quantitative and dynamic analysis of pagetic and nonpagetic bone tissue. Arthritis Rheum 23:1095–1103, 1980.
42. Rubinstein MA, Smelin A, Freedman AL: Osteoblasts and osteoclasts in bone marrow aspiration. Arch Intern Med 92:684–696, 1953.
43. Belanger LF: Osteocytic osteolysis. Calcif Tissue Res 4:1–12 , 1969.
44. Lee WR: Bone formation in Paget's disease. A quantitative microscopic study using tetracycline marks. J Bone Joint Surg 49B:146–153, 1967.
45. Belanger LF, Jarry L, Uhthoff HK: Osteocytic osteolysis in Paget's disease. Rev Can Biol 27:37–44, 1968.
46. Meunier P, Bernard J, Vignon G: The measurement of periosteocytic enlargement in primary and secondary hyperparathyroidism. Isr J Med Sci 7:482–485, 1971.
47. Eyring EJ, Eisenberg E: Congenital hyperphosphatasia: A clinical, pathological and biochemical study of two cases. J Bone Joint Surg 50A:1099–1117, 1968.
48. Thompson RC Jr, Gaull GE, Horwitz SJ, Schenk RK: Hereditary hyperphosphatasia. Studies of three siblings. Am J Med 47:209–219, 1969.
49. Woodhouse NJY, Fisher MJ, Sigurdsson G, et al: Paget's disease in a 5-year old: Acute response to human calcitonin. Br Med J 4:267–268, 1972.
50. Whalen JP, Horwith M, Krook L, et al: Calcitonin treatment in hereditary bone dysplasia with hyperphosphatasemia: A radiographic and histologic study of bone. AJR 129:29–35, 1977.
51. Dunn V, Condon VR, Rallison ML: Familial hyperphosphatasemia: Diagnosis in early infancy and response to human thyrocalcitonin therapy. AJR 132:541–545, 1979.
51a. Harinck HIJ, Bijvoet OLM, Vellenga CJLR, et al: Relation between signs and symptoms in Paget's disease of bone. Q J Med NS 58:133–151, 1986.
52. Blotman F, Suquet P, Labauge R, Simon L: L'hemodetournet carotidien externe par le crane pagetique. *In* Hioco DJ (ed): La Maladie de Paget. Symposium International. Paris, Laboratoire Armour Montagu, 1974, pp 79–87.
53. Vignon G: La douleur dans la maladie de Paget. *In* Hioco DJ (ed): La Maladie de Paget. Symposium International. Paris, Laboratoire Armour Montagu, 1974, pp 17–26.
54. Khairi MR, Wellman HN, Robb JA, Johnston CC: Paget's disease of bone—symptomatic lesions and bone scan. Ann Intern Med 79:348–351, 1973.
55. Vellenga CJLR, Pauwels EKJ, Bijvoet OLM, et al: Untreated Paget disease of bone studied by scintigraphy. Radiology 153:799–805, 1984.
56. Fogelman I, Carr D: A comparison of bone scanning and radiology in the assessment of patients with symptomatic Paget's disease. Eur J Nucl Med 5:417–421, 1980.
57. Steindler A: Lectures on the Interpretation of Pain in Orthopedic Practice. Springfield, IL, Charles C Thomas, 1959.
58. Franck WA, Bress NM, Singer FR, Krane SM: Rheumatic manifestations of Paget's disease of bone. Am J Med 56:592–603, 1974.
59. Schuller A: Ueber circumscripte Osteoporose des Schadels. Med Klin 25:631–632, 1929.
60. Kasabach HH, Gutman AB: Osteoporosis circumscripta of the skull and Paget's disease. Fifteen new cases and a review of the literature. Am J Roentgenol Radium Ther 37:577–603, 1937.
61. Wycis H: Platybasia; a case secondary to advanced osteitis deformans (Paget's disease) with severe neurological manifestations, successful surgical results. J Neurosurg 1:299–305, 1944.
62. Epstein BS, Epstein JA: The association of cerebellar tonsillar herniation with basilar impression incident to Paget's disease. AJR 107:535–542, 1969.
63. Dohrmann PJ, Elrick WL: Dementia and hydrocephalus in Paget's disease: A case report. J Neurol Neurosurg Psychiatry 45:835–837, 1982.
64. Waltner JG: Stapedectomy in Paget's disease. Histological and clinical studies. Arch Otolaryngol 82:355–358, 1965.
65. Sparrow NL, Duvall AJ: Hearing loss and Paget's disease. J Laryngol Otol 81:601–611, 1967.
66. Davies DG: Paget's disease of the temporal bone. A clinical and histopathological study. Acta Otolaryngol [Suppl] 242, 1968 .
67. Eretto P, Krohel GB, Shihab ZM, et al: Optic neuropathy in Paget's disease. Am J Ophthalmol 97:505–510, 1984.

68. Smith BJ, Eveson JW: Paget's disease of bone with particular reference to dentistry. J Oral Pathol 10:233–247, 1981.
69. Wyllie WG: The occurrence in osteitis deformans of lesions of the central nervous system, with a report of four cases. Brain 46:336–351, 1923.
70. Hartman JT, Dohn DF: Paget's disease of the spine with cord or nerve root compression: Report of 6 cases. J Bone Joint Surg 48A:1079–1084, 1966.
70a. Weisz GM: Lumbar canal stenosis in Paget's disease. Clin Orthop Rel Res 206:223–227, 1986.
71. Siegelman SS, Levine SA, Walpin L: Paget's disease with spinal cord compression. Clin Radiol 19:421–425, 1968.
72. Kadir S, Kalisher L, Schiller AL: Extramedullary hematopoiesis in Paget's disease of bone. AJR 129:493–495, 1977.
73. Samuels MA, Schiller AL: Case records of the Massachusetts General Hospital. N Engl J Med 304:1411–1421, 1981.
74. Altman RD, Collins B: Musculoskeletal manifestations of Paget's disease of bone. Arthritis Rheum 23:1121–1127, 1980.
75. Bitar E: Maladie osseuse pagetoide avec ossification des ligaments prevertebraux chez un homme jeune. Rev Med Moyen-Orient 18:477–480, 1961.
76. Layani F, Francon J, Wattebled R: Apropos de l'association cinq fois constatee de spondylorthrie ankylosante et de maladie de Paget. Sem Hop Paris 37:1037–1046, 1961.
77. Brewerton DA, Hart FD, Nicholls A, et al: Ankylosing spondylitis and HL-A27. Lancet 1:904–906, 1973.
78. Schlosstein L, Terasaki PI, Bluestone R, Pearson CM: High association of an HL-A antigen W27 with ankylosing spondylitis. N Engl J Med 288:704–706, 1973.
79. Machtey I, Rodnan GP, Benedek T: Paget's disease of the hip joint. Am J Med Sci 251:524–531, 1966.
80. Roper B: Paget's disease involving the hip joint. Clin Orthop Rel Res 80:33–38, 1971.
81. Merkow RL, Pellicci PM, Hely DP, Salvati EA: Total hip replacement for Paget's disease of the hip. J Bone Joint Surg 66A:752–758, 1984.
82. McDonald DJ, Sim FH: Total hip arthroplasty in Paget's disease. J Bone Joint Surg 69-A:766–772, 1987.
83. Meyers M, Singer F: Osteotomy for tibia vara in Paget's disease under cover of calcitonin. J Bone Joint Surg 60A:810–814, 1978.
84. Collins DH: Pathology of Bone. London, Butterworth, 1966, pp 228–248.
85. Allen ML, John RL: Osteitis deformans—fissure fractures—their aetiology and clinical significance. Am J Roentgenol Radium Ther 38:109–115, 1937.
86. Harris ED, Krane SM: Paget's disease of bone. Bull Rheum Dis 18:506–511, 1968.
87. Dove J: Complete fractures of the femur in Paget's disease of bone. J Bone Joint Surg 62B:12–17, 1980.
88. Grainger R, Laws J: Paget's disease—active or quiescent. Br J Radiol 30:120–124, 1957.
89. Wick MR, Siegal GP, Unni GP, et al: Sarcomas of bone complicating osteitis deformans (Paget's disease): Fifty years' experience. Am J Surg Pathol 5:47–59, 1981.
90. Brenton DP, Isenberg DA, Bertram J: Osteosarcoma complicating familial Paget's disease. Postgrad Med J 56:238–243, 1980.
91. Nassar VH, Gravanis MB: Familial osteogenic sarcoma occurring in pagetoid bone. Am J Clin Pathol 76:235–239, 1981.
92. Huvos AG: Osteogenic sarcoma of bones and soft tissues in older persons. A clinicopathologic analysis of 117 patients older than 60 years. Cancer 57:1442–1449, 1986.
93. McKenna RJ, Schwinn CP, Soong KY, Higinbotham NL: Osteogenic sarcoma arising in Paget's disease. Cancer 17:42–66, 1964.
94. Schajowicz F, Araujo ES, Berenstein M: Sarcoma complicating Paget's disease. J Bone Joint Surg 65B:299–307, 1983.
95. Smith J, Botet JF, Yeh SDJ: Bone sarcomas in Paget's disease: A study of 85 patients. Radiology 152:583–590, 1984.
96. Haibach H, Farrell C, Dittrich FJ: Neoplasms arising in Paget's disease of bone: A study of 82 cases. Am J Clin Pathol 83:594–600, 1985.
97. Lauchlan SC, Walsh MJ: Reticulum cell sarcoma complicating Paget's disease. Can Med Assoc J 88:891–892, 1963.
98. Riffat MG: Myelome plasmocytaire et maladie osseuse de Paget. Lyon Med 219:1035–1038, 1968.
99. von Albertini A: Uber Sarkombildung auf dem Boden der Ostitis deformans Paget. Virchows Arch Pathol Anat Physiol 268:259–273, 1928.
100. Goorin AM, Abelson HT, Frei E III: Osteosarcoma: Fifteen years later. N Engl J Med 313:1637–1643, 1985.
101. Jacobs TP, Michelsen J, Polay JS, et al: Giant cell tumor in Paget's disease of bone. Familial and geographic clustering. Cancer 44:742–747, 1979.
102. Upchurch KS, Simon LS, Schiller AL, et al: Giant cell reparative granuloma of Paget's disease of bone: A unique clinical entity. Ann Intern Med 98:35–40, 1983.
103. Case Records of the Massachusetts General Hospital. Case 1-1986. N Engl J Med 314:105–113, 1986.
104. Riggs BL, Arnaud CD, Goldsmith RS, et al: Plasma kinetics and acute effects of pharmacologic doses of porcine calcitonin in man. J Clin Endocrinol Metab 33:115–127, 1971.
105. Singer FR, Keutmann HT, Neer RM, et al: Pharmacological effects of salmon calcitonin in man. *In* Talmage RV, Munson PL (eds): Calcium, Parathyroid Hormone and the Calcitonins. Amsterdam, Excerpta Medica, 1972, pp 89–96.
106. Burckhardt PM, Singer FR, Potts JT Jr: Parathyroid function in patients with Paget's disease treated with salmon calcitonin. Clin Endocrinol 2:15–22, 1973.
107. Chapuy MC, Zucchelli P, Meunier PJ: Parathyroid function in Paget's disease of bone. Mineral Electrolyte Metab 6:112–118, 1981.
108. Krane SM, Brownell GL, Stanbury JB, Corrigan H: The effect of thyroid disease on calcium metabolism in man. J Clin Invest 35:874–887, 1956.
109. Dow EC, Stanbury JB: Strontium and calcium metabolism in metabolic bone diseases. J Clin Invest 39:885–903, 1960.
110. Avioli LV, Berman M: Role of magnesium metabolism and the effects of fluoride therapy in Paget's disease of bone. J Clin Endocrinol Metab 28:700–710, 1968.
111. Fogelman I, Bessent RG, Turner J, et al: The use of whole body retention of ^{99m}Tc-diphosphonate in the

diagnosis of metabolic bone disease. J Nucl Med 19:270–275, 1978.
112. Smith ML, Fogelman I, Ralston S, et al: Correlation of skeletal uptake of ^{99m}Tc-diphosphonate and alkaline phosphatase before and after oral diphosphonate therapy in Paget's disease. Metab Bone Dis Rel Res 5:167–170, 1984.
113. Aubert JP, Milhaud G: Methode de mesure des principales voies du metabolisme calcique chez l'homme. Biochim Biophys Acta 39:122–139, 1960.
114. Aubert JP, Bronner F, Richelle LJ: Quantitation of calcium metabolism, theory. J Clin Invest 42:885–897, 1963.
115. Pendergrass HP, Potsaid MS, Castronovo FP Jr: Clinical use of ^{99m}Tc-diphosphonate (HEDSPA). A new agent for skeletal imaging. Radiology 107:557–562, 1973.
116. Fogelman I, Carr D, Boyle IT: The role of bone scanning in Paget's disease. Metab Bone Dis Rel Res 4, 5:243–254, 1981.
117. Lee JY: Bone scintigraphy in evaluation of Didronel therapy for Paget's disease. Clin Nucl Med 6:356–358, 1981.
118. Lee W, Marshall JH, Sissons HA: Calcium accretion and bone formation in dogs: An experimental comparison between the results of Ca-45 kinetic analysis and tetracycline labeling. J Bone Joint Surg 47B:157–180, 1965.
119. Harris WH, Heaney RP: Skeletal Renewal and Metabolic Bone Disease. Boston, Little, Brown, 1970.
120. Taylor WH: Low serum magnesium concentration in Paget's disease of bone (osteitis deformans). Ann Clin Biochem 22:591–595, 1985.
121. Guillard-Cumming DF, Beard DJ, Douglas DL, et al: Abnormal vitamin D metabolism in Paget's disease of bone. Clin Endocrinol 22:559–566, 1985.
122. Nimni ME: Collagen: Structure, function, and metabolism in normal and fibrotic tissues. Semin Arthritis Rheum 13:1–86, 1983.
123. Krane SM: Skeletal metabolism in Paget's disease of bone. Arthritis Rheum 23:1087–1094, 1980.
124. Cheung HS, Singer FR, Mills B, Nimni ME: In vitro synthesis of normal bone (type I) collagen by bones of Paget's disease patients. Proc Soc Exp Biol Med 163:547–552, 1980.
125. Simon LS, Krane SM, Wortman PD, et al: Serum levels of type I and III procollagen fragments in Paget's disease of bone. J Clin Endocrinol Metab 58:110–120, 1984.
126. Cheah KSE: Collagen genes and inherited connective tissue disease. Biochem J 229:287–303, 1985.
127. Cunningham LW, Ford JD, Segrest JP: The isolation of identical hydroxylysyl glycosides from hydrolysates of soluble collagen and from human urine. J Biol Chem 242:2570–2571, 1967.
128. Segrest JP, Cunningham LL: Variations in human O-hydroxyl glycoside levels and their relationship to collagen metabolism. J Clin Invest 49:1497–1509, 1970.
129. Pinnell SR, Fox R, Krane SM: Human collagens: Differences in glycosylated hydroxylysines in skin and bone. Biochim Biophys Acta 229:119–122, 1971.
130. Krane SM, Kantrowitz FG, Byrne M, et al: Urinary excretion of hydroxylysine and its glycosides as an index of collagen degradation. J Clin Invest 59:819–827, 1977.
131. Eyre DR: Collagen: Molecular diversity in the body's protein scaffold. Science 207:1315–1322, 1980.
132. Misra DP: Crosslink in bone collagen in Paget's disease. J Clin Pathol 28:305–308, 1975.
133. Eyre DR, Koob TJ, Van Ness KP: Quantitation of hydroxypyridinium crosslinks in collagen by high-performance liquid chromatography. Anal Biochem 137:380–388, 1984.
134. Quelch KJ, Cole WG, Melick RA: Non-collagenous proteins in normal and pathological human bone. Calcif Tissue Int 36:545–549, 1984.
135. Baron R, Neff L, Louvard D, Courtoy PJ: Cell-mediated extracellular acidification and bone resorption: Evidence for a low pH in resorbing lacunae and localization of a 100-kD lysosomal membrane protein at the osteoclast ruffled border. J Cell Biol 101:2210–2222, 1985.
136. Baron R, Neff L, Roy C: Evidence for a high and specific concentration of (Na^+K^+)ATPase in the plasma membrane of the osteoclast. Cell 46:311–320, 1986.
137. Vaes G: On the mechanism of bone resorption: The action of parathyroid hormone on the excretion and synthesis of lysosomal enzymes and on the extracellular release of acid by bone cells. J Cell Biol 39:676–697, 1968.
138. Vaes G: Collagenase, lysosomes, and osteoclastic bone resorption. *In* Woolley DE, Evanson JM (eds): Collagenase in Normal and Pathological Connective Tissues. London, J Wiley, 1980, pp 185–207.
139. Sakamoto S, Goldhaber P, Glimcher MJ: The further purification and characterization of mouse bone collagenase. Calcif Tissue Res 10:142–151, 1972.
140. Sakamoto S, Goldhaber P, Glimcher MJ: Mouse bone collagenase. Effect of heparin on the amount of enzyme released in tissue culture and on the activity of the enzyme. Calcif Tissue Res 12:247–258, 1973.
141. Sakamoto S, Sakamoto M, Goldhaber P, Glimcher MJ: Mouse bone collagenase. Purification of the enzyme by heparin-substituted Sepharose 4B affinity chromatography and preparation of specific antibody to the protein. Arch Biochem Biophys 188:438–449, 1978.
142. Harris ED, Welgus HG, Krane SM: Regulation of mammalian collagenases. Coll Rel Res 4:493–512, 1984.
143. Editorial: Paget's disease of bone. Calcif Tissue Int 38:309–312, 1986.
144. Gardner B, Gray H, Hedayati H: Bone collagenase in osteolytic stress of rats and humans. Surg Forum 21:467–468, 1970.
145. Sinex FM, Van Slyke DD: The source and state of the hydroxylysine of collagen. J Biol Chem 216:245–250, 1955.
146. Stetten MR: Some aspects of the metabolism of hydroxyproline studied with the aid of isotopic nitrogen. J Biol Chem 181:31–37, 1949.
147. Adams E: Metabolism of proline and of hydroxyproline. Int Rev Connect Tissue Res 5:1–91, 1970.
148. Kivirikko KI: Urinary excretion of hydroxyproline in health and disease. Int Rev Connect Tissue Res 5:93–163, 1970.
149. Ziff M, Kibrick A, Dresner E, Gribetz HJ: Excretion of hydroxyproline in patients with rheumatic and non-rheumatic diseases. J Clin Invest 35:579–587, 1956.
150. Askenasi R: A new rapid method for measuring hydroxylysine and its glycosides in hydroxylysates

and physiological fluids. Biochim Biophys Acta 304:375–383, 1973.
151. Askenasi R: Urinary hydroxylysine and hydroxylysine glycoside excretion in normal and pathological states. J Lab Clin Med 83:673–679, 1974.
152. Askenasi R, DeBacker M, Devos A: The origin of urinary hydroxylysine glycosides in Paget's disease of bone and in primary hyperparathyroidism. Calcif Tissue Res 22:35–40, 1976.
153. Krane SM, Simon LS: Organic matrix defects in metabolic and related bone disease. *In* Veis A (ed): The Chemistry and Biology of Mineralized Connective Tissue. New York, Elsevier/North Holland, pp 185–203, 1981.
154. Dull TA, Henneman PH: Urinary hydroxyproline as an index of collagen turnover in bone. N Engl J Med 268:132–134, 1963.
155. Khairi MRA, Wellman HN, Robb JA, Johnston CC Jr: Paget's disease of bone (osteitis deformans): Symptomatic lesions and bone scan. Ann Intern Med 79:348–351, 1973.
156. Kelleher PC: Urinary excretion of hydroxyproline, hydroxylysine and hydroxylysine glycosides by patients with Paget's disease of bone and carcinoma with metastases in bone. Clin Chim Acta 92:373–379, 1979.
157. Bijvoet OLM, van der Sluys Veer J, Jansen AP: Effects of calcitonin on patients with Paget's disease, thyrotoxicosis, or hypercalcemia. Lancet 1:876–881, 1968.
158. Gilbertson TJ, Brunden MN, Gruszczyk SB, et al: Serum total hydroxyproline assay: Effects of age, sex and Paget's bone disease. J Clin Chem Clin Biochem 21:129–132, 1983.
159. Benoit FL, Watten RH: Renal tubular transport of hydroxyproline peptides: Evidence for reabsorption and secretion. Metabolism 17:20–33, 1968.
160. Meilman E, Urivetsky MM, Rapoport CM: Urinary hydroxyproline peptides. J Clin Invest 42:40–50, 1963.
161. Scriver CR: Glycyl-proline in urine of humans with bone disease. Can J Physiol Pharmacol 42:357–364, 1964.
162. Alderman MH, Frimpter GW, Isaacs M, Scheiner E: Glycylproline peptiduria in familial hyperostosis of obscure nature. Metabolism 18:692–699, 1969.
163. Krane SM, Munoz AJ, Harris ED Jr: Collagen-like fragments: Excretion in urine of patients with Paget's disease of bone. Science 147:713–716, 1967.
164. Krane SM, Munoz AJ, Harris ED Jr: Urinary polypeptides related to collagen synthesis. J Clin Invest 99:716–729, 1970.
165. Haddad JG Jr, Couranz S, Avioli LV: Nondialyzable urinary hydroxyproline as an index of bone collagen formation. J Clin Endocrinol Metab 30:282–287, 1970.
166. Prockop DJ, Kivirikko KI, Tuderman L, Guzman NA: The biosynthesis of collagen and its disorder. N Engl J Med 301:13–23, 77–85, 1979.
167. Szymanowicz A: Polymorphism of urinary 4-hydroxyproline-containing polypeptides. J Chromatog 225:55–63, 1981.
168. Goldberg B, Taubman MB, Sherr CJ: Secretion and extracellular processing of procollagen by cultured human fibroblasts. Proc Natl Acad Sci USA 70:361–365, 1973.
169. Taubman MB, Goldberg B, Sherr CJ: Radioimmunoassay for human procollagen. Science 186:1115–1117, 1974.
170. Taubman MB, Hammerman S, Goldberg B: Radioimmunoassay of procollagen in serum of patients with Paget's disease of bone. Proc Soc Exp Biol Med 152:284–287, 1976.
171. Krane SM, Harris ED Jr, Singer FR, Potts JT Jr: Acute effects of calcitonin on bone formation in man. Metabolism 22:51–58, 1973.
172. Rohde H, Vargas L, Hahn E, et al: Radioimmunoassay for type III procollagen peptide and its application to human liver disease. Eur J Clin Invest 9:451–459, 1979.
173. Fleischmajer R, Timpl R, Tuderman L, et al: Ultrastructural identification of extension aminopropeptides of type I and III collagens in human skin. Proc Natl Acad Sci USA 78:7360–7364, 1981.
174. Fleischmajer R, Olsen BR, Timpl R, et al: Collagen fibril formation during embryogenesis. Proc Natl Acad Sci USA 80:3354–3358, 1983.
174a. Wilder-Smith CH, Holz-Gottswinter G, Ziegler R: Procollagen-III peptide serum levels in Paget's disease of the bone. Klin Wochenschr 65:174–178, 1987.
175. Paglia LM, Wilczek J, DeLeon LD, et al: Inhibition of procollagen cell-free synthesis by amino-terminal extension peptides. Biochemistry 18:5030–5034, 1979.
176. Paglia LM, Wiestner M, Duchene M, et al: Effects of procollagen peptides on the translation of type II collagen messenger ribonucleic acid and on collagen biosynthesis in chondrocytes. Biochemistry 20:3523–3527, 1981.
177. Ashton BA, Smith R: Plasma α_2HS-glycoprotein concentration in Paget's disease of bone: Its possible significance. Clin Sci 58:435–438, 1980.
178. Ashton BA, Holling H-J, Triffit JT: Plasma proteins present in human cortical bone: Enrichment of the αHS-glycoprotein. Calcif Tissue Res 22:27–33, 1976.
179. Price PA, Parthemore JG, Deftos LJ, Nishimoto SK: New biochemical marker for bone metabolism. Measurement by radioimmunoassay of bone GLA protein in the plasma of normal subjects and patients with bone disease. J Clin Invest 66:878–883, 1980.
180. Deftos LJ, Parthemore JG, Price PA: Changes in plasma bone GLA protein during treatment of bone disease. Calcif Tissue Int 34:121–124, 1982.
181. Brown JP, Delmas PD, Malaval L, Meunier PJ: Serum bone GLA-protein: A specific marker of bone formation in postmenopausal osteoporosis. *In* Christiansen C, Arnaud, CD, Nordin BEC, et al (eds): Osteoporosis. Proceedings of the Copenhagen International Symposium on Osteoporosis, Department of Clinical Chemistry, Glostrop Hospital, Denmark, 1984, pp 127–131.
182. Preston CJ, Coulton LA, Couch M, Kanis JA: Serum osteocalcin levels in Paget's disease treated with diphosphonates. Calcif Tissue Int 36:S76, 1984.
183. Slovik DM, Gundberg CM, Neer RM, Lian JB: Clinical evaluation of bone turnover by serum osteocalcin measurements in a hospital setting. J Clin Endocrinol Metab 59:228–230, 1984.
184. Delmas PD, Demiaux B, Malawal L, et al: Serum bone GLA-protein is not a sensitive marker of bone turnover in Paget's disease of bone. Calcif Tissue Int 38:60–61, 1986.
185. Wilkinson MR, Wagstaff RN, Delbridge L, et al: Serum osteocalcin concentrations in Paget's disease of bone. Arch Intern Med 146:268–271, 1986.

185a. Papapoulos SE, Frolich M, Mudde AH, et al: Serum osteocalcin in Paget's disease of bone: Basal concentrations and response to bisphosphonate treatment. J Clin Endocrinol Metab 65:89–94, 1987.
186. Gundberg CM, Lian JB, Gallop PM, Steinberg JJ: Urinary-carboxyglutamic acid and serum osteocalcin as bone markers: Studies in osteoporosis and Paget's disease. J Clin Endocrinol Metab 57:1221–1225, 1983.
187. Malaval L, Delmas PD, Meunier PJ: Measurement of serum osteonectin by radioimmunoassay. Proc Am Soc Bone Mineral Res 7:265, 1985.
188. Neuman WF, Neuman MW: The Chemical Dynamics of Bone Mineral. Chicago, University of Chicago Press, 1958.
189. Kenny AD: Citric acid production by bone. *In* Greep RO, Talmage RV (eds): The Parathyroids. Springfield, IL, Charles C Thomas, 1961, pp 275–291.
190. Nisbet JA, Helliwell S, Nordin BEC: Relation of lactic acid and citric acid metabolism to bone resorption in tissue culture. Clin Orthop Rel Res 70:220–230, 1970.
191. Costello LC, Stacey R, Stevens R: Hypocitricemic effects of calcitonin, parathyroidectomy and surgical stress. Horm Metab Res 3:120–125, 1971.
192. Watson L: Citrate metabolism in hyperparathyroidism. Proc R Soc Med 52:349–351, 1959.
193. Harrison HE: The interrelation of citrate and calcium metabolism. Am J Med 20:1–3, 1956.
194. Hodgkinson A: The relation between citric acid and calcium metabolism with particular reference to primary hyperparathyroidism and idiopathic hypercalciuria. Clin Sci 24:167–178, 1963.
195. Shorr E, Almy TP, Sloan MH, et al: The relation between the urinary excretion of citric acid and calcium; its implications for urinary calcium stone formation. Science 96:587–588, 1942.
196. Kissin B, Kreeger N: Serum citric acid in Paget's disease. Am J Med Sci 228:301–305, 1954.
197. Natelson S, Pincus JB, Lugovoy JK: Microestimation of citric acid: A new colorimetric reaction for pentabromacetone. J Biol Chem 175:745–750, 1948.
198. Brodwall EK, Westlie L, Myhre E: The renal excretion and tubular reabsorption of citric acid in renal tubular acidosis. Acta Med Scand 192:137–139, 1972.
199. McComb RB, Bowers GN Jr, Posen S: Alkaline Phosphatase. New York, Plenum Press, 1979, pp 865–902.
200. Sussman HH: Structural analysis of a human alkaline phosphatase. *In* Stigbrand T, Fishman WH (eds): Human Alkaline Phosphatases. New York, Alan R Liss, 1984, pp 87–103.
201. Kay HD: Plasma phosphatase in osteitis deformans and in other disease of bone. Br J Exp Pathol 10:253–256, 1929.
202. Stinson RA, Seargent LE: Comparative studies of pure alkaline phosphatase from five human tissues. Clin Chim Acta 110:261–272, 1981.
203. Posen S, Grunstein HS: Turnover rate of skeletal alkaline phosphatase in humans. Clin Chem 28:153–154, 1982.
204. Wellman HN, Schauwecker D, Robb JA, et al: Skeletal scintimaging and radiography in the diagnosis and management of Paget's disease. Clin Orthop Rel Res 127:55–62, 1977.
205. Woodard HQ: The clinical significance of serum acid phosphatase. Am J Med 27:902–910, 1959.
206. Porretta CA, Dahlin DC, Janes JM: Sarcoma in Paget's disease of bone. J Bone Joint Surg 39A:1314–1329, 1957.
207. Hill PG, Sammons HG: An assessment of 5′-nucleotidase as a liver-function test. Q J Med 36:457–468, 1967.
208. Sullivan TJ, Gutman EB, Gutman AB: Theory and application of the serum "acid" phosphatase determination in metastasizing prostatic carcinoma; early effects of castration. J Urol 48:426–458, 1942.
209. Woodard HQ: Factors leading to elevations in serum acid glycerophosphatase. Cancer 5:236–241, 1952.
209a. Lau K-HW, Ohishi T, Wergedal JE: Characterization and assay of tartrate-resistant acid phosphatase activity in serum: potential use to assess bone resorption. Clin Chem 33:458–462, 1987.
210. O'Reilly TJ, Race J: Osteitis deformans. Q J Med 25:471–497, 1932.
211. Reifenstein EC Jr, Albright F: Paget's disease: Its pathologic physiology and the importance of this in the complications arising from fracture and immobilization. N Engl J Med 231:343–355, 1944.
212. Moehlig RC, Adler S: Carbohydrate metabolism disturbance in osteoporosis and Paget's disease. Surg Gynecol Obstet 64:747–757, 1937.
213. Ridlon HC: Urinary calculi associated with Paget's disease of bone. J Urol 87:499–503, 1962.
214. Gutman AB, Parsons WB: Hyperparathyroidism simulating or associated with Paget's disease. Ann Intern Med 12:13–25, 1938.
215. Posen S, Clifton-Bligh P, Wilkinson M: Paget's disease of bone and hyperparathyroidism: Coincidence or causal relationship? Calcif Tissue Res 26:107–109, 1978.
216. Ooi TC, Spiro TP, Ibbertson HK: Coexisting Paget's disease of bone and hyperparathyroidism. N Engl J Med 91:134–136, 1980.
217. Rosenkrantz JA, Gluckman EC: Coexistence of Paget's disease of bone and multiple myeloma. AJR 78:30–38, 1957.
218. Chapuy M-C, Zucchelli P, Meunier PJ: Parathyroid function in Paget's disease of bone. Mineral Electrolyte Metab 6:112–118, 1981.
218a. Siris ES, Clemens TP, McMahon D: Parathyroid function in Paget's disease of bone. J Bone Mineral Res 4:75–79, 1989.
219. Talbott JH, Coombs FS: Metabolic studies on patients with gout. JAMA 110:1977–1982, 1938.
220. Serre H, Mirowze J: L'osteose pagetique des goutteux et des diabetique. Presse Med 60:595–598, 1952.
221. Weiss TE, Segaloff A: Gouty Arthritis and Gout. Springfield, IL, Charles C Thomas, 1959, p 115.
222. Wright JT: Unusual manifestations of gout. Australas Radiol 10:365–374, 1966.
223. Fennelly JJ, Hogan A: Pseudouridine excretion—a reflection of high RNA turnover in Paget's disease. Ir J Med Sci 141:103–107, 1972.
223a. Lluberas-Acosta G, Hansell JR, Schumacher HR Jr: Paget's disease of bone in patients with gout. Arch Intern Med 146:2389–2392, 1986.
224. Radi I, Epiney J, Reiner M: Chondrocalcinose et maladie osseuse de Paget. Rev Rhum Mal Osteoartic 37:385–388, 1970.
225. Edholm OG, Howarth S, McMichael J: Heart failure and bone blood flow in osteitis deformans. Clin Sci 5:249–260, 1945.

226. Rutishauser E, Veyrat R, Rouiller C: La vascularisation de l'os pagetique—etude anatomopathologique. Presse Med 62:654–657, 1954.
227. Rhodes BA, Greyson ND, Hamilton CR: Absence of anatomic arteriovenous shunts in Paget's disease of bone. N Engl J Med 287:686–689, 1975.
228. Demmler K: Die vaskularisation des Pagetknochens. Dtsch Med Wochenschr 99:91–95, 1974.
229. Heistad DD, Abboud FM, Schmid PG, et al: Regulation of blood flow in Paget's disease of bone. J Clin Invest 55:69–78, 1975.
230. Wootton R, Reeve J, Veall N: The clinical measurement of skeletal blood flow. Clin Sci Mol Med 50:261–268, 1976.
231. Wootton R, Tellez M, Green JR, Reeve J: Skeletal blood flow in Paget's disease of bone. Metab Bone Dis Rel Res 3:263–270, 1981.
232. Walton R, Green JR, Reeve J, Wootton R: Reduction of skeletal blood flow in Paget's disease with etidronate therapy. Bone 6:29–30, 1985.
233. Haworth S: Cardiac output in osteitis deformans. Clin Sci 12:271–275, 1953.
234. Lequime J, Denolim H: Circulatory dynamics in osteitis deformans. Circulation 12:215–219, 1955.
235. Arnalich F, Plaza I, Sobrino JA, et al: Cardiac size and function in Paget's disease of bone. Int J Cardiol 5:491–505, 1984.
236. Harrison CV, Lennox B: Heart block in osteitis deformans. Br Heart J 10:167–172, 1948.
237. King M, Huang JM, Glassman E: Paget's disease with cardiac calcification and complete heart block. Am J Med 46:302–304, 1969.
237a. Strickberger SA, Schulman SP, Hutchins GM: Association of Paget's disease of bone with calcific aortic valve disease. Am J Med 82:953–956, 1987.
238. Acar J, Delbarre F, Waynberger M: Les complications cardio-vasculaires de la maladie osseuse de Paget. Arch Mal Coeur 61:849–868, 1968.
239. Larmande A, Margaillan A: Maladie de Paget et syndrome de Groenblad-Strandberg. Bull Soc Fr Ophthalmol 70:206–215, 1957.
240. Shaffer B, Copelan HW, Beerman H: Pseudoxanthoma elasticum. Arch Dermatol 76:622–630, 1957.
241. Moretti GF, Texier L, Staeffen J: Elastorrhexie systematisee et maladie de Paget. Unite histologique des lesions du tissu elastique. Sem Hosp Paris 38:3813–3818, 1962.
242. Paton D: The Relation of Angioid Streaks to Systemic Disease. Springfield, IL, Charles C Thomas, 1972.
243. Clarkson JG, Altman RD: Angioid streaks. Surv Ophthalmol 26:235–246, 1982.
244. Robey PG, Newson DA: Biosynthesis of proteoglycans present in primate Bruch's membrane. Ophthalmol Vis Sci 24:898–905, 1985.
245. Francis MJO, Smith R: Evidence of a generalised connective tissue defect in Paget's disease of bone. Lancet 1:841–842, 1974.
246. Somayaji BN: Malabsorption syndrome in Paget's disease of bone. Br Med J 4:278–280, 1968.
247. Milhaud G, Tsien-Ming L, Nesralla H, et al: Studies on the mode of action and the therapeutic use of thyrocalcitonin. *In* Taylor S (ed): Calcitonin. Proceedings of the Symposium on Thyrocalcitonin and the C Cells. London, W Heinemann, 1968, pp 347–360.
248. Bijvoet OLM, Jansen AP: Thyrocalcitonin in Paget's disease. Lancet 2:471–472, 1967.
249. Canniggia A, Gennari C: Azione della tirocalcitonina nell'uomo. Minerva Med 59:279–295, 1968.
250. Singer FR, Schiller AL, Pyle EB, Krane SM: Paget's disease of bone. *In* Avioli LV, Krane SM (eds): Metabolic Bone Disease, vol II. New York, Academic Press, 1978, pp 5[illegible]8–564.
251. Singer FR: Human calcitonin treatment of Paget's disease of bone. Clin Orthop Rel Res 127:86–93, 1977.
252. Nuti R, Vattimo A: Synthetisches human-calcitonin bei osteodystrophia deformans (Paget) und osteoporose. Dtsch Med Wochenschr 106:149–152, 1981.
253. Bijvoet OLM, van der Sluys Veer J, Wildiers J, Smeenk D: Effects of longterm calcitonin administration to patients. *In* Taylor S, Foster G (eds): Calcitonin 1969. Proceedings of the Second International Symposium. London, W Heinemann, 1970, pp 531–539.
254. Shai F, Baker RK, Wallach S: The clinical and metabolic effects of porcine calcitonin on Paget's disease of bone. J Clin Invest 50:1927–1940, 1971.
255. Woodhouse NJY, Bordier P, Fisher M, et al: Human calcitonin in the treatment of Paget's bone disease. Lancet 1:1139–11[illegible]3, 1971.
256. Oreopoulos DG, Husdan H, Harrison J, et al: Metabolic balance studies in patients with Paget's disease receiving salmon calcitonin over long periods. Can Med Assoc J 123: 851–855, 1977.
257. Spinks TJ, Joplin GF, Evans IMA, et al: Long-term measurement of skeletal and lean body mass in Paget's disease of bone treated with synthetic human calcitonin. Calcif Tissue Int 34:459–464, 1982.
258. Fornasier VL, Stapleton K, Williams CC: Histologic changes in Paget's disease treated with calcitonin. Human Pathol 9:[illegible]55–461, 1978.
259. Lesh JB, Aldred JP, Bastian JW, Kleszynski RR: Clinical experience with porcine and salmon calcitonin. *In* Taylor S (ed): Endocrinology, 1973. Proceedings of the Fourth International Symposium. London, W Heinemann, 1974, pp 409–424.
260. Bouvet JP: Traitement de la maladie de Paget por la thyrocalcitonine de saumon. Nouv Presse Med 6:1447–1450, 197[illegible]
261. Woodhouse NJY, Crosbie WA, Mohamedally SM: Cardiac output in Paget's disease: Response to long-term salmon calcitonin therapy. Br Med J 4:686, 1975.
262. Chen J-R, Rhee RSC, Wallach S, et al: Neurologic disturbances in Paget's disease of bone: Response to calcitonin. Neurology 29:448–457, 1979.
263. El Sammaa M, Linthicum FH Jr, House HP, House JW: Calcitonin as treatment for hearing loss in Paget's disease. Am J Otolaryngol 7:241–243, 1986.
264. Doyle FH, Pennock J, Greenberg PB, et al: Radiological evidence of a dose-related response to long-term treatment of Paget's disease with human calcitonin. Br J Radiol 47:1–8, 1974.
265. Nagant de Deuxchaisnes C, Maldague B, Malghem J, et al: The action of the main therapeutic regimes on Paget's disease of bone, with a note on the effect of vitamin D deficiency. Arthritis Rheum 23:1215–1234, 1980.
266. Wooton R, Reeve J, Spellacy E, Tellez-Yudilevich M: Skeletal blood flow in Paget's disease of bone and its response to calcitonin therapy. Clin Sci Mol Med 54:69–74, 1978.

267. Myers M, Singer F: Osteotomy for tibia vara in Paget's disease under cover of calcitonin. J Bone Joint Surg 60A:810–814, 1978.
268. Waxman AD, Ducker S, McKee D, et al: Evaluation of ^{99m}Tc diphosphonate kinetics and bone scans in patients with Paget's disease before and after calcitonin treatment. Radiology 125:761–764, 1977.
269. Waxman A, McKee D, Siemsen J, Singer F: Gallium scanning in Paget's disease of bone. AJR 134:303–306, 1980.
269a. Mills BG, Masuoka LS, Graham CC Jr, et al: Gallium-67 citrate localization in osteoclast nuclei of Paget's disease of bone. J Nucl Med 29:1083–1087, 1988.
270. Singer FR, Aldred JP, Neer RM, et al: An evaluation of antibodies and clinical resistance to salmon calcitonin. J Clin Invest 51:2331–2338, 1972.
271. Haddad JG Jr, Caldwell JG: Calcitonin resistance: Clinical and immunologic studies in subjects with Paget's disease of bone treated with porcine and salmon calcitonins. J Clin Invest 51:3133–3141, 1972.
272. MacIntyre I, Evans IMA, Hobitz HHG, et al: Chemistry, physiology and therapeutic applications of calcitonin. Arthritis Rheum 23:1139–1147, 1980.
273. Singer FR, Fredericks RS, Minkin C: Salmon calcitonin therapy for Paget's disease of bone. The problem of acquired clinical resistance. Arthritis Rheum 23:1148–1154, 1980.
274. DeRose J, Singer FR, Avramides A, et al: Response of Paget's disease to porcine and salmon calcitonins. Am J Med 56:858–866, 1974.
275. Martin TJ: Treatment of Paget's disease with the calcitonins. Aust NZ J Med 9:36–43, 1979.
275a. Levy F, Muff R, Dotti-Sigrist S, Dambacher MA, Fisher JA: Formation of neutralizing antibodies during intranasal synthetic salmon calcitonin treatment of Paget's disease. J Clin Endocrinol Metab 67:541–545, 1988.
276. Dietrich FM, Fischer JA, Bijvoet OLM: Formation of antibodies to synthetic human calcitonin during treatment of Paget's disease. Acta Endocrinol 92:468–476, 1979.
277. Woodhouse NJY, Mohamedally SM, Saed-Nejad F, Martin TJ: Development and significance of antibodies to salmon calcitonin in patients with Paget's disease on long-term treatment. Br Med J 2:927–929, 1977.
278. Hosking DJ, Denton LB, Cadge B, Martin TJ: Functional significance of antibody formation after long-term salmon calcitonin therapy. Clin Endocrinol 10:243–252, 1979.
279. Rojanasathit S, Rosenberg E, Haddad JG Jr: Paget's bone disease: Response to human calcitonin in patients resistant to salmon calcitonin. Lancet 2:1412–1415, 1974.
280. Dube WJ, Goldsmith RS, Arnaud SB, Arnaud CD: Hyperparathyroidism secondary to long-term therapy of Paget's disease of bone with calcitonin. *In* Talmage RV, Munson PC (eds): Calcium, Parathyroid Hormone and the Calcitonins. Amsterdam, Excerpta Medica, 1972, pp 113–115.
281. Ziegler R, Holz G, Raue F, et al: Therapeutic studies with human calcitonin. *In* MacIntyre I (ed): Human Calcitonin and Paget's Disease. Bern, H Huber, 1977, pp 167–178.
282. Chapuy MC, David L, Meunier PJ: Parathyroid function during treatment with salmon calcitonin. Horm Metab Res 12:486–487, 1980.
283. Heynen G, Franchimont P, Gaspar S, et al: Variations des taux seriques de parathormone au cours traitement de la maladie de Paget par calcitonine humaine ou de saumon. Ann Endocrinol 42:265–275, 1981.
284. Evans RA, Dunstan CR, Wong SYP, Hills E: Long-term experience with a calcium-thiazide treatment for Paget's disease of bone. Miner Electrolyte Metab 8:325–333, 1982.
285. Evans IMA, Banks L, Doyle FH, et al: Paget's disease of bone—the effect of stopping long-term human calcitonin and recommendations for future treatment. Metab Bone Dis Rel Res 2:87–92, 1980.
286. Nagant de Deuxchaisnes C, Devogelaer JP, Huaux JP, et al: Effect of a nasal spray of salmon calcitonin in normal subjects and in patients with Paget's disease of bone. *In* Pecile A (ed): Calcitonin. Amsterdam, Elsevier, 1985, pp 329–343.
286a. Nagant de Deuxchaisnes C, DeVogelaer JP, Huaux JP, et al: New modes of administration of salmon calcitonin in Paget's disease. Nasal spray and suppository. Clin Orthop Rel Res 217:56–71, 1987.
287. Fleisch H: Bisphosphonates: Mechanisms of action and clinical applications. *In* Peck WA (ed): Bone and Mineral Research Annual 1. Amsterdam, Excerpta Medica, 1983, pp 319–357.
288. Smith R, Russell RGG, Bishop M: Diphosphonates and Paget's disease of bone. Lancet 1:945–947, 1971.
289. Altman RD, Johnston CC, Khairi MRA, et al: Influence of disodium etidronate on clinical and laboratory manifestations of Paget's disease of bone (osteitis deformans). N Engl J Med 289:1379–1384, 1973.
290. Smith R, Russell RGG, Bishop MC, et al: Paget's disease of bone. Experience with a diphosphonate (disodium etidronate) in treatment. Q J Med 42(NS):235–256, 1973.
291. Guncaga J, Lauffenburger T, Lentner C, et al: Diphosphonate treatment of Paget's disease of bone. Horm Metab Res 6:62–69, 1974.
292. DeVries HR, Bijvoet OLM: Results of prolonged treatment of Paget's disease of bone with disodium ethane-1-hydroxy-1,1-diphosphonate (EHDP). Neth J Med 17:281–298, 1974.
293. Russell RGG, Smith R, Preston C, et al: Diphosphonates in Paget's disease. Lancet 1:894–898, 1974.
294. Khairi MRA, Johnston CC Jr, Altman RD, et al: Treatment of Paget's disease of bone (osteitis deformans). JAMA 230:562–567, 1974.
295. Kantrowitz FG, Byrne MH, Schiller AL, Krane SM: Clinical and biochemical effects of diphosphonates in Paget's disease of bone. Arthritis Rheum 18:4, 1975.
296. Meunier P, Chapuy M-C, Courpron P, et al: Effets cliniques, biologiques et histologiques de l' ethane-1-hydroxy 1,1 diphosphonate (EHDP) dans la maladie de Paget. Rev Rhum Mal Osteoartic 42:699–705, 1975.
297. Reiner M, Jung A, Seiler A, et al: Le traitement de la maladie de Paget par les diphosphonates. Schweiz Med Wochenschr 105:1701–1703, 1975.
298. Caniggia A, Gennari C, Guideri R, et al: Terapi del morbo di Paget con difosfonato (disodio etidronato). Minerva Med 67:1–15, 1976.
299. Jung A, Mermillod B, Schenk R, et al: Traitement de 10 cas symptomatiques de maladie de Paget par l'etidronate (EHDP). Schweiz Med Wochenschr 106:1667–1673, 1976.

300. Finerman GAM, Gonick HC, Smith RK, Mayfield JM: Diphosphonate treatment of Paget's disease. Clin Orthop Rel Res 120:115–124, 1976.
301. Canfield R, Rosner W, Skinner J, et al: Diphosphonate therapy of Paget's disease of bone. J Clin Endocrinol Metab 44:96–106, 1977.
302. Khairi MRA, Altman RD, DeRosa GP, et al: Sodium etidronate in the treatment of Paget's disease of bone. A study of long-term results. Ann Intern Med 87:656–663, 1977.
303. Stein I, Shapiro B, Ostrum B, Beller ML: Evaluation of sodium etidronate in the treatment of Paget's disease of bone. Clin Orthop Rel Res 122:347–358, 1977.
304. Ibbertson HK, Henley JW, Fraser TR, et al: Paget's disease of bone—clinical evaluation and treatment with diphosphonate. Aust NZ J Med 9:31–35, 1979.
305. Henley JW, Croxson RS, Ibbertson HK: The cardiovascular system in Paget's disease of bone and the response to therapy with calcitonin and diphosphonate. Aust NZ J Med 9:390–397, 1979.
306. Nagant de Deuxchaisnes C, Rombouts-Lindemans C, Huaux JP, et al: Roentgenologic evaluation of the diphosphonate EHDP and of combined therapy (EHDP and calcitonin) in Paget's disease of bone. *In* MacIntyre I, Szelke M (eds): Molecular Endocrinology. Amsterdam, Elsevier/North Holland, 1979, pp 405–433.
307. Fromm GA, Schajowicz F, Casco C, et al: The treatment of Paget's disease of bone with sodium etidronate. Am J Med Sci 277:29–37, 1979.
308. Murphy WA, Whyte MP, Haddad JG Jr.: Healing of lytic Paget bone disease with diphosphonate therapy. Radiology 134:635–637, 1980.
309. Johnston CC Jr, Khairi MRA, Meunier PJ: Use of etidronate (EHDP) in Paget's disease of bone. Arthritis Rheum 23:1172–1176, 1980.
310. Siris ES, Canfield RE, Jacobs TP, Baquiran DC: Long-term therapy of Paget's disease of bone with EHDP. Arthritis Rheum 23:1177–1184, 1980.
311. Alexandre C, Meunier PJ, Edouard C, et al: Effects of ethane-1 hydroxy-1,1-diphosphonate (5 mg/kg/day dose) on quantitative bone histology in Paget's disease of bone. Metab Bone Dis Rel Res 4, 5:309–316, 1981.
312. Norman DA, Zerwekh JE, Pak CYC: An apparent 1,25-dihydroxyvitamin D–independent stimulation of intestinal calcium absorption in patients with Paget's disease of bone during a short-term diphosphonate therapy. Metabolism 30:290–292, 1981.
313. Perry HM III, Avioli LV: Effect of sodium etidronate and phenytoin on pagetic bone. Calcif Tissue Int 33:285–286, 1981.
314. Davoine GA, Jung A, Courvoisier B: Traitement de la maladie osseuse de Paget: Diphosphonates ou calcitonine. Schweiz Med Wochenschr 111:518–524, 1981.
315. Siris ES, Canfield RE, Jacobs TP, et al: Clinical and biochemical effects of EHDP in Paget's disease of bone: Patterns of response to initial treatment and to long-term therapy. Metab Bone Dis Rel Res 4, 5:301–308, 1981.
316. Renier JC, Bontoux-Carre E, Bontoux L, et al: Le traitement de la maladie de Paget par l'ethane-1, hydroxy-1,1-diphosphonate (EHDP). Rev Rhum Mal Osteoartic 49:87–92, 1982.
317. Coindre JM, Edouard CM, Arlot ME, Meunier PJ: Etude histomorphometrique de l'os non pagetique chez le pagetique. Resultats avant et apres diphosphonates. Rev Rhum Mal Osteoartic 49:103–109, 1982.
318. Krane SM: Etidronate disodium in the treatment of Paget's disease of bone. Ann Intern Med 96:619–625, 1982.
319. Johnston CC Jr, Altman RD, Canfield RE, et al: Review of fracture experience during treatment of Paget's disease of bone with etidronate disodium. Clin Orthop Rel Res 172:186–194, 1983.
320. Alexandre CM, Chapuy MC, Vignon E, et al: Treatment of Paget's disease of bone with ethane-1, hydroxy-1,1-diphosphonate (EHDP) at a low dosage (5 mg/kg/day). Clin Orthop Rel Res 174:193–205, 1983.
321. Evans RA, Hills E, Dunstan CR, Wong SYP: Pathologic fracture due to severe osteomalacia following low-dose diphosphonate treatment of Paget's disease of bone. Aust NZ J Med 13:277–279, 1983.
322. Evans RA, MacDonald D: Diphosphonates and painful feet. Aust NZ J Med 13:175–176, 1983.
323. Holz G, Delling G, Ziegler R: Etidronsaure-therapie bei morbus Paget des skelettes. Dtsch Med Wochenschr 108:1954–1958, 1983.
324. Smith ML, Fogelman I, Ralston S, et al: Correlation of skeletal uptake of ^{99m}Tc-diphosphonate and alkaline phosphatase before and after oral diphosphonate therapy in Paget's disease. Metab Bone Dis Rel Res 5:167–170, 1984.
325. Basle MF, Rebel A, Renier JC, et al: Bone tissue in Paget's disease treated by ethane-1,hydroxy-1,1-diphosphonate (EHDP). Structure, ultrastructure, and immunocytology. Clin Orthop Rel Res 184:281–288, 1984.
326. Boyce BF, Smith L, Fogelman I, et al: Focal osteomalacia due to low-dose disphosphonate therapy in Paget's disease. Lancet 1:821–824, 1984.
327. Perry HM III, Droke DM, Avioli LV: Alternate calcitonin and etidronate disodium therapy for Paget's bone disease. Arch Intern Med 144:929–933, 1984.
328. Altman RD: Long-term follow-up of therapy with intermittent etidronate disodium in Paget's disease of bone. Am J Med 79:583–590, 1985.
329. Dewis P, Prasad BK, Anderson DC, Willets S: Clinical experience with the use of two disphosphonates in the treatment of Paget's disease. Ann Rheum Dis 44:34–38, 1985.
330. Preston CJ, Yates AJP, Beneton MNC, et al: Effective short term treatment of Paget's disease with oral etidronate. Br Med J 292:79–80, 1986.
331. Gibbs CJ, Aaron JE, Peacock M: Osteomalacia in Paget's disease treated with short term, high dose sodium etidronate. Br Med J 292:1227–1229, 1986.
332. Mautalen C, Gonzalez D, Blumenfeld EL, et al: Spontaneous fractures of uninvolved bones in patients with Paget's disease during unduly prolonged treatment with disodium etidronate (EHDP). Clin Ortho Rel Res 207:150–155, 1986.
332a. Meunier PJ, Chapuy M-C, Delmas P: Intravenous disodium etidronate therapy in Paget's disease of bone and hypercalcemia of malignancy. Am J Med 82(Suppl 2A):71–78, 1987.
332b. Gray RES, Yates AJP, Preston CJ, et al: Duration of effect of oral diphosphonate therapy in Paget's disease of bone. Q J Med NS 64:755–767, 1987.
332c. Lawson-Matthew PJ, Guilland-Cumming DF, Yates AJP, et al: Contrasting effects of intravenous and

oral etidronate on vitamin D metabolism in man. Clin Sci 74:101–106, 1988.
332d. Ravault A, Meunier PJ: Suivi au long cours de 88 pagetiques traités par l'etidronate disodique en cures discontinues a faible posologie. Rev Rheum 56:293–302, 1989.
333. Meunier PJ, Chapuy MC, Alexandre C, et al: Effects of disodium dichloromethylene diphosphonate on Paget's disease of bone. Lancet 2:489–492, 1979.
334. Douglas DL, Duckworth T, Kanis JA, et al: Biochemical and clinical responses to dichloromethylene diphosphonate (Cl_2MDP) in Paget's disease of bone. Arthritis Rheum 23:1185–1192, 1980.
335. Vergnon JM, Cheix F, Vauzelle JL, et al: Localisations sarcomateuses multifocales dans un cas de maladie osseuse de Paget. Effets du dichloromethylene diphosphonate. Nouv Presse Med 10:2353–2360, 1981.
336. Arlot ME, Meunier PJ: Effects of two diphosphonates (EHDP and Cl_2MDP) on serum uric acid in pagetic patients. Calcif Tissue Int 33:195–198, 1981.
337. Harris ST, Neer RM, Segre GV, et al: Secondary hyperparathyroidism associated with dichloromethylene diphosphonate treatment of Paget's disease. J Clin Endocrinol Metab 55:1100–1107, 1982.
338. Delmas PD, Chapuy MC, Vignon E, et al: Long-term effects of dichloromethylene diphosphonate in Paget's disease of bone. J Clin Endocrinol Metab 54:837–844, 1982.
339. Delmas PD, Chapuy MC, Meunier PJ: Paradoxical acute hypercalcemic effect of salmon calcitonin in patients having Paget's disease of bone after treatment with dichloromethylene diphosphonate. Horm Metab Res 16:258–261, 1984.
340. Adami S, Guarrera G, Salvagno G, et al: Sequential treatment of Paget's disease with human calcitonin and dichloromethylene diphosphonate. Metab Bone Dis Rel Res 5:265–267, 1984.
341. Yates AJP, Percival RC, Gray RES, et al: Intravenous clodronate in the treatment and retreatment of Paget's disease of bone. Lancet 1:1474–1477, 1985.
342. Kanis JA, Preston CJ, Beard DJ, et al: Comparative effects of an antiviral drug, inosiplex, and diphosphonate in Paget's disease of bone. Bone 6:69–72, 1985.
342a. McCloskey EV, Yates AJP, Beneton MNC, et al: Comparative effects of intravenous diphosphonates on calcium and skeletal metabolism in man. Bone 8(Suppl):535–541, 1987.
343. Frijlink WB, Bijvoet OLM, te Velde J, Heynen G: Treatment of Paget's disease with (3-amino-1-hydroxypropylidene)-1,1-bisphosphonate(A.P.D.).Lancet 1:799–803, 1979.
344. Bijvoet OLM, Frijlink WB, Jie K, et al: APD in Paget's disease of bone. Role of the mononuclear phagocyte system? Arthritis Rheum 23:1193–1204, 1980.
345. Nagant de Deuxchaisnes C, Rombouts-Lindemans C, Huaux JP, et al: Treatment of Paget's disease with the diphosphonate APD. A biological and radiological study. *In* Donath A, Courvoisier B (eds): Symposium CEMO IV Diphosphonates and Bone. Brussels, Editions Medicine et Hygiene, 1982, pp 303–327.
346. Adami S, Frijlink WB, Bijvoet OLM, et al: Regulation of calcium absorption by 1,25,dihydroxy-vitamin D–studies of the effects of a bisphosphonate treatment. Calcif Tissue Int 34:317–320, 1982.
347. Heynen G, Delwaide P, Bijvoet OLM, Franchimont P: Clinical and biological effects of low doses of (3 amino-1 hydroxypropylidene)-1,1-bisphosphonate (APD) in Paget's disease of bone. Eur J Clin Invest 11:29–35, 1982.
348. Mautalen CA: Treatment of Paget's bone disease with the bisphosphonate APD. Henry Ford Hosp Med J 31:244–248, 1983.
349. Mautalen CA, Casco CA, Gonzalez D, et al: Side effects of disodium aminohydroxypropylidenediphosphonate (APD) during treatment of bone diseases. Br Med J 288:828–829, 1984.
350. Vellenga CJLR, Mulder JD, Bijvoet OLM: Radiological demonstration of healing in Paget's disease of bone treated with APD. Br J Radiol 58:831–837, 1985.
351. Vellenga CJLR, Pauwels EKJ, Bijvoet OLM, et al: Quantitative bone scintigraphy in Paget's disease treated with APD. Br J Radiol 58:1165–1172, 1985.
352. Mautalen CA, Gonzalez D, Ghiringhelli G: Efficacy of the bisphosphonate APD in the control of Paget's bone disease. Bone 6:429–432, 1985.
353. Cantrill JA, Buckler HM, Anderson DC: Low dose intravenous 3-amino-1-hydroxypropylidene-1,1-bisphosphonate (APD) for the treatment of Paget's disease of bone. Ann Rheum Dis 45:1012–1018, 1986.
353a. Harinck HIJ, Bijvoet OLM, Blanksma HJ, Dahlinghaus-Nienhuys PJ: Efficacious management with APD in Paget's disease of bone. Clin Orthop Rel Res 217:79–98, 1987.
353b. Thiebaud D, Jaeger P, Burckhardt P: Paget's disease of bone treated in five days with AHPrBl (APD) per os. J Bone Min Res 2:45–52, 1987.
353c. Vega E, Gonzalez D, Ghiringhelli G, Mautalen C: Intravenous aminopropylidene bisphosphonate (APD) in the treatment of Paget's bone disease. J Bone Min Res 2:267–271, 1987.
353d. Harinck HIJ, Papapoulos SE, Blanksma HJ, et al: Paget's disease of bone: Early and late responses to three different modes of treatment with aminohydroxypropylidene bisphosphonate (APD). Br Med J 295:1301–1305, 1987.
353e. Thiebaud D, Jaeger P, Gobelet C: A single infusion of the bisphosphonate AHPrBP (APD) as treatment of Paget's disease of bone, Am J Med 85:207–212, 1988.
353f. Adami S, Salvagno G, Guarrera G, et al: Treatment of Paget's disease of bone with intravenous 4-amino-1-hydroxybutylidene-1,1-bisphosphonate. Calcif Tissue Int 39:226–229, 1986.
353g. Delmas PD, Chapuy M-C, Edouard C, Meunier PJ: Beneficial effects of aminohexane diphosphonate in patients with Paget's disease of bone resistant to sodium etidronate. Am J Med 83:276–282, 1987.
353h. Atkins RM, Yates AJP, Gray RES, et al: Aminohexane diphosphonate in the treatment of Paget's disease of bone. J Bone Min Res 2:273–279, 1987.
354. Ryan WG, Schwartz TB, Perlia CP: Effects of mithramycin on Paget's disease of bone. Ann Intern Med 70:549–557, 1969.
355. Ryan WG, Schwartz TB, Northrup GJ: Treatment of Paget's disease with mithramycin—further experiences. Semin Drug Treat 2:57–64, 1972.
356. Lebbin D, Ryan WG: Outpatient treatment of Paget's disease of bone with mithramycin. Ann Intern Med 81:635–637, 1974.

357. Ryan WG: Treatment of Paget's disease of bone with mithramycin. Clin Orthop Rel Res 127:106–110, 1977.
358. Ryan WG, Schwartz TB, Fordham EW: Mithramycin and long remission of Paget's disease of bone. Ann Intern Med 92:129–130, 1980.
359. Ryan WG, Schwartz TB: Mithramycin treatment of Paget's disease of bone. Exploration of combined mithramycin-EHDP therapy. Arthritis Rheum 23:1155–1161, 1980.
360. Condon JR, Reith SBM, Nassim JR, et al: Treatment of Paget's disease of bone with mithramycin. Br Med J 1:421–423, 1971.
361. Elias EG, Evans JT: Mithramycin in the treatment of Paget's disease of bone. J Bone Joint Surg 54:1730–1736, 1972.
362. Aitken JM, Lindsay ER: Mithramycin in Paget's disease. Lancet 1:1177–1178, 1973.
363. Epstein S: Mithramycin in Paget's disease. S Afr Med Tyd 48:1328–1330, 1974.
364. Ajlouni K, Thiel GB: Mithramycin effects on calcium, phosphorus and parathyroid hormone in osseous Paget's disease. Am J Med Sci 269:13–18, 1975.
365. Pembrook RC, Chung CH, Carvallo AP: Effects of mithramycin and calcitonin in cardiovascular complications of Paget's disease of bone. Conn Med 39:209–214, 1975.
366. Lentle BC, Russell AS, Heslip PG, Percy JS: The scintigraphic findings in Paget's disease of bone. Clin Radiol 27:129–135, 1976.
367. Thiel GB, Ajlouni K: Effect of mithramycin on hydroxyproline metabolism in Paget's disease. J Lab Clin Med 90:803–809, 1977.
368. Hadjipavlou AG, Tsoukas GM, Siller TN, et al: Combination drug therapy in treatment of Paget's disease of bone. J Bone Joint Surg 59A:1045–1051, 1977 .
369. Russell AS, Chalmers IM, Percy JS, Lentle BC: Long term effectiveness of low dose mithramycin for Paget's disease of bone. Arthritis Rheum 22:215–218, 1979.
370. Heath DA: The role of mithramycin in the management of Paget's disease. Metab Bone Dis Rel Res 4, 5:343–345, 1981.
371. Bilezikian JP, Canfield RE, Jacobs TP, et al: Response of 1,25-dihydroxyvitamin D_3 to hypocalcemia in human subjects. N Engl J Med 299:437–441, 1978.
372. Posen S, Grunstein HS: Turnover rate of skeletal alkaline phosphatase in humans. Clin Chem 28:153–154, 1982.
373. Fennelly JJ, Groarke JF: Effect of actinomycin D on Paget's disease of bone. Br Med J 1:423–426, 1971.
374. Fennelly JJ: Clinical and biochemical studies of Paget's disease of bone with emphasis on the effects of RNA inhibitors actinomycin D and mithramycin. Ir J Med Sci 140:431–448, 1971.
375. Somerville PJ, Evans RA: Actinomycin D in the treatment of Paget's disease of bone. Med J Aust 2:13–16, 1975.
376. Gill AB, Stein I: Bone metabolism: Its principles and its relations to orthopaedic surgery. J Bone Joint Surg 18:941–956, 1936.
377. Ghormley RK, Hinchey JJ: The use of aluminum acetate in the treatment of malacic diseases of bone. J Bone Joint Surg 26:811–817, 1944.
378. Helfet AJ: Paget's disease; considerations in its diagnosis and treatment. S Afr Med J 26:703–706, 1952.
379. Kolb FO: Paget's disease. Changes occurring following treatment with newer hormonal agents. Calif Med 91:245–250, 1959.
380. McGavack TH, Seegers W, Riefenstein EC: The influence of anabolic steroid therapy on the clinical and metabolic aspects of Paget's disease. J Am Geriatr Soc 9:533–567, 1961.
381. Rosenkrantz JA, Wolf J, Kaicher JJ: Paget's disease (osteitis deformans). Review of one hundred eleven cases. Arch Intern Med 90:610–633, 1952.
382. Maurice PF, Lynch TN, Bastomsky CH, et al: Metabolic evidence for suppression of Paget's disease of bone by aspirin. Trans Assoc Am Physicians 75:208–219, 1962.
383. Henneman PH, Dull TA, Avioli LV, et al: Effects of aspirin and corticosteroids on Paget's disease of bone. Trans Stud Coll Physicians Phila 31:10–25, 1963.
384. Galmiche P, Levy P: Etudes des variations de quelques parametres biologiques au cours de la maladie de paget (phosphatases, hydroxyproline) avant et apres traitement par l'aspirine. Rev Rhum Mal Osteoartic 3[illegible]:185–192, 1967.
385. Berman L: The endocrine treatment of Paget's disease. Endocrinology 16:109–119, 1932.
386. Watson EM: Treatment of Paget's disease by adrenal cortical preparations. Can Med Assoc J 41:561–566, 1939.
387. Charvat J, Belohradsky K: Uspesny pokus o leceni Pagetovy kostni choroby. Cas Lek Cesk 91:45, 1952.
388. Neugebauer R: Ein Beitrag zur Kklinik und Therapie des morbus Paget. Wien Med Wochenschr 103:827, 1953.
389. Albright F, Henneman PH: The suppression of Paget's disease with ACTH and cortisone. Trans Assoc Am Physicians 68:238–246, 1955.
390. Rapaport E, Kuida H, Dexter L, et al: The cardiac output in Paget's disease before and after treatment with cortisone. Am J Med 22:252–257, 1957.
391. Purves MJ: Some effects of administering sodium fluoride to patients with Paget's disease. Lancet 2:1188–1189, 1962.
392. Bernstein DS, Guri C, Cohen P, et al: The use of sodium fluoride in metabolic bone disease. J Clin Invest 42:916, 1963.
393. Rich C, Ensinck J, Ivanovich P: The effects of sodium fluoride on calcium metabolism of subjects with metabolic bone disease. J Clin Invest 43:545–556, 1964.
394. Higgins BA, Nassim JR, Alexander R, Hilb A: Effect of sodium fluoride on calcium, phosphate and nitrogen balance in patients with Paget's disease. Br Med J 1:1159–116[illegible], 1965.
395. Lukert BP, Bolinger RE, Meek JC: The effect of fluoride on Ca^{45} kinetics in Paget's disease. J Clin Endocrinol Metab 35:387–391, 1972.
396. Goldsmith RS: Treatment of Paget's disease with phosphate. Semin Drug Treat 2:69–75, 1972.
397. Condon JR: Glucagon in the treatment of Paget's disease of bone. Br Med J 4:719–721, 1971.
398. Christiansen C, Tonnesen KH: Zinc-protamine-glucagon in the treatment of Paget's disease of bone. Acta Med Scand 196:495–496, 1974.
399. Singer FR, Schiller AI, Pyle EB, Krane SM: Paget's disease of bone. *In* Avioli LV, Krane SM (eds): Metabolic Bone Disease. New York, Academic Press, 1978, pp 558–559.
400. Condon JR, Surtees J, Robinson V: Control of osteitis deformans using glucagon, calcitonin, and mithramycin. Postgrad Med J 57:84–88, 1981.

401. Theodors A, Askari AD, Wieland RG: Colchicine in the treatment of Paget's disease of bone: A new therapeutic approach. Clin Ther 3:365–373, 1983.
402. Hosking DJ, Bijvoet OLM, van Aken J, Will EJ: Paget's bone disease treated with diphosphonate and calcitonin. Lancet 1:615–617, 1976.
403. Jaeger P, Bischoff-Delaloye A, Burckhardt P: Le traitement combinede la maladie de Paget de l'os par la calcitonine et le diphosphonate EHDP. Schweiz Med Wochenschr 11:1893–1897, 1981.
404. Vellenga CJLR, Pauwels EKJ, Bijvoet OLM, et al: Bone scintigraphy in Paget's disease treated with combined calcitonin and diphosphonate (EHDP). Metab Bone Dis Rel Res 4:103–111, 1982.
404a. Rico H, Hernandez ER, Younes M, et al: Biochemical assessment of acute and chronic treatment of Paget's bone disease with calcitonin and calcium with and without bisphosphonate. Bone 9:63–66, 1988.
404b. O'donoghue DS, Hosking DS: Biochemical response to combination of disodium etidronate with calcitonin in Paget's disease. Bone 8:219–225, 1987.
405. Singer FR, Mills BG: The etiology of Paget's disease of bone. Clin Orthop Rel Res 127:37–42, 1977.
406. Kanis JA, Heynen G, Walton RJ: Plasma calcitonin in Paget's disease of bone. Clin Sci Mol Med 52:329–332, 1977.
407. Rebel A, Malkani K, Basle M: Anomalies nucleaires de la maladie osseuse de Paget. Nouv Presse Med 3:1299–1301, 1974.
408. Dubois DM, Coblentz JM, Pleet AB: Subacute sclerosing panencephalitis. Unusual nuclear inclusions and lengthy clinical course. Arch Neurol 31:355–363, 1974.
409. Mills BG, Singer FR: Nuclear inclusions in Paget's disease of bone. Science 194:201–202, 1976.
410. Schulz A, Delling G, Ringe JD, Ziegler R: Morbus Paget des knochen Untersuchugen zur Ultrastruktur des Osteoclasten und ehrer Cytopathogenese. Virchows Arch A [Pathol Anat] 376:309–328, 1977.
411. Gherardi G, LoCascio V, Bonucci E: Fine structure of nuclei and cytoplasm of osteoclasts in Paget's disease of bone. Histopathology 4:63–74, 1980.
412. Howatson AF, Fornasier VL: Microfilaments associated with Paget's disease of bone: Comparison with nucleocapsids of measles virus and respiratory syncytial virus. Intervirology 18:150–159, 1982.
413. Harvey L, Gray T, Beneton MNC, et al: Ultrastructural features of the osteoclasts from Paget's disease of bone in relation to a viral etiology. J Clin Pathol 35:771–779, 1982.
413a. Higo Y, Ohno T: An ultrastructural study of osteoclasts in Paget's disease of bone. J Clin Electron Microscopy 16:879–880, 1983.
414. Vacher-Lavenu M-C, Louvel A, Daudet-Monsac M, et al: Inclusions tubulofilamenteuses intranucleaires dans les cellules multinuclees des tumeurs a cellules geantes des os. Etude ultrastructurale d'une serie de 31 tumeurs. C R Acad Sci Paris 293:639–644, 1981.
415. Beneton MNC, Harris SC, Kanis JA: Paramyxovirus-like inclusions in two cases of pychodysostosis. Bone 8:211–217, 1987.
416. Mills BG, Yabe H, Singer FR: Osteoclasts in human osteopetrosis contain viral nucleocapsid-like nuclear inclusions. J Bone Min Res 3:101–106, 1988.
417. Rebel A, Basle M, Pouplard A, et al: Viral antigens in osteoclasts from Paget's disease of bone. Lancet 1:344–346, 1980.
418. Mills BG, Singer FR, Weiner LP, Holst PA: Immunohistological demonstration of respiratory syncytial virus antigens in Paget's disease of bone. Proc Natl Acad Sci USA 78:1209–1213, 1981.
419. Mills BG, Singer FR, Weiner LP, et al: Evidence for both respiratory syncytial virus and measles virus antigens in the osteoclasts of patients with Paget's disease of bone. Clin Orthop Rel Res 183:303–311, 1984.
420. Basle MF, Russell WC, Goswami KKA, et al: Paramyxovirus antigens in osteoclasts from Paget's bone tissue detected by monoclonal antibodies. J Gen Virol 66:2103–2110, 1985.
421. Basle MF, Fournier JG, Rosenblatt S, et al: Measles virus RNA detected in Paget's disease bone tissue by in situ hybridization. J Gen Virol 67:907–913, 1986.
422. Holland J, Spindler K, Horodyski F, et al: Rapid evolution of RNA genomes. Science 215:1577, 1982.
423. Mills BG, Singer FR, Weiner LP, Holst PA: Long-term culture of cells from bone affected by Paget's disease. Calcif Tissue Int 29:79–87, 1979.
424. Mills BG, Holst PA, Stabile EK, et al: A viral antigen-bearing cell line derived from culture of Paget's bone cells. Bone 6:193–200, 1985.
425. Buxbaum JN, Kammerman S: Immunoglobulin abnormalities in Paget's disease of bone. Clin Exp Immunol 55:200–204, 1984.
426. Renier JC, Seret P, Basle MF, Hurez D: Traitement de la maladie de Paget par vaccination antirougeoleuse et par etidronate a fortes doses. Presse Med 14:1430, 1985.

16

MICHAEL P. WHYTE
WILLIAM A. MURPHY

Osteopetrosis and Other Sclerosing Bone Disorders

Though most are rare, there is a great variety of disorders of bone formation and skeletal homeostasis that result in either focal or generalized osteosclerosis (Tables 16–1 and 16–2). Some are mere radiologic curiosities; others are difficult clinical problems.[1-9] Some provide insight into the mechanisms of mineral metabolism and skeletal homeostasis, for example, the syndrome of osteopetrosis–renal tubular acidosis–cerebral calcification, which has recently been identified as an inborn error of metabolism characterized by carbonic anhydrase II deficiency (section II). Hereditary, neoplastic, hematologic, infectious, endocrinologic, metabolic, and dietary disorders may cause osteosclerosis.[2] Cumulatively, the number of affected subjects is significant.

The purpose of this chapter is to provide a current general review of osteopetrosis and the other principal osteosclerotic dysplasias, and to discuss briefly some of the secondary causes of increased skeletal mass.*

I. OSTEOPETROSIS

Osteopetrosis (marble bone disease) was first described in 1904 by Albers-Schönberg;[10] more than 300 cases have been reported. Two principal forms are well characterized: an autosomal dominant (benign) type (McKusick 16660) with few or no symptoms,[11] and an autosomal recessive (malignant) type (McKusick 25970) that is generally fatal during infancy or early childhood.[12] An especially rare "intermediate" form that is inherited as an autosomal recessive trait (McKusick 25971) manifests during childhood with some of the clinical problems associated with the malignant type, but does not appear to shorten life expectancy.[13,14] Recently, deficiency of the carbonic anhydrase II isoenzyme has been found to explain a fourth type (McKusick 25973)—the autosomal recessive syndrome of osteopetrosis with renal tubular acidosis and cerebral calcification (section II). Malignant osteopetrosis with neuronal storage disease has been described in several subjects.[15] A few reports describe the sporadic association of "osteopetrosis" with features consistent with ectodermal dysplasia including ichthyosis, cataracts, and brittle hair.[16-20] Histologic studies of one such case, however, reveal that the osteosclerosis is not osteopetrosis but an unusual axial type of osteosclerosis.[21]

Although several genetic defects cause osteopetrosis in humans, the pathogenesis of all true forms involves defective osteoclast function wherein skeletal tissue is improperly resorbed—including the calcified cartilaginous primary spongiosa deposited during endochondral bone formation.[22-24]

A. Clinical Presentation

In the malignant form of osteopetrosis, symptoms begin during infancy.[12] Nasal "stuffiness" is often an early observation and can be attributed to malformation of the paranasal and mastoid sinuses. Subsequently, there is failure to thrive, and palsies of the optic, oculomotor, and facial nerves result from compression of their axons by narrowed cranial foramina. Dentition is delayed, and

*Throughout the text we refer to each heritable disorder by the classification number given by McKusick.[1] Since recognition of the radiologic features of the osteosclerotic skeletal disorders is essential for making a correct diagnosis, the reader is referred to several books (references 2 to 8) and a review (reference 9) that also depict these findings.

Table 16–1. Disorders That Cause Generalized Osteosclerosis

Dysplasias
Craniodiaphyseal dysplasia
Craniometaphyseal dysplasia
Dysosteosclerosis
Endosteal hyperostosis
Van Buchem disease
Sclerosteosis
Frontometaphyseal dysplasia
Infantile cortical hyperostosis (Caffey disease)
Melorheostosis
Metaphyseal dysplasia (Pyle disease)
Mixed sclerosing bone dystrophy
Oculodento-osseous dysplasia
Osteodysplasia of Melnick and Needles
Osteoectasia with hyperphosphatasia (hyperostosis corticalis)
Osteopathia striata
Osteopetrosis
Osteopoikilosis
Progressive diaphyseal dysplasia (Engelmann disease)
Pyknodysostosis
Metabolic
Carbonic anhydrase II deficiency
Fluorosis
Heavy metal poisoning
Hypervitaminosis A, D
Hyper-, hypo-, and pseudohypoparathyroidism
Hypophosphatemic osteomalacia
Milk-alkali syndrome
Renal osteodystrophy
Other
Axial osteomalacia
Fibrogenesis imperfecta ossium
Ionizing radiation
Lymphoma
Mastocytosis
Multiple myeloma
Myelofibrosis
Osteomyelitis
Osteonecrosis
Paget's disease
Sarcoidosis
Skeletal metastases
Tuberous sclerosis

bones are fragile. Short stature, a large head, frontal bossing, nystagmus, "adenoid appearance," hepatosplenomegaly, and genu valgum may be present. Some patients develop hydrocephalus;[25] sleep apnea can occur. Retinal degeneration may contribute to loss of vision.[26] Recurrent infection with spontaneous bruising and bleeding can be explained by myelophthisis. Hypersplenism and hemolysis may exacerbate the anemia. Death results during the first decade of life from pneumonia, sepsis, hemorrhage, and/or severe anemia.[12]

In the intermediate form, affected children have short stature and may develop macrocephaly, cranial nerve deficits, ankylosed teeth (which predisposes them to osteomyelitis of the jaw), recurrent fractures, and a mild or occasionally moderately severe anemia.[13,14]

In the benign form, osteosclerosis may occur as a developmental defect. Most patients are asymptomatic.[11] However, the long bones are brittle, and pathologic fractures may occur occasionally. Deafness, facial palsy, osteomyelitis of the jaw, visual or auditory impairment, psychomotor delay, carpal tunnel syndrome,[27] and osteoarthritis have also been reported.[11] Recent studies indicate that there are at least two types of benign osteopetrosis.[28,29]

B. Laboratory Findings

Standard biochemical parameters of mineral homeostasis are usually unremarkable. Serum calcium levels in malignant osteopetrosis tend to reflect the dietary intake.[30] However, in the malignant form, secondary hyperparathyroidism with increased serum levels of calcitriol (1,25-dihydroxyvitamin D) appears to be a common finding,[31] and hypocalcemia may occur with rachitic disease. Serum acid phosphatase activity, apparently derived from osteoclasts, is often elevated. Detailed investigation of leukocyte function in malignant osteopetrosis has revealed defects in circulating monocytes and granulocytes.[32,33]

C. Radiologic Features

Generalized osteosclerosis is the principal radiologic feature of osteopetrosis.[2-9] Abnormal skeletal growth, modeling, and remodeling are associated with a symmetrical increase in bone mass. The skeleton may be uniformly dense, or the osteopetrosis may manifest as alternating dense and lucent bands. The latter finding is most commonly appreciated in the pelvis and near the ends of the long bones (Fig. 16–1). In the appendicular skeleton, metaphyses and diaphyses are often widened. Erosion of the distal phalanges occurs rarely and is more characteristic of pyknodysostosis (section III). Transverse pathologic fracture of long bones is common (Fig. 16–2). As noted, rachitic changes have been described.[34] In the axial skeleton, the cranium is usually thick and

Table 16–2. Types of Osteosclerosis

Cortical and Trabecular Bone (Both)
Carbonic anhydrase II deficiency
Dysosteosclerosis
Osteopetrosis
Pyknodysostosis
Cortical Bone (Predominantly)
Autosomal dominant osteosclerosis
Diffuse idiopathic skeletal hyperostosis
Endosteal hyperostosis (van Buchem disease and sclerosteosis)
Hypertrophic osteoarthropathy
Pachydermoperiostosis
Progressive diaphyseal dysplasia (Engelmann disease)
Trabecular Bone (Predominantly)
Dysplastic
Osteomesopyknosis
Hematologic
Mastocytosis, myelofibrosis, polycythemia vera, sickle cell disease
Metabolic
Fluorosis, hyperparathyroidism, renal osteodystrophy, X-linked hypophosphatemic rickets, vitamin D toxicity
Neoplastic Disorders
Metastatic disease
Myeloma, lymphoma, leukemia

dense, with the base having the greatest osteosclerosis (Fig. 16–3), and there is underpneumatization of the paranasal and mastoid sinuses. Vertebrae may exhibit lucent central bands (Fig. 16–4) or show a "bone-in-bone" (endobone) configuration on lateral view. A recent series of studies of benign osteopetrosis from Denmark[28,29] indicates two types characterized by progressive osteosclerosis with either pronounced diffuse sclerosis of the skull and other bones (type I) or more selective sclerosis of the base of the skull together with typical endobone formation (type II).

In osteopetrosis, skeletal scintigraphy retains its usual utility to demonstrate fractures, osteomyelitis, and so on.[35] Magnetic resonance imaging of a few affected subjects has revealed a weaker signal from marrow spaces in the malignant form than in the benign form.[36] Accordingly, this technique may prove to be useful to monitor patients treated by bone marrow transplantation (see later).

D. Histopathologic Findings

Although the radiologic features of osteopetrosis are usually diagnostic, the failure of osteoclasts to resorb skeletal tissue provides a histologic finding that is also characteristic (Fig. 16–5); that is, presence of "islands" of calcified cartilage (unresorbed primary spongiosa) within bony trabeculae.[22-24,37-39] Osteoclasts have been reported to occur in increased, normal, or decreased numbers. In the malignant form of osteopetrosis, these cells are generally populous and are appropriately positioned at bone surfaces.[40] Their nuclei, however, are especially numerous and ultrastructural abnormalities may be present, including absence of ruffled borders and clear zones, which are typical features of normal osteoclasts that are actively resorbing bone.[37,38] Marrow spaces are often crowded with fibrous tissue.[37,40] In the benign form of osteopetrosis, osteoid may be increased, and osteoclasts can be scant and lack ruffled borders.[39]

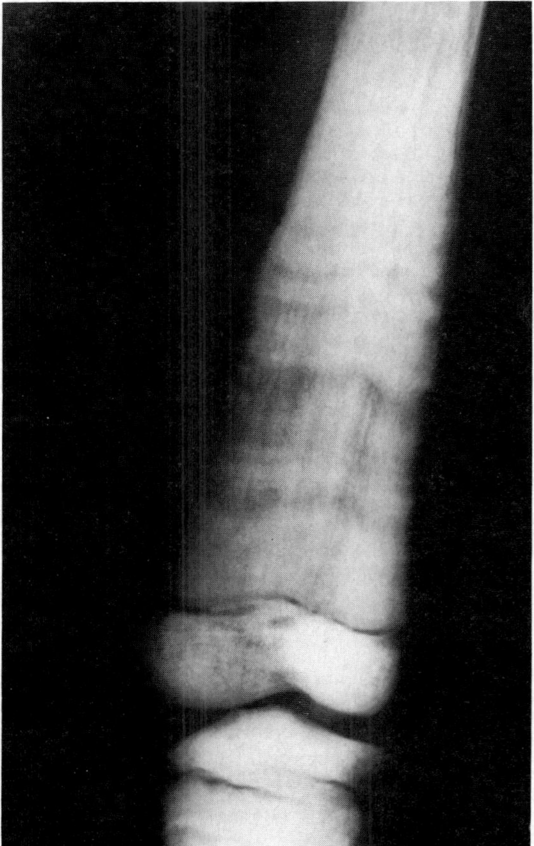

Figure 16–1. Osteopetrosis. AP radiograph of the distal femur of a 10-year-old boy shows a widened metadiaphyseal region with characteristic alternating dense and lucent bands.

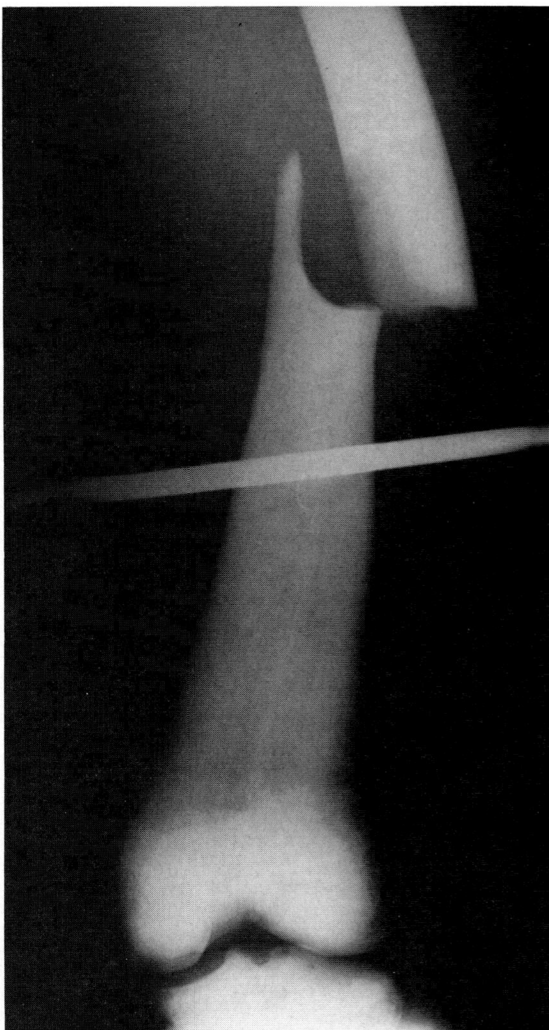

Figure 16–2. Osteopetrosis. AP radiograph of the distal femur of a 22-year-old man shows homogeneous osteosclerosis with a transverse pathologic fracture of the midshaft.

E. Etiology and Pathogenesis

Although all forms of human osteopetrosis appear to be heritable, the defective autosomal gene loci of the types discussed thus far are unknown. Primary immune defects may occur in osteopetrosis, but do not seem to be as common as believed previously.[24] In all cases, there is defective osteoclast-mediated bone resorption.[22-24] The myelophthisic disease in the malignant form is probably multifactorial and results from marrow crowding by bone, fibrous tissue, and numerous osteoclasts.[40] Skeletal fragility may be due to defective remodeling of woven bone to compact bone and/or to a paucity of collagen fibrils that connect osteons.[24]

A defect in the osteoclast stem cell or in its microenvironment or an abnormality in the mature osteoclast itself could account for osteopetrosis. In the osteopetrosis of carbonic anhydrase II deficiency, abnormal skeletal remodeling would appear to be secondary to deficiency of this isoenzyme in osteoclasts; however, definitive studies are needed (section II). Biosynthesis of an abnormal parathyroid hormone,[41] defective cellular production of interleukin-2,[42] and subnormal generation of superoxide, which may be necessary for bone resorption,[33] may all be pathogenetic mechanisms that cause osteopetrosis. The association of osteopetrosis with neuronal storage disease characterized by accumulation of ceroid lipofuscin indicates that some patients may have a primary lysosomal defect.[15] Recently, virus-like inclusions nearly identical to those of the nucleocapsids of Paramyxoviridae viruses and antigens of respiratory syncytial virus and measles virus have been noted in some of the osteoclasts of several sporadic cases of benign osteopetrosis.[43] Their significance is uncertain. The molecular defect has not been determined for any human type of osteopetrosis.[23,24]

F. Treatment

Since the various forms of osteopetrosis differ in inheritance pattern, prognosis, and therapeutic approach, correct diagnosis (which may involve careful assessment of disease progression) is crucial. The prognosis depends on the form of osteopetrosis involved—the intermediate forms are relatively benign,[13,14] and infants or young children with carbonic anhydrase II deficiency can have radiologic findings consistent with malignant osteopetrosis, yet sequential studies may reveal gradual spontaneous resolution of the osteosclerosis (section II).

Transplantation of allogeneic bone marrow in a few cases of malignant osteopetrosis has been followed by remarkable clinical improvement and reversal of neurologic, hematologic, radiologic, and histopathologic abnormalities.[44-48] Demonstration that osteoclasts, but not osteoblasts, were of donor origin

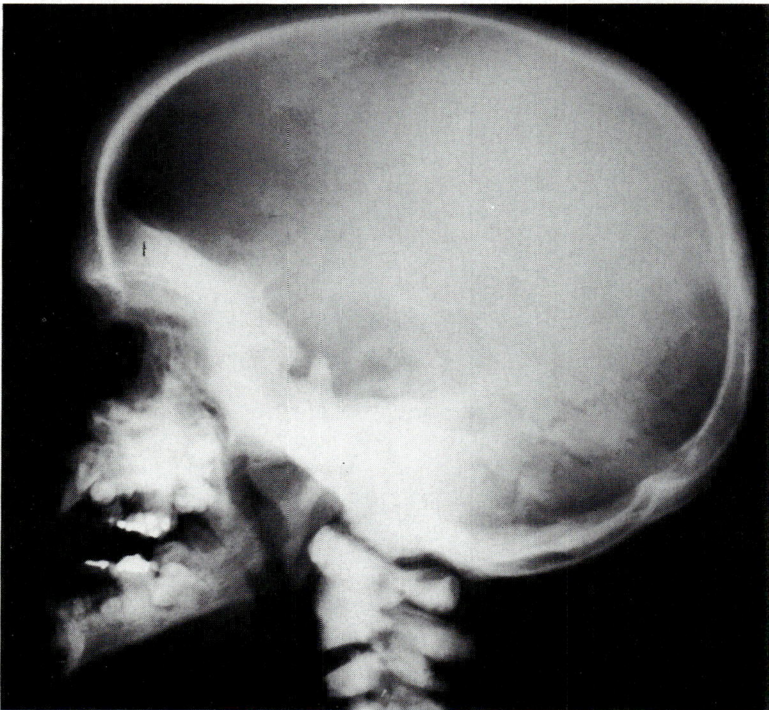

Figure 16–3. Osteopetrosis. Lateral radiograph of the skull of a 13-year-old boy shows osteosclerosis, especially apparent at the base.

after bone marrow transplantation has corroborated the hypothesis that osteoclast-mediated bone resorption is defective in the osteopetroses, and that osteoclasts are normally derived from precursor cells in the marrow.[47] Transplantation of HLA-nonidentical marrow warrants further study.[49] Since a great variety of defects appear to cause osteopetrosis, it is understandable that marrow transplantation is not helpful in all subjects.[24] Indeed, patients with severe sclerosis of the marrow cavity seem to fare less well with this procedure.[23,50] Accordingly, bone biopsy may be helpful to predict the outcome of marrow transplantation.

Treatment with large oral doses of calcitriol together with a calcium-deficient diet occasionally results in improvement in the malignant form of osteopetrosis that is as dramatic as that following successful bone marrow transplantation.[30,50] Here, calcitriol appears to act therapeutically by stimulating osteoclast activity. A long-term trial of this regimen in an adult with an apparently intermediate form of osteopetrosis has led to improved hematopoietic function and decreased skeletal mass.[51] In an early report, Dent, Smellie, and Watson reported some success with a calcium-deficient diet alone.[52] Conversely, supplementation of dietary calcium can correct the rachitic disease that occurs in some subjects with hypocalcemia.

Large doses of glucocorticoids appear to be beneficial for malignant osteopetrosis and are especially helpful in stabilizing patients with hepatomegaly and pancytopenia.[53,54] Prednisone therapy together with a low-calcium, high-phosphate diet has recently been reported to be a potentially effective alternative treatment to marrow transplantation for malignant osteopetrosis.[55] Long-term infusion of parathormone was efficacious for one infant,[41] perhaps by increasing endogenous calcitriol levels.

Osteomyelitis of the jaw can be treated with hyperbaric oxygenation.[56] Surgical decompression of the facial and optic nerves (evaluated best by computed tomography rather than by radiologic views of the optic foramen) may be successful.[25,26]

Conventional radiographic study at 20 weeks' gestation has failed to diagnose malignant osteopetrosis *in utero*.[57] Early prenatal diagnosis with ultrasound has thus far also been unsuccessful.[53]

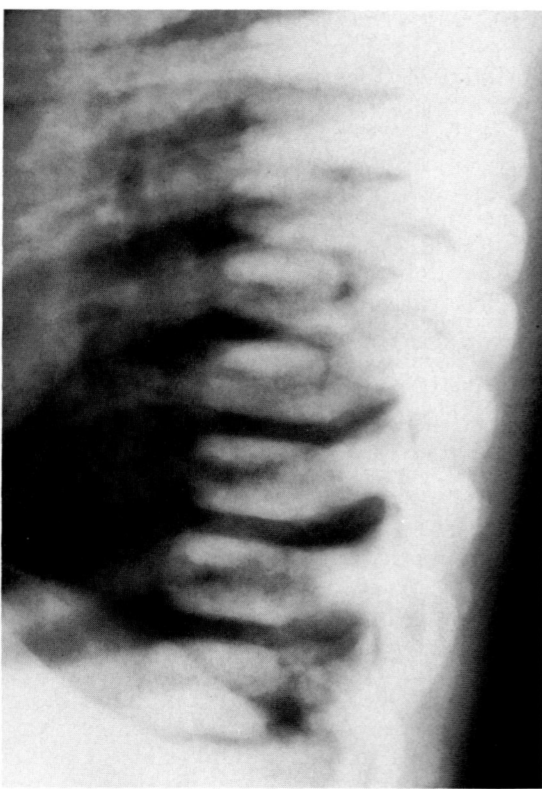

Figure 16–4. Osteopetrosis. Lateral radiograph of the lower thoracic spine of an 8-year-old boy shows osteosclerosis of ribs and vertebrae. Note the characteristic central lucent bands in each vertebra.

II. CARBONIC ANHYDRASE II DEFICIENCY

In 1972, three independent publications[58-60] described a new autosomal recessive syndrome characterized by radiologic changes of osteopetrosis in subjects with renal tubular acidosis. Cerebral calcification and histopathologic changes typical of osteopetrosis in such subjects were first reported in 1980.[61-62] Three years later,[63] deficiency of carbonic anhydrase II isoenzyme was identified as the primary biochemical defect in this newly identified inborn error of metabolism (McKusick 25973).

A. Clinical Presentation

Descriptions of more than 20 patients reveal that there may be considerable clinical variability among affected families.[64,65] Consanguinity is a common finding in kindreds from the Arabian peninsula.[66] Perinatal history is generally unremarkable. The disorder may manifest in infancy or early childhood with developmental delay, failure to thrive, or fracture. Investigation of short stature may also lead to the diagnosis. Patients commonly, but not always, have mental subnormality. Dental malocclusion and compression of the optic nerve are additional complications. A "mixed" renal tubular acidosis is usually present and may account for apathy, muscle

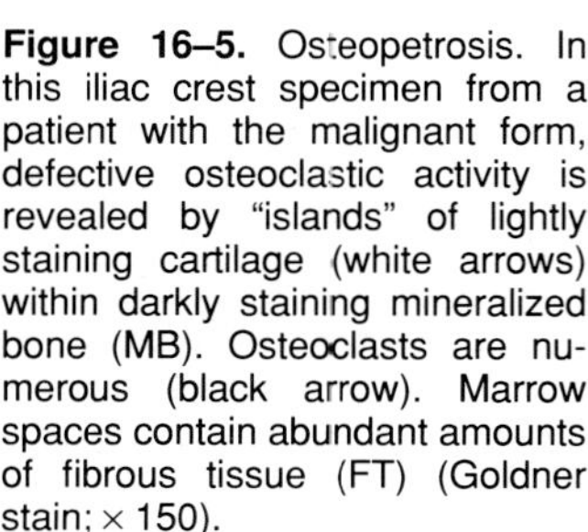

Figure 16–5. Osteopetrosis. In this iliac crest specimen from a patient with the malignant form, defective osteoclastic activity is revealed by "islands" of lightly staining cartilage (white arrows) within darkly staining mineralized bone (MB). Osteoclasts are numerous (black arrow). Marrow spaces contain abundant amounts of fibrous tissue (FT) (Goldner stain; × 150).

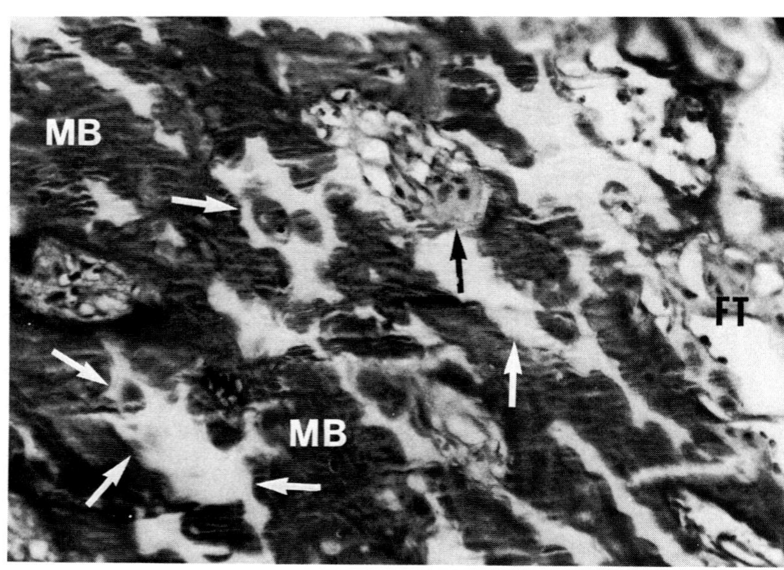

weakness, and hypotonia. Intermittent hypokalemic paralysis has been reported. Although the bones of most patients do not fracture, recurrent breaks in long bones may cause significant morbidity.[64] The disorder, however, appears to be compatible with long life.[61,65]

B. Laboratory Findings

Anemia, if present, is usually mild and apparently of nutritional origin. Bone marrow aspiration reveals normal findings. Metabolic acidosis has been noted as early as the neonatal period,[66] and both proximal and distal renal tubular acidosis have been reported.[67] Occurrence of a distal (type I) renal tubular acidosis seems to be the better established of the two; however, further studies are needed to define more precisely the defect in acid-base homeostasis.[67,68] Aminoaciduria and glycosuria are absent.[64]

C. Radiologic Features

The radiologic features of carbonic anhydrase II deficiency are similar to those of other forms of osteopetrosis, except that the osteosclerosis may diminish spontaneously over years (Figs. 16–6*A*, *B*) and basal ganglia calcification may appear.[61] Radiologic abnormalities were noted at the time of clinical presentation in all patients described, although one subject was noted to have only very subtle findings at birth.[66] Computed tomography has shown that the cerebral calcification is developmental (appearing between 2 and 5 years of age), increases during childhood, occurs in the gray matter of the cortex and basal ganglia, and is similar if not identical to that seen in idiopathic hypoparathyroidism or pseudohypoparathyroidism.[69]

D. Histopathologic Findings

Autopsy studies have not been reported. Specimens of bone taken from four subjects from two families have been examined histopathologically.[59,61] Changes characteristic of osteopetrosis[61] were noted in each of the three sisters first found to have carbonic anhydrase II deficiency (Fig. 16–7).

E. Etiology and Pathogenesis

Carbonic anhydrases catalyze the initial step in the reaction $CO_2 + H_2O \rightarrow H_2CO_3 \rightarrow H^+ + HCO_3^-$ and function importantly, therefore, in acid-base regulation. Carbonic anhydrase II has been identified in a variety of cell types and tissues including erythrocytes, eye, brain, kidney, cartilage, liver, lung, skeletal muscle, pancreas and gastric mucosa[70,71] and is the most catalytically active isoenzyme of the carbonic anhydrase family.[72] The other carbonic anhydrase isoenzymes have a more restricted tissue distribution.

Studies of erythrocyte lysates indicated that deficiency of carbonic anhydrase II accounts for the syndrome of osteopetrosis, renal tubular acidosis, and cerebral calcification.[63] Using red cell lysates of patients with this syndrome, Sly et al. purified carbonic anhydrase II by high-performance liquid chromatography, assayed carbonic anhydrase II esterase and carbon dioxide hydrase activity, and performed immunochemical studies of carbonic anhydrase isoenzymes; these studies all revealed a deficiency of carbonic anhydrase II but not of carbonic anhydrase I.[63] Carbonic anhydrase II deficiency has been demonstrated in all of 21 patients with the syndrome from 12 unrelated kindreds of diverse geographic and ethnic background.[64] Autosomal recessive inheritance for this disorder is supported by the observation that carbonic anhydrase II levels are approximately half-normal in obligate heterozygous parents of patients.[63-66]

Although deficiency of carbonic anhydrase II remains to be shown in tissues of patients with this disorder, the presence of osteopetrosis and renal tubular acidosis suggests a global deficiency of carbonic anhydrase II and an important physiologic role for this isoenzyme in the skeleton and kidney. Indeed, a variety of animal and *in vitro* studies indicate that carbonic anhydrase is important for osteoclast function, perhaps by conditioning the pericellular pH. Inhibition of carbonic anhydrase activity can block bone resorption *in vivo* and in organ culture.[73] Carbonic anhydrase II is the carbonic anhydrase isoenzyme present in osteoclasts.[74] The observation that enzyme-deficient patients respond appropriately to acetazolamide challenge with bicarbonaturia has provided evidence that a carbonic anhydrase isoenzyme in addition to carbonic anhydrase II functions im-

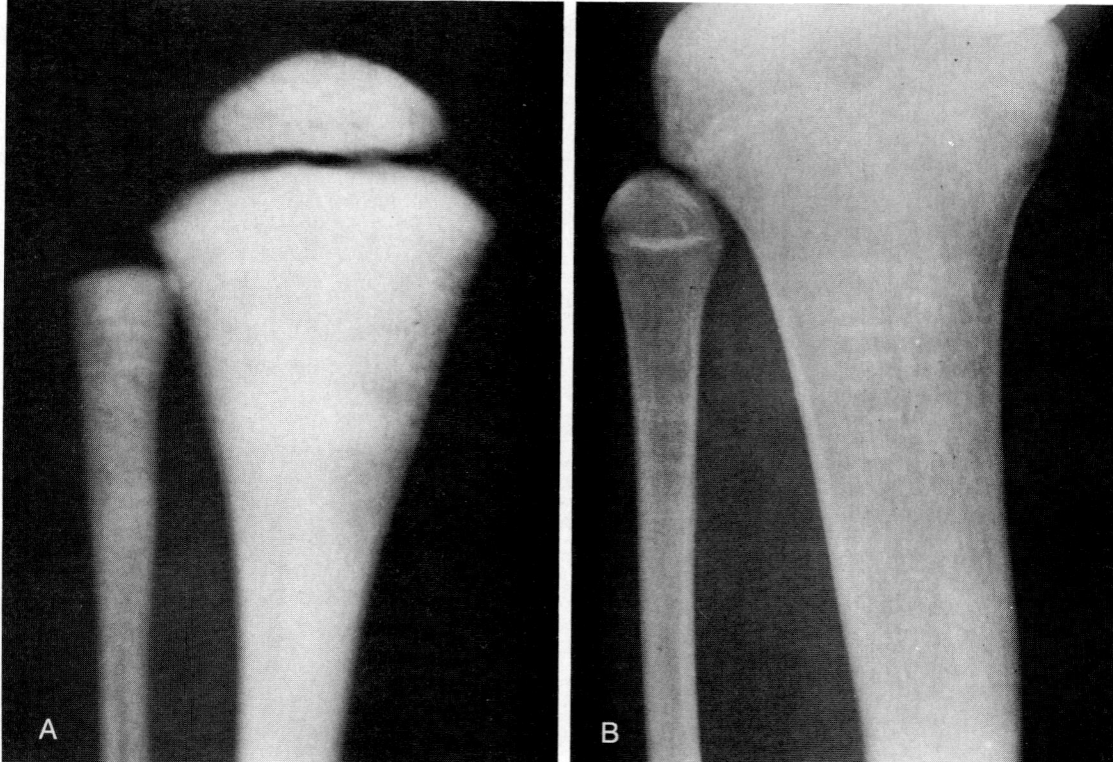

Figure 16–6. Carbonic anhydrase II deficiency. *A*, AP radiograph of the proximal tibia and fibula of a 2-year-old girl shows features of osteopetrosis including widening of the metaphysis, diffuse osteosclerosis, and alternating radiodense and radiolucent bands. *B*, AP radiograph of proximal tibia and fibula of the same patient, now age 17, shows nearly complete resolution of features of osteopetrosis. A few very faint sclerotic lines remain in what appears to be otherwise normal bone.

portantly in the kidney.[67] Whether cerebral calcification is a direct or indirect effect of carbonic anhydrase II deficiency is unclear.

Recent identification of a mouse model for this disorder indicates a selective deficiency of carbonic anhydrase II in a widespread tissue distribution.[75]

The molecular defect that accounts for carbonic anhydrase II deficiency is unknown. Localization of the gene for carbonic anhydrase II to chromosome 8 in humans should enable rapid progress in our understanding of the molecular basis for this disorder.[76] It seems likely that some of the clinical and biochemical heterogeneity observed among affected kindreds will be explained by a variety of allelic defects in the carbonic anhydrase II gene.

F. Treatment

Prenatal diagnosis has not been reported. Renal tubular acidosis in carbonic anhydrase II deficiency has been treated briefly with bicarbonate supplementation, but the long-term outcome of this therapy has not been assessed.[66] Transfusion of carbonic anhydrase II–replete erythrocytes to one patient failed to correct her systemic acidosis. This finding indicates that the renal acidification defect is not the result of carbonic anhydrase II deficiency in erythrocytes, but that carbonic anhydrase II deficiency is likely in the kidney as well.[77] This observation also suggests that bone marrow transplantation is unlikely to correct the renal defect.

Congenital Sclerosing Osteomalacia with Cerebral Calcification

In 1985, two daughters of nonconsanguineous parents were reported to have a unique, perinatal lethal osteosclerotic disorder (McKusick 25966) that radiographically mimics carbonic anhydrase II deficiency.[78] The condition presented at birth with "craniofacial

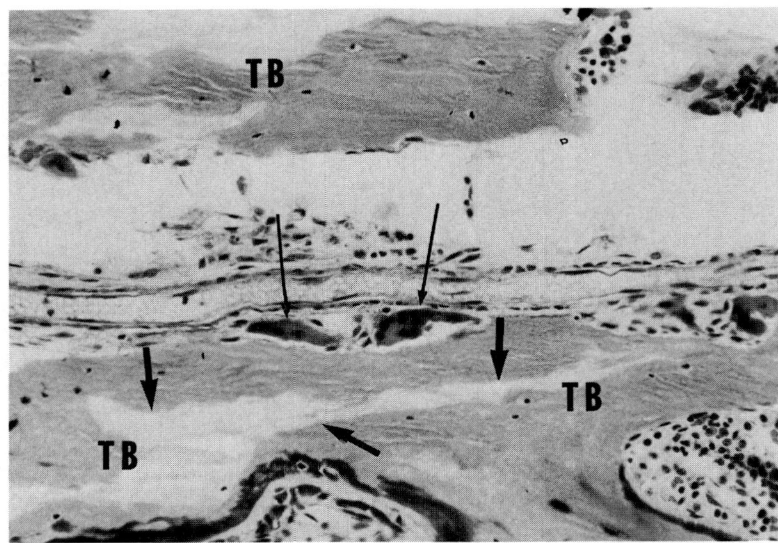

Figure 16–7: Carbonic anhydrase II deficiency. In this iliac crest specimen, defective osteoclastic function and true osteopetrosis is revealed by the presence of cartilage "islands" (short arrows) that reflect unresorbed primary spongiosa in trabecular bone (TB). Osteoclasts (long arrows) are present (Goldner stain; × 50).

dysostosis" and microthorax. Radiographic studies revealed generalized osteosclerosis and diffuse cerebral calcification consistent with carbonic anhydrase II deficiency. However, histologic studies following tetracycline labeling demonstrated osteomalacia rather than osteopetrosis. Carbonic anhydrase II levels in erythrocyte lysates were shown to be normal in one of the daughters and the parents.[78]

III. PYKNODYSOSTOSIS

Pyknodysostosis (McKusick 26580), first delineated in 1962,[79,80] is the disorder that is believed to have affected the French impressionist painter Henri de Toulouse-Lautrec (1864–1901).[81] More than 100 cases from 50 kindreds have been described. Pyknodysostosis is inherited as an autosomal recessive trait;[82-84] parental consanguinity has been described for about 30% of patients. Most reported cases have originated in Europe or the U.S., but the condition has been encountered in the peoples of Israel and Indonesia, in Asian Indians, and in African blacks; it is especially common in the Japanese.[85]

A. Clinical Presentation

Pyknodysostosis is usually diagnosed during infancy or childhood because of a disproportionate short stature together with additional dysmorphic features including a relatively large cranium with fronto-occipital prominence, small facies, obtuse mandibular angle, small chin, dental malocclusion with persistence of carious deciduous teeth, high-arched palate, proptosis, bluish sclerae, and a pointed and beaked nose.[6,82] The anterior fontanel is often palpably open, as are other major cranial sutures. The hands are small and square, the fingers are short and clubbed from acro-osteolysis or aplasia of terminal phalanges, and the nails are hypoplastic. Recurrent deforming fractures (usually of the lower limbs), a narrowed thorax, pectus excavatum, kyphoscoliosis, increased lumbar lordosis, and genu valgum may occur. Mental retardation is present in about 10% of cases.[82] Adult height ranges between 4′3″ and 4′11″. Atypical patients have been described, for example, with visceral manifestations and with rickets.[86]

B. Laboratory Findings

Patients are not anemic. Serum calcium and inorganic phosphate levels and alkaline phosphatase activity are generally normal.

C. Radiologic Features

Many of the radiologic findings of pyknodysostosis are similar to those of osteopetrosis; for example, both conditions are characterized by generalized osteosclerosis and recurrent fractures.[87,88] However, pyknodysostosis is differentiated from osteopetrosis by the following additional features: wormian bones; delayed closure of sutures and fontanels (prominently the anterior); obtuse mandibular angle; gracile clavicles that are hypoplastic at the distal ends; partial absence of the hyoid bone; and hypoplasia or aplasia of the distal phalanges and ribs.[89] Radiodense striations and endobones (bone-within-bone) do not occur.[2,5-8] In pyknodysostosis, the osteosclerosis is uniform, becomes apparent in childhood, and increases with age. However, it is not accompanied by the considerable modeling defects of osteopetrosis, although the long bones have thick cortices with narrow medullary cavities. In the skull, the calvarium and base are sclerotic and the orbital ridges are dense (Fig. 16–8). There is hypoplasia of facial bones, sinuses, and terminal phalanges (Fig. 16–9). Vertebrae are sclerotic (transverse processes are uninvolved) and may have anterior and posterior concavities. Lumbosacral spondylolisthesis is not uncommon, and lack of segmentation of the atlas and axis can occur. Madelung deformity may be present in the forearms.

D. Histopathologic Findings

Histopathologic studies reveal normal cortical bone structure in pyknodysostosis, yet decreased osteoblastic and osteoclastic activity.[90] A depressed rate of skeletal turnover has been described.[91] Electron microscopy of bone from two subjects showed findings consistent with defective degradation of skeletal collagen—perhaps due to an abnormality in the bone matrix itself, or in osteoclast function.[92] Indeed, in pyknodysostosis, osteoclasts have been found to contain cytoplasmic vacuoles that are somewhat large and are usually filled with bone collagen fibrils. These findings suggest defective extracellular or intracellular degradation of collagen.[92] Ultrastructural study of cartilage has revealed abnormal inclusions in chondrocytes.[93]

E. Etiology and Pathogenesis

The precise genetic defect in pyknodysostosis is unknown. Deletion of the short arm of a G chromosome (probably 22) has been reported;[82] however, family members of pyknodysostosis patients who did not have the condition also had this abnormality. Trisomy X with a reduced rate of bone remodeling was found in one patient.[94]

A study of calcium homeostasis using ^{47}Ca and ^{45}Ca in one subject revealed a normal exchangeable calcium pool and rate of bone accretion and calcium excretion.[95] However, when the increased skeletal mass was considered in this individual, both the rate of bone accretion and the size of the exchangeable calcium pool appeared to be reduced.[90]

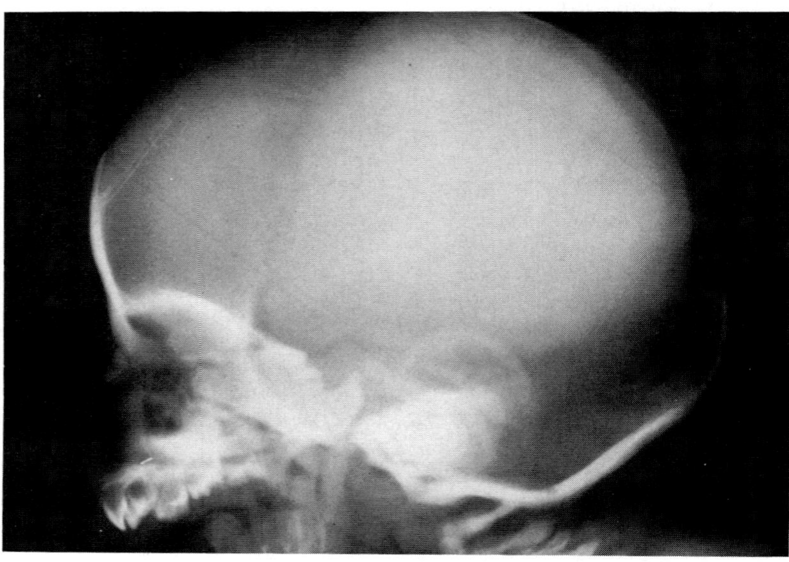

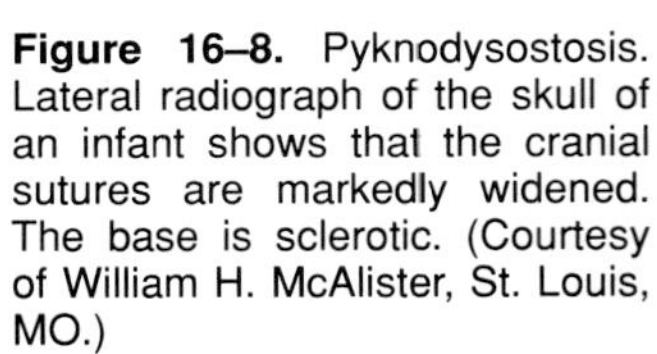

Figure 16–8. Pyknodysostosis. Lateral radiograph of the skull of an infant shows that the cranial sutures are markedly widened. The base is sclerotic. (Courtesy of William H. McAlister, St. Louis, MO.)

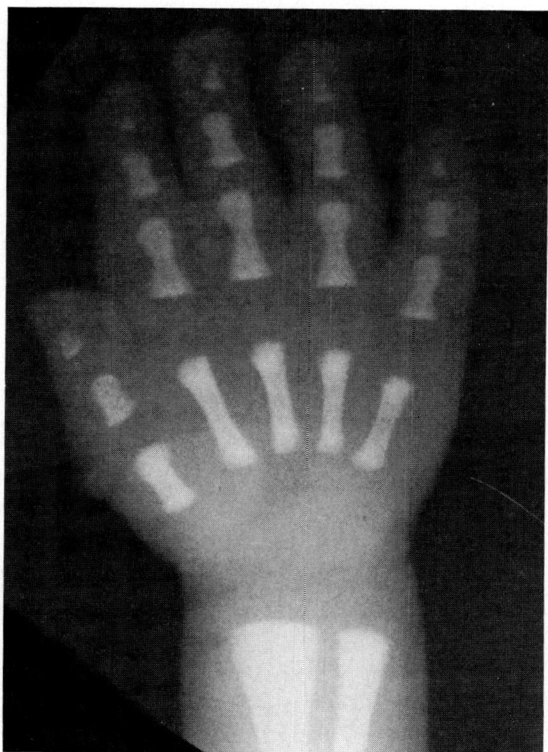

Figure 16–9. Pyknodysostosis. PA radiograph of the hand shows that the bones are sclerotic and the distal phalanges are hypoplastic. (Courtesy of William H. McAlister, St. Louis, MO.)

Accordingly, decreased bone resorption may account for the osteosclerosis in pyknodysostosis. Similar kinetic studies, using ^{85}Sr, have also been described.[80] Calcium absorption from the gastrointestinal tract has been reported to be markedly increased in pyknodysostosis. Paramyxovirus-like inclusions, like those discovered in Paget's bone disease, have been found in the osteoclasts of two brothers with pyknodysostosis.[96]

F. Treatment

There is no effective medical therapy for pyknodysostosis. Fractures of the long bones are usually transverse and heal at a satisfactory rate; however, massive callus formation and delayed union have been reported.[97] Internal fixation of long bones is made difficult by their hardness. Patients are, however, generally able to walk independently. Extraction of teeth is difficult and several patients have suffered fracture of the mandible.[82] Osteomyelitis of the jaw responds to combined surgical and antibiotic therapy.[98]

IV. OSTEOMESOPYKNOSIS

Osteomesopyknosis (McKusick 16645) was first described in 1979[99] and named in 1980.[100] This condition is inherited as an autosomal dominant trait. Fewer than 20 cases have been reported.[99-103]

Patients are usually discovered incidentally during adolescence or early adulthood by radiographic study; low-back pain appears to be a common complaint. The youngest individual with documented lesions was 10 years of age.[103] One affected woman was infertile from "ovarian sclerosis."[101] Physical examination is generally unremarkable except for tenderness of the back. Routine biochemical studies have been reported to be normal in all but one patient who had renal tubular acidosis.

Osteomesopyknosis resembles pyknodysostosis radiologically, but is characterized by patchy osteosclerosis localized to the spine, the pelvis, and the proximal parts of long bones (Fig. 16–10). The osteosclerosis is especially prominent in the vertebral endplates. Lesions appear to be well demarcated by computed axial tomography.[103] Bone scintigraphy has been reported to be normal.[103] Radiographic abnormalities may be unchanged for more than a decade.[101] Histopathologic studies of osteomesopyknotic bone have not been described.

V. PROGRESSIVE DIAPHYSEAL DYSPLASIA (Camurati-Engelmann Disease)

Progressive diaphyseal dysplasia (McKusick 13130) was first described in 1920 by Cockayne.[104] Camurati noted in 1922 that the disorder could be inherited.[105] Engelmann reported the severe form in 1929 and it became known as Engelmann's disease.[106] This is a developmental disorder that is inherited as an autosomal dominant trait, but with variable clinical and radiologic penetrance.[107-109] More than 100 cases have been reported.[109] New bone formation occurs gradually along both the endosteal and periosteal surfaces of tubular bones. In espe-

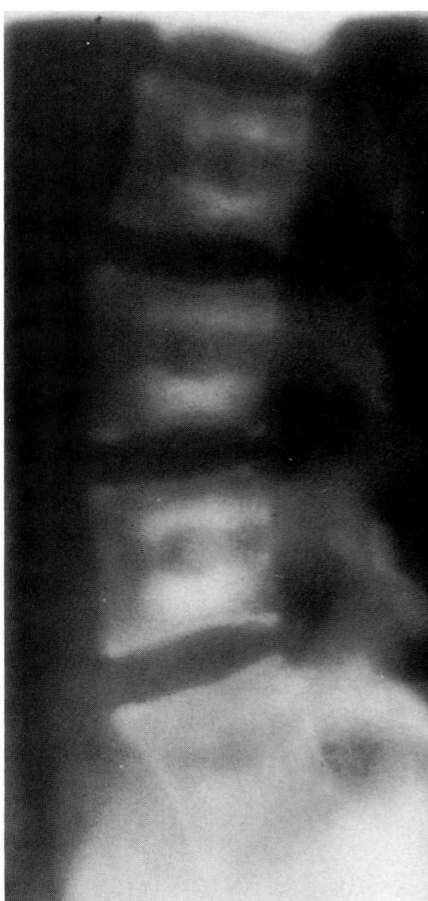

Figure 16–10. Osteomesopyknosis. Lateral radiograph of the lumbar spine of a 14-year-old girl reveals radiodense areas within the vertebral bodies; that is, a bone-in-bone pattern. (Courtesy of Dr. H. Labelle. Reprinted from Proschel R, et al: J Bone Joint Surg 67A: 652–653, 1985.)

cially severe cases, osteosclerosis is generalized and affects the skull and axial skeleton. Some adult carriers have no radiographic abnormalities. Severe cases were described by Engelmann;[106] mild forms (believed to be transmitted as an autosomal recessive trait) were first reported by Ribbing.[107,110] All races appear to be affected.

A. Clinical Presentation

Leg pain, muscle wasting, decreased subcutaneous fat in the extremities, and a limping or broad-based and waddling gait during childhood are characteristic features of progressive diaphyseal dysplasia. Unless appropriate radiologic studies are performed, the condition may be mistaken for a muscular dystrophy.[111,112] Severely affected individuals have a characteristic body habitus (Fig. 16–11*A*, *B*) that also includes an enlarged head, prominent forehead, proptosis, and cranial nerve palsies when the skull is involved. Some patients have delayed puberty due to hypothalamic hypogonadotropic hypogonadism (M.P.W., personal observation). Increased intracranial pressure can occur. Physical examination may reveal palpable bony enlargement and hepatosplenomegaly and elicit diffuse skeletal tenderness to palpation. Some patients have Raynaud's phenomenon and evidence of vasculitis.[113]

B. Laboratory Findings

Routine biochemical parameters of bone and mineral metabolism are usually unremarkable in progressive diaphyseal dysplasia, although modestly subnormal circulating calcium levels and hypocalciuria (findings that appear to reflect a markedly positive calcium balance) occur with severe disease.[114] Circulating alkaline phosphatase activity, urinary hydroxyproline, and erythrocyte sedimentation rate are increased in some patients. Mild anemia and leukopenia may also be present.[113]

C. Radiologic Features

Gradually spreading cortical hyperostosis of long bone diaphyses, secondary to proliferation of new bone on both the periosteal and endosteal surfaces, is the primary radiologic feature of progressive diaphyseal dysplasia.[2-8] Sclerosis is nearly symmetrical and occurs in the diaphyseal and metaphyseal regions of long bones—the epiphyses are spared (Fig. 16–12). Diaphyseal width slowly increases. Computed tomography has shown that endosteal involvement is more extensive than periosteal thickening.[115] Characteristically, the shafts of long bones have irregular surfaces (Fig. 16–13). The age of onset, rate of progression, and degree of diaphyseal sclerosis vary considerably among patients. Tibiae and femora are involved most frequently; less commonly the humeri, radii, ulnae, and, occasionally, the short tubular bones. Progressive sclerosis of the vertebrae, skull, scapulae, clavicles, and pelvis may also occur. Cranial involvement,

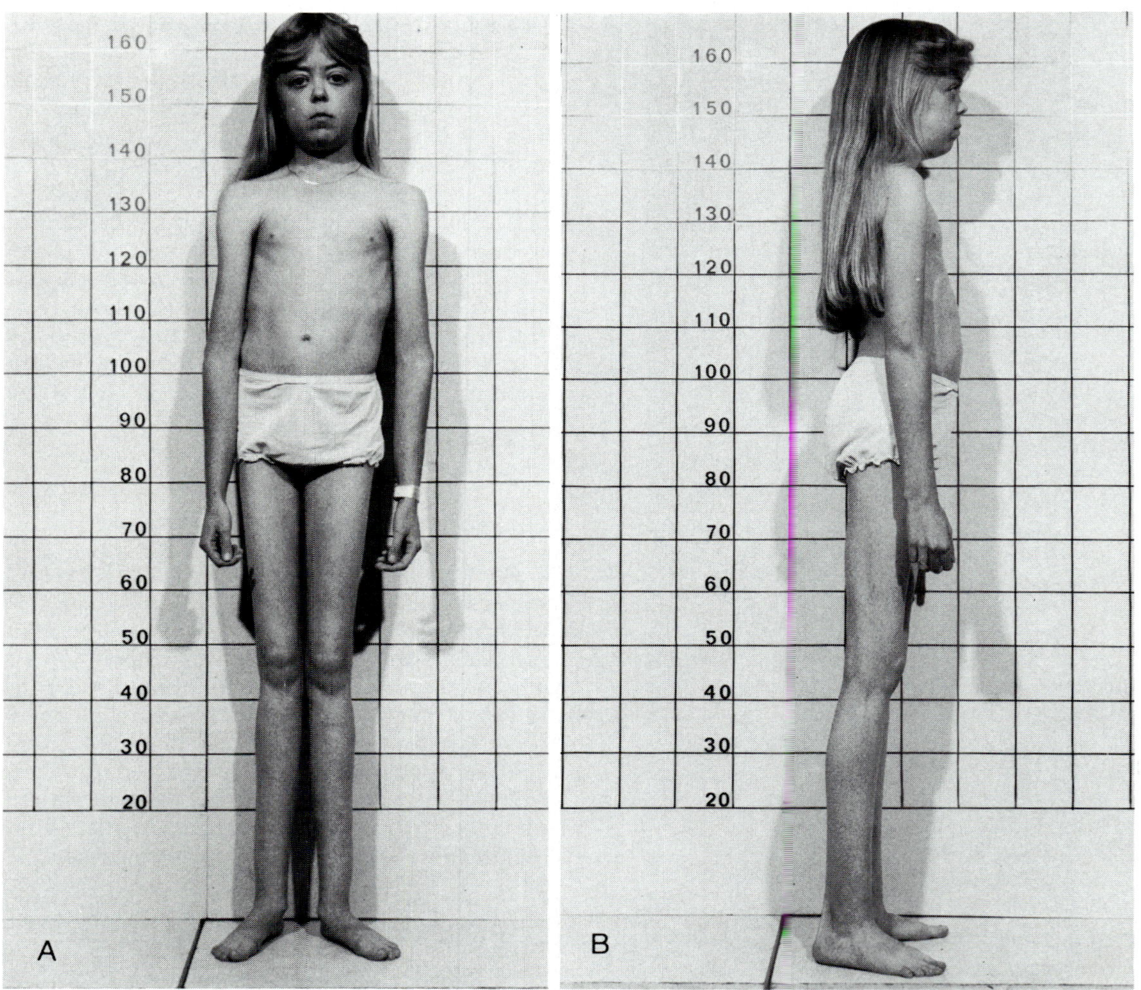

Figure 16–11. Progressive diaphyseal dysplasia. *A* and *B*, This prepubescent 17-year-old girl with severe disease involvement has the characteristic body habitus including a paucity of muscle and subcutaneous fat in the limbs, thickening of the long bones, and cranial enlargement. Reproduced with permission from Whyte MP: Rare disorders of skeletal formation and homeostasis. In Becker KL (ed): Principles and practice of endocrinology and metabolism. Philadelphia: J.B. Lippincott, (in press.)

which appears as calvarial hyperostosis and sclerosis of the base of the skull (Fig. 16–14), may cause diagnostic confusion with mild forms of craniodiaphyseal dysplasia. With maturation of the new bone, the affected areas become more sclerotic. In severely affected children, osteopenia may accompany the new bone formation.

Focally increased radionuclide accumulation occurs during bone scintigraphy. In the milder forms of progressive diaphyseal dysplasia, which develop in adolescents or young adults, radiographic and scintigraphic studies may show skeletal abnormalities limited to long bones of the lower extremities (Fig. 16–15). Comparison of the scintigraphic, radiologic, and clinical findings of four cases at different stages of the disease revealed generally concordant scintigraphic and radiographic findings. In some patients, however, bone scans were rather unremarkable despite distinct abnormalities present radiographically; here, the disease process may be quiescent.[116] Conversely, markedly increased skeletal radioisotope accumulation, despite minimal radiologic abnormalities, appears to reflect active (early) disease.[116]

Sequential radiologic findings reveal a variable course, but progressive bony in-

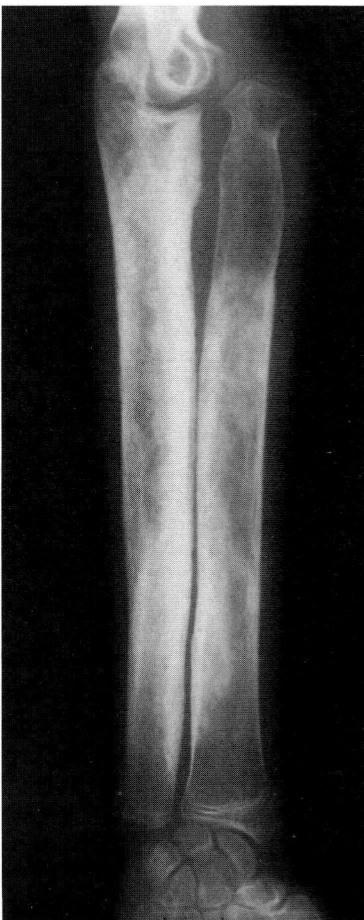

Figure 16–12. Progressive diaphyseal dysplasia. AP radiograph of the left forearm of a 19-year-old woman with severe disease shows osteopenia with superimposed sclerosis of the diaphyses of the radius and ulna from proliferation of bone on the periosteal and endosteal surfaces.

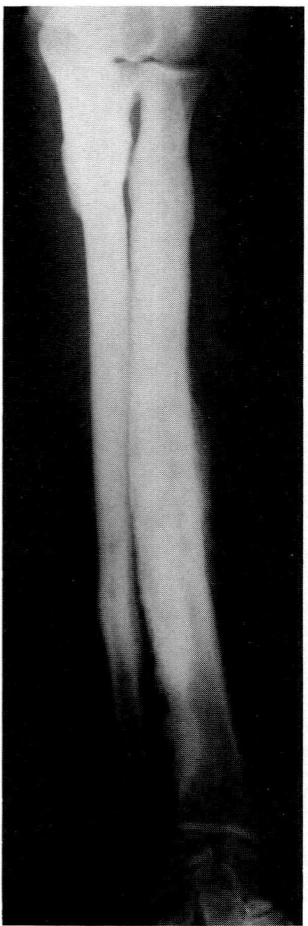

Figure 16–13. Progressive diaphyseal dysplasia. AP radiograph of the left forearm of a 41-year-old man (father of patient shown in Fig. 16–10) shows dense sclerosis resulting in thickening of the radial and ulnar cortices.

volvement of the disorder is the rule. Arrest of the disease appears to occur in some cases.[114]

D. Histopathologic Findings

New bone formation is present in areas affected by progressive diaphyseal dysplasia. Peripheral to true cortex, there appears to be centripetal maturation and "cancellous compaction" of disorganized (woven) bone.[107] In muscle, electron microscopy has revealed atrophy of isolated muscle fibers, accumulation of endomysial collagen fibrils, and thickening of perivascular basement membrane—myopathic and vascular changes that are similar in sporadic and familial cases.[111] Type II muscle fiber atrophy was noted in one subject with clinical evidence of myopathy but without degenerative changes on electron microscopy.[112]

E. Etiology and Pathogenesis

The autosomal gene defect in progressive diaphyseal dysplasia has not been mapped. Some especially mild cases may reflect a separate, autosomal recessive disorder, that is, "Ribbing's disease."[107,110,117] However, mild clinical forms of Engelmann's disease can be transmitted as an autosomal dominant trait

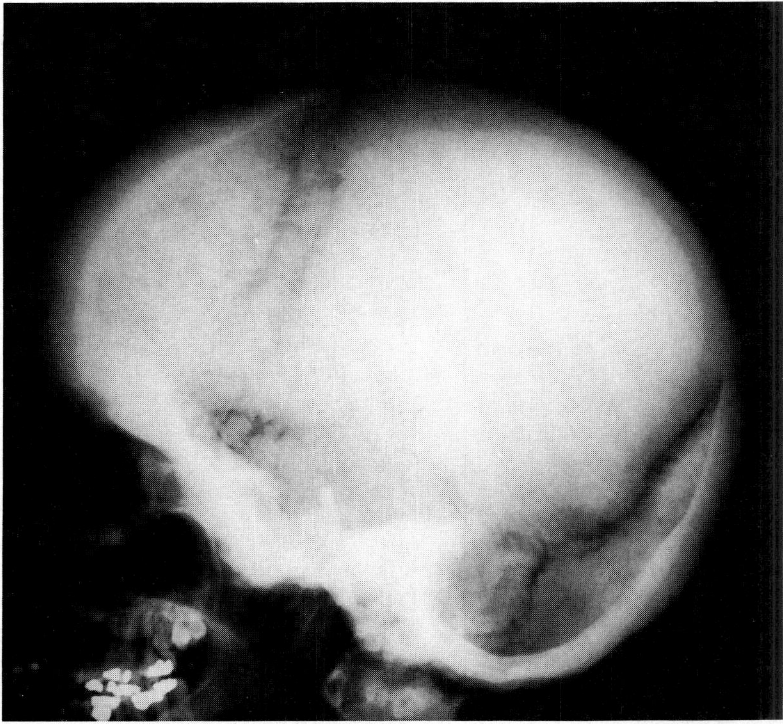

Figure 16–14. Progressive diaphyseal dysplasia. Lateral radiograph of the skull of a 19-year-old girl shows diffuse sclerosis of the cranial vault and base of the skull. Frontal bossing is present.

(M.P. Whyte and W.A. Murphy, unpublished observation). Some argue that clinical and laboratory findings in the full-blown condition and its responsiveness to glucocorticoid therapy indicate that progressive diaphyseal dysplasia is a systemic disorder that should be included within the spectrum of the inflammatory connective tissue diseases.[113] Recently, greatly increased blood flow to affected bone was noted in two of four patients.[118]

F. Treatment

Radiologic studies show that the progression of Engelmann's disease is slow and unpredictable.[115] Skeletal symptoms may remit during adolescence. Since 1967, glucocorticoid therapy (prednisone given in small doses on an alternate-day schedule) has been recognized to relieve bone pain;[119] histologic improvement of affected bone has also been described.[120-123] Intermittent courses of diphosphonate (disodium etidronate) therapy have improved symptoms in one patient in whom radiographic changes were progressing.[124] However, one of the authors (M.P.W.) has not observed symptomatic improvement in several patients treated with disodium etidronate. One adolescent with disease limited to her legs experienced complete relief of pain following a biopsy (cortical window) of the diaphysis of an affected tibia,[107] and this has been observed in other cases as well (M.P.W., unpublished observation).

VI. ENDOSTEAL HYPEROSTOSIS

Endosteal hyperostosis, first reported by van Buchem and colleagues in 1955,[125-127] is also called hyperostosis corticalis generalisata (McKusick 23910). The disorder is heritable, either as an autosomal recessive form that is clinically severe (van Buchem disease) or as an autosomal dominant condition that is more benign (Worth type).[128,129] Endosteal hyperostosis does not appear to be as common as the literature would suggest. In 1977, review of 41 reported cases revealed that only six fit uniform diagnostic criteria;[130] most had clinical and radiologic features of other craniotubular disorders, especially sclerosteosis or craniodiaphyseal dysplasia.

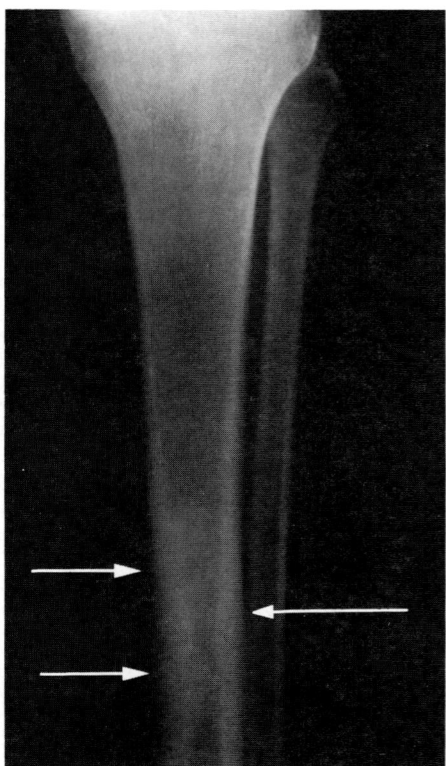

Figure 16–15. Progressive diaphyseal dysplasia. AP radiograph of the left leg of a 39-year-old man with a mild form of Engelmann's disease shows focal sclerosis and cortical thickening of the mid-tibia (arrows).

A. Clinical Presentation

Van Buchem disease has been reported in children and adults. The sex distribution appears to be equal. All adult patients have a markedly thickened mandible with wide angle, yet there is no prognathism, and dental malocclusion is uncommon. Progressive asymmetrical enlargement of the mandible occurs during puberty. Patients often live normally without complaints; however, recurrent facial paralysis, deafness, and optic atrophy due to narrowing of the cranial foramina are common and may begin during infancy.[131] There is no predisposition to fracture. Palpably thickened clavicles and ribs may be present. Long bones may be painful to pressure, but range of motion appears to be normal. Sclerosteosis (section VII) had until recently[132] been differentiated from van Buchem disease because excessive height and syndactyly are present in the former condition.

B. Laboratory Findings

Alkaline phosphatase activity in serum is of bone origin, and may be increased in the autosomal recessive form of endosteal hyperostosis. Serum levels of calcium and inorganic phosphate are normal.

C. Radiologic Features

The principal radiologic feature of van Buchem disease is endosteal cortical thickening, which results in dense homogeneous diaphyseal cortices that narrow the medullary canal (Fig. 16–16*A*, *B*). Long bones are properly shaped, but appear dense because of widening of the cortex from selective *endosteal* hyperostosis. The mandible becomes enlarged. Generalized osteosclerosis occurs because of involvement of most other bones, including the base of the skull (Fig. 16–17), facial bones and mandible (Fig. 16–18), vertebrae, pelvis, and ribs (Fig. 16–19).

D. Histopathologic Findings

Van Buchem and coworkers suggested that the disorder is due to excessive formation of normal bone tissue.

E. Etiology and Pathogenesis

Recent evidence indicates that van Buchem disease and sclerosteosis (section VII) represent homozygosity for the same genetic defect wherein the pleotropic variation may be explained by the epistatic effects of modifying genes.[132]

F. Treatment

Surgical decompression of narrowed foramina may be helpful in some patients with cranial nerve palsy.[133] There is no effective medical treatment.

VII. SCLEROSTEOSIS

Sclerosteosis (cortical hyperostosis with syndactyly), like van Buchem disease (section VI), is an autosomal recessive craniotubular

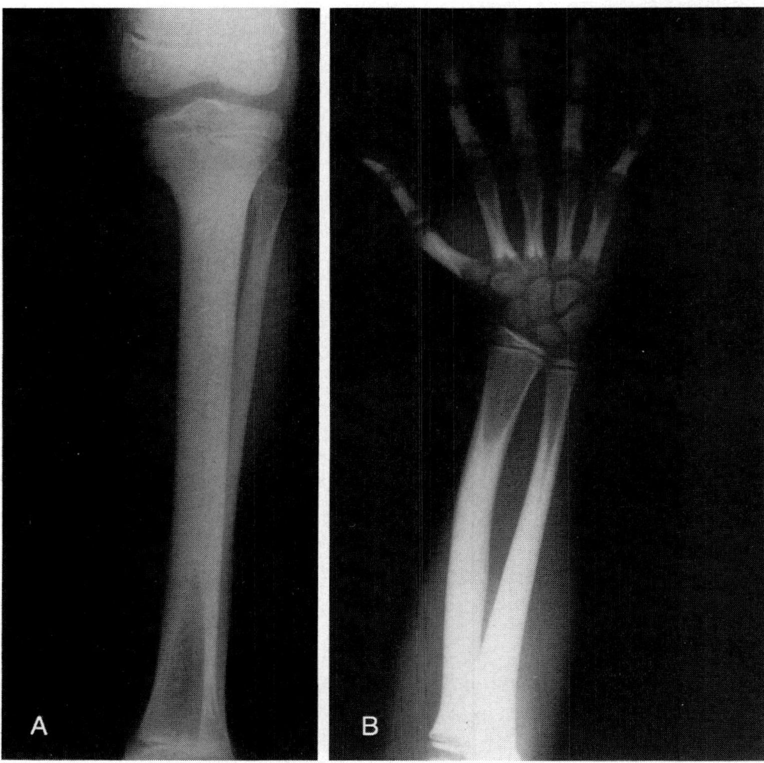

Figure 16–16. Endosteal hyperostosis. *A*, AP radiograph of the left leg of a 9-year-old boy shows bones that are of normal width yet have very thick cortices that constrict the medullary canal. *B*, Similar changes are present in his left forearm and hand.

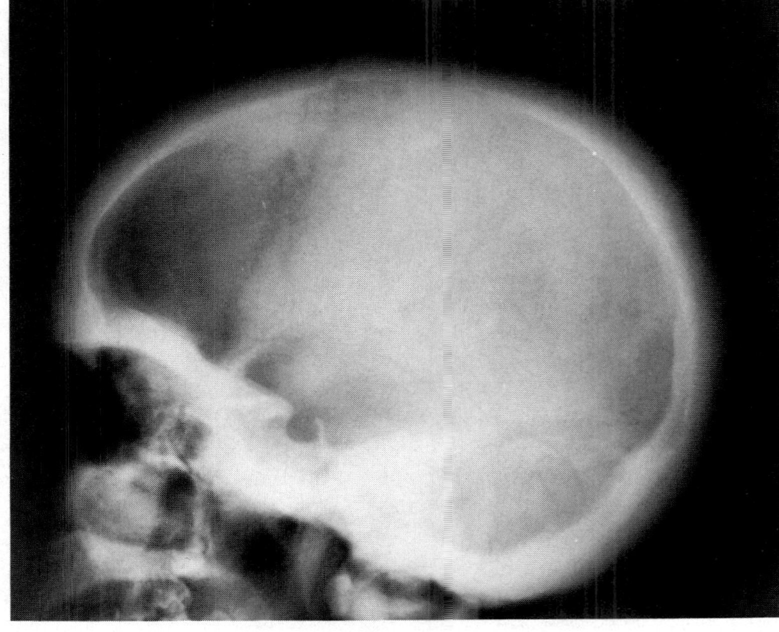

Figure 16–17. Endosteal hyperostosis. Lateral radiograph of the skull of the boy depicted in Figure 16–16 shows dense sclerosis of the cranial vault.

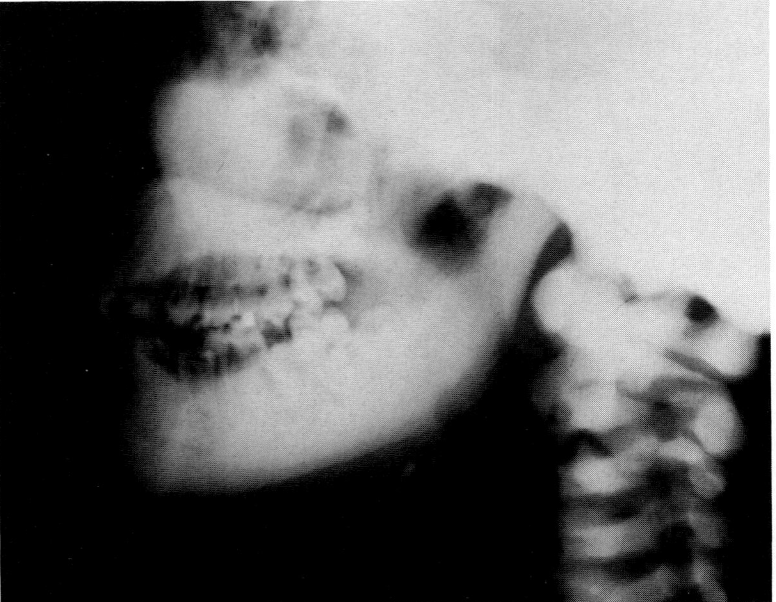

Figure 16–18. Endosteal hyperostosis. Lateral radiograph of the mandible and facial bones of the boy depicted in Figures 16–16 and 16–17 shows dense sclerosis of all osseous structures.

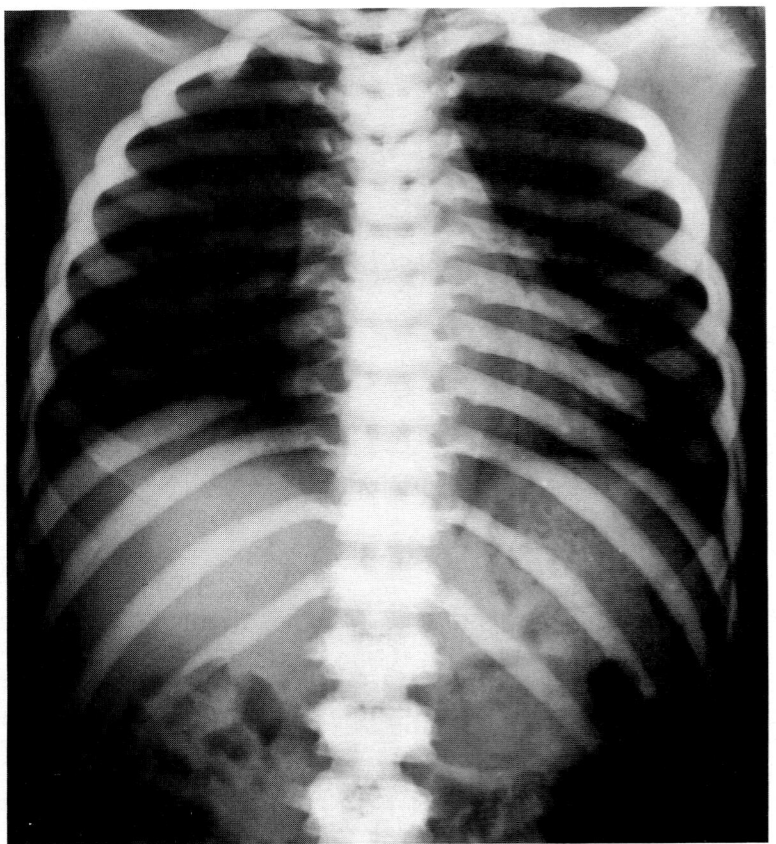

Figure 16–19. Endosteal hyperostosis. AP radiograph of the ribs of the boy depicted in Figures 16–16 to 16–18 shows homogeneous dense osteosclerosis of all ribs (note: the central portions of the vertebrae are also sclerotic).

hyperostosis; it is usually reported in the Afrikaner population of South Africa (McKusick 26950). Reported patients who live elsewhere often have Dutch ancestry.[134] Sclerosteosis was initially distinguished from van Buchem disease in 1958 by some radiographic differences and by the presence of syndactyly.[135,136]

A. Clinical Presentation

Syndactyly may be the only clinical finding in sclerosteosis at birth.[137] During early childhood, there is overgrowth and sclerosis of the skeleton, especially the skull, with attendant facial disfiguration.[137] Patients are tall and heavy beginning in childhood. "Gigantism" has been used to describe their appearance. The jaw has a very square appearance. Deafness and facial palsy from cranial nerve entrapment may be among the presenting clinical manifestations. Some patients develop raised intracranial pressure and headache from a small cranial cavity. Brain stem compression may also occur. Syndactyly due to cutaneous or bony fusion of the index and middle fingers is a characteristic finding, but of variable severity. Fingernails are dysplastic. Intelligence is not affected. Life expectancy may be shortened.[138,139]

B. Radiologic Features

The skeleton, except for possible syndactyly, is normal in early childhood. The major radiologic feature is progressive osteosclerosis and widening of the skull and mandible (including prognathism).[140] The ribs, pelvis, vertebral pedicles, and tubular bones are somewhat dense. Modeling defects occur in the long bones where the cortices are thickened. Syndactyly, usually of the index and long fingers, is common (Fig. 16–20*A*, *B*).

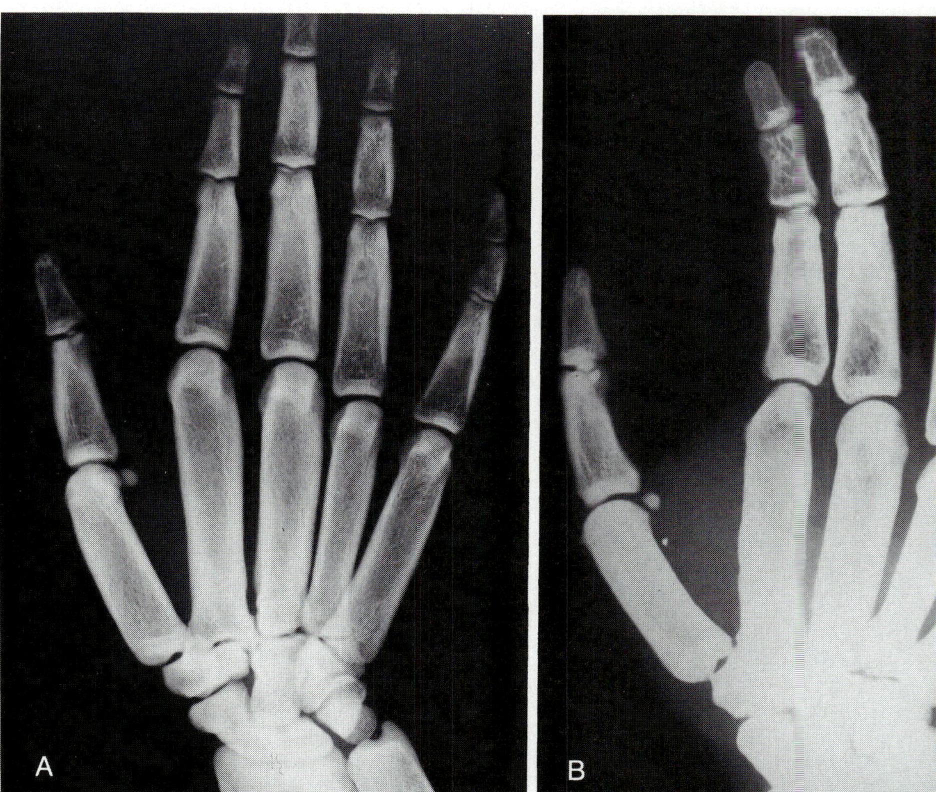

Figure 16–20. Sclerosteosis. *A*, PA radiograph of the hand of a 36-year-old man shows thickened, sclerotic tubular bones. *B*, PA radiograph of the hand of a 38-year-old man shows syndactyly of second and third fingers in addition to osteosclerotic tubular bone. (Radiographs courtesy of Dr. Peter Beighton, Capetown, South Africa.)

Cranial CT findings in sclerosteosis have recently been reported in detail and have revealed that fusion of the ossicles as well as narrowing of the internal auditory canals and cochlear aqueducts account for the deafness.[141]

C. Histopathologic Findings

A recent multidisciplinary study of an American kindred with sclerosteosis included histomorphometric analysis of calvarium following *in vivo* tetracycline labeling.[139] Dense thickened trabeculae were associated with active-appearing osteoblasts, increased total bone volume, elevated relative osteoid volume, and increased linear extent of bone formation and appositional rate. Osteoclastic bone formation seemed to be depressed.[139]

D. Etiology and Pathogenesis

Osteoblast hyperactivity, with failure of osteoclasts to compensate, appears to account for the osteosclerosis of sclerosteosis.[139] No abnormality of pituitary function or of calcium homeostasis has been found.[142] A detailed assessment of the pathogenesis of the neurologic defects is available.[139]

Recent review of 50 patients with sclerosteosis in South Africa and 15 subjects with van Buchem disease in Holland revealed similar clinical and radiographic features that were more severe in sclerosteosis. Accordingly, Beighton and coworkers suggested that both disorders share the same faulty gene(s), but that the phenotypic variation is due to the epistatic effect of modifying genes.[132]

E. Treatment

There is no direct medical treatment for sclerosteosis. Syndactyly usually requires surgical intervention, but is especially difficult to correct if there is bony fusion. Patients are not prone to fracture. Surgery to correct prognathism is complicated by dense mandibular bone (section VI). A thorough discussion of the management of the neurologic dysfunction was published in 1983.[139]

VIII. OSTEOPOIKILOSIS

Osteopoikilosis (McKusick 16670) literally translated means "spotted bones." This radiologic curiosity is inherited as an autosomal dominant trait with a high degree of penetrance.[143] In some kindreds, affected subjects also have connective tissue nevi (dermatofibrosis lenticularis disseminata), in which case the condition is then called the Buschke-Ollendorff syndrome;[144] family members may have either manifestation alone. The bony lesions are asymptomatic. However, if the condition is not recognized as a benign skeletal dysplasia, patients may be subjected to diagnostic studies for other important disorders including metastatic disease to the skeleton.[145]

A. Clinical Presentation

Osteopoikilosis is often diagnosed when radiologic study is performed for unrelated reasons. However, musculoskeletal pain has been described in some cases.

The cutaneous nevi are most commonly noted on the lower trunk or extremities and appear before puberty. They may, however, be congenital. This dermatosis appears as small asymptomatic papules. Occasionally, they appear as yellow or white disks, or plaques, deep nodules, or streaks.[144,146]

B. Radiologic Features

The principal radiologic feature of osteopoikilosis is focal bony sclerosis composed of numerous small overgrowths in the cancellous portions of the skeleton. Commonly affected sites are the metaepiphyseal regions of the long bones (Fig. 16–21), the ends of the short tubular bones, and the carpal, tarsal, and pelvic bones (Fig. 16–22). These foci are of variable shape, but tend to be round or oval. Once manifest, they are stable in size and shape for decades.[2-9] They are not associated with focal radionuclide accumulation on bone scintigraphy.[145] Metastatic lesions may mimic osteopoikilosis.[147]

C. Histopathologic Studies

Examination of the skin lesions from 12 patients of two unrelated kindreds with osteopoikilosis revealed excessive amounts of unusually broad interlacing elastin fibers in the dermis.[144] The epidermis was unremarkable. Electron microscopy showed markedly

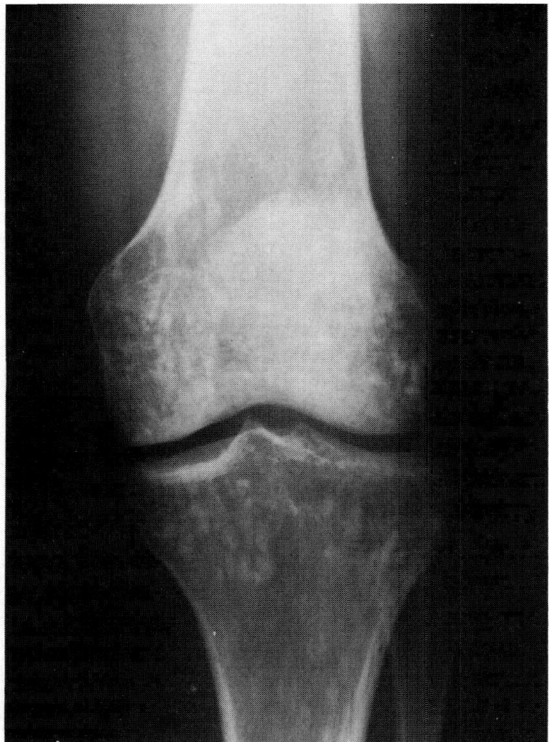

Figure 16–21. Osteopoikilosis. AP radiograph of left knee of a 39-year-old woman shows multiple sclerotic foci of variable shape located in the metaepiphyseal regions of the distal femur and proximal tibia.

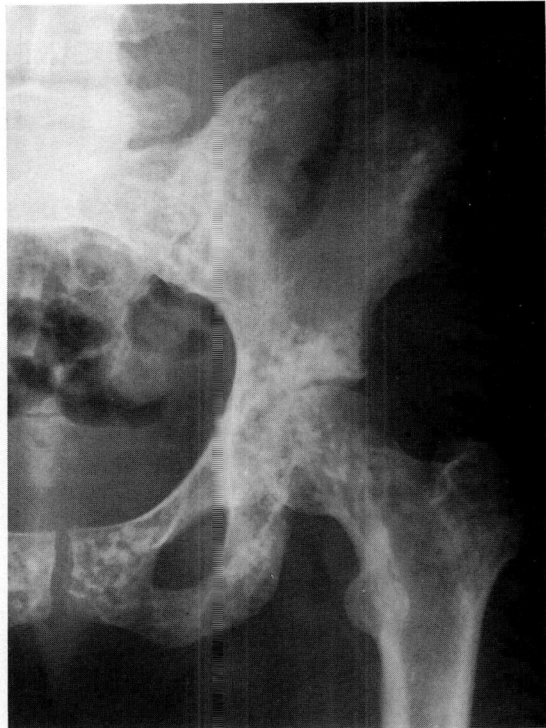

Figure 16–22. Osteopoikilosis. AP radiograph of left hemipelvis of this 39-year-old woman shows multiple small sclerotic foci throughout the innominate bone and the metaepiphyseal region of the left femur.

branched elastin fibers. These nevi can be degraded by pancreatic elastase and contain large amounts of desmosine.[144]

The bony lesions are thickened trabeculae that merge with surrounding normal bone, or islands of cortical bone with haversian systems. Remodeling of mature lesions is inactive.[148]

D. Treatment

Osteopoikilosis is a radiologic curiosity; it does not require treatment.

IX. OSTEOPATHIA STRIATA

Osteopathia striata refers to a radiographic curiosity characterized by asymptomatic linear striations at the ends of long bones and in the ilium.[2-9] These findings occur alone, or in a variety of syndromes; for example, (1) osteopathia striata with cranial sclerosis (McKusick 16650), inherited as an autosomal dominant trait,[149-153] (2) osteopathia striata inherited as an X-linked recessive trait with focal dermal hypoplasia (McKusick 30560),[154-155] or, (3) osteopathia striata with pigmentary dermopathy (including white forelock), in which X-linked dominant inheritance seems likely (McKusick 31128) and the bony abnormalities have been shown to be developmental in early childhood.[156] Osteopathia striata also occurs as a component of a sclerosing bone disorder even more radiologically complex called mixed sclerosing bone dystrophy (section XI).

A. Clinical Presentation

When osteopathia striata occurs as an isolated finding, patients are generally asymptomatic and it is a radiologic curiosity. Musculoskeletal complaints of some sort may initiate the radiologic studies that lead to the diagnosis. When there is cranial sclerosis, cranial nerve palsies and palatine malformations are common.[152,157] In one affected family with cranial sclerosis, the diagnosis was reported to have been made when a pregnant family member underwent ultrasound examination that disclosed an increased fetal biparietal diameter.[158] Osteopathia striata with focal dermal hypoplasia (Goltz's syndrome) is a serious disorder in which affected boys have widespread linear lesions of dermal hypoplasia through which adipose tissue can herniate. Affected patients also manifest a variety of skeletal defects in the limbs.[154,155] Osteopathia striata with dermopathy and white forelock[156] may be associated with developmental deafness (M.P.W., personal observation).

B. Radiologic Features

Gracile linear striation of bone is the principal radiologic feature of osteopathia striata.[2-9]

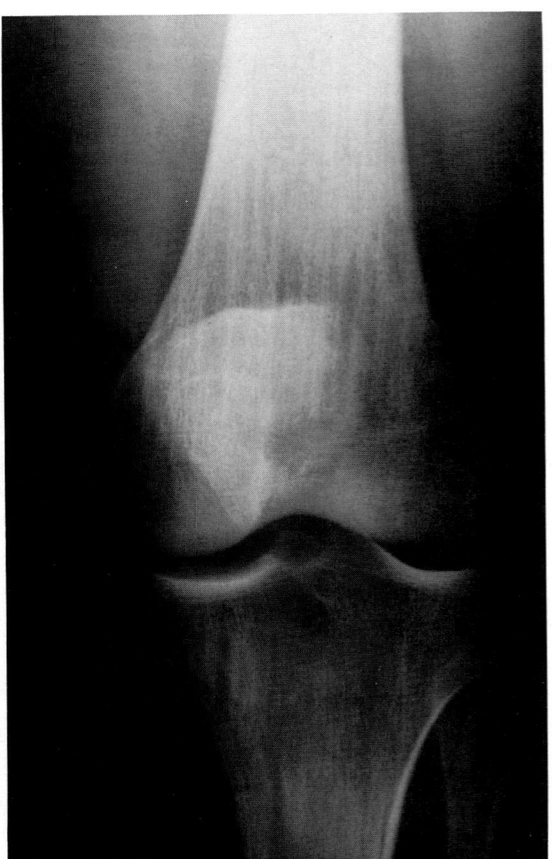

Figure 16–23. Osteopathia striata. AP radiograph of left knee of a 25-year-old woman shows vertical linear striations in the metaepiphyseal regions of the distal femur and proximal tibia.

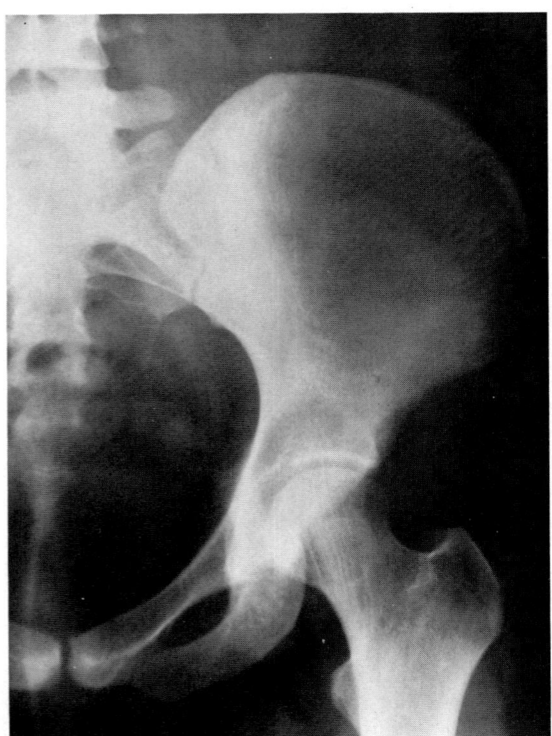

Figure 16–24. Osteopathia striata. AP radiograph of the left hemipelvis of this 25-year-old woman shows linear striations that are distributed in a fanlike pattern in the iliac wing.

This abnormality develops in the cancellous portions of the skeleton, particularly the metaepiphyseal ends of the long bones (Fig. 16–23) and the periphery of the iliac bones (Fig. 16–24). Involvement of the carpal, tarsal, and tubular bones of the hands and feet is less common and more subtle. Once manifest, the striations are stable in appearance for years. They do not show focal radionuclide accumulation on bone scintigraphy.[145]

C. Histopathologic Findings

Histopathologic studies have not been reported.

D. Treatment

There is no medical treatment for osteopathia striata.

X. MELORHEOSTOSIS

Melorheostosis (MuKusick 15595), translated from the Greek, means flowing hyperostosis of the limbs. The radiologic appearance of affected long bones has been likened to melted wax dripping down the side of a candle. The disorder was first described in 1922.[159] About 200 cases have been reported.[160] As with Ollier disease and fibrous dysplasia, no mendelian basis for melorheostosis has been established.[161,163]

A. Clinical Presentation

Melorheostosis usually presents during childhood. Monomelic involvement is most common. Bilateral disease is asymmetric. Pain and stiffness are the predominant symptoms. Affected joints may become contracted and deformity also occurs. Cutaneous changes can overlie affected skeletal regions. Of 131 patients reported in one study, 17% had a dermatosis characterized by linear scleroderma-like areas,[164] sometimes with hypertrichosis.[165] Fibromas, fibrolipomas, lymphangiectasis, capillary hemangiomas, and arterial aneurysms may occur.[166] The soft tissue abnormalities are often discovered earlier than the underlying hyperostosis. Therefore, it has been suggested that the linear scleroderma might represent the primary abnormality that extends deep into the skeleton.[167] In affected children, soft tissue contractures and premature fusion of epiphyses can cause leg length inequality as a principal clinical feature;[168] however, pain is less frequent than in adults. The skeletal changes appear to progress most rapidly during childhood; during the adult years they can stabilize or gradually extend.[169]

B. Laboratory Findings

Routine laboratory studies in melorheostosis, for example serum calcium and inorganic phosphate levels and alkaline phosphate activity, are normal.

C. Radiologic Features

Dense, eccentric, irregular hyperostosis of the cortex and adjacent medullary canal of a single bone or of several adjacent bones is the principal radiologic feature of melorheostosis.[2-9,162] Any bone or anatomic region may be involved, but the condition is more common in the lower extremities (Figs. 16–25 and 16–26). Ectopic bone may develop in soft tissue adjacent to involved skeletal areas, particularly near joints. Melorheostotic bone accumulates radionuclide during bone scintigraphy.[145,170]

D. Histologic Findings

Unlike the skin lesions of true scleroderma, the sclerodermatous skin lesions of melorheostosis contain normal-appearing collagen. Therefore, the condition has been called "linear melorheostotic scleroderma."[165,167,171] A melorheostotic skeletal lesion consists of endosteal thickening during infancy and periosteal bone formation during adulthood.[162] Affected bone is sclerotic and thickened with irregular lamellae that obliterate haversian systems. Fibrosis of intertrabecular spaces can occur.[162]

E. Etiology and Pathogenesis

The appearance of melorheostosis and soft tissue lesions in the distribution of sclerotomes, myotomes, and dermatomes suggests that a segmentary embryogenetic defect accounts for this sporadic mesodermal disorder.[160,162]

F. Treatment

Surgical correction of contractures in children with melorheostosis is difficult; recurrent deformity is usual. The calcium channel-blocking agent nifedipine has been reported to alleviate pain in one patient.[172]

XI. MIXED SCLEROSING BONE DYSTROPHY

Mixed sclerosing bone dystrophy is the term offered by Walker in 1964 to describe two patients in whom radiologic features of melorheostosis, osteopoikilosis, and osteopathia striata were present in combination.[173] Subsequently, cranial sclerosis and/or other skeletal defects were recognized to occur in addition (section IX) in some affected individuals.[174-178] Although this is clearly a very heterogeneous disorder, review of the litera-

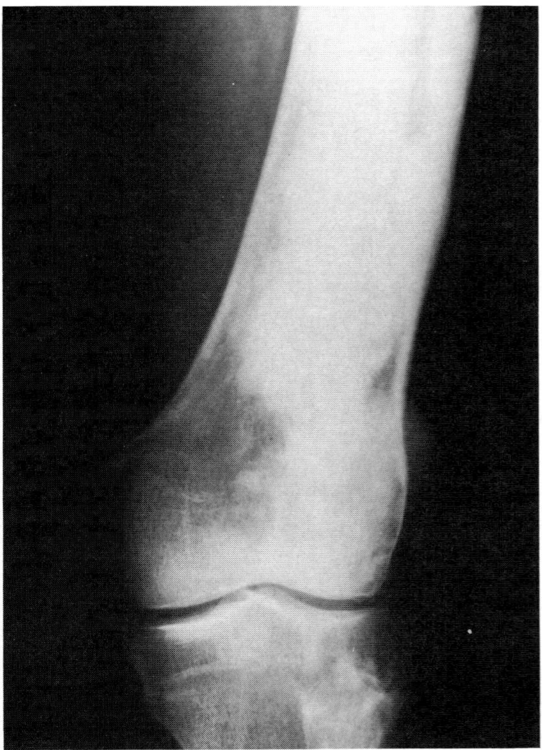

Figure 16–25. Melorheostosis. AP radiograph of the left knee of a 42-year-old woman shows asymmetric eccentric distribution of cortical thickening and dense medullary hyperostosis of the distal femur.

ture in 1981 enabled proposal of a tentative classification that might help to identify possible subgroups.[177]

A. Clinical Presentation

Patients with mixed sclerosing bone dystrophy who have components of cranial sclerosis and/or melorheostosis (sections IX and X) may be symptomatic from complications typically associated with these findings. The skull may be enlarged (Fig. 16–27*A*, *B*), and cranial nerve entrapment may occur. Skeletal pain may be present.

B. Radiologic Features

Two or more patterns of osteosclerosis described thus far—that is, osteopoikilosis, osteopathia striata, melorheostosis, focal osteosclerosis, cranial sclerosis, generalized cortical hyperostosis, or progressive diaphyseal dysplasia—are found in one subject (Figs. 16–28 and 16–29). Often, only a portion of the skeleton is involved.[173,177,178] Skeletal scintigraphy will reveal increased radionuclide uptake in areas of greatest osteosclerosis.[177,178]

C. Histopathologic Findings

Although some patients with mixed sclerosing bone dystrophy who demonstrate generalized osteosclerosis have been reported to have "osteopetrosis," detailed histopathologic study of iliac crest bone from several subjects has failed to show remnants of primary spongiosa and has thereby excluded absence of osteoclast-mediated bone resorption.[177,178]

D. Etiology and Pathogenesis

Delineation of mixed sclerosing bone dystrophy as an entity suggests a common pathogenetic mechanism for these disorders when they occur separately. However, whereas osteopoikilosis and osteopathia striata have been shown clearly to be heritable, mixed sclerosing bone dystrophy, like melorheostosis, has been reported only as a sporadic disorder.

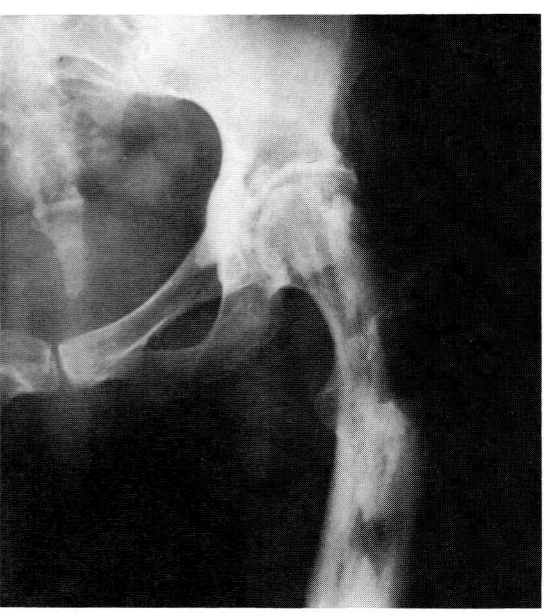

Figure 16–26. Melorheostosis. AP radiograph of the left hemipelvis of a 42-year-old woman shows dense, eccentric, irregular hyperostosis of acetabulum and proximal femur.

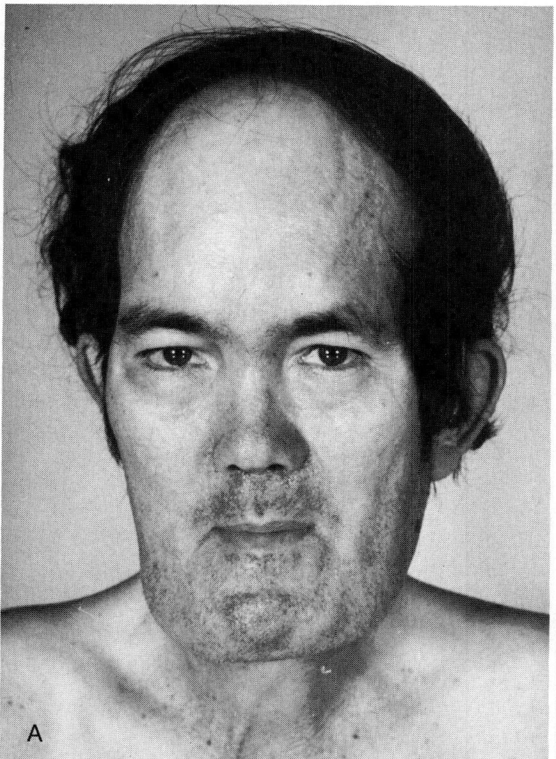

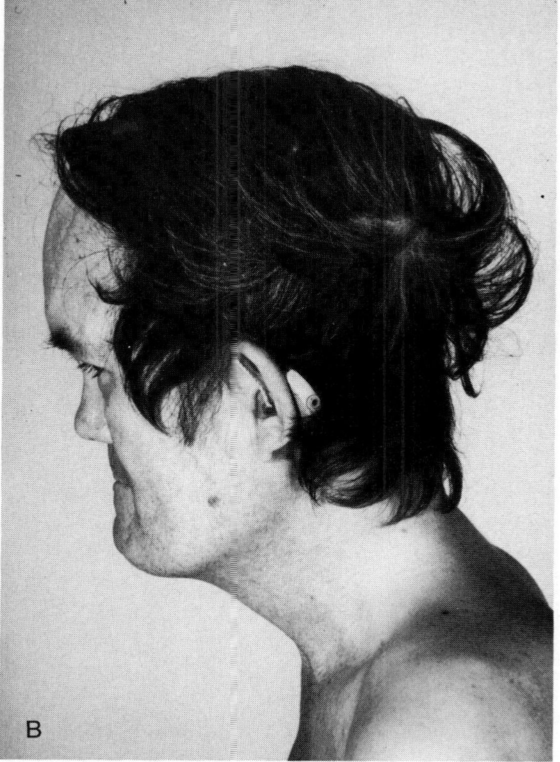

Figure 16–27. Mixed sclerosing bone dystrophy. *A* and *B*, This 49-year-old man has a very large head with prominent jaw and forehead. (From Pacifici R, et al: Calcif Tissue Int 38:175–185, 1986.)

E. Treatment

There is no effective medical treatment for mixed sclerosing bone dystrophy. Surgical correction of contractures or of neurovascular compression by osteosclerotic lesions may be necessary.

XII. FIBRODYSPLASIA OSSIFICANS PROGRESSIVA

Fibrodysplasia ossificans progressiva (myositis ossificans progressiva) is characterized by a variety of congenital skeletal abnormalities together with recurrent painful episodes of progressive heterotopic formation of true bone in fascia, aponeuroses, ligaments, tendons, and connective tissue of voluntary muscles; smooth muscle is spared. Since the disorder was first described in 1692,[179] more than 500 cases have been reported.[180,181] It appears to be transmitted as an autosomal dominant trait, but with very variable expressivity (McKusick 13510). Most cases, however, are sporadic.[1] Caucasians are reported most commonly; however, the disorder has been described in blacks.[179]

A. Clinical Presentation

Fibrodysplasia ossificans progressiva usually becomes manifest during the first decade of life,[181] but the age at presentation is highly variable. There are reports of involvement *in utero* and beginning as late as early adulthood. The diagnosis may be made at birth by the presence of a variety of congenital skeletal anomalies—the most characteristic being hallux valgus with microdactyly (Fig. 16–30). Microdactyly of the thumb may also be present. There may be synostosis and hypoplasia of the phalanges. Recurrent episodes of tender, rubbery, painful soft tissue swellings (that are sometimes associated with minor trauma) are followed by calcification and then heterotopic true bone formation. Early on,

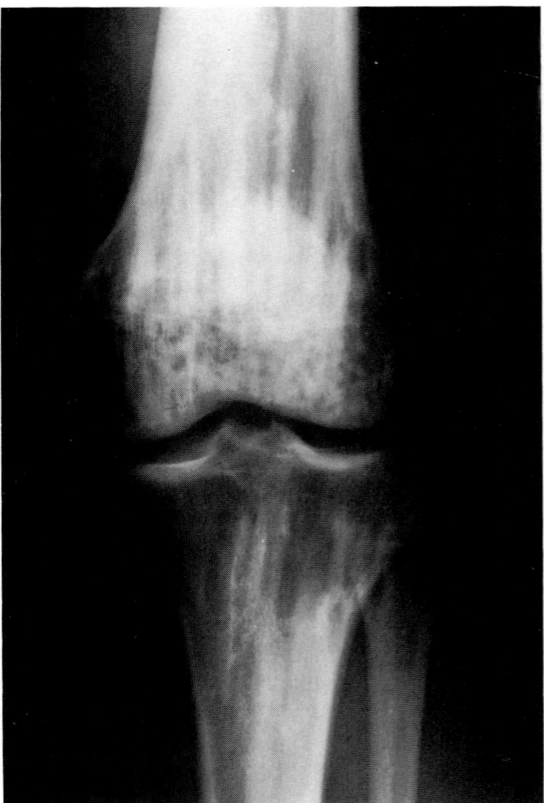

Figure 16–28. Mixed sclerosing bone dystrophy. AP radiograph of the man shown in Figure 16–27; the left knee shows osteopoikilosis of the distal femoral epiphysis, osteopathia striata of the distal femoral and proximal tibial metaepiphyses, and melorheostosis of the distal femoral diaphysis.

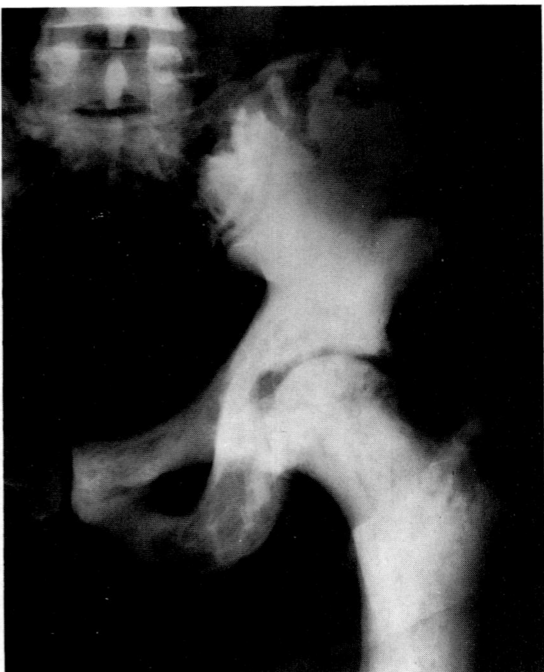

Figure 16–29. Mixed sclerosing bone dystrophy. AP radiograph of the man shown in Figure 16–27; the left hemipelvis shows focal osteosclerosis of the ilium and a melorheostosis pattern of the proximal femur.

torticollis with involvement of the sternocleidomastoid muscle is noted or the muscles of the shoulder girdle and dorsum of the trunk are affected. Fever may occur during these times and mimic an infectious process. Progressive episodes of heterotopic bone formation result in decreased range of motion, especially in the neck and shoulders. Involvement of the muscle of the mandible may lead to severe limitation of jaw movement and impair nutrition. Involvement of the musculature of the thorax may deform the chest (Fig. 16–31*A*, *B*) and thereby cause restrictive lung disease and predispose the patient to pneumonia. Scoliosis may occur more frequently in these patients.[182] Although secondary amenorrhea is not unusual, successful reproduction has been reported.[183] Deafness and alopecia occur in increased frequency.

B. Laboratory Findings

Serum alkaline phosphatase activity in fibrodysplasia ossificans progressiva may be increased. Other routine biochemical studies are usually normal.

C. Radiologic Features

A combination of anomalies of the skeleton and soft tissue ossification is the radiologic feature of fibrodysplasia ossificans progressiva.[184,185] There is progressive ossification of fascia, tendons, aponeuroses, and other tissues. The neck (Fig. 16–32*A*) and shoulders (Fig. 16–32*B*) tend to be involved earlier than the lower extremities (Fig. 16–33). Paraspinal muscles are especially prone to ossification. Ankylosis of the spine, rib cage, and joints

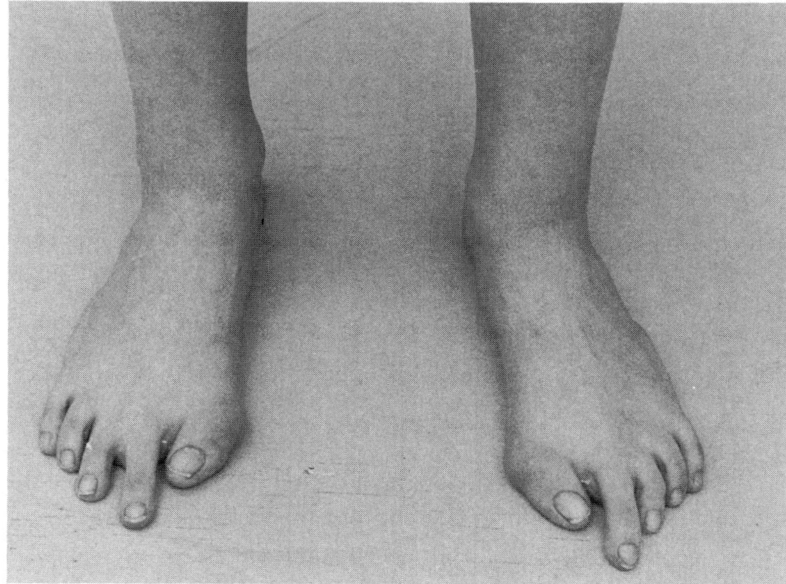

Figure 16–30. Fibrodysplasia ossificans progressiva. Typical hallux valgus deformity with microdactyly is present in this 14-year-old boy.

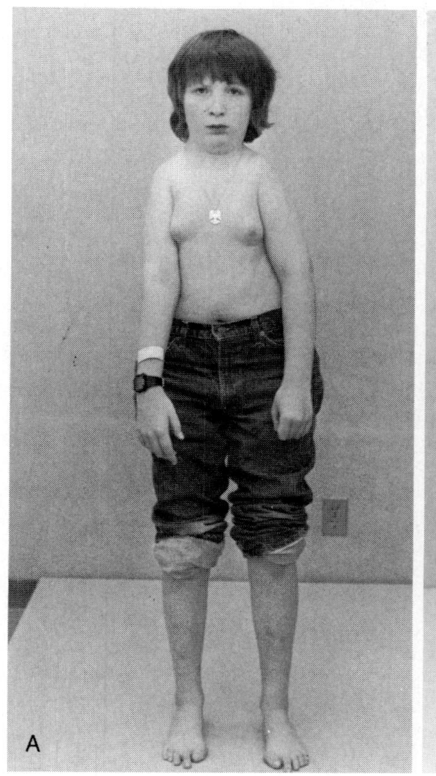

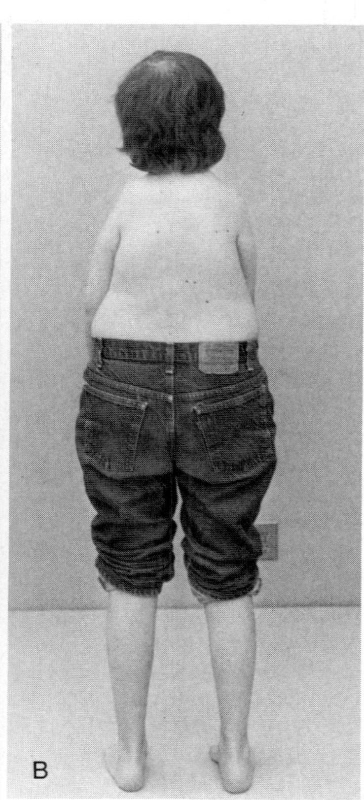

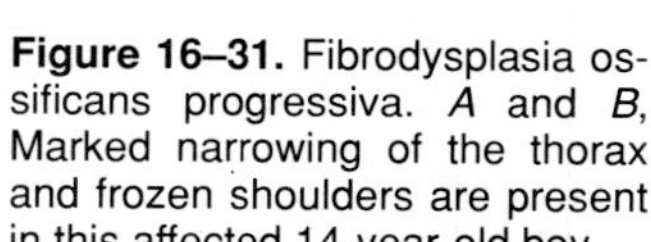

Figure 16–31. Fibrodysplasia ossificans progressiva. *A* and *B*, Marked narrowing of the thorax and frozen shoulders are present in this affected 14-year-old boy.

limits mobility. During severe inflammation, portions of the skeleton are osteopenic. Otherwise, bones are generally well mineralized. Many skeletal anomalies of the extremities occur. Chief among them are disturbances of the formation of the great toe (Fig. 16–34). Computed tomography to detect soft tissue calcification appears to be the best radiologic technique to diagnose an early lesion.[186] Skeletal scintigraphy with ^{99m}technetium methylene diphosphonate will also be abnormal before ossification will be detected radiologically. New areas of disease activity can be detected early by this technique.[187]

D. Histopathologic Findings

Early lesions of fibrodysplasia ossificans progressiva are characterized by edema of fascial planes. The soft tissue mass is an edematous muscle or group of muscles. Multifocal interconnecting nodules then form that are composed of fibroblasts. Later, osteoid, bone, and occasionally cartilage are present at the center of a fibrous connective tissue matrix.[188,189] Fasciae, tendons, ligaments, and joint capsules may be involved. True ossification develops and is characterized macroscopically by dense, flat, irregular areas of bone within the connective tissue of fascial planes, and this ossification extends partly or completely around a muscle.[190] Cancellous bone can eventually form. As the lesions mature, hematopoietic tissue will appear within the areas of trabecular bone.[191] Muscle fibers may undergo secondary degenerative and atrophic change.

E. Etiology and Pathogenesis

The autosomal gene defect that causes fibrodysplasia ossificans progressiva is unknown. Paternal age appears to contribute importantly to the incidence of new dominant mutations.[181,192] Most cases appear to be sporadic.[1,192] The pathogenesis is poorly understood. It is unclear whether the disorder is due to a connective tissue abnormality that secondarily affects muscle or a primary abnormality in muscle itself. The term fibrodysplasia ossificans progressiva is favored by those who believe that connective tissue is primarily affected and its invasion and proliferation within skeletal muscle causes

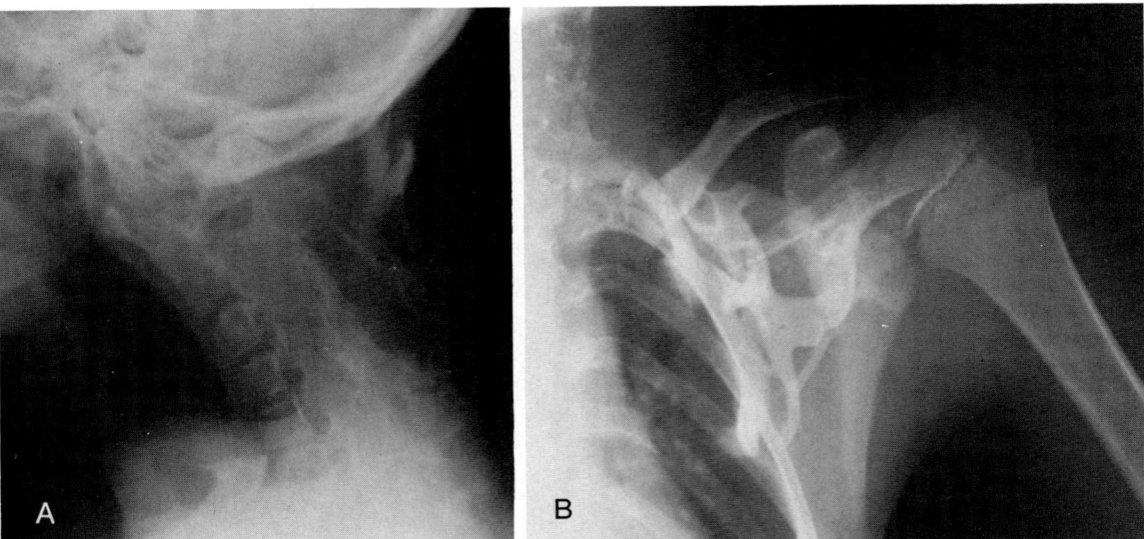

Figure 16–32. Fibrodysplasia ossificans progressiva. *A*, Lateral radiograph of the neck of a 6-year-old boy shows ossification of dorsal soft tissues and ankylosis of all cervical apophyseal joints. *B*, AP radiograph of the shoulder of the same patient shows extensive soft tissue ossification.

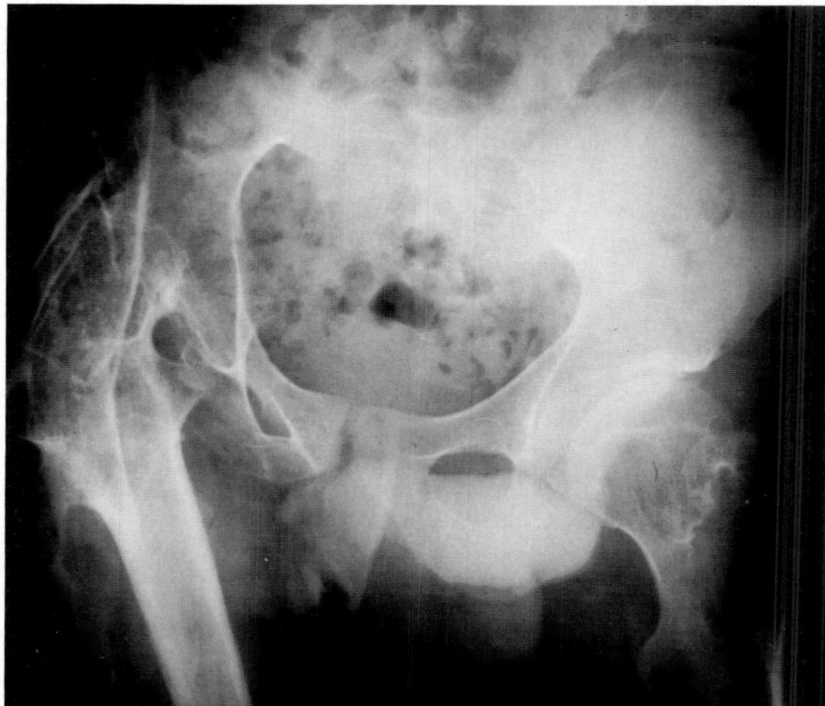

Figure 16–33. Fibrodysplasia ossificans progressiva. AP radiograph of the pelvis of a 17-year-old boy shows extensive ossification about the right hip (note that the femoral head is dislocated and that the joint is ankylosed by the ossified periarticular tissue).

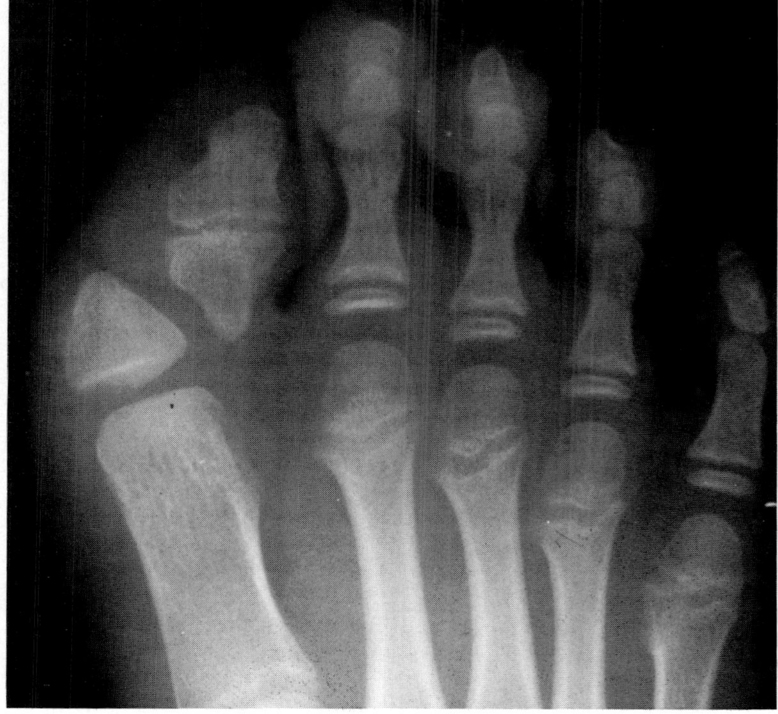

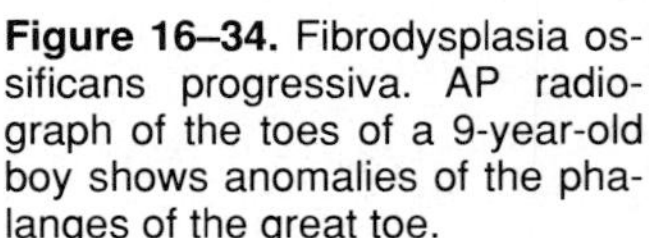

Figure 16–34. Fibrodysplasia ossificans progressiva. AP radiograph of the toes of a 9-year-old boy shows anomalies of the phalanges of the great toe.

atrophy and heterotopic bone formation. In support of this hypothesis, computed tomography has shown that characteristic swelling of muscular fascial planes occurs before development of ectopic ossification. Multifocal sites of new bone formation develop adjacent to and extend around muscles.[190] Some scholars in the field, however, see the fundamental disorder as an abnormality in skeletal muscle (myositis), since histologic and electromyographic abnormalities may occur prior to connective tissue proliferation in skeletal muscle.[193]

F. Treatment and Prognosis

There is no satisfactory medical treatment for fibrodysplasia ossificans progressiva. Therapy with adrenocorticotropic hormone or corticosteroids, calcium binders in the diet, or EDTA infusion has not been successful.[194] Treatment with the diphosphonate disodium etidronate (EHDP) has resulted in a variable response.[195] Use of warfarin to inhibit gamma-carboxylation of osteocalcin in an effort to prevent ectopic bone formation has been of no noticeable clinical benefit.[196] Surgical release procedures may be necessary to treat joint contractures or neurovascular entrapment or to increase the mandibular range of motion. Computed tomography is useful to guide surgical intervention by identifying soft tissue changes and ossification that is not yet apparent by conventional radiography.[190] Removal of lesions may be followed by recurrence and thus exacerbate the condition. In some cases, EHDP appeared to delay the mineralization of newly formed bone matrix following surgery.[195]

Despite widespread ectopic ossification involvement, some patients live into the fifth decade. Most patients, however, die from respiratory complications secondary to restricted pulmonary ventilation due to chest wall involvement.[181]

XIII. AXIAL OSTEOMALACIA

Axial osteomalacia is a rare disorder characterized by coarsening of the trabecular pattern on radiologic examination of the axial but not appendicular skeleton (see Chapter 11). The disorder was first described in 1961 by Frame and coworkers; the axial skeletons of the three patients they reported were noted to have "a unique coarsening and sponge-like appearance" on radiographs.[197] The skulls and appendicular skeletons of these patients were unremarkable. Osteoidosis was found on examination of undecalcified sections of bone. Fewer than 20 cases have been described. No mendelian pattern of transmission has been established, but autosomal dominant transmission seems possible (McKusick 10913).

A. Clinical Presentation

Most patients with axial osteomalacia have been middle-aged or elderly men. A few affected middle-aged women have also been described. Radiologic manifestations, however, are likely to be present much earlier in life.[198] The disorder may be discovered incidentally; more frequently there is dull, vague, and chronic axial skeletal pain (often in the cervical region) that prompts radiologic study. Family histories have generally been reported to be negative for skeletal disease, but radiographic surveys have usually not been performed. Axial osteomalacia has been reported once to be familial—affecting a black mother and son in whom polycystic liver and kidneys were also present.[198] Two patients had features of ankylosing spondylitis.[199]

B. Laboratory Studies

Four cases of axial osteomalacia have been described in which serum inorganic phosphate levels tended to be low.[199] In others, defective bone mineralization occurred despite normal serum levels of calcium and inorganic phosphate and increased alkaline phosphatase activity (bone isoenzyme). Serum levels of 25(OH)D and 1,25$(OH)_2$D were unremarkable in one patient.[198] One patient was found to be in strongly positive calcium and phosphorus balance.[200] Symptoms, elevated serum creatine phosphokinase activity, and muscle biospy features consistent with myopathy have been reported in one patient.[198]

C. Radiologic Features

The radiologic features of axial osteomalacia are essentially limited to the spine (Fig. 16–35)

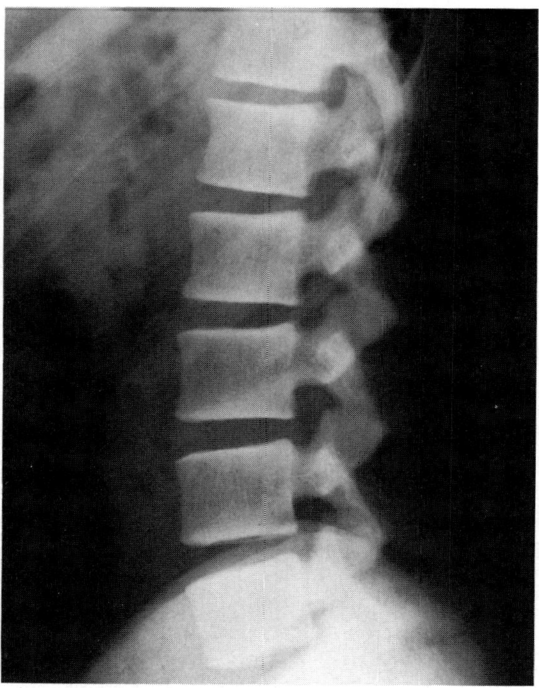

Figure 16–35. Axial osteomalacia. Lateral radiograph of the lumbar spine of a 35-year-old man shows generalized osteosclerosis due to thickening of the trabeculae. (From Whyte MP et al: Am J Med 71:1041–1049, 1981.)

and pelvis (Fig. 16–36); the trabecular pattern is somewhat coarse and resembles that found in other types of osteomalacia.[6] Looser's zones, however, have not been reported. Radiographic changes appear to be most pronounced in the cervical spine and ribs, and to a lesser extent in the lumbar spine. The appendicular skeleton is unaffected on radiologic survey.

D. Histopathologic Findings

In axial osteomalacia, osseous collagen has a normal lamellar pattern as shown by polarized light microscopy of rib specimens. Osteoidosis is present; that is, the width and extent of osteoid seams on trabecular bone surfaces and in cortical spaces may be increased (see Chapters 10 and 11). Biopsy of ribs and iliac crest following tetracycline labeling has confirmed the presence of osteomalacia, since most fluorescent "labels" are single, wide, and irregular.[198] Iliac crest specimens have distinct corticomedullary junctions, yet the cortices may have both increased width and porosity. Trabeculae can have varied thickness, and total bone volume may be increased. Osteoclasts can be few, but histochemical studies show normal levels of acid phosphatase activity. Osteoblasts are flat and inactive-appearing ("lining") cells with reduced rough endoplasmic reticulum and Golgi zones and increased cytoplasmic glycogen. Nevertheless, they may stain intensely for alkaline phosphatase activity. Evidence of secondary hyperparathyroidism is absent.[198] Histologic changes of osteomalacia following tetracycline labeling[201] help to distinguish axial osteomalacia from fibrogenesis imperfecta ossium[202] (section XIV). Christman and colleagues, in 1981, reported three cases of axial osteomalacia and two cases of fibrogenesis imperfecta ossium and contrasted the clinical, biochemical, radiologic, and histopathologic features of the disorders (section XIV).[202]

E. Etiology and Pathogenesis

Frame and colleagues suggested that axial osteomalacia was due to "unknown defects of local cellular origin."[197] Electron microscopic studies of iliac crest tissue from one patient[198] showed osteoblasts with an inactive appearance, yet the presence of intact matrix vesicles within unmineralized osteoid. The possibility that this is a heritable disorder deserves further study.

F. Treatment

There is no effective medical therapy for axial osteomalacia. In one patient treated with stilbestrol and methyltestosterone, no improvement in symptoms or radiologic features was noted.[200] Similarly, vitamin D_2 therapy (as much as 20,000 units/day for three years) resulted in no change in symptoms or radiologic pattern.[200] In a study of four cases, calcium and vitamin D_2 therapy resulted in some small improvement in skeletal histology, but there was no symptomatic benefit; it was concluded that this treatment was of no practical value.[199] Since the symptoms and radiologic findings in one patient did not change during an 18-year period,[200] and another patient remained well during five years of observation,[202] a relatively benign

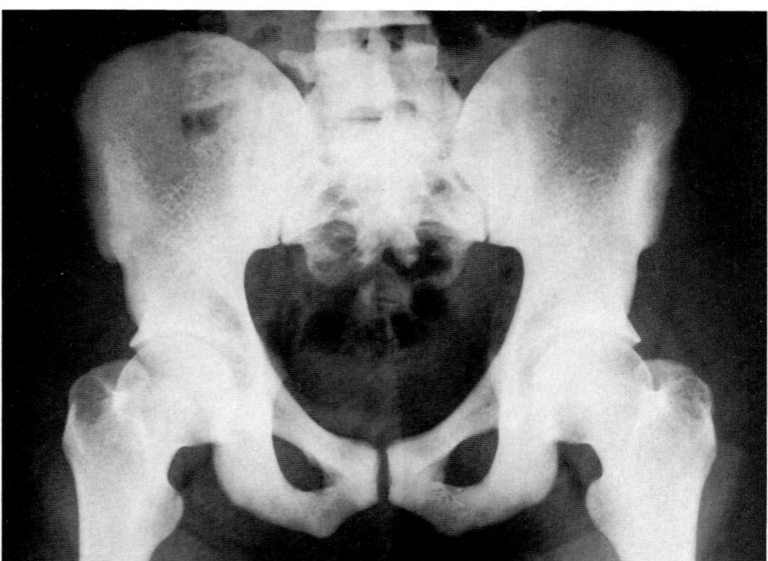

Figure 16–36. Axial osteomalacia. AP radiograph of the pelvis of a 35-year-old man shows generalized osteosclerosis. (From Whyte MP, et al: Am J Med 71:1041–1049, 1981.)

natural history for axial osteomalacia seems possible. Treatment with vitamin D_2 and mineral supplementation would seem risky, since the disorder appears to be due to a defect in the bone tissue itself, rather than in mineral homeostasis.

XIV. FIBROGENESIS IMPERFECTA OSSIUM

Fibrogenesis imperfecta ossium, first described by Baker and Turnbull in 1950,[203] is a very rare condition.[203-212] In 1986, Lang and coworkers described one case and summarized the findings in six others.[212] Although radiologic studies suggest a generalized decrease in bone mass, the coarse and dense appearance of trabeculae explain why it is discussed among the osteosclerotic disorders.

A. Clinical Presentation

Fibrogenesis imperfecta ossium is an acquired disorder that presents clinically in middle-age or late adult life. Both men and women are affected. There is gradual onset of intractable skeletal pain and progressive immobility. The disease then runs a rapidly progressive and debilitating course, with spontaneous fractures a prominent feature. Marked bony tenderness is usual. Patients generally become bedridden. One patient suffered acute agranulocytosis.[207] Another subject with radiologic changes that simulated fibrogenesis imperfecta ossium had macroglobulinemia.[213]

B. Laboratory Findings

Serum levels of calcium and inorganic phosphate in fibrogenesis imperfecta ossium are normal; alkaline phosphatase activity is increased. Urinary levels of hydroxyproline may be normal or elevated.[212] There is generally no evidence of renal tubular dysfunction or aminoaciduria. Monoclonal gammopathy appears to be common.[210]

C. Radiologic Features

The radiologic features of fibrogenesis imperfecta ossium are found throughout the skeleton except in the skull. At first these may be only osteopenia and a slightly abnormal appearance of trabecular bone.[212] The changes are then generally consistent with osteomalacia; that is, alteration of the cancellous bone pattern, irregular bone density, and cortical thinning. There is a generalized decrease in skeletal density, yet the remaining trabeculae appear coarse and dense ("fishnet" pattern). Corticomedullary junctions become indistinct, and cortices appear to be replaced by an abnormal trabecular pattern. A mixed lytic and sclerotic pattern may be present.[212]

Pseudofractures can occur. Fracture deformities may be present, although the contour of bones is generally normal. A "rugger jersey" spine is present in some patients and should not be confused with similar radiographic findings in patients with renal osteodystrophy (see Chapter 13). Periosteal reaction may occur along the shafts of long bones. The radiographic changes of fibrogenesis imperfecta ossium closely resemble those of axial osteomalacia; however, the disorders are distinguishable by different distributions of radiographic abnormalities (generalized versus axial). Furthermore, there are different histopathologic findings.[202]

D. Histopathologic Findings

The basic lesion of fibrogenesis imperfecta ossium appears to be similar throughout the skeleton, but the amount of affected bone varies widely from site to site. Cortical bone, for example, in the diaphyses of the femora and tibiae, may show the least abnormality. Osteoblasts and osteoclasts may be abundant, and osteoid seams are thick. There is an abnormal mineralization pattern. Tetracycline labeling reveals the presence of osteomalacia.[212] Characteristically, abnormal collagen is found where lamellar bone should be present (collagen in other tissues is unremarkable). On polarized light microscopy, bone collagen fibrils are not birefringent. Electron microscopy reveals them to be thin and randomly organized in a "tangled pattern," rather than in a lamellar distribution. Narrow and irregular bands of normal collagen fibrils may occasionally traverse regions of abnormal bone matrix. Only a few scattered areas of lamellar bone may be noted. In some areas of abnormal matrix, unusual circular bodies of 300 to 500 nm diameter are present.[209] This abnormal bone matrix does not calcify properly, and wide osteoid seams are present. Unless biopsy specimens are viewed with polarized light or electron microscopy, this disorder may be mistaken for osteoporosis or the more common forms of osteomalacia.[212]

E. Etiology and Pathogenesis

The etiology of fibrogenesis imperfecta ossium is unknown. The disorder has been reported only sporadically and, therefore, genetic factors have not been implicated. Although the specific biochemical defect is unknown, the condition appears to be an acquired disorder of collagen synthesis in lamellar bone that, in some way, inhibits mineralization of the osseous matrix. Only the skeleton seems to be affected. There does not appear to be a defect in subperiosteal bone formation or in collagen in nonosseous tissues. In one subject who also had monoclonal gammopathy, a toxin produced by bone marrow was postulated.[210]

F. Treatment

There is no effective medical therapy for fibrogenesis imperfecta ossium. Although the clinical course is generally one of deterioration, brief periods of clinical improvement can occur.[212] Vitamin D_2 (or active metabolites) with calcium supplements have been tried without significant benefit. Calcification of soft tissues and of tendons and ligaments occurred in one subject who was treated with large doses of vitamin D_2. Sodium fluoride, synthetic salmon calcitonin, and 24,25-dihydroxyvitamin D have also been used without apparent benefit.[212] Courses of melphalan and prednisone were followed by dramatic remission in one subject who had a monoclonal gammopathy.[210]

XV. FLUOROSIS

Fluoride may cause osteosclerosis when ingested or inhaled chronically in various forms in relatively large amounts.[214-217] Endemic fluorosis occurs in some regions (e.g., Punjab, India) from contaminated well water.[215] Men are more commonly affected than women, perhaps because their water consumption, as they perform manual labor, is greater. Leafy vegetables and tea grown in soil with a high content of fluoride, certain wines, and cooking salt represent other dietary sources of excessive amounts of fluoride.[217] However, fluorosis has also been reported as an occupational hazard, for example, in conjunction with aluminum or fertilizer production.[214] Prolonged administration of the nonsteroidal anti-inflammatory agent niflumic acid,[217] or sodium fluoride in attempted therapy for postmenopausal osteoporosis,[216] represent other potential causes (see Chapter 12).

A. Clinical Presentation

Diffuse bone pain, stiffness, decreased joint mobility, and brownish discoloration and mottling of the teeth are the principal signs and symptoms in fluorosis.[217] A "plantar fasciitis syndrome" characterized by painful and swollen feet has been described, but stress fracture of the calcaneus has recently been shown to be a likely cause of this pain.[218] Cranial nerve palsies, radiculopathies, and plexopathies can result from ligamentous calcification, exostoses, and osteophytes.

B. Laboratory Findings

Serum alkaline phosphatase activity may be increased in fluorosis, which could reflect osteoblast stimulation by a secondary hyperparathyroidism. Mineral balance studies have shown calcium retention.[219] Urinary hydroxyproline levels can similarly be increased. Assay of fluoride in blood or urine can provide biochemical support for the diagnosis.

C. Radiologic Features

Fluorosis may result in osteosclerosis and radiologic changes consistent with osteomalacia.[218] In general, it is the cancellous portions of the skeleton that become sclerotic with coarsened trabeculae (Figs. 16–37*A*, *B*). Characteristically, however, various ligaments also calcify. Irregularity at the insertion of muscles at the iliac spine and calcification of ligaments in the pelvis, vertebrae, and interosseous membranes are early radiologic signs.[6] Later, there may be generalized osteosclerosis. Osteomalacia may develop, since fluoride stimulates osteoid synthesis, yet mineral deposition may be impaired.[220] In this circumstance, stress fractures in the proximal femur or calcaneus have been reported during fluoride therapy for osteoporosis.[218]

D. Etiology and Pathogenesis

Fluoride appears to cause osteosclerosis by a combination of mechanisms including

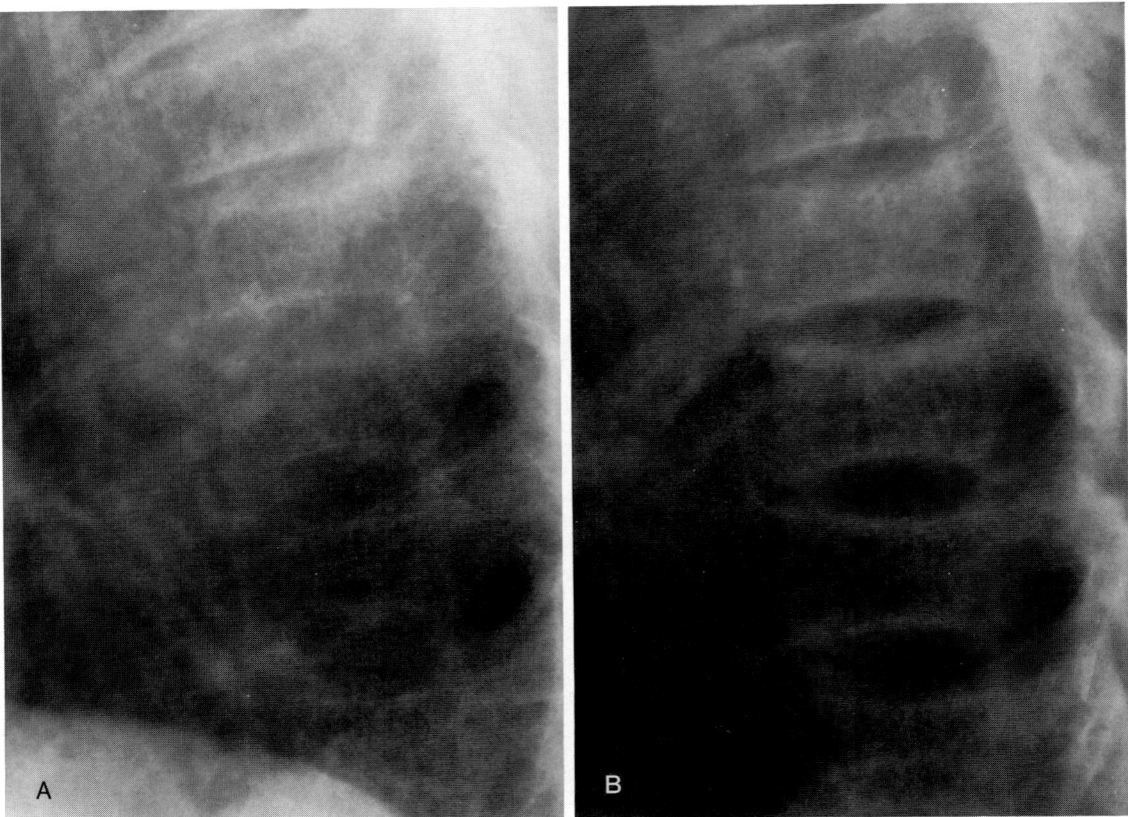

Figure 16–37. Fluorosis. *A*, Lateral radiograph of the lower thoracic spine of an 82-year-old woman with osteoporosis shows demineralized vertebral bodies. *B*, Lateral radiograph of lower thoracic spine of the same patient, now age 87, shows mild osteosclerosis of vertebral bodies after five years of sodium fluoride therapy.

direct stimulation of osteoblast mitogenic activity,[217] formation of fluorapatite crystals that are relatively resistant to osteoclastic resorption, and inducement of secondary hyperparathyroidism.[217,220]

E. Treatment

Treatment of fluorosis includes reduction of excessive intake of fluoride and, if osteomalacia is present, calcium and vitamin D supplementation to mineralize the fluoride-induced osteoidosis and to reduce secondary hyperparathyroidism.[218]

XVI. PACHYDERMOPERIOSTOSIS

Pachydermoperiostosis (hypertrophic osteoarthropathy: primary or idiopathic) was first described in 1868.[221] The condition is characterized by clubbing of the digits (Fig. 16–38), hyperhidrosis with thickening of the skin of especially the face and forehead, and periosteal new bone formation distally in the limbs. Autosomal dominant transmission with variable expression is established,[222] but autosomal recessive inheritance also appears to occur (McKusick 16710).

A. Clinical Presentation

Men appear to be more severely affected by pachydermoperiostosis than are women, and blacks have it more often than others. Symptoms usually begin during adolescence, although earlier and later presentations have been reported.[222] Some subjects have all three major findings (pachyderma, cutis verticis gyrata, periostitis); others have one or two features. These abnormalities develop for about a decade and then become quiescent.[223] Gradual progressive enlargement of the hands and feet results in a paw-like appearance. Some patients appear to be acromegalic.[224] Often there are arthralgias of the ankles, knees, wrists, elbows, and, occasionally, the small joints. Symptoms consistent with pseudogout may occur; chondrocalcinosis with calcium pyrophosphate crystals in synovial fluid has been reported in one patient.[225] Acro-osteolysis has also been described.[226] Stiffness and restricted motion of both appendicular and axial skeleton may occur. Cranial or spinal nerves may be compressed. When there are cutaneous changes, they may include coarsening, thickening, furrowing, pitting, and oiliness of the skin of the face and scalp. Some patients fatigue easily. Myelophthisic anemia with extramedullary hematopoiesis may occur.[227] Life expectancy is normal.[6]

B. Laboratory Findings

Synovial fluid in pachydermoperiostosis generally does not indicate inflammation.

C. Radiologic Features

Severe periostitis causing thickening of the distal aspect of tubular bones of the limbs—especially the tibia, fibula, radius, and ulna—is the major abnormality in pachydermoperiostosis. The clavicles, metacarpals, tarsal/metatarsals, phalanges, pelvis, and base of the skull may also be affected. The spine is rarely

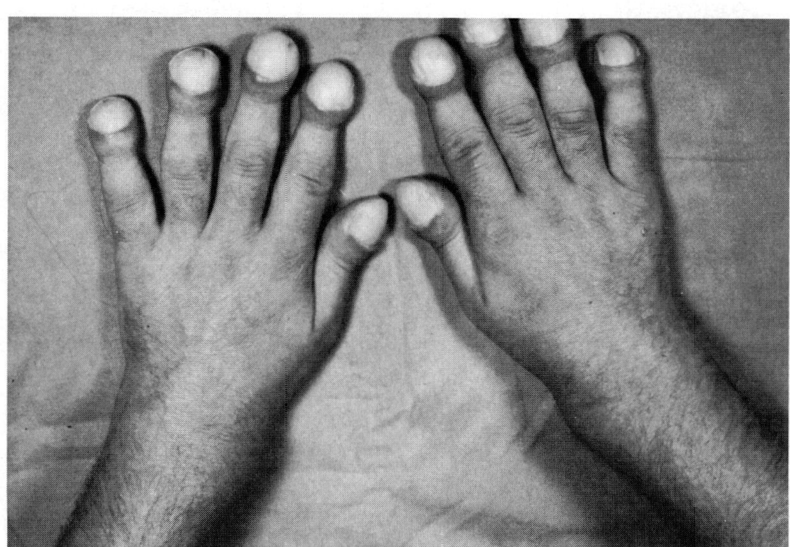

Figure 16–38. Pachydermoperiostosis. Characteristic marked clubbing of the fingers of a 33-year-old man.

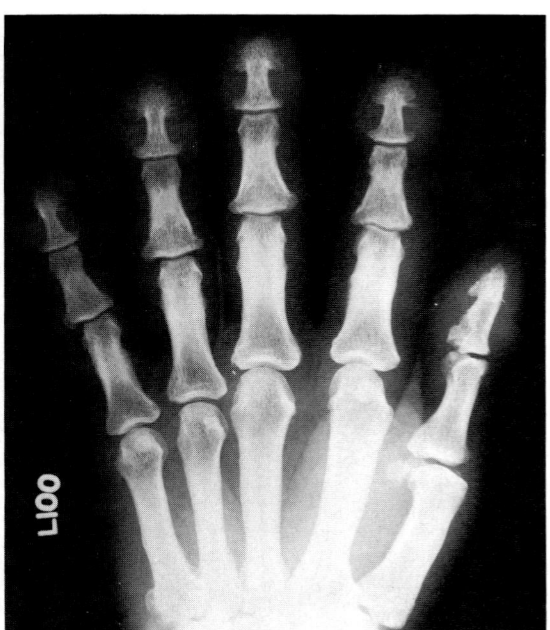

Figure 16–39. Pachydermoperiostosis. PA radiograph of the hand of the patient shown in Figure 16–38 shows clubbing of fingertips with associated hypertrophy of the distal phalangeal tufts (note also the widened tubular bones, particularly the middle phalangeal bases).

involved.[6] Clubbing is apparent radiographically (Fig. 16–39). Sclerosis and expansion of the diaphyseal region of tubular bones results from periosteal thickening. These changes are widespread and symmetric. In long-standing cases, ankylosis of joints—especially hands and feet—may occur.[6] Acro-osteolysis has also been reported with pachydermoperiostosis.[226,228]

The major consideration in the differential diagnosis is secondary hypertrophic osteoarthropathy (pulmonary or otherwise). The radiologic features are, however, somewhat different for primary and secondary disease. In pachydermoperiostosis, periosteal proliferation is more extreme, has an irregular appearance, and often extends to the epiphysis (Fig. 16–40*A*). In hypertrophic pul-

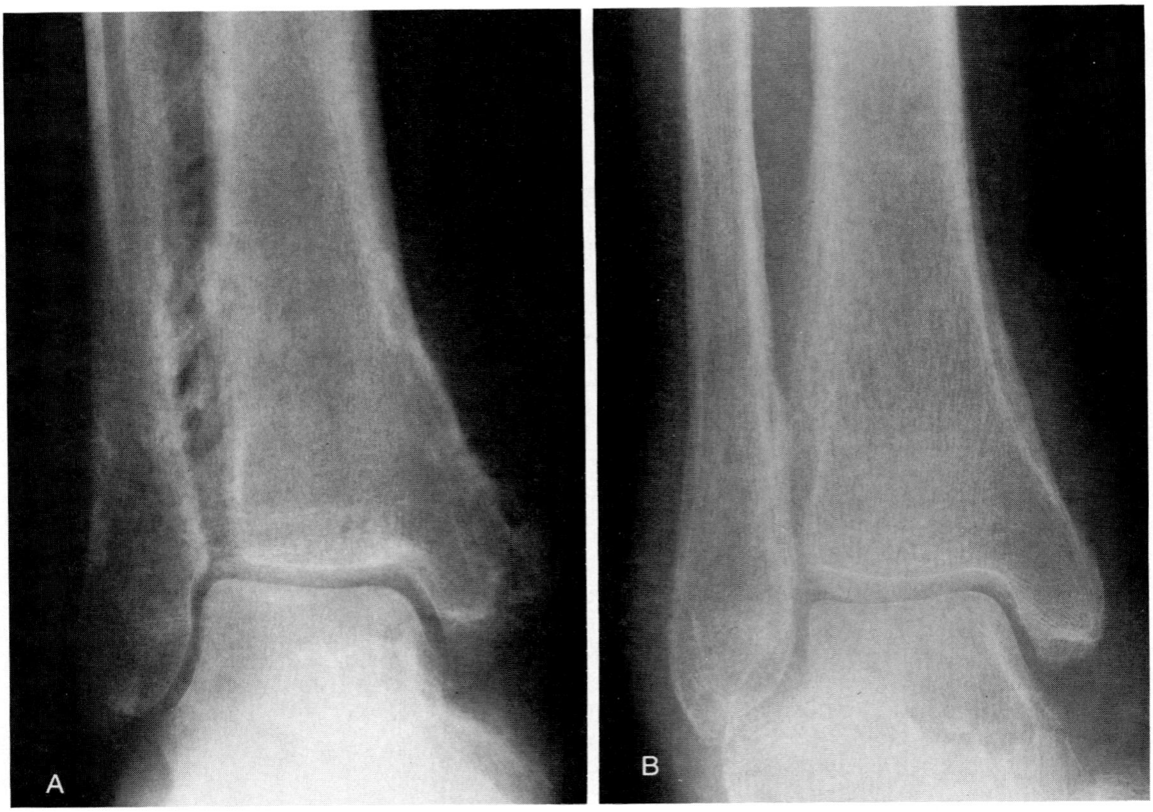

Figure 16–40. *A*, Pachydermoperiostosis. AP radiograph of the distal leg and ankle of the patient in Figure 16–38 shows extensive shaggy periosteal reaction along the interosseous membrane between the tibia and fibula (note also the extensive proliferative bone formation along the medial malleolus). *B*, Hypertrophic pulmonary osteoarthropathy. AP radiograph of distal leg and ankle of a 30-year-old woman shows smooth, layered periosteal new bone formation along the medial aspect of the distal tibia (note that the medial malleolus [epiphysis] is not involved).

monary osteoarthropathy, the periosteal reaction has a smoother, undulating appearance (Fig. 16–40*B*).[229] Skeletal scintigraphy in both conditions reveals regular and symmetrical diffuse uptake along the cortical margins of long bones, especially in the legs, which produces a "double stripe" sign.[230]

D. Histopathologic Findings

Periosteal deposition of bone in pachydermoperiostosis results in a roughened cortical surface.[231] The new bone undergoes cancellous compaction and may be difficult to distinguish from original cortex.[231] Synovial membrane shows mild cellular hyperplasia and thickening of subsynovial blood vessels.[232] Electron microscopy shows a layered basement membrane.

E. Etiology and Pathogenesis

The genetic defect of pachydermoperiostosis is unknown. Blood flow is decreased to involved areas of bone in pachydermoperiostitis, but is increased in cases of secondary clubbing.[222,233,234] The arthralgias appear to stem from the associated periostitis.

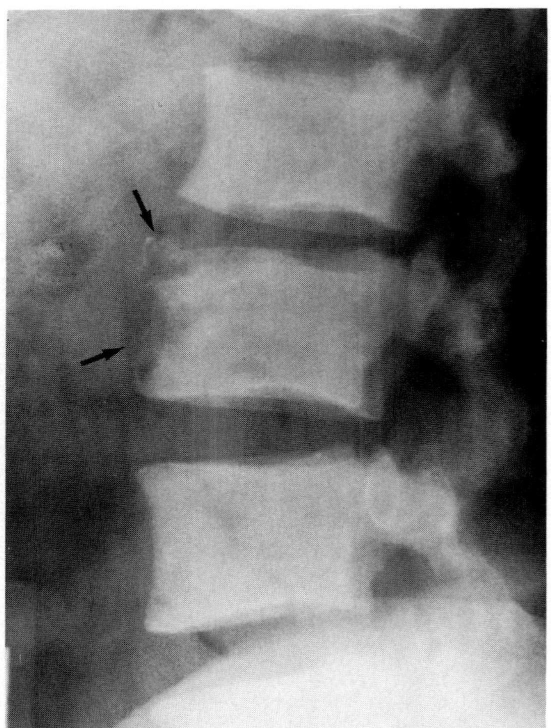

Figure 16–41. Disseminated prostatic carcinoma. Lateral radiograph of the lumbar spine of a 47-year-old man with widespread prostatic carcinoma shows characteristic radiodense vertebrae. Except for the margins of L3 (arrows), the osteosclerosis is quite uniform.

XVII. OTHER DISORDERS

As summarized in Tables 16–1 and 16–2, in addition to the primarily dysplastic osteosclerotic disorders discussed herein, a relatively large number of other conditions result in either focal or generalized increases in skeletal mass. Although limitation of space does not permit a detailed discussion of these entities here (the reader will find references 1 to 9 to be especially helpful sources of information), some generalities should be noted.

Sarcoidosis of the skeleton is typically associated with cystic and coarsely reticulated bone. Rarely, however, sclerotic lesions involve the axial skeleton or long tubular bones. These changes may occur well after the pulmonary disease is arrested.[235] Although multiple myeloma typically presents with generalized osteopenia or with osteolytic changes, widespread osteosclerosis can occur.[236,237] Lymphoma, myelosclerosis, and mastocytosis are additional hematologic causes of increased bone mass. Metastatic carcinoma—primarily prostate (Fig. 16–41)—commonly causes osteosclerosis. Osteosclerosis is a typical radiologic feature of Paget's bone disease.[238] Diffuse osteosclerosis is also a relatively frequent radiologic finding in secondary hyperparathyroidism (as with renal disease), but can occur in primary hyperparathyroidism as well.[239] Intoxication with either vitamin A[240] or D,[241] heavy metal poisoning,[242] milk-alkali syndrome,[243] ionizing radiation,[2,6] osteomyelitis,[244] and osteonecrosis[2,6] are additional etiologic factors.

Acknowledgments: This work was made possible by grant 15958 from the Shriners Hospitals for Crippled Children and grant RR-00036 from the General Clinical Research Center Branch, Division of Research Facilities and Resources, National Institutes of Health.

References

1. McKusick VA: Mendelian Inheritance in Man. 8th ed. Baltimore, The Johns Hopkins University Press, 1988.

2. Frame B, Honasoge M, Kottamasu SR: Osteosclerosis, Hyperostosis, and Related Disorders. New York, Elsevier, 1987.
3. Wynne-Davies R, Hall CM, Apley AG: Atlas of Skeletal Dysplasias, Edinburgh, Churchill Livingstone, 1985.
4. Taybi H: Radiology of Syndromes and Metabolic Disorders. 2nd ed. Chicago, Year Book Medical Publishers, 1983.
5. Papadatos CJ, Bartsocas CS: Skeletal Dysplasias. New York, Alan R. Liss, 1982.
6. Resnick D, Niwayama G: Diagnosis of Bone and Joint Disorders. 2nd ed. Philadelphia, WB Saunders, 1988.
7. Beighton P, Cremin BJ: Sclerosing Bone Dysplasias. Berlin, Springer-Verlag, 1980.
8. Maroteaux P: Bone Diseases in Children. Philadelphia, JB Lippincott, 1979.
9. Jacobson HG: Dense bone—too much bone: Radiological considerations and differential diagnosis (parts I and II). Skeletal Radiol 13:1–20, 97–113, 1985.
10. Albers-Schönberg H. Rontgenbilder einer seltenen, Knochenerkrankung. Muench Med Wochenschr 51:365, 1904.
11. Johnston CC Jr, Lavy N, Lord T, et al: Osteopetrosis: a clinical, genetic, metabolic, and morphologic study of the dominantly inherited, benign form. Medicine 47:149–167, 1968.
12. Loria-Cortes R, Quesada-Calvo E, Cordero-Chaverri E: Osteopetrosis in children: A report of 26 cases. J Pediatr 91:43–47, 1977.
13. Kahler SG, Burns JA, Aylsworth AS: A mild autosomal recessive form of osteopetrosis. Am J Med Genet 17:451–464, 1984.
14. Horton WA, Schimek RN, Iyama T: Osteopetrosis: Further heterogeneity. J Pediatr 97:580–585, 1980.
15. Jagadha V, Halliday WC, Becker LE, Hinton D: The association in infantile osteopetrosis and neuronal storage disease in two brothers. Acta Neuropathol 75:233–240, 1988.
16. Dowd PM, Munro DD: Ichthyosis and osteopetrosis. J R Soc Med 76:423–426, 1983.
17. Cote GB, Katsantoni A: Osteosclerosis and ectodermal dysplasia. Prog Clin Biol Res 104:161–162, 1982.
18. Nishiyama S, Hashimoto S: Osteosclerosis in Netherton's disease. Nippon Isaku Hoshasen Gakki Zasshi 37:437–443, 1977.
19. Johnson F, Flores C, Dodgson WB: Central osteosclerosis in an infant with bamboo hair (Netherton syndrome). Skeletal Radiol 2:185–186, 1978.
20. Blau EB: Ectodermal dysplasia, osteosclerosis, atrial septal defect, malabsorption, neutropenia, growth, and mental retardation: The Côte-Katsantoni syndrome? Am J Med Genet 26:729–732, 1987.
21. Civitelli R, McAlister WH, Teitelbaum SL, et al: Central osteosclerosis with ectodermal dysplasia. J Bone Min Res 4:863–875, 1989.
22. Brown DM, Dent PB: Pathogenesis of osteopetrosis: A comparison of human and animal spectra. Pediatr Res 5:181–191, 1971.
23. Marks SC Jr: Congenital osteopetrotic mutations as probes of origin, structure, and function of osteoclasts. Clin Orthop 189:239–263, 1984.
24. Marks SC Jr: Osteopetrosis—multiple pathways for the interception of osteoclast function. Appl Pathol 5:172–183, 1987.
25. Lehman RAW, Reeves JD, Wilson WB, et al: Neurological complications of infantile osteopetrosis. Ann Neurol 2:378–384, 1977.
26. Al-Mefty O, Fox JL, Al-Rodhan N, et al: Optic nerve decompression in osteopetrosis. J Neurosurg 68:80–84, 1988.
27. Rakic M, Elhosseiny A, Ramadan F, et al: Adult-type osteopetrosis presenting as carpal-tunnel syndrome. Arthritis Rheum 29:926–928, 1986.
28. Bollerslev J, Andersen PE Jr: Radiological, biochemical, and hereditary evidence of two types of autosomal dominant osteopetrosis. Bone 9:7–13, 1988.
29. Bollerslev J: Autosomal dominant osteopetrosis: Bone metabolism and epidemiologic, clinical, and hormonal aspects. Endocrine Rev 10:45–67, 1989.
30. Key LL, Carnes D, Holtrop M, et al: Treatment of congenital osteopetrosis with high dose calcitriol. N Engl J Med 310:409–415, 1984.
31. Reeves J, Arnaud S, Gordon S, et al: The pathogenesis of infantile malignant osteopetrosis: Bone mineral metabolism and complications in five infants. Metab Bone Dis Relat Res 3:135–142, 1981.
32. Reeves JD, August CS, Humbert JR, et al: Host defense in infantile osteopetrosis. Pediatrics 64:202–206, 1979.
33. Beard CJ, Key L, Newburger PE, et al: Neutrophil defect associated with malignant infantile osteopetrosis. J Lab Clin Med 108:498–505, 1986.
34. Oliveira G, Boechat MI, Amaral SM, et al: Osteopetrosis and rickets: An intriguing association. Am J Dis Child 140:377–378, 1986.
35. Park H-M, Lambertus J: Skeletal and reticuloendothelial imaging in osteopetrosis: Case report. J Nucl Med 18:1091–1095, 1977.
36. Rao VM, Dalinka MK, Mitchell DG, et al: Osteopetrosis: MR characteristics at 1.5T'. Radiology 161:217–220, 1986.
37. Shapiro R, Glimcher MJ, Holtrop ME, et al: Human osteopetrosis. J Bone Joint Surg 62A:384–399, 1980.
38. Revell PA: Pathology of Bone. Berlin, Springer-Verlag, 1986.
39. Silvestrini G, Ferraccioli GF, Quaini F, et al: Adult osteopetrosis: Study of two brothers. Appl Pathol 5:184–189, 1987.
40. Teitelbaum SL, Coccia PF, Brown DM, Kahn AJ: Malignant osteopetrosis: A disease of abnormal osteoclast proliferation. Metab Bone Dis Relat Res 3:99–105, 1981.
41. Glorieux FH, Pettifor JM, Marie PJ, et al: Induction of bone resorption by parathyroid hormone in congenital malignant osteopetrosis. Metab Bone Dis Rel Res 3:143–150, 1981.
42. Key LL, Ries WL, Schiff R: Osteopetrosis associated with interleukin-2 deficiency. J Bone Mineral Res 2[Suppl II]:85, 1987.
43. Mills BG, Yabe H, Singer FR: Osteoclasts in human osteopetrosis contain viral-nucleocapsid-like nuclear inclusions. J Bone Mineral Res 3:101–106, 1988.
44. Fischer A, Griscelli C, Friedrich W, et al: Bone-marrow transplantation for immunodeficiencies and osteopetrosis: European survey, 1968–1985. Lancet 2:1080–1084, 1986.
45. Sieff CA, Chessells JM, Levinsky RJ, et al: Allogeneic bone-marrow transplantation in infantile malignant osteopetrosis. Lancet 1:437–441, 1983.
46. Sorell M, Kapoor N, Kirkpatrick D, et al: Marrow transplantation for juvenile osteopetrosis. Am J Med 70:1280–1287, 1981.
47. Coccia PF, Krivit W, Cervenka J, et al: Successful bone-marrow transplantation for infantile malignant osteopetrosis. N Engl J Med 302:701–708, 1980.

48. Kaplan FS, August CS, Fallon MD, et al: Successful treatment of infantile malignant osteopetrosis by bone-marrow transplantation. A case report. J Bone Joint Surg [Am] 70:617–623, 1988.
49. Orchard PJ, Dickerman JD, Mathews CHE, et al: Haploidentical bone marrow transplantation for osteopetrosis. Am J Pediatr Hematol Oncol 9:335–340, 1987.
50. Key LL Jr: Osteopetrosis: A genetic window into osteoclast function. *In* Cases in Metabolic Bone Disease, vol 2, no 3. New York, Triclinica Communications, 1987.
51. Delmas PD, Chapuy MC, Viala JJ, et al: Improvement of adult congenital osteopetrosis with high doses of calcitriol (abstract 93). J Bone Mineral Res 2[Suppl 1], 1987.
52. Dent CE, Smellie JM, Watson L: Studies in osteopetrosis. Arch Dis Child 40:7–15, 1965.
53. Ozsoyla S: High dose intravenous methylprednisolone in treatment of recessive osteopetrosis (letter). Arch Dis Child 62:214–215, 1987.
54. Reeves JD, Hoffer WE, August CS, et al: The hematopoietic effects of prednisone therapy in four infants with osteopetrosis. J Pediatr 94:210–211, 1979.
55. Dorantes LM, Mejia AM, Dorantes S: Juvenile osteopetrosis: Effects on blood and bone of prednisone and low calcium, high phosphate diet. Arch Dis Child 61:666–670, 1986.
56. Osborn R, Boland T, DeLuchi S, et al: Osteomyelitis of the mandible in a patient with malignant osteopetrosis. J Oral Med 40:76–80, 1985.
57. Golbus MS, Loerper MA, Hall BD: Failure to diagnose osteopetrosis in utero (letter). Lancet 2:1246, 1976.
58. Sly WS, Lang R, Avioli L, et al: Recessive osteopetrosis: New clinical phenotype (abstract). Am J Hum Genet 24:34, 1972.
59. Guibaud P, Larbre F, Freycon MT, et al: Osteopetrose et acidose renale tubulaire deux cas de association dans une fratrie. Arch Fr Pediatr 29:269–286, 1972.
60. Vainsel M, Fondu P, Cadranel S, et al: Osteopetrosis associated with proximal and distal tubular acidosis. Acta Paediatr Scand 61:429–434, 1972.
61. Whyte MP, Murphy WA, Fallon MD, et al: Osteopetrosis, renal tubular acidosis and basal ganglia calcification in three sisters. Am J Med 69:64–74, 1980.
62. Ohlsson A, Stark G, Sakati N: Marble brain disease: Recessive osteopetrosis, renal tubular acidosis and cerebral calcification in three Saudi Arabian families. Dev Med Child Neurol 22:72–84, 1980.
63. Sly WS, Hewett-Emmett D, Whyte MP, et al: Carbonic anhydrase II deficiency identified as the primary defect in the autosomal recessive syndrome of osteopetrosis with renal tubular acidosis and cerebral calcification. Proc Natl Acad Sci USA 80:2752–2756, 1983.
64. Sly WS, Whyte MP, Sundaram V, et al: Carbonic anhydrase II deficiency in 12 families with the autosomal recessive syndrome of osteopetrosis with renal tubular acidosis and cerebral calcification. N Engl J Med 313:139–145, 1985.
65. Cochat P, Loras-Duclaux I, Guibaud P: Deficit en anhydrase carbonique II: Osteopetrose, acidose renale tubulaire et calcifications intracraniennes. Revue de la literature a partir des trois observations. Pediatrie 42:121–128, 1987.
66. Ohlsson A, Cumming WA, Paul A, et al: Carbonic anhydrase II deficiency syndrome: Recessive osteopetrosis with renal tubular acidosis and cerebral calcification. Pediatrics 77:371–381, 1986.
67. Sly WS, Whyte MP, Krupin T, et al: Positive renal response to acetazolamide in carbonic anhydrase II–deficient patients. Pediatr Res 19:1033–1036, 1985.
68. Bourke E, Delaney VB, Mosawi M, et al: Renal tubular acidosis and osteopetrosis in siblings. Nephron 28:268–272, 1981.
69. Cumming WA, Ohlsson A: Intracranial calcification in children with osteopetrosis caused by carbonic anhydrase II deficiency. Radiology 157:325–327, 1985.
70. Tashian RE, Hewett-Emmett D, Goodman M: On the evolution and genetics of carbonic anhydrase I, II, and III. *In* Rattazzi ME, Scandalios JG, Whitt GS, (eds): Isoenzymes: Current Topics In Biological and Medical Research, vol 7. New York, Alan R. Liss, 1983, pp 79–100.
71. Tashian RE: Evolution and regulation of the carbonic anhydrase enzymes. *In* Rattazzi ME, Scandalios JG, Whitt GS (eds): Isoenzymes: Current Topics in Biological and Medical Research, vol 2. New York, Alan R. Liss, 1977, pp 21–62.
72. Sanyal G, Swenson ER, Pessah NI, et al: The carbon dioxide hydration activity of skeletal muscle carbonic anhydrase: Inhibition by sulfonamides and anions. Mol Pharmacol 22:211–220, 1982.
73. Raisz LG, Simmons HA, Thompson WJ, et al: Effects of a potent carbonic anhydrase inhibitor in bone resorption in organ culture. Endocrinology 122:1083–1086, 1988.
74. Sundquist KT, Leppilampi M, Järvelin K, et al: Carbonic anhydrase isoenzymes in isolated rat peripheral monocytes, tissue macrophages, and osteoclasts. Bone 8:33–38, 1987.
75. Lewis SE, Erickson RP, Barnett LB, et al: N-ethyl-N-nitrosourea–induced null mutation at the mouse Car-2 locus: An animal model for human carbonic anhydrase II deficiency syndrome. Proc Natl Acad Sci USA 85:1962–1966, 1988.
76. Lee BL, Venta PJ, Tashian RE: DNA polymorphism in the 5-prime flanking region of the human carbonic anhydrase II gene on chromosome 8. Hum Genet 69:337–339, 1985.
77. Whyte MP, Hamm LL III, Sly WS: Transfusion of carbonic anhydrase–replete erythrocytes fails to correct the acidification defect in the syndrome of osteopetrosis, renal tubular acidosis, and cerebral calcification (carbonic anhydrase II deficiency). J Bone Mineral Res 3:385–388, 1988.
78. Whyte MP, McAlister WH, Kim GS, et al: Congenital sclerosing osteomalacia with cerebral calcification: A new, recessively-inherited, syndrome which radiographically mimics carbonic anhydrase II deficiency (abstract). Am J Hum Genet 37:A–82, 1985.
79. Maroteaux P, Lamy M: La pycnodysostose. Presse Med 70:999, 1962.
80. Andrén L, Dymling J-F, Hogeman KE, et al: Osteopetrosis, acro-osteolytica: A syndrome of osteopetrosis, acro-osteolysis and open sutures of the skull. Acta Chir Scand 124:496–507, 1962.
81. Maroteaux P, Lamy M: The malady of Toulouse-Lautrec. JAMA 191:715–717, 1965.
82. Elmore SM: Pycnodysostosis: A review. J Bone Joint Surg 49A:153–162, 1967.
83. Meneses de Almeida L: Contribution a l'etude genitique de la pycnodysostose. Ann Genet 15:99–101, 1972.

84. Meneses de Almeida L: A genetic study of pycnodysostosis. *In* Papadatos CJ, Bartsocas CS (eds): Skeletal Dysplasias. New York, Alan R. Liss, 1982, pp 195–198.
85. Sugiura Y, Yamada Y, Koh J: Pycnodysostosis in Japan: Report of six cases and a review of Japanese literature. Birth Defects Orig Art Ser X:78–98, 1974.
86. Santhanakrishnan BR, Panneerselvam S, Ramesh S, et al: Pycnodysostosis with visceral manifestation and rickets. Clin Pediatr (Phila) 25:416–418, 1986.
87. Maroteaux P, Faure C: Pycnodysostosis. Prog Pediatr Radiol 4:403, 1973.
88. Roth VG: Pyknodysostosis presenting with bilateral subtrochanteric fracture: Case report. Clin Orthop Rel Res 117:247–253, 1976.
89. Wolpowitz A, Matisson A: A comparative study of pycnodysostosis, cleidocranial dysostosis, osteopetrosis and acro-osteolysis. S Afr Med J 48:1011, 1974.
90. Soto TJ, Mautalen CA, Hojman D, et al: Pycnodysostosis, metabolic and histologic studies. Birth Defects: Orig Art Ser V:109–115, 1969.
91. Bressot C, Meunier PJ, Bard J, et al: La pycnodysostose. Analyse histomorphometrique et dynamique de l'os dans une nouvelle observation. Rev Rhum 47:425–430, 1980.
92. Everts V, Aronson DC, Beertsen W: Phagocytosis of bone collagen by osteoclasts in two cases of pycnodysostosis. Calcif Tissue Int 37:25–31, 1985.
93. Stanescu R, Stanescu V, Maroteaux P: Ultrastructural abnormalities in chondrocytes in pycnodysostosis. Nouveautes Medicales 437:247, 1975.
94. Lacey SH, Eyring EJ, Shaffer TE: Pycnodysostosis: A case report of a child with associated trisomy X. J Pediatr 77:1033, 1970.
95. Cabrejas ML, Fromm GA, Roca JF: Pycnodysostosis. Some aspects concerning kinetics of calcium metabolism and bone pathology. Am J Med Sci 271/2:215, 1976.
96. Beneton MNC, Harris S, Kanis JA: Paramyxovirus-like inclusions in two cases of pycnodysostosis. Bone 8:211–217, 1987.
97. Meredith SC, Simon MA, Laros GS, et al: Pycnodysostosis: A clinical, pathological, and ultramicroscopic study of a case. J Bone Joint Surg 60A:1122–1128, 1978.
98. Van Merkesteyn JPR, Bras J, Vermeeren JIJF, Van Der Saar A, Van Eps LWS: Osteomyelitis of the jaws in pycnodysostosis. Int J Oral Maxillofac Surg 16:615–619, 1987.
99. Simon D, Cazalis P, Dryll A, et al: Une osteosclerose axiale de transmission dominante autosomique nouvelle entite? Rev Rhum 46:375–382, 1979.
100. Maroteaux P: L'osteomesopycnose. Une nouvelle affection condensante de transmission dominante autosomique. Arch Franc Pediatr 37:153–157, 1980.
101. Stoll CG, Collin D, Dreyfus J: Brief clinical report. Osteomesopyknosis An autosomal dominant osterosclerosis. Am J Med Genet 8:349–353, 1981.
102. Maroteaux P, Stanescu V, Stanescu R: Four recently described osteochondrodysplasias. *In* Papadatos CJ, Bartsocas CS (eds): Skeletal Dysplasias. New York, Alan R. Liss, 1982, pp 345–350.
103. Proschel R, Labelle H, Bard C, et al: Osteomesopyknosis. J Bone Joint Surg 67A:652–653, 1985.
104. Cockayne EA: A case for diagnosis. Proc R Soc Med 13:132–136, 1920.
105. Camurati M: Di un rar caso di osteite simmettrica ereditaria delgi arti inferiori. Chir Organi Mov 6:662, 1922.
106. Engelmann G: Ein Fall von Osteopathia hyperostotica (sclerotisans) multiplex infantilis. Footscho Geb Roentgen 39:1101–1106, 1929.
107. Fallon MD, Whyte MP, Murphy WA: Progressive diaphyseal dysplasia (Engelmann's Disease). Report of a sporadic case of the mild form. J Bone Joint Surg 62–A:465–472, 1980.
108. Hundley JD, Wilson FC: Progressive diaphyseal dysplasia. Review of the literature and report of seven cases in one family. J Bone Joint Surg 55A:461–474, 1973.
109. Sparkes RS, Graham CB: Camurati-Engelmann disease. Genetics and clinical manifestations with a review of the literature. J Med Genet 9:73–85, 1972.
110. Ribbing S: Hereditary, multiple, diaphyseal sclerosis. Acta Radiol 31:522–536, 1949.
111. Naveh Y, Ludatshcer R, Alon U, et al: Muscle involvement in progressive diaphyseal dysplasia. Pediatrics 76:944–949, 1985.
112. Yoshioka H, Mino M, Kiyosawa N, et al: Muscular changes in Engelmann's disease. Arch Dis Child 55:716–719, 1980.
113. Crisp AJ, Brenton DP: Engelmann's disease of bone—a systemic disorder? Ann Rheum Dis 41:183–188, 1982.
114. Smith R, Walton RJ, Corner BD, et al: Clinical and biochemical studies in Engelmann's disease (progressive diaphyseal dysplasia). Q J Med 46:273–294, 1977.
115. Kaftori JK, Kleinhaus U, Neveh Y: Progressive diaphyseal dysplasia (Camurati-Engelmann): Radiographic follow-up and CT findings. Radiology 164:777–782, 1987.
116. Kumar B, Murphy WA, Whyte MP: Progressive diaphyseal dysplasia (Engelmann's disease): Scintigraphic-radiologic-clinical correlations. Radiology 140:87–92, 1981.
117. Shier CK, Krasicky GA, Ellis BI, Kottamasu SR: Ribbing's disease: Radiographic-scintigraphic correlation and comparative analysis with Engelmann's disease. J Nucl Med 28:244–248, 1987.
118. Green JR, Reeve J, Tellez M, et al: Skeletal blood flow in metabolic disorders of the skeleton. Bone 8:293–297, 1987.
119. Royer P, Vermeil G, Apostolides P, et al: Maladie d'Engelmann resultat du traitement par la prednisone. Arch Frac Pediatr 24:693–702, 1967.
120. Minford AMB, Hardy GJ, Forsythe WI, et al: Englemann's disease and the effect of corticosteroids: A case report. J Bone Joint Surg 63B:597–600, 1981.
121. Lindstrom JA: Diaphyseal dysplasia (Engelmann) treated with corticosteroids. Birth Defects Orig Art Ser X:504–507, 1974.
122. Naveh Y, Alon U, Kaftori JK, et al: Progressive diaphyseal dysplasia: Evaluation of corticosteroid therapy. Pediatrics 75:321–323, 1985.
123. Allen DT, Saunders AM, Northway WH Jr, et al: Corticosteroids in the treatment of Engelmann's disease: Progressive diaphyseal dysplasia. Pediatrics 46:523–531, 1970.
124. Guan DW, Moinuddin M, Pitcock J, et al: Intermittent diphosphonate in Engelmann's disease; a 5 year follow-up (abstract). J Bone Min Res 1:117, 1986.
125. Van Buchem FSP, Hadders HN, Ubbens R: An uncommon familial systemic disease of the skeleton. Hyperostosis corticalis generalisata familiaris. Acta Radiol 44:109–116, 1955.

126. Van Buchem FSP, Hadders HN, Hansen JF, et al: Hyperostosis corticalis generalisata: Report of seven cases. Am J Med 33:387–397, 1962.
127. Van Buchem FSP, Prick JJG, Jaspar HHJ: Hyperostosis Corticalis Generalisata Familiaris (Van Buchem's Disease). Amsterdam, Excerpta Medica, 1976.
128. Perez-Vicente JR Jr, Rodriquez de Castro E, Lafuente J, et al: Autosomal dominant endosteal hyperostosis. Report of a Spanish family with neurological involvement. Clin Genet 31:161–169, 1987.
129. Nakamura T, Yamada N, Nonaka R, et al: Autosomal dominant form of endosteal hyperostosis with unusual manifestations of sclerosis of the jaw bones. Skeletal Radiol 16:48–51, 1987.
130. Eastman JR, Bixler D: Generalized cortical hyperostosis (Van Buchem disease): Nosologic considerations. Radiology 125:297–304, 1977.
131. Fryns JP, Van den Berghe H: Facial paralysis at the age of 2 months as the first clinical sign of van Buchem disease (endosteal hyperostosis). Eur J Pediatr 147:99–100, 1988.
132. Beighton P, Barnard A, Hamersma H, et al: The syndromic status of sclerosteosis and van Buchem disease. Clin Genet 25:175–181, 1984.
133. Ruckert EW, Caudill RJ, McCready PJ: Surgical treatment of van Buchem disease. J Oral Maxillofac Surg 43:801–805, 1985.
134. Freire de Paes Alves A, Rubim JLC, Cardoso L, et al: Sclerosteosis a marker of Dutch ancestry? Rev Brasil Genet 4:825–834, 1982.
135. Truswell AS: Osteopetrosis with syndactyly. A morphologic variant of Albers-Schonberg's disease. J Bone Joint Surg 40B:208–218, 1958.
136. Hansen HG: Sklerosteose. *In* Opitz H, Schmid F (eds): Handbuch der Kinderheilkunde, vol 6. Berlin, Springer, 1967, pp 351–355.
137. Beighton P, Durr L, Hamersma H: The clinical features of sclerosteosis: A review of the manifestations in twenty-five affected individuals. Ann Intern Med 84:393–397, 1976.
138. Barnard AH, Hamersma H, Kretzmar JH, et al: Sclerosteosis in old age. S Afr Med J 58:401–403, 1980.
139. Stein SA, Witkop C, Hill S, et al: Sclerosteosis: Neurogenetic and pathophysiologic analysis of an American kinship. Neurology 33:267–277, 1983.
140. Beighton P, Cremin BJ, Hamersma H: The radiology of sclerosteosis. Br J Radiol 49:934–939, 1976.
141. Hill SC, Stein SA, Dwyer A, et al: Cranial CT findings in sclerosteosis. AJNR 7:505–511, 1986.
142. Epstein S, Hamersma H, Beighton P: Endocrine function in sclerosteosis. S Afr Med J 55:1105–1110, 1979.
143. Berlin R, Hedensio B, Lilja B, et al: Osteopoikilosis—a clinical and genetic study. Acta Med Scand 18:305–314, 1967.
144. Uitto J, Starcher BC, Santa-Cruz DJ, et al: Biochemical and ultrastructural demonstration of elastin accumulation in the skin of the Buschke-Ollendorff syndrome. J Invest Derm 76:284–287, 1981.
145. Whyte MP, Murphy WA, Seigel BA: 99m Tc-pyrophosphate bone imaging in osteopoikilosis, osteopathia striata, and melorheostosis. Radiology 127:439–443, 1978.
146. Verbor J, Graham R: Buschke-Ollendorf syndrome—disseminated dermatofibrosis with osteopoikilosis. Clin Expt Dermatol 11:17–26, 1986.
147. Ghandur-Mnaymnch L, Broder LE, Mnaymneh WA: Lobular carcinoma of the breast metastatic to bone with unusual clinical, radiologic, and pathologic features mimicking osteopoikilosis. Cancer 53:1801–1803, 1984.
148. Lagier R, Mbakop A, Bigler A: Osteopoikilosis: A radiological and pathological study. Skeletal Radiol 11:161–168, 1984.
149. Bass HN, Weiner JR, Goldman A, et al: Osteopathia striata syndrome: Clinical, genetic, and radiologic considerations. Clin Pediatr 19:369–373, 1980.
150. Rabinow M, Unger F: Syndrome of osteopathia striata, macrocephaly, and cranial sclerosis. Am J Dis Child 138:821–823, 1984.
151. Horan FT, Beighton PH: Osteopathia striata with cranial sclerosis: An autosomal dominant entity. Clin Genet 13:201–206, 1978.
152. Jones MD, Mulcahy ND: Osteopathia striata, osteopetrosis, and impaired hearing. A case report. Arch Otolaryngol 87:116–118, 1968.
153. Paling MR, Hyde I, Dennis NR: Osteopathia striata with sclerosis and thickening of the skull. Br J Radiol 54:344–348, 1981.
154. Happle R, Lenz W: Striation of bones in focal dermal hypoplasia: Manifestation of functional mosaicism? Br J Dermatol 96:133–138, 1977.
155. Knockaert D, Dequeker J: Osteopathia striata and focal dermal hypoplasia. Skeletal Radiol 4:223–227, 1979.
156. Whyte MP, Murphy WA: Osteopathia striata associated with familial dermopathy and white forelock: Evidence for postnatal development of osteopathia striata. Am J Med Genet 5:227–234, 1980.
157. Kornreich L, Grunebaum M, Ziv N, et al: Osteopathia striata, cranial sclerosis with cleft palate and facial nerve palsy. Eur J Pediatr 147:101–103, 1988.
158. Winter RM, Crawford MD, Meire HB, et al: Osteopathia striata with cranial sclerosis: Highly variable expression within a family including a cleft palate in two neonatal cases. Clin Genet 18:462–474, 1980.
159. Leŕi A, Joanny J: Une affection non decrite des os. Hyperostose "en coulée" sur toute la longueur d'un membre ou "melorheostose." Bul Mem Soc Hop Paris 46:1141–1145, 1922.
160. Murray RO, McCredie J: Melorheostosis and sclerotomes: A radiological correlation. Skeletal Radiol 4:57–71, 1979.
161. Morris JM, Samilson RL, Corley CL: Melorheostosis: Review of the literature and report of an interesting case with a nineteen-year follow-up. J Bone Joint Surg 45A:1191–1206, 1963.
162. Campbell CJ, Papademetriou T, Bonfiglio M: Melorheostosis: A report of the clinical, roentgenographic, and pathological findings in fourteen cases. J Bone Joint Surg 50A:1281–1304, 1968.
163. Beauvais P, Faure C, Montagne JP, et al: Leri's melorheostosis: Three pediatric cases and a review of the literature. Pediatr Radiol 6:152–159, 1977.
164. Soffa DJ, Sire DJ, Dodson JH: Melorheostosis with linear sclerodermatous skin changes. Radiology 114:577–578, 1975.
165. Miyachi Y, Horio T, Yamada A, et al: Linear melorheostotic scleroderma with hypertrichosis. Arch Dermatol 115:1233–1234, 1979.
166. Applebaum RE, Caniano DA, Sun C-C, et al: Synchronous left subclavian and axillary artery

aneurysms associated with melorheostosis. Surgery 99:249–253, 1986.
167. Muller SA, Henderson ED: Melorheostosis with linear scleroderma. Arch Dermatol 88:142–145, 1963.
168. Younge D, Drummond D, Herring J, et al: Melorheostosis in children: Clinical features and natural history. J Bone Joint Surg 61B:415–418, 1979.
169. Colavita N, Nicolais S, Orazi C, Falappa PG: Melorheostosis: Presentation of a case followed up for 24 years. Arch Orthop Trauma Surg 106:123–125, 1987.
170. Janousek J, Preston DF, Martin NL, et al: Bone scan in melorheostosis. J Nucl Med 17:1106–1108, 1976.
171. Wagers LT, Young AW Jr, Ryan SF: Linear melorheostotic scleroderma. Br J Dermatol 86:297–301, 1972.
172. Semble EL, Poehling GG, Prough DS, et al: Successful symptomatic treatment of melorheostosis with nifedipine. Clin Exp Rheumatol 4:277–280, 1986.
173. Walker GF: Mixed sclerosing bone dystrophies. J Bone Joint Surg 46B:546–552, 1964.
174. Abrahamson MN: Disseminated asymptomatic osteosclerosis with features resembling osteopoikilosis and osteopathia striata. J Bone Joint Surg 50A:991–996, 1968.
175. Ewald FC: Unilateral mixed sclerosing bone dystrophy associated with unilateral lympangiectasis and capillary haemangioma. J Bone Joint Surg 54A:878–880, 1972.
176. Kanis JA, Thompson JG: Mixed sclerosing dystrophy with regression of melorheostosis. Br J Radiol 48:400–402, 1975.
177. Whyte MP, Murphy WA, Fallon MD, et al: Mixed-sclerosing-bone dystrophy: Report of a case and review of the literature. Skeletal Radiol 6:95–102, 1981.
178. Pacifici R, Murphy MA, Teitelbaum SL, et al: Mixed-sclerosing-bone-dystrophy: 42-year follow-up of a case reported as osteopetrosis. Calcif Tissue Int 38:175–185, 1986.
179. Connor JM, Beighton P: Fibrodysplasia ossificans progressiva in South Africa: Case reports. S Afr Med J 61:404–406, 1982.
180. Rogers JG, Geho WB: Fibrodysplasia ossificans progressiva: A survey of forty-two cases. J Bone Joint Surg 61A:909–914, 1979.
181. Connor JM, Evans DAP: Fibrodysplasia ossificans progressiva: The clinical features and natural history of 34 patients. J Bone Joint Surg 64B:76–83, 1982.
182. Hsu LCS, Hsu KY, Leong JCY: Severe scoliosis associated with fibrodysplasia ossificans progressiva. Spine 11:643–644, 1986.
183. Fox S, Khoury A, Mootabar H, Greenwald EF: Myositis ossificans progressiva and pregnancy. Obstet Gynecol 69:453–455, 1987.
184. Cremin B, Connor JM, Beighton P: The radiological spectrum of fibrodysplasia ossificans progressiva. Clin Radiol 33:499–508, 1982.
185. Thickman D, Bonakdar A, Clancy M, et al: Fibrodysplasia ossificans progressiva. AJR 139:935–941, 1982.
186. Voynow JA, Charney EB: Fibrodysplasia ossificans progressiva presenting as osteomyelitis-like syndrome. Clin Pediatr 25:373–375, 1986.
187. Fang MA, Reinig JW, Hill SC, et al: Technetium-99m MDP demonstration of heterotopic ossification in fibrodysplasia ossificans progressiva. Clin Nucl Med 11:8–9, 1986
188. Sumiyoshi K, Tsuneyoshi M, Enjoji M: Myositis ossificans: A clinicopathologic study of 21 cases. Acta Pathol Jpn 35:1109–1122, 1985.
189. Maxwell WA, Spicer SS, Miller RL, et al: Histochemical and ultrastructural studies in fibrodysplasia ossificans progressiva (myositis ossificans progressiva). Am J Path 87:483–498, 1977.
190. Reinig JW, Hill SC, Fang M, et al: Fibrodysplasia ossificans progressiva: CT appearance. Radiology 159:153–157, 1986.
191. Cramer SF, Ruehl A, Mandel MA: Fibrodysplasia ossificans progressiva. Cancer 48:1016–1021, 1981.
192. Rogers JG, Chase GA: Paternal age effect in fibrodysplasia ossificans progressiva. J Med Genet 16:147–148, 1979.
193. Lutwak L: Myositis ossificans progressiva: Mineral, metabolic, and radioactive calcium studies of the effects of hormones. Am J Med 37:269–293, 1964.
194. Smith R: Myositis ossificans progressiva: A review of current problems. Semin Arthritis Rheum 4:369–380, 1975.
195. Smith R, Russell RGG, Woods CG: Myositis ossificans progressiva: Clinical features of eight patients and their response to treatment. J Bone Joint Surg 58B:48–57, 1976.
196. Moore SE, Jump AA, Smiley JD: Effect of warfarin sodium therapy on excretion of 4-carboxy-L-glutamic acid in scleroderma, dermatomyositis, and myositis ossificans progressiva. Arthritis Rheum 29:344–351, 1986.
197. Frame B, Frost HM, Ormond RS, et al: Atypical axial osteomalacia involving the axial skeleton. Ann Intern Med 55:632–639, 1961.
198. Whyte MP, Fallon MD, Murphy WA, et al: Axial osteomalacia: Clinical, laboratory and genetic investigation of an affected mother and son. Am J Med 71:1041–1049, 1981.
199. Nelson AM, Riggs BL, Jowsey JO: Atypical axial osteomalacia: Report of four cases with two having features of ankylosing spondylitis. Arthritis Rheum 21:715–722, 1978.
200. Condon JR, Nassim JR: Axial osteomalacia. Postgrad Med J 47:817–820, 1971.
201. Arnstein AR, Frame B, Frost HM: Recent progress in rickets and osteomalacia. Ann Intern Med 67:1296–1330, 1967.
202. Christman D, Wenger JJ, Dosch JC, et al: L'osteomalacie axiale analyse comparee avec la fibrogenese imparfaite. J Radiol 62:37–41, 1981.
203. Baker SL, Turnbull HM: Two cases of hitherto undescribed disease characterized by a gross defect in the collagen of the bone matrix. J Pathol Bacteriol 62:132–134, 1950.
204. Baker SL, Dent CE, Friedman M, et al: Fibrogenesis imperfecta ossium. J Bone Joint Surg 48–B:804–825, 1966.
205. Thomas WC Jr, Moore T: Fibrogenesis imperfecta ossium. Trans Am Clin Climatol Assoc 80:54–62, 1968.
206. Golding FC: Fibrogenesis imperfecta. J Bone Joint Surg 50B:619–622, 1968.
207. Golde D, Greipp P, Sanzenbacher L, et al: Hematologic abnormalities in fibrogenesis imperfecta ossium. J Bone Joint Surg 53A:365, 1971.
208. Frame B, Frost HM, Pak CYC, et al: Fibrogenesis imperfecta ossium, a collagen defect causing osteomalacia. N Engl J Med 285:769–772, 1971.
209. Swan CHJ, Shah K, Brewer DB, et al: Fibrogenesis imperfecta ossium. Q J Med 45:233–253, 1976.

210. Stamp TCB, Byers PD, Ali SY, Jenkins MV, Willoughby JMT: Fibrogenesis imperfecta ossium: Remission with melphalan. Lancet 1:582–583, 1985.
211. Byers PD, Stamp TCB, Stoker DJ: Fibrogenesis imperfecta (case report 296). Skeletal Radiol 13:72–76, 1985.
212. Lang R, Vignery AM, Jensen PS: Fibrogenesis imperfecta ossium with early onset: Observations after 20 years of illness. Bone 7:237–246, 1986.
213. Stanley P, Baker SL, Byers PD: Unusual bone trabeculation in a patient with macroglobulinaemia simulating fibrogenesis imperfecta ossium. Br J Radiol 44:305–313, 1971.
214. Roholm K: Fluorine Intoxication. London, HK Lewis, 1937.
215. Jolly SS, Singh BM, Mathur OC: Endemic fluorosis in Punjab (India). Am J Med 47:553–563, 1969.
216. Vischer TL (ed): Fluoride in Medicine. Bern, Hans Huber, 1970.
217. Krishnamachari KAVR: Skeletal fluorosis in humans: A review of recent progress in the understanding of the disease. Prog Food Nutr Sci 10:279–314, 1986.
218. Schnitzler CM, Solomon L: Histomorphometric analysis of a calcaneal stress fracture: A possible complication of fluoride therapy for osteoporosis. Bone 7:193–198, 1986.
219. Srikantia SG, Siddiqu AH: Metabolic studies in skeletal fluorosis. Clin Sci 28:477–485, 1965.
220. Kanis JA, Meunier PJ: Should we use sodium fluoride to treat osteoporosis? A review. Q J Med 53:145–164, 1984.
221. Friedreich N: Hyperostose des gesammten Skelettes. Virchows Arch [Pathol Anat] 43:83–87, 1868.
222. Rimoin DL: Pachydermoperiostosis (idiopathic clubbing and periostosis). Genetic and physiologic consideration. N Engl J Med 272:923–931, 1965.
223. Herman MA, Massaro D, Katz S: Pachydermoperiostosis—clinical spectrum. Arch Intern Med 116:919–923, 1965.
224. Harbison JB, Nice CM Jr: Familial pachydermoperiostosis presenting as an acromegaly-like syndrome. Am J Roentgenol Radium Ther Nucl Med 112:532–536, 1971.
225. Appelboom T, Busscher H, Famaey JP: Chondrocalcinosis as a possible cause of arthritis in pachydermoperiostosis (letter). Arthritis Rheum 21:174, 1978.
226. Guyer PB, Brunton FJ, Wren MWG: Pachydermoperiostosis with acro-osteolysis: A report of five cases. J Bone Joint Surg 60B:219–223, 1978.
227. Neiman HL, Gompels BM, Martel W: Pachydermoperiostosis with bone marrow failure and gross extramedullary hematopoiesis. Report of a case. Radiology 110:553–554, 1974.
228. Hedayati H, Barmada R, and Skosey JL: Acrolysis in pachydermoperiostosis (primary or idiopathic hypertrophic osteoarthropathy). Arch Intern Med 140:1087–1088, 1980.
229. Ali A, Tetalman M, Fordham EW: Distribution of hypertrophic pulmonary osteoarthropathy. AJR 134:771–780, 1980.
230. DeVries N, Datz FL, Manaster BJ: Case report 399: Pachydermoperiostosis (primary hypertrophic osteoarthropathy). Skeletal Radiol 15:658–662, 1986.
231. Vogl A, Goldfischer S: Pachydermoperiostosis: Primary or idiopathic hypertrophic osteoarthropathy. Am J Med 33:166–187, 1962.
232. Lauter SA, Vasey FB, Hüttner I, et al: Pachydermoperiostosis: Studies on the synovium. J Rheumatol 5:85–95, 1978.
233. Fam AG, Chin-Sang H, Ramsay CA: Pachydermoperiostosis: Scintigraphic, thermographic, plethysmographic, and capillaroscopic observations. Ann Rheum Dis 42:98–102, 1983.
234. Kerber RE, Vogl A: Pachydermoperiostosis: Peripheral circulatory studies. Arch Intern Med 132:245–248, 1973.
235. Abdelwahab IF, Norman A: Osteosclerotic sarcoidosis. Am Roentgenol 150:161–162, 1988.
236. Shim MS, Mowry RW, Bodie FL: Osteosclerosis (punctate form) in multiple myeloma. South Med J 72:226–228, 1979.
237. Edelman RR, Kaufman H, Kolodny G: Case report 350. Skeletal Radiol 15:160–163, 1986.
238. Hamdy RC: Paget's Disease of Bone: Assessment and Management. East Sussex, UK, Praeger Publishers, 1981.
239. Van Holsbeeck M, Roex L, Favril A, et al: Osteosclerosis in primary hyperparathyroidism. Fortschr Röntgenstr 147:690–691, 1987.
240. Frame B, Jackson CE, Reynolds WA, Umphrey JE: Hypercalcemia and skeletal effects in chronic hypervitaminosis A. Ann Intern Med 80:44–48, 1974.
241. Dewind LT: Hypervitaminosis D with osteosclerosis. Arch Dis Child 36:373–380, 1961.
242. Murphy WA, Seligman PA, Tillack T, et al: Osteosclerosis, osteomalacia, and bone marrow aplasia: A combined late complication of thorotrast administration. Skeletal Radiol 3:234–238, 1979.
243. Punsar S, Somer T: The milk-alkali syndrome. A report of three illustrative cases and a review of the literature. Acta Med Scand 173:435–449, 1963.
244. Jacobsson S, Hollender L, Lindberg S, Lansson A: Chronic sclerosing osteomyelitis of the mandible. Scintigraphic and radiographic findings. Oral Surg. 45:167–174, 1978.

DAVID W. ROWE
JAY R. SHAPIRO

17

Osteogenesis Imperfecta

This chapter is being written at a time of significant progress in our understanding of the biochemical and genetic basis of osteogenesis imperfecta based on expanding knowledge of the biochemistry of type I collagen and the application of new techniques of molecular biology to define certain mutations at the gene level. The objectives of this chapter are to provide an overall view of this disease from a clinical perspective, to review specific aspects of connective tissue biology and biochemistry that apply to heritable disorders of bone, and to relate these with clinical examples to serve as a basis for understanding OI and related clinical syndromes. It is the intent of the authors to project the excitement that is currently present in this field. Thus, with OI as the prototype, we wish to provide a basis for the clinical application of basic research, and to suggest how these recent findings relate to other more common inherited or acquired disorders of the skeleton.

I. GENERAL CONSIDERATIONS

A. Historical Overview

The history of OI can be traced to Egyptian times as evidenced by a skeleton preserved at the British Museum.[1] The more modern history of the disease has been summarized by U.H. Weil[2] and is recorded in the comprehensive text on OI by Smith, Francis, and Houghton.[3] The first recorded case of OI is attributed to Malebranche,[4] who described a subject who appeared "like a man broken on a wheel." The first detailed clinical description of OI is to be found in a thesis for the degree of Doctor of Medicine presented by Olause Jacob Eckman,[5] Chief Surgeon to the Swedish Royal Cavalry Regiment, at the University of Uppsala. Describing a form of congenital osteomalacia, Eckman provided a comprehensive report of OI in three successive generations afflicted with fragilitas ossium and skeletal deformities. The association of fractures with joint laxity was noted by Velpeau,[6] with blue sclerae by Spurway[7] and Eddowes,[8] and with deafness by Adair-Deighton.[9] Bauer suggested that OI could result from a generalized mesenchymal disorder.[10] Extensive clinical and genetic analyses of OI have been compiled by Seedorf[11] and Smars.[12]

Over the years a series of eponyms have been associated with the OI syndrome. The terms "OI congenita" and "OI tarda" were introduced by Looser[13] to indicate the age of onset of fractures and, by inference, the severity of the disease. These terms are imprecise and should be discarded in view of recent research in OI that aims toward an integrated clinical and biochemical definition of the syndrome.

B. Clinical Heterogeneity

OI is genetically and clinically a heterogeneous disorder of bone and connective tissue characterized by osteoporosis, fragile bones, hyperextensible joints, dentinogenesis imperfecta (DI), bluish coloration of the sclerae, and adult-onset hearing loss. Genetic heterogeneity and variable expressivity are principles of clinical genetics that are illustrated in OI.[14] Genetic heterogeneity implies that a limited number of clinical phenotypes will result from a larger number of gene defects; variable expressivity refers to quantitative and qualitative variation within each phenotype. For example, the incidence of fractures or the extent of skeletal deformity will vary considerably among kindreds or among members of an affected family. Variable gene expression may result from tissue-specific modifier genes, the inherent genetic background of the host, or environmental factors.

For many years, genetic heterogeneity and variable expressivity were obstacles to the precise definition of OI phenotypes. Nevertheless, useful classifications have emerged that permit separation of most cases into subgroups according to the frequency of fractures, the extent of skeletal deformities, the presence or absence of DI, blue sclerae, and hearing loss, and the mode of inheritance.[15] Each of these classifications combines variable clinical signs of the disease with mendelian patterns of inheritance. However, these schemata are not fully reliable because (1) classification based on scleral color is inaccurate, since it is difficult to measure and may change with age; (2) approximately 10% of the cases defy classification because of overlapping clinical features; and (3) inheritance may be indeterminate. Thus, reliance on clinical criteria for recurrence risk counseling in a family without a prior history of the disease will be hazardous until precise biochemical diagnosis can differentiate between a new mutation and co-dominant or recessive inheritance.

A currently popular classification of OI was proposed by Sillence et al.[16,17] and has subsequently been expanded and modified[18,19] (Table 17–1). Although a convenient tool in the absence of relevant biochemical data, this nosology may be inadequate in specific cases, since OI is sporadic in one third of cases and in two thirds of families.[20] Bauze et al.[21] have classified OI into three groups based on the extent of skeletal deformity: mild, moderate, or severe. Assignment of individual subjects may be open to dispute depending on observer, age, trauma, and so on.

C. Distinctive OI Phenotypes

The following discussion presents clinical phenotypes in order of decreasing severity

Table 17–1. Clinical Features of OI Phenotypes*

Type	Phenotype	Pattern of Inheritance
I	Mild OI, relatively few fractures, nondeforming, mild scoliosis. Blue sclerae, adult hearing loss. Dentinogenesis imperfecta (type IB) in 25%.	AD
IIA	Lethal OI. Multiple intrauterine fractures, broad short femora, continous beading of ribs, defective mineralization of the calvarium.	AD: new mutations
IIB	As IIA, except that ribs are thin, with or without continuous beading, and the calvarium is better mineralized.	AR
IIC	Less frequent than type A or B. Femora and humeri are longer, undermodeled, and irregular. Calvarium is poorly mineralized.	AR (data limited)
III	Severe OI with frequent fracture rate and marked deformity. Marked growth retardation. Scoliosis severe and may progress to compromised pulmonary function. White or blue sclerae.	AD (75%) AR (25%)
IV	Moderately severe disease. Heterogenous phenotype, white or blue sclerae. Fractures may be frequent and are associated with obvious skeletal deformity. Scoliosis is moderately severe. Dentinogenesis imperfecta (type IVB) in 25%, adult hearing loss.	AD

Key: AD: autosomal dominant; AR: autosomal recessive.

*Modified from Sillence DO: Osteogenesis imperfecta: Nosology and genetics. Ann NY Acad Sci 543:1–15, 1988.

rather than in the numerical order used in the Sillence classification.

1. Neonatal Lethal OI (Sillence Type II; Bauze Severe OI)

Lethal OI represents the most extreme form of this disease. Skeletal mass is markedly decreased. Neonates suffer multiple gestational fractures causing shortened and deformed limbs and may sustain cerebral trauma and even dismemberment during delivery. The common radiologic appearance is of a large, deformed cranium; broad, crumpled extremities (concertina deformity); a characteristic beading of the ribs; and fractured vertebrae (Fig. 17–1). However, a spectrum of radiologic severity has been demonstrated. These children are hypotonic, feed poorly, and develop respiratory insufficiency shortly after birth. The majority succumb within days or weeks from pulmonary failure.

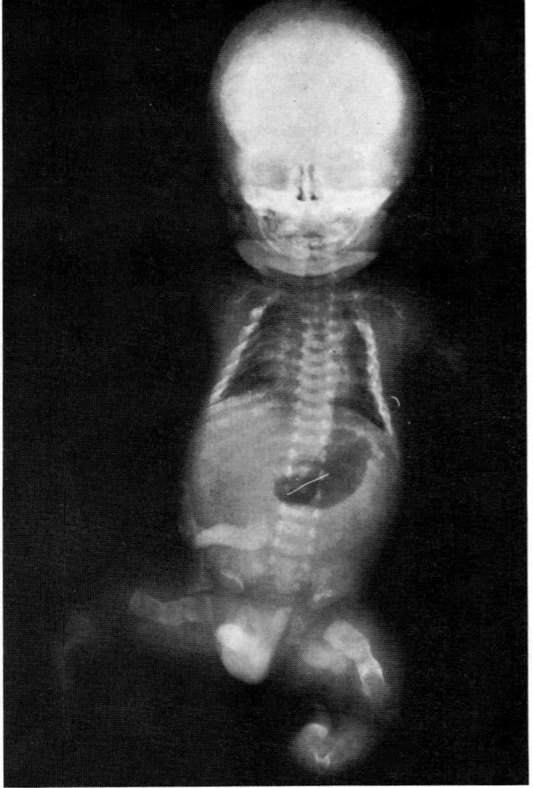

Figure 17–1. Lethal OI (Sillence type II, Bauze—severe). This radiograph illustrates the "broad-boned" type of lethal OI and the markedly defective mineralization of the calvarium and extremities. The accordion-pleated deformity of the femurs is present. Also characteristic is the beaded appearance of the ribs, a result of intrauterine fracture with callus formation. Slender long bones may also be seen in certain patients with lethal OI.

Lethal OI affects approximately 10% of patients and 20% of families.[20] The birth of multiple affected siblings to apparently normal parents is well documented and interpreted to indicate recessive inheritance in most cases.[16,22,22a] However, new autosomal dominant mutations have been suggested as an etiologic factor in lethal OI.[23,23a] This impression is supported by recent biochemical information demonstrating that new mutations may frequently underlie this form of OI.[24,25] In a comprehensive analyis of 71 affected infants, most cases occurred as sporadic events in which biochemical analysis of the parents strongly supported the abnormality in the affected infant as a new mutation.[26] In the families with more than one affected infant, pedigree and biochemical data are most consistent with germinal mosaicism of one parent. A recurrence risk of 6% to 8% was obtained when all cases were analyzed, reflecting the germinal mosaicism of a dominant trait rather than recessive or co-dominant inheritance. Because there is a finite risk of recurrence in a family with one affected infant, subsequent pregnancies should be examined by ultrasound at the 16th to 18th week of gestation to determine whether the skeleton of the fetus is deformed or normal.

2. Severe Nonlethal OI (Sillence Type III or Progressive Deforming; Bauze Severe OI)

Fractures, deformity of long bones, molding of the calvarium, and elongated vertebrae pedicles[27] are recognized at birth in this form of OI. The natural history is one of marked growth retardation, frequent and deforming fractures of the long bones (Fig. 17–2), and scoliosis with deformity of the chest wall that may ultimately lead to pulmonary insufficiency. These individuals are wheelchair-bound. Joint laxity is more marked than in other nonlethal types. The sclerae are typically white, annulus juvenilis or senilis is common, and hearing loss may appear earlier than in other types owing to a greater degree of cranial deformity. Some patients have DI and represent a subcategory.

Severe OI occurs in approximately 20% of affected patients and 15% of affected fami-

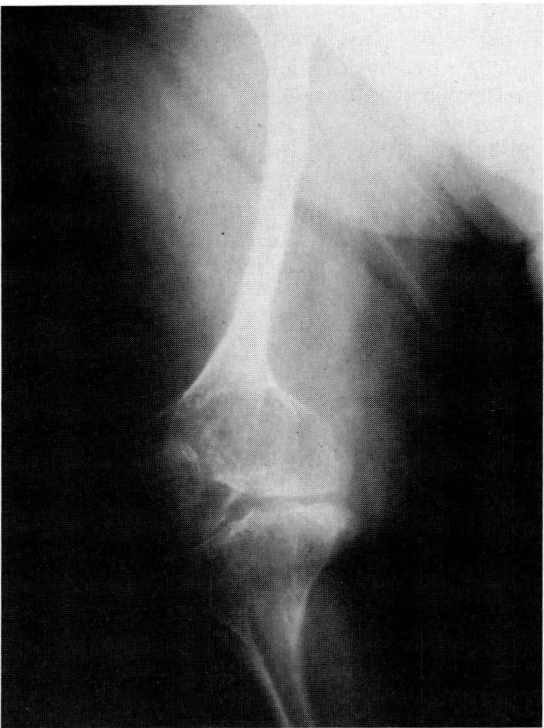

Figure 17–2. Severe, nonlethal OI (Sillence type III, Bauze—severe). This depicts the narrow diaphysis seen in severe nonlethal OI, which classically broadens to a bulbous metaphyseal-epiphyseal zone. The epiphyseal zones are severely hypomineralized and dysplastic. Whorls of partially calcified cartilage give the "popcorn" appearance. Cystic changes may predominate in some patients.

lies.[20] It is now well recognized that apparently normal parents may produce more than one affected offspring, a finding compatible with autosomal recessive inheritance.[28] Type III OI has been reported in dizygotic twins.[29] However, for reasons that are not clear, perhaps due to diminished fetal viability, the majority of severe cases are sporadic. The frequency of miscarriage has not been determined in these families. For the same reasons as noted previously, the sporadic case could also represent a new mutation, emphasizing the need for precise biochemical markers. Prenatal diagnosis of type III OI has been made in the second trimester and thus would be of value in families with a previously affected individual.[30]

3. Moderate and Deforming OI (Sillence Type IV; Bauze Mild OI)

This form of OI presents a spectrum of characteristics that range between the severely deforming and the mildly affected. As defined by Sillence, the distinguishing features common to these subjects are blue sclerae in infancy, which decrease to a lighter hue in childhood and a normal color in adults. Individuals with white sclerae are the minority in moderate OI, and we have observed adult patients with moderately severe skeletal disease typical of this phenotype OI with blue sclerae. Thus, we believe that classification of individual cases based on scleral color may be arbitrary and may prove inconsistent with biochemical data.

Despite the difficulties in defining scleral color, there exist other clinical characteristics of this form of OI. A moderate degree of growth retardation is usually present. Deformity of the extremities frequently necessitates bracing or a cane to assist ambulation (Fig. 17–3). Severe scoliosis may occur. Joint laxity is common. Hearing loss occurs, and

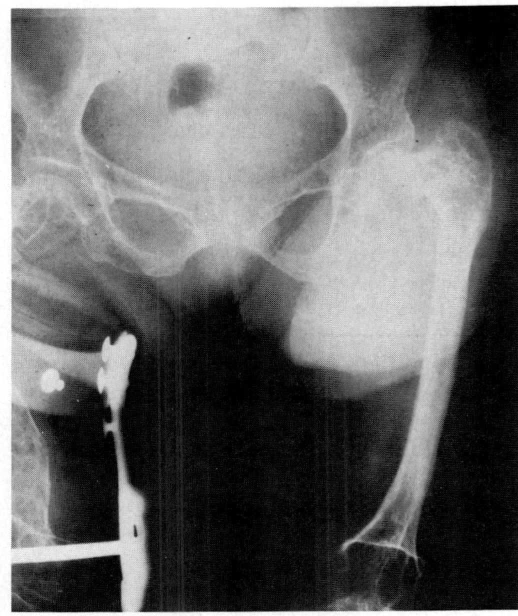

Figure 17–3. Moderately severe disease (Sillence type IV, Bauze—moderate OI). Both deformity and hypomineralization are apparent. The epiphyseal zones are dysplastic and show cystic irregularities. Scoliosis is present in these patients. Peripheral skeletal deformities frequently require bracing.

approximately 20% require hearing aids. DI is most often found in this group, and such individuals have been identified as type IVB, in contrast to type IVA, who lack dental changes.[19] Patterson et al.[31] have observed that the distinguishing features of this phenotype, when compared with type I OI, are a greater frequency of fractures at birth (28.3% versus 12.3%) but no difference in later years and a lesser tendency to bruising. The authors' experience is that these patients develop more skeletal deformity than that noted in individuals with type I OI.

This group is also genetically heterogeneous. The majority demonstrate autosomal dominant inheritance, but the occurrence of sporadic cases suggests that new mutations may occur. Increased paternal age may contribute to a new mutation.[32] Furthermore, the presence of patients having first-degree relatives with minor connective tissue findings suggests that a co-dominant mechanism may exist.

4. Mild Nondeforming OI (Sillence Type I; Bauze Mild OI)

This type includes about 60% of patients.[17] Bone fragility and osteoporosis are mild compared with other types and usually produce no skeletal deformity (Fig. 17–4). Fractures are rarely present at birth (approximately 10% are affected) and usually occur when the child ambulates. Fracture incidence declines markedly after puberty. These patients demonstrate mild growth retardation and mild scoliosis. Triangular facies are common, all have blue sclerae, and 25% have DI. The last finding has been used to subdivide this form of OI into group IA (with DI) and group IB (without DI).[19] A limited degree of joint laxity is common. Hearing impairment affects approximately 70%, only 10% of whom will require a hearing aid.

Mild OI is inherited as an autosomal dominant trait. When it occurs as a new mutation, the phenotype is subsequently transmitted as a dominant. The disease appears to breed true; for example, only rarely has there been marked variation in severity from the pattern established within a family.

5. Related Skeletal/Connective Tissue Syndromes

Several patients have been reported with multiple fractures suggestive of OI, associated with clinical features of the other heritable disorders of connective tissue. These may represent co-dominant inheritance of two gene defects. OI associated with Ehlers-Danlos syndrome (EDS) was reported by Biering and Iverson[33] in a child with blue sclerae, lax skin, bilateral hip dislocations, and fractures of vertebrae and both femurs. This child's father also had lax skin. In another family, features of both OI and arthrochalasis multiplex (EDS VII) were present and a biochemical explanation for these findings was demonstrated.[34] OI was observed in 23 members of an Irish kindred composed of 102 individuals in four generations.[35] The propositus had multiple fractures, osteoporosis, blue sclerae, Marfan's habitus, and aortic and mitral regurgitation. He apparently inherited the OI gene from his father and the marfanoid complex from his mother. His siblings were

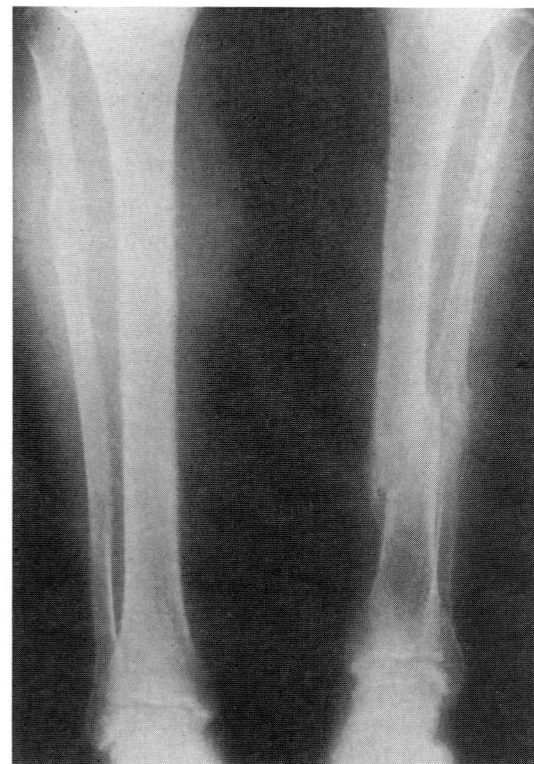

Figure 17–4. Mild and nondeforming OI (Sillence type I, Bauze—moderate OI). This radiograph illustrates the ability of these patients to heal a significant fracture without incurring a deformity. Hypomineralization is less marked than in other types, and the epiphyseal zones are normal.

affected with scoliosis, pectus excavatum, ligamentous laxity, arachnodactyly, osteoporosis, and the helmet-shaped skull of OI. An "arthropathic form" of OI has been suggested in a 14-year-old girl who developed severe osteoporosis and generalized destructive joint disease resulting in ankyloses.[36] Similarity to OI was suspected because of a relative increase in type III collagen synthesized by cultured skin fibroblasts. Arthrogryposis multiplex has been reported in association with OI.[37]

6. *Heritable Osteoporosis*

The evaluation of large numbers of adult osteoporotic patients has focused attention on a subset in which osteoporosis is apparently transmitted from generation to generation. This is consistent with the observation that a family history of osteoporosis ranks as a major risk factor for the disorder.[38,39] The relationship of mother/daughter or sibling/sibling bone mineral content, however, remains unclear.[40-42] Owing to the limited number of studies addressing this question, separation of familial from environmental factors remains difficult. Notable, however, is the observation that certain families with apparent transmissibility of osteoporosis also demonstrate clinical evidence of a connective tissue dysplasia.[43] They may present with mild scoliosis, joint laxity and skin hyperelasticity, short stature, and mitral valve prolapse, but they do not have osteogenesis imperfecta or the Ehlers-Danlos syndrome. If one considers the marked effect of race and sex on bone density, it is possible that other genetic determinants affecting either collagen or another of the extracellular matrix components could influence the development of osteoporosis in both men and women (see Chapter 12).

D. Differential Diagnosis

1. *In Neonates and Infants*

Several connective tissue syndromes that usually appear as sporadic or recessive disorders must be considered in the newborn period. The congenital lethal form of hypophosphatasia can present as severe bone disease, the result of a generalized failure of normal ossification. Osteopenia, micromelia, fractures, and a soft calvarium are present.[44] Death may occur owing to respiratory failure. The level of alkaline phosphatase is diagnostically low in blood, bone, and viscera, whereas it is high in normal growing infants or in those with traumatic fractures. Serum calcium is high-normal or elevated, and urinary phosphoethanolamine excretion is increased in this disorder in contrast to OI. Radiologically the infant develops rachitic changes with broadened epiphyses, bowing of the extremities, and prominent costochondral junctions.

The heritable chondrodystrophies can resemble lethal or severe OI because of affected infants' small size, facial features, short limbs, and hypotonia. In achondroplasia, typical skeletal manifestations should be apparent in the newborn period and include characteristic craniofacial abnormalities with bossing and flattening of the bridge of the nose, extremely short extremities, and broad long bones having an abrupt widening at their metaphyseal ends.[44] A horizontal acetabular roof and narrowing of the interpeduncular distance in the lumbar vertebrae are also found. In spite of severe micromelia, there is less marked reduction in height than in severe OI. Congenital spondyloepiphyseal dysplasia is characterized by short stature due to abnormal growth of the spine and extremities with normal-appearing hands and feet.[45] Delayed bony maturation of the spine associated with a trapezoid appearance of vertebral bodies due to shortened length of their posterior borders is typical. Skeletal fragility and limb deformity are not features of this disorder, which is inherited as either an autosomal dominant trait or a new mutation. Thanatophoric dwarfism is the prototype of the chondrodystrophies that are incompatible with survival beyond the neonatal period.[46] Extreme micromelia is associated with increased head circumference. The thorax is narrow, and the ribs are short with flaring. The epiphyses of long bones are absent at birth. Vertebral bodies are decreased in height with normally developed pedicles, which produces an H-shaped deformity. Finally, lethal OI should be differentiated from achondrogenesis, a chondrodysplasia incompatible with survival. Dwarfism is severe, skull volume is increased, and there is micromelia. Vertebral ossification is markedly impaired. The ribs are short, with lateral spur formation and irregular ossification. The disorder is transmitted as an autosomal recessive. In general, neonatal fractures are not a feature of other connective tissue dysplasias including diastrophic dwarfism, metatropic dwarfism, and punctate chondrodysplasia. These syndromes are characterized by the presence of severe micromelia.

2. In Childhood

It is frequently necessary to differentiate OI from the "battered baby" syndrome.[47,48] The presence of soft tissue trauma, metaphyseal fractures, and periarticular calcifications or evidence of psychosocial deprivation should alert the physician to the possibility of abuse as a cause of recurrent fractures. Blue sclerae, wormian bones, and a parental history of fractures are clues to the presence of OI that are frequently overlooked when children are seen in an emergency setting. In a family with an isolated case of mild OI, it may be difficult to convince well-meaning social agencies that child abuse is not present.

Childhood hypophosphatasia can be confused with severe OI (type III). Affected children have radiologic features of rickets including growth retardation, poor cranial ossification with bossing, early shedding of teeth, rachitic rosary of the chest cage, fractures, and widened epiphyses. The serum alkaline phosphatase remains low, and urinary phosphoethanolamine excretion is elevated. There is autosomal recessive inheritance. Congenital hyperphosphatasia can be manifested clinically by the second year of life with painful deformities of the extremities and pathologic fractures.[49] It is characterized by a 20- to 40-fold elevation of the serum alkaline phosphatase and high urinary hydroxyproline excretion. Bones of the skull are irregularly thickened; the long bones demonstrate evidence of markedly increased remodeling. Treatment with calcitonin may arrest the high rate of bone turnover and, in some children, prove lifesaving. This rare disorder, which has been reported in siblings, is transmitted as an autosomal recessive trait.

Homocystinuria is a heritable disorder of connective tissue characterized by a marfanoid appearance associated with the early onset of osteoporosis with fractures of the vertebrae and extremities.[50] Children typically develop inferior subluxation of the lens, chest wall deformities, kyphoscoliosis, slender extremities, tall stature, and mental retardation. For unexplained reasons, they are subject to lethal thromboses of major vessels. Several EDS variants have been recognized in children that do not conform to the currently recognized phenotypes.[51] These are usually mild sporadic cases, with excessive joint laxity, mitral valve prolapse, and, occasionally, osteoporosis with fractures in adulthood. As noted earlier, OI and the EDS may coexist in the same kindred.

Juvenile osteoporosis may be confused with OI when appearing at a young age.[52] Cases of this disorder have been noted as early as 4 or 5 years of age. However, in the majority there is a peripubertal onset of vertebral demineralization with fracture, pain, and loss of height. Pain in the extremities may result from metaphyseal fractures, which are uncommon in OI. To date, no biochemical markers of this disorder have been found. As in OI, the disease tends to remit following puberty.

Malabsorption syndromes in children may be associated with osteomalacia, fractures, and growth retardation. Therefore, an evaluation of the osteopenic child should include consideration of occult gastrointestinal disease. Additional possibilities presenting as osteopenia include lymphoma or leukemia with fractures and endocrine disorders including hyperthyroidism, Cushing's disease, and hyperparathyroidism.

3. In Adults

The presence of mild OI in the adult is frequently recognized after the diagnosis is made in an infant or child. For example, the occurrence of vertebral or extremity fractures in the premenopausal female may call attention to blue sclerae or a family history consistent with the dominant transmission of skeletal fragility. The authors are increasingly aware of patients or kindreds in whom the initial diagnosis is osteoporosis (see Chapter 12), but the presence of a systemic connective tissue lesion is suggested by scoliosis, hyperextensible joints, blue sclerae, and short stature. An understanding of the nature of these patients' disorders will depend on the elucidation of their biochemical lesion.

Mild adult hypophosphatasia with growth retardation, rickets, hyperthyroidism, hyperparathyroidism and hypogonadism, chronic renal disease, and unrecognized malabsorption must be considered in this differential diagnosis.[53]

E. Prevalence and Incidence

OI has been reported in all ethnic groups and races without a geographic predilection. The incidence of OI is underestimated because many mildly affected subjects go undetected throughout childhood and adult life, whereas severely affected fetuses, stillborn or those dying shortly after birth, may be misdiagnosed. Thus, the most reliable estimates of the frequency of OI are based on the recognition of fractures occurring in the newborn period. OI has a reported incidence of 1:20,000 to 1:60,000 live births, with a general prevalence in several reports from 1 to 5×10^{-5}.[17,54-59]

II. DETAILED CLINICAL FEATURES OF OI

A. The Skeletal System

1. *Clinical Course of Long Bone Fractures*

Although OI is a systemic disorder of connective tissue, fragile bones are the dominant clinical manifestation. The morbidity and mortality associated with OI are directly related to the degree of skeletal fragility.[60] Connective tissue involvement in other organs carries relatively little morbidity. Patients with the most severe forms of OI suffer fractures *in utero* and may succumb shortly after birth, or they may survive with the handicap of severe skeletal deformity throughout their lives. Marked fragility carries the risk of death, particularly from head trauma. The less severely affected patients are always osteoporotic, with variable amounts of deformity. We do not fully understand the relationship between the described gene defects and the diverse clinical phenotypes in OI, or why healing occurs without deformity in certain patients and with severe deformity in others.

In the milder types of OI, type I, and the less severe cases of type IV disease, there may be minimal skeletal deformity (see Fig. 17–4). Probably most common is anterior bowing of the distal tibia. Whereas fractures may be present at birth in approximately 10% of milder cases, they usually occur between the age of 6 months and 3 years as the child starts to stand and walk. Boys tend to experience more fractures than those incurred by girls.[61] Occasionally, the first fracture occurs at an older age, and rarely in the teens. Metaphyseal and epiphyseal architecture are normal in mild OI. Astley[62] noted small metaphyseal fractures in seven of 41 OI children with gross skeletal abnormalities. Most fractures in children involve the lower extremities, particularly the proximal or distal femur. Older children may injure the distal forearm or fingers and toes. Skeletal deformities are more prominent in the type IV patient, in whom osteopenia and scoliosis are more severe (see Fig. 17–3). As children first stand, we have watched the proximal femur change within a few months from no deformity to a "shepherd's crook" deformity, presumably as the result of microfractures. As a consequence, unlike the type I patient, those with type IV are frequently dependent on crutches or canes to assist in walking.

Children with severe OI (type III) are born with obvious cranial deformities and fractures of the clavicles, extremities, or ribs. These may not be recognized for weeks or until callus has formed. Irritability or failure to thrive may be the only symptom of fractures in the nursery. Here, fractures occur with minimal stress and heal with residual deformity. Non-union may occur but is uncommon. Repeated fractures and microfractures induce progressive deformity and may require immobilization of a limb or the trunk in a body spica cast, aggravating osteopenia and increasing the susceptibility to new fractures. In more severe cases, one sees progressive angulation of the neck of the femur, a "saber shin–like" anterior angulation of the lower tibia, and lateral bowing or rotation of the humerus, radius, and ulna. Once developed, these deformities represent areas highly susceptible to fracture with minimal trauma. In severe OI, the diaphysis of long bones frequently is very narrow, widening to an enlarged and dysplastic metaphyseal-epiphyseal area.[63] Clusters of small, scalloped, irregularly calcified radiolucencies at the ends of long bones have been termed "popcorn" calcifications.[64] The association of these lesions with disappearance of the normal horizontal growth plate suggests a posttraumatic disturbance in endochondral ossification (see Fig. 17–2).

Endochondral bone formation is markedly deficient in the neonatal lethal form of OI. The long bones typically appear broad and are severely osteopenic with multiple intrauterine fractures simulating an "accordion-pleated" or "concertina bone" appearance. In addition to cranial fractures, rib fractures *in utero* produce a characteristic radiographic beaded appearance (see Fig. 17–1). Sillence et al.[22] have proposed that three variants of lethal OI may be recognized radiologically: group A, characterized by markedly shortened broad and rectangular crumpled limbs, strikingly impaired cranial ossification, and short thick ribs with prominent beading; group B, in which radiographic findings are similar to those in group A, but ribs showed only occasional beading; group C, in which long bones were slender with multiple fractures and inadequate modeling, and beading of the ribs was less prominent than in group A.[64a] The spectrum of radiographic findings has been expanded further to five groups. Group 1 is more severe than group B with calvaria and long bone showing no modeling. Group 5 is less severe than group C with normal long bone modeling and metaphyseal flaring. The severity of the radiographic appearance correlates with the length of survival after birth.[65]

In the nonlethal forms of OI there is marked variation in fracture rate even within individual families. Fractures are 5- to 10-fold more frequent before puberty. Moorfield and Miller[66] found that an average of 91% of fractures occurred prior to puberty, whereas after puberty, fractures apparently require more than trivial trauma. The factors responsible for this increase in bone strength after puberty are unknown. Obviously a change in hormonal milieu is crucial, since following the menopause the fracture rate starts to climb again in each of the phenotypes. Decreased calcium stores and the postmenopausal loss of estrogen may play a role. As reported by Patterson et al.[61] the fracture rate in postmenopausal females with OI is about 7-fold that in the general population, for example, 26 fractures per 100 patient years for ages 50 to 70 years versus 3.5 to 4.8 fractures per 100 patient years in comparably aged females. Males over age 50 also experience an increase in fracture rate, but less than that in the females. Fractures in OI are frequently transverse, at times subperiosteal, and usually in alignment, depending on the thickness of cortex and the nature of the trauma. Certain patients may suffer a fracture with merely a change in position: milder cases require substantial trauma to cause fracture. The authors have examined patients with obvious (mild) OI as children who after puberty played contact sports with little injury. Contrary to a common perception, fractures in OI are painful, although minor fractures may resolve with minimal discomfort.[12]

Three skeletal complications may occur following a fracture: (1) severe angulation, which may limit function if not properly corrected; (2) non-union, which although uncommon tends to involve long bones and may prove disabling; and (3) hyperplastic callus, which occurs in less than 1% of OI fractures.[67] This is a rapidly developing inflammatory overgrowth of new bone that occurs unexpectedly. Associated with an elevated erythrocyte sedimentation rate, local erythema, and warmth, hyperplastic callus presents as a tender mass at the site of a healing fracture. It appears more commonly in boys and usually involves the femur.

2. Spine

Scoliosis is a frequent complication of OI. It may be present at an early age and is directly related to the severity of the disease and, probably, the degree of joint laxity. King and Bobechko[68] found the incidence of scoliosis to vary from 28% in the milder forms to 43% in type III OI, whereas Falvo et al.[69] found a 92% incidence in OI congenita. Weakness of the paraspinal musculature may promote asymmetric growth of the spine, particularly in young children. Either thoracic scoliotic curves or a double primary curve may develop. The majority as reported by Renshaw et al.[70] measure from 10 to 20 degrees; curves in excess of 20 degrees are found in type III patients. In the adult, scoliosis frequently increases in severity and becomes increasingly disabling as thoracic volume declines.[71] Osteopenia and lax paraspinal ligaments lead to vertebral crush fractures ("codfish" deformity), which are more common in adults than in children. Vertebral fractures in childhood are more likely to be a feature of juvenile osteoporosis than of OI.[72] Neurologic sequelae of scoliosis and vertebral collapse are usually not present. Upper cervical cord compression has been reported as a cause of death in lethal OI.[73]

3. Skull

Deformity of the skull occurs frequently in OI. Typically, the circumference of the head is increased, although, in some, circumference may only appear increased relative to the small size of the trunk. In mild cases, the face may present a triangular appearance. Softening or early fractures of the mandible may produce a type III malocclusion with protrusion of the mandible.[74] In three families, 13 subjects with OI had radiolucent or radiopaque lesions of the maxilla or mandible.[75] In more severe cases, because ossification of the skull is deficient or delayed, softening leads to flattening in the anteroposterior diameter, particularly in the hypotonic, bedridden infant with little head control. Closure of the fontanels may be delayed for several years. Molding may lead to prominence of the frontal and occipital bones, simulating the bossing seen in rickets. Softening of the calvarium causes the "helmet" or "tam-o'shanter" deformity with a palpable occipital overhang.[76] Prominence of the eyes and flattening of the forehead may combine to produce the characteristic "sunset sign" appearance of the severely affected child.

The majority of severe cases of OI present with multiple wormian bones. Cremin et al.[77] have described these as detached portions of the primary ossification centers in adjacent membranous bones. Significant persistence of wormian bones is defined as more than 10 in number that are greater than 6 mm × 4 mm in size. They are frequently located in the occipital area and may persist for several years. Although wormian bones are an important diagnostic feature of OI, they are also found occasionally in normally growing skulls, and in other heritable disorders of connective tissue: cleidocranial dysostosis, Menkes syndrome, Prader-Willi syndrome, and progeria.

Either basilar impression or platybasia may occur when there is extreme softening at the base of the skull.[78,79] These may be responsible for variable hydrocephalus with dilation of the third and lateral ventricles, upper and lower motor neuron lesions, cranial nerve abnormalities, and cerebellar dysfunction. Cortical atrophy in OI may be a consequence of macrocephaly.[80] Distortion of venous sinuses seen on CT scans may be the cause of chronic headaches experienced by severely affected patients. Rarely, decompression of the posterior fossa may be required. Trauma to the skull or face, although uncommon in OI, is a constant hazard after an accidental fall from a wheelchair or following an automobile accident.

4. *Other Skeletal Abnormalities*

Additional skeletal abnormalities include protrusio acetabuli, coxa vara deformity, genu valgum, and planovalgus deformities of the feet. Various deformities of the chest wall (pectus excavatum and carinatum, asymmetry of the rib cage) accompany scoliosis of the spine.[81] Marked elongation of the pedicles of vertebrae and posterior rib angulation have been observed in type III OI.[27]

B. Other Connective Tissues

1. *Joint Hypermobility*[81a]

Clinical criteria related to joint hypermobility have been presented by Beighton and Horan.[82] To a variable extent, approximately 70% of OI patients may demonstrate significant joint hypermobility due to underdevelopment of the ligaments. Lax joints are more common in the more severely affected subjects. This is most evident in the younger patients and usually involves the distal rather than the larger proximal joints that are affected in Marfan's syndrome and EDS. There is no relationship of joint mobility to scleral color. The OI infant may appear loose-jointed and floppy. Although sprains and dislocations are not frequent in OI, with sufficient stress, troublesome dislocations may occur at the hip, knee, ankle, or shoulder. Muscle tone is poor in the more severely affected subjects, secondary either to disuse or to the underlying connective tissue abnormality also present within the tendons. Pes planus is a common finding in the OI patient.

2. *Skin*

Diminished skin thickness is probably a consequence of diminished collagen production.[83] Skin tensile strength is decreased when type I collagen production is diminished.[84] Skin laxity is usually mild, and substantially less than the hyperelasticity characteristic of EDS. In contrast to the friability of skin in EDS, wound healing in OI is usually normal. Elastosis perforans serpiginosa, an unusual lesion common to other connective tissue disorders such as EDS and pseudoxanthoma elasticum, has been reported in OI.[85] This lesion appears as a keratotic papule that grows to a serpiginous macule, usually on the arms or trunk. On healing, such lesions may leave thin broad scars, and occasionally keloids may be found.[86]

3. Teeth

Dentin, the organic matrix of teeth, is composed of type I collagen and proteoglycans. The opalescent brown teeth characteristic of DI are the result of insufficient support of the overlying normal enamel.[87] With the continued trauma of eating, the enamel fractures, exposing the underlying dentin, and the tooth wears to the level of the gum (Fig. 17–5). Permanent teeth are usually less severely affected. Dentin, which contains the same genetic collagen as that in bone (type I), has increased relative amounts of hydroxylysine to lysine in OI patients without obvious DI,[88] a finding consistent with the overmodified collagen molecule found in the connective tissues in severe OI. When viewed by scanning electron microscopy, the dentin has an irregular tubular organization, which contrasts with the highly ordered tubular pattern of normal dentin.[89] Radiographic characteristics of DI include a normal density and thickness of enamel, an exaggerated constriction at the junction between crown and roots, and pulp chambers that may initially be larger than normal, but which become obliterated by abnormal dentin.[90]

Approximately 25% in each clinical phenotype are also found to have DI. Smith et al.[91] have found DI to be relatively uncommon in patients with mild disease and more common in those with severe bone disease. Genetic evaluation of families with dominantly inherited OI has revealed that when DI is present in a family, all affected individuals will have both skeletal and dental disease.[90] However, there is no relationship between the severity of skeletal disease and the presence of DI in affected families. Rare families have been reported to have DI and blue sclerae, but no bone disease.[92]

C. Other Organs Containing Type I Collagen

1. Eye

Although blue sclerae have been recognized as a prominent clinical sign in OI since 1831, pathogenesis still remains uncertain.[93] Type I collagen is found in the cornea, sclera, choroid, iris, and ciliary body.[94,95] A thin scleral coat permitting blue coloration has not been a consistent finding. Ruedeman[96] found a deficiency of scleral collagen and an increased density of PAS-fuscin stain, suggesting a relative increase in the mucoid component of the sclera. Eicholtz and Muller[97]

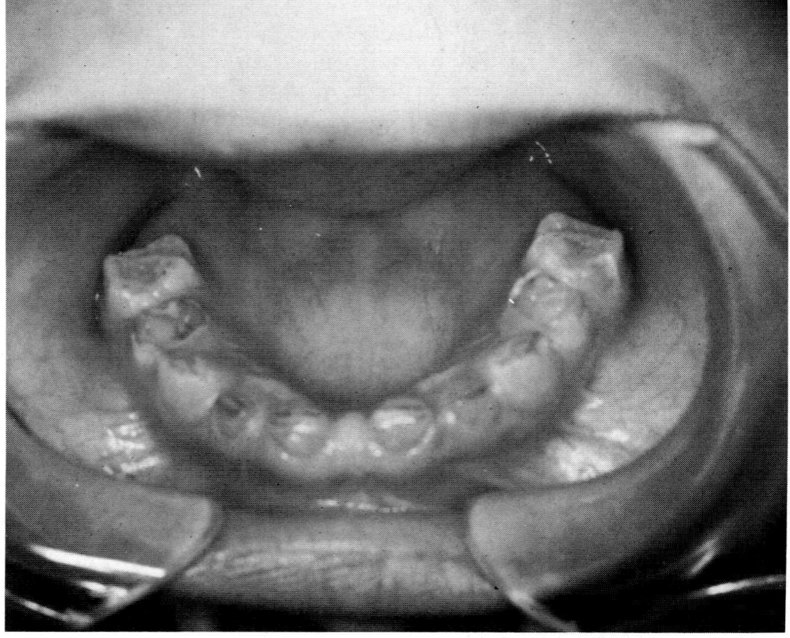

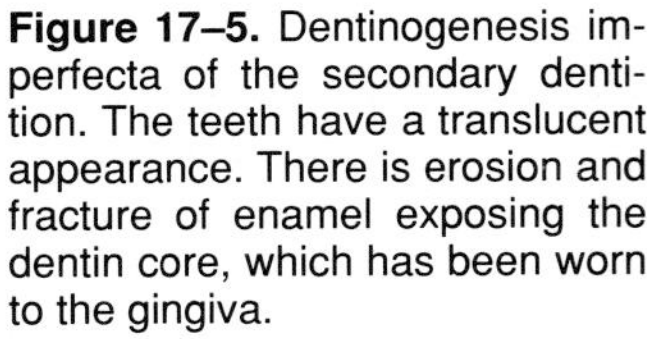

Figure 17–5. Dentinogenesis imperfecta of the secondary dentition. The teeth have a translucent appearance. There is erosion and fracture of enamel exposing the dentin core, which has been worn to the gingiva.

examined blue sclerae by electron microscopy and found that although the sclera was of normal thickness, the scleral cells had distended endoplasmic reticulum, and in one case there was deposition of dense material between scleral lamellae. Chan et al.[98] have examined the eyes of four children with lethal OI. Corneal fiber dimeter was diminished by about 25%, whereas the diameter of the scleral fibers was smaller by 50%. Bowman's and Bruch's membranes were poorly developed. Clinical evidence for a structural defect in the scleral coat is suggested by diminished ocular rigidity as measured by tonometry. This finding correlated directly with the degree of bluishness and was not seen in patients with white sclerae.[99]

Blue sclerae have been observed in each of the clinical types of OI.[99,100] In type IV OI, sclerae tend to lighten with age, and in type III OI, white sclerae are commonly observed in the presence of severe bone disease. Our experience is that blue sclerae are not unique to any one phenotype, and thus should not be used to define clinical subgroups. Blue sclerae are also observed in other heritable disorders of connective tissue (EDS, certain variants of the Marfan syndrome, Menkes syndrome) and may occur in otherwise normal subjects.

Clinical evidence of diminished corneal thickness has been reported by Pedersen and Bramsen.[101] This was not confirmed by Kaiser-Kupfer et al.[99] Corneal collagen fibers have also been reported to be thin and irregularly arranged by Haebera et al.[102] Several ocular abnormalities have been observed in a small number of patients with blue sclerae, such as keratoconus or keratoglobus, corneal perforations, megalocornea, and breaks in Descemet's membrane.[103] Most commonly observed is arcus juvenilis or senilis, which may be seen in the absence of blue sclerae.[12] Myopia, which is commonly observed in other connective tissue disorders (Marfan's syndrome, homocystinuria), is not associated with OI.

2. Ear

The otologic and maxillofacial features of OI have been summarized by Bergstrom.[104] Functional deafness requiring the use of a hearing aid appears during the second or third decade in approximately 10% of OI patients. However, the incidence of subtle defects in auditory function approaches 90% in older subjects. There has been a dispute as to the nature of this defect and the functional disturbance that leads to progressive loss of hearing in some patients but not in others. For many years the anatomic defect in OI was considered identical to otosclerosis; these are now recognized as distinct entities.[105] Biochemical differences in the ossicle bones between OI and otosclerosis have been reported.[106-108] Pedersen[109] has demonstrated that in contrast to OI, diminished skeletal bone mineral content is not present in otosclerosis. Furthermore, the histopathologic character of the temporal bone is qualitatively similar to that of the peripheral skeleton in OI. Deficient ossification occurs in the tympanic ring, ossicles, cochlea, and otic capsule, and there may be intracochlear hemorrhage.[110] Microfractures occur in the incus and stapes, and the stapes may be reduced to thin fibrous threads. The stapes footplate may be embedded in vascular fibrous tissue, which has led to an association with otosclerosis.[111]

Recent studies suggest that sensorineural hearing loss is more common than conductive loss. A characteristic audiologic pattern of sensorineural hearing loss, consisting of a high-pitched sensorineural loss starting at 6000 dB that increases at high frequencies, is found in the OI patient. With aging, the loss involves lower frequencies.[112] Testing of hearing and middle ear function in 55 patients with OI revealed sensorineural hearing loss in 49% of patients less than 30 years of age and 94% of those over 30. In contrast, conductive loss was present in only 4% of patients and mixed hearing loss in 10%. Another characteristic feature was revealed by tympanometry. OI patients demonstrated increased compliance of the tympanic membrane suggestive of discontinuity or excessive mobility of the middle ear components.[112,113] However, Reidner et al.[114] have described conductive hearing loss and a stiff middle ear system in OI.

There are few data regarding the effectiveness of stapedectomy in OI. In an uncontrolled study, Pedersen[109] found that no technical problems were encountered during surgery, and that both short- and long-term gains in acuity occurred following stapedectomy. However, whereas surgery may improve hearing initially, the long-term value of the procedure remains to be proved.

3. Heart

The myocardium contains an extensive collagen network and the heart valves are largely collagen. Types I, III, and V collagens are found throughout these structures, although the last two are found primarily in vascular components of heart muscle, the valves, and perimyocytic supporting fibers.[115] Detailed biochemical analysis of heart valves or aortic connective tissue in OI has not been performed.

There are several reports of mitral valve prolapse and aneurysms of the aortic root in OI; however, these occur much less frequently than in either EDS or Marfan's syndrome.[116,117] Only rarely are these lesions clinically important, and they do not appear related to either the severity of skeletal disease or the presence of blue sclerae. A patient with mitral and aortic insufficiency experienced mitral valve dehiscence due to extreme friability of the mitral annulus.[118] Recently three large series have utilized echocardiography to investigate these lesions in patients with OI and their relatives.[119-121] The results were similar in each. Auscultatory findings of mitral valve prolapse occur in approximately 1% to 2% of OI patients; echocardiographic evidence will be found in 10%, contrasted with 5% in the general population. Dilation of the aortic root occurs in 10% to 12% of the OI population and is unrelated to the presence of mitral valve disease. The murmur of aortic regurgitation is heard in approximately 2% of patients. Unlike in Marfan's syndrome, progression of aortic root dilation has not been observed in OI. Aortic dilation appears to occur within certain families; familial clustering of mitral valve prolapse has not been established.[121-123]

4. Pulmonary Function in OI

Impaired pulmonary function occurs in the neonate with severe skeletal deformities, and in a gradually progressive manner in children or adults with severe scoliosis. In the lethal form of OI, death appears to be the result of pulmonary insufficiency; detailed pathologic descriptions fail to indicate the cause of this lesion. The authors have observed pulmonary hypoplasia in a neonate with lethal OI.[124] This child had evidence of a mutant alpha$_1$(I) procollagen. Rodriguez et al.[125] have also observed pulmonary hypoplasia in lethal OI. Pulmonary function is variable in children and adults with type III OI; certain patients may develop right ventricular failure in association with restrictive lung disease and hypoxemia.[126]

D. Endocrine and Metabolic Function in OI

1. Short Stature

Size at birth appears to reflect severity of the disease.[127] Growth retardation becomes apparent during the first two years.[128] Diminished growth of the skeleton is found in each OI phenotype, and the majority of patients fall below the 3rd percentile for height. Normal height is attained only in rare patients with mild disease. Albright and Grunt[128] and Wynne-Davies and Gormley[54] observed that diminished height, although in part related to the severity of deformities, occurred independently of the frequency of fractures. In the severely affected, growth may virtually cease after the age of 3 or 4 years: type III adults may be no taller than three feet. In less severely affected subjects, there may be a small growth spurt prior to puberty. At that age, scoliosis, the effects of long bone fractures, and deformities may magnify what is an intrinsic defect in the response of OI bone to normal growth stimuli.

Mediators of somatic growth, growth hormone and somatomedin C, have been measured in different types of nonlethal OI.[129] Provocative tests of growth hormone reserve, including overnight sampling of growth hormone secretion, have yielded normal values. Also, the meaning of decreased levels of somatomedin C in subjects with short stature remains open to question, since several investigators have failed to correlate either normal or low somatomedin C with rates of growth, or with the growth response to growth hormone in normal or growth hormone–deficient children.[130,131] We have observed low somatomedin C levels unresponsive to exogenous growth hormone in young children with type III OI; normal basal levels were subsequently found. Growth hormone treatment of two children with type III OI for 6 months failed to produce an increase in growth rate.

2. Thyroid Function

Increased perspiration, frequently mentioned by the families of OI patients, has led to the determination of oxygen consumption rates and thyroid function. Cropp[132] observed basal body temperature in OI subjects to be 37.2° C versus 36.6° C in normals. Also, prepubertal OI patients were found to have significantly higher oxygen consumption and higher calculated metabolic rates than normal. These findings require confirmation as do reports of increased thyroid function in OI. Distiller et al.[133] have found raised thyroid hormone levels that were attributed to a disturbance in serum thyroid-binding globulins in their subjects. Evaluation of thyroid function by Shapiro et al.[129] has demonstrated normal levels of thyroid hormone, and a normal response of these to the administration of thyrotropin-releasing hormone (TRH).

Malignant hyperpyrexia has been associated with OI as a result of infrequent individual case reports of hyperpyrexia appearing with anesthesia.[134] A metabolic link to OI is undetermined at this time.

3. Miscellaneous Laboratory Tests

There are no specific abnormalities in clinical tests that are characteristic of OI. The fraction of serum alkaline phosphatase derived from bone may be elevated following a fracture. An elevation in serum acid phosphatase has been reported[135,136] but has not been confirmed in later studies.[137,138] Aminoaciduria with increased excretion of serine, threonine, valine, ethanolamine, and phosphoethanolamine has been observed in both individual patients and affected families.[139] Kinnett and Bullough[140] have observed increased excretion of phosphoethanolamine and cystine in several OI patients. However, urinary free amino acid excretion was found to be normal.[140a] The authors have found that serum parathyroid hormone levels are normal, as are serum determinations of vitamin D metabolites. Increased levels of serum copper and ceruloplasmin have been reported,[141] but serum and urinary determinations of copper and zinc have been found to be normal.

4. Clotting

Easy bruising is common in OI and in several of the heritable disorders of connective tissue, particularly in EDS. Whereas several reports have documented abnormal blood platelets,[142] clinically significant bleeding is rarely a complication. Abnormal platelet thromboplastin generation, macroplatelets, and abnormal platelet granulation have been observed.[143] A study of hemostasis in 58 subjects with mild OI revealed that 35% had increased capillary fragility, 33% decreased platelet retention, and 23% reduced factor VII antigen. Reduced ristocetin co-factor, deficient platelet aggregation by collagen, and prolonged bleeding time were less common.[144]

5. OI and Pregnancy

Most women with mild OI tolerate pregnancy without difficulty; however, severe skeletal deformities complicate pregnancy and delivery for both the mother and fetus.[145,146] The incidence of maternal fractures is not increased during pregnancy. Premature rupture of membranes, characteristic of EDS, does not occur in OI. Successful pregnancy and delivery have occurred in patients with type III OI, but these are likely to be complicated by cephalopelvic disproportion. The decision as to whether a patient should have a cesarean section should depend on maternal preference and the physician's judgment. Previously unrecognized pelvic fractures, susceptibility to perineal lacerations, and a bleeding tendency may necessitate cesarean section. Uterine rupture has been observed complicating a second pregnancy following an uneventful first pregnancy.[146]

6. Prenatal Diagnosis of OI

Prenatal diagnosis of type II OI has been accomplished with the use of ultrasonography performed at about the 18th week of gestation.[147-150] At that time one may visualize fractures, beading of ribs, foreshortening and bowing of long bones, or an enlarged head. Nonlethal but severe OI has been detected in the second trimester and thus is useful when another family member has the disease.[30,151] Diagnosis may not be possible in mild, dominantly inherited OI, in which severe deformity of the fetus is not likely to be observed.

III. PATHOPHYSIOLOGY OF OI

Diseases such as OI that alter the dynamics of bone turnover need to be clarified at the histomorphologic and metabolic level before their genetic mutations can be integrated with specific phenotypes. Underlying this is the awareness that various gene defects will be expressed in a limited number of similar clinical phenotypes. In the following section, a pathophysiologic concept of OI is developed based on (1) histomorphology and ultrastructure of bone and collagen, (2) determinations of bone mass using techniques available in a modern clinical setting, and (3) review of demonstrated molecular lesions in various phenotypes. The methods for evaluating and interpreting the various gene lesions affecting type I collagen synthesis are presented in detail.

A. Skeletal Histopathology in OI

The interpretation of skeletal pathologic changes in OI has been complicated by virtue of (1) the clinical heterogeneity, which confuses clinicopathologic correlation, (2) the fact that few bone biopsies have been obtained from areas not involved by fracture, or not doubly labeled with tetracycline for histomorphometry, and (3) the differences in techniques used for processing samples of bone for histologic analysis. The interpretation of a bone biopsy must include consideration of factors that may alter its histomorphometry, such as age, level of activity, exposure to androgenic and estrogenic hormones, or other forms of therapy.[152] Furthermore, unapparent abnormalities of collagen in other connective tissues have not been sought. As a result, there are no histologic markers that unequivocally distinguish the pathologic changes in OI from those in other osteopenic syndromes. Nevertheless, there are several features at the tissue level that assist in the differentiation of the various OI phenotypes.

1. Lethal (Type II) OI

The striking feature in this group is the paucity of type I collagen in the extracellular matrix. As a result, lamellar bone formation is severely impaired. This can be best seen at the epiphysis, where, in normal individuals, vertically oriented columns of chondrocytes differentiate into osteoblasts. In lethal disease, there is an abrupt failure of normal ossification with persistence of hypercellular, cartilaginous metaphyseal tissue surrounded by immature woven bone (Fig. 17–6). The maturation of lamellar bone is also markedly retarded in medullary and cortical zones as evidenced by the presence of multiple pregestational fractures showing partial heal-

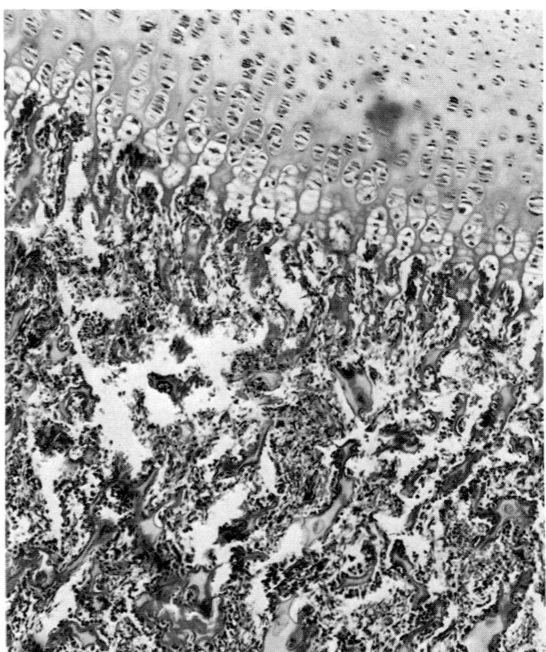

Figure 17–6. Bone biopsy of epiphyseal growth plate from a patient with lethal OI. The columns of maturing chondrocytes appear only slightly irregular. There is abrupt failure of endochondral bone formation proximal to the growth plate, leaving poorly ossified irregular lamellae with a central cartilage core.

ing.[153,154] In contrast to other forms of OI, the osteoblasts appear diminished in number. At the electron microscopic level, there are a reduced number of extracellular type I collagen fibers that are markedly decreased in diameter, but there is a normal banding pattern. Osteoblasts show large, dilated rough endoplasmic reticulum that probably represents retained mutant and overmodified type I collagen. This finding may be explained by the faulty secretion of type I collagen in this form of OI.[155]

2. Severe Nonlethal (Type III) OI

Severe osteopenia is present from birth. Bone cortices are markedly thinned. Variable amounts of immature or woven bone may be present depending on the severity of the disease.[156] As a consequence of defective periosteal growth and remodeling, the shafts of long bones are slender, widening to a bulbous metaphyseal-epiphyseal zone. The periosteum and perichondrium appear normal by conventional microscopy. The trabeculae are thin, disorganized, and separated by wide spaces of intervening marrow. Hyperosteocytosis is prominent in this phenotype (Fig. 17–7), but a consistent morphologic abnormality of osteoblast, osteocyte, or osteoclast has not been reported. Secondary centers of ossification are distorted, and the epiphysis may contain several small whorls of partially calcified cartilaginous material surrounded by woven bone that disrupt the endplate. Electron microscopy has revealed that whereas bone and dermal collagen fiber diameter is normal, there are fibers that show fraying and breakage. Using scanning electron miscroscopy on bone samples from three patients with severe OI, Teitelbaum et al.[157] found that the collagen fibers were diminished in size compared with normals and were arranged in thin sheets suggesting defective bundle formation. Falvo[69] also found bone collagen fibers to have diminished diameter but normal periodicity. Fraying and breakage of type I collagen is not unique to OI, having been observed in other heritable disorders of collagen including type IV EDS.[158]

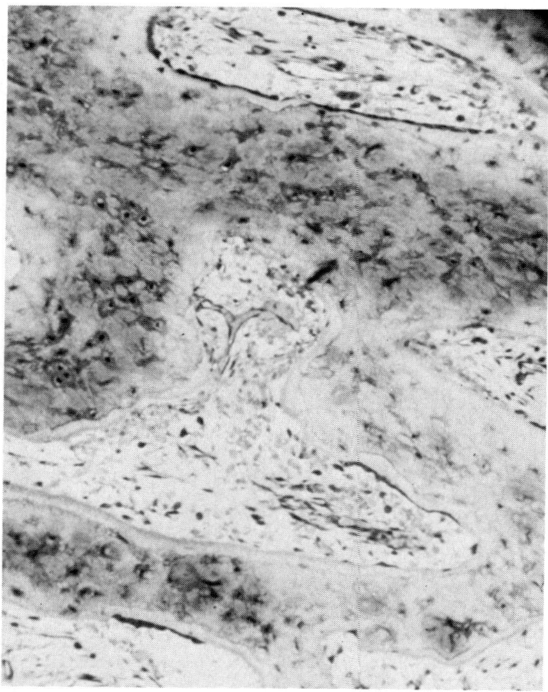

Figure 17–7. Toluidine blue stain of an iliac crest biopsy in type III OI. The characteristic findings are diminished trabecular volume, hyperosteocytosis, and an irregular pattern of lamellar staining.

3. Mild OI With or Without Deformity (Types I and IV; Bauze Mild or Moderate OI)

The mild and moderately severe forms of OI share histopathologic as well as phenotypic features. However, the type IV patients present skeletal findings of advanced osteoporosis with cortical thinning ranging from moderate to severe. Considering overlap in phenotype, individual cases range from nearly normal in type I patients to severe cortical and medullary bone loss in type IV. Microscopically, one sees a decreased number of trabeculae of diminished width, whereas the depth of osteoid seams and osteoid volume are usually normal. Children with the "tarda" variety of OI were found to have low trabecular bone volume associated with an increased bone turnover rate.[159] A decrease in the function of individual osteoblasts was observed in spite of increased formation at the tissue level. An apparent increase in unmineralized osteoid in some patients may be a consequence of a marked decrease in trabecular bone volume.[160] The staining of bone matrix with PAS or toluidine blue may be abnormal. The absolute number of osteocytes is increased, and an increased number of osteoclasts may be seen in some biopsies.

Histomorphometric analyses by Falvo and Bullough[160] have demonstrated a decreased fractional area of bone, an absolute increase in the number of osteocytes, and an increased number of resorption surfaces. In agreement with Baron et al.,[159] calculation of static and dynamic parameters of bone function after tetracycline labeling indicated an increase in the rate of bone turnover despite the apparent decrease in the synthesis of bone matrix by individual osteoblasts. Ste. Marie et al.[161] reported histomorphometric analysis of iliac crest bone following tetracycline labeling from 12 patients with type I or IV OI. In the adults, trabecular bone volume was considerably decreased, and the thickness index of osteoid seams was diminished. Trabecular osteoblastic surfaces were increased in four adults; parameters of resorption were slightly increased. Jones et al.[162] have described decreased type I collagen fiber diameter (0.04–0.06 μm versus 0.06–0.08 μm in normals) from skin in OI; Shapiro et al.[163] have also reported decreased fiber diameter and the presence of marked irregularity of individual fiber outline in a patient with coexistent mild OI and Paget's disease of bone.

B. Bone Mineral Content in OI

Methods available for the quantization of bone mineral content *in vivo* include (1) radiogramometry based on the measurement of metacarpal cortical-medullary width[164]; (2) single-photon (^{125}I) densitometry, which measures predominantly cortical bone in the radius[165]; (3) computed tomographic (CT) determination of trabecular bone mineral content of vertebral bodies T12 to L4[166]; (4) dual-photon absorptiometry (DPA), which employs gadolinium-153 to measure both cortical and trabecular bone in the lumbar spine[167]; and (5) digital radiography of the axial or vertebral bone.[168] The last three methods have only recently been introduced into routine clinical use and they appear to be the most accurate for quantitating bone mineral content (see Chapters 9 and 12).

Patterson[169] measured metacarpal medullary-cortical widths in adults with dominantly inherited mild OI ranging in age from 20 to 70 years. Although the hand bones were slender, cortical bone widths were normal. Kurtz et al.[170] reported that all OI subjects were osteopenic for their age when vertebral bone mineral content was measured by CT scan. The demineralization was roughly proportional to the severity of the OI. Type I OI patients appeared to lose bone mineral at a rate two to three times greater than nonaffected subjects. Demineralization was most severe in type III patients. Studies by the authors of a limited number of clinically unaffected relatives by both single-photon densitometry and vertebral CT have failed to disclose evidence of osteopenia. Thus, although a limited number of quantitative studies confirm that osteopenia is a constant radiologic feature of OI, it appears that the extent of bone mineral depletion may vary markedly among phenotypes.

C. Summary and Speculation

The preceding data indicate that there is insufficient type I collagen in bone and suggest that different factors underlie deficient matrix accumulation. There may be either underproduction or excessive turnover of collagen and other matrix components. There is little to suggest that OI involves a defect in normal mineralization. The woven bone seen in more severely affected cases has not been chemically characterized but suggests defective osseous maturation possibly due to improper collagen fiber formation. The hypercellularity frequently found within OI bone may reflect an effort by the osteoblast to compensate for the inadequate bone matrix synthesis through some as yet undefined mechanism. Since formation and turnover are coordinated through a bone coupling factor(s),[171] the increased number of osteoclasts and osteoblasts seen in association with measurements of enhanced bone turnover may be secondary to the production of a defective bone collagen or faulty association of collagen and glycosaminoglycans in extracellular matrix.

IV. STRUCTURE AND BIOSYNTHESIS OF TYPE I COLLAGEN AS RELATED TO OI

It is now apparent that various mutations within the type I collagen genes underlie the pathophysiology of OI. The challenge to the clinician and molecular biologist in the next decade will be the integration of clinical and molecular disciplines to obtain more accurate diagnosis, improved genetic counseling, and effective therapy. As a starting point for the clinician, a review of the essential structural and regulatory elements of bone collagen pertinent to OI is presented. A general discussion of type I collagen is given elsewhere in this book.

At least 15 genetically distinct steps must be successfully carried out[172] between the first step of transcribing the gene and the final extracellular incorporation of the collagen molecule into a crosslinked microfibril. Many of these involve multiple sites within procollagen mRNA or the translated protein. This degree of complexity undoubtedly accounts for the genetic heterogeneity associated with the heritable disorders of connective tissue. In this section, the major steps in this process are discussed with emphasis on how a regulatory or structural gene defect could result in altered collagen production or stability, and ultimately in the fragile skeleton of OI.

A. Structure of Collagen and Its Gene

1. Collagen, the Protein

Although there are a minimum of 10 genetically distinct collagenous proteins,[173,174] type I is the most prevalent and germane to diseases of bone. It is principally found in bone, tendons, skin, ligaments, dentin, and sclera, and to a lesser extent in lung, blood vessels, and other visceral supporting tissues. Therefore, the heritable disorders involving type I collagen predominantly affect bone, ligaments, and skin, cause minimal involvement of visceral structures, and have no effect on cartilage (type II collagen) or basement membranes (type IV collagen). Type I collagen molecules are organized in a three-dimensional arrangement of crosslinks in fibers as interwoven fasicles surrounded by tissue-specific proteoglycans. Little is known of the precise organization of these macromolecular complexes. Therefore, attention has been focused on defining the biochemical nature of the individual fiber components in the absence of knowledge regarding those properties that normally facilitate their interaction. Thus, in the following discussion, the reader should bear in mind that a thorough understanding of the heritable connective diseases will be appreciated only when these basic interactions are unraveled.

The microfibril is the basic organizational unit of the collagen fiber.[175,176] It consists of five collagen molecules arranged in a three-dimensional cylindrical structure and in which individual molecules are placed in quarter stagger relative to their neighbors.[177] The overlapping periodic arrangement of the collagen molecules is reponsible for the cross striations observed at 640 Å in collagen fibers by electron microscopy.[178] Each collagen molecule within the microfibril is a rod-shaped structure composed of three polypeptide chains (alpha chains) arranged in a tight triple helical conformation. The type I collagen molecule is a heterotrimer composed of two identical $alpha_1$ chains and another structurally different $alpha_2$ chain, each containing 1000 amino acids. The triple helical conformation is the result of the repeating triplet Gly-X-Y that occurs approximately 330 times. The X position is filled with a proline; the Y position may be proline or hydroxyproline. Hydroxyproline is a posttranslational modification of the procollagen alpha chains unique to collagen that adds conformational stability to the helix at physiologic temperatures.[179] Certain lysine residues are hydroxylated and several of these are also mono- or diglycosylated with glucose and galactose. In the extracellular space, lysine and hydroxylysine residues participate in the covalent crosslinkage of adjacent collagen molecules. The formation of these crosslinks ultimately determines the strength of collagenous tissues; however, the formation of normal crosslinks requires that the preceding intra- and extracellular steps of fiber formation were accomplished correctly.[180]

Since the recurring Gly-X-Y triplet is invariant in all collagens, it can be inferred that this sequence is required for normal triple helical conformation. In fact, the presence of the glycine in the first position permits the chain to maintain a tightly coiled state; a substitution of any other amino acid for a glycine will disrupt the highly ordered structure of the helix.[181] Under experimental conditions, when the temperature is elevated to 41.5° C, the triple helix of normal collagen will begin to melt or uncoil. However, if the collagen molecule contains a mutation that disrupts its tight helical configuration, the melting temperature may be less than physiologic levels.[182-184]

Not only is the correct primary amino acid sequence of the alpha chain essential to the formation of the triple helix; it also contributes polar and nonpolar charges (domains) on the exterior of the triple helix that are essential for orderly fibril formation.[176,181] Fibril aggregation occurs spontaneously *in vitro* without the aid of enzymes or other extracellular proteins.[185-187] Ultimately, the stability of the microfibril is derived from enzyme-generated covalent crosslinks that form once the collagen molecules are arranged in register within the microfibril.[180] It is also assumed that noncollagenous proteins and glycosaminoglycans interact with the microfibril, leading to a fiber composed of many microfibrils[188-190] and further stabilized by covalent crosslinks. Thus, the formation of a collagen fiber with normal tensile strength represents the composite effect of many layers of organization that ultimately depend on the correct amino acid sequence of the collagen alpha chains. Depending on the type, size, and location of mutation within an alpha chain, there may be sufficient disruption of the triple helix to impair formation of the microfibril and crosslinks.[191,192] However, other mutations may not affect microfibril assembly but instead act to specifically reduce the extent of crosslinking. The location, size, and type of such molecular defects may determine whether the subsequent phenotype resembles either OI (disordered helix) or Marfan's syndrome (altered crosslink formation).

2. Collagen, the Gene

The structure of the human collagen genes has been defined in great detail.[193-195] Like other genes, it is not continuous but has regions that code for mRNA (exons) and intervening regions that are not present in mature mRNA (introns; see Fig. 17–8, step A). There is one copy of each collagen gene per haploid set of chromosomes; alpha$_1$(I) is located on chromosome 17, whereas alpha$_2$(I) is on chromosome 7.[196,197] The enormous size and complexity of these collagen genes have limited the study of human diseases of connective tissue. In contrast to the beta globin gene of hemoglobin, which is 2.0 Kb in size with three exons, the collagen genes contain 50 to 51 exons spaced over a range of 18 to 49 Kb. The size of the exons ranges from 54 to 450 bp: most are less than 100 bp in size. Within the helical coding region, most of the exons code for amino acids in multiples of 18 that begin with glycine and end with the Y position codon.[198,199] The relative position and size of each exon are fairly constant between collagen genes, but the intron size varies widely. The gene also codes for the precursor procollagen propeptides (see later) and contains a transcription control region (promoter) at the 5′ end of the gene and transcriptional termination signals at the 3′ end of the gene.[193,200,201]

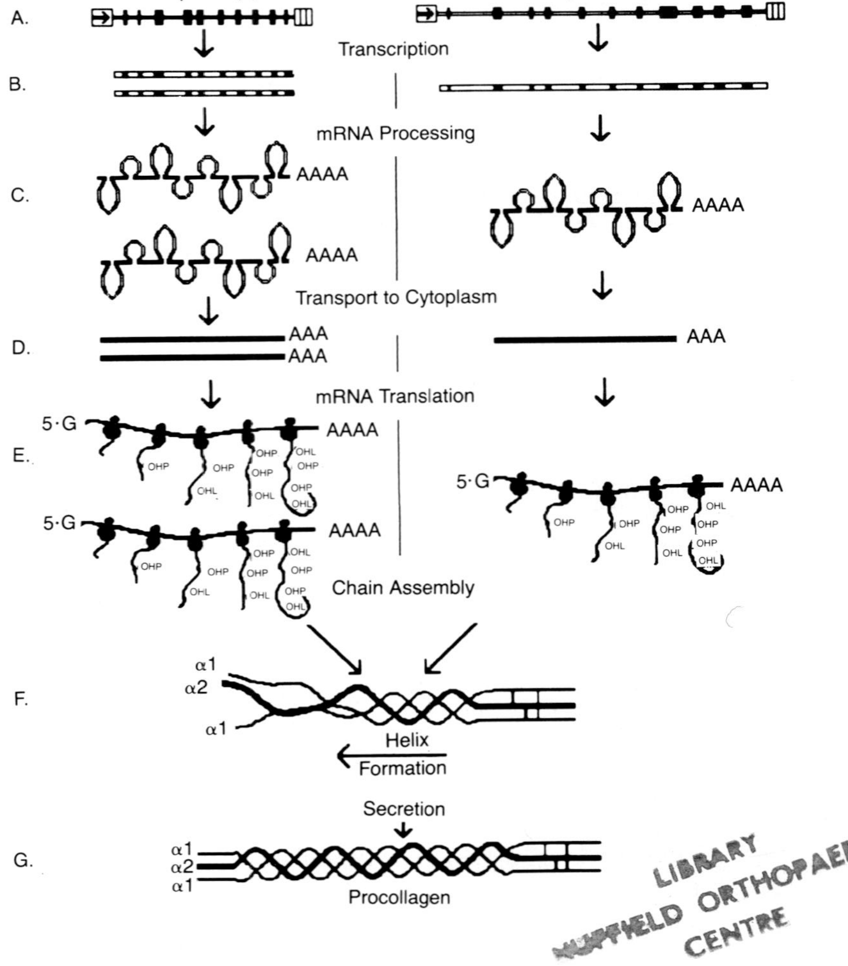

Figure 17–8. Normal type I collagen biosynthesis. There is one collagen allele per haploid set of chromosomes (step A), which transcribe two alpha$_1$(I) and one alpha$_2$(I) mRNA molecules (step B). Within the nucleus, the initial transcripts are spliced and polyadenylated to a mature mRNA (step C) prior to transport to the cytoplasm for translation (steps D and E). The alpha$_2$(I) and alpha$_2$(I) procollagen chains are synthesized in a 2:1 ratio that reflects the relative proportion of their respective mRNAs. The posttranslational modifications of the chain begin when the chain is being transcribed and continue until the molecule is completely assembled (step E). Molecular assembly begins at the C-terminal propeptide and extends to the N-terminal propeptide (step F). Once completed, the procollagen molecule is secreted from the cell (step G), in which subsequent steps incorporate it into a mature collagen fibril.

B. Collagen Biosynthesis and Assembly

1. Gene Transcription and mRNA Processing

Similar to other eukaryotic genes, the collagen promoter contains a TATA sequence that directs the start of transcription 30 bases "downstream" (Fig. 17–8, step A). Sequences up to 150 bases 5′ to the TATA region are highly conserved within mammalian species and appear to be crucial to the transcriptional activity of the gene.[201-204] Mutations in any of these regions would diminish the activity of the gene, although those mRNAs transcribed from the gene would be structurally normal. These upstream regions presumably contain hormone-binding sites that control the varied responses that are induced in bone collagen production by such hormones as parathyroid hormone (PTH), 1,25(OH)$_2$ vitamin D, extracellular fluid (EGF), and insulin.[205-208] One characteristic of collagen is that while the same structural genes are active in both mesenchymal and bone cells, it is the bone cell that produces the most collagen, apparently in a highly regulated manner. Furthermore, only type I collagen is produced by bone cells, whereas other collagen types (III and V) in addition to type I are produced by mesenchymal fibroblastic cells. This implies that factors unique to bone cells regulate these genes, since the primary gene sequence is identical in all cell types. One such element within the collagen gene complex that may account for the specialized regulation of type I collagen in osteoblasts is a tissue-specific gene enhancer.[209] Other genes are known to contain enhancer sequences either upstream from the start site or within the body of the gene that permit it to be active in certain specialized cells but not in others.[210,211] Recently an enhancer element located in the first intron of type I collagen has been identified.[212] It can be anticipated that a wide range of bone-specific disorders may result if these controlling sequences within the type I collagen genes were altered by mutations.

Although there is one copy for each type I collagen allele, twice as much alpha$_1$(I) mRNA is present in the nucleus and cytoplasm as the alpha$_2$(I) mRNA (Fig. 17–8, step B). At this point it is not known if this difference in alpha chain ratio is due to more active transcription of the alpha$_1$(I) gene or a shortened half-life or altered processing of the alpha$_2$(I) mRNA. The primary mRNA transcript of the gene contains both introns and exons that, while within the nucleus, are processed into mature mRNA (Fig. 17–8, step C). For type I collagen, this requires that 49 to 50 splicing events must occur to remove all the introns. This process recognizes mRNA sequences that flank the boundaries of the intron in addition to sequences within the body of the intron.[213,214] Although specific mutations causing altered splicing of a collagen gene have yet to be positively identified, a variety of alterations can be anticipated that resemble those identified in the hemoglobinopathies. In these disorders, mRNA species that are incompletely spliced either are not transported to the cytoplasm or cannot act as a normal translational template.[215,216] In either case, the amount of normal protein produced by the affected allele is reduced or absent, resulting in a null allele. However, the protein made from the mRNA transcribed from the other allele is normal. Polyadenylation must also be completed before a functional mRNA is transported to the cytoplasm.[217]

2. Procollagen Assembly and Secretion

Fully processed nuclear procollagen mRNA is transported to the cytoplasm and translated into a procollagen alpha chain in the rough endoplasmic reticulum[218] (Fig. 17–8, step D). The initial size of the polypeptide chain is approximately 1750 amino acids composing four specific domains:

1. A hydrophobic leader sequence that directs the nascent procollagen chain into the Golgi apparatus, during which time the leader sequence is cleaved.[219] It is within the Golgi apparatus that the posttranslational hydroxylation steps are initiated, which continue until helix formation is complete (Fig. 17–8, step E).
2. The N-terminal propeptide, a 200–amino acid region that may regulate procollagen mRNA translation,[220] and may also affect the size of a collagen fiber.[221] The likelihood of translational regulation of procollagen mRNA is strongly suggested by a highly conserved nucleotide sequence within the 5′ nontranslated region of procollagen mRNA.[222]
3. The helical domain, described previously.

4. The C-terminal domain, which contains the information that directs the initial alignment of the three pro alpha chains.[223] The completed pro alpha chains spontaneously adopt a triple helical conformation in a C→N terminal direction after the procollagen chains have been aligned and stabilized by intrachain disulfide bonds present in the C-terminal domain (Fig. 17–8, step F). Until the triple helix is complete, specific proline and lysine residues can be posttranslationally modified by hydroxylation and, in the case of lysine, glycosylation with glucose and galactose.[224] If the rate of helix formation is slowed, then the posttranslational modification process will continue, causing overhydroxylation and excessive glycosylation of lysine residues in the helical domain distal, or N-terminal, to the point of helix stability.[225] This polarity of posttranslational modification provides an indirect localization of a mutation.

The completed procollagen molecule is secreted from the cell by an exocytotic process that is poorly understood (Fig 17–8, step G). Mutant molecules with helical instability are inefficiently secreted from the cell and thus undergo intracellular degradation.[155] Specific extracellular procollagen peptidases cleave the N- and C-terminal propeptides, permitting the helical segment of the molecule to enter into the formation of the microfibril.[226] Lysyl oxidase, acting on specific lysine residues within the microfibril, initiates the formation of covalent crosslinks between procollagen molecules.[180]

Mutations within procollagen that alter its susceptibility to enzymatic cleavage of collagen have been described.[227] In contrast to most enzymatic diseases that have a recessive inheritance, these structural mutations affect the procollagen substrate for these enzymes. Dominant inheritance patterns occur because one half of the molecules that accumulate in the tissue contain the abnormality. Mutations that primarily affect this aspect of collagen biosynthesis do not result in OI but are associated with EDS and Marfan's syndrome. However, "overlap syndromes" with features of OI and EDS have been described that appear to result from mutations that destabilize the helix and affect the cleavage of the N-terminal propeptide.[34] Crosslinking may also be secondarily compromised when the unstable collagen molecule aggregates into an imperfect microfibril.[191,192]

C. Regulation of Bone Collagen Synthesis and Degradation

Although bone collagen synthesis and degradation are highly regulated by the calcitropic hormones,[205] cytokines, and growth factors,[228] the influence of these factors on collagen synthesis in OI is unknown. In a manner yet to be defined, the osteoblast can increase collagen production when sensing mechanical stress, while bone resorption occurs rapidly upon removal of mechanical or gravitational force.[229] The factor(s) mediating the increased bone turnover in certain forms of OI does not appear to be a primary or secondary alteration in calcitropic hormones. Clearly, areas for future research will be the mechanisms by which cytokines and locally acting growth factors and the structurally compromised collagen molecule each influence total collagen synthesis by the osteoblast.

V. BIOCHEMICAL AND MOLECULAR METHODS USED IN THE STUDY OF OI

Cultured dermal fibroblasts have served as osteoblasts from affected individuals as useful tissues in which to study abnormalities in the synthesis or structure of type I collagen. Although the regulation of type I collagen in the fibroblast is not the same as that of the osteoblast, genetic abnormalities of bone collagen are presumed to be accurately reflected by the collagen synthesized by the fibroblast. This is not surprising, since there is only one copy of each type I collagen gene per haploid cell, and therefore a mutation in the gene would be expressed in all cells that make type I collagen. Initial studies in OI characterized the abnormalities of type I collagen synthesis in OI, whereas newer techniques of gene cloning and endonuclease analysis have revealed the primary nucleotide alterations of collagen genes.[230] Because these methods are becoming the basis for understanding the defects in all heritable connective tissue diseases, it is necessary that the clinician appreciate their underlying principles.

A. Analysis of Collagen and Procollagen

When dermal fibroblasts are cultured with radiolabeled proline, the radioactive collagen and procollagen bands can be identified by their electrophoretic mobility within polyacrylamide gels. From this analysis, amino acid deletions or insertions within the protein may be detected (see following). Quantization of the density of bands on the autoradiograph can be used to estimate the production rate of type I collagen and its alpha chains. For example, diminished total synthesis can reveal a nonfunctional allele for one of the alpha chains.[231] It can also indicate unbalanced production of alpha chains, for example, if there is a population of molecules composed of three $alpha_1$(I) chains [$alpha_1$(I) trimer] rather than the normal heterotrimer of two $alpha_1$(I) and one $alpha_2$(I) chains.[232] Evidence for impaired secretion of procollagen molecules can be obtained by separately analyzing the medium and cell layer for their content of procollagen molecules.[155]

Polyacrylamide gel electrophoresis of procollagen alpha chains can demonstrate the presence of a gene deletion or insertion when it is greater than 30 amino acids.[182,233] Since each collagen allele is diploid, the presence of such a mutation often results in a widened or duplicate alpha chain band that represents both the normal and deleted alleles. Evidence for even smaller mutations within the collagen helix can be obtained.[225] Since a mutation may delay the rate of helix formation, this results in excessive posttranslational hydroxylation and glycosylation of lysine residues, which, in turn, results in a slowing of the migration rate within the acrylamide gel. A mutation of this type can be localized to a specific region of the helix if the collagen chains are cleaved into smaller fragments with cyanogen bromide and separated by electrophoresis. Since the collagen helix forms in a C→N terminal direction, those cyanogen bromide fragments having delayed migration must have been positioned N-terminal to the mutation site, whereas those with a normal gel migration rate should be positioned C-terminal to the site of mutation. Recent advances in protein microsequencing techniques may soon permit the identification of subtle mutations in type I collagen, particularly when the mutation can be localized to a specific cyanogen bromide fragment.[234]

The consequences of a mutation that destabilizes the triple helix can be demonstrated by measuring the thermal stability of the molecule.[34,183] The intact collagen helix is resistant to proteolytic enzymes such as pepsin or trypsin. However, when the temperature is elevated toward 41.5° C, the helix starts to unfold (denature) and becomes susceptible to the action of these enzymes. Thus, collagen molecules containing a mutation that destabilizes the helix will be degraded by these enzymes at or below physiologic temperatures.[182-184]

B. Molecular Hybridization

Under proper experimental conditions, complementary strands of nucleic acid will anneal or hybridize in a very precise manner.[235] The minimum length of homology between two strands is 50 to 100 nucleotide bases, although hybridization between even shorter lengths is possible. A cloned segment of DNA is made radioactive and is used to detect the presence of a complementary strand of DNA or RNA within a mixture of many other base sequences. The hybridization probe can be either genomic DNA (containing introns and exons) or complementary DNA (cDNA produced by reverse transcription of mRNA) and used to detect a specific DNA or mRNA base sequence. Both forms of cloned DNA to type I collagen genes are now available from a number of research laboratories. They were constructed in a bacterial plasmid from RNA extracted from cultured fibroblasts or isolated from a genomic "library" constructed in lambda phage. Recently, hybridization probes constructed with RNA have been introduced that have proved to have even greater sensitivity in detecting a complementary base sequence than that found for probes made from DNA.[236] The exquisite specificity of these probes is illustrated by the use of synthetic oligonucleotides for the detection of point mutations present in the hemoglobinopathies.[237,238] Using oligonucleotides of 19 to 21 bases, it is possible to detect the presence of a single nucleotide mutation within the total hemoglobin genomic DNA (containing over 10^9 bases) in patients with sickle cell disease or beta-thalassemia. This hybridization technique will be valuable for detecting the presence of a single base mutation within the large collagen genes and should permit highly precise genetic diagnosis.

At present, the following methods can be undertaken with existing molecular hybridization probes.

1. Southern and Northern Hybridization

A mixture of either DNA or RNA can be separated by molecular size within agarose gels and subsequently transferred and fixed to a nitrocellulose membrane. The membrane is incubated with a radiolabeled hybridization probe under defined conditions. After extensive washing, a complementary strand of RNA or DNA is identified by exposing the membrane to an x-ray film. When DNA is identified by this procedure, it is referred to as a Southern blot (after the originator's name), whereas RNA blots are termed "northern." In each case, only complementary sequences will be hybridized from a complex mixture of unrelated sequences. This method is also used to indicate the size of a particular complementary RNA species or restriction fragment of DNA (see next). The limit of resolution by this method is 50 to 100 bases.

2. Restriction Fragment Length Polymorphism (RFLP)

A recent application of the Southern hybridization technique that will have an important impact on the study of dominantly inherited forms of OI is that of RFLP.[239] Restriction fragments of DNA are generated by commercially available specific bacterial nucleases that cleave DNA through highly defined sequences 4 to 6 bases in length. Since these sites occur infrequently within genomic DNA, their presence can be used to map DNA in a highly reproducible manner.[230] The method of RFLP is based on the fact that certain restriction cleavage sites within genomic DNA are lost owing to silent base changes within the cleavage sequence. These variations are polymorphic within a population; however, within a family these base changes are transmitted as mendelian dominants. If a specific polymorphic site can be linked to the OI phenotype, then RFLP analysis of chorionic villus DNA can be used as a genetic marker for prenatal diagnosis.[240] The method does not itself indicate the site of the mutation, but it does demonstrate that the mutation is located within the gene adjacent to, or surrounding, the polymorphic site. Thus, the demonstration of a polymorphism linked to a specific OI phenotype would focus research effort to that alpha chain gene.

3. Analysis of Mutations Within Collagen mRNA

A method of greater sensitivity than that of the northern hybridization utilizes a probe that is radiolabeled at one end. After this probe is hybridized to its complementary strand (usually RNA), it is treated with the enzyme S1 nuclease. Because this enzyme cleaves only single-stranded DNA and RNA but not double-stranded DNA or a DNA/RNA duplex, the size of the protected (hybridized) radioactive probe after enzyme treatment or the presence of cleaved fragment will identify a region of hybridization mismatch. This method can detect a 3– to 4–base pair defect, but probably not a single-base mutation. Thus, although the S1 nuclease procedure represents a significant advance in sensitivity over the northern or Southern blot, even greater precision is needed to detect many of the point mutations present in genetic diseases. At this time, the only way to determine a 1–base pair mutation is via direct sequencing of the genomic DNA (see later). Other methods under development for analyzing the structure of collagen mRNA include R-loop mapping[241] and RNase protection.[242,243]

4. Quantitation of a Specific mRNA

The most commonly used method is referred to as a dot blot hybridization.[244] RNA extracted from tissue is diluted to different concentrations and fixed onto nitrocellulose membrane. After the RNA is hybridized to a specific radiolabeled cDNA, the intensity of the radioactive spot on the x-ray film is compared with the signal from an RNA standard. This permits calculation of the quantity of the specific RNA in the unknown sample. This method can be applied to RNA located within the cytoplasm or the nucleus of cultured cells and is valuable in studying regulatory mutations of collagen.[242]

C. DNA Sequencing

The advent of rapid DNA sequencing techniques now makes it possible to determine the amino acid sequence of a protein from the nucleotide sequence of its gene rather than by direct amino acid analysis of the protein. In this manner, vast knowledge about mutations present in the hemoglobinopathies has been gained by sequencing the entire hemoglobin gene.[245] However, this approach is not feasible for a complex gene such as collagen, for not only is the coding portion of the gene 10 times longer than beta globin, but the gene is diluted an additional 5- to 10-fold by intervening sequences. The first step is to localize the mutation within the expressed mRNA, or genomic DNA, using techniques of RNase protection or denaturing gradient acrylamide gel electrophoresis.[246] Although it is too early to state which of these approaches will ultimately prove useful, it is clear that precise localization of these mutations will be required before mutation-specific oligonucleotides can be generated and applied to unraveling the complexities of OI and the other heritable disorders of connective tissue.

An extremely powerful technique termed the polymerase chain reaction (PCR) has been recently applied to identification of mutations within specific domains of a gene. The procedure allows amplification of a 500 to 1000 bp segment from DNA obtained from a few cells, which can then be cloned or sequenced directly. The method is very rapid in determining the presence of a suspected mutation within genomic DNA and thus will have great utility in genetic diagnosis.[247]

VI. MOLECULAR PATHOPHYSIOLOGY OF OI

A sufficient number of cases of OI have been studied at the protein and molecular level to present an outline of the mutations of type I collagen that are associated with skeletal disease[25,248] (Table 17–2). Although many putative variants have been defined, the available data do not eliminate mutations affecting other components of the extracellular matrix. In the following discussion, the phenotypes are presented in decreasing order of clinical severity.

A. Lethal (Type II) OI

The majority of research effort has been spent with cultured dermal fibroblasts derived from this type of OI. The best studied case, first identified by Penttinen et al.,[249] has been shown to contain a 651–base pair deletion within the mid-portion of one of the $alpha_1$(I) alleles (Fig. 17–9, step A). This abnormality was first detected in the collagen $alpha_1$ chains by the presence of a doublet in the $alpha_1$(I) chain region by polyacrylamide gel electrophoresis.[155] Subsequently a doublet was demonstrated in the $alpha_1$(I) mRNA.[201] When the $alpha_1$(I) gene was analyzed, it could be shown that one allele lacked a certain restriction site, whereas another restriction fragment was shortened by about 500 bases.[250] The region of DNA containing the deletion has now been isolated and sequenced by two laboratories.[251,252] The analysis indicates that three exons and associated intervening sequences have been deleted, resulting in an mRNA lacking 252 bases, which, in turn, code for a procollagen chain deficient in 84 amino acids (Fig. 17–9, steps D and E).

Mutations that interrupt the helix weaken the stability of all the procollagen molecules containing at least one of the abnormal procollagen alpha chains.[182] The concept is referred to as the "suicide model" and proposes that three out of four procollagen molecules will have incorporated one or two of the abnormal $alpha_1$(I) alleles and will therefore be structurally unsound (Fig. 17–9, step G).[253] The important findings that have been derived from this case are:

1. The destabilized collagen helix is more susceptible to thermal denaturation, which renders the molecule susceptible to tissue proteases.[34,182,183]

2. Interruption of the helix decreases the rate of secretion of abnormal molecules from the cell, leading to dilation of the rough endoplasmic reticulum.[155] Thus, a reduced amount of collagen accumulates in the extracellular space, and that which is secreted is structurally unsound and susceptible to extracellular proteolytic digestion.[254]

3. Interruption of the helix leads to posttranslational overmodification of the lysine residues in the helical domain, N-terminal to the point at which the helix is disrupted.[255] This important point has been used to great advantage by Bonadio and Byers[256] to map the apparent mutations that interrupt the helix in other cases of lethal OI. Although the physiologic significance of these changes is uncertain, it may affect the quality of fibril formation or the generation of intermolecular crosslinks.[191,192,257]

Despite these dramatic findings, most cases of lethal OI do not have an $alpha_1$ chain

Table 17–2. Mutations/Gene Linkage Reported in OI Phenotypes

Phenotype	Collagen Type	Mutation	Reference
Type I	a1(I)	Functional deletion col 1 A1	Barsh (1)
	a1(I)	< mRNA a1(I)	Rowe (2)
	a1(I)	N terminal gly → cyst	Shapiro (3)
	a1(I), a2(I)	RFLP linkage to both	Sykes (4)
	a1(I), a2(I)	RFLP linkage to both	Beighton (5)
	a1/a2 mRNA ratio	Diminished collagen Production, ratios both Normal and reduced	Bateman (6)
Type II	Type I/III	Elevated III/I ratio	Pentinnen (7)
	a1(I)	Deletion 327–401	Barsh (8)
	a1(I)	Gly 988 → cyst	Cohn (9)
	a1(I)	Gly 391 → arg	Batemen (10)
	a1(I)	Gly 748 → cyst	Vogel (11)
	a1(I)	Gly 904 → cyst	Constantinou (12)
	a1(I)	Gly 664 → arg	Bateman (13)
	a1(I)	C,N-terminal mutants	Bateman (6)
	a1(I)	No structural mutation	Bateman (6)
	a1(I)	Gly 691 → cyst	Steinman (14)
	a2(I)	19 bp deletion, exon 10–11 Intervening sequence	Kuivaniemi (15)
	a2(I)	Gly 907 → aspar	Baldwin (16)
Type III	1(I)	Gly 526 → cyst	Starman (14)
	a1(I)	CB 8 charge change (#124–401)	Byers (17)
	a2(I)	Gly (CB4) → cyst	Byers (17)
	a1(I)/a2(I) ratio	Reduced type I, normal mRNA ratios	Bateman (6)
	a1(I) or a2(I)	No structural defect	Bateman (6)
		Overmodification	Bonadio (18)
	> a1(I) mRNA	> Type I production	Bateman (6)
	a1(I), a2(I)	< Type I production With slow migration of Both chains	Hollister (19)
	a2(I)	Only a1(I) trimer	Nichols (20)
	a2(I)	Above, 4 bp deletion C terminal	Pihlajaniemi (26)
Type IV	a2(I)	18 aa deletion (CB4)	Byers (21)
	a2(I)	Above localized to exon 12	Rowe (22)
	a1(I)	Gly ?? → cyst	DeVries (23)
	a2(I)	Gly 1012 → arg	Byers (24)
	a2(I)	10 aa deletion mid-helix	Wenstrup (25)

References
1. Proc Natl Acad Sci USA 79:3838–3842, 1982.
2. J Clin Invest 76:604–611, 1985.
3. J Bone Min Res 1989.
4. Lancet 2:69–73, 1986.
5. Ann NY Acad Sci 543:40–45, 1988.
6. Ann NY Acad Sci 543:95–105, 1988.
7. Proc Natl Acad Sci USA 72:586–589, 1975.
8. Proc Natl Acad Sci USA 82:2870–2874, 1985.
9. Proc Natl Acad Sci USA 83:6045–6047, 1986.
10. J Biol Chem 262:7021–7027, 1987.
11. J Biol Chem 263:19249–19255, 1988.
12. J Clin Invest 83:574–584, 1989.
13. J Biol Chem 263:11627–11630, 1988.
14. Ann NY Acad Sci 543:47–61, 1988.
15. J Biol Chem 263:11407–11413, 1988.
16. J Biol Chem 264:3002–3006, 1989.
17. Ann NY Acad Sci 543:117–128, 1988.
18. Nature 316:363–366, 1985.
19. Ann NY Acad Sci 543:62–72, 1988.
20. Lancet 1:1193, 1979.
21. J Clin Invest 71:689–697, 1983.
22. East Coast Conn Tissue Conf Hartford, CT, March 3, 1989.
23. J Biol Chem 261:9056–9064, 1986.
24. J Biol Chem 78:1449–1455, 1986.
25. J Clin Invest 78:1449–1455, 1986.
26. J Biol Chem 259:12941–12944, 1984.

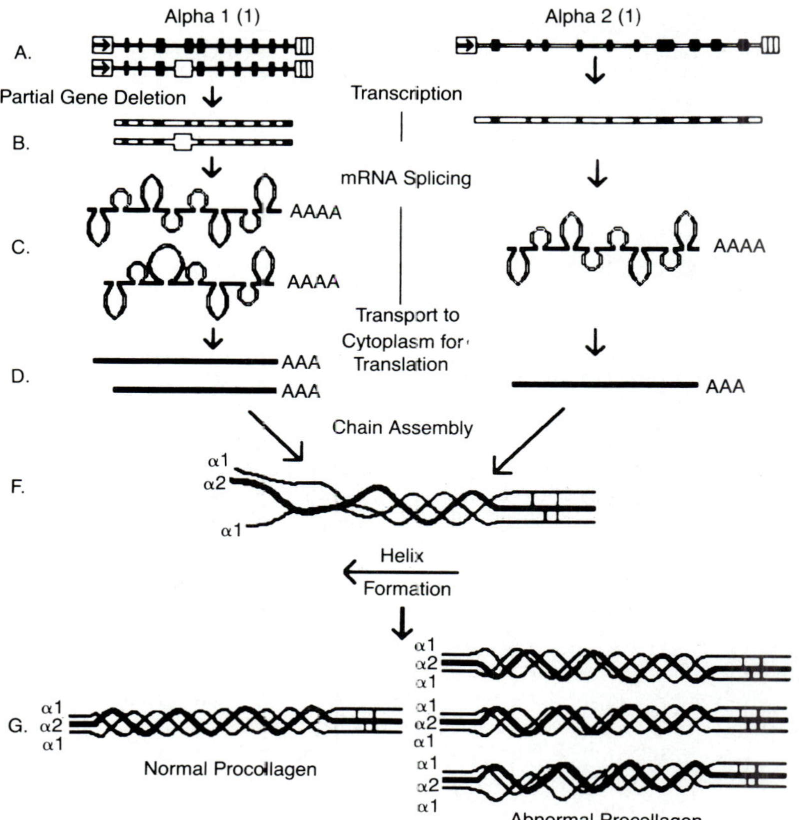

Figure 17–9. Type II OI. Deletion within one $alpha_1$(I) collagen allele. In this figure, both the normal and abnormal alleles of the diploid cell are depicted, whereas only one of the two normal $alpha_2$(I) alleles is shown. A deletion within one of the $alpha_1$(I) alleles (step A) leads to an initial transcript (step B) and mature mRNA (step D) that is shortened relative to the product of the normal allele. The mRNAs are translated into pro alpha chains that initiate assembly in a C→N direction (step F). Any molecule that incorporated the translated product of the shortened $alpha_1$(I) mRNA will disrupt the stability of the helix distal to the location of the deletion. Since the procollagen molecules will incorporate either one or two of the abnormal chains, three quarters of the resulting procollagen population will be structurally unsound (step G).

doublet, indicating that the mutation is below the resolution of this type of analysis. However, most cases do show a delay of alpha chain migration, suggesting posttranslational overmodification of lysine residues.[225] Byers has mapped the location of the putative mutation in some of these cases by determining which cyanogen bromide peptide has delayed migration on acrylamide gels. This analysis suggests that mutations in the C-terminal or mid-helical domains of the $alpha_1$(I) chain are common to the lethal form of OI. These findings were confirmed by Batemen et al.[258,259] and clearly shown to be the result of excessive hydroxylation and glycosylation of hydroxylysine residues consequent to the delay in helix formation.

The data suggested that a mutation below the size of biochemical detectability was disrupting the formation of the helix. This possibility has been well demonstrated by two cases in which a cysteine substitution was found within type I collagen molecules. This mutation was detected because cysteine is not normally present in the helical domain of type I collagen, and when it is present within two chains of the same molecule, it causes the chain to run as a dimer under nonreducing conditions. Besides cysteine, the other possible substitutions of first-position glycine include arginine, alanine, serine, aspartic and glutamic acids, tryptophan, and valine. An arginine substitution has recently been reported by Bateman et al.[260] In the case described by Steinmann et al.,[183] the cysteine mutation was found in a patient with type II OI; in the case of Nicholls et al.,[261] the child had a mild form of the disease. Recent nucleotide sequencing of the cloned DNA obtained from the lethal case demonstrated that the cysteine was a substitution for a first-position glycine.[262] In the mild case, there was no evidence of thermal destabilization of the molecules containing the mutation, suggesting that the cysteine was probably in an X or Y position.[263]

In a remarkable series of experiments, mouse cell culture DNA containing an $alpha_1$(I) cysteine for celycine mutation was microinjected into fertilized mouse eggs and reimplanted for development *in utero*. Several offspring demonstrated a phenotype consistent with skeletal changes in lethal OI.[263a]

In summary, the unifying abnormality in most forms of lethal OI appears to be the deletion of genetic material or a point mutation of a first-position glycine that has a deleterious effect on the stability of the helix. As a rule, the severity of the disease may be related to the location of the mutation. The more C-terminal within the helix, the greater the length of unstable helix. It should be anticipated that there will be a spectrum of clinical severity ranging from perinatal lethal to severe type III OI reflecting the locus of the mutation and the length of the destabilized collagen helix.

In several of the patients studied to date, the structural mutations found in the lethal cases of OI have not been found in either parent. These probably represent new mutational events rather than recessive inheritance as previously suggested from clinical data. However, genetic counseling must be tempered by the possibility that it represents a germ-line mutation in one of the parents.[26] The presence of a genetic compound is suggested by other cases. In the best example, the child had a deletion within the alpha$_2$(I) chain from the maternal allele while the other alpha$_2$(I) allele was not producing an mRNA transcript.[264] As noted previously, most isolated mutations within the alpha$_2$ chain do not result in lethal OI. However, it is probable that this case was lethal because all of the alpha$_2$(I) molecules produced contained a deletion. The father, who contributed the nonfunctional alpha$_2$(I) allele, did not have obvious clinical stigmata of OI. A second probable example of a genetic compound resulting in lethal OI occurred in a family with type I OI.[265] In both cases, had the same mutation been present in a different genetic background, the result might have been a milder form of the disease. The recurrence risk in a genetic compound would be the same as that occurring with the new mutation, since the milder trait by itself would not result in severe disease. It is also probable that a genetic compound could occur by the combination of asymptomatic mutations within either of the alpha chains contributed from either parent. In this case, there would be a 25% recurrence risk. Clearly, accurate genetic counseling will require precise definition of the mutation(s) present in the affected infant and screening the parents and even subsequent fetal tissues for the same mutations.

B. Severe (Type III) OI

Although this is the most severe of the nonlethal forms of OI, a clear biochemical basis for the disease has not yet emerged. In the best studied case (Fig. 17–10), the affected child failed to synthesize alpha$_2$(I) chains and instead produced a type I alpha collagen trimer.[232,266] However, the cultured fibroblasts do contain alpha$_2$(I) mRNA, and nascent procollagen alpha$_2$(I) chains can be demonstrated intracellularly.[267,268] An S1 nuclease analysis of the collagen mRNA from this case demonstrated a 4–base pair deletion.[269] This type of deletion places the remainder of the mRNA codons out of the correct reading phase (frameshift mutation) so that all the amino acids distal to the mutation are nonsense.[270] The location of this mutation is in the C-terminal propeptide that is essential for initial procollagen chain assembly. Since both alleles are affected (the child was the product of a consanguineous union), no alpha$_2$(I) chains are found within the procollagen molecule. The alpha$_1$(I) trimer is able to form a helix although it is less stable than the heterotrimer, and it shows biochemical evidence of excessive posttranslational modification.[271] It is interesting to note that another case with deficient alpha$_2$(I) chain synthesis has been described in a patient with Ehlers-Danlos syndrome and no bone disease.[272] This finding points out that the type I collagen genes are not necessarily expressed in a similar manner in all tissues and urges caution in extending results from cultured fibroblasts as necessarily reflective of events within bone.

No other cases resembling this mutation have been observed, nor have deletions similar to those described under lethal OI been reported within either alpha chain. However, evidence of overmodification of the lysine residues (delayed alpha chain migration) suggestive of a mutation that disrupts the stability of the helix has been found.[273,274] Byers has mapped these lesions to the N-terminal domain of the alpha$_1$(I) chain or the C-terminal region of the alpha$_2$(I) chain.[275]

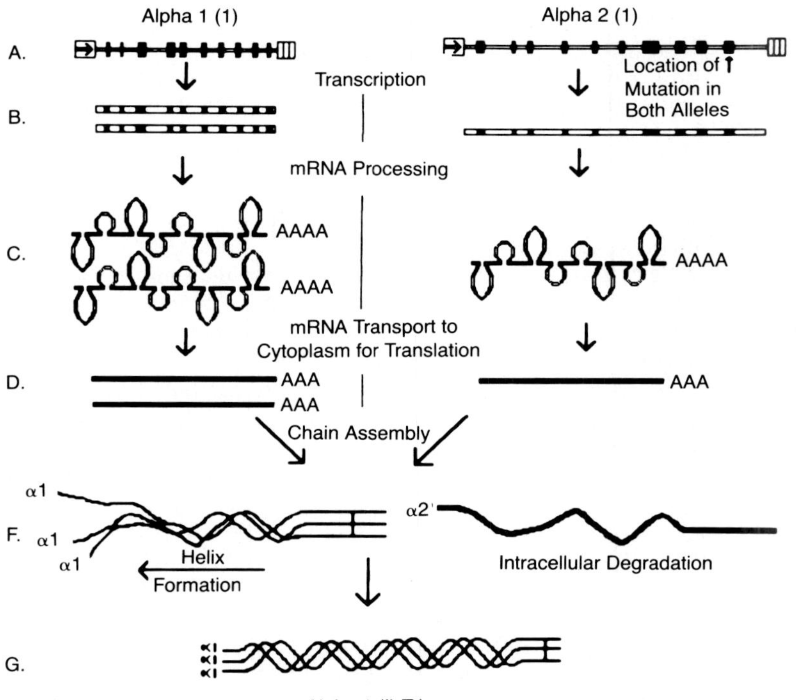

Figure 17–10. Type III OI. Failure of alpha$_2$(I) production. Both alpha$_2$(I) alleles of the diploid cell contain the same mutation, which is a 4–base pair deletion, which places the remainder of the coding region out of phase. The process of transcription and mRNA processing is unaffected. Because the frameshift mutation changes the amino acids within the alpha$_2$(I) C-terminal propeptide that is required for chain assembly, this chain does not become incorporated into the procollagen molecule (step F). The result is an alpha$_1$(I) trimer that is not sufficient to replace the function of the normal heterotrimer. The unincorporated alpha$_2$(I) chains are degraded intracellularly. The parents of this infant are obligate heterozygotes for this mutation and do synthesize a mixture of normal and homotrimer molecules. They do not have OI but may have premature osteoporosis.

A bovine model of OI that resembles type III OI may also give insight into the molecular abnormalities of the OI type. In one form of bovine OI (Texas variant), a defect in accumulation of osteonectin within bone has been demonstrated,[276] although the cultured bone cells are able to synthesize this protein. A second variant, the Australian form of bovine OI, shows normal osteonectin and bone sialoprotein, but depletion of bone proteoglycan has occurred in the Texas variant.[277] With the recent molecular cloning of the osteonectin gene, it will become possible to discern the role of important noncollagenous protein of wormian bone.

In certain cases the inheritance of severe nonlethal OI appears to be autosomal recessive.[28] However, undisclosed genetic compounds could be present. Not only could a compound mutation affecting the two collagen chains exist, but mutations affecting other noncollagenous bone proteins and proteoglycans could be involved.[278] Until precise methods of diagnosis are available, it is safest to counsel a 25% risk of recurrence.

C. Mild Deforming (Type IV) OI

Patients with this type of OI have been shown to synthesize two populations of type I collagen. One contains pro alpha$_2$ chains that migrate normally in polyacrylamide gels; the other contains slowly migrating chains. The slow chain contains a mutation within the alpha$_2$(I) chain located in one case, toward the N-terminal domain of the helix (Fig. 17–11). In this patient, a deletion of approximately 18 amino acids was detected by the presence of a doublet of the alpha$_2$ chain on acrylamide gel electrophoresis.[233] The effect of such mutations is to lower the melting temperature of molecules containing alpha$_1$(I) and alpha$_2$(I) chains.[279,280] In another case, a deletion of about 10 amino acids from the middle of the triple helical domain caused delayed migration of both the mutant pro alpha$_2$ and pro alpha$_1$ chains due to posttranslational overmodification. A cysteine for glycine substitution has also been reported in type IV disease.[281]

The inheritance of this form is stated to be autosomal dominant, although many sporad-

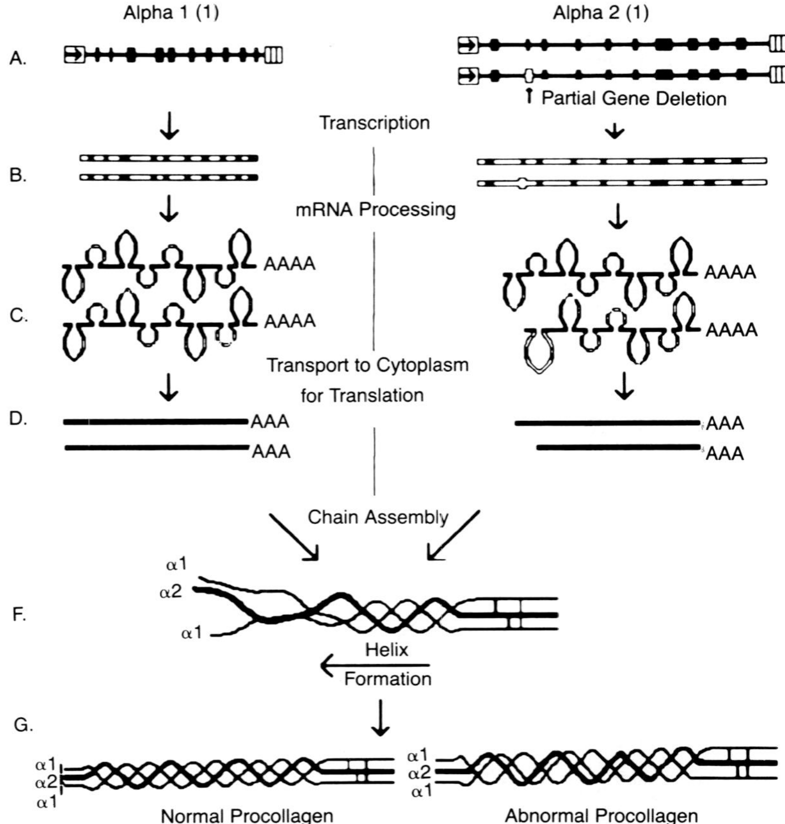

Figure 17–11. Type IV OI. Deletions within the helical domain of the alpha$_2$(I) gene. In this illustration, both alleles of the alpha$_2$(I) gene of the diploid cell are shown, whereas only one of the two normal alpha$_1$(I) alleles is depicted (step A). The two alpha$_2$(I) alleles give rise to two populations of mRNA, which are either normal or shortened in length (steps C and D). Similarly, two populations of alpha$_2$(I) molecules of different size are synthesized that become incorporated into the procollagen molecule (step F). Those molecules containing the abnormal alpha$_2$(I) chains have reduced helical stability. Since only 50% of the total procollagen population contains the abnormal alpha$_2$(I) chain, the severity of OI with this type of mutation is less severe than when the mutation is within the alpha$_1$(I) chain.

ic cases can be documented. Since many families with this form of OI do have a strong dominant pedigree, it has been possible to use RFLP for accurate genetic diagnosis. (Please refer to section V.B.2 for the basis of RFLP in biochemical diagnosis of genetic diseases). In the best-studied case, a family with type IV OI in three generations showed linkage to the pro alpha$_2$(I) gene on chromosome 7.[282] Analysis of this family indicates a deletion of about 10 amino acids within the N-terminal region of the alpha$_2$ chain[280] is present in affected individuals.

D. Mild Nondeforming (Type I) OI

The abnormality common to type I OI leads to a decrease in the production of type I collagen rather than a structural mutation of the protein (Fig. 17–12). The mutation is expressed in fibroblasts in cell culture as an elevation in the ratio of type III to type I collagen.[283] Recent studies utilizing RFLP analysis indicate that mutations may affect both the alpha$_1$(I) and the alpha$_2$(I) procollagen genes.[284-286] Underlying the reduction in type I collagen synthesis in one of these variants is one silent allele for the alpha$_1$(I) chain that results in half-normal alpha$_1$(I) mRNA levels. Since a stable collagen molecule requires two alpha$_1$(I) chains,[287] the net production of type I collagen is limited by the availability of the alpha$_1$(I) chains.[231] Among possible mechanisms to account for a silent allele is an abnormality of mRNA splicing. When this occurs in the beta globin gene in beta-thalassemia, an accumulation of the abnormally spliced mRNA can be demonstrated in the nucleus with a concomitant reduction in the cytoplasmic beta globin mRNA.[215,216] In type I OI, we have found reduced levels of alpha$_1$(I) mRNA in the cytoplasm[283] and accumulation of alpha$_1$(I) mRNA in the nucleus.[242] We hypothesize that these findings represent a splicing mutation of the alpha$_1$(I) collagen mRNA. Biochemical identification of the mutation linked to the pro alpha$_1$(I) gene in type I (mild) OI has not been reported.

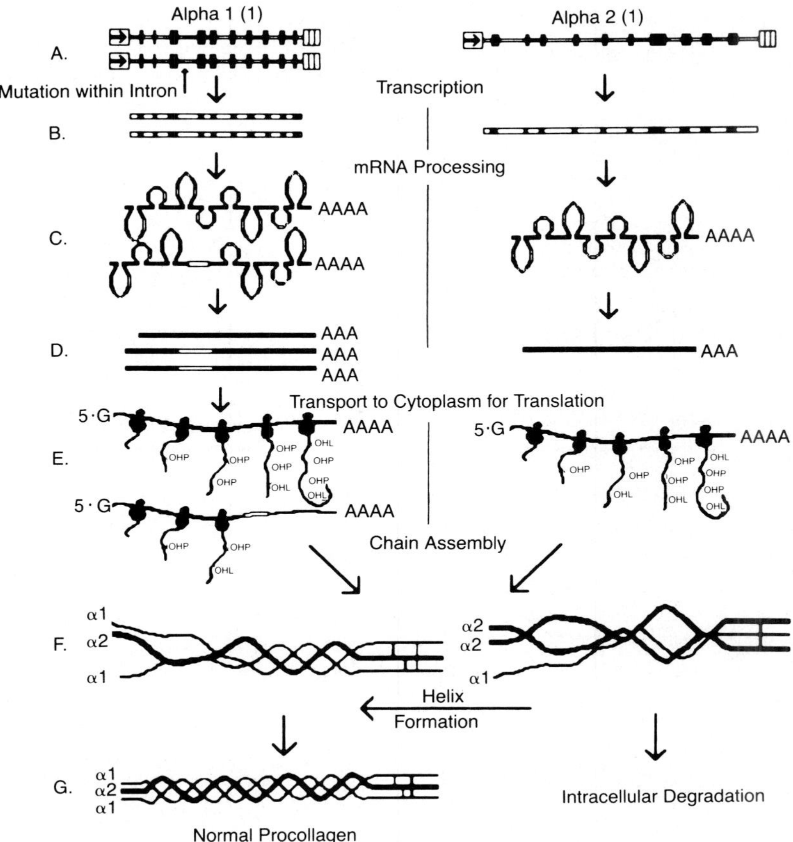

Figure 17–12. Type I OI. Functionally inactive alpha$_1$(I) allele. Both the normal and abnormal alleles of the alpha$_1$(I) gene present in the diploid cell are shown, whereas only one of the normal alpha$_2$(I) alleles is illustrated (step A). In this mutation, those mRNAs transcribed from the allele that contains a mutation that alters the steps of mRNA maturation do not readily enter the cytoplasm for translation (step E). This reduces the total amount of alpha$_1$(I) mRNA within the cytoplasm. Instead the abnormal mRNA accumulates within the nucleus (steps C and D). Those abnormally processed mRNAs that reach the cytoplasm do not produce a normal alpha$_1$(I) chain because the intron contains stop codons that prevent the completion of the chain (step E). The net effect is the synthesis of alpha$_1$(I) and alpha$_2$(I) procollagen chains in a 1:1 ratio instead of a 2:1 ratio. Since a stable type I collagen molecule requires two alpha$_1$(I) chains, the output of normal molecules is reduced by 50% (steps F and G). The alpha$_2$(I) chains present in excess are degraded intracellularly, since a molecule composed of two or three alpha$_2$(I) chains is unstable (steps F and G).

Dominant inheritance is usually present in most families with type I OI although the variability in severity may be such that mildly affected individuals may go undetected. Since the biochemical findings are quite distinctive, once the abnormality can be demonstrated in affected individuals, it can be used to identify mildly affected family members. Family studies indicate that the disease can result as a new mutation that is then transmitted as a dominant trait.

E. Syndromes with Shared Features

An interesting family with a dominantly inherited syndrome of joint and skin laxity, blue sclerae, and increased fracture history was reported by Sippola et al.[34] The molecular basis for the disorder was a small deletion at the extreme N-terminal portion of the alpha$_2$(I) chain. The effect of this mutation is an alteration in the rate of conversion of procollagen to collagen. This type of change has been observed in EDS VII and is due to a mutation that affects the N-terminal procollagen peptidase cleavage site of the alpha$_2$(I) chain.[227] Apparently the deletion present in this family places the cleavage site out of register with other determinants for the procollagen peptidase. The abnormality also destabilizes a small portion of the collagen helix, which may account for the bone fragility. Two different cases with this phenotype have now been described that result from an abnormality of RNA processing that causes skipping of exons that either delete or misalign the N-propeptide cleavage site.[288,289] It is likely that other overlap syndromes that manifest findings of EDS and Marfan's syndrome will have mutations that either destabilize the helix or affect the rate of collagen synthesis and also affect other functional aspects of the collagen molecule.

F. Heritable Osteoporosis

Pedigrees demonstrating familial transmission or clustering of osteopenia have been identified.[43] Subjects with this phenotype also display scoliosis and mild joint laxity. From the experience gained studying the milder forms of OI, there is reason to believe that abnormalities of type I collagen (or other matrix components) may be present in certain of these families. For example, the parents of the child with type III OI who lacked alpha$_2$(I) chain production each carried one of these abnormal alleles. Although they had never experienced fracturing, there was radiographic evidence of osteoporosis.[25] Based on experience in the beta-thalassemias, the amount of normal globin mRNA produced from an allele containing a splicing mutation can be extremely variable.[290] Thus it can be expected that variable degrees of osteopenia, reflecting the underlying defect of collagen mRNA processing, could account for the transition in phenotype between type I OI and heritable osteoporosis.

VII. THERAPY

The physician involved in the treatment of OI assumes responsibility not only for acute events (e.g., fractures) but also for chronic care including physical and psychological support for both the patient and the family. This must be a team effort: excellent orthopedic care in the absence of competent physical therapy will prove inadequate. A general pediatrician or internist should also be part of the team to evaluate the growth and development of the child with OI and care for the medical complications that appear in adulthood. Among the latter are pulmonary infection and respiratory insufficiency in severely affected patients of any age, dental care for those with DI, evaluation and treatment of hearing loss, and detection of secondary diseases that may aggravate the skeletal disorder such as diabetes mellitus, thyroid disease, or parathyroid disease.

Health professionals who treat this disease must appreciate the psychological needs of parents and the patient who is facing yet another crisis precipitated by a major fracture.[291] Families frequently relate stories of medical personnel who are insensitive to their pain or disability, or who do not appreciate the specific needs required by an individual with brittle bones. Parents are willing to teach the health team how they have learned to deal with these problems, but often find that the caregiver does not heed this advice. It is particularly important for the health professionals to listen and learn from their patients with OI.

A. Medical Therapy

A variety of hormones and mineral supplements considered effective in strengthening bone in postmenopausal osteoporosis and Paget's disease of bone have been administered to patients with OI. These have been summarized by Albright,[292] who noted that 70% of the articles on medical treatment of OI claimed positive results for 20 different agents. It is not surprising that each ultimately proved ineffective, since none attacks the primary defect in OI, that is, a failure to produce normal type I collagen. Modification of the collagen gene *in vivo* will be the ultimate curative therapy for OI. At this time, there is no effective hormonal, mineral, or vitamin therapy for any type of osteogenesis imperfecta.

From the pathophysiology of OI as revealed by the histomorphologic and molecular studies described previously, it is now evident that the rationale for the previous therapeutic trials was not well founded. Salmon calcitonin was intended to suppress bone resorption and thereby favor bone formation.[293] Controlled studies of calcitonin therapy have failed to confirm a significant effect on fracture rate or bone morphology.[294,295] Whereas it is true that certain forms of OI do have evidence of increased bone turnover, it is likely that defective bone collagen is the stimulus for this process. Inhibiting increased bone turnover would only lead to accumulation of more abnormal bone collagen and a compensatory fall in bone formation.

Several agents have been administered in an effort to increase bone formation. Clinical evidence suggests that anabolic steroids and estrogen therapy primarily decrease bone resorption; and effect on bone formation is probably minimal.[296] Ascorbic acid is a co-factor for prolyl hydroxylase, essential for the formation of stable collagen polymer. Recent *in vitro* studies have demonstrated that it increases collagen synthesis by increasing gene transcription and stabilizing collagen mRNA[297]; however, there is no evidence that there is ascorbic acid resistance in OI or that supplemental ascorbic acid can increase collagen synthesis.[298] Growth hormone can increase bone formation *in vivo*[299]; however, its primary rationale for use has been to increase stature (see later). Fluoride therapy appears to increase bone mass in osteoporosis by stimulating proliferation of new osteoblasts.[300] Since a hypercellular bone matrix is frequently found in OI, it is unlikely that fluoride will be of value in most cases of OI. Indeed, two trials indicate that it is not effective in OI.[128,301] Nevertheless, a therapy that could increase the production of type I collagen would be of value in those cases in which there is underproduction of an otherwise normal collagen mRNA. Before any trials of anabolic steroids or growth hormone are initiated, it will be important to restrict the trial to a patient group that is homogeneous for the inactive $alpha_1$(I) collagen allele.

Other agents have had an even less credible basis for their use. Calcium and vitamin D suplementation,[302] although not harmful when used in moderation, are inappropriate, since abnormalities in calcitropic hormones or calcium homeostasis have not been demonstrated. Magnesium supplements were intended to correct a postulated, but never confirmed, defect in pyrophosphate metabolism.[303] Furthermore, there is little evidence for an abnormality of matrix calcification in OI. The flavonoids, (+) catechins, were intended to revert collagen and glycosaminoglycan synthesis toward "normal."[304] Since these studies have not defined a specific abnormality, their use should be suspect. Flavonoids will decrease collagen production *in vitro*.[305,306]

With the increased availability of human growth hormone, there has been more interest in treating OI patients with severe growth retardation. Pharmacologic tests of growth hormone secretion in OI have demonstrated inconsistent variation of somatomedin C or growth hormone (see earlier). Of equal concern is the consequence of increasing the body mass on an imperfect skeleton, since the severest form of OI almost certainly results from defects in the structure of collagen rather than its reduced synthesis. Furthermore, the destruction of the growth plate that occurs in the severe forms of OI may be worsened by somatomedin C, which normally stimulates cartilage proliferation. It might be anticipated that this form of therapy could enhance the development of the "popcorn" deformity found in severe OI.

Any future medical therapies must have a solid theoretical basis and be evaluated in a biochemically homogeneous group of patients. Furthermore, no longer can a change in fracture rate be used as the sole criterion of efficacy. Instead, accurate measurements of bone mineral content using dual-photon absorptiometry or computed tomography will be necessary to provide periodic quantitative and nonbiased assessments during therapy. Once positive changes are revealed by these techniques, then reliance on fracture rate or change in bone morphology will be possible.

B. Surgical Therapy

The primary goal in the surgical therapy of OI should be directed toward reducing deformity and promoting normal function.[307] This means that fractures must be carefully managed to diminish the possibility of deformity while limiting the period of immobilization. Aggressive surgical therapy should be considered to maintain limbs in as near a functional condition as possible. Muscle strength should be maintained between episodes of fracture. This requires the anticipation of deformity following fractures or with weight-bearing, and the consideration of bone-straightening procedures even in severe, wheelchair-bound patients.[307a] Usually, realignment of a deformed limb requires the insertion of either a pin or rod once the deformity has been corrected by manual (osteoclasis) or surgical (osteotomy) techniques. Proper timing of the rodding procedure is important; early rather than late correction of deformity is advisable. This may mean inserting rods by age 3 to 5 years, depending on the child's mobility and extent of deformity. Rodriquez and Bailey[308] have described the internal fixation of the femur using an extensible intramedullary rod, with separate bone fragments being threaded onto the rod after the femur has been realigned. Percutaneous rodding allowing more frequent changes during growth has also been used.[309] Complications of rodding procedures include restriction of joint motion (although most patients gain nearly full range of motion at large joints), migration of the ends of the rod requiring reoperation, bending of the rod, non-union of the fractured fragments, and, rarely, development of hyperplastic callus.

Moorfield and Miller[66] have summarized the long-range results of corrective limb surgery in 31 OI adults studied an average of 19 years postoperatively. Preoperative complications of fracture included limb length discrepancy, exuberant callus, and common peroneal and radial nerve palsy. Eighteen patients were nonambulatory prior to surgery, and 13 used braces or crutches. At follow-up, only eight patients remained nonambulatory and wheelchair-bound, 18 were able to walk with braces or crutches, and five were independent. Of the 28 patients who had undergone a total of 174 operations (6.2 per patient), follow-up x-ray and clinical examinations revealed improvement of the deformity in 17, and no improvement in 11. The overall complication rate was 18%. Once rodded, many children are able to ambulate, sometimes walking for the first time, albeit using crutches or a brace. The positive impact on the child's psychosocial development may easily justify the surgical trauma and the risk of additional surgery. Upper limb surgery also involves insertion of a pin or rod (Sofield rod, Rush pins) following multiple osteotomies or external fracture and realignment of the limb. Rodding of the radius or ulna is more difficult than of the humerus, but is required less frequently.[310]

The surgical management of deformities of the spine has been reviewed by Benson and Newman.[71] Because mechanical support (Milwaukee brace, plaster bracing) is not generally useful in OI patients, these authors recommend the use of posterior correction, with fusion or the use of Harrington instrument inserted at an early age if the scoliosis exceeds 50 degrees. However, the complication rate is high. Yong-Hing and MacEwen[311] have reported that of 29 patients with posterior spinal fusion without bracing and 20 with bracing, there were five pseudoarthroses, two fractured rods, one case of rod protrusion through the skin, and seven cases of hooks being displaced. The general impression is that severe scoliosis resulting in pulmonary insufficiency cannot be reversed by surgical means.[311a]

C. Orthotic Therapy

In addition to the primary bone abnormality in OI, immobilization and the absence of weight-bearing further impede an improvement in skeletal mass and muscle strength in these patients. Furthermore, OI children have lax ligaments, which contribute to the instability of large joints. During cycles of fracture and repair, time spent on weight-bearing and exercise is lost. The prolonged use of body casts, and a reluctance on the part of the family or physician to urge physical therapy, cost dearly in the effort to maintain skeletal mass. For example, the stimulus for new bone formation provided by pubertal hormone secretion may be negated while an adolescent spends weeks or months recovering from a major fracture. Individualized orthotic care and rehabilitative therapy are key to gaining confidence and promoting independent activity once fractures have healed. As stressed by Binder et al.,[312] positioning of the infant with OI is critical to maintaining the strength of respiratory, spinal, and neck muscles. We have found swimming in a tub or heated pool to be one of the most useful procedures, and this can be started as early as 6 months of age in many children. A variety of exercises can be employed to assist muscle strengthening prior to ambulation. We have encouraged children to move in any manner and by any means as early as possible so that weight-bearing may strengthen limb and trunk muscles. However, ambulation is usually delayed depending on the extent of deformity and susceptibility to fracture.

Bleck[313] has proposed the principle of compression of the incompressible fluid muscle as one way of increasing the stress on bone. Plastic orthoses that conform to limb contour have been designed to promote more effective weight-bearing. The principle is to brace the child when ambulation is first anticipated. Binder et al.[312] have designed ultra-light polypropylene braces, extending to the pelvis and fitted for ischial weight-bearing (Fig. 17–13). The braces are initially cylindrical; knee joints are added after a year or so. The child's adaptability to these braces is quite remarkable. Trials indicate that children will readily adapt to mechanical support and will become fully active in braces: the positive psychological effect on both the child and family is remarkable. During a limited study, no exercise-related fractures occurred in four children

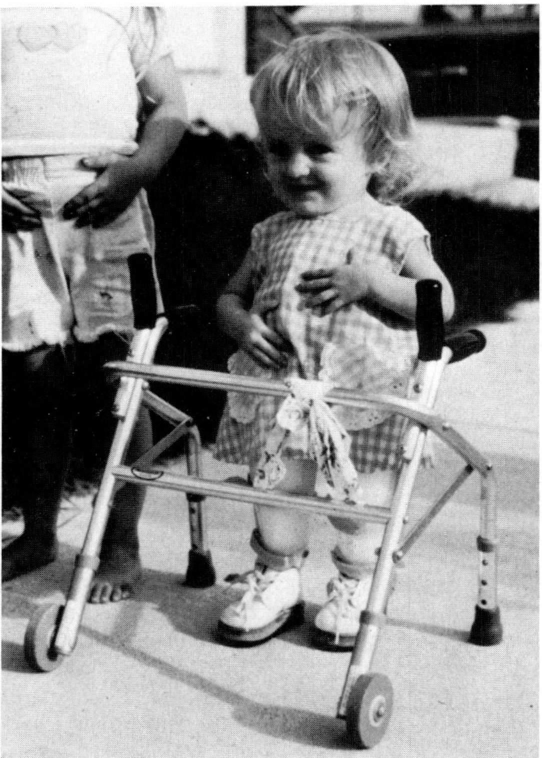

Figure 17–13. This 3-year-old child is standing in lightweight polypropylene braces, using a walker for support. Creative application of orthotic principles is essential to promote early ambulation, peer acceptance, normal schooling, and normal social development in the child with severe OI.

while they were in braces.[312] Weight-bearing walkers and A-frame orthoses have been designed to permit stress on the lower limbs without full weight-bearing. Children confined to a wheelchair require special support to minimize the risk of scoliosis. Additional work on this subject using controlled studies will be required before the effect of early weight-bearing on long bones or the spine in OI can be adequately assessed.

D. Psychological Supports

The stress of repeated hospitalizations and the need to adapt to prolonged immobility in the hospital or at home places an incredible strain on family life. Little attention has been devoted by the medical community toward an understanding of why some families succeed and others fail in this difficult task. Unlike with many other chronic illnesses, these families must rear a child with an exceptional intellectual potential, but whose disease will always limit the child's ability to compete with healthy peers. Continuing efforts to maximize physical and intellectual development are required to assure the achievement of independent living in spite of a significant physical handicap.[314,315] One avenue that we have found particularly useful is exposure of OI children to microcomputers as career aids. There are both community and national organizations such as the Osteogenesis Imperfecta Foundation, Inc. (Clearwater, FL) that are concerned with many of these issues. The physician who cares for an OI individual should make contact with the local OI group to learn of the resources available for his or her patient.

VIII. FUTURE DIRECTIONS IN OI

Because OI has such a severe and long-term impact on the patient and family, it is important that the clinician be aware of emerging diagnostic and therapeutic modalities. It is hard for the family to face their daily disappointments with OI if their physician is not enthusiastic about future developments that may affect the lives of their OI patients. The insights gained into the molecular basis of OI that have developed within the past five years are astounding. Recent advances in molecular technologies have led many investigators to feel that the tools to define any type of gene mutation are now available.[243,246] When these methods are applied to the problem of OI, the following developments can be anticipated.

A. Diagnosis

Rapid methods for detecting a previously defined molecular abnormality within the total cell genome are now possible with biochemically synthesized oligonucleotides specific for the mutated and normal DNA sequence.[237] This approach will permit identification of subjects carrying (or free of) a specific mutation in the collagen gene. The technique of gene amplification using the novel polymerase chain reaction will be particularly useful in detecting specific mutations.[238] Furthermore, application of gene amplification and mutation-specific oligonucleotides[247,316] to placental chorionic biopsy material will permit accurate diagnosis essential to informed genetic counseling. This will resolve the dilemma of the sporadic case as either a new or genetic compound mutation. In the latter case, the collagen sequence probes will uncover the subclinical expression in heterozygous parents carrying a subtle mutation in the collagen gene.

B. Therapy

In cases in which OI results from underproduction of a normal collagen, agents that stimulate collagen synthesis may have value. Not only would this benefit the child or adult with type I OI, but it might also aid the OI patient with a compound mutation when one of the abnormal alleles has an abnormality in mRNA processing. Precise definition of the molecular abnormality may suggest the optimal time to initiate sex hormone or growth hormone therapy in the prepubertal child with increasing deformities or scoliosis.

Dealing with a structural gene lesion will be more difficult. Gene therapy is ultimately going to have to be developed for this problem. Already insertion of foreign genes into animals using engineered retrovirus vectors[317] and microinjection of ova[318] has resulted in permanent expression of the foreign gene. The method has been used to correct a heritable defect in myelin basic protein associated with the Shiver (shi) mutation in mice.[319] As for OI, it is now possible to recreate a mutation in an animal model by insertion of an abnormal collagen gene in a developing embryo.[263a,320] Such an animal model will facilitate the study of various modes of therapy including the potential for correcting the defect postnatally by inactivation of the mutant gene or by insertion of additional copies of the normal gene. Eventually, it may be possible to detect the presence of OI during organogenesis and to introduce a corrective gene that prevents the development of the disease.

References

1. Gray PH: A case of osteogenesis imperfecta associated with dentinogenesis imperfecta dating from antiquity. Clin Radiol 20:106–108, 1969.
2. Weil UH: Osteogenesis imperfecta: Historical background. Clin Orthop 159:6–10, 1981.
3. Smith R, Francis MJO, Houghton GR: The Brittle Bone Syndrome. London, Butterworth, 1983, pp 5–7.
4. Malebranche N: Traite de la Recherche de las Verite. 4th ed, liv 2. Paris, 1674, chapter 7.
5. Eckman OJ: Dissertatio medica descriptinonem et casus aliquot osteomalaciae sistens. Dissertatio Medica Upsaliae, 1788.
6. Velpeau AALM: Subclavicular dislocation of the humerus. Gaz des Hopit Oiuils Et Militaires 62:265–266, 1847.
7. Spurway J: Hereditary tendency to fracture. Br Med J 2:844, 1896.
8. Eddowes A: Dark sclerotics and fragilitas ossium. Br Med J 2:222, 1900.
9. Adair-Deighton CA: Four generations of blue sclerotics. J Ophthalmol 10:188–189, 1912.
10. Bauer KH: Erbliche unvolkkommene Knochenohne dyskrasische Ursache als Krankhafte Eigenthumlichkeit drier Geschwister. Ann Ges Heilk Jahrg 4,H 1:58–61, 1940.
11. Seedorf KS: Osteogenesis imperfecta. A study of clinical features and heredity based on fifty-five Danish families comprising one hundred and eighty affected members (thesis). Opera ex Domo Biologiae Hereditariae Humane Universitatis Hafniensis, 20. Einar Munksgaard, Copenhagen, 1949.
12. Smars G: Osteogenesis Imperfecta in Sweden: Clinical, Genetic, Epidemiological and Socio-medical Aspects. Stockholm, Svenska Bokforlaget, 1961.
13. Looser E: Zur Kenntnis der Osteogenesis imperfecta congenita und tarda. Mitteilunger aus der Grenz. Der Med Chirurg 15:161–207, 1906.
14. Pyeritz RE: The Marfan phenotype: Pleiotrophy and variability as clues to genetic heterogeneity. *In* Akerson WA, Bornstein P, Glimcher MJ (eds): AAOS Symposium on Heritable Disorders of Connective Tissue. St. Louis, CV Mosby, 1982, pp 114–121.
15. Ibsen KH: Distinct varieties of osteogenesis imperfecta. Clin Orthop 159:279–290, 1967.
16. Sillence DO, Senn A, Danks DM: Genetic heterogeneity in osteogenesis imperfecta. J Med Genet 16:101–116, 1979.
17. Sillence D: Osteogenesis imperfecta: An expanding panorama of variants. Clin Orthop 159:11–25, 1981.
18. Shapiro JR, Rowe D: Collagen genes and brittle bones. Ann Intern Med 99:700–704, 1983.
19. Levin LS, Salinas CF, Jorgenson RJ: Classification of osteogenesis imperfecta by dental characteristics. Lancet 1:332–333, 1978.
20. Lubs HA, Travers H: Genetic counseling in osteogenesis imperfecta. Clin Orthop 159:36–41, 1981.
21. Bauze RJ, Smith R, Francis MJO: A new look at osteogenesis imperfecta. A clinical, radiological and biochemical study of forty-two patients. J Bone Joint Surg 57B:1–12, 1975.
22. Sillence DO, Barlow KK, Garber AP, et al: Osteogenesis imperfecta type II: Delineation of the phenotype with reference to genetic heterogeneity. Am J Med Genet 17:407–423, 1984.
22a. Tsipouras P, Shields EP, Silberberg D, Fraser FC: Genetics of osteogenesis imperfecta, type II. Pediatr Res 15:570 (abstract), 1981.
23. Langness U, Behnke H: Klinch genetik der genetics osteogenesis imperfecta. Dtsch Med Wochenschr 95:209–212, 1970.

23a. Young ID, Harper PS: Recurrence risk in osteogenesis imperfecta congenita. Lancet 1:432, 1980.
24. Byers PH, Bonadio JF, Steinmann B: Osteogenesis imperfecta: Update and perspective. Am J Med Genet 17:429–435, 1984.
25. Prockop DJ: Mutations in collagen genes: Consequences for rare and common diseases. J Clin Invest 75:783–787, 1985.
26. Byers PH, Tsipouras P, Bonadio JF, et al: Perinatal lethal osteogenesis imperfecta (OI type II)—a biochemically heterogeneous disorder usually due to new mutations in the genes for type I collagen. Am J Hum Genet 42:237–248, 1988.
27. Versfeld GA, Beighton PH, Katz K, Solomon A: Costovertebral anomalies in osteogenesis imperfecta. J Bone Joint Surg 67B:602–604, 1985.
28. Sillence DO, Barlow KK, Cole WG, et al: Osteogenesis imperfecta type III. Delineation of the phenotype with reference to genetic heterogeneity. Am J Med Genet 23:821–832, 1986.
29. Zeitoun MM, Ibraham AH, Kassem AS: Osteogenesis imperfecta in dizygotic twins. Arch Dis Child 38:289–291, 1963.
30. Robinson LP, Worthen NJ, Lachman RS, et al: Prenatal diagnosis of osteogenesis imperfecta type III. Prenat Diagn 7:7–15, 1987.
31. Patterson CR, McAllion S, Miller R: Heterogeneity of osteogenesis imperfecta type I. J Med Genet 20:203–205, 1983.
32. Carothers AD, McAllion SJ, Patterson CR: Risk of dominant mutation in older fathers: Evidence from osteogenesis imperfecta. J Med Genet 23:227–230, 1986.
33. Biering A, Iverson T: Osteogenesis imperfecta associated wtih Ehlers-Danlos syndrome. Acta Paediatr 44:279–286, 1955.
34. Sippola M, Kaffe S, Prockop DJ: A heterozygous defect for structurally altered proα2 chain of type I in procollagen in a mild variant of osteogenesis imperfecta. The altered structure decreases the thermal stability of procollagen and makes it resistant to procollagen N-proteinase. J Biol Chem 259:14094–15100, 1984.
35. Carey MC, Fitzgerald O, McKiernan E: Osteogenesis imperfecta in twenty-three members of a kindred with heritable features contributed by a nonspecific skeletal disorder. Q J Med 27:437–449, 1968.
36. Penttinen R, Sippola E, Kouvalainen K, et al: An arthropathic form of osteogenesis imperfecta. Acta Pediatr Scand 69:263–267, 1980.
37. Sharma NL, Anand JS: Osteogenesis imperfecta with arthrogryposis multiplex congenita. J Indian Med Assoc 43:124–126, 1964.
38. Johnson CC, Hui SL, Wiske R, et al: Bone mass at maturity and subsequent rate of loss as determinants of osteoporosis. *In* DeLuca HF, Jee S, Johnson C, Parfitt A (eds): Osteoporosis: Recent Advances in Pathogenesis and Treatment. Baltimore, University Park Press, 1981, pp 285–291.
39. Lane JM, Healey J: NIH Consensus Conference on Osteoporosis. Bethesda, 1984, p 79 (abstract).
40. Moller M, Horsman A, Harvald B, et al: Metacarpal morphometry in monozygotic and dizygotic elderly twins. Calcif Tissue Res 25:197–201, 1978.
41. Sowers MR, Burns TL, Wallace RB: Familial resemblance of bone mass in adult women. Genet Epidemiol 3:85–93, 1986.
42. Lutz J: Bone mineral, serum calcium, and dietary intakes of mother/daughter pairs. Am J Clin Nutr 44:99–106, 1986.
43. Shapiro JR, Rowe DW, Burn V: Familial osteoporosis pedigrees. J Bone Mineral Res 2 [Suppl 1]:344A, 1987.
44. Fallon MD, Teitelbaum SL, Weinstein RS, et al: Hypophosphatasia: Clinicopathological comparison of the infantile, childhood, and adult forms. Medicine 63:12–24, 1984.
45. Langer LO: Spondyloepiphysial dysplasia tarda. Radiology 82:833–839, 1964.
46. Sundkvist L: Thanatophoric dysplasia. A report of 3 cases. Acta Pathol Microbiol Immunol Scand 91A:335–341, 1983.
47. Silverman FN: The roentgen manifestations of unrecognized skeletal trauma in infants. AJR 69:413–427, 1953.
48. Hurwitz A, Castells S: Misdiagnosed child abuse and metabolic diseases. Pediatr Nurs 13:33–36, 1987.
49. Bachiocco R: Congenital hyperphosphatemia. Ital J Orthop Traumatol 9:533–539, 1983.
50. Mudd SH, Skovby F, Levy HL, et al: The natural history of homocystinuria due to cystathionine B–synthase deficiency. Am J Hum Genet 37:1–31, 1985.
51. Beighton P, Price A, Lord J, Dickson E: Variants of the Ehlers-Danlos syndrome: Clinical, biochemical, haematological, and chromosomal features in 100 patients. Ann Rheum Dis 28:228–245, 1969.
52. Evans RA, Dunstan CR, Hills E: Bone metabolism in idiopathic juvenile osteoporosis: A case report. Calcif Tissue Int 35:5–8, 1983.
53. Lane JM, Vigorita V, Falls M: Osteoporosis: Current diagnosis and treatment. Geriatrics 39:40–47, 1984.
54. Wynne-Davies R, Gormley J: Clinical and genetic patterns in osteogenesis imperfecta. Clin Orthop 159:26–35, 1981.
55. Orioli IM, Castilla EE, Barbosa-Neto JG: The birth prevalence rates for the skeletal dysplasias. J Med Genet 23:328–332, 1986.
56. Gunnar S: Osteogenesis Imperfecta in Sweden. Stockholm, Scandinavian University Books, 1961.
57. Komai T, Kunii H, Ozaki Y: A note on the genetics of Van der Hoeve's syndrome, with special reference to a large Japanese kindred. Am J Hum Gen 8:110–119, 1956.
58. Heiberg A: Osteogenesis imperfecta in Norway. A clinical and genetic study. Clin Genet 23:233 (abstract), 1983.
59. Robert JM, Gremeau JL, Notter A, Guilhot J: Hereditary bone fragility. Lyon Medical 219:881–982, 1968.
60. Beighton P, Spranger J, Versveld G: Skeletal complications in osteogenesis imperfecta. A review of 153 South African patients. S Afr Med J 64:565–568, 1983.
61. Patterson CR, McAllion S, Stellman JL: Osteogenesis imperfecta after the menopause. N Engl J Med 310:1694–1696, 1984.
62. Astley R: Metaphyseal fractures of osteogenesis imperfecta. Br J Radiol 52:441–451, 1979.
63. Bullough PG, Davidson DD, Lorenzo JC: The morbid anatomy of the skeleton on osteogenesis imperfecta. Clin Orthop 159:42–57, 1981.
64. Goldman AB, Davidson D, Pavlov H, Bullough PG: "Popcorn" calcifications: A prognostic sign in osteogenesis imperfecta. Radiology 136:351–358, 1980.

64a. Spranger J: Osteogenesis imperfecta: A pasture for splitters and lumpers. Am J Med Genet 17:425–428, 1984.
65. Sillence DO: Osteogenesis imperfecta: Nosology and genetics. Ann NY Acad Sci 543:1–15, 1988.
66. Moorefield WG, Miller GR: Aftermath of osteogenesis imperfecta: The disease in adulthood. J Bone Joint Surg 62A:113–119, 1980.
67. Roberts JB: Bilateral hyperplastic callus formation in osteogenesis imperfecta. J Bone Joint Surg 58A:1164–1166, 1976.
68. King JD, Bobechko WP: Scoliosis in osteogenesis imperfecta. Proc West Orthop Assoc J Bone Joint Surg 57A:136, 1971.
69. Falvo KA, Root L, Bullough PG: Osteogenesis imperfecta: Clinical evaluation and management. J Bone Joint Surg 56A:783–793, 1974.
70. Renshaw TS, Cook RS, Albright JA: Scoliosis in osteogenesis imperfecta. Clin Orthop Rel Res 145:163–167, 1979.
71. Benson DR, Newman DC: The spine and surgical treatment in osteogenesis imperfecta. Clin Orthop 159:147–153, 1981.
72. Smith R: Idiopathic juvenile osteoporosis. Am J Dis Child 133:889–891, 1979.
73. Pauli RM, Gilbert EF: Upper cervical cord compression as a cause of death in osteogenesis imperfecta type II. J Pediatr 108:579–581, 1986.
74. Schwartz S, Tsipouras P: Oral findings in osteogenesis imperfecta. Oral Surg 57:161–167, 1984.
75. Levin LS, Wright JM, Byrd DL, et al: Osteogenesis imperfecta with unusual skeletal lesions: Report of three families. Am J Med Genet 21:257–269, 1985.
76. Maroteaux P: Bone Diseases of Children. Philadelphia, JB Lippincott, 1979, p 108.
77. Cremin B, Goodman H, Spranger J, Beighton P: Wormian bones in osteogenesis imperfecta and other disorders. Skeletal Radiol 8:35–38, 1982.
78. Pozo JL, Crockard HA, Ransford AO: Basilar impression in osteogenesis imperfecta. A report of three cases in one family. J Bone Joint Surg 66B:233–238, 1984.
79. Frank E, Berger T, Tew JM Jr: Basilar impression and platybasia in osteogenesis imperfecta tarda. Surg Neurol 17:116–119, 1982.
80. Tsipouras P, Barbas G, Mathews WS: Neurologic correlates of osteogenesis imperfecta. Arch Neurol 43:150–152, 1986.
81. King JD, Bobechko WP: Osteogenesis imperfecta: An orthopedic description and surgical review. J Bone Joint Surg 53B:72–89, 1971.
81a. Wordsworth P, Ogilvie D, Smith R, Sykes B: Joint mobility with particular reference to racial variation and inherited connective tissue disorders. Br J Rheumatol 26:9–12, 1987.
82. Beighton P, Horan FT: Dominant inheritance of generalized articular hypermobility. J Bone Joint Surg 52B:145–147, 1970.
83. Follis RH Jr: Maldevelopment of the corium in the osteogenesis imperfecta syndrome. Bull Johns Hopkins Hosp 93:225–233, 1953.
84. Oxlund H, Pedersen U, Danielsen CC, et al: Reduced strength of skin in osteogenesis imperfecta. Eur J Clin Invest 15:408–411, 1985.
85. Reed WB, Pidgeon JW: Elastosis perforans serpiginosa with osteogenesis imperfecta. Arch Dermatol 89:342–344, 1964.
86. Scott D, Stiris G: Osteogenesis imperfecta tarda. A study of 3 families with special reference to scar formation. Acta Med Scand 145:237–257, 1953.
87. Witkop CJ Jr: Hereditary defects of dentin. Dent Clin North Am 19:25–45, 1975.
88. Gage JP, Francis MJ, Whitaker GE, Smith R: Dentine is biochemically abnormal in osteogenesis imperfecta. Clin Sci 70:339–346, 1986.
89. Levin LS, Brady JM, Melnick M: Scanning electron microscopy of teeth in dominant osteogenesis imperfecta: Support for genetic heterogeneity. Am J Med Genet 5:189–199, 1980.
90. Levin LS: The dentition in the osteogenesis imperfecta syndromes. Clin Orthop 159:64–74, 1981.
91. Smith R, Francis MJO, Houghton GR: The Brittle Bone Syndrome. London, Butterworth, 1983, p 49.
92. Beighton P: Familial dentinogenesis imperfecta, blue sclerae, and wormian bones without fractures. J Med Genet 18:124–128, 1981.
93. Bell J: Blue sclerotics and fragility of bone. Treasury of Human Inheritance, vol II, part III. Cambridge, Cambridge University Press, 1928.
94. Schmut O: The organization of tissues of the eye by different collagen types. Graefes Arch Clin Exp Ophthalmol 207:189–199, 1978.
95. Trelstad RL, Kang AH: Collagen heterogeneity in the avian eye: Lens, vitreous body, cornea, and sclerae. Exp Eye Res 18:395–406, 1974.
96. Reudeman AD: Osteogenesis imperfecta congenita and blue sclerotics. Arch Ophthalmol 49:6–16, 1953.
97. Eicholtz W, Muller D: Elektronenmikroskopische Befunde an der Hornhaut und sklera bei Osteogenesis imperfecta. Klin Monatsbl Augenheilkd 161:646–653, 1972.
98. Chan CC, Green WR, de la Cruz ZC, Hillis A: Ocular findings in osteogenesis imperfecta congenita. Arch Ophthalmol 100:1458–1463, 1982.
99. Kaiser-Kuper MI, McCain L, Shapiro JR, et al: Low ocular rigidity in patients with osteogenesis imperfecta. Invest Ophthalmol Vis Sci 20:807–812, 1981.
100. Smith R, Francis MJO, Sykes MB: The eye and collagen in osteogenesis imperfecta. Birth Defects 12:563–568, 1976.
101. Pedersen U, Bramsen T: Central corneal thickness in osteogenesis imperfecta and otosclerosis. J Otorhinolaryngol Relat Spec 46:38–41, 1984.
102. Haebara H, Yamasaki Y, Kyogoku M: An autopsy case of osteogenesis imperfecta congenita. Histochemical and electron microscopical studies. Acta Pathol Jpn 19:377–394, 1969.
103. Smith, Francis MJO, Houghton GR: The Brittle Bone Syndrome. London, Butterworth, 1983, p 43.
104. Bergstrom L: Osteogenesis imperfecta: Otologic and maxillofacial aspects. Laryngoscope 87 [suppl 6]:1–42, 1977.
105. Altmann F, Kornfeld M: Osteogenesis imperfecta and otosclerosis. New investigations. Ann Otol Rhinol Laryngol 76:89–104, 1967.
106. Riley FC, Brown DM, Jowsey J: Osteogenesis imperfecta: Morphologic and biochemical studies of connective tissue. Pediatr Res 9:757–768, 1973.
107. Soifer N, Altmann F, Endahl GL, et al: Biochemical studies of otosclerosis: Protein and enzymes in stapedes and cortical bone. Acta Otolaryngol 68:78–84, 1969.
108. Holdsworth CE, Endahl GL, Soifer N, et al: Comparative biochemical study of otosclerosis and osteogenesis imperfecta. Arch Otolaryngol 98:336–339, 1973.

109. Pedersen U: Osteogenesis imperfecta clinical features, hearing loss, and stapedectomy. Biochemical osteodensitometric, corneometric and histological aspects in comparison with otosclerosis. Acta Otolaryngol 415(S):1–36, 1985.
110. Igarashi M, King AL, Schwenzfeier CW, et al: Inner ear pathology in osteogenesis imperfecta congenita. J Laryngol Otol 94:697–705, 1980.
111. Zajtchuk JT, Lindsay JR: Osteogenesis imperfecta congenita and tarda: A temporal bone report. Ann Otol 84:350–358, 1975.
112. Shapiro JR, Pikus A, Weiss GG, Rowe DW: Hearing and middle ear function in osteogenesis imperfecta. JAMA 247:2120–2126, 1982.
113. Carruth JAS, Lutman ME, Stephens SDG: An audiological investigation of osteogenesis imperfecta. J Laryngol Otol 92:853–860, 1978.
114. Reidner ED, Levin S, Holliday MJ: Hearing patterns in dominant osteogenesis imperfecta. Arch Otolaryngol 106:737–740, 1980.
115. Hammer D, Leier CV, Baba N, et al: Altered collagen composition in a prolapsing mitral valve with ruptured chordae tendinae. Am J Med 67:863–866, 1979.
116. Heckman B, Steinberg I: Congenital heart disease (mitral regurgitation) in osteogenesis imperfecta. AJR 103:601–607, 1968.
117. Cohen IM, Vieweg WVR, Alpert JS, et al: Osteogenesis imperfecta tarda: Cadiovascular pathology. West J Med 126:228–231, 1977.
118. Koentges D, van de Werf F, Stalpaert J, et al: Aortic and mitral valve replacement in osteogenesis imperfecta. Report of a case. Acta Cardiol 41:147–153, 1986.
119. White NJ, Winearls CG, Smith R: Cardiovascular abnormalities in osteogenesis imperfecta. Am Heart J 106:1416–1420, 1983.
120. Levin LS, Pyeritz RE, Young RJ, et al: Dominant osteogenesis imperfecta: Heterogeneity and variation in expression. Am Soc Hum Genet 32:66 (abstract), 1981.
121. Hortop J, Tsipouras P, Hanley J, et al: Cardiovascular involvement in osteogenesis imperfecta. Circulation 73:54–61, 1986.
122. Weisinger B, Glassman E, Spencer FC, Berger A: Successful aortic valve replacement for aortic regurgitation associated with osteogenesis imperfecta. Br Heart J 37:475–477, 1975.
123. Heppner RL, Babitt HI, Bianchine JW, Warbasse JR: Aortic regurgitation and aneurysm of sinus of Valsalva associated with osteogenesis imperfecta. Am J Cardiol 31:654–657, 1973.
124. Shapiro JR, Burn VE, Chipman SD, et al: Pulmonary hypoplasia and osteogenesis imperfecta type II with defective synthesis of α1(I) procollagen. Bone (in press).
125. Rodriquez JI, Perera A, Regadera J, et al: Lethal osteogenesis imperfecta. Anatomopathologic study of 8 autopsy cases. Ann Esp Pediatr 17:18–33, 1982.
126. Falvo KA, Klain DB, Krauss AN, et al: Pulmonary function studies in osteogenesis imperfecta. Am Rev Respir Dis 108:1258–1260, 1973.
127. Elias S, Simpson JL, Griffin LP: Intrauterine growth retardation in osteogenesis imperfecta (letter). JAMA 239:23, 1978.
128. Albright JA, Grunt JA: Studies of patients with osteogenesis imperfecta. J Bone Joint Surg 53A:1415–1425, 1971.
129. Shapiro JR, Bercu B, Levine J: Thyroid function in osteogenesis imperfecta. Unpublished data, 1985.
130. Reiter ED, Lovinger RD: The use of a commercially available somatomedin-C radioimmunoassay in patients with disorders of growth. J Pediatr 99:720–724, 1981.
131. Denn HJ, Kelett JG, Hala RM, et al: The effect of growth hormone treatment on somatomedin levels in growth hormone-deficient children. J Clin Endocrinol Metab 55, 1167–1173, 1982.
132. Cropp GJA: Hypermetabolism in osteogenesis imperfecta. *In* Frame B, Parfitt AM, Duncan H (eds): Clinical Aspects of Metabolic Bone Disease. Amsterdam, Excerpta Medica, 1973, pp 308–313.
133. Distiller LA, Sagel J, Jacobson S: Thyroid function in osteogenesis imperfecta. Horm Metab Res 7:173–175, 1975.
134. Rampton AJ, Kelly DA, Shanahan EC, Ingram GS: Occurrence of malignant hyperpyrexia in a patient with osteogenesis imperfecta. Br J Anaesth 56:1443–1446, 1984.
135. Gebala AA: Acid hyperphosphatasia in three families with osteogenesis imperfecta. Lancet 2:1084–1085, 1956.
136. Kessel AW, Signy AG: Acid hyperphosphatasia in three families with osteogenesis imperfecta. Lancet 271:1217–1219, 1956.
137. Jacobsen JG, Matienzo JAP, Forbes AP, Rourke GM: Serum acid phosphatase in osteogenesis imperfecta. Metabolism 10:483–488, 1961.
138. Gionsberg DM: Normal serum acid phosphatase levels in osteogenesis imperfecta. Ann Intern Med 56:141–143, 1962.
139. Chowers I, Czaczkes JW, Ehrenfeld EN, Landau S: Familial aminoaciduria in osteogenesis imperfecta. JAMA 181:771–775, 1962.
140. Kinnett JG: Bullough PG: Urinary amino acids in osteogenesis imperfecta. Metab Bone Dis Rel Res 1:299–302, 1979.
140a. Cole WG, Kirby DM: Urinary-free amino acids in osteogenesis imperfecta. Bone 7:13–15, 1986.
141. Matkovic V, Kleerekoper M, LeVier RR, et al: Trace elements in osteogenesis imperfecta. Calcif Tissue Int 28:158, 1979.
142. Siegel BM, Friedman IA, Schwartz SO: Hemorrhagic disease in osteogenesis imperfecta. Am J Med 22:315–321, 1957.
143. Estes JW: Platelet size and function in the heritable disorders of connective tissue. Ann Intern Med 68:1237–1249, 1968.
144. Evensen SA, Myhre L, Stormorken H: Haemostatic studies in osteogenesis imperfecta. Scand J Haematol 33:177–179, 1984.
145. Key TC, Horger EO: Osteogenesis imperfecta as a complication of pregnancy. Obstet Gynecol 51:67–71, 1978.
146. Young BK, Gorstein F: Maternal osteogenesis imperfecta. Obstet Gynecol 31:461–470, 1968.
147. Shapiro JE, Phillips JA, Byers PH, et al: Prenatal diagnosis of lethal perinatal osteogenesis imperfecta (OI type II). J Pediatr 100:127–133, 1982.
148. Heller RH, Winn KJ, Heller RM: The prenatal diagnosis of osteogenesis imperfecta congenita. Am J Obstet Gynecol 121:572–573, 1975.
149. Ogita S, Kamei T, Matsumoto M, et al: Prenatal diagnosis of osteogenesis imperfecta congenita by means of fetography. Eur J Pediatr 123:179–186, 1976.

150. Milsom I, Mattison LA, Dahlen-Nilsson I: Antenatal diagnosis of osteogenesis imperfecta by real time ultrasound: Two case reports. Br J Radiol 55:310–312, 1982.
151. Carpenter MW, Abuelo D, Neave C: Midtrimester diagnosis of severe deforming osteogenesis imperfecta with autosomal dominant inheritance. Am J Perinatol 3:80–83, 1986.
152. Albright JP, Albright JA, Crelin ES: Osteogenesis imperfecta tarda. The morphology of rib biopsies. Clin Orthop 108:204–213, 1975.
153. Follis RH Jr: Osteogenesis imperfecta congenita: A connective tissue diathesis. J Pediatr 41:713–721, 1952.
154. Remigio PA, Grinvalsky HT: Osteogenesis imperfecta congenita. Association with conspicuous extraskeletal connective tissue dysplasia. Am J Dis Child 119:524–528, 1970.
155. Byers PH, Barsh GS: Reduced secretion of structurally abnormal type I procollagen in a form of osteogenesis imperfecta. Proc Natl Acad Sci USA 78:5142–5147, 1981.
156. Rowe DW, Shapiro JR, Poirer M, et al: Diminished Type I collagen synthesis and reduced alpha 1 (I) collagen messenger RNA in cultured fibroblasts from patients with dominantly inherited (Type I) osteogenesis imperfecta. J Clin Invest 76:604–610, 1985.
157. Teitelbaum SL, Kraft WJ, Lang R, Avioli LV: Bone collagen aggregation abnormalities in osteogenesis imperfecta. Calcif Tissue Res 17:75–79, 1974.
158. Holbrook KA, Byers PH: Structural abnormalities in the dermal collagen and elastic matrix from the skin of patients with inherited connective tissue disorders. J Invest Dermatol 79(S1):7–16, 1982.
159. Baron R, Gertner JM, Lang R, Vignery A: Increased bone turnover with decreased bone formation by osteoblasts in children with osteogenesis imperfecta tarda. Pediatr Res 17:204–207, 1983.
160. Falvo KA, Bullough PG: Osteogenesis imperfecta: A histometric analysis. J Bone Joint Surg 55A:275–286, 1973.
161. Ste. Marie LG, Charhon SA, Edouard C, et al: Iliac bone histomorphometry in adults and children with osteogenesis imperfecta. J Clin Pathol 37:1081–1089, 1984.
162. Jones CJ, Cummings C, Ball J, Beighton P: Collagen defect of bone in osteogenesis imperfecta (Type I). An electron microscopic study. Clin Orthop 183:208–214, 1984.
163. Shapiro JR, Triche T, Rowe DW, et al: Osteogenesis imperfecta and Paget disease of bone. Arch Intern Med 143:2250–2257, 1983.
164. Meema S, Meema HE: Radiogrammometry at four bone sites in normal middle-aged women. Clin Orthop 121:309–310, 1976.
165. Shapiro JR, Moore WT, Jorgensen H, et al: Osteoporosis: Evaluation of diagnosis and therapy. Arch Intern Med 135:563–567, 1975.
166. Genant HK, Cann CE, Ettinger B, Gordon GS: Quantitative computed tomography of vertebral spongiosa: A sensitive method for detecting early bone loss after oophorectomy. Ann Intern Med 97:699–705, 1982.
167. Mazess RB: Noninvasive bone measurements. *In* Kunin AS, Simmons DJ (eds): Skeletal Research, vol 2. New York, Academic Press, 1983, pp 277–343.
168. Reiderer SJ: Digital radiography. Crit Rev Biomed Eng 12:163–200, 1985.
169. Patterson CR: Metacarpal morphometry in adults with osteogenesis imperfecta. Br Med J 1:213–214, 1978.
170. Kurtz D, Moorish K, Shapiro JR: Vertebral bone mineral content in osteogenesis imperfecta. Calcif Tissue Int 37:14–18, 1985.
171. Farley JR, Baylink DJ: Purification of a skeletal growth factor from human bone. Biochemistry 21:3502–3507, 1982.
172. Prockop DJ, Kivirikko KI: Heritable diseases of collagen. N Engl J Med 311:376–386, 1984.
173. Burgeson RE: Genetic heterogeneity of collagens. J Invest Dermatol 79(S)1:255–305, 1982.
174. Cheah KS: Collagen genes and inherited connective tissue disease. Biochem J 229:287–303, 1985.
175. Miller A: Molecular packing in collagen fibrils. TIBS 7:13–18, 1982.
176. Piez KA: Molecular and aggregate structures of the collagens. *In* Piez KA, Reddi AH (eds): Extracellular Matrix Biochemistry. New York, Elsevier, 1984, pp 1–39.
177. Brodsky B, Eikenberry E: Supramolecular collagen assemblies. Ann NY Acad Sci 460:73–84, 1985.
178. Meek KH, Chapman JA, Hardcastle RA: The staining pattern of collagen fibrils. Improved correlation with sequence data. J Biol Chem 254:1071–1074, 1979.
179. Jimenez SA, Harsch MA, Murphy L, Rosenbloom J: Effects of temperature on conformation, hydroxylation, and secretion of chick tendon procollagen. J Biol Chem 249:4480–4486, 1974.
180. Cronlund AL, Smith BD, Kagan HM: Binding of lysyl oxidase to fibrils of type I collagen. Connect Tissue Res 14:109–119, 1985.
181. Nemethy G: Interactions between poly(Gly-Pro-Pro) triple helices: A model for molecular packing in collagen. Biopolymers 22:33–36, 1983.
182. Williams CJ, Prockop DJ: Synthesis and processing of a type I procollagen containing shortened pro $\alpha1$(I) chains by fibroblasts from a patient with osteogenesis imperfecta. J Biol Chem 258:5915–5921, 1983.
183. Steinmann B, Rao VH, Vogel A, et al: Cysteine in the triple-helical domain of one allelic product of the $\alpha1$(I) gene of type I collagen produces a lethal form of osteogenesis imperfecta. J Biol Chem 259:11129–11138, 1984.
184. Constantinou CD, Vogel BE, Jeffrey JJ, Prockop DJ: The A and B fragments of normal type I procollagen have a similar thermal stability to proteinase digestion but are selectively destabilized by structural mutations. Eur J Biochem 163:247–251, 1987.
185. Trelstad RL: Multistep assembly of type I collagen fibrils. Cell 28:197–198, 1982.
186. Gelman RA, Poppke DC, Piez KA: Collagen fibril formation in vitro. J Biol Chem 254:11741–11745, 1979.
187. Helseth D, Veis A: Collagen self-assembly in vitro. Differentiating specific telopeptide-dependent interactions using selective enzyme modification and the addition of free amino telopeptide. J Biol Chem 256:7118–7128, 1981.
188. Hedman K, Johansson S, Vartio T, et al: Structure of the pericellular matrix: Association of heparan and chondroitin sulfates with fibronectin-procollagen fiber. Cell 28:663–671, 1982.
189. Fisher LW, Termine JD, Dejter SW, et al: Proteoglycans and developing bone. J Biol Chem 258:6588–6594, 1983.

190. Termine JD, Kleinman HD, Whitson WS, et al: Osteonectin, a bone specific protein linking mineral to collagen. Cell 26:99–105, 1981.
191. Fujaii K, Tanzer ML: Osteogenesis imperfecta: Biochemical studies of bone collagen. Clin Orthop 124:271–277, 1977.
192. Petrovic OM, Miller J: An unusual pattern of peptide-bound lysine metabolism in collagen from an infant with perinatal osteogenesis imperfecta. J Clin Invest 73:1569–1575, 1984.
193. Myers JC, Dickson LA, deWet WJ, et al: Analysis of the 3′ end of the human pro-α2(I) collagen gene. J Biol Chem 258:10128–10135, 1983.
194. Chu M-L, deWet W, Bernard M, et al: Human pro α1(I) collagen gene structure reveals evolutionary conservation of a pattern of introns and exons. Nature 310:337–340, 1984.
195. Barsh GS, Roush CL, Gelinas RE: DNA and chromatin structure of the human α1(I) collagen gene. J Biol Chem 259:14906–14913, 1984.
196. Solomon E, Hiorns L, Sheer D, Rowe D: Confirmation that the type I collagen gene on chromosome 17 is COL1A1 (α1(I)), using a human genomic probe. Ann Hum Genet 48:39–42, 1984.
197. Junien C, Weil D, Myers JC, et al: Assignment of the human proα2(I) collagen structural gene (COL1A2) to chromosome 7 by molecular hybridization. Am J Hum Genet 34:381–387, 1982.
198. Yamada Y, Avvedimento VE, Mudryj M, et al: The collagen gene: Evidence for its evolutionary assembly by amplification of a DNA segment containing an exon of 54 bp. Cell 22:887–892, 1980.
199. Wozney J, Hanahan D, Tate V, et al: Structure of the proα2(I) collagen gene. Nature 294:129–135, 1981.
200. Aho S, Tate T, Boedtker H: Multiple 3′ ends of the chicken proα 2(I) collagen gene. Nucleic Acid Res 11:5443–5451, 1983.
201. Chu M-L, deWet W, Bernard M, Ramirez F: Fine structural analysis of the human pro-α1(I) collagen gene. Promoter structure, A1uI repeats, and polymorphic transcripts. J Biol Chem 260:2315–2320, 1985.
202. Mathis DJ, Chambon P: The SV40 early region and TATA box is required for accurate in vitro initiation of transcription. Nature 290:310–316, 1981.
203. Everett RD, Baty D, Chambon P: The repeated GC-rich motifs upstream from the TATA box are important elements of the SV40 early promoter. Nucleic Acid Res 11:2447–2465, 1983.
204. Schmidt A, Yamada Y, de Crombrugghe B: DNA sequence comparison of the regulating signals at the 5′ end of the mouse and chick α2 type II collagen genes. J Biol Chem 259:7411–7415, 1984.
205. Kream BE, Smith MD, Canalis E, Raisz LG: Characterization of the effect of insulin and collagen synthesis in fetal rat bone. Endocrinology 116:296–302, 1986.
206. Rowe DW, Kream BE: Regulation of collagen synthesis in fetal rat calvaria by 1,25 dihydroxyvitamin D_3. J Biol Chem 257:8009–8015, 1982.
207. Kream BE, Rowe DW, Gworek SC, Raisz LG: Parathyroid hormone alters collagen synthesis and procollagen mRNA levels in fetal rat calvaria. Proc Natl Acad Sci USA 77:5654–5658, 1980.
208. Canalis E, Raisz LG: Effect of epidermal growth factor on bone formation in vitro. Endocrinology 104:862–869, 1979.
209. Ninomiya Y, Schowalter AM, Olsen BR: Collagen genes with cartilage differentiation. *In* Trelstad RL (ed): The Role of Extracellular Matrix and Development. New York, Alan R. Liss, 1984, pp 255–275.
210. Khoury G, Gruss P: Enhancer elements. Cell 33:313–314, 1983.
211. Queen C, Baltimore D: Immunoglobulin gene transcription is activated by downstream sequence elements. Cell 33:741–748, 1983.
212. Rossi P, deCrumbrugghe B: Identification of a cell-specific transcription of enhancer in the first intron of the mouse α2 (type I) collagen gene. Proc Natl Acad Sci USA 84:5590–5594, 1987.
213. Sharp PA: Speculations on RNA splicing. Cell 23:643–646, 1981.
214. Keller W: The RNA lariat: A new ring to the splicing of mRNA precursors. Cell 39:423–425, 1984.
215. Fukumaki Y, Ghosh PK, Benz EJ, et al: Abnormally spliced messenger RNA in erythroid cells from patients with β^+ thalassemia and monkey cells expressing a cloned β^+ thalassemic gene. Cell 28:585–593, 1982.
216. Maquat LE, Kinniburgh AJ: A β^0-thalassemic β-globin RNA that is labile in bone marrow cells is relatively stable in HeLa cells. Nucleic Acids Res 13:2855–2867, 1985.
217. Higgs DR, Goodbourn SE, Lamb J, et al: α-Thalassaemia caused by a polyadenylation signal mutation. Nature 306:398–400, 1983.
218. Veis A, Leibovich SJ, Evans J, Kirk TZ: Supramolecular assemblies of mRNA direct the coordinated synthesis of type I procollagen chains. Proc Natl Acad Sci USA 82:3693–3697, 1985.
219. Palmiter RD, Davidson JM, Gagnon J, et al: NH_2-terminal sequence of the chick proα1(I) chain synthesized in the reticulocyte lysate system. Evidence for a transient hydrophobic leader sequence. J Biol Chem 254:1433–1436, 1979.
220. McPherson JM, Horlein D, Abbott-Brown D, Bornstein P: Inhibition of protein synthesis in vitro by procollagen derived fragments is associated with changes in protein phosphorylation. J Biol Chem 257:8557–8560, 1982.
221. Miyahra M, Hayashi K, Beger J, et al: Formation of collagen fibrils by enzymic cleavage of precursors of type I collagen in vitro. J Biol Chem 259:9891–9898, 1984.
222. Yamada Y, Mudryj M, deCrombrugghe B: A uniquely conserved regulatory signal is found around the translation initiation site in three different collagen genes. J Biol Chem 258:14914–14919, 1983.
223. Yamada Y, Kuhn K, deCrombrugghe B: A conserved nucleotide sequence, coding for a segment of the C-propeptide, is found at the same location in different collagen genes. Nucleic Acids Res 11:2733–2744, 1983.
224. Kivirikko KI, Myllyla R: Collagen glycosyltransferases. Int Rev Connect Tissue Res 8:23–72, 1979.
225. Byers PH, Bonadio JF: Lethal mutations in type I collagen: Relationships in the type I molecule. Birth Defects 20:65–77, 1984.
226. Leung MK, Fessler LI, Greenberg DB, Fessler JH: Separate amino and carboxyl procollagen peptidases in chick embryo tendon. J Biol Chem 254:224–232, 1979.
227. Steinmann B, Tuderman L, Peltonen L, et al: Evidence for a structural mutation of procollagen type I in a patient with the Ehlers-Danlos syndrome type VII. J Biol Chem 285:8887–8893, 1980.

228. Raisz LG, Kream BE: Regulation of bone formation. N Engl J Med 309:29–35, 83–89, 1983.
229. Black J: Tissue response to exogenous electromagnetic signals. Orthop Clin North Am 15:15–31, 1984.
230. Borresen AL, Berg K, Tsipouras P, et al: DNA polymorphisms in collagen genes; potential use in the study of disease. Prog Clin Biol Res 177:37–51, 1985.
231. Barsh GS, David KE, Byers PH: Type I osteogenesis imperfecta: A nonfunctional allele for pro α1(I) chains of type I procollagen. Proc Natl Acad Sci USA 79:3838–3842, 1982.
232. Nicholls AC, Pope FM, Schloon H: Biochemical heterogeneity of osteogenesis imperfecta: New variant. Lancet 1:1193, 1979.
233. Byes PH, Shapiro JR, Rowe DW, et al: Abnormal α2-chain in type I collagen from a patient with a form of osteogenesis imperfecta. J Clin Invest 71:689–697, 1983.
234. Hunkapiller M, Kent S, Caruthers M, et al: A microchemical facility for the analysis and synthesis of genes and proteins. Nature 310:105–111, 1984.
235. Miller WL: Recombinant DNA and the pediatrician. J Pediatr 99:1–15, 1981.
236. Green MR, Maniatis T, Melton DA: Human β-globin pre-mRNA synthesis in vitro is accurately spliced in xenopus oocyte nuclei. Cell 32:681–694, 1983.
237. Conner BJ, Reyes AA, Morin C, et al: Detection of sickle cell β-globin allele by hybridization with synthetic oligonucleotides. Proc Natl Acad Sci USA 80:278–282, 1983.
238. Wu DY, Ugozzoli L, Pal BK, Wallace RB: Allele-specific enigmatic amplification of beta-globulin genomic DNA for diagnosis of sickle cell anemia. Proc Natl Acad Sci USA 86:2757–2760, 1989.
238a. Studencki AB, Wallace RB: Allele-specific hybridization using oligonucleotide probers of very high specific activity: Discrimination of the human β^A- and β^S-globin genes. DNA 3:7–15, 1984.
239. Antonarakis SE, Phillips JA, Kazazian HH: Genetic diseases: Diagnosis by restriction endonuclease analysis. J Pediatr 100:845–856, 1982.
240. Tsipouras P, Schwartz R, Goldberg J, et al: Prenatal prediction of osteogenesis imperfecta (OI type IV): Exclusion of inheritance using a collagen gene probe. J Med Genet 24:406–409, 1987.
241. deWet W, Sippola M, Tromp G, et al: Use of R-loop mapping for the assessment of human collagen mutations. J Biol Chem 261:3857–3862, 1986.
242. Genovese C, Rowe D: Analysis of cytoplasmic and nuclear messenger RNA in fibroblasts from patients with type I osteogenesis imperfecta. Methods Enzymol 145:223–235, 1987.
243. Veres G, Gibbs RA, Scherer SE, Caskey CT: The molecular basis of the sparse fur mouse mutation. Science 237:415–417, 1987.
244. Thomas PS: Hybridization of denatured RNA and small DNA fragments transferred to nitrocellulose. Proc Natl Acad Sci USA 77:5201–5205, 1980.
245. Orkin SH, Kazazian HH Jr, Antonarakis SE, et al: Linkage of β-thalassaemia mutations and β-globin gene polymorphisms with DNA polymorphisms in human β-globin gene cluster. Nature 296:627–631, 1982.
246. Myers RM, Maniatis T: Recent advances in the development of methods for detecting single-base substitutions associated with human genetic diseases. Cold Spring Harbor Symp Quant Biol 51:275–284, 1986.
247. Orkin SH: Genetic diagnosis by DNA analysis: Progress through amplification. N Engl J Med 317:1023–1025, 1987.
248. Smith R: The molecular genetics of collagen disorders. Clin Sci 71:129–135, 1986.
249. Penttinen R, Lichenstein J, Martin GR, McKusick VA: Abnormal collagen metabolism in cultured cells in osteogenesis imperfecta. Proc Natl Acad Sci USA 72:586–589, 1975.
250. Chu M-L, Williams CJ, Pepe G, et al: Internal deletion in a collagen gene in perinatal lethal form of osteogenesis imperfecta. Nature 304:78–80, 1983.
251. Chu M-L, Gargiulo V, Williams CT, Ramirez F: Multiexon deletion in an osteogenesis imperfecta variant with increased type III collagen mRNA. J Biol Chem 260:691–694, 1985.
252. Barsh GS, Roush CL, Bonadino J, et al: Intron-mediated recombination may cause a deletion in an α1 type I chain in a lethal form of osteogenesis imperfecta. Proc Natl Acad Sci USA 82:2870–2874, 1985.
253. Prockop DJ, Chu M-L, deWet W, et al: Mutations in osteogenesis imperfecta leading to synthesis of abnormal type I procollagens. Ann NY Acad Sci 460:289–297, 1985.
254. van der Rest M, Hayes A, Marie P, et al: Lethal osteogenesis imperfecta with amniotic band lesions: Collagen studies. Am J Med Genet 24:433–446, 1986.
255. Bonadio J, Holbrook KA, Gelinas RE: Altered triple helical structure of type I procollagen in lethal perinatal osteogenesis imperfecta. J Biol Chem 260:1734–1742, 1985.
256. Bonadio J, Byers PH: Subtle structural alterations in the chains of type I procollagen produce osteogenesis imperfecta type II. Nature 316:363–366, 1985.
257. Traub W, Steinmann B: Structural study of a mutant type I collagen from a patient with lethal osteogenesis imperfecta containing an intramolecular disulfide bond in the triple-helical domain. FEBS Lett 198:213–216, 1986.
258. Bateman JF, Mascara T, Chan D, Cold WG: Abnormal type I collagen metabolism by cultured fibroblasts in lethal perinatal osteogenesis imperfecta. Biochem J 217:103–115, 1984.
259. Bateman JF, Chan D, Mascara T, et al: Collagen defects in lethal perinatal osteogenesis imperfecta. Biochem J 240:699–708, 1986.
260. Bateman JF, Chan D, Walker ID, et al: Lethal perinatal osteogenesis imperfecta due to the substitution of arginine for glycine at residue 391 of the α1(I) chain of type I collagen. J Biol Chem 262:7021–7027, 1987.
261. Nicholls AC, Pope FM, Craig D: An abnormal collagen α chain containing cysteine in autosomal dominant osteogenesis imperfecta. Br Med J 288:112–113, 1984.
262. Cohn DH, Byers PH, Steinmann B, Gelinas RE: Lethal osteogenesis imperfecta resulting from a single nucleotide change in one human pro α1(I) collagen allele. Proc Natl Acad Sci USA 83:6045–6047, 1986.
263. Steinmann B, Nicholls A, Pope FM: Clinical variability of osteogenesis imperfecta reflecting molecular heterogeneity: Cysteine substitutions in the α1(I) collagen chain producing lethal and mild forms. J Biol Chem 261:8958–8964, 1986.

263a. Stacey A, Bateman J, Choi T, Mascara T, Cole W, Jaenish R: Perinatal lethal osteogenesis imperfecta in transgenic mice bearing an engineered mutant pro-α1(I) collagen gene. Nature 332:131–136, 1988.

264. deWet WJ, Pihlajaniemi T, Myers JC, et al: Synthesis of a shortened pro-α2(I) chain and decreased synthesis of pro-α2(I) chains in a proband with osteogenesis imperfecta. J Biol Chem 258:7721–7728, 1983.

265. Gillerot Y, Druart JM, Koulischer L: Lethal perinatal osteogenesis imperfecta in a family with a dominantly inherited type I. Eur J Pediatr 141:119–122, 1983.

266. Nicholls AC, Osse G, Schloon HG, et al: The clinical features of homozygous α2(I) collagen deficient osteogenesis imperfecta. J Med Genet 21:257–262, 1984.

267. Chu ML, Rowe DW, Nicholls AC, et al: Presence of translatable mRNA for pro α2(I) chains in fibroblasts from a patient with osteogenesis imperfecta whose type I collagen does not contain α2(I) chains. Coll Relat Res 4:389–394, 1984.

268. Deak SA, Nicholls FM, Pope FM, Prockop DJ: The molecular defect in a nonlethal variant of osteogenesis imperfecta. Synthesis of pro-α2(I) chains which are not incorporated into trimers of type I procollagen. J Biol Chem 258:15192–15197, 1983.

269. Dickson LA, Pihlajaniemi T, Deak S, et al: Nuclease S1 mapping of a homozygous mutation in the carboxyl propeptide coding region of the pro α2(I) collagen gene in a patient with osteogenesis imperfecta. Proc Natl Acad Sci USA 81:4524–4528, 1984.

270. Pihlajaniemi T, Dickson LA, Pope FM: Osteogenesis imperfecta: Cloning of a pro-α2(I) collagen gene with a frameshift mutation. J Biol Chem 259:12941–12944, 1984.

271. Deak SB, van der Rest M, Prockop DJ: Altered helical structure of a homotrimer of α1(I) chains synthesized by fibroblasts from a variant of osteogenesis imperfecta. Coll Relat Res 5:305–313, 1985.

272. Hata R-I, Kurata S-I, Shinkai H: Existence of malfunctioning proα2(I) collagen genes in a patient with a proα2(I)-chain-defective variant of Ehlers-Danlos syndrome. Eur J Biochem 174:231–237, 1988.

273. Stoss H, Pontz BF, Pesch HJ, Ott R: Heterogeneity of osteogenesis imperfecta. Biochemical and morphological findings in a case of type III according to Sillence. Eur J Pediatr 145:34–39, 1986.

274. Bonaventure J, Cohen-Solal L, Lasselin C, et al: Abnormal procollagen synthesis in fibroblasts from three patients of the same family with a severe form of osteogenesis imperfecta (type III). Biochem Biophys Acta 889:23–34, 1986.

275. Byers PH, Bonadio JA: The molecular basis of clinical heterogeneity in osteogenesis imperfecta. *In* Lloyd J, Scriber C (eds): International Review of Pediatrics: Metabolic and Genetic Diseases. London, Butterworth, 1985, pp 56–90.

276. Termine JD, Robey PG, Fisher LW, et al: Osteonectin, bone proteoglycan, and phosphophoryn defects in a form of bovine osteogenesis imperfecta. Proc Natl Acad Sci USA 81:2213–2217, 1984.

277. Fisher LW, Denholm LJ, Conn KM, Termine JD: Mineralized tissue protein profiles in the Australian form of bovine osteogenesis imperfecta. Calcif Tissue Int 38:16–20, 1986.

278. Turakainen H: Altered glycosaminoglycan production in cultured osteogenesis-imperfecta skin fibroblasts. Biochem J 213:171–178, 1983.

279. Wenstrup RJ, Hunter AGW, Byers PH: Osteogenesis imperfecta type IV: Evidence of abnormal triple helical structure of type I collagen. Hum Genet 74:47–53, 1986.

280. Wenstrup RJ, Tsipouras P, Byers PH: Osteogenesis imperfecta type IV. Biochemical confirmation of genetic linkage to the pro α2(I) gene of type I collagen. J Clin Invest 78:1449–1455, 1986.

281. deVries WN, deWet WJ: The molecular defect in an autosomal dominant form of osteogenesis imperfecta: Synthesis of type I procollagen containing cysteine in the triple-helical domain of pro-α1(I) chains. J Biol Chem 261:9056–9064, 1986.

282. Tsipouras P, Myers JC, Ramirez F, Prockop DJ: Restriction fragment length polymorphism associated with the pro α2(I) gene of human type I procollagen. Application to a family with an autosomal dominant form of osteogenesis imperfecta. J Clin Invest 72:1262–1267, 1983.

283. Rowe DW, Shapiro JE, Poirier M, Schlesinger S: Diminished type I collagen synthesis and reduced α1(I) collagen messenger RNA in cultured fibroblasts from patients with dominantly inherited (type I) osteogenesis imperfecta. J Clin Invest 76:604–611, 1985.

284. Wallis G, Beighton P, Boyd C, Mathew CG: Mutations linked to the pro α2(I) collagen gene are responsible for several cases of osteogenesis imperfecta type I. J Med Genet 23:411–416, 1986.

285. Sykes B, Ogilvie D, Wordsworth P, et al: Osteogenesis imperfecta is linked to both type I collagen structural genes. Lancet 2:69–72, 1986.

286. Grobler-Rabie AF, Wallis G, Brebner DK, et al: Detection of a high frequency Rsa I polymorphism in the human pro α2(I) collagen gene which is linked to an autosomal dominant form of osteogenesis imperfecta. EMBO J 4:1745–1748, 1985.

287. Tkocz C, Kuhn K: The formation of triple-helical collagen molecules from α1 or α2 polypeptide chains. Eur J Biochem 1:454–462, 1969.

288. Weil D, Bernard M, Combates N, et al: Identification of a mutation that causes exon skipping during collagen pre-mRNA splicing in an Ehlers-Danlos syndrome variant. J Biol Chem 263:8561–8564, 1988.

289. Kuivaniemi H, Sabol C, Tromp G, et al: A 19-base pair deletion in the pro-α2(I) gene of type I procollagen that causes in-frame RNA splicing from exon 10 to exon 12 in a proband with atypical osteogenesis imperfecta and in his asymptomatic mother. J Biol Chem 263:11407–11413, 1988.

290. Orkin SH, Kazazian HH Jr, Antonarakis SE, et al: Abnormal RNA processing due to the exon mutation in β^E thalassemia. Nature 300:768–769, 1982.

291. Shea-Landry GL, Cole DE: Psychosocial aspects of osteogenesis imperfecta. Can Med Assoc J 135:977–981, 1986.

292. Albright JA: Systemic treatment of osteogenesis imperfecta. Clin Orthop 159:88–96, 1981.

293. Rosenberg E, Lang R, Boisseau V, et al: Effect of long-term calcitonin therapy on the clinical course of osteogenesis imperfecta. J Clin Endocrinol Metab 44:346–355, 1977.

294. August GP, Shapiro JR, Hung W: Calcitonin therapy of children with osteogenesis imperfecta. J Pediatr 91:1001–1005, 1977.

295. Pedersen U, Charles P, Hansen HH, Elbrond O: Lack of effects of human calcitonin in osteogenesis imperfecta. Acta Orthop Scand 56:260–264, 1985.

296. Cattell HS, Clayton B: Failure of anabolic steroids in the treatment of osteogenesis imperfecta. J Bone Joint Surg 50A:123–141, 1968.
297. Rowe LB, Schwarz RI: Role of procollagen mRNA levels in controlling the rate of procollagen synthesis. Mol Cell Biol 3:241–249, 1983.
298. Kurtz D, Eyring EJ: Effects of vitamin C on osteogenesis imperfecta. Pediatrics 54:56–61, 1974.
299. Kruse HP, Kuhlencordt F: On an attempt to treat primary and secondary osteoporosis with human growth hormone. Horm Metab Res 7:488–491, 1975.
300. Farley JR, Wegedal JE, Baylink DJ: Fluoride directly stimulates proliferation and alkaline phosphatase activity of bone-forming cells. Science 222:330–332, 1983.
301. Shoenfeld Y, Fried A, Ehrenfeld NE: Osteogenesis imperfecta. Review of the literature and presentation of 29 cases. Am J Dis Child 129:679–687, 1975.
302. Gertner J, Baron R, Vigery A, Lasng R: Cyclical therapy of osteogenesis imperfecta with fluoride and 25 hydroxyvitamin D. Calcif Tissue Int 31:62 (abstract), 1980.
303. Granada JL, Falvo KA, Bullough P: Pyrophosphate levels and magnesium oxide therapy in osteogenesis imperfecta. Clin Orthop 126:228–231, 1977.
304. Cetta G, Balduini C, Valli M, et al: Influence of a flavonoid on some abnormalities of connective tissues in osteogenesis imperfecta. Perspect Inher Metab Dis 3:181–183, 1979.
305. Becker Y, Stevely W, Hamburger Y, et al: Effect of flavonoid (+) cyanidanol-3 on procollagen biosynthesis and transport in normal and ataxia telangiectasis cultured skin fibroblasts. Connect Tissue Res 8:77–84, 1981.
306. Blumenkrantz N, Asboe-Hansen G: Effect of (+) catechin on connective tissue. Scand J Rheumatol 7:55–60, 1978.
307. Root L: The treatment of osteogenesis imperfecta. Orthop Clin North Am 15:775–790, 1984.
307a. Cole WG: Orthopaedic treatment of osteogenesis imperfecta. Ann NY Acad Sci 543:157–166, 1988.
308. Rodriquez RP, Bailey RW: Internal fixation of the femur in patients with osteogenesis imperfecta. Clin Orthop 159:126–133, 1981.
309. Middleton RW, Frost RB: Percutaneous intramedullary rod interchange in osteogenesis imperfecta. J Bone Joint Surg 69B: 429–432, 1987.
310. Root L: Upper limb surgery in osteogenesis imperfecta. Clin Orthop 159:141–146, 1981.
311. Yong-Hing K, MacEwen GD: Scoliosis associated with osteogenesis imperfecta: Results of treatment. J Bone Joint Surg 64B:36–43, 1982.
311a. James JIP: Scoliosis. Edinburgh, Churchill Livingstone, 1976, pp 116–146.
312. Binder H, Hawks L, Graybill G, et al: Osteogenesis imperfecta: Rehabilitation approach with infants and young children. Arch Phys Med Rehabil 65:537–541, 1984.
313. Bleck EE: Nonoperative treatment of osteogenesis imperfecta: Orthotic and mobility management. Clin Orthop 159:111–122, 1981.
314. Dubowski FM: Children with osteogenesis imperfecta. Nurs Clin North Am 11:709–715, 1976.
315. Werner P, Metz L, Dubowski F: Nursing care of an osteogenesis imperfecta infant and child. Clin Orthop 159:108–110, 1981.
316. Kogan S, Doherty M, Gitschier J: An improved method for prenatal diagnosis of genetic diseases by analysis of amplified DNA sequences. N Engl J Med 317:985–990, 1987.
317. Stuhlmann H, Cone R, Mulligna RC, Jaenisch R: Introduction of a selectable gene into different animal tissue by a retrovirus recombinant vector. Proc Natl Acad Sci 81:7151–7155, 1984.
318. Brinster RL, Chen HY, Warren R, et al: Regulation of metallothionein-thymidine kinase fusion plasmids injected into mouse eggs. Nature 296:39–41, 1982.
319. Readhead C, Popko B, Takahashi N, et al: Expression of a myelin basic protein gene in transgenic shiverer mice: Correction of the dysmyelinating phenotype. Cell 48:703–712, 1987.
320. Schneike A, Dziadek M, Bateman J, et al: Introduction of the human pro $\alpha 1(I)$ collagen gene into pro $\alpha 1(I)$-deficient Mov-13 mouse cells leads to formation of functional mouse-human hybrid type I collagen. Proc Natl Acad Sci USA 84:764–768, 1987.

18

LEONARD J. DEFTOS

The Thyroid Gland in Calcium and Skeletal Metabolism

The thyroid gland plays a very important role in skeletal metabolism. This effect is mediated by two distinct classes of hormones: the thyroid hormones proper, thyroxine (T_4) and triiodothyronine (T_3), and the peptide hormone of neural crest origin, calcitonin. The gene encoding for calcitonin also regulates the production of other peptides that may regulate skeletal metabolism. The effects of T_4 and T_3 on the skeleton have been well known for many decades. In contrast, it is more recently that the existence of calcitonin and its influence on skeletal homeostasis have been uncovered. The thyroid hormones and calcitonin exert their effects on each of the three organ systems that influence skeletal metabolism: the skeleton itself, the kidney, and the gastrointestinal tract. By their actions, these hormones affect the growth, maturation, and homeostasis of the skeletal system. In addition, these hormones also influence the metabolism of the mineral and organic constituents of bone, especially calcium, phosphate, and collagen.

The importance of the thyroid hormones and calcitonin on skeletal metabolism can be appreciated by considering the effects produced by conditions characterized by hormonal excess and deficiency, respectively.

I. THE THYROID HORMONES: T_3 AND T_4

A. Thyroid Hormone Deficiency

1. Growth and Maturation

One of the most dramatic illustrations of the importance of thyroid hormones in the growth and maturation of the skeleton can be seen in cretins, who are congenitally deficient in thyroid hormone. There is a marked delay in the appearance of ossification in epiphyseal centers. Although all epiphyseal centers are probably involved, the most diagnostically useful in the newborn are the proximal tibial and distal femoral epiphyses.[1] Intrauterine thyroid hormone deficiency can be postulated when the distal femoral epiphysis is absent in a newborn who weighs 3000 g or more or when the distal femoral and proximal tibial epiphyses are absent in a newborn weighing 2500 to 3000 g at birth.[2] It is of note that infants born of hypothyroid mothers do not exhibit delays in ossification.[3]

Although thyroid hormone deficiency results in delayed skeletal maturation, the skeleton does eventually mature. When an epiphyseal center does ossify in the hypothyroid child, it does so in an irregular pattern of multiple foci. When these foci coalesce, there results a "stippled" appearance, which is known as epiphyseal dysgenesis.[4] The onset of thyroid deficiency can be dated by the occurrence of dysgenesis in a particular center of ossification. For example, the finding of stippled epiphyses in the femoral head of a child indicates that thyroid deficiency began before the ninth to twelfth month, since this center usually begins to ossify at this time.[5]

In addition to delays in ossification, the hypothyroid dwarf retains infantile skeletal proportions. This is in contrast to the pituitary dwarf who may have proportions consistent with his or her skeletal age. The ratio of bone age to chronological age in hypothyroid infants and children is often less than 0.5. In older children or in patients with a short duration of thyroid deficiency, a lesser degree of skeletal retardation will occur.[6]

The importance of thyroid hormones in skeletal maturation and growth can be further demonstrated by experimental studies. Skeletal maturation in the rat can be accelerated by very small doses of T_3.[7] Furthermore, physiologic concentrations of either T_3 or T_4 can promote the maturation in tissue culture of isolated limb buds.[8] These effects of the thyroid hormones on skeletal maturation do not require the presence of sex hormones.

The growth retardation of thyroidectomized animals may also be contributed to by a secondary deficiency of secreted growth hormone, due perhaps to "pituitary myxedema." Very little growth can be produced in the hypophysectomized rat by thyroxin alone, whereas growth hormone can stimulate growth in the thyroidectomized rat. However, thyroid hormones do play some primary role in skeletal growth, since T_4 can potentiate the growth action of growth hormone.[9]

Thyroid hormones can also affect the growth and maturation of teeth. In rats made thyroid deficient by either thyroidectomy or propylthiouracil, the rate of tooth eruption and the size of tooth structures are impaired. Enamel is thinned and there is a decrease in the vascularity of the pulp.[10] These changes can be reversed by thyroid hormone replacement. In hypothyroid children, delayed dentition is characteristic. In addition, the loss of deciduous teeth is delayed and the growth of the roots is also slowed.[11]

2. Skeletal Metabolism

The metabolism of the skeleton is markedly retarded in thyroid deficiency. This is reflected in most of the parameters that can be used to evaluate skeletal activity.

Histopathology. The delay in ossification of epiphyseal centers has been mentioned earlier. When it does occur, epiphyseal ossification takes place in a fragmentary manner that results in a porous appearance of the bone. The decrease in activity of bone cells is also testified to by the low level of alkaline phosphatase in patients with myxedema.[12]

Radiologic Changes. The characteristic x-ray appearance of epiphyseal dysgenesis has already been discussed. Although there is a generalized decrease in the cellular activity of bone in hypothyroidism, this is not reflected by significant changes in x-ray findings. This is probably due to several reasons. Since bone resorption and bone formation are closely coupled processes, they are both decreased in hypothyroidism and there may be little net change in bone density. Furthermore, there must be substantial changes in bone density before there are any x-ray changes.[13] However, in some patients with hypothyroidism, an increase in bone density can be demonstrated by x-ray studies.

Metabolic Studies. All of the indices that can be used to measure the dynamics of bone turnover demonstrate a decreased activity in hypothyroidism. There is a decrease in the excretion of calcium and phosphorus in both the urine and feces of patients with hypothyroidism.[14] The excretion of hydroxyproline in the urine of hypothyroid subjects is also reduced.[15] Experimental studies have demonstrated that the decreased excretion of hydroxyproline is due to a decreased rate of degradation of both soluble and insoluble collagen.[16] Injected doses of ^{45}Ca are incorporated into bone more slowly in thyroid-deficient patients.[17] Finally, essentially all of these abnormalities can be reversed by thyroid hormone replacement.[18]

3. Calcium Metabolism

Overt disorders of calcium metabolism are not usually seen in patients with hypothyroidism. In most studies, blood calcium has usually been within normal limits despite the presence of a decrease in calcium and skeletal turnover.[19] However, a tendency to hypocalcemia can exist, and in a recent study, hypothyroid patients were found to have lower blood calcium levels than a control group of normal subjects. In addition, increased parathyroid hormone secretion was also observed in these patients, consistent with the presence of secondary hypoparathyroidism due to the hypocalcemia. The possibility that such a subtle form of secondary hypoparathyroidism can develop in hypothyroidism awaits further evaluation. If true, this phenomenon might also explain in part the increase in the intestinal absorption of calcium reported in hypothyroidism.[20]

Although not a consistent finding, in some hypothyroid patients there is a decreased calcium tolerance.[21] When challenged with either an oral or intravenous calcium load, hypothyroid subjects exhibit a greater rise in blood calcium than do control subjects. This has been explained on the basis of a decreased calcium deposition in bone due to the decreased skeletal metabolism of thyroid hormone deficiency. However, a concurrent deficiency in calcitonin may also play a role when this phenomenon occurs in athyreotic and thyroidectomized patients who are deficient in calcitonin as well as T_3 and T_4. The absence of the hypocalcemic action of calcitonin may interfere with the subject's ability to regulate a calcium challenge. Such calcium intolerance has also been observed in children with congenital thyroid dysgenesis.[22] Finally, hypercalcemia and nephrocalcinosis occasionally have been reported in cretins,[23] and hypocalciuric hypercalcemia has recently been reported in adult hypothyroidism.[24]

4. *Clinical Sequelae*

The skeletal consequences of hypothyroidism have been mentioned in the preceding sections. To summarize, there is a retardation of growth and maturation of skeleton. Evidence of this is greatest in growing subjects who exhibit (1) short stature, (2) retarded bone age, (3) epiphyseal dysgenesis, and (4) abnormal dentition. In older subjects, the skeletal changes are more subtle and may include an increase in bone density; similarly, overt calcium abnormalities are rare, although there may be a tendency to hypocalcemia and consequent secondary hyperparathyroidism.

B. Thyroid Hormone Excess

The effects of thyroid hormone excess on the skeletal system are essentially the opposite of the effects of thyroid hormone deficiency. There is an increase in the parameters of skeletal metabolism.

1. *Growth and Maturation*

There is a marked acceleration in the growth and maturation of bone in the young child with hyperthyroidism. Several mechanisms have been suggested as the cause of this process, including increased secretion of growth hormone, increased secretion of insulin, and increased secretion of gonadal steroids. However, the evidence for an increased secretion of these other hormones is not convincing, and a primary anabolic effect of the thyroid hormones may be an adequate explanation for the enhanced growth and maturation of bone seen in hyperthyroidism.[25] In the experimental animal, T_4 stimulates the proliferation of cartilage as well as epiphyseal maturation and closure.[26] Although an excess of thyroid hormone does not lead to hypernormal growth in the experimental animal, it can cause an early eruption of teeth and an increased rate of amelogenesis.[27]

2. *Skeletal Metabolism*

Histopathology. An increase in skeletal activity in hyperthyroid states can be demonstrated by many techniques. There is an increase in the number of osteoblasts and osteoclasts and an increase in plasma alkaline phosphatase and bone Gla protein (BGP).[28] Increased cellularity can be accompanied by increased vascularity and connective tissue proliferation to such an extent that, in rare cases, the findings are indistinguishable from those of osteitis fibrosa cystica.[29] More sophisticated techniques, including microradiography and tetracycline labeling, reveal increased bone resorption, and this effect is a direct action of thyroid hormone.[30] Although there can be increased bone formation as well, the rate of bone resorption seems to exceed the rate of bone formation.[27] In some patients with hyperthyroidism, there is an increase in the number and length of osteoid borders but not the width. However, in contrast to osteomalacia, the increased osteoid is always associated with bone-forming surfaces and these regions are calcified in a normal fashion.[27] Therefore, the increased osteoid is a result of the increased rate of bone formation.

Radiologic Changes. With the exception of the changes seen in thyroid acropathy, x-ray findings are not common in hyperthyroidism. Despite the excessive bone resorption and the negative calcium and phosphorus balance, a decrease in bone density is not commonly seen in hyperthyroidism. Hyperthyroidism may exaggerate the development of osteoporosis, since the incidence of such bone disease is seen with increased frequency in hyperthyroid women in the older age group.[31,32]

A form of hypertrophic osteoarthropathy can be seen in patients with hyperthyroidism.[33] The bony abnormalities consist of subperiosteal swelling, which can have the radiologic appearance of bubbles. There is increased vascularity in the affected regions. In contrast to hypertrophic pulmonary osteoarthropathy, there is no marked new bone formation, and the symptoms are minimal except for slight stiffness. The bone changes are usually seen in the metacarpals and proximal phalanges, although the distal phalanges and the proximal ends of the radius and ulna may be involved. A soft, diffuse swelling of adjacent tissues accompanies the bony changes. Although no etiologic factor has been definitely established for thyroid acropachy, this rare syndrome is often associated with pretibial myxedema and exophthalmos. It may occur at any time in relationship to hyperthyroidism, but thyroid acropachy is seldom seen during the active phases of the disease and most commonly occurs weeks to years after the hyperthyroidism has been treated.[34]

Metabolic Studies. The changes in skeletal turnover that occur in hyperthyroidism can be demonstrated by a wide variety of metabolic parameters. Studies of the effect of thyroid hormone on intestinal calcium absorption are contradictory. In some patients with hyperthyroidism, increased absorption has been demonstrated. However, in some patients, calcium absorption is normal; and in some subjects with clinical and experimental hyperthyroidism, calcium absorption is decreased.[27,35-37] These contradictory studies cannot be clearly resolved at this time. The absorption of calcium chloride, which is used in clinical and experimental studies, may not reflect the absorption of food calcium. Furthermore, the absorption of calcium may be influenced by the decreased intestinal transit time seen in hyperthyroidism.[18]

3. Calcium Metabolism

There is an increase in both urinary and fecal excretion of calcium and phosphorus in both spontaneous and experimental hyperthyroidism.[14] In some patients, the fecal calcium may be higher than the dietary calcium intake. This may be due to a decrease in calcium absorption caused by thyroid hormone excess.[38] There is even an increase in the calcium excreted by the sweat glands.[39] The effect of all these abnormalities in calcium metabolism is often the negative calcium balance that is commonly seen in hyperthyroidism. Despite the increased urinary excretion of calcium, urinary stones are not common.

Both the plasma level and the urinary excretion of hydroxyproline are increased in spontaneous and experimental hyperthyroidism.[14] The hydroxyproline indices can be well correlated with indices of thyroid activity in hyperthyroid subjects as well as hypothyroid and normal subjects.[18,40] The increase in the urinary excretion of collagen is caused by increased rates of degradation of both soluble and insoluble collagen (see Chapter 8); collagen synthesis does not seem to be increased but may even be decreased.[16] Nondialyzable urinary hydroxyproline, which seems to represent the breakdown of the most recently synthesized collagen, contributes less to the total urinary hydroxyproline in hyperthyroidism.[41] There may even be tubular secretion of hydroxyproline-containing peptides in hyperthyroidism.[42] In hyperthyroidism there is a rapid decrease in the plasma level of administered doses of ^{45}Ca and strontium. This probably reflects a rapid uptake of the isotope by the skeletal system, which is undergoing increased bone formation as well as resorption.[17] The increased uptake of bone-seeking isotopes gradually returns toward normal after treatment.[18]

In view of the excessive bone destruction that takes place in hyperthyroidism, it is not surprising that disorders of mineral metabolism are not uncommon in hyperthyroid states. The increased urinary and fecal excretion of calcium as well as phosphate has been mentioned. Furthermore, there is a significant occurrence of hypercalcemia in hyperthyroidism. In some series, an incidence of 16% to 23% has been reported. In addition, hyperthyroid patients who are not hypercalcemic tend to have blood calcium levels toward the upper limits of the normal range.[43] In most cases the hypercalcemia is mild and not clinically important and resolves coincidently with treatment of the hyperthyroidism.[44] In addition, the elevated levels of plasma alkaline phosphatase that are seen in hyperthyroidism return to normal after treatment.[18]

The hypercalcemia of hyperthyroidism can probably be best explained on the basis of increased bone resorption.[45] Alternative explanations have been offered,[46] including the view that there is increased parathyroid hormone secretion in hyperthyroidism.[47] There is, in fact, a reported incidence of frank hyperparathyroidism in patients with hyperthyroidism with 17 reported cases of an associated parathyroid adenoma;[48] however, coincidental occurrence of these two disease states cannot be ruled out. Despite some evidence to support this view, it has been shown that hypercalcemia can occur even in parathyroidectomized animals with experimental hyperthyroidism. In fact, the best evidence suggests that parathyroid function is actually suppressed in hyperthyroidism, presumably owing to the tendency toward hypercalcemia.[20]

Although the majority of patients with hyperthyroidism have plasma phosphate levels within the normal range,[18] the values in hyperthyroid patients tend to be slightly higher. A mean plasma phosphorus of 4.01 mg has been reported in hyperthyroid patients and a mean value of 3.2 mg in normal subjects.[27] Similar results have also been reported.[18] Since serum calcium levels tend to be higher in patients with hyperthyroidism, the decrease in plasma phosphate may be a reflection of suppressed parathyroid hormone secretion by the increased plasma calcium concentrations. This view is also supported by the finding that the tubular reabsorption of phosphorus is increased in patients with hyperthyroidism[27,49] and returns toward normal after treatment.[50]

Although alternative explanations exist for these findings,[46] further support for the concept of functional hypoparathyroidism in hyperthyroidism comes from the observation that patients with hyperthyroidism have increased sensitivity to exogenous parathyroid hormone.[51] Although the histologic character of the parathyroid gland has been reported as normal in patients with hyperthyroidism,[52] this may not be a reliable index of secretory activity. In fact, direct support to indicate that there is functional hypoparathyroidism in patients with hyperthyroidism has come from the recent demonstration of decreased levels of PTH (along with increased serum phosphorous) in such patients.[20]

4. *Clinical Sequelae*

Clinically significant skeletal disease is uncommon in hyperthyroidism despite the increased rate of bone resorption and compensatory increase in bone formation. Probably because of the relatively mild increase in bone turnover, skeletal sequelae such as severe demineralization, subperiosteal erosions, and cysts are not as commonly seen in hyperthyroidism as they are in hyperparathyroidism. When it does occur, the treatment of clinically significant skeletal disease is the treatment of the hyperthyroidism itself. There has, however, been recent evidence to suggest that the administration of excessive doses of thyroxin for treatment of real or imagined hypothyroidism could produce increased bone resorption and contribute to the development of osteoporosis in susceptible individuals[53-55,55a,55b] (see Chapter 12).

II. PHYSIOLOGY AND PATHOPHYSIOLOGY OF CALCITONIN

Calcitonin is a potent hypocalcemic peptide whose discovery has opened a new chapter in skeletal metabolism[56-58] (see Chapter 4). Its major biological action is to inhibit bone resorption.[58] Accordingly, it has been used as a therapeutic agent in disease states that are characterized by increased bone resorption, such as Paget's disease (see Chapter 15), hypercalcemia of malignancy (see Chapter 21), and osteoporosis (see Chapter 12). The chemistry and mechanisms of action of calcitonin are presented in detail in Chapter 4.

A. Measurement of Human Calcitonin

The significance of calcitonin in human physiology is not well defined. A major impediment to the study of this hormone in humans has come from the conflicting results that have been reported about the measurement of this hormone in normal subjects. The first measurements of calcitonin in normal subjects were made by bioassay procedures in which basal concentrations of 200 to 1700 pg of calcitonin per milliliter of plasma were reported.[59,60] However, it became apparent that this method was subject to artifacts.[61] The first reported radioimmunoassay for human calcitonin was sufficiently sensitive only to record normal calcitonin levels as being less than 2000 pg/ml.[62] Using an immunoassay of improved sensitivity, it was reported[63] that plasma calcitonin could be readily measured in the peripheral blood of normal adults and that its range was 20 to 400 pg/ml; there were not significant differences in calcitonin between normals and either chronic hypo- or hypercalcemic subjects. A similar method demonstrated that most normal subjects had undetectable (less than 100 pg/ml) basal values of plasma calcitonin.[64] Some patients were found to have higher values, but artifacts were shown to operate in the radioimmunoassay for human calcitonin, which could have given spuriously high results. Although calcitonin gradients were demonstrated across the thyroid vein in some subjects, the possibility of an immunoassay artifact could not be definitely eliminated.[65] This finding was also observed in other laboratories.[66] Subsequently, it was reported in additional studies[67] that basal calcitonin levels were less than 100 pg/ml (undetectable) in most normal subjects and never greater than 350 to 380 pg/ml.[68,69]

Several other laboratories have also reported conflicting results of basal calcitonin measurements. One laboratory reported a mean ± SD of 270 ± 240 pg/ml,[70-72] another laboratory reported that most normals have values of 50 to 150 pg/ml.[73] Using an immunometric assay, the same group reported normal calcitonin at 150 ± 140 pg/ml.[74] The Mayo Clinic has reported normal calcitonin values as 50 to 500 pg/ml with only 5% undetectable, and as less than 500 pg/ml;[75,76] this group also reported a direct correlation between basal calcitonin and calcium, a result not confirmed by others.[77,78] Silva et al.[79] have reported a normal mean of 180 ± 97 pg/ml and, in contrast to Tashjian et al.,[63] observed higher values in hypercalcemic subjects of 281 ± 91 and even a higher mean value of 510 pg/ml (110–2700 pg/ml) in a subsequent study.[77] Silva et al.[77] also reported that normal women seemed to have lower basal concentrations than did men, with 82% having values of < 200 pg/ml and 24% having values < 50 pg/ml in contrast to the male range of 63 to 450 pg/ml with only 4% < 50 pg/ml. Melvin et al.[68] reported that 22 of 25 thyroidectomized patients had undetectable plasma calcitonin, whereas several laboratories have reported detectable levels of calcitonin in thyroidectomized patients. Patients with chronic renal failure had higher concentrations than normal with a mean of 690 ±260 pg/ml and a range of 300 to 1200 pg/ml; dialysis and parathyroidectomy had no effect on plasma calcitonin.[80] Heynen and Franchimont[78] also found that patients with chronic renal failure had higher than normal plasma calcitonin, 500 to 3800 pg/ml (mean 1341 as compared with normals (10–580 pg/ml, mean 108) and even hypercalcemics (100–2000 pg/ml, mean 824). However, in contrast to Silva et al.,[80] they noted a significant increase in calcitonin following dialysis. In addition, calcitonin was undetectable (< 10 pg/ml) in 103 of 166 normal subjects. Furthermore, Heynen and Franchimont[78] observed that higher than normal basal levels of calcitonin are seen in patients with Paget's disease (range 0–1200 pg/ml, mean ± SEM 428 ± 151) and patients with pernicious anemia (range 0–1880 pg/ml, mean ± SEM 787 ± 173 pg/ml). Beceiro et al.[70] reported intermittently elevated levels of calcitonin in hypercalcemic states, and Bieler et al.[81] observed that normals have undetectable (< 50 pg/ml) basal values of plasma calcitonin.

There exist reports of increased plasma calcitonin over normal (270 ± SD 240 pg/ml) in umbilical cord blood (1890 ± SD 1000 pg/ml) and maternal plasma (660 ± SD 40 pg/ml) at term.[71] These results have led to the suggestion that calcitonin may be an important developmental hormone. This hypothesis is supported by recent observations that calcitonin is increased above adult levels in young children.[82]

Just as there is controversy about the measurement of basal levels of calcitonin in adults, disagreement exists about measurement of the hormone during provocative tests of secretion. Calcium infusion has been the most reliable provocative test for calcitonin secretion in experimental animals and in humans with medullary carcinoma of the thyroid.[83] However, its effect in normal adults has not been well defined. Tashjian et al.[63] reported that calcium infusion produced no detectable rise of calcitonin in 38% of normal adults; the remainder exhibited a mean calcitonin increase following calcium infusion of 100 pg/ml, and the increase in plasma calcitonin never exceeded either 550[68] or 700 pg/ml.[84] Heynen and Franchimont[78] and Silva et al.[77] reported that approximately 80% of their subjects showed an increase in plasma calcitonin following calcium infusion with stimulated values similar to those reported by Melvin et al.[68] Beceiro et al.[70] reported that normal subjects exhibit a post–calcium infusion rise in calcitonin of up to 1000 pg/ml.[71] Sizemore et al.[85] reported that calcium infusion caused only a 20% to 30% increase in plasma calcitonin in normal adults but that oral calcium, even though it did not produce as great a rise in blood calcium as did calcium infusion, resulted in a 30% to 300% increase in plasma hormone concentration.[85] In contrast, Melvin et al.[68] and Silva et al.[79] reported that oral calcium was less effective than calcium infusion in stimulating plasma calcitonin. The latter group observed an average maximal increase in plasma calcitonin of 230% following calcium infusion with a detectable rise occurring within 20 minutes of the start of the infusion; they also observed a 50% reduction in plasma calcitonin following EDTA-induced hypocalcemia.[77,79] Heynen and Franchimont[78] did not give details about the increase they observed in calcitonin following oral calcium in two of five patients; in three of five patients, EDTA infusion decreased calcitonin. Austin et al.[86] have demonstrated that oral calcium administration results in an increased serum calcitonin only when there is an increase in blood calcium,[86] whereas with an immunoconcentration assay Body et al.[87] have stated that some normal subjects have a postprandial increase in calcitonin without a change in serum calcium. In a group of patients with pseudohypoparathyroidism, idiopathic hypoparathyroidism, and osteomalacia, calcium infusion led to a marked rise in plasma calcitonin.[88,89] The calcitonin levels found after calcium infusion in these patients approached the levels seen in some patients with medullary thyroid carcinoma. In some patients, the administration of pentagastrin also resulted in an increase in plasma calcitonin. It is likely that the hypocalcemia in these patients resulted in increased storage of calcitonin in the parafollicular cells and that the induced hypercalcemia resulted in the release of these increased calcitonin stores, producing a blood level that could be readily detected by existing assay systems. Baker et al.[69] have also demonstrated intermittently elevated levels of calcitonin in pyknodysostosis.

There are several possible explanations for these discrepancies regarding the measurement of plasma calcitonin. Many of the reported measurements are made at or near the detection limits of the assay procedures. It is well known that artifacts are likely to operate under such conditions.[64-66,78] Attempts have been made in some studies to control for such artifacts by the use of adsorption or filtration procedures.[65,69,72,78,84] Although such procedures have been useful in demonstrating the operation of artifacts, they may introduce additional artifacts of their own.[83] Another potential explanation for these discrepancies in calcitonin measurements may result from the immunochemical heterogeneity of plasma calcitonin. Since there are several immunologic species of calcitonin in peripheral plasma, it may be that different antisera (in different laboratories) have varying affinities for the various circulating calcitonin species. As has been well documented with parathyroid hormone,[83] such a circumstance could result in varying estimations of calcitonin in the same plasma sample.

To further study the secretion of calcitonin, several laboratories have utilized immune concentration procedures to improve functional assay sensitivity.[90-92] The further application of extant and newer assays for calcitonin should help to define the importance of this hormone in humans. Of special importance is to design procedures to measure the biological activity of calcitonin in blood.[93]

With the development of newer methods for the accurate measurement of calcitonin, many of the earlier controversies have been resolved.[94] It is now firmly established that immunoreactive calcitonin circulates in human peripheral blood. Most laboratories agree that basal calcitonin concentrations are usually under 100 pg/ml. Women have lower blood calcitonin than do men, and this may contribute to the greater incidence of osteoporosis in females (see Chapter 12). Calcitonin levels are highest in neonates and gradually decrease to adult levels. Many laboratories have reported a further progressive decrease in calcitonin throughout adulthood to old age, but this has not been a universal finding. If present, such a progressive decline with age of calcitonin secretion could also contribute to the age-related loss of bone mass commonly seen in humans, especially females. As discussed later in this chapter, several disorders of calcitonin secretion have been defined and others have been postulated.

B. Role of Calcitonin in Mineral Metabolism

The physiologic role of calcitonin with respect to calcium homeostasis or skeletal metabolism has not been established in humans. Athyreotic adults do not seem to have a clearly defined abnormality in skeletal metabolism as assessed by short-term studies. However, these studies should be interpreted with reservation. For example, it is difficult to determine if adults who have been thyroidectomized are truly calcitonin-deficient.[95] Thyroidectomy or ablation with radioiodine may leave remnants of thyroid tissue. There may also be extrathyroidal sources of calcitonin. Both plasma and urinary calcitonin have been described in presumably athyreotic adults.[96]

In addition, the role of a potentially damaged parathyroid has not been carefully considered in such studies, nor have there been long-term studies conducted to establish the presence or absence of mineral abnormalities in athyreotic adults. Bone disease is common among athyreotic cretins, but it is generally ascribed to deficiencies of T_3 and T_4. However, a role for calcitonin deficiency in the pathogenesis of thyroid-related bone disease has not been ruled out,[22] and differences in bone density have been attributed to calcitonin deficiency rather than thyroid replacement status in thyroidectomized patients.[97]

Calcitonin may play a role in blood-calcium homeostasis. Some thyroidectomized patients demonstrate a decreased tolerance to oral and parenteral calcium challenge, and patients with medullary thyroid carcinoma (MTC) and high levels of calcitonin demonstrate an increased calcium tolerance.[98] In animals, feeding increases and fasting decreases plasma calcitonin.[99] These and other observations in animals notwithstanding, most human studies have failed to demonstrate a postprandial increase in plasma calcitonin that cannot be accounted for by an increase in blood calcium.[86]

Abnormalities in calcium or bone have not been consistently found in patients with MTC characterized by increased plasma calcitonin. However, it is possible that the escape of bone from the biological effect of calcitonin has minimized such changes, perhaps in a homeostatically appropriate manner.[100] It remains possible that an increase in parathyroid hormone secretion in such patients, either in a compensatory manner or due to genetic factors, obviates the effect of calcitonin. There is even evidence in very careful studies of a presumed calcitonin effect on bone in MTC patients.[101] The hypocalcemic effect of calcitonin appears to decrease with age, according to animal studies. Thus, it has been suggested that calcitonin plays a role in the growth and development of bone.[102] Elevated levels of plasma calcitonin in neonates tend to support this view.[71,72] In normal animals, the elimination of calcitonin leads only to a transient rise in steady-state blood calcium levels.[103]

Pregnancy, suckling, and lactation result in an increase in plasma calcitonin in rats.[104-106] This may protect the fetus and neonate against postprandial hypercalcemia and promote the assimilation of calcium into the developing skeleton. The elevated calcitonin may also attenuate any increased bone resorption that occurs to provide calcium in milk (lactation), thus benefiting the mother as well. In general, in humans as well as bovines, basal plasma calcitonin is lower in females than in males, and females have decreased calcitonin reserve during provocative testing.[107] In bovines, a high-calcium diet can bring female plasma calcitonin levels up to male levels.[108] This disparity associated with gender may play some role in the pathogenesis of bone diseases in females. Females with primary hyperparathyroidism are unable to increase their plasma calcitonin in the face of this hypercalcemic (and bone hyperresorptive) challenge, whereas hyperparathyroid males can do so.[109] This may explain the higher incidence of bone disease found in hyperparathyroid females.[110] Calcitonin deficiency may also be involved in the pathogenesis of postmenopausal osteoporosis, since calcitonin secretion in females decreases with increasing age.[111]

Calcitonin may have multiple paracrine functions in addition to the endocrine activities described. Calcitonin or a calcitonin-like peptide has been identified in a variety of normal and malignant cells, including the pituitary, pancreas, gastrointestinal tract, thymus, lungs, testes, adrenals, ovaries, and parathyroids.[112-120] A variety of paracrine substances, including somatostatin, substance P, and beta-endorphin, have similar distributions.[121-125] These other paracrine substances function as neurotransmitters. In addition, there are a variety of processes and sites upon which calcitonin has been demonstrated to exert an inhibitory action,[126-138] including the lung, heart, gastrointestinal tract, gallbladder, salivary gland, pancreas, pituitary, and brain. Whereas calcitonin may act as an endocrine hormone at some of these sites, it may actually be synthesized in many of these same tissues as well. Thus, calcitonin may have a general paracrine function of inhibiting cell function. This may represent a manifestation of calcitonin's role in biological communication. In unicellular organisms, hormones act as intracellular regulators; in oligocellular organisms, hormones can act as a paracrine mediator of cell-to-cell communication; in multicellular organisms, hormones have an endocrine effect. Applying this developmental sequence to calcitonin, it may be that in neural tissue calcitonin is a neurotransmitter,[139,140] and in more complex organisms calcitonin becomes an endocrine hormone.[141] Whereas this evolutionary sequence might explain the widespread distribution of calcitonin, its paracrine, neurocrine, and endocrine functions may still be mediated by the same mechanism—the translocation of calcium and phosphate, either intracellularly or intercellularly.[142]

C. Calcitonin Secretion in Osteoporosis

Among the calcemic hormones, evidence has accumulated to implicate calcitonin in the development of the age-related loss of bone mass and in the pathogenesis of osteoporosis: the main skeletal effect of calcitonin is to inhibit bone resorption; a main skeletal defect in osteoporosis is increased bone resorption.[143] In both sexes, calcitonin secretion progressively declines with age, and calcitonin secretion is consistently less in women than in men.[111,144] Calcium-stimulation studies of calcitonin secretion in women with osteoporosis suggest a deficient calcitonin response in comparison to normal women (Chapter 12).[145,146,146a,146b] Lower calcitonin levels have been observed in hypogonadal men with osteoporosis.[147] This view is supported by the recent demonstration of decreased bone mass in totally thyroidectomized subjects.[97] Thus, age- and gender-related calcitonin loss may contribute to age- and gender-related bone loss. In addition to studies of endogenous calcitonin secretion, studies of calcitonin treatment indicate a role for this hormone in osteoporosis. The administration of calcitonin in some but not all studies has been reported to retard, and perhaps reverse, the progressive and accelerated loss of bone mass occurring in osteoporosis;[148-152] this has occurred not only in osteoporotic patients but also in the normal bone of patients with Paget's disease treated with calcitonin. Some experimental and clinical studies suggest that calcitonin may actually increase bone formation. Although more studies are needed to fully evaluate these observations, they provide further impetus for evaluating the role of calcitonin in bone loss and osteoporosis.[153]

Calcitonin and gonadal steroids may be linked in the pathogenesis and treatment of osteoporosis.[154] The mechanism of action of estrogen replacement therapy in the treatment of osteoporosis has not been elucidated. The major therapeutic effect of estrogen replacement therapy is to inhibit bone resorption.[155] Estrogens may also act to promote the gastrointestinal absorption of calcium, but this effect has not been consistently seen, and any increased calcium absorption may be negated by increased calcium excretion in the urine.[147,156] The most puzzling aspect of the ability of estrogens to inhibit bone resorption is their mechanism of action. Despite some reports to the contrary, most investigators have failed to show the presence of estrogen receptors in bone.[157] Thus, estrogens appear to exert their skeletal effects indirectly. Estrogens may inhibit the sensitivity of bone to other bone-active substances like parathyroid hormone and $1{,}25(OH)_2D_2$.[158] However, considerable evidence is accumulating to indicate that estrogens may also act by stimulating the secretion of calcitonin. In some studies, pregnancy and use of oral contraceptives have been reported to increase plasma calcitonin levels in women.[154,155] Higher levels of calcitonin have also been found in women during the middle of the menstrual cycle in some, but not all, reports.[159,160] The administration of estrogens has been reported to increase plasma calcitonin in young and elderly women.[161,162] It has been suggested that their relative calcitonin deficiency may play some role in the pathogenesis of other bone diseases in females.[143] Evidence for this view is provided by studies of plasma calcitonin in primary hyperparathyroidism. Some females with primary hyperparathyroidism are unable to increase their plasma calcitonin concentrations in the face of this hypercalcemia (and bone hyperresorptive) challenge, as are males.[109] This may account for the greater severity of bone disease reported for females with primary hyperparathyroidism.[158]

Finally, recent preliminary evidence has been presented to suggest a role for calcitonin secretion in preventing osteoporosis in blacks. It has been well documented that this racial group shows little incidence for osteoporosis, but no endocrine basis for this had been elucidated.[143,163] Studies have now appeared of calcitonin measurements (only basal measurement) in blacks compared with Caucasians indicating that Caucasians are calcitonin-deficient compared with blacks.[164,165] This new observation, along with the previously discussed data, provides a powerful impetus for studying the role of calcitonin and other related hormones in the pathogenesis of bone loss and osteoporosis.

III. MEDULLARY THYROID CARCINOMA

Medullary thyroid carcinoma (MTC) is a tumor of the calcitonin-producing cells (C cells) of the thyroid gland. The thyroidal C cells are now generally accepted to be of neural crest origin. These cells migrate to the ultimobranchial bodies from the neural crest. In submammals, the cells form a distinct organ, the ultimobranchial organ, which becomes the residence of the C cells and their secretory product, calcitonin. In mammals, the C cells become incorporated into the thyroid gland and perhaps other sites. The neural crest origin of C cells offers an explanation for the association of MTC with other tumors of neural crest origin and also appears to explain the production by these tumors of a wide variety of bioactive substances.

A second clinical syndrome involving tumors of multiple endocrine glands has become elucidated during the last three decades. This syndrome has been designated MEN (multiple endocrine neoplasia) type II. Medullary thyroid carcinoma (MTC), a neoplastic disorder of the calcitonin-secreting cells of the thyroid gland, is the signal tumor of MEN type II. In the early reports of MTC as part of a multiple endocrine disorder, the associated lesions were pheochromocytomas, hyperparathyroidism, and a syndrome consisting of multiple mucosal neuromas (MMN) and marfanoid habitus. It is now appreciated that two distinct clinical syndromes can be defined by these associated endocrinopathies, MEN type IIa (Table 18–1) and MEN type IIb (Table 18–2). MEN type IIa consists of MTC, pheochromocytoma, and hyperparathyroidism (Sipple's syndrome); MEN type IIb (or MEN type III) consists of MTC, pheochromocytoma, and MMN and the marfanoid habitus (mucosal neuroma syndrome) (Table 18–3). The component tumors of MEN type IIa and MEN type IIb vary in their incidence and prevalence. Medullary thyroid carcinoma is the central tumor in this disorder and will be discussed first.

Table 18–1. Components of MEN Type IIa and Their Approximate Frequency of Occurrence in Patients with MEN Type IIa

Component	Frequency (%)
Medullary thyroid carcinoma	97
Hyperparathyroidism	50
Pheochromocytoma	30

From Deftos LJ, Cartherwood BD: Syndromes involving multiple endocrine glands. *In* Greenspan FS, Forsham PH (eds): Basic and Clinical Endocrinology. Los Altos, CA, Lange, 1988.

Table 18–2. Components of MEN Type IIb and Their Approximate Frequency of Occurrence in Patients with MEN Type IIb

Component	Frequency (%)
Multiple mucosal neuromas	100
Medullary thyroid carcinoma	90
Marfanoid habitus	65
Pheochromocytoma	45

From Deftos LJ, Cartherwood BD: Syndromes involving multiple endocrine glands. *In* Greenspan FS, Forsham PH (eds): Basic and Clinical Endocrinology. Los Altos, CA, Lange, 1988.

A. Embryology

Medullary thyroid carcinoma is a tumor of cells that are of neural crest origin. These neural crest cells migrate into the developing thyroid anlage in humans and other mammals and reside in proximity to the thyroid follicles, and are, therefore, called parafollicular cells. The parafollicular cells are epithelial in appearance; they are very difficult to identify in the normal human thyroid with standard histologic procedures. Using an immunoperoxidase procedure, McMillan et al.[166] demonstrated that these cells reside in the central region of the lobes of the normal thyroid gland. In medullary thyroid carcinoma, these calcitonin-secreting cells (C cells) undergo malignant transformation and produce an excess of calcitonin.

B. Histopathology

Medullary carcinoma of the thyroid is made up of sheets and nests of granular cells with eosinophilic staining properties. Most of the cells are closely packed and polygonal in shape. A second type of cell, spindle-shaped, has also been described in these tumors.[167] The presence of dense amyloid stroma that separates the cells is one of the most characteristic features of medullary thyroid carcinoma. The amyloid is usually a conspicuous feature of the tumor, but in some cases may be difficult to find. When detected, however, the presence of amyloid in a thyroid tumor is

Table 18–3. Summary of Clinical Features in 41 Patients with MEN III

Clinical Features	Number of Patients with Findings			Number of Patients with Inadequate Information
	Positive	*Probable*	*Negative*	
Family history	14	2	15	10
Neuroma	41			
Oral	37		4	
Ocular	24		16	1
Others	4		36	1
"Bumpy" lips	35	2		4
Pheochromocytoma	19	4	18	
Unilateral	7			
Bilateral	12			
Medullary thyroid carcinoma	38		2	1
Marfanoid habitus	26	5		10
Hypertrophied corneal nerves	23			18
Skeletal defects	24		4	13
Gastrointestinal tract abnormalities	23		10	8

From Khairi MRA, et al: Medicine 54:89–112, 1975, as reproduced in Deftos LJ: Medullary Thyroid Carcinoma. New York, Karger, 1983.

of great value to the pathologist in establishing the diagnosis. However, since it may be difficult to find, the absence of amyloid, particularly when only small amounts of tissue are available for examination, should not exclude the diagnosis of medullary thyroid carcinoma. Electron photomicrographs show the tumor to be rich in secretory (calcitonin) granules. Because the tumor can have a variable histologic appearance, immunohistologic identification of calcitonin-containing cells is necessary for definitive diagnosis.[168] Such immunohistologic studies can have prognostic value.[169] Calcitonin-rich tumors are associated with a better prognosis than are calcitonin-poor tumors.

This tumor of the thyroid has been shown to secrete a wide variety of peptides and bioactive substances. In addition to calcitonin, these substances include ACTH, histaminase, prostaglandins, and serotonin. The measurement of some of these secretory products in the blood of affected patients is only occasionally useful for the diagnosis of the disease. However, the biological activity of these secreted substances presumably accounts for some of the clinical features seen in patients with medullary thyroid carcinoma.[68,94,170,171]

C. Clinical Features

1. The Patient with MTC

There are several possible explanations for the lack of dramatic effects of calcitonin excess in the patient with MTC. A most obvious possibility is that the calcitonin produced by MTC is not biologically active. This hypothesis is not tenable, since the biological activity of calcitonin isolated from MTC has been conclusively demonstrated. Furthermore, structurally identical synthetic human calcitonin is biologically active. Another possibility is that the biological activity of calcitonin is counteracted by the presence of its antagonist, PTH. A significant percentage of patients with MTC do have high levels of PTH that can block the action of calcitonin at several organ sites. However, even patients with MTC and normal levels of PTH do not seem to exhibit any effects that might be expected of calcitonin excess. A most attractive explanation for the apparent lack of calcitonin effect in patients with MTC has been suggested by the work of Raisz et al.[100] and of Tashjian et al.[172] They observed that *in vitro* preparations of bone cells that were continually exposed to calcitonin became unresponsive to the hormone. This was not entirely due to a progressive loss of biological activity of the incubating hormone. Tashjian et al.[172] extended these results by demonstrating a decrease in the number of receptors for calcitonin on the bone cells. These observations suggest that the lack of a prominent calcitonin response in patients with MTC may be the result of down-modulation at the receptor level to maintain homeostasis. If such a receptor mechanism exists, it represents an additional homeostatic system for regulating hormone action.

The patient with MTC can present to the physician in a variety of ways. Since the tumor is relatively uncommon, the physician must be aware of its protean manifestations in order to make the correct diagnosis in the patient and to additionally consider the diagnosis in the patient's relatives. It is important to keep in mind that the patient with MTC may have no signs or symptoms of the tumor. The patient may be asymptomatic but referred to the physician because a relative was found to have MTC. The following symptoms and signs should suggest the possibility of MTC. The most common sign is an enlargement in the thyroid gland, and the most common symptom is diarrhea.

Bone Disease. Except for the presence of metastases, bone x-ray features are usually normal as are plasma alkaline phosphatase and urinary hydroxyproline, indices of bone formation and resorption, respectively, in the patient with MTC. Balance and kinetic studies of bone metabolism are also normal. The lack of bone changes has been surprising when one considers the high levels in these patients of plasma calcitonin, which is biologically active. Several explanations can be offered for the apparent lack of inhibition of bone resorption by the high levels of the hormone. In some patients, the potential effect of calcitonin may be countered by associated hyperparathyroidism and high levels of parathyroid hormone, the physiologic antagonist to calcitonin on bone. Another possible explanation for the lack of a calcitonin effect on bone in patients with MTC may be due to a decrease in the number of receptors for the hormone.[100,172]

In some patients there are, however, bony changes that may be due to the abnormal concentration of plasma calcitonin. Despite the lack of x-ray changes, bone biopsy in affected patients does reveal a decrease in the number of osteoclasts and a decrease in osteocytic osteolysis.[101] More dramatic than these subtle histologic changes were the observations made by Verdy et al.[173] They studied a patient with MTC over the course of a 5-year period. During that time, the patient's skeletal survey changed from normal to a picture of abnormally dense bones. However, calcitonin excess was not the only explanation for these x-ray changes. The patient also gave birth to four children who also had dense bones. Two of the children had normal plasma calcitonin concentrations. These observations suggest that the abnormally dense bones could have been a manifestation of a genetic bone disease rather than calcitonin excess. These dramatic findings notwithstanding, most patients with MTC do not have bone abnormalities unless caused by tumor metastases.

Blood and Urinary Minerals. In most patients with MTC the concentration of calcium and phosphate in peripheral blood is normal. This finding may be surprising, since the administration of calcitonin can produce hypocalcemia and hypophosphatemia. Decreased calcitonin receptors and/or a compensating increase in PTH may explain these blood chemistries that usually occur in MTC. There are, however, some studies that do suggest altered mineral metabolism in MTC. Miravet et al.[174] observed a resistance to the effects of parathyroid extract and 25(OH)D in MTC. Paterson[175] similarly reported resistance to the effect of vitamin D in a patient with hypoparathyroidism and MTC. There is experimental evidence that calcitonin inhibits the formation of $1,25(OH)_2D$[176] and promotes the formation of $24,25(OH)_2D$.[177] $25(OH)D_3$ has been reported to interfere with the phosphaturic effect of calcitonin,[178] and MTC can be characterized by a slight hyperphosphatemia.[179] Magnesium is normal.[179] Some patients with MTC may be slightly hypocalcemic and demonstrate greater tolerance to calcium challenge.[68] However, the hypocalcemia may be due to a commonly accompanying diarrhea.[180] The renal excretion of electrolytes is normal in patients with MTC. However, Krane et al.[181] have demonstrated that the kidneys in patients with MTC are responsive to further doses of calcitonin. They observed that the administration of salmon calcitonin to such patients produced an increase in the urinary excretion of calcium. This effect was contrasted with the absence of a decrease in urinary hydroxyproline, which signified the lack of a bone effect of the hormone. Thus, in patients with MTC, the kidney maintains its responsiveness to calcitonin, whereas bone may not.

Kidney Stones. The incidence of kidney stones in patients with MTC is usually explained by the common association with MTC of hyperparathyroidism and the consequent hypercalcemia and hypercalciuria.[182] However, there is some clinical evidence to suggest that the increased calcitonin may result in the hyperabsorption of calcium from the gastrointestinal tract and that this abnormality is responsible for the nephrolithiasis.[183] Experimental studies of the effect of calcitonin on the absorption of calcium have produced inconsistent and inconclusive results.[184-188] However, clinical studies in patients with MTC demonstrate increased calcium absorption. When the tumor is removed, calcium absorption returns toward normal. These events occur independently of any changes in parathyroid hormone or blood calcium. Although additional studies are necessary to confirm this pathophysiologic consequence of hypercalcitoninemia, the current data suggest that kidney stones may be another feature of MTC due to the abnormal concentrations of calcitonin.[182]

Diarrhea. Diarrhea occurs in approximately one third of patients with the tumor, and it can even precede the diagnosis.[179,188] The diarrhea is characterized by a rapid transit time of both the large and small intestine.[187,188] This may produce a diabetic glucose tolerance test.[188] There is excessive loss of fluids and electrolytes due to their poor absorption.[189] These abnormalities occur primarily in the ileum, and jejunal function seems to be normal.[189] Malabsorption, as evaluated by B_{12} and xylose absorption, does not occur, and steatorrhea is mild or absent; however, cellulose and starch are apparent in the stool.[188] Intestinal biopsy is normal or mildly abnormal; in the latter circumstance there is mild inflammation and some villous atrophy, but the epithelium is usually normal. However, the radiologic appearance of the gastrointestinal tract can sometimes be confused with ulcerative or granulomatous colitis.[190,191] There are two general groups of factors that can contribute to the diarrhea commonly seen in patients with MTC—humoral factors and anatomic factors. Many of the various bioactive substances produced by MTC have been implicated in the pathogenesis of the diarrhea seen with this tumor. Such peptide hormones are (1) calcitonin; (2) ACTH and MSH; (3) neurotensin; (4) somatostatin; (5) beta-endorphin; and (6) nerve growth factor. However, the relationship between diarrhea and these various agents is not always direct, and in many patients other causes must be sought for the diarrhea. The various anatomic abnormalities discussed subsequently that can be found in the gastrointestinal tract of patients with MTC may also account for the diarrhea. These anatomic lesions can reflect and perhaps even produce fundamental abnormalities in gastrointestinal innervation that can produce abnormal motility.

Removal of the tumor may decrease the diarrhea associated with MTC. The presumed mechanism is a decrease in the concentration of a tumor responsible for the diarrhea. The diarrhea of MTC may respond, at least partially, to standard antidiarrheal regimens of atropine-like agents.[184,185,188] There are some anecdotal reports of the value of nutmeg (*Myristica fragrans*) in the treatment of the diarrhea of MTC.[192,193] Specific antitumoral substances, such as aspirin and indomethacin for prostaglandins, may be beneficial in some patients. If alcohol ingestion accentuates the diarrhea, it should be eliminated. If an anatomic lesion, such as ganglioneuromatosis, is thought to contribute to the diarrhea, surgery is not likely to be effective, since the lesion is likely to be diffusely distributed.

Peptic Ulcer Disease. It is not possible to determine from existing data if ulcer disease is directly associated with MTC.[194] Hill et al.[170] observed that five of 44 patients with MTC had peptic ulcer disease and two of them had multiple ulcers. They reiterated the relationship proposed by Pearse,[195,196] Pearse et al.,[197] and Weichert[198] between ulcerogenic tumors[198] and MTC and its associated tumors. It was suggested that MTC may produce an ulcerogenic factor. However, only one patient with MTC and increased plasma gastrin has been reported.[185] The majority of patients showed decreased plasma gastrin due to feedback inhibition caused by calcitonin.[75] Ljungberg[199] and Walker[200] also reported the occurrence of ulcers in patients with MTC. The increased incidence of ulcer disease may also be due to hyperparathyroidism associated with MTC.

Carcinoid Syndrome. There is a significant incidence of carcinoid tumors in patients with MTC.[201,202] The occurrence of carcinoid tumors should be noted for the following reasons: (1) the cells of carcinoid tumors and MTC are of neural crest origin; (2) the histologic appearance of MTC can resemble carcinoid tumors; (3) carcinoid tumors can produce calcitonin; and (4) MTC can produce serotonin. These observations provide additional support for the embryologic, histologic, and functional relationship of the tumors that occur in MEN.[94,203]

Hypertension. The presence of pheochromocytomas in MTC can account for hypertension in these patients. However, the clinical and biochemical features of the hypertension may differ from those observed in patients with nonfamilial pheochromocytomas.

The hypertension may not be sustained, and the routine tests may be nondiagnostic.[94,203]

Cushing's Syndrome. A small percentage of patients with MTC exhibit the ectopic production of ACTH by the tumor.[204] This can produce the rapidly progressive Cushing's syndrome associated with ectopic ACTH production. Hypokalemic alkalosis is the dominant feature of this type of Cushing's syndrome, since the clinical course is not long enough for the more classic somatic features of Cushing's syndrome to develop. However, some MTCs that ectopically secrete ACTH run a more indolent course. In such patients, the more classic picture of Cushing's syndrome may develop.[203]

2. Pheochromocytoma

There are several distinct features of pheochromocytomas occurring in association with MTC.[94] Bilateral and multifocal pheochromocytomas are very common in this clinical setting and have an incidence of greater than 70% (Table 18–3). This contrasts with a bilateral incidence of usually less than 10% for sporadic pheochromocytomas. Pheochromocytomas are much more likely to occur in patients with familial rather than sporadic MTC. The thyroid tumor may antedate the pheochromocytomas by as much as two decades. Furthermore, a second pheochromocytoma may become manifest after removal of the first. Thus, there is a greater incidence of pheochromocytomas in older patients with MTC. If hyperparathyroidism also exists, it, too, is likely to be diagnosed before the pheochromocytoma. Adrenal medullary hyperplasia may be a predecessor of the pheochromocytomas seen with MTC, just as C cell hyperplasia may be a predecessor of MTC and chief cell hyperplasia a predecessor of primary hyperparathyroidism in these patients. The increase in adrenal medullary mass results from diffuse and/or multifocal proliferation of adrenal medullary cells, primarily those found within the head and body of the glands. Diagnostic tests for pheochromocytomas should be pursued vigorously because the biochemical as well as clinical manifestations of this tumor may be subtle.[94,203,203a] In this regard, it should be emphasized that the diagnosis of metastatic pheochromocytoma in MEN type IIa is probably best achieved by ^{123}I MIBG scintigraphy.[204a]

3. Hyperparathyroidism

The exact incidence of hyperparathyroidism in patients with MTC is difficult to establish.[94] Hyperparathyroidism is considerably more common in MEN type IIa than in MEN type IIb (Tables 18–1 and 18–2). Recent literature suggests that hyperplasia is more common than adenoma. Despite these uncertainties, the concurrence of hyperparathyroidism and MTC in MEN is well established, and although it cannot be quantitated, the presence of one tumor should always make the presence of the other suspect. Hyperparathyroidism does not easily fit into a unitary concept of embryogenesis, since parathyroid cells are not classically considered to be of neural crest origin. However, some authorities have suggested a neural crest origin for the parathyroid gland. An alternative explanation for the hyperparathyroidism is a functional relationship between it and MTC. According to this hypothesis, the abnormal concentrations of calcitonin produce hyperparathyroidism that is secondary to the hypocalcemic actions of the calcitonin. Although this type of functional relationship between the neoplasias may exist, the most convincing evidence supports a genetic relationship between MTC and hyperparathyroidism.[94,203]

4. Multiple Mucosal Neuromas (MMN)

The presence of neuromas with a centrofacial distribution is the most consistent component of this syndrome.[194] The most common location of neuromas is in the oral cavity. The most prominent microscopic feature of the neuromas is an increase in the size and number of nerves. The lips, tongue, and buccal mucosa are the most common sites for the oral mucosal neuromas, but other sites can be involved. The oral lesions are almost invariably present by the first decade and can even be present at birth. Mucosal neuromas can be present in the eyelids, conjunctiva, and cornea. The medullated corneal nerves are thickened and traverse the cornea and anastomose in the pupillary area. These hypertrophied nerve fibers are seen readily with the slit lamp but occasionally may be evident on direct funduscopic examination.[94,194]

Gastrointestinal abnormalities are part of the mucosal neuroma syndrome. The most common of these is gastrointestinal ganglioneuromatosis. The ganglioneuromatosis is best observed in the small and large intestine but has also been noted in the esophagus and stomach. The anatomic lesions can be associated with the functional difficulties in swallowing, megacolon, diarrhea, and constipation, respectively. Similar lesions can be present at other mucosal surfaces.

5. Marfanoid Habitus

A marfanoid habitus is seen commonly in the MMN syndrome.[194] It refers to a tall, slender body with an abnormal upper to lower body segment ratio and poor muscle development. The extremities are thin and long, and there may be lax joints and hypotonic muscles. Associated with the marfanoid habitus may be dorsal kyphosis, pectus excavatum, pectus carinatum, pes cavus, and a high-arched palate. In contrast to patients with true Marfan's syndrome, no patients with MMN have been reported who have aortic abnormalities, ectopia lentis, homocystinuria, or mucopolysaccharide abnormalities. The clinical features of MMN syndrome are summarized in Table 18–3.

D. Diagnosis

The diagnosis of medullary thyroid carcinoma should be considered in any patient with a thyroid tumor. It should be especially suspected in the relatives of patients who have the disease and in patients who have thyroid tumor with histologic appearance that is atypical and does not conform to the features described for tumors of those thyroid cells responsible for iodine metabolism. The possibility of ACTH-producing medullary thyroid carcinoma should be considered in patients with otherwise unexplained Cushing's syndrome.

The most reliable (nonsurgical) method for establishing the diagnosis of medullary thyroid carcinoma is the measurement of blood calcitonin. The large majority of patients with medullary thyroid carcinoma have increased basal concentrations of plasma calcitonin before there is any clinical evidence of the presence of the tumor. Therefore, especially in familial cases, the presence of high levels of calcitonin may be a very early clue to the presence of this malignancy. In the initial immunoassay studies, all patients with this tumor had basal concentrations of calcitonin that were clearly distinguishable from normal and, therefore, diagnostic of the presence of the tumor.[63] However, subsequent studies demonstrated that some patients with this tumor had basal levels of calcitonin that could not be distinguished from normal; provocative tests of calcitonin secretion were necessary to establish the presence of tumor in these patients.[67,205-207] Furthermore, it is now apparent that in some of these patients, basal plasma calcitonin may be intermittently elevated.[207] In these types of patients, provocative tests of calcitonin secretion may be useful in confirming the presence of this disease.

The first provocative test for establishing the presence of medullary thyroid carcinoma in suspect patients without abnormally elevated basal levels of calcitonin was a 2- to 4-hour calcium infusion. Virtually all patients show a markedly increased level of plasma calcitonin following this procedure. Furthermore, in some patients with basal levels of the hormone that are not abnormal, the postinfusion values are diagnostic of the presence of tumor. This provocative testing can lead to the diagnosis of the tumor in its earliest stages.[208] In some patients, more convenient and shorter infusion of calcium may establish the diagnosis. This response to calcium indicates that the secretion of calcitonin by these malignant parafollicular cells is stimulated by the same ion that influences secretion of calcitonin by normal C cells.[83]

The effects of gastrin, a peptide that has been shown to stimulate the secretion of calcitonin in the porcine species and in some patients with hypocalcemia, has also been evaluated in patients with this tumor. This peptide, speculated to be a physiologic stimulus for calcitonin secretion, has also been shown to be useful as a provocative agent for calcitonin secretion in patients with medullary thyroid carcinoma; in fact, one report describes gastrin infusion as a more reliable diagnostic procedure than calcium infusion.[209] Gastrin has been combined with calcium as a provocative test for MTC.[209,210]

In summary, the measurement of calcitonin by radioimmunoassay thus offers a precise, reliable, and relatively simple test for establishing the diagnosis of medullary thyroid carcinoma.[62,83,94] Provocative tests for calcitonin secretion, either calcium and/or gastrin infusion, are important ancillary procedures that can lead to even earlier diagnosis. Since false-negative results can occur with either procedure, both should probably be used for excluding the diagnosis in the subject at risk because of family history. In many instances, plasma measurements of calcitonin can establish the presence of medullary carcinoma even before there is any clinical evidence of the disease. Total thyroidectomy, performed because of increased calcitonin detected in the blood prior to any sign or symptom or detectable thyroid abnormality, has led to detection of microscopic foci of medullary carcinoma in the removed thyroid tissue.[68] Calcitonin measurement can also be useful in relatives of these patients.[94]

Several other bioactive substances have been identified as secretory products of medullary carcinoma of the thyroid.[203] Histaminase measurements may be especially helpful in identifying the presence of metastatic disease.[171] However, the presence of these other substances does not seem to occur with enough consistency to make their measurement diagnostically useful. Prostaglandins, serotonin, and ACTH may be responsible for some signs and symptoms associated with the tumor. Thyroid scintigraphy with ^{99m}Tc (V) dimer-captosuccinic acid may be useful in identifying MTC.[211,212]

E. Treatment

Suppression of tumor growth by thyroid hormone cannot be expected in these patients.[94] The most effective treatment for patients with medullary thyroid carcinoma is surgical removal of the tumor.[68,170] In advanced cases, surgery is often palliative and directed at the symptoms due to local obstruction by the tumor of large veins or of the trachea. With the introduction of the immunoassay for calcitonin, however, the disease can be detected very early in some individuals from affected kindred; consequently, surgery in these cases may be curative.

Total thyroidectomy should be undertaken because of the multifocal distribution of the disease, especially in the familial form.[203] Wide excision of lymph nodes is recommended, but radical neck dissection has not been fully evaluated. Surgical management is influenced by the presence of other associated endocrinopathies. For example, when pheochromocytomas are present, it may be expeditious to perform bilateral adrenalectomy first. This permits direct examination of the liver for the presence of metastases from the thyroid carcinoma. If such metastases are present, direct attack on the tumor may not be justified. Bilateral adrenalectomy may also be indicated in the patients with Cushing's disease due to the production of ACTH by a medullary thyroid tumor if the medullary carcinoma is already metastatic and, therefore, cannot be removed. There is no extensive experience with radiotherapy or chemotherapy in the treatment of this disease,[170] although some case reports of ^{125}I and adriamycin treatment have recently appeared.[213] Whatever forms of therapy are used, the immunoassay for calcitonin can be used to monitor treatment.[214]

IV. OTHER CALCITONIN DISORDERS

A. Ectopic Calcitonin Production

Several laboratories have observed that other forms of cancer are also characterized by the increased production of calcitonin.[79,215-221] It was at first considered that the other forms of cancer derived from cells that were embryologically related to the C cells of the thyroid, which are neural crest in origin. However, such a wide variety of cancers has been associated with increased calcitonin production that such a hypothesis no longer seems tenable. Ectopic calcitonin production has been reported with a wide variety of nonthyroidal neoplasms, which include the following: intestinal, bronchial, and gastric carcinoids; pheochromocytoma; melanoma; carcinoma of the lung, especially oat cell; pancreatic carcinoma; maxillary carcinoma; prostatic carcinoma; uterine carcinoma; bladder carcinoma; breast carcinoma; and leukemia. Thus, calcitonin may be a more general marker for the malignant transformation of cells, although neural crest cells may predominate in such calcitonin-producing tumors. The measurement of calcitonin not only may serve as a diagnostic marker for such tumors but may also be a guide to therapy. Because of these observations, the detection of an elevated plasma level of calcitonin does not necessarily mean the presence of medullary thyroid carcinoma. The patient must now be evaluated for other malignant disorders.

B. Disorders of Calcium Metabolism

1. Hypercalcemia

A number of clinical and experimental studies in humans have demonstrated that plasma calcitonin (CT) increases in response to acute hypercalcemia.[222-225] However, an increase in plasma CT, perhaps as a compensatory homeostatic response, has not been clearly established in chronic hypercalcemic states. As noted in Chapter 21, elevated basal levels of CT have been reported in some patients with malignancy and hypercalcemia, but it has been difficult in these studies to differentiate among hypercalcemia, ectopic CT production by the tumor, and impaired renal function as the cause of increased plasma CT.[221,226] In hypercalcemia due to hyperparathyroidism, most studies have failed to demonstrate any consistent abnormalities in plasma CT, although normal, elevated, and decreased levels of the hormone have been reported.[227-232] However, there has been histologic evidence of C cell hyperplasia that is inconsistent with the increased CT secretion in some hyperparathyroid patients.[233-235]

The most likely explanation of the increased plasma CT in such patients is that chronic hypercalcemia has a stimulatory effect on hormone secretion, which results in a state of secondary hypercalcitoninemia characterized by C cell hyperplasia.[233,236] Similar to studies in normal subjects,[223,225] females with primary hyperparathyroidism seem to have lower plasma CT levels than do males with primary hyperparathyroidism, and they do not demonstrate an increase in plasma CT to correlate with the increase in blood Ca as do the males. This suggests a decreased CT reserve, which may play some role in the greater incidence and severity of bone disease reported to occur in females with primary hyperparathyroidism.[158] Thus, the secretion of CT in primary hyperparathyroidism seems variable and may be influenced by factors such as the duration and severity of the hyperparathyroidism.

One could speculate further concerning the homeostatic role of secondary hypercalcitoninism in the pathogenesis of clinical and biochemical manifestations of primary hyperparathyroidism. However, longitudinal studies will be necessary to establish any pathophysiologic or pathogenetic importance of secondary hypercalcitoninism in primary hyperparathyroidism. Similarly, studies of larger populations may show that other factors influence plasma CT in a manner not evident in our studies. Nevertheless, although the secretion of CT in primary hyperparathyroidism is variable, there is some evidence for a homeostatic role for CT in some patients with this disorder.[132]

2. Hypocalcemia

The effect of calcium challenge on calcitonin secretion has been studied in hypocalcemic patients.[89] Calcium infusion (and, to a lesser degree, pentagastrin) in patients with hypocalcemia of several causes results in abnormal increase of plasma calcitonin, presumably due to release of hypocalcemia-induced increased stores of the hormone.

3. Nephrolithiasis

Intestinal hyperabsorption of calcium mediated through increased synthesis of calcitriol [1,25$(OH)_2D_3$] plays a major role in the generation of hypercalciuria in both absorptive hypercalciuria (AHC) and renal hypercalciuria (RHC)[237-241] (see Chapter 23). Because a putative physiologic role for calcitonin is its antihypercalcemic effect, adaptive alterations in its regulation and secretion might be anticipated in states of increased enteral calcium absorption. Indeed, although not clearly present in all patients, selected individuals with either absorptive hypercalciuria or renal hypercalciuria appear to have increased calcitonin secretory capacity as assessed by basal calcitonin measurements[242] and calcitonin secretion in response to a calcium infusion.[243] The significance or role of increased calcitonin secretory capacity in this setting is unclear. Based primarily on animal studies, an enterocalcitonin secretory axis has been postulated whereby some enteral factor, perhaps gastrin, stimulates calcitonin secretion. However, most clinical studies in humans demonstrate that any enterally mediated increase in calcitonin secretion is mediated by changes in blood calcium.[86] Recently, newer calcitonin assay procedures have demonstrated a postprandial increase in calcitonin, independent of changes in serum calcium, thus reintroducing the possibility of an enterocalcitonin axis in humans.[244] If calcitonin secretory capacity is an adaptive response to the challenge of increased intestinal absorption of calcium, alterations in calcitonin would be anticipated in individuals with absorptive hypercalciuria. In this setting, calcitonin could be attenuating the calcium challenge by its well-known antihypercalcemic effect or a more speculative inhibitory effect on intestinal transport of calcium.[245,246]

An alternative consideration is that augmented calcitonin secretion is a primary defect in some individuals. Hypercalciuria could develop through direct renal calciuretic action of calcitonin; this would also explain the lowered TmP_i/GFR reported in some patients with absorptive hypercalciuria.[241] Elevated levels of $1,25(OH)_2D_3$ could be explained by direct stimulation of renal 25-dihydroxy-1-hydroxylase activity by calcitonin.[247] Some support for this view comes from the report of elevated levels of $1,25(OH)_2D_3$ in patients with medullary carcinoma of the thyroid and increased plasma calcitonin.[248] In relationship to increased urinary excretion of calcium, it should be noted that hypercalciuria is less common in females, and females are relatively calcitonin-deficient compared with males.[144] Furthermore, a notable incidence of hypercalciuria occurs in patients with calcitonin excess due to medullary thyroid carcinoma, but the role of concomitant hyperparathyroidism in the generation of hypercalciuria has not been excluded.[249] It may thus be possible that calcitonin secretion plays some role in the pathogenesis of hypercalciuria.

C. Pediatric Disorders

1. Congenital Thyroid Dysgenesis

Children with congenital thyroid dysgenesis (CTD) have lower than normal levels of plasma CT in the basal state and during provocative testing with two known CT secretagogues, calcium and pentagastrin.[22] Because CT can act to lower blood calcium, this CT deficiency may explain why the children with congenital cretinism are less able than the normal children to rapidly correct the hypercalcemia induced by the calcium infusion.[250] In addition, the pattern of stimulated CT secretion in the congenital cretin group is also different from that observed in the normal children. In normal children, the peak plasma CT response occurs within a consistent time period after the initiation of each infusion. In the CTD group, the peak response is erratic and occurs later than in the normal group. Thus, children with CTD not only have significantly lower plasma CT concentrations than normal children but also have CT secretory responses that differ qualitatively from those observed in normal children.[97]

The CT deficiency in these children with hypothyroidism may be the result of either quantitative or qualitative C cell abnormalities. There are no data regarding C cell numbers in congenital thyroid dysgenesis. However, the thyroid does play an important role in the embryogenesis of C cells in mammals. These C cells are derived from neural crest elements present in the fourth pair of pharyngeal pouches.[251] During embryogenesis in mammals, these neural crest elements migrate to the developing thyroid and become disseminated among the follicular cells. A physiologic interaction between the C cells and the thyroid follicular cells has been suggested.[252] The similarity of the poor secretory response observed in both the children with congenital cretinism and the patient with the lingual thyroid suggests that the CT deficiency in these children may be due not only to the absence of thyroid tissue but also to the failure of normal thyroidal migration and failure of incorporation of C cells into a normally situated thyroid gland.

The demonstration of CT deficiency in children is of particular interest because there is evidence that CT may play an important role in the regulation of skeletal metabolism during childhood. Tashjian et al.[253] have demonstrated C cells in the normal neonatal thyroid gland to be relatively greater in number and to have greater CT content than those of the normal adult. Elevated levels of plasma CT have been described in neonates[254-256] and in cord blood compared with matched maternal blood.[257]

Despite CT deficiency or undersecretion, children with thyroid dysgenesis have no obvious disorder of calcium metabolism, and the typical skeletal abnormalities of this disease appear to be corrected by thyroid hormone replacement. Nonetheless, an unappreciated mineral abnormality may be present in these children. These data suggest that comprehensive evaluation of calcium homeostasis and skeletal metabolism should be considered to determine any pathophysiologic consequence of decreased calcitonin secretion in children with congenital thyroid dysgenesis.[97]

2. Williams Syndrome

Children with Williams syndrome (WS) have decreased calcitonin secretion and a slower than normal clearance of calcium following an intravenous calcium bolus.[258,259] Because calcitonin acts to lower serum calcium levels, a deficiency of calcitonin would explain why children with WS have subnormal calcium clearance. It might also explain the tendency of WS patients to develop infantile hypercalcemia. However, it is highly unlikely that all of the diverse features of this syndrome are due to calcitonin deficiency. An intriguing but purely speculative hypothesis that might relate the association of central nervous system dysfunction and abnormalities of calcium metabolism in patients with WS is that these patients might have an underlying genetic disturbance resulting in the abnormal production of two of the peptides regulated by the calcitonin gene, calcitonin itself and calcitonin gene-related peptide (CGRP).

D. Renal Disease

Although there are increases in immunoassayable calcitonin with both acute and chronic renal failure,[260-263] there is considerable disagreement regarding the significance of the increases (see Chapter 13). It has been reported that when patients with renal disease are dialyzed or receive calcium infusion, their already elevated calcitonin increases further.[109,263-267] Other studies indicate no increase in these patients upon dialysis or calcium infusion.[261-272] It is still not clear whether the elevation represents an abnormality of hormone secretion, metabolism, or both. However, since the kidney is active in the metabolism of the hormone, it is likely that the abnormality is metabolic, at least in part.[94,206] This is supported by the fact that the metabolic clearance rate of calcitonin in renal failure is decreased.[268] Moreover, resolution of the renal failure is associated with a return to normal calcitonin levels.[263,265,269] Since the secretion and/or metabolism of calcitonin is abnormal in renal disease and since renal osteodystrophy is characterized by, among other features, increased bone resorption, then calcitonin, which acts to inhibit bone resorption, may be implicated in the pathogenesis of uremic osteodystrophy.[262,263] In support of this view is the observation that lesser bone involvement in renal disease is associated with the greatest increases in plasma calcitonin, which may be compensatory to the increased bone resorption.[270] Both hormone secretion and hormone metabolism may be involved in the mechanism of hypercalcitoninemia seen in renal failure. Since calcium levels are typically low in these patients, there is no obvious reason for increased secretion of calcitonin. However, serum gastrin is increased in renal failure, and pentagastrin is a potent calcitonin secretagogue.[271] Additionally, other chronic hypergastrinemic states, such as pernicious anemia, are reported to have hypercalcitoninemia. However, in renal disease,[78] there is no correlation between levels of calcitonin and plasma gastrin.

It has been noted that the calcitonin found in the plasma of patients with renal disease has a relatively small proportion of calcitonin monomer, unlike other hypercalcitoninemic states (such as MTC) in which the monomeric form of calcitonin seems to be dominant.[266] The dominant form of calcitonin in patients with renal disease is of a much higher molecular weight and unknown biological significance. There even appear to be differences between the species of calcitonin in the blood of patients with acute renal failure versus dialysis patients.[269] In the patient undergoing dialysis, monomeric and other small species of calcitonin may be lost through the dialysis, thus decreasing plasma calcitonin concentration. Conversely, the calcium load of the dialysis may represent a challenge sufficient to stimulate all calcitonin species, with the larger less likely to be removed via dialysis. It is possible that the abnormal immunochemical forms of calcitonin found in renal disease are less biologically active. In rats, activity as measured by radioimmunoassay is reduced and calcitonin response to calcium challenge is blunted when the animal tested has acute renal failure.[269] It may be that established renal failure is characterized by low levels of biologically active calcitonin with high levels of inactive hormone, whereas early renal failure might be characterized by calcitonin deficiency alone.[94,203]

E. Bone Disease

Calcitonin secretion is abnormal in patients with pyknodysostosis and may be altered in other hyperostotic states as well.[69] Reduced calcitonin reserve in females may account for the greater severity of osteitis fibrosa cystica in women with primary hyperparathyroidism.[109,272] If osteoporosis is due to elevated bone resorption, then, as detailed in Chapter 12, calcitonin deficiency may play a role in this disease as well.[148,273-278] This view is supported by studies in which calcitonin has been of therapeutic benefit.[147,275,276]

V. RECENT DEVELOPMENTS: NEWLY APPRECIATED SECRETORY PRODUCTS OF THYROID C CELLS

Two new groups of substances are related to calcitonin secretion: the chromogranins, particularly chromogranin A (Chr A), and the peptides encoded for by the calcitonin gene, especially CGRP (calcitonin gene-related peptide) and PDN-21 (katacalcin).[280] Chr A is a 70,000 to 80,000 dalton protein that is present in essentially every endocrine tissue studied.[279-286] Chr A was originally identified as the major soluble protein of catecholamine storage vesicles of the adrenal medulla and sympathetic nerves.[287-294] Immunochemical and biochemical techniques have subsequently localized it in the pituitary gland, pancreas, hypothalamus, thymus, thyroid gland, intestine, and parathyroid gland of several species including humans.[282-284,295] In retrospect, in its parathyroidal location, Chr A is probably indistinguishable from parathyroid secretory protein (PSP).[295-298] In addition to being present in endocrine tissues, Chr A is also present in nonendocrine tissues like the lung and intestine that contain endocrine cells.[281,283,284,286,299]

Chr A is also present in abnormally increased amounts in malignant endocrine tissues and in malignant nonendocrine tissues that produce hormones.[281,283,299] In both normal and malignant endocrine tissue, Chr A is co-secreted with its associated hormones, for example, with parathyroid hormone in hyperparathyroidism, with calcitonin in medullary thyroid carcinoma, with catecholamines in pheochromocytomas, and with a variety of peptide hormones including calcitonin in lung cancer.[282-284,299] Because Chr A is so widely distributed among endocrine tissues in several animal species and because it is contained within the same storage vesicles and cosecreted with the hormonal product(s) of these various tissues, it is very likely that Chr A plays some role in the biosynthesis, storage, and secretion of the various hormones with which it is associated.[283,284,290,293,295,300-303] In addition, the secretion of Chr A provides another method of assessing the secretory activity of these various hormone-producing tissues, especially since there is structural heterogeneity of Chr A from different tissues.[285] Thus, Chr A has emerged as a marker for a wide variety of hormone-producing tumors, such as pituitary tumors, pancreatic tumors, parathyroid tumors, adrenal tumors, and thyroid tumors, and the wide variety of tumors that produce hormones ectopically, such as carcinoma of the lung and gastrointestinal tract.

Calcitonin is a well-established marker for medullary thyroid carcinoma and other tumors such as carcinoma of the lung.[94,203] During the last several years, it has become apparent from studies with recombinant DNA technology that the calcitonin gene encodes for putative peptides other than calcitonin.[304-307] This scheme demonstrates the potential presence of eight consequent peptides. Of these peptides, biological activity has been demonstrated for CGRP (calcitonin gene-related peptide) and PDN-21 (katacalcin), and it is thus likely that they are true hormones.[308-310] Thus, the techniques of molecular biology have demonstrated the complexity of mRNA processing and have correctly predicted the existence of new peptide hormones.[309] More important, however, has been the demonstration that at least two of the new peptide sequences predicted by the calcitonin gene, CGRP and PDN-21, are contained in and secreted by tumors associated with abnormal calcitonin production, most notably medullary thyroid carcinoma.[280,306,311]

References

1. Lowery GH, Aster RH, Carr EA, et al: Early diagnostic criteria of congenital hypothyroidism. J Dis Child 96:131–136, 1958.
2. Fisher DA: Thyroid function tests in childhood. Pediatric aspects. *In* Werner SC, Ingbar SH (eds): The Thyroid. 3rd ed. New York, Harper and Row, 1971, pp 292, 807.
3. Krane SM: Review of body systems. II. Skeletal system; neuromuscular systems; reproductive tract; blood; adrenal cortex; adrenal medulla; pituitary myxedema. *In* Werner SC, Ingbar SH (eds): The Thyroid. 3rd ed. New York, Harper and Row, 1971, pp 763-769.
4. Wilkins LW: Hormonal influences on skeletal growth. Ann NY Acad Sci 60:763–770, 1955.
5. Wilkins LW: Growth hormone. *In* Blizzard RM, Migeon CJ (eds): The Diagnosis and Treatment of Endocrine Disorders in Childhood and Adolescence. Springfield, IL, Charles C Thomas, 1962, pp 93-99.
6. Tapp E: Effects of hormones on bone in growing rats. J Bone Joint Surg 48B:526, 1966.
7. Walker DG: An assay of the skeletogenic effect of L-triiodothyronine and its acetic acid analogue in immature rats. Bull Johns Hopkins Hosp 101:101–105, 1957.
8. Fell HB, Mellanby E: Effect of L-triiodothyronine on the growth and development of embryonic chick limb-bones in tissue culture. J Physiol (London) 133:89–95, 1956.
9. Reikstniece E, Asling CW: Thyroxine augmentation of growth hormone–induced endochondral osteogenesis (31460). Proc Soc Exp Biol Med 123:258–263, 1966.
10. Baume LJ, Beck H, Evans HM: Hormonal control of tooth eruption. II. The response of the incisors of hypophysectomized rats to growth hormone, thyroxin or the combination of both. J Dent Res 33:104, 1954.

11. Jenkins GN: Mucosal neuromas. *In* The Physiology of the Mouth. Philadelphia, Davis, 1966, pp 199-204.
12. Talbot NB: Influence of thyroid hormone on serum phosphatase. Endocrinology 24:872, 1939.
13. Whedon GE, Neumann WF, Jenkins DW: *In* Progress in the Development of Methods in Bone Densitometry. March 25–27, 1965, Washington, DC. Sponsored by NIAMD and the American Institute of Biological Sciences. Published by Scientific and Technical Information Division of NASA, 1966.
14. Aub JC, Bauer W, Heath C, Ropes M: Studies of calcium and phosphorus metabolism. III. The effects of the thyroid hormone and thyroid disease. J Clin Invest 7:97–102, 1929.
15. Kivirikko KI, Laitinen O, Lamberg BA: Value of urine and serum hydroxyprolene in the diagnosis of thyroid disease. J Clin Endocrinol Metab 1347:25–31, 1965.
16. Kivirikko KI: Urinary excretion of hydroxyproline in health and disease. Int Rev Connect Tissue Res 5:93–98, 1971.
17. Krane SM, Brownell GL, Stanbury JB, Corrigan H: The effect of thyroid disease on calcium metabolism in man. J Clin Invest 35:874–880, 1956.
18. Smith DA, Fraser SA, Wilson GM: Hyperthyroidism and calcium metabolism. Clin Endocrinol Metab 2:333–337, 1973.
19. Krane SM: Skeletal system, neuromuscular system, emotions and mentation. *In* Werner SC, Ingbar SH (eds): The Thyroid. 3rd ed. New York, Harper and Row, 1971, pp 598–603.
20. Bouillon R, DeMoor P: Parathyroid function in patients with hyper or hypothyroidism. J Clin Endocrinol Metab 38:999–1003, 1974.
21. Gittes RF, Irwin GL: Roles of thyroxine and thyrocalcitonin in the response to hypercalcemia in rats. Endocrinology 79:1033–1038, 1966.
22. Carey DE, Jones KL, Parthemore JG, Deftos LJ: Calcitonin secretion in congenital nongoitrous cretinism. J Clin Invest 65:892–895, 1980.
23. Bateson EM, Chandler S: Nephrocalcinosis in cretinism. Br J Radiol 38:581–587, 1965.
24. Zaloga G, Eil C, O'Brian JT: Reversible hypocalciuric hypercalcemia associated with hypothyroidism. Am J Med 77:1101–1104, 1984.
25. Silberberg M, Silberberg R: Growth and development of the long bones of castrated mice under the influence of thyroxine. Anat Rec 98:181–186, 1947.
26. Silberberg M, Silberberg R: Influence of the endocrine glands on growth and aging of the skeleton. Arch Pathol 36:512–517, 1943.
27. Adams PH, Jowsey J, Kelly PJ, et al: Effects of hyperthyroidism on bone and mineral metabolism in man. QJ Med 36:1–6, 1967.
28. Price PA, Parthemore JG, Deftos LJ: A new biochemical marker for bone metabolism. J Clin Invest 66:878–883, 1980.
29. von Recklinghausen F: Die fibrose oder deformirende Ostitis, die Osteomalacie und die osteoplatische Carcinose in ihren gegenseitigen Beziehungen. Berlin, Festschr. Rudolf Virchow Reimer, 1891, pp 1–7.
30. Raisz LG, Kream BE: Regulation of bone formation. Part I. N Engl J Med 309:83–88, 1983.
31. Laake H: Osteoporosis in association with thyrotoxicosis. Acta Med Scand 15:229–235, 1955.
32. Fraser SA, Anderson JB, Smith DA, et al: Osteoporosis and fractures following thyrotoxicosis. Lancet 1:981–987, 1971.
33. Freedberg IM: Skin and connective tissue. *In* Werner SC, Ingbar SH (eds): The Thyroid. 3rd ed. New York, Harper and Row, 1971, pp 515–521.
34. Gimlett TMD: Localized myxoedema and thyroid acropachy. *In* Pitt-Rivers R, Trotter WR (eds): The Thyroid Gland, vol 2. London, Butterworth, 1964, pp 198–206.
35. Friedlander JA, Williams GA, Bowser EN, et al: Amino acid transport by rat parathyroid glands in vivo: Effect of low calcium diet. Proc Soc Exp Biol Med 120:20–26, 1965.
36. Krawitt EL: Duodenal calcium transport in hyperthyroidism (32108). Proc Soc Exp Biol Med 125:417–422, 1967.
37. Lewin I, Samackson J: Changes in calcium metabolism following the correction of hyperthyroidism and hypermetabolism in man. J Lab Clin Med 76:1016–1021, 1972.
38. Peerenboom H, Keck E, Kruskemper HL, et al: The defect of intestinal calcium transport in hyperthyroidism and its response to therapy. Clin Endocrinol Metab 59:936–940, 1984.
39. Harden RM, Harrison MT, Alexander WD, et al: Phosphate excretion and parathyroid function in thyrotoxicosis. J Endocrinol 28:281–287, 1964.
40. Kivirikko KI, Koivulsalo M, Laitinen O, et al: Effect of thyroxine on the hydroxyproline in rat urine and skin. Acta Physiol Scand 57:462–468, 1963.
41. Haddad J, Birge S, Couranz S, et al: Non-dialyzable urinary hydroxyproline: An index of bone formation? Clin Res 17:285–291, 1969.
42. Benoit FL, Watten RH: Renal tubular transportation of hydroxyproline peptides—evidence for reabsorption and secretion. Metab Clin Exp 17:20–26, 1968.
43. Baxter JD, Bondy PK: Hypercalcemia of thyrotoxicosis. Ann Intern Med 65:429–436, 1966.
44. Epstein FH, Freedman LR, Levitin H: Hypercalcemia, nephrocalcinosis and reversible renal insufficiency associated with hyperthyroidism. N Engl J Med 259:782–788, 1958.
45. Sataline LR, Powell C, Hamwi GJ: Suppression of the hypercalcemia of thyrotoxicosis by corticosteroids. N Engl J Med 267:646–652, 1962.
46. Parfitt AM, Dent LE: Hyperthyroidism and hypercalcemia. Found J Med 39:171–177, 1970.
47. Engfeldt B, Hertquist SO: The functional relation between the thyroid and parathyroids and the effect of the thyroid on bone tissue. Acta Endocrinol 15:109–113, 1954.
48. Breuer RI, McPherson HT: Hypercalcemia in concurrent hyperthyroidism and hyperparathyroidism. Arch Intern Med 118:310–315, 1966.
49. Malamos B, Sfikakis P, Pandos P: Renal handling of phosphate in thyroid disease. J Endocrinol 45:269–275, 1969.
50. Parsons V, Anderson J: The maximum renal tubular reabsorptive rate of inorganic phosphate in thyrotoxicosis. Clin Sci 27:313–319, 1964.
51. Harrison MT, Harden RM, Alexander WD: Some effects of parathyroid hormone in thyrotoxicosis. J Clin Endocrinol Metab 24:214–220, 1964.
52. Askanazy M, Rutishauser E: Die Knocken der Basedow-kranken. Beitrag zur latenten Osteodystrophia Fibrosa. Virchows Arch Pathol Anat Physiol 291:653–658, 1933.
53. Fallon MD, Perry III HM, Bergfeld M, et al: Exogenous hyperthyroidism with osteoporosis. Arch Intern Med 143:442–447, 1983.
54. Beigel Y, Arie R, Halable E, et al: Hypocalcemia, a

possible manifestation of thyrotoxicosis. PG Med J 59:317–322, 1983.
55. Daly JG, Greenwood RM, Hinsworth RL: Serum calcium concentration in hyperthyroidism at diagnosis and after treatment. Clin Endocrinol 19:397, 1983.
55a. Kabadi UM: Optimal daily levothyroxine dose in primary hypothyroidism. Arch Intern Med 149:2209–2212, 1989.
55b. Perry HM: Thyroid replacement and osteoporosis. Arch Intern Med 146:41–42, 1986.
56. Copp DH, Cameron EC, Chaney BA, et al: Evidence for calcitonin—a new hormone from the parathyroid that lowers blood calcium. Endocrinology 70:638–643, 1962.
57. Deftos LJ: Calcitonin. *In* Gray CH, James VHT (eds): Hormones in Blood, vol 2. London, Academic Press, 1979, pp 97–141.
58. Hirsch PF, Garthier GF, Munson PL: Thyroid hypocalcemic principle and recurrent laryngeal nerve injury as factors affecting the response to parathyroidectomy in rats. Endocrinology 73:244–250, 1963.
59. Sturtridge WC, Kumar MA: Assay of calcitonin in human plasma. Lancet 1:725-726, 1968.
60. Gudmundsson TV, Woodhouse NJY, Osafo TD, et al: Plasma-calcitonin in man. Lancet 1:443-445, 1969.
61. Bell PH, Dziobkowski C, Barg WF, et al: Plasma calcitonin in man. Lancet 2:104–105, 1970.
62. Clark MB, Byfield PGH, Boyd GW, et al: A radioimmunoassay for human calcitonin M. Lancet 2:74, 1969.
63. Tashjian AHT Jr, Howland BG, Melvin KEW, et al: Immunoassay of human calcitonin. Clinical measurement, relation to serum calcium and studies in patients with medullary carcinoma. N Engl J Med 283:890–894, 1970.
64. Deftos LJ: Immunoassay for human calcitonin. I. Method. Metab Clin Exp 20:1122–1127, 1971.
65. Deftos LJ, Bury AE, Habener JF, et al: Immunoassay for human calcitonin. II. Clinical studies. Metab Clin Exp 20:1129–1135, 1971.
66. MacIntyre I, Foster GV, Woodhouse NJY, et al: Calcitonin. *In* Talmage RV, Munson PL (eds): Calcium, Parathyroid Hormone and the Calcitonins. Amsterdam, Excerpta Medica Foundation, 1972, pp 83-88.
67. Melvin KEW, Miller HH, Tashjian AHT Jr: Early diagnosis of medullary carcinoma of the thyroid gland by means of calcitonin assay. N Engl J Med 285:1115–1121, 1971.
68. Melvin KEW, Tashjian AHT Jr, Miller HH: Studies in familial medullary thyroid carcinoma. Recent Prog Horm Res 28:344-399, 1972.
69. Baker RK, Wallach S, Tashjian AH Jr: Plasma calcitonin in pycnodysostosis. Intermittently high basal levels and exaggerated responses to calcium and glucagon infusions. J Clin Endocrinol Metab 37:46–55, 1973.
70. Beceiro J, Quais S, Hill CS Jr, et al: Serum calcitonin levels in medullary carcinoma of thyroid (MCT), hypercalcemia associated with malignancy and carcinoid tumors. Clin Res 19:367, 1971.
71. Samaan NA, Hill CS, Beceiro JR, et al: Immunoreactive calcitonin in medullary carcinoma of the thyroid and in maternal and cord serum. J Lab Clin Med 81:671–677, 1973.
72. Klein GL, Wadlington EL, Collins ED, et al: Calcitonin levels in sera of infants and children: Relations to age and periods of bone growth. Calcif Tissue Int 36:635–638, 1984.
73. Hesch RD, Hufner M, Hausenhager R: Inhibition of gastric secretion by calcitonin in man. Horm Metab Res 3:140–146, 1971.
74. Hesch RD, Woodhead S, Huffner M, et al: Gastrointestinal stimulation of calcitonin in adults and newborns. Horm Metab Res 5:235–240, 1973.
75. Sizemore GW, Go VLW, Kaplan EL, et al: Relations of calcitonin and gastrin in the Zollinger-Ellison syndrome and medullary carcinoma of the thyroid. N Engl J Med 288:614–644, 1973.
76. Markey WS, Ryan WG, Economou SG, et al: Familial medullary carcinoma and parathyroid adenoma without pheochromocytoma. Report of two cases. Ann Intern Med 78:898–903, 1973.
77. Silva OL, Snider RH, Becker KD: Radioimmunoassay of calcitonin in human plasma. Clin Chem 20:337–342, 1974.
78. Heynen G, Franchimont P: Human calcitonin radioimmunoassay in normal and pathological conditions. Eur J Clin Invest 4:213–222, 1974.
79. Silva OL, Becker KC, Primack A, et al: Ectopic production of calcitonin measurement of physiological levels of calcitonin in human plasma. Lancet 2:443–444, 1973.
80. Silva OL, Becker KC, Selawry HP: Human calcitonin and serum-phosphate. Lancet 1:1055, 1974.
81. Bieler EU, van Rooyen RJ, deBruin EJP, et al: A radioimmunoassay technique for human calcitonin (HC) in plasma avoiding the nonspecific interferences of plasma proteins on the tracer binding. Horm Metab Res 5:231–236, 1973.
82. Bijvoet OLM, van der Sluys Veer J, Greven HM, et al: Influence of calcitonin on renal excretion of sodium and calcium. *In* Talmage RV, Munson PL (eds): Calcium, Parathyroid Hormone and the Calcitonins. Amsterdam, Excerpta Medica Foundation, 1972, pp 284-289.
83. Potts JT Jr, Deftos LJ: Parathyroid hormone, calcitonin, vitamin D, bone and bone mineral metabolism. *In* Bondy PK (ed): Duncan's Diseases of Metabolism. 7th ed. Philadelphia, WB Saunders, 1974, pp 1225-1231.
84. Jackson CE, Tashjian AHT Jr, Block MA: Diagnostic dependability of calcitonin assay in family studies for medullary thyroid carcinoma. J Lab Clin Med 78:817–823, 1971.
85. Sizemore GW, Leffler J, Fisher J, et al: Physiological aspects of human calcitonin secretion. Clin Res 20:441, 1972.
86. Austin LA, Heath H III, Go VLW: Regulation of calcitonin secretion in normal man by changes of serum calcium within the physiologic range. J Clin Invest 64:1721–1724, 1979.
87. Body JJ, Heath H III: Estimates of circulating monomeric calcitonin: Physiological studies in normal and thyroidectomized man. J Clin Endocrinol Metab 57:897-902, 1983.
88. Deftos LJ, Murray TM, Powell DA, et al: Radioimmunoassay of plasma calcitonin in hypo and hypercalcemic states in man. *In* Talmage RV, Munson PL (eds): Calcium, Parathyroid Hormone and the Calcitonins. Amsterdam, Excerpta Medica Foundation, 1972, p 140.
89. Deftos LJ, Powell D, Parthemore JG, et al: Secretion of calcitonin in hypocalcemic states in man. J Clin Invest 52:3109–3115, 1973.
90. Mohsen S, Moukhtar AJ, Tharaud D, et al: Endocrinologie—extraction et concentration de la calcitonine plasmatique humaine par des anticorps

couples sur support solide. CR Hebd Seanc Acad Sci Ser D 276:3445–3451, 1973.
91. Tashjian AHT Jr, Voelkel EF: Human calcitonin: Application of affinity chromatography. *In* Jaffe BM, Behrman HR (eds): Methods of Hormone Radioimmunoassay. New York, Academic Press, 1974, pp 199–213.
92. Body JJ, Heath HD: Nonspecific increases in plasma immunoreactive calcitonin in healthy individuals: Discrimination from medullary thyroid carcinoma by a new extraction technique. Clin Chem 30:511–514, 1984.
93. Salmon DM, Azria M, Zanelli J: Quantitative cytochemical responses to exogenous administered calcitonins in rats kidney and bone cells. Mol Cell Endocrinol 33:293–304, 1983.
94. Deftos LJ: Medullary Thyroid Carcinoma. New York, S. Karger, 1983, pp 1–114.
95. Blahos J: Calcitonin activity assessed by calcium tolerance test in patients with thyroid disorders. Endokrinologie 64:191–195, 1975.
96. Silva OL, Wisneski LA, Cyrus J, et al: Calcitonin in thyroidectomized patients. Am J Med Sci 275:159–164, 1978.
97. McDermott MT, Kidd GS, Blue B, et al: Reduced bone mineral content in totally thyroidectomized patients: Possible effect of calcitonin deficiency. J Clin Endocrinol Metab 56:936–939, 1983.
98. Melvin KEW, Tashjian AH Jr, Cassidy CE, et al: Cushing's syndrome caused by ACTH- and calcitonin-secreting medullary carcinoma of the thyroid. Metabolism 19:831–838, 1970.
99. Roos BA, Cooper CW, Frelinger AL, et al: Acute and chronic fluctuations of immunoreactive and biologically active plasma calcitonin in the rat. Endocrinology 103:2180–2186, 1978.
100. Raisz LG, Au WYW, Friedman J, et al: Inhibition of bone resorption in tissue culture by thyrocalcitonin. *In* Taylor S: Calcitonin. Proceedings, Symposium on Thyrocalcitonin and C-cells. London, Heinemann, 1968, pp 215–222.
101. Melvin KEW, Tashjian AH Jr, Bordier P: The metabolic significance of calcitonin-secreting thyroid carcinoma. *In* Clinical Aspects of Metabolic Bone Disease. Amsterdam, Excerpta Medica, 1973, pp 193–201.
102. Deftos LJ, Glowacki J: Mechanisms of Bone Disease. *In* Frohlich ED (ed): Pathophysiology. Altered Regulatory Mechanisms in Disease. 3rd ed. Philadelphia, JB Lippincott, 1984, pp 445–467.
103. Kalu DN, Hadzi-Georgopoulos A, Foster GV: Evidence for physiological importance of calcitonin in the regulation of plasma calcium in rats. J Clin Invest 55:722–727, 1975.
104. Cooper CW, Obie JF, Toverud SU, et al: Elevated serum calcitonin and serum calcium during suckling in the baby rat. Endocrinology 101:1657–1664, 1977.
105. Taylor TG, Lewis PE, Balderstone O: Role of calcitonin in protecting the skeleton during pregnancy and lactation. J Endocrinol 66:297–298, 1975.
106. Toverud SU, Harper C, Munson PL: Calcium metabolism during lactation. Enhanced effects of thyrocalcitonin. Endocrinology 99:371–378, 1976.
107. Sizemore GW, Heath H: Immunochemical heterogeneity of calcitonin in plasma of patients with medullary thyroid carcinoma. J Clin Invest 55:111–118, 1975.
108. Deftos LJ, Habener JF, Mayer GP, et al: An immunoassay for bovine calcitonin. J Lab Clin Med 79:480–490, 1972.
109. Parthemore JG, Deftos LJ: Calcitonin secretion in primary hyperparathyroidism. J Clin Endocrinol Metab 49:223–226, 1979.
110. Pak CYC, Steward A, Kaplan R, et al: Photon absorptiometric analysis of bone density in primary hyperparathyroidism. Lancet 2:78, 1975.
111. Deftos LJ, Weisman MH, Williams GW, et al: Influence of age and sex on plasma calcitonin in human beings. N Engl J Med 302:1351–1353, 1980.
112. Becker KL, Silva OL: Hypothesis. The bronchial Kulchitsky (K) cell as a source of humoral biologic activity. Med Hypothesis 7:943, 1981.
113. Blaustein A: Calcitonin secreting struma-carcinoid tumor of the ovary. Hum Pathol 10:222–228, 1979.
114. Catherwood BD, Deftos LJ: Presence by radioimmunoassay of a calcitonin-like substance in porcine pituitary glands. Endocrinology 106:1886–1891, 1980.
115. Deftos LJ, Burton D, Catherwood BD, et al: Demonstration by immunoperoxidase histochemistry of calcitonin in the anterior lobe of the rat pituitary. J Clin Endocrinol Metab 47:457–460, 1978.
116. Cooper CW, Peng TC, Obie JF, et al: Calcitonin-like immunoreactivity in rat and human pituitary glands: Histochemical, in vitro, and in vivo studies. Endocrinology 107:98–107, 1980.
117. Deftos LJ, Burton DW, Watkins WB, et al: Immunohistological studies of artiodactyl and teleost pituitaries with antisera to calcitonin. Gen Comp Endocrinol 42:9–18, 1980.
118. De Lellis RA, Wolfe JH: Calcitonin in spindle cell thymic carcinoid tumors. Arch Pathol Lab Med 100:340, 1976.
119. Israel L, Depiene A, Calmettes C, et al: The secretion of calcitonin by testicular carcinomas. Nouv Presse Med 6:3866–3870, 1977.
120. Watkins WB, Moore RY, Burton D, et al: Distribution of immunoreactive calcitonin in the rat pituitary gland. Endocrinology 106:1966–1970, 1980.
121. Alumets J, Hakanson R, Lundquist G, et al: Ontogeny and ultrastructure of somatostatin and calcitonin cells in the thyroid gland of the rat. Cell Tissue Res 206:193–201, 1980.
122. Deftos LJ, Bone HG, Parthemore JG: Immunohistological studies of medullary thyroid carcinoma and C-cell hyperplasia. J Clin Endocrinol Metab 51:857–862, 1980.
123. Deftos LJ, Catherwood BD: Dissociation between ACTH and beta endorphin immunoreactivity in cells of the rat pituitary. Life Sci 27:223–228, 1980.
124. Shibaski T, Deftos L, Guillemin R: Immunoreactive-endorphin, -adrenocorticotropin, and -calcitonin in extracts of anaplastic or differentiated (rat) medullary thyroid carcinoma. Biochem Biophys Res Commun 90:1266–1273, 1979.
125. Zeytinoglu FU, Gagel RF, Tashjian AH Jr, et al: Characterization of neurotensin production by a line of rat medullary thyroid carcinoma cells. Proc Natl Acad Sci USA 77:3741–3745, 1980.
126. Anderson A, Bergdahl L, Boquist L: Thyroid carcinoma in children. Am Surg 43:159–163, 1977.
127. Cantalamessa L, Catania A, Reschini E, et al: Inhibitory effect of calcitonin in growth hormone and insulin secretion in man. Metabolism 27:987–992, 1978.
128. Chiba S, Himori N: Effects of salmon calcitonin on SA nodal pacemaker activity and contractility in

isolated, blood-perfused atrial and papillary muscle preparations of dogs. Jpn Heart J 18:220–241, 1977.
129. Chiba T, Taminato T, Kadowaki S, et al: Effects of (Asul, 7)–331 calcitonin on gastric somatostatin and gastrin release. Gut 21:94–97, 1980.
130. Dangoumau J, Bussiere C, Noel M, et al: Influence of calcitonin on bile production in the rat. J Pharmacol 7:69–76, 1976.
131. Freed WJ, Perlow MJ, Wyatt RJ: Calcitonin. Inhibitory effect on eating in rats. Science 206:850–851, 1979.
132. Hotz J, Goebell H: Similar modes of action of calcitonin and glucagon in inhibiting pancreatic enzyme secretion in man. Klin Wochenschr 57:1265–1272, 1979.
133. Kisloff B, Moore EW: Effects of intravenous calcitonin on water, electrolyte, and calcium movement across in vivo rabbit jejunum and ileum. Gastroenterology 73:462–468, 1977.
134. Koelz HR, Drack GT, Blum AL: Effect of calcitonin on salivary amylase secretion in vivo and in vitro. Schweiz Med Wochenschr 106:298–299, 1976.
135. Pecile A, Ferri S, Braga PC, et al: Effects of intracerebroventricular calcitonin in the conscious rabbit. Experientia 31:332–333, 1975.
136. Perlow MJ, Freed WJ, Carman JS, et al: Calcitonin reduces feeding in man, monkey, and rat. Pharmacol Biochem Behav 12:609–612, 1980.
137. Strettle RJ, Bates RFL, Buckley GA: Evidence for a direct anti-inflammatory action of calcitonin. Inhibition of histamine-induced mouse Pinnal oedema by porcine calcitonin. J Pharm Pharmacol 32:192–195, 1980.
138. Werner S, Low H: Inhibitory effects of calcitonin on lipolysis and 47 calcium accumulation in rat adipose tissue in vivo. Horm Metab Res 6:30–36, 1974.
139. Fritsch H, Van S, Pearse A: Localization of somatostatin–substance P and calcitonin-like immunoreactivity in the neural ganglion of Ciona intestinalis L. Cell Tissue Res 202:262–274, 1979.
140. Fritsch H, Van S, Pearse A: Calcitonin-like immunochemical staining in the alimentary tract of Ciona intestinalis L. Cell Tissue Res 205:439–444, 1980.
141. Deftos LJ: Calcitonin in clinical medicine. *In* Stollerman GH (ed): Advances in Internal Medicine, vol 23. Chicago, Year Book Medical Publishers, 1978, pp 159–193.
142. Borle AB: Regulation of cellular calcium metabolism and calcium transport by calcitonin. J Membr Biol 21:125–146, 1975.
143. Parfitt AM: Calcitonin in the pathogenesis and treatment of osteoporosis. Triangle 22:91–102, 1983.
144. Shamonki IM, Frumar AM, Tatryn IV, et al: Age-related changes in calcitonin secretion in females. J Clin Endocrinol Metab 50:437–439, 1980.
145. Chestnut CH III, Baylink DJ, Sisom K, et al: Basal plasma immunoreactive calcitonin in postmenopausal osteoporosis. Metabolism 29:559–562, 1980.
146. Taggart H, Ivey JL, Sisom K, et al: Deficient calcitonin response to calcium stimulation in postmenopausal osteoporosis? Lancet, Feb 27:475–477, 1982.
146a. Reginster JY, Derasy R, Albert A, et al: Relationship between whole plasma calcitonin levels, calcitonin secretory capacity and plasma levels of estrone in healthy women and postmenopausal osteoporosis. J Clin Invest 83:1073–1077, 1989.
146b. Cano RP, Montoya MJ, Moruno R, et al: Calcitonin reserve in healthy women and patients with postmenopausal osteoporosis. Calcif Tissue Int 45:203–208, 1989.
147. Foresta C, Busnardo B, Ruzza G, et al: Lower calcitonin levels in young hypogonadic men with osteoporosis. Horm Metab Res 15:206–207, 1983.
148. Baud CA, de Siebenthal J, Langer B, et al: The effects of prolonged administration of thyrocalcitonin in human senile osteoporosis. Proceedings of the Second International Symposium on Calcitonin. New York, Elsevier, 1969, pp 540–546.
149. Gruber HE, Ivey JL, Thompson ER, Chestnut C, Baylink DJ: Long-term calcitonin therapy in postmenopausal osteoporosis. Min Electrolyte Metab 1:246–249, 1986.
150. Hioco D, del Pozo E, Bordier Ph, et al: The effects of prolonged administration of synthetic salmon calcitonin on calcium metabolism and bone morphology in postmenopausal osteoporosis. Proceedings of the 9th European Symposium on Calcified Tissues. Baden Near Vienna, Excerpta Medica, October 1-6, 1972, pp 135–138.
151. Jowsey JB, Riggs BL, Kelly PJ, et al: Calcium and salmon calcitonin in treatment of osteoporosis. J Clin Endocrinol Metab 47:633–639, 1978.
152. Milhaud G, Talbot JN, Coutris G: Calcitonin treatment of postmenopausal osteoporosis. Evaluation of efficacy by principal components analysis. Biomedicine 23:223–232, 1975.
153. Whedon GD: Osteoporosis. N Engl J Med 305:397–398, 1981.
154. Stevenson JC, White MC, Joplin GF, et al: Osteoporosis and calcitonin deficiency. Br Med J 285:1010–1011, 1982.
155. Stevenson JC, Hillyard C, Abeyasekera G, et al: Calcitonin and the calcium-regulating hormones in postmenopausal women: Effect of estrogens. Lancet, March 28:693–695, 1981.
156. Stevenson JC: Regulation of calcitonin and parathyroid hormone secretion by estrogens. Maturitas 4:1–7, 1982.
157. Parfitt AM: Treatment of osteoporosis: Theoretical possibilities. Clin Invest Med 5:181–183, 1980; Clin Invest Med 47:633–639, 1978.
158. Parfitt AM: The actions of parathyroid hormone on bone: Relation to bone remodeling and turnover, calcium homeostasis, and metabolic bone disease. Metabolism 25:1157–1188, 1976.
159. Baran DT, Whyte MP, Haussler, MR, et al: Effect of the menstrual cycle on calcium-regulating hormones in the normal young woman. J Clin Endocrinol Metab 50:377–379, 1980.
160. Pitkin RM, Reynolds WA, Williams GA, et al: Calcium regulating hormones during the menstrual cycle. J Clin Endocrinol Metab 47:626–632, 1978.
161. Morimoto S, Tsuji M, Okada Y, et al: The effect of estrogens on human calcitonin secretion after calcium infusion in elderly female subjects. Clin Endocrinol 13:135–143, 1980.
162. Morita R, Yamamoto I, Fukunaga M: Changes in sex hormones and calcium regulating hormones with reference to bone mass associated with aging. Endocrinol Jpn 1:15–22, 1979.
163. Orimo H, Shiraki M: Role of calcium regulating hormones in the pathogenesis of senile osteoporosis. Endocrinol Jpn 26:1–6, 1979.
164. Mulder R, Hackeng WHL, Silberbusch J: Racial difference in serum-calcitonin. Lancet 2:154–159, 1979.
165. Stevenson JC: Differential effects of aging and

menopause on calcitonin secretion. Proceedings of the International Symposium on Calcitonin, Milan, Italy, Abstract 19, 1984.

166. McMillan PJ, Hooker WM, Deftos LJ: Distribution of calcitonin-containing cells in the human thyroid. Am J Anat 140:73–78, 1974.
167. Williams ED: Medullary carcinoma of the thyroid. J Clin Pathol 20:395-401, 1967.
168. Ljungberg O, Bondeson L, Bondeson AG: Differentiated thyroid carcinoma, intermediate type: A new tumor entity with features of follicular and parafollicular cell carcinoma. Hum Pathol 15:218–228, 1984.
169. Saad MP, Ordonez NG, Guido JJ: The prognostic value of calcitonin immunostaining in medullary carcinoma of the thyroid. J Clin Endocrinol Metab 59:850–855, 1984.
170. Hill CS Jr, Ibanez ML, Samaan NA, et al: Medullary (solid) carcinoma of the thyroid gland. An analysis of the M.D. Anderson Hospital experience with patients with the tumor, its special features, and its histogenesis. Medicine (Baltimore) 52:141–171, 1973.
171. Baylink SB, Beaven MA, Buga LM, et al: Histaminase activity—a biochemical marker for medullary carcinoma of the thyroid. Am J Med 53:723–728, 1972.
172. Tashjian AH Jr, Wright DR, Ivey JL, et al: Calcitonin binding sites in bone. Relationships to biological response and escape. Recent Prog Horm Res 34:285–287, 1978.
173. Verdy M, Beaulieu R, Demers L, et al: Plasma calcitonin activity in a patient with thyroid medullary carcinoma and her children with osteoporosis. J Clin Endocrinol Metab 32:216–221, 1971.
174. Miravet L, Queille ML, Carre M, et al: Action of vitamin D metabolites on the bone of vitamin D–deficient rats. Ann Biol Anim Biochim Biophys 18:187–194, 1978.
175. Paterson CR: Vitamin D resistance in hypoparathyroidism with medullary carcinoma of the thyroid. Br Med J 1:952, 1977.
176. Rasmussen H, Wong M, Bikle D, et al: Hormonal control of the renal conversion of 25-hydroxycholecalciferol to 1,25-dihydroxycholecalciferol. J Clin Invest 51:2502–2504, 1972.
177. Avioli LV: Vitamin D, the kidney and calcium homeostasis. Kidney Int 2:241–246, 1972.
178. Popovtzer MM, Blum MS, Flis RS: Evidence for interference of 25(OH)vitamin D_3 with phosphaturic action of calcitonin. Am J Physiol E232:515–521, 1977.
179. Rasmussen B: Magnesium and phosphate in the serum of patients with medullary carcinoma of the thyroid. Clin Chim Acta 89:279–283, 1978.
180. Aach R, Kissane J: Medullary carcinoma of the thyroid with hypocalcemia and diarrhea. Am J Med 46:961–971, 1969.
181. Krane SM, Harris ED Jr, Singer FR, et al: Acute effects of calcitonin on bone formation in man. Metabolism 22:51–58, 1973.
182. Chong GL, Beahrs OH, Sizemore GW: Medullary carcinoma of the thyroid gland. Cancer 35:695–704, 1975.
183. Bone HG, Snyder WH, McMillan P, et al: Hyperabsorption of calcium in C-cell proliferative disorders. Proc 60th Ann Meeting Endocr Soc A70:109, 1978.
184. Cramer CF, Parkes CO, Copp DH: The effect of chicken and hog calcitonin on some parameters of Ca, P, and Mg metabolism in dogs. Can J Physiol Pharmacol 47:181–184, 1969.
185. Cramer CF: Effect of salmon calcitonin on in vivo calcium absorption in rats. Calcif Tissue Res 13:169–172, 1973.
186. Milhaud G, Moukhtar MS: Thyrocalcitonin. Effects on calcium kinetics in the rat. Proc Soc Exp Biol Med 123:207–209, 1966.
187. Kaplan EL, Peskin GW: Physiologic implications of medullary carcinoma of the thyroid gland. Surg Clin North Am 51:125–137, 1971.
188. Bernier JJ, Rambaud JC, Cattan D, et al: Diarrhea associated with medullary carcinoma of the thyroid. Gut 10:980–985, 1969.
189. Isaacs P, Whittaker SM, Turnberg LA: Diarrhea associated with medullary carcinoma of the thyroid. Studies of intestinal function in a patient. Gastroenterology 67:521–526, 1974.
190. Pearson KD, Wells SA, Keiser HR: Familial medullary carcinoma of the thyroid, adrenal pheochromocytoma, and parathyroid hyperplasia. Radiology 107:249–256, 1973.
191. Wallace S, Hill CS, Paulus DD Jr, et al: The radiologic aspects of medullary (solid) thyroid carcinoma. Radiol Clin North Am 8:463–474, 1970.
192. Barrowman JA, Bennett A, Hillenbrand R, et al: Diarrhea in thyroid medullary carcinoma. Role of prostaglandins and therapeutic effect of nutmeg. Br Med J 3:11–12, 1975.
193. Fawell WN, Thompson G: Nutmeg for diarrhea of medullary carcinoma of thyroid. N Engl J Med 289:108–109, 1973.
194. Khairi MRA, Dexter RN, Burzynski NJ, et al: Mucosal neuroma, pheochromocytoma, and medullary thyroid carcinoma. MEN, type III. Medicine 54:89–112, 1975.
195. Pearse AGE: The cytochemistry of the thyroid cells and their relationship to calcitonin. Proc R Soc 164:478–487, 1966.
196. Pearse AGE: Common cytochemical and ultrastructural characteristics of cells producing polypeptide hormones (the APUD series) and their relevance to thyroid and ultimobranchial C-cells and calcitonin. Proc R Soc 170:71–80, 1968.
197. Pearse AGE, Ewen SEB, Polak JM: The genesis of APUD amyloid in endocrine polypeptide tumors. Histochemical distinction for immunamyloid. Virchows Arch Abt B Zellpath 10:93–107, 1972.
198. Ellison EH, Wilson SD: The Zollinger-Ellison syndrome. Reappraisal and evaluation of 260 registered cases. Ann Surg 160:512–530, 1964.
199. Ljungberg O: On medullary carcinoma of the thyroid. A clinicopathologic entity. Acta Pathol Microbiol Scand 231:1–57, 1972.
200. Walker DM: Oral mucosal neuroma—medullary thyroid carcinoma syndrome. Br J Dermatol 88:599–603, 1973.
201. Dunn EL, Nishiyama RH, Thompson NW: Medullary carcinoma of the thyroid gland. Surgery 73:848–858, 1973.
202. Milhaud G, Calmettes C, Raymond JP, et al: Carcinoid secretant de la thyrocalcitonine. CR Hebd Seanc Acad Sci 270:2195–2198, 1970.
203. Deftos LJ: The thyroid gland in skeletal and calcium metabolism. *In* Avioli LV, Krane SM (eds): Metabolic Bone Disease. New York, Academic Press, 1978, pp 447–487.

203a. Mannelli M: Diagnostic problems in pheochromocytoma. J Endocrinol Invest 12:739–757, 1989.

204. Rosenberg EM, Hahn TJ, Orth DN, et al: ACTH-

secreting medullary carcinoma of the thyroid presenting as severe idiopathic osteoporosis and senile purpura: Report of a case and review of the literature. J Clin Endocrinol Metab 47:255–262, 1978.
204a. Spapen H, Gerlo E, Achlen E, et al: Pre- and peroperative diagnosis of metastatic pheochromocytoma in multiple endocrine neoplasia type 2a. J Endocrinol Invest 12:729–731, 1989.
205. Deftos LJ, Potts JT Jr: Plasma calcitonin (CT) measurements in medullary thyroid carcinoma (MTC) and disorders of calcium metabolism. Clin Res 18:673, 1970.
206. Jackson CE, Tashjian AHT Jr, Block MA: Detection of medullary thyroid cancer by calcitonin assay in families. Ann Intern Med 78:845–850, 1973.
207. Deftos LJ: Radioimmunoassay for calcitonin in medullary thyroid carcinoma. JAMA 227:403–409, 1974.
208. Wolfe HJ, Melvin KEW, Cervi-Skinner SJ, et al: C-cell hyperplasia preceding medullary thyroid carcinoma. N Engl J Med 289:437–442, 1973.
209. Hennessy JF, Wells SA, Ontjes DA, et al: A comparison of pentagastrin injection and calcium infusion as provocative agents for the detection of medullary carcinoma of the thyroid. J Clin Endocrinol Metab 39:487–495, 1974.
210. Hennessey JF, Gray TK, Cooper CW, et al: Stimulation of thyrocalcitonin secretion by pentagastrin and calcium in 2 patients with medullary carcinoma of the thyroid. J Clin Endocrinol Metab 36:200–206, 1973.
211. Ohta H, Yamamoto K, Endo K, et al: A new imaging agent for medullary carcinoma of the thyroid. J Nucl Med 25:323–325, 1984.
212. Hoefnagel H, Delprat CC, Marcuse HR, de Vijlder JJM: Role of thallium-201 total-body scintigraphy in follow-up of thyroid carcinoma. J Nucl Med 27:1854–1857, 1986.
213. Gottlied JA, Hill CS Jr: Chemotherapy of thyroid cancer with adriamycin. Experience with 30 patients. N Engl J Med 290:193–198, 1974.
214. Goltzman D, Potts JT Jr, Ridgway EC, et al: Calcitonin as a tumor marker. Use of the radioimmunoassay for calcitonin in the postoperative evaluation of patients with medullary thyroid carcinoma. J Clin Endocrinol Metab 290:1036–1041, 1974.
215. Milhaud G, Calmettes C, Julienne A, et al: Calcitonin secretion. *In* Talmage RV, Munson PL (eds): Calcium, Parathyroid Hormone and the Calcitonins. Amsterdam, Excerpta Medica Foundation, 1972, p 56.
216. Whitelaw AGL, Cohen SL: Ectopic production of calcitonin. Lancet 2:443–450, 1973.
217. Silva OL, Becker KC, Primack A, et al: Ectopic secretion of calcitonin by oat-cell carcinoma. N Engl J Med 290:1122–1127, 1974.
218. Deftos LJ, Rosen SW, Sartiano GP: Simultaneous ectopic production of parathyroid hormone (PTH) and calcitonin (CT). Clin Res 22:486, 1974.
219. Deftos LJ, McMillan PJ, Sartiano GP, et al: Simultaneous ectopic production of parathyroid hormone and calcitonin. Metabolism 25:543–549, 1976.
220. Milhaud G, Calmettes C, Taboulet J, et al: Letter: Hypersecretion of calcitonin in neoplastic conditions. Lancet 2:462–467, 1974.
221. Coombes RC, Hillyard C, Greenberg PB, et al: Plasma-immunoreactive-calcitonin in patients with non-thyroid tumors. Lancet 2:1080, 1974.
222. Parthemore JG, Deftos LJ, Bronzert D: The regulation of calcitonin in normal human plasma as assessed by immunoprecipitation and immunoextraction. J Clin Invest 56:835–841, 1975.
223. Heath H III, Sizemore GW: Plasma calcitonin in normal man, difference between men and women. J Clin Invest 60:1135–1140, 1977.
224. Deftos LJ: Calcitonin in clinical medicine. *In* Stollerman GH (ed): Advances in Internal Medicine, vol 23. Chicago, Year Book Medical Publishers, 1978, pp 159–164.
225. Parthemore JG, Deftos LJ: Calcitonin secretion in normal human subjects. J Clin Endocrinol Metab 47:184–189, 1978.
226. Silva OL, Becker KL, Primack A, et al: Increased serum calcitonin levels in bronchogenic cancer. Chest 69:495–504, 1976.
227. Lambert PW, Heath H, Sizemore GW: Basal and stimulated immunoreactive calcitonin values are not high in primary hyperparathyroidism (abstract). Clin Res 24:581, 1976.
228. Goldsmith REGW, Sizemore IW, Chen E, et al: Altemeier, familial hyperparathyroidism. Ann Intern Med 84:36–41, 1976.
229. Silva OL, Snider RH, Becker KL: Radioimmunoassay of calcitonin in human plasma. Clin Chem 20:337–342, 1974.
230. Adachi I, Abe K, Tanaka M, et al: Plasma human calcitonin (HCT) levels in normal and pathologic conditions and their responses to short calcium or tetragastrin infusion. Endocrinol Jpn 23:517, 1976.
231. Morita R, Fukunaga M, Yamamoto I, et al: Radioimmunoassay for human calcitonin employing synthetic calcitonin M: Its clinical application. Endocrinol Jpn 22:419–424, 1975.
232. Rojanasathit S, Haddad JG Jr: Human calcitonin radioimmunoassays: Characterization and application. Clin Chim Acta 78:425, 1977.
233. Ljunberg O, Dymling JF: Pathogenesis of C-cell neoplasia in thyroid gland. C-cell proliferation in a case of chronic hypercalcemia. Acta Pathol Microbiol Scand [A] 80:577–582, 1972.
234. Kracht J, Hachmeister U, Christ U: C-cells in the human thyroid. *In* Taylor S (ed): Calcitonin 1969. New York, Springer-Verlag, 1970, pp 274–280.
235. LiVolsi VA, Feind CR, LoGerfo P, et al: Demonstration by immunoperoxidase staining of hyperplasia of parafollicular cells in the thyroid gland in hyperparathyroidism. J Clin Endocrinol Metab 37:550–555, 1973.
236. Tashjian AHT Jr, Voelkel EF: Decreased thyrocalcitonin in thyroid glands from patients with hyperparathyroidism. J Clin Endocrinol Metab 27:1353–1358, 1967.
237. Kaplan RA, Haussler MR, Deftos LH, et al: The role of 1,25-dihydroxyvitamin D in the mediation of intestinal hyperabsorption of calcium in primary hyperparathyroidism and absorptive hypercalciuria. J Clin Invest 59:756–760, 1977.
238. Shen FH, Baylink DJ, Nielsen RL, et al: Increased serum 1,25-dihydroxyvitamin D in idiopathic hypercalciuria. J Lab Clin Med 90:955–962, 1977.
239. Coe FL, Favus MJ, Crockett T, et al: Effects of low-calcium diet on urine calcium excretion, parathyroid function and serum $1,25(OH)_2D_3$ levels in patients with idiopathic hypercalciuria and in normal subjects. Am J Med 72:25–32, 1982.
240. Gray RW, Wilz DR, Caldas AE, et al: The importance of phosphate in regulating plasma $1,25(OH)_2$-

vitamin D levels in humans: Studies in healthy subjects, in calcium stone formers, and in patients with primary hyperparathyroidism. J Clin Endocrinol Metab 45:299–306, 1977.

241. Broadus AE, Insogna KL, Lang LE, et al: A consideration of the hormonal basis and phosphate leak hypothesis of absorptive hypercalciuria. J Clin Endocrinol Metab 58:161–169, 1984.
242. Ivey JL, Roos BA, Shen FH, et al: Increased immunoreactive calcitonin in idiopathic hypercalciuria. Metab Bone Dis Rel Res 3:39–42, 1981
243. Brickman AS, Manolagas SC, Taylor B, et al: Calcitonin homeostasis in individuals with hypercalciuric nephrolithiasis. Clin Res 32:45A, 1984.
244. Cooper CW, Bolman RM III, Lineham WM, et al: Interrelationships between calcium, calcemic hormones and gastrointestinal hormones. Recent Prog Horm Res 34:259-283, 1979.
245. Barlet JP: Inhibition of calcium intestinal absorption: A possible physiological role for calcitonin in sheep. *In* Czitober H, Eschberger J (eds): Calcified Tissue 1972. Proceedings of the Ninth European Symposium on Calcified Tissues. Vienna, Facta Publications, 1979, pp 153–158.
246. Olson EB, DeLuca HF, Potts JT: Calcitonin inhibition of vitamin D–induced intestinal calcium absorption. Endocrinology 90:151–157, 1972.
247. Galante L, Coston KW, MacAuley SJ, et al: Effects of calcitonin on vitamin D metabolism. Nature 238:272–273, 1972.
248. Emmertsen KF, Melsen L, Mosekilde BI, et al: Altered vitamin D metabolism and bone remodeling in patients with medullary thyroid carcinoma and hypercalcitoninemia. Metab Bone Dis Rel Res 4:17–23, 1981.
249. Broadus AE: Mineral metabolism. *In* Felig JD, et al (eds): Endocrinology and Metabolism. New York, McGraw Hill, 1981, pp 963–1079.
250. Anast CS, Guthrie RA: Decreased calcium tolerance in nongoitrous cretins. Pediatr Res 5:668–672, 1971.
251. Weichert RF III: The neural ectodermal origin of the peptide-secreting endocrine glands. Am J Med 49:232–241, 1970.
252. Nunez EA, Gershon MD: Cytophysiology of thyroid parafollicular cells. Int Rev Cytol 52:1–80, 1978.
253. Tashjian AHT Jr: Distribution of calcitonin containing cells in the normal neonatal thyroid gland: A correlation of morphology with peptide content. J Clin Endocrinol Metab 41:1076–1081, 1975.
254. Dirksen HC, Anast CS: Interrelationship of serum immunoreactive calcitonin (iCT) and serum calcium in newborn infants (abstract). Pediatr Res 11:1180–1185, 1976.
255. David L, Anast CS: Serum immunoreactive calcitonin (iCT) in newborn (abstract). Pediatr Res 7:386, 1973.
256. Bergman L, Kjelimer I, Selstam U: Calcitonin and parathyroid hormone—relation to early neonatal hypocalcemia in infants of diabetic mothers. Biol Neonate 24:151–159, 1974.
257. Samaan NA, Anderson GD, Adam-Mayne MD: Immunoreactive calcitonin in the mother, neonate, child, and adult. Am J Obstet Gynecol 121:622–625, 1975.
258. Forbes GB, Bryson MF, Manning J, et al: Impaired calcium homeostasis in the infantile hypercalcemic syndrome. Acta Paediatr Scand 61:305–309, 1972.
259. Culler FL, Jone KL, Deftos LJ: Impaired calcitonin secretion in patients with Williams Syndrome. Pediatrics 107:720–723, 1985.
260. Ardaillou R, Beaufils M, Nivez MP, et al: Increased plasma calcitonin in early acute renal failure. Clin Sci Molec Med 49:301–304, 1975.
261. Augustin R, Hackeng WHL: Acute rise in serum calcitonin concentration during haemodialysis. Dtsch Med Wochenschr 103:508–512, 1978.
262. Cochran M, Hillyard CJ, Dew GJ, Martin TJ: Acute responsiveness to calcitonin in chronic renal failure. Br Med J 2:396–398, 1976.
263. Heynen G, Kanis JA, Oliver D, et al: Evidence that endogenous calcitonin protects against renal bone disease. Lancet 2:1322–1325, 1976.
264. Roos BA, Parthemore JG, Lee JC, Deftos LJ: Calcitonin heterogeneity. In vivo and in vitro studies. Calcif Tissue Res 22S:298–302, 1977.
265. Deftos LJ: Plasma calcitonin measurement as a marker for cancer. West J Med 124:489–490, 1976.
266. Lee JC, Catanzara A, Parthemore JG, et al: Hypercalcemia in disseminated coccidioidomycosis. N Engl J Med 297:431–433, 1977.
267. Parthemore JG, Deftos LJ: The regulation of calcitonin in normal human plasma as assessed by immunoprecipitation and immunoextraction. J Clin Invest 56:835–840, 1975.
268. Isaac R, Nivez MP, Piamba G, et al: Influence of calcium infusion on calcitonin and parathyroid hormone concentrations in normal and hemodialyzed subjects. Clin Nephrol 3:14–17, 1975.
269. Lee JC, Parthemore JG, Deftos LJ: Immunochemical heterogeneity of calcitonin in renal failure. J Clin Endocrinol Metab 45:528–533, 1977.
270. Kanis JA, Earnshaw M, Heynen G, et al: The possible role of calcitonin deficiency in the development of renal failure. Br Med J 1:209–210, 1972.
271. Korman MG, Lauer MC, Hansky J: Hypergastrinemia in chronic renal failure. Br Med J 1:209–210, 1972.
272. Heath H, Sizemore GW: Plasma calcitonin in normal man. Differences between men and women. J Clin Invest 60:1135–1140, 1977.
273. Bloch-Michel H, Milhaud G, Coutris J, et al: Traitement au long cours de l'osteoporose par la thyrocalcitonine. A propos de 7 observations. Rev Rhum Mal osteo-artic. 37:629–638, 1970.
274. Caniggia A, Gennari C, Bencini M, et al: Calcium metabolism and 47-calcium kinetics before and after long-term thyrocalcitonin treatment in senile osteoporosis. Clin Sci 38:397–407, 1970.
275. Cohn SH, Dombrowski CS, Hauser W, et al: Effects of porcine calcitonin on calcium metabolism in osteoporosis. J Clin Endocrinol Metab 33:719–728, 1971.
276. Milhaud G: Calcitonin 1975. Biomedicine 24:159–161, 1976.
277. Tamburino G, Fiore CE, Cottini E, Petralito A: Plasma calcitonin after calcium infusion in normal adults and in senile osteoporosis. IRCS Med Sci 4:41–47, 1976.
278. Riggs BL, Jowsey J, Kelly PJ, Arnaud CD: Role of hormonal factors in the pathogenesis of postmenopausal osteoporosis. Isr J Med Sci 12:615–619, 1976.
279. O'Connor DT: Human plasma chromogranin A (CgA): Detection by radioimmunoassay (RIA), and elevation in pheochromocytoma and in essential hypertension. Clin Res, May 1984.
280. Iwasaki J, Myers C, Freake HC: Concomitant secretion of katacalcin and calcitonin from perfused

human medullary thyroid carcinoma tissue. Horm Metab Res 15:572-577, 1983.
281. O'Connor DT, Deftos LJ: Human chromogranin A (CgA): Radioimmunoassay (RIA) demonstrates diagnostic plasma elevations in diverse peptide producing tumors. Clin Res, May 1984.
282. O'Connor DT, Burton D, Deftos LJ: Human chromogranin A (hCgA): Detection by immunohistochemistry in diverse polypeptide hormone-producing tumors. Proceedings, 65th Annual Meeting of the Endocrine Society, June 8–10, 1983, #186.
283. O'Connor DT, Burton D, Deftos LJ: Immunoreactive human chromogranin A in diverse polypeptide hormone producing human tumors and normal endocrine tissues. J Clin Endocrinol Metab 57:1084–1086, 1983.
284. O'Connor DT, Burton D, Parmer RJ, Deftos LJ: Human chromogranin A: Detection by immunohistochemistry in C cells and diverse polypeptide hormone producing tumors. Proceedings of the VIII International Conference on Calcium Regulating Hormones. Amsterdam, Elsevier Science Publishers, 1983.
285. O'Connor DT, Frigon RP: Chromogranin A, the major catecholamine storage vesicle soluble protein: Multiple size forms, subcellular storage, and regional distribution in chromaffin and nervous tissue elucidated by radioimmunoassay. J Biol Chem 259:3237–3247, 1984.
286. O'Connor DT: Chromogranin: Widespread immunoreactivity in polypeptide hormone producing tissues and in serum. Regul Pept 6:263–280, 1983.
287. Klein RL: Chemical composition of the large noradrenergic vesicles. *In* Clein RL, Lagerorantz H, Zimmerman H (eds): Neurotransmitter Vesicles. New York, Academic Press, 1982, pp 133–174.
288. Kobayashi S: Adrenal medulla: Chromaffin cells as paraneurones. Arch Histol Jpn 40[Suppl]:67–79, 1977.
289. Kobayashi S: Synaptic vesicles and secretory granules. A morphologist's view on their identity and difference. Biomed Res 1 [Suppl]:50–53, 1980.
290. Kobayashi S: Paraneuronic aspects of adrenal chromaffin cells. *In* Izumi F, Oka M, Kumakura K (eds): Advances in Biosciences, vol 36: Synthesis, Storage, and Secretion of Adrenal Catecholamines. Elmsford, NY, Pergamon Press, 1982, pp 21–28.
291. Lloyd RV, Wilson BS: Specific endocrine tissue marker defined by a monoclonal antibody. Science 222:628–630, 1983.
291a. Schneider FH, Smith AD, Winkler H: Secretion from the adrenal medulla: Biochemical evidence for exocytosis. Br J Pharmacol Chemother 31:94–104, 1967.
292. Winker H, Westhead E: The molecular organization of adrenal chromaffin granules. Neuroscience 5:1803–1823, 1980.
293. Smith AD, Winkler H: Purification and properties of an acidic protein from chromaffin granules of bovine adrenal medulla. Biochem J 103:483–492, 1967.
294. Smith WJ, Kirshner N: A specific soluble protein from the catecholamine storage vesicles of bovine adrenal medulla. Molec Pharmacol 3:52–62, 1967.
295. Cohn DV, Zangerle R, Fisher-Colbrie R, et al: Similarity of secretory protein I from parathyroid gland to chromogranin A from the adrenal medulla. Proc Natl Acad Sci USA 79:6056–6059, 1982.
296. Bhargava G, Sherwood LM: Phosphorylation of both parathyroid secretory protein and adrenal chromogranin A, similar proteins involved with secretory function in different tissues. Clin Res 31:469A, 1983.
297. Cohn DV, Elting J: Biosynthesis, processing and secretion of parathormone and secretory protein-I. Recent Prog Horm Res 39:181, 1983.
298. Habener JF, Kempner BW, Rich A, Potts JT Jr: Biosynthesis of parathyroid hormone. Recent Prog Horm Res 33:249, 1977.
299. O'Connor DT, Burton D, Deftos LJ: Chromogranin A: Immunohistology reveals its universal occurrence in normal polypeptide hormone producing endocrine glands. Life Sci 33:1657-1663, 1983.
300. Kempner B, Habener JF, Rich A, Potts JT Jr: Parathyroid secretion: Discovery of major calcium-dependent protein. Science 184:167, 1981.
301. Majzoub JA, Dee PC, Habener JF: Cellular and cell-free processing of parathyroid secretory proteins. J Biol Chem 257:3581–3588, 1982.
302. Ravazzola M, Orci L, Habener JF, Potts JT Jr: Parathyroid secretory protein. Lancet 2:371, 1978.
303. Blaschko H, Comline RS, Schneider FH, et al: Secretion of a chromaffin granule protein, chromogranin, from the adrenal gland after splanchnic stimulation. Nature 215:58–59, 1967.
304. Amara S, Jonas V, Rosenfeld MG, et al: Alternative RN processing in calcitonin gene expression. Nature 298:240-244, 1982.
305. Amara SG, Jonas V, O'Neil JA, et al: Calcitonin OOOH-terminal cleavage peptide as a model for identification of novel neuropeptides predicted by recombinant DNA analysis. J Biol Chem 257:2129-2135, 1982.
306. Ali-Rachedi A, Varndel IM, Facer P, et al: Immunocytochemical localization of katacalcin, a calcium-lowering hormone cleaved from the human calcitonin precursor. J Clin Endocrinol Metab 57:680-682, 1983.
307. Allison J, Hall L, MacIntyre I, et al: The construction and partial characterization of plasmids containing complementary DNA sequences to human calcitonin precursor polyprotein. Biochem J 199:725-731, 1981.
308. Craig RK, Hall L, Edbrooke HR, et al: Partial nucleotide sequence of human calcitonin precursor mRNA identifies flanking cryptic peptides. Nature 295:345, 1982.
309. Fisher DA, Kikkawa DO, Rivier JE, et al: Stimulation of noradrenergic sympathetic outflow by calcitonin gene-related peptide. Nature 305:534–536, 1983.
310. Hillyard CJ, Myers C, Abeysekera G, et al: Measurement in man of a new plasma calcium-lowering hormone. Lancet 16:846, 1983.
311. Roos BA, O'Neil JA, Muszynski M, Birnbaum RS: Noncalcitonin secretory products of calcitonin gene expression. Proceedings of the VIII International Conference on Calcium Regulating Hormones, Kobe, Japan, October 16–24, 1983.

19

HENRY J. MANKIN
SAMUEL H. DOPPELT
ANDREW E. ROSENBERG
JOHN A. BARRANGER

Metabolic Bone Disease in Patients with Gaucher's Disease

I. HISTORY AND PATHOGENESIS

In 1882, Philippe Charles-Ernest Gaucher[1] first described a 32-year-old woman with splenomegaly who became the index case of the disorder that now bears his name. He ascribed the morbid condition of the spleen and the infiltration with large, foamy nonleukemic cells (subsequently to be known as Gaucher's cells [Fig. 19–1]) to a primary neoplastic process ("epithelioma of the spleen"). Following the original description, additional cases were reported from numerous centers in Europe and the United States emphasizing the nonneoplastic and generalized nature of the process (which was found to involve not only the spleen, but the liver, bone marrow, lymph nodes, skin, and other viscera).[2–9] Subsequently, the Gaucher's cells were identified as histiocytes and macrophages[8a] containing increased amounts of a lipid material,[9a] ultimately defined as a glucocerebroside—glucosylceramide, present in the form of microtubular structures in the lysosomal bodies of the phagocytic cells of the reticuloendothelial system.[2,10,11] Although originally thought to be neoplastic or infectious, the genetic nature of the disorder was defined in the early part of the 20th century, and subsequent studies have shown that all forms of Gaucher's disease are transmitted as an autosomal recessive trait. Type 1 disease has a high rate of prevalence in Ashkenazi Jews in whom the carrier frequency is estimated to be as high as 1 in 12.[12–16]

In 1965, in a landmark discovery, Brady et al.[17] proved the pathogenetic process in patients with type 1 disease to be a relative deficiency in concentration of a lysosomal enzyme required for the hydrolysis of glucosylceramide to glucose and ceramide. This material, an acid beta-glucosidase also known as glucosylceramide hydrolase or glucocerebrosidase, can now be measured in the cells of the peripheral blood, bone marrow, or amniotic fluid, and a reduction in the concentration of the enzyme is diagnostic for the disease (a marked decline indicative of the clinical disease state, and a lesser degree of decrease characteristic of the carrier state).[14,18–20] Gaucher's disease is no longer considered to be a single entity, and currently at least three separate clinically distinct phenotypes have been described (Table 19–1).[21–23] These result from different mutations in the gene responsible for the production of the glucocerebrosidase. As can be noted by examination of Table 19–1, the nonneuronopathic phenotype (type 1) is the most common and predilects Ashkenazi Jews (10 times more frequently than Gentiles). The acute neuronopathic phenotype (type 2) is much less common and has no ethnic predilection.[14,21] The subacute neuronopathic form of the disease is uncommon but has been noted around the world in different ethnic groups. An apparent genetic isolate of a phenotype with similar symptoms has been discovered in Sweden.[24,25]

Of considerable interest to investigators and clinicians in the field is the remarkable lack of correlation of the phenotypic expression of the disease or severity of the presentation (particularly for bone disease) with either the concentration of residual beta-glucosidase in the cells or the tissue-plasma concentrations of glucosylceramide.[26,27] Part of the difficulty lies with the recent finding that glucocerebrosidase is only one of several tissue

---

Supported in part by a grant from the National Gaucher's Foundation.

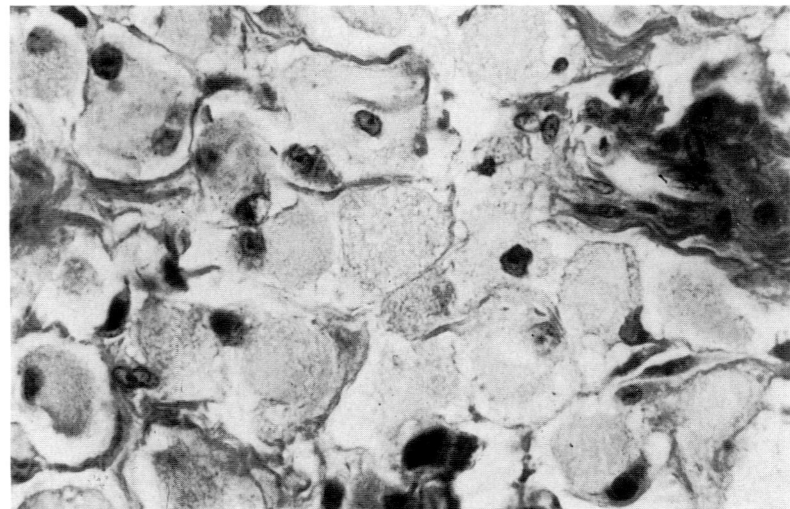

Figure 19–1. The Gaucher's cell: a swollen histiocyte or macrophage, containing large quantities of glucosylceramide. The nucleus is small and often eccentrically placed, and the cytoplasm is foamy and stains poorly (H and E; ×450).

beta-glucosidases;[28–32] and there are several isozymes of both beta-glucosidase and glucocerebrosidase.[26,33]

Recent studies have examined the properties of the various isolated glucocerebrosidases in an attempt to establish a biochemical explanation for the differences in phenotypic expression. The enzyme obtained from human placenta has been purified to homogeneity and found to have a molecular mass of 67,000 daltons.[34] It is a glycoprotein of the complex type containing sialic acid, galactose, and N-acetylglucosamine in the terminal portion of the oligosaccharide chain.[35] The amino acid composition of the purified protein is consonant with its properties as a hydrophobic molecule tightly associated with membranes. Monospecific polyvalent and monoclonal antibodies have been prepared against the molecule and have been used to study the biosynthesis of the enzyme in order to distinguish the abnormalities present in the three known phenotypes.[22,36–38] Normal peripheral cells have three bands of cross-reactive material to glucocerebrosidase at 66,000, 63,000, and 59,000 daltons, and this pattern is consistently seen in cells from patients with nonneuronopathic type 1 Gaucher's disease, but not in patients with the neuronopathic type 2 and type 3 disorders in which the 59,000 dalton form is absent (Fig. 19–2). Since additional studies have demonstrated that the major form of glucocerebrosidase in brain tissue is the 59,000 dalton species, this may be an explanation of some of the differences in the type 2 and type 3 forms of the disorder.

Furthermore, the type 2 and type 3 forms of the disorder react differently with monoclonal antibodies to the enzyme, suggesting that these are different mutations in the gene. This concept is supported by studies of the biosynthesis of the glucocerebrosidase in porcine kidney cells[38] and human fibroblasts,[37,38] which show that the different molecular species of the enzyme are related to several precursors

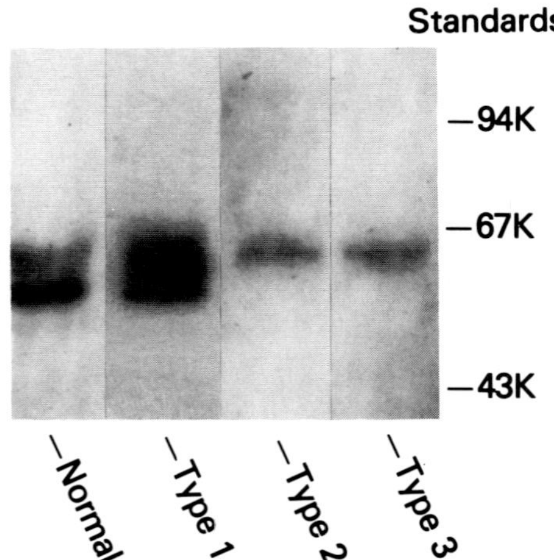

Figure 19–2. Pattern of glucocerebrosidase identified in blots from polyacrylamide gels, which separate the several different molecular species of the enzyme (polymorphism). Extracts from fibroblasts from control subjects and the three phenotypes of Gaucher's disease are identified with antibody to the pure enzyme. Note that normal cells have three cross-reactive bands at 66,000, 63,000, and 59,000 daltons. Patients with type 1 Gaucher's disease have the same species, but in patients with types 2 and 3 disease, the 59,000 dalton mature processed form is absent.

Table 19–1. Phenotypes of Gaucher's Disease

Names	Clinical Characteristics	Pathology	Biochemistry	Genetics
Type 1 Nonneuronopathic chronic "adult"	Heterogeneous presentation Marked differences in age of onset of clinical signs and symptoms (from birth to 80 yrs) Marked differences in rate of progression of signs and symptoms Marked differences in number of organ systems involved and rate of progression in organ systems No neurologic involvement in preponderance of cases Common signs: Hepatomegaly Splenomegaly Osseous lesions: Osteopenia Lytic lesions Osteonecrosis Failed remodeling Rare signs: Pulmonary infiltration Pulmonary hypertension PAO_2<50 Renal involvement Cirrhosis and liver failure Pericarditis	Gaucher's cells and variable degree of fibrosis in all organs; perivascular Gaucher's cells in brain Reticuloendothelial cell storage predominates	Deficiency of glucocerebrosidase Accumulation of glucocerebrosidase in all organs, except brain Cross-reactive material to normal enzyme present	Autosomal recessive Incidence among Askenazim: 1/600–1/2500 Incidence among general population: suspect many allelic mutations different from types 2,3
Type 2 Acute neuropathic "infantile"	Stereotypic presentation Onset of clinical signs at about 3 months Death before 2 years Common signs: Hepatosplenomegaly Hypertonic posture and retroflexion of head Strabismus Trismus Brain stem signs Seizures	Gaucher's cells in all tissues including both perivascular and parenchyma of brain Areas of mild gliosis and neuronophagia, especially occipital cortex	Deficiency of glucocerebrosidase Accumulation of glucocerebroside in all tissues including brain CRM present, but altered	Autosomal recessive Incidence: rare No ethnic predilection Distinctly different allelic mutation separate from types 1,3
Type 3 Subacute neuronopathic "juvenile"	Heterogeneous presentation Variable age of onset of systemic signs; variable progression Onset of neurologic signs in childhood or adolescence Common signs: Hepatosplenomegaly Osseous involvement Slowly progressive dementia Myoclonus Supranuclear ophthalmoplegia	Gaucher's cells in all tissues, but without marked changes in brain	Deficiency of glucocerebrosidase Accumulation of glucocerebroside in all tissues including brain, but to a lesser extent than in type 2 CRM present, but altered	Autosomal recessive Incidence: rare Norrbottnian subgroup No other ethnic predilection Distinctly different allelic mutation separate from types 1,2

and products encountered in the assembly process. It has been demonstrated that the mutations observed in type 1 Gaucher's disease alter the active site but that processing of the catalytically altered enzyme to the 59,000 dalton form is allowed. The mutations in the two neuronopathic forms of the disease differ in that they result in a product that not only has a diminished enzyme activity, but also appears to prevent posttranslational processing of the precursor to the mature form, which is the principal enzyme encountered in brain (Fig. 19–3). Although mutations at multiple loci have not been ruled out, genetic

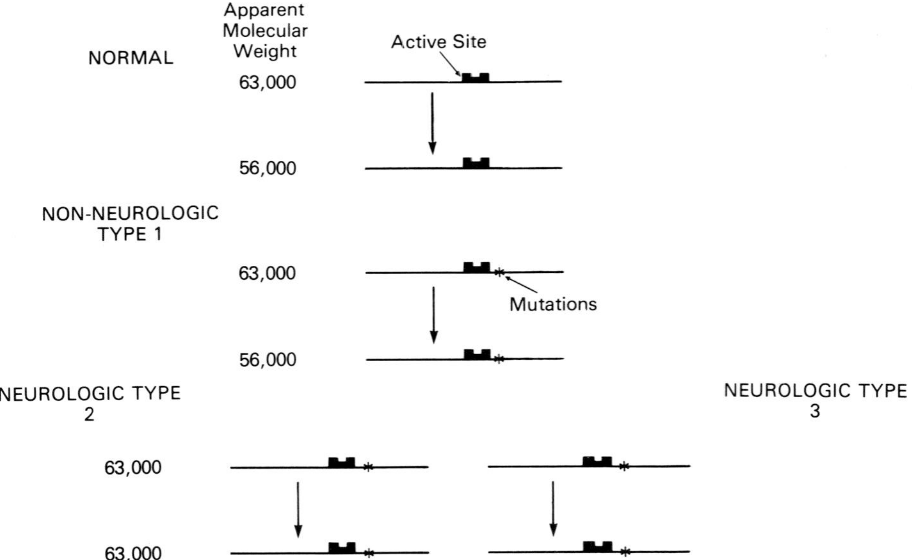

Figure 19–3. Schematic representation of the mutations in the gene for glucocerebrosidase leading to three different phenotypes of Gaucher's disease based on mutations in the synthesis of the forms of the enzyme (see text).

complementation studies in somatic cell hybrids suggest the simplest explanation for these data is allelic mutations.[39,40]

Significant progress has been made in the approach to defining and understanding the molecular genetic bases for the clinical differences in Gaucher's disease. A cDNA containing the sequences for the complete structural protein of glucocerebrosidase has been isolated[41] and the gene has been mapped to chromosome 1q21.[42,43] Genomic DNA has been described,[44] expression of the gene has been accomplished in bacteria,[45] and the complete primary structure of the gene product (protein sequence) has been defined. These advances have made it possible to consider novel approaches to the management of patients with Gaucher's disease, including gene transfer or enzyme replacement; and studies involving both of these approaches are currently in progress.

II. CLINICAL MANIFESTATIONS OF TYPE 1 GAUCHER'S DISEASE

Type 1 Gaucher's disease is the most common form of the disorder and, in fact, the most frequently encountered lipidosis. The manifestations of the disease can be more or less directly attributed to the slow accumulation of histiocytes and macrophages laden with glucosylceramide in the various organ systems. For obvious reasons, the problems in the hematopoietic system tend to dominate the picture for patients with this disorder and often lead to the primary complaints for which the patient seeks medical care.

A. Skin and Conjunctivae

A patchy yellow-brownish to gray flaky macular rash has been occasionally described in patients with Gaucher's disease, and although it was at one time attributed to infiltration of the subcuticular layers with Gaucher's cells,[14,16,46] recent studies have suggested that the pigment is either hemosiderin or melanin and not directly related to the biochemical disorder.[47] The finding is not a prominent one and is often absent or overlooked. A more constant finding is the conjunctival abnormality that appears as asymptomatic vascularized pinguecula-like lesions starting at the outer or inner canthus and fanning out in triangular fashion toward the cornea (Fig. 19–4).[46,48,49] A high percentage of the patients with type 1 disease have this abnormality even in childhood. The evidence that the lesions contain Gaucher's cells is meager, and since the lesions are present in a high percentage of normal individuals at later ages, the value of this finding as a diagnostic aid is limited.[50]

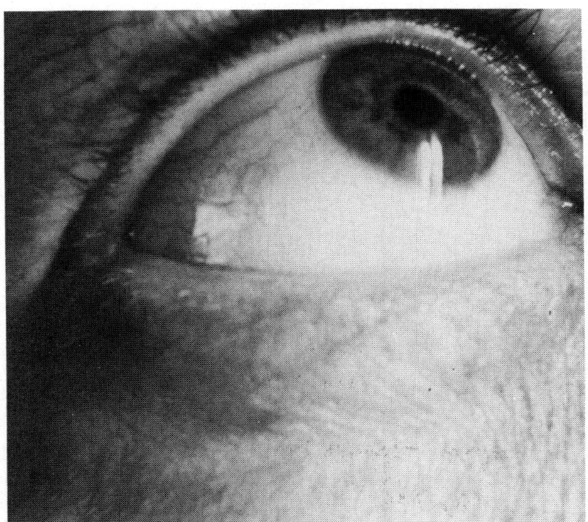

Figure 19–4. Pinguecula-like lesion of the conjunctiva in a patient with type 1 Gaucher's disease.

B. Visceral Manifestations

The major presenting finding in most patients with type 1 Gaucher's disease is splenomegaly, and the spleen may grow to enormous proportions.[14,15,31,51–53] Splenic rupture is rare. Infarction may be the presenting complaint in an otherwise asymptomatic patient, or the patient may be aware of abdominal enlargement, disturbed posture, or a dull aching pain in the left side of the abdomen.[14,53] Hepatomegaly is also common in patients, and the liver may become so large as to seriously restrict chest excursion and/or descend into the pelvis.[14,51,52,54] Hepatic function may be minimally impaired early in the disease, but a not uncommon sequel later in life is a mild to moderate hepatic dysfunction. In some cases, cirrhosis and portal hypertension may occur and lead to portal hypertension and esophageal varices.[54–57] Lymphadenopathy is infrequent in Gaucher's disease, and only a small fraction of the patients present with palpable lymph nodes.[58] Chronic renal disease[14,59,60] or pulmonary fibrosis[61] occurs rarely. An occasional patient with Gaucher's disease presents with evidence of hypertrophic pulmonary osteoarthropathy.

C. Hematopoietic System

As might be expected with a disorder involving the spleen and bone marrow, the principal findings in patients with Gaucher's disease are related to alterations in the hematopoietic system.[14,15,62,63] Patients complain of easy fatigability and generalized weakness and frequently display a pallor on initial physical examination. If hypersplenism is the dominant factor, a pancytopenia is often noted with unusually low leukocyte counts, a hypochromic anemia, and low platelet counts on examination of the peripheral blood.[14] Most patients with chronic Gaucher's disease have hematocrits below 30 and platelet counts under 100,000.[14,15,62] The sedimentation rate is often elevated and is frequently over 100 mm/hour. If a splenectomy has been performed, the pancytopenic state is corrected and immature forms are often present in the peripheral blood smear.[53] Late in the course, marrow failure is sometimes seen.

Bleeding times are often significantly increased in patients with Gaucher's disease, and the most consistent complaints are those of the bleeding diatheses associated with thrombocytopenia and at times a significant hypoprothrombinemia.[55,56] Epistaxis, conjunctival hemorrhages, petechiae, and ecchymosis in the skin and bleeding gums are common in patients with Gaucher's disease; the more severely affected individuals may develop retinal hemorrhages, subdural hematoma, hemopericardium with resultant tamponade, gastrointestinal bleeding, and bleeding esophageal varices.[8,14,15,57,62,63]

D. Laboratory Data

As indicated earlier, patients with Gaucher's disease often show evidence of pancytopenia on examination of the peripheral blood. The tartrate-resistant acid phosphatase activity is usually elevated.[64,65] Examination of the bone marrow shows the presence of Gaucher's cells in most of the patients and is diagnostic of the disease.[51,52,66,67] Measurement of the leukocyte beta-glucosidase activity and assay of serum levels of glucosylceramide can be performed to determine not only the presence of the disease but the carrier state and can also be performed on the amniotic fluid to determine the presence of the disease or carrier state in the fetus.[14,18–20] In splenomegalic patients with type 1 Gaucher's disease who are over 50 years of age, abnormal immunoglobulins are often present and may present as a diffuse polyclonal, biclonal, or monoclonal gammopathy.[68–72] Since patients with Gaucher's disease have a higher than normal incidence of myeloma[73,74] and amyloidosis,[75] the differential diagnosis of this finding is often difficult.

E. Malignancy in Patients with Gaucher's Disease

Sporadic reports in the literature have supported the impression among physicians who treat patients with Gaucher's disease that the incidence of myeloma,[73,74] leukemia,[52,76–78] and Hodgkin's lymphoma[79] is somewhat higher than in the general population. No known cause for this finding can be identified, and the frequency does not correlate with splenectomy. The diagnosis may be difficult because Gaucher's patients often have peripheral leukopenia or leukocytosis, abnormal peripheral blood smears, lymphadenopathy, hepatosplenomegaly, an altered immunoglobulin profile, and abnormal bone marrow cellular distribution.

III. BONE MANIFESTATIONS IN GAUCHER'S DISEASE

As noted in section I, most of the clinical manifestations of Gaucher's disease can be more or less directly related to the storage of excessive quantities of glucosylceramide in the macrophages of the reticuloendothelial system. Splenomegaly and hypersplenism, hepatomegaly and chronic hepatic insufficiency, myeloid packing with Gaucher's cells, and the pancytopenia can all be explained pathophysiologically by the now well-documented failure of patients with all three types of Gaucher's disease to synthesize sufficient quantities of functional glucocerebrosidase and the slow accumulation of the substrate in the lysosomal bodies of the phagocytic cells.

In addition to the visceral disease, a careful study of any group of patients with Gaucher's disease will show that almost all affected individuals have some abnormalities of the skeleton. As will be discussed later in greater detail, however, the pathogenetic mechanisms for the bone changes, which are often severe and may dominate the clinical picture, are far less clear; and indeed the mechanism of such diverse and significant disorders as Gaucher's crisis, osteonecrosis, diffuse or localized bone loss, osteosclerotic areas, and failure to remodel remains relatively unexplained. Furthermore, the severity of the alterations in bony structure generally do not correlate well with any single or multiple factors, such as extent of visceral involvement, bone marrow depression, degree of enzyme deficit, or concentration of circulating glucosylceramide.

The purpose of this portion of the chapter is to describe in detail the changes that occur in the skeletons of patients with Gaucher's disease, their clinical and radiographic presentation and management. A final section is devoted to presentation of some metabolic data that, although preliminary and incomplete, allow some speculation in the Discussion section as to pathogenetic mechanisms by which at least some of the processes occur.

A. Failure of Remodeling

The most common and the least symptomatic skeletal abnormality in patients with Gaucher's disease is failure of remodeling of the distal femora, proximal tibiae, and, at times, other bony parts.[14,21,31,51,80–83] This sometimes striking but not, as popularly believed, pathognomonic abnormality is present early in the affected individual's life, often becoming manifest prior to or at the time of the preschool growth spurt and developing progressively throughout the period of rapid skeletal growth. About 80% of the adults with the disease show the finding, and radiographic study of the distal femora and proximal tibiae is reasonably reliable as a screening tool for the disease.[14,81]

As has been clearly defined over the last several decades, the cylindrical bones of the mammalian embryo undergo a process of "tubulation" early in development, by which the shafts of the long bones narrow, while the metaphyseal and epiphyseal ends remain wide to participate in the development of the joint.[84] In postnatal life, the physis adds bone to the widened metaphysis, which then participates in the "remodeling" process mediated through osteoclastic activity in the ring of Ranvier, during which the bone is symmetrically narrowed in width to produce a "herald trumpet" appearance. A failure of the remodeling process results in bones that have very wide metaphyseo-diaphyseal regions and, therefore, an "Erlenmeyer flask" appearance. Such a change may be associated with a number of skeletal disorders including

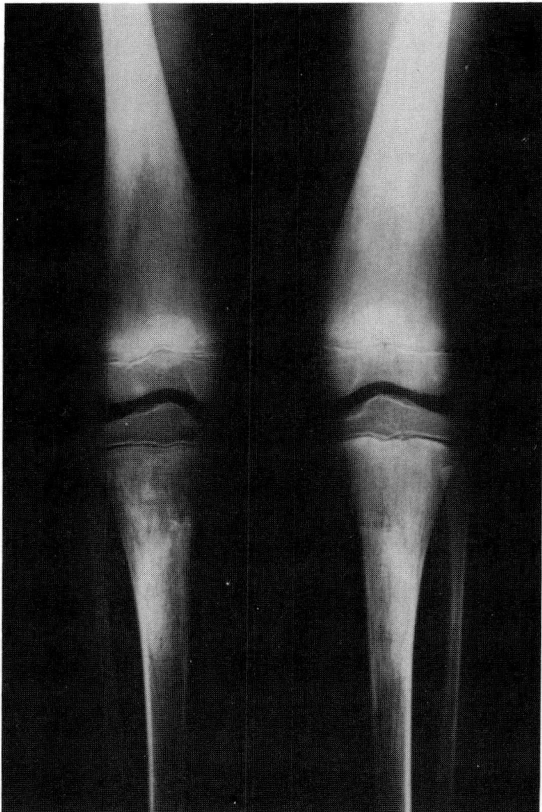

Figure 19–5. Radiograph of the distal femora and proximal tibiae of patient with type 1 Gaucher's disease illustrating the typical Erlenmeyer flask deformities affecting all of the bones. The normal tubulation that appears in the form of a "herald trumpet" is absent and, instead, the bones show the gradual narrowing typical but not pathognomonic of the disease.

Pyle's disease, craniometaphyseal dysplasia, osteopetrosis, and some of the hemoglobinopathies, but the most frequent cause is Gaucher's disease.[31,51]

The failure of remodeling seen in patients with Gaucher's disease characteristically occurs in the distal femur, to a somewhat lesser extent in the proximal tibia and proximal humerus, and is absent or only slightly evident in the distal tibia and radius.[31,81,82] The finding is always bilateral and, in the absence of additional skeletal abnormalities or surgical factors, is strikingly symmetrical. Radiographically, the finding is well described by its popular name—in contrast to the more abrupt and angular "herald trumpet" appearance of the normal metaphyseal region, the anteroposterior view of the distal femur suggests an "Erlenmeyer flask," with a gentle, gradual narrowing of the metaphyseal diameter from the joint to the diaphysis (Fig. 19–5).

B. Diffuse and Localized Bone Loss

Many of the patients with Gaucher's disease are found on routine radiographs or CT to have a significant decrease in bone density, which may be either diffuse or localized.[14,81,85] The diffuse decrease in density is common, occasionally severe in extent, and generally greater in individuals who either have extensive visceral disease or are in the older age ranges.[31,83,86,87] The bone changes on standard radiographic examination may be difficult to distinguish at any single site from other osteopenic states such as osteomalacia, osteoporosis, and hyperparathyroidism but may be readily differentiated from these disorders if the entire skeleton is studied. (See Chapter 12.) Almost always patients with diffuse bone loss will show other features of Gaucher's disease of the bones, including the Erlenmeyer flask deformity, localized lytic lesions, and areas of osteosclerosis. The cause of the localized or diffuse bone loss in Gaucher's disease is poorly understood. Metabolic studies performed in the past in patients with these lesions have failed to show a consistent pattern, and the histologic findings on biopsy studies do not vary greatly from the typical marrow packing with Gaucher's cells, except perhaps in degree, from that seen in patients with relatively normal-appearing bones (Fig. 19–6).[51,52,83]

Radiographically, the diffuse bone loss is characterized by marked thinning of the cortices of the long bones and a decreased number and size of the trabecular markings. The axial skeleton and more proximal parts of the appendicular skeleton are usually more severely involved (Fig. 19–7). The diffuse bone loss causes the skeleton to be significantly more fragile than normal, and fractures of the vertebrae, ribs, hips, or shafts of the long bones may occur with minimal trauma.[80,85] Patients are generally asymptomatic until fractures or infarctions supervene but may complain of mild aching in the bones and loss of height with advancing years.

The localized areas of bone loss present as poorly outlined, small to moderately sized lytic areas most often located in the diaphyses of the long bones and the vertebrae.[81–83,86–89] Characteristically, the lesions show marked

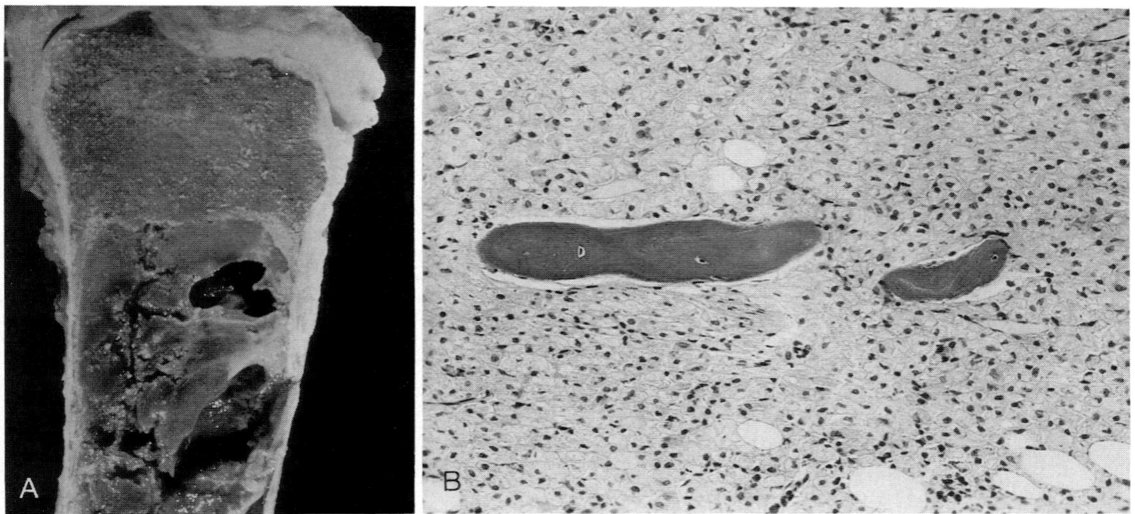

Figure 19–6. Gross and histologic appearance of the lytic areas in the tibia of a 25-year-old female patient with Gaucher's disease who required an amputation. *A*, The gross appearance of a split section of the proximal tibia with a zone of marked bone lysis and absent trabeculae at and below the metaphyseal-epiphyseal junction. *B*, Low power photomicrograph of a section from the severely osteopenic region. Note the small trabeculae surrounded by sheets of Gaucher's cells. Osteoclasts are absent and there is no evidence of osteoblastic activity (H and E; ×180).

thinning of the cortices, endosteal scalloping, and a virtually complete absence of trabecular markings (Fig. 19–8). Only rarely do the lesions demonstrate a sclerotic margination and, in the absence of fracture, fail to demonstrate a soft tissue extension. Expansion of the bone is relatively uncommon but may at times be striking in degree (Fig. 19–9). The lesions can be confused with those of myeloma or metastatic carcinoma. Pathologic fracture may occur through one of the lytic lesions of Gaucher's disease and represent a major problem in management, based on the relatively slow healing of the fracture and the difficulty in applying internal fixation devices (see later). Non-union, malunion, and adjacent joint disability are common.[80]

C. Osteosclerotic Lesions

Patients with Gaucher's disease frequently show areas of increased density in the medullary cavities of the long bones and the pelvis.[31,51,90] The finding ranges in extent from a diffuse increase affecting the entire diaphyseal region and involving the entire medulla and endosteal side of the cortex, to small patches or islands in the otherwise normal or more frequently osteopenic bone.[81,83,86] The cause of the change is not well understood,

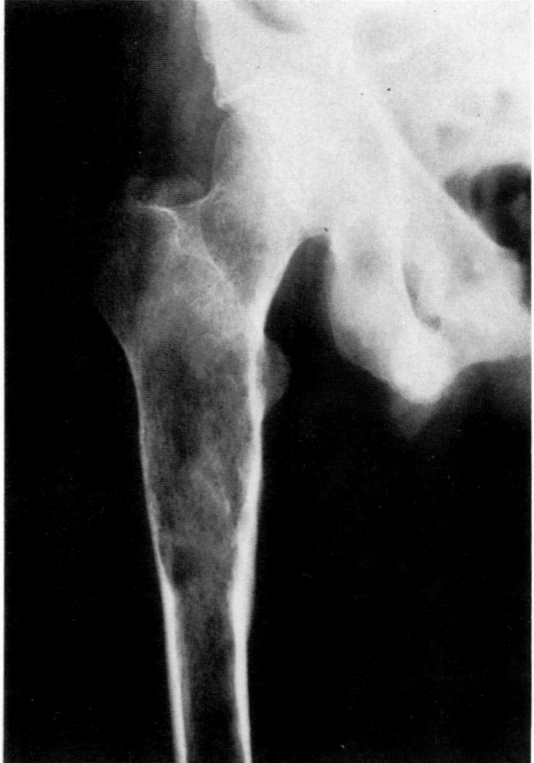

Figure 19–7. Radiograph of the proximal femur of a 66-year-old woman showing the typical changes of diffuse osteopenia. Note the absence of trabeculae and the thin cortices. The bone is moderately expanded in the subtrochanteric area.

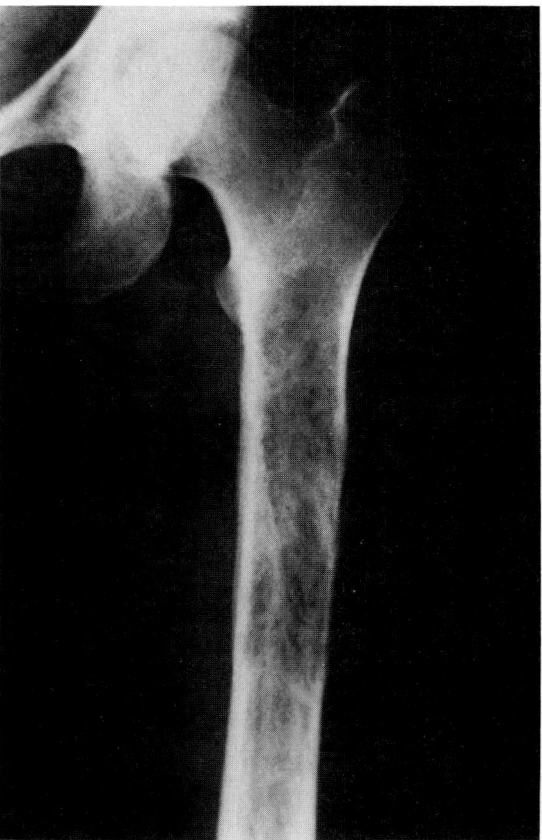

Figure 19–8. Radiograph of the proximal half of the femur of a 36-year-old woman with Gaucher's disease illustrating the localized bone loss, which shows extensive local cortical destruction and absence of trabeculae. Such a segment is at high risk for fracture.

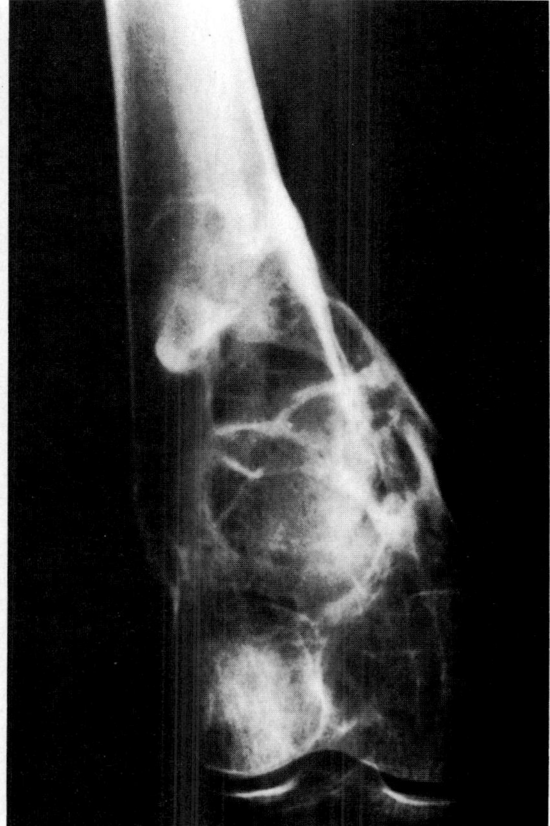

Figure 19–9. A lytic area in the distal femur of a 44-year-old woman with type 1 disease showing enormous expansion of the bone. The patient has suffered a pathologic fracture through the weakened bony structure.

but most authorities agree that the process probably represents the end stage of a diffuse or localized medullary osteonecrosis and, in fact, may result from a "Gaucher's crisis" (see later).[83,86,90] Histologic study of the material is likely to show medullary infarction with dead bone, fat necrosis, and calcareous detritus (Fig. 19–10), the last probably representing an insoluble calcium soap that results from the combination of ionic calcium bound to a free fatty acid released either from a dead marrow lipocyte or from a Gaucher's cell (the ceramide moiety consists of a sphingosine linked to a fatty acid). In some sites, viable bone may be noted surrounding the dead trabeculae, indicating an attempt at revascularization and new bone formation, but osteoblast rimming is usually absent.

Patients with osteosclerotic lesions of the long or flat bones are usually asymptomatic at the time of presentation, but one occasionally can obtain a history of a prior "crisis" occurring at the site of the bony abnormality. The lesions appear to be more prevalent in patients with more severe bone disease (as manifested by marked Erlenmeyer flask deformities and numerous sites of bone loss), but not necessarily in those with more serious systemic disease or decreased enzyme levels. The extent of the change on radiograph varies widely from a single area of increased density in the supra-acetabular region (often running medially and cephalad to the iliac side of the sacroiliac joint) (Fig. 19–11) to a diffuse change in density of many of the bones, relatively easily confused with osteopetrosis or Paget's disease (Fig. 19–12). The bone scan is often positive in regions of osteosclerosis but at times is normal or even subnormal, suggesting the possibility of a large medullary infarct.[91]

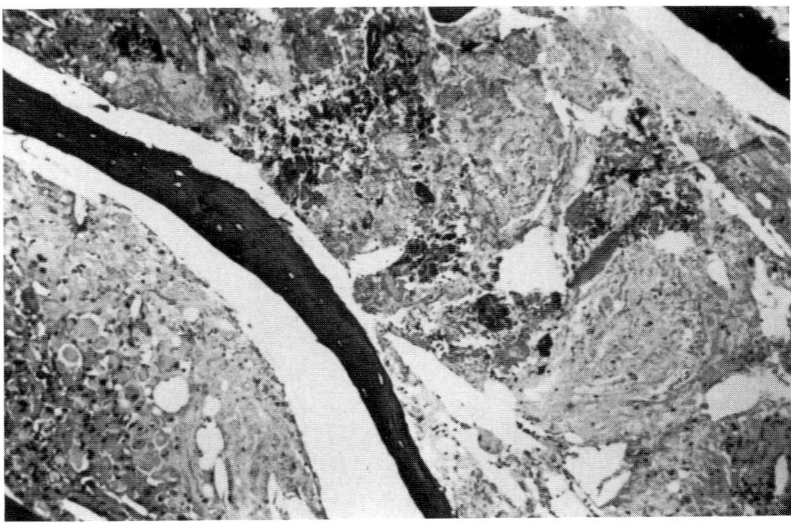

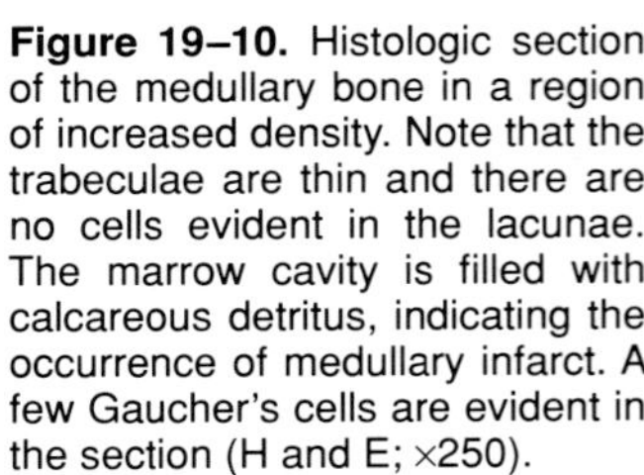

Figure 19–10. Histologic section of the medullary bone in a region of increased density. Note that the trabeculae are thin and there are no cells evident in the lacunae. The marrow cavity is filled with calcareous detritus, indicating the occurrence of medullary infarct. A few Gaucher's cells are evident in the section (H and E; ×250).

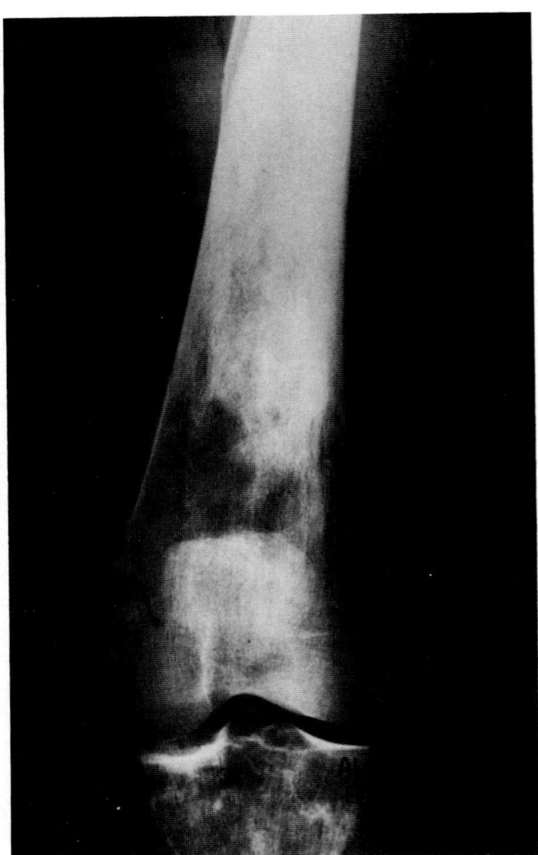

Figure 19–11. Radiograph of the distal femur in a patient with type 1 Gaucher's disease showing the diffuse increase in bone density at the junction of the middle and distal thirds.

D. Corticomedullary Osteonecrosis

Perhaps the most chronically disabling of the musculoskeletal problems that arise in patients with Gaucher's disease is corticomedullary osteonecrosis, usually of the femoral head, proximal humerus, or, less commonly, a

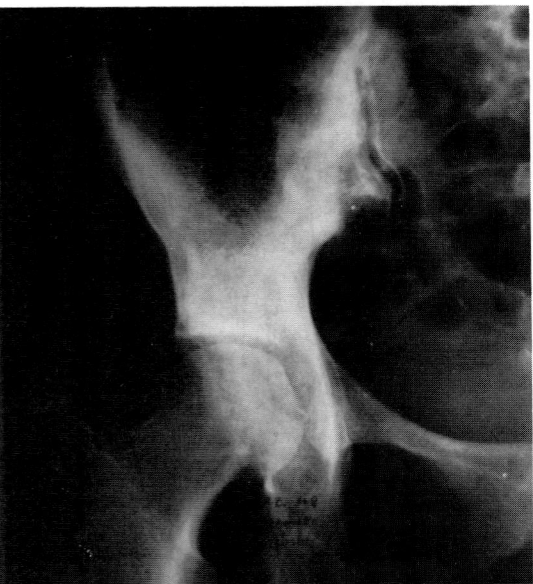

Figure 19–12. Radiograph of the bony pelvis showing an area of increased density running from the supra-acetabular region to the region of the sacroiliac joint. The patient was asymptomatic.

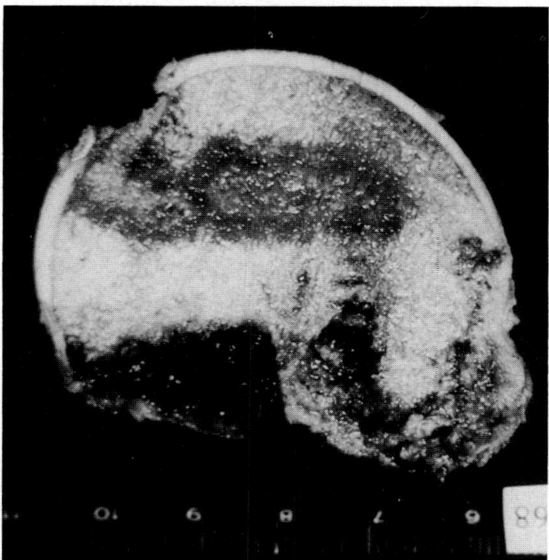

Figure 19–13. Cross section of a femoral head demonstrating a massive infarct in an adult patient with type 1 Gaucher's disease.

femoral or tibial condyle, talus, or capitellum.[14,31,80–83,85–87,92,92a,96] The process does not always affect the articular portion of a bone but may occur as a small or large corticomedullary infarct in the shaft of any of the long bones. (The term "corticomedullary" is an awkward one and not often used to further define osteonecrosis; the purpose of introducing it is to distinguish this process from the more common but far less disabling osteosclerotic lesions believed to be caused by "medullary" infarction, which does not affect the cortex or the overlying joint.) The process appears to affect patients with Gaucher's disease at any age but is more common in younger individuals with the peak ages from 8 to 35 years.[53,54,76,92] Women and men are equally affected, and the incidence of osteonecrosis does not appear to correlate with the percentage of Gaucher's cells in the marrow, severity of the enzyme deficit, or systemic illness or even other types of change in the bones (with the exception of Gaucher's crises). Several studies have suggested a direct correlation of osteonecrosis to splenectomy,[68,84,84a] but in recent analyses of large series of patients, this finding could not be substantiated.[53,57] Corticomedullary osteonecrosis tends to be bilateral (in over 50% of the patients who have osteonecrosis of one proximal femur, changes will be present in the opposite side) and often multifocal.

The cause of corticomedullary osteonecrosis in patients with Gaucher's disease is unknown. The most frequently observed pathologic pattern, that of a wedge-shaped infarction of the weight-bearing portion of the femoral head, is one that is common to many genetic and acquired disorders (including fracture and dislocation, hemoglobinopathies, dysbarism, certain connective tissue disorders, and corticosteroid treatment),[11] and for some of these at least, pathogenetic mechanisms have been postulated and are reasonably well substantiated and accepted.[16,97] To date, despite considerable study of pathologic material obtained at the time of surgical replacement of the femoral heads, the cause and pathogenesis of the massive necrosis of the subchondral cortical and medullary segment in patients with Gaucher's disease remain unknown. One must postulate an occlusion of the vascular supply of the femoral or humeral heads, probably at the arteriolar or even greater sized vessel level, but why this should occur in patients whose major problem is one of storage of glucosylceramide in marrow cells is currently obscure.

Corticomedullary osteonecrosis of a segment of a long bone may be clinically "silent," but that involving the subchondral portion of a femoral or humeral head is usually not (Fig. 19–13). If the lesion results from a "Gaucher's crisis" (see later), the pain and disability at the outset may be rapid in appearance and severe; if not, the onset may be insidious and only slowly progressive.[16,54,68,78,80] Patients complain of pain in the affected joint, more severe with weight-bearing, and a diminished range of motion. If the upper end of the femur is affected, the principal complaint may be a limp, especially in children, in whom the lesion may be relatively painless.[96] Examination early in the course usually shows only a modest decrease in range of motion (usually most noticeable in internal rotation in flexion) and a flexion contracture, but later there may be a severe concentric limitation of motion, fixed pelvic obliquity, Trendelenburg gait, and shortening of the extremity. Although some of the hip lesions may remain stationary in extent or appear to "heal" (at least on serial radiographs), the usual clinical pattern is that of a slow but inexorable progression with increasing disability with time. The lesions of the shoulder are far less likely to progress, and once a level of disability is reached in which the upper

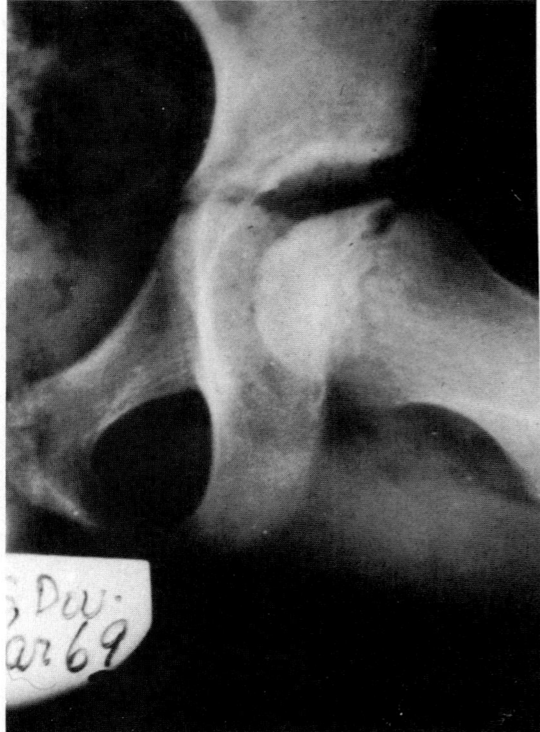

Figure 19–14. Radiograph of the upper end of the femur of a child with type 1 Gaucher's disease showing changes of early osteonecrosis. Note the increased density, the slight deformity of the femoral head, and the increased cartilage space.

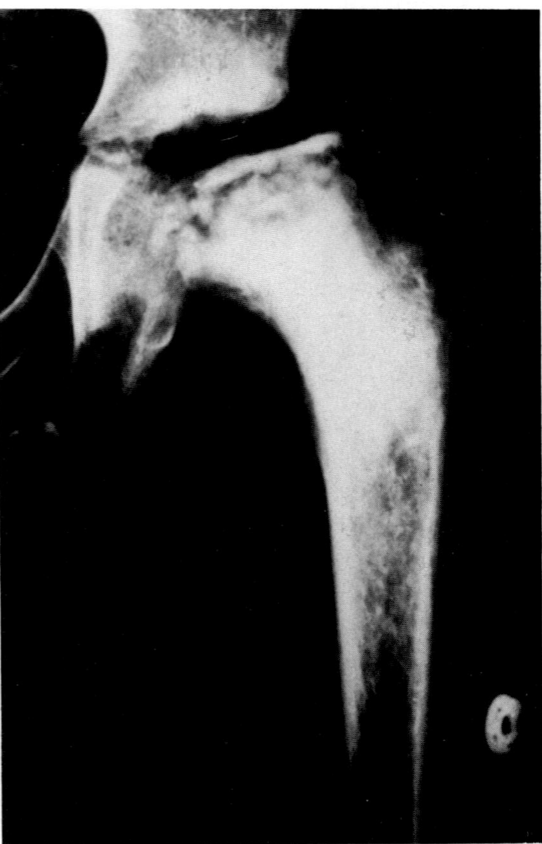

Figure 19–15. Severe collapse of the capital femoral epiphysis in Gaucher's osteonecrosis in a pre-teen-aged-child.

ranges of motion are reduced, the patient usually notes no progression of symptoms despite alterations of appearance of the part on sequential radiographs.

Radiographic changes are similar to and often indistinguishable from those seen in children with Legg-Calvé-Perthes' disease[88,96,96a] and in adults with either "idiopathic" or the "specific" osteonecroses associated with dysbarism, sickle cell disease, lupus erythematosus, corticosteroid administration, and so on.[13,16,97] In the pre-teen child, the femoral head is likely to demonstrate a decrease in size of the epiphyseal center with increase in the cartilage space (Fig. 19–14), progressive fragmentation and flattening of the capital segment (Fig. 19–15), and finally partial reconstitution of the bony architecture and axial height, but usually with some deformity of the proximal femur and acetabulum (Fig. 19–16). In the older child or adult, the pattern includes the early-appearing wedge-shaped segment of increased density (Fig. 19–17), subsequent subchondral fracture and collapse, and ultimately, narrowing of the cartilage space and progressive changes of secondary osteoarthritis (Fig. 19–18).

The bone scan in patients with Gaucher's disease is often helpful in defining the disease prior to the onset of radiologic changes. Although the scan initially is likely to show decreased activity (as seen in Gaucher's crises), within a few weeks a moderate to marked increase in activity can be noted over the affected femoral or humeral head (Fig. 19–19). The increase in activity remains throughout the course of the disorder, even in those patients whose lesions remain quiescent and seemingly nonprogressive.

As indicated earlier, many of the children with capital femoral corticomedullary osteonecrosis and adult patients with limited disease of the humeral heads, shafts of the long bones, and less common sites such as capitellum

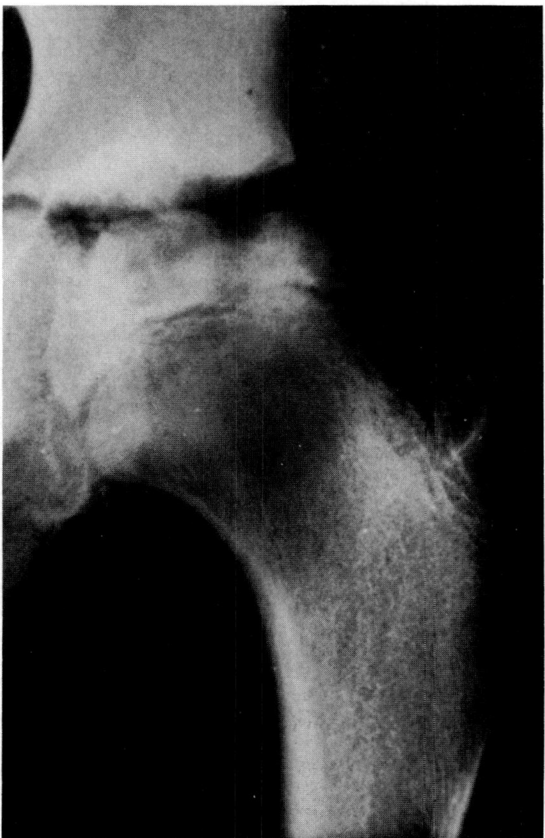

Figure 19–16. Partial reconstitution of the osteonecrotic femoral head in a child with Gaucher's disease. Note that the head and acetabulum are deformed.

Figure 19–17. Early changes of osteonecrosis in an adult showing the wedge-shaped, partially deformed segment. At this point, this 21-year-old woman was severely disabled.

or head of the talus may have a relatively benign course, with subsidence of symptoms after a period of conservative management and eventual apparent revascularization and "healing" of the process as monitored by serial radiographic observations. For the adult with hip disease, the course is usually far more progressive, and patients often require hemiarthroplasty joint replacement surgery to achieve relief from the progressive pain and disability.[20,80,86,92]

In consideration of total joint replacement surgery in patients with Gaucher's disease, it should be noted that the course of the surgery may be stormy and the results not as successful as might be anticipated by the surgeon who has limited experience with patients with the disease.[58,80,93,98,99] Because of the almost always present thrombocytopenia, patients with Gaucher's disease may bleed excessively during the operative procedure, and if chronic liver disease is present, reduced prothrombin activity may materially worsen this problem. Even in the hematologically normal patient, a propensity for bleeding is present. Although the reason for this is not well defined, it presents an additional complication in management.[100,101] As has been noted, patients with Gaucher's disease may have a significant reduction in bone mass and a resultant increase in the incidence of intraoperative and postoperative fractures. Fractures of the shafts of the bones during or subsequent to the joint replacement surgery may lead to very serious problems in inserting the devices and their later function. Allograft implants may be necessary to provide sufficient bone stock in which to seat the prosthetic device.[67]

As will be discussed later, the risk of infection is probably greater in patients with Gaucher's disease, and the possibility of this

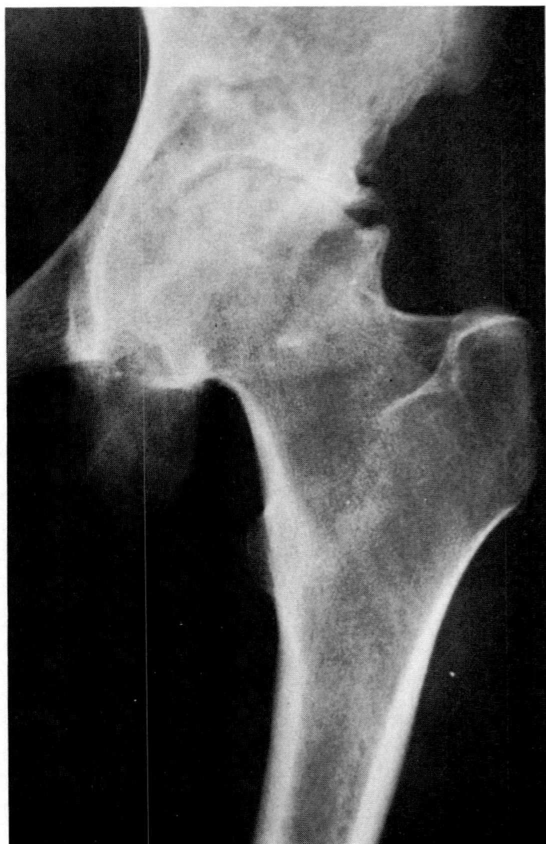

Figure 19–18. Late changes of osteonecrosis in an adult showing the extensive deformity of the femoral head and the loss of joint space.

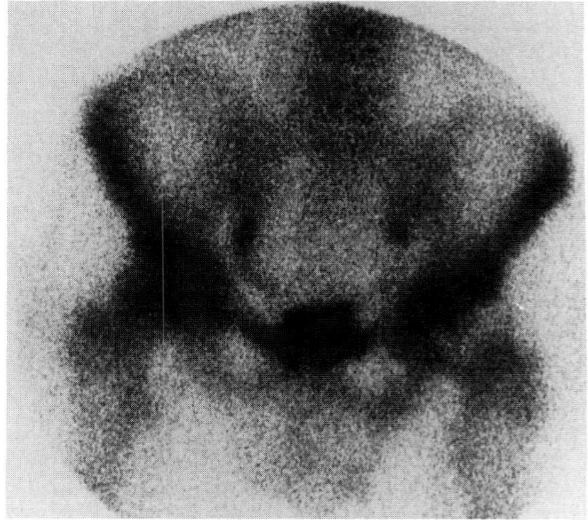

Figure 19–19. 99mTc-diphosphonate bone scan of a patient with a recent crisis. The right femoral head has begun to show some deformity on radiograph, and the bone scan, initially normal, now shows increased activity.

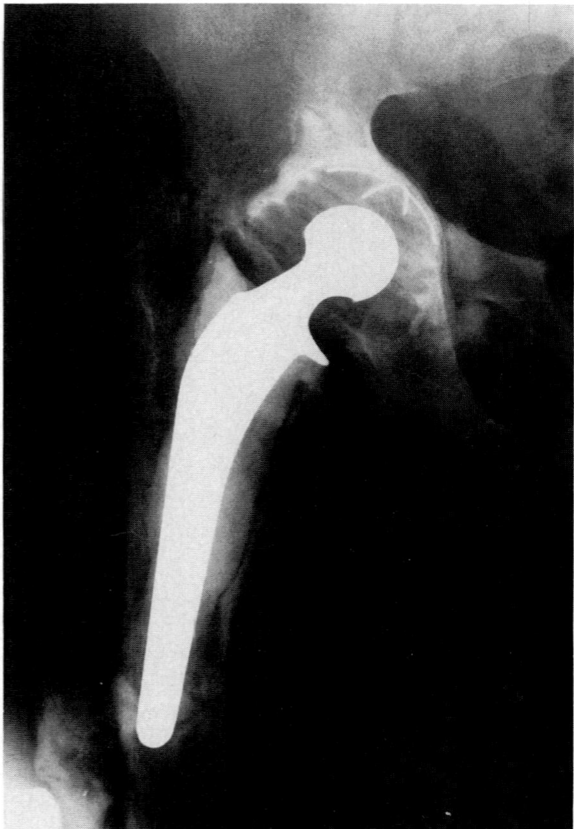

Figure 19–20. Radiograph showing loosening of a total hip replacement inserted into the hip of this 54-year-old male for osteonecrosis 20 months previously. Note the radiolucent lines surrounding both the acetabular and femoral components and the evidence for subsidence of the femoral portion.

devastating complication of joint replacement surgery looms high on the list of problems facing the patient who undergoes the surgery. Scrupulous attention to hemostasis, adequate prophylactic antibiotic coverage, and prolonged drainage of the almost inevitable hematoma are advisable.

Perhaps the most common problem in patients in whom total joint replacements have been performed is early aseptic loosening of the device (Fig. 19–20). Loosening at the cement-bone interface for hip and knee prostheses, as evidenced by progressive widening of a radiolucent line and subsequent malfunction of the device, occurs in increasing numbers of normal patients with time following the surgery. It has been estimated that approximately 15% or more of hips and even a greater percentage of knees are clinically

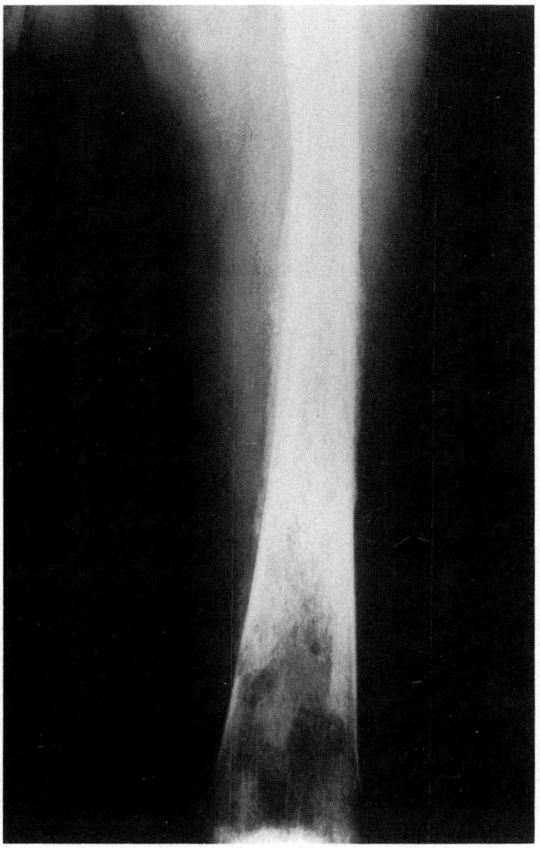

Figure 19–21. Radiograph showing the shaft of the femur 20 days following the onset of a Gaucher's crisis. Note the periosteal new bone formation around the shaft strongly suggestive of an acute osteomyelitic process.

loose by 10 years.[30,102,102a] The figures for patients with Gaucher's disease are not known, but in our series and those reported by others, the incidence of the complication is increased and the time of its occurrence considerably earlier than for normal individuals.[58,93,98,98a] We have as yet no experience with bony ingrowth devices, but since bone formation rates for patients with Gaucher's disease appear to be significantly diminished, it would seem unlikely that these cementless prosthetic implants would hold any greater promise of success.

E. Gaucher's Crisis

A relatively small number of patients with Gaucher's disease may from time to time develop an acute process affecting the bones and adjacent joints that is intensely painful, dramatic, and very disabling.[9,12,15,53,54,61,61a,63,74,103] The similarity in clinical presentation to crises seen in patients with hemoglobinopathies has resulted in the name of "Gaucher's crisis" for the disease state, but there is no evidence to suggest that the pathogenesis is similar. The cause of the process is unknown but appears to result in an acute infarction of a large segment of the bone (either corticomedullary or medullary) and is sometimes multifocal in one or several bones.[53] The process may affect the spine or pelvis, femoral heads, or shafts of the long bones and be so acute as to suggest hematogenous osteomyelitis.[9,61,85a,86,86a] In terms of pathogenesis, the authors have been struck by the frequency with which the Gaucher's crisis follows an acute viral illness, such as influenza, gastroenteritis, or in one case, a varicella infection.

Patients with Gaucher's crisis usually present with severe pain of rapid onset, localized to an anatomical part.[12,53,54] The pain is almost always so intense as to require large doses of intravenous narcotics for control. The patient appears acutely ill, often febrile (up to 104° F), flushed, diaphoretic, and unable to move from the bed. If the process affects a long or flat bone, the part may be very tender to touch and there may be significant overlying soft tissue swelling, sometimes affecting the entire extremity. Laboratory studies usually show a marked leukocytosis to as high as 30,000 (especially in the splenectomized patient), although the differential may fail to show a marked shift to the left. The hematocrit is often low, and the erythrocyte sedimentation rate is usually markedly elevated (100 or more per hour).

Initial radiographic studies are almost invariably normal. The bone scan is sometimes helpful in that, early in the course, it may show an area of reduced activity over the site of the infarct. With advancing time and usually within a few weeks, the radiographs may show alarming changes suggestive of progressive hematogenous osteomyelitis. Lytic areas in the bones and periosteal and endosteal new bone formation are common, particularly in the shafts of the long bones (Fig. 19–21). If the infarct has occurred in relation to a joint or in a vertebra, progressive collapse of the subchondral cortex may be noted.[61,104] The bone scan becomes positive at about two to five weeks (Fig. 19–19) and remains intensely active throughout the course, even when the patient becomes asymptomatic.

As noted earlier, the final pattern is often a focus of osteosclerosis in the medullary cavity of the long bones or corticomedullary osteonecrosis of the subchondral region of the proximal femur, or femoral or tibial condyle.

The duration of the Gaucher's crisis may vary depending in part on the severity and extent of the infarct, but usually the patient remains severely affected for two or more weeks and then, over several months, gradually improves. Restoration of the laboratory values to normal (for the patient) may take several months or more. The ultimate degree of disability depends on the segment affected and the extent of the process, but many patients recover completely, especially if the subchondral bone of the hips, knees, or spine is not involved.

The treatment of patients with Gaucher's crisis is generally symptomatic. Pain control by liberal doses of narcotics, intravenous fluids to maintain hydration, antipyretics other than salicylates (which are contraindicated in patients with thrombocytopenia), and oxygen are the usually instituted measures. Hyperbaric oxygen has been suggested, but only sporadic case reports are available to support the value of this technique and the authors have no experience with it. Antibiotics should not be introduced unless a specific infection is detected.

A major problem in dealing with the patient in Gaucher's crisis is distinguishing the syndrome from that of hematogenous osteomyelitis, a disease process that appears to occur with increased frequency in patients with Gaucher's disease (see later).[86,105,106] In a febrile patient with bone pain, leukocytosis and a rapid sedimentation rate, and later lytic areas and periosteal new bone on radiographs, distinguishing between the two syndromes is sometimes exceedingly difficult. The bone scan is sometimes helpful in that it almost always will show a marked increase in activity in patients with osteomyelitis even at onset of symptoms, whereas in Gaucher's crises, the scan is often normal or decreased in activity over the affected part at the time of first observation of the patient. Computed tomography is sometimes helpful in demonstrating a soft tissue abscess around the bone, and aspiration of the soft tissues in the patient with osteomyelitis may, if positive, be diagnostic but not very helpful if no purulent material is obtained.

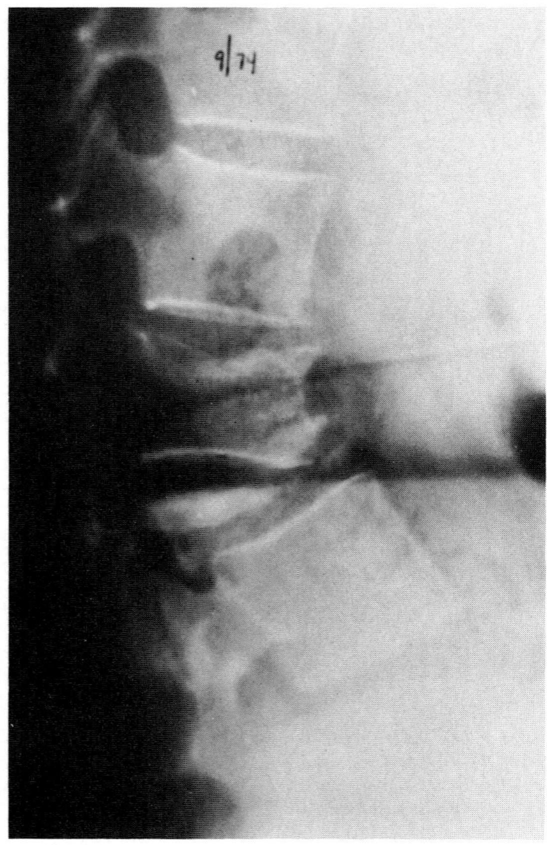

Figure 19–22. Wedge compression fracture of a vertebra in a 42-year-old woman with type 1 Gaucher's disease.

F. Other Osseous Manifestations of Gaucher's Disease

In addition to the five characteristic processes described in the preceding sections, two other less specific but none the less important problems should be included in a discussion of the osseous manifestations of Gaucher's disease. These include fractures and osteomyelitis.

As indicated in the discussion of the diffuse or segmental areas of bone loss in patients with Gaucher's disease, pathologic fractures through weakened areas of the bones are common.[14,80,83,85] These may consist of compression fractures of the vertebrae (Fig. 19–22),[89] fractures through the metaphyseal or diaphyseal portions of the long bones, or fractures of the bony pelvis (Fig. 19–23). Fractures may occur with minimal trauma and be relatively undisplaced but may represent major problems in acute management because of the

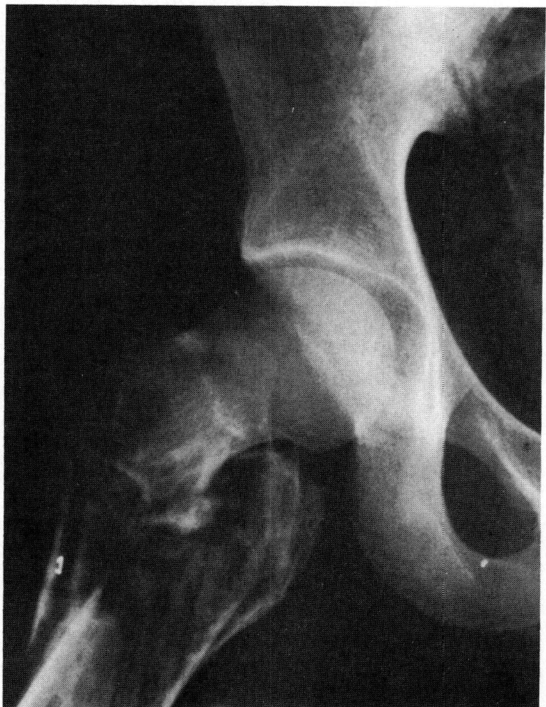

Figure 19–23. Fracture of the femoral shaft in a patient with severe osteopenia. The fracture healed very slowly despite internal fixation, and the patient was unable to bear weight for over a year.

patient's reduced ability to clot (based on the almost always present thrombocytopenia and the sometimes severe interference with prothrombin activity in patients with liver disease). The hematomas that occur at the site of the fracture in patients with Gaucher's disease may be enormous, and compartment syndromes requiring emergency decompression may result in such sites as the leg or forearm.

Because of the risk of excessive bleeding and infection and the mechanical difficulties with the use of internal fixation devices, fractures in patients with Gaucher's disease should be treated conservatively if at all possible.[80,95] Traction, casts, and braces are generally preferred to either external fixators or open operative procedures. If operative procedures are indicated in order to gain union or prevent malalignment, scrupulous attention should be paid to hemostasis and prevention of postoperative wound infection. In addition, the type of internal fixation device should be carefully chosen to place the least stress on the weakened cortices. Prophylactic antibiotics should be administered during and after the operative procedure, adequate drains inserted to prevent the accumulation of a large hematoma, and the circulation and clotting system supported by liberal administration of oxygen, fresh blood and plasma transfusions, and platelets (HLA-matched, if necessary). For obvious reasons, anticoagulants should not be utilized.

Although there is little documentation of the fact, study of large numbers of patients with Gaucher's disease suggests that they are more prone to infection than are normal individuals.[86] Hematogenous osteomyelitis and septic arthritis are not uncommon in patients with Gaucher's disease, and the incidence of postoperative wound infections appears to be higher in this group than in others. No known cause is reported for this problem. Patients with Gaucher's disease have been studied for immune deficiency states and none have been found, and the unusual susceptibility of patients with sickle cell disease to infection with salmonella is not noted in patients with Gaucher's disease. In reviewing our own experience with infection, a preponderance of coliform and anaerobic organisms has been noted in patients with Gaucher's disease, but not to the exclusion of the gram-positive organisms.

In consideration of the mechanism of the increased susceptibility of patients with Gaucher's disease to bone infection, it is possible that a bone infarct may represent a "locus minoris resistentiae" in which bacteria may settle during episodes of transient bacteremia, or the fault may possibly lie in a relative incompetence of phagocytic cells laden with excessive concentrations of glucosylceramide to appropriately respond to bacterial invasion. Both of these explanations are highly speculative, however, and currently no hard evidence exists to support the concept that the patient with Gaucher's disease handles bacterial disease differently from a normal individual.

The management of patients with Gaucher's disease and osteomyelitis is difficult. For the reasons mentioned previously, operative procedures are hazardous, and because of the poor perfusion of the dead bone, the concentration of systemically administered antibiotics is probably markedly reduced at the site of the infectious process. Acute osteomyelitis often goes on to chronic disease, and patients may have draining sinuses for years. At times, despite multiple operative procedures and introduction of large doses of appropriate antibiotics, amputation is the only method by which the process can be controlled.

G. Metabolic Bone Changes in Patients with Gaucher's Disease

Analysis of the literature has shown a paucity of metabolic studies of the bones, serum, or urine of patients with Gaucher's disease, with the possible exception of several qualitative histologic evaluations in the older literature.[14,15,51,52] In patients with often such extensive osteopenia and other manifestations that might be interpreted as demonstrating rather marked alterations in calcium and phosphorus homeostasis or uncoupling of bone formation and destruction, it is somewhat surprising that investigational efforts have been so limited. One of the first such studies is that recently reported by Stowens et al.,[83] which showed no consistent abnormalities in evaluation of serum and urine parameters, but evidence on bone morphometry of diminished bone turnover.

In the past year, our group has performed extensive biochemical, physiologic, and morphometric analyses on 15 adult patients with type 1 Gaucher's disease; although the data obtained are incomplete and also somewhat limited because of heterogeneity of the patient population in terms of extent of visceral and bony disease, some preliminary findings suggest that patients with Gaucher's disease have rather extensive abnormalities of both mineral metabolism and bony structure. Most of these studies have focused on the osteopenic states (see earlier), but some additional data will soon be forthcoming regarding the osteosclerotic changes, particularly in relation to special imaging studies using quantitative bone scans, computed tomography, and magnetic resonance imaging.

The 15 patients admitted to the MGH Clinical Research Unit were maintained on a 1000 mg calcium, low-gelatin diet. All were found to have normal values for calcium, phosphorus, and alkaline phosphatase (with the exception of those with modest increments in the last tests associated with alterations in liver function). Of considerably greater significance was the finding that 7 of the 15 patients were found to have low urinary calcium excretion despite normal creatinine clearances. Four of the 15 patients had 25-hydroxyvitamin D concentrations less than 10 ng/ml (normal: 8–55 ng/ml), and five had 1,25-dihydroxyvitamin D levels below 25 pg/ml (normal: 25–65 pg/ml). Serum carotene values were generally low, and dietary histories suggested that most of the patients ingested less than 500 mg of calcium per day. All of these data support the concept that absorption of calcium and vitamin D are probably impaired or inadequate in many patients with Gaucher's disease, possibly as a result of an intestinal absorptive defect, conceivably from an alteration in gut cell structure as a result of the disease.

The findings on forearm densitometric analyses and CT densitometric studies of the spine suggested that all of the patients had values for bone mass three or more standard deviations below the mean for age-matched controls, and these data coupled with normal values for hydroxyproline excretion and diminished retention of ^{99m}Tc-diphosphonate on quantitative bone scans support the concept of a reduction in bone remodeling. Parathyroid hormone levels were low or low-normal in 12 of the 15 patients, suggesting a partial loss of regulation of calcium homeostasis and the negative feedback loop associated with an uncoupling of the normal turnover system, and that the patients were unable to respond appropriately to chronic calcium and vitamin D deficits.

Bone morphometric studies performed in 11 of the 15 patients supported the hypothesis with markedly reduced osteoclast numbers and significantly diminished rates of bone formation. Static measurements showed low values for both surface percentage of bone covered with osteoid and relative osteoid volumes, and dynamic measurements using fluorescent analysis of double tetracycline–labeled specimens showed a prolonged mineralization lag time in several of the patients.

These findings are preliminary but suggest at least two major abnormalities occurring in many of the patients with Gaucher's disease. A decreased gastrointestinal absorption of calcium and vitamin D (or possibly a failure of polar conversion of vitamin D in the diseased liver or kidney) appears to be the cause of reduced calcium pools for bone formation and normal mineralization of the skeleton. The response to this deficit, in some of the patients at least, is extraordinary in that the PTH values are low and osteoclast populations almost absent, suggesting a failure of coupling and a distinctly abnormal response of the skeleton to a calcium-deficient state. Despite the diminished turnover rate in the skeleton, the bones show a marked reduction in bone mass consistent with the evident severe osteopenia observed in many of the patients with the disease.

IV. DISCUSSION

The bone changes in patients with Gaucher's disease are frequent in occurrence, often severe in manifestation, and not wholly explainable by the now clearly documented cause and pathogenesis of the visceral and hematologic disease. Patients with Gaucher's disease may have a relatively light "burden" of visceral disturbance, be nearly normal hematologically, and yet develop severe and very disabling problems in their osseous system as a result of osteopenia, fractures, bone crises, osteonecrosis, and osteomyelitis. Furthermore, the management of these bony disorders is not simple and often leads to complications that cause further morbidity and disability and may shorten the life span of the patient.

In rather sharp contrast with the sophisticated and successful efforts of the geneticists and molecular biologists to define the cause of the disorder, little attention has been paid to the bony manifestations, and as indicated in the foregoing and by review of the small number of literature citations, studies are few, data are sparse, and knowledge is limited. However, on the basis of radiologic evaluation, histologic study, and some very recent (and incomplete) biochemical data, we have reached a point at which it is possible to speculate on some of the ways patients with Gaucher's disease may develop bone disease and, perhaps much more important, can at least partially consider avenues of treatment by which their suffering can be alleviated.

In regard to the osteopenia, it seems evident that it is common and often severe but, unlike osteomalacia, hyperparathyroidism, and even osteoporosis, does not appear to obey the laws that govern the interaction of minerals and the bone. Specifically, without evident lesions in the gut, kidney, parathyroid gland, or bone, the patient appears to have a reduced absorption of vitamin D and calcium and an uncoupling of the rates of bone formation and bone resorption resulting in severe bone loss unassociated with parathyroid hormone response or osteoclastic resorption of the bones. These data suggest that the common denominator may lie with the monocyte, which because of the collection of substrate in the lysosomal body of the cell produces mediator substances that interfere with calcium transport, osteoclast action, and bone formation. In the absence of research data, the existence and nature of these mediators can be only speculative, but the authors are sufficiently convinced of the importance of this avenue of exploration to make it the primary focus of their current research efforts.

As regards osteonecrosis, even less knowledge is available. The bone crises, osteosclerotic foci, and disabling corticocancellous osteonecrosis speak for episodes of severe compromise of blood flow to the bone, hypoxia, and cell death. Why this should occur in patients in whom the visceral disease is only rarely characterized by infarction and in whom pathologic studies have failed to show obstructive vascular disease is obscure. Several possibilities exist. The first is the suggestion that the serum burden of glucosylceramide becomes intermittently great enough to affect the small vessels either by inducing spasm or conceivably by increasing local viscosity in a patient whose oxygen carrying capacity is already markedly compromised by a refractory hypochromic anemia. The second possibility is that the macrophages and monocytes may, under appropriate circumstances (perhaps as a result of excessive storage, viremia, or other systemic insult), disgorge their lysosomal contents of other toxins including lysosomal enzymes into their microenvironment. Macrophages in culture release lysosomal enzymes and a number of activators in response to the accumulation of glucocerebroside.[107,108] These substances are very likely to be injurious to surrounding cells and may initiate a vasospastic response. It is probable that this mechanism is responsible for the massive necrosis and subsequent fibrosis sometimes observed in the liver and spleen;[52,54] and it is certainly possible that similar mechanisms occurring in bone are responsible for some of the pathologic changes seen in the disorder. Another possible cause is related to "swelling" of the large Gaucher's cells as might occur with changes in atmospheric pressure or during a viremia. Although unlikely, it is possible that sufficient swelling can occur in a rigid bony framework to occlude small delicate vascular channels and, in the already modestly hypoxic marrow cavity, lead to infarction of a discrete segment. These hypotheses are much more difficult to test than are those related to the osteopenia, but if the disease is to be conquered, they must be further evaluated by appropriately designed studies.

Finally is the question regarding the frequency with which these patients develop osteomyelitis. Is there a macrophagic incompetence for bacteria in patients with Gaucher's disease? Is the pancytopenia alone responsible for the high infection rate? Does the marrow hypoxia play a role? Is it possible that the protective leukocytic systems may be sufficient for normal bone even in patients with severe forms of Gaucher's disease, but that the dead bone serves as a "locus minoris resistentiae" and, during a bacteremia, organisms lodge in the dead segment and proliferate without interference either by the leukocytic elements or by diffusion of parenterally administered antibiotics? These questions must also be addressed if we are to solve one of the most vexing and troublesome problems that face the patient with the disease.

In final statement, the osseous manifestations of Gaucher's disease are common and often severe and disabling. Knowledge regarding them at least at the time of this writing is sparse and limited as a result of very little attention paid to the disease by students of bone and mineral metabolism. With appropriate study and application of newer methods, some of these puzzles may be solved, and perhaps between the capabilities of the geneticist to increase production of a potent enzyme and attempts at alteration of mineral metabolism, the hapless patient with the disorder, for whom little could be done until recently, may receive some significant aid in conquering the disease.

References

1. Gaucher PCE: De l'epithelioma primitif de la rate, hypertrophe idiopathigue de la rate sans lucemie. Paris, Octave Doin, Editeur, 1882.
2. Bloem TF, Groen J, Postma C: Gaucher's disease. Q J Med 5:517–527, 1936.
3. Brill NE, Mandlebaum FS, Libman E: A case of "splenomagalie primitif" with involvement of the hematopoetic organs. Proc NY Path Soc 4:143–152, 1904.
4. Bychowski Z: Zurkasuisti der heredo-familiaren Splenomeglie. Wien Klin Wochenschir 24:1519–1522, 1911.
5. DeLange C: Uber die maligne Form der Gauchershen Krankheit. Acta Pediatr 27:34–50, 1939.
6. Mandlebaum FS, Downey H: The histopathology and biology of Gaucher's disease (large cell splenomegaly). Fol Haematol 20:139–142, 1916.
7. Pick L: Classification of diseases of lipid metabolism and Gaucher's disease. Am J Med Sci 185:453–469, 1933.
8. Reich C, Seife M, Kessler BJ: Gaucher's disease: A review and discussion of twenty cases. Medicine 30:1–20, 1951.

8a. Epstein E: Beitrag zur Pathologie der Gaucherschen Krankheit. Virchows Arch Pathol Anat 253:157–207, 1924.

9. Reuben MS: Gaucher's disease. Arch Pediatr 41:456–475, 1924.

9a. Epstein E: Beitrag zur Chemie der Gaucherschen Krankheit. Biochem Ztschr 145:398–414, 1924.

10. Brill NE: Primary splenomegaly with a report of three cases occurring in one family. Am J Med Soc 121:377–392, 1901.
11. Groen JF: The hereditary mechanism of Gaucher's disease. Blood 3:1238–1249, 1948.
12. Fried K: Population study of chronic Gaucher's disease. Isr Med J Sci 9:1396–1398, 1973.
13. Goldblatt J, Beighton P: Gaucher's disease in South Africa. J Med Genet 16:302–305, 1979.
14. Kolodny EH, Ullman MD, Mankin HJ, et al: Phenotypic manifestations of Gaucher disease: Clinical features in 48 biochemically verified type 1 patients and comment on type 2 patients. *In* Desnick RJ, Gatt S, Grabowski GA (eds): Gaucher Disease: A Century of Delineation and Research, vol 95: Progress in Clinical and Biological Research. New York, Alan R. Liss, 1982, pp 33–65.
15. Matoth Y, Fried K: Chronic Gaucher's disease. Clinical observations in 34 patients. Isr J Med Sci 1:521–530, 1965.
16. Medoff AS, Boyd ED: Gaucher's disease in 29 cases: Hematologic complications and effect of splenectomy. Ann Intern Med 40:481–492, 1954.
17. Brady RO, Kanfer JN, Shapiro D: Metabolism of glucocerebrosides. II. Evidence of an enzymatic deficiency in Gaucher's disease. Biochem Biophys Res Commun 18:221–225, 1965.
18. Beutler E, Krihl W: The diagnosis of the adult type of Gaucher's disease and its carrier state by demonstration of deficiency of beta-glucosidase activity in peripheral blood leukocytes. J Lab Clin Med 76:747–755, 1970.
19. Brady RO, Johnson WG, Uhlendorf BW: Identification of heterozygous carriers of lipid storage diseases: Current status and clinical applications. Am J Med 51:423–431, 1971.
20. Raghavan SS, Topol J, Kolodny EH: Leukocyte β-glucosidase in homozygotes and heterozygotes for Gaucher disease. Am J Hum Genet 32:158–173, 1980.
21. Brady RO, Barranger JA: Glucosyl ceramide lipidosis: Gaucher's disease. *In* Stanbury JB, Wyngaarden JB, Gredericksom SD, et al (eds): The Metabolic Basis of Inherited Disease. New York, McGraw-Hill, 1983, pp 842–856.
22. Ginns EI, Brady RO, Pirruccello S, et al: Mutations of glucocerebrosidase: Discrimination of neurologic and non-neurologic phenotypes of Gaucher's disease. Proc Natl Acad Sci USA 79:5607–5710, 1982.
23. Ginns EI, Tegelaers FPW, Barneveld R, et al: Determination of Gaucher's disease phenotypes with monoclonal antibody. Clin Chim Acta 131:283–287, 1983.

24. Dreborg S, Erikson A, Hagberg B: Gaucher's disease—Norrbottnian type 1. General clinical description. Eur J Pediatr 133:107–118, 1980.
25. Svennerholm L, Dreborg S, Erikson A, et al: Gaucher disease of the Norrbottnian type (type III), phenotypic manifestations. *In* Desnick RJ, Gatt S, Grabowski GA (eds): Gaucher's Disease: A Century of Delineation and Research. New York, Alan R. Liss, 1982, pp 67–94.
26. Barranger JA, Murray GJ, Ginns EI: Genetic heterogeneity of Gaucher's disease. *In* Barranger JA, Brady RO (eds): Molecular Basis of Lysosomal Storage Disorders. New York, Academic Press, 1984, pp 311–323.
27. Wenger DA, Olson GC: Heterogeneity in Gaucher's disease. *In* Callahan JW, Lowden JA (eds): Lysosomes and Lysosomal Storage Diseases. New York, Raven Press, 1981, pp 157–171.
28. Basu A, Glew RH, Daniels LB, et al: Activators of spleen glucocerebrosidase from controls and patients with various forms of Gaucher's disease. J Biol Chem 259:1714, 1984.
29. Choy FYM: Gaucher's disease: The effects of phosphatidylserine on glucocerebrosidase from normal and Gaucher fibroblasts. Hum Genet 67:432–436, 1984.
30. Glew RH, Daniels LB, Clark LS, et al: Enzymic differentiation of neurologic and non-neurologic forms of Gaucher's disease. J Neuropathol Exp Neurol 41:630–641, 1982.
31. Moseley JE: The reticuloendothelioses. *In* Bone Changes in Hematologic Disorders (Roentgen Aspects). New York, Grune and Stratton, 1963, p 183.
32. Peters SP, Coyle P, Glew RH: Differentiation of β-glucosidase in human tissues using sodium taurocholate. Arch Biochem Biophys 175:569–582, 1976.
33. Ginns EI, Erickson A, Tegelaers FPW, et al: Isozymes of β-glucosidase: Determination of Gaucher's disease phenotypes. *In* Rattazzi MC, Scandalios JG, Whitt GS (eds): Isozymes: Current Topics in Biological and Medical Research, vol 11: Medical and Other Applications. New York, Alan R. Liss, 1983, pp 83–93.
34. Murray GJ: Lectin-specific targeting of lysosomal enzymes to reticuloendothelial cells. Methods Enzymol 149:25–42, 1987.
35. Takasaki S, Murray GJ, Furbish FS, et al: Structure of the N-asparagine-linked oligosaccharide units of human placental β-glucocerebrosidase. J Biol Chem 259:10112–10117, 1984.
36. Choudary PV, Tsuji S, Martin BM, et al: The molecular biology of Gaucher disease and the potential for gene therapy. Cold Springs Harbor Symposium in Quantitative Biology 51, P22:1047–1052, 1986.
37. Jonsson LV, Murray GJ, Sorrell SH, et al: Biosynthesis and maturation of glucocerebrosidase in Gaucher fibroblasts. Eur J Biochem 164:171–179, 1987.
38. Erickson AH, Ginns EI, Barranger JA: Biosynthesis of liposomal enzyme glucocerebrosidase. J Biol Chem 260:14319–14324, 1985.
39. Gravel RA, Leung A: Complementation analysis in Gaucher's disease using single cell microassay techniques. Evidence for a single "Gaucher gene." Hum Genet 65:112, 1983.
40. Wenger DA, Roth S, Kuloh T, et al: Biochemical studies in a patient with subacute neuropathic Gaucher disease without visceral glucosylceramide storage. Pediatr Res 17:344–348, 1983.
41. Ginns EI, Choudary PV, Martin BM, et al: Isolation of cDNA clones for human β-glucocerebrosidase using the gt11 expression system. Biochem Biophys Res Commun 123:574–580, 1984.
42. Barnevald RA, Keijzer W, Tegelaers FPW, et al: Assignment of the gene coding for human β-glucocerebrosidase to the region q21–q31 of chromosome 1 using monoclonal antibodies. Hum Genet 64:227–231, 1985.
43. Ginns EI, Choudary PV, Tsuji S, et al: Gene mapping and leader polypeptide sequence of human glucocerebrosidase: Implications for Gaucher disease. Proc Natl Acad Sci USA 82:7101–7105, 1985.
44. Choudary PV, Ginns EI, Barranger JA: Molecular cloning and characterization of human β-glucocerebrosidase gene. DNA 4:74, 1985.
45. Choudary PV, Barranger JA, Tsuji S, Mayor J, et al: Retrovirus-mediated transfer of human glucocerebrosidase gene to Gaucher fibroblasts. Mol Biol Med 3:293–299, 1986.
46. Fleischmajer R: Gaucher's disease. *In* The Dyslipidoses. Springfield, IL, Charles C Thomas, 1960, pp 248–269.
47. Goldblatt J, Beighton P: Cutaneous manifestations of Gaucher's disease. Br J Dermatol 111:331–334, 1984.
48. Carbone AO, Petrozzi CF: Gaucher's disease: Case report with stress on eight findings. Henry Ford Hosp Med J 16:55–60, 1968.
49. Petrohilos M, Tricoulis D, Kotsiris I, Vouzoukos A: Ocular manifestations of Gaucher's disease. Am J Opthalmol 80:1006–1010, 1975.
50. East T, Savin LH: A case of Gaucher's disease with biopsy of the typical pingueculae. Br J Ophthalmol 24:611–613, 1940.
51. Jaffe HL: Gaucher's disease and certain other inborn metabolic disorders. *In* Metabolic, Degenerative and Inflammatory Diseases of Bones and Joints. Philadelphia, Lea and Febiger, 1972, pp 506–522.
52. Lee RE: Pathology of Gaucher's disease. *In* Desnick RJ, Gatt S, Grabowski GA (eds): Gaucher Disease: A Century of Delineation and Research, vol 95: Progress in Clinical and Biological Research. New York, Alan R. Liss, 1982, pp 177–217.
53. Shiloni E, Bitran D, Rachmilewitz E, Durst AL: The role of splenectomy in Gaucher's disease. Arch Surg 118:929–932, 1983.
54. James SP, Stromeyer FW, Chang C, Barranger JA: Liver abnormalities in patients with Gaucher's disease. Gastroenterology 80:126–133, 1981.
55. Brady RO, James SP, Barranger JA: The liver in lipid storage disease: Biochemical basis of pathogenesis and clinical features. Prog Liver Dis 7:331–346, 1982.
56. James SP, Stromeyer FW, Stowens DW, Barranger JA: Gaucher disease: Hepatic abnormalities in 25 patients. *In* Desnick RJ, Gatt S, Grabowski GA (eds): Gaucher Disease: A Century of Delineation and Research, vol 95: Progress in Clinical and Biological Research. New York, Alan R. Liss, 1982, pp 131–142.
57. Kozower M, Kaplan MN, Kanfer JN, et al: Esophageal varices in a 60 year old man with Gaucher's disease. Am J Dig Dis 19:565–570, 1974.
58. Katzen BT: Positive lymphangiography in Gaucher's disease. Report of a case. Radiology 115:85–86, 1975.

59. Chander PN, Nurse HM, Pirani CL: Renal involvement in adult Gaucher's disease after splenectomy. Arch Pathol Lab Med 103:440–445, 1979.
60. Siegal A, Gutman A, Shapiro MS, Griffel B: Renal involvement in Gaucher's disease. Postgrad Med J 57:398–401, 1981.
61. Schneider EL, Epstein CJ, Kaback MJ, Brandes D: Severe pulmonary involvement in adult Gaucher's disease. Report of three cases and review of the literature. Am J Med 63:475–480, 1977.
61a. Gelfand G, Bienenstock H: Hemorrhagic bursitis and bone crises in chronic adult Gaucher's disease. Arthritis Rheum 25:1369, 1982.
62. Beighton P, Sacko S: Gaucher's disease in Southern Africa. S Afr Med J 48:1295–1299, 1974.
63. Wei J, Martinez CR, Valle DL: Gaucher's disease. Johns Hopkins Med J 141:35–44, 1977.
64. Robinson DB, Glew RH: Acid phosphatase in Gaucher's disease. Clin Chem 26:371–382, 1980.
65. Tuchman LR, Goldstein G, Clyman M: Studies on the nature of the increased serum acid phosphatase in Gaucher's disease. Am J Med 27:959–962, 1959.
66. Brooks SEH, Audretsch JJ: Ultrastructural diagnosis of Gaucher's disease with negative staining technique. Arch Pathol 95:226–228, 1973.
67. Lee RE: The fine structure of the cerebroside occurring in Gaucher's disease. Proc Natl Acad Sci USA 61:484–489, 1968.
68. Pratt PW, Estren S, Kochiva S: Immunoglobulin abnormalities in Gaucher's disease. Report of 16 cases. Blood 31:633–640, 1968.
69. Schoenfeld Y, Berliner S, Pinkhas J, Beutler E: The association of Gaucher's disease and dysproteinemias. Acta Haematol 64:241–243, 1980.
70. Schoenfeld Y, Gallant LA, Shaklai M, et al: Gaucher's disease: A disease with chronic stimulation of the immune system. Arch Pathol Lab Med 106:388–391, 1982.
71. Turesson I, Rausing A: Gaucher's disease and benign monoclonal gammopathy. Acta Med Scand 197:507–512, 1975.
72. Wolf P: Monoclonal gammopathy in Gaucher's disease. Lab Med 4:28–29, 1973.
73. Pinkhas J, Djaldetti M, Yaron M: Coincidence of multiple myeloma with Gaucher's disease. Isr J Med Sci 1:537–540, 1965.
74. Ruestow PC, Levinson DJ, Catchatourian R, et al: Coexistence of IgA myeloma and Gaucher's disease. Arch Intern Med 140:1115–1116, 1980.
75. Hanasl SM, Rueknagel DL, Heidelberger KP, Raden NS: Primary amyloidosis associated with Gaucher's disease. Ann Intern Med 89:639–641, 1978.
76. Krause JR, Bures C, Lee RE: Acute leukemia and Gaucher's disease. Scand J Haematol 23:115–118, 1979.
77. Mark T, Dominquez C, Rywlin AM: Gaucher's disease associated with chronic lymphocytic leukemia. South Med J 75:361–363, 1982.
78. Shinar E, Gershon ZL, Leiserowitz R, et al: Coexistence of Gaucher disease and Philadelphia positive chronic granulocytic leukemia. Am J Hematol 12:199–202, 1982.
79. Bruckstein AH, Karanas A, Dire JJ: Gaucher's disease associated with Hodgkin's disease. Am J Med 68:610–613, 1980.
80. Amstutz HC, Carey EJ: Skeletal manifestations and treatment of Gaucher's disease. J Bone Joint Surg 48A:670–701, 1966.
81. Greenfield GB: Bone changes in chronic adult Gaucher's disease. Am J Roentgenol 110:800–807, 1970.
82. Rourke JA, Heslin DJ: Gaucher's disease: Roentgenologic bone changes over 20 year interval. Am J Roentgenol 94:621–630, 1965.
83. Stowens DW, Teitelbaum SL, Kahn AJ, Barranger JA: Skeletal complications of Gaucher's disease. Medicine 64:310–322, 1985.
84. Shapiro F, Glimcher MJ: Organization and cellular biology of the perichondrial ossification groove of Ranvier: A morphological study in rabbits. J Bone Joint Surg 59A:703–723, 1977.
84a. Rose JS, Grabowski GA, Barnett SH, Desnick RJ: Accelerated skeletal deterioration after splenectomy in Gaucher type 1 disease. Am J Roentgenol 139:1202, 1982.
85. Strickland B: Skeletal manifestations of Gaucher's disease with some unusual findings. Br J Radiol 30:246–253, 1958.
85a. Schubiner H, Letourneau M, Murray DL: Pyogenic osteomyelitis versus pseudo-osteomyelitis in Gaucher's disease. Clin Pediatr 20:667, 1981.
86. Beighton P, Goldblatt J, Sacks S: Bone involvement in Gaucher's disease: A century of delineation and research. *In* Desnick RJ, Grabowski GA (eds): Progress in Clinical and Biological Research, vol 95. New York, Alan R. Liss, 1982, pp 107–129.
86a. Yossipovitch ZH, Herman G, Makin M: Aseptic osteomyelitis in Gaucher's disease. Isr J Med Sci 1:531, 1965.
87. Goldblatt J, Sacks S, Beighton P: The orthopaedic aspects of Gaucher's disease. Clin Orthop 137:208, 1978.
88. Jackson DC, Simon G: Unusual bone and lung changes in a case of Gaucher's disease. Br J Radiol 38:698–700, 1965.
89. Schwartz AM, Homer MJ, McCauley RG: "Step-off" vertebral body: Gaucher's disease versus sickle cell hemoglobinopathy. Am J Roentgenol 132:81–85, 1979.
90. Windholz F, Foster SE: Sclerosis of bones in Gaucher's disease. Am J Roentgenol 60:246–250, 1948.
91. Cheng TH, Holman BL: Radionuclide assessment of Gaucher's disease. J Nucl Med 19:1333–1336, 1978.
92. Arkin AM, Schein AJ: Aseptic necrosis in Gaucher's disease. J Bone Joint Surg 30A:631–641, 1948.
92a. Hungerford DS, Zizic TM; Pathogenesis of ischemic necrosis of the femoral head. *In* Hungerford DS (ed): Proceedings of the Eleventh Open Scientific Meeting of the Hip Society. St. Louis, CV Mosby, 1983, pp 249–262.
93. Katz JF: Recurrent avascular necrosis of the proximal femoral epiphysis in the same hip in Gaucher's disease. J Bone Joint Surg 49A:514, 1967.
94. Levin B: Gaucher's disease. Clinical roentgenographic manifestations. Am J Roentgenol 85:685–691, 1961.
95. Siffert RS, Platt A: Gaucher disease: Orthopaedic considerations. *In* Desnick RJ, Gatt S, Grabowski GA (eds): Gaucher Disease: A Century of Delineation and Research, vol 95: Progress in Clinical and Biological Research. New York, Alan R. Liss, 1982, pp 617–626.
96. Silverstein MN, Kelly PJ: Osteoarticular manifestations of Gaucher's disease. Am J Med Sci 253:569–577, 1967.

96a. Todd RM, Keidan SE: Changes in the head of the femur in children suffering from Gaucher's disease. J Bone Joint Surg 34B:447, 1952.
97. Green DL, Bahnuuk E, Liebedt RA: Biplane radiographic measurements of reversible displacement (including clinical loosening and migration) of total joint replacements. J Bone Joint Surg 65A:1134–1143, 1983.
98. Amstutz HC: The hip in Gaucher's disease. Clin Orthop 90:83–89, 1973.
98a. Lau MM, Lichtman DM, Hamati YI, Bierbaum BE: Hip arthroplasties in Gaucher's disease. J Bone Joint Surg 63A:591–601, 1981.
99. Seinsheimer F, Mankin HJ: Acute bilateral symmetrical pathologic fractures of the lateral tibial plateaus in a patient with Gaucher's disease. Arthritis Rheum 20:1550, 1977.
100. Benjamin D, Joshua H, Dower D, et al: Circulatory anticoagulants in patients with Gaucher's disease. Acta Haematol 61:233–234, 1979.
101. Boklan BF, Sawitsky A: Factor IX deficiency and Gaucher's disease. Arch Intern Med 136:489–492, 1976.
102. Lachiewicz PF, Lane JM, Wilson PD Jr: Total hip replacement in Gaucher's disease. J Bone Joint Surg 63A:602–608, 1981.
102a. Linder L, Lindberg L, Carlsson A: Aseptic loosening of hip prostheses. A histologic and enzyme histochemical study. Clin Orthop 175:93–105, 1983.
103. Mankin HJ, Doppelt SH, Sullivan TR, Tomford WW: Osteoarticular and intercalary allograft transplantation in the management of malignant tumors of bone. Cancer 50:613–630, 1982.
104. Sacks S: Osteitis in Gaucher's disease. S Afr J Surg 9:161, 1971.
105. Miller JH, Ortega JA, Heisel MA: Juvenile Gaucher disease stimulating osteomyelitis. Am J Roentgenol 137:880, 1981.
106. Noyes FR, Smith WS: Bone crises and chronic osteomyelitis in Gaucher's disease. Clin Orthop 79:132, 1971.
107. Gery I, Davies P, Krett N, Barranger JA: Relationship between production and release of lymphocyte-activating factor (interleukin-1) by murine macrophages. 1. Effect of various agents. Cell Immunol 64:293–303, 1981.
108. Gery I, Zigler JS Jr, Brady RO, Barranger JA: Selective effects of glucocerebroside (Gaucher's storage material) on macrophage cultures. J Clin Invest 68:1182–1189, 1981.

MARK C. GEBHARDT
HENRY J. MANKIN

20

The Diagnosis and Management of Bone Tumors

Primary tumors of bone are uncommon lesions. Less than 3000 malignant tumors occur annually in the United States (about 1/100 the frequency with which patients with metastatic tumors of bone are encountered[1–3]), and although the incidence of the benign lesions is greater[4] (the frequency of some tumors such as osteocartilaginous exostoses is quite high), one could hardly consider osseous neoplasms as representing either a major field of study or, in fact, a significant health hazard. Despite this relative rarity, however, an intense and quite productive interest in the subject has developed among pathologists, radiologists, orthopedists, oncologists, and scientists interested in the musculoskeletal system.

Because neoplasms of bone may arise from all of the connective tissue components that normally constitute osseous and epiphyseal tissues and also recapitulate the phylogeny and biology of those structures, an extraordinary array of lesions has been identified—some arising from bony elements, from cartilaginous or fibrous components, from fat, from marrow elements, and from other more obscure cells of origin.[5] Each of these lesions has a specific histologic appearance and a characteristic clinical and radiographic presentation; in fact, many of the tumors have a benign and malignant counterpart and, for some, a spectrum of biological behavior, often not clearly predictable on the basis of imaging studies or routine histologic examination.

Perhaps the most exciting aspect of the current status of our knowledge of the neoplasms of bone is the apparent unparalleled success in oncologic management, partly related to improvements in surgical treatment and development of satisfactory implant systems, but also due to the introduction of protocols for the use of potent adjuvant chemotherapeutic and radiation modalities that appear to have a major effect on the primary lesion and the distant metastases. Bone tumors arise most frequently in younger individuals, and the most malignant of these principally occur during the second decade of life (not surprisingly, during or just after the final growth spurt)[4]; hence, although rare, they are psychologically and socioeconomically devastating. Children with osteosarcoma or Ewing's sarcoma who 25 years ago faced an amputation and a high probability of death from pulmonary metastases (survival rates of 15%–30% and 15%, respectively) now can look forward to a much greater likelihood of long survival (50%–80%)[6–17] and an equally great possibility of retaining a useful extremity.[8,18]

The readers of a textbook on metabolic bone disease would be unlikely to have a high degree of interest in the nuances of histologic or radiologic diagnosis of bone tumors or the intricacies of surgical, radiation, or chemotherapeutic management of patients with these rare entities; for those few who require further information, more detailed accounts can be readily obtained in texts devoted to the subject[4,5,19–24] or by study of the list of references appended to this chapter. The chapter itself is confined to a limited description of only some of the more common entities and highlights only those aspects of classification, staging, and therapeutic approaches that have general relevance to bone pathology and bone structure and will, at the same time, also illuminate some current research efforts in the field.

Table 20–1. Classification of Primary Bone Tumors

Tissue of Origin	Benign	Malignant	
Bone	Osteoid osteoma Osteoblastoma Osteoma	Juxtacortical Central Telangiectatic Low-grade medullary Paget's sarcoma Radiation-induced sarcoma	*Osteosarcoma*
Cartilage	Osteocartilaginous exostosis Enchondroma Chondroblastoma Chondromyxoid fibroma Juxtacortical chondroma	Enostotic Exostotic Mesenchymal Clear cell Dedifferentiated	*Chondrosarcoma*
Fibrous	Fibrous dysplasia Unicameral bone cyst Aneurysmal bone cyst Fibrous cortical defect Nonossifying fibroma Subperiosteal desmoid Desmoplastic fibroma	Fibrosarcoma Malignant fibrous histiocytoma	
Blood vessels	Hemangioma Glomus tumor Angiomatosis	Hemangiosarcoma Hemangiopericytoma Gorham's disease	
Fat	Lipoma	Liposarcoma Myxosarcoma	
Marrow elements	Histiocytosis	Primary Hodgkin's lymphoma of bone Primary non-Hodgkin's lymphoma of bone Ewing's sarcoma Myeloma	
Notochord	—	Chordoma	
Neural elements	Neurofibroma Neurolemmoma Neurofibromatosis Ganglioneuroma	Neurofibrosarcoma	
Unknown	—	Giant cell tumor Adamantinoma	

Adapted from Spjut HJ, Dorfman HD, Fechner RE, Ackerman LV: Atlas of Tumor Pathology, Fascicles: Tumors of Bone and Cartilage. Armed Forces Institute of Pathology, 1971.

I. CLASSIFICATION AND STAGING OF BONE TUMORS

A. Classification

Most of the systems developed for the classification of primary bone tumors utilize the putative cell or tissue of origin as their basis; hence, lesions may be divided according to the principal cell type and matrix component displayed on histologic examination of the lesions.[4,5] Thus, the bulk of primary lesions will fall into the categories of osseous, cartilaginous, fibrous, round cell (probably arising from marrow elements), and "other" components, in which the cell of origin is obscure. Such a classification is shown in Table 20–1. Note that for most of the categories there are both benign and malignant members and that within each such subcategory there are a number of types of lesions, each of which exhibits different patterns of presentation and biological behavior. Furthermore, some of the lesions of the same cell type, such as chondrosarcoma or fibrosarcoma, may present as "high" or "low" grade, depending in part on their imaging characteristics, histologic patterns, and, most important, propensity for local recurrence and distant metastases.

It should be readily apparent on the basis of this extraordinary array of lesions (some of which, such as the adamantinoma or desmoplastic fibroma, are exceedingly rare) why even the experienced clinician or pathologist often finds this field a challenging and difficult one. The more important issue is perhaps the problems that arise in management, in which errors in diagnosis may lead to over- or undertreatment, which may cost the patient dearly in morbidity and mortality.

B. Staging

One of the recent major advances in the management of tumors of the skeletal system has been the development of a staging system. A recent article by Enneking and coworkers[25] based on his studies and those of the Musculoskeletal Tumor Society details the technique of this system, which has brought some order to the chaos of the diagnosis of these lesions. Whereas formerly only a histologic diagnosis was available upon which to base prognosis and development of a management protocol, the staging system vastly expands our information regarding the lesion and permits algorithmic planning of the work-up and, much more important, the treatment. The staging system detailed in Table 20–2 is based on obtaining specific information about the tumor that defines the grade (G) of the tumor (benign = G0; low grade = G1; and high grade = G2); the anatomic site (T) determined by whether the lesion is confined to one anatomic compartment (T1) or has extended out of the original site to involve a second adjacent compartment (T2); and the absence or presence of distant metastases (M0 or M1). As can be noted, benign lesions are all classified in one group independent of the fact that the more aggressive of these (such as the chondromyxoid fibroma or osteoblastoma) often break out of the bone to become T2 and may recur after intralesional or marginal resection. The absence of the propensity for distant metastases justifies their inclusion in the benign category (G0), and they are thus classified as stage 0. Stage I lesions are low-grade tumors (G1), such as paraosteal osteosarcoma, low-grade chondrosarcoma, giant cell tumor, chordoma, and adamantinoma, all of which are capable of unrelenting local destruction, recurrence after inadequate local resection, and distant metastases (all at a slower rate and less frequently than is observed for the high-grade tumors). The category is divided into stages IA and IB by the anatomic extent of the lesion as determined by imaging studies. Those that are confined to the bone and hence are intracompartmental (T1) are included in stage IA, whereas those that have broken out of the bone to lie in the adjacent soft tissues (T2) are stage IB. Stage II lesions include the more malignant lesions, such as osteosarcoma, high-grade chondrosarcoma, high-grade fibrosarcoma, and malignant fibrous histiocytoma, all of which are prone to metastasize. These are also subdivided into two categories based on whether the lesion is intracompartmental (T1) or extracompartmental (T2). Stage III lesions include any grade and can be either intra- or extracompartmental but have evidence of distant metastasis to lung (the most common site of sarcoma metastasis), other bones, or lymph nodes.

Table 20–2. Surgical Stages

Stage	Grade	Site	Metastasis
IA	Low (G1)	Intracompartmental (T1)	None (M0)
B	Low (G1)	Extracompartmental (T2)	None (M0)
IIA	High (G2)	Intracompartmental (T1)	None (M0)
B	High (G2)	Extracompartmental (T2)	None (M0)
III	Low (G1) or High (G2)	Intracompartmental (T1) or Extracompartmental (T2)	Yes (M1)

Adapted from Enneking WF, Spanier SS, Goodman MA: A system for the surgical staging of musculoskeletal sarcoma. Clin Orthop 153:111, 1980.

The staging system is simple in application and is highly useful in assessing prognosis, dictating treatment protocols, and enhancing communication among clinicians and investigators.[25] An enchondroma confined to the medullary canal of the proximal humerus is a G0, T1, M0 and hence is a stage 0 lesion. A giant cell tumor of the distal femur that has broken out of the bone to lie in the medial quadriceps muscle compartment is a G1, T2, M0 and, therefore, a stage IB tumor. A patient with an osteosarcoma of the proximal femur that has broken out of the bone has a G2, T2, M0 lesion and hence a stage IIB sarcoma; if pulmonary metastases are present, the condition is described by the designators G2, T2, M1 and the stage is III.

The staging process is also relatively simple and should become routine for physicians evaluating patients with bone tumors. The grade of the lesion (G) is almost always determined on the basis of histologic examination, although in several recent studies, flow cytometric analysis of DNA kinetics using propidium iodide has been found to be a valuable adjunct to the grading process.[26,27] The presence or absence of distant metastases (M) is almost always determined on the basis of a careful history and physical examination, some key laboratory studies (such as an immunoelectrophoresis for myeloma or alkaline phosphatase for osteosarcoma), full lung tomograms or CT of the chest (the former study is used principally for older individuals who may show an excessive number of false-positives on the more sensitive CT), bone scan, and appropriate radiographs. In an occasional circumstance in which lymphoma or myeloma is suspected, a staging abdominal CT, bipedal lymphangiogram, liver-spleen scan, and bone marrow aspiration are often helpful in establishing the presence or absence of disseminated disease.[28] It should be noted, however, that the staging system described is applicable only to primary solid bone tumors and does not apply to marrow tumors such as Ewing's sarcoma, lymphoma, or myeloma. Rather, these diseases have their own specific staging systems.

To assess the anatomic location of the lesion (T), plain radiographs, standard tomograms, angiography, bone scan, CT of the lesion,[29] and, more recently, magnetic resonance imaging (MRI)[30–33] are often essential, although the last two recently introduced imaging techniques have begun to replace some of the more conventional studies.

In considering the timing of the staging procedures, the biopsy should probably be done last and only following careful study of all of the imaging studies and review of the material with the radiologist and pathologist.[34,35] The biopsy should be done with considerable care and planned as thoroughly as the definitive operation. Material obtained for biopsy should be examined by frozen section to be certain that the sample is adequate and the tissue is representative. Samples should be obtained for culture (some infections of bone may assume the appearance of a bone tumor), estrogen and progesterone receptors if metastatic breast carcinoma is suspected, immunoperoxidase staining after exposure to specific antibodies, and surface markers if lymphoma is the tentative diagnosis. In our laboratory, we routinely obtain a small portion of the tissue under sterile conditions for flow cytometric study,[26,27] not only for DNA kinetics, but more recently for doxorubicin (Adriamycin) binding,[36] which may be helpful in deciding on the appropriate chemotherapeutic regimen.

II. PRINCIPLES OF TREATMENT OF BONE TUMORS

It is clearly inappropriate in a chapter such as this to detail the surgical, radiation, or chemotherapeutic regimens used in the management of patients with benign, low-grade or high-grade tumors of bone. It is useful, however, to at least point out some of the modalities available, their limitations, and areas of application.

First, in consideration of surgical management, four types of operative treatments are recognized:[25] *intralesional,* in which the removal of the tumor violates the margin (such as during a curettage or piecemeal resection), leaving gross tumor; *marginal,* in which the plane of resection is on or through the pseudocapsule of the tumor; *wide,* in which the plane of resection or amputation is remote from the lesion but still within the involved compartment; and *radical,* in which the entire compartment in which the tumor lies is sacrificed. A simple curettage of an enchondroma is an "intralesional" procedure; extraperiosteal resection of a giant cell tumor of the distal femur is classified as "marginal"; cross-bone amputation through the proximal femur for an osteosarcoma of the distal femur is considered "wide"; and a hemipelvectomy for a high-grade chondrosarcoma of the upper end of the femur is clearly a "radical" procedure.

The second issue is the question of multimodality treatment. Some lesions such as metastatic carcinoma, Ewing's sarcoma, lymphoma, and myeloma are often exquisitely radiosensitive, and the use of local radiotherapy is standard in the management of many of these tumors, either alone or in combination with surgery and/or chemotherapy. The use of chemotherapy, a major advance that has materially extended the disease-free period and much improved the ultimate survival statistics for patients with certain high-grade sarcomas, is based on a postulate, at least partially proven, that patients often have micrometastases to the lungs even at the time of initial presentation. Systemic chemotherapy given prior to and/or following surgical extirpation of the lesion may reduce the likelihood that these lesions will survive and grow, and hence enhance the probability of long-term survival.

Finally, an aggressive attitude toward pulmonary metastases appears to be appropriate for patients with high-grade sarcomas. Several studies have demonstrated that the resection of pulmonary metastases and chemotherapy not only prolong survival but result in long-term remission in about 30% of the patients so treated.[37–44]

One of the major advances in recent years has been the development of methods of limb-sparing surgery, which has resulted in the retention of a useful, functional extremity in selected patients. Patients with an osteosarcoma, chondrosarcoma, or other high-grade lesion, who in past years would have been treated with an often disfiguring and disabling amputation, can now have limb salvage procedures, using metal and plastic implants, autograft (avascular or vascularized), or allograft bone parts to replace the resected segment. Although the parts are not "normal," useful function can often be maintained and the patient restored to a more acceptable psychosocial and economic status. Caution should be exhibited by the surgeon in prescribing such methods of treatment, since the survival rates following a local failure are usually poor (90% of the patients die of disease, even following amputation of or radiation to the local site),[45] but in selected individuals with small tumors not involving the vessels and nerves, it is possible to achieve adequate wide surgical margins safely and using any one of a number of devices or techniques, restoring the patient to useful upper or lower extremity function without resorting to an ablation of the part.

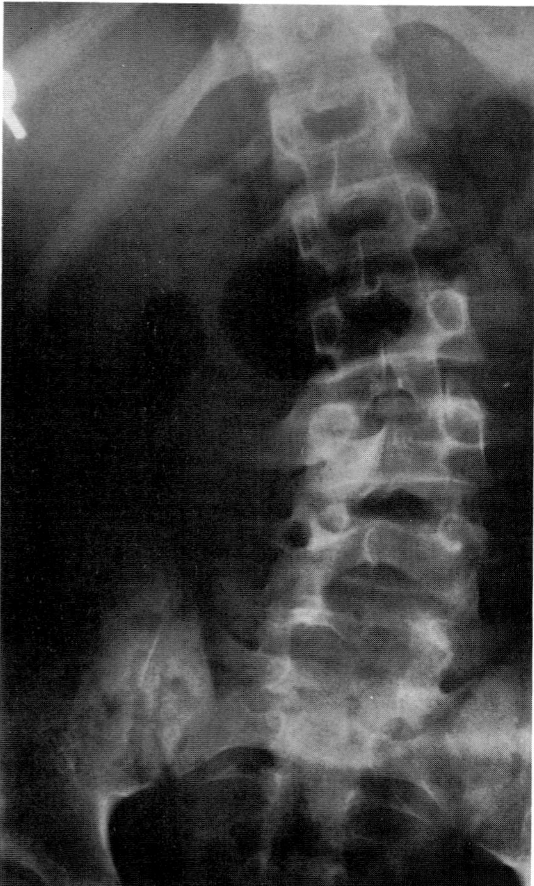

Figure 20–1. An AP radiograph of the spine in a 15-year-old boy with a painful, irritative scoliosis measuring 20 degrees. The lamina of L 4 on the right is thickened and dense with a barely perceptible rounded lucency within the reactive zone. Some internal mineralization is visible within the nidus.

III. SPECIAL TUMORS OF SPECIFIC INTEREST

A. Benign and Malignant Osseous Lesions

As noted in the section on classification and Table 20–1, bone tumors are categorized pathologically by the type of matrix they display. All osseous lesions show varying amounts of woven bone as the primary matrix component, and the aggressiveness of the lesion is generally determined by grading the cytologic characteristics of the stromal cells. For tumors in the osseous series there are two major benign lesions (the osteoid osteoma and osteoblastoma) and one major malignant category with several subsets (the osteosarcomas). These lesions must also be separated from other lesions that are probably not true neoplasms but also exhibit abnormal bone formation on pathologic section, namely, fibrous dysplasia and Paget's disease of bone. As indicated previously, it is beyond the scope of this chapter to provide a detailed description of each of these entities; instead, we will provide a brief overview of the main features of the more common lesions and sufficient bibliographic citations for the interested reader to further his or her knowledge.

An *osteoid osteoma* is a benign osseous tumor that usually presents a characteristic and quite distinctive clinical, radiographic, and pathologic picture.[46,47] The lesion is relatively common, accounting for about 10% of benign bone tumors in Dahlin's series,[4] and occurs primarily in individuals in the second or third decades of life. It is most commonly located

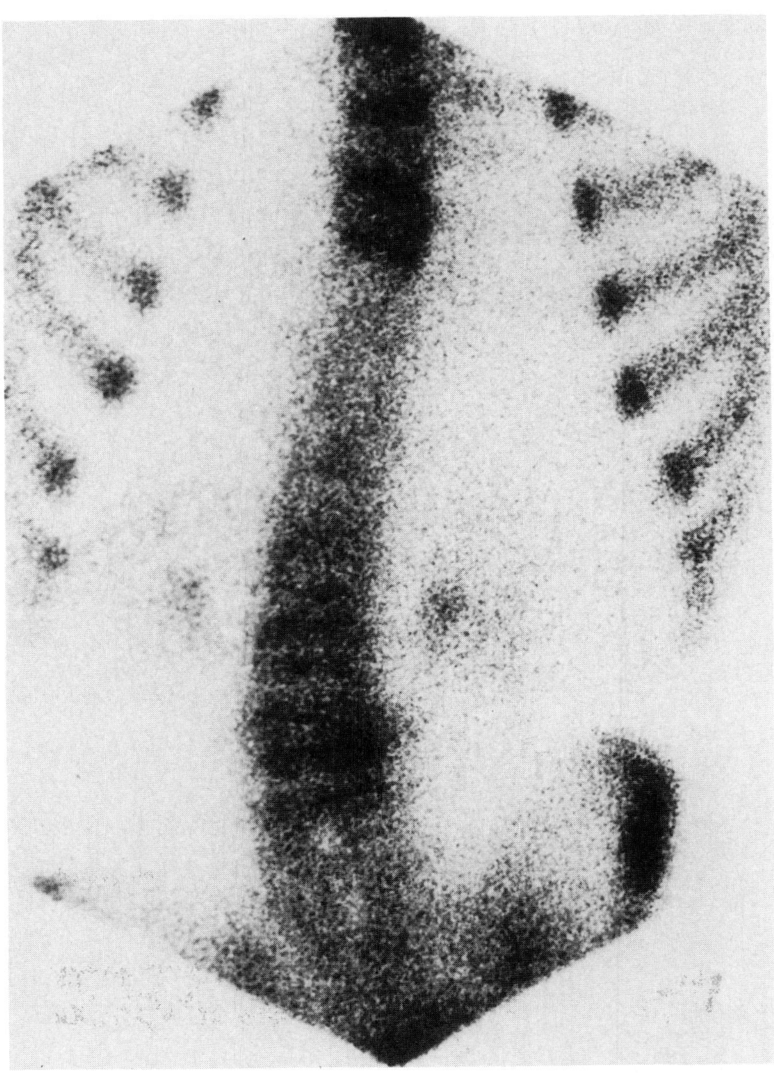

Figure 20–2. A radionuclide bone scan shows increased uptake in the L 4 lamina and is often useful in locating osteoid osteomas of the spine.

in the femur, tibia, or posterior elements of the vertebral bodies but has been reported to occur in all bones, excepting perhaps the skull, clavicle, and sternum.[47]

The clinical presentation is remarkably constant in character. The affected patient experiences a sharp, boring pain that is unrelated to activity and is often worse at night. Acetylsalicylic acid and other nonsteroidal anti-inflammatory agents usually relieve the pain completely, but temporarily so that the patient must usually take the drug every 3 to 4 hours to maintain a pain-free existence. The aspirin dependence is so striking as to suggest a prostaglandin-mediated mechanism for the pain.[48] The primary site of the lesion is usually locally tender; but in addition, the osteoid osteoma may produce a variety of associated physical findings such as muscle weakness and atrophy, sciatica-like symptoms,[49] painful scoliosis (Fig. 20–1), joint swelling, effusion, and limitation of motion or limb length inequality.

On radiographs (Fig. 20–1), the lesion is seen as an eccentrically located radiolucent, round or oval nidus, often with varying amounts of central mineralization, surrounded by a dense zone of reactive bone. This nidus, which is the true lesional tissue, is seldom greater than 1 cm in greatest dimension, but the adjacent reactive bone may be so pronounced as to obscure the lucency. It may occur in any location along the bone, but the majority are located near the cortex, and the lesion may be found to be

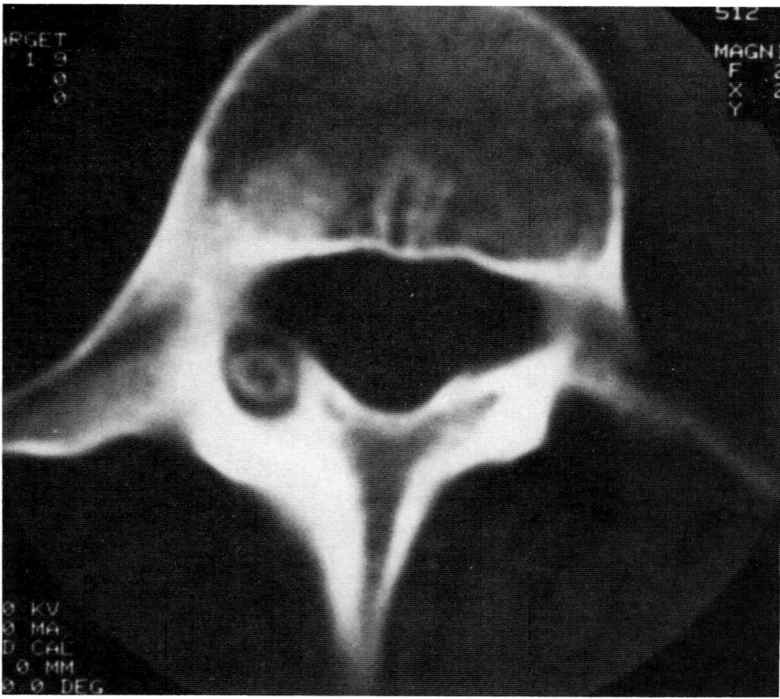

Figure 20–3. A computed tomographic cut of L 4 nicely demonstrates the nidus with the thickened lamina. A ring of mineralization within the nidus is present. This patient had an incomplete excision of the nidus with persistent symptoms. The irritative scoliosis dramatically responded to treatment with indomethacin.

periosteal, intracortical, endosteal, or rarely truly medullary. The lesions are readily detected by radionuclide bone scans (Fig. 20–2) because of their vascularity and the surrounding active bone production or by angiography, which also highlights the lesion. Plain and computed tomograms (CT)[50] are useful in detecting the presence of a nidus in lesions with excessive reactive bone (Fig. 20–3).[20]

On pathologic examination of the resected specimen, one sees an often bright red to red-gray discrete "nidus" that stands in sharp contrast to the surrounding dense sclerotic bone. Histologically, the nidus is composed of irregular trabeculae of woven bone set in a highly vascular, loosely packed benign fibrous stroma. The nidus is surrounded by varying amounts of reactive lamellar bone.[4,19,21–24,46,47,51]

The natural history of these lesions is that of continued pain that persists for years, although radiographically the lesions show no increase in size. There are case reports of spontaneous regression of symptoms, although this may take years, and the sclerosis persists after the pain subsides.[5,52] Treatment usually consists of block resection of the nidus, which relieves the symptoms, although curettage may be necessary in certain anatomic locations (small bones of the hands and feet, posterior elements of the spine). Incomplete excision may lead to persistence of the lesion and unrelenting symptoms.[19,20,52,53]

The *osteoblastoma*, although very similar to the osteoid osteoma in histologic appearance, is a distinct clinicopathologic entity. The tumors are rare (accounting for less than 3% of the benign bone tumors at the Mayo Clinic[4]) and may occur at any age but occur most frequently in patients in the second and third decades. Osteoblastomas occur in any site, but the metaphyses or diaphyses of the long bones and posterior elements of the spine are the most common sites. Although pain is usually present, it is not as severe as that associated with osteoid osteoma, nor is it relieved by aspirin. There is tenderness over the site of the lesion, and if it is located near a joint, swelling and limited range of motion may be present. Spinal lesions are often indistinguishable from osteoid osteoma, and they may cause an irritative scoliosis or disk-like pain syndrome.

On radiographs, osteoblastomas appear as well-circumscribed lytic but occasionally blastic lesions usually considerably larger than the osteoid osteoma.[54] Instead of a thick reactive zone, the central sheets of osteoid tissue are usually surrounded by a thin periosteal shell of new reactive bone, which contains the lesion. Although usually benign in appearance and biological behavior, the lesions may be quite expansile and demonstrate cortical erosion and irregular margins, making the distinction from a low-grade malignant lesion difficult. Special studies such as the bone scan and computed tomogram help to better define the nature and extent of the lesion.

Histologically the findings are similar to the osteoid osteoma in that sheets of immature woven bone are seen, lying in a benign fibrovascular stroma.[4,55–57] The defined architectural characteristic of the osteoid osteoma is absent, which is sometimes helpful in distinguishing the two lesions. The principal cell, the osteoblast, shows no evidence of malignancy, which separates the lesion from its malignant counterpart, the osteosarcoma, or from an even rarer entity, the "aggressive osteoblastoma," which has a more malignant pattern on histologic and radiographic study and acts biologically as a low-grade sarcoma.[57–59]

Osteoblastomas tend to recur if inadequately resected so that most authorities advocate treatment by en bloc (marginal) excision of the lesion if this is possible without impairment of reasonable function.[20,57,58] Curettage and bone grafting is employed for less accessible lesions, recognizing that the recurrence rate will be higher than with complete excision. Radiotherapy is avoided because of the risk of subsequent radiation-induced sarcoma. Recurrent lesions must be viewed with caution to ensure that one is not dealing with either an "aggressive" osteoblastoma or an osteosarcoma, both of which will require wide local resections or occasionally amputative surgery to eliminate the lesion.

The malignant counterpart of the osseous tumors is the *osteosarcoma* (osteogenic sarcoma), which comprises a group of diseases varying somewhat in clinical presentation and aggressiveness (Table 20–3). Osteosarcoma is the most common primary malignant tumor of bone (excluding myeloma) and accounts for about 38% of malignant bone neoplasms[4]; of the group, the most frequent lesion (and the focus of this discussion) is the classic central osteosarcoma. This highly malignant tumor predominantly affects adolescents and is slightly more frequent in males than in females. A second peak incidence occurs in the fifth and sixth decades, probably relating to the occurrence of osteosarcoma in Paget's disease or in previously radiated bone.[4] (See Chapter 15.) The tumor is most commonly found in the metaphyseal regions of the distal femur, proximal tibia, proximal humerus, or proximal femur, although any bone may be involved. Rapid bone growth has been postulated as an etiologic factor in osteosarcoma because of the frequently metaphyseal location of the tumor (near growth centers in adolescents)[60] during or just after the growth spurt; and studies have suggested that the patients with osteosarcomas are significantly taller than their cohorts.

Table 20–3. Types of Osteosarcoma

Primary Osteosarcoma
Classic central osteosarcoma
Low-grade medullary osteosarcoma
Telangiectatic osteosarcoma
Multicentric osteosarcoma
Osteosarcoma in jaws
Secondary Osteosarcoma
Paget's disease
Postradiation
In other benign lesions
Juxtacortical Osteosarcoma
Parosteal osteosarcoma
Periosteal osteosarcoma

There are no specific clinical characteristics peculiar to osteosarcoma. Most patients complain of local pain and limp and may describe a traumatic episode that coincided with the onset of symptoms. Physical findings usually include local tenderness, the presence of a firm mass outside of but affixed to the involved bone, and some limitation of motion of the adjacent joint. Lesions near the knee may present with a joint effusion, and in advanced cases, a pathologic fracture may occur.[4,60] Laboratory tests are of limited value, although both the erythrocyte sedimentation rate and alkaline phosphatase may be elevated.

The radiographs of central osteosarcoma are often diagnostic. The tumors are large, centrally placed, most often metaphyseal, destructive or productive lesions demonstrating ill-defined internal margins and marked cortical destruction. A soft tissue mass is invariably present. Periosteal reaction in the form of a "Codman's triangle" or "sunburst" perpendicular striations may be evident. On occasion it may be difficult to distinguish the findings from those of a Ewing's sarcoma or even more rarely a benign or low-grade process such as a stress fracture, osteoblastoma, aneurysmal bone cyst, or giant cell

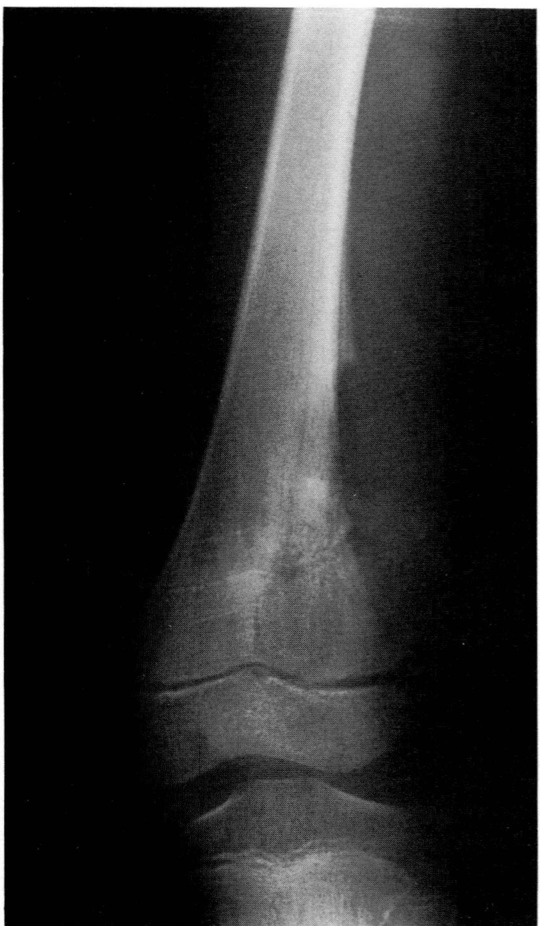

Figure 20–4. This 6-year-old boy has a destructive, eccentrically placed lesion of his distal femoral metaphysis. There is destruction of the lateral cortex with periosteal reaction (Codman's triangle) proximally. Blastic changes are visible within the bony lesion and in the large soft tissue mass that is characteristic of the ossification seen in osteosarcoma. The lesion does not appear to cross the growth plate.

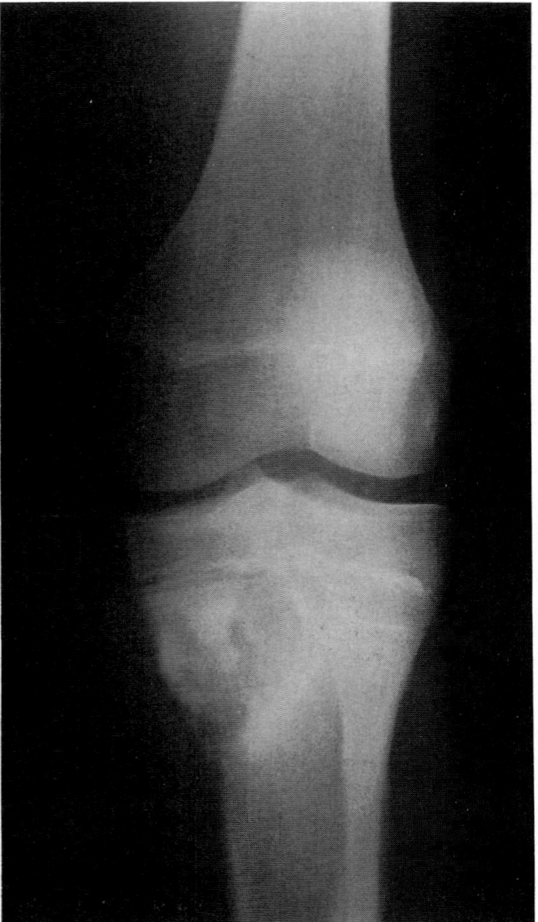

Figure 20–5. This AP radiograph of a 15-year-old boy shows a blastic, lytic lesion of the proximal tibial metaphysis. On casual inspection it appears fairly well delineated, and although evident by physical examination, a soft tissue mass is hard to distinguish on this radiograph.

tumor (Figs. 20–4 and 20–5). Special studies such as tomograms, bone scan, CT, angiograms, and magnetic resonance imaging (MRI) are helpful in making these distinctions as well as providing essential anatomic information relative to the staging of the lesion and to planning of surgical therapy (Figs. 20–6 and 20–7). All patients must have either full lung tomograms or computed tomograms of the lungs to search for pulmonary metastases, which are present in 10% to 20% of patients at the time of initial diagnosis.[61]

The gross pathology of classic osteosarcoma[4,62] parallels the radiographic findings in that there is replacement of the marrow cavity with malignant osseous or, at times, chondroid or fibrous tissue (Fig. 20–8). The tumor may extend for a considerable distance within the medullary cavity and even present "skip" metastases, remote from the primary lesion and with normal intervening marrow.[63] The tumor perforates and destroys the surrounding cortex and comes to lie as a contiguous soft tissue mass that extends along muscle planes and often into the adjacent joint along the capsule or cruciate ligaments.[64] Histologically the tumor consists of pleomorphic and anaplastic sarcoma cells with frequent bizarre forms showing considerable nuclear hyperchromatism and numerous normal and

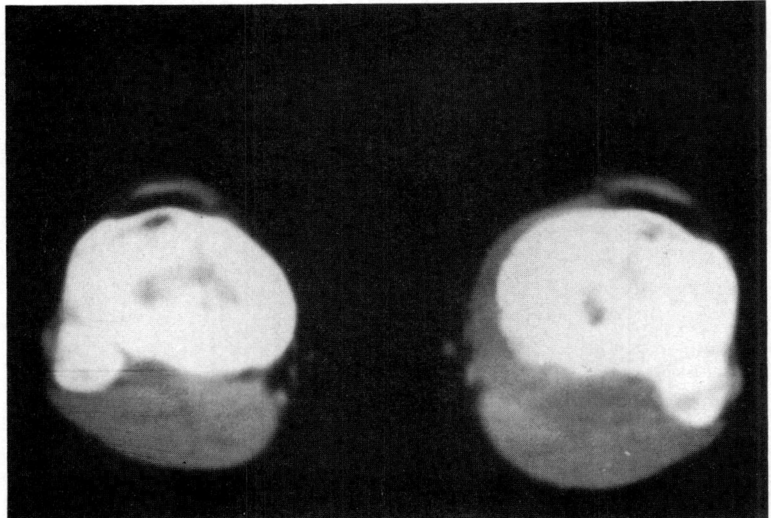

Figure 20–6. A computed tomogram of the lesion in Figure 20–5 shows a large, poorly mineralized soft tissue mass enveloping the anteromedial proximal tibia with extension behind the tibia toward the fibula. The distinction of the soft tissue mass is made easier by comparing the left tibia with the unaffected right side.

abnormal mitoses. The cells may be synthesizing cartilage or fibrous tissue, but to support the diagnosis of osteosarcoma, malignant osteoid production should be evident. Unlike myositis ossificans, osteosarcomas are usually more mature and mineralized centrally and more anaplastic and malignant-appearing peripherally so that the edge of the soft tissue mass is probably the most appropriate place to biopsy.[35]

The prognosis for patients with osteosarcoma is variable and depends on the location and size of the primary, the presence or absence of metastatic disease, and the pathologic subtype (variant) of osteosarcoma (Table 20–3). Classic osteosarcoma treated by amputation alone has a 15% to 30% 5-year disease-free survival in most historic reviews.[65–68] Proximal lesions fare less well than distal lesions, and larger lesions are associated with a worse prognosis than smaller lesions.[61] The presence of metastatic disease at time of discovery of

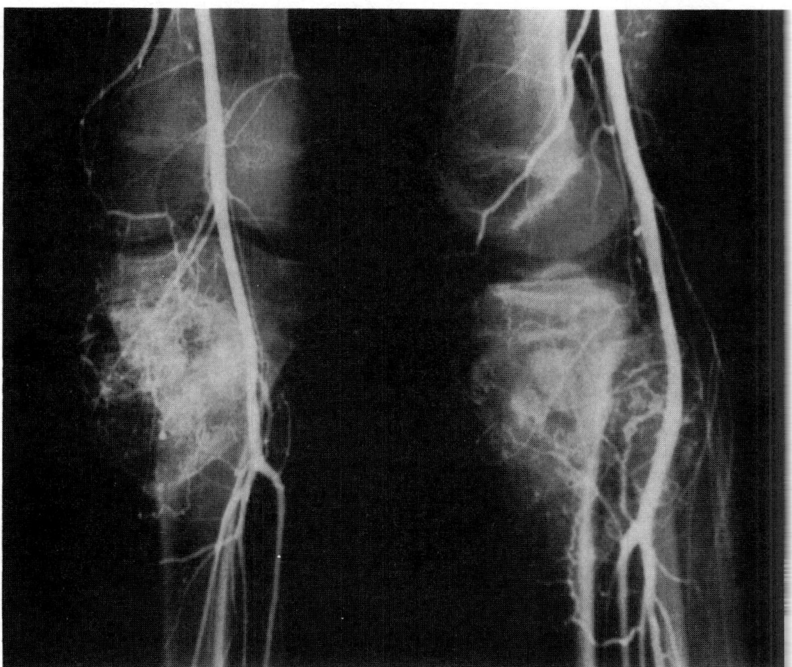

Figure 20–7. AP and lateral arteriographic views show the extent of the soft tissue mass, which displaces the popliteal vessel laterally and posteriorly, although there is no encasement of the vessel by tumor.

the primary is an ominous sign. Telangiectatic osteosarcomas, radiation-induced sarcomas, and sarcomas of Paget's disease carry a worse prognosis than classic osteosarcomas, whereas juxtacortical,[69–71] low-grade intramedullary, and osteosarcomas of the jawbone have a more favorable prognosis for survival.[68]

The current favored treatment of classic osteosarcoma involves two basic principles: surgical eradication of the primary tumor and treatment of putative micrometastatic deposits with systemic chemotherapy.[72] The primary tumor is most frequently managed by amputation following a thorough staging protocol as outlined previously. With modern prosthetic devices, this allows rapid restoration to functional activities of daily living and participation in some athletic activities, both of which are of major importance in decreasing the grief, anxiety, and psychological pain that accompany the loss of a limb (especially in the adolescent). Because of the development of improved methods of limb restoration in recent years, several treatment centers have performed limb-sparing operations in appropriate patients for whom adequate margins could be obtained while still preserving sufficient muscle and neurovascular structures to allow good function. Controversy remains as to whether preoperative treatment of the tumor with chemotherapy and/or radiotherapy prior to the resection improves the overall result and especially reduces the risk of local recurrence after limb-sparing surgery. To date, no studies have documented a superiority for preoperative treatment compared with resection followed by adjuvant chemotherapy with the same drugs. Reconstructions following limb-sparing surgery usually involve replacing the resected segment of bone and all or a portion of the adjacent joint with allograft bone transplants,[73] custom metallic prostheses,[18,74–78] or an arthrodesis using massive autograft[79] or allograft bone segments.[80,81] The ultimate functional outcome of these resections is as yet unknown, but they are obviously less durable than amputations, do not allow as much athletic freedom, and are associated with a much higher complication rate. The local recurrence rate following limb-sparing surgery is reported for some series to be as high as 30% and thus is of great concern, since the mortality rate for patients with a local recurrence is well over twice that of the group in which the tumor is eradicated.[45] In more recent studies from large tumor centers, however, the local recurrence rate

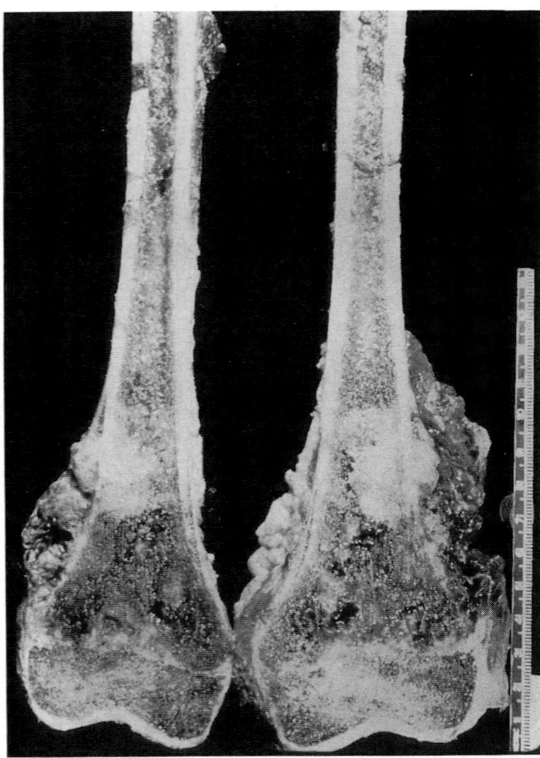

Figure 20–8. This gross specimen from a 10-year-old girl with osteosarcoma, treated by high above-knee amputation, shows replacement of the metaphysis and of the bone by tumor, which is destructive in some areas and densely mineralized in others. The periosteal elevation (Codman's triangle) is visible, but the response is insufficient to adequately contain the soft tissue mass. The proximal marrow cavity is free of tumor, but the tumor does cross the growth plate to enter the epiphysis of the bone.

does not appear to be significantly different in resected versus amputated patients (selected patients) as long as adjuvant chemotherapy is administered. Of considerable concern is the recent report of a poorer disease-free survival in all patients undergoing limb-sparing surgery (even those in whom no local recurrence is reported).[17] All of these findings have supported the concept that limb-sparing surgery be utilized for a selected population of osteosarcoma patients who meet strict tumor and psychological criteria.[82] The ultimate safety and efficacy of the procedure is as yet largely unknown.

A further area of controversy in the treatment of osteosarcoma is related to the role of adjuvant chemotherapy.[10,83,84] Early results employing agents such as high-dose methotrexate (HD-MTX) and doxorubicin (Adriamycin) were very encouraging compared with historic controls.[9,85] Most centers, employing a variety of chemotherapeutic protocols, report actuarial disease-free survival (DFS) results in the 50% to 60% range,[8,9,62,84–86] whereas one institution reported a projected disease-free survival of 80% to 90%.[87] Recently, however, the Mayo Clinic, in review of results in patients treated without chemotherapy, found that the survival rates had improved over time[88,89] with a recent analysis suggesting a 2-year disease-free survival and projections of 37.8% and survival rates of 56.5%, which is not statistically different from results for other centers employing routine adjuvant chemotherapy. In response to these somewhat iconoclastic and rather startling findings, a recent study was designed to randomly assess the worth of adjuvant chemotherapy, and preliminary results from this group strongly support the use of chemotherapy as an adjuvant in control of the disease.[11]

Pulmonary metastatic disease, when it occurs as a site of initial relapse, is managed in most treatment centers when possible by thoracotomy and wedge resection of the lung. Although pulmonary metastases remain an ominous sign, approximately 30% to 40% of patients initially made disease-free can be salvaged by wedge resection combined with chemotherapy if the lungs are the only site of recurrence.[37–44,90] These data support the need for close monitoring of osteosarcoma patients by serial chest radiographs and CT scans in order to provide an early detection system for metastatic disease.

B. Benign and Malignant Fibrous Lesions

Several different types of lesions are placed within the category of benign fibrous lesions (Table 20–1), but all (except the aneurysmal bone cyst and desmoplastic fibroma) are common lesions arising mainly in children, and their main import lies in distinguishing them from other, more aggressive lesions. The reader is referred to the major textbooks[4,5,19–24] for more complete details on the pathology of these lesions, but a brief description of the clinical and radiographic findings of these lesions will be presented.

The *fibrous cortical defect* and *nonossifying fibroma* are the most common of the benign fibrous lesions of bone, and most authorities suggest that they represent developmental defects rather than true neoplasms[22,24,91] in part based on their bland histologic appearance and also on their pattern of spontaneous disappearance with age. The two are histologically identical and differ mainly in size and location: the fibrous cortical defect occurring as a relatively small lesion in the metaphyseal cortex of a long bone of a young child, and the nonossifying fibroma being larger, occurring in older individuals and extending into the medullary cavity. Jaffe believed the latter represented a true neoplasm, whereas he considered the former a disturbance of growth,[22] and this view was supported by Caffey, who demonstrated the spontaneous disappearance of fibrous cortical defects with age in serial radiographic studies. The fibrous cortical defect probably begins as a defect of the growth plate[22,91] or fibrous periosteum.[92] The nonossifying fibroma may represent a true neoplasm arising from within the medullary cavity[22] or possibly occurs secondary to a developmental vascular disturbance[93] or intraosseous hemorrhage.[24] The distal femur is the most common site, followed by the proximal and distal tibia, proximal humerus, and distal radius and ulna.[91–93] On occasion, the lesions are multiple and must be distinguished from brown tumors of hyperparathyroidism. A normal serum calcium and the absence of diffuse osteopenia in multiple nonossifying fibromas aid in the distinction, but the histologic appearance may be quite similar to the brown tumor of hyperparathyroidism. The lesions occur mainly in the first and second decades of life and have been noted to appear in 42% of girls who had skeletal surveys in that age group.[92] The usual appearance for a fibrous cortical defect is a well demarcated, eccentrically placed metaphyseal radiolucent lesion often with slight cortical bulging, dense bony margination, and internal loculation (Fig. 20–9). The greatest dimension of the lesion is almost always aligned with the long axis of the bone. With growth, the lesions migrate away from the growth plate and eventually "fill in," with bone appearing in adult life as a dense cortical "scar."[93,94] Nonossifying fibromas are larger, less well demarcated, and commonly unloculated in appearance and extend into the medullary cavity of the bone.[22] The lesions usually cause no symptoms unless a pathologic fracture has occurred, although on occasion a large nonossifying fibroma may be painful for no apparent reason.

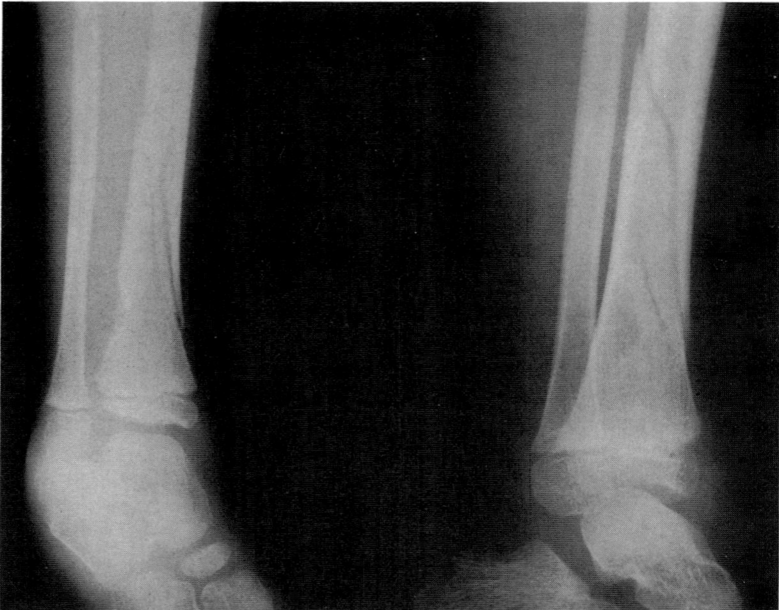

Figure 20–9. This 8-year-old boy had an asymptomatic fibrous cortical defect that was not recognized until he fell and sustained a pathologic fracture. The lesion itself is small, lytic, and well marginated by a rim of reactive bone. It has the characteristic appearance of fibrous cortical defect.

Spontaneous regression of these lesions is the rule, and a biopsy is usually not necessary for lesions that are of classic appearance on radiographs. Treatment by curettage and auto- or allograft packing is reserved for larger lesions that threaten the integrity of the bone, those that cannot be clearly diagnosed radiographically, or those that do not regress following pathologic fracture.[20,95] The occurrence of malignant degeneration is extremely rare; only a few case reports have appeared in the literature.[24] At times, the *periosteal desmoid* or *developmental defect of the distal femoral metaphysis,* a fibrous lesion occurring at the posteromedial aspect of the distal femur at the site of insertion of the adductor magnus,[96] may mimic a malignant tumor, but even in these cases an experienced bone radiologist can usually identify these as such and avoid a biopsy.

Fibrous dysplasia is a disorder of the skeleton in which the medullary cavity of parts of one, several, or, at times, many bones is replaced by a peculiar fibro-osseous tissue. Although often discussed along with neoplasms of bone, it is probably a developmental defect of bone-forming mesenchyme.[22,97,98] The exact cause is unknown, but there is no evidence for hereditary transmission of the syndrome. The disease, particularly when florid, is usually detected in childhood, but small solitary lesions may go unrecognized until even late adulthood.[97,98] The bony lesions occur mainly in the metaphysis and diaphysis of the long bones, but the process may extend from one end of the bone to the other. It typically appears on radiographs as a lytic, "ground-glass" textured lesion, associated with thinning of the cortex and expansion of the width of the bone (Fig. 20–10). Endosteal scalloping is frequently seen, and pathologic fractures and resultant deformities of the bones such as the "shepherd's crook" of the proximal femur may be observed. Tiny purposeless trabeculae are seen within the lesion.[97] The femur, tibia, ribs, and facial bones are the most frequent sites affected, and although any bone may be involved, spinal lesions are rare.[22,24] Skull changes include thickening of the occiput, obliteration of the sphenoid and frontal sinuses,[99] and occasionally a peculiar increase in density of one half of the skull or hemihypertrophy cranii. Displacement of the orbits inferiorly and laterally and geographic lytic bone lesions are also seen.

Three forms of the disease are recognized: a monostotic form, a polyostotic form, and Albright's disease. The monostotic form[100] is usually recognized in the second and third decades and is equally distributed between the sexes. The lesion may go unnoticed until pathologic fracture occurs, or at times a clinical deformity calls attention to the lesion.

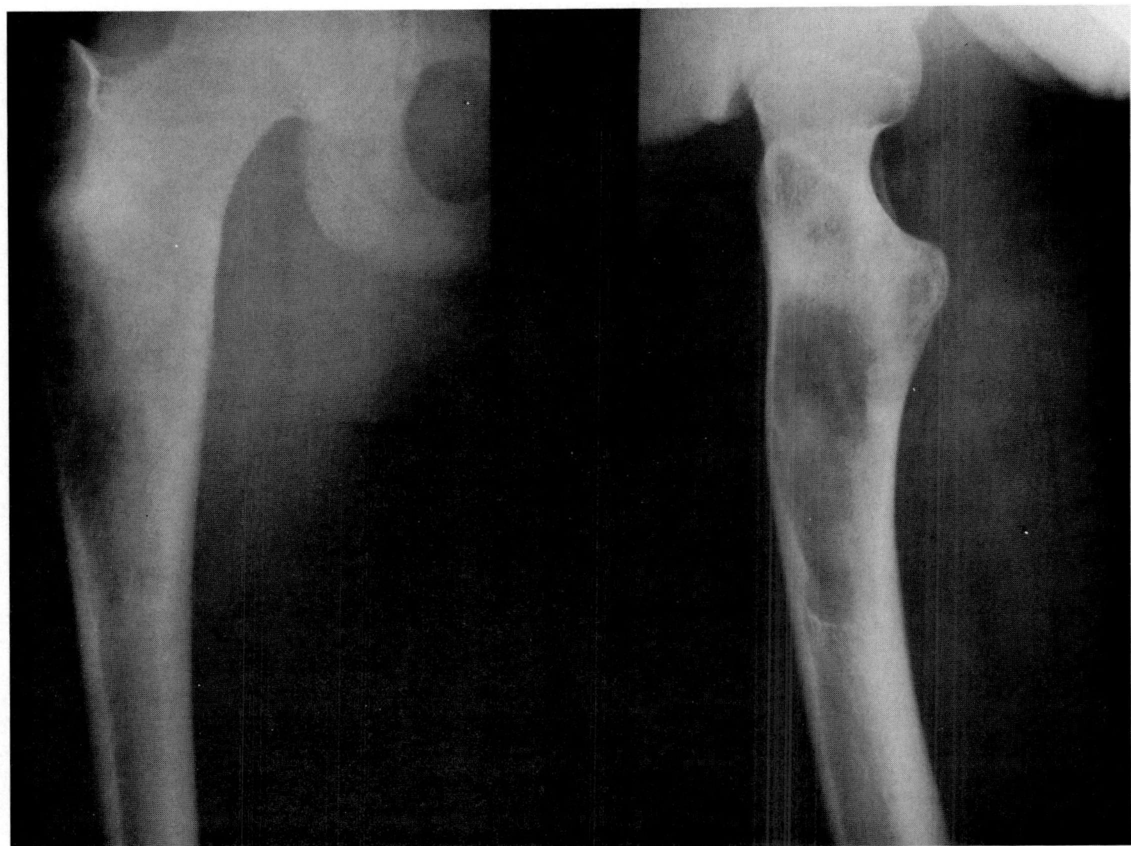

Figure 20–10. This 17-year-old patient had a large, lytic lesion of the proximal femur. Areas of lysis intermix with other areas that appear "ground glass." The cortex is thinned, and the bone is slightly expanded. These findings are consistent with monostotic fibrous dysplasia.

Pain is usually not present in the absence of fracture. Cranial lesions may cause hearing or visual loss.[101] There is some evidence that the monostotic lesions may stabilize with age as a result of increasing sclerosis at the margins of the lesions,[97,98] but the disease does not spontaneously disappear, nor does increased activity on bone scan lessen with advancing years. Skin lesions are not often associated with this form of the disease.

The polyostotic form is usually noted at a younger age because of more severe involvement of the skeleton[99] and is more prevalent in females.[97] The age at diagnosis, presentation, and clinical course are extremely variable.[99] Lesions may be distributed within one extremity (monomelic) or throughout the body. Pathologic fractures, limb deformities (bowing, malunited fractures), and inequalities in extremity length are common. Craniofacial involvement occurs in about half of the patients. Although lesions may increase in size, it is unusual for new lesions to arise in areas that were previously normal. Puberty does not seem to favorably affect the incidence of pathologic fracture, the occurrence of new lesions, or the regression of existing bony lesions in polyostotic fibrous dysplasia.[99] Characteristic skin lesions (café-au-lait spots) are often distributed in relation to the bony lesions. These are lightly pigmented macules with irregular borders (coast of Maine), in distinction from the smoother bordered skin lesions of neurofibromatosis (coast of California). Albright's syndrome[102] consists of the triad of polyostotic fibrous dysplasia, multiple café-au-lait spots, and primarily an extraordinary gonadal abnormality characterized by precocious puberty. Although precocious puberty is the most common endocrine disorder, others have been described including acromegaly, hyperthyroidism, vitamin D–resistant rickets, and Cushing's syndrome.[97,103] Sexual precocity is much less commonly observed in male patients.[98,104] Short stature due to premature closure of the growth plates occurs, as well as the other bony sequelae of polyostotic disease.

The differential diagnosis of polyostotic fibrous dysplasia includes hyperparathyroidism with brown tumors, neurofibromatosis, multiple enchondromatoses (Ollier's disease), and metastasis. The radiographs are usually sufficient for distinction, but laboratory values such as serum calcium, phosphorus, alkaline phosphatase, and parathormone levels may be helpful. The histologic picture in fibrous dysplasia is usually characteristic and consists of a fibrous stroma containing wisps of purposeless tiny trabeculae of woven bone, without osteoblastic rimming. Occasionally areas of cystic change or cartilage metaplasia are seen.[97,99] Repeated biopsies show no evidence of maturation of the woven bone trabeculae over time.[99]

Treatment consists of stabilizing fractures and of preventing or correcting deformities.[97,99] Monostotic lesions may require biopsy to confirm the diagnosis and internal fixation or bone grafting to prevent pathologic fracture, whereas the diagnosis is usually evident by radiographic appearance alone in the polyostotic form. Fractures usually heal well by closed treatment, although open reduction and internal fixation may be necessary. Limb length inequalities require careful assessment and epiphyseodesis or other corrective procedures at the appropriate time. Osteotomies of the proximal femur or tibia may be necessary to correct the shepherd's crook deformities and tibial bowing, and this is usually augmented with internal fixation and bone grafting (autograft or allograft). Our preference is to employ allograft bone, at times using large cortical struts, to lessen the chances of resorption of the graft by the fibrous dysplastic process and to provide structural support for large lesions in weight-bearing sites. Malignant degeneration to a fibrosarcoma, osteosarcoma, or chondrosarcoma is extremely rare but has been reported, usually following radiation of one of the bony lesions.[105] For this reason as well as the fact that it does not appear to be very effective in controlling the disease, radiotherapy has no role in the treatment of the skeletal involvement.[97]

Two lesions of bone, the *unicameral or simple bone cyst* and the *aneurysmal bone cyst*, are probably misnomers, because neither is a true cyst, although they do present as well-demarcated, fluid-filled lytic lesions of bone. The *unicameral bone cyst* is a common lesion of childhood, usually presenting in patients of the first and second decades with open growth plates. The cause is unclear, but is presumed to be either a disorder of the physis[4] or a transient circulatory compromise resulting from venous anomalies of the affected bone.[94,106] In children the cysts abut the growth plate in the metaphysis of the long bones and predilect the proximal humerus (55%) and proximal femur (26%).[106] They are seen to "grow away" from the physis as the child grows, and eventually at least some of the lesions fill in spontaneously. In adults the lesions are more commonly seen in the calcaneus and flat bones (especially the pelvis). Symptoms are usually not present unless a pathologic fracture occurs, or they may be discovered serendipitously. Radiographs reveal a well-delineated lytic lesion that is never wider than the growth plate (Fig. 20–11*A*). The cortex is thinned but intact, and there may be thin incomplete septae within the cyst, especially if there has been a previous pathologic fracture. Aspiration of the cyst reveals a clear fluid that is chemically similar to serum or extracellular fluid, unless it is bloody because of recent fracture.[106] The lesions do not require treatment unless a pathologic fracture has occurred or is considered to be highly likely on the basis of thinning of the cortex. It is best to observe the cysts for a time following fracture because a small percentage of them will heal following such an event.[107] The occurrence of malignancy in a preexisting cyst is distinctly unusual.[108] Treatment methods have included curettage and bone grafting,[106,109] subtotal resection with or without bone grafting,[110,111] or, more recently, injecting the cysts with methylprednisolone acetate.[112–114] The two surgical treatments are associated with a substantial recurrence rate, and the last is a formidable procedure for a benign lesion. Neither should be performed until the growth plate has laid down a zone of normal bone between the plate and the cyst (the so-called latent cyst). Injecting the cyst with methylprednisolone appears to be quite successful, although the mechanism by which this treatment acts is not clear (Figs. 20–11*B*, *C*). Repeated injections may be necessary to achieve the reported success rates of greater than 80%.[112]

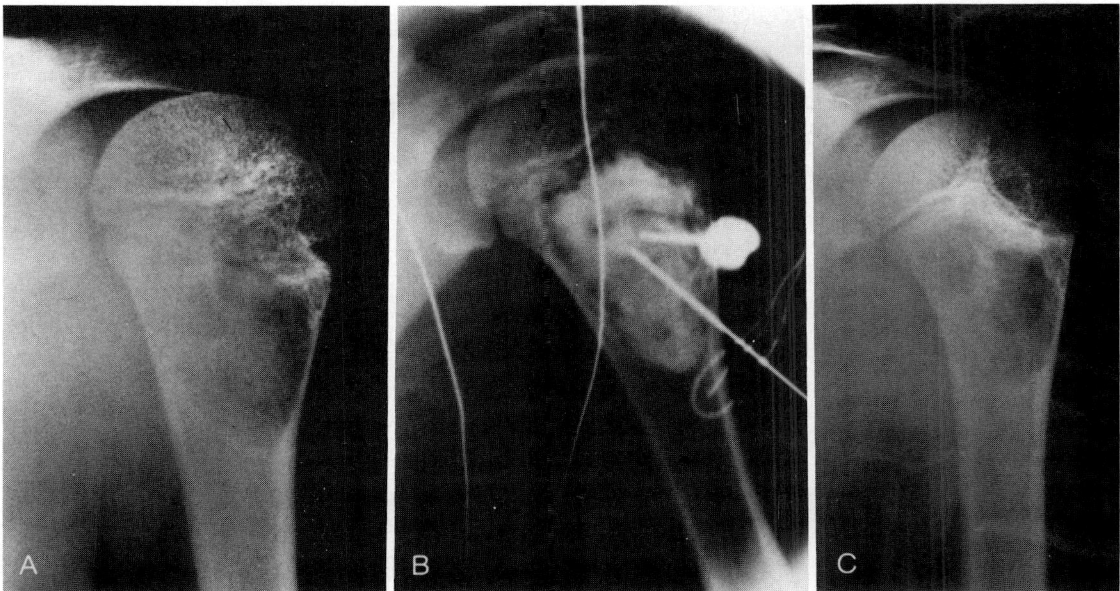

Figure 20–11. *A*, Typical appearance of a unicameral bone cyst of the proximal humerus. The lesion is juxtaposed to the growth plate and is lytic, is well marginated, and thins the lateral cortex. There is containment of the lesion by periosteum, and although the lesion widens the metaphysis, it is not wider than the width of the growth plate. *B*, The cyst was aspirated and clear fluid was recovered. Contrast material was instilled to document the presence of a cystic cavity prior to steroid injection. *C*, Three months after injection, the cyst is filling in, but as yet the process is incomplete.

The *aneurysmal bone cyst* is another lesion of unknown cause occurring in patients usually less than 20 years of age. It predilects the long bones and spine.[115,116] Pain and swelling are noted occasionally following a traumatic event, and radiographs reveal an eccentrically placed, expansible lesion that is purely lytic and trabeculated, appearing as a "blow-out" of the cortical surface. The cysts may appear quite aggressive and mimic a giant cell tumor of telangiectatic osteosarcoma, but close inspection will invariably reveal intact periosteal bone surrounding the lesion.[116,117] Pathologically they are composed of spongy, anastomosing cavernous spaces filled with unclotted blood that lack a true endothelium.[4] Despite the name of the lesion and the extraordinary bleeding that occurs with biopsy or curettage of the lesion, aneurysmal bone cysts appear relatively hypovascular on angiograms. There is considerable debate among pathologists regarding the true nature of the aneurysmal bone cyst: some feel it is a distinct entity (primary aneurysmal bone cyst), and others feel it almost always represents a vascular degenerative process superimposed on another underlying lesion such as fibrous dysplasia, giant cell tumor, or chondroblastoma.[4,116,117] Treatment is by curettage and grafting or marginal resection depending on the location of the cyst.[116–118]

Malignant fibroblastic tumors include the *fibrosarcoma* and the *malignant fibrous histiocytoma of bone*. Both of these pathologic entities are rare in bone in contrast with similarly named and histologically identical tumors of soft tissue; the fibrosarcomas account for less than 4% of the malignant bone lesions in the Mayo Clinic series.[4] *Fibrosarcoma of bone*[24] most often presents as a central, destructive lesion of long bones, with a distribution similar to osteosarcoma.[22,119] All age groups are affected, but fibrosarcomas occur most commonly in patients in their fourth to seventh decades of life.[22,24,120] Secondary fibrosarcomas may arise in patients in whom the bony site has been affected by Paget's disease, fibrous dysplasia, chronic osteomyelitis, giant cell tumor of bone, or bone infarcts or has been previously subjected to irradiation.[24,120,121] Because they are somewhat more slow-growing than osteosarcomas, symptoms may be present for several months before the diagnosis is made, and it is not unusual for patients to present with pathologic fractures.[24,120] Radiographs show a purely lytic, destructive lesion of the central metaphyseal region of the bone associated with cortical destruction and a soft tissue mass. The lack of production of a mineralized matrix makes it difficult to distinguish fibrosarcomas from other malignant lesions that occur in the older age groups, such as lymphoma, myeloma, and metastatic disease. Low-grade lesions may be difficult to distinguish from giant cell tumor of bone or desmoplastic fibroma.[122]

Histologically these lesions are composed of malignant fibroblastic stromal cells interspersed with variable amounts of collagen fibers. They vary from low to high grade[22,119] but do not show evidence of malignant bone or cartilage production as seen in osteosarcomas or chondrosarcomas.[22]

Treatment is by wide or radical resection or amputation depending on the stage of the lesion.[20] Radiotherapy and adjuvant chemotherapy appear to be of little value, although these modalities may be employed for palliation or advanced (metastatic) disease.[20] Five-year survival rates vary from 28%[119,120] to 34%.[123,124]

The *malignant fibrous histiocytoma of bone (MFH)* is a recently recognized variant that is distinguished from fibrosarcoma pathologically by its storiform or radiating pattern of malignant fibroblast-like cells and the presence of large, bizarre, sometimes multinucleated cells with grooved nuclei, prominent nucleoli, and an acidophilic cytoplasm thought to be malignant histiocytes.[21,125] The clinical and radiographic presentation is similar to that of fibrosarcoma,[124] but unlike other sarcomas of bone, the MFH has a higher incidence of lymph node metastases.[126] Treatment is similar to that discussed for osteosarcoma, with the possible addition of radiotherapy to the regional lymph nodes. Systemic adjuvant chemotherapy appears to be of value.[127–129]

C. Benign and Malignant Cartilage Tumors

Perhaps the most difficult and perplexing groups of lesions that affect the skeleton are the cartilage tumors. As might be expected from an understanding of the various roles that cartilage plays in the development of the skeleton, a rather large array of clinicopathologically distinct cartilage tumors compose the group, and each has its own pattern of presentation, appearance, and biological behavior. Furthermore, particularly for the hyaline group, the distinction between benign and malignant lesions is often extremely difficult to make, and with the malignant group, deciding whether a lesion is low grade (and unlikely to metastasize) or high grade is extraordinarily taxing. Some of the cartilage lesions are thought to be "premalignant" in that there appears to be a high propensity for the development of malignant chondrosarcomas over time, but it is still unclear whether the benign lesions actually undergo malignant degeneration or whether malignant lesions arise from a separate adjacent clone of cells distinct from the benign lesions.[130]

In dealing with cartilage tumors, several axioms are helpful in assessing the potential of a tumor to be malignant. These include:

1. The larger the tumor and the more proximally located the lesion, the most likely it is to be malignant. Conversely, small lesions in distal sites are less likely to be (or become) malignant.[20]
2. Chondrosarcomas are rare under the age of 30 years.
3. Chondrosarcomas of the hands and feet are extremely rare, and most cartilage tumors of these sites are benign.
4. Patients with multiple lesions (such as hereditary multiple osteocartilaginous exostosis and enchondromatosis) are more likely to develop malignancies than are patients with solitary benign lesions.
5. Regardless of all of the above, a patient with continued pain in relation to a cartilage tumor should be fully evaluated for the possibility of a chondrosarcoma.

Evaluation of patients with suspected cartilage tumors frequently requires a "full-scale" workup including bone scans, computed tomographic evaluations, arteriograms, and histologic determinations and flow cytometric studies[26,27] of the biopsy material to arrive at a correct diagnosis. There is some evidence that MRI may be of particular value in assessing the biological nature of the cartilage tumors[131] because of variations in the biochemistry of the lesions with advancing grade.[132,133]

The *benign cartilage tumors* can be divided into enostotic and exostotic lesions. The enostotic lesions include the enchondroma, the chondroblastoma, and the chondromyxoid fibroma; the exostotic lesions are the osteocartilaginous exostosis and the juxtacortical chondroma.[20] The *enchondroma* is a benign central

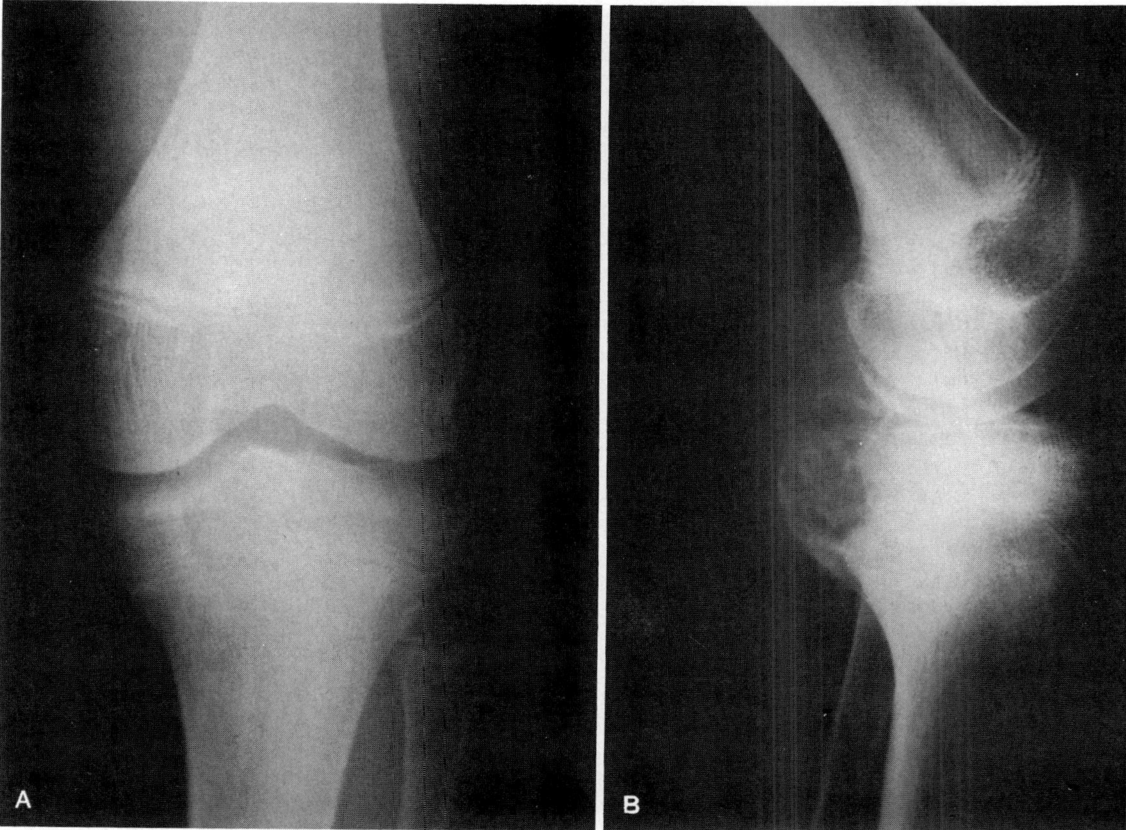

Figure 20–12. *A* and *B*, AP and lateral radiographs of the knee in a 14-year-old with pain. There is a lytic lesion of the epiphysis containing stippled calcifications. The periosteal shell is intact.

lesion of hyaline cartilage occurring in the medullary cavity of long and short tubular bones and flat bones[4,5,20] and is the most common bone tumor of the hand.[4] Enchondromas may be discovered at any age but are usually asymptomatic and not detected until adulthood when they are either noted as incidental findings or less commonly result in a pathologic fracture. As indicated, the differentiation of this lesion from chondrosarcoma is difficult, and a history of increasing size or persistent pain should be viewed with suspicion. On radiographs, enchondromas appear as lucent, centrally placed lesions located in the metaphysis or diaphysis of the bone. There may be thinning of the cortex and poor margination in some areas, but marked endosteal scalloping, cortical destruction, or extension into the soft tissues is not present. Areas of rounded or stippled calcifications are usually present in adults. The lesions usually show increased activity on bone scans.[20] Pathologically they are composed of nodules of benign hyaline cartilage that are usually surrounded by a thin rim of reactive bone.[4,20,134]

The major therapeutic challenge for the management of an enchondroma is usually establishing that one is dealing with a benign lesion. They may be observed if they are causing no symptoms or deformity and if the weakening of the bony structure does not increase the risk of pathologic fracture. Treatment by curettage, phenolization of the cavity, and bone grafting is sometimes necessary and usually results in complete eradication of the lesion.[20]

Multiple enchondromatosis (Ollier's and Mafucci's syndrome)[135,136] is an uncommon disorder in which multiple benign cartilage tumors are widely dispersed through the skeleton. The disease is usually noted in childhood and may be more severe on one side of the body. Commonly gross distortion of the extremities or hands is observed, and the aim

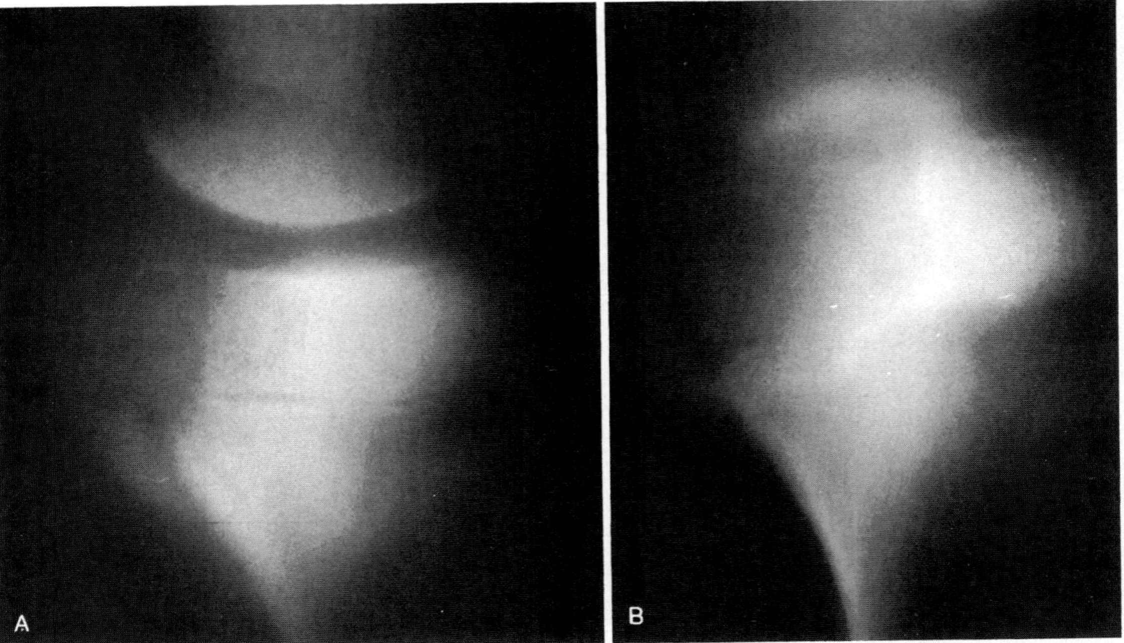

Figure 20–13. *A* and *B*, The lateral tomographic cuts show the extent of the lesion more clearly. It has destroyed the subchondral bone plate and crossed the physis to involve the proximal tibial metaphysis.

of early management during childhood is correcting or preventing deformities. In later life the chief concern is that of development of a chondrosarcoma, and careful observation for change in symptoms, size, or character of the lesions is mandatory throughout their lifetime.[20,130,134]

The *chondroblastoma* is of special interest to those dealing with joint disease because of its predilection for the epiphyseal ends of long bones. It is a rare lesion of cartilage most frequently encountered in adolescent males with open growth plates and is most often located in the proximal and distal femur, proximal humerus, and proximal tibia.[137–139] Symptoms include localized pain, tenderness, swelling and limitation of range of motion of the associated joint, and often an effusion.[139] On radiographs, the chondroblastoma appears as a round to oval lucency usually within an epiphysis and characteristically containing stippled calcifications (Figs. 20–12*A, B*). The tumors usually show sclerotic margins and rarely any cortical destruction, although distortion of the joint contour may be present (Figs. 20–13*A, B*). In adults the lesions may be found in areas of the bones other than the epiphysis and are sometimes more aggressive in behavior. Histologically the lesion is composed of sheets of polygonal cells believed to be chondroblasts, which are surrounded in areas by a reticulin matrix that may mineralize. There are scattered multinucleated giant cells and areas of chondroid matrix.[4,24] Treatment is by curettage and bone grafting,[140] a procedure that is often difficult because of the location of the lesion between the articular cartilage and growth plate. The recurrence rate is approximately 25%,[20,137] and in rare instances there may be spread of the tumor to the lungs.[137,141,142]

The *chondromyxoid fibroma* will be only briefly mentioned because it is extremely rare. It is a benign lesion occurring in the metaphyseal region of the long bones and occasionally the pelvis[143–145] that predilects individuals in the second decade. The femur and tibia are the most common sites. It may be difficult to distinguish from a nonossifying fibroma, but unlike the latter, it often expands through the cortex of the bone, producing a periosteal shell of reactive bone in the adjacent soft tissues. The recurrence rate, approximately 40% following curettage, is higher than any of the other benign cartilage tumors, and at times marginal excision is more appropriate.[145]

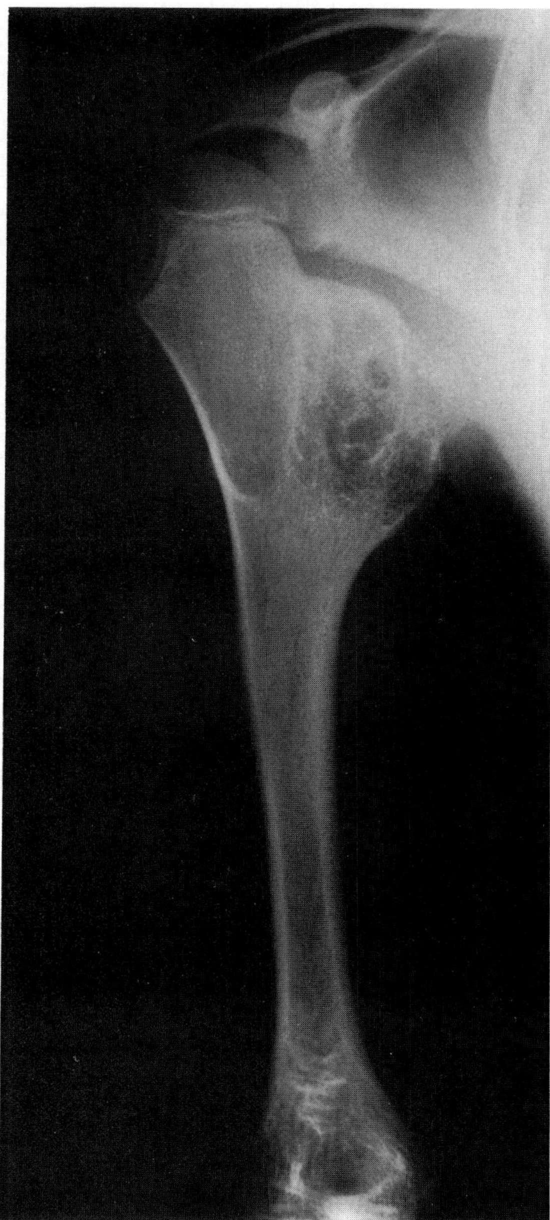

Figure 20–14. This radiograph of the humerus of a 10-year-old boy shows a large, sessile, solitary osteochondroma that wrapped nearly 180 degrees around the bone. It is important to note that the cortex of the lesion is continuous with that of the host bone and that the medullary cavities communicate.

Although probably not a true neoplasm, the *solitary osteocartilaginous exostosis* is a very frequently encountered lesion of the skeletal system. It probably arises from a genetic defect in the embryonic cartilage anlage,[146] or the restraining periosteum and ring of Ranvier.[22] Similar lesions may be induced by irradiation of the immature skeleton.[24,147–149] Osteocartilaginous exostoses appear as sessile or pedunculated outgrowths from the metaphyseal ends of the bone, which usually appear to be growing from the joint. They may occur in any bone that is embryonically preformed in cartilage, although the long bone sites predominate. Detection often does not occur until the second decade because the lesions are asymptomatic unless they fracture through a narrowed stalk, entrap or press on an adjacent nerve, or cause a painful bursa. The lesions are almost always readily diagnosed on routine radiographs (Fig. 20–14), but one should carefully distinguish them from more aggressive juxtacortical lesions (such as the parosteal osteosarcoma) by the finding that for the exostoses, the bony cortices of the host bone and the lesion are continuous and their marrow cavities communicate (not so for the others, which appear to be engrafted on the underlying cortex). The pathologic tissue is at the tip or cap of the bony excrescence and appears histologically as a disordered growth plate of varying thickness.[22] The lesion grows by endochondral ossification and, like the true growth plate, usually ceases to do so at maturity. Continued or renewed growth is a worrisome sign, but malignant degeneration of a solitary osteocartilaginous exostosis is extremely rare (much less than 0.1%).[20–22] If needed for relief of symptoms, they may be removed at their base with care to remove the entire cartilaginous cap and perichondrium.[20] Recurrence is unusual.[22,150]

Hereditary multiple osteocartilaginous exostosis (diaphyseal aclasis) is a genetic disorder, transmitted as an autosomal dominant trait characterized by multiple exostotic lesions that cause distortion of the skeleton and a variable degree of functional impairment.[20,22,151] Treatment is directed toward preventing or correcting the associated bony deformities such as short stature, bowing or knock-knee deformities of the lower extremity, and ulnar club hand.[151–154] Unlike the solitary form, this syndrome is associated with an increased incidence of malignant degeneration, and patients must be followed carefully for changes in size, symptoms, or increased radionuclide activity on bone scans of any of the lesions.[20]

The neoplasms that compose the category of the *chondrosarcomas* vary widely in their clinicopathologic presentation and biological behavior. For this reason they are perhaps the most difficult of bone lesions to manage. Chondrosarcomas may be central or peripheral and are further classified into primary and secondary (to enchondromas or osteochondromas) groups. In addition, there are the rarer chondrosarcoma variants such as the mesenchymal chondrosarcoma,[155–158] the dedifferentiated chondrosarcoma,[159–161] and the clear cell chondrosarcoma,[162] which are so infrequently encountered that they will not be included in the review.

Primary chondrosarcoma is a malignant neoplasm of hyaline cartilage that occurs most frequently as an enostotic lesion in individuals in the third to sixth decades of life.[5,20,163–166] The tumors are rare, accounting for approximately 10% to 12% of all malignant bone tumors.[4,24] They may arise in any bone preformed in cartilage but have a predilection for the more proximal portions of the skeleton such as the proximal femur and humerus, pelvis, and scapula.[4,24] The patient often complains of dull, aching pain or may note a slowly enlarging mass, but the lesion, especially if located in the pelvis, may grow to a large size before it is detected. Pathologic fracture is rare, but adjacent neuromuscular structures may be compressed by the lobular soft tissue mass that often extends from the lesion. The staging procedure for chondrosarcomas is as outlined in the previous section and should include a bone scan to exclude lesions in other sites and to assess the extent of the primary neoplasm, a CT scan or MRI and arteriogram to evaluate the soft tissue extent in relation to adjacent vital structures, and a chest radiograph and tomographic study to exclude metastatic disease.[167] The principles of the biopsy are particularly crucial in chondrosarcomas because tumor "spill" can easily lead to recurrent soft tissue implants. It is important not to violate normal tissue planes and adjacent neurovascular structures and to avoid entering the bone if possible. If it is necessary to enter the bone to obtain diagnostic tissue, such bony defects should be plugged with methylmethacrylate to prevent further tumor spill and hematoma.[167]

The radiographic appearance of enostotic chondrosarcoms is that of a large, central metadiaphyseal lesion with scalloping and erosion of the cortex from within and often a marked periosteal response giving the cortex a thickened, expanded appearance in lower grade lesions (Figs. 20–15 and 20–19). The more aggressive lesions show evidence of cortical destruction and transgression with an associated lobular soft tissue mass. There may be a variable amount of calcification arranged in ringlike structures or amorphous masses within the lesion and the soft tissue mass. The extent of the lesion is determined by CT, bone scans, and arteriograms (Figs. 20–16, 20–17, and 20–20).

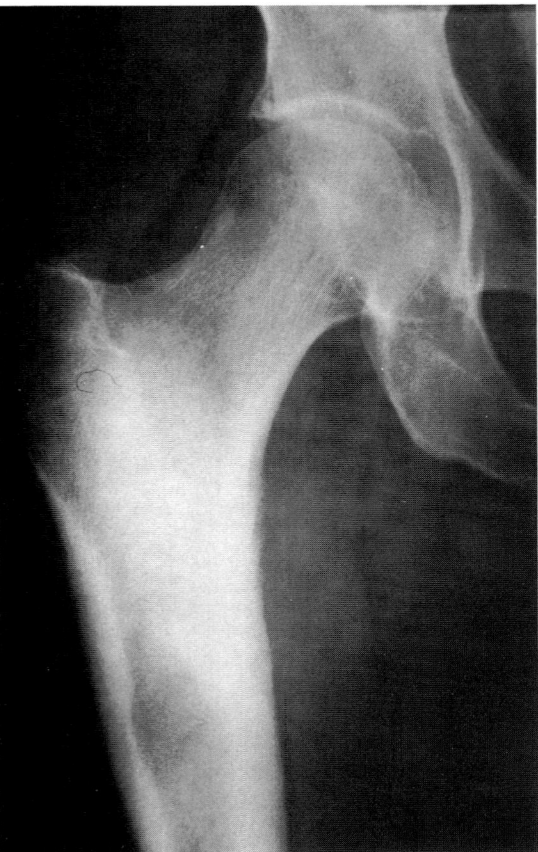

Figure 20–15. This AP hip radiograph shows a lesion of the proximal femur that is lytic and scallops the lateral cortex from within. The thickened cortex and reactive medullary bone surrounding the lesion is evidence of relatively slow growth. A biopsy showed that this was a chondrosarcoma, grade 2/3.

Exostotic lesions are not as common as the central lesions and may occur in a slightly younger age group.[24] They appear to arise from a preexisting osteochondroma usually in the proximal femur, humerus, or pelvis,[5,165] although this relationship to their benign counterparts is extremely difficult to document. The lesions occur with greater frequency in patients with hereditary multiple osteocartilaginous exostoses, and although

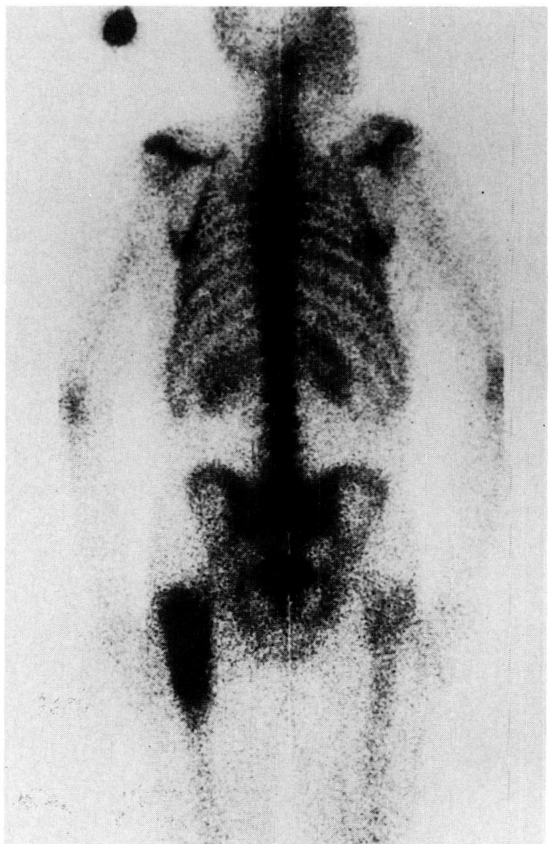

Figure 20–16. A radionuclide bone scan shows increased uptake of tracer in the lesion without evidence of other lesions.

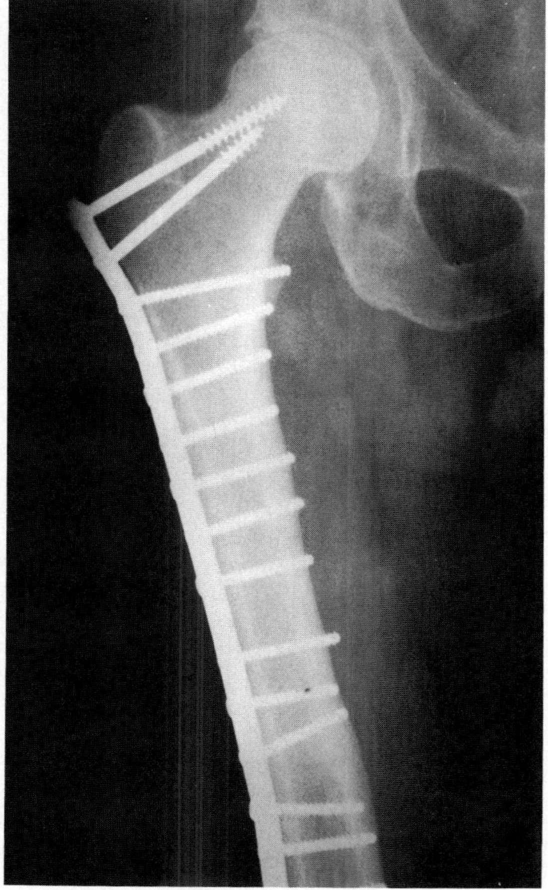

Figure 20–18. Postoperative radiograph two years after wide resection and allograft bone replacement of the proximal femur. The host-donor osteosynthesis site has healed, and although there is some narrowing of the joint space, he has no pain and is ambulating well.

malignant degeneration of a solitary exostosis is extremely rare (less than 0.1%), estimates of malignant degeneration in the disseminated genetic form of the disease have ranged from 10% to 28%.[4,24] It should be stressed that these figures are tentative, but they do indicate that patients with the multiple form require close observation in the adult years.

The pathologic details of the central and exostotic chondrosarcomas are similar and will not be stressed; rather, they are well described in several excellent reviews.[5,20,163–166] Grossly they appear as large translucent nodules of malignant cartilage that on histologic examination are composed of hyaline or myxoid cartilaginous tissue. The evidence of malignancy is not as striking as in the other

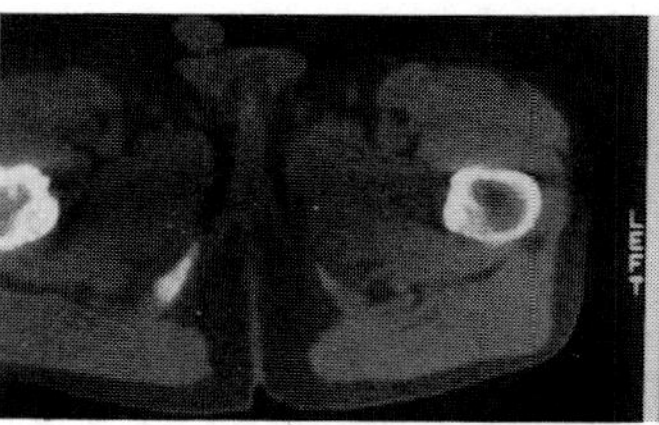

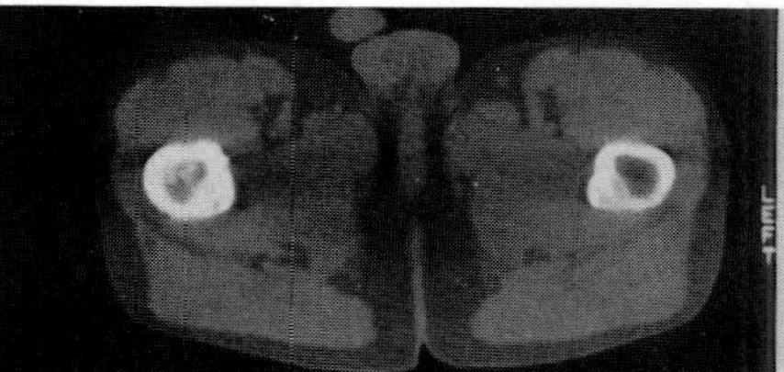

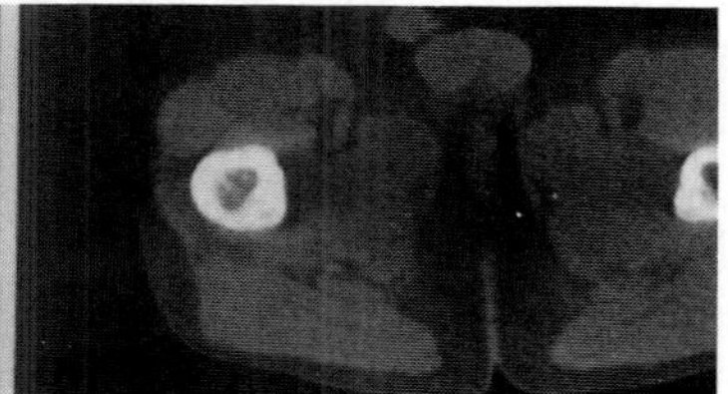

Figure 20–17. A computed tomogram demonstrates the increased density of the partially mineralized chondrosarcoma, which has replaced the normal medullary cavity. There is no appreciable soft tissue mass.

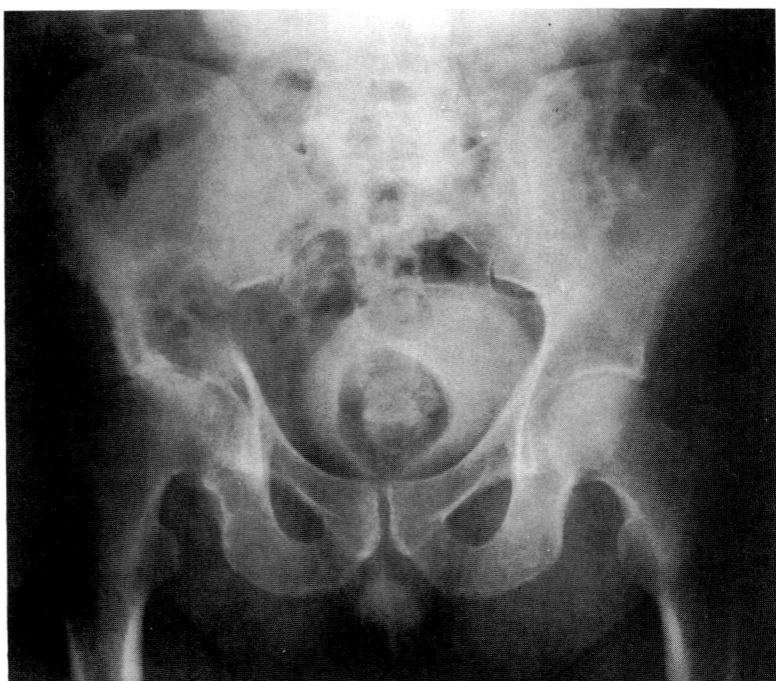

Figure 20–19. AP radiograph of the pelvis in a 67-year-old man with grade 3/3 chondrosarcoma of the right supra-acetabular region. It has destroyed the medial wall of the ilium and there is a protrusio acetabuli.

bone sarcomas, but they may be graded (low, medium, high) based on the cellularity, pleomorphism, and mitotic rate seen on histologic sections. Recently our laboratory has examined biochemical parameters in an attempt to grade these lesions and has found that malignant cartilage contains an unusual concentration of nonstructural protein and that the higher grade lesions have a greater concentration of water.[132,133] This latter finding has been confirmed by NMR spectrometric analysis of chondrosarcomas[131] and indicates that MRI may be of value in grading these lesions noninvasively. In general there are no major differences in the biochemical composition of malignant cartilage compared with normal, but analytical studies appear to support a more immature form in that the water content is higher and the proteoglycan subunits are deficient in keratan sulfate.[132,168] Additional studies from our laboratory have demonstrated that flow cytometric analysis of DNA patterns after incubation with propidium iodide is of considerable value as an adjunct in assessing the grade of the lesions.[27]

The treatment of chondrosarcoma is primarily surgical. Resection of the lesion should be with a wide margin, and several studies have indicated that the adequacy of the margin correlates clearly with the ultimate patient outcome.[164,166,167] Low-grade and certain accessible high-grade chondrosarcomas may be effectively treated by limb-sparing procedures, but it is obviously essential that tumor-free margins be obtained. Reconstruction may be achieved with a metallic implant, allograft bone segment,[73] or arthrodesis depending on the site of the primary lesion, the nature of the lesion, and the preference of the patient and surgeon (Figs. 20–18 and 20–21). Large, high-grade lesions often require ablative operations to adequately remove the tumor. Standard radiation therapy is thought to be of limited value for chondrosarcoma, but recent reports have supported improved control of surgically inaccessible lesions (such as in the spine and cranium) with proton beam. Similarly, as could be logically predicted by the low DNA synthetic rate for many of these lesions,[132,169] chemotherapy appears to be of limited value in the management of patients with chondrosarcoma, although it is often advocated for high-grade or metastatic lesions. In all, the survival rates for chondrosarcoma are better than for osteosarcoma (5-year, 59%–67%; 10-year, 46%–50%)[164,166] but vary considerably with the grade of the lesion. Ten-year survival figures for grades 1, 2, and 3 have

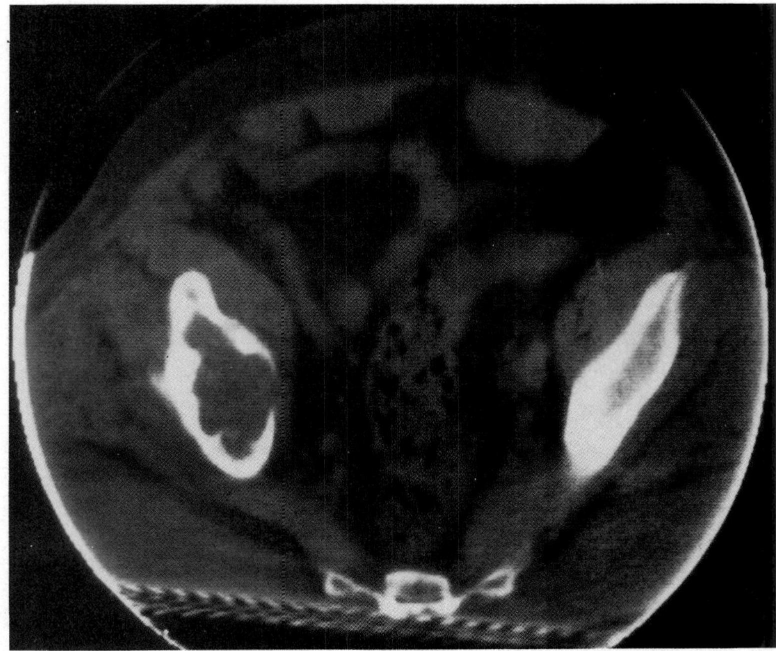

Figure 20–20. A computed tomograph shows the destruction of the medial pelvic cortex and marrow replacement by chondrosarcoma as well as the presence of a medial soft tissue mass.

been reported to be 77% to 87%, 50% to 59%, and 27% to 36% respectively. These studies as well as our own[167] point out that the adequacy of resection is crucial to patient outcome.

D. Round Cell Tumors and Myeloma

Histologic examination of the tissue from a number of malignant lesions of the skeleton demonstrates the presence of a uniform field consisting of small round cells with hyperchromatic nuclei and scant cytoplasm. Characteristically these tumors are purely lytic on radiographs and display a "permeative" or "moth eaten" pattern of bony destruction, without evidence of mineralized matrix production. The list of lesions that can produce such patterns is long but includes principally Ewing's sarcoma, malignant lymphoma of bone, metastatic neuroblastoma,[170,171] embryonal rhabdomyosarcoma, myeloma, small cell osteosarcoma,[172] mesenchymal chondrosarcoma,[173] and metastatic small cell carcinoma of the lung.[170] At times the nonneoplastic process of osteomyelitis and histiocytosis must be included in the differential diagnosis. Since the treatment of each of these neoplasms differs somewhat from the others, patients suspected of having a round cell sarcoma pattern must be accurately and completely staged. Workup should include staging abdominal CT scan, lung tomography, bipedal lymphangiogram, gallium scan, liver-spleen scan, intravenous pyelogram, and bone marrow biopsy. In addition to the routine laboratory tests, a urinary VMA and HVA quantitation should be obtained in appropriately aged patients, and serum and urine immunoelectrophoresis and Bence-Jones protein determinations should be ordered in patients suspected of having myeloma. Special attention should be paid at the time of biopsy to obtaining sufficient tissue to allow cultures, special staining (PAS, reticulum stains, and so on), electron microscopy, and determination of surface markers.

Ewing's sarcoma is the prototypical round cell lesion of bone. The highly malignant sarcoma accounts for about 6% to 10% of all malignant bone tumors and is the most lethal of the group.[4,105] The tumor is very rarely encountered in black or Chinese populations[60,170] and is more prevalent in males (60/40%). The peak age incidence is the second decade of age with over a third of the lesions occurring between the ages of 10 and 15 years. The tumor is rare in individuals below the age of 5 and over the age of 30 years.[21,170] Primary lesions may occur in almost any bone, but there is a striking preponderance of pelvic and lower extremity sites

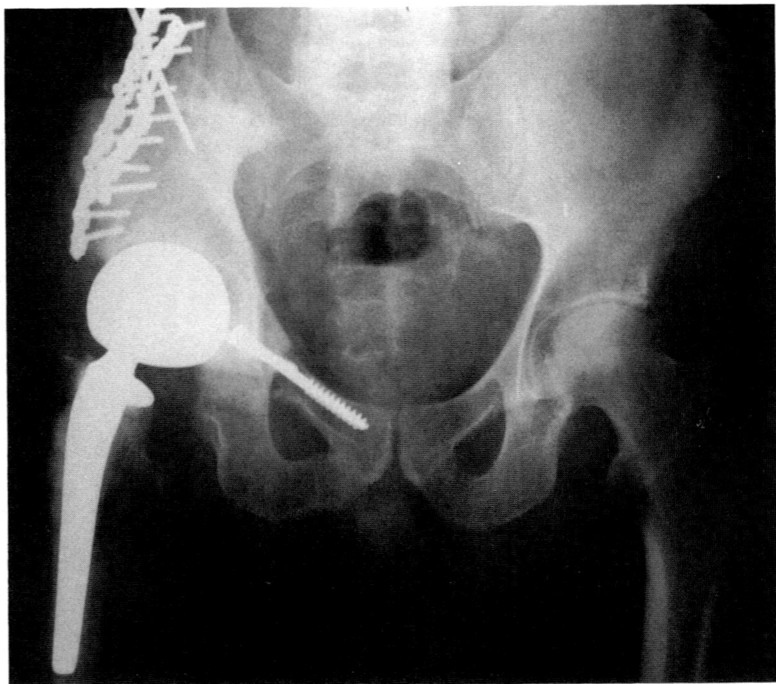

Figure 20–21. A wide resection of the ilium, acetabulum, and proximal femur was performed en bloc, and a reconstruction using an allograft pelvic segment and a metallic proximal femur component was carried out.

in all major studies.[4,21,170] In the long bones, the lesion predilects the metaphyseal ends of the bone, but it may also be located in the diaphysis, a site that is unusual for other malignant tumors.[5,21]

In contrast to most other bone tumors, patients with Ewing's sarcoma may present with systemic symptoms and signs suggestive of acute illness including fever, malaise, sweats, an elevated sedimentation rate, anemia and leukocytosis.[20,174] There is almost always a painful swelling or mass that may appear erythematous and be warm to touch. The serum LDH may be elevated and appears to have prognostic significance.[175] Pathologic fractures are present in 2% to 5% of patients at the time of diagnosis.[5,21]

Radiographs of a Ewing's tumor almost always show a permeative, lytic destructive lesion of bone with occasional areas of reactive bone formation within the lesion and in the adjacent periosteum (Figs. 20–22 and 20–23). Cortical transgression by the malignant process is almost invariably present and produces the appearance of a large soft tissue mass and a layered periosteal bony response (described by the term "onion skin"). The extent of the soft tissue mass is best appreciated on the CT scan or MRI (Fig. 20–24). At times it is difficult to distinguish the radiographic findings from those of osteosarcoma or even infection.

Histologically, Ewing's sarcoma consists of sheets of closely packed, round cells about the size of histiocytes with scant cytoplasm, indistinct cell borders, and hyperchromatic nuclei. Mitotic activity is variable, and there may be large areas of necrosis. The architecture may take on several forms, from diffuse broad fields of tumor, to lobular patterms separated by fibrous septa, or various organoid patterns.[170] Special stains (PAS) and electron microscopy are useful in demonstrating glycogen granules within the cells, but this finding is not constant or specific for Ewing's sarcoma. The exact origin of these cells is not clear, but studies employing immunohistochemical and cytochemical techniques lead one to believe that they are of mesenchymal or possibly endothelial origin.[5]

The prognosis for patients with Ewing's sarcoma treated by surgery or radiotherapy alone is poor. In a large series from the Mayo Clinic,[174] the overall 5- and 10-year survival rate was 16.2% and 13.9% respectively for those patients who did not present with metastatic disease. Patients with proximal lesions fare worse than those with distal lesions, and pelvic lesions have the worst prognosis.[170,174] Other unfavorable prognostic

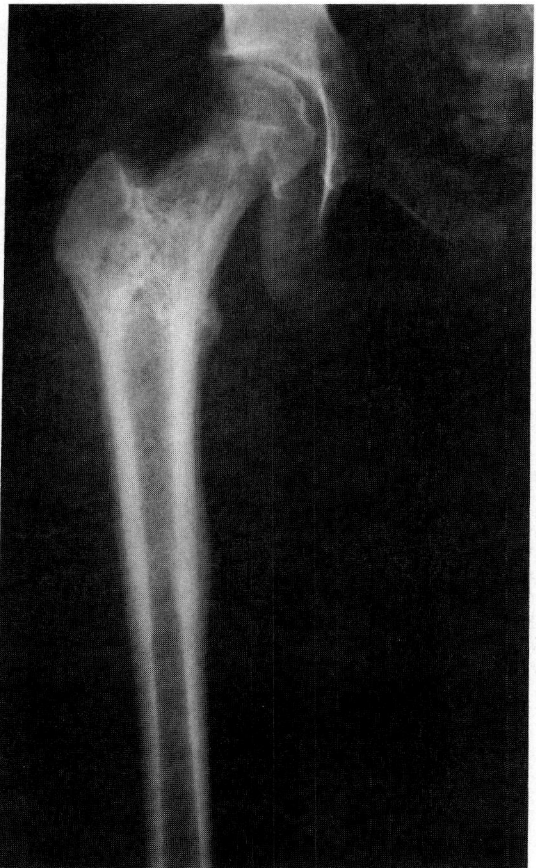

Figure 20–22. AP radiograph of the femur in a 16-year-old girl with Ewing's sarcoma. Physical examination and CT disclosed a large soft tissue mass. The cortex appears thickened but is weakened by a permeative intramedullary and intracortical process extending from the femoral neck to the midshaft area. The classic "onion skin" appearance of the periosteal response is evident.

factors include elevations of the sedimentation rate and serum LDH, pathologic fracture, and the presence of metastases at diagnosis.[174,175] The lungs, other bones, and lymph nodes are the most common sites of metastases,[21] and fully 20% of the patients present with distant spread at the time of initial discovery.

The current treatment of nonmetastatic Ewing's sarcoma is heavily based on combined drug and radiation therapy, and this has markedly improved the survival statistics. The use of doxorubicin (Adriamycin), cyclophosphamide (Cytoxan), vincristine, and actinomycin-D in combination with radiation has resulted in a 3-year survival that approached 50% in a large multi-institutional Intergroup Ewing's Sarcoma Study,[170,175] and 79% (53 of 67 patients) survival at 12 to 118 months of follow-up in a recent report from Memorial Sloan Kettering.[15] In most of these studies, radiation therapy has been employed to achieve local control with reasonable success for primaries in the vertebral body, ribs, tibia, and fibula (>90%), whereas lesions of the humerus, femur, and pelvis had a much higher rate of local relapse (15%–20%).[12,176,177] The doses employed vary from 5500 to 7000 cGy and are not without some morbidity in terms of growth arrest, fracture,[178] soft tissue fibrosis, nerve damage,[179] and late development of radiation-induced sarcoma.[180,181,181a] For these reasons, in recent years it has been suggested that resective surgery be added to the treatment regimen,[174,182–185] particularly if functional loss can be minimized. Lesions of the ribs, fibula, scapula, and clavicle may be considered resectible; and in other patients it may be possible to employ reconstructive modalities, such as metallic implants and allograft bone transplants to achieve functional results for certain other lesions of the upper and lower extremities.[185] An improved survival has been demonstrated in one center by performing pelvic resections in conjunction with induction chemotherapy and postoperative radiation.[186] Amputations may be required for distal lesions in very young children, for patients with extremely large tumors, and for certain pathologic fractures.[187]

Perhaps the most confusing lesions of bone with regard to nomenclature and differential diagnosis are the *malignant lymphomas of bone*. It has only been relatively recently that this group of lesions has been clearly separated from Ewing's sarcoma and other round cell lesions of bone. The first of these to be described and most often localized to bone is the reticulum cell sarcoma now termed diffuse histiocytic lymphoma[188]; but the terminology of lymphomas is rapidly changing with advances in histologic analysis and immunologic techniques.[189] The diffuse histiocytic lymphoma is now considered to be a disease of transformed B lymphocytes.[28] Other types of lymphomas may involve bone primarily, such as Hodgkin's lymphoma and the lymphocytic lymphomas.[4] It has been estimated that between 5% and 25% of lymphomas are entirely localized to bone as a primary site, but this number is diminishing as staging techniques improve.[21,188] Lymphoma

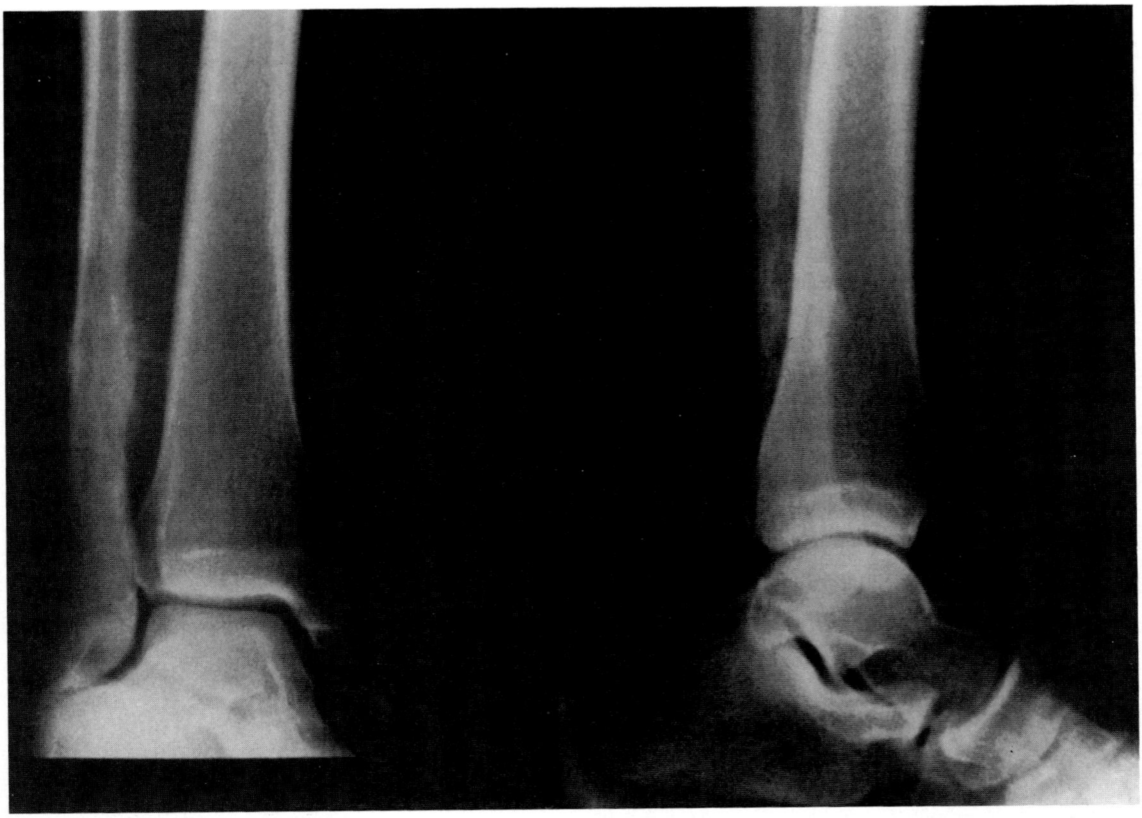

Figure 20–23. AP and lateral radiographs of a distal fibular Ewing's sarcoma showing the permeative changes in the medullary cavity, cortical destruction, and "star burst" perpendicular striations of periosteal response. It would be difficult to distinguish this from an osteosarcoma radiographically.

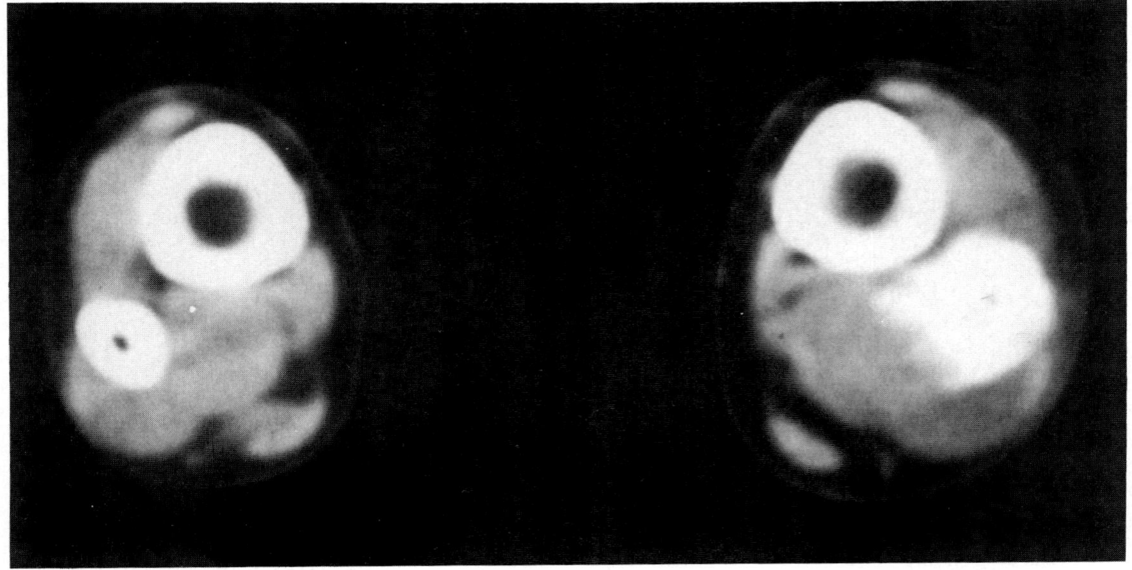

Figure 20–24. The computed tomogram image shows a large soft tissue mass encircling the distal fibula.

of bone is most prevalent in the middle to older age groups and, although uncommon in childhood and teens, may be an important differential consideration for patients thought to have Ewing's sarcoma. The lesions may occur at any site in the skeleton, but the pelvis, femur, humerus, ribs, and tibia are the most common.[4,21,190] Pain, swelling, and the presence of a mass are the usual presenting symptoms, although occasionally fever and weight loss are noted.[21,190] Laboratory work is useful in eliminating the possibility of leukemia, infection, and myeloma. A staging workup including ^{99m}technetium-diphosphonate bone scan, gallium scan, bipedal lymphangiogram, intravenous pyelogram, abdominal CT scan, and bone marrow aspiration often reveals that the lesion is not localized to bone and that systemic disease is present at the time of diagnosis.[21,188]

The radiographic appearance of the lymphomas of bone is very similar to that of Ewing's tumor in that the lesion presents as a purely lytic, permeative lesion with no margination and little periosteal response. Patchy sclerosis may be present. The cortex is usually partially destroyed, and soft tissue extension is evident on computed tomograms. The histologic appearance of lymphomas is variable but always of a diffuse type[21,188] containing a mixture of cell types.[187] The reticulum cell is a large cell usually containing a nucleus with a grooved nuclear membrane; the cytoplasm is abundant, and the cell membrane is distinct. Special silver stains demonstrate the presence of reticulin fibers around the individual cells. It is often difficult to subclassify the lymphomas of bone into the categories found at other sites.[21,187]

The management of lymphoma of bone is similar to that of lymphoma in other sites, namely, chemotherapy with or without local radiotherapy.[188] Treatment of the primary lesion is usually by radiotherapy, employing 4500 to 6000 cGy, although local recurrences have been reported in a high percentage of patients treated in this manner.[191] Radiotherapy alone appears to be sufficient for disease purely localized to bone,[188] but this is often difficult to ascertain, and opinion is divided regarding the use of chemotherapy in these circumstances.[20,21,188,192] Careful staging is mandatory. Surgery is usually reserved for pathologic fracture.[187] The 5-year survival is approaching 50% or greater,[190] with less favorable results for patients with regional spread[188] or Hodgkin's lymphoma of bone.[187]

By far the most common primary malignant tumor of bone is *multiple myeloma or plasmacytoma*. It is usually excluded from discussions of bone tumors because it is considered to more closely resemble the marrow cancers, such as the leukemias. The plasma cell is the cell of origin, and the malignant process is one of a family of disorders termed monoclonal gammopathies. This group of disorders includes benign as well as malignant conditions all characterized by proliferation of a single clone of plasma cells, which elaborate increased concentrations of gamma globulins.[193] Multiple myeloma is usually a diffuse disorder affecting the entire bone marrow, but occasionally a single lesion is observed with no apparent involvement of the remainder of the skeleton. This entity, termed *solitary plasmacytoma*, usually develops into a disseminated disorder with time, and many authorities doubt that a localized monostotic process ever really exists as such.[194]

The clinical presentation is variable, ranging from a low-grade diffuse bone pain to an acute episode of severe pain associated with a pathologic fracture. Although a single focus of bone involvement may be the first sign of myeloma, most patients are found to have diffuse disease after careful staging. Any bone may be involved, but the spine, ribs, skull, pelvis, and proximal long bones are the most common sites of bony lesions.[194] A pathologic fracture of a vertebra, rib, or hip may occur with minimal or no trauma. Anorexia, weight loss, malaise, and easy fatigability usually antedate the discovery of the disease by several months. Physical findings are those of chronic illness and anemia; hepatosplenomegaly may be present.[193] The most characteristic findings on radiographs are a profound osteoporosis and small punctate or rounded radiolucencies in the skeleton, sometimes becoming confluent to produce large lytic lesions with severe thinning of the cortices and distortion of the normal architecture of the bone. Multiple "punched out" lesions may be observed in the skull. Not all lesions show increased uptake on radionuclide bone scans; therefore, skeletal surveys are indicated to search for other sites of involvement.[193,194]

Laboratory studies are very helpful at arriving at a diagnosis. A normochromic, normocytic anemia and elevated sedimentation rate are present in approximately 90% of patients with diffuse disease.[21,193] The serum calcium may be elevated in patients with extensive osseous involvement (partly on the basis of binding to globulin), and the serum uric acid is commonly elevated.[193] The serum protein electrophoresis is helpful in that some 80% of patients have a nonspecific increase in the globulin fraction; immunoelectrophoresis demonstrates the presence of an abnormal "M-component" in 90% of affected patients, usually migrating with the IgG or IgA fractions, which is virtually diagnostic of multiple myeloma. Urine analyses for Bence-Jones proteins are positive in less than 50% of patients, but a protein electrophoresis of the urine is abnormal in over 60% of patients. The bone marrow biopsy is the diagnostic test for myeloma, demonstrating a pathognomonic increase in the percentage of plasma cells, and over 8% is considered suspicious; over 20% is diagnostic. The peripheral blood smear may show sufficient numbers of the myeloma cells to justify the diagnosis of plasma cell leukemia.[193] Biopsy of the bone lesions is usually unnecessary, but if performed, the tissue obtained will be found to contain sheets of plasma cells without a matrix or stromal tissue. The plasma cells may appear quite mature or frankly anaplastic.[21]

The prognosis for patients with myeloma is poor with most succumbing to the disease within a few years of diagnosis.[193,195] The bony lesions can be controlled by radiation therapy, employing internal fixation with metallic implants (with or without polymethyl methacrylate) or prostheses to stabilize or treat impending or established pathologic fractures.[20] The current chemotherapeutic agents of choice include corticosteroids, melphalan,[196] and cyclophosphamide, but remissions obtained by their administration are often only temporary.[195]

E. Giant Cell Tumor of Bone

Perhaps the most intriguing and surgically challenging of the osseous tumors is the *giant cell tumor of bone*, an uncommon neoplasm accounting for approximately 4% of bone tumors.[4] Although unlikely to metastasize, it is locally aggressive, and its metaphyseo-epiphyseal location makes treatment difficult. It is a lesion of early adulthood, occurring mainly in the 18- to 45-year age group; it is extremely rare prior to closure of the growth plates and is more common in women. The principal sites of predilection are the distal femur, proximal tibia, distal radius, proximal humerus and femur, and proximal fibula.[197] Giant cell tumors of the spine are fortunately rare and seem to occur predominantly in the sacrum.[4] Giant cell tumors of the bones of the hands are uncommon but ominous, since they are more frequently associated with multicentric disease and metastasis to the lungs.[198,199] When the tumor is found in the skull, it may indicate underlying Paget's disease.[22]

The biological nature of giant cell tumor of bone has not been completely defined; it is considered a benign lesion by some authorities because of its low metastatic rate (probably less than 5%),[200,201] whereas others consider the tumor to be a low-grade malignancy because of its local aggressiveness, its capacity to recur after inadequate treatment, and its recognized, albeit rare, ability to metastasize. Further confusion arises because the exact cell of origin has not been completely determined. The multinucleated giant cell has the histologic hallmarks of an osteoclast,[202] hence the tumor has been labeled osteoclastoma by the British. Studies employing time-lapse cinemicrography have demonstrated that the giant cells arise from fusion of the stromal cells. The stromal cells appear to take origin from the cells of the bone marrow, and parathormone receptors have been found to be present on their cell membrane in tissue culture.[203]

The patient usually presents with complaints of dull aching pain around the affected joint, often exacerbated by a traumatic episode. The symptoms may have been present for several months.[22,197,204] A mass may be present and joint dysfunction and significant muscle atrophy may ensue in lesions that are long-standing.[204] A pathologic fracture may occur through the weakened bone; and in lesions that are rapidly progressive, warmth and erythema of the skin and occasionally pulsations of the mass may be appreciated.[19] The growth rate appears to be accelerated during pregnancy, although a recent study of several tumors on our service has failed to detect the presence of estrogen or progesterone receptors on the cell membrane. Lesions in the spine or sacrum may mimic disk protrusions or lead to intestinal and urologic symptoms.

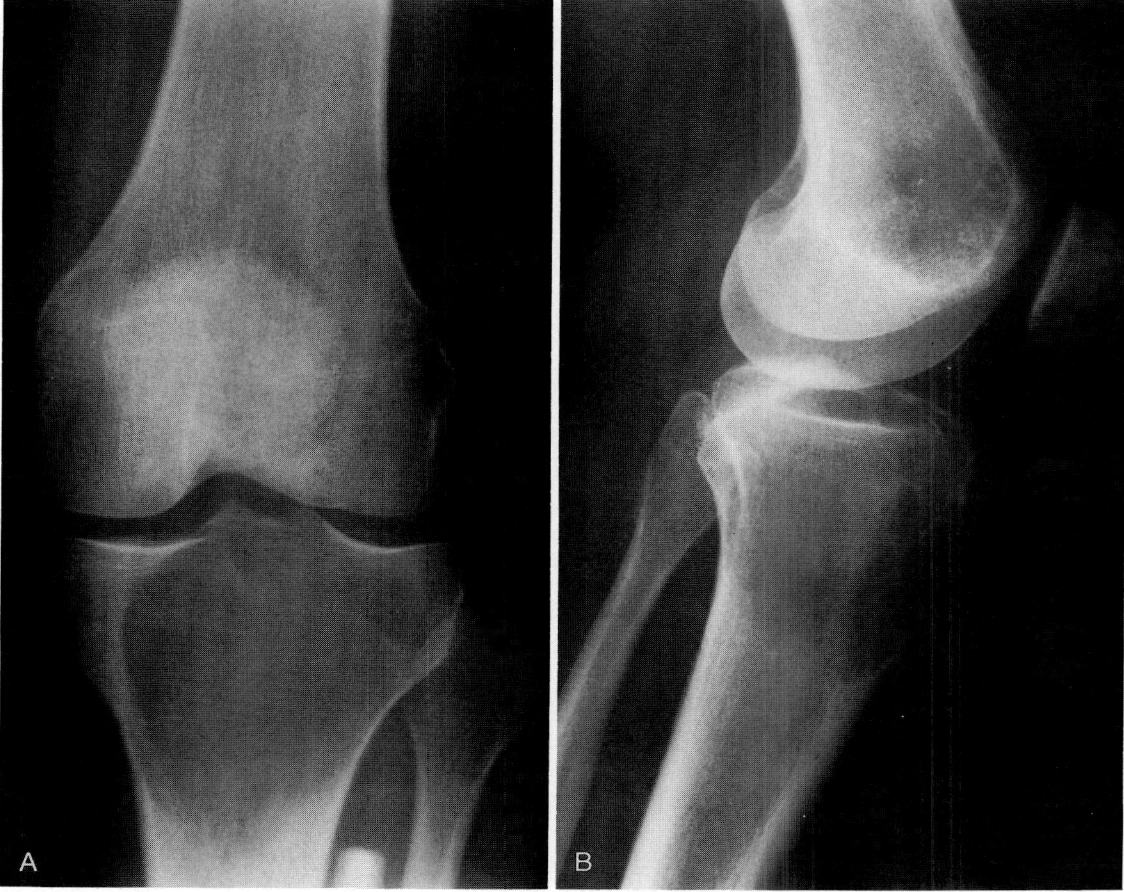

Figure 20–25. *A* and *B*, AP and lateral radiographs of the proximal tibia in a 25-year-old man with a giant cell tumor of the proximal tibia. It is a purely lytic geographic lesion that is well demarcated but poorly marginated. There is a small subchondral fracture of the medial tibial plateau but no evidence of a soft tissue mass.

On plain radiographs, the tumor is lytic and eccentrically placed in the metaphyseo-epiphyseal region of a long bone (Fig. 20–25*A*, *B*). This location in a patient with closed physes is essentially diagnostic of giant cell tumor of bone. The lesion extends to and sometimes through the subchondral bone plate, and pathologic fracture may allow tumor to enter the adjacent joint. The cortex is almost always expanded and thinned with some areas of destruction; but the tumor, which may extend well into the adjacent soft tissues, is usually contained by a periosteal shell of bone that may be difficult to detect radiographically. The lesion is purely lytic, although ridges in the thinned cortex or healing of a pathologic fracture may give the appearance of septa.[22,197] The medullary border of the tumor is usually well delineated, but not marginated by a rim of reactive bone. Close inspection of this border reveals a zone where the tumor permeates the existing trabeculae for a small distance around the perimeter of the lesion. The intense vascularity of the lesion is appreciated by angiography and radionuclide scans, and computed tomograms or magnetic resonance images demonstrate the extent of the lesion within the bone and soft tissues.

On gross inspection, the undisturbed tumor is fleshy tan in color and quite soft, but areas of the lesion may show hemorrhage, necrosis, and lipid degeneration, providing a variegated appearance and color pattern.[22,197,204] Histologically, the lesional tissue is highly vascular, the majority of the cells appearing as rounded, ovoid, or spindled cells with well-defined vesicular nuclei containing prominent

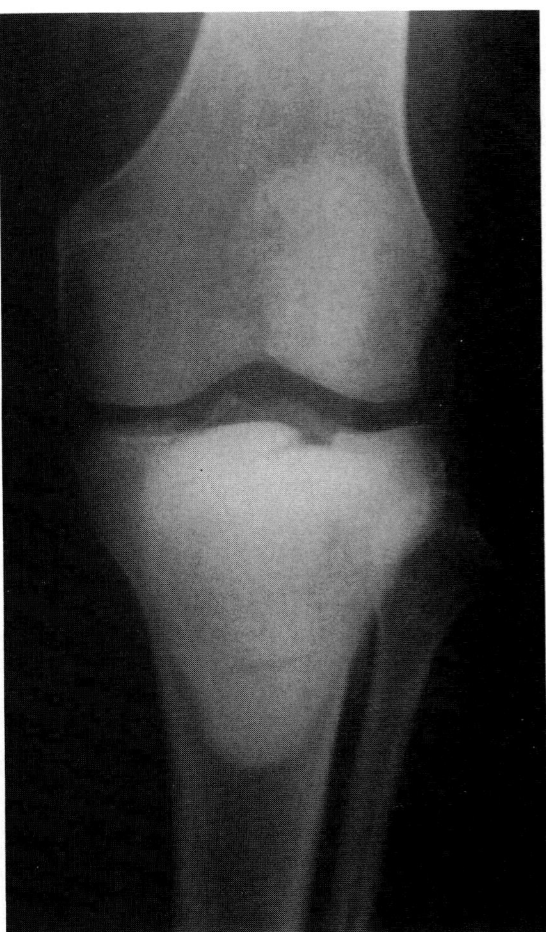

Figure 20–26. This lesion was treated with aggressive curettage, phenolization of the cavity, bone grafting of the subchondral bone, and packing with polymethylmethacrylate. Although the tumor extended down to the subchondral surface, resective therapy was felt to be too aggressive as initial treatment.

nucleoli. The most striking feature is the presence of numerous, randomly distributed, multinucleated giant cells, often with 50 to 150 or more nuclei in a centripetal arrangement that show a remarkable similarity to the nuclei of the stromal cells.[22] Considerable variation is often present in the histologic appearance of different sites from the same tumor, and *many other lesions of bone contain giant cells*, so that correct diagnosis at times may be difficult to obtain, especially on small amounts of tissue or necrotic areas.

The giant cell tumor is a difficult lesion to treat because of its local aggressiveness and its proximity to major, often weight-bearing joints. Although less than 5% of the tumors metastasize[200,201] (and then usually after radiotherapy or local recurrence), the local recurrence rate following incomplete (intralesional) surgery is quite high (over 50% in some series).[197,204] Marginal resective surgery is probably curative,[20] but the location of the tumor makes this difficult without sacrificing the joint. When the lesion occurs in the proximal fibula, resective surgery is appropriate and curative[20,197]; but in the distal femur, proximal tibia, and other common sites, the giant cell tumor represents a major dilemma for the orthopedic oncologist. If the lesion is small and well marginated and the subchondral cortex is at least 3 mm in thickness, intralesional treatment is appropriate; the authors have utilized for this purpose a thorough curettage, washing of the cavity with 50% phenol, and the implantation of polymethylmethacrylate (Fig. 20–26). The recurrence rate following acrylic implantation is reported to be markedly reduced compared with packing with either auto- or allograft bone.[205] Other centers have employed liquid nitrogen to freeze the cavity and extend the area of cell kill following curettage. This is associated with a 10% recurrence rate, but complications such as fracture and nonunion are common.[192,206] When the tumor is large, is poorly marginated, has destroyed the subchondral bone, or has a soft tissue mass or a pathologic fracture, we prefer to treat it by en bloc (marginal or wide) resection and implantation of a fresh frozen cadaveric allograft bone in which the cartilage is treated with 8% DMSO as a cryopreservative, and the donor ligaments and tendinous insertions are utilized to reconstruct resected motors and joint stabilizers.[73] Other options for treatment include the use of metallic prostheses or arthrodesis to reconstruct the surgical defect.[20] Amputation is infrequently necessary for multiple recurrent disease.

Giant cell tumors of the axial skeleton represent a special problem in management.[20] The lesions of the spine, sacrum, or pelvis are sometimes impossible to resect without injury to the adjacent anatomic structures, and control of hemorrhage from the lesions represents a major problem. For these lesions, some centers have advocated selective angiographic embolization of the lesional area followed in some cases by intralesional surgery.[207] The use of supervoltage radiation is usually successful in eradicating the tumor but introduces the problems of radiation necrosis (a major problem in the pelvis if it involves the

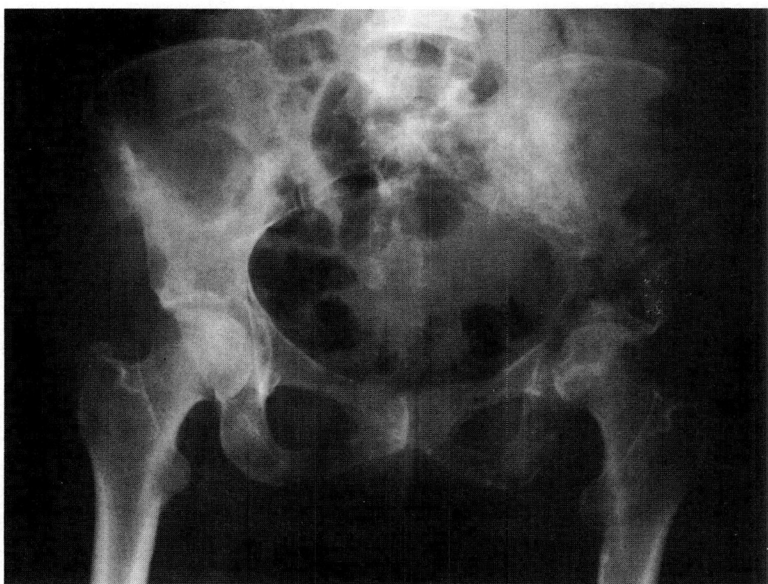

Figure 20–27. Metastatic carcinoma of the breast involving the left hemipelvis. There is a mixed blastic lytic response involving the entire ilium with a pathologic fracture of the acetabulum.

acetabulum) and the threat of radiation-induced sarcoma, which has been reported to be quite high.[197,204,208,209] In the small number of patients in whom pulmonary metastases occur, the lesions should be resected surgically with good expectation of cure.[19,20,200,201]

F. Metastatic Carcinoma

In contrast to the rarity of the primary bone tumors, *metastatic carcinoma to bone* is perhaps 100-fold more common, especially in the elderly age groups. This age distribution of bone lesions is helpful in differential diagnosis. Primary tumors of bone are almost unheard of in newborns and early childhood and, with the exception of histiocytosis, are rare before the age of 10 years. Within this early period, metatastic neuroblastoma, Wilm's tumor, and leukemias account for the majority of malignant lesions of the osseous system. In contrast, metastatic lesions are less common than primary lesions until the age of 45 years and beyond when it becomes increasingly more likely that a destructive lesion will be a metastatic deposit. Thus, a patient in the sixth decade of life who presents with an aggressive-appearing bone tumor should be considered to have a metastasis until proven otherwise, and the workup should be planned accordingly.

The number of lesions present at diagnosis is another consideration in evaluating these patients. With the exception of Ollier's disease, hereditary multiple osteocartilaginous exostosis, and fibrous dysplasia, primary bone tumors are usually solitary, in sharp contrast to metastatic disease, which often involves multiple osseous sites. In fact, only 9% of 212 autopsies with metastatic bone disease[210] and 25% of a large clinically assessed series[211] had solitary lesions. Thus, any patient, particularly a mature adult, who presents with polyostotic disease should be considered to have either myeloma or metastasis.[23] With the exception of metastatic carcinoma of the lung, secondary carcinomatous deposits are rare distal to the knees and elbows,[212,213] and the vast majority of the bony metastases affect the axial skeleton, proximal femora, ribs, and skull.[4,5,23] Characteristically, osseous metastases are centrally placed within the bone, erode the cortex symmetrically with little expansion, and rarely present with a soft tissue mass (Fig. 20–27). Pathologic fractures, especially of the spine and femora, are common.[22,210]

The mechanism by which tumors metastasize, an area of intense current research beyond the scope of this review, involves more than random access of tumor cells into the vascular system. Rather it appears to be an active process involving a series of steps wherein certain clones of cells have the ability to spread and select specific organs in which to establish a clinical metastatic deposit.[214] Several animal studies confirm the clinical

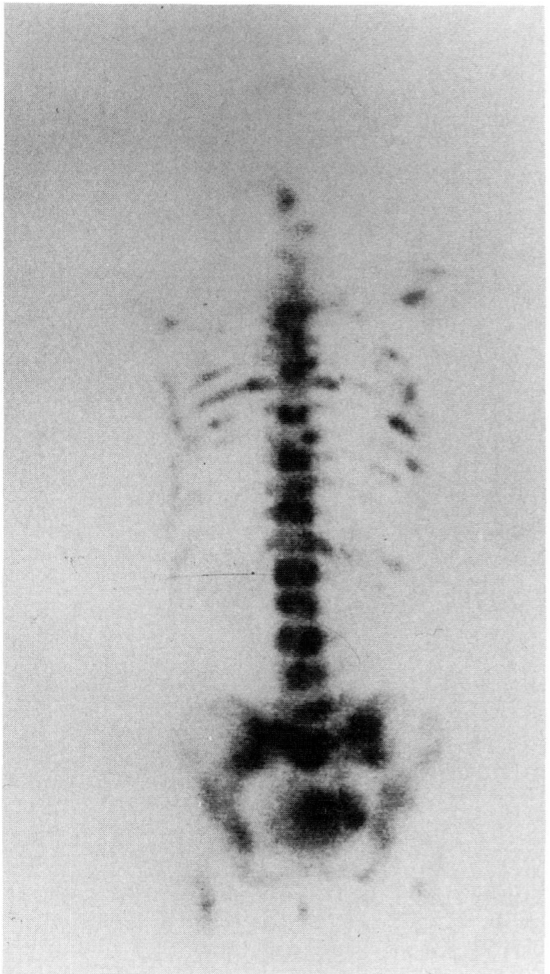

Figure 20–28. A bone scan of the patient in Figure 20–27 shows evidence of wide metastatic disease.

impression that whereas almost any tumor can spread to bone, certain solid tumors seem to have a propensity for bony metastasis. Once the tumor cells reach the bone, they effect either a blastic or a lytic response, although it is often a mixture of both. The mechanisms of bone formation and destruction are largely unknown, but the latter is an active process mediated by osteoclasts or other cell types. The tumor probably stimulates osteoclastic bone resorption by releasing factors such as prostaglandins (carcinomas) or osteoclast-activating factors (myeloma, lymphoma).[214–216] There is also evidence that certain neoplastic cells or monocytic cells can directly resorb bone (reviewed in ref. 216). Bone formation, which yields blastic metastases, is due either to intramembranous bone formation of the fibrous stroma of the tumor (e.g., prostatic carcinoma) or to a reactive osteoblastic response of the surrounding host bone.[215]

In males, the most frequent primary carcinoma that spreads to bone is the prostate.[217] Over 60% of these lesions are located in the axial skeleton,[218] presumably due to the dissemination of the tumor cells through the valveless venous plexus of Batson,[219] whereas involvement of the ilium, sternum, and other bones appears to occur as a late event after other organs are involved.[220] The vast majority of prostatic bone lesions are very destructive and often evoke a profound sclerotic response in the surrounding normal bone, which may at times mimic the radiographic appearance of Paget's disease of bone. The serum alkaline phosphatase is elevated (and may be so in any patient with widespread metastatic disease), but a serum acid phosphatase elevation is virtually diagnostic for prostatic malignancy.[221] The bone scan is helpful in localizing the often multiple sites of skeletal involvement and usually shows extensive activity in the axial skeleton.[23,222] Factors associated with a poor prognosis include age (greater than 65 years), severe bone pain, presence of soft tissue metastases, anemia, and elevation of the serum LDH, AST, and alkaline and acid phosphatase.[221]

In women, breast carcinoma is the most frequent primary source of metastatic disease to bone.[210,223] As in prostatic carcinoma, the axial skeleton and proximal long bones are the sites most frequently affected, and a sclerotic response to the lesion is frequent (Fig. 20–27). Radionuclide bone scans are useful in detecting lesions prior to the occurrence of radiographic changes and often reveal the presence of multiple sites of involvement (Fig. 20–28).[222] Pathologic fractures are common.

In both sexes, carcinoma of the lung is the second most common cause of metastatic bone disease. The lesions are usually lytic and very destructive on radiographs, often widely distributed throughout the skeleton.[218] These lesions frequently cause pathologic fractures and may be associated with a surrounding soft tissue mass. Other lesions that commonly spread to bone include carcinoma originating in the gastrointestinal tract,[224] renal cell carcinoma, and thyroid carcinoma.[223] Renal cell carcinoma often first presents with a bone lesion, and the primary site is discovered only when the biopsy shows the characteristic clear cell histology or the urine contains occult blood.[225,226] These lesions are quite vascular and produce a lytic, destructive bony lesion with a considerable expansion of the cortex to give a "soap bubble" appearance. Of considerable interest is the frequency with which these tumors present at long intervals after resection of the primary and seeming cure. Especially in patients with solitary bony lesions, aggressive treatment of the metastasis is warranted because long-term remissions are reported.[23,225] Metastases from thyroid carcinoma may be solitary or multiple, but not all lesions are detectable by radionuclide scanning.[227] The bony lesions may respond spectacularly to total thyroidectomy, iodine, and thyroid-stimulating hormone.[23] For this reason, an aggressive approach including chemotherapy is also justified on the basis of the possibility of long-term survival of the patients.[217]

The treatment of skeletal metastases from primary carcinomas will differ considerably according to a variety of factors.[217,228–230] The site and size of the metastatic deposit and the threat to skeletal integrity or adjacent vital structures, such as the spinal cord, may dictate emergency surgery or aggressive treatment to avoid calamity. Otherwise, the main orthopedic goals are to provide pain relief, prevent pathologic fractures, and maintain mobility of the patient to obviate problems of hypercalcemia and bed sores. Prophylactic fixation of long bone fractures, especially in the lower extremity, is indicated for large lesions (>2.5 cm), lytic destruction of 50% or more of the cortex, and persistent pain with weight-bearing despite local radiotherapy.[228] Established fractures of the long bones are also addressed surgically if the patient is metabolically able to withstand the procedure and has a reasonable (greater than 6 weeks) life expectancy. In the long bones, open reduction followed by plate or intramedullary fixation is usually employed; and if there is an extensive bony defect, methylmethacrylate packing aids in achieving immediate stability. Prosthetic replacements are employed about the hip and shoulder. There is no evidence that such fixations interfere with the ability to deliver local radiotherapy or that radiation in therapeutic doses adversely affects the strength of the cement. In one series, the use of cement improved the pain relief, ambulatory ability, and survival of patients compared with those whose fixations did not include cement.[231] Following the stabilization, local radiation therapy, hormonal manipulations, or chemotherapy is directed toward eradicating or controlling the bony lesion. Some tumors may regress remarkably with appropriate systemic management; and the use of anti-estrogens in hormonally responsive breast cancer and estrogens in patients with prostatic carcinoma may produce long-lasting remissions in symptoms and regression of the lesions on radiographs.[217,229] Radiation therapy is usually very effective in dealing with solitary or even multiple lesions that are likely to cause a fracture if left untreated.[230] As indicated earlier, there are circumstances, particularly for solitary lesions metastatic from the kidney or thyroid, in which aggressive, resective, or even ablative surgery is indicated in the hope of obtaining a cure.

Lesions of the spine present often complex treatment dilemmas.[232] Asymptomatic lesions are treated with systemic chemotherapy or hormonal therapy in appropriate primary cancers, reserving local radiation therapy to painful deposits or upper cervical lesions where progression could be catastrophic. Compression fractures without neurologic compromise can be managed with radiation and bracing or traction. Established fractures with neurologic compromise are initially managed with high-dose steroids to diminish the spinal cord edema, followed by either surgical decompression or radiotherapy. Since the compression is usually anterior, it may be more advantageous to perform an anterior decompression and fixation rather than a destabilizing laminectomy. If the latter is performed, stabilization with Harrington rods is employed.[232]

The overall survival rate of 306 patients who underwent surgery for metastatic lesions of the femur was 59% at 6 months and 48% at 12 months.[231] In this series, patients with breast cancer fared slightly better than the other primaries, with 6- and 12-month survival figures of 74% and 64% respectively. These somewhat dismal survival data for metastatic bone disease support attempts to aggressively prevent and stabilize fractures to limit the discomfort of these unfortunate patients.

References

1. Larsson S-E, Lorentzon R: The geographic variation of the incidence of malignant primary bone tumors in Sweden. J Bone Joint Surg 56A:592–600, 1974.

2. Mankin HJ: Advances in the diagnosis and treatment of bone tumors. N Engl J Med 300:543–545, 1979.
3. Silverberg E: Cancer statistics. CA 34:7023, 1984.
4. Dahlin DC: Bone Tumors: General Aspects and Data on 6,221 Cases. Springfield, IL, Charles C Thomas, 1978.
5. Spjut HJ, Dorfman HD, Fechner RE, Ackerman LV: Atlas of Tumor Pathology, Fascicle 5: Tumors of Bone and Cartilage. Armed Forces Institute of Pathology, 1971.
6. Bleyer WA, Haas JE, Feigl P, et al: Improved three-year disease-free survival in osteogenic sarcoma: Efficacy of adjunctive chemotherapy. J Bone Joint Surg 64B:233–238, 1982.
7. Edmonson JH, Green SJ, Ivins ET, et al: Methotrexate as adjuvant treatment for primary osteosarcoma. N Engl J Med 303:642–643, 1980.
8. Goorin AM, Frei E III, Abelson AT: Adjuvant chemotherapy for osteosarcoma. A decade of experience. Surg Clin North Am 61:1379–1389, 1981.
9. Jaffe N, Frei E III, Tragis D, Bishop Y: Adjuvant methotrexate and citrovorum factor treatment of osteogenic sarcoma. N Engl J Med 291:994–1006, 1974.
10. Lange B, Levine AS: Is it ethical not to conduct a prospectively controlled trial of adjuvant chemotherapy in osteosarcoma? Cancer Treat Rep 66:1699–1704, 1982.
11. Link M, Goorin AM, Miser A, et al: The role of adjuvant chemotherapy in the treatment of osteosarcoma (OS) of the extremity: Preliminary results of the Multi-Institutional Osteosarcoma Study (MIOS). Proc Am Soc Clin Oncol 4:237, 1985.
12. Perez CA, Tefft M, Nesbit ME, et al: Radiation therapy in the multimodal management of Ewing's sarcoma of bone: Report of the Intergroup Ewing's Sarcoma Study. Natl Cancer Inst Monogr 56:263–271, 1981.
13. Rosen G: Preoperative (neoadjuvant) chemotherapy for osteogenic sarcoma: A ten year experience. Orthopaedics 8: 659–664, 1985.
14. Rosen G, Caparros B, Huvos AG, et al: Preoperative chemotherapy for osteogenic sarcoma. Selection of postoperative adjuvant chemotherapy based on the response of the primary tumor to preoperative chemotherapy. Cancer 49:1221–1230, 1982.
15. Rosen G, Juergens H, Caparros B, et al: Combination chemotherapy (T-6) in the multidisciplinary treatment of Ewing's sarcoma. Natl Cancer Inst Monogr 56:289–299, 1981.
16. Rosen G, Nirenberg A: Chemotherapy for osteogenic sarcoma: An investigative method, not a recipe. Cancer Treat Rep 66:1687–1697, 1982.
17. Winkler K, Beron G, Kotz R, et al: Neoadjuvant chemotherapy for osteogenic sarcoma: Results of a cooperative German-Austrian study. J Clin Oncol 2:614–617, 1984.
18. Marcove RC, Rosen G: En bloc resections for osteogenic sarcoma. Cancer 45:3040–3044, 1980.
19. Enneking WF: Musculoskeletal Tumor Surgery. New York, Churchill Livingstone, 1983.
20. Evarts CM: Surgery of the Musculoskeletal System, vol 4. New York, Churchill Livingstone, 1980, pp 1–416.
21. Huvos AG: Bone Tumors. Diagnosis, Treatment and Prognosis. Philadelphia, WB Saunders, 1979.
22. Jaffe HL: Tumors and Tumorous Conditions of the Bones and Joints. Philadelphia, Lea and Febiger, 1958.
23. Lichtenstein L: Bone Tumors. St. Louis, CV Mosby, 1977.
24. Schajowicz F: Tumors and Tumorlike Lesions of Bone and Joints. New York, Springer-Verlag, 1981.
25. Enneking WF, Spanier SS, Goodman MA: A system for the surgical staging of musculoskeletal sarcoma. Clin Orthop Rel Res 153:106–120, 1980.
26. Alho A, Connor JF, Mankin HJ, et al: Assessment of malignancy of cartilage tumors using flow cytometry. J Bone Joint Surg 65A:779–785, 1983.
27. Mankin HJ, Connor JF, Schiller AL, et al: Grading of bone tumors by analysis of nuclear DNA content using flow cytometry. J Bone Joint Surg 67A:404–413, 1985.
28. Sweet DL, Mass DP, Simon MA, Shapiro CM: Histiocytic lymphoma (reticulum-cell sarcoma) of bone. Current strategy for orthopaedic surgeons. J Bone Joint Surg 63A:79–84, 1981.
29. Rosenthal DI: Computed tomography of orthopaedicneoplasms.OrthopClinNorthAm16:461–470,1985.
30. Brady TJ, Gebhardt MC, Pykett IL, et al: NMR forearms in healthy volunteers and patients with giant cell tumor of bone. Radiology 144:548–552, 1982.
31. Brady TJ, Pykett IL, McGuire MH, et al: NMR imaging of leg tumors. Radiology 149:181–187, 1983.
32. Gebhardt MC, Rosenthal D, Mankin HJ, Brady TJ: NMR imaging of soft tissue sarcoma of the leg. Orthopaedics 8:369–372, 1985.
33. Pykett IL, Newhouse JH, Buonanno FS: Principles of nuclear magnetic resonance imaging. Radiology 143:157–168, 1982.
34. Mankin HJ, Lange TA, Spanier SS: The hazards of biopsy in patients with primary bone tumors and soft tissue tumors. J Bone Joint Surg 64A:1121–1127, 1982.
35. Simon MA: Biopsy of musculoskeletal tumors. J Bone Joint Surg 64A:1253–1257, 1982.
36. Mankin HJ, Gregg P, Perlmutter N, et al: Assessment of in-vitro adriamycin binding of osteosarcoma by flow cytometry: A preliminary report. Unpublished.
37. Goorin AM, Delorey MJ, Lack EE, et al: Prognostic significance of complete surgical resection of pulmonary metastases in patients with osteogenic sarcoma. J Clin Oncol 2:425–431, 1984.
38. Han MT, Telander RL, Pairolero PC, et al: Aggressive thoracotomy for pulmonary metastatic osteogenic sarcoma in children and young adolescents. J Pediatr Surg 16:928–933, 1982.
39. Huth JF, Holmes EC, Vernon SE, et al: Pulmonary resection for metastatic sarcoma. Am J Surg 140:9–16, 1980.
40. Marion J, Buyers V, Bruer K, et al: Role of metastatectomy without chemotherapy in the management of osteosarcoma in children. Cancer 45:1664–1668, 1980.
41. Putnam JB Jr, Roth JA, Wesley MN, et al: Survival following aggressive resection of pulmonary metastases from osteogenic sarcoma: Analysis of prognostic factors. Ann Thorac Surg 36:515–523, 1983.
42. Rosen G, Huvos AG, Mosende C, et al: Chemotherapy and thoracotomy for metastatic osteogenic sarcoma. Cancer 41:841–849, 1978.
43. Roth JA, Putnam JBJ, Wesley MN, Rosenberg SA: Differing determinants of prognosis following resection of pulmonary metastases from osteogenic and soft tissue sarcoma patients. Cancer 55:1361–1366, 1985.

44. Schaller RTJ, Haas J, Schaller J: Improved survival in children with osteosarcoma following resection of pulmonary metastases. J Pediatr Surg 17:546–550, 1982.
45. Campanacci M, Cervellati G: Osteosarcoma: A review of 345 cases. Ital J Orthop 1:5–22, 1975.
46. Jaffe HL: "Osteoid osteoma." A benign osteoblastic tumor composed of osteoid and atypical bone. Arch Surg 31:709–728, 1935.
47. Sherman MS: Osteoid osteoma. Review of the literature and report of thirty cases. J Bone Joint Surg 29A:918–930, 1947.
48. Makley JT, Dunn M: A mechanism for pain mediation in osteoid osteoma. Orthop Trans 6:72, 1982.
49. Rushton JG, Mulder DW, Lipscomb PR: Neurologic symptoms with osteoid osteoma. Neurology 5:794–797, 1955.
50. Herrlin K, Ekelund L, Lovdahl R, Persson B: Computed tomography in suspected osteoid osteomas of tubular bones. Skeletal Radiol 9:92–97, 1982.
51. Jackson RP, Reckling FW, Mantz FA: Osteoid osteoma and osteoblastoma: Similar histologic lesions with different natural histories. Clin Orthop 128:303–313, 1977.
52. Golding JSR: The natural history of osteoid osteoma with a report of 20 cases. J Bone Joint Surg 36B:218–229, 1954.
53. Sim FH, Dahlin DC, Beabout JW: Osteoid osteoma: Diagnostic problems. J Bone Joint Surg 57A:154–159, 1975.
54. McLeod R, Dahlin DC, Beabout JW: The spectrum of osteoblastoma. Am J Roentgenol 126:321–335, 1976.
55. Lichtenstein L, Sawyer WR: Benign osteoblastoma. Further observations and report of twenty additional cases. J Bone Joint Surg 46A:755–765, 1964.
56. Marcove RC, Alpert M: A pathologic study of benign osteoblastoma. Clin Orthop 30:175–181, 1963.
57. Tonai M, Campbell CJ, Ahn GH, et al: Osteoblastoma: Classification and report of 16 patients. Clin Orthop 167:222–235, 1982.
58. Marsh BW, Bonfiglio M, Brady LP, Enneking WF: Benign osteoblastoma. Range of manifestations. J Bone Surg 37A:1–9, 1975.
59. Schajowicz F, Lemos C: Malignant osteoblastoma. J Bone Joint Surg 58B:202–211, 1976.
60. Levine AS: Cancer in the Young. New York, Masson Publishing, 1982, pp 575–602.
61. McKenna RJ, Schwinn CP, Soong KY, Higginbotham NL: Sarcomata of the osteogenic series (osteogenic sarcoma, fibrosarcoma, chondrosarcoma, parosteal osteogenic sarcoma, and sarcomata arising in abnormal bone). J Bone Joint Surg 48A:1–26, 1966.
62. Cortes EP, Holland JF, Glidewell O: Adjuvant therapy of operable primary osteosarcoma—cancer and leukemia group B experience. Recent Results Cancer Res 68:16, 1979.
63. Enneking WF, Kogan A: The implications of "skip" metastases in osteosarcoma. Clin Orthop 111:33–41, 1975.
64. Simon MA, Hecht JD: Invasion of joints by primary bone sarcomas in adults. Cancer 50:1649–1655, 1982.
65. Dahlin DC, Coventry MB: Osteogenic sarcoma. A study of six hundred cases. J Bone Joint Surg 49A:101–110, 1967.
66. Friedman MA, Carter SK: The therapy for osteogenic sarcoma: Current status and thoughts for the future. J Surg Oncol 4:482–491, 1972.
67. Marcove RC, Mike V, Hajek JV, et al: Osteogenic sarcoma under the age of twenty-one. A review of one hundred and forty-five operative cases. J Bone Joint Surg 52A:411–423, 1970.
68. Simon R: Clinical prognostic factors in osteosarcoma. Cancer Treat Rep 62:193–197, 1978.
69. Enneking WF, Springfield DS, Gross M: The surgical treatment of parosteal osteosarcoma in long bones. J Bone Joint Surg 67A:125–135, 1985.
70. Unni KK, Dahlin DC, Beabout JW, Ivins JC: Parosteal osteogenic sarcoma. Cancer 37:2466–2475, 1976.
71. Unni KK, Dahlin DC, Beabout JW: Periosteal osteogenic sarcoma. Cancer 37:2476–2485, 1976.
72. Goorin AM, Abelson HT, Frei E III: Osteosarcoma: A decade later. N Engl J Med 313:1637–1643, 1985.
73. Mankin HJ, Doppelt SH, Tomford WW: Clinical experience with allograft implantation. The first ten years. Clin Orthop 174:69–86, 1983.
74. Burrows HJ, Wilson JN, Scales JT: Excision of tumors of humerus and femur, with restoration by internal prosthesis. J Bone Joint Surg 57B:148–159, 1975.
75. Eckardt JJ, Eilber FR, Dorey FJ, Mirra JM: The UCLA experience in limb salvage for malignant tumors. Orthopaedics 8:612–626, 1985.
76. Gebhardt MC, Lane JM, McCormack RR, et al: Limb salvage in bone sarcomas—Memorial Hospital experience. Orthopaedics 8:626–640, 1985.
77. Malawar M: Surgical technique and results of limb sparing surgery for high grade bone sarcomas of the knee and shoulder. Orthopaedics 8:597–611, 1985.
78. Sim FH, Ivins JC, Pritchard DJ: Total joint arthroplasty. Applications in the management of bone tumors. Mayo Clin Proc 54:583–589, 1979.
79. Enneking WF, Shirley PD: Resection-arthrodesis for malignant and potentially malignant lesions about the knee using an intramedullary rod and local bone grafts. J Bone Joint Surg 59A:223–236, 1977.
80. Dunham WK, Calhoun JC: Resection arthrodesis of the knee for sarcoma. Preliminary results. Orthopaedics 7:1810–1818, 1984.
81. Gebhardt MC, McGuire MH, Mankin HJ: Resection and allograft arthrodesis for malignant bone tumors of the extremity. Bristol-Meyer/Zimmer Symposia: International Symposium on Limb Salvage in Musculoskeletal Oncology, 1985.
82. Lawrence WC: Limb-sparing treatment of adult soft-tissue sarcomas and osteosarcomas. Bethesda, MD, National Institutes of Health Consensus Development Conference Statement, 5:1984.
83. Carter SK: Adjuvant chemotherapy in osteogenic sarcoma: The triumph that isn't? J Clin Oncol 2:147–148, 1984.
84. Edmonson JH, Green SJ, Ivins JC, et al: A controlled pilot study of high-dose methotrexate as post-surgical adjuvant treatment of primary osteosarcoma. J Clin Oncol 2:152–156, 1984.
85. Cortes EP, Holland JF, Wang JJ, et al: Amputation and adriamycin in primary osteosarcoma. N Engl J Med 291:998–1000, 1974.
86. Sutow WW, Sullivan MP, Fernbach DJ, et al: Adjuvant chemotherapy in primary treatment of osteogenic sarcoma: A Southwest Oncology Group Study. Cancer 36:1598–1602, 1975.
87. Rosen G, Marcove RC, Huvox AG, et al: Primary osteogenic sarcoma: Eight-year experience with adjuvant chemotherapy. J Cancer Res Clin Oncol 106:55–67, 1983.

88. Taylor WF, Ivins JC, Dahlin DC, et al: Trends and variability in survival from osteosarcomas. Mayo Clin Proc 53:695–700, 1978.
89. Taylor WF, Ivins JC, Pritchard DJ, et al: Trends and variability in survival among patients with osteosarcoma: A 7-year update. Mayo Clin Proc 60:91–104, 1985.
90. Rosenberg SA, Flye MW, Conkle D, et al: Treatment of osteogenic sarcoma. II. Aggressive resection of pulmonary metastases. Cancer Treat Rep 63:753–756, 1979.
91. Cunningham JB, Ackerman LV: Metaphyseal fibrous defects. J Bone Joint Surg 38A:797–808, 1956.
92. Caffey J: On fibrous defects in cortical walls of growing tubular bones: Their radiographic appearance, structure, prevalence, natural course and diagnostic significance. Adv Pediatr 8:13–51, 1955.
93. Hatcher CH: The pathogenesis of localized lesions in the metaphysis of long bones. Ann Surg 122:1016–1030, 1945.
94. Broder HM: Possible precursor of unicameral bone cyst. J Bone Joint Surg 50A:549–552, 1982.
95. Devlin JA, Bowman HE, Mitchell CL: Non-osteogenic fibroma of bone. A review of the literature with the addition of six cases. J Bone Joint Surg 37A:472–486, 1955.
96. Dunham WK, Marcus NW, Enneking WF, Haun C: Developmental defects of the distal femoral metaphysis. J Bone Joint Surg 62A:801–806, 1980.
97. Grabias SL, Campbell CJ: Fibrous dysplasia. Orthop Clin North Am 8:771–783, 1977.
98. Stewart MJ, Gilmer WS, Edmonson AS: Fibrous dysplasia of bone. J Bone Joint Surg 44B:302–318, 1962.
99. Harris WH, Dudley R, Barry RJ: The natural history of fibrous dysplasia. J Bone Joint Surg 44A:207–233, 1962.
100. Henry A: Monostotic fibrous dysplasia. J Bone Joint Surg 51B:300–306, 1969.
101. Smy LL, Girgis IH, Wasef SA: Fibrous dysplasia in relation to the paranasal sinuses and the ear. J Laryngol Otol 81:1357–1371, 1967.
102. Albright F, Butler AM, Hampton AO, Smith P: Syndrome characterized by osteitic fibrosa dissemmata, areas of pigmentation and endocrine dysfunction, with precocious puberty in females. Report of five cases. N Engl J Med 216:727–746, 1937.
103. Danon M, Robboy MO, Kim S, et al: Cushing's syndrome, sexual precocity, and polyostotic fibrous dysplasia (Albright's syndrome) in infancy. J Pediatr 87:917–921, 1975.
104. Warwick CK: Polyostotic fibrous dysplasia—Albright's syndrome. A review of the literature and report of four male cases, two of which were associated with precocious puberty. J Bone Joint Surg 31B:175–183, 1949.
105. Huvos AG, Higginbotham NL, Miller TR: Bone sarcomas arising in fibrous dysplasia. J Bone Joint Surg 54A:1047–1056, 1972.
106. Cohen J: Unicameral bone cysts. A current synthesis of reported cases. Orthop Clin North Am 8:715–736, 1972.
107. Galasko CSB: The fate of simple bone cysts which fracture. Clin Orthop 101:302–304, 1974.
108. Grabias S, Mankin HJ: Chondrosarcoma arising in histologically proved unicameral bone cyst. A case report. J Bone Joint Surg 56A:1501–1509, 1974.
109. Neer CS, Francis KC, Marcove RC, et al: Treatment of unicameral bone cyst. A follow-up study of one hundred seventy-five cases. J Bone Joint Surg 48A:731–745, 1966.
110. Fahey J, O'Brien E: Subtotal resection and grafting in selected cases of solitary unicameral bone cysts. J Bone Joint Surg 55A:59–60, 1973.
111. McKay D: Treatment of unicameral bone cysts by subtotal resection without grafts. J Bone Joint Surg 59A:515–519, 1978.
112. Capanna R, Dal Monte A, Gitelis S, Campanacci M: The natural history of unicameral bone cyst after steroid injection. CORR 166:204–211, 1982.
113. Scaglietti O, Marchetti PG, Bartolozzi P: The effects of methylprednisilone acetate in the treatment of bone cysts. Results of three years followup. J Bone Joint Surg 61B:200–204, 1979.
114. Scaglietti O, Marchetti PG, Bartolozzi P: Final resuls obtained in the treatment of bone cysts with methylprednisilone acetate (Depo-Medral) and a discussion of results achieved in other bone lesions. CORR 165:33–42, 1982.
115. Campana R, Albisinni U, Picci P, et al: Aneurysmal bone cyst of the spine. J Bone Joint Surg 67A:527–531, 1985.
116. Slowick FA, Campbell CJ, Kettlekamp DB: Aneurysmal bone cyst. An analysis of thirteen cases. J Bone Joint Surg 50A:1142–1151, 1968.
117. Koskinen VS, Visuri TI, Holmstrom T, Roukkula MA: Aneurysmal bone cyst. Evaluation of resection and curettage in 20 cases. Clin Orthop 118:136–146, 1976.
118. Clough JR, Price CHG: Aneurysmal bone cyst: Pathogenesis and long term results of treatment. CORR 97:52–63, 1973.
119. Pritchard DJ, Sim FH, Ivins JC, et al: Fibrosarcoma of bone and soft tissues of the trunk and extremities. Orthop Clin North Am 8:869–881, 1977.
120. Eyer-Brook AL, Price CHG: Fibrosarcoma of bone. Review of fifty cases from the Bristol Bone Tumor Registry. J Bone Joint Surg 51B:20–37, 1973.
121. Dorfman HD, Norman A, Wolft H: Fibrosarcoma complicating bone infarction in a Caisson worker. J Bone Joint Surg 48A:528–532, 1966.
122. Gebhardt MC, Campbell CJ, Schiller AL, Mankin HJ: Desmoplastic fibroma of bone. A report of eight cases and review of the literature. J Bone Joint Surg 67A:732–747, 1985.
123. Huvos AG, Higginbotham NL: Primary fibrosarcoma of bone. A clinicopathologic study of 133 patients. Cancer 35:837–847, 1975.
124. Taconis WK, Van Rijssel TG: Fibrosarcoma of long bones. A study of the significance of areas of malignant fibrous histiocytoma. J Bone Joint Surg 67B:111–116, 1985.
125. Dahlin DC, Unni KK, Matsuno T: Malignant (fibrous) histiocytoma of bone—fact or fancy. Cancer 39:1508–1516, 1977.
126. Spanier SS, Enneking WF, Enriquez P: Primary malignant fibrous histiocytoma of bone. Cancer 36:2084–2098, 1975.
127. Bacci G, Springfield DS, Campana R, et al: Adjuvant chemotherapy for malignant fibrous histiocytoma in the femur and tibia. J Bone Joint Surg 67A:620–625, 1985.
128. Urban C, Rosen G, Huvos AG, et al: Chemotherapy of malignant fibrous histiocytoma of bone. A report of five cases. Cancer 51:795–802, 1983.
129. Yuen WWH, Saw D: Malignant fibrous histiocytoma of bone. J Bone Joint Surg 67A:482–486, 1985.

130. Unni KK, Dahlin DC: Premalignant tumors and conditions of bone. Am J Surg Pathol 3:47–60, 1977.
131. Penning BJ, Rosenthal DI, Gebhardt MC, et al: T1 versus water content in human chondrosarcoma. Presented at the Society of Magnetic Resonance in Medicine, Third Annual Meeting, New York, August 13–17, 1984.
132. Mankin HJ, Cantley KP, Lippiello L, et al: The biology of human chondrosarcoma. I. Description of the cases, grading and biochemical analysis. J Bone Joint Surg 62A:160–176, 1980.
133. Mankin HJ, Cantley KP, Schiller AL, Lippiello L: The biology of human chondrosarcoma. II. Variation in chemical composition among types and subtypes of benign and malignant cartilage tumors. J Bone Joint Surg 62A:176–194, 1980.
134. McFarland GB Jr, Morden ML: Benign cartilaginous lesions. Orthop Clin North Am 8:749–751, 1977.
135. Lewis RJ, Ketcham AS: Mafucci's syndrome: Functional and neoplastic significance. Case report and review of the literature. J Bone Joint Surg 55A:1465–1479, 1973.
136. Maroteaux P: Bone Disease in Children. Philadelphia, JB Lippincott, 1979, pp 93–97.
137. Huvos AG, Marcove RC: Chondroblastoma of bone. A critical review. Clin Orthop 95:300–311, 1973.
138. Jaffe HL, Lichenstein L: Benign chondroblastoma of bone. A reinterpretation of the so-called calcifying or chondromatous giant cell tumor. Am J Pathol 18:909–983, 1942.
139. Schajowicz F, Gallardo H: Epiphyseal chondrosarcoma of bone. A clinico-pathologic study of thirty-two cases. J Bone Joint Surg 52B:205–226, 1970.
140. Springfield DS, Campana R, Gherlinzoni F, et al: Chondroblastoma. A review of seventy cases. J Bone Joint Surg 67A:748–755, 1985.
141. Green P, Whittaker RP: Benign chondroblastoma. Case report with pulmonary metastasis. J Bone Joint Surg 57A:418–419, 1975.
142. Huvos AG, Higginbotham NL, Marcove RC, O'Leary P: Aggressive chondroblastoma. Review of the literature on aggressive behavior and metastases with a report of one new case. Clin Orthop 126:266–272, 1977.
143. Gherlinzoni F, Rock M, Picci P: Chondromyxoid fibroma. The experience at the Instituto Ortopedico Rizzoli. J Bone Joint Surg 65A:198–204, 1983.
144. Ralph LL: Chondromyxoid fibroma of bone. J Bone Joint Surg 44B:7–24, 1962.
145. Schajowicz F, Gallardo H: Chondromyxoid fibroma (fibromycoid chondroma) of bone. A clinico-pathologic study of thirty-two cases. J Bone Joint Surg 53B:198–216, 1971.
146. D'Ambrosia R, Ferguson AB Jr: The formation of osteochondroma by epiphyseal transplantation. Clin Orthop 61:103–115, 1968.
147. Jaffe N, Reid HL, Cohen M, et al: Radiation induced osteochondroma in long-term survivors of childhood cancer. Int J Radiat Oncol Biol Phys 9:665–670, 1983.
148. Katzman H, Waugh T, Berdon W: Skeletal changes following irradiation of childhood tumors. J Bone Joint Surg 51A:825–842, 1969.
149. Murphy FD, Blount WP: Cartilaginous exostoses following irradiation. J Bone Joint Surg 44A:662–668, 1962.
150. Morton KS: On the question of recurrence of osteochondroma. J Bone Joint Surg 46B:723–725, 1964.
151. Jaffe HL: Hereditary multiple exostosis. Arch Pathol 36:335–357, 1943.
152. Shapiro F, Simon S, Glimcher MJ: Hereditary multiple exostoses. J Bone Joint Surg 61A:815–824, 1979.
153. Solomon L: Bone growth in diaphyseal acalsis. J Bone Joint Surg 43B:700–716, 1961.
154. Solomon L: Hereditary multiple exostosis. J Bone Joint Surg 45B:292–304, 1963.
155. Dahlin DC, Henderson ED: Mesenchymal chondrosarcoma. Further observations in a new entity. Cancer 15:401–410, 1962.
156. Dowling EA: Mesenchymal chondrosarcoma. J Bone Joint Surg 46A:747–754, 1964.
157. Huvos AG, Rosen G, Dabaska M, Marcove RC: Mesenchymal chondrosarcoma. A clinicopathologic analysis of 35 patients with emphasis on treatment. Cancer 51:1230–1237, 1983.
158. Salvador AH, Beabout JW, Dahlin DC: Mesenchymal chondrosarcoma—observations on 30 new cases. Cancer 28:605–615, 1971.
159. Dahlin DC, Beabout JW: Dedifferentiation of low grade chondrosarcoma. Cancer 28:461–466, 1971.
160. McFarland GB Jr, McKinley LM, Reed RJ: Dedifferentiation of low-grade chondrosarcoma. Clin Orthop 112:157–164, 1977.
161. Mirra JM, Marcove RC: Fibrosarcomatous dedifferentiation of primary and secondary chondrosarcoma. J Bone Joint Surg 56A:285–296, 1974.
162. Unni KK, Dahlin DC, Beabout JW, Sim FH: Chondrosarcoma: Clear-cell variant. J Bone Joint Surg 58A:676–683, 1976.
163. Barnes R, Catto M: Chondrosarcoma of bone. J Bone Joint Surg 48B:729–764, 1969.
164. Gitelis S, Gertoni FCPP, Campanacci M: Chondrosarcoma of bone. The experience at the Instituto Ortopedico Rizzoli. J Bone Joint Surg 63A:1248–1257, 1981.
165. Henderson ED, Dahlin DC: Chondrosarcoma of bone—a study of two hundred and eighty-eight cases. J Bone Joint Surg 45A:1450–1458, 1963.
166. Pritchard DJ, Lunke RJ, Taylor WF, et al: Chondrosarcoma: A clinicopathologic and statistical analysis. Cancer 45:149–157, 1980.
167. Eriksson AI, Schiller A, Mankin HJ: The management of chondrosarcoma of bone. Clin Orthop 153:44–66, 1980.
168. Rosenberg L, Francis K, Gallo G, et al: Isolation and characterization of proteoglycan subunit and proteoglycan aggregate from human chondrosarcoma. Orthop Trans 1:47–48, 1977.
169. Cuvelier CA, Roels HJ: Cytometric studies of the nuclear content in cartilaginous tumors. Cancer 44:1374–1463, 1979.
170. Kissane JM, Askin FB, Nesbit MEJ, et al: Sarcomas of bone in childhood: Pathologic aspects. NCI Monogr 56:29–41, 1981.
171. Yunis EJ, Walpusk JA, Agostini RM, Hubbard JD: Glycogen in neuroblastomas. A light- and electron-microscopic study of 40 cases. Am J Surg Pathol 3:313–323, 1979.
172. Sim FH, Unni KK, Beabout JW, et al: Osteosarcoma with small cells simulating Ewing's tumor. J Bone Joint Surg 61A:207–215, 1979.
173. Kissane JM, Askin FB, Foulkes M, et al: Ewing's sarcoma of bone: Clinicopathologic aspects of 303 cases from the Intergroup Ewing's Sarcoma Study. Hum Pathol 14:773–779, 1983.

174. Pritchard DJ, Dahlin DC, Dauphine RT, Beabout JW: Ewing's sarcoma. A clinicopathological and statistical analysis of patients surviving five years or longer. J Bone Joint Surg 55A:10–16, 1975.
175. Glaubiger DL, Makuch RW, Schwarz J: Influence of prognostic factors on survival in Ewing's sarcoma. Natl Cancer Inst Monogr 56:285–288, 1981.
176. Kinsella TJ, Lichter AS, Miser J, et al: Local treatment of Ewing's sarcoma: Radiation therapy versus surgery. Cancer Treat Rep 68:695–701, 1984.
177. Tepper J, Glaubiger D, Lichter A, et al: Local control of Ewing's sarcoma of bone with radiotherapy and combination chemotherapy. Cancer 46:1969–1973, 1980.
178. Springfield DS, Pagliarulo C: Fracture of long bones previously treated for Ewing's sarcoma. J Bone Joint Surg 67A:477–481, 1985.
179. Jentzsch K, Binder H, Cramer H, et al: Leg function after radiotherapy for Ewing's sarcoma. Cancer 47:1267–1278, 1982.
180. Greene MH, Glaubiger DL, Mead GD, Fraumeni JFJ: Subsequent cancer in patients with Ewing's sarcoma. Cancer Treat Rep 63:2043–2046, 1979.
181. Li FP, Cassady R, Jaffe N: The risk of second tumors in survivors of childhood cancer. Cancer 35:1230–1235, 1975.
181a. Strong LC, Herson J, Osborn BM, Sutow WW: Risk of radiation-related subsequent malignant tumors in survivors of Ewing's sarcoma. JNCI 62:1401–1406, 1979.
182. Bacci G, Picci P, Gitelis S, et al: The treatment of localized Ewing's sarcoma: The experience of the Instituto Ortopedico Rizzoli in 163 cases treated with and without chemotherapy. Cancer 49:1561–1570, 1982.
183. Gehan EA, Nesbit MEJ, Vietti TJ, et al: Prognostic factors in children with Ewing's sarcoma. Natl Cancer Inst Monogr 56:273–278, 1981.
184. Lewis RJ, Marcove RC, Rosen G: Ewing's sarcoma. J Bone Joint Surg 59A:325–331, 1977.
185. Marcove RC, Rosen G: Radical en bloc excision of Ewing's sarcoma. Clin Orthop 153:86–91, 1980.
186. Li W, Lane JM, Rosen G, et al: Pelvic Ewing's sarcoma. Advances in treatment. J Bone Joint Surg 65A:738–747, 1983.
187. Pritchard DJ: Small Cell Tumors of Bone. St. Louis, CV Mosby, Instructional Course Lectures, vol 33, 1984, pp 26–39.
188. Reimer RR, Chabner BA, Young RC, et al: Lymphoma presenting in bone. Results of histopathology, staging and therapy. Ann Int Med 87:50–55, 1977.
189. Hait WN, Faber L, Cadman E: Non-Hodgkin's lymphoma for the nononcologist. JAMA 253:1431–1435, 1985.
190. Boston HC Jr, Dahlin DC, Ivins JC, Cupps RE: Malignant lymphoma (so-called reticulum cell sarcoma) of bone. Cancer 34:1131–1137, 1974.
191. Shorji H, Miller TR: Primary reticulum cell sarcoma of bone. Significance of clinical features upon the prognosis. Cancer 28:1234–1244, 1971.
192. Conrad EU, Lane JM, Marcove RC, et al: Giant cell tumors treated with cryosurgery. Orthop Trans 9: 468–469, 1985.
193. Kyle RA: Multiple myeloma. Review of 869 cases. Mayo Clinic Proc 50:29–40, 1975.
194. Griffiths DL: Orthopaedic aspects of myelomatosis. J Bone Joint Surg 48B:703–728, 1966.
195. Kyle RA: Long-term survival in multiple myeloma. N Engl J Med 308:314–316, 1983.
196. Cornwell GG III, Pajak TF, Kochwa S, et al: Comparison of oral melphalan, CCNU, and BCNU with and without vincristine and prednisone in the treatment of multiple myeloma. Cancer 50:1669–1675, 1982.
197. Goldenberg RR, Campbell CJ, Bonfiglio M: Giant cell tumor of bone. An analysis of two hundred and eighteen cases. J Bone Joint Surg 52A:619–664, 1970.
198. Averill RM, Smith J, Campbell CJ: Giant cell tumors of the bones of the hand. J Hand Surg 5:39–50, 1980.
199. Peimer CA, Schiller AL, Mankin HJ, Smith RS: Multicentric giant cell tumor of bone. J Bone Joint Surg 62A:652–656, 1980.
200. Bertoni F, Present D, Enneking WF: Giant cell tumor of bone with pulmonary metastases. J Bone Joint Surg 67A:890–900, 1985.
201. Rock MG, Pritchard DJ, Unni KK: Metastasis from histologically benign giant cell tumors of bone. J Bone Joint Surg 66A:269–274, 1984.
202. Schajowicz F: Giant-cell tumors of bone (osteoclastoma). A pathological and histochemical study. J Bone Joint Surg 43A:1–29, 1961.
203. Goldring SR, Dayer JM, Russell RGG, et al: Cells cultured from human giant cell tumor of bone respond to parathyroid hormone. Calcif Tissue Res [Suppl] 22:269–274, 1977.
204. Dahlin DC, Capps RE, Johnson EWJ: Giant cell tumor: A study of 195 cases. Cancer 25:1061–1070, 1970.
205. Persson BM, Wouters HW: Curettage and acrylic cementation in surgery of giant cell tumors of bone. CORR 126:125–133, 1976.
206. Marcove R: A 17-year review of cryosurgery in the treatment of bone tumors. Clin Orthop 163:231–234, 1982.
207. Wallace S, Granmaylia M, DeSantos LA, et al: Arterial occlusion of pelvic bone tumor. Cancer 43:322–328, 1979.
208. Bell RS, Harwood AR, Goodman SB, Fornasier VL: Supervoltage radiotherapy in the treatment of difficult giant cell tumors of bone. Clin Orthop 174:208–216, 1983.
209. Harwood AR, Fornasier UL, Rider WD: Supervoltage irradiation in the management of giant-cell tumor of bone. Radiology 125:223–226, 1977.
210. Johnston AD: Pathology of metastatic tumors in bone. Clin Orthop 73:8–32, 1970.
211. Lodwick GS: The radiographic diagnosis of metastatic cancer in bone. *In* Tumors of Bone and Soft Tissue, University of Texas MD Anderson Hospital and Institute. Chicago, Yearbook Medical Publishers, 1965, pp 253–268.
212. Bryan RS, Soule EH, Dobyns JH, et al: Metastatic lesions of the hand and forearm. Clin Orthop 101:167–170, 1974.
213. Healey JH, Miedema B, Turnbull A, Lane JM: Treatment of metastasis to the hands and feet. Orthop Trans 9:447–448, 1985.
214. Springfield DS: Mechanisms of metastasis. Clin Orthop 169:95–102, 1982.
215. Galasco CSB: Mechanisms of lytic and blastic metastatic disease of bone. Clin Orthop 169:20–27, 1982.
216. Gebhardt MC, Lippiello L, Bringhurst FR, Mankin HJ: Prostaglandin E2 synthesis by human primary and metastatic bone tumors in culture. Clin Orthop 196:300–305, 1985.

217. Bhardwaj S, Halland JF: Chemotherapy of metastatic cancer in bone. Clin Orthop 169:28–37, 1982.
218. Krishramunthy GT, Tubis M, Hiss J, Blahd WN: Distribution pattern of metastatic bone disease. A need for total body skeletal image. JAMA 237:2504–2506, 1977.
219. Batson OV: The role of the vertebral veins in metastatic process. Ann Intern Med 16:38–45, 1942.
220. Saitoh H, Hida M, Shimbo T, et al: Metastatic patterns of prostatic cancer. Correlation between sites and number of organisms involved. Cancer 54:3078–3084, 1984.
221. Berry WR, Laszlo J, Cox E, et al: Prognostic factors in metastatic and hormonally unresponsive carcinoma of the prostate. Cancer 44:763–775, 1979.
222. Blair RJ, McAfee JG: Radiological detection of skeletal metastases: Radiographs versus scans. Int J Radiat Oncol Biol Phys 1:1201–1205, 1976.
223. Meyor PC: A statistical and histological survey of metastatic carcinoma in the skeleton. Br J Cancer 11:509–518, 1957.
224. Ihle PM, McBeath AA: Bone metastasis from colonic cancer. A case report. J Bone Joint Surg 55A:398–399, 1973.
225. Bowers TA, Murray JA, Charnsangarej C, et al: Bone metastases from renal carcinoma. J Bone Joint Surg 64A:749–754, 1982.
226. Silverberg SG, Evans RH, Koehler AL: Clinical and pathological features of initial metastatic presentations of renal cell carcinoma. Cancer 21:1126–1132, 1969.
227. McCormack KR: Bone metastases from thyroid carcinoma. Cancer 19:181–184, 1966.
228. Harrington KD: New trends in the management of lower extremity metastases. Clin Orthop 169:53–61, 1982.
229. Sherry HS, Levy RN, Siffert RS: Metastastic disease of bone in orthopaedic surgery. CORR 169:44–52, 1982.
230. Shocken JD, Luther WB: Radiation therapy for bone metastasis. CORR 169:38–43, 1982.
231. Haberman ET, Sachs R, Stern RE, et al: The pathology and treatment of metastatic disease of the femur. Clin Orthop 169:70–82, 1982.
232. Boland PJ, Land JM, Sundaresan N: Metastatic disease of the spine. Clin Orthop 169:95–102, 1982.

GREGORY R. MUNDY

21

Hypercalcemia of Malignancy

Hypercalcemia is a very frequent complication of malignant disease. It occurs in approximately 30% of patients with advanced breast cancer and possibly up to 20% of patients with lung cancer, the two most common forms of malignant disease seen in Western communities. This chapter reviews the pathophysiology, the types of malignant disease that are associated with hypercalcemia, the clinical features of hypercalcemia associated with malignant disease, and finally the management of patients with hypercalcemia associated with malignancy.

I. PATHOPHYSIOLOGY

Types of Malignancies Associated with Hypercalcemia. Although hypercalcemia is seen frequently in common malignancies such as lung cancer and breast cancer, there are other common forms of malignancies in which hypercalcemia is rare.[1] There is not a direct relationship between the presence of bone metastases and the occurrence of hypercalcemia. For example, tumors of the gastrointestinal tract and female genitalia are frequently associated with metastatic bone disease but rarely are associated with hypercalcemia. The tumors most frequently associated with hypercalcemia are squamous cell carcinomas of the lung, head, neck, breast cancer of all varieties, hematologic malignancies including myeloma and T cell lymphomas, renal cancer, and some unusual malignancies such as the VIPomas and cholangiocarcinomas. Unlike other ectopic hormone syndromes, hypercalcemia is rare in oat cell carcinoma of the lung. The relative frequencies of the types of malignant disease associated with hypercalcemia are demonstrated in Table 21–1.

Pathophysiology of Hypercalcemia. Hypercalcemia associated with malignant disease is due to a combination of complex pathophysiologic events affecting fluxes of calcium across the skeleton, kidney, and gut. The primary cause is the release of calcium from bone into the extracellular fluid by increased osteoclastic bone resorption. However, it is also clear that renal factors are important. Under most circumstances, increased entry of calcium from bone will be filtered by the kidneys so that homeostatic control of the extracellular fluid calcium concentration is maintained. However, in malignant disease, a number of events occur in the kidney that interfere with this homeostatic regulation of calcium. These include (1) volume depletion, with impairment of glomerular filtration rate, which in turn leads to increased renal tubular sodium and calcium reabsorption in the proximal convoluted tubules; and (2) increased renal tubular calcium reabsorption independent of volume depletion. It is likely that in some tumors associated with the hypercalcemia of malignancy, factors produced by the tumors are renotropic and increase calcium reabsorption from the renal tubules, probably in a manner similar to that of parathyroid hormone. The relative importance of these renal effects varies from tumor to tumor. In myeloma, hypercalcemia is an unusual occurrence in the absence of impaired glomerular filtration. However, in solid tumors associated with hypercalcemia, glomerular filtration is usually adequate, and increased renal tubular

Table 21–1. Malignancies Associated with Hypercalcemia

Types of Malignancy	Percentage of Total
Lung	35
Breast	25
Hematologic (myeloma, lymphoma)	14
Head and neck	6
Renal	3
Prostate	3
Unknown primary	7
Others	

calcium reabsorption occurs presumably because of increased humoral effects of calcium-retaining factors on the renal tubules.[2,3]

Although these renal effects may be important in enhancing hypercalcemia, it is unlikely that renal calcium reabsorption alone can produce hypercalcemia. Hypercalcemia is due primarily to an increase in bone resorption, which is on most occasions due to the production by tumor cells of factors that stimulate osteoclast activity. These factors are undergoing intense investigation and vary with different types of tumors. A clearer understanding of the hypercalcemia of malignancy can be gained by dividing patients with this syndrome into three clinical groups on the basis of the differing pathogenic mechanisms that are responsible for increasing the entry of calcium from bone into the extracellular fluid.

A. Hematologic Malignancies

1. Myeloma

In myeloma, osteolytic bone lesions are almost invariable, and hypercalcemia occurs in 20% to 40% of patients. As already indicated, hypercalcemia rarely occurs unless the patient has impaired glomerular filtration. Patients with myeloma are predisposed to renal failure because of Bence-Jones proteinuria, urinary tract infection, and uric acid nephropathy. The bone destruction is due to a local factor released by the myeloma cells called osteoclast-activating factor (OAF), which is the same or similar to a lymphokine released by normal activated lymphocytes.[4,5] Release of this factor results in activation of adjacent osteoclasts, which in turn are responsible for resorbing the bone and causing the characteristic bone lesions. The evidence that osteoclast activating factor is responsible is based on a series of cell and organ culture experiments showing that myeloma cells produce this factor *in vitro*.[6–9] It has been shown that a number of lymphokines and monokines resorb bone *in vitro*, including lymphotoxin, tumor necrosis factor, and interleukin-1.[10,11] The role of these factors in myeloma has not yet been investigated. (See Comment at end of chapter.)

2. Lymphomas

Some types of lymphomas are also associated with bone lesions and hypercalcemia.[12] A syndrome of adult T cell lymphoma has been reported in which bone lesions and hypercalcemia have been an almost universal finding.[13] This condition has occurred in clusters in Japan, the West Indies, and the southern United States. The disease is due to a human type C retrovirus that is carried by mature T lymphocytes of the helper-inducer type. It also appears that some tumors have the capacity to synthesize 1,25-dihydroxyvitamin D, a powerful bone-resorbing factor, which could also play a role in the osteolytic bone lesions seen in this condition.[14] Some patients have increased serum 1,25-dihydroxyvitamin D.[15–18] It is unclear what the relationship is between the lymphokine produced by these cells and the factor produced by myeloma cells, which are the neoplastic progeny of a different subset of lymphocytes.

Occasionally other types of lymphomas that are non–virus-associated cause hypercalcemia. The mechanism in these conditions remains to be clarified.

B. Solid Tumors with Metastasis

In many patients with hypercalcemia there is extensive bone destruction due to osteolytic bone metastasis. Many tumors may cause hypercalcemia in association with bone metastasis, but the tumor most frequently associated with osteolytic bone destruction and hypercalcemia is breast cancer. Although it is possible that in some of these patients hypercalcemia is due to a humoral systemic factor produced by the tumor cell and the presence of the metastases is irrelevant, it is clear that in some cases the extent of bone metastasis is related to the hypercalcemia. This is most apparent in breast cancer, in which hypercalcemia almost never occurs early in the course of the disease or in the absence of extensive bone metastasis.[1]

The cellular mechanism of bone destruction in metastatic cancer may be twofold. Although increased osteoclastic activity is an important mechanism for bone destruction, it is also likely that tumor cells may have a direct erosive effect themselves.[19] *In vitro*, tumor cells have the capacity to resorb bone directly related to the release of lysosomal enzymes.[20–22] Manipulations of tumor cells *in vitro* that stimulate lysosomal enzyme release also are associated with increased resorption of devitalized bone substrates.[21,22] A metastatic tumor could stimulate osteoclastic bone resorption by multiple mechanisms, including the local production of prostaglandins of the E series, or the production of lymphokines such as osteoclast-activating factor or interleukin-1 by the monocytes and lymphocytes that accumulate at the site of the metastatic deposit as part of the cell-mediated immune response to the presence of the tumor. Although all of these mechanisms are possible and most have been demonstrated *in vitro*, their relative importance in the clinical situation or *in vivo* is entirely unknown.

Occasionally patients with breast cancer develop hypercalcemia when they are treated with estrogens or anti-estrogens. This can occur even when the tumor responds favorably to the presence of hormonal manipulations as far as tumor growth and progression are concerned. We have found that when breast cancer cells with estrogen receptors are treated with estrogens or anti-estrogens *in vitro*, they release large amounts of prostaglandins of the E series in parallel with bone-resorbing activity.[23] These effects can be inhibited by treatment of the cells with prostaglandin synthesis inhibitors such as indomethacin. It is possible, therefore, that estrogen- or anti-estrogen–induced hypercalcemia that occurs clinically may be due to release of prostaglandins locally by metastatic tumor cells that activate adjacent osteoclasts to increase the release of calcium from bone into the extracellular fluid.

The mechanisms by which tumor cells metastasize to bone surfaces has not been clearly defined, although *in vitro* techniques have been developed to clarify some of the molecular mechanisms involved.[24–26] Tumor cells metastasize by being shed from the primary site, possibly related to the production of proteolytic enzymes by the tumor tissue itself. Once shed from the primary site, tumor cells can enter the circulation and then spread to vascular organs such as the red bone marrow. Once within the marrow cavity, the tumor cells migrate through wide-channeled marrow sinusoids. They may be attracted out of the sinusoids toward endosteal bone surfaces to cause bone destruction by the release of local osteoclast-stimulating agents or by direct effect of the tumor cells themselves. We have found *in vitro* that tumor cell migration can be enhanced by the conditioned medium that is harvested from resorbing or remodeling bone.[24,25] In addition, tumor cell migration can be stimulated by fragments of type I collagen, which are chemotactic for tumor cells.[26] It is possible that these fragments of collagen could be released from bone by the action of tumor cells at endosteal bone surfaces and cause the attraction of the tumor cells toward bone, where they could then, in turn, stimulate resorption either by a direct effect of the tumor cells themselves as indicated previously or by releasing local factors that stimulate osteoclasts that lie along endosteal bone surfaces.

It is clear that much work needs to be done to understand the cellular and molecular events by which tumor cells are selectively attracted toward bone in patients with metastatic disease and then how they are capable of destroying bone to produce the osteolytic deposit.

C. Solid Tumors Associated with Increased Bone Resorption and Hypercalcemia

Hypercalcemia occurs in some cases in the absence of bone metastasis or in the presence of minimal bone metastasis. In these situations it is clear that the tumor cells are producing a humoral factor that stimulates osteoclastic bone resorption to increase the entry of calcium into the extracellular fluid. There is a great amount of current research aimed at identifying and characterizing the humoral factors responsible for increasing osteoclastic bone resorption. A number of candidates have been suggested over the years.

1. Transforming Growth Factors

Transforming growth factors are a family of polypeptide stimulators of cell growth and replication that have biological properties that overlap with those of epidermal growth factor (EGF).[27] These polypeptides are acid-soluble and acid-stable compounds that are probably produced by all tumors. They represent a family of factors and not all have the same biological properties. However, the one property that they all have in common is their capacity to maintain the transformed phenotype in cells that are normally nonneoplastic. This is assayed *in vitro* by their capacity to stimulate soft agar colony formation of fibroblasts, which do not grow otherwise in anchorage-independent conditions.[28] We have studied purified preparations of the transforming growth factors and found that they are powerful stimulators of osteoclastic bone resorption. Transforming growth factors belong to two general classes, one that depends on occupancy of the EGF receptor for its biological effects (TGF-alpha),[29] and one that functions independently of the EGF receptor (TGF-beta).[30]

We have found that large molecular weight transforming growth factors of the alpha series are responsible for the increased bone resorption that occurs in some animal models of the hypercalcemia of malignancy. The evidence is based on co-purification of the transforming growth factor of the alpha series with bone-resorbing activity harvested from tumor extracts and conditioned media from the cultured cells.[31] Moreover, specific antisera, which block the activity of the transforming growth factors by occupying the EGF receptor, inhibit activity of the tumor-derived bone-resorbing factor.[32] However, it is clear that this particular variety of transforming growth factor cannot account for all of the increased bone resorption that occurs in tumors associated with the hypercalcemia of malignancy. Recently, we have shown that synthetic TGF-alpha resorbs bone *in vitro*,[33] and we and others have shown that human recombinant TGF-alpha also resorbs bone *in vitro*.[34–36]

2. Parathyroid Hormone

It is clear that parathyroid hormone (PTH) cannot account for the hypercalcemia of malignancy associated with nonparathyroid tumors. In most current immunoassays, immunoreactive parathyroid hormone concentrations are suppressed.[1,37] Moreover, a specific cDNA probe for parathyroid hormone that employs base pair hybridization of cloned PTH DNA to detect mRNA for parathyroid hormone shows that most tumors associated with the hypercalcemia of malignancy do not contain detectable PTH mRNA.[38] We have found only one tumor out of 30 associated with hypercalcemia that contained PTH mRNA, and in this case the evidence suggested that PTH mRNA was not translated or secreted by the tumor cells (Jacobs and Mundy, unpublished observations). These data indicate that nonparathyroid tumors rarely synthesize parathyroid hormone, and it is apparent that parathyroid hormone is at most a rare cause of the hypercalcemia of malignancy.

3. Prostaglandins

Although prostaglandins may be responsible for increased bone resorption occurring in some patients with metastatic cancer, it is unlikely that they could be responsible for the humoral hypercalcemia associated with human malignancies. No circulating bone-resorbing prostaglandin has been described that is powerful enough to induce hypercalcemia. Moreover, prostaglandin production by tumors does not correlate well with calcium levels in those situations in which a humoral mechanism is responsible. Nevertheless, it is possible that prostaglandins of the E series can be responsible for the hypercalcemia that has been described in several animal models.[39,40] Drugs that inhibit prostaglandin synthesis such as indomethacin are generally ineffective in the treatment of cancer associated with hypercalcemia.[41]

4. Other Factors

Other factors, which have not been shown to stimulate bone resorption, have been implicated in the hypercalcemia of malignancy.

PTH-like Factors. Many tumors associated with hypercalcemia produce factors that engage the parathyroid hormone receptor, although they are clearly not parathyroid hormone. The assays used to identify these factors are based on stimulation of adenylate cyclase activity in canine renal membranes or on cultured rat osteosarcoma cells or measurement of increased G6PD content in renal tubular cells.[42–44] These effects are inhibited by specific antagonists of parathyroid hormone, and therefore it is reasoned that these factors are interacting with parathyroid hormone receptors. It is likely that they may be responsible for clinical manifestations of the hypercalcemia of malignancy including increased renal phosphate wasting, increased cyclic AMP generation, and increased reabsorption of calcium by the kidneys.

Colony-Stimulating Activity. Recently, some workers have shown that tumors associated with hypercalcemia also produce factors that have colony-stimulating activity for cells of the monocyte-macrophage family.[45–48] Nude mice carrying these tumors may develop leukocytosis, and it has been postulated that a colony-stimulating factor that could affect cells of the monocyte-phagocyte series (the presumed precursors of osteoclasts) could also be associated with leukocytosis as well as increased osteoclast activity and hypercalcemia. However, these factors have not been clearly identified or characterized as yet, and preliminary studies suggest that they probably do not co-purify with bone-resorbing activity. Moreover, this mechanism could not account for hypercalcemia in more than a small number of cases, since most patients with hypercalcemia do not have leukocytosis.

II. CLINICAL FEATURES

The clinical features of hypercalcemic patients with malignant disease are similar to the clinical features associated with hypercalcemia due to other causes. These have been well described before on numerous occasions. The most outstanding clinical features of hypercalcemia are neurologic and gastrointestinal. The neurologic features include lethargy, confusion, nightmares, stupor, and in extreme cases coma followed by death. The most prominent gastrointestinal features are nausea and vomiting associated with anorexia and occasionally constipation. Constipation is a much rarer symptom in patients with malignancy than it is in patients with primary hyperparathyroidism. Other organ systems may also be affected, particularly the urinary tract. Hypercalcemia is always associated with loss of concentrating ability and insensitivity to antidiuretic hormone. In some patients there may also be impaired renal function, particularly when the serum phosphorus is high or when the patient has myeloma. Renal stones, which are common in patients with hyperparathyroidism, are rare in patients with the hypercalcemia of malignancy, presumably because hypercalcemia is not of long-standing enough duration for this complication to occur.

Although the clinical features of hypercalcemia due to malignancy are similar to the features of hypercalcemia due to other causes, nevertheless there are some special features of hypercalcemia associated with malignancy. Hypercalcemia may develop very rapidly, and for this reason symptoms may be apparent at relatively lower serum calcium concentrations. For instance, patients with primary hyperparathyroidism of long-standing duration may tolerate a serum calcium that is in the range of 15 mg/100 ml without noticeable symptoms. In contrast, patients with malignant disease who have been normocalcemic but develop hypercalcemia very rapidly may become symptomatic with much lesser elevations in the serum calcium. Another point is that the symptoms of hypercalcemia that are so distressing for the patient, in particular gastrointestinal symptoms, may be confused with other causes in patients with malignant disease. For example, patients treated with cytotoxic drug therapy or irradiation therapy frequently develop nausea and vomiting, and the symptoms caused by hypercalcemia can be confused with those due to these therapies.

III. TREATMENT

A. Indications for Treatment

Patients in whom the serum calcium is greater than 13 mg/100 ml or patients who are symptomatic should be treated urgently. Asymptomatic patients with corrected total serum calcium less than 12 mg/100 ml should be followed very carefully. In the hypercalcemia of malignancy, hypercalcemia is progressive and may develop very rapidly over a period of a few weeks. This contrasts with primary hyperparathyroidism, in which hypercalcemia may remain constant for many years. This observation influences our treatment decision. Even in asymptomatic patients with minor elevations in the serum calcium, we advise treatment, since it is likely that more severe and possibly life-threatening hypercalcemia will develop rapidly. Similar elevations in the serum calcium in primary hyperparathyroidism may not cause any symptoms if the serum calcium has been constant for years, and in that situation active treatment may not be necessary (see Chapter 14).

B. Choice of Treatment

The treatment of hypercalcemia of malignancy may be considered under two categories:

1. Urgent treatment for those patients who are symptomatic or who have a serum calcium greater than 13 mg/100 ml.
2. Chronic treatment, for those patients who have mild hypercalcemia and are ambulant.

Before therapy for hypercalcemia is commenced, treatment of the underlying malignancy should be considered. In many patients and particularly in patients with myeloma, chemotherapy that is effective against the underlying malignancy will relieve the hypercalcemia. In addition, any drugs that can potentiate or precipitate hypercalcemia, such as thiazide diuretics, estrogens, or anti-estrogens (in the case of breast cancer), should be discontinued, and immobilization, which enhances bone loss, should be avoided if possible.

1. Urgent Treatment for Hypercalcemia

The agents available for the urgent treatment of hypercalcemia are intravenous saline, calcitonin and glucocorticoids, loop diuretics, and parenteral phosphate.

Intravenous Saline. The treatment of choice is intravenous saline. Saline is recommended because a sodium diuresis is accompanied by a calcium diuresis. Saline should be delivered with some care because some patients may become hypernatremic, particularly if they are obtunded and do not have an intact thirst mechanism. The pathophysiology of saline-induced hypernatremia is probably related to the loss of concentrating ability and relative resistance to antidiuretic hormone that occurs with hypercalcemia. This results in continued excretion of free water and subsequent increase in the serum sodium concentration when large volumes of isotonic saline are administered, particularly to the obtunded patient who does not have normal thirst sensation. Hypernatremia can be readily reversed by the administration of hypotonic fluids.

Calcitonin and Glucocorticoids. Calcitonin and glucocorticoids are relatively safe and effective in the acute treatment of hypercalcemia, particularly if the hypercalcemia is due to a hematologic malignancy.[49] They have the advantage that they can be used at the same time as rehydration and they can be used in patients with poor renal function. They are effective in about 80% of patients and work within 4 to 6 hours. Salmon calcitonin should be administered in doses of 200 to 400 MRC units each 12 hours subcutaneously, and hydrocortisone 100 mg intravenously each 6 hours. They are least effective in patients with primary hyperparathyroidism or parathyroid carcinoma in our experience, but there are notable exceptions recorded in the literature,[50] and their safety and relative efficacy make them worthy of trial.

Furosemide. Although furosemide has been widely used, it is unlikely to be effective unless it is used in very large doses (100 mg every hour),[51] and when used in this way it is not very convenient. The administration of furosemide in this manner requires the patient to be housed on an intensive care unit with careful monitoring of all fluids and electrolytes. In addition the patient must be fully rehydrated before these doses of furosemide are commenced, because this diuretic may promote extracellular fluid volume depletion, which will worsen hypercalcemia rather than relieve it. There is no evidence that furosemide in smaller doses has any beneficial effect on hypercalcemia, and it will worsen it if the patient is not fully rehydrated. The evidence that even in larger doses it has substantive effects beyond that of the fluid load is weak. Furosemide may be indicated for those unusual patients with hypercalcemia who are fluid overloaded, but here the indication for treatment with furosemide is for fluid overload and not because of its efficacy in lowering the serum calcium.

Intravenous Phosphate. Parenteral phosphate is very effective in lowering the serum calcium.[52] However, this therapy is dangerous because it lowers the serum calcium by depositing calcium in soft tissues, including the lungs, heart, and kidney.[53] The mortality associated with this form of therapy may be high, and we believe it should be reserved for desperate situations in which no other therapy is possible or effective.

Dialysis. Peritoneal or hemodialysis has been occasionally used for the treatment of hypercalcemia.[54] It may be transiently effective for lowering the serum calcium but has no effect on the increased bone resorption that is the primary cause of hypercalcemia. The mortality is usually high in these patients and this is probably due to the moribund state of patients who have severe hypercalcemia combined with renal failure. We recommend dialysis only for those patients who have severe renal failure combined with hypercalcemia, but it should only be used with the understanding that its beneficial effects will be temporary and that other forms of therapy will be necessary.

2. Chronic Treatment

The agents available for the chronic treatment of malignant hypercalcemia include oral phosphate, corticosteroids, diphosphonates, mithramycin, and indomethacin. An ideal form of therapy for the chronic management of hypercalcemia would be an orally administered agent without side-effects that could maintain normocalcemia during the last few months of the patients' lives. Most of these patients have underlying widespread disease and are within the last 6 months of life. The aim of treatment is to keep the patient relatively symptom-free and ambulant as long as possible.

Oral Phosphate. Oral phosphate is a relatively reliable form of therapy since it usually lowers the serum calcium, particularly in patients who have a serum phosphorus of less than 3.7 mg/100 ml. However, its usefulness is limited because it cannot be used safely in patients with impaired renal function, and many patients cannot tolerate it because of diarrhea. Moreover, we have found that some patients treated with oral phosphate "escape" from the beneficial effects (lowering of serum calcium) with prolonged therapy.[41] This "escape" is not always related to the serum phosphorus concentration. In other words, this escape phenomenon cannot be explained simply by the increase in serum phosphorus that oral phosphate therapy causes.

Corticosteroids. Corticosteroids work in about 30% of all patients with hypercalcemia of malignancy.[41] They are probably most effective in patients with hematologic malignancies. They are very useful in most patients who respond, since many of these patients have only a short life span left to them. When needed for a period that is usually less than 6 months, the well-known side-effects of corticosteroid therapy are not a problem. In addition, these agents are given orally and can be taken by patients who will respond before therapy is commenced. Some patients with breast and lung cancer respond, but some do not. Nevertheless, at the current time, we advise an early trial because if the patient is a responder, corticosteroid therapy is an extremely convenient form of treatment.

Indomethacin. Indomethacin is rarely effective and should not be used as routine treatment.[41] Despite several earlier case reports suggesting efficacy, later experiences have been almost uniformly negative. Our own data suggest that less than 5% of patients with malignancy and hypercalcemia will respond to indomethacin. It appears unlikely that prostaglandins are responsible for the humoral hypercalcemia of malignancy, except in a few rare situations. One of these possible situations is estrogen-induced hypercalcemia. Indomethacin has not been used in this situation, but it may be effective for reasons indicated earlier in this review.[23] Although there have not been extensive studies of other prostaglandin synthesis inhibitors, it seems unlikely that these will prove to be more effective than indomethacin.

Mithramycin. Mithramycin is an effective agent but it is also toxic. It is not convenient to use in ambulant patients because it must be given by intravenous infusion. Nevertheless it is usually effective. In our experience, it works in more than 80% of patients in whom it is administered.[41] Its toxicity is probably greater than indicated in the literature and involves hepatocellular damage, bleeding unrelated to thrombocytopenia, nausea, anorexia and vomiting, and marrow suppression.[55] One of the problems we have noticed with mithramycin is that it is difficult to space infusions of mithramycin appropriately. We have had the experience of a patient being treated with mithramycin successfully but then developing acute severe hypercalcemia again over a few hours, which proved to be fatal before the patient could be retreated.[41] Mithramycin probably works because it is toxic to bone cells and inhibits their capacity to cause bone resorption.[56]

Diphosphonates. The diphosphonates are newer agents that may become very useful in the treatment of hypercalcemia. The diphosphonates inhibit bone resorption[57,58] and may be used not only for treating patients with hypercalcemia of malignancy, but also for relieving bone pain in normocalcemic patients with osteolytic disease. The diphosphonates that have been used are EHDP (etidronate), APD, and Cl_2MDP (clodronate). EHDP has been used both orally and intravenously. It is rarely effective orally and should not be used in this manner.[41] However, it is effective in a variable number of patients when administered intravenously. It is difficult to know at the present time how frequently it will work intravenously, but current experience suggests that approximately 60% to 70% of patients will respond after a 48-hour period of treatment with intravenous infusions of EHDP.[59] This agent is still being evaluated in investigative studies at the present time. On the other hand, clodronate is very effective whether used intravenously or orally.[60–62] However, because of unexpected side-effects including the development of acute leukemia in several patients on long-term therapy, this drug is not being used at the present time. It is possible that the development of acute leukemia was unrelated to the drug, and should this become apparent by further observation of the many patients who received this drug, then it may be reintroduced. It is very effective in reversing hypercalcemia and relieving bone pain as well as in the treatment of Paget's disease (see Chapter 15). The other diphosphonate that has received widespread use is APD.[63,64] This useful agent is almost uniformly effective when given intravenously. It is also frequently effective when used orally.[41] It has few side-effects, although some patients have developed mouth ulcers with the oral preparation, fever, and leukocytosis. These have not been important complications. It is not available at the present time in the United States but has been used extensively by European investigators.

The diphosphonates are possibly the most exciting agents on the horizon for the treatment of hypercalcemia and increased bone resorption associated with malignant disease, and it is possible that over the next few years newer agents of this class will be developed that will be even more effective and freer of side-effects than those that have been used to date.

New Agents. Two cytotoxic agents that have been suggested as effective therapeutic agents for the treatment of hypercalcemia are gallium nitrate[65] and *cis*-platinum.[66] Both of these agents are drugs that are used as chemotherapeutic agents in patients with malignant disease and probably have a similar mode of action to mithramycin, that is, they are probably cytotoxic to osteoclasts and inhibit bone resorption by inhibiting osteoclast activity. It has been suggested that *cis*-platinum may also work by lowering the serum magnesium, which would predispose to hypocalcemia, but this seems unrelated to effectiveness in the hypercalcemia of cancer. These agents are still being evaluated at the present time, so their place in the treatment of hypercalcemia of malignancy cannot be assessed. They also both have the disadvantage that they are associated with severe side-effects, particularly impairment of renal function. Because renal function is often impaired prior to treatment in patients with hypercalcemia, this may limit their widespread usefulness. Since these cytotoxic drugs do seem to be effective in lowering the serum calcium, it is likely that other cytotoxic drugs with similar modes of action may also turn out to be useful in this situation.

Comment. Since this manuscript was written, there have been major advances in the identification of tumor products that can mediate hypercalcemia. The PTH-related protein has been purified,[67–69] molecularly cloned,[70–71] and tested extensively in vitro and in vivo.[72–75] This protein binds to and activates the PTH receptor[69] and seems to have all the biologic effects of PTH. It causes hypercalcemia after single bolus injection, repeated injections, or infusions.[72–75] It also stimulates bone resorption in vitro and in vivo[72, 75] and enhances renal tubular calcium reabsorption.[72, 75] It is not clear yet whether it has additional effects unrelated to those of PTH, although its identification in keratinocytes,[76] in placentas, in sheep fetal parathyroid glands,[77] and in rat lactating breast[78] suggests this is likely. Neutralizing antibodies to this factor have lowered the plasma calcium concentration in some animal models of hypercalcemia of malignancy.[65] It does not account for all of the features of humoral hypercalcemia of malignancy. For example, decreased bone formation, decreased 1,25-dihydroxyvitamin D production, and metabolic alkalosis are features of the humoral hypercalcemia of malignancy but not of primary hyperparathyroidism. It appears likely that the complete syndrome of humoral hypercalcemia of malignancy is caused by multiple mediators working in concert. For example, transforming growth factor α is frequently produced by the same tumors that produce PTH-rP and may be responsible for those features of the hypercalcemic syndrome that cannot be ascribed to PTH-rP. It is now apparent that some of these factors, such as TGFα, TNF, TGF, and interleukin-1, can modulate bone cell and renal tubular cell response to PTH and PTH-rP.[80, 81]

This topic has been reviewed a number of times recently.[82–84]

In myeloma, the major mediator responsible for increased osteoclast activity appears to be lymphotoxin. Myeloma cells express lymphotoxin messenger RNA and release lymphotoxin biologic activity.[85] They also release bone-absorbing activity, the majority of which can be inhibited by neutralizing antibodies to lymphotoxin. Lymphotoxin itself causes hypercalcemia when infused into normal intact mice.[85] Both interleukin-1α and PTH-rP have been implicated in the hypercalcemia that occurs in some T-cell lymphomas as well as solid tumors.[86, 87]

Acknowledgments: Some of the studies described in this paper were supported by grants CA 29537, AM 28149, and RR 01346 from the National Institutes of Health. The concepts presented in this review were developed over the years through discussions with numerous coworkers including Kenneth Ibbotson, Sharyn D'Souza, Alexandre Valentin, Donald Bertolini, Maxine Gowen, and Daniel Twardzik.

The author is grateful to Nancy Garrett for typing this manuscript and to Catherine Delea for her careful editing of the final version.

References

1. Mundy GR, Martin TJ: Hypercalcemia of malignancy—pathogenesis and treatment. Metabolism 31:1247–1277, 1982.
2. Ralston SH, Fogelman I, Gardiner MD, et al: Relative contribution of humoral and metastatic factors to the pathogenesis of hypercalcaemia in malignancy. Br Med J 288:1405–1408, 1984.
3. Caverzasio J, Rizzoli R, Fleisch H, Bonjour J-P: PTH-like changes of renal calcium and phosphate (Pi) reabsorption induced by Leydig cell tumor in thyroparathyroidectomized (TPTX) Fischer rats. Calcif Tissue Int [Suppl 2]:S26, 1984.
4. Horton JE, Raisz LG, Simmons HA, et al: Bone resorbing activity in supernatant fluid from cultured human peripheral blood leukocytes. Science 177:793–795, 1972.
5. Raisz LG, Luben RA, Mundy GR, et al: Effect of osteoclast activating factor from human leukocytes on bone metabolism. J Clin Invest 56:408–413, 1975.
6. Mundy GR, Luben RA, Raisz LG, et al: Bone resorbing activity in supernatants from lymphoid cell lines. N Engl J Med 290:867–871, 1974.
7. Mundy GR, Raisz LG, Cooper RA, et al: Evidence for the secretion of an osteoclast stimulating factor in myeloma. N Engl J Med 291:1041–1046, 1974.
8. Gailani S, McLimans WF, Mundy GR, et al: Controlled environment culture of bone marrow explants from human myeloma. Cancer Res 36:1299–1304, 1976.
9. Josse RG, Murray TM, Mundy GR, et al: Observations on the mechanism of bone resorption induced by multiple myeloma marrow culture fluids and partially purified osteoclast activating factor. J Clin Invest 67:1472–1481, 1981.
10. Gowen M, Wood DD, Ihrie EJ, et al: An interleukin 1 like factor stimulates bone resorption in vitro. Nature 306:378–380, 1983.
11. Bertolini DR, Nedwin G, Bringman T, Mundy GR: Stimulation of bone resorption and inhibition in vitro by human tumour necrosis factors. Nature 319:516–518, 1986.
12. Mundy GR, Rick ME, Turcotte R, et al: Pathogenesis of hypercalcemia in lymphosarcoma cell leukemia: Role of an osteoclast activating factor–like substance and mechanism of action for glucocorticoid therapy. Am J Med 65:600–606, 1978.
13. Bunn PA, Schechter GP, Jaffe E, et al: Clinical course of retrovirus-associated adult T cell lymphoma in the United States. N Engl J Med 309:257–264, 1983.
14. Fetchick DA, Bertolini DR, Sarin P, et al: Production of 1,25 hydroxyvitamin D by human T cell lymphotropic virus-transformed lymphocytes. J Clin Invest 78:592–596, 1986.
15. Breslau NA, McGuire JL, Zerwekh JE, et al: Hypercalcemia associated with increased serum calcitriol levels in three patients with lymphoma. Ann Intern Med 100:1–7, 1984.
16. Rosenthal N, Insogna KL, Godsall JW, et al: Elevations in circulating 1,25-dihydroxyvitamin D in three patients with lymphoma-associated hypercalcemia. J Clin Endocrinol Metab 60:29–33, 1985.
17. Zaloga GP, Eil C, Medbery CA: Humoral hypercalcemia in Hodgkin's disease. Arch Intern Med 145:155–157, 1985.
18. Davies M, Hayes ME, Mawer EB, Lumb GA: Abnormal vitamin D metabolism in Hodgkin's lymphoma. Lancet 1:1186–1188, 1985.
19. Galasko CSB: Mechanisms of bone destruction in the development of skeletal metastases. Nature 263:507–508, 1976.
20. Eilon G, Mundy GR: Direct resorption of bone by human breast cancer cells in vitro. Nature 276:726–728, 1978.
21. Eilon G, Mundy GR: Inhibition of microtubule assembly on bone mineral release and enzyme release by human breast cancer cells. J Clin Invest 67:69–86, 1981.
22. Eilon G, Mundy GR: Association of increased cyclic AMP content in cultured human breast cancer cells and release of hydrolytic enzymes and bone resorbing activity. Cancer Res 43:5792–5794, 1983.
23. Valentin A, Eilon G, Saez S, et al: Estrogens and antiestrogens stimulate release of bone resorbing activity by cultured human breast cancer cells. J Clin Invest 75:726–731, 1985.
24. Orr W, Varani J, Gondek GD, et al: Chemotactic responses of tumor cells to products of resorbing bone. Science 203:176–179, 1979.
25. Orr FW, Varani J, Gondek MD, et al: Partial characterization of a bone derived chemotactic factor for tumor cells. Am J Pathol 99:43–52, 1980.
26. Mundy GR, De Martino S, Rowe DW: Collagen and collagen fragments are chemotactic for tumor cells. J Clin Invest 68:1102–1105, 1981.
27. Sporn MB, Todaro GJ: Autocrine secretion and malignant transformation of cells. N Engl J Med 303:878–880, 1980.
28. Kahn P, Shin S-I: Cellular tumorigenicity in nude mice: Test of associations among loss of cell surface fibronectin, anchorage independence, and tumor forming ability. J Cell Biol 82:1–16, 1979.
29. Todaro GJ, Fryling C, De Larco JE: Transforming growth factors produced by certain human tumor cells: Polypeptides that interact with epidermal growth factor receptors. Proc Natl Acad Sci USA 77:5258–5262, 1980.
30. Roberts AB, Anzano MA, Lamb LC, et al: Isolation from murine sarcoma cells of novel transforming growth factors potentiated by EGF. Nature 295:417–419, 1982.
31. Ibbotson KJ, D'Souza SM, Ng KW, et al: Tumor derived growth factor increases bone resorption in a tumor associated with the humoral hypercalcemia of malignancy. Science 221:1292–1294, 1983.
32. Ibbotson KJ, D'Souza SM, Smith DD, et al: EGF receptor antiserum inhibits bone resorbing activity produced by a rat Leydig cell tumor associated with the humoral hypercalcemia of malignancy. Endocrinology 116:469–471, 1985.

33. Ibbotson KJ, Harrod J, Gowen M, et al: Human recombinant transforming growth factor α stimulates bone resorption and inhibits formation in vitro. Proc Natl Acad Sci USA 83:2228–2232, 1986.
34. Ibbotson KJ, Twardzik DR, D'Souza SM, et al: Stimulation of bone resorption in vitro by synthetic transforming growth factor-alpha. Science 228:1007–1009, 1985.
35. D'Souza SM, Ibbotson KJ, Mundy GR: Failure of PTH antagonists to inhibit in vitro bone resorbing activity produced by two animal models of the humoral hypercalcemia of malignancy. J Clin Invest 74:1104–1107, 1984.
36. Tashjian AH, Voelkel EF, Lazzaro M, et al: Alpha and beta transforming growth factors stimulate prostaglandin production and bone resorption in cultured mouse calvaria. PNAS 82:4535–4538, 1985.
37. Mundy GR, Ibbotson KJ, D'Souza SM, et al: The hypercalcemia of cancer. Clinical implications and pathogenic mechanisms. N Engl J Med 310:1718–1727, 1984.
38. Simpson EL, Mundy GR, D'Souza SM, et al: Absence of parathyroid hormone messenger RNA in nonparathyroid tumors associated with hypercalcemia. N Engl J Med 309:325–330, 1983.
39. Tashjian AH, Voelkel EF, Levine L, et al: Evidence that the bone resorption stimulating factor produced by mouse fibrosarcoma cells is prostaglandin E_2: A new model for the hypercalcemia of cancer. J Exp Med 136:1329–1343, 1972.
40. Voelkel EF, Tashjian AH, Franklin R, et al: Hypercalcemia and tumor prostaglandins: The VX_2 carcinoma model in the rabbit. Metabolism 24:973–986, 1975.
41. Mundy GR, Wilkinson R, Heath DA: Comparative study of available medical therapy for hypercalcemia of malignancy. Am J Med 74:421–432, 1983.
42. Stewart AF, Insogna KL, Goltzman D, et al: Identification of adenylate cyclase stimulating activity and cytochemical glucose-t-phosphate dehydrogenase–stimulating activity in extracts of tumors from patients with humoral hypercalcemia of malignancy. Proc Natl Acad Sci USA 80:1454–1458, 1983.
43. Goltzman D, Stewart AF, Broadus AE: Malignancy associated hypercalcemia: Evaluation with a cytochemical bioassay for parathyroid hormone. J Clin Endocrinol Metab 53:899–904, 1981.
44. Strewler GJ, Williams RD, Nissenson RA: Human renal carcinoma cells produce hypercalcemia in the nude mouse and a novel protein recognized by parathyroid hormone receptors. J Clin Invest 71:769–774, 1983.
45. Lee MY, Baylink DJ: Hypercalcemia, excessive bone resorption, and neutrophilia in mice bearing a mammary carcinoma. Proc Soc Exp Biol Med 172:424–429, 1983.
46. Oshawa N, Ueyama Y, Morita K, et al: Heterotransplantation of human functioning tumors to nude mice. *In* Nomura T, Oshawa N, Tamaoki N, Fujiwara F (eds): Proceedings of the Second International Workshop on Nude Mice. Tokyo, University of Tokyo Press, 1977, pp 395–405.
47. Kondo Y, Sato K, Ohkawa H, et al: Association of hypercalcemia with tumors producing colony-stimulating factor(s). Cancer Res 43:2368–2374, 1983.
48. Sato K, Mimura H, Han DC, et al: Production of bone resorbing activity and colony stimulating activity in vivo and in vitro by a human squamous cell carcinoma associated with hypercalcemia and leukocytosis. J Clin Invest 78:145–154, 1986.
49. Binstock ML, Mundy GR: Effects of calcitonin and glucocorticoids in combination in hypercalcemia of malignancy. Ann Intern Med 93:269–272, 1980.
50. Au WYW: Calcitonin treatment of hypercalcemia due to parathyroid carcinoma—synergistic effect of prednisone on long-term treatment of hypercalcemia. Arch Intern Med 135:1594, 1975.
51. Suki WN, Yium JJ, Von Minden M, et al: Acute treatment of hypercalcemia with furosemide. N Engl J Med 283:836–840, 1970.
52. Fulmer DH, Dimich AB, Rothschild EO, et al: Treatment of hypercalcemia, comparison of intravenously administered phosphate sulfate and hydrocortisone. Arch Intern Med 129:923–930, 1972.
53. Carey RW, Schmitt GW, Kopaid HH: Massive extraskeletal calcification during phosphate treatment of hypercalcemia. Arch Intern Med 122:150–155, 1968.
54. Miach PJ, Dawborn JK, Martin TJ, et al: Management of the hypercalcemia of malignancy by peritoneal dialysis. Med J Aust 1:782–784, 1975.
55. Mundy GR, Rodan SB, Majeska RJ, et al: Unidirectional migration of osteosarcoma cells with osteoblast characteristics in response to products of bone resorption. Calcif Tissue Int 34:542–546, 1982.
56. Minkin C: Inhibition of parathyroid hormone stimulated bone resorption in vitro by the antibiotic mithramycin. Calcif Tiss Res 13:249–257, 1973.
57. Fleisch H, Russell RGG, Francis MD: Diphosphonates inhibit hydroxyapatite dissolution in vitro and bone resorption in tissue culture and in vivo. Science 165:1262–1264, 1969.
58. Russell RGG, Muhlbauer RC, Bisaz S, et al: The influence of pyrophosphate, condensed phosphates, phosphonates, and other phosphate compounds on the dissolution of hydroxyapatite in vitro and on bone resorption induced by parathyroid hormone in tissue culture and in thyroparathyroidectomized rats. Calcif Tiss Res 6:183–196, 1970.
59. Ryzen E, Rude RK, Singer FR, et al: Intravenous didronel (etidronate disodium) in the treatment of hypercalcemia of malignancy. Calcif Tiss Int 36:483 (abstract), 1984.
60. Chapuy MC, Meunier PJ, Alexandre CM, et al: Effects of disodium dichloromethylene diphosphonate on the hypercalcemia produced by bone metastases. J Clin Invest 65:1243–1247, 1980.
61. Siris ES, Sherman WH, Baquiran DC, et al: Effects of dichloromethylene diphosphonate on skeletal mobilization of multiple myeloma. N Engl J Med 302:310–315, 1980.
62. Jacobs TP, Siris ES, Bilezikian JP, et al: Hypercalcemia of malignancy. Treatment with intravenous dichloromethylene diphosphonate. Ann Intern Med 94:312–316, 1981.
63. Fuijlink WB, Bijvoet OLM, te Velde J, et al: Treatment of Paget's disease with (3-amino-1-hydroxypropylidene)-1,1-bisphosphonate (A.P.D.). Lancet 1:799–803, 1979.
64. Van Breukelen FJM, Bijvoet OLM, Van Oosterom AT: Inhibition of osteolytic bone lesions by (3-amino-1-hydroxypropylidene)-1,1-bisphosphonate (A.P.D.). Lancet 1:803–805, 1979.
65. Warrell RP, Brockman RS, Coonley CJ, et al: Gallium nitrate inhibits calcium resorption from bone and is effective treatment for cancer-related hypercalcemia. J Clin Invest 73:1487–1490, 1984.

66. Abramson EC, Kukla LJ, Bowser EN, et al: A model for human hypercalcemia of malignancy in athymic nude mouse. Calcif Tissue Int 35:A61, 1983.
67. Mosely JM, Kubota M, Diefenbach-Jagger H, et al: Parathyroid hormone-related protein purified from a human lung cancer cell line. Proc Natl Acad Sci USA 84:5048–5052, 1987.
68. Stewart AF, Wu T, Goumas D, et al: N-terminal amino acid sequence of two novel tumor-derived adenylate cyclase-stimulating proteins: Identification of parathyroid hormone-like and parathyroid hormone-unlike domains. Biochem Biophys Res Commun 146:672–678, 1987.
69. Strewler GJ, Stern PH, Jacobs JW, et al: Parathyroid hormone-like protein from human renal carcinoma cells: Structural and functional homology with parathyroid hormone. J Clin Invest 80:1803–1807, 1987.
70. Suva LJ, Winslow GA, Wettenhall REH, et al: A parathyroid hormone-related protein implicated in malignant hypercalcemia: Cloning and expression. Science 237:893–896, 1987.
71. Mangin M, Wegg AC, Dreyer BE, et al: Identification of a cDNA encoding a parathyroid hormone-like peptide from a human tumor associated with humoral hypercalcemia of malignancy. Proc Natl Acad Sci USA 85:597–601, 1988.
72. Kemp BE, Moseley JM, Rodda CP, et al: Parathyroid homone-related protein of malignancy: Active synthetic fragments. Science 238:1568–1570, 1987.
73. Horiuchi N, Caulfield MP, Fisher JE, et al: Similarity of synthetic peptide from human tumor to parathyroid hormone in vivo and in vitro. Science 238:1566–1567, 1987.
74. Stewart AF, Mangin M, Wu T, et al: Synthetic human parathyroid hormone-like protein stimulates bone resorption and causes hypercalcemia in rats. J Clin Invest 81:596–600, 1988.
75. Yates AJP, Gutierrez GE, Smolens P, et al: Effects of a synthetic peptide of a parathyroid-hormone-related protein on calcium homeostasis, renal tubular calcium reabsorption and bone metabolism. J Clin Invest 81:932–938, 1988.
76. Merendino JJ, Insogna KL, Milstone LM, et al: A parathyroid hormone-like protein from cultured human keratinocytes. Science 231:388–390, 1986.
77. Rodda CP, Heath JA, Ebeling PR, et al: Regulation of fetal calcium metabolism: Evidence for a novel parathyroid hormone-related protein promoting placental calcium transport. J Bone Min Res 3:51, 577, 1988.
78. Thiede MA, Rodan GA: Expression of a calcium-mobilizing parathyroid hormone-like peptide in lactating mammary tissue. Science 242:278–280, 1988.
79. Kukreja SC, Shevrin DH, Wimbiscus SA, et al: Antibodies to parathyroid hormone-related protein lower serum calcium in athymic mouse models of malignancy-associated hypercalcemia due to human tumors. J Clin Invest 82:1798–1802, 1988.
80. Gutierrez GE, Mundy GR, Derynck R, et al: Inhibition of parathyroid hormone-responsive adenylate cyclase in clonal osteoblast-like cells by transforming growth factor α and epidermal growth factor J Biol Chem 262:15845–15850, 1987.
81. Gutierrez GE, Mundy GR, Katz MS: Modulation of osteoblast responsiveness to PTH by growth regulatory peptides. J Bone Min Res 2:113, 1987.
82. Mundy GR: Calcium Homeostasis and Its Disorders. London, M. Dunitz, 1989.
83. Mundy GR: The hypercalcemia of malignancy revisited. J Clin Invest 82:1–6, 1988.
84. Broadus AE, Mangin M, Ikeda K, et al: Humoral hypercalcemia of cancer. Identification of a novel parathyroid hormone-like peptide. N Engl J Med 319:556–563, 1988.
85. Garrett IR, Durie BGM, Nedwin GE, et al: Production of the bone resorbing cytokine lymphotoxin by cultured human myeloma cells. N Engl J Med 317:526–532, 1987.
86. Sato K, Fujii Y, Kasono K, et al: Production of interleukin-1 alpha and a parathyroid hormone-like factor by a squamous cell carcinoma of the esophagus (EC-GI) derived from a patient with hypercalcemia. J Clin Endocrinol Metab 67:592–601, 1988.
87. Motokura T, Fukumoto S, Takahashi S, et al: Expression of parathyroid hormone-related protein in a human T cell lymphotrophic virus type I-infected T cell line. Biochem Biophys Res Commun 154:1181–1188, 1988.

22

NORMAN H. BELL

Sarcoidosis and Related Disorders

Sarcoidosis is a protean systemic disease of unknown cause in which noncaseous granulomas are found in affected organs. The lymph nodes, lungs, eyes, and skin are the most common sites of involvement.[1,2]

Whereas sarcoidosis may occur in any tissue, some 90% of patients have lesions in the lungs, thoracic lymph nodes, or both.[2] This observation has led to the idea that the disease begins in the respiratory tract and associated lymphatic system. As will be seen, utilization of bronchoalveolar lavage to obtain cells and cellular products from bronchial washings has permitted an investigation and analysis of the immune inflammatory response in this disease.

I. IMMUNOLOGY AND PATHOLOGY

A. Alveolitis

Available evidence indicates that pulmonary sarcoidosis begins as an alveolitis, that is, an accumulation of inflammatory cells within the alveolus.[3,4] In patients with active pulmonary disease, large numbers of lymphocytes are present within the alveolar interstitium and on the alveolar surfaces.[5,6] Most of the cells are T lymphocytes, many of which are activated,[5,7] and the majority were identified as T-helper cells in studies with monoclonal antibodies.[7] In active pulmonary sarcoidosis, the increased number of T lymphocytes occurs because of an increased rate of their replication.[8–11] This enhanced rate of proliferation occurs in part because of synthesis and release by the activated T lymphocytes of the lymphokine interleukin-2, a T lymphocyte growth factor.[9,10] In addition, recent evidence indicates that antigen-driven, alveolar macrophage-modulated T cell proliferation may also be a factor.[11] Thus, antigen-pulsed alveolar macrophages from sarcoid patients induce a greater increment in proliferation of T lymphocytes than do cells from normal subjects. On the other hand, patients with sarcoid have a deficiency of T lymphocytes in the peripheral circulation.[5,8]

In active pulmonary sarcoid, the activated T lymphocytes spontaneously produce a number of factors in addition to interleukin-2 that are important in the development and maintenance of the inflammatory process. These include macrophage chemotactic factor,[12] leukocyte inhibitory factor,[5] gamma-interferon,[13] but not interleukin-1.[14] The macrophages that occur in granulomas are derived from monocytes that originate in the bone marrow and reach the site of inflammation by way of the peripheral circulation.[12] By release of monocyte chemotactic factor, the activated alveolar T lymphocytes recruit peripheral monocytes, thereby providing maintenance of granuloma formation. Neutrophils are seldom found in the sarcoid lung, and their absence may be accounted for in part by leukocyte inhibitory factor.[5] Also, serum lysozyme, an enzyme that inhibits the migration of neutrophils,[15] is increased in sarcoidosis.[16]

There is evidence that enhanced antibody production by pulmonary B cells in sarcoid lesions may account for the hypergammaglobulinemia that commonly occurs in the disease.[17] In this regard, it was proposed that the activated T lymphocytes stimulated B cells in the lungs to differentiate into immunoglobulin-producing cells. It was found that the number of pulmonary B lymphocytes from patients with active sarcoid that secreted immunoglobulins was markedly increased and that there was a significant positive correlation between the percentage of T cells and the percentage of B cells secreting IgG.[18] These results provide an explanation for the paradoxical observation that circulating lymphocytes of patients with sarcoidosis do not release increased amounts of immunoglobulins despite hypergammaglobulinemia in the peripheral circulation.[16]

Alveolar macrophages from bronchoalveolar lavage of patients with sarcoidosis and hypercalcemia caused by increased circulating 1,25-dihydroxyvitamin D were shown to convert [^{3}H]-25-hydroxyvitamin D_3 to [^{3}H]-1,25-dihydroxyvitamin D_3 *in vitro*.[19–22] Production of 1,25-dihydroxyvitamin D in this system was enhanced in a dose-dependent fashion by gamma-interferon.[21,22] Since gamma-interferon is produced spontaneously by activated T cells and alveolar macrophages in sarcoid,[13] this lymphokine may be important in the pathogenesis of synthesis of 1,25-dihydroxyvitamin D.

Receptors for 1,25-dihydroxyvitamin D_3 are present in activated peripheral T lymphocytes from normal human subjects,[23] and 1,25-dihydroxyvitamin D_3 was shown to inhibit proliferation and to suppress interleukin-2 activity[24] and gamma-interferon synthesis[25] by phytohemagglutin-stimulated human peripheral lymphocytes. 1,25-Dihydroxyvitamin D_3 was shown to inhibit activated T helper-inducer lymphocyte activity from normal human subjects *in vitro*.[26] If receptors for 1,25-dihydroxyvitamin D are present in activated pulmonary T lymphocytes and if 1,25-dihydroxyvitamin D_3 inhibits proliferation of activated T cells and their secretion of interleukin-2 and gamma-interferon in granulomas of patients with sarcoid, production of 1,25-dihydroxyvitamin D by alveolar macrophages could provide a compensatory mechanism to inhibit the inflammatory process. Regardless of the potential role of 1,25-dihydroxyvitamin D in modification of inflammation, it is evident that nonrenal production of 1,25-dihydroxyvitamin D is responsible for the abnormal vitamin D and mineral metabolism that occurs in sarcoidosis.[27]

B. Granulomas

In sarcoidosis, the granulomas are made up of collections of inflammatory and immune effector cells. In developing granulomas, loosely arranged epithelioid cells, derived from macrophages, are surrounded by a ring of lymphocytes. There are no giant cells. In more mature granulomas, numerous epithelioid cells are present with giant cells and are surrounded by a few lymphocytes. Thus, initially the number of macrophages, monocytes, and lymphocytes is greater than the number of epithelioid cells, whereas later the number of epithelioid cells increases as the number of macrophages, monocytes, and lymphocytes declines.[4] In pulmonary sarcoidosis, when alveolitis predominates, few or no granulomas are present. In contrast, when extensive granulomas occur, alveolitis is minimal or absent.[5,28] Alveolitis, therefore, is thought to precede the development of granulomas in sarcoid.[4–17]

Once formed, granulomas either undergo resolution with little in the way of residual morphologic alterations or progress to fibrosis.[29,30] The fibrotic process begins as a deposition of collagen around the periphery of the granuloma.[3,28] It is assumed but not established that collagen is derived from fibroblasts that surround the granuloma.[28] As fibrosis develops, the fibroblasts proliferate so that there is eventual destruction of the granuloma and fibrosis and destruction of the normal structures of the lung.[31,32] Thus, pulmonary sarcoidosis either resolves leaving little in the way of impairment of function, as occurs in some 80% of patients, or progresses to fibrosis with the development of pulmonary insufficiency and cor pulmonale, as occurs in the remaining 20% of patients.

II. ABNORMAL CALCIUM METABOLISM

In sarcoidosis, the characteristic changes in calcium metabolism that occur are increases in serum and urinary calcium and, as shown by balance studies and investigations with radiolabeled calcium, enhanced intestinal absorption of calcium.[33–36] Increases in turnover of ^{47}Ca were found in patients with sarcoidosis and hypercalcemia that were similar to changes produced by pharmacologic doses of vitamin D in normal subjects and patients with hypoparathyroidism.[35] Hypercalcemia and hypercalciuria in sarcoidosis occur spontaneously and are produced by small doses of vitamin D that are without effect in normal subjects[33–35] as well as by brief irradiation with ultraviolet light.[37] The importance of ultraviolet radiation in the pathogenesis of the abnormal vitamin D and mineral metabolism in sarcoidosis is underscored by the seasonal incidence of hypercalcemia, which usually occurs during the summer months,[38] and by the demonstration that the abnormal calcium metabolism is reversed by omission of vitamin D from the diet and prevention of exposure to sunlight.[39]

Abnormal metabolism of calcium also occurs in patients with sarcoid who are normocalcemic.[40,41] Enhanced intestinal absorption of calcium, determined in studies with labeled calcium, was found and correlated with increased renal excretion of calcium.[40] Thus, hypercalciuria in sarcoid occurs in the absence of hypercalcemia and results from increased intestinal absorption of calcium.[40,41] Since increases in urinary hydroxyproline, an index of bone resorption, also occur in sarcoidosis,[42] it is likely that excess urinary calcium also may be derived from the skeleton.

In sarcoidosis, it is clear that hypercalciuria is present in greater frequency than hypercalcemia.[40,43] The true incidence of hypercalciuria is difficult to establish, since there is known seasonal variation in the serum calcium[38] and considerable variation in urinary calcium in normal subjects. Further, urinary calcium varies with race and body habitus. Thus, we demonstrated that normal nonobese black subjects and obese white individuals have secondary hyperparathyroidism with increased circulating 1,25-dihydroxyvitamin D and urinary cyclic adenosine 3′,5′-monophosphate and decreased urinary calcium as compared with nonobese white men and women.[44,45]

III. PATHOGENESIS

A. Normal Physiology of Vitamin D

Because of its relevance to abnormal calcium metabolism in sarcoidosis and related disorders, the metabolism of vitamin D is briefly discussed. A more comprehensive and detailed description is provided in Chapter 5.

Vitamin D_3 is synthesized in the skin from 7-dehydrocholesterol, provitamin D, with previtamin D_3 as an intermediate. On exposure to ultraviolet light, 7-dehydrocholesterol absorbs one photon of light energy at the site of conjugated double bonds in the B-ring, $\Delta^{5,7}$-diene, which produces rearrangement of the double bonds and cleavage of the double bond between carbons 9 and 10 to form provitamin D_3. Since some 80% of the 7-dehydrocholesterol is in the stratum spinosum and stratum basale, the major site of photochemical conversion of provitamin D to previtamin D_3 is at that site.[46]

Previtamin D_3 is thermally unstable and undergoes isomerization to vitamin D_3 (cholecalciferol), a conversion that is temperature-dependent and takes place over a period of days.[46] Vitamin D_3, which is thermally stable, is preferentially transported from the dermis bound to vitamin D–binding protein and is removed by the capillary bed that is adjacent to the deeper layer of skin. Vitamin D–binding globulin has a high affinity for vitamin D_3 but little, if any, affinity for previtamin D_3 so that previtamin D_3 remains in the dermis for eventual conversion to vitamin D_3.

Vitamin D_2 (ergocalciferol) and vitamin D_3 in the diet are absorbed in the proximal small intestine, a step requiring bile acids, by the lymphatic system. They are transported to the liver in chylomicrons and are released into the systemic circulation bound to vitamin D–binding protein. Vitamins D_2 and D_3 are hydroxylated in the liver to their respective metabolites of 25-hydroxyvitamin D by action of the enzyme vitamin D 25-hydroxylase.[47] 25-Hydroxyvitamin D is transported to the kidney where it is hydroxylated further to 1,25-dihydroxyvitamin D,[48] the most biologically active metabolite of vitamin D that acts to enhance the intestinal absorption of calcium[49] and the skeletal release of the ion.[50] 1,25-Dihydroxyvitamin D also acts to reduce the concentration of its precursor 25-hydroxyvitamin D[51] by enhancing its metabolic clearance.[52]

The synthesis of 1,25-dihydroxyvitamin D by the kidney normally is tightly regulated by parathyroid hormone. Values are low in hypoparathyroidism, are elevated in primary hyperparathyroidism, and are increased by administration of parathyroid extract in normal subjects and in patients with hypoparathyroidism.[53,54] 1,25-Dihydroxyvitamin D is the major determinant of calcium absorption in humans, and adaptation to changes of calcium intake is mediated by changes in circulating parathyroid hormone and 1,25-dihydroxyvitamin D.[55] Thus, serum parathyroid hormone and 1,25-dihydroxyvitamin D increase when dietary calcium is restricted and decrease when dietary calcium is augmented.

B. Abnormal Vitamin D Metabolism

Increased intestinal absorption of calcium, hypercalcemia, and hypercalciuria in sarcoid are caused by increased circulating 1,25-dihydroxyvitamin D.[27,56–59] Values are either

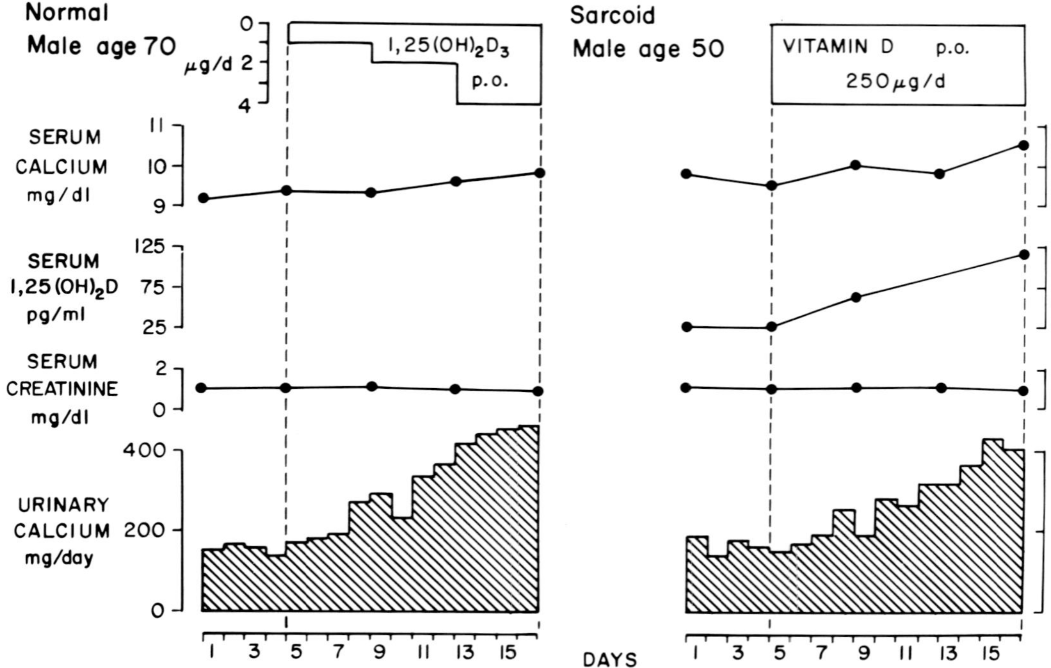

Figure 22–1. Effects on serum and urinary calcium of 1,25-dihydroxyvitamin D_3 in a normal subject and of vitamin D in a patient with sarcoidosis. Note (1) that the increases in urinary calcium produced by exogenous 1,25-dihydroxyvitamin D_3 in the normal subject were similar to the increases produced by endogenous 1,25-dihydroxyvitamin D in the patient and (2) that the serum calcium increased and remained within the normal range in both of them.

increased or at the upper range of normal in hypercalcemic patients, and serum immunoreactive parathyroid hormone is either suppressed or in the low-normal range.[27,56–58,60] In small doses, 10,000 units a day for 12 days, vitamin D increases serum 1,25-dihydroxyvitamin D and urinary calcium in normocalcemic patients with sarcoid and a history of hypercalcemia, but does not alter serum 1,25-dihydroxyvitamin D or urinary calcium in patients with normal calcium metabolism.[56] As shown in Figure 22–1, increases in urinary calcium produced by 1,25-dihydroxyvitamin D in a normal subject were the same as the increases in urinary calcium produced by small doses of vitamin D in a normocalcemic patient with sarcoidosis who had a history of hypercalcemia. In larger doses, 100,000 units a day for 4 days, vitamin D increased serum 1,25-dihydroxyvitamin D and serum calcium in some patients with sarcoid who had normal calcium metabolism (Fig. 22–2), but did not change the serum concentration of the metabolite or serum calcium in normal subjects.[61] This defect in the regulation of circulating 1,25-dihydroxyvitamin D provides the mechanism for increased sensitivity to vitamin D that is so characteristic of the disorder.

Enhanced dermal production of vitamin D_3 by sunlight during summer months produces seasonal variation in serum calcium in patients with sarcoid[38] and accounts for the fact that increases in serum 1,25-dihydroxyvitamin D and hypercalcemia usually occur in the summer in the northern hemisphere (Fig. 22–3).[56–58] This occurs because the production of 1,25-dihydroxyvitamin D is not regulated in sarcoid so that the concentration of 1,25-dihydroxyvitamin D is more likely to be influenced by the concentration of the substrate 25-hydroxyvitamin D. In normal subjects as a result of differences in the time of exposure to sunlight, there is seasonal variation in serum 25-hydroxyvitamin D but not in serum 1,25-dihydroxyvitamin D.[62,63] This lack of change in circulating 1,25-dihydroxyvitamin D occurs because the renal synthesis of the metabolite is closely regulated.

Serum 1,25-dihydroxyvitamin D also may be increased in patients who do not have hypercalcemia.[41,61] In these individuals, increases in fractional intestinal absorption of calcium

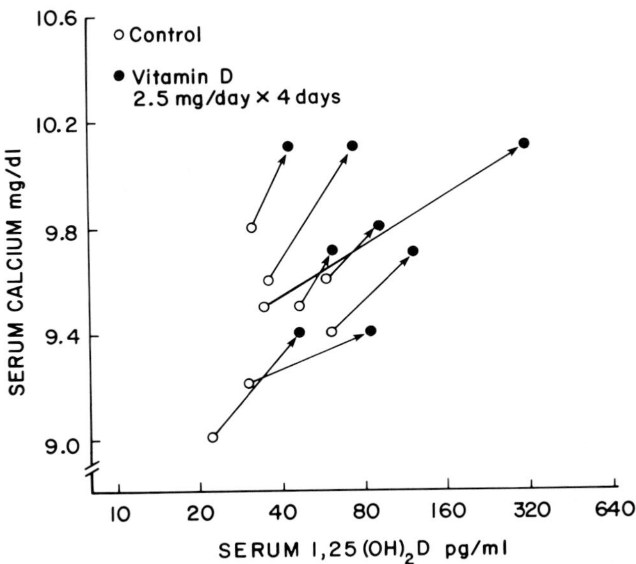

Figure 22–2. Effects of vitamin D, 2.5 mg (100,000 units) a day for 4 days in eight patients with sarcoidosis and normal calcium metabolism. Note (1) that the serum 1,25-dihydroxyvitamin D and serum calcium increased in each of them and (2) that the serum 1,25-dihydroxyvitamin D is drawn on a semilog plot. (Modified from Stern PH, DeOlazabal J, Bell NH: J Clin Invest 66:852, 1980.)

occur in association with hypercalciuria.[41] In sarcoidosis, hypercalcemia usually occurs in patients with some degree of renal insufficiency and limitation in the ability of the kidneys to excrete the excess calcium resulting from increased intestinal absorption and skeletal release of the ion.[56] Hypercalcemia is also related to calcium intake and can be corrected or prevented by restriction of dietary calcium.[34,35]

Demonstration of increased circulating 1,25-dihydroxyvitamin D, hypercalcemia, and suppression of serum immunoreactive parathyroid hormone in an anephric patient with sarcoid was the first indication of extrarenal synthesis of 1,25-dihydroxyvitamin D.[27] As noted already, conversion of [^{3}H]-25-hydroxyvitamin D_3 to [^{3}H]-1,25-dihydroxyvitamin D_3 by cultured pulmonary alveolar macrophages from patients with sarcoidosis was observed.[19–21] The structure of the putative 1,25-dihydroxyvitamin D_3 produced by the macrophages was confirmed by mass spectral analysis.[20] Kinetic analysis of the synthesis of 1,25-dihydroxyvitamin D_3 by pulmonary alveolar macrophages from five patients with sarcoidosis revealed a K_m that varied from 52 to 210 nM.[21] This range is similar to values obtained with mammalian renal tissues including homogenates of mouse kidney,[64] mouse kidney cells in culture,[65] rat renal cortical cells,[66] and partially purified 25-hydroxyvitamin D 1α-hydroxylase from rat kidney.[67]

On the other hand, the 25-hydroxyvitamin D 1α-hydroxylase activity in pulmonary alveolar macrophages from patients with sarcoidosis differs from the renal enzyme in a number of important respects. In contrast to the kidney,[64–67] stimulation of 25-hydroxyvitamin D 24-hydroxylase activity in the macrophages occurs only at very high concentrations of 1,25-dihydroxyvitamin D_3.[22] This means that there is little competition for the substrate 25-hydroxyvitamin D to be converted to 24,25-dihydroxyvitamin D, which has only modest biological activity, and that 1,25-dihydroxyvitamin D will not undergo further hydrolysis to 1,24,25-trihydroxyvitamin D, which has less biological activity than 1,25-dihydroxyvitamin D.[68,69] Also, unlike the mammalian kidney,[65,70] there is only modest inhibition of 25-hydroxyvitamin D 1α-hydroxylase activity by 1,25-dihydroxyvitamin D_3 in the pulmonary alveolar macrophages.[22] Activity is inhibited by dexamethasone added directly to the culture system, and the inhibition is dose-dependent.[21,22] These *in vitro* findings account in part for the clinical observations that production of 1,25-dihydroxyvitamin D in sarcoidosis is not regulated and is inhibited by glucocorticoids.[27,56–58] It remains to be demonstrated whether the activated pulmonary alveolar macrophage possesses a 25-hydroxyvitamin D 1α-hydroxylase enzyme with an associated cytochrome P-450 system similar to that in the kidney.

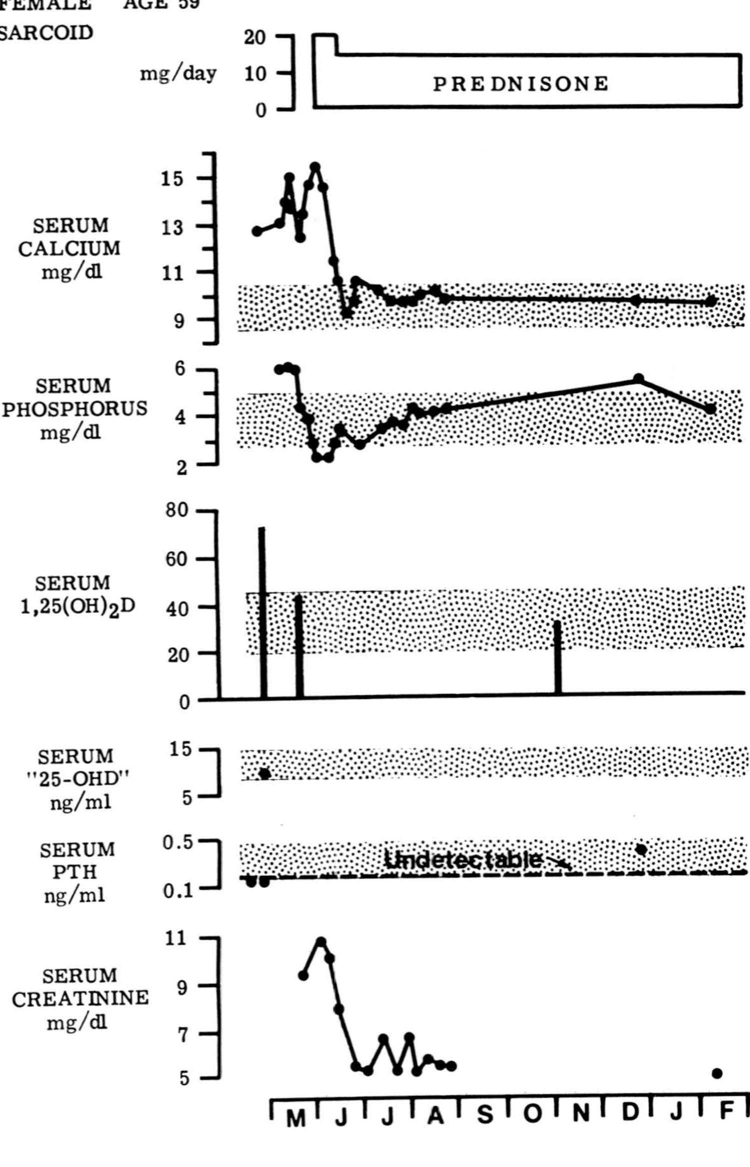

Figure 22–3. Effects of prednisone on serum calcium, phosphorus, 1,25-dihydroxyvitamin D, 25-hydroxyvitamin D, immunoreactive parathyroid hormone, and creatinine in a patient with sarcoid who had renal failure as a result of hypercalcemia. Note (1) that initially the serum 1,25-dihydroxyvitamin D was elevated or at the upper limit of normal, the serum calcium was elevated, the serum immunoreactive parathyroid hormone was undetectable, and the serum 25-hydroxyvitamin D was at the lower range of normal and (2) that prednisone reduced the serum 1,25-dihydroxyvitamin D to normal, corrected the hypercalcemia, and lowered the serum creatinine.

IV. CLINICAL MANIFESTATIONS

A. Calcium Metabolism

The true incidence of abnormal calcium metabolism—hyperabsorption of calcium, hypercalcemia, and hypercalciuria—is difficult to assess because of variation in urinary calcium in the general population such as occurs, for example, in obesity and in blacks.[44,45] Hypercalcemia probably occurs in less than 10% of patients with sarcoid, but this, too, is difficult to assess because of seasonal variation in the serum calcium.[38] Hypercalcemia of clinical importance probably occurs in less than 5% of patients.

The symptoms related to abnormal calcium metabolism may be categorized relative to the gastrointestinal tract, the kidney, and the central nervous system. Anorexia, nausea, and vomiting may lead to dehydration and weight loss. Hypercalcemia and hypercalciuria may result in nephrogenic diabetes insipidus with polydipsia, polyuria, frequency, and nocturia.[71] The renal concentrating defect is reversible upon correction of the abnormal calcium metabolism. Renal stones may produce renal colic, hematuria, dysuria, urgency, and frequency. Hypercalcemia may be asymptomatic or produce generalized symptoms of muscle weakness, easy fatigue, and lethargy and, if severe and prolonged, may produce a variety of mental disturbances and even coma. In sarcoidosis, however, the hypercalcemia usually does not exceed 14 or 15 mg/100 ml and usually does not produce a hypercalcemic crisis.

Nephrolithiasis and nephrocalcinosis may produce pyelonephritis. Hypercalcemia may also produce impaired renal function. The author has seen two patients with sarcoid referred because of anemia who were found to have chronic renal failure as a result of hypercalcemia. The anemia in them was caused by renal insufficiency. Clinical findings in patients with sarcoid related to abnormal calcium metabolism include calcium deposits in the conjunctivae and costovertebral angle tenderness in patients with urinary tract infections and kidney stones.

B. Other Systems

1. Lungs

Over 90% of patients have pulmonary involvement of sarcoid that includes the hilar lymph nodes.[1,2] Thus, less than 10% of patients have a normal radiograph of the chest. Changes based on radiographic findings are classified into four categories. In stage 1, there is bilateral hilar adenopathy, which may be associated with paratracheal lymph node enlargement. In stage 2, there is bilateral hilar lymphadenopathy, which is associated with parenchymal infiltration. In stage 3, there is widespread parenchymal infiltration without hilar adenopathy. In stage 4, there is irreversible fibrosis, formation of bullae, hilar retraction, and emphysema. Pulmonary function studies show restrictive impairment. Vital capacity, residual volume, and total lung capacity are reduced, and the ratio of forced expiratory volume in one second to vital capacity is normal or increased. Lung compliance is diminished, and hypoxemia occurs as a result of impaired diffusing capacity because of a disturbance in ventilation-perfusion. Airway obstruction is also common. In patients with progressive disease, severe pulmonary hypertension and cor pulmonale occur.

Patients may either be asymptomatic or, with mild disease, have shortness of breath on exertion. With more extensive involvement, dyspnea, dry cough, and wheezing may be present.

2. Skin

Skin lesions in sarcoidosis include erythema nodosum, plaques, maculopapular rash, scars, and lupus pernio.[1,2] The erythema nodosum occurs on the calves, knees, buttocks, and sometimes the arms. It often is associated with systemic symptoms including fever, malaise, and joint pains. Lupus pernio occurs as bluish indurated lesions involving the nose, cheeks, and lips. It commonly occurs in patients with chronic disease and is associated with pulmonary fibrosis, uveitis, and bone lesions. Maculopapular eruptions occur with acute uveitis or parotid gland enlargement and there is involvement of the trunk, face, arms, thighs, calves, ears, and fingers. Sarcoidosis may involve scars and produce a keloid reaction. Alopecia is also a dermatologic complication of sarcoidosis.

3. Eyes

Any part of the eye may be involved in sarcoidosis.[1,2] The most common lesion is uveitis, which may be subacute or chronic. Subacute uveitis or iridocyclitis characteristically has a sudden onset with redness and watering of the eyes and cloudy vision and photophobia. Chronic uveitis has a slow onset and may progress to glaucoma, adhesions between the iris and the lens, cataract formation, and blindness. Symptoms include pain and blurred vision. Choroidoretinitis, conjunctivitis, and conjunctival follicles also occur. Keratoconjunctivitis sicca results from granulomatous infiltration of the lacrimal glands with impaired formation of tears.

4. Reticuloendothelial System

Peripheral lymphadenopathy occurs in about 25% of patients with sarcoidosis.[1,2] Commonly affected sites include the axillary, inguinal, iliac, lumbar, and epitrochlear nodes.

Involved glands are usually nontender, painless, discrete, and moderately enlarged. Splenomegaly is about half as common and is usually asymptomatic. Hypersplenism, however, may occur and be associated with pancytopenia, thrombocytopenia, purpura, and hemolytic anemia.

5. Liver

The liver is enlarged in about 20% of patients with sarcoidosis, but granulomas are found in some three quarters of patients.[1,2] In general, liver involvement is more frequent in acute disease and less common in chronic disease. Intrahepatic obstruction rarely occurs but when present is associated with jaundice, pruritus, hepatosplenomegaly, and portal hypertension.

6. Heart

Clinically apparent myocardial involvement occurs in 3% to 5% of patients with sarcoidosis.[1,2] Any part of the heart may be involved as well as the aorta, pulmonary arteries, superior vena cava, and pulmonary veins. Conduction disturbances, arrhythmias, congestive heart failure, and sudden death may occur. Occasionally, patients present with a picture that resembles that of an acute myocardial infarction.

7. Kidneys

In sarcoidosis, the kidneys are most often affected by hypercalcemia and hypercalciuria but other manifestations are found.[1,2] Thus, granulomatous infiltration occurs and may produce mild albuminuria and abnormal urinary sediment. In addition, diminished renal concentrating ability, alteration in tubular function, impaired renal tubular reabsorption of water, and abnormal urinary acidification occur. Occasionally the involvement is so extensive as to produce severe impairment of renal function. In addition, membranous and proliferative glomerular disease sometimes occurs and is associated with proteinuria or the nephrotic syndrome.

8. Nervous System

The nervous system is involved in sarcoidosis in about 5% of patients.[1,2] The sites include cranial nerves, meninges, hypothalamus, and pituitary gland. The facial nerve is the one most frequently affected and also the most common neurologic abnormality. Involvement of the optic nerve with blurred vision, field defects, and abnormalities also occurs. Endocrine abnormalities include diabetes insipidus and disturbances of the hypothalamus causing obesity, lethargy, sleep disturbances, hypogonadism, and amenorrhea. Seizures, granulomatous masses that produce localizing signs and symptoms, granulomatous involvement of the meninges that produces meningitis, and peripheral neuropathy occur.

9. Musculoskeletal System

Granulomatous invasion of bones occurs most commonly in the hands and feet and may present as diffusely expanded bone with cysts of various sizes, round and well-defined punched out areas, or a lattice-like appearance.[1,2] The joints may be involved in sarcoidosis and the most commonly affected ones are the knees, ankles, elbows, wrists, and small joints of the hands. The joints are usually warm, tender, swollen, and painful with associated effusions. The joint disease may be associated with fever, erythema nodosum, and hilar adenopathy. The muscles may also be involved, and patients may be either asymptomatic or have multiple nodules and polymyositis associated with severe muscle pain and tenderness with involvement of the proximal shoulder and pelvic girdle muscles. Sarcoidosis may also be associated with chronic myopathy manifested by muscle wasting and weakness and by an isolated myopathy.

10. Gastrointestinal Tract

Involvement of the gastrointestinal tract is rare in sarcoidosis.[1,2] However, an association has been noted between sarcoidosis and celiac disease.[72] In five patients with both disorders, gastrointestinal symptoms preceded those of sarcoid in three of them, and in the other two the onset of symptoms of the two diseases occurred at the same time. There is evidence that gluten-induced abnormalities of the small intestine in celiac disease may have an immunologic basis. Increases in circulating gamma globulins, particularly IgA, occur in both diseases, and the Kveim reaction may be positive in celiac disease and primary biliary cirrhosis, a disorder in which granulomas also occur. Finally, the genotype HLA-B8 is common to sarcoid and adult celiac disease.

Table 22–1. Differential Diagnosis of Hypercalcemia

Increased resorption of bone
Primary hyperparathyroidism
Secondary hyperparathyroidism
Chronic renal failure
Post renal transplant
Malignancy associated
Without skeletal metastases
With skeletal metastases
Hematologic
Multiple myeloma
Thyrotoxicosis
Immobilization
Vitamin A intoxication
Increased intestinal absorption of calcium
Increased circulating $1,25(OH)_2D$
Sarcoid
Tuberculosis
Other granulomatous diseases
Lymphoma and solid tumors
Hypercalcemia without associated disease
$1,25(OH)_2D_3$ intoxication
Vitamin D intoxication
Milk-alkali syndrome
Miscellaneous causes
Thiazides
Adrenal insufficiency
Familial hypercalciuric hypercalcemia

V. DIFFERENTIAL DIAGNOSIS

As outlined in Table 22–1, the differential diagnosis of abnormal calcium metabolism in sarcoidosis includes other diseases in which hypercalcemia and hypercalciuria occur.

A. Primary Hyperparathyroidism

In primary hyperparathyroidism, hypercalcemia, hypercalciuria, and increased circulating 1,25-dihydroxyvitamin D are caused by increased secretion of parathyroid hormone and may be associated with increased intestinal absorption of calcium.[73] Depending on the radioimmunoassay used, serum immunoreactive parathyroid hormone is usually abnormally elevated,[74] together with nephrogenous cyclic adenosine 3′,5′-monophosphate.[75] Since parathyroid hormone acts to enhance the tubular reabsorption of calcium,[76] urinary calcium is lower than it otherwise might be for a given value of serum calcium. Urinary calcium may therefore not be increased. Since hypercalcemia suppresses renal 25-hydroxyvitamin D 1α-hydroxylase,[77] serum 1,25-dihydroxyvitamin D may not be abnormally elevated.

It is sometimes difficult to distinguish hypercalcemia caused by primary hyperparathyroidism from hypercalcemia caused by sarcoidosis. Serum immunoreactive parathyroid hormone and urinary cyclic adenosine 3′,5′-monophosphate are not consistently elevated in primary hyperparathyroidism and are not consistently suppressed in sarcoidosis. Further, radiographs of the chest are not always abnormal in sarcoidosis. Serum angiotensin-converting enzyme is usually increased in patients with sarcoidosis and hypercalcemia but may be increased in patients with primary hyperparathyroidism as well.[78] Because of the occasional difficulty in diagnosis, a few patients with sarcoidosis have been diagnosed in the course of parathyroid exploration when granulomas were observed in excised lymph nodes or other tissue. Finally, some patients may have both diseases. One potentially useful test is the response to corticosteroids. Glucocorticoids suppress serum 1,25-dihydroxyvitamin D in sarcoidosis[41,56–59] and transiently increase serum 1,25-dihydroxyvitamin D in primary hyperparathyroidism.[79] A more detailed description of the clinical and laboratory findings in primary hyperparathyroidism is presented in Chapter 14.

B. Secondary Hyperparathyroidism

Hypertrophy of the parathyroids may cause hypercalcemia in the course of chronic renal failure both before and after renal transplantation.[80] Hypercalcemia caused by increased circulating 1,25-dihydroxyvitamin D associated with chronic renal failure was described in patients with sarcoidosis[27,81] and tuberculosis.[82] In the face of end-stage renal disease, the distinguishing features are that serum immunoreactive parathyroid hormone is increased and serum 1,25-dihydroxyvitamin D is abnormally low or undetectable in hypercalcemia caused by secondary hyperparathyroidism, whereas serum immunoreactive parathyroid hormone is suppressed or undetectable in hypercalcemia resulting from abnormal elevation of serum 1,25-dihydroxyvitamin D.[27,79,82] Further, glucocorticoids correct hypercalcemia caused by increased circulating 1,25-dihydroxyvitamin D and lower the serum 1,25-dihydroxyvitamin D.[27,81,82]

C. Malignancies

Hypercalcemia occurs in a variety of malignancies and results from invasion and destruction of the skeleton as well as from the production of bone-resorbing factors by malignant cells.[83] In some 55% of patients with malignancies, hypercalcemia occurs in association with solid tumors including squamous cell carcinoma of the kidney and ovary and is caused by synthesis and secretion of one or more factors that stimulate osteoclastic bone resorption, the so-called humoral hypercalcemia of malignancy. Skeletal metastases may be present. In addition to hypercalcemia, the syndrome is characterized by renal phosphate wasting, increases in urinary cyclic adenosine 3′,5′-monophosphate, and suppression of circulating immunoreactive parathyroid hormone and serum 1,25-dihydroxyvitamin D.[84] The features that distinguish the syndrome from hypercalcemia that occurs with sarcoidosis are the low serum phosphorus and serum 1,25-dihydroxyvitamin D and increased urinary cyclic adenosine 3′,5′-monophosphate that occur in patients with malignancies.

In some 25% of patients, hypercalcemia develops late in the course of tumors that are associated with widespread skeletal metastases.[83] In instances such as these, serum immunoreactive parathyroid hormone, serum 1,25-dihydroxyvitamin D, and urinary cyclic adenosine 3′,5′-monophosphate are suppressed. The low serum 1,25-dihydroxyvitamin D and the clinical picture of cancer with metastases serve to distinguish the disorder from hypercalcemia associated with sarcoidosis.

In some 15% to 20% of patients with malignancies, hypercalcemia is caused by synthesis and secretion of factors that produce localized bone resorption.[83] One such is osteoclast-activating factor that is produced by myeloma cells.[85] In these and related diseases, hypercalcemia is associated with suppression of serum immunoreactive parathyroid hormone, serum 1,25-dihydroxyvitamin D, and urinary cyclic adenosine 3′5′-monophosphate. The low serum 1,25-dihydroxyvitamin D is a distinguishing feature that is different from hypercalcemia associated with sarcoidosis.

Hodgkin's disease, histiocytic lymphoma, T cell leukemia-lymphoma, B cell leukemia, seminoma, plasma cell granuloma and leiomyoblastoma in association with hypercalcemia resulting from increased circulating 1,25-dihydroxyvitamin D are described at the end of the chapter.

A more detailed description of the clinical and laboratory findings in malignancies is presented in Chapter 21.

D. Thyrotoxicosis

Hypercalcemia sometimes occurs in thyrotoxicosis[86] and is attributed to a direct skeletal effect of thyroid hormones.[87] The clinical picture together with laboratory findings of increases in serum T_3 and T_4 and suppression of serum thyroid-stimulating hormone are features that distinguish this illness from hypercalcemia associated with sarcoidosis.

E. Immobilization

Hypercalcemia may occur in association with immobilization as the result of quadriplegia, paraplegia, or prolonged bed rest. It is associated with suppression of serum immunoreactive parathyroid hormone, serum 1,25-dihydroxyvitamin D, and urinary cyclic adenosine 3′,5′-monophosphate.[88] The clinical picture and low serum 1,25-dihydroxyvitamin D are findings that distinguish this illness from hypercalcemia associated with sarcoidosis.

F. Vitamin A Intoxication

Hypercalcemia rarely occurs as a result of vitamin A intoxication. The diagnosis is made from the history, the finding of increased serum values for vitamin A (usually above 100 μg/100 ml), and the clinical picture.

G. Other Granulomatous Diseases

Hypercalcemia associated with tuberculosis, disseminated coccidioidomycosis, candidiasis, histoplasmosis, leprosy, and silicone-induced granulomas is discussed at the end of the chapter.

H. 1,25-Dihydroxyvitamin D Intoxication

Hypercalcemia may also occur in patients who are receiving 1,25-dihydroxyvitamin D_3.[89] The hypercalcemia develops spontaneously even after a dose has been established that maintains the serum calcium in the normal range. As shown in Figure 22–4, the hypercalcemia is associated with abnormal increases in serum 1,25-dihydroxyvitamin D and suppression of serum immunoreactive parathyroid hormone. It has been reported to occur in

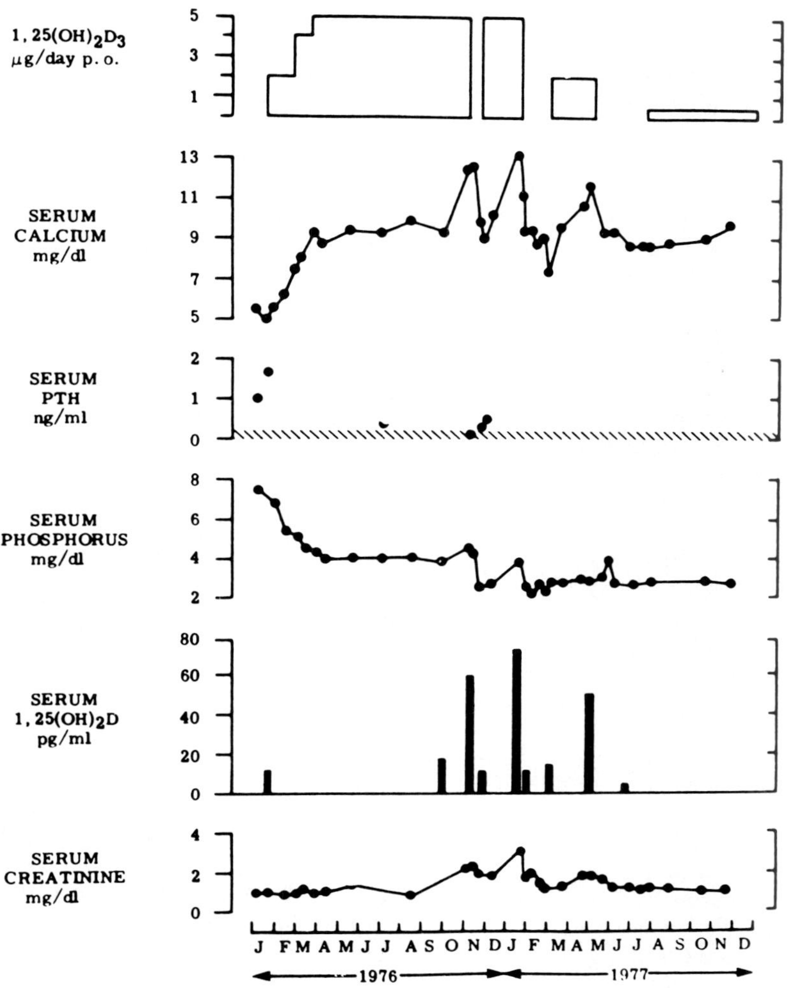

Figure 22–4. Effects of 1,25-dihydroxyvitamin D_3 on serum calcium, phosphorus, immunoreactive parathyroid hormone, and serum creatinine in a 51-year-old man with pseudohypoparathyroidism. Note (1) that the hypercalcemia was associated with increases in serum 1,25-dihydroxyvitamin D and (2) that the hypercalcemia was corrected by stopping treatment and was prevented by reducing the dose of 1,25-dihydroxyvitamin D_3. (From Bell NH, Stern PH: N Engl J Med 298:1241, 1978.)

a number of disorders including renal failure, osteoporosis, hypoparathyroidism, and pseudohypoparathyroidism. The diagnosis is made from the history.

I. Vitamin D Intoxication

Hypercalcemia and hypercalciuria that are corrected by corticosteroids and are associated with suppression of serum immunoreactive parathyroid hormone and urinary cyclic adenosine 3′5′-monophosphate occur in vitamin D intoxication.[90] In patients with vitamin D intoxication, the abnormal calcium metabolism is caused by excess circulating 25-hydroxyvitamin D. Thus, serum 25-hydroxyvitamin D is markedly increased and serum 1,25-dihydroxyvitamin D is either normal or only modestly elevated.[91] The diagnosis of vitamin D intoxication is made by the history of excessive intake of vitamin D and is confirmed by the finding of markedly elevated serum 25-hydroxyvitamin D, 200 ng/ml or higher.

J. Milk-Alkali Syndrome

Hypercalcemia sometimes occurs as the result of excessive intake of calcium and antacids for treatment of peptic ulcer.[92] The illness seldom occurs at the present time, since drugs that block histamine receptors have proved to be so effective. The diagnosis is made by history. It is likely that some of the patients originally described with the syndrome, many of whom had renal insufficiency, may have had primary hyperparathyroidism.[93]

K. Miscellaneous Disorders

Thiazides sometimes produce hypercalcemia and do so in part by increasing the renal tubular reabsorption of calcium.[94,95] The diagnosis is made by history. Adrenal insufficiency may cause hypercalcemia. It is caused by severe salt loss and dehydration as the result of deficiency of aldosterone. The hypercalcemia results from increases in serum albumin and increased calcium binding to albumin. Thus, the ionized calcium is not elevated so that the hypercalcemia is of no pathophysiologic consequence.[96] Hypercalcemia also occurs in association with a familial disorder in which the urinary calcium is reduced, so-called familial hypocalciuric hypercalcemia.[97] The family history and low urinary calcium serve to distinguish this disorder from hypercalcemia associated with sarcoidosis.

L. Idiopathic Hypercalciuria

Hypercalciuria in association with nephrolithiasis may occur as the result of renal loss of calcium (renal hypercalciuria) or of enhanced intestinal absorption of calcium (absorptive hypercalciuria)[98] (see Chapter 23). In renal hypercalciuria, renal loss of calcium produces secondary hyperparathyroidism, increases in serum 1,25-dihydroxyvitamin D and urinary cyclic adenosine 3′,5′-monophosphate, and enhanced intestinal absorption of calcium. In absorptive hypercalciuria, increased intestinal absorption of calcium leads to suppression of serum immunoreactive parathyroid hormone, serum 1,25-dihydroxyvitamin D, and urinary cyclic adenosine 3′,5′-monophosphate. Thus, renal hypercalciuria produces biochemical changes that are found in normocalcemic patients with sarcoidosis and hypercalciuria. Other evidence for sarcoidosis must be obtained in a given patient to distinguish the two disorders from each other. Also, glucocorticoids lower serum 1,25-dihydroxyvitamin D in sarcoid but not in normal subjects or patients with absorptive hypercalciuria.[41]

VI. TREATMENT

A. Glucocorticoids

The abnormal vitamin D and calcium metabolism in sarcoidosis consistently respond to treatment with glucocorticoids. Serum and urinary calcium are decreased to normal and fecal calcium is increased.[33–36] Glucocorticoids thus inhibit the intestinal absorption and turnover of calcium as determined with labeled calcium.[33,36] Increased circulating 1,25-dihydroxyvitamin D is lowered to values that are within or even below the normal range,[27,56–59] and serum immunoreactive parathyroid hormone increases as the serum calcium declines.[56–60] Glucocorticoids also reduce serum 1,25-dihydroxyvitamin D and the intestinal absorption of calcium even in patients with sarcoid and a normal serum calcium.[41] In contrast, values in normal subjects do not change.[99] Glucocorticoids act to reverse the abnormal calcium metabolism in sarcoid by correcting the altered metabolism of vitamin D. They may also act by inhibiting the peripheral actions of 1,25-dihydroxyvitamin D as well.[100]

Glucocorticoids may be effective in reducing serum 1,25-dihydroxyvitamin D in sarcoidosis by suppressing the inflammatory response. They inhibit the proliferation of T lymphocytes,[101,102] the production of T cell growth factor,[103] and the production of macrophage migration inhibitory factor.[104] Since sarcoidosis is a granulomatous disease that is perpetuated by activated T lymphocytes, glucocorticoids could act by inhibiting the growth, development, and maintenance of granulomas. In this regard it is interesting to note that glucocorticoids lower serum angiotensin-converting enzyme in patients with sarcoidosis and hypercalcemia,[78] that serum angiotensin-converting enzyme is present in sarcoid granulomas,[105] and that it is produced by peripheral monocytes in this disease.[106]

B. Other Therapy

Other modes of therapy that may be effective in treatment of abnormal calcium metabolism in sarcoidosis include reduction of calcium intake,[35] administration of sodium phytate or edetate disodium, which bind dietary calcium and prevent its absorption,[34,107] and omission of dietary vitamin D and exposure to ultraviolet light.[39]

The prostaglandin synthesis inhibitor flurbiprofen was used to successfully treat hypercalcemia in one patient with sarcoidosis.[108] Unlike glucocorticoids, which reduce serum 1,25-dihydroxyvitamin D, flurbiprofen corrected the hypercalcemia but did not influence the increased circulating 1,25-dihydroxyvitamin D. If the effectiveness of flurbiprofen is confirmed, it could be a useful alternative means to treat abnormal calcium metabolism in sarcoidosis.

Since glucocorticoids do cause substantial loss of bone in patients with sarcoidoses,[108a] hydroxychloroquine has been tried successfully, reversing the abnormal vitamin D metabolism and skeletal disability that resulted from the disease.[108b]

VII. OTHER DISEASES

The diseases that are reported to be associated with hypercalcemia caused by increases in serum 1,25-dihydroxyvitamin D are listed in Table 22–2. Each of them is discussed here in some detail.

A. Tuberculosis

Hypercalcemia and hypercalciuria occur in pulmonary as well as miliary tuberculosis,[82,109–116] and hypercalcemia is associated with suppression of serum immunoreactive parathyroid hormone.[110–112] Patients with tuberculosis are abnormally sensitive to vitamin D, and the hypercalcemia is reversed by glucocorticoids.[109,111,115] Hypercalcemia in pulmonary tuberculosis is caused by increased circulating 1,25-dihydroxyvitamin D.[82,116] Further, regulation of serum 1,25-dihydroxyvitamin D is abnormal in normocalcemic patients with pulmonary tuberculosis.[117] Thus, we observed a modest but significant increase in mean serum 1,25-dihydroxyvitamin D in a group of 11 patients given vitamin D, 100,000 units a day for 4 days, but no change in mean serum 1,25-dihydroxyvitamin D in a group of normal subjects. These findings show that the abnormalities in the metabolism of vitamin D and calcium in pulmonary tuberculosis are similar to those that occur in sarcoidosis.

The clinical course of hypercalcemia in tuberculosis, however, differs from that in sarcoidosis in several important respects. As noted already, hypercalcemia in sarcoid often develops following exposure to sunlight during the summer months and may be the cause for hospitalization.[56–59] The abnormal calcium metabolism frequently persists, usually requires treatment with glucocorticoids, and may be associated with nephrolithiasis, nephrocalcinosis, and recurrent urinary tract infections. As a consequence, renal failure may develop and even result in death. In contrast, hypercalcemia in tuberculosis usually develops after several months of antituberculous therapy and is readily managed by hydration, and impairment of kidney function is short-lived and does not require hospitalization.[116] Thus, the prognosis for the abnormal calcium metabolism in the two diseases is quite different.

It is not known whether 1,25-dihydroxyvitamin D is synthesized by the tuberculous granuloma. The findings that the occurrence of hypercalcemia in tuberculosis varies with the extent of the disease[111] and that hypercalcemia and increased circulating 1,25-dihydroxyvitamin D occurred in a patient with tuberculosis and end-stage renal disease[82] are consistent with this possibility. The delay in onset of hypercalcemia that usually develops in the course of treatment suggests that abnormal production of 1,25-dihydroxyvitamin D may be related in some way to antituberculous therapy. However, no changes in serum 25-hydroxyvitamin D or 1,25-dihydroxyvitamin D were found in a long-term study of eight patients with pulmonary tuberculosis during their treatment with rifampin and isoniazid.[118]

B. Other Granulomatous Diseases

Hypercalcemia was reported in histoplasmosis,[119] disseminated candidiasis,[120] disseminated coccidioidomycosis,[121] berylliosis,[122] leprosy,[123] and silicone-induced granulomas.[124] Increased serum 1,25-dihydroxyvitamin D was demonstrated in patients with disseminated candidiasis,[120] leprosy,[123] and silicone-induced granulomas[124] and is assumed to be the cause for the abnormal calcium metabolism in these granulomatous diseases. Hypercalcemia and elevated 1,25-dihydroxyvitamin D were corrected by treatment with salmon calcitonin, saline, furosemide, and mithramycin in the patient with candidiasis and by prednisone in the patients with leprosy and silicone-induced granulomas. The cause for abnormal calcium metabolism in the other diseases was not determined. A low serum 1,25-dihydroxyvitamin D was demonstrated in a patient with hypercalcemia and disseminated coccidioidomycosis[125] and in another patient with hypercalcemia and leprosy.[126] This indicates that hypercalcemia may also result from mechanisms not related to abnormal vitamin D metabolism in these disorders.

We found hypercalcemia, hypercalciuria, and suppression of immunoreactive parathyroid hormone caused by increased circulating 1,25-dihydroxyvitamin D in a patient with rheumatoid arthritis.[127] The patient showed lack of regulation of serum 1,25-dihydroxyvitamin D in response to small doses of vitamin D. The abnormal calcium metabolism and increased serum 1,25-dihydroxyvitamin D were returned to normal by prednisone. It is not established whether the abnormal metabolism of vitamin D in this patient is related to rheumatoid arthritis.

C. Lymphoma and Solid Tumors

Hypercalcemia that is associated with increases in serum 1,25-dihydroxyvitamin D and responds to glucocorticoids occurs in patients with histiocytic lymphoma,[128,129] T cell leukemia-lymphoma,[128] B cell lymphoma,[130] Hodgkin's disease,[131–134] and plasma cell granuloma.[135] The hypercalcemia is associated with suppression of serum immunoreactive parathyroid hormone. Studies carried out in one of the patients with histiocytic lymphoma indicated that the hypercalcemia was associated with hyperabsorption of calcium and hypercalciuria.[128] T cell lymphoma resulting from human T cell lymphotrophic virus (HTLV-1) is characterized by lymphocytosis, hepatosplenomegaly, hypercalcemia, and a rapidly progressive course.[136] One patient with the disease, as noted, had hypercalcemia caused by increased circulating 1,25-dihydroxyvitamin D.[128] Other patients with T cell leukemia were found who had hypercalcemia and suppressed serum 1,25-dihydroxyvitamin D.[137] Thus, the hypercalcemia in them was not caused by abnormal vitamin D metabolism.

Human T lymphocytes from cord blood of normal infants infected with HTLV-1 by incubation of the lymphocytes with lymphoma cells carrying the virus secrete HTLV-1 proteins and exhibit morphologic and functional properties of the lymphoma cell.[138,139] Cord blood lymphocytes transformed by this means were shown to convert [^{3}H]25-hydroxyvitamin D_3 to [^{3}H]1,25-dihydroxyvitamin D_3.[140] The putative 1,25-dihydroxyvitamin D_3 caused release of ^{45}Ca from long bones of fetal rats in tissue culture, displaced [^{3}H]1,25-dihydroxyvitamin D_3 from the receptors of rat osteosarcoma cells in the same manner as authentic 1,25-dihydroxyvitamin D_3, and had the same retention times as authentic 1,25-dihydroxyvitamin D_3 on high-pressure liquid chromatography in a number of different solvent systems. The identity of the metabolite was confirmed as 1,25-dihydroxyvitamin D_3 by mass spectral analysis.[140] It remains to be demonstrated, however, that lymphocytes from patients with lymphoma produce 1,25-dihydroxyvitamin D. The question arises also whether activated lymphocytes synthesize 1,25-dihydroxyvitamin D in sarcoidosis.

Hypercalcemia with increased serum 1,25-dihydroxyvitamin D was reported in a patient with metastatic leiomyoblastoma of the jejunum.[141] No skeletal lesions were detected. Moderate renal insufficiency developed, and the abnormal vitamin D and calcium metabolism persisted despite subtotal parathyroidectomy. The hypercalcemia and abnormally elevated 1,25-dihydroxyvitamin D were reversed by prednisone, phenytoin, and phenobarbital.

Hypercalcemia with increased circulating 1,25-dihydroxyvitamin D was reported in a patient with seminoma.[142] These abnormal findings were reversed by partial resection of the tumor and chemotherapy.

A sterol tentatively identified as 1,24-dihydroxyvitamin D_3 was observed in extracts of serum and tumor in a patient with small cell carcinoma of the lung and hypercalcemia.[143] The sterol co-migrated with authentic 1,25-dihydroxyvitamin D_3 on high-pressure liquid chromatography and displaced [^{3}H]1,25-dihydroxyvitamin D_3 bound to the chick intestinal receptor in a manner similar to that of the authentic sterol. Further, the sterol and synthetic 1,24-dihydroxyvitamin D_3 showed identical biological activity in producing release of ^{45}Ca from mouse calvariae in tissue culture. The results provide evidence that the hypercalcemia in this patient resulted from increased production of 1,24-dihydroxyvitamin D_3. This important investigation is the first indication that an endogenously produced sterol other than 1,25-dihydroxyvitamin D may be responsible for abnormal calcium metabolism in a clinical disorder.

D. Hypercalcemia Without Associated Disease

Three patients were reported in whom hypercalcemia occurred in association with increased circulating 1,25-dihydroxyvitamin D, low-normal or undetectable serum immunoreactive parathyroid hormone and urinary cyclic adenosine 3′,5′-monophosphate, hypercalciuria, nephrolithiasis, and no apparent systemic disease.[144–146] All of them were males. In two of the patients, hypercalcemia was corrected by glucocorticoids. The site of the production of 1,25-dihydroxyvitamin D is not known. The fact that serum 1,25-dihydroxyvitamin D is unregulated strongly suggests a nonrenal source for the metabolite.

E. Hypercalcemia of Infancy

Hypercalcemia, hypercalciuria, and increased intestinal absorption of calcium associated with anorexia, vomiting, impaired renal function, mental retardation, and failure to thrive occurs in newborn infants.[147–153] Patients show increased sensitivity to vitamin D,[148,149] and the hypercalcemia and abnormal calcium metabolism are corrected by glucocorticoids.[148,149,151] The illness usually occurs in the first 2 years of life and is self-limited. There is an association with the Williams syndrome in which supravalvular aortic stenosis, an elfin facies, and mental retardation are found in association with a number of other congenital defects.[153–157] White children with the syndrome show an exaggerated increase in serum 25-dihydroxyvitamin D after vitamin D challenge compared with normal children.[158] This is attributed to a lack of increase in serum 1,25-dihydroxyvitamin D in the patients and lack of feedback reduction of circulating 25-hydroxyvitamin D.[51,52]

In four infants with elfin facies and hypercalcemia, increases in serum 1,25-dihydroxyvitamin D were observed.[159] Values declined with time, and hypercalcemia was successfully treated with a low-calcium diet. In another child with hypercalcemia, the serum 1,25-dihydroxyvitamin D was abnormally low.[157,160] This indicates that hypercalcemia in the syndrome of hypercalcemia of infancy may result not only from elevation of circulating 1,25-dihydroxyvitamin D but from other causes as well. In the infants with abnormal elevations of circulating 1,25-dihydroxyvitamin D, the source of the metabolite is not known. Restriction of calcium intake, hydration, and glucocorticoids are effective means of treating children with hypercalcemia and abnormal vitamin D metabolism in this disorder.[150,152,158,159]

References

1. Sharma OP: Sarcoidosis: Clinical Management. London, Butterworths, 1984, pp 22–124.
2. James DG, Williams WJ: Sarcoidosis and Other Granulomatous Disorders. Philadelphia, WB Saunders, 1985, pp 38–162.
3. Takahashi M: Histopathology of sarcoidosis and its immunological basis. Acta Pathol Jpn 20:171–182, 1970.
4. Rosen Y, Athanassiades TJ, Moon S, et al: Nongranulomatous interstitial pneumonitis in sarcoidosis: Relationship to the development of epithelioid granulomas. Chest 74:122–125, 1978.
5. Hunninghake GW, Fulmer JD, Young RC, et al: Localization of the immune response in sarcoidosis. Am Rev Respir Dis 120:49–57, 1979.
6. Weinberger SE, Kelman JA, Elson NA, et al: Bronchoalveolar lavage in interstitial lung disease. Ann Intern Med 89:459–466, 1978.
7. Hunninghake GW, Crystal RG: Pulmonary sarcoidosis: A disorder mediated by excess helper T-lymphocyte activity at sites of disease activity. N Engl J Med 305:429–434, 1981.
8. Daniele R, Dauber JH, Rossman MD: Immunologic abnormalities in sarcoidosis. Ann Intern Med 92:406–416, 1980.
9. Hunninghake GW, Bedell GN, Zavala DC, et al: Role of interleukin-2 release by lung T-cells in active pulmonary sarcoidosis. Am Rev Respir Dis 128:634–638, 1983.
10. Pinkston P, Bitterman PB, Crystal RG: Spontaneous release of interleukin-2 by lung T-lymphocytes in active pulmonary sarcoidosis. N Engl J Med 308:793–800, 1983.
11. Venet A, Hance AJ, Saltini C, et al: Enhanced alveolar macrophage-mediated antigen-induced T lymphocyte proliferation in sarcoidosis. J Clin Invest 75:293–301, 1985.
12. Hunninghake GW, Gadek JE, Young RC Jr: Maintenance of granuloma formation in pulmonary sarcoidosis by T lymphocytes within the lung. N Engl J Med 302:594–598, 1980.
13. Robinson BWS, McLemore TL, Crystal RG: Gamma interferon is spontaneously released by alveolar macrophages and lung T lymphocytes in patients with pulmonary sarcoidosis. J Clin Invest 72:1488–1495, 1985.
14. Wewers MD, Saltini C, Sellers S, et al: Evaluation of alveolar macrophages in normals and individuals with active pulmonary sarcoidosis for the spon-

taneous expression of the interleukin-1 beta gene. Cell Immunol 107:479–488, 1987.

15. Gordon LI, Douglas SD, Kay NE, et al: Modulation of neutrophil function by lysozyme: Potential feedback system of inflammation. J Clin Invest 64:226–232, 1979.
16. Gee JB, Godel PT, Zorn SK, et al: Sarcoidosis and mononuclear phagocytes. Lung 155:243–253, 1978.
17. Hunninghake GW, Crystal RG: Mechanisms of hypergammaglobulinemia in pulmonary sarcoidosis: Site of increased antibody production and role of T lymphocytes. J Clin Invest 67:86–92, 1981.
18. Katz P, Fauci AS: Inhibition of polyclonal B-cell activation by suppressor monocytes in patients with sarcoidosis. Clin Exp Immunol 32:554–562, 1978.
19. Adams JS, Sharma OP, Gacad MA, et al: Metabolism of 25-hydroxyvitamin D_3 by cultured pulmonary alveolar macrophages in sarcoidosis. J Clin Invest 72:1856–1860, 1983.
20. Adams JS, Singer FR, Gacad MA, et al: Isolation and structural identification of 1,25-dihydroxyvitamin D_3 produced by cultured alveolar macrophages in sarcoidosis. J Clin Endocrinol Metab 60:960–966, 1985.
21. Adams JS, Gacad MA: Characterization of 1α-hydroxylation of vitamin D_3 sterols by cultured alveolar macrophages from patients with sarcoidosis. J Exp Med 161:755–765, 1985.
22. Reichel H, Koeffler HP, Barbers R, Norman AW: Regulation of 1,25-dihydroxyvitamin D_3 production by cultured alveolar macrophages from normal human donors and from patients with pulmonary sarcoidosis. J Clin Endocrinol Metab 65:1201–1209, 1987.
23. Provvedini DM, Tsoukas CD, Deftos LJ, et al: 1,25-Dihydroxyvitamin D_3 receptors in human leukocytes. Science 221:1181–1183, 1983.
24. Tsoukas CD, Provvedini DM, Monalagas SC: 1,25-Dihydroxyvitamin D_3: A novel immunoregulatory hormone. Science 224:1438–1440, 1984.
25. Reichel H, Koeffler HP, Tobler A, Norman AW: 1α,25-Dihydroxyvitamin D_3 inhibits γ-interferon synthesis by normal human peripheral blood lymphocytes. Proc Natl Acad Sci USA 84:3385–3389, 1987.
26. Lemire JM, Adams JS, Kermani-Arab V, et al: 1,25-Dihydroxyvitamin D_3 suppresses human T helper/inducer lymphocyte activity in vitro. J Immunol 134:3032–3035, 1985.
27. Barbour GL, Coburn JW, Slatopolsky E, et al: Hypercalcemia in an anephric patient with sarcoidosis: Evidence for extrarenal generation of 1,25-dihydroxyvitamin D_3. N Engl J Med 305:440–443, 1981.
28. Solar P, Basset F: Morphology and distribution of the cells of a sarcoid granuloma: Ultrastructural study of serial sections. Ann NY Acad Sci 278:147–160, 1976.
29. Mitchell DN, Scadding JG: Sarcoidosis. Am Rev Respir Dis 110:774–802, 1974.
30. Mitchell DN, Scadding JG, Heard BE, et al: Sarcoidosis: Histopathological definition and clinical diagnosis. J Clin Pathol 30:395–408, 1977.
31. DiBenedetto RJ, Ribaudo C: Bronchopulmonary sarcoidosis. Am Rev Respir Dis 94:952–955, 1966.
32. Scadding JG: The late stages of pulmonary sarcoidosis. Postgrad Med J 46:530–536, 1970.
33. Anderson J, Dent CE, Harper C, Philpott GR: Effect of cortisone on calcium metabolism in sarcoidosis with hypercalcemia, possible antagonistic actions of cortisone and vitamin D. Lancet 2:720–724, 1954.
34. Henneman PH, Dempsey EF, Carroll EL, Albright F: The cause of hypercalciuria in sarcoid and its treatment with cortisone and sodium phytate. J Clin Invest 35:1229–1242, 1956.
35. Bell NH, Gill JR Jr, Bartter FC: On the abnormal calcium metabolism in sarcoidosis: Evidence for increased sensitivity to vitamin D. Am J Med 36:500–513, 1964.
36. Bell NH, Bartter FC: Studies of ^{47}Ca metabolism in sarcoidosis: Evidence for increased sensitivity of bone to vitamin D. Acta Endocrinol 54:173–180, 1967.
37. Dent CE: Calcium metabolism in sarcoidosis. Postgrad Med J 46:471–473, 1970.
38. Taylor RL, Lynch HJ, Wysor WG Jr: Seasonal influence of sunlight on the hypercalcemia of sarcoidosis. Am J Med 34:221–227, 1963.
39. Hendrix JZ: Abnormal skeletal mineral metabolism in sarcoidosis. Ann Intern Med 64:797–805, 1966.
40. Reiner M, Sigurdsson G, Nunziata MA, et al: Abnormal calcium metabolism in normocalcaemic sarcoidosis. Br Med J 2:1473–1476, 1976.
41. Zerwekh JE, Pak CYC, Kaplan RA, et al: Pathogenetic role of 1α,25-dihydroxyvitamin D in sarcoidosis and absorptive hypercalciuria: Different response to prednisolone therapy. J Clin Endocrinol Metab 51:381–386, 1980.
42. Studdy PR, Bird R, Neville E, et al: Biochemical findings in sarcoidosis. J Clin Pathol 33:528–533, 1980.
43. Goldstein RA, Israel HL, Becker KL, Moore CF: The infrequency of hypercalcemia in sarcoidosis. Am J Med 51:21–30, 1971.
44. Bell NH, Greene A, Epstein S, et al: Evidence for alteration of the vitamin D-endocrine system in blacks. J Clin Invest 76:470–473, 1985.
45. Bell NH, Epstein S, Greene A, et al: Evidence for alteration of the vitamin D-endocrine system in obese subjects. J Clin Invest 76:370–373, 1985.
46. Holick MF, McNeill SC, McLaughlin JA, et al: Physiologic implications of the formation of previtamin D_3 in the skin. Trans Assoc Am Physicians 92:54–63, 1979.
47. Ponchon A, DeLuca HF: "Activation" of vitamin D by the liver. J Clin Invest 48:1273–1279, 1969.
48. Fraser DR, Kodicek E: Unique biosynthesis by kidney of a biological active vitamin D metabolite. Nature 228:764–766, 1970.
49. Holick MF, Schnoes HK, DeLuca HF, et al: Isolation and identification of 1,25-dihydroxycholecalciferol. A metabolite of vitamin D active in intestine. Biochemistry 10:2799–2804, 1981.
50. Raisz LG, Trummel CL, Holick MF, DeLuca HF: 1,25-dihydroxycholecalciferol: A potent stimulator of bone resorption in tissue culture. Science 175:768–769, 1972.
51. Bell NH, Shaw S, Turner RT: Evidence that 1,25-dihydroxyvitamin D_3 inhibits the hepatic production of 25-hydroxyvitamin D in man. J Clin Invest 74:1540–1544, 1984.
52. Halloran BP, Bikle DD, Levens MJ, et al: Chronic 1,25-dihydroxyvitamin D_3 administration in the rat reduces the serum concentration of 25-hydroxyvitamin D by increasing metabolic clearance rate. J Clin Invest 78:622–628, 1986.
53. Haussler MR, Baylink DJ, Hughes MR, et al: The assay of 1α,25-dihydroxyvitamin D_3, physiologic and

pathophysiologic modulation of circulating hormone levels. Clin Endocrinol 5:151s–165s, 1976.

54. Lambert PW, Hollis BW, Bell NH, Epstein S: Demonstration of a lack of change in serum 1α,25-dihydroxyvitamin D in response to parathyroid extract in pseudohypoparathyroidism. J Clin Invest 66:852–855, 1980.
55. Gallagher JG, Riggs BL, Eisman J: Intestinal calcium absorption and serum vitamin D metabolites in normal subjects and osteoporotic patients. J Clin Invest 64:729–736, 1979.
56. Bell NH, Stern PH, Pantzer E, et al: Evidence that increased circulating 1α,25-dihydroxyvitamin D is the probable cause for abnormal calcium metabolism in sarcoidosis. J Clin Invest 64: 218–225, 1979.
57. Papapoulos SE, Clemens TL, Fraher LJ, et al: 1,25-Dihydroxycholecalciferol in the pathogenesis of the hypercalcemia of sarcoid. Lancet 1:627–630, 1979.
58. Koide Y, Kugai N, Kimura S, et al: Increased 1,25-dihydroxycholecalciferol as a cause of abnormal calcium metabolism in sarcoidosis. J Clin Endocrinol Metab 52:494–498, 1981.
59. Sandler LM, Winearls CG, Fraher LJ, et al: Studies of the hypercalcemia of sarcoidosis: Effect of steroids and exogenous vitamin D_3 on the circulating concentration of 1,25-dihydroxyvitamin D. Q J Med 210:165–180, 1984.
60. Cushard WG Jr, Simon AB, Canterbury JM, et al: Parathyroid function in sarcoidosis. N Engl J Med 286:395–398, 1972.
61. Stern PH, DeOlazabal J, Bell NH: Evidence for abnormal regulation of circulating 1α,25-dihydroxyvitamin D in patients with sarcoidosis and normal calcium metabolism. J Clin Invest 66:852–855, 1980.
62. McLaughlin M, Ruggart PR, Fairney A, et al: Seasonal variation in serum 25-hydroxycholecalciferol in healthy people. Lancet 1:536–538, 1974.
63. Chesney RW, Rosen JF, Hamstra AJ, et al: Absence of seasonal variation in serum concentrations of 1,25-dihydroxyvitamin D despite a rise in 25-hydroxyvitamin D in summer. J Clin Endocrinol Metab 53:139–142, 1981.
64. Fukase M, Avioli LV, Birge SJ, et al: Abnormal regulation of 25-hydroxyvitamin D_3-1α-hydroxylase activity by calcium and calcitonin in renal cortex from hypophosphatemic (Hyp) mice. Endocrinology 114:1203–1207, 1984.
65. Fukase MS, Birge SJ Jr, Rifas L, et al: Regulation of 25-hydroxyvitamin D_3-1-hydroxylase in serum-free monolayer cultures of mouse kidney. Endocrinology 110:1073–1075, 1982.
66. Turner RT, Bottemiller BL, Howard GA, et al: In vitro metabolism of 25-hydroxyvitamin D_3 by isolated rat kidney cells. Proc Natl Acad Sci USA 77:1537–1540, 1980.
67. Warner M: Catalytic activity of partially purified renal 25-hydroxyvitamin D hydroxylases from vitamin D-deficient and vitamin D-replete rats. J Biol Chem 257:12995–13000, 1982.
68. Holick MF, Kleiner-Bossaller A, Schnoes HK, et al: 1,24,25-Trihydroxyvitamin D_3: A metabolite of vitamin D_3 effective on intestine. J Biol Chem 248:6691–6696, 1973.
69. Stern PH: A monolog on analogues: In vitro effects of vitamin D metabolites and consideration of the mineralization question. Calcif Tissue Int 33:1–4, 1981.
70. Omdahl JL: Modulation of kidney 25-hydroxyvitamin D_3 metabolism by 1α,25-dihydroxyvitamin D_3 in thyroparathyroidectomized rats. Life Sci 19:1943–1948, 1976.
71. Gill JR Jr, Bartter FC: On the impairment of renal concentrating ability in prolonged hypercalcemia and hypercalciuria in man. J Clin Invest 40:716–722, 1961.
72. Douglas JG, Gillon J, Logan RFA, et al: Sarcoidosis and coeliac disease: An association? Lancet 2: 13–15, 1984.
73. Kaplan RA, Haussler MR, Deftos LJ, et al: The role of 1α,25-dihydroxyvitamin D in the mediation of the intestinal hyperabsorption of calcium in primary hyperparathyroidism and absorptive hypercalciuria. J Clin Invest 59:756–760, 1977.
74. Mallette LE, Tuma SN, Berger RE, Kirkland JL: Radioimmunoassay for the middle region of human parathyroid hormone using an homologous antiserum with a carboxy-terminal fragment of bovine parathyroid hormone as a radioligand. J Clin Endocrinol Metab 54:1017–1024, 1982.
75. Broadus AE, Mahaffey JE, Bartter FC, Neer RM: Nephrogenous cyclic adenosine monophosphate as a parathyroid function test. J Clin Invest 60:771–783, 1977.
76. Widrow SH, Levinsky NG: The effect of parathyroid extract on renal tubular calcium reabsorption in the dog. J Clin Invest 41:2151–2159, 1962.
77. Hulter HN, Halloran BP, Toto RD, Peterson JC: Long-term control of plasma calcitriol concentrations in dogs and humans: Dominant role of plasma calcium concentration in experimental hyperparathyroidism. J Clin Invest 76:695–702, 1985.
78. DeRemee RA, Lufkin EG, Rohrbach MS: Serum angiotensin-converting enzyme activity: Its use in the evaluation and management of hypercalcemia associated with sarcoidosis. Arch Intern Med 145:677–679, 1985.
79. Braun JJ, Juttman, Visser TJ, Birkenhager JC: Short-term effect of prednisone on serum 1,25-dihydroxyvitamin D in normal individuals and in hyper- and hypoparathyroidism. Clin Endocrinol 17:21–28, 1982.
80. Stanbury SW: Bone disease in uremia. Am J Med 44:714–724, 1968.
81. Maesaka JK, Batuman V, Pablo NC, Shakamuri S: Elevated 1,25-dihydroxyvitamin D levels: Occurrence with end-stage renal disease. Arch Intern Med 142:1206–1207, 1982.
82. Gkonos PJ, London R, Hendler ED: Hypercalcemia and elevated 1,25-dihydroxyvitamin D levels in a patient with end-stage renal disease and active tuberculosis. N Engl J Med 311:1683–1685, 1984.
83. Mundy GR, Ibbotson KJ, D'Souza SM: Tumor products and the hypercalcemia of malignancy. J Clin Invest 76:391–394, 1985.
84. Stewart AF, Horst R, Deftos LJ, et al: Biochemical characterization of patients with cancer-associated hypercalcemia. Evidence for humoral and nonhumoral groups. N Engl J Med 303:1377–1383, 1980.
85. Mundy GR, Raisz LG, Cooper RA, et al: Evidence for the secretion of an osteoclast stimulating factor in myeloma. N Engl J Med 291:1041–1046, 1974.
86. Parfitt AM, Dent CE: Hyperthyroidism and hypercalcemia. Q J Med 39:171–187, 1970.
87. Mundy GR, Shapiro JL, Bandelin JG, et al: Direct stimulation of bone resorption by thyroid hormones. J Clin Invest 58:529–534, 1976.
88. Stewart AF, Adler M, Byers CM, et al: Calcium

homeostasis in immobilization: An example of resorptive hypercalciuria. N Engl J Med 306:1136–1140, 1982.
89. Bell NH, Stern PH: Hypercalcemia and increases in serum hormone value during prolonged administration of 1α,25-dihydroxyvitamin D. N Engl J Med 298:1241–1243, 1978.
90. Streck WF, Waterhouse C, Haddad JG: Glucocorticoid effects in vitamin D intoxication. Arch Intern Med 139:974–977, 1979.
91. Hughes MR, Baylink DJ, Jones PG, et al: Radioligand receptor assay for 25-hydroxyvitamin D_2/D_3 and 1α,25-dihydroxyvitamin D_2/D_3: Application to hypervitaminosis D. J Clin Invest 58:61–70, 1976.
92. McMillan DE, Freeman RB: The milk-alkali syndrome: A study of the acute disorder with comments on the development of the chronic condition. Medicine 44:485–501, 1965.
93. Burnett CH, Commons RR, Albright F, et al: Hypercalcemia without hypercalciuria or hypophosphatemia, calcinosis and renal insufficiency: A syndrome following prolonged intake of milk and alkali. N Engl J Med 240:787–794, 1949.
94. Parfitt AM: Chlorothiazide-induced hypercalcemia in juvenile osteoporosis and hyperparathyroidism. N Engl J Med 281:55–59, 1969.
95. Koppel MH, Massry SG, Shinaberger JH, et al: Thiazide-induced rise in serum calcium and magnesium in patients on maintenance hemodialysis. Ann Intern Med 72:895–901, 1970.
96. Walser M, Robinson BHB, Duckett JW Jr: The hypercalcemia of adrenal insufficiency. J Clin Invest 42:456–465, 1963.
97. Marx SJ, Brandi M-L: Familial primary hyperparathyroidism. Bone Mineral Res 5:375–407, 1987.
98. Zerwekh JE, Pak CYC: Vitamin D metabolism in idiopathic renal nephrolithiasis. *In* Kumar R (ed): Vitamin D: Basic and Clinical Concepts. Boston, Martinus Nijhoff Publishing, 1984, pp 747–764.
99. Hahn TJ, Halstead LR, Baran DT: Effects of short term glucocorticoid administration on intestinal calcium absorption and circulating vitamin D metabolite concentrations in normal man. J Clin Endocrinol Metab 52:111–115, 1981.
100. Seeman E, Kumar R, Hunder GG, et al: Production, degradation and circulating levels of 1,25-dihydroxyvitamin D in health and in chronic glucocorticoid excess. J Clin Invest 66:664–669, 1980.
101. Hedfors E: Influence of steroid therapy on lymphocyte response in sarcoidosis. Clin Immunol Immunopathol 4:96–100, 1975.
102. Fauci AS, Dale DC, Balow JE: Glucocorticosteroid therapy: Mechanisms of action and clinical considerations. Ann Intern Med 84:304–315, 1976.
103. Gillis S, Crabtree GR, Smith KA: Glucocorticoid-induced inhibition of T cell growth factor production I. The effect on mitogen-induced lymphocyte proliferation. J Immunol 123:1624–1631, 1979.
104. Balow JE, Rosenthal AS: Glucocorticoid suppression of macrophage migration inhibitory factor. J Exp Med 137:1031–1041, 1973.
105. Silverstein E, Perschuk LP, Friedland J: Immunofluorescent localization of angiotensin converting enzyme in epithelioid and giant cells of sarcoidosis granulomas. Proc Natl Acad Sci USA 76:6646–6648, 1979.
106. Okabe T, Yamagata K, Fujisawa, et al: Increased angiotensin-converting enzyme in peripheral blood monocytes from patients with sarcoidosis. J Clin Invest 75:911–914, 1985.
107. Bell NH, Bartter FC: Transient reversal of hyperabsorption of calcium and of abnormal sensitivity of vitamin D in a patient with sarcoidosis during episode of nephritis. Ann Intern Med 61:702–710, 1964.
108. Littlewood T, Hunter A, Beck P, et al: Treatment of hypercalcemia in sarcoidosis with flurbiprofen. Br Med J 287:1762–1763, 1983.
108a. Rizzato G, Tosi G, Mella C, et al: Researching osteoporosis in prednisone treated sarcoid patients. Sarcoidosis 4:45–48, 1987.
108b. DeSimone DP, Brillant HL, Basilez J, et al: Granulomatous infiltration of the talus and abnormal vitamin D and calcium metabolism in a patient with sarcoidosis: Sucessful treatment with hydroxychloroquine. Am J Med 87:694–696, 1989.
109. Shai F, Baker RK, Addrizzo JR, et al: Hypercalcemia in mycobacterial infection. J Clin Endocrinol Metab 34:251–256, 1972.
110. Bradley GW, Sterling GM: Hypercalcaemia and hypokalaemia in tuberculosis. Thorax 33:464–467, 1978.
111. Abbasi AA, Chemplavil JK, Farah S, et al: Hypercalcemia in active pulmonary tuberculosis. Ann Intern Med 90:324–328, 1979.
112. Need AG, Phillips PJ, Chiu FTS, et al: Hypercalcemia associated with tuberculosis. Br Med J 1:831, 1980.
113. Kitrou MP, Phytou-Pallikari A, Tzannes SE, et al: Hypercalcemia in active pulmonary tuberculosis. Ann Intern Med 96:55, 1982.
114. Sharma OP, Lamon J, Winsor D: Hypercalcemia and tuberculosis (letter). JAMA 222:582, 1972.
115. Braman SS, Goldman Al, Schwarz MI: Steroid-responsive hypercalcemia in disseminated bone tuberculosis. Arch Intern Med 132:269–271, 1973.
116. Bell NH, Shary J, Shaw S, et al: Hypercalcemia associated with increased circulating 1,25-dihydroxyvitamin D in a patient with pulmonary tuberculosis. Calcif Tissue Int 37:588–591, 1985.
117. Epstein S, Stern PH, Bell NH, et al: Evidence for abnormal regulation of circulating 1α,25-dihydroxyvitamin D in patients with pulmonary tuberculosis and normal calcium metabolism. Calcif Tissue Int 36:541–544, 1984.
118. Williams SE, Wardman AG, Taylor GA, et al: Long-term study of the effect of rifampin and isoniazid on vitamin D metabolism. Tubercle 66:49–54, 1985.
119. Walker JV, Baran D, Yakub YN, et al: Histoplasmosis with hypercalcemia, renal failure and papillary necrosis. JAMA 237:1350–1352, 1977.
120. Kantarjian HM, Saad MF, Estey EH, et al: Hypercalcemia in disseminated candidiasis. Am J Med 74:721–724, 1983.
121. Lee JC, Cantanzaro A, Parthemore JG, et al: Hypercalcemia in disseminated coccidioidomycosis. N Engl J Med 297:431–433, 1977.
122. Stoeckle JD, Hardy HL, Weber AL: Chronic beryllium disease; long-term follow-up of sixty cases and selective review of the literature. Am J Med 46:545–561, 1969.
123. Hoffman VN, Korzeniowski OM: Leprosy, hypercalcemia, and elevated serum calcitriol levels. Ann Intern Med 105:890–891, 1986.
124. Kozeny GA, Barbato AL, Bansal VK, et al: Hypercalcemia associated with silicone-induced granulomas. N Engl J Med 311:1103–1105, 1984.

125. Parker MS, Dokoh S, Woolfenden JM, et al: Hypercalcemia in coccidioidomycosis. Am J Med 76:341–344, 1984.
126. Ryzen E, Singer FR: Hypercalcemia in leprosy. Arch Intern Med 145:1305–1306, 1985.
127. Gates S, Shary J, Turner RT, et al: Abnormal calcium metabolism caused by increased circulating 1,25-dihydroxyvitamin D in a patient with rheumatoid arthritis. J Bone Mineral Res 1:221–226, 1986.
128. Breslau NA, McGuire JL, Zerwekh JE, et al: Hypercalcemia associated with increased serum calcitriol levels in three patients with lymphoma. Ann Intern Med 100:1–7, 1984.
129. Rosenthal N, Insogna KL, Godsall JW, et al: Elevations in circulating 1,25-dihydroxyvitamin D in three patients with lymphoma-associated hypercalcemia. J Clin Endocrinol Metab 60:29–33, 1985.
130. Mudde AH, Van Den Berg H, Boshuis PG, et al: Ectopic production of 1,25-dihydroxyvitamin D by B-cell lymphoma as a cause of hypercalcemia. Cancer 59:1543–1546, 1987.
131. Davies M, Hayes ME, Mawer EB, et al: Abnormal vitamin D metabolism in Hodgkins lymphoma. Lancet 1:186–188, 1985.
132. Zaloga GP, Eil C, Medbery CA: Humoral hypercalcemia in Hodgkin's disease: Association with elevated 1,25-dihydroxycholecalciferol levels and subperiosteal bone resorption. Arch Intern Med 145:155–157, 1985.
133. Schaefer K, Saupe J, Pauls A, Von Herrath D: Hypercalcemia and elevated serum 1,25-dihydroxyvitamin D_3 in a patient with Hodgkin's lymphoma. Klin Wochenschr 64:89–91, 1986.
134. Linde R, Basso L: Hodgkin's disease with hypercalcemia detected by thallium-201 scintigraphy. J Nucl Med 28:112–115, 1987.
135. Helikson MA, Havey AD, Zerwekh JE, et al: Plasma-cell granuloma producing calcitriol and hypercalcemia. Ann Intern Med 105:379–381, 1986.
136. Sarin PS, Gallo RC: Human T lymphotropic viruses in adult T-cell leukemia lymphoma and acquired immunodeficiency syndrome. J Clin Immunol 4:415–423, 1984.
137. Grossman B, Schecter GP, Horton JE, et al: Hypercalcemia associated with T cell lymphoma-leukemia. Am J Clin Pathol 75:149–155, 1981.
138. Popovic M, Sarin PS, Robert-Guroff M, et al: Isolation and transmission of human retrovirus (human T-cell leukemia virus). Science 219:856–859, 1983.
139. Broder S, Bunn PA, Jaffe ES, et al: T-cell lymphoproliferative syndrome associated with human T-cell leukemia/lymphoma virus. Ann Intern Med 100:543–557, 1984.
140. Fetchick DA, Bertolini DR, Sarin PS, et al: Production of 1,25-dihydroxyvitamin D by human T-cell lymphotrophic virus-I transformed lymphocytes. J Clin Invest 78:592–596, 1986.
141. Maislos M, Sobel R, Shany S: Leiomyoblastoma associated with intractable hypercalcemia and elevated 1,25-dihydroxycholecalciferol levels. Arch Intern Med 145:565–567, 1985.
142. Grote TH, Hainsworth JD: Hypercalcemia and elevated serum calcitriol in a patient with seminoma. Arch Intern Med 147:2212–2213, 1987.
143. Shigeno C, Yamamoto I, Dokoh S, et al: Identification of 1,24(R)-dihydroxyvitamin D_3-like bone-resorbing lipid in a patient with cancer-associated hypercalcemia. J Clin Endocrinol Metab 61:761–768, 1985.
144. Schaeffer PC, Fadem SZ, Lifschitz M, et al: Hypercalcemia due to high serum 1α,25-dihydroxycholecalciferol. Clin Res 26:533A (abstract), 1978.
145. Frame B, Parfitt AM: Corticosteroid-responsive hypercalcemia with elevated serum 1-alpha,25-dihydroxyvitamin D. Ann Intern Med 93:449–451, 1980.
146. Silver J, Popovtzor MM: Hypercalcemia with elevated dihydroxycholecalciferol levels and hypercalciuria; a parathyroid concentration-independent mechanism. Arch Intern Med 144:162–163, 1984.
147. Stapleton T, MacDonald WB, Lightwood R: Management of "idiopathic" hypercalcaemia of infancy. Lancet 1:932–934, 1956.
148. Morgan HG, Mitchell RG, Stowers JM, Thomson J: Metabolic studies on two infants with idiopathic hypercalcaemia. Lancet 1:925–931, 1956.
149. Forfar JO, Balf CL, Maxwell GM, Tompsett SL: Idiopathic hypercalcaemia of infancy: Clinical and metabolic studies with special reference to the aetiological role of vitamin D. Lancet 1:981–988, 1956.
150. Fellers FX, Schwartz R: Etiology of the severe form of idiopathic hypercalcemia of infancy: A defect in vitamin D metabolism. N Engl J Med 259:1050–1058, 1958.
151. Smith DW, Blizzard RM, Harrison HE: Idiopathic hypercalcemia: A case report with assays of vitamin D in the serum. Pediatrics 24:258–269, 1959.
152. Kenny FM, Aceto T Jr, Purisch M, et al: Metabolic studies in a patient with idiopathic hypercalcemia of infancy. J Pediatr 62:531–537, 1963.
153. Black JA, Bonham Carter RE: Association between aortic stenosis and facies of severe infantile hypercalcaemia. Lancet 2:745–749, 1963.
154. Garcia RE, Friedman WF, Kabach MM, Rowe RD: Idiopathic hypercalcemia and supravalvular aortic stenosis: Documentation of a new syndrome. N Engl J Med 271:117–120, 1964.
155. Wiltse HE, Goldbloom RB, Anita AU, et al: Infantile hypercalcemia syndrome in twins. N Engl J Med 275:1157–1160, 1966.
156. Williams JCP, Barratt-Boyes BG, Lowe JB: Supravalvular aortic stenosis. Circulation 24:1311–1318, 1961.
157. Jones KL, Smith DW: The Williams elfin facies syndrome: A new perspective. J Pediatr 86:718–723, 1975.
158. Taylor AB, Stern PH, Bell NH: Abnormal regulation of circulating 25-hydroxyvitamin D in the Williams syndrome. N Engl J Med 306:972–975, 1982.
159. Garabedian M, Jacqz E, Guillozo H, et al: Elevated plasma 1,25-dihydroxyvitamin D concentrations in infants with hypercalcemia and an elfin facies. N Engl J Med 312:948–952, 1985.
160. Aarskog O, Aksnes L, Markestad T: Vitamin D metabolism in idiopathic infantile hypercalcemia. Am J Dis Child 135:1021–1024, 1981.

CHARLES Y.C. PAK

23

Kidney Stones: Pathogenesis, Diagnosis, and Therapy

Current Status of the Field

The recent introduction of nephrostolithotomy[1] and extracorporeal shock wave lithotripsy[2] has revolutionized the treatment of nephrolithiasis. Most stones can now be removed with greater ease and less morbidity.

Because of these improved methods of stone removal, there has been a tendency to disparage the need for medical diagnosis and treatment.[3] However, it is clear that the medical approach cannot be ignored if ultimate control of nephrolithiasis is to be achieved. First, there is no evidence that removal of stones, no matter now easily achieved, would prevent recurrence of stones. In contrast, it is now possible to identify the cause of stone formation in the vast majority of patients and to inhibit new stone formation in most patients with appropriate medical treatments.[4] Second, most renal stones are spontaneously passed and may not require intervention for their removal. However, spontaneous stone passage is often associated with severe colic; this morbidity could be averted by medical prevention of new stone formation. Third, medical treatment could potentially correct extrarenal manifestations of the stone disease,[4] whereas surgical approach concentrates on stone removal alone.

This chapter reviews advances in the medical area. Each of the principal causes of stone disease is discussed separately, with consideration of pathophysiology, diagnostic criteria, and medical prevention.

Epidemiology and Chemical Composition

Nephrolithiasis is common, affecting 1% to 5% of the population in the industrialized countries, with an annual incidence of 0.1% to 0.3%. Stones originating in the bladder are rare in industrialized countries except in association with a foreign body (e.g., indwelling catheter), although they were common in antiquity and are still frequent in certain countries in Southeast Asia.

In industrialized countries, most stones are calcareous stones, composed mainly of calcium oxalate occurring alone (35% of all stones) or in combination with hydroxyapatite (35%). The remaining calcareous stones (5%) are represented by those composed principally of hydroxyapatite or brushite ($CaHPO_4 \cdot 2H_2O$). Non-calcareous stones, comprising up to 25% of all stones, are composed of uric acid, magnesium ammonium phosphate, cystine, and rarely xanthine, sodium urate, 2,8-dihydroxyadenine, or triamterene.

Stones composed principally of calcium oxalate are generally more common in men than in women, with a particular susceptibility for middle-aged, white men. Struvite stones and predominantly calcium phosphate stones are more common in women. Chemical composition of the stone may sometimes provide the diagnosis (e.g., cystine stones for cystinuria, struvite stones for urinary tract infection with urea-splitting organisms, and uric acid stones for gouty diathesis). The finding of calcium phosphate as the predominant phase suggests the diagnosis of distal renal tubular acidosis or primary hyperparathyroidism. However, the identification of the most common, calcium oxalate stones, has a limited diagnostic value, since they could result from a wide variety of metabolic and environmental disturbances.

Diagnostic Separation Based on "Physiologic" Derangements

It is now known that patients with renal calculi suffer from a wide variety of physiologic disturbances,[5] which are believed to

Table 23–1. Classification of Nephrolithiasis

Calcareous Renal Calculi
Hypercalciuria
Absorptive
Renal
Resorptive
Renal phosphate leak
Excessive 1,25$(OH)_2$ vitamin D synthesis
Combined renal tubular disturbances
Hyperuricosuria
Primary urate overproduction
Dietary purine overindulgence
Hyperoxaluria
Primary
Secondary
Inhibitor deficiency
Hypocitraturia
Other
Gouty diathesis
Noncalcareous Renal Calculi
Gouty diathesis
Uric acid stones
Cystinuria
Cystine stones
Infection with urea-splitting organisms
Struvite stones

be pathogenetically important in stone formation. It is presumed that these physiologic disturbances could result from environmental influences as well as from metabolic factors (of hormonal or genetic origin). These derangements have served as the basis of a refined classification of nephrolithiasis[6] and a more rational approach to medical treatment.[7]

According to this classification scheme (Table 23–1), calcareous renal calculi are due to hypercalciuria, hyperuricosuria, hyperoxaluria, inhibitor deficiency (hypocitraturia), and gouty diathesis. Non-calcareous calculi result from gouty diathesis, cystinuria, and urinary tract infection (with urea-splitting organisms). Some of these derangements are heterogeneous in origin. Thus, hypercalciuria may be due to an excessive intestinal calcium absorption, renal calcium or phosphate leak, or high 1,25$(OH)_2$ vitamin D synthesis.

In the category of inhibitor deficiency, hypocitraturia will be described in detail, because of increasing recognition of its importance in stone formation. Other simple (small molecular weight) and complex (macromolecular) inhibitors of the crystallization of calcium salts have been identified in urine, including pyrophosphate,[8] glycopeptides,[9] glycosaminoglycans,[10] ribonucleic acids, and glycoproteins.[11] There is some evidence that the renal excretion of these substances may be disturbed in certain patients with nephrolithiasis; however, this suggestion has not been fully substantiated. A recent finding that a particular glycoprotein from patients with calcium nephrolithiasis may be abnormal structurally and functionally is most intriguing but requires substantiation.[11] It is expected that these inhibitors may have diagnostic utility, if methods could be developed for simple and reliable assays. They may have clinical relevance if therapeutic approaches could be found for augmenting the amount of the activity of these inhibitors in urine.

Each cause of nephrolithiasis will now be considered *in toto* from the perspective of pathophysiology, diagnosis, and treatment.

I. HYPERCALCIURIA

A. Causal Role of Hypercalciuria in Calcium Stone Formation

Hypercalciuria could cause or contribute to calcium stone formation by the following mechanisms. First, it increases saturation of urine with respect to stone-forming calcium salts.[12] An induced hypercalciuria from a high calcium intake invariably increases the urinary saturation of calcium oxalate. Second, hypercalciuria may reduce the inhibitor activity in urine against the crystallization of stone-forming calcium salts by binding negatively charged inhibitors (such as citrate and glycosaminoglycans) and inactivating them.[13] Finally, the correction of hypercalciuria by thiazide[14] or sodium cellulose phosphate[15] has been shown to produce amelioration of stone disease.

B. Pathophysiology of Hypercalciuria

The association of hypercalciuria with calcium nephrolithiasis has long been recognized. The term "idiopathic hypercalciuria" has been used to denote this entity.[16] The recent progress in pathophysiologic elucidation mandates that this term be discarded. Our own view is to consider hypercalciuria of nephrolithiasis to comprise several entities of heterogeneous origin.[17] This approach permits incorporation of prevailing major theories of hypercalciuria.

Absorptive Hypercalciuria Type I and II

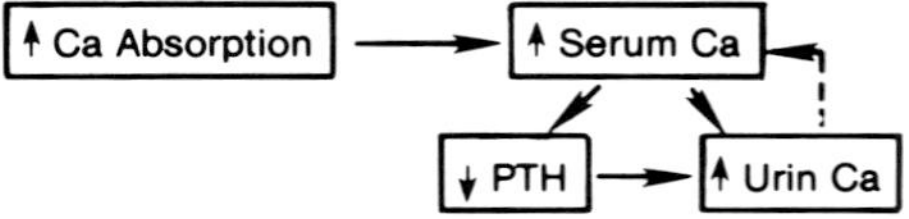

Renal Hypercalciuria

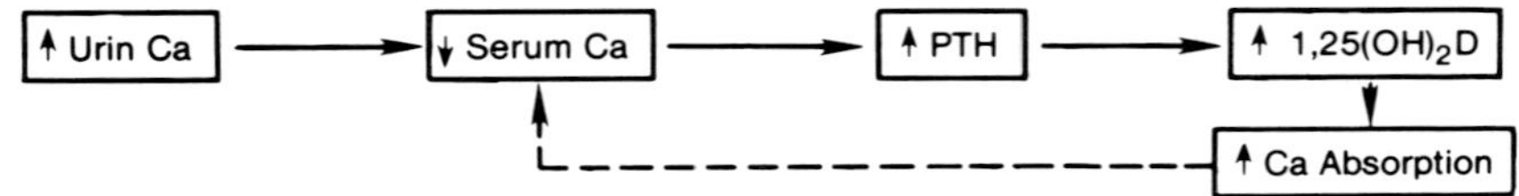

Resorptive Hypercalciuria

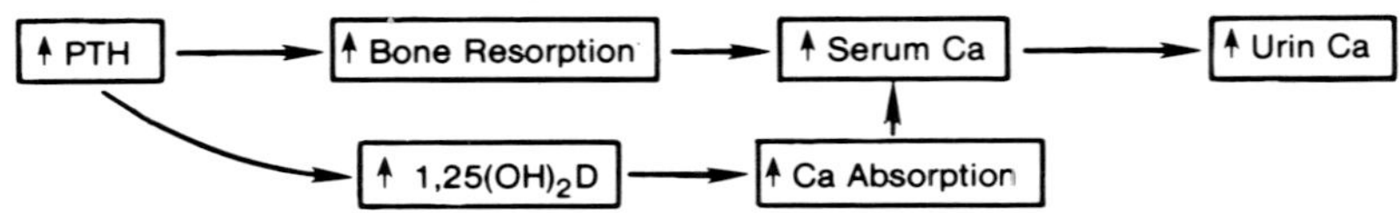

Figure 23–1. Schemes for absorptive hypercalciuria type I and type II, renal hypercalciuria, and resorptive hypercalciuria. Dashed line indicates compensatory inhibition. (After Pak CYC: Kidney stones. *In* Foster SW, Wilson JD (eds): Williams Textbook of Endocrinology. Philadelphia, WB Saunders, 1985.)

1. Absorptive Hypercalciuria (Fig. 23–1)

The primary abnormality in absorptive hypercalciuria is the intestinal hyperabsorption of calcium, presumed to occur independently of 1,25(OH)$_2$ vitamin D.[18] The consequent increase in the circulating concentration of calcium enhances the renal filtered load and suppresses parathyroid function. Hypercalciuria ensues from the increased filtered load and the reduced tubular reabsorption of calcium consequent to parathyroid suppression. The excessive renal loss of calcium compensates for the high calcium absorption from the intestinal tract and helps to maintain serum calcium in the normal range. This condition excludes those with a primary renal phosphate leak or an excessive 1,25(OH)$_2$ vitamin D production.

The exact cause for the enhancement of intestinal calcium absorption is not known. It may be a primary jejunal disease,[18,19] since the high calcium absorption has been disclosed only in the jejunum, and the absorption of magnesium and phosphate has been shown to be normal. The primary nature of this disturbance is indicated by persistence of intestinal hyperabsorption of calcium during treatment with adrenocorticosteroids (which lowers intestinal calcium absorption in sarcoidosis),[20] thiazide (which lowers urinary calcium),[21] and orthophosphate (which reduces serum concentration of 1,25(OH)$_2$ vitamin D).[22] Moreover, this disturbance appears to be inherited as an autosomal dominant trait.[23]

There is no evidence that the skeleton is adversely affected in this condition, consistent with the lack of parathyroid stimulation, hypophosphatemia, or 1,25(OH)$_2$ vitamin D excess. Normal values have been reported for serum osteocalcin, alkaline phosphatase activity, urinary hydroxyproline, and bone density in the radius (shaft) and lumbar vertebrae.[17] No clinically evident bone disease has been attributed to absorptive hypercalciuria. Calcium conservation is intact even when the intestinal calcium absorption is reduced by sodium cellulose phosphate. The absorbed calcium (lumen-to-blood) exceeds urinary calcium by an amount equivalent to the estimated net secreted calcium.

In this classic presentation of absorptive hypercalciuria, evidence for a "primary" renal calcium leak is lacking. Fasting urinary calcium may be secondarily increased in patients with absorptive hypercalciuria from the primary enhancement of intestinal calcium absorption. If the duration of fast is inadequate and the absorbed calcium is incompletely cleared by the kidneys, the high calcium absorption may cause fasting hypercalciuria by increasing the renal filtered load of calcium and by suppressing parathyroid function, thus impairing renal tubular reabsorption of calcium.[24] However, fasting hypercalciuria can be eliminated by a prolongation of fast or by prior administration of sodium cellulose phosphate (which binds calcium in the intestinal tract and reduces calcium absorption) without provoking hyperparathyroidism. A lack of a generalized disturbance in renal proximal tubular function is shown by normal calciuric response to carbohydrate load[25] and by normal natriuretic response to thiazide.[26]

2. *Renal Hypercalciuria (Fig. 23–1)*

The primary abnormality in renal hypercalciuria is believed to be the impairment of the renal tubular reabsorption of calcium (Fig. 23–1). The consequent reduction in the circulating concentration of calcium stimulates parathyroid function. There may be an excessive mobilization of calcium from bone and an enhanced intestinal absorption of calcium because of the parathyroid hormone (PTH) excess and the ensuing stimulation of the renal synthesis of 1,25$(OH)_2$ vitamin D. These effects restore serum calcium toward normal. Unlike primary hyperparathyroidism, serum calcium is normal, and the state of hyperparathyroidism is secondary.

Some patients with hypercalciuric nephrolithiasis, albeit a minority in most series, have been shown to have biochemical presentation supporting operation of this scheme. The occurrence of high serum PTH or urinary cyclic AMP, and elevated serum 1,25$(OH)_2$ vitamin D and intestinal calcium absorption, have been shown in such patients in the setting of normal serum calcium and fasting hypercalciuria (indicative of renal calcium leak).[18] The correction of renal calcium leak by thiazide restores normal serum 1,25$(OH)_2$ vitamin D and fractional calcium absorption commensurate with the correction of hyperparathyroidism.[21] These findings support the contention that 1,25$(OH)_2$ vitamin D synthesis is enhanced from secondary parathyroid stimulation and that intestinal calcium absorption is high owing to 1,25$(OH)_2$ vitamin D excess.

The occurrence of a primary renal calcium leak is supported by three lines of evidence. First, fasting hypercalciuria is associated with parathyroid stimulation and is poorly corrected by the inhibition of intestinal calcium absorption (and removing the effect of absorbed calcium) with sodium cellulose phosphate.[24] Second, there is a unique natriuretic response to thiazide. When thiazide is given to block reabsorption of calcium and sodium in the distal (renal) tubule, impaired proximal tubular function would be manifested as an exaggerated renal excretion of these cations. In our study, the exaggerated natriuretic and calciuric response to hydrochlorothiazide was encountered only in patients with documented renal hypercalciuria with secondary hyperparathyroidism.[26] Third, an exaggerated calciuric response to 100 g of glucose was encountered in patients with renal hypercalciuria with secondary hyperparathyroidism, not in those with absorptive hypercalciuria.[25] Ingestion of readily metabolizable carbohydrate (without calcium) normally augments renal calcium excretion, believed to be due to an alteration in renal proximal tubular function.[27]

It has been suggested that renal calcium leak is secondary to an excessive dietary intake of sodium.[28] However, in one preliminary study, institution of a low sodium intake (9 mEq/day) did not eliminate fasting hypercalciuria in patients with renal hypercalciuria.

That renal calcium leak (and secondary hyperparathyroidism) had been long-standing is shown by changes disclosed in bone density. Although clinical bone disease is rare, bone density as measured by photon absorptiometry in the distal third of the radius is reduced in the group with renal hypercalciuria (as compared with age- and sex-matched controls).[29] These results indicate that secondary hyperparathyroidism exerts deleterious effects on the skeleton. The lack of a more serious involvement is probably due to the compensatory intestinal hyperabsorption of calcium that results from the PTH-induced renal synthesis of 1,25$(OH)_2$ vitamin D. This compensation is often inadequate, since urinary calcium usually exceeds absorbed calcium indicative of negative calcium balance.

3. *Resorptive Hypercalciuria (Fig. 23–1)*

Resorptive hypercalciuria is characterized by primary hyperparathyroidism. The initial event is excessive resorption of bone resulting from hypersecretion of PTH. Intestinal absorption of calcium is frequently elevated because of PTH-dependent stimulation of renal synthesis of 1,25(OH)$_2$ vitamin D.[30] These effects increase the circulating concentration and the renal filtered load of calcium. The occurrence of hypercalciuria in primary hyperparathyroidism seems paradoxical, since the primary renal effect of PTH is to stimulate tubular reabsorption of calcium. However, hypercalciuria is often encountered in primary hyperparathyroidism because PTH-dependent augmentation of renal tubular reabsorption of calcium is "overcome" by an increase in the renal filtered load and by a suppressive effect of hypercalcemia on calcium reabsorption.

4. *Fasting Hypercalciuria with Normal Parathyroid Function*

In some patients with normocalcemic hypercalciuric nephrolithiasis, the diagnosis of absorptive or renal hypercalciuria cannot be made with certainty.[6] This unclassified hypercalciuria is largely represented by fasting hypercalciuria without parathyroid stimulation. This picture points to neither absorptive hypercalciuria nor renal hypercalciuria. The lack of hyperparathyroidism suggests the diagnosis of absorptive hypercalciuria, but fasting urinary calcium is high. The fasting hypercalciuria indicates that a renal leak of calcium is present; however, secondary stimulation of parathyroid function is lacking. In our latest series, unclassified hypercalciuria was disclosed in 27.6% of patients with recurrent renal calculi referred to us for evaluation, compared to 33.4% with absorptive hypercalciuria and 2.7% with renal hypercalciuria.

In our experience, this ambiguous presentation is often caused by incomplete exclusion of the effects of absorbed calcium in patients with absorptive or renal hypercalciuria. When calcium restriction is not maintained and the duration of fast is insufficient, there may be incomplete renal clearance of calcium absorbed from the intestinal tract. Under such circumstances, patients with absorptive hypercalciuria may present with fasting hypercalciuria, and those with renal hypercalciuria may not show parathyroid stimulation (because of the suppressive effect of absorbed calcium). A prior treatment with sodium cellulose phosphate to remove the effects of absorbed calcium may disclose underlying absorptive hypercalciuria or renal hypercalciuria. In the former, sodium cellulose phosphate restores normal fasting urinary calcium without causing hyperparathyroidism, whereas in renal hypercalciuria the treatment may unmask parathyroid stimulation.

In some patients, however, fasting hypercalciuria with normal parathyroid function cannot be accounted for by an underlying absorptive or renal hypercalciuria. Typically, parathyroid function remains normal and fasting hypercalciuria persists despite an inhibition of calcium absorption by sodium cellulose phosphate. Fasting hypercalciuria with normal parathyroid function, exclusive of classic absorptive hypercalciuria or renal hypercalciuria, may be due to the following conditions (Fig. 23–2).

5. *Renal Phosphate Leak (Absorptive Hypercalciuria Type III) (Fig. 23–2)*

In this condition, hypophosphatemia ensuing from renal phosphate leak has been implicated for the intestinal hyperabsorption of calcium by stimulating the renal synthesis of 1,25(OH)$_2$ vitamin D.[31] This scheme is supported by findings of (1) low tubular threshold concentration of phosphate (TmP) and hypophosphatemia in patients with hypercalciuric nephrolithiasis without parathyroid stimulation, (2) ability of induced hypophosphatemia from limitation of intestinal phosphate absorption to stimulate the renal synthesis of 1,25(OH)$_2$ vitamin D, and (3) significant inverse correlation between serum 1,25(OH)$_2$ vitamin D and serum phosphorus concentration.[32] Moreover, the presence of hypophosphatemia and/or high serum 1,25(OH)$_2$ vitamin D provides an explanation (other than PTH excess) for the reported occurrence of fasting hypercalciuria, poor calcium conservation, reduced bone density, and abnormal histomorphometric picture of bone[33] in hypercalciuric patients with normal parathyroid function.

In our experience, renal phosphate leak is an uncommon cause of calcium nephrolithiasis. Two patients who satisfied the diagnostic criteria of this entity were shown to have later surgically proven primary hyperparathyroidism. Thus, renal phosphate leak may sometimes represent an early phase of primary hyperparathyroidism.

FASTING HYPERCALCIURIA WITH NORMAL PTH

1. Absorptive Hypercalciuria Type III

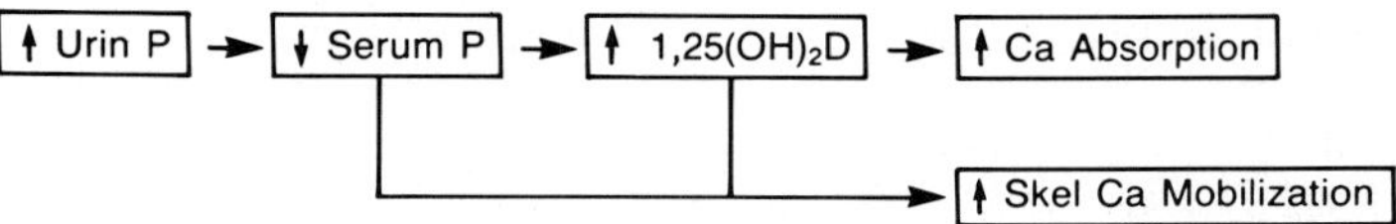

2. Primary Enhancement of 1,25(OH)₂D Production

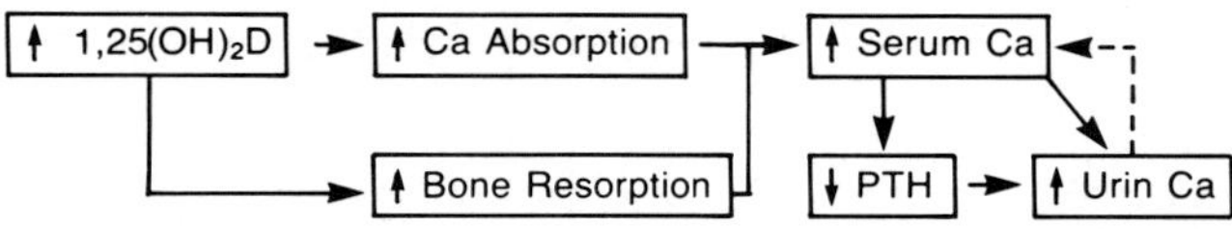

3. Combined Renal Tubular Disturbances

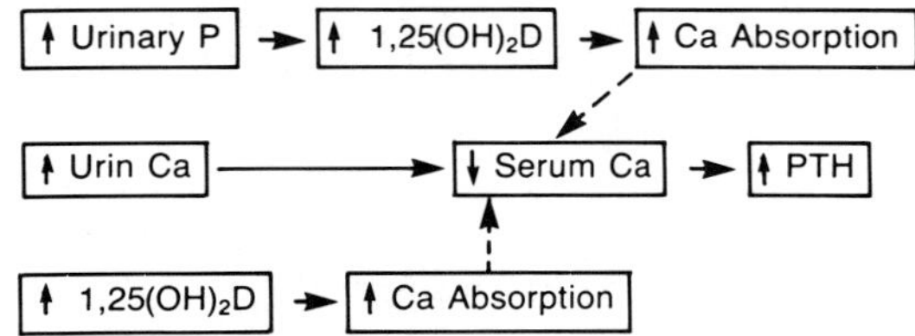

Figure 23–2. Schemes for renal phosphate leak (absorptive hypercalciuria type III), primary enhancement of $1,25(OH)_2$ vitamin D production, and combined renal tubular disturbances.

6. Primary Enhancement of $1,25(OH)_2$ Vitamin D Synthesis (Fig. 23–2)

Many of the biochemical characteristics of absorptive hypercalciuria can be explained by an overproduction of $1,25(OH)_2$ vitamin D, whether it occurs independently of or secondarily to the renal phosphate leak. These include intestinal hyperabsorption of calcium and parathyroid suppression. The parathyroid suppression can secondarily produce the high fasting urinary calcium sometimes encountered, because of the loss of PTH-dependent stimulation of the renal tubular reabsorption of calcium.[34] This conclusion is supported by the biochemical similarity of absorptive hypercalciuria to the state induced in normal subjects by exogenous $1,25(OH)_2$ vitamin D therapy.[34] Thus, the picture of fasting hypercalciuria with suppressed parathyroid function could occur from a primary increase in $1,25(OH)_2$ vitamin D synthesis, as a form of an acquired renal calcium leak.

Fasting hypercalciuria could also be due to the $1,25(OH)_2$ vitamin D–dependent stimulation of bone resorption.[35] Exogenous $1,25(OH)_2$ vitamin D has been shown to augment urinary calcium excretion even when patients are placed on a low-calcium diet, as well as to increase urinary hydroxyproline (a marker of bone resorption) and serum osteocalcin (a marker of bone formation and turnover).[36]

The scheme for excessive $1,25(OH)_2$ vitamin D production is supported by the finding of high serum $1,25(OH)_2$ vitamin D in some patients with absorptive hypercalciuria and the demonstration of accelerated *in vivo* $1,25(OH)_2$ vitamin D synthesis in patients with absorptive hypercalciuria selected from high extremes of serum $1,25(OH)_2$ vitamin D levels.[37] This condition probably represents a variable fraction of those presenting with absorptive hypercalciuria, and should be distinguished from classic absorptive hypercalciuria (previously described) in which a pathogenetic role of $1,25(OH)_2$ vitamin D is not implicated.

7. Combined Renal Tubular Disturbances (Fig. 23–2)[4]

The occurrence of fasting hypercalciuria with normal parathyroid function could be explained by multiple disturbances in renal proximal tubular function, characterized by varying degrees of calcium leak, a disturbance in phosphate transport, and accelerated $1,25(OH)_2$ vitamin D synthesis.[38] This unifying scheme could explain the pathogenesis of

Table 23–2. Diagnostic Criteria

	Serum				Urinary								
	Ca	*P*	*PTH*	*1,25*	*Ca* Fasting	*Ca* Load	*Ca* Restricted	*UA*	*Ox*	*Cit*	*pH*	α	BD
AH-I	N	N	N	N	N	↑	↑	N	N	N	N	↑	N
AH-II	N	N	N	N	N	↑	N	N	N	N	N	↑/N	N
RH	N	N	↑	↑	↑	↑	↑	N	N	N	N	↑	↓
P-leak	N	↓	N	↑	↑	↑	↑	N	N	N	N	↑	↓
1,25-excess	N	N	N	↑	↑	↑	↑	N	N	N	N	↑	N
Combined	N	N/↓	N	↑	↑	↑	↑	N	N	N	N	↑	N/↓
HUCU	N	N	N	N	N	N	N	↑	N	N	N	N	N
EH	N/↓	N/↓	N/↑	N	↓	↓	↓	↓	↑	↓	N	↓	↓
Hypocit	N	N	N	N	N	N	N	N	N	↓	N	N	N
RTA	N	N	N/↑	N	↑	N	N/↑	N	N	↓	N/↑	↓	↓
Gouty diathesis	N	N	N	N	N	N	N	N/↑	N	N	↓	N	N
Struvite stones	N	N	N	N	N	N/↑	N/↑	N	N	↓	↑	N	N

Fasting samples represent 2-hour collections obtained in morning following an overnight fast. Ca load samples were obtained over a 4-hour period subsequent to oral ingestion of 1 g Ca. Fractional Ca absorption (α) was obtained from fecal recovery of radioactivity following oral administration of radiocalcium with 100 mg Ca. Bone density (BD) was obtained in distal third of radius by photon absorptiometry.

PTH, immunoreactive parathyroid hormone; ↑, high; ↓, low; N, normal; 1,25, 1,25(OH)$_2$D; UA, uric acid; Ox, oxalate; Cit, citrate; AH-I, absorptive hypercalciuria type I; AH-II, absorptive hypercalciuria type II; RH, renal hypercalciuria; P-leak, renal phosphate leak; 1,25-excess, primary 1,25(OH)$_2$D excess; Combined, combined renal tubular disturbances; HUCU, hyperuricosuric calcium nephrolithiasis; EH, enteric hyperoxaluria; Hypocit, idiopathic hypocitraturic calcium nephrolithiasis; RTA, incomplete renal tubular acidosis.

both renal and absorptive hypercalciurias from the general defect originating in the kidney. The predominance of the renal calcium leak would lead to renal hypercalciuria with secondary hyperparathyroidism. On the other hand, the prominence of 1,25(OH)$_2$ vitamin D synthesis, occurring independently of or secondarily from renal phosphate leak, would produce a picture of absorptive hypercalciuria by enhancing intestinal calcium absorption and masking parathyroid stimulation. The occurrence of both renal calcium leak and renal phosphate leak or increased 1,25(OH)$_2$ vitamin D synthesis may produce a picture of fasting hypercalciuria without parathyroid stimulation. Thus, renal hypercalciuria need not be accompanied by hyperparathyroidism, and absorptive hypercalciuria results secondarily from 1,25(OH)$_2$ vitamin D–dependent stimulation of intestinal calcium absorption.

C. Diagnostic Criteria (Table 23–2)

Absorptive hypercalciuria type I is characterized by normocalcemia; normophosphatemia; normal fasting urinary calcium (< 0.11 mg/100 ml glomerular filtrate [GF]); exaggerated urinary calcium following an oral calcium load (> 0.2 mg/mg creatinine); normal or suppressed parathyroid function (normal serum immunoreactive PTH); and urinary calcium on a restricted diet (400 mg calcium and 100 mEq sodium/day) of more than 200 mg/day. These values reflect increased intestinal calcium absorption, resultant parathyroid suppression, and hypercalciuria.

Absorptive hypercalciuria type II is characterized by the same biochemical features as those of type I except for normocalciuria (< 200 mg/day) on a restricted diet (400 mg calcium and 100 mEq sodium/day). If these patients are placed on a diet of 1000 mg calcium and 100 mEq sodium/day, urinary calcium exceeds 4 mg/kg/day or 250 mg/day.

Renal hypercalciuria has the following features: normocalcemia; high fasting urinary calcium (> 0.11 mg/100 ml GF); and enhanced parathyroid activity (high serum immunoreactive PTH and/or 24-hour urinary cyclic AMP > 5.4 nM/100 ml GF). These results indicate a renal leak of calcium with compensatory parathyroid stimulation. Either serum PTH or urinary cyclic AMP, or both, must be elevated to confirm the diagnosis of renal hypercalciuria. In most patients urinary cyclic AMP, which is high in the fasting state, decreases to the normal range following an oral calcium load, a finding indicative of the suppressibility of parathyroid stimulation. Bone density may be low in patients with renal hypercalciuria, and in some, osteopenia may occur.[29]

Table 23–3. Medical Treatment Programs

Indication	Treatment	Physiologic Action	Physicochemical Action
Absorptive hypercalciuria type I (also 1,25$(OH)_2$D excess)	Sodium cellulose phosphate	↓ Intestinal Ca absorption ↓ Urinary Ca	↓ Urinary saturation of Ca oxalate ↓ Ca phosphate saturation
	Thiazide	= Intestinal Ca absorption ↓ Urinary Ca (transient) ↓ Urinary citrate	↓ Urinary saturation of Ca salts
Absorptive hypercalciuria type II	Low Ca diet	↓ Intestinal Ca absorption ↓ Urinary Ca	↓ Urinary saturation of Ca oxalate and Ca phosphate
Renal hypercalciuria (also combined renal tubular disturbances)	Thiazide	↓ Urinary Ca (sustained) ↓ Intestinal Ca absorption	↓ Urinary saturation of Ca salts
Renal phosphate leak	Orthophosphate	↓ 1,25$(OH)_2$D ↓ Intestinal Ca absorption ↓ Urinary Ca ↑ Urinary citrate and pyrophosphate	↓ Urinary saturation of Ca oxalate ↑ Inhibitor activity
Hyperuricosuric Ca nephrolithiasis	Allopurinol	↓ Urinary uric acid	↓ Urate-induced crystallization of Ca salts
	Potassium citrate	↑ Urinary citrate	↓ Urinary saturation of Ca oxalate ↓ Urate-induced crystallization of Ca salts
Enteric hyperoxaluria	↓ Oxalate intake	↓ Urinary oxalate	↓ Urinary saturation of Ca oxalate
	Potassium citrate	↑ Urinary citrate ↑ Urinary pH	↓ Urinary saturation of Ca oxalate ↑ Inhibitor activity
	Magnesium gluconate	↑ Urinary Mg	↓ Urinary saturation of Ca oxalate
	Calcium citrate	↑ Urinary citrate ↑ Urinary pH	↑ Inhibitor activity
Hypocitraturic Ca nephrolithiasis	Potassium citrate	↑ Urinary citrate ↑ Urinary pH ↓/= Urinary Ca	↓ Urinary saturation of Ca oxalate ↑ Inhibitor activity
Gouty diathesis	Potassium citrate	↑ Urinary pH ↓ Undissociated uric acid ↑ Urinary citrate	↓ Urinary saturation of uric acid ↓ Ca oxalate crystallization
Cystinuria	D-penicillamine or MPG	Mixed disulfide with cysteine ↓ Urinary cystine	↓ Urinary saturation of cystine
Infection stones	Acetohydroxamic acid	↓ Urease activity ↓ NH_4^+ ↓ pH	↓ Urinary saturation of struvite

↓ decrease; ↑ increase; = no change.

Primary hyperparathyroidism may be recognized by the presence of hypercalcemia, hypophosphatemia, hypercalciuria, and increased or inappropriately high serum PTH and/or urinary cyclic AMP. Bone density in the radial diaphysis is often low. Hypercalcemic symptoms, peptic ulcer, or bone disease (osteitis, pathologic fractures, osteoporosis) may be present.

Fasting hypercalciuria with normal parathyroid function depicts normocalcemic hypercalciuric patients with calcium nephrolithiasis in whom the diagnosis of absorptive or renal hypercalciurias cannot be made with certainty.[6] It is represented by normocalcemia, high fasting urinary calcium (> 0.11 mg/100 ml GF), and normal serum PTH. This presentation is accountable by an incomplete clearance of absorbed calcium in patients with an underlying absorptive or renal hypercalciuria. A more complete elimination of the effect of absorbed calcium by prior treatment with sodium cellulose phosphate may provide further clarification.[24] In patients with persistent fasting hypercalciuria and normal serum PTH (despite preparation with sodium cellulose phosphate), one should suspect renal phosphate leak (previously called absorptive hypercalciuria type III), primary 1,25$(OH)_2$ vitamin D excess, or combined disturbances in renal proximal tubular function. In renal phosphate leak, serum phosphorus and renal threshold concentration of phosphorus are less than 2.5 mg/100 ml, and remain low despite examination in an inpatient setting and avoidance of dietary phosphate excess.[22,31]

D. Treatment of Hypercalciuric Calcium Nephrolithiasis (Table 23–3)

1. Absorptive Hypercalciuria Type I

There is currently no treatment program that is capable of correcting the basic abnormality of absorptive hypercalciuria type I, although several drugs are available that have been shown to restore normal calcium excretion. *Sodium cellulose phosphate* best meets the criteria for optimal therapy.[15] When given orally, this nonabsorbable, ion exchange resin binds calcium and inhibits calcium absorption. However, this inhibition is caused by limiting the amount of intraluminal calcium available for absorption, and not by correcting the basic disturbance in calcium transport.

This mode of action accounts for the three potential complications of sodium cellulose phosphate therapy.[39] First, it may cause negative calcium balance and parathyroid stimulation if it is used in patients with normal intestinal calcium absorption or with renal or resorptive hypercalciuria. Second, the treatment may cause magnesium depletion by binding magnesium as well. Third, sodium cellulose phosphate may produce secondary hyperoxaluria, by binding divalent cations in the intestinal tract, reducing divalent cation-oxalate complexation, and making more oxalate available for absorption. These complications may be overcome by using the drug only in documented cases of absorptive hypercalciuria type I, by applying oral magnesium supplementation (1.0–1.5 g magnesium gluconate twice daily, separately from sodium cellulose phosphate), and by imposing a moderate dietary restriction of oxalate.

When these precautions are followed,[39] sodium cellulose phosphate at a dosage of 10 to 15 g/day (given with meals) has been shown to reduce urinary calcium and the saturation of calcium salts (calcium phosphate as well as calcium oxalate), to maintain stable bone density, and to be clinically effective.

Thiazide is not considered a selective therapy for absorptive hypercalciuria, since it does not decrease intestinal calcium absorption in this condition.[18] However, this drug has been widely used to treat this disorder, because of its hypocalciuric action.

Our studies indicate that thiazide may have a limited long-term effectiveness in absorptive hypercalciuria type I.[40] Thiazide is usually effective in reducing urinary calcium during the first 2 years of treatment. Thereafter, however, urinary calcium generally returns to the pretreatment range (Fig. 23–3). In contrast, intestinal calcium absorption persistently remains elevated throughout thiazide treatment. Preliminary studies suggest that thiazide may cause accretion of calcium in bone during the early years of therapy.[41] Bone density, determined in the distal third of the radius by single-photon absorptiometry, increased significantly during thiazide treatment in absorptive hypercalciuria, with an annual increment of 1.34%. With continued treatment, however, the rise in bone density stabilized as the hypocalciuric effect of thiazide became attenuated. The results suggest that thiazide treatment may eventually cause a low-turnover state of bone, which interferes with a continued calcium accretion in the skeleton. The "rejected" calcium would then be excreted in urine. In contrast, bone density was not significantly altered in renal hypercalciuria, in which thiazide was shown to cause a decline in intestinal calcium absorption commensurate with a reduction in urinary calcium.

Thus, thiazide is often ineffective in correcting hypercalciuria in absorptive hypercalciuria after more than 2 years of treatment[40]

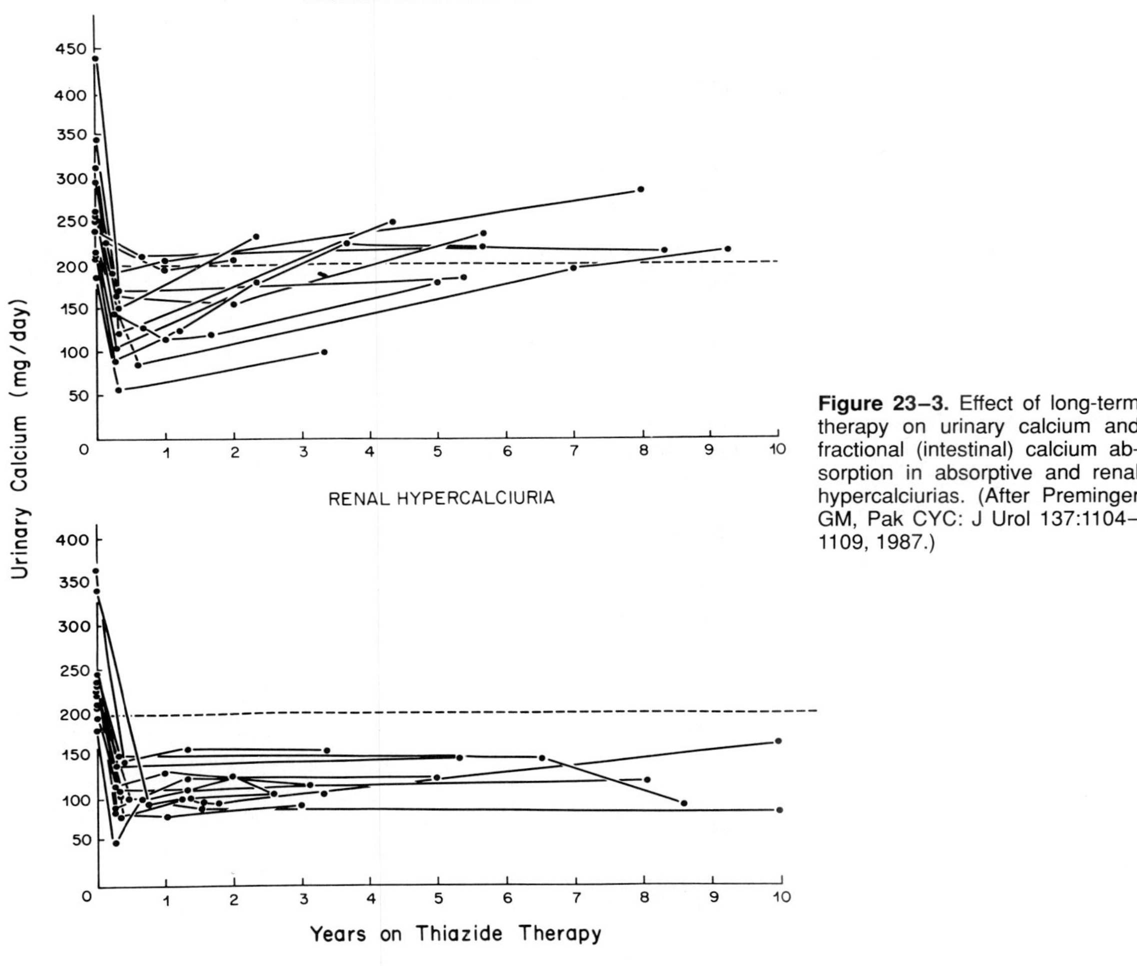

Figure 23–3. Effect of long-term therapy on urinary calcium and fractional (intestinal) calcium absorption in absorptive and renal hypercalciurias. (After Preminger GM, Pak CYC: J Urol 137:1104–1109, 1987.)

(Fig. 23–3). Another problem with thiazide is the induction of hypocitraturia.[14,42] In our own experience, thiazide used alone is relatively ineffective in the management of stone disease in patients with absorptive hypercalciuria type I probably owing to these changes.

It is recognized that sodium cellulose phosphate does not correct the basic intestinal calcium transport defect in absorptive hypercalciuria type I, and that thiazide treatment may eventually be ineffective in correcting hypercalciuria or is attendant with certain complications. We recommend the following guidelines in the use of these two agents until more selective therapies are found.

We recommend that sodium cellulose phosphate be used in patients with severe absorptive hypercalciuria type I (urinary calcium > 300 mg/day) or those resistant to or intolerant of thiazide therapy. In patients with absorptive hypercalciuria type I who may be at risk for bone disease (growing children, elderly patients, or postmenopausal women), thiazide might be the first choice. When thiazide becomes ineffective in lowering urinary calcium, this treatment may be temporarily substituted by sodium cellulose phosphate or orthophosphate (for approximately 6 months). Restoration of hypocalciuric response to thiazide generally ensues then, permitting resumption of thiazide therapy.

We would recommend that *potassium citrate* (e.g., 20 mEq twice/day) always be used with thiazide (e.g., trichlormethiazide 4 mg/day or hydrochlorothiazide 25–50 mg twice/day) in order to prevent hypokalemia and augment citrate excretion.[43]

2. Absorptive Hypercalciuria Type II

The features of absorptive hypercalciuria type II[6] are identical to those of absorptive hypercalciuria type I, except that normocalciuria (< 200 mg/day) can be induced by a diet of 400 mg calcium and 100 mEq sodium/day. In addition, many patients show disdain for drinking fluids and thus excrete concentrated urine. A *low calcium intake* (400–600 mg/day) and *high fluid intake* (sufficient to achieve a minimum urine output of greater than 2 liters/day) would seem ideally indicated, since normocalciuria could be restored by dietary calcium restriction alone, and increased urine volume has been shown to reduce urinary saturation of calcium oxalate, brushite, and monosodium urate, and inhibit spontaneous nucleation of calcium oxalate.[44]

3. Renal Hypercalciuria

Thiazide is ideally indicated for the treatment of renal hypercalciuria.[18,21] This diuretic has been shown to correct the renal leak of calcium by augmenting calcium reabsorption in the distal tubule directly, and by causing extracellular volume depletion and stimulating proximal tubular reabsorption of calcium. The ensuing correction of secondary hyperparathyroidism restores normal serum $1,25(OH)_2$ vitamin D and intestinal calcium absorption. In a recent study, thiazide has been shown to produce a sustained correction of hypercalciuria, commensurate with a restoration of normal serum $1,25(OH)_2$ vitamin D and intestinal calcium absorption (and stability of bone density) during up to 10 years of therapy.[40] Thus, thiazide action in renal hypercalciuria differs from that previously described for absorptive hypercalciuria.

Physicochemically, the urinary environment becomes less saturated with respect to calcium oxalate and brushite during thiazide treatment, largely because of the reduced calcium excretion.[45] These effects are shared by hydrochlorothiazide 50 mg twice daily, chlorthalidone 50 mg/day, or trichlormethiazide 4 mg/day. Potassium citrate (30–60 mEq/day in divided doses) should be used as well in order to avert hypokalemia and to increase urinary citrate.[42,43] Concurrent use of triamterene, a potassium-sparing agent, should be undertaken with caution because of recent reports of triamterene stone formation.[46] Amiloride may be used with thiazide, since it alone has sometimes been shown to exert a hypocalciuric action, to exaggerate the hypocalciuric action of thiazide, and to prevent hypokalemia.[47] However, amiloride itself does not augment citrate excretion. Thus, in patients with hypercalciuric nephrolithiasis presenting with hypocitraturia, in whom the use of potassium citrate is contemplated, it is probably wise to use thiazide alone without a potassium-sparing diuretic.

4. Primary Hyperparathyroidism

There is no established medical treatment for the nephrolithiasis of primary hyperparathyroidism. Although *orthophosphates* have been recommended for disease of mild to moderate severity,[48] their safety or efficacy has not yet been proved. They should be used only when parathyroid surgery cannot be undertaken.

Estrogen is a reasonable alternative in postmenopausal women with primary hyperparathyroidism in whom surgery is refused or contraindicated.[49] This treatment (e.g., conjugated estrogen 0.625 mg/day, 25 days of each month) has been shown to reduce serum calcium concentration (by inhibiting PTH-induced bone resorption) and thereby reduce urinary calcium.

Parathyroidectomy is the optimal treatment for the nephrolithiasis of primary hyperparathyroidism. Following removal of abnormal parathyroid tissue, urinary calcium is restored to normal commensurate with a decline in serum concentration of calcium and in intestinal calcium absorption.[50] The urinary environment becomes less saturated with respect to calcium oxalate and brushite, and its limit of metastability (formation product ratio, a measure of inhibitor activity) for these calcium salts increases.[51] There is typically a reduced rate of new stone formation, unless urinary tract infection is present.

5. Renal Phosphate Leak

Orthophosphate (neutral or alkaline salt of sodium and/or potassium, 0.5 g phosphorus three to four times/day) would seem to be the logical treatment because of its potential for the inhibition of $1,25(OH)_2$ vitamin D synthesis.[22] However, there is currently no convincing evidence that this treatment restores normal intestinal calcium absorption in this condition. Orthophosphate reduces urinary calcium probably by directly enhancing the renal tubular reabsorption of calcium. Urinary phosphorus is markedly increased during therapy, a finding reflecting the absorbability of soluble phosphate. Physicochemically, orthophosphate reduces urinary saturation of calcium oxalate but increases that of brushite.[45] Moreover, the urinary inhibitor activity is increased, probably owing to the stimulated renal excretion of pyrophosphate and citrate. Although contrary reports have appeared, this treatment program has been reported to cause soft tissue calcification and parathyroid stimulation.[52] It is contraindicated in nephrolithiasis complicated by urinary tract infection.

6. Primary 1,25(OH)$_2$ Vitamin D Excess

There is no known treatment that is capable of correcting this disturbance. Adrenocorticosteroids do not reduce serum 1,25(OH)$_2$ vitamin D or calcium absorption in hypercalciuric nephrolithiasis unlike in sarcoidosis.[20] Whereas orthophosphate has been shown to reduce serum 1,25(OH)$_2$ vitamin D, our limited studies indicated persistent hyperabsorption of calcium from the intestinal tract.[22]

Since the skeleton may be adversely affected because of the bone resorptive capacity of 1,25(OH)$_2$ vitamin D, thiazide may be preferable to sodium cellulose phosphate in controlling hypercalciuria. Eventual attenuation of the hypocalciuric action to thiazide is likely as in absorptive hypercalciuria type I.

A potentially useful agent is one that either inhibits the synthesis or facilitates the clearance of 1,25(OH)$_2$ vitamin D.[53]

7. Combined Disturbance in Renal Proximal Tubular Function

Since renal calcium leak is presumed to be an invariant feature, coexisting with either phosphate leak or excessive 1,25(OH)$_2$ vitamin D synthesis, thiazide treatment should be attempted first. If this treatment is ineffective in controlling hypercalciuria or should hypercalcemia develop, orthophosphate or sodium cellulose phosphate may be added to the treatment program.

II. HYPERURICOSURIA

The association of hyperuricosuria with calcium nephrolithiasis is well known, and has received the appellation of hyperuricosuric calcium nephrolithiasis.

A. Causal Role of Hyperuricosuria in Calcium Stone Formation

Recurrent calcium nephrolithiasis can occur in subjects with hyperuricosuria with no other discernible cause of nephrolithiasis, and with normal urinary pH (> 5.5). The following scheme has been proposed.[54] The urinary environment may be supersaturated with respect to monosodium urate because of a high urinary content of uric acid and a favorable urinary pH (> pk_a for the first proton of uric acid of 5.47) in which adequate dissociation of uric acid occurs. Either a colloidal or crystalline monosodium urate could theoretically form in such an environment. It can then initiate the crystallization of calcium oxalate by direct induction of heterogeneous nucleation of calcium oxalate or by removing urinary macromolecules through adsorption, thereby attenuating their inhibitor activity.[55]

This scheme is supported by studies using artificial monosodium urate and naturally occurring urinary macromolecules. Moreover, the induction of hyperuricosuria by oral purine loading has been shown to facilitate spontaneous precipitation of calcium oxalate in urine, providing further credence to this scheme.[56] Unfortunately, the presence of colloidal or crystalline monosodium urate in urine has not been conclusively demonstrated, and the role of monosodium urate in heterogeneous nucleation has not been consistently found.

The uric acid may cause the crystallization of calcium oxalate by the same mechanisms described for monosodium urate.[57] Although uric acid is less efficient than monosodium urate in inducing heterogeneous nucleation of calcium oxalate, its crystallization dimensions are more compatible with epitaxy (crystalline overgrowth of calcium oxalate). Moreover, uric acid has been shown to remove naturally occurring urinary macromolecular inhibitors, thereby attenuating their activity.[55]

B. Pathophysiology of Hyperuricosuria

Uric acid is an end product of purine metabolism. It cannot be degraded in humans because of the absence of uricase, unlike the situation in lower mammalian species. A major site of disposal of uric acid is the kidney, in which both secretion and reabsorption occur.

Hyperuricosuria may ensue when the serum concentration and the renal filtered load of uric acid are increased from the provision of an excessive amount of substrate, for example, a high dietary intake of purine-rich foods[58] or an accelerated cellular degradation and release of nucleic acids, or a disturbance in the enzymatic pathway for purine biosynthesis that causes overproduction of purine substrates for uric acid synthesis. A high urinary uric acid may occur transiently when renal tubular reabsorption of uric acid is impaired, for example, during early stages of extracellular volume expansion (from sodium load) and following administration of uricosuric agents such as probenecid. In the steady state, however, normal urinary uric acid is restored, because of the decline in serum concentration and renal filtered load of uric acid, even though the renal tubular reabsorption of uric acid remains impaired.[59]

Hyperuricosuria may be the only recognizable physiologic abnormality in patients with calcium nephrolithiasis. It occurs alone in approximately 10% of patients with renal calculi,[6] and may coexist with various forms of hypercalciuria previously enumerated.

The most common cause for hyperuricosuria in patients with hyperuricosuric calcium nephrolithiasis is probably "dietary overindulgence" with purine-rich foods.[58] Such individuals have a history of a liberal intake of meat, poultry, and fish, and estimated purine intake is higher than in the control group. Hyperuricosuria may be produced by an oral purine load and ameliorated by dietary purine deprivation.[56,58]

However, some patients with hyperuricosuric calcium nephrolithiasis (approximately 30%) have hyperuricosuria as a result of uric acid overproduction. Hyperuricosuria persists despite long-term purine deprivation. No further studies have been performed to elucidate the nature of this apparent urate overproduction.

C. Diagnostic Criteria (Table 23–2)

Hyperuricosuric calcium nephrolithiasis (pure presentation) is characterized by hyperuricosuria (urinary uric acid > 600 mg/day on mean of three samples and on at least two of the three samples); normocalcemia; normal fasting and calcium load response, normal urinary calcium and oxalate (< 44 mg/day); and calcium nephrolithiasis. Hyperuricosuria, defined functionally here by the upper normal limit of 600 mg/day, correlates with the urinary supersaturation with respect to monosodium urate and with the propensity for calcium stone formation.[60] (Other laboratories employ a higher upper limit for urinary uric acid: e.g., 750 mg/day for women and 800 mg/day for men.) Urinary pH is typically greater than 5.5. Hyperuricosuria may be the only abnormality in patients with calcium stones, or it may coexist with various forms of hypercalciuria.

Potassium citrate may be particularly useful in patients with mild-moderate hyperuricosuria (< 800 mg/day) in whom hypocitraturia is also present. However, allopurinol is probably preferred in patients with more marked hyperuricosuria, especially if hyperuricemia coexists.

D. Treatment of Hyperuricosuric Calcium Nephrolithiasis (Table 23–3)

Allopurinol (300 mg/day) is the physiologically meaningful drug of choice in hyperuricosuric calcium oxalate nephrolithiasis resulting from uric acid overproduction, because of its ability to reduce uric acid synthesis and lower urinary uric acid.[61] Its use in hyperuricosuria associated with dietary purine overindulgence is also reasonable, since dietary purine restriction is often impractical. Physicochemical changes ensuing from restoration of normal urinary uric acid include an increase in the urinary limit of metastability of calcium oxalate.[56] Thus, the spontaneous nucleation of calcium oxalate is retarded by treatment, probably via inhibition of monosodium urate–induced stimulation of calcium oxalate crystallization.[54] Because of the potential exaggeration of monosodium urate–induced calcium oxalate crystallization from excessive sodium intake, a moderate sodium restriction (< 150 mEq/day) is also advisable.

Potassium citrate represents an effective alternative to allopurinol in the treatment of this condition.[62] Citrate added to a synthetic medium metastably supersaturated with respect to calcium oxalate was shown to inhibit the heterogeneous nucleation of calcium oxalate by monosodium urate.[62] When potassium citrate (60 mEq/day in divided doses) was given to patients with hyperuricosuric calcium oxalate nephrolithiasis, urinary citrate rose significantly. The induced hypercitraturia not only reduced urinary saturation of calcium oxalate (by complexing calcium), but also inhibited urate-induced crystallization of calcium oxalate.

III. HYPEROXALURIA

The main cause of moderate-severe hyperoxaluria causing calcium oxalate nephrolithiasis is ileal disease (enteric hyperoxaluria). This entity will therefore be the principal focus of this section.

A. Causal Role of Hyperoxaluria in Calcium Stone Formation

Hyperoxaluria probably facilitates calcium oxalate stone formation by increasing urinary saturation of calcium oxalate. This conclusion is supported by its identification as an important risk factor for stone formation and its frequent association with calcium oxalate nephrolithiasis.

B. Pathophysiology of Hyperoxaluria

Oxalate is derived both from *in vivo* synthesis and from intestinal absorption. Once synthesized or absorbed, it is not further degraded *in vivo*. Its principal route of excretion is the kidney. Data on renal handling of oxalate are limited and conflicting. Of the 30 mg of oxalate that is excreted normally, 80% to 90% may be accounted by *in vivo* synthesis and the remainder is derived from the diet.

Hyperoxaluria resulting from a primary derangement in renal handling of oxalate has not been recognized. Rather, the abnormality typically results from the increased serum concentrations and renal filtered loads due to high substrate availability, for example, administration of methoxyflurane or ascorbic acid; enzymatic disturbance(s) in the oxalate biosynthetic pathway, as in primary hyperoxaluria (rare); or increased intestinal absorption of oxalate.

Increased intestinal absorption is the cause of hyperoxaluria in enteric hyperoxaluria.[63] Common denominators are ileal disease (Crohn's disease, ileal resection, bypass), fat malabsorption, and presence of functioning colon. Two factors probably act in concert to cause intestinal hyperabsorption of oxalate. First, intestinal transport of oxalate may be primarily increased because of the action of bile salts and fatty acids on the permeability of intestinal mucosa to oxalate. Second, the total amount of oxalate absorbed may also be increased because of an enlarged intraluminal pool of oxalate available for absorption. The intestinal fat malabsorption characteristic of ileal disease may exaggerate soap formation with divalent cations, limit the amount of "free" divalent cations to complex oxalate, and thereby raise the available oxalate pool.

In addition to the disturbance in oxalate metabolism, the intestinal absorption and renal excretion of calcium are often decreased in enteric hyperoxaluria, probably a reflection of the loss of the intestinal site of calcium absorption from disease or resection, of intraluminal binding of calcium by nonabsorbed fatty acids, or of vitamin D deficiency associated with fat malabsorption. Urine output may be substantially reduced consequent to fluid loss from the intestinal tract. Urinary citrate may be low because of hypokalemia and metabolic acidosis.[64,65] Low urinary magnesium may result from impaired intestinal magnesium absorption.

The cause of the formation of calcium oxalate stones in enteric hyperoxaluria is multifactorial and includes hyperoxaluria as well as some of the other disturbances enumerated. Saturation of urine with respect to calcium oxalate may be increased because of high oxalate concentration, and low urinary citrate and magnesium (which reduces complexation of calcium and oxalate, respectively), even though urinary calcium may be low. Low urine volume exaggerates urinary supersaturation. Moreover, inhibitor activity against crystallization of calcium salts is reduced because of low renal excretion of citrate.

C. Diagnostic Criteria (Table 23–2)

Hyperoxaluria, defined as urinary oxalate > 44 mg/day, is associated with calcium oxalate stones. If urinary oxalate is > 80 mg/day, primary or enteric hyperoxaluria is probably present. In primary hyperoxaluria, urinary glycolate or glycerate may be increased in addition to oxalate. Moreover, oxalosis (tissue deposition of calcium oxalate), anemia, and renal failure are common in primary hyperoxaluria. In enteric hyperoxaluria, there is a history of small bowel disease, ileal bypass, or resection.[66] Urinary calcium is typically low (< 100 mg/day). Serum calcium and magnesium may be low or low-normal, and parathyroid function may be stimulated. Serum bicarbonate and urinary citrate may be reduced. Even in the absence of intestinal disease, a mild to moderate hyperoxaluria (urinary oxalate 44–80 mg/day) may occur with vitamin C therapy, overindulgence in oxalate-rich foods (particularly spinach) or severe dietary calcium deprivation. Mild hyperoxaluria may also occur in patients with increased calcium absorption, such as those suffering from absorptive hypercalciuria.

D. Treatment of Hyperoxaluric Calcium Nephrolithiasis (Table 23–3)

The cause for stone formation in enteric hyperoxaluria is multifactorial. The treatment should therefore be directed at correcting the various disturbances present, including hyperoxaluria, hypocitraturia and low urinary pH, hypomagnesiuria, and low urine volume.

Oral administration of large amounts of calcium (0.25–1.0 g four times/day) or magnesium has been recommended for the control of calcium nephrolithiasis of ileal disease. Although urinary oxalate may decrease (probably from binding of oxalate by divalent cations), the concurrent rise in urinary calcium may obviate the beneficial effect of this therapy, at least in some patients.[67] Cholestyramine does not cause a sustained reduction in oxalate excretion. A limitation of dietary oxalate intake and partial replacement of dietary fat with medium-chain fatty acids may be helpful in those patients who also have malabsorption.

The treatment of low urinary citrate and pH with potassium citrate is considered in section IV-D under chronic diarrheal syndrome. Hypomagnesiuria is due to impaired intestinal absorption of magnesium. It contributes to calcium oxalate stone formation because of reduced complexation of oxalate by magnesium and consequent rise in the urinary saturation of calcium oxalate. Oral magnesium supplementation could partially correct hypomagnesiuria, although it may provoke further diarrhea. In our experience, magnesium gluconate (0.5–1 g three times/day) is better tolerated than magnesium oxide or hydroxide. Magnesium chloride is contraindicated, since it will exaggerate metabolic acidosis.

A high fluid intake is recommended to assure adequate urine volume. Control of excessive intestinal fluid loss with an antidiarrheal agent may be necessary before a sufficient urine output could be achieved.

Calcium citrate may theoretically have a role in the management of enteric hyperoxaluria. This treatment may lower urinary oxalate by binding oxalate in the intestinal tract. It may raise urinary citrate and pH by providing an alkali load.[68] Finally, it may correct the malabsorption of calcium and adverse effects on the skeleton by providing an efficiently absorbed calcium.

IV. HYPOCITRATURIA

A. Causal Role of Hypocitraturia in Calcium Stone Formation

Hypocitraturia probably represents an important risk for the formation of calcium stones based on the known capacity of citrate to inhibit the crystallization of stone-forming calcium salts. Citrate reduces urinary saturation of calcium oxalate or calcium phosphate by forming a soluble complex with calcium and thereby reducing calcium ion activity.[41,69] Although citrate is an effective inhibitor of calcium phosphate crystal growth,[70] it has only a modest inhibitor activity against calcium oxalate crystal growth.[71] Moreover, citrate directly inhibits spontaneous nucleation of calcium oxalate.[69] A recent study suggests that citrate is a potent inhibitor of the agglomeration of preformed calcium oxalate crystals.[72]

B. Pathophysiology of Hypocitraturia

Urinary citrate excretion is a function of filtration, reabsorption, peritubular transport, and synthesis by the renal tubular cell.[73] Approximately 80% to 90% of filtered citrate is normally reabsorbed. Citrate secretion is negligible in humans. Peritubular transport (citrate flux between peritubular blood and tubular cell) and tubular synthesis do not directly influence citrate excretion in urine; they do so by affecting the renal tissue content of citrate and ultimately the filtered load of citrate.

Although the exact physiologic mechanism of renal handling of citrate has not been elucidated, several factors influence its excretion. Citrate excretion may be enhanced by alkalosis,[74] PTH,[75] vitamin D, growth hormone, and estrogen. On the other hand, citrate excretion may be impaired by acidosis,[76] hypokalemia,[42] androgen, and urinary tract infection (probably from bacterial enzymatic degradation of citrate). Among these factors, acid-base status probably plays the most important role in the handling of citrate. For example, acidosis reduces urinary citrate by both enhancing renal tubular reabsorption and impairing peritubular uptake and synthesis of citrate. This mechanism accounts for the occurrence of hypocitraturia in renal tubular acidosis (complete or incomplete distal),[77] chronic diarrheal states (including enteric hyperoxaluria)[65,78] hypokalemia (from intracellular acidosis),[42] thiazide therapy (from hypokalemia),[42] and high animal protein diet (from elevated acid-ash content).[79] The urinary citrate may also be low following strenuous physical exercise (from acquired acidosis)[80] and high sodium intake (probably from sodium-induced potassium loss).

In our series, hypocitraturia occurred with other causes of nephrolithiasis in approximately 50% of patients, and existed as a sole abnormality in 5%.[64]

Distal acidification defect (type I) is the only form of renal tubular acidosis that is associated with nephrolithiasis. The stone formation is the result of high urinary pH and calcium and low urinary citrate. Calcium phosphate crystallization is promoted because of increased urinary saturation (from increased dissociation of phosphate and hypercalciuria) and reduced inhibitor activity (from hypocitraturia). The crystallization of calcium oxalate may be enhanced as well owing to increased saturation (from hypercalciuria and reduced citrate complexation of calcium) and impaired inhibitor activity (from hypocitraturia). Thus, the predominant stone constituent is calcium phosphate (hydroxyapatite). Calcium oxalate is also present in the stone typically, albeit as a minor constituent. Nephrocalcinosis may be often found with nephrolithiasis.

There is no evidence that nephrolithiasis is associated with proximal renal tubular acidosis (type II) or with hyporeninemic hypoaldosteronism (type IV). Urinary citrate may be low because of acidosis. However, urinary calcium is often low owing to bicarbonaturia in type II and renal insufficiency in type IV. Moreover, urinary pH is normal in type IV.

Distal renal tubular acidosis should not be confused with calcium oxalate nephrolithiasis of chronic diarrheal syndrome. In the latter case, metabolic acidosis is secondary to intestinal alkali loss from frequent diarrhea. Stone (calcium) formation is consequent to low urinary citrate and volume. Underlying gastrointestinal disorders producing this syndrome include postgastrectomy state, inflammatory disease of the small bowel, bowel resection or bypass, and colitis. In states of malabsorption of fat, hyperoxaluria and low urinary magnesium may be present as well, contributing to calcium oxalate stone formation. Uric acid lithiasis may develop owing to low urinary pH.

C. Diagnostic Criteria (Table 23–2)

Hypocitraturic calcium nephrolithiasis in the pure presentation refers to the condition in which hypocitraturia (urinary citrate < 320 mg/day) is present alone without other physiologic derangements (such as hypercalciuria, hyperuricosuria).[64] Hypocitraturia often coexists with other abnormalities. It may be caused by distal renal tubular acidosis,[77] metabolic acidosis of chronic diarrheal states,[65] or thiazide-induced hypokalemia.[42] Complete distal renal tubular acidosis is characterized by hyperchloremic metabolic acidosis (high serum chloride, low serum potassium and carbon dioxide) and high urinary pH (> 6.8) in the absence of infection of the urinary tract. There is also an incomplete form of renal tubular acidosis characterized by normal serum electrolytes but an impaired ability to acidify the urine following ammonium chloride load. Both complete and incomplete forms may be associated with hypercalcemia, hypocitraturia, calcium nephrolithiasis, and nephrocalcinosis. A typical stone analysis shows preponderance of hydroxyapatite with calcium oxalate as a minor constituent.

Chronic diarrheal states capable of producing hypocitraturia and calcium nephrolithiasis include ileal disease or resection, gastrectomy, ulcerative colitis, or colectomy. The degree of hypocitraturia is generally proportional to the severity of intestinal fluid loss. In severe diarrheal states, urinary citrate may be very low (< 50 mg/day). Besides hypocitraturia, there may be serum electrolyte abnormalities of acquired metabolic acidosis (due to intestinal fluid loss) and low urinary pH. Same patients may show full features of enteric hyperoxaluria.

In thiazide-induced hypocitraturia, serum potassium is low or low-normal, and urinary citrate low (< 320 mg/day). Serum carbon dioxide may be high, serum chloride low, and urinary calcium normal, due to thiazide action.

D. Treatment of Hypocitraturic Calcium Nephrolithiasis (Table 23–3)

1. Renal Tubular Acidosis (Distal)[77]

Potassium citrate therapy is capable of correcting both metabolic acidosis and hypokalemia. Moreover, it may restore normal urinary citrate, although large doses (up to 120 mEq/day) may be required in severe acidotic states. Urinary calcium typically declines with the correction of acidosis. The overall rise in urinary pH is small, since urinary pH is high to begin with; the urinary pH is generally below 7.5 during treatment unless there is complication by a urinary tract infection.

Thus, potassium citrate treatment produces a sustained decline in the urinary saturation of calcium oxalate (from reduction in urinary calcium and in citrate complexation of calcium). The urinary saturation of calcium phosphate does not increase because the rise in phosphate dissociation is relatively small (due to a modest rise in pH) and is adequately compensated by a decline in ionic calcium concentration. Moreover, inhibitor activity against the crystallization of calcium oxalate and calcium phosphate is augmented by the direct action of citrate.

If there is substantial renal sodium leak, alkali might be provided as a mixed sodium-potassium salt. However, renal sodium wasting is not prominent in most patients with renal tubular acidosis presenting with stones.

2. Chronic Diarrheal Syndrome[78]

In patients with mild-moderate severity of intestinal fluid loss in whom hypocitraturia is not severe (urinary citrate being in the range of 100–300 mg/day), potassium citrate (60 mEq in three to four divided doses in a liquid form) is generally effective in restoring normal urinary citrate and pH. Urinary calcium generally remains low. In those with severe hypocitraturia (with urinary citrate < 100 mg/day), even excessive doses of potassium citrate (up to 120 mEq/day) may be ineffective in restoring normal urinary citrate.

We recommend that a liquid preparation of potassium citrate be used rather than a slow-release tablet preparation in these states, because some of these patients may have intestinal adhesions and may be more prone to obstruction from a tablet preparation. Furthermore, a slow release medication may be poorly absorbed owing to rapid intestinal transit.

We suggest a frequent dose schedule (three to four times/day) for the liquid preparation because of relative short duration of biological action. In other hypocitraturic conditions, the solid slow-release preparation is preferable or is better tolerated. A less frequent dose schedule (twice/day) is acceptable for the solid preparation because of its slow-release characteristic.

3. Thiazide-Induced Hypocitraturia

Hypokalemia resulting from thiazide may cause hypocitraturia probably by causing intracellular acidosis, and may thereby attenuate the beneficial hypocalciuric effect of therapy on renal stone formation.[43]

It has been suggested that potassium citrate may be less effective than potassium chloride in correcting the thiazide-induced hypokalemia, because of the poor reabsorbability of citrate from the renal tubules.[81] However, severe chloride depletion is uncommon in patients with thiazide-induced hypocitraturia. Thus, in our study, potassium citrate was as effective as potassium chloride in correcting thiazide-induced hypokalemia.[43] Moreover, the addition of potassium citrate to thiazide therapy raised urinary pH and citrate.

4. *Idiopathic Hypocitraturic Calcium Nephrolithiasis*[82]

This entity, idiopathic hypocitraturic calcium oxalate nephrolithiasis, includes hypocitraturia occurring alone with calcium stones, and hypocitraturia occurring in conjunction with absorptive and renal hypercalciurias and hyperuricosuric calcium oxalate nephrolithiasis. Stones formed are predominantly composed of calcium oxalate.

Potassium citrate treatment has been shown to produce a sustained increase in urinary citrate excretion.[82] Urinary pH could be maintained at 6.5 to 7.0. Along with these changes, the urinary saturation of calcium oxalate declined significantly to normal limits.

V. GOUTY DIATHESIS

A. Causal Role of Low Urinary pH in Formation of Calcium or Uric Acid Stones

Persistent passage of unusually acid urine (pH < 5.5) may cause both uric acid and calcium stones.[83] Because urinary pH is close to or less than the dissociation constant of uric acid, the concentration of undissociated uric acid is high, leading to uric acid crystallization. The uric acid so formed may cause the crystallization of calcium oxalate by the same mechanism described for monosodium urate. Although uric acid is less efficient than monosodium urate in inducing heterogeneous nucleation of calcium oxalate (on a weight basis), its crystalline dimensions are more compatible with epitaxy.[57] Moreover, uric acid has been shown to remove naturally occurring urinary macromolecular inhibitors, thereby attenuating their activity.[55]

B. Pathophysiology of Gouty Diathesis

1. *Gouty Diathesis*

We have previously utilized the term gouty diathesis[83] to describe the overall clinical entity of uric acid lithiasis. The invariant feature was the persistent passage of unusually acid urine (pH < 5.5) in which uric acid is sparingly soluble. Some patients had gouty arthritis or hyperuricemia. Stone analysis disclosed uric acid alone or in combination with calcium oxalate and/or calcium phosphate.

In some patients, we have found these features of gouty diathesis except for the lack of uric acid on stone analysis. The stone analysis has disclosed only the presence of calcium oxalate and/or calcium phosphate. No obvious cause has been detected for the unusually low urinary pH, such as excessive intestinal alkali loss or a consumption of an animal protein–rich diet. It was presumed that urate-induced crystallization of calcium salts accounted for calcium nephrolithiasis.[54,57]

It is our contention that gouty diathesis represents varying phases of primary gout; the occurrence of hyperuricemia and gouty arthritis represents the full manifestation of the syndrome, whereas the picture of low urinary pH and uric acid/calcium nephrolithiasis without hyperuricemia or gouty arthritis reflects a forme frust or an early phase of classic gout. Stone symptoms may precede articular symptoms in 40% of gouty patients, occasionally by more than 10 years.

2. *Primary Gout*

In primary gout, the principal abnormality, identifiable in all patients, is a persistently acid urinary pH.[84,85] In fasting morning specimens, the urinary pH is 5.0 or less in about half of these patients, in comparison with 15% of normal subjects.[85] The abnormality is also manifest by a loss of the normal alkaline tide in the gouty population. In spite of a relatively large amount of literature on the subject, the basis of this tendency to a persistently acid urine remains unclear.[86–89] The data indicate that patients with gout excrete relatively more titratable acid and relatively less ammonia than do normal subjects,[90] but it is unclear whether the defect in ammonia production is primary, whether it is dependent on a primary abnormality in the excretion of titratable acid, or whether both abnormalities reflect an unknown fundamental defect in acid-base regulation. Many patients, but not all, present with hyperuricosuria as well due to urate overproduction. Such patients are at particular risk for uric acid nephrolithiasis.

3. Others

Other causes of uric acid nephrolithiasis include certain inborn errors of uric acid metabolism, secondary causes of urate overproduction, chronic diarrheal states, and use of uricosuric agents. Three well-studied enzymatic disorders of uric acid metabolism are hypoxanthine-guanine phosphoribosyl transferase deficiency (Lesch-Nyhan syndrome), phosphoribosyl pyrophosphate synthetase overactivity, and glucose-6-phosphatase deficiency (type I glycogen storage disease). Affected patients have extreme rates of uric acid overproduction. In myeloproliferative disorders, leukemia, neoplasia, or hemolytic anemia, hyperuricemia and hyperuricosuria occur because of an increased rate of nucleoprotein turnover. As many as 50% of patients with myeloproliferative disorders may form uric acid stones, which often is the initial clinical manifestation.

Certain drugs such as probenecid and high-dose salicylates, as well as x-ray contrast agents, may produce an acute uricosuria by inhibiting net uric acid reabsorption and increasing the fractional excretion of uric acid. The chronic administration of these agents, however, results in a new steady state, in which the rate of uric acid excretion should be no greater than the pretreatment rate. Thus, the risk of stone formation occurs early, and not late, except in the setting of urate overproduction. Several gastrointestinal disorders have been associated with a high incidence of uric acid lithiasis. The three most common conditions are ulcerative colitis, regional enteritis, and the presence of ileostomy.[91–93] The pathogenesis of uric acid stones in these disorders is related to variable degrees of dehydration and bicarbonate loss resulting in an unusually acid and concentrated urine. The excretion rate of uric acid is usually normal in these patients.

In the preceding entities, calcium nephrolithiasis could also occur.

C. Diagnostic Criteria (Table 23–2)

The invariant feature in gouty diathesis is the persistent passage of unusually acid urine (pH < 5.5).[83,94] The cause for low urinary pH cannot be readily ascertained. Same patients may give a positive personal or family history of gouty arthritis. Some patients may present with hyperuricemia or hypertriglyceridemia. Stones formed may be uric acid alone, calcium oxalate–phosphate alone, or the mixture of the two. Some patients may form uric acid on one occasion and calcium stones on another occasion. Uric acid stones are radiolucent.

D. Treatment of Gouty Diathesis (Table 23–3)

Potassium citrate is the treatment of choice for this condition. In our study this treatment at a dosage of 30–80 mEq/day in divided doses significantly increased urinary pH from the low mean value of 5.30 to above 6.19, but less than 7.[83] Owing to the resulting enhanced dissociation of uric acid, the amount of undissociated uric acid significantly decreased to the range encountered in normal subjects without stones (< 150 mg/day). Thus, potassium citrate therapy significantly increased the solubility of uric acid, preventing uric acid stone formation. Moreover, potassium citrate therapy inhibited the complication of calcium stones by reducing urinary saturation of calcium oxalate and retarding the crystallization of calcium oxalate.

It is acknowledged that sodium alkali therapy would be as effective as potassium citrate in preventing uric acid nephrolithiasis, since it possesses a similar capacity for raising urinary pH. However, complication of calcium stones, albeit rare, may occur with sodium alkali therapy.

In patients who present with hyperuricemia or marked hyperuricosuria, allopurinol (e.g., 300 mg/day) is recommended.

VI. CYSTINURIA

Cystine stones develop in patients with homozygous cystinuria.[95] Homozygous cystinuria is characterized by urinary cystine excretion of more than 250 mg/g creatinine, excessive renal excretion of other dibasic amino acids (lysine, ornithine, and arginine) and varying intestinal absorptive defects for these amino acids.[95] The only recognized clinical manifestation is cystine lithiasis, which may develop any time during life, with peak times for expression during the second and third decades.

A. Physicochemical Basis for Cystine Stone Formation

Cystine stone formation has been ascribed to the low solubility of cystine in the aqueous environment of urine. In the setting of excessive urinary concentration of cystine (as in homozygous cystinuria), the solubility limit for cystine is often exceeded, creating a supersaturated environment conducive to cystine crystallization.

1. *Factors Affecting Cystine Solubility*

It has long been known that cystine solubility is pH-dependent, with lowest solubility at low range of urinary pH, gradual increased solubility with rising pH to 7.5, and rapid increase in solubility above pH 7.5.

Dent and Senior[96] showed that the solubility curve of cystine was the same whether it was obtained in urine from normal subjects or from cystinuric patients, and that it was unaffected by the presence of urea or sodium chloride. Studies by Ettinger and Kolb[97] indicated that cystine solubility was greater in urine samples with a specific gravity exceeding 1.01 than in samples with a specific gravity of less than this value. The results suggested that some components of urine might influence cystine solubility. Our own studies have disclosed that the enhanced solubility of cystine in urine is accountable by mineral electrolytes and macromolecules.[98]

Because of the solvent action of electrolytes and macromolecules, the maximum solubility of cystine determined in *urine*[98] is considerably greater than that derived in simple solution (5 mM Na), but less than that derived by Dent and Senior.[96] Thus, the saturation of cystine in individual urine samples cannot be estimated by comparing the original cystine concentration with a defined cystine solubility curve. The comparison of urinary cystine value in a given specimen with the curve of Dent and Senior[96] would underestimate urinary cystine saturation, whereas comparison with the cystine solubility curve in a 5 mM Na solution would overestimate it. It may be more accurately measured as the ratio of original cystine concentration and the directly determined cystine solubility in urine.[98]

2. *Determinants of Cystine Crystallization*

The main determinant of cystine crystallization is urinary supersaturation. There is no known inhibitor of cystine crystallization. If the urine sample is supersaturated with respect to cystine, precipitation of cystine invariably occurs. It is virtually impossible to maintain a metastably supersaturated solution.[98] Thus, there is a stronger cause and effect relationship between excessive cystine excretion and stone formation than for any other form of stone disease (e.g., between hypercalciuria and calcium nephrolithiasis).

Although cystine stones often coexist with calcium stones (up to 40%),[99] no epitaxy or heterogeneous nucleation has been disclosed between cystine and calcium salts.[98]

B. Pathophysiology of Cystinuria

1. *Renal Transport Defects in Cystinuria*

Normally, cystine is filtered and almost completely reabsorbed in the proximal nephron, leaving less than 20 mg in urine each day. In cystinuria, serum concentration of cystine and hence the renal filtered load of cystine are reduced. Exaggerated cystine excretion under this circumstance suggests a disturbance in renal handling of cystine. Prevailing evidence indicates multiple transport defects[100] for cystine, characterized by impaired tubular reabsorption and back diffusion.

A similar transport defect for other dibasic amino acids is present. However, exaggerated renal excretion of these amino acids and cystine probably cannot be explained by a single transport defect as originally suggested by Dent and Rose.[101] Increasing the filtered load of one of these amino acids does not necessarily augment the excretion of others.[95]

2. *Intestinal Transport Defect for Cystine in Cystinuria*

There is also a defect in the intestinal transport for dibasic amino acids in cystinuria. Cystinuria has been classified into three types based on varying intestinal transport disturbances for these amino acids.[102] The intestinal transport has been assessed from the *in vitro* uptake of radiolabeled amino acid by specimens of jejunal mucosa obtained by peroral biopsy, and from plasma cystine elevation following oral cystine load. In type I cystinuria, there is no uptake of cystine, lysine, or arginine by jejunal mucosa and there is no plasma cystine elevation following oral cystine load. Thus, there is total abrogation of intestinal transport for these dibasic amino acids. In types II and III, the intestinal transport of dibasic amino acids is disturbed, but less severely than in the type I presentation. Thus, in type II cystinuria, some cystine uptake by jejunal mucosa prevails but at a markedly reduced level, and oral cystine loading does not increase plasma cystine level. In type III cystinuria, cystine and lysine uptake by jejunal mucosa is variably reduced but not obliterated, and the increment in plasma cystine following oral cystine load is blunted but present. Studies by Rosenberg et al.[102] have disclosed that all three types of cystinuria in the homozygous state present with excessive renal excretion of all four dibasic amino acids. However, in the heterozygous state, type I cystinuria is characterized by normal cystine (nonelevated) excretion, whereas type II and type III presentations show elevation in cystine and lysine excretion (although not quite up to the level encountered in the homozygous state) probably owing to a prevailing (although reduced) intestinal uptake of these amino acids.

C. Diagnostic Criteria

The urinary sediment (preferably in fresh first morning void) should be examined for the presence of typical hexagonal cystine crystals. The urine sample should also be screened for "qualitative" cystine by the cyanide-nitroprusside test. A positive reaction suggests that cystine excretion exceeds 75 mg/liter. A false-positive test may be encountered in patients with homocystinuria and acetonuria. On roentgenologic examination, cystine calculi are radiopaque (although not as much) like calcareous calculi, but are more rounded and homogeneous in appearance. They may attain a staghorn size.

If these studies are suggestive of the presence of cystinuria, urinary cystine excretion should be quantitated. Urinary cystine exceeding 250 mg/g creatinine is usually diagnostic of homozygous cystinuria. Stones passed or removed should be analyzed. The presence of cystine provides a definitive diagnosis of cystinuria.

D. Treatment of Cystine Nephrolithiasis (Table 23–3)

1. *Dietary Manipulation*

A low-methionine diet has often been recommended for the control of cystine nephrolithiasis because of the well-known requirement of this essential amino acid for cystine production.[103] Whereas this dietary maneuver may reduce cystine excretion, a rigid methionine restriction is impractical. The compliance is often poor to a diet devoid of or severely restricted in flesh meat, poultry, fish, and dairy products. Moreover, there may be long-term adverse consequences of such a diet on other organ systems such as the skeleton. Thus, it is our practice to recommend avoidance of excessive intake of these food items, but not necessarily to severely restrict them.

A recent report[104] suggests that cystine excretion is dependent on dietary sodium intake, by a mechanism poorly described. Thus, a direct correlation has been described between urinary cystine and urinary sodium in four cystinuric patients. This study implies that a reduction in dietary sodium intake by 150 mEq/day (8.8 g sodium chloride) could reduce urinary cystine by 650 μM (156 mg)/day. Although we would agree that an avoidance of dietary sodium excess would be advisable, it should be noted that (1) such a rigid dietary sodium restriction is difficult to achieve practically, (2) the reduction in cystine excretion is modest, (3) there may be an opposing effect of reduced solvent action of sodium on cystine solubility from a low-sodium diet, and (4) the above-mentioned study of Jaeger et al.[104] was done on an uncontrolled diet with a variable intake of proteins.

2. Conservative Measures

In patients with moderate cystinuria (250–500 mg/day) with cystine calculi, conservative measures of high fluid intake and alkali should be attempted first. The aim of fluid therapy is to increase urine volume sufficiently in order to reduce cystine solubility below the solubility limit. At least 3 liters of fluid (ten 10 oz glassfuls) should be provided, including two glasses with each meal and at bedtime. The patients should be expected to awake at night to urinate; they should drink two more glasses of fluids before returning to bed. Additional fluids should be consumed if there is excessive sweating or intestinal fluid loss. A minimum urine output of 2 liters/day on a consistent basis should be sought, a goal attainable by most patients with proper and persistent instruction. Stone dissolution has been reported following high fluid intake.[105]

All types of fluid are generally permissible, with the possible exception of milk (with high methionine content) and brewed tea (with high oxalate content increasing risk for calcium oxalate nephrolithiasis, which sometimes complicates cystine nephrolithiasis). Fruit juices (grapefruit, orange, cranberry, apple, grape) may be particularly advantageous, because they provide not only water but alkali. For example, 600 ml of orange juice (one glassful with breakfast and again with dinner) may provide enough citrate to increase urinary pH by 0.5 unit.

The object of alkali therapy is to increase urinary pH to enhance cystine solubility. However, excessive alkali therapy is not indicated.[101] Substantial increase in cystine solubility does not occur until the urinary pH exceeds 7.5. The provision of alkali, no matter how much, rarely raises urinary pH above 7.5. When urinary pH increases above 7.0, with alkali therapy, the complication of calcium phosphate nephrolithiasis may ensue because of the enhanced urinary supersaturation of hydroxyapatite in an alkaline environment.

We recommend that a modest amount of alkali be provided in order to maintain urinary pH at a high-normal range (6.5–7.0). Potassium alkali are advantageous over sodium alkali, because they do not cause hypercalciuria and are less likely to cause the complication of calcium stones[83,106] and are devoid of sodium-induced enhancement of cystine excretion.[104] Citrate is preferable to bicarbonate because it produces a more constant and persistent elevation in urinary pH. The slow-release citrate preparation is probably superior to the readily available liquid preparation in this regard. It is our common practice to use potassium citrate (wax matrix tablets) at a typical dosage of 30 mEq twice a day. The dosage may be adjusted depending on the results of urinary pH.

3. Glutamine

In 1979, Miyagi et al.[107] reported that glutamine given orally or intravenously significantly reduced cystine excretion in a patient with cystinuria. This effect was attributed to the secretion of glutamine into the proximal tubular lumen in exchange for cystine. Unfortunately, van den Berg et al.[108] were unable to confirm this finding in their study of five cystinuric patients.

In a recent report, however, Jaeger et al.[104] showed that glutamine administration (2.1 g/day in three divided doses orally) reduced cystine excretion when the sodium intake was high (300 mEq/day) but not when it was normal (150 mEq/day).

The reduction in cystine excretion is equivalent to that produced by an avoidance of an excessive sodium intake. Thus, glutamine has little value in patients maintained on a sodium-restricted diet.

4. D-Penicillamine

The object of D-penicillamine treatment is to reduce total cystine excretion by complexing cysteine, the monomeric form of cystine. It may be added to the conservative treatment program when the latter is ineffective in controlling stone formation in patients with moderate cystinuria. In patients with severe cystinuria (> 500 mg/day), in whom customary conservative program alone is not likely to be effective, D-penicillamine therapy (*with* conservative measures) may be begun to start with.

D-penicillamine (ββ-dimethyl-cysteine)[109] shares with cysteine a free sulfhydryl group. Thus, it readily undergoes thiol-disulfide exchange with cystine to form penicillamine-cysteine disulfide, which has a much higher aqueous solubility than cystine. Following oral administration, a sufficient amount of D-penicillamine could appear in urine to complex cysteine and thereby lower cystine excretion.

The dose of D-penicillamine should not be arbitrary but should be based on that amount required to reduce urinary cystine concentration to below its solubility limit (generally < 250 mg/liter). The extent of the decline in cystine excretion is proportional to the D-penicillamine dosage. Each increment in D-penicillamine dosage of 250 mg/day might be expected to reduce urinary cystine by 75 to 100 mg/day. Accordingly, assuming that a minimum desired urine output of 2 liters/day has been achieved, the minimum effective D-penicillamine dose might be 1250 mg/day when cystine excretion is 1000 mg/day or 750 mg/day when urinary cystine is 800 mg/day. The medication is generally given in divided doses before meals, since its absorption may be impaired when mixed with certain foods.

There is substantial evidence that D-penicillamine can favorably modify the course of cystine nephrolithiasis.[110] If adequate amounts of the drug could be given to lower urinary cystine to desired levels, one should expect a reduction in rates of stone passage and new stone formation. When there is a sufficient fall in cystine excretion to produce urinary undersaturation, dissolution of existing cystine stones could occur.

Unfortunately, a substantial number of patients develop adverse reactions to D-penicillamine treatment.[111] Side-effects include gastrointestinal complications (nausea, emesis, diarrhea, loose stools, anorexia, abdominal pain, bloating, or flatus), impairment in taste and smell (probably due to chelation of zinc), dermatologic complications (pharyngitis, oral ulcers, rash, ecchymosis, pruritus, urticaria, pemphigus, elastosis perforans serpiginosa, skin wrinkling), hypersensitivity reactions (laryngeal edema, dyspnea, respiratory distress, fever, chills, arthralgia, weakness, fatigue, myalgia, adenopathy), hematologic abnormalities (leukopenia, agranulocytosis, thrombocytopenia, anemia, eosinophilia), abnormal liver function tests, and renal complication (proteinuria, nephrotic syndrome, glomerulonephritis). In up to 50% of patients, the cessation of D-penicillamine therapy may be required because of these side-effects. In some of them, D-penicillamine therapy may be reinstituted by desensitization. This technique entails restarting treatment at a low dosage of D-penicillamine of 10 to 25 mg/day, with a gradual increase in dosage at 3-day intervals until the desired dosage is reached to be achieved over a period of about 1 month.

During long-term therapy, D-penicillamine may cause vitamin B_6 deficiency by binding pyridoxine. Before the appearance of significant symptoms (dizziness, seizures, glossitis, seborrheic dermatitis), it may be prudent to provide pyridoxine supplementation (50 mg/day) in patients receiving large doses of D-penicillamine (> 1 g/day) chronically.

When serious side-effects preclude D-penicillamine use, the only available recourse currently is to further increase fluid intake, reduce sodium intake, provide more alkali, and impose a more rigid methionine restriction.

5. Alpha-mercaptopropionylglycine (MPG)

This investigational drug, once approved, may serve as a reasonable alternative to D-penicillamine, especially in the setting of toxic reactions to the latter drug. MPG shares similar chemical properties with D-penicillamine. The reduction in urinary cystine produced by MPG is similar to that obtained during D-penicillamine therapy.[112] Thus, the same comments regarding dosage schedule previously given for D-penicillamine apply to the MPG treatment. Available data from Japan and Europe suggest that MPG is as effective as D-penicillamine in inhibiting cystine stone formation.[113]

The major advantage of MPG appears to be its apparent reduced toxicity. A recent review of the literature disclosed 10 reports entailing 120 cystinuric patients undergoing clinical trial with MPG. Minor gastrointestinal problems occurred in 35 patients, rash in 14, urticaria in three, pemphigus foliaceus in one, fever in seven, and nephrotic syndrome in two patients. These adverse reactions were generally less common and less serious than those reported with D-penicillamine. Although serious side-effects such as pemphigus and nephrotic syndrome have also been encountered during MPG therapy, they occurred less frequently. Thus, among 120 patients taking MPG, only two apparently had to stop taking the medication because of adverse reactions.

Our own experience is compatible with these findings.[112] Since 1980, we have organized and have been conducting a multiclinic trial with MPG as an investigational new drug in the United States, in order to assess the therapeutic role of MPG as an alternative to D-penicillamine in the management of cystine nephrolithiasis. The primary objective was to determine the safety and efficacy of MPG in patients with known toxic reactions to D-penicillamine.

Among 49 patients who took D-penicillamine first and later received MPG, 41 patients (83.7%) developed side-effects to D-penicillamine and 37 (75.5%) to MPG. Adverse reactions involved all organ systems. Frequent adverse reactions to D-penicillamine were nausea in 36.7%, proteinuria in 12.2%, and fatigue in 16.3%. These reactions were also observed during MPG therapy, but less frequently. Thus, nausea was encountered in 24.5% of patients, emesis in 10.2%, anorexia in 8.2%, rash in 14.3%, proteinuria in 10.2%, and fatigue in 14.3%.

Moreover, serious side-effects were less common during MPG therapy. Thus, 69.4% of patients required cessation of D-penicillamine treatment, whereas only 30.6% had to stop taking MPG. Among 34 patients who could not tolerate D-penicillamine, 22 could be maintained on MPG.

MPG was effective in reducing cystine excretion. During long-term treatment with MPG (average dose of 1193 mg/day), urinary cystine was maintained at 350 to 560 mg/day and urinary saturation of cystine was kept undersaturated. Commensurate with these changes, MPG produced remission of stone formation in 63% to 71% of patients and reduced individual stone formation rate in 81% to 94%.

Thus, MPG, once it becomes available, would seem to have a definite therapeutic role in the management of cystine nephrolithiasis, especially in patients who have developed toxic reactions to D-penicillamine.

VII. INFECTION WITH UREA-SPLITTING ORGANISMS

A. Causal Role of Infection and Pathophysiology of Struvite Stone Formation

Infection of the urinary tract with urea-splitting organisms may be associated with renal stones of struvite (magnesium ammonium phosphate) and of calcium carbonate apatite.[114] The critical determinant is the formation of ammonia in urine due to enzymatic degradation of urea by bacterial urease. The ammonia undergoes hydrolysis to form ammonium and hydroxyl ions. The resulting alkalinity of urine augments dissociation of phosphate to form triphosphate ions, and reduces the solubility of struvite. Although struvite stones may form *de novo* from infection alone, they also occur as a complication of other causes of renal calculi, such as hypercalciuria.

B. Diagnostic Criteria (Table 23–2)

Lithiasis due to infection is disclosed by the presence of magnesium ammonium phosphate on stone analysis. Such struvite stones are often associated with pyuria, positive urine culture for urea-splitting organisms (*Proteus*, certain species of *Staphylococcus*, *Pseudomonas*, and *Klebsiella*), and high urinary pH (> 7.5).[114] Struvite stones are radiopaque and sometimes may attain a large (staghorn) size; they usually occur as mixtures with calcium carbonate apatite and tricalcium phosphate or less commonly with calcium oxalate. Some patients with struvite stones may have hypercalciuria. Urinary citrate may be low owing to bacterial enzymatic degradation of citrate.

C. Treatment of Struvite Stones (Table 23–3)

If long-standing effective control of infection with urea-splitting organisms can be achieved, new stone formation may be averted and some dissolution of existing stones may be achieved. Unfortunately, such control is difficult to obtain with antibiotic therapy. If there is an existing struvite stone, it is difficult to completely eradicate the infection because the stone often harbors the organisms within its interstices. Even if "sterilization" of urine can be achieved by antibiotic therapy, reinfection could occur by harbored organisms. For these reasons, surgical removal of struvite stones is usually recommended.

In recent clinical trials, acetohydroxamic acid, a urease inhibitor, has been shown to reduce urinary saturation of struvite and to retard stone formation.[114] However, 30% of the patients experienced minor side-effects and 15% developed deep venous thrombosis.

Additional long-term studies must be done to determine the benefit/risk ratio.[115]

References

1. Segura JW, Patterson DE, LeRoy AJ, et al: Percutaneous lithotripsy. J Urol 130:1051–1054, 1983.
2. Chaussy C, Brendel W, Schmiedt E: Extracorporeally induced destruction of kidney stones by shock waves. Lancet 2:1265–1267, 1980.
3. Resnick MI, Pak CYC: Is the metabolic work-up of urolithiasis necessary? J Urol 137:960–961, 1987.
4. Pak CYC: Kidney stones. *In* Foster DW, Wilson JD (eds): Williams Textbook of Endocrinology. Philadelphia, WB Saunders, 1985, pp 1256–1273.
5. Pak CYC, Skurla C, Harvey J: Graphic display of urinary risk factors for renal stone formation. J Urol 134:867–870, 1985.
6. Pak CYC, Britton F, Peterson R, et al: Ambulatory evaluation of nephrolithiasis: Classification, clinical presentation and diagnostic criteria. Am J Med 69:19–30, 1980.
7. Pak CYC, Peters P, Hurt G, et al: Is selective therapy of recurrent nephrolithiasis possible? Am J Med 71:615–622, 1981.
8. Fleisch H, Bisaz S: Isolation from urine pyrophosphate, a calcification inhibitor. Am J Physiol 203:671–675, 1962.
9. Kitamura T, Zerwekh JE, Pak CYC: Partial biochemical and physicochemical characterization of organic macromolecules in urine from patients with renal stones and control subjects. Kidney Int 21:379–386, 1981.
10. Bowyer RC, Brockis JG, McCulloch RK: Glycosaminoglycans as inhibitors of calcium oxalate crystal growth and aggregation. Clin Chim Acta 95:23–28, 1979.
11. Nakagawa Y, Abram V, Parks JH, et al: Urine glycoprotein crystal growth inhibitors. Evidence for a molecular abnormality in calcium oxalate nephrolithiasis. J Clin Invest 76:1455–1462, 1985.
12. Pak CYC, Holt K: Nucleation and growth of brushite and calcium oxalate in urine of stone-formers. Metabolism 25:665–673, 1976.
13. Preminger GM, Sakhaee K, Pak CYC: Alkali action on the urinary crystallization of calcium salts: Contrasting responses to sodium citrate and potassium citrate. J Urol 139:240–242, 1988.
14. Yendt ER, Cohanim M: Prevention of calcium stones with thiazides. Kidney Int 13:397–409, 1978.
15. Pak CYC, Delea CS, Bartter FC: Successful treatment of recurrent nephrolithiasis (calcium stones) with cellulose phosphate. N Engl J Med 290:175–180, 1974.
16. Henneman PH, Benedict PH, Forbes AP: Idiopathic hypercalciuria. N Engl J Med 259:801–807, 1958.
17. Pak CYC: Pathogenesis of hypercalciuria. *In* Peck WA (ed): Bone and Mineral Research/4. New York, Elsevier, 1985, pp 303–334.
18. Pak CYC: Physiological basis for absorptive and renal hypercalciurias. Am J Med 237:F415–F423, 1979.
19. Brannan PG, Morawski S, Pak CYC, et al: Selective jejunal hyperabsorption of calcium in absorptive hypercalciuria. Am J Med 66:425–428, 1979.
20. Zerwekh JE, Pak CYC, Kaplan RA, et al: Pathogenetic role of 1,25-dihydroxyvitamin D in sarcoidosis and absorptive hypercalciuria: Different response to prednisolone therapy. J Clin Endocrinol Metab 51:381–386, 1980.
21. Zerwekh JE, Pak CYC: Selective effects of thiazide therapy on serum 1α,25-dihydroxyvitamin D and intestinal calcium absorption in renal and absorptive hypercalciurias. Metabolism 29:13–17, 1980.
22. Barilla DE, Zerwekh JE, Pak CYC: A critical evaluation of the role of phosphate in the pathogenesis of absorptive hypercalciuria. Mineral Electrolyte Metab 2:302–309, 1979.
23. Pak CYC, McGuire J, Peterson R, et al: Familial absorptive hypercalciuria in a large kindred. J Urol 126:717–719, 1981.
24. Pak CYC, Galosy RA: Fasting urinary calcium and adenosine 3′,5′-monophosphate: A discriminant analysis for the identification of renal and absorptive hypercalciuria. J Clin Endocrinol Metab 48:260–265, 1979.
25. Barilla DE, Townsend J, Pak CYC: An exaggerated augmentation of renal calcium excretion following oral glucose ingestion in patients with renal hypercalciuria. Invest Urol 14:486–488, 1978.
26. Sakhaee K, Nicar MJ, Brater DC, et al: Exaggerated natriuretic and calciuric response to hydrochlorothiazide in renal hypercalciuria but not in absorptive hypercalciuria. J Clin Endocrinol Metab 61:825–829, 1985.
27. Lemann J, Piering WF, Lennon EJ: Possible role of carbohydrate-induced calciuria in calcium oxalate kidney-stone formation. N Engl J Med 280:232–237, 1969.
28. Muldowney FP, Freaney R, Moloney MF: Importance of dietary sodium in the hypercalciuria syndrome. Kidney Int 22:292–296, 1982.
29. Lawoyin S, Sismilich S, Browne R, et al: Bone mineral content in patients with primary hyperparathyroidism, osteoporosis, and calcium urolithiasis. Metabolism 28:1250–1254, 1979.
30. Kaplan RA, Haussler MR, Deftos LF, et al: The role of 1α,25-dihydroxyvitamin D in the mediation of intestinal hyperabsorption of calcium in primary hyperparathyroidism and absorptive hypercalciuria. J Clin Invest 59:756–760, 1977.
31. Shen FH, Baylink DJ, Nielson RL, et al: Increased serum 1,25-dihydroxyvitamin D in idiopathic hypercalciuria. J Lab Clin Med 90:955–962, 1977.
32. Gray RW, Wilz DR, Caldas AE, et al: The importance of phosphate in regulating plasma 1,25-$(OH)_2$ vitamin D levels in humans: Studies in healthy subjects, in calcium-stone formers and in patients with primary hyperparathyroidism. J Clin Endocrinol Metab 45:299–306, 1977.
33. Bordier R, Ryckewart A, Gueris J, et al: On the pathogenesis of so-called idiopathic hypercalciuria. Am J Med 63:398–409, 1977.
34. Broadus AE, Erickson SB, Gertner JM, et al: An experimental human model of 1,25-dihydroxyvitamin D–mediated hypercalciuria. J Clin Endocrinol Metab 59:202–206, 1984.
35. Reynolds JJ, Holick MF, DeLuca HF: The role of vitamin D metabolites on bone resorption. Calcif Tissue Res 12:295–301, 1973.
36. Zerwekh JE, Sakhaee K, Pak CYC: Short term 1,25-dihydroxyvitamin D_3 administration raises serum osteocalcin in patients with postmenopausal osteoporosis. J Clin Endocrinol Metab 60:615–617, 1985.

37. Broadus AE, Insogna KL, Lang R, et al: Evidence for disordered control of 1,25-dihydroxyvitamin D production in absorptive hypercalciuria. N Engl J Med 311:73–80, 1984.
38. Coe FL, Favus MJ, Crockett T, et al: Effects of low-calcium diet on urine calcium excretion, parathyroid function and serum 1,25-$(OH)_2D_3$ levels in patients with idiopathic hypercalciuria and in normal subjects. Am J Med 72:25–32, 1982.
39. Pak CYC: A cautious use of sodium cellulose phosphate in the management of calcium nephrolithiasis. Invest Urol 19:187–190, 1981.
40. Preminger GM, Pak CYC: Eventual attenuation of hypocalciuric response to hydrochlorothiazide in absorptive hypercalciuria. J Urol 137:1104–1109, 1987.
41. Pak CYC, Nicar MJ, Northcutt C: The definition of the mechanism of hypercalciuria is necessary for the treatment of recurrent stone formers. Contrib Nephrol 33:136–151, 1982.
42. Nicar MJ, Peterson R, Pak CYC: Use of potassium citrate as potassium supplement during thiazide therapy of calcium nephrolithiasis. J Urol 131:430–433, 1984.
43. Pak CYC, Peterson R, Sakhaee K, et al: Correction of hypocitraturia and prevention of stone formation by combined thiazide and potassium citrate therapy in thiazide-unresponsive hypercalciuric nephrolithiasis. Am J Med 78:284–288, 1985.
44. Pak CYC, Sakhaee K, Crowther C, et al: Evidence justifying a high fluid intake in treatment of nephrolithiasis. Ann Intern Med 93:36–39, 1980.
45. Pak CYC, Galosy RA: Propensity for spontaneous nucleation of calcium oxalate. Quantitative assessment of urinary FPR-APR discriminant score. Am J Med 69:681–689, 1980.
46. Ettinger B, Oldroyd NO, Sorgel F: Triamterene nephrolithiasis. JAMA 244:2443–2445, 1980.
47. Leppla D, Browne R, Hill K, et al: Effect of amiloride with or without hydrochlorothiazide on urinary calcium and saturation of calcium salts. J Clin Endocrinol Metab 57:920–924, 1983.
48. Broadus AE, Magee JS, Mallette LE, et al: A detailed evaluation of oral phosphate therapy in selected patients with primary hyperparathyroidism. J Clin Endocrinol Metab 56:953–961, 1983.
49. Gallagher JC, Nordin BEC: Treatment with oestrogens of primary hyperparathyroidism in post-menopausal women. Lancet i:503–507, 1972.
50. Kaplan RA, Synder WH, Stewart A, et al: Metabolic effect of parathyroidectomy on asymptomatic primary hyperparathyroidism. J Clin Endocrinol Metab 42:415–426, 1976.
51. Pak CYC: Effect of parathyroidectomy on crystallization of calcium salts in urine of patients with primary hyperparathyroidism. Invest Urol 17:146–148, 1979.
52. Dudley FJ, Blackburn CRB: Extraskeletal calcification complicating oral neutral-phosphate therapy. Lancet 2:628–630, 1970.
53. Zerwekh JE, Harvey JA, Pak CYC: Administration of pharmacologic amounts of 25(s),26-dihydroxyvitamin D reduces serum 1,25-dihydroxyvitamin D levels in rats. Endocrinology 121:1671–1677, 1987.
54. Pak CYC, Holt K, Zerwekh JE: Attenuation by monosodium urate of the inhibitory effect of glycosaminoglycans on calcium oxalate nucleation. Invest Urol 17:138–140, 1979.
55. Zerwekh JE, Holt K, Pak CYC: Natural urinary macromolecular inhibitors: Attenuation of inhibitory activity by urate salts. Kidney Int 23:838–841, 1983.
56. Pak CYC, Barilla DE, Holt K, et al: Effect of oral purine load and allopurinol on the crystallization of calcium salts in urine of patients with hyperuricosuric calcium urolithiasis. Am J Med 65:593–599, 1978.
57. Coe FL: Hyperuricosuric calcium oxalate nephrolithiasis. *In* Massry SG, Ritz E, Jahn H (eds): Phosphate and Minerals in Health and Disease. New York, Plenum Press, 1980, pp 439–450.
58. Coe FL, Kavalach AG: Hypercalciuria and hyperuricosuria in patients with calcium nephrolithiasis. N Engl J Med 291:1344–1350, 1974.
59. Breslau NA, Pak CYC: Lack of effect of salt intake on urinary uric acid excretion. J Urol 129:531–532, 1983.
60. Pak CYC, Waters O, Arnold L, et al: Mechanism for calcium urolithiasis among patients with hyperuricosuria: Supersaturation of urine with respect to monosodium urate. J Clin Invest 59:426–431, 1977.
61. Coe FL: Hyperuricosuric calcium oxalate nephrolithiasis. Kidney Int 13:418–426, 1978.
62. Pak CYC, Peterson R: Successful treatment of hyperuricosuric calcium oxalate nephrolithiasis with potassium citrate. Arch Intern Med 146:863–868, 1986.
63. Earnest DL, Williams HE, Admirand WH: A physicochemical basis fo treatment of enteric hyperoxaluria. Trans Assoc Am Physicians 88:224–234, 1975.
64. Nicar MJ, Skurla C, Sakhaee K, et al: Low urinary citrate excretion in nephrolithiasis. Urology 21:8–14, 1983.
65. Rudman D, Dedonis JL, Fountain MT, et al: Hypocitraturia in patients with gastrointestinal malabsorption. N Engl J Med 303:657–661, 1980.
66. Smith LH, Fromm H, Hofmann AF: Acquired hyperoxaluria, nephrolithiasis, and intestinal disease. N Engl J Med 286:1371–1375, 1972.
67. Barilla DE, Notz C, Kennedy D, et al: Renal oxalate excretion following oral oxalate loads in patients with ileal disease and with renal and absorptive hypercalciurias: Effect of calcium and magnesium. Am J Med 64:576–585, 1978.
68. Harvey JA, Zobitz MM, Pak CYC: Calcium citrate: Reduced propensity for the crystallization of calcium oxalate in urine resulting from induced hypercalciuria of calcium supplementation. J Clin Endocrinol Metab 61:1223–1225, 1985.
69. Nicar MJ, Hill K, Pak CYC: Inhibition by citrate of spontaneous precipitation of calcium oxalate, *in vitro*. J Bone Mineral Res 2:215–220, 1987.
70. Bisaz S, Felix R, Neiman W: Quantitative determination of inhibitors of calcium phosphate precipitation in whole urine. Mineral Electrolyte Metab 1:74–83, 1978.
71. Meyer JL, Smith LH: Growth of calcium oxalate crystals. II. Inhibition by natural urinary crystal growth inhibitors. Invest Urol 13:36–39, 1975.
72. Kok DJ, Papapoulos SE, Bijvoet OLM: Excessive crystal agglomeration with low citrate excretion in recurrent stone-formers. Lancet 1:1056–1058, 1986.
73. Baruch SB, Barich RL, Eun CK, et al: Renal metabolism of citrate. Med Clin North Am 59:569–582, 1975.

74. Simpson DP: Regulation of renal citrate metabolism by bicarbonate ion and pH: Observations in tissue slices and mitochondria. J Clin Invest 16:225–238, 1967.
75. Smith LH, Werness PG, Lee KE, et al: Inhibitors of crystal growth and aggregation in calcium urolithiasis. Clin Res 26:727A, 1979.
76. Morrissey JF, Ocha M, Lotspeich WD, et al: Citrate excretion in renal tubular acidosis. Ann Intern Med 55:159–166, 1963.
77. Preminger GM, Sakhaee K, Skurla C, et al: Prevention of recurrent calcium stone formation with potassium citrate therapy in patients with distal renal tubular acidosis. J Urol 134:20–23, 1985.
78. Pak CYC, Fuller C, Sakhaee K, et al: Long-term treatment of calcium nephrolithiasis with potassium citrate. J Urol 134:11–19, 1985.
79. Pak CYC, Breslau NA, Harvey JA: Nutrition and metabolic bone disease. *In* Scarpelli DG, Migaki G (eds): Nutritional Diseases: Research Directions in Comparative Pathobiology. New York, Alan R. Liss, 1986, 15:215–240.
80. Sakhaee K, Nigam S, Snell P, et al: Assessment of the pathogenetic role of physical exercise in renal stone formation. J Clin Endocrinol Metab 65:974–979, 1987.
81. Kassirer JP, Berkman PM, Lawrenz DR, et al: The critical role of chloride in the correction of hypokalemic alkalosis in man. Am J Med 38:172–189, 1965.
82. Pak CYC, Fuller C: Idiopathic hypocitraturic calcium oxalate nephrolithiasis successfully treated with potassium citrate. Ann Intern Med 104:33–37, 1986.
83. Pak CYC, Sakhaee K, Fuller C: Successful management of uric acid nephrolithiasis with potassium citrate. Kidney Int 30:422–428, 1986.
84. Holmes EW: Uric acid nephrolithiasis. *In* Coe FL, Brenner BM, Stein JH (eds): Contemporary Issues in Nephrology, vol 5. Edinburgh, Churchill Livingstone, 1980, pp 188–207.
85. Yu TF, Gutman AB: Uric acid nephrolithiasis in gout. Predisposing factors. Ann Intern Med 67:1133–1148, 1967.
86. Gutman AB, Yu TF: Uric acid nephrolithiasis. Am J Med 756–779, 1968.
87. Henneman PH, Wallach S, Dempsey EF: Metabolic defect responsible for uric acid stone formation. J Clin Invest 41:537–542, 1962.
88. Gutman AB, Yu TF: Urinary ammonium excretion in primary gout. J Clin Invest 44:1474–1481, 1965.
89. Plante GE, Durivage J, Lemieux G: Renal excretion of hydrogen in primary gout. Metabolism 17:377–385, 1968.
90. Gutman AB, Yu TF: A three-component system for regulation of renal excretion of uric acid in man. Trans Assoc Am Physicians 74:353–365, 1961.
91. Deren JJ, Porush JG, Levitt MF, et al: Nephrolithiasis as a complication of ulcerative colitis and regional ileitis. Ann Intern Med 56:843–853, 1962.
92. Maratka Z, Nedbal J: Urolithiasis as a complication of the surgical treatment of ulcerative colitis. Gut 5:214–217, 1964.
93. Bennett RC, Jepson RP: Uric acid stone formation following ileostomy. Aust NZ J Surg 36:153–158, 1966.
94. Pak CYC: The problem of idiopathic stone formers presenting with no metabolic disorder: Pathogenesis and management. *In* Contributions to Nephrology, Third International Symposium on Recent Advances in Pathogenesis and Treatment of Nephrolithiasis. Basel, S. Karger 58:164–171, 1987.
95. Thier SO, Segal S: Cystinuria. *In* Stanbury JB, Wyngaarden JB, Frederickson DS (eds): The Metabolic Basis of Inherited Disease. New York, McGraw-Hill, 1972, pp 1504–1519.
96. Dent CE, Senior B: Studies on the treatment of cystinuria. Br J Urol 27:317–332, 1955.
97. Ettinger B, Kolb FP: Factors involved in crystal formation in cystinuria. In vivo and in vitro crystallization dynamics and a simple, quantitative colorimetric assay for cystine. J Urol 106:106–110, 1971.
98. Pak CYC, Fuller CJ: Assessment of cystine solubility in urine and of heterogeneous nucleation. J Urol 129:1066–1070, 1983.
99. Bostrom H, Hambraeus L: Cystinuria in Sweden. Acta Med Scand [Suppl] 411:7–128, 1964.
100. Broadus A, Thier S: Metabolic basis of renal stone disease. N Engl J Med 300:839–845, 1979.
101. Dent CE, Rose GA: Amino acid metabolism in cystinuria. Q J Med 20:205–219, 1951.
102. Rosenberg LE, Downing S, Durant JL, et al: Cystinuria: Biochemical evidence for three genetically distinct diseases. J Clin Invest 45:365–371, 1966.
103. Kolb FO, Earll JM, Harris HA: Disappearance of cystinuria in a patient treated with prolonged low methionine diet. Metabolism 16:378–381, 1967.
104. Jaeger P, Portmann L, Saunders A, et al: Anticystinuric effects of glutamine and of dietary sodium restriction. N Engl J Med 315:1120–1123, 1986.
105. Dent CE, Friedmann M, Green TT, Watson LCA: Treatment of cystinuria. Br Med J 1:403–408, 1965.
106. Sakhaee K, Nicar M, Hill K, et al: Contrasting effects of potassium citrate and sodium citrate therapies on urinary chemistries and crystallization of stone-forming salt. Kidney Int 24:348–352, 1983.
107. Miyagi K, Nakada F, Ohshiro S: Effect of glutamine on cystine excretion in a patient with cystinuria. N Engl J Med 301:196–198, 1979.
108. van den Berg C, Jones JD, Wilson DM, Smith LH: Glutamine therapy of cystinuria. Invest Urol 18:155–157, 1980.
109. Perrett D: The metabolism and pharmacology of d-penicillamine in man. J Rheumatol [Suppl 7] 8:41–50, 1981.
110. Crawhall JC: Experience with penicillamine in the treatment of cystinuria. J Rheumatol [Suppl 7] 9:100–102, 1981.
111. Halperin EC, Thier SO, Rosenberg LE: The use of d-penicillamine in cystinuria: Efficacy and untoward reactions. Yale J Biol Med 54:439–446, 1981.
112. Pak CYC, Fuller C, Sakhaee K, et al: Management of cystine nephrolithiasis with alpha-mercaptopropionylglycine (Thiola). J Urol 136:1003–1008, 1986.
113. Linari F, Maragella M, Fruttero B, Bruno M: The natural history of cystinuria: A 15 year follow-up in 106 patients. *In* Smith L, Robertson W, Finlayson B (eds): Urolithiasis, Clinical and Basic Research. New York, Plenum Press, 1981, pp 145–154.
114. Griffith DP: Struvite stones. Kidney Int 13:372–382, 1978.
115. Williams JJ, Rodman JS, Peterson CM: A randomized double-blind study of acetohydroxamic acid in struvite nephrolithiasis. N Engl J Med 311:760–764, 1984.

24

CONSTANTINE S. ANAST
THOMAS O. CARPENTER
L. LYNDON KEY, Jr.

Metabolic Bone Disorders in Children

I. RICKETS

Although signs of rickets were described in antiquity, rickets was first described as a clinical entity in the mid-17th century by English physicians.[1] The first detailed description of rickets was presented in the reading of a thesis in 1645 for the degree of M.D. by an English student from Oxford, then 25 years of age, named Daniel Whistler.[2] This description of rickets attracted little attention and credit, for the first description is usually given to Francis Glisson, another Englishman, whose account published in 1650 was a fuller and more detailed study of rickets.[3] In the mid-19th century, the industrial revolution in Europe and North America produced a high incidence of rickets attributed to smoke emitted by factories and consequent air pollution that prevented ultraviolet light from reaching the skin of children. Although the effectiveness of cod-liver oil in the treatment of rickets had been reported, it was ignored to a large extent during the latter half of the 19th century. It was not until the second decade of this century that vitamin D was identified and it was established that the major cause of rickets in children and of osteomalacia in adults was a deficiency in vitamin D.[1] The use of vitamin D steroids for prevention and treatment largely eliminated vitamin D–deficiency rickets. Shortly thereafter it was recognized that a small number of patients did not respond to the usual doses of vitamin D, and the terms "vitamin D–resistant" and "vitamin D–refractory" rickets were used to characterize such individuals.[4] Subsequent work demonstrated that vitamin D–refractory rickets was not one entity but included a number of disorders of various pathogenesis. During the last decade the application of modern technology has markedly increased our understanding of the biochemistry and physiology of vitamin D, which in turn has provided important and new insights into the pathogenesis of various vitamin D–refractory disorders.

A. Pathophysiology

As noted in Chapter 2, the crystalline phase of bone mineral is a hydroxyapatite with the basic formula $Ca_{10}(PO_4)_6(OH)_2$. Rickets may be defined as a disorder in a growing person in which osteoblastic activity and the production of bone matrix continues but in which there is a lag in the rate of mineralization of bone matrix (osteoid) and in preosseous cartilage matrix at the zone of provisional calcification, which results in the accumulation of an abnormal amount of unmineralized matrix.[5] The formation of apatite depends on adequate concentrations of extracellular calcium and phosphate (see Chapter 2). Therefore, rickets or unmineralized matrix occurs when there is a deficiency of either or both of these minerals in the extracellular fluid. Vitamin D plays an important role in maintaining normal concentrations of extracellular calcium and phosphate except, perhaps, when these minerals are supplied parenterally. A deficiency of calcium and/or phosphate may result in extracellular fluid from dietary deficiency or gastrointestinal malabsorption of calcium, phosphate, and/or vitamin D, from insufficient sunlight exposure, from a renal tubular leak of phosphate, and from various abnormalities in vitamin D metabolism.

It is important to point out that some controversy exists as to whether bone mineralization is controlled simply by the plasma mineral ion product or whether vitamin D metabolites and possibly parathyroid hormone play contributory roles (see Chapters 2, 3, and

5). In favor of the former is the observation that mineralization and growth of bone are normal in vitamin D–deficient rats infused with calcium and phosphate in quantities that maintain normal plasma concentrations of these minerals.[6,7] On the other hand, there is some evidence to suggest 24,25-dihydroxyvitamin D is a bone active metabolite and that a combination of 1,25-dihydroxyvitamin D and 24,25-dihydroxyvitamin D is more effective than either metabolite alone in increasing the rate of bone mineralization in human vitamin D deficiency.[8,9] Other observations have questioned the pivotal role of 1,25-dihydroxyvitamin D in rickets since (1) the level of this metabolite may be low-normal or elevated in human vitamin D–deficient rickets,[10–12] and (2) in rats made vitamin D–deficient, the fall in bone appositional rate could be corrected by the administration of 25-hydroxyvitamin D but not 1,25-dihydroxyvitamin D.[13,14] These and other observations have led to the speculation that the mineralization of bone is not simply controlled by the mineral ion product but is also directly regulated by the interplay of three humoral factors, namely, 1,25-dihydroxyvitamin D, 24,25-dihydroxyvitamin D, and parathyroid hormone.[9] Consistent with this possibility is the report of infants with normal serum calcium and phosphate levels who had evidence of subclinical rickets as reflected by low serum 25-hydroxyvitamin D levels and x-ray changes at the metaphysis of the wrist compatible with the diagnosis of rickets.[15]

The histologic characteristics of rickets are well known[5] and are described in some detail in Chapter 11. Bone resorption continues but the deposition of bone mineral in newly formed matrix is reduced, resulting in demineralized bone trabeculae and cortex. At the epiphyseal region there is a markedly expanded zone of proliferating cartilage with increased osteoid tissue and invasion by wide, tortuous vessels. The epiphyseal cartilage is transformed into uncalcified chondro-osteoid rather than into calcified bone. Due to the defect in mineralization, rachitic bone is weakened and bends or twists easily under the weight of the body and the pull of muscles. This may result in fractures and a variety of orthopedic deformities including genu valgum, genu varum, coxa vara, tibial and femoral torsion, pelvic deformities, chest deformations, scoliosis, and kyphosis. Angulation and bending of bone may result from fractures. Poor mineralization of the skull may result in craniotabes in the infant. The overproduction and lateral spread of unmineralized chondro-osteoid is the cause of the characteristic knobby widening at the ends of the long bones and of the expanded costal cartilage forming the rachitic rosary. With increasing severity the costal cartilages are pulled in by muscle, leading to a pigeon breast deformity. The lower rib cage is flared out, and due to reduced rigidity of the ribs a depression (Harrison's groove) is produced at the sites of insertion of the diaphragm. Bossing of the skull results from increased unmineralized osteoid in the frontal and parietal bones.

As indicated previously, rachitic bone can be thin and fragile. On the other hand, it can also be thick as a result of excessive production of osteoid that is usually the result of long-standing rickets in which there are alternating periods of activity and healing. This results in the formation of a series of new cortices from the periosteum, one enveloping the other.

B. Classification

Over 30 causes of rickets and osteomalacia have been reported.[16] A number of classification schemes have been employed to categorize the various forms of rickets. The intent is not to discuss all of the reported forms but, instead, to concentrate on those that most frequently present clinically as well as on some interesting and more recently reported causes of rickets. For purposes of this discussion, the following classification scheme will be followed:

1. Nutritional rickets including deficiencies in vitamin D, calcium, and phosphate.
2. Rickets secondary to renal phosphate tubulopathies.
3. Rickets associated with gastrointestinal malabsorption.
4. Rickets secondary to abnormalities in vitamin D metabolism.
5. Rickets secondary to end-organ resistance to vitamin D.

C. Radiographic Findings

The radiographic findings in rickets have been well defined. A number of changes occur at the cartilage-shaft junction that, although not pathognomonic, are characteristic of rickets. One of the early signs is a widening of the space between the calcified plate at the end of the metaphysis and the center of ossification in the epiphysis. This is the result of proliferation of uncalcified cartilage and osteoid. Cupping is another characteristic finding and frequently is best seen at either end of the fibula or the lower end of the ulna. Cortical spurs, composed of unmineralized matrix, are linear shadows that extend as prolongations of the shadows of the cortex along the sides of the proliferative cartilage. Fraying consists of thin shadows that extend from the end of the shaft into the transparent cartilage and is usually seen in moderate to severe rickets. The cortex appears thin and frequently is invisible in the atrophic form of rickets. In the hypertrophic form of rickets there is thickening of the cortex, which is usually greater on one side. The hypertrophic form is usually seen in long-standing rickets in which there are alternating periods of activity and healing.

D. Biochemical Findings

The biochemical findings in rickets commonly include depressed serum calcium and/or phosphate with an elevated serum alkaline phosphatase activity. Exceptions to the increase in alkaline phosphatase activity include rickets associated with hypophosphatasia and vitamin D–deficient rickets in severely malnourished children. As secondary hyperparathyroidism develops, the serum immunoreactive parathyroid hormone (iPTH) level increases, and this, in turn, leads to a generalized aminoaciduria as well as an increase in urinary cyclic AMP. There are usually abnormalities in circulating vitamin D metabolites. The normal values for the D metabolites vary to some extent in different laboratories (see Chapter 5). The values for normal adults in our laboratory are 10 to 80 ng/ml of 25-hydroxyvitamin D, 1 to 4 ng/ml of 24,25-dihydroxyvitamin D, and 15 to 70 pg/ml of 1,25-dihydroxyvitamin D. The levels of 25-hydroxyvitamin D vary with the season and vitamin D intake. There does not appear to be any consistent age-related difference in serum 25-hydroxyvitamin D levels in children and adults. A number of laboratories have reported higher serum levels of 1,25-dihydroxyvitamin D levels in children than in adults. However, there is no unanimity among these reports regarding possible age-related differences in serum 1,25-dihydroxyvitamin D during childhood. One laboratory reported higher values in infants and early childhood than in later childhood, a second reported no age-related difference, whereas a third reported gradually increasing values throughout childhood with significantly higher values in adolescents between the ages of 12 and 16 years than in children less than 12 years of age. In another report, an increase in serum 1,25-dihydroxyvitamin D_3 was noted at Tanner pubertal stages II and III in both girls and boys.

The biochemical as well as clinical findings vary according to the type of rickets that is present. The specific findings are discussed in the following section on the various forms of rickets.

E. Nutritional Rickets

1. *Vitamin D Deprivation*

During the past several years there has been a resurgence of nutritional rickets associated with breast feeding and special dietary practices including macrobiotic and other vegetarian diets.[11,17–20] Rickets has been reported in infants ages 4 to 20 months who had received unsupplemented breast milk exclusively for periods ranging from 7 to 14 months.[18] The majority of the infants were from families that were strict vegetarians. Many of the patients who developed rickets were receiving only unsupplemented breast milk, whereas others were diagnosed a few months after foods low in vitamin D content were added to the diet. The patients and their mothers had minimal exposure to sunlight because of protective clothing or unsafe neighborhood conditions prohibiting outdoor activity. The diagnosis of rickets was usually made in winter or early spring. There are relatively small quantities of vitamin D and vitamin D metabolites in human breast milk. The contents of vitamin D and 25-hydroxyvitamin D in human breast milk will vary with the sunlight exposure and vitamin D intake of the mother. It has been estimated that breast milk provides as little as 10 IU vitamin D in the winter and 20 IU/day in the summer. It has been suggested that there may be variations in the individual requirement for vitamin D that may, in part, explain why rickets develops in some infants with low vitamin D intake in breast milk but not in others.[5,21]

Rickets is observed in children receiving macrobiotic and vegetarian diets, especially when there is an avoidance of animal food, including milk and fish.[11,17,18] It has been estimated that children receiving macrobiotic diets ingest approximately 33 IU of vitamin D per day, 319 mg calcium/day, and 506 mg phosphorus/day. The vitamin D intake is even lower (5 IU) in children receiving macrobiotic diets in which there is extensive animal food avoidances. The foods prominent in the macrobiotic diet include refined cereal grains, vegetables, beans, seeds, and nuts. Although exposure to sunlight may have been a factor in preventing rickets in some of the children, there are no data to suggest that parents who adhere to macrobiotic philosophy are more or less likely to expose their children to sunlight. As indicated previously, another factor that might account for the lack of rickets in some children receiving macrobiotic diets may be related to the variations in the individual requirement for vitamin D.

It is pertinent that studies in Ireland suggest that nutritional rickets in humans cannot always be explained on the basis of deficient D intake alone, whether derived from diet or ultraviolet light.[22] An increase in rickets from 1939 to 1942 was observed in Ireland, which coincided with the increase in the extraction rate of flour from 70% to 100%. The authors point out that ultraviolet light exposure may be normal in the number of situations in which rickets and osteomalacia are prevalent. Thus, rickets and osteomalacia have been found in Asians in Britain whose outdoor exposure did not differ from that of their white counterparts. The traditional Asian diet contains much unleavened, high-extraction cereal as chappity and a variety of pulses. Severe osteomalacia has also been found in seaworkers in Kasmir who spend many days in the outdoors but whose diets are exclusively vegetarian, consisting almost entirely of rice, lentils, and whole-wheat flour. The authors, therefore, conclude that the epidemiologic evidence suggests that high-extraction and whole-meal cereal may be rachitogenic. The mechanism of the possible rachitogenic action of cereals is uncertain, but it seems unlikely that dietary phytate, by itself, is responsible. It has been suggested that the interruption of the enteral hepatic circulation of vitamin D metabolites by constituents of high extraction of cereals and pulses may be important in the causation of nutritional vitamin D deficiency. Lignin, an important component of wheat fiber, combines with bile acids and increases their excretion. It has been postulated that should vitamin D become attached to the fiber-bile complex, which is chemically likely, it may be transported to the gut. High-fiber diets, therefore, may lead to enough wastage of vitamin D and its metabolites derived mainly from UV radiation to produce rickets or osteomalacia.[22]

Physical findings at the time of diagnosis of rickets in infants and children include frontal bossing, rachitic rosary, long bone fractures, flaring of the wrists and ankles, Harrison's grooves, bowed legs, potbelly, leg tenderness, and large fontanelles. Lower respiratory infections may be observed in some infants and small children with vitamin D deficiency rickets. It is of interest that a deficiency of vitamin D has been reported to be associated with recurrent infections.[23] Some studies suggest that vitamin D deficiency may reduce the body's ability to react to nonspecific stimuli. The peripheral blood leukocytes in humans and the peripheral blood macrophages and bone marrow polymorphonuclear leukocytes of vitamin D–deficient mice have been shown to have impaired, spontaneous migration and decreased phagocytic ability.[24,25] Impaired macrophage phagocytosis in vitamin D–deficient mice was corrected *in vitro* by incubating the cells with 1,25-dihydroxyvitamin D.

Anemia, thrombocytopenia, and bone marrow hypocellularity together with extramedullary hematopoiesis have been reported in infants with severe vitamin D deficiency rickets.[26] Hypochromia was observed in some infants and macrocytosis in others. Mild reticulocytosis or reticulocytopenia was present in each of the infants. Normal or elevated iron and folic acid levels were observed, indicating that these substances were not responsible for the red blood cell abnormalities. Repeated attempts to obtain bone marrow from different sites resulted only in hypocellular specimens that showed increased osteoblast counts. In these studies, there were no marked changes in the diets before and during vitamin D therapy. Hematologic improvement followed vitamin D treatment and suggests that the presence of myeloid metaplasia, also known as myelofibrosis, was most likely the result of vitamin D deficiency. Possible explanations for the association of myeloid metaplasia and vitamin D deficiency include chronic occlusion of bone marrow vessels and possibly malnutrition. However, malnutrition was not a constant feature in the patients with myeloid metaplasia.

The biochemical findings of vitamin D deficiency rickets are of interest. The serum calcium and/or phosphate concentrations are usually depressed. However, normal concentrations of both of these minerals have been reported in infants and children with subclinical rickets[15] as well as in patients in whom there is evidence of spontaneous healing of the rickets.[27] The serum alkaline phosphatase activity is increased with the exception of vitamin D–deficient malnourished children, in whom there may be a lesser or no increase above normal of alkaline phosphatase activity.[28,29] Vitamin D deficiency rickets has been divided into three stages based on clinical and laboratory data[30] and, more recently, into four stages.[27] The clinical and radiologic signs of rickets are mild in stage I and moderate to severe in stages II to IV, with some recalcification of osteoid indicating spontaneous healing in the patients in stage IV. In stage I, the serum calcium is low, whereas the serum phosphorus and iPTH levels are normal. Stage I is thought to be transient, persisting for only a few days. In stage II, the serum calcium is normal, the serum phosphorus depressed, and the serum iPTH elevated. The reasons for the normal serum iPTH in the presence of hypocalcemia in stage I and the presence of elevated iPTH in the presence of normocalcemia in stage II are uncertain. It has been suggested that secondary hyperparathyroidism develops during the transient period of stage I and proceeds to stage II, in which the serum calcium returns to normal as a consequence of mobilization of calcium from bone and increased renal calcium reabsorption. Furthermore, it has been postulated that the continuous hypersecretion of parathyroid hormone, despite normocalcemia in stage II, may be related to the serum 1,25-dihydroxyvitamin D levels, which are insufficient to suppress parathyroid secretion. However, controversy exists as to whether circulating 1,25-dihydroxyvitamin D levels influence parathyroid hormone secretion. In stage III the serum calcium and phosphorus levels are both depressed, whereas the serum iPTH level is elevated. The findings in stage III are thought to reflect a greater deficiency of vitamin D that results in bone hyporesponsiveness to parathyroid hormone. In stage IV the serum calcium, phosphorus, and iPTH levels are all normal and there is histologic evidence that suggests that spontaneous healing is occurring in this stage. Evaluation of the data of the patients in all four stages revealed a positive correlation between serum iPTH and urinary cyclic AMP and a negative relationship between both of these indices of parathyroid activity to serum phosphate concentration. Furthermore, there are data to suggest that there is a correlation between urinary phosphate excretion and the severity of vitamin D–deficient rickets as assessed by clinical, radiologic, and chemical data.[31]

The serum 25-hydroxyvitamin D concentrations are depressed in vitamin D deficiency rickets and are usually less than 10 to 12 ng/ml.[10,11,19,20,32] The 1,25-dihydroxyvitamin D levels may be either low, normal, or elevated in vitamin D deficiency.[10,11,19,20,32] The reason for the normal or elevated circulating 1,25-dihydroxyvitamin D levels is uncertain but, according to one hypothesis, may simply reflect the complex interaction of circulating vitamin D metabolites and calcium and phosphate concentrations in the bone mineralization process. A striking increase in circulating 1,25-dihydroxyvitamin D levels in vitamin D–deficient patients may be observed as early as 24 hours after the first orally administered dose of vitamin D.[19] It has, therefore, been postulated that either a brief exposure to sunlight or the ingestion of a small amount of vitamin D may account for the elevated circulating 1,25-dihydroxyvitamin D levels in initial blood samples obtained at the time of the diagnosis.[20] In one study of patients with vitamin D deficiency, the circulating 24,25-dihydroxyvitamin D levels were found to be depressed, normal, or increased,[19] whereas in another study the 24,25-dihydroxyvitamin D levels were depressed.[20] In the latter study, but not in the former, there was a significant correlation between the serum 25-hydroxyvitamin D levels and the serum 24,25-dihydroxyvitamin D as well as the serum 1,25-dihydroxyvitamin D levels.

Vitamin D_2 is used in the treatment of nutritional vitamin D deficiency rickets. In our clinic we prescribe 1000 to 2000 IU of vitamin D_2 per day. In recent reports in the literature, the dose has ranged from 400 to 4000 IU of vitamin D_2 per day in infants and children.[11,19,20] The administration of these relatively low dosages of vitamin D_2 decreased the probability of toxic effects and does not mask non-nutrient forms of rickets. Healing requires 6 to 12 weeks of therapy. Normal serum calcium and phosphorus levels have been achieved after 1 to 2 weeks of therapy in some studies but not until 4 weeks of therapy in others.[11,19,20] Although the serum alkaline phosphatase activities fall, they remain above the upper limits of normal for age as long as 8 to 12 weeks after the initiation of therapy. In two studies of infants less than 24 months of age, the administration of 400 IU and 1700 to 4000 IU of vitamin D_2 daily resulted in an increase in serum 25-hydroxyvitamin D to within the normal range after 1 week of therapy.[11,19,20] On the other hand, in another study the serum 25-hydroxyvitamin D remained low while the serum calcium and phosphorus increased to normal and the alkaline phosphatase activity declined after 4 weeks of daily administration of 2000 IU of vitamin D_2 to vitamin D–deficient children, the majority of whom were between 4 and 6 months of age.[19] In general, the change in serum 24,25-dihydroxyvitamin D follows the pattern of change of 25-hydroxyvitamin D.[19,20]

Of great interest is the marked increase in circulating 1,25-dihydroxyvitamin D that is seen after the initiation of vitamin D_2 or 25-hydroxyvitamin D therapy. The increase in circulating 1,25-dihydroxyvitamin D may be seen as early as 24 hours after treatment is started and subsequently may rise to levels that are 2- to 3-fold greater than the upper limit of normal.[10,11,19,20,32] Elevated serum 1,25-dihydroxyvitamin D levels may persist for several weeks during treatment even after the serum calcium, serum phosphorus, and iPTH levels are normal. This suggests that hypocalcemia, hypophosphatemia, and elevated parathyroid hormone concentrations are not the only factors responsible for the elevation of 1,25-dihydroxyvitamin D levels found in these vitamin D–deficient children after, and possibly before, treatment. The parallel decline toward normal of serum 1,25-dihydroxyvitamin D and alkaline phosphatase raises the possibility that the stimulation of 1,25-dihydroxyvitamin D synthesis may be directly related to the state of skeletal mineralization in these patients.[19] It has been suggested that the duration of the raised 1,25-dihydroxyvitamin D concentrations coincides with the period of increased net retention and correction of skeletal deficits in calcium and phosphorus that is known to occur in response to treatment of rickets.[20]

Alternative therapies of vitamin D deficiency rickets include the administration of intermediate amounts of oral vitamin D_2 or very large doses of vitamin D_2 ("stoss" therapy).[5] Intermediate doses of vitamin D_2 (8000–16,000 IU/day) are administered for 3 weeks, at which time there should be clearly demonstrable biochemical and roentgenologic evidences of healing. Following this course, the dose is reduced to the usual prophylactic amounts of 400 IU/day. In patients for whom compliance is an issue, a single oral or IM dose of 600,000 IU of vitamin D_2 will result in healing of rickets. This form of therapy has not been associated with complications, even in infants.[5] One of the advantages of the "stoss" treatment is that it reduces the possibility of low-calcium tetany occurring during treatment. When relatively small doses of vitamin D are given to rachitic infants, there may be a reduction in serum calcium and resultant tetany in the initial phases of healing because of the rise of inorganic phosphate in extracellular fluid and the deposition of calcium in osteoid before the complete effect of vitamin D on the mobilization of calcium is obtained. On the other hand, when a relatively large dose of vitamin D is given, the effect on calcium homeostasis is obtained early and the danger of hypocalcemia is lessened.

An adequate calcium intake is necessary to avoid severe hypocalcemia following the inception of vitamin D_2 therapy and to ensure healing. Dietary intake or calcium supplementation to ensure 50 mg/kg/day of elemental calcium is recommended. In our experience, dietary calcium is usually adequate. However, supplementation is recommended in all cases when symptomatic hypocalcemia is present prior to the onset of therapy or when symptoms develop during therapy.

2. Phosphate Deprivation

Rickets secondary to dietary phosphate deprivation is seen in infants and most commonly is observed in the neonatal period in low birth weight infants who are fed human milk.[33–36] Human milk has been prescribed as a food source for premature infants for a variety of reasons including immunologic protection against infection, encouragement of maternal-infant bonding, and protection of the premature infant against necrotizing enterocolitis.

Eighty per cent of bone mineralization in the fetus normally occurs during the last trimester, when the fetal requirements are 60 to 75 mg/kg/day phosphorus and 100 to 120 mg/kg/day calcium.[37,38] Human milk contains only 11 to 20 mg/100 ml of phosphorus, and therefore a premature infant fed 100 to 200 ml of human milk daily will obtain only 25% to 75% of the phosphorus assimilated by a fetus of similar gestational age *in utero*. Moreover, in the reported cases of rickets in preterm infants receiving human milk, the phosphorus content of the milk was relatively low, ranging from 3.1 to 11 mg/100 ml.[33–35]

Characteristically, preterm infants with rickets secondary to phosphate deprivation have hypophosphatemia, hypercalcemia, hypercalciuria, normal or depressed serum parathyroid hormone levels, normal 25-hydroxyvitamin D levels, and elevated 1,25-dihydroxyvitamin D levels. The hypophosphatemia is the stimulus for the production of 1,25-dihydroxyvitamin D, which, in turn, increases the intestinal absorption of calcium. In the presence of hypophosphatemia, only limited amounts of calcium can be deposited in bone and hypercalcemia results, which, in turn, inhibits parathyroid hormone secretion. The rate of bone resorption and calcium release from bone is increased as an effect of both low serum phosphorus and increased 1,25-dihydroxyvitamin D.[39] Therefore, both a direct bone effect and a gut effect tend to increase the serum calcium and the glomerular filtered load of calcium. A low serum phosphate may also directly inhibit the renal tubular reabsorption of calcium.[40] It seems likely that each of these factors contributes to the hypercalciuria that is characteristically found in phosphate deprivation rickets.

Phosphate deprivation rickets in the preterm infant does not respond to vitamin D therapy, but responds promptly to an increase in the ingestion of inorganic phosphate. This can be accomplished either by supplementing human milk with 20 to 25 mg/kg/day of phosphorus as potassium phosphate, or by switching from human milk to a proprietary formula with a high phosphate content. The phosphate supplements may reduce the serum calcium to subnormal values and require the addition of calcium supplements in a dosage of 30 mg/kg/day of calcium. Phosphate and calcium supplements can be used prophylactically to prevent the development of rickets in preterm infants fed human milk.

It is of interest that a low phosphate content (5.4 mg/100 ml) was reported in the breast milk of a woman with X-linked hypophosphatemia.[41] Her full-term infant developed early signs of rickets at the end of the third month of life, which responded to phosphate and vitamin D intake. In addition, the baby had inherited the X-linked mutation from his mother.

Rickets and osteomalacia may occur in patients receiving chronic antacid therapy, such as aluminum hydroxide, which binds phosphate, making it unavailable for absorption by the gastrointestinal tract.[42,43] There are reports suggesting that phosphate depletion, resulting from regular hemodialysis against the standard, phosphate-free dialysate, may play an important contributory role in the development of osteomalacia in patients undergoing hemodialysis.[44]

3. *Calcium Deprivation*

Although uncommon, rickets due to dietary calcium deficiency has been reported in infants and children.[45–50] Two 12-month-old infants, one in the United States[45] and the other in Canada,[46] each developed rickets while receiving low-calcium formulas (21–180 mg Ca/day) for treatment of gastrointestinal disorders. Rickets has been observed in rural South Africa[47–49] in children between 4 and 14 years of age who were receiving very low calcium intakes with a mean SE of 125 ± 40 mg/day. Three sisters, from a poor family in India, with a history of deficiency dietary calcium, were found to have rickets at 14, 16, and 18 years of age, respectively.[50] In all of these cases, vitamin D deficiency was not thought to play a pathogenetic role, and the rickets healed when adequate dietary calcium was provided.

The clinical findings in the infants with rickets secondary to calcium deficiency include rachitic rosary, enlargement at the ends of the long bones, large anterior fontanelle, and retarded growth and motor development.[45,46] The clinical manifestations in the older children include limb deformities most prominent in the lower extremities, difficulty in walking, a waddling gait, skeletal pain, and stunted growth. Muscular weakness was absent in the children in South Africa,[47,48] but was noted in the sisters with rickets reportedly secondary to calcium deficiency in India.[50] The radiographic findings are similar to those of vitamin D deficiency and may include cortical erosions of secondary hyperparathyroidism.

In patients with rickets secondary to calcium deficiency, the serum calcium levels are low to low-normal, the serum alkaline phosphatase activity is increased, and the serum phosphate and TRP are depressed with the exception of some children in South Africa[47–49] who had normal serum phosphate and TRP values. In children in whom measurements were made, the serum 25-hydroxyvitamin D level was normal, whereas serum 1,25-dihydroxyvitamin D was elevated. The serum iPTH and urinary cyclic AMP were increased, and there was generalized aminoaciduria.[45–50] The following could account for the biochemical findings in rickets secondary to calcium deficiency: calcium deficiency, hypocalcemia, secondary hyperparathyroidism, hyperphosphaturia, generalized aminoaciduria, increased urinary cyclic AMP, and hypophosphatemia. The increase in circulating parathyroid hormone and the depressed serum calcium and phosphorus levels would act to stimulate the synthesis of 1,25-dihydroxyvitamin D and account for the increased circulating level of this metabolite. The increase in circulating parathyroid hormone and 1,25-dihydroxyvitamin D would mobilize calcium from bone and thereby increase serum calcium, which would account for the normal serum calcium in some patients. It has been speculated that in patients in whom secondary hyperparathyroidism fails to correct hypocalcemia, there may be unresponsiveness of bone to parathyroid hormone due to lack of calcium needed for efficient functioning of cells that normally respond to parathyroid hormone, or, alternatively, the movement of calcium from bone into the general circulation may be blocked by excessive osteoid tissue.

It is of interest that some of the children with rickets secondary to calcium deficiency in South Africa had normal serum calcium, serum phosphorus, serum 25-hydroxyvitamin D, and TRP values in association with elevated serum immunoreactive parathyroid hormone and 1,25-dihydroxyvitamin D levels.[48] The reason for the normal serum phosphorus and TRP values in the presence of elevated serum immunoreactive parathyroid hormone is uncertain. Similarly, the reason for the finding of rickets in the children with normal serum calcium and phosphorus levels is not apparent.

Metabolic acidosis has been reported in some children with calcium deprivation rickets.[45,50] In one study, the low serum bicarbonate levels were accompanied by urine pH values of 6.4 to 6.8 and decreased urine titrable acidity.[50] After the initiation of calcium treatment, the acidosis corrected in parallel with an increase in urine titrable acidity and a decrease in urine pH. The apparent renal tubular acidosis was most likely a manifestation of secondary hyperparathyroidism, since parathyroid hormone decreases proximal tubular reabsorption of bicarbonate.[51]

Bone histomorphometric studies in three children with dietary calcium deficiency revealed severe osteomalacia as well as features of increased bone resorption.[49] All three children were hypocalcemic and had normal serum phosphate levels. Correction of dietary calcium intake led to normal serum calcium levels, reduced alkaline phosphatase levels, and normalization of bone histologic features.

Treatment consists of increasing dietary calcium, which is best accomplished by including milk in the diet. In addition, calcium supplements providing 30 to 45 mg/kg/day of calcium may be prescribed. Radiographic evidence of healing may be observed within 3 to 4 weeks after the initiation of treatment; the biochemical findings usually return to normal by 2 to 3 months.[45–50]

F. Rickets Secondary to Renal Phosphate Tubulopathies

In this group of disorders, a defect in the tubular reabsorption of phosphate leads to hypophosphatemic rickets and osteomalacia. Several mendelian disorders or phenotypes have been described, including (1) X-linked hypophosphatemic rickets; (2) autosomal dominant hypophosphatemic and autosomal recessive hypophosphatemic rickets; (3) acquired primary hypophosphatemic rickets; (4) autosomal dominant hypophosphatemic bone disease; (5) hereditary hypophosphatemic rickets with hypercalciuria; and (6) the

Fanconi syndrome. This discussion deals primarily with X-linked hypophosphatemia.

1. *X-Linked Hypophosphatemic Rickets (XLH)*

X-linked hypophosphatemic rickets (XLH) is also known as familial hypophosphatemic rickets and vitamin D–resistant rickets (VDRR). The disorder is inherited as an X-linked dominant trait and is characterized by hypophosphatemia and decreased renal tubular phosphate reabsorption (see Chapter 7). The inherited trait may vary in degree of manifestations from severe to mild bone disease associated with hypophosphatemia to hypophosphatemia alone without evidence of active or former rickets. With an abnormal gene residing on an X chromosome, an affected female is heterozygous (X′X), whereas an affected male, lacking the normal allele, is hemizygous (X′Y). The male progeny of an affected male are all normal, since they receive the Y chromosome from their fathers. On the other hand, the female progeny of an affected male receive the single X′ chromosome of the father and are, therefore, all affected. The inheritance of an X-linked trait would predict that half of the progeny of an affected female would be normal and half affected, without regard to sex.

The severity of bone disease does not correlate with the degree of hypophosphatemia. Whereas hypophosphatemic males nearly always have chronic rickets or postrachitic deformities, hypophosphatemic females tend to have less severe skeletal involvement.[52,53] Indeed, in XLH kindreds, several females, but rarely a male, have been observed to be hypophosphatemic with no evidence of active or previous rickets.[53–56] Thus the hypophosphatemic females usually are less severely affected than are males and may have no deformities or impairment of growth. The less severe disease in the female and the variable phenotype from one heterozygous XLH female to another may be explained by the Lyon phenomenon, that is, random inactivation of one X chromosome.[57]

The accumulated evidence suggests that hypophosphatemia is almost uniformly inherited in XLH, whereas overt bone disease varies considerably. Hypophosphatemia, then, is an important, but not the sole, determinant of bone disease and provides the best discriminant for identifying the trait.[58]

Clinical Findings. The children with XLH usually present in the second year of life, or later, with bow legs and short stature.[5,58] Other early manifestations include late dentition, sagittal cranial synostosis, and "sitting" deformity of the legs. Rachitic rosary, deformity of the upper extremities, and active rickets of the spine and pelvis occur less frequently than in vitamin D deficiency and vitamin D dependency rickets.

Past studies of children with XLH have suggested that growth failure is limited to the legs.[59–61] In these studies the lower segment was determined by measuring the distance between the top of the symphysis pubis and the floor when the patient was standing upright. The upper segment was then determined by subtracting the length of the lower segment from the total height. In a more recent study, the upper segment has been determined by measuring the sitting height and the lower segment by subtracting the sitting height from the total length.[62] These measures, which are thought to be better defined and more reproducible, were compared with normal values compiled by Tanner and Whitehouse,[63] who have defined the normal limits of the difference between these two measures. The results indicated that in children with XLH, the average values for the upper and lower segments were both reduced, the latter to a greater extent. However, the difference between the lower and upper segments was abnormally low in only four of 16 children with XLH, indicating a mild degree of disproportion. There was no relationship between the height and the degree of disproportion, a finding that was also considered to be consistent with a relatively mild degree of disproportion. The interindividual differences in proportion were fairly large and apparently more pronounced than the preferential effect of the rickets on the leg length.

Spontaneous dental abscesses are a common finding in XLH in both primary and permanent caries-free dentitions.[64–66] Dental abnormalities are characterized by dentin defects of interglobular dentin and by enlarged pulp chambers. These defects permit the contamination of the dental pulp by oral fluids, particularly if there is an associated enamel defect.

Spinal canal stenosis is observed in some patients as the disorder progresses.[67–69] This complication is thought to be secondary to bone overgrowth and osteoid masses within the spinal canal as well as to interference with normal growth. The more severely affected patients are susceptible to spinal cord compromise resulting in back pain and lower limb weakness for which surgical intervention may be necessary. The age of the patients when spine changes become evident is uncertain. A study of lumbar spine radiographs of 17 adult patients with XLH rickets demonstrated narrower spinal canals when compared with a group of normal individuals.[68] In another study, a narrow spinal canal was noted in one patient at 5 years of age, in another at 12 years, and in another severely affected 19-year-old patient who had a normal canal width at 5 years of age.[69]

Of importance are the striking negative findings in this disorder, which include a lack of muscle weakness, tetany, and convulsions, which are common features of both vitamin D deficiency and vitamin D dependency rickets.

In this section we have discussed the clinical findings in children with XLH at the usual age of presentation (the second or third year of life) and thereafter. Recent studies have added to our knowledge of the natural history and treatment of this disorder during the early months of life, and this is discussed separately in a later section.

Laboratory Findings. The characteristic serum biochemical findings in XLH rickets include hypophosphatemia, normocalcemia, and an elevated alkaline phosphatase level. Other serum electrolytes, blood pH, bicarbonate, and BUN are normal. In the untreated state, urinary calcium excretion is usually low and urinary phosphate excretion high. The tubular reabsorption rate (TRP) and the maximum reabsorption rate of phosphate (TmP/GFR) are decreased. The TRP and TmP/GFR values are intermediate in obligate female heterozygotes relative to normal and mutant hemizygote subjects.[70] Indeed, the TRP in female heterozygotes overlaps the normal range as predicted by the Lyon hypothesis (which implies random inactivation of one X chromosome early in development) if phosphate transport in the kidney is closely coupled to the effect of an X-linked mutation. The urinary excretion of cyclic AMP is normal,[70] and there is neither aminoaciduria nor glycosuria.

The serum iPTH level is usually normal,[58] although slightly elevated levels have been reported in some untreated subjects.[71,72] Secondary hyperparathyroidism with an increase in circulating iPTH levels may be observed after the institution of phosphate therapy.

In the untreated state, the serum 25-hydroxyvitamin D levels are normal. Normal serum 24,25-dihydroxyvitamin D levels have been reported in untreated children with XLH,[73] whereas in a study of untreated adult patients, the serum 24,25-dihydroxyvitamin D levels, although generally within the normal range, were significantly lower than in normal subjects.[74]

Normal and low levels of serum 1,25-dihydroxyvitamin D have both been reported in untreated patients with XLH.[74–79] In one study, the serum 1,25-dihydroxyvitamin D levels were found to be similar to growth rate–matched controls but significantly lower than the levels of age-matched controls who were growing at a normal rate.[77] In another study of untreated children, the mean serum 1,25-dihydroxyvitamin D level was higher than the age-matched controls.[80] However, in this study, with the exception of one slightly elevated value, the individual values were within the normal limits. Treatment with pharmacologic doses of vitamin D or 25-hydroxyvitamin D and phosphate results in an increase in serum 25-hydroxyvitamin and 24,25-dihydroxyvitamin D[73,74] and a decrease in 1,25-dihydroxyvitamin D.[73,74,80] It is possible that the relatively lower levels of 1,25-dihydroxyvitamin D reported in some patients with XLH may have been the result of vitamin D and phosphate treatment, rather than a primary biochemical manifestation of the disorder *per se*. Although patients with X-linked hypophosphatemic rickets may have normal serum 1,25-dihydroxyvitamin D levels, elevated levels of this metabolite would be expected in the presence of hypophosphatemia. In this regard, therefore, the normal circulating levels of this metabolite are inappropriately low in the presence of hypophosphatemia and reflect the presence of a relative deficiency of this active metabolite in XLH.

Radiologic Findings. In the first few years of life, radiologic findings characteristic of rickets are seen at the metaphyseal ends of the long bones, including the proximal and distal tibia and the distal femur, radius, and ulna.[5,58] The abnormalities include fraying, widening, and cupping of the metaphyseal ends of these long bones. The changes in the wrist may improve with time, possibly owing to the slower growth of the bones of the forearm. The changes in the lower extremities persist and may progress, and conceivably, weight-bearing may be an important factor in the further development of the metaphyseal lesions. Consequently, in later childhood, the bony changes at the distal radius and ulna are not marked, whereas the abnormalities in the lower extremities are prominent.[5] Therefore, x-ray films of the knee and ankle joints are more informative than are those of the wrist in the diagnosis and follow-up of XLH rickets in later childhood. In later stages of XLH, x-ray examination of the proximal tibia frequently shows a web-shaped defect of the medial portion of the metaphyseal surface that has been attributed to the stress of weight-bearing.

On radiologic examination, the shafts of the long bones frequently appear unusually thick but normally mineralized. The trabecular bone structure is coarse and may appear unusually dense. Bone mineral analysis of the radius by ^{125}I-computer tomography has been evaluated in children with XLH previously treated with pharmacologic doses of vitamin D.[81] In these children, the trabecular bone density of the radius at 10% of the ulna length was normal. An increased cross-sectional area of the diaphysis of the radius at 30% ulna length was observed, consistent with the radiographic description of an increased thickness of the long bones; the cortical width of the diaphysis of the radius at 30% ulna length was decreased, but the total amount of compact bone mineral in the cross-sectional area was normal because of the enlargement of the bone; the bone density was decreased consistent with a normal amount of compact bone mineral in a relatively larger area. Microradiographic and histologic examinations of the fibula were carried out in this study and revealed grossly abnormal mineralization of bone tissue with a perilacunae mineral deficit. It was concluded that (1) the amount of compact bone and trabecular bone is not decreased in children with XLH, and (2) the normal mineral content determined by CT and the impaired mineralization of bone material found by microradiography indicates an overabundance of incompletely mineralized bone.

A recent study of 26 patients with XLH demonstrated calcification of tendon and ligament insertions and of joint capsules in 69% of the subjects.[82] The ages of the patients ranged from 1 to 62 years. Nineteen of the patients had not been treated, whereas seven had been receiving vitamin D or oral phosphorus supplements or both. Regardless of therapy or lack of therapy, the prevalence and extent of the calcification increased with age but there was no correlation with sex. The disorder was observed in 45% of 11 patients who were under 20 years of age (and in none of the four who were under 10 years of age); in 78% of nine patients who were between 20 and 40 years; and in 100% of six patients who were over 40 years of age. Calcific deposits were most commonly found in the hand and sacroiliac joints and somewhat less frequently in the hip joints, iliolumbar ligaments, tendon insertions at the lesser trochanter, and lumbar annulus fibrosus ligaments. The disease process was actually observed at all sites examined with the exception of the thoracic interspinal ligaments. Calcifications occurred bilaterally at each affected capsule or insertion. Patients under 20 years of age did not have symptoms secondary to calcifications, whereas older subjects had symptoms related to joint dysfunction, which was consistent with increased radiographic severity of the disorder. An exception was the absence of symptomatic expression of the disease in the hands and wrists. Histologic examination in a selected patient revealed intratendinous lamellar bone without inflammatory cells. The pathophysiologic mechanism of this calcification disorder is unknown but it appears to be a distinct component of XLH.

Bone Histomorphometric Studies. Histologic findings characteristic of rickets are found at the epiphyseal region. There is a markedly expanded zone of proliferating cartilage with increased osteoid tissue and invasion by wide, tortuous blood vessels.[58]

Transileal biopsies demonstrate altered bone remodeling in children with untreated XLH.[75,76,83,84] Trabecular and cortical osteomalacia are both present, as demonstrated by excessive thickness of osteoid borders and decreased bone mineralization. When compared with normal age-matched controls, the trabecular calcified bone volume is not decreased and there is no evidence of excessive osteoclastic resorption.[84] Both trabecular and cortical bone have an increase in osteoid tissue (as reflected by the increase in osteoid volume, osteoid surface, and mean osteoid seam thickness) and a decreased mineralization front. A decrease in osteoblast calcification rate and a marked prolongation of the mineralization lag time and of the formation is revealed by dual tetracycline labeling (see Chapters 10 and 11). The birth rate of new basic multicellular remodeling units (BMU) in the intracortical haversian system is markedly reduced, resulting in a markedly depressed bone formation rate at the level of the whole tissue.[84] Marie and Glorieux concluded from their studies that the combination of the decrease in birth rate of new BMU in the prolonged formation period appears to be characteristic of XLH rickets.[84]

In association with osteomalacia, hypomineralized periosteocytic lesions have been consistently observed in the calcified sections of cortical bone from patients with XLH.[85–87] Electron microscopic studies suggest that these lesions result from impaired mineralization of bone matrix. These lesions are rather unique and apparently have not been observed in other states of osteomalacia associated with chronic hypophosphatemia.

Pathophysiology. The pathophysiology of XLH rickets is incompletely understood. In this discussion, we consider the possibility of defects in the (1) renal tubular transport of phosphate; (2) intestinal transport of calcium and phosphate; (3) synthesis and metabolism of 1,25-dihydroxyvitamin D; and (4) osteoblasts.

Phosphate reabsorption takes place in both the proximal and distal tubules, in the loop of Henle, and probably in the early collecting tubule. Two important factors that regulate tubular phosphate transport are parathyroid hormone and dietary phosphate intake. Micropuncture studies indicate that when parathyroid hormone is infused into a normal animal, the major site of reduced phosphate transport is the early proximal nephron.[88] However, in a euparathyroid animal that undergoes parathyroidectomy, the major increases in tubular phosphate reabsorption occur distally in the pars recta and distal convoluted tubule.[88] Dietary phosphate restriction leads to a rapid decrease (1–3 days) in urinary phosphate excretion, even when the plasma phosphate concentration remains normal.[89] Available evidence indicates that the adaptation to a low phosphate intake occurs primarily in the early proximal nephron. The response to phosphate deprivation is quantitatively much greater than the response to parathyroid hormone. Whereas parathyroid hormone alters phosphate reabsorption two to five times, phosphate deprivation and excess can alter this process several hundred times.[89] Parathyroid hormone is not necessary for the adaptive process to occur. Thus, the increase in tubular phosphate reabsorption in response to dietary phosphate restriction is observed in animals that receive parathyroid hormone as well as in parathyroidectomized animals. It is not known whether phosphate deprivation and parathyroid hormone act on the same or on different phosphate transport systems within the nephron.

The accumulated evidence indicates that there is a selective disorder in renal phosphate transport in patients with XLH. The hypophosphatemic disorder is consistently associated with increased renal excretion and decreased net renal tubular reabsorption of phosphate.[58] There is impaired ability to conserve phosphate in response to phosphorus deprivation as reflected in a decrease in urinary phosphate excretion and an increase in TmP/GFR that are significantly less in male patients with XLH than in normal controls.[79] Studies in the Hyp mouse, which represent a homologue of the disease process in human XLH, have demonstrated a defect in phosphate transport in purified kidney brush border membrane vesicles.[90,91]

Controversy exists concerning the role of parathyroid hormone in the defect in phosphate transport in XLH. In one study, the infusion of a parathyroid hormone into affected male hemizygotes resulted in essentially no change in the tubular reabsorption of phosphate, whereas the responses in female heterozygotes overlapped with normal.[70] On the other hand, hypercalcemia induced by calcium infusion was attended by an increase in the value of tubular reabsorption of phosphate in both male and female patients with XLH. From these observations the authors concluded that renal phosphate transport involves two components, one that is modulated by parathyroid hormone and the other by calcium ion. It was suggested that in XLH there is a lack of the parathyroid hormone–sensitive component in male hemizygotes, whereas female heterozygotes retain a variable proportion of this transport. Consistent with this possibility is the observation that subtotal parathyroidectomy in XLH, sufficient to cause hypocalcemia of several weeks' duration, resulted in no significant improvement in tubular reabsorption of phosphate and did not correct the hypophosphatemia. In contrast to these observations, Lyles and Drezner reported that following the administration of parathyroid extract, there was a decrease in TmP/GFR that was not significantly different in XLH patients and in normal controls.[78] The discrepancy in the results of the two studies may, in part, be related to the difference in populations that were studied. In the first study, little or no renal phosphate response to parathyroid hormone was observed in three male hemizygotes, whereas an overlap in phosphate excretion in response to parathyroid hormone was found between heterozygote females and normal controls. In the second study, in which a normal renal phosphate response to parathyroid hormone was documented, four of the five patients were female heterozygotes and the mean, but not the individual, values for the change in TmP/GFR were reported.

In a third study, parathyroid hormone was infused into affected hemizygotes and normal controls following calcium infusion that reduced endogenous circulating parathyroid hormone levels.[92] Under this condition the infusion of parathyroid hormone caused an exaggerated phosphaturic response when compared with controls, whereas the increase in urinary cyclic AMP was the same as in the control subjects. The authors concluded that the reduced TRP in XLH is the result of an increase in renal phosphaturic responsiveness to parathyroid hormone at normal or even reduced concentrations. They also suggested that if hemizygotes were hyperresponsive to the phosphaturic effect of normal concentrations of circulating parathyroid hormone, then the induction of even greater concentrations of circulating parathyroid hormone might not induce a greater magnitude of phosphaturia.

In two studies, treatment of XLH patients with 1,25-dihydroxyvitamin D resulted in a decrease in serum parathyroid hormone and an elevation of the TmP/GFR in both hemizygous males and heterozygous females.[75,93] In one of the studies, an inverse linear correlation was found between the mean serum parathyroid hormone level and the mean TmP/GFR before and after treatment, whereas no correlation was found between TmP/GFR and serum calcium.[93] In one XLH patient with autonomous secondary hyperparathyroidism secondary to phosphate therapy, the administration of 1,25-dihydroxyvitamin D had no effect on serum parathyroid hormone and phosphate concentrations or on the TmP/GFR. Although not conclusive, the results of these studies are consistent with the thesis that parathyroid hormone modulates, to some extent, the tubular handling of phosphate.

In XLH patients, the intestinal absorption of calcium is generally reduced, but usually not to the extent that is observed in vitamin D deficiency.[58] As a result, urinary calcium excretion is low but the calcium balance is usually slightly positive, although less so than that observed in normally growing children. In one study, calcium absorption by a calcium tolerance test was thought to be normal.[94] However, it is difficult to relate these findings to those of several older calcium balance studies in which significant reduction in calcium absorption was observed. Whether intestinal phosphate absorption is altered in XLH is uncertain. Balance studies reveal that phosphate absorption is decreased, but not to the extent of the reduction of calcium absorption. The administration of small doses of 1,25-dihydroxyvitamin D results in a marked increase in the intestinal absorption of phosphate under conditions in which there is little or no effect upon renal tubular phosphate reabsorption.[95] The results of this study, as well as the inability to demonstrate an abnormality in phosphate uptake in jejunal biopsies from hypophosphatemic subjects,[96] suggest that there is no intrinsic defect in the intestinal absorption of phosphate.

Whereas patients with XLH have low to normal serum 1,25-dihydroxyvitamin D levels, elevated levels of this metabolite would be expected in the presence of hypophosphatemia. This suggests a possible abnormality in vitamin D metabolism patients with XLH. In response to a low-phosphate diet, the serum 1,25-dihydroxyvitamin D levels rose progressively in normal subjects, whereas no change was observed in XLH patients.[79] In response to parathyroid hormone, the serum 1,25-dihydroxyvitamin D levels increased by 218% in normal controls as compared with only 68% in XLH patients.[78] The increase in urinary cyclic AMP in response to parathyroid hormone was not significantly different in the two groups. Thus, results of these studies indicate that the generation of 1,25-dihydroxyvitamin D is impaired in XLH in response to both parathyroid hormone and phosphate deprivation. The following results obtained in studies of the Hyp mice are also consistent with an abnormality in the synthesis of 1,25-dihydroxyvitamin D: (1) the renal mitochondrial 25-hydroxyvitamin D1α-hydroxylase activity is depressed in Hyp mice when compared with normal littermates[97]; and (2) the activity of this enzyme is significantly elevated in renal homogenates of Hyp mice when compared with normal mouse kidney but substantially less than that in renal homogenates prepared from phosphate-depleted mice.[98]

Seino et al. recently reported that 25-hydroxyvitamin D1α-hydroxylase activity in a homogenate of renal tissue was significantly elevated in a 10-year-old boy with XLH as compared with seven age-matched controls[99] and suggested that the normal or low 1,25-dihydroxyvitamin D concentration in XLH patients could be due to accelerated catabolism of the metabolite. In view of the studies of Hyp mice and phosphate-depressed mice discussed previously, the increased renal 25-hydroxyvitamin D1α-hydroxylase activity observed in the patient with XLH, as compared with normal controls, remains uncertain until comparative studies can be made on renal homogenates obtained from phosphate-deprived patients. However, Seino and coworkers presented the following additional evidence in support of accelerated catabolism of 1,25-dihydroxyvitamin: (1) the plasma clearance of 1,25-dihydroxyvitamin D after a bolus of this metabolite was greater at 11 hours in Hyp mice as compared with normal littermates[100]; and (2) following the administration of 1α-hydroxyvitamin D (0.4–2.0 mg/kg/day) to patients with XLH, the rise in serum 1,25-dihydroxyvitamin D is significantly less than that observed in patients with hypoparathyroidism or pseudohypoparathyroidism who receive a significantly smaller dose of 1α-hydroxyvitamin D (0.1–0.2 mg/kg/day).[101] The possibility that the metabolic clearance rate of circulating 1,25-dihydroxyvitamin D is increased in XLH is of interest and worthy of additional studies.

Histomorphometric studies suggest the possibility that abnormal differentiation and function of the osteoblasts contribute to the osteomalacic lesion in XLH.[83,84,102] Although the defect of mineralization and impaired osteoblastic function might be the consequence of the chronic hypophosphatemic state, it has been suggested that a primary disorder of the bone cell line cannot be excluded. A direct correlation between the mineralization front activity and the serum level of 1,25-dihydroxyvitamin D has been observed in patients before and during treatment with 1,25-dihydroxyvitamin D.[75] The lack of correlation of the mineralization front activity with other factors, such as serum phosphorus, suggested that the action of 1,25-dihydroxyvitamin D on bone may be direct and that a relative deficiency of this metabolite may be a factor in the pathogenesis of the rachitic and osteomalacic lesion in XLH. It has been further speculated that the alleged osteoblast defect in XLH causes the osteoblast to fail to react to normal concentrations of 1,25-dihydroxyvitamin D and it is only by inducing supraphysiologic concentrations that this resistance is overcome.[83]

Marie and Glorieux have suggested that in addition to the proposed defective osteoblastic function there may be a specific abnormality in the osteocyte similar to or arising from the proposed defect in osteoblast function.[85] The frequency of hypomineralized periosteocytic lesions is unrelated to the severity of osteomalacia in untreated XLH patients. Moreover, these lesions are absent in other osteomalacic states associated with chronic hypophosphatemia. Lastly, it has been suggested that members of families afflicted with XLH who have hypophosphatemia but no evidence of skeletal disease may have the renal but not the osteoblast defect.[83]

Treatment. Large doses of vitamin D alone (10,000–25,000 IU/day for infants and up to 300,000 IU/day for older children) were originally used for treatment of XLH rickets.[103–106] With this mode of therapy there was a slight increase in serum phosphate and a decrease in serum alkaline phosphatase activity, but rarely to normal values. There was usually significant although often not complete healing of the rachitic lesions in the growth plates radiographically. With large doses of vitamin D alone, skeletal deformities frequently remained problems and there was little evidence of improved growth. Moreover, patients receiving large doses of vitamin D alone were at risk for vitamin D intoxication with hypercalciuria and permanent renal damage.

Subsequently, with increased knowledge of the pathogenetic role of phosphate deficiency in XLH rickets, phosphate therapy was introduced. One to 5 g of oral elemental phosphorus per day increases the serum phosphate concentration into the normal or low-normal range for a significant portion of the day. Phosphate therapy alone induced mineralization of the growth plate, but had little effect on the endosteal bone surface.[83] Unfortunately, phosphate therapy decreases the serum ionized calcium level, which, in turn, results in the development of secondary hyperparathyroidism with attendant characteristic bone changes, hyperaminoaciduria, and further impairment of the tubular reabsorption of phosphate.

Vitamin D (4000–50,000 IU/day) was introduced as an adjunct to phosphate therapy in an effort to prevent secondary hyperparathyroidism. Treatment with phosphate in conjunction with vitamin D results in radiographic healing of the rachitic lesions in the growth plates comparable to that observed with phosphate treatment alone.[83,107] However, radiographic studies and bone histomorphometric analysis have demonstrated that similar to phosphate treatment alone, treatment with phosphate in conjunction with vitamin D induced mineralization of the growth plate but had little effect on the endosteal bone surface.[83]

More recent studies demonstrated that combined therapy with oral phosphate and either 1,25-dihydroxyvitamin D or 1α-hydroxyvitamin D greatly improves mineralization of endosteal bone as well as that of the growth plate.[76,83] These metabolites have a shorter circulating half-time than does vitamin D, which is an advantage if episodes of hypercalcemia should occur. Currently the recommended mode of therapy for XLH rickets is oral phosphate combined with either 1,25-dihydroxyvitamin D or 1α-hydroxyvitamin D.[76,83,95,108–110] One to 4 g of phosphorus per day, as a neutral phosphate salt, is best given in five divided doses at 3.5- to 4-hour intervals. It is necessary to give the phosphate salt at frequent intervals because following an oral dose, the plasma concentration of phosphate reaches a peak in about 90 minutes and usually returns to baseline within 4 hours. Initially the patient may develop diarrhea with phosphate therapy but usually develops tolerance to the treatment within 1 or 2 weeks. It is advisable to start treatment with a relatively small dose of phosphate and gradually increase the dose over a 1- to 2-week period. In addition, 1,25-dihydroxyvitamin D or 1α-hydroxyvitamin D is administered in doses that usually range from 0.5 to 2.0 μg/day (10–40 ng/kg/day). This mode of therapy leads to an increase in serum phosphate concentration with no change,[83,108] or, as reported in one study,[109] a decrease in TmP/GFR. This is in contrast to reported increases in TmP/GFR during the chronic administration of relatively large doses of 1α-hydroxyvitamin D alone.[111,112] The combined treatment with phosphate and 1,25-dihydroxyvitamin D or 1α-hydroxyvitamin D results in a significant increase in the intestinal absorption of both phosphate and calcium. The beneficial effect on phosphate homeostasis with this mode of therapy is attributed to the increase in intestinal phosphate absorption. The serum calcium concentration may remain unchanged or rise to a modest degree (< 1.0 mg/100 ml) with successful therapy while the serum alkaline phosphatase activity decreases.

The aim of the combined therapy is to ameliorate the rickets by increasing the serum phosphate concentration above 3 to 3.5 mg/100 ml while maintaining a serum calcium level in the normal range. It is important to be aware of the complications of this combined therapy. Phosphate therapy can lead to secondary hyperparathyroidism; treatment with the vitamin D metabolites can lead to hypercalciuria, hypercalcemia, and reduced creatinine clearance. Hypercalciuria usually develops before hypercalcemia. It is, therefore, necessary to balance the doses of phosphate and the vitamin D metabolites so that hyperparathyroidism, on the one hand, and hypercalciuria, on the other, are avoided. One approach is to begin phosphate therapy and a small dose of 1,25-dihydroxyvitamin D or 1α-hydroxyvitamin D (0.25–0.50 μg/day). At 3- to 4-week intervals, serum parathyroid hormone, calcium, phosphate, creatinine, and fasting urinary calcium and creatinine levels are measured. If the serum calcium is normal or less than normal, and the urinary calcium to creatinine ratio is within the normal range (< 0.25), the dose of the vitamin D metabolite is progressively increased until the serum parathyroid hormone level is normal and the fasting urinary calcium to creatinine ratio is below the upper limit of normal.

Combined treatment with phosphate and 1,25-dihydroxyvitamin D or 1α-hydroxyvitamin D results in a healing effect of both the growth plate and trabecular bone lesions radiographically. Treatment with phosphate and conventional doses of 1,25-dihydroxyvitamin D (mean dose of 32 ng/kg/day or 1 μg/day) or 1α-hydroxyvitamin D (mean dose of 1.27 μg/day) leads to an increase in serum phosphate in the majority of patients with no alteration in the renal phosphate threshold.[76,83,108] Histomorphometric analysis of bone from these patients reveals improvement but usually not normalization of the osteomalacic lesions as defined by an excess of osteoid tissue, a decreased extent of the calcification front, and a low mineralization rate at the trabecular bone surface. In a recent study,[110] patients with XLH were treated with phosphate and relatively high dosages of 1,25-dihydroxyvitamin D (68.2 ± 10.0 ng/kg/day). On high dosages of 1,25-dihydroxyvitamin D, the serum levels of this metabolite rose into supraphysiologic ranges in association with an increase in serum phosphate, and in contrast to patients who received conventional doses of 1,25-dihydroxyvitamin D, there was an increase in TmP/GFR and complete healing of the osteomalacic lesions. In this study, complications of hypercalcemia and hypercalciuria necessitated reduction of 1,25-dihydroxyvitamin D to conventional doses (28 ± 4 ng/kg/day). This resulted in a decrease in serum phosphate and $TmPO_4$/GFR, but healing of the osteomalacia was maintained for 11 months after the reduction in 1,25-dihydroxyvitamin D dose when the last follow-up bone biopsies were obtained. The results of this study suggest that high-dose 1,25-dihydroxyvitamin D in conjunction with phosphate induces complete healing of the osteomalacia, which is then maintained for at least 11 months by smaller doses of 1,25-dihydroxyvitamin D. Further studies are required to determine whether shorter courses of high-dose 1,25-dihydroxyvitamin D can promote bone healing without complications and to determine whether subsequent treatment with smaller doses of 1,25-dihydroxyvitamin D can maintain normal bone mineralization for even longer periods of time.

It has been suggested that the effects of 1,25-dihydroxyvitamin D on bone mineralization are exerted through its osteoblastic effect[113] and that in XLH, the osteoblast fails to react to normal concentrations of 1,25-dihydroxyvitamin D.[83] The healing effect that combined therapy with phosphate and 1,25-dihydroxyvitamin D has on the osteomalacic lesions in XLH, in contrast to the effect of combined treatment with phosphate and vitamin D, may be due to the action of supraphysiologic concentrations of 1,25-dihydroxyvitamin D on the osteoblast.[83,110]

There are two reports of the treatment of a total of four children with XLH rickets with large doses of 1α-hydroxyvitamin D alone.[111,112] Treatment with 1α-hydroxyvitamin D led to an increase in serum phosphate and a modest increase in TmP/GFR. The occurrence of hypercalcemia was controlled by reducing the dose of 1α-hydroxyvitamin D. There was improvement in the bone lesions radiographically, but bone histomorphometric analysis was not reported. Growth data were given for only one patient in whom growth increased from 3.4 cm in the seven months before treatment to 5.6 cm during seven months of treatment.[112] However, this patient was stated to have mild disease, and the follow-up period was only of seven months' duration. The results of these studies are, therefore, difficult to interpret, and the possibility of hypercalcemia and hypercalciuria with high-dose 1α-hydroxyvitamin D remains a concern.

In another study, Drezner et al. treated four patients with 2.25 to 3.0 μg of 1,25-dihydroxyvitamin D alone.[75] This resulted in a modest increase of TmP/GFR, an increase in serum phosphate, a fall in plasma alkaline phosphatase activity, a decrease in plasma iPTH, and a positive calcium and phosphate balance. Bone histomorphometric analysis revealed that despite normalization of mineralization front activity, the treatment with 1,25-dihydroxyvitamin D alone had only variable effects on the wide osteoid seams and the excess osteoid-covered trabecular bone surface present in initial biopsies. Indeed, in two of three patients, 1,25-dihydroxyvitamin D treatment resulted in no change in the extent of osteoid. Moreover, in all of the subjects studied, bone age exceeded 16 years, longitudinal growth had ceased, and there was no evidence of rickets. Therefore, it was not possible to determine whether the rachitic lesions characteristic of XLH respond to treatment with 1,25-dihydroxyvitamin D alone or whether the treatment promotes catch-up growth in affected subjects. The accumulated evidence indicates that neither vitamin D plus phosphate nor 1,25-dihydroxyvitamin D alone is as effective as the combination of 1,25-dihydroxyvitamin D or 1α-hydroxyvitamin D plus phosphate in the treatment of XLH rickets as assessed by quantitative histomorphometric analysis of bone biopsy material.

Alon and Chan recently reported the adjunct use of thiazide-amiloride diuretic therapy with a low-sodium diet in patients with XLH rickets under treatment with phosphate plus 1,25-dihydroxyvitamin D.[114] They found that the adjunct diuretic therapy resulted in an increase in serum phosphate, an increase in TmP/GFR, the maintenance of normal serum parathyroid hormone concentrations, and a reduction in urinary calcium, and, with the exception of one episode of hypercalcemia, the serum calcium levels remained within the normal range. Radiographic findings improved in five of the patients who had radiologic evidence of active rickets prior to the adjunct diuretic therapy. Linear height velocity improved in four children and did not change in two during the adjunct therapy. The authors suggest that the addition of hydrochlorothiazide-amiloride may be especially beneficial in children who are particularly intolerant of the high intake of oral phosphate and/or in those children especially prone to hypercalciuria. However, the possible adverse effects of the adjunct thiazide therapy coupled with the low-sodium diet must be weighed against the possible beneficial effects in treatment of XLH rickets. Additional long-term control studies are needed to resolve this issue.

Effect of Treatment on Growth. Growth retardation is a serious problem in children with XLH rickets and it is important that this factor be taken into consideration when evaluating various modes of therapy. Steendijk and Latham[115] examined the stature of untreated XLH patients, ages 1 to 13 years, using the method of standard deviation of the mean for chronologic age.[116] They found that the mean height of the patients was approximately 2 standard deviations below the normal mean (i.e., at the 3rd percentile). The upper limit of height was approximately equal to the normal mean, and half of the patients fell within the normal range. The standard deviation for height was equal to the standard deviation for height in a normal sample of population. No correlation was found between the deficit in height and age, sex, or deficit in serum phosphate level.

The relative effectiveness of various forms of therapy on growth reported in the literature is difficult to evaluate owing to a number of confounding variables, such as severity of the disorder including skeletal abnormalities, initial degree of growth retardation, methods of evaluating stature, age at time of initiation of therapy, duration of treatment, compliance, length of follow-up, doses of vitamin D, vitamin D metabolites and phosphate, and complications of therapy such as vitamin D intoxication and phosphate-induced secondary hyperparathyroidism. In addition, the reported studies usually contain little information regarding the stature of unaffected family members so that it is not possible to appraise the genetic potential of the patient. Moreover, in a number of reports, only one mode of therapy is evaluated and, therefore, there is no comparison to another mode of therapy by the same investigators.

With these problems taken into consideration, the accumulated evidence suggests that phosphate therapy plays a prime role in the correction of the short stature, since this will heal the epiphyseal or rachitic lesion. Thus, Glorieux and colleagues[83] report that 1.2 to 3.6 g/day of oral phosphate alone resulted in growth rates of approximately 8 to 9 cm/year, and the addition of either 25,000 to 50,000 IU of vitamin D or 1.0 μg of 1,25-dihydroxyvitamin D per day did not alter this pattern. Chesney et al.[109] evaluated growth in children with XLH rickets who each received 1.5 to 3.6 g/day of oral phosphate plus a mean dose of 37,500 IU/day of vitamin D followed by the same dose of phosphate plus a mean dose of 0.65 μg of 1,25-dihydroxyvitamin D per day. No significant difference in the height velocity (cm/year) was found in six patients who were evaluated for at least 12 months while receiving each form of therapy. In this study, stature was also examined using the method of standard deviation of the mean for chronologic age.[116] Using this method, the following were observed: (1) there was no difference in the mean height in patients receiving no therapy or 20,000 IU of vitamin D per day; (2) there was a significant increase in the mean height in the patients after receiving vitamin D plus oral phosphate and 1,25-dihydroxyvitamin D plus oral phosphate; (3) no significant differences in height were found between periods of vitamin D plus phosphate and 1,25-dihydroxyvitamin D plus phosphate therapy. By contrast, there is a report of increased growth rate in four children when they were changed from phosphate plus 10,000 to 60,000 IU of vitamin D per day to phosphate plus 17 to 80 ng/kg/day of 1,25-dihydroxyvitamin D.[95] However, in two of the four patients, this finding is difficult to interpret, since adolescent growth spurt may have contributed to the increased growth rate during 1,25-dihydroxyvitamin D therapy.

Currently oral phosphate in conjunction with either 1,25-dihydroxyvitamin D or 1α-hydroxyvitamin D is most often used in the treatment of XLH because of the superior effect these metabolites have on the trabecular bone lesions when compared with therapy with vitamin D and phosphate. However, there is as yet no conclusive evidence that any one of these three modes of therapy is superior to the others in promoting linear growth. In most studies using these forms of therapy, growth has increased from a range of less than the 3rd to the 10th percentile to a range of the 3rd to the 25th percentile in the majority of patients with an increase to the 50th percentile or greater in a smaller number of patients. In a few children, for reasons that are uncertain, there has been little or no increase in the rate of growth. It is apparent that additional well-controlled and informative studies are needed to more clearly define optimal therapy for promoting growth in XLH.

XLH Rickets in the Neonatal Period and Early Infancy. XLH rickets is usually diagnosed during the second and third years of life. However, there are reports of studies carried out in the neonatal period and early months of life of infants born in XLH kindreds in which either the mother or the father was affected.[117–121] In these studies the following criteria were used in an attempt to establish the diagnosis: (1) decreased serum phosphate level; (2) elevated serum alkaline phosphatase activity; (3) reduced TRP; (4) abnormal radiographic findings; and (5) abnormal physical findings. All infants who subsequently proved to be affected appeared normal at birth, and there were neither clinical nor radiologic signs of rickets. Linear growth was apparently normal during the first 6 to 12 months of life with a tendency to slow down to a varying degree thereafter. The serum phosphate level was low at birth in some infants, and in most it was depressed by 6 weeks of age. However, in some infants a low serum phosphate concentration was not observed until 3 to 8 months of life. The serum alkaline phosphatase activity was normal at birth but steadily increased to abnormally high levels that were reached between 1 and 3 months of age. In studies in which urinary phosphate was investigated, a low TRP was observed between 2 and 6 months of age with the exception of one preterm infant in whom a low TRP was observed at 9 days of age. A low serum phosphate in the presence of a normal TRP observed in some infants was attributed to a decreased gastrointestinal absorption of phosphate, although this was not measured.

Radiographic signs of rickets were reported at 10 weeks of age in one infant, but in the majority of infants, radiographic abnormalities did not appear until 3 to 6 months of age. In one study, signs of rickets were carefully looked for by physical examination from birth on. In the three infants studied, there was a suspicion of rachitic rosary and enlarged metaphysis between 2 and 6 months of age with confirmation of these findings between 4½ and 8 months of age. Bowing of the legs of these infants was suspected between 6 and 10 months of age, but the authors were aware that slight pathologic bowing of an infant's legs is difficult to distinguish from physiologic variations.

In three infants described in two reports,[119,121] combined treatment with 1α-hydroxyvitamin D and phosphate was initiated at 6 to 8 weeks of life. The serum phosphate was low, the alkaline phosphatase was elevated, and the x-ray findings were normal in each infant. During treatment, the serum phosphate usually ranged between 3 and 4 mg/100 ml, whereas the alkaline phosphatase decreased toward normal. In two infants, both girls, the x-ray findings remained normal, and they were growing at the 50th and 75th percentile at 26 and 30 months of age, respectively. In the third child, a boy, x-ray evidence of rickets developed at 12 months of age but healed with the adjustment of the dosage of 1α-hydroxyvitamin D and phosphate. At 5 years of age he was growing at the 50th percentile. There were no apparent bone deformities in any of these children.

In three other reports, treatment was withheld until there was radiologic evidence of rickets. In one study, treatment with 1α-hydroxyvitamin D and phosphate was initiated at 6 months of age in three full-term infants with biochemical and radiologic abnormalities of rickets.[118] Healing of the rickets occurred within a year and all three were growing at the 10th percentile. In a fourth infant who was preterm, treatment was initiated at 3 months of age. Height remained at less than the 3rd percentile and rickets did not heal until 3½ years of age. In a second study, treatment with large doses of vitamin D alone was initiated at 3 months of age in an infant with biochemical and radiologic abnormalities of rickets.[117] With treatment the rickets healed radiographically, the alkaline phosphatase declined to normal, and serum phosphate ranged between 3 and 4 mg/100 ml. At 18 months of age the child was growing at the 50th percentile. In a third study, treatment with vitamin D plus phosphate was initiated when x-ray evidence of rickets appeared in three infants at 10 weeks, 19 weeks, and 8 months of age.[120] In two of the infants there was radiologic evidence of healing at 12 to 14 months of age. However, one of the infants developed bowed legs, which required osteotomies. At 9 years of age this child was growing at the 10th to the 20th percentile, whereas the other was growing at the 50th percentile at 7 years of age. With treatment, the serum alkaline phosphatase activity declined to normal while the serum phosphate level ranged between the low and low-normal range. In the third infant in whom treatment was initiated at 8 months of age, both biochemical and radiologic evidence of rickets persisted and the child was growing at less than the 3rd percentile at 19 months of age.

In summary, in 11 infants in whom therapy was initiated during the early months of life, one was growing at the 75th percentile, four at the 50th percentile, one at the 10th to the 20th percentile, three at the 10th percentile, and two at less than the 3rd percentile. Thus, growth was proceeding well in most of the infants. The infants in whom treatment was initiated at 6 to 8 weeks of life, before there was radiographic evidence of rickets, have apparently done especially well. It has been suggested that an infant born to a family with one affected parent should be followed closely with periodic biochemical determinations and x-ray examination. It has been further suggested that treatment should be initiated in infants with biochemical abnormalities before the appearance of radiographic evidence of rickets. However, the results of studies reported to date present some problems in interpretation and do not permit definitive conclusions owing to: (1) the limited number of infants that have been studied, (2) the known variations in the severity of the disorder, and (3) possible differences in compliance, especially as relates to phosphate, which may produce gastrointestinal disturbances in the infants. Additional well-controlled studies are needed to better define the possible beneficial effects of early diagnosis and treatment of XLH rickets.

2. Autosomal Recessive and Autosomal Dominant Hypophosphatemic Rickets

Not all cases of hypophosphatemic vitamin D–resistant rickets are inherited as an X-linked trait. An autosomal recessive transmission pattern of hypophosphatemic rickets has been reported.[122] In this genetic variant, hypophosphatemic rickets was associated with increased bone density, early fusion of cranial sutures, nerve deafness with narrowing of the internal auditory canal, and optic atrophy with normal optic foramina. The relationship of these clinical findings to the hypophosphatemic rickets is uncertain.

A phenotype similar to X-linked hypophosphatemia in its severity has been described in which the inheritance was consistent with autosomal dominant transmission.[5] Sporadic cases have been observed[56,123] that could be due to (1) a single patient who is homozygous for an autosomal gene; (2) a new mutation on the dominant X chromosome or previously unrecognized autosomal locus; (3) phenocopy; or (4) an acquired disease postnatally.

3. Acquired Primary Hypophosphatemic Rickets

In addition to genetic hypophosphatemic rickets, acquired forms of hypophosphatemic rickets and osteomalacia have been observed.[5,124,125] The onset is later in childhood or in adulthood, and the cases are sporadic with no family history. The patients usually grow normally during early childhood. The clinical findings often include bone pain and muscle weakness, and eventually deformities may develop. In contrast to genetic hypophosphatemia, marked muscle weakness may be a clinical feature of acquired hypophosphatemic rickets. Similar to genetic hypophosphatemia, the serum calcium is normal, the serum phosphate depressed, and the tubular reabsorption of phosphate reduced. The serum phosphate is often less than 2 mg/100 ml and the muscle weakness has been attributed to this marked hypophosphatemia. There is neither acidosis nor generalized aminoaciduria. In some cases, there may be a mild degree of glycosuria. Hyperglycinuria has also been observed in acquired hypophosphatemic rickets.

Several cases of acquired hypophosphatemic rickets have been found to be associated with skeletal and soft tissue mesenchymal tumors, and the term "oncogenic rickets" has been applied to these cases. For a more detailed discussion of oncogenic rickets, see Chapter 11 by Dr. Parfitt. It is possible that a mesenchymal tumor may be a pathogenetic factor in most if not all cases of acquired hypophosphatemic rickets, but because the tumors are often benign and may be of small size, they may have not been discovered.

4. Autosomal Dominant Hypophosphatemic Bone Disease

Hypophosphatemic bone disease (HBD) is an inherited disorder of phosphate homeostasis.[126,127] Although the disorder is in some ways similar to X-linked hypophosphatemia, there are distinct differences between the two disorders.

Hypophosphatemic bone disease is an autosomal dominant disorder, when not sporadic, in contrast to the X-linked dominant inheritance of X-linked hypophosphatemia. In both disorders, serum immunoreactive parathyroid hormone and calcium levels are within normal ranges while the serum phosphate concentration is depressed. Although the degree of hypophosphatemia is similar, the renal handling of phosphate differs in the two conditions. The percentage TRP is normal in the fasting state in hypophosphatemic bone disease in contrast to reduced values in X-linked hypophosphatemic males and many females. The theoretic renal phosphate threshold (TmP/GFR) and the maximum rate of tubular reabsorption of phosphate (TmP_i) are decreased in both disorders, and negative phosphate reabsorption can occur in both conditions. The urinary cyclic AMP response to parathyroid hormone infusion is adequate in both disorders. However, the phosphaturic response to parathyroid hormone under endogenous conditions is quantitatively normal in hypophosphatemic bone disease, but depressed in X-linked hypophosphatemia. It is of interest that compared with normal, the onset of the phosphaturic response after parathyroid hormone infusion is delayed in hypophosphatemic bone disease.

Growth retardation and bone disease are both less severe in hypophosphatemic bone disease than in X-linked hypophosphatemia at equivalent serum phosphate concentrations. In both conditions, osteomalacia is present in the metaphyseal and diaphyseal cortical bone, but in contrast to X-linked hypophosphatemia, rachitic changes at the epiphyseal plate are mild or absent in hypophosphatemic bone disease. The clinical manifestations of hypophosphatemic bone disease appear in late infancy and include bowing of the lower limbs and modest short stature. The x-ray findings include coarsened trabeculation in metaphysis and diaphysis of long bone and sclerosis in the distal medial metaphysis of the femora. Rachitic bone changes at the epiphysis are either absent or very mild. In childhood and adolescence, height is decreased but growth velocity is normal in hypophosphatemic bone disease. This implies that the shortness of the patients is the result of impaired growth during infancy without subsequent catch-up growth. Hypophosphatemia with a depressed TmP/GFR without osteomalacia or shortened stature may be observed in one parent. Normal mineralization of endosteal trabecular bone was found in one parent with persistent hypophosphatemia.

The serum 1,25-dihydroxyvitamin D levels are normal in hypophosphatemic bone disease. In contrast to patients with X-linked hypophosphatemia, patients with hypophosphatemic bone disease respond favorably to modest doses of 1,25-dihydroxyvitamin D without phosphate therapy. In one 38-month-old girl, treatment with 1 μg/day of 1,25-dihydroxyvitamin D increased the serum phosphate, improved tubular reabsorption of phosphate, and healed the bone deformity. On the other hand, 1,25-dihydroxyvitamin D therapy did not correct the hypophosphatemia or the TmP/GFR in her hypophosphatemic father. Since clinical studies imply that the shortness of stature in patients with hypophosphatemic bone disease is a result of an impairment during infancy, early treatment may be necessary to achieve normal stature.

It is apparent that hypophosphatemic bone disease differs from X-linked hypophosphatemia, both in bone metabolism and in renal handling of phosphate, despite comparable hypophosphatemia in each. Scriver et al.[127] suggest that the explanation for the different phenotypes is that independent gene products, each responsible for a different aspect of phosphate homeostasis, are affected by the two mutations. They further suggest that different mechanisms for the tubular reabsorption of phosphate seem to be affected in these two disorders and the human nephron may possess two mechanisms for the tubular reabsorption of phosphate, namely (1) one that is more sensitive to inhibition by parathyroid hormone, which is under the control of an X-linked gene, and (2) another less sensitive to parathyroid hormone, which is under the control of an autosomal gene.

Finally, although the degree of hypophosphatemia is similar in both disorders, the fact that the bone disease is more severe in X-linked hypophosphatemia implies that extracellular phosphate is not the sole determinant of homeostasis in the bone compartment. Scriver et al. have postulated that the X-linked gene is expressed in bone and affects phosphate transport in that compartment. They conclude that a mutation affecting an X-linked secondary active type of phosphate transfer in the bone compartment may be a feature of X-linked hypophosphatemia that would not be expressed in hypophosphatemic bone disease.[127]

5. Hereditary Hypophosphatemic Rickets with Hypercalciuria

A hereditary syndrome of hypophosphatemic rickets has recently been described that is associated with hypercalciuria in contrast to the low or normal urinary calcium excretion in the previously described hypophosphatemic syndrome.[128] The mode of inheritance of this syndrome appears to be autosomal recessive, and the clinical manifestations of rickets and short stature begin in early childhood. The characteristic laboratory findings include increased renal phosphate clearance, hypophosphatemia, normocalcemia, hypercalciuria, increased gastrointestinal absorption of calcium and phosphorus, elevated serum 1,25-dihydroxyvitamin D levels, and suppressed parathyroid function. Treatment with 1 to 2.5 g of elemental phosphorus per day as a neutral phosphate salt reverses all of the clinical and biochemical abnormalities with the exception of the decreased TmP/GFR.

It has been suggested that the primary defect in this syndrome is a renal phosphate leak resulting in hypophosphatemia, which, in turn, leads to an increase in circulating 1,25-dihydroxyvitamin D. The elevated 1,25-dihydroxyvitamin D increases the gastrointestinal absorption of calcium and phosphate. The increase in intestinal absorption of calcium results in parathyroid suppression and hypercalciuria.

The elevated serum 1,25-dihydroxyvitamin D distinguishes this syndrome from X-linked hypophosphatemia. The low serum concentrations of 1,25-dihydroxyvitamin D are not elevated in the presence of hypophosphatemia in X-linked hypophosphatemia. Two possible explanations have been proposed to account for the difference in circulating 1,25-dihydroxyvitamin D levels in these two syndromes. The first is that there are different anatomic sites for the renal tubular defect in phosphate reabsorption, one of which (X-linked hypophosphatemia) is associated with a deranged response of renal 1α-hydroxylase to a low phosphate signal. The second possible explanation proposes that there is an identical site for phosphate reabsorption and that in the presence of phosphate depletion there is a normal stimulatory and effector system for 1α-hydroxylation in hereditary hypophosphatemic rickets with hypercalciuria but not in X-linked hypophosphatemic rickets.

6. Fanconi Syndrome

In the Fanconi syndrome, rickets is found in association with multiple defects of the proximal renal tubule. In this syndrome there is renal wastage of amino acids, glucose, bicarbonate, leading to metabolic acidosis, and phosphate, leading to hypophosphatemia. In addition, there may be sodium wasting, uricosuria, proteinuria, and hyperkaluria, leading to hypokalemia. The serum calcium level is normal to low, whereas the urinary calcium excretion varies. The clinical manifestations include impaired linear growth and rickets. The Fanconi syndrome is frequently idiopathic but is also found in association with inborn errors of metabolism that affect proximal renal tubule function. These include glycogen storage disease, galactosemia, cystinosis, tyrosinemia, hereditary fructose intolerance, and hepatolenticular degeneration. The Fanconi syndrome may also be caused by toxic agents including mercury, lead, cadmium, streptozotocin, and outdated tetracycline.

Although the hypophosphatemia can account for the rickets, it is possible that acidosis plays a contributing role, since bone serves as a buffer for excess hydrogen ion. The excess acid is buffered by bone calcium carbonate leading to dissolution of bone mineral and possible hypercalciuria. It is also possible that acidosis and/or other proximal tubular dysfunction impairs the production of 1,25-dihydroxyvitamin D. Studies in rats and chicks suggest that metabolic acidosis impairs the synthesis of 1,25-dihydroxyvitamin D.[129–131] Exogenous cyclic AMP will restore 1α-hydroxylase activity in acidotic rats, suggesting that the mechanism of suppression of the enzyme activity is due to an inhibition of parathyroid hormone–dependent adenylate cyclase activity in the proximal convoluted tubule. However, studies in normal humans indicate that induced acidosis does not impair vitamin D metabolism.[132,133] In a recent study of patients with the Fanconi syndrome, there were marked abnormalities in the circulating concentrations of 25-hydroxyvitamin D, 1,25-dihydroxyvitamin D, or 24,25-dihydroxyvitamin D.[134] This finding is similar to that in patients with X-linked hypophosphatemia in that the serum 1,25-dihydroxyvitamin D levels are normal but not elevated in the presence of hypophosphatemia.

The rickets is treated with a combination of increased phosphate intake and pharmacologic doses of vitamin D. Depending on the age of the patient, the dose of phosphorus is 1 to 3 g/24 hours. The initial dose of vitamin D is 4000 to 5000 IU/day. This may be increased gradually to a maximum dose of 2000 to 4000 IU/kg/day. Most patients require on the order of 25,000 IU of vitamin D per day or 0.1 to 0.2 mg/day of dihydrotachysterol. Alkali therapy is used to correct the metabolic acidosis.

G. Rickets Associated with Gastrointestinal Malabsorption

Vitamin D deficiency rickets, secondary to malabsorption of vitamin D, can occur in disorders of the gastrointestinal tract that cause malabsorption and steatorrhea (see Chapter 11). This is most likely to occur in patients in whom there is limited skin exposure to ultraviolet light, such as in individuals who live in northern climates and debilitated patients who remain indoors. The clinical, biochemical, and radiographic findings are similar to those described in section I-E under vitamin D deprivation. Gastrointestinal disorders that may cause malabsorption and rickets include Crohn's disease, celiac disease, sprue, and pancreatic insufficiency. Although rickets is reportedly unusual in patients with cystic fibrosis of the pancreas, we recently observed vitamin D deficiency rickets as a manifestation of cystic fibrosis in a 9-month-old child.[135] Fat malabsorption, due to primary intestinal disease with normal pancreatic lipase, may lead to severe calcium malabsorption due to the precipitation of calcium in the gut as insoluble calcium soaps of long-chain fatty acids.[5] Rickets and/or osteomalacia may be observed several years after partial gastrectomy. The reason for this is uncertain, since partial gastrectomy rarely results in clinically apparent steatorrhea. It has been suggested that following a partial gastrectomy, impaired absorption of vitamin D may be secondary to impaired coordination of digestion and absorption as well as to an increase in the intestinal transit time.

Failure of vitamin D absorption with low circulating levels of 25-hydroxyvitamin D may be treated with oral vitamin D doses of 5000 to 10,000 IU/day; in some severe cases, doses as large as 25,000 to 50,000 IU of oral vitamin D may be needed. In cases of very severe malabsorption, 1,25-dihydroxyvitamin D_3 in dosages of 0.1 to 0.2 μg/kg/day may be beneficial. 1,25-Dihydroxyvitamin D has an advantage over vitamin D because some 1,25-dihydroxyvitamin D_3 is absorbed through a water-soluble mechanism directly into the portal system.

H. Abnormalities in Vitamin D Metabolism

1. Vitamin D–Dependent Rickets, Type I

Vitamin D–dependent rickets type I is a rare autosomal recessive disorder in which there is a defect in 25-hydroxyvitamin D 1α-hydroxylase, the enzyme that converts 25-hydroxyvitamin D to 1,25-dihydroxyvitamin D. This disorder is also known as hereditary pseudo–vitamin D deficiency rickets (PDR) and autosomal recessive vitamin D dependency (ARVDD).

The clinical course of vitamin D–dependent rickets type I is similar to that of ordinary vitamin D deficiency rickets.[136–144] The onset of symptoms usually appears within the first 4 to 12 months of age. As in ordinary vitamin D deficiency, hypotonia, weakness, and growth failure are common manifestations. There may be a history of convulsions or tetany, and, in some children, this may be the presenting clinical feature. A history of an adequate intake of vitamin D is usually obtained.

The biochemical features are similar to those of ordinary vitamin D deficiency rickets and include hypocalcemia, elevated serum immunoreactive parathyroid hormone, elevated serum alkaline phosphatase activity, and generalized aminoaciduria. Hypocalcemia is a cardinal feature of vitamin D–dependent rickets. There is grossly impaired intestinal transport of calcium, and urinary calcium is low.[140,142,143] The serum phosphate concentration may be normal or low; values below 2.2 mg/100 ml have been reported in a few patients with vitamin D–dependent rickets type I. The intestinal absorption and retention of phosphate may be reduced to a variable degree.[143,145] The urinary excretion of phosphate may be increased when expressed as milligrams of phosphate per milligram of creatinine[145] or when urinary phosphate is examined in relation to serum phosphate concentration. A decrease in renal tubular reabsorption of phosphate and of amino acids leading to generalized aminoaciduria is likely due to the increase in circulating parathyroid hormone. On the other hand, normal values for the renal tubular reabsorption of phosphate, phosphate excretion index, and phosphate clearance have also been reported.[140,146–148]

Measurement of circulating vitamin D metabolites has provided insight into the pathogenesis of vitamin D–dependent rickets type I. The serum 25-hydroxyvitamin D levels are normal in untreated patients and elevated in patients receiving therapeutic doses of vitamin D or 25-hydroxyvitamin D.[141,143,144,147,149] This indicates that the intestinal absorption of vitamin D and the production of 25-hydroxyvitamin D by the liver are not impaired in this disorder.

The most important finding is that circulating levels of 1,25-dihydroxyvitamin D are low in untreated patients with vitamin D–dependent rickets type I.[147,150,151] The serum 1,25-dihydroxyvitamin D levels remain low or low-normal in D–dependency type I patients successfully treated with pharmacologic doses of vitamin D or 25-hydroxyvitamin D.[149,150,152] These findings are all consistent with a defect in the 25-hydroxyvitamin D 1α-hydroxylase enzyme.

The calcemic response to parathyroid hormone is usually absent or reduced in vitamin D–dependent rickets type I, consistent with the diminished bone responsivity to parathyroid hormone in vitamin D deficiency.[141,148,153,154] The phosphaturic but not the urinary cyclic AMP response to parathyroid hormone is blunted in untreated patients.[147,155] The phosphaturic response to parathyroid hormone is restored when the circulating 1,25-dihydroxyvitamin D levels are increased following treatment with this metabolite. These findings suggest that 1,25-dihydroxyvitamin D has an effect on tubular phosphate resorption and plays a permissive role in the phosphaturic effect of parathyroid hormone. In normal subjects, the serum concentration of 1,25-dihydroxyvitamin D increases after the infusion of parathyroid extract. However, no response was observed in a patient with vitamin D–dependent rickets, suggesting that renal 25-hydroxyvitamin D 1α-hydroxylase is unresponsive to the stimulatory effect of parathyroid hormone in this disorder.[155]

Vitamin D–dependent rickets type I responds to treatment with pharmacologic doses of vitamin D and 25-hydroxyvitamin D. The dose of vitamin D required for adequate treatment varies but usually ranges from 20,000 to 100,000 IU/day, and some patients may require as much as 150,000 IU/day; doses of 100 to 1000 μg/day of 25-hydroxyvitamin D appear to be adequate.[143,148,149,153,154] Treatment with vitamin D and 25-hydroxyvitamin D increases the serum 25-hydroxyvitamin D and 24, 25-dihydroxyvitamin D levels, while the levels of 1,25-dihydroxyvitamin D remain in the low-normal range. It has been suggested that the therapeutic action of large doses of vitamin D and 25-hydroxyvitamin D may be related partly, if not totally, to the maintenance of high serum concentrations of 25-hydroxyvitamin D or 24,25-dihydroxyvitamin D, or both.[149] Treatment with 1α-hydroxyvitamin D_3, an analogue of 1,25-dihydroxyvitamin D_3, in doses of 1 to 3 μg/day is effective in the treatment of this disorder.[144,154] Treatment with 1,25-dihydroxyvitamin D appears to be optimal, and patients with vitamin D–dependent rickets type I respond to small doses of this metabolite.[147,154,156,157] The reported initial dose of

1,25-dihydroxyvitamin D in children is 0.5 to 1.0 μg/day; the maintenance dose varies from 0.25 to 2.0 μg/day.[147]

Although most cases of vitamin D–dependent rickets type I present during the first year of life, some patients may not present until later childhood.[145,158,159] The disorder in the patients who present in later childhood appears to be milder, since they have responded to 10,000 IU/day or less of vitamin D.

2. Rickets Associated with Liver Disorders

Rickets with low circulating levels of 25-hydroxyvitamin D is found in some patients with liver disorders. Some cholestatic disorders in children, such as biliary atresia and biliary hypoplasia, may result in steatorrhea. The steatorrhea is the result of decreased hepatic secretion of conjugated bile acids, which results in a decreased intraluminal concentration of bile acids within the small intestine. The steatorrhea leads to increased fecal fat excretion and reduced intestinal absorption of vitamin D and low circulating 25-hydroxyvitamin D levels. In addition, low circulating 25-hydroxyvitamin D levels and rickets may occur secondary to reduced conversion of vitamin D to 25-hydroxyvitamin D, as a result of hepatocellular damage. Rickets associated with hepatobiliary disorders may be treated with 25-hydroxyvitamin D in doses of 1 to 3 μg/kg/day.

Defects in vitamin D metabolism are observed in other disorders, including (1) as previously discussed, X-linked hypophosphatemic rickets, in which there is impaired responsiveness of the renal 25-hydroxyvitamin D 1α-hydroxylase to either phosphorus depletion or parathyroid hormone; (2) oncogenic rickets or osteomalacia, in which low levels of circulating 1,25-dihydroxyvitamin D are found in the presence of hypophosphatemia; and (3) rickets associated with anticonvulsant therapy. The last two conditions are discussed in Chapter 11 by Dr. Parfitt.

I. End-Organ Refractoriness to 1,25-Dihydroxyvitamin D (Vitamin D–Dependent Rickets Type II)

Vitamin D–dependent rickets type II is a relatively rare disorder in which the clinical, radiologic, and most of the biochemical features are similar to those found in vitamin D–dependent rickets type I.[160–168] Similar to the type I disorder, the clinical findings include growth failure, hypotonia, muscle weakness, convulsions, and bony deformities of the classic vitamin D deficiency rickets. The biochemical findings that occur in common in vitamin D–dependent rickets type I and type II include hypocalcemia, hypophosphatemia, elevated serum alkaline phosphatase activity, elevated serum immunoreactive parathyroid hormone, and increased urinary excretion of cyclic AMP and amino acids. In contrast to vitamin D–dependent rickets type I, in which impaired 25-hydroxyvitamin D-1α-hydroxylase activity results in decreased 1,25-dihydroxyvitamin D levels, patients with the type II disorder have markedly elevated serum 1,25-dihydroxyvitamin D levels that may range from 140 to 745 pg/ml. The elevated circulating 1,25-dihydroxyvitamin D levels in patients with vitamin D–dependent rickets type II is consistent with end-organ refractoriness to this metabolite. In the untreated state, the serum 25-hydroxyvitamin D and 24,25-dihydroxyvitamin D levels tend to be within the normal range. However, in one patient in whom serum 24,25-dihydroxyvitamin D was measured in the untreated state on multiple occasions, the levels were undetectable.[163]

In many of the patients, rickets is noted between 4 and 16 months of age. Although widening of the wrists and ankles was observed at birth in one patient, radiographs were not obtained until 18 months of age when the diagnosis of rickets was made.[163] It is possible, therefore, that vitamin D–dependent rickets type II may be present at birth in some infants. On the other hand, in another patient, symptoms of bone pain did not appear until 12 years of age and the diagnosis of vitamin D–dependent rickets type II was made at 14 years of age.[168] Many, but not all, of the patients are resistant to therapy with pharmacologic doses of vitamin D and vitamin D metabolites including 1,25-dihydroxyvitamin D.

A unique feature in many patients with vitamin D–dependent rickets type II is total body and scalp alopecia. The alopecia may be evident at birth. Scalp biopsy has revealed findings typical of alopecia totalis with no abnormal lymphocytic infiltration.[161]

Available evidence indicates that an autosomal recessive inheritance is the most likely mode of transmission of vitamin D–dependent rickets type II. Consanguinity has been reported in several kindreds with this disorder. No clinical, radiologic, or biochemical abnormalities have been observed in unaffected first-degree relatives.

A number of studies have been carried out to investigate the pathogenesis of vitamin D–dependent rickets type II. The steps required for the action of 1,25-dihydroxyvitamin D at the cellular level include entry of hormone into the cell, binding of hormone to a cytosol-receptor protein, entry of the cytosol-receptor hormone complex into the nucleus, and interaction of the cytosol-receptor hormone complex with nuclear receptor sites, which result in increased transcription of structural genes and subsequent appearance of new messenger RNA and protein in the cytoplasm.

An interaction of 1,25-dihydroxyvitamin D with cultured skin fibroblasts has been reported in several studies. Specifically the following have been demonstrated in cultured skin fibroblasts from normal individuals: (1) immunoassayable 1,25-dihydroxyvitamin D_3 receptors in extracts of the cultured fibroblasts[169]; (2) cytosol binding of $[^3H]$1,25-dihydroxyvitamin D[170]; (3) nuclear binding of $[^3H]$1,25-dihydroxyvitamin D_3 following whole cell uptake of this metabolite[171]; (4) stimulation of 25-hydroxyvitamin D-24-hydroxylase activity by 1,25-dihydroxyvitamin D_3 in normal fibroblast monolayers[172]; and (5) inhibition of fibroblast cell growth by 1,25-dihydroxyvitamin D_3.[173]

These techniques have been employed in several studies to investigate possible receptor defects in patients with vitamin D–dependent rickets type II.[172–181] The results of these studies will be briefly summarized:

1. Extracts from cultured fibroblasts of normal subjects and patients with vitamin D–dependent rickets type II were evaluated for receptors by immunoassay with a monoclonal antibody to the chick 1,25-dihydroxyvitamin D receptor. The results demonstrated that a protein sedimenting at 3.7 S and recognizable by the antibody exists in comparable concentrations in cells from both normal and resistant patients, regardless of the hormone-binding abnormalities of the cells. It has been suggested that the clinical manifestations of 1,25-dihydroxyvitamin D_3 resistance in D–dependent rickets type II are rarely, if ever, due to the absence of receptor, which suggests structural variations in the receptor molecule rather than deficient receptor synthesis. The remainder of the discussion is based on the supposition that patients with D–dependent rickets type II have immunoassayable receptors comparable to normal in the skin fibroblasts.

2. Absent or markedly reduced cytosolic receptor binding of 1,25-dihydroxyvitamin D has been observed in several patients. In the presence of immunoassayable receptors, the defect in receptor binding suggests internal changes in the receptor molecule, which might include molecular instability or lack of conformational changes inducible by 1,25-dihydroxyvitamin D.

3. Normal cytosolic receptor binding of 1,25-dihydroxyvitamin D, but reduced or absent nuclear uptake of 1,25-dihydroxyvitamin D, suggests reduced capacity to bind to nuclear sites or DNA.

4. Normal cytosolic receptor binding and nuclear uptake of 1,25-dihydroxyvitamin D is suggestive of a postreceptor defect. The failure of 1,25-dihydroxyvitamin D to stimulate 24-hydroxylase activity in these fibroblasts is also consistent with a postreceptor defect.

In a recent study, cells were cultured from explants of long bone of one patient with vitamin D–dependent rickets type II and from a normal control subject.[182] The cultured cells showed morphologic features of fibroblasts but contained alkaline phosphatase activity without detectable acid phosphatase activity, indicating an osteoblastic origin for some or all of the cultured cells. Both cytosolic binding and nuclear uptake of 1,25-dihydroxyvitamin D were demonstrated in the fibroblasts from the normal subject. In the patient with vitamin D–dependent rickets type II, there was normal cytosol binding of 1,25-dihydroxyvitamin D but unmeasurable uptake of 1,25-dihydroxyvitamin D into nuclei. These findings were indistinguishable from those obtained with fibroblast cultured from the skin of the same patient.

Alopecia is a unique feature of many patients with vitamin D–dependent rickets type II. Whether the alopecia represents a separate but linked genetic abnormality or in some way is related to an effect of 1,25-dihydroxyvitamin D is uncertain. It is of interest that nuclear uptake of 1,25-dihydroxyvitamin D has been demonstrated in the outer root sheaths of the rat hair follicle.[183] In a recent study, saturable binding of 1,25-dihydroxyvitamin D to cytosol receptor protein was demonstrated in the epidermal keratinocytes and dermal fibroblasts grown from normal human skin.[173] In this study, specific saturable binding of 1,25-dihydroxyvitamin D to cytosol receptor protein could not be demonstrated in either epidermal keratinocytes or dermal fibroblasts grown from a patient with vitamin D–dependent rickets type II.

Megadoses of vitamin D and vitamin D metabolites have been used in the treatment of vitamin D–dependent rickets type II.[160–167,172–182] Doses as large as 7 million IU/day of vitamin D_2, 5000 μg/day of 25-hydroxyvitamin D, 150 μg/day of 1α-hydroxyvitamin D, and 35 μg/day of 1,25-dihydroxyvitamin D have been administered. With these forms of therapy, circulating levels of 1,25-dihydroxyvitamin D that were 10 to 100 times normal were achieved. Some patients responded to these pharmacologic doses of vitamin D and vitamin D metabolites, but many did not. Patients with alopecia appear to be more resistant to treatment than are patients without alopecia.

As pointed out previously, the induction of 24,25-dihydroxyvitamin D synthesis by 1,25-dihydroxyvitamin D has been found to be impaired in cultured skin fibroblasts obtained from patients with vitamin D–dependent rickets type II. This raises the question of whether the *in vivo* induction of 24,25-dihydroxyvitamin D synthesis by vitamin D and vitamin D metabolites is impaired in these patients. In vitamin D–deficient patients treated with small doses of vitamin D,[184] and in patients with vitamin D–dependent rickets type I treated with small doses of 1α-hydroxyvitamin D,[185] marked increases in serum 24,25-dihydroxyvitamin D concentrations occurred independently of significant changes in serum concentrations of its precursor. By contrast, in several patients with vitamin D–dependent rickets type II treated with pharmacologic doses of 25-hydroxyvitamin D (which raised the serum 25-hydroxyvitamin D level to five times normal), 1α-hydroxyvitamin D, or 1,25-dihydroxyvitamin D, the serum 24,25-dihydroxyvitamin D level did not rise above normal.[172,177,178] On the other hand, treatment of one patient with vitamin D–dependent rickets type II with 7 million IU/day of vitamin D_2 resulted in a serum 24,25-hydroxyvitamin D level that was approximately 10 times greater than normal in the presence of a serum 1,25-dihydroxyvitamin D level that was 180 times greater than normal. It is possible that the markedly elevated serum 25-hydroxyvitamin D level in this patient accounts for the increase in serum 24,25-dihydroxyvitamin D level. Additional studies are needed to better clarify the relation of impaired induction of 24-hydroxylase activity in fibroblasts *in vitro* to the *in vivo* formation of 24,25-dihydroxyvitamin D in patients with D–dependent rickets type II.

There is a report of two children with vitamin D–resistant rickets type II and alopecia in whom severe rickets persisted for several years while they were being treated with 50,000 to 60,000 IU/day of vitamin D_2.[179] When the two children reached and passed the age of 7 to 9 years, they showed apparently spontaneous unexplained healing of the rachitic changes. The alopecia was unchanged; the bone healing was accompanied by normalization of serum phosphorus and by significant reduction of alkaline phosphatase activity. The process was not brought about by any change in vitamin D therapy or mineral supplementation, which had been the same for several years. The mechanism responsible for the unexpected healing in these children is uncertain. Apparently a mechanism that was not operative during the first years of life began to function in later years and led to the healing process. Skin fibroblast receptor studies during the end of the healing process in one patient and at the time of severe rickets in the other revealed severe defects in both, namely, nondetectable binding both in cytosol and in whole cell nuclear receptor assays. Thus, healing was apparently not due to a mechanism that restored receptor binding to normal. It is possible that metabolites of vitamin D, other than 1,25-dihydroxyvitamin D, played a role in the spontaneous healing process. It has been suggested that spontaneous healing may have occurred in other cases reported in the literature in which the healing process was ascribed to specific treatment regimens, such as megadoses of vitamin D_2 or 24,25-dihydroxyvitamin D_3.[162,164]

In contrast to the preceding, there is a report of healing of rickets and catch-up growth between 27 months and 6 years of age in a patient with D–dependent rickets type II and alopecia who was treated with 4 to 5 μg/day of 1α-hydroxyvitamin D.[178] While the child was on this therapy, relapse occurred shortly after the age of 6 years and persisted in spite of increasing doses of 1α-hydroxyvitamin D. During the relapse, the child maintained circulating 1,25-dihydroxyvitamin D levels comparable to those found previously when she received and had responded to similar therapy. It was concluded that a change in a degree of resistance to 1,25-dihydroxyvitamin D occurred during the evolution of her disease.

More recently, long-term administration of parenteral calcium has been shown to completely correct skeletal abnormalities and serum biochemical alterations in this disorder.[185a]

II. OSTEOPENIA IN CHILDHOOD: AN APPROACH TO THE CHILD WITH RADIOGRAPHIC EVIDENCE OF DECREASED BONE MASS

Osteopenia should be recognized as a general term for diminished bone mass, as determined radiographically, with no inference to histologic, biochemical, or etiologic features. Osteopenia is present in osteoporosis and in osteomalacia. *Osteoporosis* literally means sparse or "porous" bone, and implies that an abnormally decreased amount of bone tissue is present per unit volume of the skeleton. The diminished amounts of skeletal matrix are appropriately mineralized. Osteoporosis may result from any imbalance between bone matrix production and degradation such that the net accumulation of bone matrix is diminished.

Osteomalacia, meaning soft or "malleable" bone, refers to skeletal tissue with undermineralized osteoid. There may be overproduction of matrix, further diminishing the proportion of osteoid that is actually mineralized. Osteomalacia connotes a defect in the mineralization of appropriately or even excessively produced bone matrix, whereas osteoporosis refers to defective accumulation of bone matrix, resulting in the paucity of available osteoid for mineralization. Historical usage of the term "osteomalacia" has been reserved for descriptions of trabecular bone, whereas the term "rickets" refers to the analogous process occurring at the epiphyseal growth plate in growing bone (see Chapter 11).

Since osteopenia is a radiographic feature of both osteomalacia and osteoporosis, differentiation between the two may not be possible radiographically. In an adult or in a child who is growing poorly, the characteristic features of rickets may be absent, such that any distinct diagnosis requires histologic examination. Furthermore, it has been suggested that certain cases of childhood bone disease, particularly hypophosphatemic hypercalciuria, manifest osteomalacia but not rickets.[186] However, undermineralization and excess osteoid production are generally thought to occur more commonly at both trabecular and epiphyseal sites rather than isolated to one area alone. Osteoporosis may occur in conjunction with osteomalacia, although more so in the elderly. (See Chapter 12). Even where a paucity of osteoid is present, it may become poorly mineralized.

A. Presentation of Osteopenia in Childhood

Although it is considerably less common in childhood than in adulthood, children do come to the attention of a physician with evidence of osteopenia. Osteomalacia in children usually presents with the physical findings associated with concomitant rickets. Alterations in blood chemistry (calcium, phosphorus, and alkaline phosphatase) may also indicate the presence of osteomalacia. When isolated osteopenia does face the physician, differentiation between osteomalacia and osteoporosis must be sought so that a rational therapy, if available, suited to the appropriate pathophysiologic process can be instituted.

Presentations of such children vary widely. Some patients suffer repetitive fracturing throughout early life. Infants with osteopenic disorders have been inappropriately diagnosed as having "battered children syndrome." Older children may complain of back pain, develop kyphosis deformities,[187] and refuse to walk. In addition to disorders in which osteopenia may be a major feature, there are numerous conditions in which osteopenia may be an associated finding and not the primary manifestation of the disease. In others, osteopenia is incidentally noted on radiographs obtained following accidental trauma, or for the determination of skeletal age.

B. Major Childhood Osteopenias

This section is concerned with those disorders in which osteopenia may bring the patient to the physician's attention.

1. Inborn Errors of Metabolism and Other Genetically Related Conditions

a. Osteogenesis Imperfecta

This term describes a heterogeneous group of diseases that are clinically manifested by osseous fragility. Incidence is estimated as 1 in 15,000 live births.[188] The skeletal lesion, attributed to the production of abnormal bone matrix resulting from defective collagen synthesis or assembly,[189] is discussed in Chapter 17.

b. Homocystinuria[190]

"Homocystinuria" refers to several disorders of methionine metabolism resulting in increased blood and urinary homocystine. The prototype disorder, due to cystathionine synthase deficiency, is discussed here, although variants include defective synthesis of cobalamin coenzyme or deficiency of methyltetrahydrofolate reductase. Characteristic clinical features include dislocated lens, mild to moderate mental retardation, seizures, and a malar flush. The most common finding of ectopia lentis leads to diagnosis in many cases. Other features are not as constant. Vascular thrombosis is a common fatal event.

Skeletal abnormalities resemble those in Marfan's syndrome, including kyphosis, scoliosis, pectus excavatum and carinatum, and arachnodactyly. There is a consistent, marked osteoporosis, which may predispose the skeleton to disfiguration. The spine appears to be the most common site of osteoporosis, rather than long bones.

Diagnosis is made by the presence of homocysteine or homocystine in urine. The urinary cyanide-nitroprusside reaction is a reasonable screen, although false-positive and false-negative results occur. Management has included low-methionine diets and large amounts of pyridoxine as well as supportive management of complications.

The skeletal defect is thought to result from homocystine interference with collagen crosslinking. Two mechanisms have been implicated, one involving impaired aldehyde formation of the side-chain amino group of lysine (preventing access of lysyl oxidase to lysine residues) and the other involving a more complex crosslinking defect. D-penicillamine is thought to inhibit crosslinking by similar mechanisms.

c. Lysinuric Protein Intolerance[191,192]

Osteopenia is an almost constant feature of this inherited disorder of amino acid transport. Episodic vomiting, anorexia, hepatomegaly, protein aversion, or unexplained osteopenia may bring the child to the physician's attention. A definitive dietary history is essential, since subtle protein avoidance may escape parental notice. Variable neurologic features (related to episodic hyperammonemia) may occur, including seizures, stupor, coma, and even death. Hence, early diagnosis is important.

The pathophysiologic mechanism involves defective transport of dibasic amino acids (ornithine, lysine, and arginine) at the intestine, in the renal tubule, and into the hepatocyte. Circulating levels of dibasic amino acids are decreased, and defective hepatocellular transport of arginine and ornithine effectively limits urea cycle activity. Protein is therefore inadequately metabolized to urea, generating hyperammonemia. Renal tubular reabsorption of dibasic amino acids is impaired, often resulting in increased urinary excretion. Characteristically massive lysine excretion occurs. Generalized aminoaciduria may be present, obscuring the dibasic aminoaciduria and potentially misleading the physician.

Physical findings include muscular atrophy and thin extremities and may involve increased centripetal fat distribution. Variable liver enlargement occurs, and splenomegaly may occur.

Diagnosis is confirmed by hyperammonemia following an intravenous alanine infusion. Other laboratory abnormalities include elevations in AST and ALT, and very marked elevations in LDH. Granulocytopenia, thrombocytopenia, and a slight normochromic anemia have been reported.

Therapy has been most successful with dietary supplementation of citrulline, which is adequately transported into the hepatocyte and fuels the urea cycle, enhancing protein metabolism. Citrulline promotes markedly improved protein tolerance, improved well-being, and increased mineralization of the skeleton. Liver abnormalities persist, however, and the long-term prognosis of the condition has not been established.

Osteopenia is evident on radiographs. Histomorphometric analysis in one patient revealed markedly decreased volume of bone, with normal osteoid volume and osteoid surface.

This osteoporosis could theoretically be due to a specific deficiency of lysine, an essential component of collagen. A severe restriction of protein intake, however, is well known to result in osteoporosis and seems to be a sufficient explanation.

d. Menkes Kinky Hair Syndrome[193]

Menkes kinky hair syndrome is an X-linked disorder characterized by defective intestinal absorption of copper and defective accumulation of copper in tissues. Copper-dependent enzyme systems are deficient, resulting in abnormal hair, neuronal degeneration, and hypothermia. Arterial degeneration is thought to be related to defective elastin synthesis. Osteoporosis is due to defective collagen synthesis. Elastin and collagen require the copper-dependent enzyme lysyl oxidase for conversion of the amino side-chain of lysine to an aldehyde, thereby allowing normal cross-linkage to occur.

Skeletal changes associated with copper deficiency (i.e., infants receiving prolonged total parenteral nutrition and infants of very low birth weight) are often indistinguishable from rickets seen in premature children and may include subperiosteal new bone formation and metaphyseal spurs.[194–196]

e. Osteoporosis with Hypouricemia and Hypercalciuria

Sperling and colleagues have described a kindred with an unusual syndrome involving three adults, a 9-year-old boy, and a 4-year-old girl.[197] The boy showed overt radiographic osteopenia with thin epiphyseal and metaphyseal cortices. The girl was not examined radiographically. Both children were healthy, well-developed, and of normal stature. Of the three adults, two had moderate to severe complaints of bone pain. Although no fractures had been evident, radiographic examination revealed compression fractures of vertebrae in the adult propositus. All five individuals had hypouricemia and hypercalciuria. The propositus had a marked increase in renal uric acid clearance, which could be suppressed by pyrazinamide. No other metabolic abnormalities were detected.

f. Turner's Syndrome

Turner's syndrome, strictly speaking, is a chromosomal defect and not a specific inborn error of metabolism. The reported frequency of osteopenia in Turner's syndrome varies from 31% to 86%.[198] Hypogonadism is known to be associated with osteopenia, but girls with Turner's syndrome often have evidence of osteopenia long before puberty. The abnormalities could be associated with missing X chromosomal material or related to absence of estrogen early in life. Patients treated with estrogen have a lesser degree of demineralization as assessed by photon absorption,[199] although others have suggested that long-term estrogen therapy is not useful.[200] There are no well-controlled long-term studies of therapeutic estrogen in this syndrome. The osteoporosis is generally asymptomatic in childhood; however, a predisposition to severe adulthood osteoporosis is of concern (see Chapter 12).

Microradiographic analysis of iliac crest biopsies demonstrated increased bone resorptive surfaces in six of eight patients with Turner's syndrome.[201] These six patients had decreased bone density, whereas the remaining girls had normal bone density. In this study, parameters of bone formation, cortical thickness, trabecular thickness, and osteoid width were normal in all patients.

2. Acquired

a. Transient Osteoporosis of Childhood

Transient osteoporosis of childhood, often referred to as idiopathic juvenile osteoporosis, usually becomes evident just before puberty.[202,203] Additional reports[204,205] suggest that this entity may occur throughout childhood (age of onset 19 months to 23 years). Kooh et al.[205] have noted the usual transient nature of the condition, and thus we prefer their term, "transient osteoporosis of childhood." A note of caution: rarely such individuals have sustained osteoporosis.

Patients with transient osteoporosis of childhood present most commonly because of pain in the weight-bearing skeleton, specifically in the thoracolumbar spine, ankles, distal tibia, or knee (either distal femur or proximal tibia). Abnormalities in gait may be evident. There is no family history of similar bone disease. Radiographic evaluation shows generalized osteopenia. Vertebral compression fractures in the thoracolumbar area and metaphyseal compression fractures may occur.[202–207] Marked osteopenia in the metaphyseal region of new bone formation (referred to as neo-osseous porosis)[202–205,208] is said to be pathognomonic of transient osteoporosis of childhood. In late stages of this disorder, narrowed bones, similar to those in osteogenesis imperfecta, have been observed.[206–208]

The trabecular bone has reduced numbers

of osteoblasts in almost all biopsies reported.[204,208,209] Although there are increased areas of trabecular surface showing the irregular appearance characteristic of resorption, little osteoclastic activity is seen.[204,205,208] This suggests that transient osteoporosis of childhood results from reduced osteoblastic activity that is unable to keep pace with a normal (or even reduced) resorption rate. Furthermore, tetracycline labeling of trabecular bone may be abnormal.[205] Of interest, cortical bone does not seem to be involved in this process—osteoblasts are present, and this bone is normally labeled with tetracycline.[205]

Serum calcium, phosphorus, and alkaline phosphatase are usually normal, and urinary calcium excretion has been reported as normal, increased, and low.[202–208] Increased hydroxyproline excretion and a negative calcium balance[203,205,207] are characteristic of transient osteoporosis of childhood. A positive calcium balance, however, may be seen in recovering or healed patients.[203–205,207] Despite negative calcium balance, no generalized abnormalities in gastrointestinal absorption have been found.[203,204] Assessment of specific mucosal transport of divalent cations has not been performed.

The negative calcium balance could be related to decreased serum 1,25-dihydroxyvitamin D levels, which were observed in one patient with transient osteoporosis of childhood.[206] Calcitriol supplementation led to improvement of the osteopenia and normal 1,25-dihydroxyvitamin D. In contrast, we have noted normal circulating levels of 1,25-dihydroxyvitamin D in three patients during the active phase of their disease (unpublished data). Another patient[209] had an elevated 1,25-dihydroxyvitamin D level (300 pg/ml) that became normal as the condition resolved. Circulating immunoreactive parathyroid hormone has been reported as elevated relative to the serum calcium[210] but was not elevated in three patients we sampled.

Traditional management has consisted of providing adequate dietary calcium (greater than 1.0 g elemental calcium per day) and vitamin D to maintain a normal serum level of 25-hydroxyvitamin D. The active disease resolves spontaneously in nearly all patients, but in approximately 25% there is residual deformity yielding altered gait or markedly reduced stature. Some patients are confined to wheelchairs and are up to 35 mm shorter than their anticipated adult height.[203] However, in the majority of patients, growth resumes and the normal pubertal growth spurt is observed.[202–210]

The diagnosis of transient osteoporosis of childhood may be elusive in mild cases or in younger age groups.[204,205,208] Patients with kyphosis in childhood may also have undiagnosed transient osteoporosis of childhood.[208,211,212] The importance of establishing the diagnosis, since no specific treatment is currently available, is to assure appropriate genetic counseling for patients with osteogenesis imperfecta, and to avoid an inappropriate accusation of child abuse.

b. Malnutrition

Celiac disease and protein-calorie malnutrition may result in osteopenia. Poor matrix formation may occur that is, in general, appropriately mineralized. Copper deficiency may also result in skeletal deformities, including osteoporosis. Impaired activity of the copper-dependent enzyme lysyl oxidase results in defective crosslinking of collagen. Lysyl oxidase catalyzes the conversion of the side-chain amino group of lysine to an aldehyde, which is, in turn, involved in the crosslinking reaction. Copper deficiency is rare but may occur during total parenteral nutrition[213] in generalized malnutrition and in cases of prolonged diarrhea. Hospital diets may be low in copper content.[214] Certain dried milk formulas in Japan and Europe are not supplemented with copper; at least one case of copper deficiency osteopenia has resulted from the use of such a formula in Japan.[215] As noted earlier, lesions that resemble rickets may be seen on radiographs.[194–196]

c. Immobilization

This well-known cause of osteoporosis is poorly understood. Severe trauma, myelodysplasia, and juvenile rheumatoid arthritis (JRA) are predisposing conditions for this problem in children, although the etiologic factor of osteopenia in JRA is not certain[216] (see Chapter 12).

d. Hypercortisolism

As detailed in Chapter 12, an excess of endogenous glucocorticoids may result in osteopenia and decreased growth in children, although other features of hypercortisolism are also usually evident. Management includes treatment of endogenous Cushing's disease, attempts to maintain therapy of chronic disease with calcium supplements, alternate-day steroid therapy, and use of vitamin D or one of its metabolites. The recent marketing of a new diene derivative of prednisolone (deflazacort), which possesses all the anti-inflammatory and therapeutic potential of prednisone with much less effect on the skeleton and statural growth in children, should add a new dimension to our therapeutic approach (see Chapter 12). Calcitonin, which is decreased in steroid-treated patients,[217] has also been used effectively to prevent bone loss in animal models treated with large doses of glucocorticoids.[218]

e. Leukemia

Leukemia has presented with osteoporosis before abnormal cellular forms were evident in the peripheral circulation. An impressive and worrisome account of acute leukemia presenting as childhood osteoporosis is offered by Friedman and Dent.[202]

C. Childhood Diseases in Which Osteopenia May Occur as an Associated Finding

Many other disorders in childhood, not mentioned in the preceding, may be complicated by osteopenia. In such conditions, osteopenia is seen but is usually not the presenting feature. Osteopenia has been reported in various endocrinopathies including thyrotoxicosis, acromegaly, diabetes mellitus, and hyperparathyroidism (see Chapter 12). Hypogonadism may contribute to osteopenia; such is the mechanism speculated for the osteopenia seen in Klinefelter's and Noonan's syndromes, as well as in hyperprolactinemia. Lactating adolescent mothers have been shown to have decreased bone mass. Heparin therapy is associated with osteopenia, as is mastocytosis. Increased erythropoietic activity enlarges the marrow spaces and results in osteopenia, a severe problem in certain patients with thalassemia. Osteopenia has also been noted in Down's syndrome, in Wilson's disease, and in other severe chronic diseases such as cystic fibrosis.

D. Investigation of the Child with Osteopenia

We approach the child with unexplained fractures or osteopenia with the preceding entities in mind. Many of the diagnoses are strongly suggested by history or careful physical examination. For instance, a family history of early onset deafness or dental problems may suggest osteogenesis imperfecta, whereas a distaste for milk may suggest lysinuric protein intolerance.

A decreased serum calcium and phosphate and increased serum alkaline phosphatase activity indicate that osteomalacia is a component of the disorder. Determination of urinary calcium and phosphate excretion and measurement of serum immunoreactive parathyroid hormone and vitamin D metabolites may also be helpful. Mineral balance studies are of interest from an investigational standpoint.

In the absence of any evidence of a primary osteomalacia, serum copper, bicarbonate, uric acid, urine and serum amino acid levels, and occasionally chromosomal analysis (in females) is performed. A search for evidence of Cushing's syndrome should be performed if even subtle cushingoid manifestations are present. If the child is severely affected, yet with no features of any specific disorder, a bone marrow aspirate may be necessary and could be performed during a bone biopsy procedure if employed. More often than not, no definitive diagnosis is evident and one is left with distinguishing between transient osteoporosis of childhood and mild osteogenesis imperfecta. A provisional diagnosis of one or the other of these two disorders is usually made based on whatever characteristic clinical features of these conditions are present in the child.

Such patients should be evaluated where complete medical and orthopedic services are available. Bone histology with tetracycline labeling as presented in Chapter 10 may be useful. Serial determination of bone density as detailed in Chapter 9, using photon absorptiometry, is useful in monitoring the course of disease (see Chapter 12). Any experimental therapy should employ careful monitoring of bone histopathology. Even with careful attention to detail, it may be difficult to ascertain whether any improvements in transient osteoporosis of childhood result from therapy or merely reflect the natural history of the condition. Indeed, definitive diagnosis may not be apparent until the course is observed for some time.

References

1. Cone TE Jr: History of rickets in America. *In* Cone TE (ed): 200 Years of Infant Feeding in America. Columbus, Ohio, Ross Laboratories, 1976, pp 57–73.

2. Whistler D: De morbo puerile anglorum patrio idiomate indigenae vocant the rickets. Leyden, Lugduni Batavorum, 1645.
3. Glisson F: De rachitide sive morbo puerili gui vulgo, the rickets dictur. London, 1650.
4. Albright F, Butler AH, Bloomberg E: Rickets resistant to vitamin D therapy. Am J Dis Child 54:529–547, 1937.
5. Harrison HE, Harrison HC: Rickets and osteomalacia. *In* Harrison HE, Harrison HC (eds): Disorders of Calcium and Phosphate Metabolism in Childhood and Adolescence. Philadelphia, WB Saunders, 1979, pp 141–256.
6. Underwood JL, DeLuca HF: Vitamin D is not directly necessary for bone growth and mineralization. Am J Physiol 246:E493–E498, 1984.
7. Weinstein RS, Underwood JL, Hutson MS, DeLuca HF: Bone histomorphometry in vitamin D–deficient rats infused with calcium and phosphorus. Am J Physiol 246:E499–E505, 1984.
8. Bordier P, Ramussen H, Marie P, et al: Vitamin D metabolites and bone mineralization in man. J Clin Endocrinol Metab 46:284–294, 1978.
9. Rasmussen H: The role of 1,25(OH)D_3 in the pathogenesis of osteomalacia. *In* Frame B, Potts JT Jr (eds): Clinical Disorders of Bone and Mineral Metabolism. Amsterdam, Excerpta Medica, 1983, pp 82–89.
10. Chesney RU, Zimmerman J, Hamstra A, et al: Vitamin D metabolite concentrations in vitamin D deficiency. Are calcitriol levels normal? Am J Dis Child 135:1025–1028, 1981.
11. Venkataraman PS, Tsang RC, Buckley DD, et al: Elevation of serum 1,25-dihydroxyvitamin D in response to physiologic doses of vitamin D in vitamin D–deficient infants. J Pediatr 103:416–419, 1983.
12. Markestad T, Halvorsen S, Halvorsen SK: Plasma concentrations of vitamin D metabolites before and during treatment of vitamin D–deficiency rickets in children. Acta Paediatr Scand 73:225–231, 1984.
13. Harrison JE, Hitchman AJW, Jones G, et al: Plasma vitamin D metabolite levels in phosphorus deficient rats during the development of vitamin D deficient rickets. Metabolism 32:1121–1127, 1982.
14. Tam CS, Jones G, Heerscke JNM: The effect of vitamin D restriction and repletion on bone apposition in the rat and its dependence on parathyroid hormone. Endocrinology 109:1448–1453, 1981.
15. Pettifor JM, Isdale JM, Sahakian J, Hansen J: Diagnosis of subclinical rickets. Arch Dis Child 55:155–157, 1980.
16. Dent CE, Stamp TCB: Vitamin D rickets and osteomalacia. *In* Avioli LV, Krane SM (eds): Metabolic Bone Diseases. New York, Academic Press, 1977, pp 237–305.
17. Dwyer JT, Dietz DH Jr, Hass G, Siskind R: Risk of nutritional rickets among vegetarian children. Am J Dis Child 133:134–140, 1979.
18. Edidin DV, Levitsky LL, Schey W, et al: Resurgence of nutritional rickets associated with breast feeding and special dietary practices. Pediatrics 65:232–235, 1980.
19. Garabedian M, Vainset M, Mallet E, et al: Circulating vitamin D metabolite concentrations in children with nutritional rickets. J Pediatr 103:381–386, 1983.
20. Castile RG, Marks LJ, Stickler GB: Vitamin D deficiency rickets: Two cases with faulty infant feeding practices. Am J Dis Child 129:964–966, 1975.
21. O'Hara-May J, Widdowson EM: Diets and living conditions of Asian boys in Coventry with and without signs of rickets. Br J Nutr 36:23–26, 1976.
22. Robertson I, Ford JA, McIntosh WB, Dunnigan MG: The role of cereals in the aetiology of nutritional rickets: The lesson of the Irish National Nutrition Survey 1943–8. Br J Nutr 45:17–22, 1981.
23. Stroder J: Immunity in vitamin D deficient rickets. *In* Norman AW (ed): Vitamin D and Problems Related to Uremic Bone Disease: Proceedings Second Workshop on Vitamin D, Wiesbaden, West Germany, October 1974. Berlin, de Gruyter, 1975, pp 675–687.
24. Lorente F, Fontan G, Jara P, et al: Defective neutrophil motility in hypovitaminosis D rickets. Acta Paediatr Scand 65: 695–699, 1976.
25. Bar-Shavit Z, Noff D, Edelstein S, et al: 1,25-dihydroxyvitamin D and the regulation of macrophage function. Calcif Tissue Int 33:673–676, 1981.
26. Yetgin S, Ozsoylu S: Myeloid metaplasia in vitamin D deficiency rickets. Scand J Haematol 28:180–185, 1982.
27. Kruse K, Bartels H, Kracht U: Parathyroid function in different stages of vitamin D deficiency rickets. Eur J Pediatr 141:158–162, 1984.
28. Raghuramulu N, Reddy V: Serum 25-hydroxyvitamin D levels in malnourished children with rickets. Arch Dis Child 55:285–287, 1980.
29. Reddy V, Srikantia SG: Serum alkaline phosphatase in malnourished children with rickets. J Pediatr 71:595–597, 1967.
30. Fraser D, Kooh SW, Scriver CR: Hyperparathyroidism as the cause of hyperaminoaciduria and phosphaturia in human vitamin D deficiency. Pediatr Res 1:425–435, 1967.
31. Hochberg Z, Hardoff D: Quantitative assessment of nutritional rickets by urinary phosphorus excretion. Short communication. Acta Paediatr Scand 70:579–580, 1981.
32. Mallet E, Nguyen T, Garabedian M, Bassuyau JP: Circulating parathyroid hormone and dihydroxylated vitamin D metabolites after oral 25-hydroxycholecalciferol in infantile rickets. Horm Metab Res 14:503–504, 1982.
33. Rowe JD, Wood DH, Rowe DW, Raisz LG: Nutritional hypophosphatemic rickets in a premature infant fed breast milk. N Engl J Med 300:292–296, 1979.
34. Sagy M, Birenbaum E, Balin A, et al: Phosphate depletion syndrome in a premature infant fed human milk. J Pediatr 96:683–685, 1980.
35. Kovar IZ, Mayne PD, Robbe I: Hypophosphatemic rickets in the pre-term infant: Hypocalcemia after calcium and phosphorus supplementation. Arch Dis Child 58:629–631, 1983.
36. Lapatsanis P, Makaronis G, Vretos C, Doxiadis S: Two types of nutritional rickets in infants. Am J Clin Nutr 29:1222–1226, 1976.
37. Heaney RP, Skillman TG: Calcium metabolism in normal human pregnancy. J Clin Endocrinol Metab 33:661–670, 1971.
38. Ziegler EE, O'Donnell AM, Nelson SE, et al: Body composition of the reference fetus. Growth 40:329–341, 1976.

39. Gray PW, Wilz DR, Caldus AE, et al: The importance of phosphate in regulating plasma 1,25(OH)$_2$ vitamin D levels in humans: Studies in healthy subjects in calcium-stone formers and in patients with primary hyperparathyroidism. J Clin Endocrinol Metab 45:299–306, 1977.
40. Goldfarb S, Westby GR, Goldberg M, et al: Renal tubular effects of chronic phosphate depletion. J Clin Invest 59:770–779, 1977.
41. Reade TM, Scriver CR: Hypophosphatemic rickets and breast milk. N Engl J Med 300:1397, 1979.
42. Bloom WL, Flinchum D: Osteomalacia with pseudofractures caused by the ingestion of aluminum hydroxide. JAMA 174:1327–1330, 1960.
43. Lotz M, Ney R, Bartter FC: Osteomalacia and debility resulting from phosphorus depletion. Trans Assoc Am Physicians 77:281–295, 1964.
44. Pierides AM, Ellis HA, Kerr DNS: Phosphate-deficiency osteomalacia during regular hemodialysis. Lancet 2:746, 1976.
45. Maltz HE, Fish MB, Holliday MA: Calcium deficiency rickets and the renal response to calcium infusion. Pediatrics 46:865–870, 1970.
46. Kooh SW, Fraser D, Reilly BJ, et al: Rickets due to calcium deficiency. N Engl J Med 297:1264–1266, 1977.
47. Pettifor JM, Ross P, Wang J, et al: Rickets in children of rural origin in South Africa: Is low dietary calcium a factor? Pediatrics 92:320–324, 1978.
48. Pettifor JM, Ross FP, Travers R, et al: Dietary calcium deficiency: A syndrome associated with bone deformities and elevated serum 1,25-dihydroxyvitamin D concentrations. Metab Bone Rel Res 2:301–305, 1981.
49. Marie PJ, Pettifor JM, Ross FP, Glorieux FH: Histological osteomalacia due to dietary calcium deficiency in children. N Engl J Med 307:584–588, 1982.
50. Sulochana G, Balakrishnan S: Calcium deficient puberty rickets with acidosis responding to large dose of oral calcium. J Indian Med Assoc 79:140–142, 1982.
51. Muldowney FP, Donohoe JF, Carroll DV, et al: Parathyroid acidosis in uremia. Q J Med 41:321–342, 1972.
52. Winters RW, Graham JB, Williams TF, et al: A genetic study of familial hypophosphatemia and vitamin D–resistant rickets. Trans Assoc Am Physicians 70:234–242, 1957.
53. Winters RW, Graham JB, Williams TF, et al: A genetic study of familial hypophosphatemia and vitamin D resistant rickets with a review of the literature. Medicine 37:97–142, 1958.
54. Graham JB, McFalls VW, Winters RW: Familial hypophosphatemia with vitamin D–resistant rickets. II. Three additional kindreds of sex-linked dominant type with a genetic analysis of four such families. Am J Hum Genet 11:311–326, 1959.
55. Williams TF, Winters RW: Familial (hereditary) vitamin D–resistant rickets with hypophosphatemia. *In* Stanbury JB, Wyngaarden JB, Fredrickson DS (eds): The Metabolic Basis of Inherited Disease. 3rd ed. New York, McGraw-Hill, 1972, pp 1465–1485.
56. Burnett CH, Dent CE, Harper C, Warland BJ: Vitamin D–resistant rickets: Analysis of 24 pedigrees with hereditary and sporadic cases. Am J Med 36:222–232, 1964.
57. Lyon MF: Sex chromatin and gene action in the mammalian X-chromosome. Am J Hum Genet 14:135–148, 1962.
58. Rasmussen H, Anast C: Familial hypophosphatemic rickets and vitamin D–dependent rickets. *In* Stanbury JB, Wyngaarden JB, Fredrickson DS: The Metabolic Basis of Inherited Disease. 5th ed. New York, McGraw-Hill, 1983, pp 1743–1773.
59. Steendijk R: Studies on growth in refractory rickets. J Pediatr 60:340–345, 1962.
60. Pederson HE, McCarroll HR: Vitamin D resistant rickets. J Bone Joint Surg 33A:203–220, 1951.
61. McNair SL, Stickler GB: Growth in familial hypophosphatemic vitamin D–resistant rickets. N Engl J Med 281:511–516, 1969.
62. Steendijk R, Herweijer TJ: Height, sitting height and leg length in patients with hypophosphatemic rickets. Acta Paediatr Scand 73:181–184, 1984.
63. Tanner JM, Whitehouse RH: Growth charts for sitting height and subischeal leg length (LSHG49 & LSHB51). Hertford, England, Creaseys Ltd, Castlemead.
64. Gallo LG, Merle SG: Spontaneous dental abscesses in vitamin D–resistant rickets: Report of case. J Dent Child 46:55–57, 1979.
65. Rakocz M, Keating J III, Johnson R: Management of the primary dentition in vitamin D–resistant rickets. Br Dent J 154:136–138, 1983.
66. Tulloch EN, Andrews FFH: The association of dental abscesses with vitamin D resistant rickets. Br Dent J 154:136–138, 1983.
67. Cartwright DW, Latham SC, Masel JP, Yelland JDN: Spinal canal stenosis in adult with hypophosphatemic vitamin D–resistant rickets. Aust NZ J Med 9:705–708, 1979.
68. Cartwright DW, Masel JP, Latham SC: The lumbar spinal canal in hypophosphatemic vitamin D–resistant rickets. Aust NZ J Med 11:154–157, 1981.
69. Masel JP, Cartwright DW, Latham SC: Hypophosphatemic vitamin D–resistant rickets—a cause of spinal stenosis in adults. Aust Radiol 25:264–271, 1981.
70. Glorieux F, Scriver CR: Loss of a parathyroid hormone–sensitive component of phosphate transport in X-linked hypophosphatemia. Science 175:997–1000, 1972.
71. Reitz RE, Weinstein RL: Parathyroid hormone secretion in familial vitamin D–resistant rickets. N Engl J Med 289:941–945, 1973.
72. Lewy JE, Cabana EC, Repetto HA, et al: Serum parathyroid hormone in hypophosphatemic vitamin D–resistant rickets. J Pediatr 81:294–298, 1972.
73. Mguyen TM, Guillozo H, Garabedian M, et al: Serum concentration of 24,25-dihydroxyvitamin D in normal children and children with rickets. Pediatr Res 13:973–976, 1979.
74. Mason RS, Rohl PG, Lissner D, Posen S: Vitamin D metabolism in hypophosphatemic rickets. Am J Dis Child 136:909–913, 1982.
75. Drezner MK, Lyles KW, Haussler MR, Harrelson JM: Evaluation of a role for 1,25-dihydroxyvitamin D_3 in the pathogenesis and treatment of X-linked hypophosphatemic rickets and osteomalacia. J Clin Invest 66:1020–1032, 1980.
76. Rasmussen H, Pechet M, Anast C, et al: Long-term treatment of familial hypophosphatemic rickets with oral phosphate and 1α-hydroxyvitamin D_3. J Pediatr 99:16–25, 1981.

77. Lyles KW, Clark AG, Drezner MK: Serum 1,25-dihydroxyvitamin D levels in subjects with X-linked hypophosphatemic rickets and osteomalacia. Calcif Tissue Int 34:125–130, 1982.
78. Lyles KW, Drezner MK: Parathyroid hormone effects on serum 1,25-dihydroxyvitamin D levels in patients with X-linked hypophosphatemic rickets: Evidence for abnormal 25-hydroxyvitamin D-1-hydroxylase activity. J Clin Endocrinol Metab 54:638–644, 1982.
79. Insogna KL, Broadus AE, Gertner JM: Impaired phosphorus conservation and 1,25-dihydroxyvitamin D generation during phosphorus deprivation in familial hypophosphatemic rickets. J Clin Invest 71:1562–1569, 1983.
80. Delvin EE, Glorieux FH: Serum 1,25-dihydroxyvitamin D concentration in hypophosphatemic vitamin D–resistant rickets. Calcif Tissue Int 33:173–175, 1981.
81. Exner GU, Prader A, Elsasser U, et al: Hypophosphatemic vitamin D resistant rickets (phosphate diabetes): Bone mineral problems studied by ^{125}I-computed tomography and microradiography. Helv Paediatr Acta 35:39–49, 1980.
82. Polisson PP, Martinez S, Khoury M, et al: Calcification of entheses associated with X-linked hypophosphatemic osteomalacia. N Engl J Med 313:1–6, 1985.
83. Glorieux FH, Pierre JM, Pettifor JM, Delvin EE: Bone response to phosphate salts, ergocalciferol, and calcitriol in hypophosphatemic vitamin D–resistant rickets. N Engl J Med 303:1023–1031, 1980.
84. Marie PJ, Glorieux FH: Histomorphometric study of bone remodeling in hypophosphatemic vitamin D–resistant rickets. Metab Bone Dis Rel Res 3:31–38, 1981.
85. Marie PJ, Glorieux FH: Relation between cortical periosteocytic lesions and bone mineralization in vitamin D–resistant rickets. Transactions of 27th Annual Meeting of Orthopaedic Research Society, Las Vegas, February 1984.
86. Frost HM: Some observations on bone mineral in a case of vitamin D–resistant rickets. Henry Ford Hosp Med Bull 6:300–310, 1958.
87. Choufoer JH, Steendjik R: Distribution of the perilacunar hypomineralized areas in cortical bone of patients with familial hypophosphatemic (vitamin D–resistant) rickets. Calcif Tissue Int 27:101–104, 1979.
88. Lau K, Goldfarb S, Goldberg M: The effects of parathyroid hormone on renal phosphate handling. *In* Massry SG, Fleisch H (eds): Renal Handling of Phosphate. New York, Plenum, 1980, pp 115–135.
89. Bonjour JP, Fleisch H: Tubular adaptations to the supply and requirement of phosphate. *In* Massry SG, Fleisch H (eds): Renal Handling of Phosphate. New York, Plenum, 1980, pp 243–264.
90. Tenenhouse HS, Scriver CR, McInnes RR, Glorieux FH: Renal handling of phosphate in vivo and in vitro by the X-linked hypophosphatemic male mouse: Evidence for a defect in the brush border membrane. Kidney Int 14:236–244, 1978.
91. Tenenhouse HS, Scriver CR: The defect in transcellular transport of phosphate in the nephron is located in brush-border membranes in X-linked hypophosphatemia (Hyp mouse model). Can J Biochem 56:640–646, 1978.
92. Short E, Morris RC Jr, Sebastian A, Spencer M: Exaggerated phosphaturic response to circulating parathyroid hormone in patients with familial X-linked hypophosphatemic rickets. J Clin Invest 58:152–163, 1976.
93. Alon U, Chan JCM: Effects of parathyroid hormone and 1,25-dihydroxyvitamin D_3 on tubular handling of phosphate in hypophosphatemic rickets. J Clin Endocrinol Metab 58:671–675, 1984.
94. Condon Jr, Nassium JR, Rutter A: Defective intestinal phosphate absorption in familial and non-familial hypophosphatemia. Br Med J 3:138–141, 1970.
95. Chan JCM, Lovinger RD, Mamunes P: Renal hypophosphatemic rickets: Growth acceleration after long-term treatment with 1,25-dihydroxyvitamin D_3. Pediatrics 66:445–454, 1980.
96. Glorieux FH, Morin CL, Travers R, et al: Intestinal phosphate transport in familial hypophosphatemic rickets. Pediatr Res 10:691–696, 1976.
97. Tenenhouse HS: Investigation of the mechanism for abnormal renal 25-hydroxyvitamin D_3-1-hydroxylase activity in the X-linked Hyp mouse. Endocrinology 115:634–639, 1984.
98. Lobaugh B, Drezner MK: Abnormal regulation of renal 25-hydroxyvitamin D-1α-hydroxylase activity in the X-linked hypophosphatemic mouse. J Clin Invest 71:400–403, 1983.
99. Seino Y, Satomura K, Yamaoka K, et al: Activity of renal 25-hydroxyvitamin D-1α-hydroxylase in a case of X-linked hypophosphatemic rickets. Eur J Pediatr 142:219–222, 1984.
100. Seino Y, Yamaoka K, Ishida M, et al: Plasma clearance for high doses of exogenous 1,25-dihydroxy [23,24(n)-^{3}H] cholecalciferol in X-linked hypophosphatemic mice. Biomed Res 3:683–687, 1982.
101. Seino Y, Shimotsuji T, Ishida M, et al: Vitamin D metabolism in hypophosphatemic vitamin D–resistant rickets. Contrib Nephrol 22:101–106, 1980.
102. Frame B, Arnstein AR, Frost HM, Smith JR: Resistant osteomalacia. Studies with tetracycline bone labeling and metabolic balance. Am J Med 38:134–144, 1965.
103. Tapia J, Stearns G, Ponsetti IV: Vitamin D–resistant rickets. J Bone Joint Surg 64A:935, 1964.
104. Stickler GB, Beabout JW, Riggs BL: Vitamin D–resistant rickets: Clinical experience with 41 typical familial hypophosphatemic patients and 2 atypical nonfamilial cases. Mayo Clin Proc 45:197–218, 1970.
105. Stearns G: A guide to the adequacy of therapy in resistant rickets due to familial or essential hypophosphatemia. J Bone Joint Surg 46A:959–964, 1964.
106. Pierce DS, Wallace WM, Herndon CH: Long-term treatment of vitamin D–resistant rickets. J Bone Joint Surg 46A:978–997, 1964.
107. Glorieux FH, Scriver CR, Reade TM, et al: Use of phosphate and vitamin D to prevent dwarfism and rickets in X-linked hypophosphatemia. N Engl J Med 287:481–487, 1972.
108. Costa T, Marie PJ, Scriver CR, et al: X-linked hypophosphatemia: Effect of calcitriol on renal handling of phosphate, serum phosphate, and bone mineralization. J Clin Endocrinol Metab 52:463–472, 1981.

109. Chesney RW, Mazess RB, Rose P, et al: Long-term influence of calcitriol (1,25-dihydroxyvitamin D) and supplemental phosphate in X-linked hypophosphatemic rickets. Pediatrics 71:559–567, 1983.

110. Hanell RH, Lyles KW, Harrelson JM, et al: Healing of bone disease in X-linked hypophosphatemic rickets/osteomalacia: Indication and maintenance with phosphorus and calcitriol. J Clin Invest 75:1858–1868, 1985.

111. Seino Y, Shimotxuji T, Ishii T, et al: Treatment of hypophosphatemic vitamin D–resistant rickets with massive doses of 1α-hydroxyvitamin D_3 during childhood. Arch Dis Child 55:49–53, 1980.

112. Muraki K, Nishi Y, Tsuda K, et al: A case of hypophosphatemic vitamin D–resistant rickets treated with initial massive doses of 1α-hydroxyvitamin D_3 alone. Acta Paediatr Scand 72:763–768, 1983.

113. Meunier PJ, Edouard C, Arlot M, et al: Effects of 1,25-dihydroxyvitamin D on bone mineralization. *In* MacIntyre I, Szelke M (eds): Molecular Endocrinology. Amsterdam, Elsevier/North-Holland, 1979, pp 283–292.

114. Alon U, Chan JCM: Effects of hydrochlorothiazide and amiloride in renal hypophosphatemic rickets. Pediatrics 75:754–763, 1985.

115. Steendijk R, Latham SC: Hypophosphatemic vitamin D–resistant rickets; an observation on height and serum inorganic phosphate in untreated cases. Helv Paediatr Acta 26:179–184, 1971.

116. Tanner JM: Physical growth and development. *In* Forfar JO, Arneil GC (eds): Textbook of Pediatrics. New York, Churchill Livingstone, 1978, pp 249–303.

117. Schoen EJ: The question of normal height in patients with vitamin D–resistant rickets. JAMA 195:524–526, 1966.

118. Moncrieff MW: Early biochemical findings in familial hypophosphatemic, hyperphosphaturic rickets and response to treatment. Arch Dis Child 57:70–72, 1982.

119. Lapatsanis PD, Sbyrakis S, Megreli C, Edelstein S: The management of siblings with familial hypophosphatemic rickets. Helv Paediatr Acta 38:373–381, 1983.

120. Schimert G, Fanconi A: Early history of familial hypophosphatemic vitamin D–resistant rickets. Report of three cases observed since birth. Helv Paediatr Acta 38:383–398, 1983.

121. Roxa M, Miguel MA, Galbe M, et al: Early treatment of familial hypophosphatemic rickets. Arch Dis Child 58:1020–1022, 1983.

122. Stamp TCB, Baker LRI: Recessive hypophosphatemic rickets, and possible aetiology of the "vitamin D–resistant" syndrome. Arch Dis Child 51:360–365, 1976.

123. Winters RW, McFalls VW, Graham JB: "Sporadic" hypophosphatemia and vitamin D–resistant rickets. Pediatrics 25:959–966, 1960.

124. Riggs BL, Sprague RG, Jowsey J, Maher FT: Adult-onset vitamin-D-resistant hypophosphatemic osteomalacia. Effect of total parathyroidectomy. N Engl J Med 281:762–766, 1969.

125. Ojwang PJ, Gitau W, Shah MV: Adolescent hypophosphatemic rickets. East Afr Med J 59:416–419, 1982.

126. Scriver CR, MacDonald W, Reade T: Hypophosphatemic nonrachitic bone disease: An entity distinct from X-linked hypophosphatemia in the renal defect, bone involvement, and inheritance. Am J Med Genet 1:101–117, 1977.

127. Scriver CR, Reade T, Halal F, et al: Autosomal hypophosphatemic bone disease responds to $1,25(OH)_2D_3$. Arch Dis Child 56:203–207, 1981.

128. Tieder M, Modai D, Samuel R, et al: Hereditary hypophosphatemic rickets with hypercalciuria. N Engl J Med 312:611–617, 1985.

129. Sauveur B, Garabedian M, Fellot C, et al: The effect of induced metabolic acidosis on vitamin D_3 metabolism in rachitic chicks. Calcif Tissue Res 23:121–124, 1977.

130. Lee SW, Russell J, Avioli LV: 25-hydroxycholecalciferol to 1,25-dihydroxycholecalciferol: Conversion impaired by systemic metabolic acidosis. Science 195:994–995, 1977.

131. Kawashima H, Kraut JA, Kurokawa K: Metabolic acidosis suppresses 25-hydroxyvitamin D_3-1α-hydroxylase in the rat kidney. J Clin Invest 70:135–140, 1982.

132. Weber HP, Gray RW, Dominguez JH, Lemann J Jr: The lack of effect of chronic metabolic acidosis on 25-hydroxyvitamin D metabolism and serum parathyroid hormone in humans. J Clin Endocrinol Metab 43:1047–1055, 1976.

133. Adams ND, Gray RW, Lemann J Jr: The calciuria of increased fixed acid production in humans: Evidence against a role for parathyroid hormone and $1,25(OH)_2$-vitamin D. Calcif Tissue Int 28:233–238, 1979.

134. Chesney RW, Kaplan BS, Phelps M, et al: Renal tubular acidosis does not alter circulating values of calcitriol. J Pediatr 104:51–55, 1984.

135. Abraham EH, Gerdes JS, Castille RG, et al: Vitamin D deficiency rickets with abnormal liver function tests and myopathy as the presenting manifestations of cystic fibrosis. Pediatr Res 15A:625, 1981.

136. Prader A, Illig R, Heierli E: Eine besondere Form der primaren Vitamin D–resistenten Rachitis mit Hypocalcamie und autosomaldominantem Erbgang: die hereditaire Pseudo-mangelrachitis. Helv Paediatr Acta 16:452–464, 1961.

137. Dent CE: Rickets (and osteomalacia): Nutritional and metabolic (1919–69). Proc R Soc Med 63:401–408, 1970.

138. Scriver CR: Vitamin D dependency. Pediatrics 45:361–363, 1970.

139. Hamilton R, Harrison J, Fraser D, et al: The small intestine in vitamin D–dependent rickets. Pediatrics 45:364–373, 1970.

140. Dent CE, Friedman M, Watson L: Hereditary pseudo-vitamin D–deficiency rickets. J Bone Joint Surg 50B:708–719, 1968.

141. Fanconi A, Prader A: Pseudo-vitamin D–deficiency rickets. *In* Burland WL, Barltrap D (eds): Mineral Metabolism in Pediatrics. Oxford, Blackwell, 1969, p 19.

142. Matsuda L, Sugai M, Ohsawa T: Laboratory findings in a child with pseudo-vitamin D–deficiency rickets. Helv Paediatr Acta 24:329–336, 1969.

143. Hamilton R, Harrison J, Fraser D, et al: The small intestine in vitamin D–dependent rickets. Pediatrics 45:364–373, 1970.

144. Reade TM, Scriver CR, Glorieux FH, et al: Response to crystalline 1α-hydroxyvitamin D_3 in vitamin D–dependency. Pediatr Res 9:593–599, 1975.

145. Rosen JF, Finberg L: Vitamin D–dependent rickets: Actions of parathyroid hormone and 25-hydroxycholecalciferol. Pediatr Res 6:552–562, 1972.
146. Birtwell WM, Magsamen BF, Fenn PA, et al: An unusual hereditary osteomalacic disease—pseudo-vitamin D–deficiency. Am J Bone Joint Surg 52A:1222–1228, 1970.
147. Delvin EE, Glorieux FH, Marie PH, et al: Vitamin D–dependency: Replacement therapy with calcitriol. J Pediatr 99:26–34, 1981.
148. Soriano RR, Einhorn A, Stark H, et al: Deficiency-type rickets due to decreased sensitivity to vitamin D. J Pediatr 68:227–236, 1966.
149. Balsan S, Garabedian M, Lieberherr M, et al: Serum 1,25-dihydroxyvitamin D concentrations in two different types of pseudo-deficiency rickets. *In* Norman AW, Schaefer K, Herrath DV, et al (eds): Vitamin D Basic Research and Its Clinical Application. Berlin, Walter de Gruyter, 1979, p 1143.
150. DeLuca HF: Vitamin D metabolism and function. Arch Intern Med 138:836–847, 1978.
151. Haussler MR: Biochemical mechanism of action of 1α-25-hydroxyvitamin D_3 in the intestine. Proc Second Workshop on Vitamin D. New York, de Gruyter, 1975.
152. Scriver CR, Reade TM, DeLuca HF, et al: Serum 1,25-dihydroxyvitamin D levels in normal subjects and in patients with hereditary rickets or bone disease. N Engl J Med 299:976–979, 1977.
153. Balsan S, Garabedian M, LeBouadec L: La richitisme vitaminoresistant pseudocareitial hypocalcemique. Arch Fr Pediatr 29:287–304, 1972.
154. Prader A, Kind HP, DeLuca HF: Pseudovitamin D deficiency (vitamin D dependency). *In* Rickel H, Stern J (eds): Inborn Errors of Calcium and Bone Metabolism. Baltimore, University Park Press, 1976, pp 115–123.
155. Aarskog D, Aksnes L, Markestad T: Effect of parathyroid hormone on cAMP and 1,25-dihydroxyvitamin D formation and renal handling of phosphate in vitamin D–dependent rickets. Pediatrics 71:59–63, 1983.
156. Fraser D, Kooh SW, Kind HP, et al: Pathogenesis of hereditary vitamin D–dependent rickets: An inborn error of vitamin D metabolism involving defective conversion of 25-hydroxycholecalciferol to 1α,25-dihydroxyvitamin D. N Engl J Med 289:817–822, 1973.
157. Balsan S, Garabedian M, Sorgniard R, et al: 1,25-dihydroxyvitamin D_3 and 1α-hydroxyvitamin D_3 in children: Biologic and therapeutic effects in nutritional rickets and different types of vitamin D resistance. Pediatr Res 9:586–593, 1975.
158. Strewler GJ, Bernstein DS, Pletka PL: Pseudo-vitamin D–deficiency rickets (PDR) and relative hypoparathyroidism: A report of a family. J Clin Endocrinol Metab 37:220–229, 1973.
159. Cowen J, Harris F: Late presentation of vitamin D–dependent rickets. Arch Dis Child 55:964–966, 1980.
160. Brooks MH, Bell NH, Love L, et al: Vitamin D–dependent rickets type II: Resistance of target organs to 1,25-dihydroxyvitamin D. N Engl J Med 298:996–999, 1978.
161. Rosen JF, Fleischman AR, Finberg L, et al: Rickets with alopecia: An inborn error of vitamin D metabolism. J Pediatr 94:729–735, 1979.
162. Liberman UA, Halabe A, Samuel R, et al: End-organ resistance to 1,25-dihydroxycholecalciferol. Lancet 1:504–506, 1980.
163. Sockalosky JJ, Ulstrom RA, DeLuca HF, et al: Vitamin D–resistance rickets: End-organ unresponsiveness to $1,25(OH)_2D_3$. J Pediatr 96:701–703, 1980.
164. Tsuchiya Y, Nobutake M, Cho H, et al: An unusual form of vitamin D–dependent rickets in a child: Alopecia and marked end-organ hyposensitivity to biologically active vitamin D. J Clin Endocrinol Metab 51:684–690, 1980.
165. Marx SJ, Spiegel AM, Brown EM, et al: A familial syndrome of decrease in sensitivity to 1,25-dihydroxyvitamin D. J Clin Endocrinol Metab 47:1303–1310, 1978.
166. Zerwekh JE, Glass K, Jowsey J, et al: A unique form of osteomalacia associated with end organ refractoriness to 1,25-dihydroxyvitamin D and apparent defective synthesis of 25-hydroxyvitamin D. J Clin Endocrinol Metab 49:171–175, 1979.
167. Marx SJ, Swart EG Jr, Hamstra AJ, et al: Normal intrauterine development of the fetus of a woman receiving extraordinarily high doses of 1,25-dihydroxyvitamin D_3. J Clin Endocrinol Metab 51:1138–1142, 1980.
168. Kudoh T, Kumagai T, Uetsuji N, et al: Vitamin D dependent rickets: Decreased sensitivity to 1,25-dihydroxyvitamin D. Eur J Pediatr 137:307–311, 1981.
169. Dokoh S, Haussler MR, Pike JW: Development of a radioligand immunoassay for 1,25-dihydroxycholecalciferol receptors utilizing monoclonal antibody. Biochem J 221:129–136, 1984.
170. Feldman D, Chen T, Hirst M, et al: Demonstration of 1,25-dihydroxyvitamin D_3 receptors in human skin biopsies. J Clin Endocrinol Metab 51:1463–1465, 1980.
171. Eil C, Marx SJ: Nuclear uptake of 1,25-dihydroxy $[^3H]$ cholecalciferol in dispersed fibroblasts cultured from normal human skin. Proc Natl Acad Sci USA 78:2562–2566, 1981.
172. Griffin JE, Zerwekh JE: Impaired stimulation of 25-hydroxyvitamin D-24-hydroxylase in fibroblasts from a patient with vitamin D dependent rickets, type II: A form of receptor-positive resistance to 1,25-dihydroxyvitamin D_3. J Clin Invest 72:1190–1199, 1983.
173. Clemens TL, Adams JS, Horiuchi N, et al: Interaction of 1,25-dihydroxyvitamin D_3 with keratinocytes and fibroblasts from skin of a subject with vitamin D–dependent rickets type II: A model for the study of the mode of action of 1,25-dihydroxyvitamin D_3. J Clin Endocrinol Metab 56:824–830, 1983.
174. Beer S, Tieder M, Kohelet D, et al: Vitamin D resistant rickets with alopecia: A form of end organ resistance to 1,25-dihydroxyvitamin D. Clin Endocrinol (Oxf) 14:395–402, 1981.
175. Eil C, Liberman UA, Rosen JF, et al: A cellular defect in hereditary vitamin D dependent rickets type II: Defective nuclear uptake of 1,25-dihydroxyvitamin D in cultured skin fibroblasts. N Engl J Med 304:1588–1591, 1981.
176. Feldman D, Chen T, Cone C, et al: Vitamin D resistant rickets with alopecia: Cultured skin fibroblasts exhibit defective cytoplasmic receptors and unresponsiveness to $1,25(OH)_2D_3$. J Clin Endocrinol Metab 55:1020–1022, 1982.

177. Liberman UA, Eil C, Marx SJ: Resistance to 1,25-dihydroxyvitamin D. Association with heterogeneous defects in cultured skin fibroblasts. J Clin Invest 71:192–200, 1983.

178. Balsan S, Garabedian M, Liberman UA, et al: Rickets and alopecia with resistance to 1,25-dihydroxyvitamin D: Two different clinical courses with two different cellular defects. J Clin Endocrinol Metab 57:803–811, 1983.

179. Hochberg Z, Benderli A, Levy J, et al: 1,25-dihydroxyvitamin D resistance, rickets, and alopecia. Am J Med 77:805–811, 1984.

180. Chen TL, Hirst MA, Cone CM, et al: 1,25-dihydroxyvitamin D resistance, rickets, and alopecia: Analysis of receptors and bioresponse in cultured fibroblasts from patients and parents. J Clin Endocrinol Metab 59:383–388, 1984.

181. Pike JW, Dokoh S, Haussler MR, et al: Vitamin D_3-resistant fibroblasts have immunoassayable 1,25-dihydroxyvitamin D_3 receptors. Science 224:879–881, 1984.

182. Liberman UA, Eil C, Holst P, et al: Hereditary resistance to 1,25-dihydroxyvitamin D: Defective function of receptors for 1,25-dihydroxyvitamin D in cells cultured from bone. J Clin Endocrinol Metab 57:958–962, 1983.

183. Stumpf WE, Sar M, Reid FA, et al: Target cells for 1,25-dihydroxyvitamin D_3 in intestinal tract, stomach, kidney, skin, pituitary, and parathyroid. Science 206:1188–1190, 1979.

184. Stanbury SW, Taylor CM, Lumb GA, et al: Formation of vitamin D metabolites following correction of human vitamin D deficiency. Mineral Electrolyte Metab 5:212–227, 1981.

185. Nguyen TM, Guillozo H, Garabedian M, et al: Serum concentrations of 24,25-dihydroxyvitamin D in normal children and in children with rickets. Pediatr Res 13:973–976, 1979.

185a. Balsan S, Garabedian M, Larchet M, et al: Long-term nocturnal calcium infusions can cure rickets and promote normal mineralization in hereditary resistance to 1,25-dihydroxyvitamin D. J Clin Invest 77:1661–1667, 1986.

186. Glorieux FH, Insogna KL, Travers R, et al: Hypophosphatemic rickets with or without osteomalacia in correlation with circulating calcitriol levels. Proc 7th Annual Meeting American Society of Bone and Mineral Research, no. 131, 1985.

187. Bradford DS, Brown DM, Moe JH, et al: Scheuermann's kyphosis: A form of osteoporosis? Clin Orthop Rel Res 118:10–15, 1976.

188. Sillence DO, Senn A, Danks DM: Genetic heterogeneity in osteogenesis imperfecta. J Med Genet 16:101–116, 1979.

189. Prockop DJ, Kivirikko KI: Heritable diseases of collagen. N Engl J Med 311:376–386, 1984.

190. Mudd SH, Levy HL: Disorders of transsulfuration. *In* Stanbury JB, Wyngaarden JB, Fredrickson DS, et al (eds): The Metabolic Basis of Inherited Disease. 5th ed. New York, McGraw-Hill, 1983, pp 522–559.

191. Simell O, Perheentupa J, Rapola J, et al: Lysinuric protein intolerance. Am J Med 59:229–240, 1975.

192. Carpenter TO, Levy HL, Holtrop ME, et al: Lysinuric protein intolerance presenting as childhood osteoporosis. N Engl J Med 312:290–294, 1985.

193. Danks DM: Hereditary disorders of copper metabolism in Wilson's disease and Menkes' disease. *In* Stanbury JB, Wyngaarden JB, Fredrickson DS, et al (eds): The Metabolic Basis of Inherited Disease. 5th ed. New York, McGraw-Hill, 1983, pp 1251–1268.

194. Sutton AM, Harvie A, Cockburn F, et al: Copper deficiency in the infant of very low birthweight. Arch Dis Child 60:644–651, 1985.

195. Grunebaum M, Horodniceanu C, Steinberg R: Radiographic manifestations of bone changes in copper deficiency. Pediatr Radiol 9:101–104, 1980.

196. Heller RM, Kirchner SG, O'Neill JA, et al: Skeletal changes of copper deficiency in infants receiving prolonged parenteral nutrition. J Pediatr 92:947–949, 1978.

197. Sperling O, Weinberger A, Oliver I, et al: Hypouricemia, hypercalciuria, and decreased bone density: A hereditary syndrome. Ann Intern Med 80:482–487, 1974.

198. Beals RK: Orthopedic aspects of the XO (Turner's) syndrome. Clin Orthop Rel Res 97:19–30, 1973.

199. Shore RM, Chesney RW, Mazess RB, et al: Skeletal demineralization in Turner's syndrome. Calcif Tissue Int 34:519–522, 1982.

200. Smith MA, Wilson J, Price WH: Bone demineralization in patients with Turner's syndrome. J Med Genet 19:100–103, 1982.

201. Brown DM, Jowsey J, Bradford DS: Osteoporosis in ovarian dysgenesis. J Pediatr 84:816–820, 1974.

202. Dent CE, Friedman M: Idiopathic juvenile osteoporosis. Q J Med 34:177–220, 1965.

203. Brenton DP, Dent CE: Idiopathic juvenile osteoporosis. *In* Bickel H, Stern J (eds): Inborn Errors of Calcium and Bone Metabolism. Lancaster, MTP Press, 1976, pp 222–238.

204. Smith R: Idiopathic osteoporosis in the young. J Bone Joint Surg 62B:417–427, 1980.

205. Kooh SW, Cumming SA, Fraser D, et al: Transient childhood osteoporosis of unknown cause. *In* Frame B, Parfitt AM, Duncan H (eds): Clinical Aspects of Metabolic Bone Disease. Amsterdam, Excerpta Medica, 1973, pp 329–332.

206. Marder HK, Tsang RC, Hug G, et al: Calcitriol deficiency in idiopathic juvenile osteoporosis. Am J Dis Child 136:914–917, 1982.

207. Teotia M, Teotia SPS, Singh RK: Idiopathic juvenile osteoporosis. Am J Dis Child 133:894–900, 1979.

208. Smith R: Idiopathic juvenile osteoporosis. Am J Dis Child 133:889–891, 1979.

209. Leroy D, Garabedian M, Guillozo H, et al: Evolution des concentrations serigues en metabolites de la vitamine D anbd ans un cas d'osteoporose juvenile idiopathique. Arch Fr Pediatr 38:165–170, 1981.

210. Jowsey J, Johnson KA: Juvenile osteoporosis: Bone findings in seven patients. J Pediatr 81:511–517, 1972.

211. Jones ET, Hensinger RN: Spinal deformity in idiopathic juvenile osteoporosis. Spine 6:1–4, 1981.

212. Montgomery SP, Erwin WE: Scheuermann's kyphosis—long-term results of Milwaukee brace treatment. Spine 6:5–8, 1981.

213. Allen TM, Manoli A, LaMont RL: Skeletal changes associated with copper deficiency. Clin Orthop Rel Res 168:206–210, 1982.

214. Klevay LM: Diets deficient in copper and zinc? Med Hypotheses 5:1323–1326, 1979.

215. Tanaka Y, Hatano S, Nishi Y, et al: Nutritional copper deficiency in a Japanese infant on formula. J Pediatr 96:255–257, 1980.

216. Stapleton FB, Hanissian AS, Miller LA: Hypercalciuria in children with juvenile rheumatoid arthritis: Association with hematuria. J Pediatr 107:235–239, 1985.
217. LoCascio V, Adami S, Avioli LV, et al: Suppressive effect of chronic glucocorticoid treatment on circulating calcitonin in man. Calcif Tissue Int 23:309–310, 1982.
218. Thompson JS, Palmieri GMA, Eliel LP, et al: Effect of calcitonin on glucocorticoid bone loss. J Bone Joint Surg 54A:1490–1494, 1972.

Index

Note: Page numbers in *italics* refer to illustrations; page numbers followed by t refer to tables.